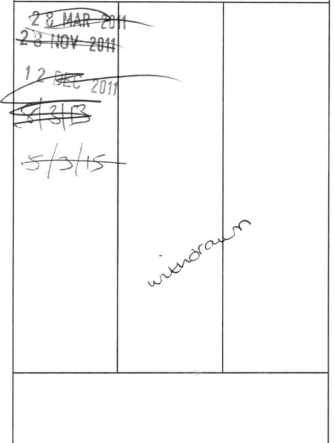

# Kirsner's Inflammatory Bowel Diseases

Sixth Edition

*Commissioning Editor:* Rolla Couchman
*Project Development Manager:* Joanne Scott
*Project Manager:* Rory MacDonald
*Illustration Manager:* Mick Ruddy
*Design Manager:* Jayne Jones
*Illustrator:* Paul Bernson

# Kirsner's Inflammatory Bowel Diseases
## Sixth Edition

Edited by

# R Balfour Sartor MD

Professor of Medicine, Microbiology and Immunology
Division of Gastroenterology and Hepatology
Director, Multidisciplinary Center for IBD Research and Treatment
University of North Carolina School of Medicine
Chapel Hill, North Carolina, USA

# William J Sandborn MD

Professor of Medicine, Mayo Medical School
Head of the IBD Interest Group
Director of the IBD Clinical Research Unit
Mayo Clinic
Rochester, Minnesota, USA

SAUNDERS

Edinburgh  London  New York  Oxford  Philadelphia  St. Louis  Sydney  Toronto  2004

SAUNDERS
An imprint of Elsevier Inc.

© 2000, 1995, 1988, 1980, 1975
© 2004, Elsevier Inc. All rights reserved.

ISBN 0-7216-0001-8

**British Library Cataloguing in Publication Data**
A catalogue record for this book is available from the British Library

**Library of Congress Cataloging in Publication Data**
A catalog record for this book is available from the Library of Congress

**Notice**
Medical knowledge is constantly changing. Standard safety precautions must be followed, but as new research and clinical experience broaden our knowledge, changes in treatment and drug therapy may become necessary or appropriate. Readers are advised to check the most current product information provided by the manufacturer of each drug to be administered to verify the recommended dose, the method and duration of administration, and contraindications. It is the responsibility of the practitioner, relying on experience and knowledge of the patient, to determine dosages and the best treatment for each individual patient. Neither the Publisher nor the editors/ contributors assume any liability for any injury and/or damage to persons or property arising from this publication.
The Publisher

Printed in the United States of America.

The
publisher's
policy is to use
**paper manufactured
from sustainable forests**

# Contents

# List of Contributors

**Paul Angulo MD**
Associate Professor of Medicine
Division of Gastroenterology and Hepatology
Mayo Medical School, Clinic and Foundation
Minnesota, MN, USA

**Kirsten A Arseneau MS**
Instructor of Research in Internal Medicine
Digestive Health Center of Excellence
University of Virginia
Charlottesville, VA, USA

**Robert N Baldassano MD**
Director, Center for Pediatric IBD
The Children's Hospital of Philadelphia
Associate Professor, University of Pennsylvania School of Medicine
Philadelphia, PA, USA

**Terry Barrett MD**
Director, Division of Dermatopathology
Associate Professor of Dermatology and Pathology
John Hopkins Medical Institutions
Baltimore, MD, USA

**Charles Bernstein MD**
Head, Section of Gastroenterology
Director, Inflammatory Bowel Disease Clinical and Research Centre
University of Manitoba
Winnipeg, Manitoba, Canada

**Vibeke Binder MD**
Chief Physician, Consultant Gastroenterologist
Department of Gastroenterology
Herlev University Hospital
Herlev, Denmark

**Richard S Blumberg MD**
Chief, Gastroenterology Division
Brigham and Women's Hospital
Harvard Medical School
Boston, MA, USA

**Johan Bohr MD PhD**
Consultant Gastroenterologist
Division of Gastroenterology
Örebro University Hospital
Örebro, Sweden

**Michael Cantor MD**
Fellow, Inflammatory Bowel Disease Fellowship
Inflammatory Bowel Disease Clinical and Research Centre
University of Manitoba
Winnipeg, Manitoba, Canada

**Judy H Cho MD**
Assistant Professor of Medicine
Gastroenterology Section, Department of Medicine
University of Chicago
Chicago, IL, USA

**Robert R Cima MD**
Assistant Professor of Surgery
Mayo Clinic
Rochester, MN, USA

**Stephen M Collins MBBS FRCP(UK) FRCPC**
Professor of Medicine
Division of Gastroenterology
McMaster University Medical Centre
Hamilton, Ontario, Canada

**Jean-Frédéric Colombel MD**
Professor of Hepatogastroenterology
Department of Hepatogastroenterology
Hôpital Huriez
Lille, France

**Janice C Colwell RN MS CWOCN**
Clinical Nurse Specialist
University of Chicago Hospitals
Chicago, IL, USA

**Fabio Cominelli MD PhD**
David D Stone, Professor of Internal Medicine, Microbiology and Immunology
Director, Digestive Health Center of Excellence
University of Virginia Health Center
Charlottesville, VA, USA

**Geert R D'Haens MD PhD**
Consultant Gastroenterologist for IBD
Division of Gastroenterology
University Hospital Gasthuisberg
Leuven, Belgium

**Axel U Dignass MD**
Assistant Professor of Medicine
Division of Hepatology and Gastroenterology
Virchow Hospital
Berlin, Germany

**Iris Dotan MD**
Head of Inflammatory Bowel Disease Center
Department of Gastroenterology
Tel Aviv Sourasky Medical Center
Tel Aviv, Israel

**Douglas A Drossman MD**
Professor of Medicine and Psychiatry
Division of Gastroenterology and Hepatology
University of North Carolina
Chapel Hill, NC, USA

**Lars Eckmann MD**
Associate Professor of Medicine
Department of Medicine
University of California, San Diego
La Jolla, CA, USA

**Anders Ekbom MD**
Professor of Medicine
Clinical Epidemiology Unit, Department of Medicine
Karolinska Hospital
Stockholm, Sweden

**Richard A Farrell MD**
Assistant Professor of Medicine
Department of Gastroenterology
Beth Israel Deaconness Medical Center
Boston, MA, USA

**Brian G Feagan MD**
Professor of Medicine, Epidemiology and Biostatistics
University of Western Ontario
London, Ontario, Canada

**George D Ferry MD**
Professor of Pediatrics
GI and Nutrition Department
Baylor College of Medicine and Texas Children's Hospital
Houston, TX, USA

**Alessandro Fichera MD**
Assistant Professor of Surgery
Department of Surgery
The University of Chicago
Chicago, IL USA

**Elliot K Fishman MD**
Professor of Radiology and Oncology
John Hopkins University School of Medicine
Baltimore, MD, USA

**David Forcione MD**
Senior Clinical Fellow
Gastrointestinal Unit
Massachusetts General Hospital
Boston, MA, USA

**Ivan J Fuss MD**
Staff Scientist
Mucosal Immunity Section
National Institutes of Health
Bethesda, MD, USA

**D Neil Granger PhD**
Professor of Molecular and Cellular Physiology
Department of Molecular and Cellular Physiology
Louisiana State University Health Sciences Center
Shreveport, LA, USA

**Matthew B Grisham PhD**
Professor of Molecular and Cellular Physiology
Department of Molecular and Cellular Physiology
Louisiana State University Health Sciences Center
Shreveport, LA, USA

**Stephen B Hanauer MD**
Professor of Medicine and Clinical Pharmacology;
Section Chief, Gastroenterology and Nutrition
University of Chicago
Chicago, IL, USA

**Karen M Horton MD**
Associate Professor of Radiology
Department of Radiology
Johns Hopkins University School of Medicine
Baltimore, MD, USA

**Jean-Pierre Hugot MD PhD**
Fondation Jean Dausset CEPH
Department of Paediatric Gastroenterology
Hôpital Robert Debre
Paris, France

**Steven H Itzkowitz MD**
The Dr Burrill B Crohn Professor of Medicine
Director, The Dr Henry D Janowitz Division of Gastroenterology
Mount Sinai School of Medicine
New York, NY, USA

**Gunnar Järnerot MD PhD FRCP**
Professor of Gastroenterology
Division of Gastroenterology
Örebro University Hospital
Örebro, Sweden

**Derek P Jewell MA DPhil FRCP FMedSci**
Professor of Gastroenterology
Gastroenterology Unit
Radcliffe Infirmary
Oxford, UK

**Bronwyn Jones MD**
Professor of Radiology
Department of Radiology
Johns Hopkins University School of Medicine
Baltimore, MD, USA

**Thomas A Judge MD**
Assistant Professor of Medicine
University of Medicine and Dentistry of New Jersey
Newark, NJ, USA

**Martin F Kagnoff MD**
Professor of Medicine
Department of Medicine
University of California, San Diego
La Jolla, CA, USA

**Ishaan S Kalha MD**
Fellow, Gastroenterology
Division of Gastroenterology
University of Texas Medical School
Houston, TX, USA

**Sunanda V Kane MD MSPH**
Assistant Professor of Medicine
Center for Advanced Medicine
University of Chicago
Chicago, IL, USA

**Loren C Karp BSc MA**
Researcher and Specialist
Inflammatory Bowel Disease Center
Cedars-Sinai Medical Center
Los Angeles, CA, USA

**Gary R Lichtenstein MD**
Professor of Medicine
Director, Centre for Inflammatory Bowel Disease
Gastrointestinal Division, Department of Medicine
Hospital of the University of Pennsylvania
Philadelphia, PA, USA

**Keith D Lindor MD**
Professor of Medicine
Division of Gastroenterology and Hepatology
Mayo Medical School, Clinic and Foundation
Rochester, MN, USA

**Herbert Lochs MD**
Professor of Medicine
The Internal Medicine Clinic Specializing in Gastroenterology,
    Hepatology and Endocrinology
Humboldt University
Berlin, Germany

**Robert Löfberg MD PhD**
Director
Inflammatory Bowel Disease Unit
Karolinska Institute
Stockholm, Sweden

**Edward Loftus Jr MD**
Associate Professor of Medicine
Mayo Medical School
Consultant, Division of Gastroenterology and Hepatology
Mayo Clinic
Rochester, MN, USA

**P Kay Lund MD PhD**
Professor in Cell and Molecular Physiology, Pediatrics and Nutrition
University of North Carolina at Chapel Hill
Chapel Hill, NC, USA

**Thomas T MacDonald PhD FRCPath**
Professor of Immunology
Division of Infection, Inflammation and Repair
University of Southampton School of Medicine
Southampton, UK

**James L Madara MD**
Richard T Crane Professor
Dean, Division of Biological Sciences and the Pritzker School of Medicine
The University of Chicago
Chicago, IL, USA

**Uma Mahadevan MD**
Clinical Assistant Professor of Medicine
Director of Clinical Research, UCSF Center for Colitis and Crohn's Disease
Division of Gastroenterology
University of California
San Francisco, CA, USA

**Petar Mamula MD**
Assistant Professor of Pediatrics
The Children's Hospital of Philadelphia
University of Pennsylvania School of Medicine
Philadelphia, PA, USA

**James F Marion MD**
Assistant Clinical Professor of Medicine
Divison of Gastroenterology
Mount Sinai School of Medicine
New York, NY, USA

**Jonathan E Markowitz MD**
Attending Physician
The Children's Hospital of Philadelphia
University of Pennsylvania School of Medicine
Philadelphia, PA, USA

**Lloyd Mayer MD**
Professor and Chairman
Immunobiology Centre
Mount Sinai School of Medicine
New York, NY, USA

**Robin S McLeod MD FRCSC FACS**
Professor of Surgery and Health Policy Management
Head, Division of General Surgery
Mount Sinai Hospital
Toronto, Ontario, Canada

**Fabrizio Michelassi MD**
Professor of Surgery
Department of Surgery
The University of Chicago
Chicago, IL, USA

**Pia Munkholm MD DMSci**
Consultant Physician
Department of Gastroenterology
Herlev University Hospital
Herlev, Denmark

**Markus Neurath MD**
Associate Professor of Medicine
Laboratory of Immunology
University of Mainz
Mainz, Germany

**Timothy R Orchard MA MD MRCP**
Consultant Physician
Department of Gastroenterology
St Mary's Hospital NHS Trust
London, UK

**John H Pemberton MD**
Professor of Surgery
Mayo Clinic
Rochester, MN, USA

**Sylvia L F Pender PhD**
Lecturer, Division of Infection, Inflammation and Repair
University of Southampton School of Medicine
Southampton, UK

**Mark A Peppercorn MD**
Director, Center for Inflammatory Bowel Disease
Beth Israel Deaconess Medical Center
Professor of Medicine
Harvard Medical School
Boston, MA, USA

**Theresa T Pizarro PhD**
Assistant Professor of Internal Medicine
Digestive Health Center of Excellence
University of Virginia
Charlottesville, VA, USA

**Daniel K Podolsky MD**
Mallinckrodt Professor of Medicine, Harvard Medical School
Chief, Gastrointestinal Unit
Massachusetts General Hospital
Boston, MA, USA

**Daniel H Present MD**
Clinical Professor of Medicine
Department of Medicine
Division of Gastroenterology
Mount Sinai School of Medicine
New York, NY, USA

**Robert Riddell MD MBBS**
Professor of Pathology
University of Toronto
Mount Sinai Hospital
Toronto, Ontario, Canada

**Yehuda Ringel MD**
Assistant Professor of Medicine Department of Medicine
Division of Gastroenterology and Hepatology
University of North Carolina at Chapel Hill
Chapel Hill, NC, USA

**Paul Rutgeerts MD PhD FRCP**
Professor of Medicine
University Hospital Gasthuisberg
Department of Internal Medicine
Leuven, Belgium

**William J Sandborn MD**
Professor of Medicine, Mayo Medical School
Head of the IBD Interest Group
Director of the IBD Clinical Research Unit
Mayo Clinic
Rochester, MN, USA

**Robert S Sandler MD MPH**
Professor of Medicine and Epidemiology
Division of Gastroenterology and Hepatology
University of North Carolina at Chapel Hill
Chapel Hill, NC, USA

**Bruce E Sands MD**
Director, Clinical IBD Research
Gastrointestinal Unit
Massachusetts General Hospital
Boston, MA, USA

**R Balfour Sartor MD**
Professor of Medicine, Microbiology and Immunology
Division of Gastroenterology and Hepatology
Director, Multidisciplinary Center for IBD Research and Treatment
University of North Carolina School of Medicine
Chapel Hill, NC, USA

**Joseph H Sellin MD**
Professor of Medicine
Division of Gastroenterology
University of Texas Medical School
Houston, TX, USA

**Shanthi V Sitaraman MD PhD**
Assistant Professor
Department of Medicine and Department of Pathology and
    Laboratory Medicine
Emory University School of Medicine
Atlanta, GA, USA

**Scott B Snapper MD PhD**
Assistant Professor of Medicine
Gastrointestinal Unit
Center for the Study of Inflammatory Bowel Disease
Harvard Medical School
Massachusetts General Hospital
Boston, MA, USA

**Hillary Steinhart MD MSc FRCP(C)**
Associate Professor of Medicine, University of Toronto
Samuel Lunenfeld Research Institute
Mount Sinai Hospital
Toronto, Ontario, Canada

**Warren Strober MD**
Head, Mucosal Immunity Section
National Institutes of Health
Bethesda, MD, USA

**Lloyd R Sutherland MD CM BA MSc FRCPC FACP**
Professor of Medicine
Canadian Journal of Gastroenterology
Calgary, Alberta, Canada

**Cyrus P Tamboli MD FRCPC**
Resident, Department of Internal Medicine
Division of Gastroenterology
University of Iowa Hospitals and Clinics
Iowa City, IA, USA

**Stephen R Targan MD**
Director, Cedars-Sinai Division of Gastroenterology, Inflammatory Bowel
   Disease Center, and Immunobiology Institute, Cedars Sinai Medical Center
Professor in Residence, UCLA School of Medicine
Los Angeles, CA, USA

**William J Tremaine MD**
Professor of Medicine
Division of Gastroenterology and Hepatology
Mayo Foundation
Rochester, MN, USA

**Curt Tysk MD PhD**
Associate Professor of Gastroenterology
Department of Gastroenterology
Örebro University Hospital
Örebro, Sweden

**Sander van Deventer MD PhD**
Professor and Head
Department of Gastroenterology
Academic Medical Centre
Amsterdam, Netherlands

**Kent C Williams MD**
GI Fellow
GI and Nutrition Department
Baylor College of Medicine
Texas Children's Hospital
Houston, TX , USA

**Feng Xiao Li MD PhD**
Research Associate
Department of Community Health Sciences
Centre for Health and Policy Studies
University of Calgary
Calgary, Alberta, Canada

**Ellen M Zimmerman MD**
Associate Professor of Medicine
Division of Gastroenterology
University of Michigan
Ann Arbor, MI, USA

# Foreword

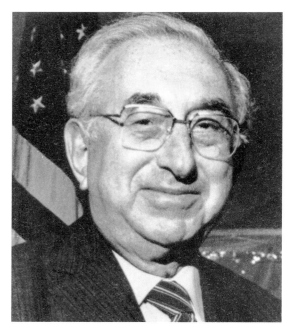

Evolution of our understanding of inflammatory bowel diseases: From the mystical to the cellular and now the molecular.

*Science (IBD) is moving but slowly, slowly creeping on from point to point*

*Alfred Lord Tennyson (1809–1892)*

It is of interest in an era of increasing biomedical sophistication to recall that a relatively short time ago, early in the 20th century, 'simple' ulcerative colitis was an obscure 'medical curiosity' emerging slowly from an unknown past. Crohn's disease was yet unidentified as a separate entity, although careful review of the IBD literature documented its early presence, masquerading as 'intestinal tuberculosis'. Into the 1930s, the etiology and pathogenesis of ulcerative colitis and Crohn's disease were unknown, and investigative hypotheses were scarce. Therapeutic resources were limited and treatment was primitive. At a time of limited biomedical knowledge and minimal clinical awareness, unsubstantiated views prevailed, including 'vague reactions to foods' (sugar, margarine, corn flakes), deficiency of a 'protective factor' in pig intestine, and psychiatric disease.

The position of inflammatory bowel diseases in the medical world today is vastly different. Ulcerative colitis, and Crohn's disease are now recognized worldwide, are frequent subjects at medical meetings and increasingly provide the focus of important clinical and laboratory research. Indeed, few diseases in gastroenterology present as varied an array of investigative opportunities. This dramatic change began in the mid-20th century with the increasing support of biomedical research and the subsequent growth of the basic sciences, highlighted by the discoveries of sulfonamides in the 1930s, antibiotics in the 1940s, and ACTH and adrenocorticosteroids in the 1950s. The entry of young physicians into gastroenterology during the 1930s and 40s, trained in the rigors of basic research and controlled clinical study, contributed to this advance. Progress accelerated following the establishment of the General Medicine Study Section of the National Institutes of Health in 1956, which subsequently provided a major source for support of research in gastroenterology, the growth of academic medicine and the establishment of the Crohn's and Colitis Foundation of America. By the 1970s, sufficient new clinical and scientific information on IBD had been accumulated to justify a comprehensive publication on ulcerative colitis and Crohn's disease, the 1975 First Edition of *Inflammatory Bowel Diseases*, a volume of approximately 400 pages, with contributions from 25 authors. Subsequent editions of *Inflammatory Bowel Diseases*, appearing approximately every five years, documented the increasing depth and sophistication of clinical and scientific knowledge of ulcerative colitis and Crohn's disease. The Third Edition of *Inflammatory Bowel Diseases* in 1985, involving 44 authorities, had doubled in size and included chapters on the nature of intestinal defenses, the M cell, early information on immunologic and genetic aspects of ulcerative colitis and Crohn's disease, as well as advances in the pathology, radiology and endoscopy of IBD, and its improving medical and surgical treatment. Psychiatric and other early 20th century hypotheses had been replaced by concepts based in the disciplines of epidemiology, microbiology, immunology, and genetics.

Into the 1990s, with more investigators involved, knowledge of the inflammatory bowel diseases increased exponentially. Etiologic possibilities, as outlined by Balfour Sartor, now were more definitive, including persistent pathogenic microbial infection, enhanced intestinal mucosal permeability, 'dysbiosis' or the altered balance of protective bacteria versus aggressive commensals, and 'dysregulated' immune responses, leading to loss of oral tolerance to commensal bacteria and aggressive cellular activation. Academically based IBD centers generated more focused research and controlled therapeutic trials. IBD research in the laboratory had advanced from the study of tissues and epithelial cells to cellular biology and cellular constituents. Chapters now included the biologic nature of IBD tissue reactions, the gut mucosal immune system and more advanced immunological and genetic mechanisms. Ulcerative colitis and Crohn's disease had become regular features of national and international medical meetings, attracting large audiences.

The 1999 5th Edition included more than 70 authorities submitting increasingly diverse chapters on epithelial cell function in health and disease (including heat shock proteins and trefoil peptides), cytokines, chemokines, growth factors, eicosanoids and other bioactive molecules in clinical IBD and experimental intestinal inflammation, leukocyte-endothelial interactions, altered intestinal neuromuscular function and the nature of oral tolerance. Genetic studies had identified susceptibility loci for ulcerative colitis and, most importantly, a locus (now identified as NOD-2) on chromosome 16 for Crohn's disease, particularly involving the ileum, the first gene linked with susceptibility to Crohn's disease. Transgenic and recombinatorial science now facilitated the creation of a variety of experimental animal models seeking to approximate human IBD, thereby enabling the more comprehensive study of intestinal tissue injury. The molecular nature of inflammation now became a prime area of investigation, with therapeutic dividends. After one hundred years of intermittent immunologic research led to the identification of tumor necrosis factor (TNF), an antibody to TNF proved to be a highly effective treatment, though not a cure, for Crohn's disease. Newly recognized bioactive molecules, IL-1, IL-2R, CAMS, addressins, defensins, flagellins, granulysins, selectins, claudins, annexins, guanilyns, laminins, intimins, aquaporins and microsins now filled the IBD literature. Into the 21st century, additional bioactive molecules relevant to intestinal inflammation were identified at a rapid pace: adaptins, fibrillarins, syndecan-1, stromelysin, integrins, galanin-1, tropomyosin, fibroblast growth factor, epidermal growth factor, permeability-enhancing factor, neurotrophins, survivins, ubiquitins, and zonulins.

The many pro-inflammatory and immunoregulation molecules, countless cytokines, and other biological substances, generated a series of novel biologic therapeutic agents (CP571, IDEC-131, OPC 6535, LDP02, CDP870 J695), creating a formidable, if not intimidating, array of terms and pathways for the IBD physician and investigator alike. How do these molecules relate to IBD and to each other? Where are the signaling mechanisms and pathways determining their coordinated action? Are they different in ulcerative colitis and Crohn's disease? Does $NF_kB$ have both pro-inflammatory and anti-inflammatory actions, also involving trace elements (boron, selenium, vanadium, zinc)? Are there other dominant pro-inflammatory molecules analogous to TNF which can be successfully blocked? What is the possible role of the Peyer's patch microenvironment in the regulation of T cell function? Since the intestinal bacterial flora play a critical role in the pathogenesis of IBD, what might be the abnormalities in the commensal mucosal flora or the defects in the intestinal epithelial barrier leading to chronic intestinal inflammation? The role of human regulatory T cells? The 5q31 cytokine gene cluster? The role of the M cell in the entry of protective or detrimental antigens? The pivotal regulatory role of $AP_{20}$ in intestinal inflammation? The role of the intestinal epithelial barrier in the development of intestinal immunity? The possibility of increasing the production of local secretory IgA antibodies as a protection against bacterial infec-

tion and inflammation? The possible involvement of nitric oxide in the inflammatory responses and immune reaction of IBD? The possible role of maternal immunologic memory in predisposing children to IBD and the genetic regulation of the intestinal epithelium? Important clinical issues similarly await resolution: the nature of the environment associated with urban industrialization and its relationship to IBD; and the role of today's 'hygienic home environment' in the vulnerability to IBD among children? Jewell and his colleagues recently have pointed out 'the importance of NOD-2/CARD 15 and the HLA region in determining clinical subgroups of Crohn's disease, which may provide the initial basis for the construction of a molecular classification of Crohn's disease.'

The discovery of new therapeutic approaches, in addition to currently available methotrexate, cyclosporine, antimicrobial compounds, thalidomide, and the adhesion molecule inhibitor heparin, including: growth factors, anti $NF_kB$ transcriptional agents, the prostaglandin receptor EP4, anti-A4 integrin antibody, inhibitors of stress-activated MAP kinases, antisense oligonucleotides vasoactive intestinal polypeptide and heterologous hemopoietic stem-cell transplantation. Sartor has raised the possibility of more effective local treatment of IBD via 'targeted delivery of biologically active immunosuppressive molecules by recombinant bacteria colonizing mucosal surfaces'. More immediately available microenvironmental approaches include the resurrection of 'old' treatment probiotics, live microbial food ingredients (lactobacilli, bifidobacteria species) and prebiotics (germinated barley and non-absorbed carbohydrates) and their newly recognized actions: production of antimicrobials and short chain fatty acids, inhibition of microbial adherence to the intestinal epithelium and restoration of normal intestinal permeability. In classic Karl Popper fashion, the expanding IBD research has generated many new important IBD questions and new research opportunities, necessitating a new IBD 'road map'. Despite the extraordinary progress in scientific information, more fundamental knowledge awaits discovery, as the pace and the dimensions of IBD research continue to increase.

The impressive scientific advances in IBD, illuminating fundamental biologic and physiologic aspects of intestinal function, accentuate the importance of the 6th Edition of *Inflammatory Bowel Diseases*, and also defines its purpose: to clarify the new intestinal biology, translate its relevance to the clinical situation, and provide a launching pad for the remarkable advances towards etiology and the cure of IBD yet to come. *Inflammatory Bowel Diseases* - Sixth Edition, provides the currently indispensable 'road map' guiding IBD physicians, and scientists through the multicomplex, IBD labyrinth. Co-editors, Dr R Balfour Sartor, Professor of Medicine, Microbiology and Immunology at the University of North Carolina, and Dr William J Sandborn, Professor of Medicine at the Mayo Clinic, have assembled a superb panel of national and international authorities and a 'cutting edge' array of IBD scientific and clinical topics. This book, *Inflammatory Bowel Diseases*, since 1975, has played a vital part in assembling and expertly analyzing for the medical world the evolving 'basic' science and the expanding clinical information and will continue this role, befitting the status of *Inflammatory Bowel Diseases* as 'the best book in the IBD field.'

Dr. Joseph B. Kirsner
The Louis Block Distinguished Service
Professor of Medicine
The University of Chicago

# Preface

Very few medical textbooks have so thoroughly dominated, and even defined a field, as has *Inflammatory Bowel Diseases* by Joe Kirsner. Originally co-edited with Roy Shorter of Mayo Clinic, this book, beginning with its first edition in 1975, encapsulated the science and art of caring for patients with Crohn's disease and ulcerative colitis. Thus it is with considerable respect, and indeed some awe and trepidation, that we eagerly embraced the opportunity to assume the editorship of this preeminent textbook and the obligation to transition it to reflect the changing, increasingly complex pathophysiology and treatment of these diseases.

Our editorial principle has been 'evolution, not revolution', in an effort to maintain the unique character of the original book while advancing its format and scope to encompass the important recent developments in basic and clinical investigations and to emphasize translational areas. We added multiple new chapters, including clinical pharmacology, epithelial/immune and epithelial/bacterial interactions, T lymphocyte dysregulation, T lymphocyte trafficking, fibrogenesis, serology and laboratory markers of disease activity, assessment of disease activity and clinical trial design, pouchitis, and pharmacoeconomics, and split genetics and colon cancer into basic and clinical components. In the process of changing the character of the contents, 30 new primary authors have contributed chapters. These authors are a blend of established thought leaders and younger investigators who have brought new concepts to the field, but all authors share the common characteristics of having a global perspective and being the premier investigator in their respective field. We thank the individual authors for their considerable efforts to create concise yet authoritative chapters and for their good humor in our exhortations to meet deadlines and to make suggested alterations. This adherence to deadlines and the timely production schedule by Elsevier have resulted in the most current textbook on IBD, with a lapse of only 7 months from final submission to publication. Thus, recent trends in treatment and the latest concepts in pathogenesis are reflected in this book.

The cover encapsulates the evolving concepts of applying new insights into the pathogenesis of ulcerative colitis and Crohn's disease to their diagnosis and treatment. This book discusses the interactions between mucosal innate and acquired immune responses and between enteric commensal microflora and environmental triggers that lead to disease in genetically susceptible hosts. Novel mechanisms of diagnosis provide earlier and more precise diagnosis of disease, and novel biologic treatments bring new opportunities to induce a remission, and hopefully maintain disease quiescence. The individual chapters collectively develop the theme of genetic and molecular heterogeneity that results in distinct phenotypes of disease. The subclassification of both Crohn's disease and ulcerative colitis should define clinically relevant populations of patients that selectively and predictably respond to individual therapeutic agents, resulting in highly effective and minimal cost treatment. Ultimately, preclinical diagnosis will lead to a way to prevent onset of clinical disease and associated complications in genetically susceptible individuals.

Finally, we must thank our family members, especially Em and Kenna, who have encouraged and supported this undertaking and in the process have endured many lonely weekends and holidays as the task was completed. We dedicate this book to these family members; to Joe Kirsner, for his guidance and confidence in our ability to continue his superb tradition, to our colleagues, fellows and students who provide continued stimulation and important questions; to the authors for their eloquent and comprehensive contributions, to the publishers for their strong support and professional production; and to the patients who have entered the clinical studies which have advanced our knowledge of the pathogenesis, epidemiology, diagnosis, and treatment of these diseases. We hope that our readers will profit by this collective experience and make suggestions to improve future editions.

R. Balfour Sartor MD

William J. Sandborn MD
September 2003

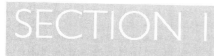

# MUCOSAL PROTECTION AND HOMEOSTASIS

# Intestinal epithelial barrier function: characteristics and responses to neutrophil transepithelial migration

James L Madara and Shanthi V Sitaraman

## INTRODUCTION

The defining characteristics of intestinal epithelium are 'vectorial transport' (energy-dependent absorption and secretion) and the ability to form a physical barrier that restricts passive movement of solutes from the intestinal lumen to the underlying tissue. This chapter considers intestinal epithelial structure as it relates to barrier function and subsequently analyzes what is currently known concerning the state of this barrier in active inflammation, such as is seen in flares of the idiopathic inflammatory bowel diseases (IBD). The focus is on cellular mechanisms of barrier function and the modulation of cellular events within the intestinal epithelium during active inflammation. This 'histopathologist view' of potential cellular interactions occurring in such states necessarily relies heavily on data obtained from reductionistic models of these events.

## RELATIVE PHYSICAL BARRIERS (BARRIERS DISCRETE FROM CELLS AND JUNCTIONS)

As detailed in the sections below, epithelial cells and junctions are the major physical barriers to passive movement of noxious compounds and particles from the lumen to the subepithelial spaces. Other important barriers that are extrinsic to the epithelium, such as mucins, secretory IgA, $HCO_3^-$, and peptides with antimicrobial functions, also exist (for reviews see [1,2]). Mucins are polydisperse glycoproteins (250–20 000 Da; 0.25–20 kDa) that are produced by goblet and other epithelial cell types. They have high viscosity, are often composed of $\sim$ 80% carbohydrate by mass, and probably protect the mucosal surface against bacteria and surface shear. More than 12 human mucin (MUC) genes have been identified.[3] Mucus behaves as a viscous

hydrated gel that undoubtedly attenuates the shear forces associated with peristaltic movement of luminal contents. Mucins can also cross-link and thereby aggregate luminal bacteria – an event that probably aids in clearance of the bacteria. One protective effect of mucins is highlighted by the fact that Muc2-deficient mice have increased epithelial turnover and enhanced gut epithelial tumorigenesis.[4] Intestinal trefoil factor (ITF), secreted by goblet cells, increases the viscosity of mucus, in addition to its ability to stimulate epithelial restitution (see below[131]).

A second example of a relative luminal barrier is secretory IgA. In general, the epithelial surfaces in the alimentary tract are bathed by the secretory immunoglobulin IgA, which binds to luminal threats such as pathogenic bacteria or antigens secreted by bacteria such as cholera toxin. IgA is a specific type of barrier that depends on antigenic sensitization.

Net $HCO_3^-$ secretion by the duodenal epithelial surface provides another type of relative barrier which relates specifically to protection against low pH. For example, whereas the pH of the gastric lumen may be 2–3, the pH at the surface of epithelial cells is at or near 7.19, owing to foveolar $HCO_3^-$ secretion.

Recently, it has been shown that gut epithelial cells may produce and secrete peptides with antimicrobial functions. For example, Paneth cells at the base of the crypt in the small intestine and ascending colon produce defensin-like peptides termed cryptdins.[5] In general such peptides are characterized by six conserved cysteine residues which constitute a unique disulfide motif which stabilizes a tertiary conformation consisting predominantly of a β sheet. These peptides have been shown to have in vitro activities against intestinal pathogens such as *Salmonella typhimurium*. In addition, intestinal epithelial cells can be induced by proinflammatory molecules such as IL-1 and TNF to secrete β-defensins through activation of NFkB.[6] An additional defense mechanism is provided by the ability of intestinal epithelial cells to respond to various agonists that induce fluid secretion, aiding in the flushing of microbes from the intestinal lumen, thus preventing their attachment to host epithelial cells or possibly dislodging adherent organisms.[7] Interestingly, recent data have shown that antimicrobial peptides are not solely restricted to the specific defense mechanism with which they were initially associated. For example, although cryptdins possess potent antimicrobial activity, a study by Lencer et al.[8] demonstrated that the exposure of cryptdins 2 and 3 (but not 1, 4, 5 or 6) to the apical surface of cultured intestinal epithelial (T84) monolayers stimulated the secretion of Cl . Cryptdin-induced Cl secretion was attributed to the formation of membrane pores probably related to those that are responsible for the killing of microorganisms.[9] The above and other (hydrophobic surface layer hypothesis; trefoil factor – see section on 'Resealing disrupted TJ', as well as chapter 3) attributes provide an array of luminal barriers above the intrinsic barrier of the epithelium which will now be discussed in detail.

# TIGHT JUNCTIONS: THE RATE-LIMITING BARRIER OF THE TRANSEPITHELIAL 'LEAK' PATHWAY

The main physical barrier that restricts transepithelial passive permeation of hydrophilic solutes is intrinsic to the epithelium. This barrier has two components: the epithelial cells (transcellular pathway) and the spaces around the epithelium, termed the paracellular pathway (Fig. 1.1). The transcellular pathway can be viewed as a low-viscosity gel (intracellular content having minimal resistance) bounded by the apical and basolateral membranes. Thus the passive movement of solutes across cells is essentially dictated by the characteristics of these two biomembranes. The resistance of model or biologic membranes is several orders of magnitude higher (106–109 ohm/cm$^2$ for model and 103–104 ohm/cm$^2$ for biologic membranes) than the resistance of small intestinal epithelia (102 ohm/cm$^2$) as a whole. Therefore, it comes as no surprise that the major permeation pathway across the epithelium is paracellular.[10–12] As the above resistance data would indicate, more than 85% of passive permeation is via the paracellular pathway, which restricts solutes based on their size, charge and hydrophilicity.[10] This pathway consists of two components, the apical junctional complex (Figs 1.1, 1.2) and the subjunctional space.

Over a century ago the apical junctional complex was visualized by light microscopy as a 0.5–2 mm apical density referred to as 'terminal bar' and thought to represent a static extracellular cement which holds neighboring cells together. The concept of the paracellular barrier has since evolved from being such an absolute and unregulated extracellular cement to a complex, dynamic and highly regulated apical junctional complex which consists of three parts: the zonula occludens, also referred to as the tight junction (TJ), or the occluding junction; the underlying zonula adherens, often referred to as the adherens junction, or the belt desmosome; and the most basally located macula adherens, also referred to as the spot desmosomes. The subjunctional space is a slit-like opening between lateral membranes of neighboring cells and, if collapsed, might affect the passive flow of solutes through the paracellular pathway. Because even macromolecules such as horseradish peroxidase can diffuse freely within the subjunctional paracellular space but are

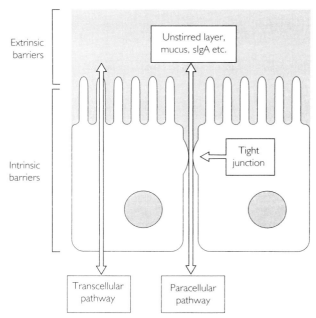

**Fig. 1.1** Schematic diagram of intestinal epithelial barriers. (From Madara JL. Epithelia: biologic principles of organization. In: Yamada T, ed. Textbook of gastroenterology. Philadelphia: Lippincott Raven; 1991, with permission.)

restricted by the TJ[10–12] it is clear that the TJ is the key barrier within this system. It is the rate-limiting barrier of the major permeation pathway of epithelial monolayers. In addition, there is considerable evidence to suggest that the TJ functions as a boundary between apical and basolateral plasma membrane domains, which differ in protein, lipid composition and physiological function, and thus the TJ also assists in creating and maintaining epithelial cell polarity. As has been the topic of several reviews[10–13] and first described by Farquhar and Palade[14] the TJ consists of an apical circumferential band varying from 100 to 600 nm in depth in which lateral membranes of adjacent cells are opposed. Electron micrographs of thin sections cut perpendicular to this zone reveal a series of punctate fusions or 'kisses' of outer membrane leaflets of adjacent cells (Fig. 1.3). These fusions are represented on freeze fracture replicas as net-like meshworks of strands and grooves, termed fibrils. In theory,[15] and on the basis of circuit analog analysis of data obtained from cultured[16] and natural[17] intestinal epithelia, there seems to be a general positive relationship between the number of fibrils and the barrier function of the individual junction.

# MOLECULAR STRUCTURE OF TIGHT JUNCTIONS

As depicted in Figure 1.2, several components of TJ have been identified in recent years, and characteristics of these proteins suggest testable hypotheses concerning the organization and regulation of TJ. The extracellular adhesive function of TJ is probably served by the transmembrane proteins occludin, claudin(s) and junctional adhesion molecule (JAM). Occludin is a 65 kDa protein that localizes to the TJ of epithelial and endothelial cells.[18] It is a 504 amino acid protein whose predicted structure contains four potential transmembrane domains, two small extracellular loops, and amino and carboxy terminals located within the cytoplasm. The hydrophobic extra-

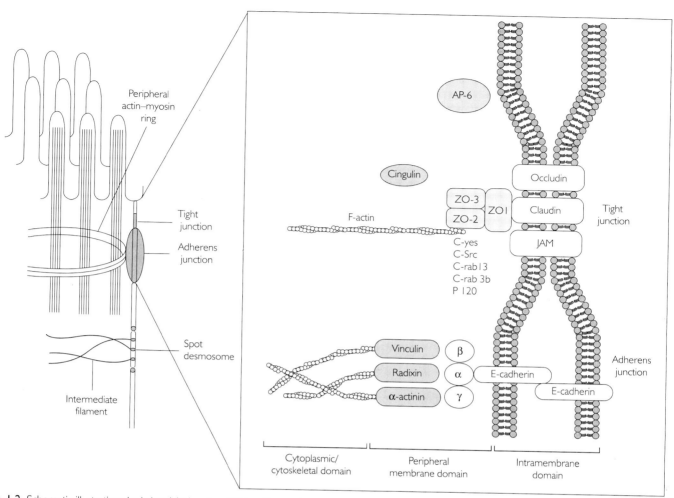

**Fig. 1.2** Schematic illustration depicting tight junction (TJ) location and structure in intestinal epithelial cells. On the left is the brush border region of a transected cell. Actin rootlets project from each microvillus into the apical cytosol. A peripheral actin–myosin ring, essentially representing a small cellular sphincter, associates with the lateral membrane at the adherens junction, which lies just below the TJ. Spot desmosomes into which the intermediate filaments insert are seen below the adherens junction. An expanded diagram of the apical junctional complex is shown on the right. The phospholipid bilayers of two neighboring cells are shown. At the TJ the integral membrane proteins occludin, claudin and JAM span the membrane and putatively seal the paracellular space by interacting in a homotypic fashion with a similar element on the adjacent cell. The cytosolic tail of these integral membrane proteins interacts with peripheral membrane proteins, including ZO-1, ZO-2 and ZO-3. F-actin filaments intimately associate with the sealing element of the TJ. The adherens junction is shown below with E-cadherin mediated cell–cell adherence. Like TJ, adherens junctions also associate with peripheral membrane proteins and cytoskeleton. At this apical junctional complex, several cytosolic molecules (c-src, c-yes etc.) thought to be important in signaling events reside.

cellular loops create a paracellular seal through association with similar loops from an adjacent cell.[19] Transfection experiments have shown that occludin localizes to TJ, and the transfected cells show a correlation between the number of parallel TJ strands, the mean width of the TJ network and transepithelial resistance.[20] However, data from a number of experiments indicate that occludin is not sufficient to generate bona fide TJ strands. The establishment of TJ strands depends on claudins, which is another recently identified protein family that has at least 18 members.[21] Like occludin, claudins possess four transmembrane domains and are localized at the site of close membrane–membrane apposition (kisses) within TJs. Expression of claudins 1 and 2 into fibroblasts lacking TJs induces the formation of TJ strands that are morphologically similar to the epithelial TJ strands,[22] and lack of claudin results in dehydration due to decreased epithelial barrier ability.[23] JAM belongs to the immunoglobulin superfamily: it has a single transmembrane domain, and its extracellular portion is thought to be folded into two immunoglobulin-like domains.

JAM has been shown to be involved in cell–cell adhesion/ junctional assembly of epithelial/endothelial cells,[24–26] as well as in the extravasation of monocytes through endothelial cells.[27]

The TJ proteins are bound to a plaque of peripheral membrane proteins, some of which are linked to cytoskeletal filaments and some of which display structural features suggesting their connection to diverse signaling pathways (see below). The cytoplasmic component of TJ has been observed as a plaque of electron-dense material adjacent to TJ in detergent extracted preparation of intestinal epithelial cells.[28] This material often localizes specifically at the sites of kiss/strands within the TJ. Some of these plaque proteins have been purified and their association with TJ has been characterized in recent years. Zonula occludens (ZO) ZO-1, ZO-2 and ZO-3 are three such PDZ domain-containing cytoplasmic plaque proteins that interact with the carboxy terminal of TJ protein. ZO are concentrated at TJs in epithelial cells through their binding to occludin, claudins and JAM, and are thought to function as a scaffold

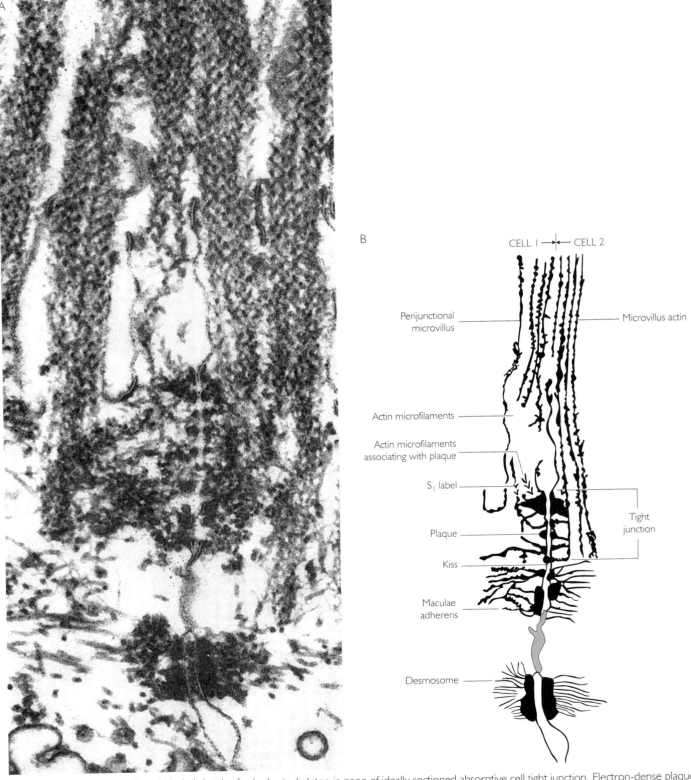

**Fig. 1.3** Electron micrograph and labeled sketch of naked cytoskeleton in zone of ideally sectioned absorptive cell tight junction. Electron-dense plaques intimately associated with 'intrajunctional kisses' on one side and with cytoskeletal elements on the other. Specifically, in sections unlabeled with S1 actin probe such cytoskeletal elements appear to be microfilaments (not shown), and in section labeled with S1 such microfilaments are shown to be actin microfilaments by characteristic arrowhead label because of S1 actin association ~ 115 000 (From Madara JL. Am J Physiol 1987; 253:C171, with permission.)

protein that recruits various proteins to TJs. ZO-1 is a 220 kDa monomer that binds the carboxy terminal domain of occludin, claudin and JAM.[29] ZO-2 is a 160 kDa protein that binds to ZO-1,[30] as does ZO-3, a 130 kDa protein.[31] Whereas ZO-2 is found exclusively in TJ, ZO-1 has been found in adherens junctions and in non-epithelial cell cadherin-based junctions.[32] Two additional cytoplasmic proteins, cingulin, a 140 kDa protein[33] and 7H6 antigen, a 155 kDa protein,[34] have also been precisely localized to TJ, although their functional significance is unknown. In addition to these proteins, small cytosolic regulatory proteins, including Rab-13, Rab-3b,[35] c-src and c-yes,[36] also localize to the region of TJ. Recently, AF-6, a novel *ras* binding protein, has been shown to interact with ZO-1 and modulate TJ function.[37] All in all, the above organization suggests a highly and uniquely regulated TJ structure, although the details of the mechanisms of regulation and physiological impact are only beginning to be recognized.

Subtle but direct anatomic associations appear to exist between the cytoskeleton and the TJ (Fig. 1.3).[28,38] As determined using both immunoelectron microscopic[38] and detergent extraction[28] techniques, actin microfilaments intimately associate with plaque-like condensations that flank the TJ. As shown in Figures 1.2 and 1.3, one characteristic feature of intestinal epithelial cells is an apical circumferential ring composed of bipolar actin filaments and myosin II.[28,38,39] This ring is also termed a contractile ring, as studies of isolated brush borders show that morphologic alterations suggestive of ring contraction can be elicited with divalent cations and adenosine triphosphate (ATP).[40,41] The perijunctional actin–myosin ring is positioned just below the TJ, where several actin-binding proteins are located and could serve as links to the plasma membrane. Interestingly, in vitro studies have shown that ZO-1 physically binds to a tetrameric form of spectrin, thus linking it to the cytoskeleton.[42] These data raise the speculative possibility that not only may the intestinal epithelial TJ be indirectly affected by tension within the perijunctional actin–myosin ring, but perhaps elements of the TJ can be directly manipulated through cytoskeletal interactions mediated by TJ-specific proteins. On the basis of such data, a tentative working model of the direct structural relationships between the cytoskeleton and the TJ is presented as an enlargement in Figure 1.2.

# REGULATION OF TIGHT JUNCTION BARRIER FUNCTION: GENERAL

It is not clear how the anatomically defined subunits of the TJ relate to TJ barrier function, although a general relationship appears to exist between fibril number and resistance. Taking into consideration a variety of indirect data, such as TJ structure–function correlation,[16,17,43] TJ ion selectivity,[13,16,44–47] TJ sieving characteristics[14] and TJ charge selectivity,[48–51] the following hypothetical model of how the TJ might function is formulated: TJ kisses/strands could be viewed as relatively impermeable structures in which discontinuities, 'channels' or pores, reside. As with channels of biomembranes, it is proposed that these channels may open and close.[16] The interior of the channel would appear to be highly hydrated and contain fixed negative charges. Assuming this model is correct, it is evident that there are numerous potential ways to modify TJ barrier function: the number of kisses/strands (i.e. TJ subunits) could be changed, the probability of channels

being in the open state could be altered, or physical characteristics of the pore interior might be changed. Evidence suggests that some of these mechanisms do indeed occur. Examples include alteration in TJ subunit number (number of strands/kisses),[46,49,52,53] and alterations in surface charge within the pores of the TJ, as suggested by altered TJ charge selectivity.[47] Although there is indirect evidence that occludin may contribute to the formation of aqueous pores within TJ, it is not clear how subunits of occludin form such pores.

As elucidated in the preceding section, TJs on the one hand are linked to the cytoskeleton, and on the other possess an array of signaling proteins. There is considerable evidence that changes in the tension of the underlying cytoskeleton and/or localized disassembly in response to signaling cascade can modulate TJ permeability. Functional links between the cytoskeleton and the TJ were first described[52] in seminal studies which took the approach of pharmacologically manipulating the cytoskeleton and subsequently assessing the alterations that occur in TJ function. In response to cytochalasin D, an agent that affects actin microfilaments, intestinal absorptive cell TJs becomes perturbed in structure and display diminished charge selectivity and resistance.[52] In parallel, the perijunctional ring becomes segmented and condensed and the brush borders become rounded – all features suggesting that, analogous to isolated brush borders, contraction of isolated segments of the ring had occurred. Supporting this view was the subsequent finding that the effects of cytochalasin D on TJ structure, TJ function and ring condensation were energy dependent and appeared to be interrelated.[53]

This hypothesis, which links functional alterations in TJs to cytoskeletal rearrangement, is further supported by the observation that the perijunctional actin–myosin ring contracts and ZO-1 redistributes to the cytoplasm in response to ADP-ribosylation of rho protein, which uncouples rho from downstream effectors.[55] This alteration in the cytoskeleton is paralleled by altered permeability of TJ.[55] Recent studies on phosphorylation of myosin light chains have provided further evidence for functional links between cytoskeleton and TJ. Phosphorylation of myosin light chain is required for the activation of myosin by actin. This phosphorylation results in ATP hydrolysis and sliding of myosin filaments over actin, causing contraction of the peripheral actin–myosin ring and increased TJ permeability. Hecht et al.[56,57] have shown that expression of constitutively active myosin light chain kinase in MDCK cells (polarized epithelial cells) results in enhanced myosin light chain phosphorylation and disruption of TJ barrier function. Thus each enterocyte harbors its own tiny internal sphincter, and it is therefore plausible that cytoskeletal tension can modulate junctional permeability just as mechanically applied lateral tension,[58] by itself, is capable of altering TJ structure.

It has long been observed that TJ structure and function can be modulated by various intracellular events. Recognition that TJ could potentially be regulated by intracellular events came from various observations. First, intracellular mediators can result in altered TJ. Using microelectrode impalement techniques, Duffey et al.[50] showed that the TJs of gallbladder epithelium increase in resistance to passive ion flow as cAMP is elevated. Concurrently, TJ gained structurally defined subunits and TJ charge selectivity was altered. $Ca^{2+}$ ionophore[46] signals and protein kinase C activation[59,60] were also been shown to modulate TJ resistance, charge selectivity and structure in various epithelia. Other mediators that have been shown to modulate TJ structure and function include G-proteins, inositol phosphate, calmodulin and tyrosine kinase (reviewed in [61]). Recently, Rac[62] and Rho,[55] members of the small G-protein family, have been shown to modulate TJ. It is not known how such intracellular activation signals might influence intestinal TJs, and there are few direct data bearing on this issue.

## REGULATION OF TIGHT JUNCTION BARRIER FUNCTION: PHYSIOLOGICAL

It was recently observed that the structure and permeability characteristics of intestinal epithelial TJs are regulated by meal-related nutrients. Thus exposure of the apical membrane of enterocytes to even 10 mmol glucose, which saturates energy-dependent transcellular transport, results in diminished transepithelial resistance[60,61] owing to altered TJ permeability (Fig. 1.4).[63] Concurrent with this permeability alteration, dilatations appear within TJs which represent sites at which junctional fibrils are pushed apart. Tracer studies not only reveal that these dilatations are the anatomic sites of enhanced permeation, but also indicate that dilatations can be permeated by oligopeptides up to 11 amino acids in length (though not by macromolecules).[63] A shared characteristic of all nutrient regulators of intestinal TJs thus far identified is that they activate $Na^+$-coupled transcellular absorption. In addition, glucose exposure induces an altered phenotype in the actin–myosin perijunctional ring suggestive of enhanced tension. The kinetics of the $Na^+$-glucose cotransporter on the apical membrane has been closely linked to the kinetics of the induced permeability change,[63,64] strongly suggesting that activation of this apical transport protein is the initial trigger that results in altered junctional permeation.[63,66] Thus, as a consequence of bulk inward water flow occurring secondary to transcellular active transportation of solutes, luminal solutes such as small molecules can be absorbed paracellularly by solvent drag. Recently, experiments in which the $Na^+$-glucose transporter SGLT-1 was stably expressed in cultured enterocytes have demonstrated that activation of this transporter results in enhanced phosphorylation of myosin light chain (the biochemical equivalent of increased cytoskeletal tension).[67,68] The pathophysiological importance of TJ is elucidated in a study wherein the forced disruption of TJ using dominant negative cadherin resulted in spontaneous Crohn's disease in mice.[69] In addition, recent studies have shown a downregulation of TJ molecules in mucosal biopsies of patients with collagenous colitis, and the authors speculate that the TJ disruption is a structural correlate of barrier dysfunction and may contribute to diarrhea by a leak flux mechanism in these patients.[70] Recently, novel observations have been made on the role of amino acid transporters in the regulation of cytoskeletal organization. Merlin et al. have shown that the amino acid transporter LAT-2 associates with CD98 and $\beta_1$ integrin at the basolateral membrane of model intestinal epithelia.[71] The expression of CD98 in polarized epithelia lacking human CD98 (MDCK cells) disrupted $\beta_1$ integrin surface distribution and cytoskeletal architecture, suggesting that CD98 can influence integrin function. These data provide a novel link between classic transport events and a critical element of barrier function and integrin-mediated influences on cytoskeletal organization.

## MUCOSAL BARRIER FUNCTION IN CROHN'S DISEASE

There is little doubt that mucosal permeability is increased in active Crohn's disease as a consequence of direct effects of proinflammatory molecules and transmigrating neutrophils. However, considerable controversy exists regarding a primary genetically determined defect in epithelial barrier function.

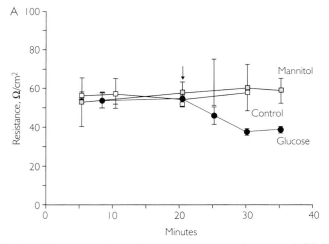
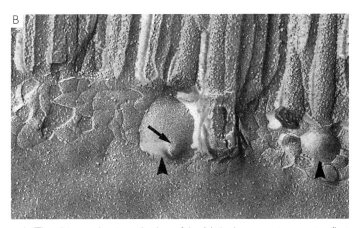

**Fig. 1.4** Tight junction barrier function is physiologically regulated. (A) decrease in TJ resistance due to activation of the $Na^+$-glucose cotransporter (but not due to mannitol – a sugar not recognized by the cotransporter) of mammalian small intestine. (B) freeze fracture image of an intestinal epithelial cell tight junction in the physiological state of low resistance. The normal uniform web-like appearance of the fusions between adjacent cells is distorted (arrows). Such physiologically elicited anatomical changes have been shown to represent the site at which enhanced epithelial permeability occurs. Given such physiological plasticity of this important barrier, it would not be surprising if it were influenced in a globally changed local milieu such as occurs in IBD. (From Atisook K, Carlson S, Madara JL. Effects of phlorizin and sodium on glucose-elicited alterations of cell junctions in intestinal epithelia. Am J Physiol 1990; 258:C77, and Pappenheimer JR. Physiological regulation of transepithelial impedance in the intestinal mucosa of rat and hamsters. J Membrane Biol 1987; 100:137, with permission.)

Several investigators have replicated Hollander's[72] original observations that a subset of asymptomatic relatives of patients with Crohn's disease have increased small intestinal permeability to inert molecules.[72–74] A pathophysiologic consequence of this increased permeability in asymptomatic relatives is the onset of Crohn's disease 8 years after evidence of increased permeability.[75] However, other studies have found no increased permeability in relatives,[76–79] which would suggest an environmental influence rather than genetic determination. Further complexity is introduced by the observation of Medding's group showing that pharmacologically relevant doses of NSAIDs selectively enhanced mucosal permeability in the subset of Crohn's disease patients and their asymptomatic relatives; this trait was conserved within families.[80,81] The discrepancies were explained in part by the observation of Soderholm et al.[82] that baseline (nonstressed) mucosal permeability was increased in Crohn's disease patients, their spouses and asymptomatic relatives, suggesting an environmental factor, but only Crohn's disease patients and their relatives showed increased responses to challenge with aspirin. These latter results indicate a genetic regulation of induced injury, but do not differentiate between an overly aggressive response to injury from defective epithelial healing (see Chapter 2). The consequence of defective mucosal barrier function, whether intrinsic or acquired, is induced uptake of luminal antigens, adjuvants and viable bacteria, which can lead to induction and perpetuation of intestinal injury.

# NEUTROPHIL MIGRATION ACROSS THE INTESTINAL EPITHELIAL BARRIER

## ACTIVE INFLAMMATION IN IBD

When viewing intestinal mucosal biopsies retrieved from patients with IBD, pathologists make several judgments: is evidence of chronicity (i.e. deranged architecture) present; is there epithelial dysplasia; are features of one of the major subcategories of IBD present (i.e. granulomas etc.); and what is the level of 'active inflammation'? The term active inflammation refers to the presence of extravascular acute inflammatory cells such as polymorphonuclear leukocytes (PMN) or neutrophils. When present extravascularly, neutrophils almost invariably infiltrate the epithelial lining of the intestine. Indeed, the classic appearance of active inflammation in IBD is the 'crypt abscess' (Fig. 1.5), a lesion characterized by marked migration of neutrophils across the crypt epithelium with the subsequent collection of aggregated neutrophils in the crypt lumen. If transepithelial migration of neutrophils continues unabated, epithelial disruption can proceed, leading ultimately to severe disease characterized by erosions and ulcerations.

Judging active inflammation by the above criteria is often useful for pathologists as the prevalence of these findings correlates, in general, with disease activity.[83] Such relationships have been studied in a rigorous fashion. For example, circulating neutrophils have been removed from IBD patients, labeled and reperfused. Thus neutrophil transepithelial migration could be quantified by the recovery of label from the intestinal lumen.[84] When neutrophil transepithelial migration was so quantified and subsequently compared with clinically defined disease activity

indices, it was found that the extent of 'active inflammation' correlated with the severity of patient symptoms.

Unfortunately, we do not yet know why neutrophils transmigrate across the intestinal epithelium in disease flares of patients with IBD. The reason for this stems not only from our continuing uncertainty as to the cause of IBD, but, even more fundamentally, our ignorance as to how neutrophils and epithelial cells interact. Below we will consider what is known about neutrophil interactions with intestinal epithelia. We can begin by asking the questions obvious from analyzing the image of a crypt abscess as shown in Figure 1.5: By what route (across cells? between cells?) do neutrophils cross epithelial cells? What effects on epithelial function, if any, accompany such simple transmigration? Do neutrophils disrupt intracellular TJs, which seal the space between epithelial cells? When neutrophils enter the crypt lumen do they interact with the apical membrane of epithelial cells? If so, are there functional sequelae?

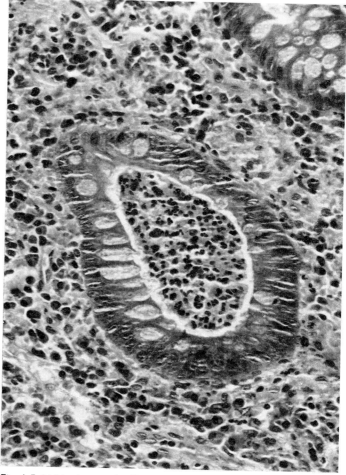

Fig. 1.5 Light micrograph of intestinal epithelial crypt abscess in a patient with active IBD. Numerous neutrophils have transmigrated across the crypt epithelium and have collected within the crypt lumen. Such events raise several issues concerning neutrophil–epithelial interactions in IBD. How do neutrophils transmigrate? How do they move across epithelia? What functional consequences does this have to the epithelium? How might neutrophils in the crypt lumen influence crypt epithelial function? etc. (Photo courtesy of Dr Charles Parkos, Emory University School of Medicine, Department of Pathology.)

# NEUTROPHIL TRANSMIGRATION

Our current understanding of neutrophil–epithelial interaction stems from extensive work done on crypt abscess formation using model intestinal epithelial cells. This reductionistic approach serves to provide initial insights into the questions outlined above, and also demonstrates the complexity of epithelial–neutrophil interaction, especially given the fact that neutrophils synthesize and release a plethora of bioactive substances (for a comprehensive review refer to the splendid text by Gallin[85]). In this model, transformed and non-transformed epithelial cell lines are cultured on permeable filters with pores of sufficient size to allow the passage of neutrophils. The epithelial cells grow as physiologically confluent columnar monolayers, which resemble crypt epithelium in both structure and function.[86,87] The experimental approach to such studies is shown diagrammatically in Figure 1.6. Intestinal epithelial monolayers grown on permeable supports are exposed to neutrophils purified from human peripheral blood, and neutrophils are either coaxed to transmigrate across the model crypt epithelium by constructing transepithelial gradients of a chemotactic molecule endogenous to the colonic lumen (N-formylated peptide derived from bacteria) or are activated by factors naturally present in the colonic lumen (N-formylated peptides and endotoxin)[88–91] (Fig. 1.7). Using this approach various stages of neutrophil transmigration, such as signals for transmigration, adhesion to the extracellular matrix, movement across the columnar epithelium and interaction with epithelial cells on the apical (luminal) surface, have been explored.

Recent observations stemming from analysis of the interactions of *Salmonella typhimurium* with cultured human intestinal epithelial cells indicate that epithelial cells possess the capacity to orchestrate transepithelial movement of neutrophils. When the apical surface of intestinal epithelial cells is colonized by *Salmonella*, the epithelial cells recognize this event and participate in the recruitment of an appropriate inflammatory response. The response to such pathogen challenge includes polarized basolateral release of the chemokine IL-8 (as well as related chemokines), coordinated with polarized apical release of another chemoattractant, pathogen-elicited epithelial chemoattractant – PEEC[92] (Fig.1.8). Surprisingly, the epithelial cell accomplishes this even before movement of the bacterium across the epithelial cell, and also before any detectable functional alterations have occurred in either the epithelial barrier function or active ion transport capacity.[93,94] Recently bacteria-derived flagellin, acting through toll-like receptor-5, has been identified as the key mediator of IL-8 secretion in the intestinal epithelia.[95,96] Flagellin has been identified within the basal media of cultured cells colonized with *Salmonella typhimurium* on the apical surface and TLR-5, interestingly, is localized at the basolateral surface of the intestinal epithelia. Under these conditions neither bacterial translocation nor internalization occurs. These data are consistent with the observation that the epithelial cells secrete IL-8 even before movement of the bacterium across the epithelial cell, and before any detectable alterations have occurred in epithelial barrier function. It appears that IL-8, by virtue of its matrix-binding characteristics, may provide a long-range chemotactic signal across the subepithelial matrix that PMN then follow, whereas PEEC induces the final step of transepithelial migration of PMN.[93] The potential importance of this observation for IBD is apparent: if the epithelium has evolved signaling cascades to initiate active inflammation in

A

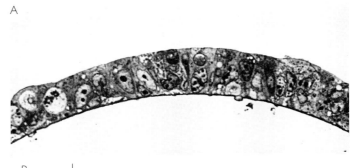

B

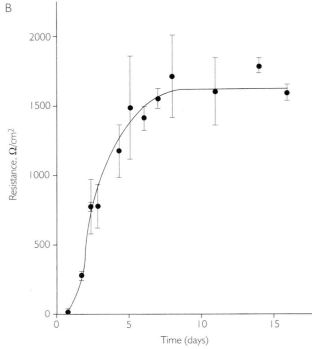

**Fig. 1.6** (A) T84 monolayers grow as columnar epithelial monolayer on permeable supports. This human-derived cell line has the ability to form high-resistance barriers (B) and displays many features of crypt epithelia, such as the ability to secrete isotonic fluid (i.e. secretory diarrhea).

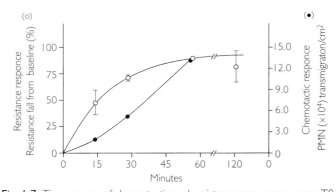

**Fig. 1.7** Time course of chemotactic and resistance responses across T84 monolayers. 107 PMN were placed in the presence of a 107 M gradient of n-formyl-met-leu-phe (fMLP). Maximal responses were achieved at 60 minutes. The resistance response occurred rapidly compared to the chemotactic response. This is to be anticipated, as resistance is a sensitive index of barrier function that is inordinately affected by the presence of a relatively small subpopulation of enhanced permeability sites. (From Nash S, Stafford J, Madara JL. J Clin Invest 1987; 80:1104, with permission.)

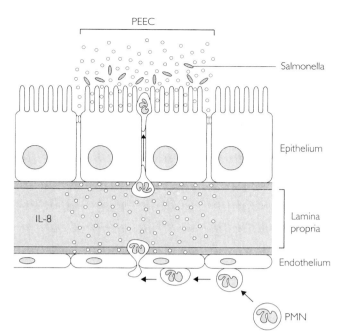

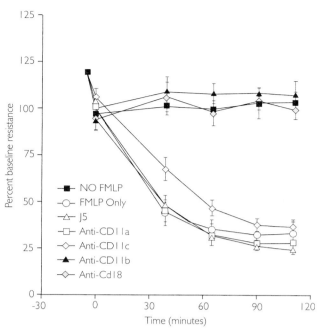

**Fig. 1.8** Schematic illustration of events in neutrophil transmigration. Emigration of PMN can be conceptually divided into three events: a) the well-characterized event of microvascular emigration, b) transmigration across the lamina propria matrix, and c) transepithelial migration (see text). Intestinal epithelial responses to the pathogen *Salmonella typhimurium* is depicted schematically. In response to apical attachment of *Salmonella*, epithelia secrete, in a polarized fashion, chemokines including IL-8 basolaterally. This polarized basolateral secretion of IL-8 is coordinated with the polarized apical release of another chemoattractant, pathogen-elicited epithelial chemoattractant (PEEC). It is conceivable, though now unknown, that such aberrant triggering of epithelial cascades contribute to the recruitment of inflammatory cells such as those seen in IBD. Known distorting effects of solvent flow in the microenvironment of the lamina propria would seem to favor long-range matrix-binding chemotactic signals for the second event. It is now known that basolateral IL-8 secretion imprints underlying matrices with gradient sufficient to stimulate neutrophil migration to the immediate subepithelial space. However, it appears that basolateral secretion of the chemoattractant IL-8 is not sufficient to stimulate the final event of transmigration. Rather, apical signals, such as PEEC, probably account for this final event.

**Fig. 1.9** Effect of antibodies to PMN adhesive molecules on the PMN transmigration-associated fall in transepithelial resistance to passive ion flow. Transmigration was stimulated by a transepithelial gradient of the chemotactic peptide FMLP. Antibody to the β subunit of $\beta_2$ integrin adhesive molecules (anti-CD18) blocks transmigration and PMN transmigration-associated effect on epithelial barrier function. Of the three subunits which associate with $\beta_2$ (CD11a, 11b, 11c), only anti-CD11b substantially prevents transmigration as assessed in this assay. J5 is an antibody control which binds to a non-integrin epitope on the PMN surface. This integrin-based adhesion of PMN to intestinal epithelial cells appears to be required for transmigration and the transmigration-associated effects on epithelial barrier function. (From Parkos CA et al. J Clin Invest 1991; 88:1605, with permission.)

response to colonization by enteric pathogens, perhaps such pathways could be triggered by inappropriate events even though the usual initiating agent (pathogen) may be missing. Indeed, the above described polarized release of IL-8 by intestinal epithelia can be simply elicited by the activation of protein kinase C.[92]

It has been demonstrated that $\beta_2$ integrins play a central role in neutrophil–epithelial adhesive interactions. $\beta_2$ integrins are heterodimeric integral membrane glycoproteins expressed only on leukocytes, and consist of a common CD18 β chain, which associates with one of four α chains, CD11a, CD11b, CD11c and CD11d. It was first noted that neutrophils derived from patients with leukocyte adhesive deficiency lacking $\beta_2$ integrins were unable to transmigrate across epithelia. Subsequently, experiments using blocking monoclonal antibodies showed that one of these integrins, CD11b/CD18, was required for transmigration (Fig. 1.9).[97] The epithelial counter-receptor for this integrin is not known. However, signals such as cytokines may potentially modulate the epithelial expression of neutrophil

ligands, and thus movement of neutrophils through the paracellular pathway also appears to be regulated. For example, pre-exposure of such intestinal epithelial monolayers to interferon-γ results in enhanced migration of neutrophils into the paracellular space, but retention within the monolayer.[98] These effects are mediated by epithelial protein synthesis, are associated with the appearance of additional adhesive ligands for neutrophils on the epithelial surface, and these new ligands appear also to be dependent on interactions with the CD11b/CD18 integrin on the neutrophil surface.[99] The paradigm for $\beta_2$ integrin-defined associations between neutrophils and intestinal epithelial cells developed from in vitro model systems has been supported by analyses of the attachment of freshly isolated human colonocytes to purified $\beta_2$ integrins.

Recent studies have shown that the integrin-associated protein CD47, a membrane glycoprotein of the immunoglobulin superfamily, plays a crucial role in neutrophil transepithelial migration. CD47 is expressed not only on the neutrophil surface, but is richly expressed on the basolateral membrane of intestinal epithelial cells. The importance of CD47 is best exemplified in CD47-deficient mice, which rapidly succumb to bacterial sepsis following intra-abdominal challenge with *Escherichia coli* owing to delayed recruitment of PMN to the site of infection.[96] Consistent with these studies, anti-CD47 antibodies prevent neutrophil transmigration while not affecting the adhesion of PMN to epithelial cells.[100,101] In transmigration assays performed in the presence of anti-CD47, this results in an accumulation of PMN within the epithelium.[100] Further, increased surface expression of CD47 enhances the rate of migration of neutrophils.[102]

Recently, a novel link between peptide transporters and neutrophil–intestinal epithelial interaction has been demonstrated. It has been largely assumed that directed neutrophil movement across columnar epithelia was probably a response to transepithelial chemoattractant gradient. As mentioned above, bacterial contamination of spaces in contact with an external environment could readily be imagined to support a lumen–tissue gradient of potent chemoattractants, such as *n*-formyl peptides. Until recently it was believed that fMLP passively diffused across TJ to create a paracellular gradient. However, it has been demonstrated that the oligopeptide transporter hPepT1, expressed in epithelial cells, is partly responsible for the apical transport of fMLP.[103] Interestingly, hPepT1 expression is normally restricted to the small intestine, where the environment is relatively sterile, whereas it is not expressed in the colon, where bacteria reside.[103] It is possible that this decreased expression may be an adaptive mechanism in response to bacterial colonization to prevent inflammatory responses to commensal bacteria. However, aberrant metaplastic expression of hPepT1 occurs in the colon in chronic IBD, including Crohn's colitis and ulcerative colitis. Forced expression of hPepT1 in colonic epithelia in vitro enhances neutrophil transmigration.[103] These finding indicate that transporters may play an active role in neutrophil transmigration, and that activation of such transporters during active inflammation may modify subsequent interaction with neutrophils. It will be important to determine whether expression of these transports during IBD is due to inappropriate regulation or a non-specific response to inflammation.

As shown in Figure 1.10, neutrophils cross intestinal epithelial monolayers by migrating between cells across intercellular TJ.[104] This chemotactic response is paralleled by impaired TJ barrier function, as indicated by a falling resistance. Other experiments have shown that these functional effects are due specifically to chemotaxis rather than chemokinesis (i.e. dependent on directed rather than random movement).[88,89] With large numbers of transmigrating PMN, TJ function is dramatically impaired. In intestinal epithelial monolayers, impairment takes the form of diminished transepithelial flux of inert tracers such as mannitol and inulin, and, during the phase in which TJs are actively being impaled by PMN, leaks to macromolecules. Upon ablation of chemotactic conditions, these barrier alterations are readily reversed. Thus, TJ reseal after transmigration ceases, again highlighting their dynamic nature. It does not appear that products released by the PMN are responsible for these defects in TJ permeability, as 1) when PMN are densely layered on to monolayers and stimulated with the chemotactic agent in the absence of a chemotactic gradient, no change in barrier function occurs; and 2) selected inhibitors of products released by PMN under chemotactic conditions do not prevent altered barrier function. It does appear that an adhesion plaque that forms before transmigration between the PMN and epithelial cells may be the 'foothold' from which the PMN is able to generate the force required to open the TJ. Thus, it has been speculated that the opening of the TJ that occurs during PMN transmigration is produced by mechanical force, just as mechanical force may underlie the TJ perturbation induced by the above-outlined pharmacologic and physiologic manipulations. The difference is

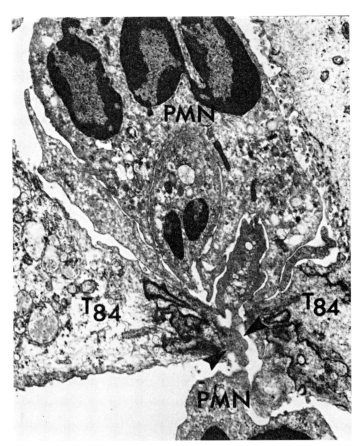

**Fig. 1.10** Electron micrograph of PMN indenting a T84 monolayer and passing through a TJ impalement site. Transmigration occurs by extension of pseudopodia through sites of epithelial discontinuity (arrowheads). (From Nash S et al. J Clin Invest 1991; 87:1474, with permission.)

that in these latter instances the speculative mechanical force may be generated by the cytoskeleton within the epithelial cell, whereas with PMN transmigration the mechanical force may be generated externally by the PMN pseudopodia. In contrast to dendritic cell pseudopodia, which have been shown to transgress the tight junction, sample luminal content and then withdraw back to a subepithelial position, PMN largely transmigrate the TJ driven by chemotactic gradients for which they possess receptors. It is also the case, however, that at low PMN transmigration densities TJ barriers remain intact.[105]

## NEUTROPHIL–EPITHELIAL INTERACTIONS

Neutrophil transmigration across model intestinal epithelium has also been shown to elicit electrogenic $Cl^-$ secretion.[106,107] Physiologic (constitutive) $Cl^-$ transport is the basis for hydration of mucosal surfaces and, when substantially upregulated, causes secretory diarrhea. Neutrophils stimulate such epithelial fluid secretion in a novel fashion. The neutrophil–epithelial interaction is depicted schematically in Figure 1.11. Upon stimulation with activating factors such as those normally present in the intestinal lumen, PMN release 5'-AMP, in a regulated fashion. This classic intracellular metabolite interfaces, in paracrine fashion, with the apical membrane of crypt cells.[107] There it is converted by an epithelial ectoenzyme, 5'-ectonucleotidase (CD73), to adenosine, a bioactive molecule which activates apical adenosine receptors of the A2b subtype. 5'-Ectonucleotidase is apically polarized in native human intestinal crypts[108]

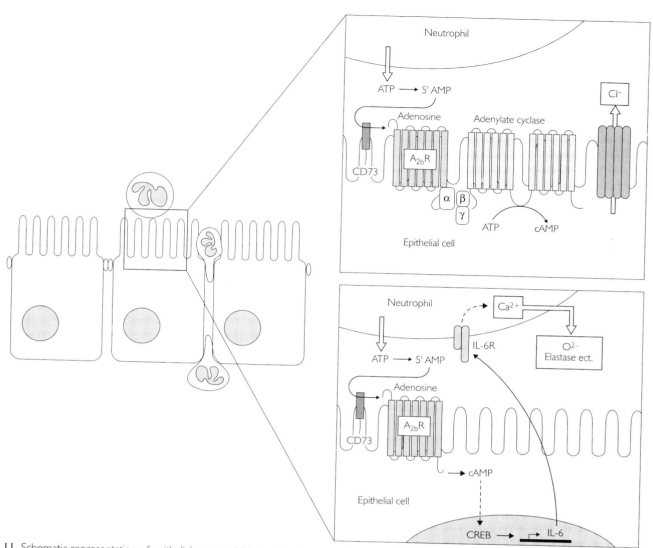

**Fig. 1.11** Schematic representation of epithelial–neutrophil interaction in a crypt abscess: an epithelial monolayer with neutrophils transmigrating to the luminal compartment is shown in the left panel. Translocation of PMN into the luminal compartment results in a paracrine signaling to the epithelial apical membrane by 5'-AMP. At the epithelial cell surface the 5'-AMP is efficiently translated into an adenosine signal by 5' ectonucleotidase (CD73). The resulting adenosine activates adenosine receptor of A2b subtype. The adenosine receptor is coupled to heterotrimeric G protein and stimulates chloride secretion by mechanisms which involve protein kinase A, and perhaps other signaling pathways (inset at the top). Adenosine also interacts with the adenosine A2b receptor and induces cAMP-mediated transcriptional activation of IL-6 secretion. IL-6 is preferentially released in the apical compartment and induces intracellular $Ca^{2+}$ flux in neutrophils, which may be involved in the release of oxygen radicals, elastase etc. from the neutrophils (inset at the bottom).

and 5'-AMP has been shown to stimulate freshly isolated crypt cells to secrete chloride.[108] The A2b adenosine receptor is coupled to G proteins, which activate adenylate cyclase. cAMP thus generated has been shown to activate chloride channels.[109,110] In addition to chloride secretion, adenosine induces a polarized secretion of IL-6 into the intestinal lumen. IL-6 thus released by epithelia can, in turn, activate a calcium response in neutrophils (Fig. 1.11), an event associated with degranulation of neutrophils.[111]

Although the findings above highlight the crosstalk that can occur between neutrophils and epithelial cells, they undoubtedly also oversimplify these interactions such as would occur in IBD. For example, whereas 5'-AMP is the major direct-acting secretagogue released by neutrophils, other neutrophil products, in purified form, are also able to stimulate Cl⁻ secretion experimentally.[112,113] Moreover, the plethora of bioactive compounds released by transmigrating neutrophils (arachidonic acid metabo-

lites, for example)[85] might interact with subepithelial cells, which in turn could release their own agonists of Cl⁻ secretion. Thus the paradigm considered in this chapter is best used to stimulate our thinking concerning the mechanisms of epithelial–neutrophil interactions which we observe, in static state, in biopsy materials derived from IBD patients.

# MECHANISMS OF DOWNREGULATION OF EPITHELIAL PROINFLAMMATORY ACTIVATION

The intestinal epithelium tolerates a wide variety of prokaryotic organisms and their products on their cell surface without eliciting an inflammatory response. Recent work by Neish et al. and others have provided insight into mechanisms by which proinflammatory signaling from pathogens can be dampened by non-pathogenic bacteria.[114] They made the discovery that cells colonized with non-pathogenic strains of *Salmonella typhimurium* were refractory to upregulation of inflammatory effector molecule or the activation of NFkB. This blockade of the proinflammatory pathway occurred by the complete inhibition of ubiquitination of phosphorylated IkB, which prevents the degradation of IkB such that NFkB cannot be translocated to the nucleus. Even without bacterial stimulation, many intestinal epithelial cell lines and native intestinal cells have delayed and incomplete NFkB degradation in response to IL-1, TNF and LPS.[115] Furthermore, Abreu et al. demonstrated that intestinal epithelial cells have low expression of TLR-4 and MD88,[116] providing an additional mechanism of buffered responses to proinflammatory bacterial products. The intestinal epithelium also dynamically alters its gene expression in response to the changing environments in both the intestinal lumen and the subepithelial domain. For example, in response to either luminal enteric pathogens or lamina propria proinflammatory cytokines, the intestinal epithelium activates the expression of a panel of genes that promote an acute inflammatory response.[117] Because uncontrolled inflammation can result in tissue damage, the intestinal epithelium defends itself by synthesizing anti-inflammatory mediators that can attenuate proinflammatory responses. One example of such a mediator is the anti-inflammatory eicosanoid lipoxin (lipoxin A4 or LXA4). Lipoxins such as LXA4 are derived from arachidonate as a result of its exposure to the unique combinations of lipoxygenases that occur during specific heterotypic cell–cell interactions such as those that take place in inflammation (e.g. epithelial–neutrophil interactions). LXA4-induced responses downregulate events associated with inflammation in a variety of in vitro and in vivo models. For example, LXA4 has been shown to downregulate NFkB activation and IL-8 secretion induced by *Salmonella* and other proinflammatory cytokines.[118] Yet another mechanism by which epithelial cells may downregulate proinflammatory signaling by cytokines such as IL-6 is by the activation of suppressor of cytokine signaling (SOCS) proteins. These proteins have been recently cloned and shown to downregulate inflammation by their specific binding to the cytokine receptor.[119] For example, in intestinal epithelia SOCS-3 is induced by IL-6, and overexpression of SOCS-3 abolishes IL-6 signaling.[120] It is clear that intestinal epithelial cells interact with lamina propria mononuclear cells in a bidirectional manner, and that this crosstalk regulates physiologic responses to commensal bacteria. For example, in in vitro systems *Bacteroides vulgatus* or LPS activate NFkB in intestinal epithelial cell monolayers, but co-cultured lymphocytes downregulate bacterial-induced NFkB activation via secreted products, which are unidentified.[121] Thus, the intestine is equipped with various mechanisms to downregulate and defend itself from pathogens and commensal luminal insults.

## POTENTIAL MODULATION OF TIGHT JUNCTIONS BY INFLAMMATORY CYTOKINES AND LUMINAL FACTORS SUCH AS BACTERIAL TOXINS

Regulation of junctional permeability not only occurs as a reversible rapid response as outlined above, but also can result from biological signals which, over time, lead to 'remodeled' epithelial cells (i.e. changes dependent on new protein synthesis and slowly reversible) with altered junctional permeation. For example, the cytokine interferon-γ can lead to enhanced permeation of junctions in cultured intestinal epithelial monolayers.[122] The importance of junctional regulations such as those outlined above is that the passive transepithelial movement of biologically active solutes derived from other cell types, or even microorganisms, may change depending on the physiological state and the microenvironment of the epithelium. Indeed, it would not be surprising if colonization of epithelial surfaces by particular microbes could result in signals which, in themselves, would modulate epithelial permeability. Recent studies have shown that toxins elaborated by (or other events associated with) *Clostridium difficile*, enteropathogenic *E. coli* (EPEC) and *Vibrio cholerae* result in altered TJ permeability, which may play an important role in the pathogenesis of diarrhea caused by these organisms. For example, toxin A derived from *Clostridium difficile* results in a loss of F-actin staining in the perijunctional ring, which occurs in parallel with enhancement of TJ permeability without the loss of cell–cell contacts.[123] This effect of toxin A on the perijunctional ring is mediated through covalent modification of the small GTP-binding protein rho.[52] Studies on the pathogenesis of EPEC-associated diarrhea have shown that myosin light chain is phosphorylated following EPEC exposure, and this parallels with an increased TJ permeability. Inhibition of myosin light chain phosphorylation restores TJ barrier function, suggesting that altered TJ permeability may contribute to diarrhea induced by EPEC.[113] Fasono et al.[105] have isolated a novel toxin elaborated by *V. cholerae* called zonula occludens toxin, or Zot. Zot decreases epithelial tissue resistance, increases TJ permeability, and increases $Na^+$ and water secretion in a time- and dose-dependent manner, suggesting that alteration of TJ permeability may, in part, contribute to diarrhea associated with EPEC.[104]

## RESEALING DISRUPTED TIGHT JUNCTIONS

Unimpeded intestinal inflammation may result in complete loss of the epithelial barrier as erosions or ulcers form. Such sites are obvious ones where free diffusion of even the largest macromolecules could occur via the resulting paracellular space. The groups of Silen and Ito showed that comparable wounds in gastric epithelia reseal by a process termed restitution, in which epithelial cells bordering the defect flatten and migrate into the wound. It was subsequently shown that restitution also occurs in intestinal epithelia.[125–127] Using wounded cultured intestinal epithelial cell models, it has been demonstrated that immediately after villous tips are denuded epithelial permeability is markedly enhanced, but within 60 minutes returns to normal.[128] Consequent upon such wounding, columnar cells bordering the wound flatten, extend lamellipodia over the denuded matrix, F-actin arcs cross the base of the lamellipodia-like extensions, and F-actin microspikes project from the leading edge of these extensions.[13,129] As wounds become smaller (< 30 mm), epithelial cells at the wound edge assume a columnar phenotype with poorly formed or absent lamellopodia. Apically localized circumferential F-actin–myosin

II rings encircle such wounds, suggesting that final closure is by a sphincter-like contraction.[130] A wide variety of growth factors (TGFβ, FGF, EGF, KGF-2) and cytokines produced by epithelial as well as lamina propria cell populations promote restitution in models of epithelial injury.[127] In addition, trefoil peptides, members of a recently recognized family of small proteins produced by goblet cells, promote restitution following secretion on to apical surfaces and interaction with receptors distinct from those of growth factors or cytokines[131] (see also Chapter 27). Although these features are similar to those occurring in professionally migrating cells such as macrophages, movement of epithelial-specific proteins such as villin to the leading edge at such sites[132] suggests that epithelial specific caveats may exist. A better understanding of these events is crucial to IBD, particularly if the rate of resealing can be influenced by exogenous stimuli which could be of therapeutic benefit.

## SUMMARY

Enhanced epithelial permeability is thought to play a role in the symptomatology (and, some speculate, the pathogenesis) of IBD. We now know that the rate-limiting barrier governing passive permeation across this epithelium, the intercellular TJ, is highly dynamic and regulated. By better understanding the nature of TJ regulation and the molecular events governing 'up'- and 'down'-regulation of the TJ one may be able to manipulate barrier function independently. Such knowledge, which could potentially affect IBD management, awaits further development in this field.

It is reasonably clear that the PMN–intestinal epithelial interactions in general, and PMN–transepithelial migration in particular, are associated with clinically defined disease activity in IBD. The above observations suggest that such transmigration is dependent on PMN–epithelial cell adhesive events and that, as a result of transmigration, epithelial secretion induced by neutrophil products may occur. Thus, definition of the epithelial counter-receptors for neutrophil adhesive interactions should potentially provide therapeutic strategies for blocking transmigration in active IBD. If such strategies were successful, data from the above-described model would predict improvement of epithelial barrier function and attenuation of secretory diarrhea – desired goals in the therapy of IBD. Similar strategies are now being developed to block PMN–endothelial interactions. However, it is doubtful that this latter approach, which lacks organ or tissue specificity, would be useful on a sustained basis. Fortunately, it appears that the cell–cell adhesion 'rules' governing transendothelial migration of PMN differ significantly from those governing transmigration of PMN across intestinal epithelia. Similarly, a better understanding of the nature of inflammation-elicited secretion may lead to new avenues for the treatment of IBD, as would a better understanding of the biology of epithelial cell spreading and migration in response to wounding.

Paradigms of active intestinal inflammation such as those considered above are necessarily simplistic in the extreme. However, they do highlight the types of molecular interactions that need to be explained if we are to better understand the complex nature of active inflammation in vivo as we see it in IBD biopsy specimens.

## REFERENCES

1. Madara JL. Epithelia: biologic principles of organization. In: Yamada T, ed. Textbook of gastroenterology, 2nd edn. Philadelphia: JB Lippincott; 1995; 141.
2. McNabb PC, Tomasi TB. Host defense mechanisms at mucosal surfaces. Ann Rev Microbiol 1981;35:477.
3. Williams SJ, Wreschner DH, Tran M, Eyre HJ, Sutherland GR, McGuckin MA. MUC13, a novel human cell surface mucin expressed by epithelial and hemopoietic cells. J Biol Chem 2001;276:18327.
4. Velcich A, Yang W, Heyer J et al. Colorectal cancer in mice genetically deficient in the mucin Muc2. Science 2002; 295:1726.
5. Ouelette AJ. Paneth cells and innate immunity in crypt microenvironment. Gastroenterology 1997;113:1779.
6. O'Neil DA, Porter EM, Elewaut D et al. Expression and regulation of the human beta-defensins hBD-1 and hBD-2 in intestinal epithelium. J Immunol 1999;163:6718–6724.
7. Hecht G. Microbes and microbial toxins: paradigms for microbial–mucosal interactions. VII. Enteropathogenic *Escherichia coli*: physiological alterations from an extracellular position. Am J Physiol Gastrointest Liver Physiol 2001;281:G1–7.
8. Lencer WI, Cheung G, Strohmeier GR et al. Induction of epithelial chloride secretion by channel-forming cryptdins 2 and 3. Proc Natl Acad Sci USA 1997;94:8585–8589.
9. Yue G, Merlin D, Selsted ME, Lencer WI, Madara JL, Eaton DC. Cryptdin 3 forms anion selective channels in cytoplasmic membranes of human embryonic kidney cells. Am J Physiol Gastrointest Liver Physiol 2002;282:G757–765.
10. Madara JL. Loosening TJs. Lessons from the intestine. J Clin Invest 1989; 83:1089.
11. Gumbiner B. The structure, biochemistry, and assembly of epithelial TJs. Am J Physiol 1987;253:C749.
12. Powell D. Barrier function of epithelia. Am J Physiol 1981;241:G275.
13. Frizzell RA, Schultz SG. Ionic conductance of extracellular shunt pathway in rabbit ileum. J Gen Physiol 1972;59:318.
14. Farquhar MG, Palade GE. Junctional complexes in various epithelia. J Cell Biol 1963;17:375.
15. Claude P. Morphologic factors influencing transepithelial permeability: A model for the resistance of the zonula occludens. J Membrane Biol 1978;39:219.
16. Madara JL, Dharmsathaphorn K. Occluding junction structure–function relationships in a cultured epithelial monolayer. J Cell Biol 1985;101:2124.
17. Marcial M, Carlson SL, Madara JL. Partitioning of paracellular conductance along the ileal crypt–villus axis: a hypothesis based on structural analysis with detailed consideration of TJ structure–function relationships. J Membrane Biol 1984;80:59.
18. Furuse M, Hirase T, Itoh M et al. Occludin: a novel intergral membrane protein localizing at the TJs. J Cell Biol 1993;123:1777.
19. Wong V, Gumbiner BM. A synthetic peptide corresponding to the extracellular domain of occludin perturbs the TJ permeability barrier. J Cell Biol 1997;136:399.
20. McCarthy KM, Francis SA, McCormack JM et al. Occludin is a functional component of the TJ. J Cell Sci 1996;109:2287.
21. Furuse M, Fujita K, Hiiragi T, Fujimoto K, Tsukita S. Claudin-1 and -2: novel integral membrane proteins localizing at tight junctions with no sequence similarity to occludin. J Cell Biol 1998;141:1539–1550.
22. Furuse M, Sasaki H, Fujimoto K, Tsukita S. A single gene product, claudin-1 or -2, reconstitutes tight junction strands and recruits occludin in fibroblasts. J Cell Biol 1998;143:391–401.
23. Furuse M, Hata M, Furuse K et al. Claudin-based tight junctions are crucial for the mammalian epidermal barrier: a lesson from claudin-1-deficient mice. J Cell Biol 2002;156:1099.
24. Williams LA, Martin-Padura I, Dejana E, Hogg N, Simmons DL. Identification and characterisation of human Junctional Adhesion Molecule (JAM). Mol Immunol 1999;36:1175–1188.
25. Bazzoni G, Martinez-Estrada OM, Mueller F et al. Homophilic interaction of junctional adhesion molecule. J Biol Chem 2000;275(40):30970–30976.
26. Liu Y, Nusrat A, Schnell FJ et al. Human junction adhesion molecule regulates tight junction resealing in epithelia. J Cell Sci 2000;113:2363–2374.
27. Martin-Padura I, Lostaglio S, Schneemann M et al. Junctional adhesion molecule, a novel member of the immunoglobulin superfamily that distributes at intercellular junctions and modulates monocyte transmigration. J Cell Biol 1998;142:117–127.
28. Madara JL. Intestinal absorptive cell TJs are linked to cytoskeleton. Am J Physiol 1987;253:C171.
29. Furase M, Itoh M, Hirase T et al. Direct association of occludin with ZO-1 and its possible involvement in the localization of occludin at TJ. J Cell Biol 1994;127:1617.
30. Gumbiner B, Lowenkopf T, Apatira D. Identification of a 160 kDa polypeptide that binds to the TJ-associated protein ZO-1. Proc Natl Acad Sci USA 1991;88:3460.
31. Haskins J, Gu L, Wittchen ES, Hibbard J, Stevenson BR. ZO-3, a novel member of the MAGUK protein family found at the tight junction, interacts with ZO-1 and occludin. J Cell Biol 1998;141:199–208.
32. Howarth AG, Hughes MG, Stevenson BR. Detection of TJ-associated protein ZO-1 in astrocytes and other non-epithelial cell types. Am J Physiol 1992;262:C461.
33. Citi S, Sabanay H, Jakes R, Geiger B, Kendrick-Jones J. Cingulin, a new peripheral component of TJ. Nature 1988;333:272.

34. Zhong Y, Enomoto K, Isomura H et al. Monoclonal antibody 7H6 reacts with a novel TJ-associated protein distinct from ZO-1, cingulin and ZO-2. J Cell Biol 1993;120:477.

35. Weber E, Berta G, Tousson A et al. Expression of polarization of a Rab3 isoform in epithelial cells. J Cell Biol 1994;125:583.

36. Tsukita S, Oishi K, Akiyama T, Yamanashi Y, Yamamoto T, Tsukita S. Specific proto-oncogenic tyrosine kinase of src family are enriched in cell-cell adherens junctions where the level of tyrosine phosphorylation is elevated. J Cell Biol 1991;13:867.

37. Yamamoto T, Harada N, Kano K et al. The ras target AF-6 interacts with ZO-1 and serves as a peripheral component of TJ in epithelial cells. J Cell Biol 1997;139:785.

38. Drenckhan D, Dermietzal R. Organization of the actin filament cytoskeleton in the intestinal brush border: a quantitative and qualitative immunoelectron microscope study. J Cell Biol 1988;107:1037.

39. Stevenson BR, Goodenough DA. Zonulae occludens in junctional complex-enriched fractions from mouse liver. Preliminary morphological and biochemical characterization. J Cell Biol 1984;98:1209.

40. Rodewald R, Newman SB, Karnovsky MJ. Contraction of isolated brush borders from the intestinal epithelium. J Cell Biol 1976;70:541.

41. Burgess DR. Reactivation of intestinal epithelial brush border motility: ATP-dependent contraction via a terminal web contractile ring. J Cell Biol 1982;95:853.

42. Nelson WJ, Shore EM, Wang AZ et al. Identification of a membrane–cytoskeletal complex containing the cell adhesion molecule uvomorulin (E-cadherin), ankyrin, and fodrin in Madin–Darby canine kidney epithelial cells. J Cell Biol 1990;110:349.

43. Claude P, Goodenough DA. Fracture faces of zonulae occludens from 'tight' and 'leaky' epithelia. J Cell Biol 1973;58:390.

44. Diamond JM, Wright EM. Biological membranes: The physical basis of ion and non-electrolyte permeability. Annu Rev Physiol 1969;31:581.

45. Cereijido M, Robbins ES, Dolan WJ, Rotunno CA, Sabatini DD. Polarized monolayers formed by epithelial cells on a permeable and translucent support. J Cell Biol 1978;77:853.

46. Palant CE, Duffey ME, Mookerjee BK, Ho S, Bentzel CJ. Ca++ regulation of TJ permeability and structure in Necturus gallbladder. Am J Physiol 1983;245:C203.

47. Rao MC, Nash NT, Field M. Differing effects of cGMP and cAMP on ion transport across flounder intestine. Am J Physiol 1984;246:C167.

48. Smyth DH, Wright EM. Streaming potentials in the rat small intestine. J Physiol (Lond) 1966;182:591.

49. Madara JL. Increases in guinea pig small intestinal transepithelial resistance induced by osmotic loads are accompanied by rapid alterations in absorptive-cell TJ structure. J Cell Biol 1983;97:125.

50. Duffey ME, Hainan B, Ho S, Bentzel CJ. Regulation of epithelial TJ permeability by cyclic AMP. Nature 1981;294:451.

51. Bakker R, Groot JA. cAMP-mediated effects of ouabain and theophylline on paracellular ion selectivity. Am J Physiol 1984;246:G213.

52. Madara JL, Barenberg D, Carlson S. Effects of cytochalasin D on occluding junctions of intestinal absorptive cells: further evidence that the cytoskeleton may influence paracellular permeability. J Cell Biol 1986;97:2125.

53. Bentzel CJ, Hainau B, Ho S et al. Cytoplasmic regulation of tight junction permeability: Effects of plant cytokinins. Am J Physiol 1988;239:C75.

54. Madara JL, Moore R, Carlson S. Alteration of intestinal TJ structure and permeability by cytoskeletal contraction. Am J Physiol 1987;253:C854.

55. Nusrat A, Giry M, Turner JR et al. Rho protein regulates TJ and perijunctional actin organization in polarized epithelia. Proc Natl Acad Sci USA 1995;92:10629.

56. Hecht G, Pestic L, Nikcevic G et al. Expression of the catalytic domain of myosin light chain kinase increases paracellular permeability. Am J Physiol 1996;271:C1678.

57. Turner JR, Angle JM, Black ED, Joyal JL, Sacks DB, Madara JL. PKC-dependent regulation of transepithelial resistance: roles of MLC and MLC kinase. Am J Physiol 1999;277:C554–562.

58. Pitelka DR, Taggart BN. Mechanical tension induces lateral movement of intramembrane components of the TJ: Studies on mouse mammary cells in culture. J Cell Biol 1983;96:606.

59. Mullin JE, O'Brien TG. Effects of tumor promoters on LLC-PK, renal epithelial TJs and transepithelial fluxes. Am J Physiol 1986;251:C597.

60. Meza I, Sabanero M, Stefani E, Cereijido M. Occluding junctions and cytoskeletal components in cultured transporting epithelium. J. Cell Biol 1980;87:746.

61. Anderson JM, Van Itallie CM. TJs and the molecular basis for the regulation of paracellular permeability. Am J Physiol 1995;269:G467.

62. Takaishi K, Matozaki T, Nakano K, Takai Y. Multiple downstream signalling pathways from ROCK, a target molecule of Rho small G protein, in reorganization of the actin cytoskeleton in Madin–Darby canine kidney cells. Genes Cells 2000;5:929–936.

63. Atisook K, Carlson S, Madara JL. Effects of phlorizin and sodium on glucose-elicited alterations of cell junctions in intestinal epithelia. Am J Physiol 1990;258:C77.

64. Atisook K, Madara JL. An oligopeptide permeates intestinal tight junctions at glucose-elicited dilatations. Gastroenterology 1991;100:719.

65. Pappenheimer JR. Physiological regulation of transepithelial impedance in the intestinal mucosa of rat and hamsters. J Membrane Biol 1987;100:137.

66. Turner JR, Cohen DE, Mrsny RJ, Madara JL. Noninvasive in vivo analysis of human small intestinal paracellular absorption: regulation by Na+-glucose cotransport. Dig Dis Sci 2000;45:2122–2126.

67. Turner JR, Rill BK, Carlson SL et al. Physiological regulation of epithelial TJ is associated with myosin light-chain phosphoryation. Am J Physiol 1997;273:C1378.

68. Nusrat A, Turner JR, Madara JL. Molecular physiology and pathophysiology of tight junctions. IV. Regulation of tight junctions by extracellular stimuli: nutrients, cytokines, and immune cells. Am J Physiol Gastrointest Liver Physiol 2000;279:G851–857.

69. Hermiston ML, Gordon JI. Inflammatory bowel disease and adenomas in mice expressing a dominant negative N-cadherin. Science 1995;270:1203–1207.

70. Burgel N, Bojarski C, Mankertz J, Zeitz M, Fromm M, Schulzke JD. Mechanisms of diarrhea in collagenous colitis. Gastroenterology 2002;123:433–443.

71. Merlin D, Sitaraman S, Liu X et al. CD98-mediated links between amino acid transport and beta 1 integrin distribution in polarized columnar epithelia. J Biol Chem 2001; 276:39282–39289.

72. Hollander D, Vadheim CM, Brettholz E, Petersen GM, Delahunty T, Rotter JI. Increased intestinal permeability in patients with Crohn's disease and their relatives. A possible etiologic factor. Ann Intern Med 1986;105:883–885 .

73. May GR, Sutherland LR, Meddings JB. Is small intestinal permeability really increased in relatives of patients with Crohn's disease? Gastroenterology 1993;104:1627–1632.

74. Secondulfo M, de Magistris L, Fiandra R et al. Intestinal permeability in Crohn's disease patients and their first degree relatives. Dig Liver Dis 2001;33:680–685.

75. Irvine EJ, Marshall JK. Increased intestinal permeability precedes the onset of Crohn's disease in a subject with familial risk. Gastroenterology 2000;119:1740–1744.

76. Teahon K, Smethurst P, Levi AJ, Menzies IS, Bjarnason I. Intestinal permeability in patients with Crohn's disease and their first degree relatives. Gut 1992;33:320–323.

77. Katz KD, Hollander D, Vanheim CM. Intestinal permeability in patients with Crohn's disease and their healthy relatives. Gastroenterology 1989;97:927–931.

78. Munkholm P, Langholz E, Hollander D et al. Intestinal permeability in patients with Crohn's disease and ulcerative colitis and their first degree relatives or increased permeability in spouses. Gut 1994;35:68–72.

79. Breslin NP, Nash C, Hilsden RJ et al. Intestinal permeability is increased in a proportion of spouses of patients with Crohn's disease. Am J Gastroenterol 2001;96:2934–2938.

80. Hilsden RJ, Meddings JB, Sutherland LR. Intestinal permeability changes in response to acetylsalicylic acid in relatives of patients with Crohn's disease. Gastroenterology 1996;110:1395–1403.

81. Zamora SA, Hilsden RJ, Meddings JB, Butzner JD, Scott RB, Sutherland LR. Intestinal permeability before and after ibuprofen in families of children with Crohn's disease. Can J Gastroenterol 1999;13:31–36.

82. Soderholm JD, Olaison G, Lindberg E et al. Different intestinal permeability patterns in relatives and spouses of patients with Crohn's disease: an inherited defect in mucosal defence? Gut 1999;44:96–100.

83. Teahon K, Smethurst P, Pearson M, Levi AJ, Bjarnason I. The effect of elemental diet on intestinal permeability and inflammation in Crohn's disease. Gastroenterology 1991;101:84.

84. Keshavarzian A, Price YE, Peters AM, Lavender JP, Wright NA, Hodgson HJ. Specificity of indium-111 granulocyte scanning and fecal excretion measurement in inflammatory bowel disease – an autoradiographic study. Dig Dis Sci 1985;30:1156–1160.

85. Gallin JI, Goldstein IM, Snyderman R, eds. Inflammation: basic principles and clinical correlation. New York: Raven Press; 1992.

86. Dhamsathaphorn K, McRoberts JA, Mandel KG et al. A human colonic tumor cell line that maintains vectorial electrolyte transport. Am J Physiol 1984; 246:G204.

87. Dhamsathaphorn K, Madara JL. Established intestinal cells as model systems for electrolyte transport studies. In: Fleisher S, Fleisher B, eds. Methods in enzymology, vol 192. Orlando: Academic Press; 1990.

88. Nash S, Stafford J, Madara JL. Effects of polymorphonuclear leukocyte transmigration on the barrier function of cultured intestinal epithelial monolayers. J Clin Invest 1987; 80:1104.

89. Nash S, Stafford J, Madara JL. The selective and superoxide-independent disruption of intestinal epithelial TJs during leukocyte transmigration. Lab Invest 1988;59:531.

90. Chadwick VA, Mellor DM, Myers DB et al. Production of peptides inducing chemotaxis and lysosomal enzyme release in human neutrophils by intestinal bacteria in vitro and in vivo. Scand J Gastroenterol 1988;23:121.

91. Parkos CA, Colgan SP, Delp C et al. Neutrophil migration across a cultured epithelial monolayer elicits a biphasic resistance response representing sequential effects on transcellular and paracellular pathways. J Cell Biol 1992;117:757.

92. McCormick BA, Hofman PM, Kim J, Carnes DK, Miller SI, Madara JL. Salmonella typhimurium attachment to human intestinal epithelial monolayers: transcellular signalling to subepithelial neutrophils. J Cell Biol 1993;123:895.

93. McCormick BA, Parkos CA, Colgan SP, Carnes DK, Madara JL. Apical secretion of a pathogen-elicited epithelial chemoattractant activity in response to surface colonization of intestinal epithelia by salmonella typhimurium. J Immunol 1998;160:455.

94. Gewirtz AT, Siber AM, Madara JL, McCormick BA. Orchestration of neutrophil movement by intestinal epithelial cells in response to Salmonella typhimurium can be uncoupled from bacterial internalization. Infect Immun 1999;67:608–617.

95. Gewirtz AT, Navas TA, Lyons S, Godowski PJ, Madara JL. Cutting edge: bacterial flagellin activates basolaterally expressed TLR5 to induce epithelial proinflammatory gene expression. J Immunol. 2001;167:1882–1885.

96. Reed KA, Hobert ME, Kolenda CE et al. The Salmonella typhimurium flagellar basal body protein FliE is required for flagellin production and to induce a proinflammatory response in epithelial cells. J Biol Chem 2002; 277:13346–13353.

97. Parkos CA, Colgan SP, Delp C, Arnaout MA, Madara JL. Neutrophil migration across a cultured intestinal epithelium: Dependence on a CD 11b/18 mediated event and enhanced efficiency in physiological direction. J Clin Invest 1991; 88:1605.

98. Colgan SP, Parkos CA, Delp C, Arnaout MA, Madara JL. Neutrophil migration across cultured epithelial monolayers is modulated by epithelial exposure to INF-gamma in a highly polarized fashion. J Cell Biol 1992;120:895.

99. Lindberg FP, Bullard DC, Caver TE, Gresham HD, Beaudet AL, Brown EJ. Decreased resistance to bacterial infection and granulocyte defects in lap-deficient mice. Science 1996;274:795.

100. Parkos CA, Colgan SP, Liang TW et al. CD 47 mediates post-adhesive events required for neutrophil migration across polarized intestinal epithelia. J Cell Biol 1996;132:437.

101. Cooper D, Lindberg FP, Gamble JR, Brown EJ, Vadas MA. Transendothelial migration involves integrin-associated protein (CD47). Proc Natl Acad Sci USA 1995;92:3978.

102. Liu Y, Merlin D, Burst SL, Pochet M, Madara JL, Parkos CA. The role of CD47 in neutrophil transmigration. Increased rate of migration correlates with increased cell surface expression of CD47. J Biol Chem. 2001;276:40156–40166.

103. Merlin D, Si-Tahar M, Sitaraman SV et al. Colonic epithelial hPepT1 expression occurs in inflammatory bowel disease: transport of bacterial peptides influences expression of MHC class I molecules. Gastroenterology 2001;120:1666–1679.

104. Nash S, Parkos C, Nusrat A, Delp C, Madara JL. In vitro model of intestinal crypt abcess: a novel neutrophil-derived secretagogue activity. J Clin Invest 1991;87:1474.

105. Nash S, Stafford J, Madara JL. Effects of polymorphonuclear leukocyte transmigration on the barrier function of cultured intestinal epithelial monolayers. J Clin Invest 1987;80:1104–1113.

106. Madara JL, Parkos C, Colgan S et al. Cl⁻ secretion in a model intestinal epithelium induced by a neutrophil derived secretagogue. J Clin Invest 1992;89:1938.

107. Madara JL, Patapoff TW, Gillece-Castro B et al. 5'-AMP is the neutrophil derived paracrine factor that elicits chloride secretion from T84 intestinal epithelial monolayers. J Biol Chem 1993;91:2320.

108. Strohmeier GR, Lencer WI, Patapoff TW et al. Surface expression, polarization, and functional significance of CD73 in human intestinal epithelia. J Clin Invest 1997;99:2588.

109. Strohmeier GR, Reppert SM, Lencer WI, Madara JL. The A2b adenosine receptor mediates cAMP responses to adenosine receptor agonists in human intestinal epithelia. J Biol Chem 1994;270:2387.

110. Sitaraman SV, Si-Tahar M, Merlin D, Strohmeier GR, Madara JL. Polarity of A2b adenosine receptor expression determines characteristics of receptor desensitization. Am J Physiol Cell Physiol 2000;278:C1230–1236.

111. Sitaraman SV, Merlin D, Wang L et al. Neutrophil–epithelial crosstalk at the intestinal luminal surface mediated by reciprocal secretion of adenosine and IL-6. J Clin Invest 2001;107:861–869.

112. Tamai H, Kachur JF, Baron DA, Grisham MB, Gaginella TS. Monochloramine, a neutrophil derived oxidant stimulates rat colonic secretion. J Pharmacol Exp Ther 1990;257:884.

113. Karayalcin SS, Sturbaum CW, Wachsman JT, Cha JH, Powell DW. Hydrogen peroxide stimaulates rat colonic prostaglandin production and alters electrolyte transport. J Clin Invest 1990;86:60.

114. Neish AS, Gewirtz AT, Zeng H et al. Prokaryotic regulation of epithelial responses by inhibition of IkappaB-alpha ubiquitination. Science 2000;289:1560–1563.

115. Jobin C, Haskill S, Mayer L, Panja A, Sartor RB. Evidence for altered regulation of I kappa B alpha degradation in human colonic epithelial cells. J Immunol 1997;158:226–234.

116. Abreu MT, Vora P, Faure E, Thomas LS, Arnold ET, Arditi M. Decreased expression of Toll-like receptor-4 and MD-2 correlates with intestinal epithelial cell protection against dysregulated proinflammatory gene expression in response to bacterial lipopolysaccharide. J Immunol 2001;167:1609–1616.

117. Jung HC, Eckmann L, Yang SK et al. A distinct array of proinflammatory cytokines is expressed in human colon epithelial cells in response to bacterial invasion. J Clin Invest 1995;95:55–65.

118. Gewirtz AT, Collier-Hyams LS, Young AN et al. Lipoxin a(4) analogs attenuate induction of intestinal epithelial proinflammatory gene expression and reduce the severity of dextran sodium sulfate-induced colitis. J Immunol 2002;168:5260–5267

119. Starr R, Willson TA, Viney EM et al. A family of cytokine-inducible inhibitors of signalling. Nature 1997;387:917–921.

120. Sitaraman SV, Merlin D, Wang L, Madara JL. Positive and negative regulation of IL-6 in intestinal epithelia. Gastroenterology 2002;122: A147.

121. Haller D, Russo MP, Sartor RB, Jobin C. IKKbeta and phosphatidylinositol 3-kinase/Akt participate in non-pathogenic Gram-negative enteric bacteria-induced RelA phosphorylation and NF-kappa B activation in both primary and intestinal epithelial cell lines. J Biol Chem 2002;277:38168–38178.

122. Madara JL, Stafford J. Interferon directly affects barrier function of cultured intestinal epithelial monolayers. J Clin Invest 1989;83:724.

123. Hecht G, Pothoulakis C, LaMont JT, Madara JL. Clostridium difficile toxin A perturbs cytoskeletal structure and TJ permeability of cultured human intestinal epithelial monolayers. J Clin Invest 1988;82:1516.

124. Yuhan R, Koutsouris A, Savkovic SD, Hecht G. Enteropathogenic Escherichia coli-induced myosin light chain phosphorylation alters intestinal epithelial permeability. Gastroenterology 1997;113:1873.

125. Di Pierro M, Lu R, Uzzau S et al. Zonula occludens toxin structure–function analysis. Identification of the fragment biologically active on tight junctions and of the zonulin receptor binding domain. J Biol Chem 2001;276:19160–19165.

126. Moore R, Carlson S, Madara JL. Rapid barrier restitution in an in vitro model intestinal epithelial injury. Lab Invest 1989;60:237.

127. Moore R, Madri J, Carlson S, Madara JL. Collagens are required for epithelial migration in restitution of native guinea pig intestinal epithelium. Gastroenterology 1992;101:119.

128. Dignass AU. Mechanisms and modulation of intestinal epithelial repair. Inflammatory Bowel Dis 2001;7:68–77.

129. Feil W, Wenzl E, Vattay P, Starlinger M, Sogukoglu T, Schiessel R. Repair of rabbit duodenal mucosa after acid injury in vivo and in vitro. Gastroenterology 1987;92:973.

130. Nusrat A, Delp C, Madara JL. Intestinal epithelial restitution: characterization of a cell culture mapping of cytoskeletal elements in migrating cells. J Clin Invest 1992;89:1501.

131. Nusrat A, Parkos CA, Liang TW, Carnes DK, Madara JL. Neutrophil migration across model intestinal epithelia: monolayer disruption and subsequent events in epithelial repair. Gastroenterology 1997;113:1489.

132. Sands BE, Podolsky DK. The trefoil peptide family. Annu Rev Physiol 1996;58:253.

133. Nusrat A, Parkos CA, Bacarra AE et al. Hepatocyte growth factor/scatter factor effects on epithelia: regulation of intercellular junctions, basolateral polarization of c-met receptor, and induction of rapid wound repair. J Clin Invest 1994;93:2056.

## CHAPTER 2

# Epithelial restitution and intestinal repair

Axel U Dignass and Daniel K Podolsky

## INTRODUCTION

The surface epithelium of the alimentary tract forms an essential barrier to a broad spectrum of potentially immunogenic and noxious factors within the intestinal lumen. The epithelium separates the luminal ecologic system of commensal and sometimes pathogenic microbial flora, digested food components, and GI tract secretory products from the underlying mucosa-associated immune system. Impaired integrity of the mucosal epithelial barrier may be present in a variety of intestinal disorders, including inflammatory bowel diseases (IBD), celiac disease, intestinal infections, radiation- and chemotherapy-associated intestinal injury, and various other diseases. Transient damage of the epithelial surface mucosa occurs even in healthy conditions and may be caused by secreted proteases, intestinal microorganisms, dietary compounds and other factors. The robust regenerative capability of the mucosal surface epithelium ensures rapid restoration of the integrity of the intestinal mucosal surface barrier even after extensive destruction. Resealing of the surface epithelium is accomplished primarily by epithelial cell migration, a process designated epithelial restitution. Migration is followed by subsequent epithelial cell proliferation, differentiation and maturation.

Healing of the intestinal surface epithelium is regulated by a complex network that includes many structurally distinct regulatory peptides. Thus growth factors and cytokines have been found to play a significant role in regulating differential epithelial cell functions to preserve normal homeostasis and integrity of the intestinal mucosa. In addition, extracellular matrix proteins and blood clotting factors, as well as non-peptide molecules including phospholipids, short-chain fatty acids (SCFA), adenine nucleotides, trace elements and pharmacological agents, modulate intestinal epithelial repair mechanisms. This chapter will summarize the current understanding of normal intestinal repair mechanisms and highlight key aspects of this process in the context of IBD.

## STRUCTURE AND FUNCTION OF THE INTESTINAL SURFACE BARRIER

The surface of the digestive tract is comprised of polarized epithelial cells that form an effective physical barrier but which also allow the exchange of nutrients between the lumen and the systemic circulation. The epithelial barrier is composed of three key compartments: pre-epithelial, epithelial and postepithelial [1-4] (Fig. 2.1). The pre-epithelial mucus barrier is formed by mucin associated with other proteins as well as lipids. It is present as a continuous gel into which a bicarbonate-rich fluid is secreted, maintaining a near neutral pH at the epithelial surface. Mucus is secreted by intestinal epithelial cells, especially specialized goblet cells, and consists of trefoil peptides, various glycoproteins, phospholipids, secretory IgA and a glycocalyx.[2,5-9] Phosphatidylcholine is the predominant surface bioactive phospholipid present within the gastrointestinal tract.[10] The tight adherence of mucin to the apical surfaces of epithelia may result from complexes formed between mucin oligosaccharides and a mucin-binding protein on the apical mucosal membrane.[11] The hydrophobic lining of the luminal surface has an important functional role. It prevents microorganisms adhering to the plasma membrane, and it also protects the mucosal epithelium against chemical and mechanical injury.[12]

Epithelial cells are the central compartment of the mucosal defense system. Whereas in the oropharynx and esophagus this layer consists of a stratified epithelium, the stomach, small and large intestine are covered with a simple single epithelial layer sealed by tight junctions.[4] When this layer is intact, the uptake of antigens and microorganism through it is highly restricted.

The mucosal surface epithelium of the alimentary tract is composed of multifunctional, rapidly proliferating epithelial cells that undergo complete turnover approximately every

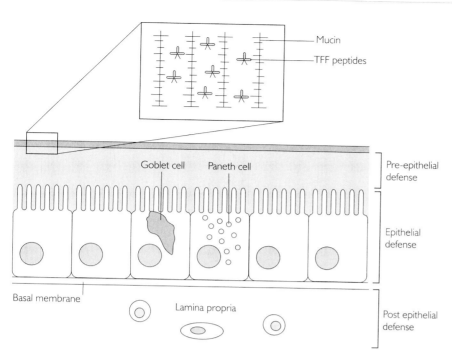

**Fig. 2.1** Schematic model of the intestinal barrier.

Mucin

TFF peptides

Pre-epithelial
defense

Goblet cell    Paneth cell

Epithelial
defense

Basal membrane

Lamina propria

Post epithelial
defense

24–96 hours.[13,14] The proliferative compartment of epithelial cells is localized in the basal third of the crypt and is segregated from a gradient of increasingly differentiated epithelial cells present along the vertical axis of the functional villus compartment.

The mucosal surface epithelium provides a barrier to a broad spectrum of factors normally present in the gastrointestinal lumen (intestinal flora, nutrients etc.), as well as noxious and immunogenic substances (pathogenic microorganisms, bacterial and dietary antigens, toxic products of digestive processes, proteases etc.) separating them from the underlying mucosa-associated immune system. However, this barrier is not impermeable, and flux through the epithelium exists via both transcellular and paracellular pathways. Interestingly, the barrier properties of the gastrointestinal mucosa vary in different parts of the intestinal tract.[15]

Although the intestinal barrier may be best thought of as a functional property of the mucosa, rather than a single feature, it does encompass some specific anatomical structures. In addition to the intestinal epithelial cells in toto, several proteins assemble into tight junctions that are present as a series of discrete membrane contacts of adjacent cells. Although additional constituents of this complex remain to be identified, they include the cytoplasmic zonula occludens proteins (ZO-1, ZO-2, ZO-3), claudins, cingulin and 7H6, as well as the transmembrane proteins occludin and cadherins. Occludins and claudins may serve as the major sealing proteins. The permeability of tight junctions may be regulated by modulating the expression of tight junction components, especially some claudins, and possibly by phosphorylation of some tight junction proteins. Calcium regulates the formation of tight junctions and the polarization of epithelial cells. It acts primarily extracellularly by activating E-cadherin molecule aggregation, thereby facilitating the binding of E-cadherin between neighboring cells, either as homodimers or as heterodimers with integrins.[16] This process is followed by an intracellular signal transduction pathway involving two G proteins that activate phospholipase

C, protein kinase C, calmodulin and mitogen-activated protein kinase.[17–19] Activation of these pathways eventually results in the formation of junctional strands. However, it is still unclear how signals are delivered from E-cadherin to the tight junction and back. Linkage of the cytoskeleton to E-cadherin through catenins, vinculin, fodrin, α-actin and spectrin suggests its involvement in the information network.[3,20]

## MECHANISMS OF INTESTINAL EPITHELIAL HEALING

Damage to the intestinal barrier occurs in various inflammatory and infectious diseases, permitting increased penetration and absorption of toxic and immunogenic factors, which lead to uncontrolled immune response and inflammation. Thus, rapid resealing of the epithelial surface barrier following injury or physiological damage is essential to the preservation of normal homeostasis. The intestinal tract is able to rapidly re-establish the continuity of the surface epithelium after extensive destruction.[21–32] Healing of the intestinal surface epithelium involves multiple processes and is regulated by a complex network of peptide and non-peptide factors, as well as direct cell–cell interactions (Fig. 2.2).

In a simplified in vitro model of epithelial repair, healing of a 'wounded' monolayer can be reduced to three distinct mechanisms. First, epithelial cells adjacent to the injured surface migrate into the wound to cover the denuded area. Those epithelial cells that migrate into the wound defect dedifferentiate, form pseudopodia-like structures, reorganize their cytoskeleton to extend into the wound, and then redifferentiate after closure of the wound defect.[33–36] This process has been termed epithelial restitution. It does not require cell proliferation and occurs within minutes to hours both in vivo and in vitro.[21–25,37,38] Subsequent epithelial cell proliferation is necessary in order to replenish the decreased cell pool. Finally, maturation and

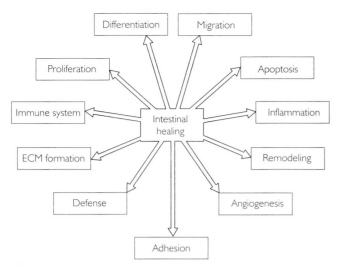

Fig. 2.2 Mechanisms with relevance for intestinal epithelial healing.

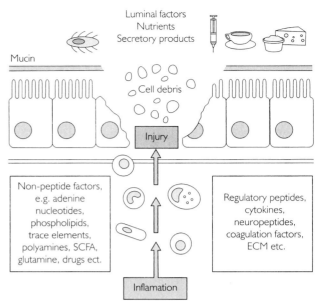

Fig. 2.3 Modulation of intestinal epithelial healing.

differentiation of undifferentiated epithelial cells is needed to restore the functional activities of the mature mucosal epithelium.

In vivo, the three described wound healing processes overlap. However, simplified in vitro models have provided the means to characterize the physiology and pathophysiology of intestinal epithelial wound healing. Superficial injuries involving exfoliation of the epithelial cells with an intact basement membrane heal by restitution. Deeper lesions or penetrating injuries require additional repair mechanisms that involve inflammatory processes, degradation and formation of extracellular matrix components, and various non-epithelial cell populations such as immunocytes, myofibroblasts, platelets and other cells that cannot be adequately studied in this model. Inflammatory processes and potentially some therapies may interfere with epithelial cell migration and proliferation and thus modulate intestinal epithelial healing.

## MODULATION OF INTESTINAL EPITHELIAL WOUND HEALING

Intestinal epithelial cell functions are modulated by a number of luminal factors, the epithelium itself and the underlying lamina propria (Fig. 2.3). Modulating factors present in the lumen include dietary compounds; products of alimentary secretions from salivary glands, the stomach, pancreas or intestinal glandular cells; secreted regulatory peptides and constituents; or products of the physiological or pathogenic intestinal microflora. Important factors produced by the epithelium itself include various regulatory peptides, products of intestinal epithelial lymphocytes (IEL), and local cell–cell interactions. Factors produced within the lamina propria include several regulatory peptides produced by the cellular constituents of the lamina propria, extracellular matrix proteins, neurotransmitters, neural interactions, and mediators that are transported via the bloodstream. In addition, dying or injured cells release a variety of mediators, including regulatory peptides, phospholipids, adenine nucleotides and others.

Although the full variety of regulatory peptide and non-peptide factors that regulate intestinal epithelial and non-

epithelial cell populations has not yet been characterized, there is an increasing appreciation of the diversity of these factors in general and the importance of a number of specific factors produced or released within the intestine (Fig. 2.4). These varied peptide and non-peptide factors modulate different functions of intestinal cell populations, including cell migration, proliferation, differentiation, adhesion and apoptosis. This network possesses multiple functional properties and exhibits pleiotropism in its cellular sources and targets. As a result, the different components of this network are highly redundant in several dimensions.[39–41]

1. Each cell type expresses or releases multiple regulatory factors.
2. Many regulatory factors are produced by several cell populations within the intestinal tract.
3. Individual cell populations express specific receptors for more than one regulatory factor.
4. Receptors for a single regulatory factor may be present on multiple different cell types, so that a single regulatory factor can exert different functional effects within the intestinal tract.
5. The functional effects of one regulatory factor may be modulated by the coexistence of other regulatory peptide or non-peptide factors or different cellular contexts.
6. Multiple structurally related members of a peptide growth factor family can interact with a single receptor and can cause comparable functional activities (e.g. EGF family peptides).
7. Many regulatory factors modulate their own expression and that of other regulatory factors and their receptors on various cellular targets.
8. Different cellular or extracellular surroundings cause different responses within this network.
9. Intestinal epithelial responses may vary in physiological and disease conditions. (This review is dedicated to the modulation of those epithelial cell functions that are relevant for healing of intestinal injury. For a more extensive description of the functional role of regulatory peptide factors the interested reader is referred to more detailed handbooks and reviews and the references therein, e.g. [30,40,42–51].)

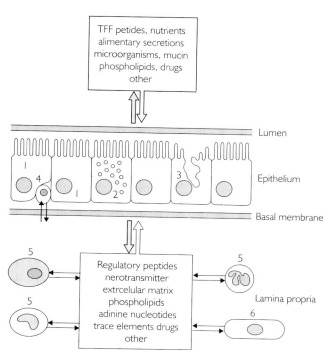

Fig. 2.4 Model of a regulatory network within the intestinal mucosa. 1, epithelial cell; 2, Paneth cell; 3, goblet cell; 4, IEL; 5, LPMNC; 6, myofibroblast.

As noted below and summarized in Tables 2.1 and 2.2, the effects of different regulatory peptides on repair are diverse, with varying effects (either positive or negative) on restitution per se, cell proliferation, cellular differentiation, extracellular matrix production and tissue remodeling.

## MODULATION OF INTESTINAL EPITHELIAL WOUND HEALING BY REGULATORY PEPTIDES

A broad spectrum of regulatory peptides expressed within the intestinal mucosa (Table 2.1) modulate different epithelial cell functions in order to preserve normal homeostasis and the integrity of the intestinal mucosa.[31,37,38,40,48,52–74] The terminology of regulatory peptides is often confusing and arbitrary. The term cytokines is now increasingly used to describe regulatory proteins that can be variously identified as regulatory peptides, peptide growth factors, interleukins, interferons and colony-stimulating or hematopoietic stem cell factors.[42,47] For the purpose of simplification, in this chapter the term regulatory peptide will be used to address these various peptide classes.

Regulatory peptide factors are usually characterized by a relatively low molecular weight (<25 kDa), and exert their effects through binding to specific high-affinity cell surface receptors present on their respective target cells.[41,75,76] In contrast to classic peptide hormones, regulatory peptides tend to act locally on adjacent cells (paracrine or juxtacrine action) or on the same cell that has expressed the peptide factor (autocrine action).[47,76,77]

Regulatory peptides can be categorized on the basis of structural homologies and disparities into several discrete families. Peptide growth factor families and selected members that modulate intestinal wound healing and their key activities with respect to intestinal wound healing are summarized in Tables 2.1 and 2.2. In addition to these growth factor families, a number of regulatory peptide factors, without structural similarities to other peptide families such as hepatocyte growth factor (HGF), vascular endothelial cell growth factor (VEGF) and platelet-derived growth factor (PDGF), have been found to be expressed within the intestinal tract and to modulate wound healing properties within the intestinal mucosa.[45,78–81] Many classic cytokines, e.g. IL-1, IL-2, IL-8, IL-10, IL-11, IL-15, IL-17 and IFN-γ, are also expressed within the intestine and modulate intestinal epithelial cell function.[38,42,52,58,62,82,83–93,93–95] In brief, IL-1, IL-2, IL-8, IL-11 and IFN-γ stimulate migration, whereas IL-2 may either stimulate or inhibit proliferation (depending on conditions), and IFN-γ inhibits migration.

Among the numerous regulatory peptides that are expressed within the intestinal mucosa, TGF-β and the EGF family peptides EGF and TGF-α play especially important roles. Intestinal EGF is produced in submaxillary glands, Brunner's glands in the duodenum, and within the exocrine pancreas.[96] TGF-α has been identified as a product of many cell types, including most epithelial cells.[97] TGF-α mRNA and bioactive protein are present in gastric, small intestinal and colonic epithelium.[98–100] Binding sites for EGF and TGF-α in the intestinal tract appear equivalent in distribution when either EGF or TGF-α has been used as the ligand in a manner consistent with the assumption that they share a common receptor.[100–103] Several other members of this family are also expressed, including amphiregulin and HB-EGF.

TGF-β is the prototypic member of the TGF-β family.[47,104,105] In both man and mouse three isoforms of TGF-β (TGF-β$_{1,2,3}$) have been detected in all gastrointestinal tract tissues and accessory organs.[106] Within the small intestine, TGF-β expression is present in lamina propria cells and the epithelium.[61,66,106] TGF-β binds to several specific cell surface TGF-β receptors. The type 1 and type 2 receptors work in a cooperative fashion: ligand binding to the type 1 receptor facilitates activation of the associated type 2 receptor, which then activates the intracellular signaling machine via SMAD proteins.[105,107–112] Many observations indicate a role for TGF-β in both inflammation as well as tissue repair and immunoregulation.[113] Direct intramuscular TGF-β$_1$ gene delivery has been reported to effectively ameliorate trinitrobenzene sulfonic acid-induced colitis.[114] In another study, a single intranasal dose of a plasmid encoding active TGF-β$_1$ prevented the development of the T-helper cell type 1 (Th1)-mediated inflammation in the TNBS model of colitis. In addition, such plasmid administration abrogated TNBS colitis after it had been established.[115] The importance of TGF-β in regulating inflammatory conditions is also supported by targeted disruption of the TGF-β$_1$ gene by gene 'knockout' technology which results in multifocal, mixed inflammatory cell infiltration, often with necrosis.[116]

A variety of studies of regulatory peptides, including EGF, TGF-α and TGF-β, on cell adhesion, migration, proliferation, differentiation, intestinal epithelial barrier function and angiogenesis, suggest that these peptides are probably relevant effect for intestinal repair. In vitro and in vivo studies have demonstrated that several growth factors and cytokines can enhance epithelial cell restitution.[30,38,50,61,78,117–126] Many of these

**Table 2.1 Peptide growth factors with potential relevance for intestinal epithelial healing**

| Growth factor family | Family members | Target cells | Biological activity |
|---|---|---|---|
| TGF-α/ EGF family | TGF-α, EGF, amphiregulin, cripto, heparin-binding EGF, heregulin | Epithelial cells, endothelial cells, macrophages/ monocytes | Stimulate proliferation and migration, stimulate differentiation and adaptation, trophic factor for mucosa, modulate expression of enzymes relevant for the production of polyamines, stimulate intestinal electrolyte and nutrient transport, stimulate expression of brush border enzymes, promote growth of intestinal neoplasia, enhance angiogenesis |
| TGF-β family | TGF-$\beta_{1-3}$, inhibin A and B, follistatin, activins A and AB | Epithelial cells, endothelial cells, immunocytes, mesenchymal cells | **Epithelial cells**: inhibit proliferation, stimulate epithelial restitution<br>**B-lymphocytes**: inhibit proliferation, suppress IgM and IgG production, stimulate IgA production<br>**T-lymphocytes**: inhibit proliferation, suppress cytokine production, inhibit generation of cytotoxic T cells<br>**Monocytes/macrophages**: chemotactic, inhibit respiratory burst, induces production of cytokines (IL-1, TGF-α)<br>**Neutrophils**: chemotactic, inhibit cytotoxic activity<br>**Fibroblasts**: inhibit proliferation, modulate collagen, fibronectin and collagenase production<br>**Endothelial cells**: inhibit proliferation, modulate angiogenesis<br>**Smooth muscle cells**: stricture formation |
| FGF family | Acidic FGF (=FGF-1), basic FGF (=FGF-2), hst oncogene (=K-FGF), FGF-5, FGF-6, KGF (=FGF-7), FGF-18, FGF-20 | Epithelial cells, endothelial cells, mesenchymal cells | Stimulate proliferation of epithelial, endothelial cells and fibroblasts, enhance angiogenesis and neovascularization, stimulate epithelial restitution, stimulate matrix formation |
| TFF peptides | TFF-1 (pS2), TFF-2 (Spasmolytic Polypeptide), TFF-3 (Intestinal Trefoil Factor; ITF) | Epithelial cells, goblet cells, smooth muscle cells | Protect intestinal mucosa against aggressive luminal factors, enhance epithelial restitution, exert antiapoptotic effects |
| IGF family | Insulin, insulin-like growth factors I and II (IGF I and II) | Epithelial cells, endothelial cells, fibroblasts | Mitogenic for epithelial and non-epithelial cells, trophic factor for intestinal mucosa, sustaining tumor growth, participation in intestinal wound healing and adaptation, participate in development of fibrosis, promote chemotaxis of endothelial cells |
| CSF family | IL-3 (=Multi-CSF), GM-CSF, M-CSF (=CSF-1) and G- CSF | Epithelial cells, immunocytes, hematopoietic cells | Stimulate hematopoietic cell proliferation, modulate immune cell populations, recruit inflammatory cells |

TGF-α, EGF, TGF-β, HGF, FGF peptides, IL-1, IL-2 and IFN-γ enhance epithelial cell restitution through a TGF-β-dependent pathway.[30,38,119] Interestingly, it appears that restitution-enhancing cytokines use different mechanisms to modulate TGF-β peptide. TGF-α, EGF, IL-1, IFN-γ and HGF increase the concentration of bioactive TGF-β. In contrast, acidic and basic FGF (FGF1 and FGF2), as well as IL-2, enhance the bioactivation of TGF-β, the expression of TGF-β mRNA and the production of latent TGF-β peptide.[38,82,119] These growth factors and cytokines act at the basolateral surfaces of the epithelium where TGF-β receptors are located.

In contrast, various members of the trefoil factor family (TFF peptide family) at the apical surface, stimulate epithelial restitution in conjunction with mucin glycoproteins through a TGF-β-independent mechanism.[30,118,122,127] TFF peptides are a family of proteins expressed in a region-selective pattern throughout the gastrointestinal tract. Trefoil peptides are characterized by a highly conserved motif designated a 'P' or trefoil domain, which consists of six cysteine residues that form three intrachain loops.[5,128–130] Members of the trefoil factor family include TFF1 (formerly pS2), TFF2 (formerly spasmolytic polypeptide, SP), and TFF3 (previously ITF, intestinal trefoil factor). TFF1 was first identified in human breast carcinoma cell lines and is usually expressed in the stomach, in Brunner's glands, and in large intestinal goblet cells near to the surface.[131,132] TFF2 is expressed in the fundus and antrum of the stomach, in Brunner's gland acini, and in distal ducts of the small intestine.[131–135] TFF3 is absent in the stomach, but is

**Table 2.2 Biological activities of selected cytokines with relevance for intestinal wound healing and repair**

| Cytokine | Migration/ restitution | Proliferation | Miscellaneous effects relevant for intestinal healing |
|---|---|---|---|
| IL-1 | + | none | Modulates cytokine expression in various cell populations |
| IL-2 | + | + (initially) − (late event) | Modulates cytokine expression in various cell populations |
| IL-8 | + | none | Chemotaxis |
| IL-10 | | | Suppresses intestinal inflammation, Impairs healing of intestinal anastomoses |
| IL-11 | + | none | Modulates ion transport and inflammation, antiapoptotic |
| IL-15 | none | + | |
| IFN-γ | + | − | Impairs intestinal epithelial barrier function, Modulates expression of tight junction molecules, Modulates cytokine expression in various cell populations |
| TNF-α | none | none | Impairs healing of intestinal anastomoses, inhibits matrix formation |

expressed in goblet cells in the small and large intestine, and in Brunner's gland acini and ducts in the small intestine.[57,136] TFF2 mRNA increases within 30 minutes after mucosal injury induced in the rat stomach, and the administration of exogenous TFF2 protects against ethanol-induced gastric injury and stimulates repair in a model of experimental colitis.[137–140] Mashimo et al.[141] showed that TFF3 knockout mice have impaired mucosal healing properties, with increased mortality and more aggressive colitis following dextran sodium sulfate exposure. Other studies suggest that modulation of repair mechanisms by trefoil peptides may be mediated by modulation of the E-cadherin–catenin complex.[142,143] Some growth factors in the FGF family (KGF-2 and FGF-20) stimulate the expression of TFF3.[144,145] In the case of KGF-2, prevention of colitis appears to be mediated through TFF3, as KGF-2 fails to prevent experimental disease in TFF3-deficient mice (Iwakiri and Podolsky, unpublished observation). Moreover, KGF enhances TFF2 expression in proximal small bowel and increases goblet cell numbers and TFF3 protein content throughout the intestine.[146]

In addition to their potent effects on epithelial restitution, a number of regulatory peptide factors also act as potent modulators of epithelial cell proliferation.[48,62,65,69,119,120,147–153] EGF and TGF-α are especially potent stimulators of intestinal epithelial proliferation. Conversely, TGF-β inhibits intestinal epithelial cell proliferation and plays an important counterbalancing role in the regulation of intestinal epithelial cell proliferation. Indeed, TGF-β is the most potent inhibitor of intestinal epithelial cell proliferation, in that it overrides the stimulatory effects of other stimulatory factors. Interestingly, a number of promigratory regulatory peptides, such as EGF, TGF-α, FGF peptides, HGF and IL-2, induce a coordinated sequential induction of TGF-β which may be important to inhibit unrestrained cell growth.[62,119,154] The growth stimulating effects of IL-2, FGF peptides, IGF and HGF are moderate compared to the effects of EGF and TGF-α, which stimulate epithelial cell proliferation up to five- to tenfold in several intestinal epithelial cell lines in vitro.[82,119,120,149] Nevertheless, these factors and various non-peptide factors may act in an additive or even a synergistic fashion to potentiate individual effects. In addition to TGF-β the TGF-β family member activin A has also recently been shown to inhibit epithelial cell proliferation, thus providing an additional mechanism to counterbalance the effects of proliferative factors present within the intestinal mucosa, and to inhibit unrestrained cell growth.[152,153]

# MODULATION OF INTESTINAL EPITHELIAL WOUND HEALING BY EXTRACELLULAR MATRIX FACTORS

Extracellular matrix factors (ECM) have been demonstrated to modulate cell adhesion, differentiation and spatial organization within the intestinal mucosa.[117,155,156] The extracellular matrix molecules on which intestinal epithelial cells reside also have the potential to stimulate intestinal epithelial cell migration.[157] The extracellular matrix influences restitution as a physical substrate and by modulating the expression, organization, and activation of select intracellular proteins such as actin, villin, focal adhesion kinase and paxillin.[155,156,158] They also regulate the expression and organization of integrins and receptors for soluble factors in the extracellular environment which influence cell motility.[156] The basement membrane components fibronectin and collagen type IV may be especially important, as their distribution is altered in migrating cells after wounding. Indeed, specific blockade by neutralizing antibodies to these matrix components impairs restitution of intestinal epithelial cells in vitro.[117,157] Loss of matrix-dependent cytoskeletal tyrosine kinase signals such as focal adhesion kinase during restitution may trigger a phenotypic switch to a dedifferentiated migrating intestinal epithelial phenotype.[159] Mahida et al. have demonstrated that intestinal myofibroblasts express the extracellular matrix proteins collagen type IV, laminin-β$_1$ and -γ$_1$ and fibronectin, and that colonic subepithelial myofibroblasts may influence epithelial cell function via these secreted ECM proteins.[160]

# MODULATION OF EXTRACELLULAR MATRIX FORMATION AND ITS ROLE IN INTESTINAL EPITHELIAL WOUND HEALING AND IBD

Degradation of the extracellular matrix and ulceration of the mucosa are major features of IBD. Matrix metalloproteinases (MMP) have been reported to be involved in the tissue remodeling, angiogenesis and promotion of leukocyte extravasation in the actively inflamed area in the bases of ulcers in both ulcerative colitis and Crohn's disease.[161] Louis et al.[162] reported that the inflamed mucosa of both Crohn's disease and ulcerative colitis shows increased production of both MMP-3 and its tissue inhibitor TIMP-1 (tissue inhibitor of matrix metalloproteinase-1). MMP-3 and TIMP-1 could not be detected in uninflamed colonic tissue, and their expression correlated with the production of IL-1β, IL-6, TNF and IL-10 in IBD patients. Another study in pediatric IBD patients also found increased expression of MMP-3, but no alterations of TIMP-1 in inflamed colonic tissue. Neither MMP-3 activity nor TIMP-1 was detectable in uninflamed colonic tissues.[163] MMP-10 (stromelysin-2) has been suggested to modulate epithelial cell migration in IBD, presumably by modification of the extracellular nature.[164] As the abundance and activation of matrix metalloproteinases is significantly increased in ulcerative colitis and Crohn's mucosa, inhibitors of these proteolytic enzymes may have therapeutic utility in the treatment of inflammatory bowel disease.[165] Treatment with a matrix metalloproteinase inhibitor had dose-dependent beneficial effects on the inflammatory alterations in rat experimental colitis.[166,167] Thus, the inhibition of MMP may represent a novel therapeutic approach for the treatment of intestinal inflammation.

The formation of strictures is a frequent complication of prolonged inflammation in patients with Crohn's disease. Stallmach et al.[168] demonstrated that fibroblasts isolated from strictures in patients with Crohn's disease produce significantly more collagen, especially type III, than fibroblasts from normal or nonstrictured but inflamed intestinal lamina propria. In other studies TGF-β₁ has been demonstrated to significantly increase collagen type III synthesis in intestinal lamina propria fibroblasts.[168] TGF-β₁-stimulated type III collagen synthesis in fibroblasts from strictures in Crohn's disease was significantly higher than that in fibroblasts from inflamed specimens obtained from the same patients. Collagen type III stimulated the adhesion and proliferation of lamina propria fibroblasts. Upregulation of insulin-like growth factor-1 (IGF-1) binding proteins (IGFBP-4, -5 and -3) in cultured colonic smooth muscle cells (SMC) support a role for IGF in tissue fibrosis and stricture formation during chronic intestinal inflammation.[169] Consistent with these studies suggesting a role for TGF-β and IGF-1 in fibrosis, transmural increases in TGF-β₁ and IGF-1 mRNA expression were observed in Crohn's disease, whereas in ulcerative colitis the increase was confined to the lamina propria and submucosa.[170,171] Both in patients with ulcerative colitis and those with Crohn's disease the distribution of TGF-β₁ and IGF-1 expression coincided with the distribution of the inflammatory infiltrate. An increase in the ratio of collagen type III to type I in both CD and UC also coincided with the inflammatory infiltrate. Collectively, these findings suggest that TGF-β₁ and IGF-1 are involved in intestinal ECM remodeling in IBD.[170]

In addition to the regulatory factors TGF-β₁ and IGF-1, other studies suggest that most cells may also play an important role in response to deep injury. Thus, Gelbmann et al. have reported a striking accumulation of mast cells in strictures in Crohn's disease, particularly in the hypertrophied and fibrotic muscularis propria.[165] Mast cells in the muscularis propria colocalized with patches of laminin. Similarly, in the submucosa, laminin was exclusively found in the basal lamina of blood vessels, where many adherent mast cells were seen. This colocalization with laminin suggests that interaction between smooth muscle cells and mast cells may be important in the process of fibrosis.[172]

# MODULATION OF INTESTINAL EPITHELIAL WOUND HEALING BY BLOOD COAGULATION FACTORS

Recent evidence suggests that blood coagulation factors are also involved in wound healing and tissue repair.[173–177] Factor XIII has been shown to promote intestinal epithelial wound healing in vitro by enhancing epithelial cell restitution through a TGF-β-independent pathway.[173] Factor XIII significantly improved healing in a rat model of colitis.[178] In addition, activated factor XIII reduces endothelial permeability and prevents the loss of endothelial barrier function under conditions of energy depletion.[179] Supplementation with factor XIII has been reported to enhance the healing of fistulae in Crohn's disease.[180]

# MODULATION OF INTESTINAL EPITHELIAL WOUND HEALING BY NON-PEPTIDE FACTORS

It is increasingly clear that a broad spectrum of non-peptide factors exerts potent effects on intestinal epithelial cell populations and modulates those epithelial cell functions that are involved in the healing of intestinal injury (Table 2.3). These non-peptide factors encompass a broad spectrum of unrelated substances including phospholipids, nutrients, adenine nucleotides, polyamines, short-chain fatty acids (SCFA), products of the intestinal microflora, trace elements, pharmacological agents and other factors. Some of these are released by injured or dying mucosal cell populations (e.g. adenine nucleotides, phospholipids), whereas others reach the intestinal mucosa via the intestinal lumen or the bloodstream. Some of these non-peptide factors exhibit growth factor-like activities and exert potent effects on cell growth and differentiation in different cell populations, including fibroblasts, vascular smooth muscle cells, endothelial cells and keratinocytes.[30,181–188] As some of these non-peptide factors are stable within the gastrointestinal tract despite high concentrations of acid, bile salts, proteases and microorganisms, and as they exhibit only limited toxicity in vivo and are available in larger quantities, they may serve as potential future targets to improve the armamentarium to promote healing of mucosal epithelial injury. For example, phospholipids

**Table 2.3 Selected non-peptide factors with relevance for intestinal epithelial wound healing**

| Factor | Mechanism of action | Reference |
|---|---|---|
| Lysophosphatidic acid (LPA) | Stimulates intestinal epithelial restitution<br>Inhibits intestinal epithelial proliferation<br>Modulates cell interactions with ECM<br>Stimulates cytoskeletol activation and remodeling | 2; 183; 198; 210–212 |
| Polyamines | Stimulate intestinal epithelial restitution and proliferation<br>Activates intestinal epithelial potassium channels<br>Modulates cytoskeleton and differentiation | 24; 193; 194; 213–215 |
| Adenine nucleotides | Stimulate intestinal epithelial restitution<br>Inhibit intestinal epithelial proliferation<br>Modulate cytoskeleton | 184; 185; 216 |
| Short chain fatty acids | Stimulate intestinal epithelial migration | 181; 217; 218 |
| Glutamine | Stimulates intestinal epithelial proliferation and migration | 187; 217; 219; 220 |
| Corticosteroids | Inhibit intestinal epithelial proliferation and migration<br>Decrease bursting strength of intestinal anastomoses | 199; 201; 202 |

and polyamines might be provided as a dietary supplement; alternatively, their overall content and biological activity can be modulated by various pharmacological agents.[182,189–195]

Lipophosphatidic acid (LPA) is a key intermediate in the early steps of phospholipid biosynthesis and is rapidly produced and released from thrombin-activated platelets and growth factor-stimulated fibroblasts. It regulates target cells by activating a specific 38–40 kDa G protein-coupled receptor that is expressed by many cells. As a product of the blood-clotting process LPA is a normal constituent of serum, where it is present in an albumin-bound form in physiologically relevant concentrations. Activated platelets, stimulated fibroblasts and, presumably, injured cells release LPA in proximity to sites of injury due to non-specific phospholipase activation.[191,196–198] Serum LPA levels range from 2 to 20 $\mu$mol. LPA promotes platelet aggregation and induces cellular tension and cell surface fibronectin assembly, important processes in wound repair. The naturally occurring phospholipid lysophosphatidic acid (LPA) significantly enhanced intestinal epithelial wound healing in vitro and in vivo.[183] LPA effects on intestinal epithelial cells are mediated through TGF-$\beta$-independent and pertussis toxin-sensitive and -insensitive G protein signaling cascades.

Interestingly, a number of agents that are currently used for the treatment of IBD may also interfere with wound healing processes. It has long been recognized that concomitant corticosteroid therapy at the time of surgical intervention is associated with impaired intestinal wound repairs and the risk of inadequate healing of intestinal anastomoses.[199–201] Impaired intestinal epithelial wound healing due to corticosteroid therapy

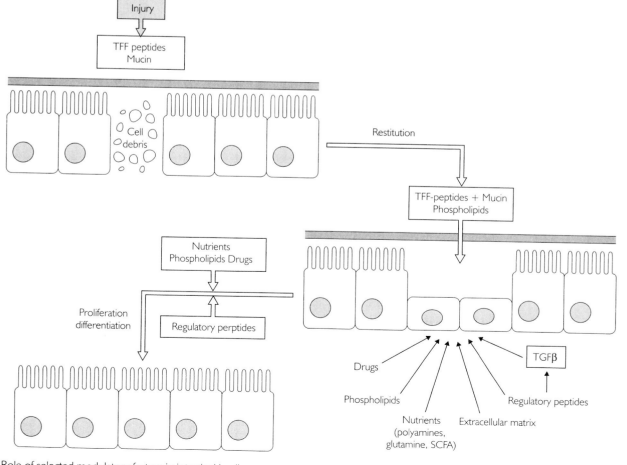

**Fig. 2.5** Role of selected modulatory factors in intestinal healing.

may result from inhibition of intestinal epithelial cell restitution and proliferation, as indicated by in vitro studies.[202]

# MODULATION OF INTESTINAL EPITHELIAL WOUND HEALING BY CELL–CELL INTERACTIONS

It is increasingly evident that intestinal epithelial wound healing is also modulated by direct cell–cell interactions with non-epithelial cells. Cell populations with special relevance in this context include intestinal myofibroblasts, immune cell populations and nerve cells.[160,203–208] Mononuclear cells promote intestinal epithelial wound repair by enhancing restitution through the secretion of various cytokines, among them IL-2 and IFN-γ. IL-2 and IFN-γ are abundantly expressed in the course of inflammatory diseases by various constituents of the intestinal immune system, including lamina propria T cells, intra-epithelial lymphocytes and macrophages. In addition, colonic subepithelial myofibroblasts have been reported to secrete predominantly bioactive TGF-$\beta_3$ and enhance restitution in wounded epithelial monolayers via a TGF-β-dependent pathway.[204] Another study has demonstrated that fibroblasts stimulate intestinal epithelial proliferation through a paracrine mechanism mediated predominantly by HGF.[209]

# PERSPECTIVES

Repeated damage and injury to the intestinal surface are intrinsic to IBD and require constant repair of the epithelium. A complex network of peptide and non-peptide factors and direct cell–cell interactions modulate healing of the intestinal epithelium (Fig. 2.5). Enhancement of intestinal repair mechanisms by regulatory peptides or other modulatory factors may provide effective approaches to the treatment of these disorders and their complications.

# REFERENCES

1. Scheiman JM. NSAIDs, gastrointestinal injury, and cytoprotection. Gastroenterol Clin North Am 1996;25:279–298.
2. Sturm A, Dignass AU. Modulation of gastrointestinal wound repair and inflammation by phospholipids. Biochim Biophys Acta 2002;1582:282–288.
3. Cereijido M, Shoshani L, Contreras RG. Molecular physiology and pathophysiology of tight junctions. I. Biogenesis of tight junctions and epithelial polarity. Am J Physiol Gastrointest Liver Physiol 2000;279:G477–G482.
4. Kraehenbuhl JP, Pringault E, Neutra MR. Review article: Intestinal epithelia and barrier functions. Aliment Pharmacol Ther 1997;11 (Suppl 3):3–8.
5. Sands BE, Podolsky DK. The trefoil peptide family. Annu Rev Physiol 1996;58:253–273.
6. Shirazi T, Longman RJ, Corfield AP, Probert CS. Mucins and inflammatory bowel disease. Postgrad Med J 2000;76:473–478.
7. Kindon H, Pothoulakis C, Thim L, Lynch-Devaney K, Podolsky DK. Trefoil peptide protection of intestinal epithelial barrier function: cooperative interaction with mucin glycoprotein. Gastroenterology 1995;109:516–523.
8. Podolsky DK, Isselbacher KJ. Composition of human colonic mucin. J Clin Invest 1983;72:142–153.
9. Poulsom R, Wright NA. Trefoil peptides: A newly recognized family of epithelial mucin-associated molecules. Am J Physiol 1993;265:G205–G213.
10. Schmitz MG, Renooij W. Phospholipids from rat, human, and canine gastric mucosa. Composition and metabolism of molecular classes of phosphatidylcholine. Gastroenterology 1990;99:1292–1296.
11. Slomiany A, Grabska M, Slomiany BL. Essential components of antimicrobial gastrointestinal epithelial barrier: specific interaction of mucin with an integral apical membrane protein of gastric mucosa. Mol Med 2001;7:1–10.
12. Frey A, Giannasca KT, Weltzin R et al. Role of the glycocalyx in regulating access of microparticles to apical plasma membranes of intestinal epithelial cells: implications for microbial attachment and oral vaccine targeting. J Exp Med 1996;184:1045–1059.
13. Lipkin M, Sherlock P, Bell B. Cell proliferation kinetics in the gastrointestinal tract of man. II. Cell renewal in stomach, ileum, colon and rectum. Gastroenterology 1963;45:721–729.
14. Potten CS, Kellet M, Roberts SA, Rew DA, Wilson GD. Measurement of in vivo proliferation in human colorectal mucosa using bromodeoxyuridine. Gut 1992;33:71–78.
15. Nejdfors P, Ekelund M, Jeppsson B, Westrom BR. Mucosal in vitro permeability in the intestinal tract of the pig, the rat, and man: species- and region-related differences. Scand J Gastroenterol 2000;35:501–507.
16. Mizuno M, Okayama N, Kasugai K et al. Acid stimulates E-cadherin surface expression on gastric epithelial cells to stabilize barrier functions via influx of calcium. Eur J Gastroenterol Hepatol 2001;13:127–136.
17. Hubner G, Alzheimer C, Werner S. Activin: a novel player in tissue repair processes. Histol Histopathol 1999;14:295–304.
18. Ma TY, Hoa NT, Tran DD et al. Cytochalasin B modulation of Caco-2 tight junction barrier: role of myosin light chain kinase. Am J Physiol Gastrointest Liver Physiol 2000;279:G875–G885.
19. Cho KR, Vogelstein B. Genetic alterations in the adenoma–carcinoma sequence. Cancer 1992;70:1727–1731.
20. Karczewski J, Groot J. Molecular physiology and pathophysiology of tight junctions III. Tight junction regulation by intracellular messengers: differences in response within and between epithelia. Am J Physiol Gastrointest Liver Physiol 2000;279:G660–G665.
21. Lacy ER. Epithelial restitution in the gastrointestinal tract. J Clin Gastroenterol 1988;10 (Suppl.):72–77.
22. Feil W, Wentzl E, Vattay P, Starlinger M, Sogukoglu R, Schiessel R. Repair of rabbit duodenal mucosa after acid injury in vivo and in vitro. Gastroenterology 1987;92:1973–1986.
23. Moore R, Carlson S, Madara JL. Rapid barrier restitution in an in vitro model of intestinal epithelial injury. Lab Invest 1989;60:237–244.
24. McCormack SA, Viar MJ, Johnson LR. Migration of IEC-6 cells: a model for mucosal healing. Am J Physiol 1992;263G:426–435.
25. Nusrat A, Delp C, Madara J. Intestinal epithelial restitution. J Clin Invest 1992;89:1501–1511.
26. Dieckgraefe BK, Stenson WF, Alpers DH. Gastrointestinal epithelial response to injury. Curr Opin Gastroenterol 1996;12:109–114.
27. Rutten MJ, Ito S. Morphology and electrophysiology of guinea pig gastric mucosal repair in vitro. Am J Physiol 1983;244G:171–182.
28. Silen W. Gastric mucosal defense and repair. In: Johnson LR, ed. Physiology of the gastrointestinal tract. New York: Raven Press; 1987:1044–1069.
29. Weinman MD, Allan CH, Trier JS, Hagen SJ. Repair of microvilli in the rat small intestine after damage with lectins contained in the red kidney bean. Gastroenterology 1989;97:1193–1204.
30. Wilson AJ, Gibson PR. Epithelial migration in the colon: filling in the gaps. Clin Sci (Colch) 1997;93:97–108.
31. Wright NA. Aspects of the biology of regeneration and repair in the human gastrointestinal tract. Philos Trans Roy Soc Lond B Biol Sci 1998;353:925–933.
32. Dignass AU. Mechanisms and modulation of intestinal epithelial repair. Inflamm Bowel Dis 2001;7:68–77.
33. Lotz MM, Rabinovitz I, Mercurio AM. Intestinal restitution: progression of actin cytoskeleton rearrangements and integrin function in a model of epithelial wound healing. Am J Pathol 2000;156:985–996.
34. Nusrat A, Delp C, Madara JL. Intestinal epithelial restitution. Characterization of a cell culture model and mapping of cytoskeletal elements in migrating cells. J Clin Invest 1992;89:1501–1511.
35. Pignatelli M. Modulation of cell adhesion during epithelial restitution in the gastrointestinal tract. Yale J Biol Med 1996;69:131–135.
36. Wang J, McCormack SA, Johnson LR. Role of nonmuscle myosin II in polyamine-dependent intestinal epithelial cell migration. Am J Physiol 1996;270:G355–G362.
37. Ciacci C, Lind SE, Podolsky DK. Transforming growth factor β regulation of migration in wounded rat intestinal epithelial monolayers. Gastroenterology 1993;105:93–101.
38. Dignass AU, Podolsky DK. Cytokine modulation of intestinal epithelial cell restitution: central role of transforming growth factor beta. Gastroenterology 1993;105:1323–1332.
39. Babyatsky MW, Podolsky DK. Growth and differentiation in the GI tract. In: Yamada T, Alpers DH, Owyang C, Powell DW, Silverstein FE, eds. Textbook of gastroenterology. New York: Lippincott; 1991:475–501.
40. Dignass AU, Podolsky DK. Growth factors in inflammatory bowel disease. In: Fiocchi C, ed. Cytokines in inflammatory bowel disease. Austin, TX: R G Landes Co.; 1996:137–155.
41. Nathan C, Sporn M. Cytokines in context. J Cell Biol 1991;113:981–986.
42. Dignass AU, Sturm A. Peptide growth factors in the intestine. Eur J Gastroenterol Hepatol 2001;13:763–770.

43. Podolsky DK. Mechanisms of regulatory peptide action in the gastrointestinal tract: trefoil peptides. J Gastroenterol 2000;35 (Suppl 12):69–74.

44. Beck PL, Podolsky DK. Growth factors in inflammatory bowel disease. Inflamm Bowel Dis 1999;5:44–60.

45. Jones MK, Tomikawa M, Mohajer B, Tarnawski AS. Gastrointestinal mucosal regeneration: role of growth factors. Front Biosci 1999;4:D303–D309.

46. Murphy MS. Growth factors and the gastrointestinal tract. Nutrition 1998;14:771–774.

47. Sporn MB, Roberts AB. Peptide growth factors and their receptors I and II. New York: Springer-Verlag; 1991.

48. Alison MR, Sarraf CE. The role of growth factors in gastrointestinal cell proliferation. Cell Biol Int 1994;18:1–10.

49. Baldwin GS, Whitehead RH. Gut hormones, growth and malignancy. Baillières Clin Endocrinol Metab 1994;8:185–214.

50. Podolsky DK. Healing the epithelium: solving the problem from two sides. J Gastroenterol 1997;32:122–126.

51. Rogler G, Andus T. Cytokines in inflammatory bowel disease. World J Surg 1998;22:382–389.

52. Fiocchi C. Intestinal inflammation: a complex interplay of immune and nonimmune cell interactions. Am J Physiol 1997;273:G769–G775.

53. Podolsky DK. Mucosal immunity and inflammation. V. Innate mechanisms of mucosal defense and repair: the best offense is a good defense. Am J Physiol 1999;277:G495–G499.

54. Drucker DJ. Epithelial cell growth and differentiation. I. Intestinal growth factors. Am J Physiol 1997;273:G3–G6.

55. Babyatsky MW, Rossiter G, Podolsky DK. Expression of transforming growth factor α and β in colonic mucosa in inflammatory bowel disease. Gastroenterology 1996;110:975–984.

56. Jaffe DL, Koyama S, Podolsky DK. Expression of multiple insulin-like growth factor II (IGF II) transcripts in adult rat intestinal epithelial cells. Gastroenterology 1990;98:A659.

57. Podolsky DK, Lynch Devaney K, Stow JL et al. Identification of human intestinal trefoil factor. Goblet cell-specific expression of a peptide targeted for apical secretion. J Biol Chem 1993;268:6694–6702.

58. Reinecker HC, Macdermott RP, Mirau S, Dignass A, Podolsky DK. Intestinal epithelial cells both express and respond to interleukin 15. Gastroenterology 1996;111:1706–1713.

59. Bajaj-Elliott M, Breese E, Poulsom R, Fairclough PD, MacDonald TT. Keratinocyte growth factor in inflammatory bowel disease. Increased mRNA transcripts in ulcerative colitis compared with Crohn's disease in biopsies and isolated mucosal myofibroblasts. Am J Pathol 1997;151:1469–1476.

60. Cai YC, Jiang Z, Vittimberga F et al. Expression of transforming growth factor-alpha and epidermal growth factor receptor in gastrointestinal stromal tumours. Virchows Arch 1999;435:112–115.

61. Dignass AU, Stow JL, Babyatsky MW. Acute epithelial injury in the rat small intestine in vivo is associated with expanded expression of transforming growth factor alpha and beta. Gut 1996;38:687–693.

62. Ciacci C, Mahida YR, Dignass A, Koizumi M, Podolsky DK. Functional interleukin-2 receptors on intestinal epithelial cells. J Clin Invest 1993;92:527–532.

63. Farrell CL, Bready JV, Rex KL et al. Keratinocyte growth factor protects mice from chemotherapy and radiation-induced gastrointestinal injury and mortality. Cancer Res 1998;58:933–939.

64. Gonzalez AM, Hill DJ, Logan A, Maher PA, Baird A. Distribution of fibroblast growth factor (FGF)-2 and FGF receptor-1 messenger RNA expression and protein presence in the mid-trimester human fetus. Pediatr Res 1996;39:375–385.

65. Hu MC, Qiu WR, Wang YP et al. FGF-18, a novel member of the fibroblast growth factor family, stimulates hepatic and intestinal proliferation. Mol Cell Biol 1998;18:6063–6074.

66. Penttila IA, van Spriel AB, Zhang MF et al. Transforming growth factor-beta levels in maternal milk and expression in postnatal rat duodenum and ileum. Pediatr Res 1998;44:524–531.

67. Young GP, Taranto TM, Jonas HA. Insulin-like growth factor and the developing and mature rat small intestine: receptors and biological actions. Digestion 1990;46:240–252.

68. Alexander RJ, Panja A, Kaplan-Liss E, Mayer L, Raicht RF. Expression of growth factor receptor-encoded mRNA by colonic epithelial cells is altered in inflammatory bowel disease. Dig Dis Sci 1995;40:485–494.

69. Barnard JA, Beauchamp RD, Coffey RJ, Moses HL. Regulation of intestinal epithelial cell growth by transforming growth factor type β. Proc Natl Acad Sci USA 1989;86:1578–1582.

70. Cordon-Cardo C, Vlodavsky I, Haimovitz-Friedman A, Hicklin D, Fuks Z. Expression of basic fibroblast growth factor in normal human tissues. Lab Invest 1990;63:832–840.

71. Kawamura N, Nobusawa R, Mashima H, Kanzaki M, Shibata H, Kojima I. Production of activin A in human intestinal epithelial cell line. Dig Dis Sci 1995;40:2280–2285.

72. Koyama S, Podolsky DK. Differential expression of transforming growth factors α and β in rat intestinal epithelial cells: mirror-image gradients from crypt to villus. J Clin Invest 1989;83:1768–1773.

73. McGee DW, Beagley KW, Aicher WK, McGhee JR. Transforming growth factor-beta and IL-1 beta act in synergy to enhance IL-6 secretion by the intestinal epithelial cell line, IEC-6. J Immunol 1993;151:970–978.

74. Munz B, Smola H, Engelhardt F et al. Overexpression of activin A in the skin of transgenic mice reveals new activities of activin in epidermal morphogenesis, dermal fibrosis and wound repair. EMBO J 1999;18:5205–5215.

75. Green AR. Peptide regulatory factors: multifunctional mediators of cellular growth and differentiation. Lancet 1989;1:705–707.

76. Sporn MB, Roberts AB. Autocrine secretion – 10 years later. Ann Intern Med 1992;117:408–414.

77. Sporn MB, Roberts AB. Transforming growth factor-β: recent progress and new challenges. J Cell Biol 1992;119:1017–1021.

78. Takahashi M, Ota S, Shimada T et al. Hepatocyte growth factor is the most potent endogenous stimulant of rabbit gastric epithelial cell proliferation and migration in primary culture. J Clin Invest 1995;95:1994–2003.

79. Nusrat A, Parkos CA, Bacarra AE et al. Hepatocyte growth factor/scatter factor effects on epithelia. Regulation of intercellular junctions in transformed and nontransformed cell lines, basolateral polarization of c-met receptor in transformed and natural intestinal epithelia, and induction of rapid wound repair in a transformed model epithelium. J Clin Invest 1994;93:2056–2065.

80. Nishimura S, Takahashi M, Ota S, Hirano M, Hiraishi H. Hepatocyte growth factor accelerates restitution of intestinal epithelial cells. J Gastroenterol 1998;33:172–178.

81. Kernochan LE, Tran BN, Tangkijvanich P, Melton AC, Tam SP, Yee HF Jr. Endothelin-1 stimulates human colonic myofibroblast contraction and migration. Gut 2002;50:65–70.

82. Dignass AU, Podolsky DK. Interleukin 2 modulates intestinal epithelial cell function in vitro. Exp Cell Res 1996;225:422–429.

83. Wilson AJ, Byron K, Gibson PR. Interleukin-8 stimulates the migration of human colonic epithelial cells in vitro. Clin Sci (Colch) 1999;97:385–390.

84. Colgan SP, Parkos CA, Delp C, Arnaout MA, Madara JL. Neutrophil migration across cultured epithelial monolayers is modulated by epithelial exposure to IFN-g in a highly polarized fashion. J Cell Biol 1993;120(3):785–798.

85. Breese EJ, Michie CA, Nicholls SW et al. Tumor necrosis factor alpha-producing cells in the intestinal mucosa of children with inflammatory bowel disease. Gastroenterology 1994;106:1455–1466.

86. Colgan SP, Resnick MB, Parkos CA et al. IL-4 directly modulates function of a model human intestinal epithelium. J Immunol 1994;153:2122–2129.

87. Fukushima K, West G, Fiocchi C. Adequacy of mucosal biopsies for evaluation of intestinal cytokine-specific mRNA. Comparative study of RT-PCR in biopsies and isolated cells from normal and inflamed intestine. Dig Dis Sci 1995;40:1498–1505.

88. Macdermott RP. Alterations of the mucosal immune system in inflammatory bowel disease. J Gastroenterol 1996;31:907–916.

89. Takahashi I, Kiyono H. Gut as the largest immunologic tissue. JPEN J Parenter Enteral Nutr 1999;23:S7–12.

90. Ziambaras T, Rubin DC, Perlmutter DH. Regulation of sucrase–isomaltase gene expression in human intestinal epithelial cells by inflammatory cytokines. J Biol Chem 1996;271:1237–1242.

91. Stadnyk AW, Sisson GR, Waterhouse CCM. IL-1 alpha is constitutively expressed in the rat intestinal epithelial cell line IEC-6. Exp Cell Res 1995;220:298–303.

92. Kucharzik T, Lugering N, Pauels HG, Domschke W, Stoll R. IL-4, IL-10 and IL-13 down-regulate monocyte-chemoattracting protein-1 (MCP-1) production in activated intestinal epithelial cells. Clin Exp Immunol 1998;111:152–157.

93. Zachrisson K, Neopikhanov V, Samali A, Uribe A. Interleukin-1, interleukin-8, tumour necrosis factor alpha and interferon gamma stimulate DNA synthesis but have no effect on apoptosis in small-intestinal cell lines. Eur J Gastroenterol Hepatol 2001;13:551–559.

94. Meijssen MA, Brandwein SL, Reinecker HC, Bhan AK, Podolsky DK. Alteration of gene expression by intestinal epithelial cells precedes colitis in interleukin-2-deficient mice. Am J Physiol 1998;274:G472–G479.

95. Fiore NF, Ledniczky G, Liu Q et al. Comparison of interleukin-11 and epidermal growth factor on residual small intestine after massive small bowel resection. J Pediatr Surg 1998;33:24–29.

96. Konturek JW, Bielanski W, Konturek SJ. Distribution and release of epidermal growth factor in man. Gut 1989;30:1194–1200.

97. Carpenter G, Wahl MI. The epidermal growth factor family. In: Sporn MB, Roberts AB, eds. Peptides growth factors and their receptors I. New York: Springer Verlag; 1991:69–171.

98. Malden LT, Novack U, Burgess AW. Expression of transforming growth factor a messenger RNA in the normal and neoplastic gastro-intestinal tract. Int J Cancer 1989;43:380–384.

99. Thomas DM, Nasim MM, Gullick WJ et al. Immunoreactivity of transforming growth factor α in the normal adult gastrointestinal tract. Gut 1992;33:628–631.

100. Montaner B, Asbert M, Perez-Tomas R. Immunolocalization of transforming growth factor-alpha and epidermal growth factor receptor in the rat gastroduodenal area. Dig Dis Sci 1999;44:1408–1416.

101. Menard D, Pothier P. Radioautographic localization of epidermal growth factor receptors in human fetal gut. Gastroenterology 1991;101:640–649.

102. Malecka-Panas E, Kordek R, Biernat W, Tureaud J, Liberski PP, Majumdar AP. Differential activation of total and EGF receptor (EGF-R) tyrosine kinase (tyr-k) in the rectal mucosa in patients with adenomatous polyps, ulcerative colitis and colon cancer. Hepatogastroenterology 1997;44:435–440.

103. Wong WM, Wright NA. Epidermal growth factor, epidermal growth factor receptors, intestinal growth, and adaptation. J Parenter Enteral Nutr 1999;23:S83–S88.

104.  Massague J. The transforming growth factor β family. Annu Rev Cell Biol 1990;6:597–641.

105.  Massague J. Receptors for the TGF-β family. Cell 1992;69:1067–1070.

106.  Barnard JA, Warwick GJ, Gold L. Localizations of TGF-β isoforms in the normal small intestine and colon. Gastroenterology 1993;105:67–73.

107.  Chen R-H, Ebner R, Derynck R. Inactivation of the type II receptor reveals two receptor pathways for the diverse TGF-β activities. Science 1993;260:1335–1338.

108.  Lopez-Casillas F, Cheifetz S, Doody J. Structure and expression of the membrane proteoglycan betaglycan, a component of the TGF-β receptor system. Cell 1991;67:785–795.

109.  Massague J. TGF-beta signal transduction. Annu Rev Biochem 1998;67:753–791.

110.  Kretzschmar M, Massague J. SMADs: mediators and regulators of TGF-beta signaling. Curr Opin Genet Dev 1998;8:103–111.

111.  Nakao A, Imamura T, Souchelnytskyi S et al. TGF-beta receptor-mediated signalling through Smad2, Smad3 and Smad4. EMBO J 1997;16:5353–5362.

112.  Persson U, Souchelnytskyi S, Franzen P, Miyazono K, ten Dijke P, Heldin CH. Transforming growth factor (TGF-beta)-specific signaling by chimeric TGF-beta type II receptor with intracellular domain of activin type IIB receptor. J Biol Chem 1997;272:21187–21194.

113.  Border WA, Ruoslathi E. Transforming growth factor β1 in disease: The dark side of tissue repair. J Clin Invest 1992;90:1–7.

114.  Giladi E, Raz E, Karmeli F, Okon E, Rachmilewitz D. Transforming growth factor-beta gene therapy ameliorates experimental colitis in rats. Eur J Gastroenterol Hepatol 1995;7:341–347.

115.  Kitani A, Fuss IJ, Nakamura K, Schwartz OM, Usui T, Strober W. Treatment of experimental (trinitrobenzene sulfonic acid) colitis by intranasal administration of transforming growth factor (TGF-)-beta1 plasmid: TGF-beta1-mediated suppression of T helper cell type 1 response occurs by interleukin (IL)-10 induction and IL-12 receptor beta2 chain downregulation. J Exp Med 2000;192:41–52.

116.  Shull MK, Ormsby I, Kier AB. Targeted disruption of the mouse transforming growth factor β1 gene results in multifocal inflammatory disease. Nature 1992;359:693–699.

117.  Goke M, Podolsky DK. Regulation of the mucosal epithelial barrier. Baillières Clin Gastroenterol 1996;10:393–405.

118.  Dignass A, Lynch-Devaney K, Kindon H, Thim L, Podolsky DK. Trefoil peptides promote epithelial migration through a transforming growth factor beta-independent pathway. J Clin Invest 1994;94:376–383.

119.  Dignass AU, Tsunekawa S, Podolsky DK. Fibroblast growth factors modulate intestinal epithelial cell growth and migration. Gastroenterology 1994;106:1254–1262.

120.  Dignass AU, Lynch Devaney K, Podolsky DK. Hepatocyte growth factor/scatter factor modulates intestinal epithelial cell proliferation and migration. Biochem Biophys Res Commun 1994;202:701–709.

121.  Paimela H, Goddard PJ, Carter K et al. Restitution of frog gastric mucosa in vitro: effect of fibroblast growth factor. Gastroenterology 1993;104:1337–1345.

122.  Poulsom R, Begos DE, Modlin IM. Molecular aspects of restitution: functions of trefoil peptides. Yale J Biol Med 1996;69:137–146.

123.  Riegler M, Sedivy R, Sogukoglu T et al. Epidermal growth factor promotes rapid response to epithelial injury in rabbit duodenum in vitro. Gastroenterology 1996;111:28–36.

124.  Riegler M, Sedivy R, Sogukoglu T et al. Effect of growth factors on epithelial restitution of human colonic mucosa in vitro. Scand J Gastroenterol 1997;32:925–932.

125.  Basson MD, Modlin JM, Flynn SD, Jena BP, Madri JA. Independent modulation of enterocyte migration and proliferation by growth factors, matrix proteins and pharmalogic agents in an in vitro model of mucosal healing. Surgery 1992;112:299–308.

126.  Blay J, Brown KD. Epidermal growth factor promotes the chemotactic migration of cultured rat intestinal epithelial cells. J Cell Physiol 1985;24:107–112.

127.  Playford RJ, Marchbank T, Goodlad RA, Chinery RA, Poulsom R, Hanby AM. Transgenic mice that overexpress the human trefoil peptide pS2 have an increased resistance to intestinal damage. Proc Natl Acad Sci USA 1996;93:2137–2142.

128.  Poulsom R. Trefoil peptides. Baillières Clin Gastroenterol 1996;10:113–134.

129.  Wong WM, Poulsom R, Wright NA. Trefoil peptides. Gut 1999;44:890–895.

130.  Thim L. Trefoil peptides: from structure to function. Cell Mol Life Sci 1997;53:888–903.

131.  Hanby AM, Poulsom R, Elia G, Singh S, Longcroft JM, Wright NA. The expression of the trefoil peptides pS2 and human spasmolytic polypeptide (hSP) in 'gastric metaplasia' of the proximal duodenum: Implications for the nature of 'gastric metaplasia'. J Pathol 1993;169:355–360.

132.  Khulusi S, Hanby AM, Marrero JM et al. Expression of trefoil peptides pS2 and human spasmolytic polypeptide in gastric metaplasia at the margin of duodenal ulcers. Gut 1995;37:205–209.

133.  Poulsom R, Chinery R, Sarraf C et al. Trefoil peptide gene expression in small intestinal Crohn's disease and dietary adaptation. J Clin Gastroenterol 1993;17:S78–S91.

134.  Poulsom R, Chinery R, Sarraf C, Lalani EN, Stamp G, Elia G, Wright N. Trefoil peptide expression in intestinal adaptation and renewal. Scand J Gastroenterol 1992;192:17–28.

135.  Jeffrey GP, Oates PS, Wang TC, Babyatsky MW, Brand SJ. Spasmolytic polypeptide: a trefoil peptide secreted by rat gastric mucous cells. Gastroenterology 1994;106:336–345.

136.  Suemori S, Lynch-Devaney K, Podolsky DK. Identification and characterization of rat intestinal trefoil factor: tissue- and cell-specific member of the trefoil protein family. Proc Natl Acad Sci USA 1991;88:11017–11021.

137.  Babyatsky MW, DeBeaumont M, Thim L, Podolsky DK. Oral trefoil peptides protect against ethanol- and indomethacin-induced gastric injury in rats. Gastroenterology 1996;110:489–497.

138.  Tran CP, Cook GA, Yeomans ND, Thim L, Giraud AS. Trefoil peptide TFF2 (spasmolytic polypeptide) potently accelerates healing and reduces inflammation in a rat model of colitis. Gut 1999;44:636–642.

139.  Playford RJ, Marchbank T, Chinery R et al. Human spasmolytic polypeptide is a cytoprotective agent that stimulates cell migration. Gastroenterology 1995;108:108–116.

140.  Chinery R, Playford RJ. Combined intestinal trefoil factor and epidermal growth factor is prophylactic against indomethacin-induced gastric damage in the rat. Clin Sci 1995;88:401–403.

141.  Mashimo H, Wu DC, Podolsky DK, Fishman MC. Impaired defense of intestinal mucosa in mice lacking intestinal trefoil factor. Science 1996;274:262–265.

142.  Efstathiou JA, Noda M, Rowan A et al. Intestinal trefoil factor controls the expression of the adenomatous polyposis coli-catenin and the E-cadherin–catenin complexes in human colon carcinoma cells. Proc Natl Acad Sci USA 1998;95:3122–3127.

143.  Liu D, el Hariry I, Karayiannakis AJ et al. Phosphorylation of beta-catenin and epidermal growth factor receptor by intestinal trefoil factor. Lab Invest 1997;77:557–563.

144.  Iwakiri D, Podolsky DK. Keratinocyte growth factor promotes goblet cell differentiation through regulation of goblet cell silencer inhibitor. Gastroenterology 2001;120:1372–1380.

145.  Jeffers M, McDonald WF, Chillakuru RA et al. A novel human fibroblast growth factor treats experimental intestinal inflammation. Gastroenterology 2002;123:1151–1162.

146.  Fernandez-Estivariz C, Gu LH, Gu L et al. Trefoil peptide expression and goblet cell number in rat intestine: effects of KGF and fasting/refeeding. Am J Physiol Regul Integr Comp Physiol 2002;284(2):R564-R573.

147.  Chakrabarty S, Fan D, Varani J. Modulation of differentiation and proliferation in human colon carcinoma cells by transforming growth factor β1 and β2. Int J Cancer 1990;46:493–499.

148.  Huang W, Trujillo JM, Chakrabarty S. Proliferation of human colon cancer cells: role of epidermal growth factor and transforming growth factor α. Int J Cancer 1992;52:978–986.

149.  Kurokowa M, Lynch K, Podolsky DK. Effects of growth factors on an intestinal epithelial cell line: transforming growth factor beta inhibits proliferation and stimulates differentiation. Biochem Biophys Res Commun 1987;142:775–782.

150.  Podolsky DK. Regulation of intestinal epithelial proliferation: a few answers, many questions. Am J Physiol 1993;264:G179–G186.

151.  Thompson MA, Cox AJ, Whitehead RH, Jonas HA. Autocrine regulation of human tumor cell proliferation by insulin-like growth factor II: an in vitro model. Endocrinology 1990;126:3033–3042.

152.  Sonoyama K, Rutatip S, Kasai T. Gene expression of activin, activin receptors, and follistatin in intestinal epithelial cells. Am J Physiol Gastrointest Liver Physiol 2000;278:G89–G97.

153.  Dignass AU, Schulte KM, Jung S, Harder-d'Heureuse J, Wiedenmann B. Activin A modulates intestinal epithelial cell function in vitro. Gastroenterology 2000;118(4):A823.

154.  Suemori S, Ciacci C, Podolsky DK. Regulation of transforming growth factor expression in rat intestinal epithelial cell lines. J Clin Invest 1991;87:2216–2221.

155.  Albers TM, Lomakina I, Moore RP. Structural and functional roles of cytoskeletal proteins during repair of native guinea pig intestinal epithelium. Cell Biol Int 1996;20:821–830.

156.  Basson MD. In vitro evidence for matrix regulation of intestinal epithelial biology during mucosal healing. Life Sci 2001;69:3005–3018.

157.  Goke M, Zuk A, Podolsky DK. Regulation and function of extracellular matrix intestinal epithelial restitution in vitro. Am J Physiol 1996;271:G729–G740.

158.  Yu CF, Sanders MA, Basson MD. Human caco-2 motility redistributes FAK and paxillin and activates p38 MAPK in a matrix-dependent manner. Am J Physiol Gastrointest Liver Physiol 2000;278:G952–G966.

159.  Liu YW, Sanders MA, Basson MD. Loss of matrix-dependent cytoskeletal tyrosine kinase signals may regulate intestinal epithelial differentiation during mucosal healing. J Gastrointest Surg 1999;3:82–94.

160.  Mahida YR, Beltinger J, Makh S et al. Adult human colonic subepithelial myofibroblasts express extracellular matrix proteins and cyclooxygenase-1 and -2. Am J Physiol 1997;273:G1341–G1348.

161.  Arihiro S, Ohtani H, Hiwatashi N, Torii A, Sorsa T, Nagura H. Vascular smooth muscle cells and pericytes express MMP-1, MMP-9, TIMP-1 and type I procollagen in inflammatory bowel disease. Histopathology 2001;39:50–59.

162.  Louis E, Ribbens C, Godon A et al. Increased production of matrix metalloproteinase-3 and tissue inhibitor of metalloproteinase-1 by inflamed mucosa in inflammatory bowel disease. Clin Exp Immunol 2000;120:241–246.

163.  Heuschkel RB, MacDonald TT, Monteleone G, Bajaj-Elliott M, Smith JA, Pender SL. Imbalance of stromelysin-1 and TIMP-1 in the mucosal lesions of children with inflammatory bowel disease. Gut 2000;47:57–62.

164. Vaalamo M, Karjalainen-Lindsberg ML, Puolakkainen P, Kere J, Saarialho-Kere U. Distinct expression profiles of stromelysin-2 (MMP-10), collagenase-3 (MMP-13), macrophage metalloelastase (MMP-12), and tissue inhibitor of metalloproteinases-3 (TIMP-3) in intestinal ulcerations. Am J Pathol 1998;152:1005–1014.

165. Baugh MD, Perry MJ, Hollander AP et al. Matrix metalloproteinase levels are elevated in inflammatory bowel disease. Gastroenterology 1999;117:814–822.

166. Di Sebastiano P, di Mola FF, Artese L et al. Beneficial effects of Batimastat (BB-94), a matrix metalloproteinase inhibitor, in rat experimental colitis. Digestion 2001;63:234–239.

167. Sykes AP, Bhogal R, Brampton C et al. The effect of an inhibitor of matrix metalloproteinases on colonic inflammation in a trinitrobenzenesulphonic acid rat model of inflammatory bowel disease. Aliment Pharmacol Ther 1999;13:1535–1542.

168. Stallmach A, Schuppan D, Lazar D, Riese HH, Riecken E. Increased collagen type III synthesis by fibroblasts isolated from strictures of patients with Crohn's disease. Gastroenterology 1992;102:1920–1929.

169. Zeeh JM, Ennes HS, Hoffmann P et al. Expression of insulin-like growth factor I receptors and binding proteins by colonic smooth muscle cells. Am J Physiol 1997;272:G481–G487.

170. Lawrance IC, Maxwell L, Doe W. Inflammation location, but not type, determines the increase in TGF- beta1 and IGF-1 expression and collagen deposition in IBD intestine. Inflamm Bowel Dis 2001;7:16–26.

171. Zimmermann EM, Li L, Hou YT, Mohapatra NK, Pucilowska JB. Insulin-like growth factor I and insulin-like growth factor binding protein 5 in Crohn's disease. Am J Physiol Gastrointest Liver Physiol 2001;280:G1022–G1029.

172. Gelbmann CM, Mestermann S, Gross V, Kollinger M, Scholmerich J, Falk W. Strictures in Crohn's disease are characterised by an accumulation of mast cells colocalised with laminin but not with fibronectin or vitronectin. Gut 1999;45:210–217.

173. Cario E, Goebell H, Dignass AU. Factor XIII modulates intestinal epithelial wound healing in vitro. Scand J Gastroenterol 1999;34:485–490.

174. English D, Garcia JG, Brindley DN. Platelet-released phospholipids link haemostasis and angiogenesis. Cardiovasc Res 2001;49:588–599.

175. Muszbek L, Yee VC, Hevessy Z. Blood coagulation factor XIII: structure and function. Thromb Res 1999;94:271–305.

176. Muszbek L, Adany R, Mikkola H. Novel aspects of blood coagulation factor XIII. I. Structure, distribution, activation, and function. Crit Rev Clin Lab Sci 1996;33:357–421.

177. Oshitani N, Kitano A, Hara J et al. Deficiency of blood coagulation factor XIII in Crohn's disease. Am J Gastroenterol 1995;90:1116–1118.

178. D'Argenio G, Grossman A, Cosenza V, Valle ND, Mazzacca G, Bishop PD. Recombinant factor XIII improves established experimental colitis in rats. Dig Dis Sci 2000;45:987–997.

179. Noll T, Wozniak G, McCarson K et al. Effect of factor XIII on endothelial barrier function. J Exp Med 1999;189:1373–1382.

180. Oshitani N, Nakamura S, Matsumoto T, Kobayashi K, Kitano A. Treatment of Crohn's disease fistulas with coagulation factor XIII. Lancet 1996;347:119–120.

181. Wilson AJ, Gibson PR. Short-chain fatty acids promote the migration of colonic epithelial cells in vitro. Gastroenterology 1997;113:487–496.

182. Sturm A, Dignass AU. Clinical relevance of phospholipids in the gastrointestinal tract. Dtsch Med Wochenschr 2000;125:192–198.

183. Sturm A, Sudermann T, Schulte KM, Goebell H, Dignass AU. Modulation of intestinal epithelial wound healing in vitro and in vivo by lysophosphatidic acid. Gastroenterology 1999;117:368–377.

184. Dignass AU, Becker A, Spiegler S, Goebell H. Adenine nucleotides modulate epithelial wound healing in vitro. Eur J Clin Invest 1998;28:554–561.

185. Kartha S, Toback FG. Adenine nucleotides stimulate migration in wounded cultures of kidney epithelial cells. J Clin Invest 1992;90:288–292.

186. Moolenaar WH, Kruijer W, Tilly BC, Verlaan I, Bierman AJ, de Laat SW. Growth factor-like action of phosphatidic acid. Nature 1986;323:171–173.

187. Rhoads JM, Argenzio RA, Chen W et al. Glutamine metabolism stimulates intestinal cell MAPKs by a cAMP- inhibitable, Raf-independent mechanism. Gastroenterology 2000;118:90–100.

188. Dowling RH. Polyamines in intestinal adaptation and disease. Digestion 1990;46 (Suppl 2):331–344.

189. Jalink K, Hordijk PL, Moolenaar WH. Growth factor-like effects of lysophosphatidic acid, a novel lipid mediator. Biochim Biophys Acta 1994;1198:185–196.

190. Moolenaar WH. Mitogenic action of lysophosphatidic acid. Adv Cancer Res 1991;57:87–102.

191. Moolenaar WH, Jalink K, van Corven EJ. Lysophosphatidic acid: a bioactive phospholipid with growth factor-like properties. Rev Physiol Biochem Pharmacol 1992;119:47–65.

192. Moolenaar WH. LPA: a novel lipid mediator with diverse biological actions. Trends Cell Biol 1994;4:213–219.

193. Wang JY, Johnson LR. Gastric and duodenal mucosal ornithine decarboxylase and damage after corticosterone. Am J Physiol 1990;258:G942–G950.

194. Wang JY, Johnson LR. Polyamines and ornithine decarboxylase during repair of duodenal mucosa after stress in rats. Gastroenterology 1991;100:333–343.

195. Wang JY, Viar MJ, McCormack SA, Johnson LR. Effect of putrescine on S-adenosylmethionine decarboxylase in a small intestinal crypt cell line. Am J Physiol 1992;263:G494–G501.

196. Eichholtz T, Alblas J, van Overveld M, Moolenaar W, Ploegh H. A pseudosubstrate peptide inhibits protein kinase C-mediated phosphorylation in permeabilized Rat-1 cells. FEBS Lett 1990;261:147–150.

197. Moolenaar WH. Lysophosphatidic acid signalling. Curr Opin Cell Biol 1995;7:203–210.

198. Moolenaar WH. Lysophosphatidic acid, a multifunctional phospholipid messenger. J Biol Chem 1995;270:12949–12952.

199. Anstead GM. Steroids, retinoids, and wound healing. Adv Wound Care 1998;11:277–285.

200. Aszodi A, Ponsky JL. Effects of corticosteroid on the healing bowel anastomosis. Am Surg 1984;50:546–548.

201. Furst MB, Stromberg BV, Blatchford GJ, Christensen MA, Thorson AG. Colonic anastomoses: bursting strength after corticosteroid treatment. Dis Colon Rectum 1994;37:12–15.

202. Jung S, Fehr S, Harder-d'Heureuse J, Wiedenmann B, Dignass AU. Corticosteroids impair intestinal epithelial wound repair mechanisms in vitro. Scand J Gastroenterol 2001;36:963–970.

203. Beltinger J, McKaig BC, Makh S, Stack WA, Hawkey CJ, Mahida YR. Human colonic subepithelial myofibroblasts modulate transepithelial resistance and secretory response. Am J Physiol 1999;277:C271–C279.

204. McKaig BC, Makh SS, Hawkey CJ, Podolsky DK, Mahida YR. Normal human colonic subepithelial myofibroblasts enhance epithelial migration (restitution) via TGF-beta3. Am J Physiol 1999;276:G1087–G1093.

205. McAlindon ME, Gray T, Galvin A, Sewell HF, Podolsky DK, Mahida YR. Differential lamina propria cell migration via basement membrane pores of inflammatory bowel disease mucosa. Gastroenterology 1998;115:841–848.

206. Powell DW, Mifflin RC, Valentich JD, Crowe SE, Saada JI, West AB. Myofibroblasts. II. Intestinal subepithelial myofibroblasts. Am J Physiol 1999;277:C183–C201.

207. Cario E, Becker A, Sturm A, Goebell H, Dignass AU. Peripheral blood mononuclear cells promote intestinal epithelial restitution in vitro through an interleukin-2/interferon-gamma- dependent pathway. Scand J Gastroenterol 1999;34:1132–1138.

208. Mahida YR, Galvin AM, Gray T et al. Migration of human intestinal lamina propria lymphocytes, macrophages and eosinophils following the loss of surface epithelial cells. Clin Exp Immunol 1997;109:377–386.

209. Goke M, Kanai M, Podolsky DK. Intestinal fibroblasts regulate intestinal epithelial cell proliferation via hepatocyte growth factor. Am J Physiol 1998;274:G809–G818.

210. Panetti TS, Magnusson MK, Peyruchaud O et al. Modulation of cell interactions with extracellular matrix by lysophosphatidic acid and sphingosine 1-phosphate. Prostaglandins 2001;64:93–106.

211. Balazs L, Okolicany J, Ferrebee M, Tolley B, Tigyi G. Topical application of the phospholipid growth factor lysophosphatidic acid promotes wound healing in vivo. Am J Physiol Regul Integr Comp Physiol 2001;280:R466–R472.

212. Hines OJ, Ryder N, Chu J, McFadden D. Lysophosphatidic acid stimulates intestinal restitution via cytoskeletal activation and remodeling. J Surg Res 2000;92:23–28.

213. Wang JY, McCormack SA, Viar MJ, Johnson LR. Stimulation of proximal small intestinal mucosal growth by luminal polyamines. Am J Physiol 1991;261:G504–G511.

214. Wang JY, Johnson LR. Luminal polyamines stimulate repair of gastric mucosal stress ulcers. Am J Physiol 1990;259:G584–G592.

215. Rao JN, Li J, Li L, Bass BL, Wang JY. Differentiated intestinal epithelial cells exhibit increased migration through polyamines and myosin II. Am J Physiol 1999;277:G1149–G1158.

216. Kartha S, Atkin B, Martin TE, Toback FG. Cytokeratin reorganization induced by adenosine diphosphate in kidney epithelial cells. Exp Cell Res 1992;200:219–226.

217. Scheppach W, Dusel G, Kuhn T et al. Effect of L-glutamine and n-butyrate on the restitution of rat colonic mucosa after acid induced injury. Gut 1996;38:878–885.

218. Ruthig DJ, Meckling-Gill KA. Both (n-3) and (n-6) fatty acids stimulate wound healing in the rat intestinal epithelial cell line, IEC-6. J Nutr 1999;129:1791–1798.

219. Dignass AU, Harder-d'Heureuse J, Jung S, Wiedenmann B. Glutamine enhances intestinal epithelial wound healing in vitro. Clin Nutr 2000;19(Suppl.1): 24.

220. Ziegler TR, Estivariz CF, Jonas CR, Gu LH, Jones DP, Leader LM. Interactions between nutrients and peptide growth factors in intestinal growth, repair, and function. J Parenter Enteral Nutr 1999;23:S174–S183.

## CHAPTER 3

# Epithelial–microbial interactions

Lars Eckmann and Martin F Kagnoff

## INTRODUCTION

The mucosa of the human colon and small intestine is a site of chronic regulated 'physiologic' inflammation. This contrasts with other mucosal sites and the skin. If the numbers of T and B lymphocytes, eosinophils, mast cells, macrophages and dendritic cells that are present in the human intestinal tract were to be present in other sites, those sites would be considered pathologically inflamed. The intestinal mucosa is continuously exposed to an abundant, and normally non-pathogenic, commensal bacterial microbiota, although intermittent encounters with bacterial pathogens also occur. These enteric bacteria maintain the state of physiologic intestinal inflammation, as the intestinal mucosa in germ-free animals is largely devoid of inflammatory cells. In addition, commensal bacteria are important for initiating and sustaining chronic intestinal inflammation in animal models, and may also play a similar role in patients with IBD.

Commensal bacteria and enteric bacterial pathogens first – and sometimes exclusively – interact with the host at the level of the intestinal epithelium, which lines the intestinal mucosa and separates the host's internal milieu from the intestinal lumen and the external environment. This places the epithelium in a central position to function as a microbial detector, signal integrator and central relay system in a communications network that transmits signals from enteric microbes and their products to cells in the underlying lamina propria. This is particularly important for microbes that do not normally invade the mucosa, including commensals, as they are not likely to have relevant contacts with other host cells. For invasive enteric microbes, the interactions with the epithelium are transient and mostly relevant during the initial stages of infection. None the less, the initial innate host response to infection is important, as the development of adaptive T and B cell-mediated immune defenses is delayed for several days after initial encounter with the pathogen. In the absence of effective innate immune defense mechanisms, many enteric pathogens cause severe disease and even death during this lag period. Moreover, initiation of adaptive immune defense requires the activation of T cells by antigen-presenting cells of the innate immune system. When viewed in this context, it is evident that innate defense mechanisms, and the role intestinal epithelial cells play in inducing them, are essential for host survival during encounters with invasive enteric pathogens.

This chapter examines the interactions of intestinal epithelial cells with enteric microbes, and the role these cells can play in initiating and sustaining mucosal immune and inflammatory responses to microbial infection. A focus is placed on in vitro and in vivo model systems used to define epithelial cell responses to microbial infection and the spectrum of intestinal epithelial responses activated by various enteric commensals and pathogens that utilize different strategies to interact with the host.

## MODEL SYSTEMS TO STUDY INTERACTIONS BETWEEN INTESTINAL EPITHELIAL CELLS AND ENTERIC MICROBES

By definition, interactions between enteric microbes and intestinal epithelial cells involve two major components, the microbe and the host epithelial cell. Several approaches and model systems are used to study these interactions, including different cell culture models, intestinal xenografts, and transgenic mouse models.

### CELL CULTURE MODELS

One of the simplest reductionist approaches is to ask: What genes are upregulated and what mediators are produced by intestinal epithelial cells when they encounter an enteric microbe in vitro? A number of cell line models have been used to address these and other questions relevant for understanding the biology of intestinal epithelial cells (Table 3.1). As many

**Table 3.1 Commonly used cell culture models of human colon epithelial cells**

| Cell lines | No. of citations in PubMed | Growth rate | Polarization on filters | Major applications | References |
|---|---|---|---|---|---|
| Caco-2 | 1,146 | Moderate | Yes | Barrier studies, gene expression | 7 |
| T84 | 477 | Slow | Yes | Ion transport | 6 |
| HT-29 | 404 | Fast | No (except for special sublines) | Cytokine studies, cell differentiation | 183 |
| SW480/SW620 | 82 | Fast | No | Cancer research | 184,185 |
| DLD-1 | 49 | Moderate | No | Immune functions | 186 |
| HCA-7 | 35 | Moderate | Yes | Growth regulation | 8 |
| HCT-8 | 26 | Fast | No | Microbial interactions | 10 |

Notes: Searches in the PubMed database were performed in November 2002 using the terms 'epithelial' and the name of the respective cell line. Major applications only refer to selected areas of research for which the specific lines were used. Many other applications have been reported for the various cell lines.

of the human intestinal epithelial cells available for such studies are lines generated from colon carcinomas, cellular responses of a single cell line to a given enteric microbe should be verified using several different cell lines, and even then the results should be interpreted with caution, as in some instances they may not accurately reflect the response of normal intestinal epithelial cells. None the less, this approach has provided large amounts of data, many of which have subsequently been confirmed with normal epithelial cells using in vivo models. In addition to studies focused on individual epithelial cell mediators, high-density cDNA arrays have been employed to probe the up-regulated expression of thousands of genes in gastrointestinal epithelial cells in response to infection with bacterial pathogens.[1–4] Notably, those studies revealed that infection of intestinal epithelial cell lines with enteric pathogens (e.g. *Salmonella*) upregulates mRNA expression of a limited number of genes, many of which are NFκB responsive.[1] mRNA expression profiles obtained using microarray analysis provide a powerful approach to characterizing and understanding epithelial cell–microbe interactions, permitting the discovery of epithelial cell products upregulated by enteric microbes, which would not have been otherwise predicted. In contrast to colon carcinoma cell lines, there are only few, if any, representative human small intestinal epithelial cell lines available for study using in vitro model systems.[5]

The ability to grow several human colon cancer-derived epithelial cell lines as a polarized model epithelium on micro-porous supports in transwell culture in vitro adds another useful tool for exploring epithelial cell–microbial interactions (Table 3.1).[6–12] This model system more closely approximates the epithelium in vivo, which is polarized into apical and basolateral domains. Thus, in vivo the intestinal epithelium variably interacts with enteric microbes at the apical and basolateral surface and vectorally secretes cytokines and innate defense molecules from the basolateral or apical membrane. Delineating apical versus basolateral secretion of epithelial cell products is important when considering intestinal epithelial cell mediators that signal effective host defense responses and defend against lumen-dwelling pathogens that are not invasive for epithelial cells, compared to enteroinvasive pathogens. Such polarized model epithelia can also be used to generate more complex cellular systems where one examines interactions between microbes, epithelial cells and an additional cell type, for example by the addition of dendritic cells or lymphocytes.[13,14] These model epithelia are generated using colon cancer cell lines, so the aforementioned cautions apply regarding the generalization of results to normal epithelium.

## INTESTINAL XENOGRAFT MODELS

Studies of epithelial cell responses to enteric microbes in humans in vivo are limited for ethical and practical reasons. Further, the very early events following natural infection with enteric microbes cannot be adequately examined. Such events are either asymptomatic (i.e. after colonization with commensal bacteria) or their detection is substantially delayed as patients present to the clinic only several hours to days after the onset of infection with enteric pathogens. Moreover, in areas where enteric microbial infections are common, patients are often infected with multiple pathogens. Human intestinal xenograft models can overcome these limitations by studying the early responses of an intact human intestinal epithelium in vivo to a range of stimuli.[10,15–20]

In this model, human fetal small intestine or colon is transplanted subcutaneously into immunodeficient mice (e.g. severe combined immunodeficient (SCID) or Rag$^{-/-}$ mice) that cannot reject the xenograft (Fig. 3.1). Initially the graft undergoes degeneration, but subsequently over a 10-week period regrows a small segment of intestine[15,16] (Fig. 3.2). The mature xenograft contains a fully regenerated intestinal mucosa characteristic of either the colon or the small intestine, and is lined by an epithelium that is strictly of human origin.[15,16] The xenografts can be injected intraluminally with enteric microbes or their products, or stimulated by systemic injection of xenograft-carrying mice with cytokines or mediators of human origin that in some cases (e.g. human IFN-γ) act only on their cognate receptors on human cells in the xenograft, and not on murine cells. Infected or cytokine-stimulated xenografts can be removed from mice and analyzed using molecular or histopathological tools. Alternatively, unstimulated xenografts can be harvested and used

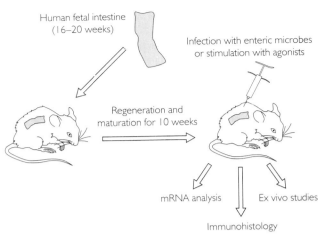

Fig. 3.1 Human intestinal xenograft model in SCID mice. Human fetal intestine is transplanted subcutaneously into adult SCID mice and allowed to develop for 10 or more weeks, after which the tissue represents a fully mature human intestine. Tissues can be used for infections with enteric microbes or stimulation with various agonists. Tissue responses are analyzed by molecular and histological approaches. In addition, tissues can be removed and studied ex vivo in modified Ussing chambers.

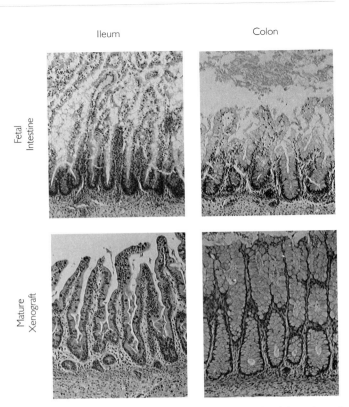

Fig. 3.2 Histology of human intestinal xenografts. Fetal intestine of 18 weeks' gestational age was transplanted subcutaneously into immuno-deficient (SCID) mice. In parallel, other portions of the freshly harvested fetal tissue were fixed, and paraffin sections were prepared and stained with hematoxylin/eosin (top panels). After 10 weeks, mature xenografts were removed and processed for histology (bottom panels). Fetal tissues show considerable degeneration of villi but not crypts in the ileum and colon (fetal colon has rudimentary villi) owing to typical delays in obtaining and transplanting tissues. Villi are fully regenerated in the mature ileal xenografts. Mature colon xenografts lose their villi and consist of fully developed crypts and a surface epithelium, both with abundant goblet cells. All photographs have the same magnification.

as a source of intact non-transformed human intestinal epithelium for ex vivo studies (e.g. the mucosa can be mounted in Ussing chambers for studies of mucosal ion secretion).

No model is useful for all studies, and this is the case also for the human intestinal xenograft models. For example, the usefulness of xenografts is limited in adoptive cell transfer studies, in which human myeloid cells would be tested for their ability to migrate into the xenograft mucosa, as the vasculature of the xenografts is of mouse origin.[15,16] The potential incompatibility of receptor–ligand interactions required for extravasation could limit the entry of human cells into the xenografts. None the less, some cytokines, such as human CXCL8 (IL-8) produced by human epithelial cells in the xenograft, chemoattract murine myeloid cells into the lamina propria and subepithelial region upon microbial infection.[10,21]

## TRANSGENIC MOUSE MODELS

Murine models have been a mainstay for studies of innate defense mechanisms and adaptive immunity because of the availability of genetic manipulations in which selected genes are overexpressed (traditional transgenic mice) or specific genes are knocked out (e.g. through Cre/lox-P mediated somatic recombination). Key for such studies as applied to intestinal epithelial cells is the development and characterization of suitable promoters and expression vectors, which allow the selective expression of specific transgenes in the intestinal epithelium. Several promoters have been used for this purpose, including the promoters for fatty acid-binding protein (FABP),[22] cytokeratin 19[23] and villin.[24] Despite their demonstrated usefulness in some applications, they also suffer from shortcomings, including the chimeric nature of epithelial expression (i.e. not all epithelial cells may express the transgene) and the occurrence of extraintestinal expression, which can limit their utility for some purposes. There is a continued need for improved promoters/expression vectors with the desired expression properties, as well as inducible expression systems to allow the controlled induction or deletion of a specific gene product. Such systems

have been generated, including the ecdysone receptor,[25] tetracycline responsive elements[26] and tamoxifen inducibility,[27] although their use for transgene expression in the intestinal epithelium is still in its infancy.

In general, murine models have not been broadly applied to studies of intestinal infection by human enteric pathogens and commensal microbes, as the pathogenesis of murine infections with such microbes often differs from findings in humans. Thus, some pathogens, such as *Salmonella*, that cause gastroenteritis in humans cause systemic disease with little if any gastroenteritis in mice, whereas other pathogens, such as *Cryptosporidium parvum* and rotavirus, that readily infect neonatal mice, do not efficiently infect the intestinal mucosa of adult mice. None the less, genetic modification can render murine models more suitable for studying epithelial innate defense responses to microbial pathogens that cause human disease. For example, the human enteric pathogen *Listeria monocytogenes* does not infect murine intestinal epithelial cells. E-cadherin is the intestinal epithelial cell receptor for *Listeria* internalin A, which is essential for bacterial invasion of these cells.[28,29] Murine E-cadherin has an amino acid mutation at position 16 that interferes with binding to internalin A.[30] However, transgenic mice have been engineered that express human E-cadherin in intestinal epithelial cells, which renders the cells susceptible to invasion by *L. monocytogenes* with resulting mucosal inflammation.[31] Thus, novel strategies can be applied to improve the utility of murine models for studies of epithelial cell-mediated innate host defense to human microbial pathogens.

# COMMON FEATURES IN THE INTERACTIONS OF INTESTINAL EPITHELIAL CELLS WITH DIFFERENT ENTERIC MICROBES

The interactions between intestinal epithelial cells and different enteric microbes can be conceptually divided into an early phase, including initial adhesion, attachment and cell signaling events, and later events such as altered epithelial gene expression and secretion of various mediators. The late consequences of epithelial cell–microbial interactions are remarkably uniform and appear to be largely independent of the specific properties of the initiating microbe.[32] For this reason, the following section will focus on the common features in the late epithelial responses to enteric microbes. In contrast, the early events in the interaction between intestinal epithelium and specific microbes are highly diverse, and depend on the nature of the specific microbe. Examples of unique aspects of epithelial cell–microbe interactions are discussed below.

## PRODUCTION OF CHEMOATTRACTANT CYTOKINES

One of the most extensively characterized areas of epithelial cell responses to enteric microbes is the regulated production of immunoregulatory and proinflammatory cytokines, which have central functions in the initiation and control of immune and inflammatory responses. A particular focus has been placed on chemokines, which are low-molecular-weight cytokines (8–10 kDa) with a broad range of activities in the recruitment and functions of different leukocyte populations at sites of microbial infection or inflammation. The chemokines can be categorized into four families based on the structural arrangement of their amino terminal cysteines and intervening amino acids (i.e. CXC, CC, CX3C and C).[33,34] Several of the CXC chemokines, including CXCL8/IL-8, have an ELR (glutamic acid, leucine, arginine) motif and function as neutrophil chemoattractants.

### Chemokines for neutrophils and macrophages

Human intestinal epithelial cells produce several CXC ELR-motif neutrophil chemoattractants in response to bacterial infection. These include CXCL8 and members of the GRO family of CXC chemokines (CXCL1, CXCL2, CXCL3), which are rapidly, but transiently, upregulated following bacterial infection of intestinal epithelial cells.[35–39] Human intestinal epithelial cells also produce another CXC ELR-motif chemokine, CXCL5 (ENA78).[38,40] However, the regulation of CXCL5 differs from that of CXCL8 and the GRO family members.[40] Although the upregulated expression of CXCL5 is delayed relative to that of CXCL8, its production is more prolonged.[38,41] These findings suggest a model in which the epithelium produces an array of chemokines that establish spatial and temporal chemokine gra-

dients in the underlying mucosa[38] for the chemotaxis of neutrophils into the mucosa (Fig. 3.3). For example, CXCL8, which is produced rapidly and in relatively large amounts by intestinal epithelial cells, but whose duration of production is short-lived, might function to rapidly chemoattract neutrophils into the proximity of epithelial cells. In contrast, CXCL5, with its delayed onset of expression, lower potency and more long-lived production, may imprint chemotactic gradients that bring neutrophils into closer contact with the epithelium, and maintain neutrophils in that location for longer periods of time. These chemokines are secreted predominantly from the basolateral domain of polarized epithelia, consistent with their functions as chemoattractants for the recruitment of neutrophils from the intestinal vasculature or lamina propria to the intestinal epithelial vicinity. In addition, neutrophils can transmigrate across the epithelium and reach the intestinal lumen (Fig. 3.3), a feature observed in patients with ulcerative colitis (see Chapter 1). Basolateral release of neutrophil chemokines is not likely to play a role in this process, as no effective chemokine gradients would exist to support transmigration. However, a neutrophil chemotactic factor is apically released from polarized epithelial cells in response to apical infection with *Salmonella*.[42] In addition to neutrophil chemoattractants, microbial infection of intestinal epithelial cells can upregulate the production of CC chemokines that act as macrophage/monocyte chemoattractants, including CCL2/MCP-1 and RANTES.[38,43,44]

### Chemokines for T cells

In addition to signaling neutrophils and macrophages, as examples of host cell types that are essential for mediating mucosal innate defense, epithelial cells produce mediators important for chemoattracting subpopulations of T cells into the intestinal mucosa which mediate mucosal adaptive immunity. CXCL9 (Mig), CXCL10 (IP-10) and CXCL11 (I-TAC) are CXC chemokines that lack the ELR motif and whose expression is upregulated by IFN-γ.[45] They function as chemoattractants for CXCR3-expressing CD4 T cells that produce IFN-γ, which mediates host resistance to a broad array of microbial pathogens.[46,47] CXCL9, 10 and 11 are expressed constitutively at low levels by normal human colon epithelium, and their cognate receptor, CXCR3, is expressed on mucosal mononuclear cells,[20] including intraepithelial lymphocytes.[14] As in other cell types, mRNA expression and secretion of CXCL9, 10 and 11 are upregulated in response to stimulation of intestinal epithelial cells with IFN-γ.[20] Whereas infection of these cells with enteroinvasive bacteria or proinflammatory cytokines minimally affects epithelial cell CXCL9, 10 or 11 production, if at all, microbial infection or proinflammatory cytokines strongly potentiate IFN-γ-induced production of CXCL10 and, to a lesser extent, that of CXCL11.[20] These findings suggest that IFN-γ-inducible CXC chemokines produced by intestinal epithelial cells may function as chemoattractants for intraepithelial and lamina propria CXCR3-expressing T cells, which may be particularly important under conditions that activate mucosal inflammation, most notably during enteric microbial infection.

The normal intestinal mucosa contains predominantly CD4 T-cell populations that produce a Th1 pattern of cytokines. None the less, it also contains a smaller subset of T lymphocytes that produce Th2 cytokines. Intestinal epithelial cells produce CCL22/MDC, a chemokine known to chemoattract Th2 cytokine-producing CD4 T cells that express the chemokine receptor CCR4.[48] Epithelial cells in healthy human colons and

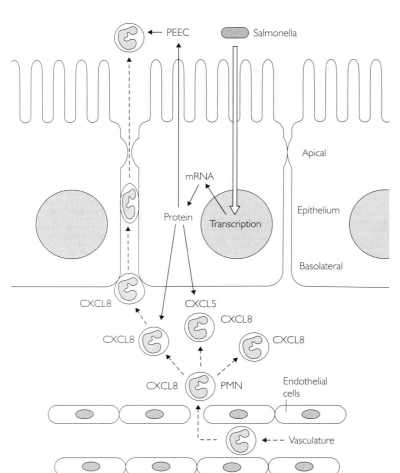

**Fig. 3.3** Model of the role of the intestinal epithelium in directing PMN migration into the mucosa in response to infection with enteric pathogens. Attachment and invasion of the invasive enteric bacteria *Salmonella* transmit signals into the nucleus of intestinal epithelial cells that induce increased transcription of an array of chemoattractant proteins. As a consequence, mRNA expression and protein secretion increase for the PMN chemoattractants CXCL8/IL-8, CXCL5/ENA-78, and pathogen-elicited epithelial chemoattractant, PEEC. CXCL8 and CXCL5 are mostly secreted from the basolateral side of the epithelium, whereas PEEC is secreted apically. Production of CXCL8 and PEEC is rapid after bacterial infection, whereas that of CXCL5 is delayed. A gradient of CXCL8 forms that promotes extravasation of PMN from the vasculature into the mucosa and, together with CXCL5, subsequent migration towards the epithelium. Epithelial cell-derived CXCL8 can bind to the extracellular matrix, including the basal membrane (BM) underneath the cells, which stabilizes the chemotactic gradient. Once PMN have reached the epithelium, a gradient of PEEC can induce their transmigration across the intercellular junctions of the epithelium into the intestinal lumen.

intestinal xenografts constitutively produce CCL22.[48] Moreover, CCL22 mRNA levels and CCL22 protein secretion are upregulated in colon epithelial cell lines infected with enteroinvasive bacteria or stimulated with proinflammatory cytokines.[48] Whereas IFN-γ synergizes with TNF to upregulate CCL22 production, the Th2 cytokines IL-4 and IL-13 downregulate TNF-induced CCL22 production. CCL22 produced by intestinal epithelial cells is basolaterally secreted and manifests functional activity with respect to chemoattracting CCR4-expressing T cells, as shown in studies using polarized model intestinal epithelium.[48] Intestinal epithelial cells do not produce another chemokine, CCL17/TARC, which acts on the same receptor. However, studies using cultured human airway epithelial cells and human fetal lung xenografts demonstrated that CCL17/TARC, but not CCL22/MDC, is abundantly expressed and regulated by human bronchial epithelial cells.[49] Although both CCL22/MDC and CCL17/TARC function as NFκB-responsive genes[48,49] and act on the same receptor, these chemokines are differentially expressed by intestinal compared to bronchial epithelium, suggesting they may have different functional roles in defense of the intestine and airways.

## Chemokines for dendritic cells

Dendritic cells (DC) play a key role in linking innate and adaptive immunity through their role in antigen uptake and presentation to T lymphocytes.[50] The interactions of DC with intestinal epithelial cells may have a central role in activating host innate immune defense and the later signaling of adaptive

immune responses to enteric microbial pathogens. The CC chemokine CCL20 (also termed MIP-3α or LARC) is chemotactic for immature DC[51] that express the receptor CCR6, which is the cognate chemokine receptor for CCL20.[52] CCL20 production is markedly upregulated in human intestinal epithelial cell lines in response to infection with invasive enteric bacteria or stimulation with the proinflammatory mediators IL-1 or TNF.[11] Moreover, CCL20 is basolaterally secreted from polarized intestinal epithelium infected with bacterial enteric pathogens or stimulated with proinflammatory cytokines.[11] Increased epithelial CCL20 expression is also observed in human intestinal xenografts stimulated with proinflammatory mediators and inflamed human intestinal mucosa, suggesting that CCL20 produced by intestinal epithelial cells may chemoattract immature DC into the inflamed or infected intestinal mucosa.[11]

DC recruited by epithelial cell-derived CCL20 in response to microbial infection may be involved in bacterial uptake across the intestinal epithelium, as DC can send their dendrites through epithelial tight junctions to sample luminal bacteria.[13,53] During this process, the integrity of the epithelial barrier is preserved because DC express tight junction proteins, such as occludin, claudin 1 and junctional adhesion molecule (JAM), and can establish tight junction-like structures with neighboring epithelial cells. Following bacterial uptake the dendrites recede and the tight junction is reformed by interactions between adjacent epithelial cells.[13,53] These studies offer a mechanism by which DC–epithelial cell interactions can link the mucosal innate and adaptive immune responses.

## PRODUCTION OF OTHER CYTOKINES

In addition to chemoattractant cytokines, intestinal epithelial cells express a range of other cytokines when infected with enteric bacteria. Inflammatory cytokines are the most prominent in this group. For example, *Salmonella* infection of cultured intestinal epithelial cells induces increased expression and secretion of TNF, which in turn can induce expression of a plethora of other chemoattractant and proinflammatory cytokines, including TNF itself.[37] Thus, TNF can amplify epithelial proinflammatory responses to bacterial infection. Intestinal epithelial cells also express IL-1α at low levels, which can be released upon cell lysis after contact with certain microbial pathogens, such as *Entamoeba histolytica*.[54] The proform of IL-1α, unlike that of IL-1β, does not require cleavage by cellular proteases for biological activity, so its release from epithelial cells can serve as a warning system to activate adjacent cells in response to microbially induced cell lysis. The actions of IL-1 can be counterregulated by IL-1 receptor antagonist (IL-1Ra), which is also expressed by intestinal epithelial cells.[55] Epithelial expression of the secretory type I isoform of IL-1Ra is upregulated in patients with Crohn's disease, and after stimulation of cultured cells with PMA and IL-1.[55] Transgenic overexpression of IL-1Ra I inhibits IL-1-induced IL-8 secretion in epithelial cells, suggesting that the balance of epithelial IL-1 and IL-1Ra expression determines the magnitude of mucosal effects induced by epithelial cell-derived IL-1.[55]

Several of the chemokines (e.g. IL-8, GROα) released by intestinal epithelial cells are chemotactic for neutrophils. In addition, epithelial cells infected with invasive enteric bacteria secrete GM-CSF and G-CSF, which induce activation, proliferation, and prolonged survival of neutrophils.[1,37] Thus, signals derived from the intestinal epithelium can not only attract neutrophils, but also sustain and activate them once they have migrated to subepithelial regions.

Although activated intestinal epithelial cells produce a large number of cytokines, the repertoire of these cells is limited. For example, cultured human intestinal epithelial cells do not express mRNA for IFN-γ, IL-2, IL-3 IL-4, IL-5, or IL-12p40.[37] In other cases, the cells express mRNA for some cytokines, such as IL-15 and IL-18, but so far no stimulation conditions have been identified under which the corresponding proteins appear to be secreted by the cells.[56,57] Despite the many functional differences between these cytokines, a common feature is that many of them have a role in regulating antigen-specific immune responses. For example, IL-12p40, IL-18 and IFN-γ are important for initiating Th1-type T-cell responses, whereas IL-4 and IL-5 regulate Th2-type T-cell functions. Therefore, the failure of epithelial cells to express these cytokines, combined with their capacity to secrete multiple cytokines with chemotactic functions for diverse leukocyte populations, suggest that these cells function primarily as initiators of inflammatory and immune responses, rather than sustaining antigen-specific responses.

## PRODUCTION OF OTHER INFLAMMATORY MEDIATORS

Intestinal epithelial cells stimulated by enteric microbes produce a range of products and inflammatory mediators other than cytokines. These mediators not only have immunoregulatory functions but also contribute to other pathophysiologic mani-

festations of infections with enteric pathogens. For example, interactions between microbial pathogens and intestinal epithelial cells may play a role in the early onset of diarrhea after infection with enteric pathogens such as *Salmonella*. Increased intestinal fluid secretion is an important host innate defense mechanism which, when coupled with increased intestinal motility, 'flushes' the pathogen from the intestinal tract. Concurrently, this allows the enteric pathogen to escape the host and infect additional hosts. Infection of intestinal epithelial cells with *Salmonella* results in increased epithelial cell chloride secretion, a parameter that reflects increased epithelial cell fluid secretion. One pathway leading to increased chloride secretion is upregulated expression of cyclooxygenase (COX)-2 and increased production of prostaglandin (PG) $E_2$ in intestinal epithelial cells infected in vitro and in vivo with *Salmonella* (Fig. 3.4) or *C. parvum*. [19,58] $PGE_2$ released by intestinal epithelial cells in response to infection acts in an autocrine/paracrine manner and activates epithelial chloride secretion, a process that occurs via a cAMP-mediated pathway.[19] In addition to inducing epithelial secretory responses, epithelial cell-derived $PGE_2$ might also play a role in maintaining the integrity of the epithelium under inflammatory conditions. Recent studies with an

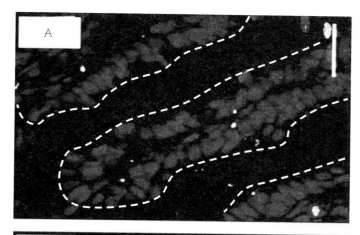

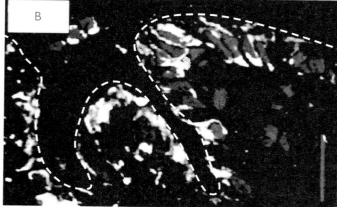

**Fig. 3.4** Induction of COX-2 expression in epithelial cells in response to *Salmonella* infection of human intestinal xenografts. Mature human fetal intestinal xenografts in SCID mice were infected luminally for 6 hours with an invasive *Salmonella* strain (B). Uninfected xenografts were used as a control (A). Frozen sections were prepared and stained by indirect immunofluorescence for COX-2. The luminal side of the epithelium is marked by dashed white lines. The scale bars represent 10 μm.

experimental colitis model have shown that mice lacking one of the PGE$_2$ receptors, EP4, which is predominantly expressed by intestinal epithelial cells,[59] have more severe inflammation and epithelial destruction.[60]

Bacterial infection of human colon epithelial cells rapidly upregulates the expression of inducible nitric oxide synthase (iNOS) and nitric oxide (NO) production.[61,62] This suggests that NO and/or its redox products are an important component of the intestinal epithelial cell response to microbial infection. In addition to epithelial invasive pathogens, NO may also mediate epithelial innate responses to minimally invasive and non-invasive pathogens, as demonstrated by interactions between NO produced by human intestinal epithelial cells and the non-invasive protozoan pathogen *Giardia lamblia*.[63] NO is cytostatic for *G. lamblia* and inhibits giardial differentiation. However, *G. lamblia* is not a passive target for host-produced NO. Rather, *G. lamblia* has strategies to evade this potential innate host defense.[63] Thus, in vitro, *G. lamblia* inhibited epithelial NO production by consuming arginine, the crucial substrate used by epithelial cell NO synthase to produce NO.[63] It will be important to determine whether such mechanisms, either alone or in concert with other innate host defense mechanisms, play a role in host defense to these enteric pathogens in vivo.

## EXPRESSION OF ANTIMICROBIAL PEPTIDES

Antimicrobial peptides and proteins are highly conserved in evolution and have an important role in intestinal epithelial cell innate defense. The defensins are one major class of antimicrobial peptides produced by human gastrointestinal epithelium.[64–66] Human defensins are divided into two major families, α and β, both of which have three disulfide bonds and a β-sheet structure. α-Defensins are produced by specialized cells, the Paneth cells, in the small intestinal crypts and consist of two members, human defensin (HD)5 and HD6.[67] In contrast, the β-defensins are ubiquitously expressed throughout the epithelium in the stomach, small intestine and colon. Although there are several reported subfamilies of β-defensins,[68,69] most currently available information regarding gastrointestinal epithelium relates to human β-defensin (hBD)-1 and hBD2.[70–73] hBD1 is constitutively expressed in the stomach, small intestine and colon, and not upregulated by proinflammatory stimuli or microbial infection, as shown in intestinal epithelial cell lines, human intestinal xenografts and human gastrointestinal tissue.[70] In marked contrast, hBD2 is minimally expressed in the epithelium of normal gastrointestinal mucosa,[70] but is upregulated through NFκB in response to infection with enteric pathogens or stimulation with proinflammatory mediators such as IL-1.[70,71]

The cathelicidins are another class of antimicrobial peptides in which a cathelin domain is linked to a peptide that has antimicrobial activity.[74] The only known cathelicidin in humans is LL-37/hCAP18. LL-37, the carboxy-terminal part of the molecule that is cleaved and has antimicrobial activity, has a linear amphipathic α-helical structure. In addition to its antimicrobial activity, LL-37 binds bacterial lipopolysaccharide (LPS) and has chemotactic activity for monocytes, neutrophils and T cells.[75,76] LL-37/hCAP18 has a restricted distribution in the human gastrointestinal tract, being expressed by the more differentiated surface and upper crypt epithelial cells in the human colon, with little or no expression within the deeper colon crypts, or within epithelial cells of the small intestine.[77] Studies using cell lines, human intestinal xenografts and human colon tissue have shown that LL-37 is constitutively produced by colon epithelium, and

that expression does not require a commensal microflora.[77] Moreover, epithelial cell LL-37 expression was not upregulated by several proinflammatory or other cytokines, including TNF, IL-1, IFN-γ, IL-6 or LPS in vitro, and was similar in both healthy and inflamed human colon.[77] None the less, studies using cell lines suggest that LL-37/hCAP18 may be modestly upregulated in intestinal epithelial cells infected with *Salmonella* or entero-invasive *Escherichia coli*.[77] Based on the above studies, a paradigm is emerging wherein the distribution and regulation of a variety of antimicrobial peptides differs in the epithelium in various regions of the human gastrointestinal tract, suggesting that the various antimicrobial peptides have distinct functional niches in mucosal innate defense.

## CENTRAL ROLE OF NFκB IN MEDIATING EPITHELIAL CELL RESPONSES TO MICROBIAL EXPOSURE

Many of the genes induced in intestinal epithelial cells after infection with invasive enteric bacteria are target genes of NFκB. Dimers of this transcription factor are held in the cytoplasm through interactions with specific inhibitors, the IκBs, which mask the nuclear localization domains of the NFκB proteins.[78] In response to microbes and their products or TNF and IL-1, IκBs are phosphorylated, which triggers their polyubiquitination and proteasomal degradation.[79,80] The inducible phosphorylation of IκBs is mediated by the IκB kinase (IKK) complex, which contains two catalytic subunits, IKKα and IKKβ. Most signal-induced phosphorylation of the IκBs relevant to activation of innate defense mechanisms is mediated by IKKβ,[81] which activates p50:RelA(p65) heterodimers in response to enteric microbes, their products, IL-1, and TNF.[82–86]

Activation of NFκB signaling via IKKβ has two major physiological functions: activation of genes whose products are important for mediating innate immune defense and inflammation,[78,87] and activation of genes whose products are important for the suppression of apoptosis.[88] Thus, many of the genes that encode cytokines, chemokines and adhesion molecules produced by intestinal epithelial cells and involved in innate defense and inflammatory reactions contain NFκB-binding sites in their promoters (e.g. CXCL8, CXCL1, CCL2, CCL20, CCL22, ICAM-1, TNF, hBD-2).[11,48,70,71,78,82] These genes, and genes that encode enzymes that produce secondary inflammatory mediators, such as NOS2 and COX-2, which also contain NFκB-binding sites in their promoters, are induced in intestinal epithelium during the course of microbial infection and mucosal inflammatory responses.[19,61,89]

NFκB is a central regulator of intestinal epithelial cell responses to infection with invasive and non-invasive pathogenic enteric bacteria.[82,90] Enteric bacterial pathogens use different strategies and mechanisms to interact with or invade intestinal epithelial cells. None the less, each of these microbes activates NFκB and NFκB target genes that are essential for epithelial innate defense responses.[82,90,91] In this way, the diverse signals activated by enteric bacterial pathogens are integrated by a common signaling pathway that culminates in the expression of a conserved set of proinflammatory genes in infected host cells. Although NFκB is important for activation of host innate defense, other signal transduction pathways are also involved, most notably MAP kinase pathways.[92–96]

A newly described pathway for the activation of NFκB employs intracellular NOD or CARD proteins, which have structural homology to apoptosis regulators and a class of plant disease-resistance gene products.[97–99] At least one of the NOD proteins (NOD1), which was thought initially to bind bacterial LPS[97,100] but now appears to interact intracellularly with bacterial peptidoglycan, activates IKK and NFκB by a pathway independent of TLR receptors. This provides a possible pathway by which bacterial products from intracellular microbes can activate NFκB, its target genes and innate epithelial cell defense mechanisms.[97,100]

## IMPORTANCE OF PATHOGEN-ASSOCIATED MOLECULAR PATTERNS (PAMP) AND THEIR RECEPTORS IN THE INTERACTIONS OF INTESTINAL EPITHELIAL CELLS AND ENTERIC BACTERIA

Invasive and non-invasive enteric bacteria can activate epithelial cell signaling cascades that are essential for the development of innate host defense (see Chapter 10). This involves a number of complex evolutionary co-evolved strategies on the part of the microbes and the host epithelial cells that are the targets of infection. PAMP associated with specific microbial products activate signaling pathways that are important for epithelial cell innate defense mechanisms. PAMP are highly conserved and characteristic of various microbes,[101] and include the bacterial cell wall components LPS, peptidoglycans and lipoteichoic acid (LTA), as well as bacterial flagellin, non-methylated bacterial DNA (also termed immunostimulatory DNA or ISS-DNA) and double-stranded (ds) RNA. PAMP are recognized by receptors called pattern-recognition receptors (PRR). PRR in turn activate host cellular signal transduction pathways that trigger innate defense mechanisms.[101,102]

Relevant to the activation of innate mucosal defense by intestinal epithelial cells, some of the members of one family of PRR, the Toll-like receptors (TLR),[102–104] are expressed by intestinal epithelial cells.[105–108] These include TLR2, which is involved in recognizing a broad range of PAMP, including peptidoglycans and bacterial lipoproteins from Gram-positive bacteria, mycobacterial cell wall components, atypical LPS from certain Gram-negative bacteria, and yeast cell wall components.[109–111] In contrast, TLR4 is mostly involved in the recognition of LPS.[112,113] TLR3, which is also expressed by intestinal epithelial cell lines, mediates responses to dsRNA.[114] The TLR family also includes TLR5, which is involved in the recognition of bacterial flagellin[115] and which is emerging as important for microbial–epithelial cell interactions, as well as TLR9 which mediates responses to non-methylated, CpG-containing bacterial DNA.[116]

Signaling through TLR activates genes whose products play a key role in further activating or mediating innate defense mechanisms. TLR signaling leads to activation of NFκB and MAP kinases.[102] All TLR appear to use a 'shared' signaling mechanism, based on recruitment of the MyD88 adaptor protein, the protein kinase IRAK[117–119] and TRAF6[120] with downstream activation of NFκB and the MAPK cascades. In addition, there may also be TLR receptor-specific signaling mechanisms that account for receptor-specific biological responses.[102,117,121–125] Thus far, the consequences of cellular activation through TLR for innate immunity has been studied most extensively in non-epithelial cell types (e.g. macrophages and DC), but emerging evidence suggests that the engagement of TLR expressed by intestinal epithelial cells (e.g. TLR4 by LPS and TLR5 by bacterial flagellin) may also play a key functional role in epithelial cell signaling of innate immune defense.[95,96,126–130]

PAMP such as bacterial LPS and unmethylated bacterial DNA are not unique to enteric pathogens and are also present in commensal microorganisms that populate the gastrointestinal tract. A key question is why does the host tolerate the presence of commensal microbes yet activate an innate immune and inflammatory responses to enteric pathogens? This apparent paradox may be explained by a combination of bacterial and host factors. On the bacterial side, pathogens, through their virulence factors, can often occupy niches within the host that are not typically accessible to commensals. Expression of PRR in those sites allows the host to sense the presence of bacterial pathogens. On the other hand, the host may not express functional PRR in locations where commensals are usually present. For example, intestinal epithelial cells, which are in permanent apical contact with luminal commensals, may not express certain TLR on the apical surface, or may not effectively signal through those receptors (e.g. some intestinal epithelial cell lines do not appear to express CD14 or MD2, important for signaling through TLR4).[131] However, bacterial products that enter the host epithelial cell consequent upon invasion by a pathogen have the potential to activate epithelial cell signaling pathways, as demonstrated by the activation of the NFκB pathway through NOD1.[97,100] The site of cellular expression of certain TLR may favor interactions with membrane-adherent or invasive pathogens, as has been suggested for TLR5.[107] Further, mechanisms that maintain the integrity and barrier functions of epithelial surfaces probably modulate the host's ability to discriminate between commensal and pathogenic microorganisms, with pathogenic microbes having strategies to breach this barrier and better activate PRR on underlying cells important for innate host defense. Interactions with adjacent T cells attenuate epithelial cell responses to apical commensal bacteria.[96] It is also possible that exposure to microbial products such as LPS or unmethylated DNA associated with commensal bacteria may activate different signaling pathways from the ones activated by enteric pathogens, and lead to the induction of different gene programs.

## APOPTOSIS OF INTESTINAL EPITHELIAL CELLS IN RESPONSE TO ENTERIC MICROBES

The intestinal epithelium normally forms a tight physical barrier between myriad microorganisms residing in the intestinal lumen and host immune and inflammatory cells in the mucosa. This barrier is not static but undergoes constant high turnover. Epithelial cells in the crypts proliferate and migrate up the small intestinal villi or towards the surface in the colon, where they undergo apoptosis and are shed into the lumen or taken up by subepithelial macrophages. This remarkably efficient and 'silent' process has no effect on barrier function or the induction of inflammatory responses under normal conditions.

Interactions with many enteric microbial pathogens can disturb the physiologic balance of proliferation and apoptosis, leading to the death of intestinal epithelial and other cells.[132] For example, the invasive enteric pathogens Salmonella and entero-invasive E. coli induce apoptosis of human intestinal epithelial cells.[133] Apoptosis of human intestinal epithelial cell lines infected by Salmonella is delayed for 18–24 hours and is accompanied by a loss of F-actin and activation of caspase 3. Bacterial products related to the activity of the *Salmonella* virulence genes *spv* and SPI-2, produced during the initial phase of intracellular infection, have a key role in the delayed execution phase of apoptosis in intestinal epithelial cell lines.[134]

Apoptosis of intestinal epithelial cells in response to bacterial infection may have a protective function by deleting infected and damaged epithelial cells and restoring epithelial cell growth regulation and epithelial integrity, which are altered during enteric infection. Delayed onset of epithelial cell apoptosis after bacterial invasion may be important to both the host and the invading pathogen. This delay provides sufficient time for host epithelial cells to generate signals important for the activation of mucosal innate and downstream acquired immune defense systems, but concurrently allows invading bacteria time to adapt to the intracellular host environment before invading deeper mucosal layers. A similar theme has emerged from studies of C. *parvum* infection of epithelial cells. C. *parvum* activates NFκB in intestinal and biliary epithelial cells,[135] which stimulates innate defense mechanisms such as production of the neutrophil chemoattractant CXCL8 and mucosal influx of neutrophils.[10] The latter prevents dissemination of the pathogen at the cost of increased mucosal damage and altered barrier function. On the other hand, NFκB has antiapoptotic functions, and delayed epithelial cell apoptosis allows sufficient time for this pathogen to undergo development and lifecycle changes essential for its replication and survival.[136,137]

In contrast to microbially induced epithelial cell apoptosis, little evidence exists that enteric microbes can directly affect epithelial cell proliferation. However, compensatory increases in proliferation typically occur in response to excessive loss of epithelium. For example, differentiated epithelial cells at the villus tips express the antiproliferative cytokine TGF-β.[138] Loss of these cells by microbially induced apoptosis would release crypt epithelial cells from a negative regulator of proliferation, thereby promoting increased growth. In addition, factors released by immune and inflammatory cells recruited to the inflamed mucosa contribute to altered proliferation and apoptosis in the intestinal epithelium. For example, TNF released by macrophages in response to LPS stimulation induces apoptosis in epithelial cells.[133]

# BACTERIAL PRODUCTS THAT ALTER EPITHELIAL CELL FUNCTIONS

The initial interactions between different enteric microbes and intestinal epithelium typically show unique features for a given microbe. This reflects the specific bacterial genes involved in the interactions and the cellular responses. Owing to the diversity of physiologically relevant enteric bacteria and their interactions with the epithelium, common themes in these interactions are emphasized and illustrated with specific examples. Most of these are taken from enteric bacterial pathogens, as they often possess distinct virulence strategies that exploit host cell functions for specific bacterial purposes. It should be noted, however, that these underlying principles can be employed to investigate and understand interactions between host epithelium and a wide range of enteric bacteria, including those with little apparent pathogenic potential.

# CLASSIC BACTERIAL TOXINS

All enteric bacteria release multiple low- and high-molecular weight products at various growth phases. Some of these are byproducts of bacterial metabolism and have little effect on the host, although they may influence other bacteria in the intestinal tract. Others have specific activities on the host, often causing intestinal or systemic disease. Classic toxins are one of the best-characterized groups of bacterial virulence factors.

## Cholera toxin and *E. coli* heat-labile toxin

Infections with *Vibrio cholerae* and enterotoxigenic *E. coli* (ETEC) are among the leading causes of diarrheal disease worldwide. Both pathogens have little capacity to invade the intestinal mucosa. Intestinal disease is caused mainly by the release of classic toxins that act on the intestinal epithelium. *V. cholerae* produces cholera toxin (CT), and ETEC secretes at least two toxins, heat-labile toxin (LT) and heat-stable toxin.[139] Both CT and LT are AB holotoxins composed of a single A subunit and five B subunits. The B subunits bind to the cell surface of epithelial cells, whereas the A subunit enters the cells and exerts enzymatic activity. CT and LT are taken up by apical endocytosis and subsequently follow a retrograde trafficking pathway through the Golgi cisternae to the endoplasmic reticulum, after which they enter the cytoplasm and bind to a G protein, Gαs, at the cell membrane.[140] Both toxins ADP-ribosylate Gαs, which activates epithelial adenylyl cyclases, leading to increased cAMP production, activation of protein kinase A and epithelial ion transporters such as the CFTR, and diarrhea. LT alone is not specific for Gαs, but requires a host cell-derived cofactor, ADP-ribosylation factor (ARF), to exert strong specificity,[141] which provides an example for coopting of a cellular protein for specific bacterial purposes.

## *Clostridium difficile* toxins

C. *difficile*, anaerobic Gram-positive spore-forming bacilli, are the leading cause of hospital-acquired diarrhea and colitis. Infection typically occurs during antibiotic treatment, which suppresses the normal intestinal microbiota and thereby diminishes normal colonization resistance against C. *difficile*.[142] Once established in the intestinal lumen, C. *difficile*, like *V. cholerae* and ETEC, causes disease through the release of two classic toxins, A and B.[143] Most strains of disease-causing C. *difficile* produce both toxins, although a small percentage produce only toxin B. Both toxins are high molecular weight (~300 kDa) proteins. Toxin A, also termed enterotoxin, induces fluid secretion, increased mucosal permeability and inflammation in animal models, whereas toxin B is a potent cytotoxin in cultured cells but has little enterotoxic activity in vivo.[143,144] Both toxins enter epithelial cells by receptor-mediated endocytosis and pass through an acidic intracellular compartment before acting on their cellular targets. They glycosylate and thereby inactivate the small GTP-binding proteins rhoA, rac and cdc42, which regulate and maintain the actin cytoskeleton.[142,143] As a consequence, protein synthesis ceases and intoxicated cells die by apoptosis. In addition, toxin A stimulates several MAP kinase pathways, including ERK, p38 and JNK, in monocytes, which precedes significant glycosylation of GTP-binding proteins.[145] In particular, activation of p38 is critical for induction of the NFκB-dependent increase in expression of proinflammatory and chemotactic cytokines in these cells.[145] Toxin A also targets mitochondria in epithelial cells, resulting in the release of reactive oxidant intermediates and subsequent activation of NFκB and chemotactic cytokine production.[146] These observations demonstrate that C. *difficile* toxins have different activities and targets in intestinal epithelial cells, thus representing an example of a bacterial virulence factor with multiple interactions with the host epithelium, rather than a single molecular target as seen for CT and LT.

## Shiga toxins

*Shigella dysenteriae* and enterohemorrhagic *E. coli* (EHEC) are important causes of foodborne outbreaks of diarrhea and enterocolitis, which can be complicated by the hemolytic uremic syndrome with a high mortality. Both pathogens produce Shiga toxins (Stx), which play a central role in disease pathogenesis.[147,148] S. *dysenteriae* produce a single chromosomally encoded toxin, Stx1, whereas EHEC typically produce two antigenically distinct toxins, Stx1 and Stx2 (of which several variants exist), whose genes are located on a toxin-converting lambdoid phage. All Stx types are holotoxins with one A subunit and five B subunits, analogous to the structures of CT and LT. Upon secretion by the bacteria, Stx binds via its B subunits to the glycolipids, globotriaosyl ceramide (Gb3) for Stx1 and most variants of Stx2 and globotetraosyl ceramide (Gb4) for Stx2e. Gb3 and/or Gb4 are present on toxin-sensitive cells such as endothelial cells, and ileal villus epithelial cells in the small intestine of rabbits.[148] Interestingly, some human intestinal epithelial cell lines lack Gb3 and Gb4, yet take up Stx,[149] indicating that alternative pathways exist which allow toxin binding and uptake in the absence of Gb3 or Gb4. During passage through the Golgi network and/or early endosomes, the enzymatically active A subunit is released from Stx holotoxin through protease-mediated cleavage.[150,151] The active A subunit cleaves an N-glycosidic bond in the 28S ribosomal RNA which blocks aminoacyl-tRNA binding to the acceptor site on the 60S ribosomal subunit and hence protein synthesis. Complete inhibition of protein synthesis leads to cell death, yet partial inhibition owing to lower Stx concentrations activates the expression of proinflammatory genes in epithelial cells.[152] Thus, Stx provides an example of a classic bacterial toxin exerting global effects on intestinal epithelial cell function, spanning the spectrum from induction of proinflammatory genes to cell death.

## OTHER BACTERIAL VIRULENCE FACTORS

Whereas classic bacterial toxins are released by the microbes and diffuse through the extracellular space within the host before they act on their targets, many other bacterial virulence factors are delivered more directly to target cells. This can be in the form of factors expressed on the surface of bacteria that attach to host cells, or as factors directly released into host cells upon bacterial attachment or uptake. These modes of delivery are host cell selective and highly effective for the bacteria, as they limit the actions of specific virulence factors to the host cell interacting with a given bacterial cell. Such actions are very specific for each factor and bacterial species, although they generally promote the establishment of a microbial niche within the host and the avoidance of detection and/or destruction of bacteria by host immune defenses. A large and diverse number of bacterial virulence factors belong in this group. For this reason, the following discussion has been divided into broad functional categories based on the cellular events affected by specific virulence factors. This categorization tends to underestimate the true complexity of the cellular events affected by specific bacterial virulence factors, as they commonly affect multiple signaling pathways and cell functions.

## Factors involved in bacterial invasion into intestinal epithelial cells

Commensal bacteria of the intestinal tract reside in the intestinal lumen and have little capacity to penetrate the epithelial barrier that separates the lumen from the lamina propria and prevents access to the circulation and systemic spread. This relative inability to invade epithelial cells is an important and characteristic feature of commensals, and reflects a lack of specialized bacterial genes needed to engage the host epithelium in crosstalk leading to attachment and uptake. In contrast, many enteric bacterial pathogens have strategies to invade and pass through the intestinal epithelium, which allows them to establish infection in the intestinal lamina propria, and potentially to spread to other sites. Despite the conserved ability to enter intestinal epithelial cells, different invasive bacteria show remarkably diverse strategies to accomplish this task, ranging from actions of single bacterial proteins to highly orchestrated events involving dozens of bacterial genes. Examples of the former include virulence factors from *Yersinia* and *Listeria*, and the latter is exemplified by invasion genes in *Salmonella*.

### *Yersinia* invasin

*Yersinia* are foodborne Gram-negative bacterial pathogens that cause a spectrum of diseases, ranging from bubonic plaque (*Y. pestis*) to limited gastroenteritis (*Y. pseudotuberculosis*, *Y. enterocolitica*). Upon ingestion, they adhere to and are taken up by intestinal epithelial cells, particularly M cells, in the small intestine. This process is initiated and mediated by a bacterial attachment factor, termed invasin, which is expressed on the surface of *Yersinia*. Invasin is necessary and sufficient to mediate bacterial uptake into epithelial cells, as *Yersinia* lacking this protein cannot invade epithelial cells and normally non-invasive *E. coli* engineered to express invasin become fully invasive.[153] Furthermore, coating of inert latex beads with invasin is sufficient to facilitate their phagocytic uptake into epithelial cells.[154] The epithelial receptors for invasin are integrins, which are heterodimeric surface proteins involved in cell adhesion to various substrates and other cells.[154] Invasin binds with high affinity to several different integrins, which share a common $\beta_1$ subunit. Integrins are normally expressed on the basolateral side of polarized enterocytes, suggesting that the cells are not readily infectible from the apical side where *Yersinia* reside initially after oral infection. However, some studies have suggested that integrins can be expressed in a limited region at epithelial tight junctions and are accessible from the apical side in those areas.[155] Contrary to enterocytes, M cells, specialized epithelial cells in the dome region of Peyer's patches, express integrins on the apical side.[156] This provides an explanation for the preferential invasion of these cells by *Yersinia*. Once invasin binds to integrin receptors on epithelial cells a cellular signaling cascade is activated, which culminates in actin reorganization and bacterial uptake into the cells. The details of this process are complex but involve tyrosine kinases (focal adhesion kinase), adaptor proteins (CAS), members of the Rho family of small GTPases

(Rac1, but not RhoA or CDC42), and actin-binding proteins (Arp 2/3, but not N-WASP).[157,158] These events are reminiscent of those involved in cell migration, suggesting that intimin-mediated bacterial uptake is an example for bacterial subversion of a physiologically occurring host cell function.

### Listeria internalins

The importance of single bacterial products for rendering bacteria invasive for epithelial cells is also documented by the invasion proteins internalin (Inl) A and B in *Listeria monocytogenes*. This foodborne pathogen can enter most mammalian cells, including intestinal epithelial cells. Invasion into the latter is mostly dependent on InlA, although InlB increases invasion efficiency.[28,159] For other cells, InlB alone is sufficient for invasion. InlA binds to E-cadherin, a cellular adhesion molecule specifically expressed by intestinal epithelial cells.[29,31] Two cellular receptors have been identified for InlB, gC1q-R,[160] which is the receptor for the globular part of the complement component C1q, and Met,[161] the receptor for hepatocyte growth/scatter factor. The former is ubiquitously expressed, whereas the latter is largely restricted to cells of the epithelial lineage. Binding of InlB to Met triggers a cascade of signaling events, including activation of PtdIns 3-kinase, Akt kinase, and the small G protein Ras, which leads to cytoskeletal rearrangements and bacterial uptake.[162] This process is accompanied by activation of NFκB, leading to increased expression of chemokines such as CXCL8. InlB alone is sufficient for activation of signaling, as InlB-coated latex beads exert the same functions as live *L. monocytogenes*.[163] The role of qC1q-R in mediating InlB functions is poorly understood at present, as this receptor lacks a transmembrane domain and an identifiable cytoplasmic region.

### Invasion genes in *Salmonella*

In contrast to *Yersinia* and *L. monocytogenes*, the invasive Gram-negative *Salmonella* employ a fairly large number of genes to achieve invasion into epithelial cells. The necessary genes are located in a chromosomal gene cluster, termed *Salmonella* pathogenicity island (SPI)1.[164] The cluster consists of at least 29 genes, which code for components of a type III secretion system, a 'molecular syringe' (also termed 'injectisome') required for the delivery of specific bacterial virulence into the host cell, and effector proteins and regulators.[165,166] Additional effector molecules coded outside the SPI1 gene cluster are also transported into the host cell by the SPI1 type III secretion system and required for invasion into epithelial cells. *Salmonella* entry into intestinal epithelial cells involves massive ruffling of the host cell membrane at the site of interaction with the bacteria and uptake into large vesicles resembling macropinosomes.[167] The underlying mechanism involves local rearrangement of the host cell actin cytoskeleton in response to different effector molecules encoded both within the SPI1 locus (e.g. SptP, SipA, SipB, SipC and SipD) and outside that locus (e.g. SopE). These effector proteins exert different functions inside host cells, which show a finely coordinated and synergistic activity for facilitating bacterial uptake into intestinal epithelial cells. For example, SptP is a phosphotyrosine phosphatase whose actions disrupt the actin cytoskeleton,[168] whereas SipA binds directly to actin in host cells and promotes its polymerization.[169] Deletion of specific SPI1 proteins abrogates *Salmonella* invasion into epithelial cells and thus attenuates virulence after oral infection.[164] The same mutants show no attenuation after systemic infection, which indicates that the functions of the virulence genes in the SPI1 locus are limited to translocation of *Salmonella* across the intestinal epithelial barrier.

## Factors that interfere with signaling events in intestinal epithelial and other host cells

Bacterial invasion into intestinal epithelial cells is one important pathogen strategy to occupy a new niche within the host not available to commensals. In addition, many bacterial pathogens have other virulence strategies that interfere with host functions important for antibacterial immune defense. Such disarming capabilities are typically directed against those effector cells, particularly monocytes/macrophages, that are needed for destruction of the pathogenic bacteria by the host. Intestinal epithelial cells are often not important effector cells directly involved in pathogen destruction, so that, in this context, the functional significance of bacterial interference with specific epithelial cell signaling pathways is not always apparent. None the less, studies in these cells have revealed interesting paradigms of host–microbe interactions in regard to interference with specific signaling pathways and cellular functions that may also apply to other cell types, and are probably important for understanding the pathogenesis of infections with a number of enteric pathogens. Two examples of such bacterial virulence factors are discussed here: SigD/SopB of *Salmonella*, and YopH of *Yersinia*.

### Salmonella *SigD/SopB*

Inositol polyphosphates (InsP$_i$) and phosphoinositides (PtdInsP$_i$) are important second messengers in mammalian cells that control a wide range of functions, ranging from cytoplasmic calcium levels to gene expression and DNA repair. Multiple forms of InsP$_i$ exist, of which some, such as InsP$_6$ and InsP$_5$, are present constitutively at high levels in intestinal epithelial cells, whereas others, such as different isomers of InsP$_4$ and InsP$_3$, are normally found at only low levels but are induced by various stimuli. Specific cellular kinases and phosphatases regulate the relative abundance of different InsP$_i$ under resting and stimulated conditions.[170] In addition, specific proteins of bacterial pathogens can exploit these pathways. For example, *Salmonella* produces a virulence protein, SigD/SopB, which has phosphatase activity for InsP$_i$ (Fig. 3.5). SigD is delivered into infected host cells via a bacterial type III secretion system and associates with the cell membrane.[171] Once inside cells, SigD dephosphorylates InsP$_5$ to a specific isomer of InsP$_4$, Ins(1,4,5,6)P$_4$, which promotes ion secretion in polarized epithelia[172,173] (Fig. 3.5). In addition, through its phosphatase activity SigD degrades the phosphoinositides PtdInsP$_3$ and PtdInsP$_2$, which normally activate the signaling kinase Akt and play a role in remodeling of the actin cytoskeleton.[174] These effects on cellular InsP$_i$ and PtdInsP$_i$ metabolism are physiologically important, because the deletion of SigD/SopB from *Salmonella* attenuates fluid secretion and mucosal inflammation upon infection in animal models.[175]

### Yersinia *YopH*

Another example of a bacterial virulence factor that interferes with specific cellular signaling pathways is the phosphatase YopH of *Yersinia*. YopH resembles structurally eukaryotic phosphatases and is one of the most powerful known phosphotyrosine phosphatases.[176] It is translocated into target cells (e.g. intestinal epithelial cells and macrophages) via a bacterially produced injectisome and dephosphorylates several cellular proteins, including p130cas, Fyb, and the scaffolding protein SKAP-

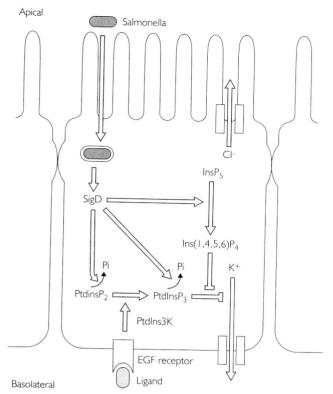

**Fig. 3.5** Model of *Salmonella* SigD effects on inositol phosphate metabolism and ion transport functions in intestinal epithelial cells. *Salmonella* enters polarized intestinal epithelial cells from the apical side and resides inside a vacuole. Intracellular bacteria release SigD, which associates with the cell membrane and dephosphorylates $PtdInsP_2$ and $PtdInsP_3$, which become inactive, and $InsP_5$, releasing $Ins(1,4,5,6)P_4$. The latter antagonizes the inhibitory effects of $PtdInsP_3$, formed by EGF receptor-activated PtdIns 3-kinase (PtdIns3K) from $PtdInsP_2$, on stimulated $K^+$ efflux from the basolateral side. Basolateral $K^+$ efflux in response to elevation of intracellular calcium levels is necessary for facilitating stimulated apical $Cl^-$ secretion, which is the key driving force for increased epithelial fluid secretion characteristic of secretory diarrhea. Thus, SigD can promote epithelial fluid secretion through the dual effects of degrading the inhibitory second messenger, $PtdInsP_3$, and of generating the stimulatory molecule $Ins(1,4,5,6)P_4$. Arrowheads depict stimulatory and capped lines inhibitory effects.

HOM, important for the formation of focal adhesions.[177] The latter are localized rearrangements of the cytoskeleton that mediate cellular attachment to substrates and uptake of particulates into cells. Phosphorylation of p130cas and other focal adhesion components is required for formation of focal adhesions, so that interference with this process by YopH blocks uptake of *Yersinia* into host cells.[177] This antiphagocytic action of YopH is particularly important for bacterial interaction with macrophages, as it prevents the uptake and hence intracellular destruction of the bacteria. Consequently, *Yersinia* resides mostly in extracellular locations within the host, despite its potent ability to invade cells via $\beta_1$ integrins (as discussed above).

## Factors affecting host cell integrity

The effects of most bacterial virulence factors directly delivered into the host cell are remarkably selective and do not compromise cell survival in general (in contrast to classic toxins, which often kill host cells). This may be related to the observation that

once bacteria have established the intimate association needed for delivery of such virulence factors, the bacteria depend, to some degree, on the host cell for continued survival. However, most bacterial enteric pathogens are not obligate intracellular pathogens, so that this dependence is relative and likely to be transient. Consequently, close interactions between intestinal epithelial cells and invasive bacteria can result in loss of host cell integrity and cell death, which is typically incidental to other events and often delayed.

This concept is illustrated by the *Salmonella* virulence gene SpvB. The gene coding for SpvB is located on a large plasmid (60–80 kb) found in many non-typhoid *Salmonella*. Bacteria carrying the plasmid are more virulent in animal models of infection and are more commonly present in *Salmonella* isolated from severe systemic than from localized intestinal infections in humans. The key plasmid virulence genes are located in the *spv* operon, which codes for one regulatory (SpvR) and four structural proteins (SpvABCD). SpvB is a mono(ADP-ribosyl)transferase that ADP-ribosylates actin in infected epithelial cells and macrophages.[178–180] This modification of actin interferes with its polymerization.[180] Consequently, in cells infected with SpvB expressing *Salmonella* or transfected with an SpvB expression vector, the actin cytoskeleton is destabilized and ultimately lost.[179,180] Specific point mutations that interfere with the enzymatic activity of SpvB and hence its ability to ADP-ribosylate actin, show attenuation in animal infection models comparable to that of plasmid-free *Salmonella*.[180] This indicates that the enzymatic activity of SpvB is the key virulence principle encoded on the *Salmonella* virulence plasmid. Although SpvB acts in both intestinal epithelial cells and macrophages, it is likely that its actions are more important pathogenetically in macrophages, as they would be expected to interfere with vesicle trafficking in these cells. Such interference would prevent the fusion of *Salmonella*-containing endosomes with lysosomes as an important step towards bacterial destruction inside the cells. None the less, disruption of the actin cytoskeleton in intestinal epithelial cells also has functional consequences, as it contributes to detachment and apoptotic death in these cells after *Salmonella* infection.[134]

# PHYSIOLOGIC IMPORTANCE OF INTERACTIONS BETWEEN INTESTINAL EPITHELIAL CELLS AND ENTERIC MICROBES

Substantial information is available regarding the repertoire of innate defense molecules produced by intestinal epithelial cells in vitro and in vivo, as the available model systems are well suited for such studies. None the less, the expression of a gene under specific circumstances is only a first step towards assigning relevance to the corresponding gene product, but is not sufficient for drawing conclusions regarding functional significance. For each gene product identified by expression studies, it is possible that it is produced at levels too low, or at the incorrect time, to significantly influence physiologic events. In addition, a given gene may be expressed in multiple cell types and at different times, which further complicates the analysis of the contribution of individual gene products in specific cell types to complex physiologic events in vivo. Such studies will ultimately require technologies to ablate the expression of specific genes in selected cell types under controlled in vivo conditions. The feasibility of this approach has been demonstrated by inducible cell lineage-specific knock-out mice using the Cre/loxP system (see above), but such studies are complex and have so far not been used to determine the role of intestinal epithelial cells in mediating host responses to enteric microbes.

Three studies provide examples suggesting that products made by intestinal epithelial cells in response to bacteria can control mucosal responses to infection. These studies took advantage of the observation that a specific secreted gene product appeared to be solely expressed in the epithelium, so that the consequences of systemic interference with that product suggested a role of the epithelium in the observed events. For example, studies of the role of CXCL8 in a rabbit model of intestinal invasion by *Shigella flexneri* showed that CXCL8, which is largely produced by intestinal epithelial cells in this model, acts as a major mediator in the recruitment of polymorphonuclear leukocytes (PMN) to the subepithelial area and in the transmigration of those cells through the epithelial lining.[181] Neutralization of CXCL8 in this model resulted in a decrease in the numbers of PMN entering the lamina propria and the epithelium, and decreased the severity of epithelial lesions in areas of bacterial invasion. However, concurrently there was increased transepithelial translocation of bacteria, as well as bacterial overgrowth in the lamina propria and increased passage of bacteria into the mesenteric blood. By mediating the eradication of bacteria at their epithelial entry site, although at the cost of severe epithelial destruction, intestinal epithelial cell-produced neutrophil chemoattractants appear to be important innate defense mechanisms to control bacterial translocation.[181]

In a second example, luminal infection of human intestinal xenografts with the invasive protozoan parasite *Entamoeba histolytica* is accompanied by mucosal infiltration with PMN and the increased expression of CXCL8 in intestinal epithelial but not other cells.[21] Blockade of the expression of CXCL8, a NFκB target gene, by injection of xenografts with an antisense oligonucleotide against the p65 subunit of NFκB, prevented PMN infiltration.[21] Although antisense p65 probably affected more than the epithelial expression of CXCL8 in this model, these data are consistent with a role of epithelium-derived mediators in controlling PMN influx into the intestinal mucosa.

Finally, a transgenic mouse model has been established in which the murine PMN chemoattractant MIP-2 is selectively overexpressed in intestinal epithelial cells.[182] The transgenic mice are characterized by increased numbers of PMN in the mucosa, as well as intraepithelial lymphocytes,[182] indicating that epithelium-derived chemokines modulate mucosal trafficking of leukocyte subpopulations.

## CONCLUSIONS

Intestinal epithelial cells actively interact with enteric commensal bacteria, pathogens and their products through membrane and cytoplasmic receptors (e.g. PRR), which results in the induction of a characteristic profile of NFκB and MAP kinase-dependent cytokines, chemokines and other proinflammatory molecules. This programmed response creates a chemotactic gradient for the entry of neutrophils, monocytes and T cells into the mucosa, which facilitate the clearance of invading pathogens and mediate dysregulated intestinal inflammation in genetically susceptible

hosts. Enteric pathogens have developed multiple strategies to evade epithelial innate defense mechanisms by exploiting and counteracting host cell signaling pathways. An improved understanding of the mechanisms governing bacterial–epithelial interactions will lead to better strategies to accelerate the clearance of enteric pathogens and restore mucosal homeostasis in idiopathic IBD.

## REFERENCES

1. Eckmann L, Smith JR, Housley MP et al. Analysis by high density cDNA arrays of altered gene expression in human intestinal epithelial cells in response to infection with the invasive enteric bacteria *Salmonella*. J Biol Chem 2000;275:14084–14094.
2. Kagnoff MF, Eckmann L. Analysis of host responses to microbial infection using gene expression profiling. Curr Opin Microbiol 2001;4:246–250.
3. Rosenberger CM, Pollard AJ, Finlay BB. Gene array technology to determine host responses to *Salmonella*. Microbes Infect 2001;3:1353–1360.
4. Bach S, Makristathis A, Rotter M et al. Gene expression profiling in AGS cells stimulated with *Helicobacter pylori* isogenic strains (cagA positive or cagA negative). Infect Immun 2002;70:988–992.
5. Pang G, Buret A, O'Loughlin E et al. Immunologic, functional, and morphological characterization of three new human small intestinal epithelial cell lines. Gastroenterology 1996;111:8–18.
6. Madara JL, Stafford J, Dharmsathaphorn K et al. Structural analysis of a human intestinal epithelial cell line. Gastroenterology 1987;92:1133–1145.
7. Peterson MD, Mooseker MS. Characterization of the enterocyte-like brush border cytoskeleton of the C2BBe clones of the human intestinal cell line, Caco-2. J Cell Sci 1992;102:581–600.
8. Kirkland SC. Dome formation by a human colonic adenocarcinoma cell line (HCA-7). Cancer Res 1985;45:3790–3795.
9. Eckmann L, Jung HC, Schurer-Maly C et al. Differential cytokine expression by human intestinal epithelial cell lines: regulated expression of interleukin 8. Gastroenterology 1993;105:1689–1697.
10. Laurent F, Eckmann L, Savidge TC et al. Cryptosporidium parvum infection of human intestinal epithelial cells induces the polarized secretion of C-X-C chemokines. Infect Immun 1997;65:5067–5073.
11. Izadpanah A, Dwinell MB, Eckmann L et al. Regulated MIP-3a/CCL20 production by human intestinal epithelium: mechanism for modulating mucosal immunity. Am J Physiol Gastrointest Liver Physiol 2001;280:G710–G719.
12. Maaser C, Eckmann L, Paesold G et al. Ubiquitous production of macrophage migration inhibitory factor by human gastric and intestinal epithelium. Gastroenterology 2002;122:667–680.
13. Rescigno M, Urbano M, Valzasina B et al. Dendritic cells express tight junction proteins and penetrate gut epithelial monolayers to sample bacteria. Nature Immunol 2001;2:361–367.
14. Shibahara T, Wilcox JN, Couse T et al. Characterization of epithelial chemoattractants for human intestinal intraepithelial lymphocytes. Gastroenterology 2001;120:60–70.
15. Savidge TC, Morey AL, Ferguson DJ et al. Human intestinal development in a severe-combined immunodeficient xenograft model. Differentiation 1995;58:361–371.
16. Shmakov AN, Morey AL, Ferguson DJ et al. Conventional patterns of human intestinal proliferation in a severe-combined immunodeficient xenograft model. Differentiation 1995;59:321–330.
17. Savidge TC, Lowe DC, Walker WA. Developmental regulation of intestinal epithelial hydrolase activity in human fetal jejunal xenografts maintained in severe-combined immunodeficient mice. Pediatr Res 2001;50:196–202.
18. Huang GT, Eckmann L, Savidge TC et al. Infection of human intestinal epithelial cells with invasive bacteria upregulates apical intercellular adhesion molecule-1 (ICAM)-1) expression and neutrophil adhesion. J Clin Invest 1996;98:572–583.
19. Eckmann L, Stenson WF, Savidge TC et al. Role of intestinal epithelial cells in the host secretory response to infection by invasive bacteria. Bacterial entry induces epithelial prostaglandin H synthase-2 expression and prostaglandin E2 and F2a production. J Clin Invest 1997;100:296–309.
20. Dwinell MB, Lugering N, Eckmann L et al. Regulated production of interferon-inducible T-cell chemoattractants by human intestinal epithelial cells. Gastroenterology 2001;120:49–59.
21. Seydel KB, Li E, Zhang Z et al. Epithelial cell-initiated inflammation plays a crucial role in early tissue damage in amebic infection of human intestine. Gastroenterology 1998;115:1446–1453.
22. Saam JR, Gordon JI. Inducible gene knockouts in the small intestinal and colonic epithelium. J Biol Chem 1999;274:38071–38082.
23. Brembeck FH, Moffett J, Wang TC et al. The keratin 19 promoter is potent for cell-specific targeting of genes in transgenic mice. Gastroenterology 2001;120:1720–1728.

24. Pinto D, Robine S, Jaisser F et al. Regulatory sequences of the mouse villin gene that efficiently drive transgenic expression in immature and differentiated epithelial cells of small and large intestines. J Biol Chem 1999;274:6476–6482.

25. No D, Yao TP, Evans RM. Ecdysone-inducible gene expression in mammalian cells and transgenic mice. Proc Natl Acad Sci USA 1996;93:3346–3351.

26. Shockett P, Difilippantonio M, Hellman N et al. A modified tetracycline-regulated system provides autoregulatory, inducible gene expression in cultured cells and transgenic mice. Proc Natl Acad Sci USA 1995;92:6522–6526.

27. Feil R, Brocard J, Mascrez B et al. Ligand-activated site-specific recombination in mice. Proc Natl Acad Sci USA 1996;93:10887–10890.

28. Gaillard JL, Berche P, Frehel C et al. Entry of L. monocytogenes into cells is mediated by internalin, a repeat protein reminiscent of surface antigens from Gram-positive cocci. Cell 1991;65:1127–1141.

29. Mengaud J, Ohayon H, Gounon P et al. E-cadherin is the receptor for internalin, a surface protein required for entry of L. monocytogenes into epithelial cells. Cell 1996;84:923–932.

30. Lecuit M, Dramsi S, Gottardi C et al. A single amino acid in E-cadherin responsible for host specificity towards the human pathogen Listeria monocytogenes. EMBO J 1999;18:3956–3963.

31. Lecuit M, Vandormael-Pournin S, Lefort J et al. A transgenic model for listeriosis: role of internalin in crossing the intestinal barrier. Science 2001;292:1722–1725.

32. Kagnoff MF, Eckmann L. Epithelial cells as sensors for microbial infection. J Clin Invest 1997;100:6–10.

33. Olson TS, Ley K. Chemokines and chemokine receptors in leukocyte trafficking. Am J Physiol Regul Integr Comp Physiol 2002;283:R7–R28.

34. Kunkel EJ, Butcher EC. Chemokines and the tissue-specific migration of lymphocytes. Immunity 2002;16:1–4.

35. Eckmann L, Kagnoff MF, Fierer J. Epithelial cells secrete the chemokine interleukin-8 in response to bacterial entry. Infect Immun 1993;61:4569–4574.

36. McCormick BA, Hofman PM, Kim J et al. Surface attachment of Salmonella typhimurium to intestinal epithelia imprints the subepithelial matrix with gradients chemotactic for neutrophils. J Cell Biol 1995;131:1599–1608.

37. Jung HC, Eckmann L, Yang SK et al. A distinct array of proinflammatory cytokines is expressed in human colon epithelial cells in response to bacterial invasion. J Clin Invest 1995;95:55–65.

38. Yang SK, Eckmann L, Panja A et al. Differential and regulated expression of C-X-C, C-C, and C-chemokines by human colon epithelial cells. Gastroenterology 1997;113:1214–1223.

39. Eckmann L, Kagnoff MF. Cytokines in host defense against Salmonella. Microbes Infect 2001;3:1191–1200.

40. Keates AC, Keates S, Kwon JH et al. ZBP-89, Sp1, and nuclear factor-kB regulate epithelial neutrophil-activating peptide-78 gene expression in Caco-2 human colonic epithelial cells. J Biol Chem 2001;276:43713–43722.

41. Keates S, Keates AC, Mizoguchi E et al. Enterocytes are the primary source of the chemokine ENA-78 in normal colon and ulcerative colitis. Am J Physiol 1997;273:G75–G82.

42. McCormick BA, Parkos CA, Colgan SP et al. Apical secretion of a pathogen-elicited epithelial chemoattractant activity in response to surface colonization of intestinal epithelia by Salmonella typhimurium. J Immunol 1998;160:455–466.

43. Reinecker HC, Loh EY, Ringler DJ et al. Monocyte-chemoattractant protein 1 gene expression in intestinal epithelial cells and inflammatory bowel disease mucosa. Gastroenterology 1995;108:40–50.

44. Casola A, Estes MK, Crawford SE et al. Rotavirus infection of cultured intestinal epithelial cells induces secretion of CXC and CC chemokines. Gastroenterology 1998;114:947–955.

45. Gasperini S, Marchi M, Calzetti F et al. Gene expression and production of the monokine induced by IFN-γ (MIG), IFN-inducible T cell a chemoattractant (I-TAC), and IFN-γ-inducible protein-10 (IP-10) chemokines by human neutrophils. J Immunol 1999;162:4928–4937.

46. Loetscher M, Gerber B, Loetscher P et al. Chemokine receptor specific for IP10 and mig: structure, function, and expression in activated T-lymphocytes. J Exp Med 1996;184:963–969.

47. Qin S, Rottman JB, Myers P et al. The chemokine receptors CXCR3 and CCR5 mark subsets of T cells associated with certain inflammatory reactions. J Clin Invest 1998;101:746–754.

48. Berin MC, Dwinell MB, Eckmann L et al. Production of MDC/CCL22 by human intestinal epithelial cells. Am J Physiol Gastrointest Liver Physiol 2001;280:G1217–G1226.

49. Berin MC, Eckmann L, Broide DH et al. Regulated production of the T helper 2-type T-cell chemoattractant TARC by human bronchial epithelial cells in vitro and in human lung xenografts. Am J Respir Cell Mol Biol 2001;24:382–389.

50. Luster AD. The role of chemokines in linking innate and adaptive immunity. Curr Opin Immunol 2002;14:129–135.

51. Greaves DR, Wang W, Dairaghi DJ et al. CCR6, a CC chemokine receptor that interacts with macrophage inflammatory protein 3a and is highly expressed in human dendritic cells. J Exp Med 1997;186:837–844.

52. Baba M, Imai T, Nishimura M et al. Identification of CCR6, the specific receptor for a novel lymphocyte-directed CC chemokine LARC. J Biol Chem 1997;272:14893–14898.

53. Rescigno M, Rotta G, Valzasina B et al. Dendritic cells shuttle microbes across gut epithelial monolayers. Immunobiology 2001;204:572–581.

54. Eckmann L, Reed SL, Smith JR et al. Entamoeba histolytica trophozoites induce an inflammatory cytokine response by cultured human cells through the paracrine action of cytolytically released interleukin-1 a. J Clin Invest 1995;96:1269–1279.

55. Bocker U, Damiao A, Holt L et al. Differential expression of interleukin 1 receptor antagonist isoforms in human intestinal epithelial cells. Gastroenterology 1998;115:1426–1438.

56. Reinecker HC, MacDermott RP, Mirau S et al. Intestinal epithelial cells both express and respond to interleukin 15. Gastroenterology 1996;111:1706–1713.

57. Kalina U, Koyama N, Hosoda T et al. Enhanced production of IL-18 in butyrate-treated intestinal epithelium by stimulation of the proximal promoter region. Eur J Immunol 2002;32:2635–2643.

58. Laurent F, Kagnoff MF, Savidge TC et al. Human intestinal epithelial cells respond to Cryptosporidium parvum infection with increased prostaglandin H synthase 2 expression and prostaglandin E2 and F2a production. Infect Immun 1998; 66:1787–1790.

59. Belley A, Chadee K. Prostaglandin E2 stimulates rat and human colonic mucin exocytosis via the EP4 receptor. Gastroenterology 1999;117:1352–1362.

60. Kabashima K, Saji T, Murata T et al. The prostaglandin receptor EP4 suppresses colitis, mucosal damage and CD4 cell activation in the gut. J Clin Invest 2002;109:883–893.

61. Witthoft T, Eckmann L, Kim JM et al. Enteroinvasive bacteria directly activate expression of iNOS and NO production in human colon epithelial cells. Am J Physiol 1998;275:G564–G571.

62. Salzman AL, Eaves-Pyles T, Linn SC et al. Bacterial induction of inducible nitric oxide synthase in cultured human intestinal epithelial cells. Gastroenterology 1998;114:93–102.

63. Eckmann L, Laurent F, Langford TD et al. Nitric oxide production by human intestinal epithelial cells and competition for arginine as potential determinants of host defense against the lumen-dwelling pathogen Giardia lamblia. J Immunol 2000;164:1478–1487.

64. Bevins CL, Martin-Porter E, Ganz T. Defensins and innate host defence of the gastrointestinal tract. Gut 1999;45:911–915.

65. Lehrer RI, Ganz T. Defensins of vertebrate animals. Curr Opin Immunol 2002;14:96–102.

66. Raj PA, Dentino AR. Current status of defensins and their role in innate and adaptive immunity. FEMS Microbiol Lett 2002;206:9–18.

67. Ouellette AJ, Bevins CL. Paneth cell defensins and innate immunity of the small bowel. Inflamm Bowel Dis 2001;7:43–50.

68. Garcia JR, Jaumann F, Schulz S et al. Identification of a novel, multifunctional beta-defensin (human β-defensin 3) with specific antimicrobial activity. Its interaction with plasma membranes of Xenopus oocytes and the induction of macrophage chemoattraction. Cell Tissue Res 2001;306:257–264.

69. Schutte BC, Mitros JP, Bartlett JA et al. Discovery of five conserved β-defensin gene clusters using a computational search strategy. Proc Natl Acad Sci USA 2002;99:2129–2133.

70. O'Neil DA, Porter EM, Elewaut D et al. Expression and regulation of the human β-defensins hBD-1 and hBD-2 in intestinal epithelium. J Immunol 1999;163:6718–6724.

71. O'Neil DA, Cole SP, Martin-Porter E et al. Regulation of human β-defensins by gastric epithelial cells in response to infection with Helicobacter pylori or stimulation with interleukin-1. Infect Immun 2000;68:5412–5415.

72. Frye M, Bargon J, Lembcke B et al. Differential expression of human α- and β-defensins mRNA in gastrointestinal epithelia. Eur J Clin Invest 2000;30:695–701.

73. Hamanaka Y, Nakashima M, Wada A et al. Expression of human β-defensin 2 (hBD-2) in Helicobacter pylori-induced gastritis: antibacterial effect of hBD-2 against Helicobacter pylori. Gut 2001;49:481–487.

74. Lehrer RI, Ganz T. Cathelicidins: a family of endogenous antimicrobial peptides. Curr Opin Hematol 2002;9:18–22.

75. Larrick JW, Hirata M, Balint RF et al. Human CAP18: a novel antimicrobial lipopolysaccharide-binding protein. Infect Immun 1995;63:1291–1297.

76. De Y, Chen Q, Schmidt AP et al. LL-37, the neutrophil granule- and epithelial cell-derived cathelicidin, utilizes formyl peptide receptor-like 1 (FPRL1) as a receptor to chemoattract human peripheral blood neutrophils, monocytes, and T cells. J Exp Med 2000;192:1069–1074.

77. Hase K, Eckmann L, Leopard JD et al. Cell differentiation is a key determinant of cathelicidin LL-37/human cationic antimicrobial protein 18 expression by human colon epithelium. Infect Immun 2002;70:953–963.

78. Baeuerle PA, Henkel T. Function and activation of NFkB in the immune system. Annu Rev Immunol 1994;12:141–179.

79. Ghosh S, May MJ, Kopp EB. NFkB and Rel proteins: evolutionarily conserved mediators of immune responses. Annu Rev Immunol 1998;6:225–260.

80. Karin M, Ben-Neriah Y. Phosphorylation meets ubiquitination: the control of NFkB activity. Annu Rev Immunol 2000;18:621–663.

81. Ghosh S, Karin M. Missing pieces in the NFkB puzzle. Cell 2002;109:S81–S96.

82. Elewaut D, DiDonato JA, Kim JM et al. NFkB is a central regulator of the intestinal epithelial cell innate immune response induced by infection with enteroinvasive bacteria. J Immunol 1999;163:1457–1466.

83. Li Q, Van Antwerp D, Mercurio F et al. Severe liver degeneration in mice lacking the IkB kinase 2 gene. Science 1999;284:321–325.

84. Li Z-W, Chu W, Hu Y et al. The IKKb subunit of IkB kinase (IKK) is essential for NFkB activation and prevention of apoptosis. J Exp Med 1999;189:1839–1845.

85. Chu W-M, Ostertag D, Li Z-W et al. JNK2 and IKKb are required for activating the innate response to viral infection. Immunity 1999;11:721–731.

86. Chu WM, Gong X, Li ZW et al. DNA-PKcs is required for activation of innate immunity by immnostimulatory DNA. Cell 2000;103:909–918.

87. Barnes PJ, Karin M. NFkB – A pivotal transcription factor in chronic inflammatory diseases. N Engl J Med 1997;336:1066–1071.

88. Karin M, Lin A. NFkB at the crossroads of life and death. Nature Immunol 2002;3:221–227.

89. Jobin C, Sartor RB. The IkB/NFkB system: a key determinant of mucosal inflammation and protection. Am J Physiol Cell Physiol 2000;278:C451–462.

90. Savkovic SD, Koutsouris A, Hecht G. Activation of NFkB in intestinal epithelial cells by enteropathogenic Escherichia coli. Am J Physiol 1997;273:C1160–C1167.

91. Keates S, Hitti YS, Upton M et al. Helicobacter pylori infection activates NFkB in gastric epithelial cells. Gastroenterology 1997;113:1099–1109.

92. Hobbie S, Chen LM, Davis RJ et al. Involvement of mitogen-activated protein kinase pathways in the nuclear responses and cytokine production induced by Salmonella typhimurium in cultured intestinal epithelial cells. J Immunol 1997;159:5550–5559.

93. Savkovic SD, Ramaswamy A, Koutsouris A et al. EPEC-activated ERK1/2 participate in inflammatory response but not tight junction barrier disruption. Am J Physiol Gastrointest Liver Physiol 2001;281:G890–G898.

94. Keates S, Keates AC, Warny M et al. Differential activation of mitogen-activated protein kinases in AGS gastric epithelial cells by cag+ and cag– Helicobacter pylori. J Immunol 1999;163:5552–5559.

95. Berin MC, Darfeuille-Michaud A, Egan LJ et al. Role of EHEC O157:H7 virulence factors in the activation of intestinal epithelial cell NFkB and MAP kinase pathways and the upregulated expression of interleukin 8. Cell Microbiol 2002;4:635–648.

96. Haller D, Russo MP, Sartor RB et al. IKKb and phosphatidylinositol 3-kinase/Akt participate in non-pathogenic Gram-negative enteric bacteria-induced RelA phosphorylation and NFkB activation in both primary and intestinal epithelial cell lines. J Biol Chem 2002; 277:38168–38178.

97. Inohara N, Ogura Y, Chen FF et al. Human Nod1 confers responsiveness to bacterial lipopolysaccharides. J Biol Chem 2001;276:2551–2554.

98. Bertin J, Nir WJ, Fischer CM et al. Human CARD4 protein is a novel CED-4/Apaf-1 cell death family member that activates NFkB. J Biol Chem 1999;274:12955–12958.

99. Inohara N, Nunez G. The NOD: a signaling module that regulates apoptosis and host defense against pathogens. Oncogene 2001;20:6473–6481.

100. Girardin SE, Tournebize R, Mavris M et al. CARD4/Nod1 mediates NFkB and JNK activation by invasive Shigella flexneri. EMBO Rep 2001;2:736–742.

101. Janeway CA Jr. The immune system evolved to discriminate infectious nonself from noninfectious self. Immunol Today 1992;13:11–16.

102. Medzhitov R. Toll-like receptors and innate immunity. Nature Rev Immunol 2001;1:135–145.

103. Rock FL, Hardiman G, Timans JC et al. A family of human receptors structurally related to Drosophila Toll. Proc Natl Acad Sci USA 1998;95:588–593.

104. Anderson KV. Toll signaling pathways in the innate immune response. Curr Opin Immunol 2000;12:13–19.

105. Cario E, Rosenberg IM, Brandwein SL et al. Lipopolysaccharide activates distinct signaling pathways in intestinal epithelial cell lines expressing Toll-like receptors. J Immunol 2000;164:966–972.

106. Cario E, Podolsky DK. Differential alteration in intestinal epithelial cell expression of Toll-like receptor 3 (TLR3) and TLR4 in inflammatory bowel disease. Infect Immun 2000;68:7010–7017.

107. Gewirtz AT, Navas TA, Lyons S et al. Cutting edge: bacterial flagellin activates basolaterally expressed TLR5 to induce epithelial proinflammatory gene expression. J Immunol 2001;167:1882–1885.

108. Cario E, Brown D, McKee M et al. Commensal-associated molecular patterns induce selective Toll-like receptor-trafficking from apical membrane to cytoplasmic compartments in polarized intestinal epithelium. Am J Pathol 2002;160:165–173.

109. Aliprantis A, Yang R-B, Mark M et al. Cell activation and apoptosis by bacterial lipoproteins through Toll-like receptor-2. Science 1999;285:736–739.

110. Underhill DM, Ozinsky A, Smith KD et al. Toll-like receptor-2 mediates mycobacteria-induced proinflammatory signaling in macrophages. Proc Natl Acad Sci USA 1999;96:14459–14463.

111. Campos MA, Almeida IC, Takeuchi O et al. Activation of Toll-like receptor-2 by glycosylphosphatidylinositol anchors from a protozoan parasite. J Immunol 2001;167:416–423.

112. Poltorak A, He X, Smirnova I et al. Defective LPS signaling in C3H/HeJ and C57BL/10ScCr Mice: Mutations in Tlr4 Gene. Science 1998;282:2082–2088.

113. Takeuchi O, Hoshino K, Kawai T et al. Differential roles of TLR2 and TLR4 in recognition of Gram-negative and Gram-positive bacterial cell wall components. Immunity 1999;11:443–451.

114. Alexopoulou L, Holt AC, Medzhitov R et al. Recognition of double-stranded RNA and activation of NFkB by Toll-like receptor 3. Nature 2001;413:732–738.

115. Hayashi F, Smith KD, Ozinsky A et al. The innate immune response to bacterial flagellin is mediated by Toll-like receptor 5. Nature 2001;410:1099–1103.

116. Hemmi H, Takeuchi O, Kawai T et al. A Toll-like receptor recognizes bacterial DNA. Nature 2000;408:740–745.

117. Muzio M, Ni J, Feng P et al. IRAK (Pelle) family member IRAK-2 and MyD88 as proximal mediators of IL-1 signaling. Science 1997;278:1612–1615.

118. Wesche H, Henzel WJ, Shillinglaw W et al. MyD88: an adapter that recruits IRAK to the IL-1 receptor complex. Immunity 1997;7:837–847.

119. Cao Z, Henzel WJ, Gao X. IRAK: a kinase associated with the interleukin-1 receptor. Science 1996;271:1128–1131.

120. Cao Z, Xiong J, Takeuchi M et al. TRAF6 is a signal transducer for interleukin-1. Nature 1996;383:443–446.

121. Burns K, Clatworthy J, Martin L et al. Tollip, a new component of the IL-1RI pathway, links IRAK to the IL-1 receptor. Nature Cell Biol 2000;2:346–351.

122. Arbibe L, Mira JP, Teusch N et al. Toll-like receptor 2-mediated NFk B activation requires a Rac1-dependent pathway. Nature Immunol 2000;1:533–540.

123. Takeuchi O, Kaufmann A, Grote K et al. Cutting edge: preferentially the R-stereoisomer of the mycoplasmal lipopeptide macrophage-activating lipopeptide-2 activates immune cells through a Toll-like receptor 2- and MyD88-dependent signaling pathway. J Immunol 2000;164:554–557.

124. Horng T, Barton GM, Medzhitov R. TIRAP: an adapter molecule in the Toll signaling pathway. Nature Immunol 2001;2:835–841.

125. Fitzgerald KA, Palsson-McDermott EM, Bowie AG et al. Mal (MyD88-adapter-like) is required for Toll-like receptor-4 signal transduction. Nature 2001;413:78–83.

126. Gewirtz AT, Simon PO Jr, Schmitt CK et al. Salmonella typhimurium translocates flagellin across intestinal epithelia, inducing a proinflammatory response. J Clin Invest 2001;107:99–109.

127. Steiner TS, Nataro JP, Poteet-Smith CE et al. Enteroaggregative Escherichia coli expresses a novel flagellin that causes IL-8 release from intestinal epithelial cells. J Clin Invest 2000;105:1769–1777.

128. Sierro F, Dubois B, Coste A et al. Flagellin stimulation of intestinal epithelial cells triggers CCL20-mediated migration of dendritic cells. Proc Natl Acad Sci USA 2001;98:13722–13727.

129. Lee CA, Silva M, Siber AM et al. A secreted Salmonella protein induces a proinflammatory response in epithelial cells, which promotes neutrophil migration. Proc Natl Acad Sci USA 2000; 97:12283–12288.

130. Reed KA, Hobert ME, Kolenda CE et al. The Salmonella typhimurium flagellar basal body protein FliE is required for flagellin production and to induce a proinflammatory response in epithelial cells. J Biol Chem 2002;277:13346–13353.

131. Abreu MT, Vora P, Faure E et al. Decreased expression of Toll-like receptor-4 and MD-2 correlates with intestinal epithelial cell protection against dysregulated proinflammatory gene expression in response to bacterial lipopolysaccharide. J Immunol 2001;167:1609–1616.

132. Weinrauch Y, Zychlinsky A. The induction of apoptosis by bacterial pathogens. Annu Rev Microbiol 1999; 53:155–187.

133. Kim JM, Eckmann L, Savidge TC et al. Apoptosis of human intestinal epithelial cells after bacterial invasion. J Clin Invest 1998;102:1815–1823.

134. Paesold G, Guiney DG, Eckmann L et al. Genes in the Salmonella pathogenicity island 2 and the Salmonella virulence plasmid are essential for Salmonella-induced apoptosis in intestinal epithelial cells. Cell Microbiol 2002;4:771–781.

135. Chen XM, Levine SA, Splinter PL et al. Cryptosporidium parvum activates nuclear factor kB in biliary epithelia preventing epithelial cell apoptosis. Gastroenterology 2001; 120:1774–1783.

136. McCole DF, Eckmann L, Laurent F et al. Intestinal epithelial cell apoptosis following Cryptosporidium parvum infection. Infect Immun 2000;68:1710–1713.

137. Laurent F, McCole D, Eckmann L et al. Pathogenesis of Cryptosporidium parvum infection. Microbes Infect 1999;1:141–148.

138. Barnard JA, Warwick GJ, Gold LI. Localization of transforming growth factor β isoforms in the normal murine small intestine and colon. Gastroenterology 1993;105:67–73.

139. Nataro JP, Kaper JB. Diarrheagenic Escherichia coli. Clin Microbiol Rev 1998;11:142–201.

140. Lencer WI. Microbes and microbial toxins: paradigms for microbial–mucosal toxins. V. cholerae: invasion of the intestinal epithelial barrier by a stably folded protein toxin. Am J Physiol Gastrointest Liver Physiol 2001;280:G781–G786.

141. Zhu X, Kahn RA. The Escherichia coli heat labile toxin binds to Golgi membranes and alters Golgi and cell morphologies using ADP-ribosylation factor-dependent processes. J Biol Chem 2001;276:25014–25021.

142. Kyne L, Farrell RJ, Kelly CP. Clostridium difficile. Gastroenterol Clin North Am 2001;30:753–777.

143. Poxton IR, McCoubrey J, Blair G. The pathogenicity of Clostridium difficile. Clin Microbiol Infect 2001;7:421–427.

144. Qa'Dan M, Ramsey M, Daniel J et al. Clostridium difficile toxin B activates dual caspase-dependent and caspase-independent apoptosis in intoxicated cells. Cell Microbiol 2002;4:425–434.

145. Warny M, Keates AC, Keates S et al. p38 MAP kinase activation by Clostridium difficile toxin A mediates monocyte necrosis, IL-8 production, and enteritis. J Clin Invest 2000;105:1147–1156.

146. He D, Sougioultzis S, Hagen S et al. *Clostridium difficile* toxin A triggers human colonocyte IL-8 release via mitochondrial oxygen radical generation. Gastroenterology 2002;122:1048–1057.

147. Tesh VL, O'Brien AD. The pathogenic mechanisms of Shiga toxin and the Shiga-like toxins. Mol Microbiol 1991;5:1817–1822.

148. O'Loughlin EV, Robins-Browne RM. Effect of Shiga toxin and Shiga-like toxins on eukaryotic cells. Microbes Infect 2001;3:493–507.

149. Philpott DJ, Ackerley CA, Kiliaan AJ et al. Translocation of verotoxin-1 across T84 monolayers: mechanism of bacterial toxin penetration of epithelium. Am J Physiol 1997;273:G1349–G1358.

150. Sandvig K, van Deurs B. Entry of ricin and Shiga toxin into cells: molecular mechanisms and medical perspectives. EMBO J 2000;19:5943–5950.

151. Johannes L. The epithelial cell cytoskeleton and intracellular trafficking. I. Shiga toxin B-subunit system: retrograde transport, intracellular vectorization, and more. Am J Physiol Gastrointest Liver Physiol 2002;283:G1–G7.

152. Thorpe CM, Hurley BP, Lincicome LL et al. Shiga toxins stimulate secretion of interleukin-8 from intestinal epithelial cells. Infect Immun 1999;67:5985–5993.

153. Pepe JC, Miller VL. *Yersinia enterocolitica* invasin: a primary role in the initiation of infection. Proc Natl Acad Sci USA 1993;90:6473–6477.

154. Isberg RR, Hamburger Z, Dersch P. Signaling and invasin-promoted uptake via integrin receptors. Microbes Infect 2000;2:793–801.

155. Tafazoli F, Holmstrom A, Forsberg A et al. Apically exposed, tight junction-associated beta1-integrins allow binding and YopE-mediated perturbation of epithelial barriers by wild-type *Yersinia* bacteria. Infect Immun 2000;68:5335–5343.

156. Schulte R, Kerneis S, Klinke S et al. Translocation of *Yersinia enterocolitica* across reconstituted intestinal epithelial monolayers is triggered by *Yersinia* invasin binding to beta1 integrins apically expressed on M-like cells. Cell Microbiol 2000;2:173–185.

157. Weidow CL, Black DS, Bliska JB et al. CAS/Crk signalling mediates uptake of *Yersinia* into human epithelial cells. Cell Microbiol 2000;2:549–560.

158. Alrutz MA, Srivastava A, Wong KW et al. Efficient uptake of *Yersinia pseudotuberculosis* via integrin receptors involves a Rac1-Arp 2/3 pathway that bypasses N-WASP function. Mol Microbiol 2001;42:689–703.

159. Bergmann B, Raffelsbauer D, Kuhn M et al. InlA- but not InlB-mediated internalization of *Listeria monocytogenes* by non-phagocytic mammalian cells needs the support of other internalins. Mol Microbiol 2002;43:557–570.

160. Braun L, Ghebrehiwet B, Cossart P. gC1q-R/p32, a C1q-binding protein, is a receptor for the InlB invasion protein of *Listeria monocytogenes*. EMBO J 2000;19:1458–1466.

161. Shen Y, Naujokas M, Park M et al. InlB-dependent internalization of *Listeria* is mediated by the Met receptor tyrosine kinase. Cell 2000;103:501–510.

162. Mansell A, Khelef N, Cossart P et al. Internalin B activates nuclear factor-kB via Ras, phosphoinositide 3-kinase, and Akt. J Biol Chem 2001;276:43597–43603.

163. Braun L, Dramsi S, Dehoux P et al. InlB: an invasion protein of *Listeria monocytogenes* with a novel type of surface association. Mol Microbiol 1997;25:285–294.

164. Marcus SL, Brumell JH, Pfeifer CG et al. *Salmonella* pathogenicity islands: big virulence in small packages. Microbes Infect 2000;2:145–156.

165. Galan JE, Collmer A. Type III secretion machines: bacterial devices for protein delivery into host cells. Science 1999;284:1322–1328.

166. Galan JE. *Salmonella* interactions with host cells: type III secretion at work. Annu Rev Cell Dev Biol 2001;17:53–86.

167. Galan JE, Zhou D. Striking a balance: modulation of the actin cytoskeleton by *Salmonella*. Proc Natl Acad Sci USA 2000;97:8754–8761.

168. Fu Y, Galan JE. The *Salmonella typhimurium* tyrosine phosphatase SptP is translocated into host cells and disrupts the actin cytoskeleton. Mol Microbiol 1998;27:359–368.

169. Zhou D, Mooseker MS, Galan JE. Role of the *S. typhimurium* actin-binding protein SipA in bacterial internalization. Science 1999;283:2092–2095.

170. Shears SB. The versatility of inositol phosphates as cellular signals. Biochim Biophys Acta 1998;1436:49–67.

171. Marcus SL, Knodler LA, Finlay BB. *Salmonella enterica* serovar Typhimurium effector SigD/SopB is membrane-associated and ubiquitinated inside host cells. Cell Microbiol 2002;4:435–446.

172. Eckmann L, Rudolf MT, Ptasznik A et al. D-myo-Inositol 1,4,5,6-tetrakisphosphate produced in human intestinal epithelial cells in response to *Salmonella* invasion inhibits phosphoinositide 3-kinase signaling pathways. Proc Natl Acad Sci USA 1997;94:14456–14460.

173. Feng Y, Wente SR, Majerus PW. Overexpression of the inositol phosphatase SopB in human 293 cells stimulates cellular chloride influx and inhibits nuclear mRNA export. Proc Natl Acad Sci USA 2001;98:875–879.

174. Terebiznik MR, Vieira OV, Marcus SL et al. Elimination of host cell PtdIns(4,5)P(2) by bacterial SigD promotes membrane fission during invasion by *Salmonella*. Nature Cell Biol 2002;4:766–773.

175. Norris FA, Wilson MP, Wallis TS et al. SopB, a protein required for virulence of *Salmonella dublin*, is an inositol phosphate phosphatase. Proc Natl Acad Sci USA 1998;95:14057–14059.

176. Zhang ZY, Clemens JC, Schubert HL et al. Expression, purification, and physicochemical characterization of a recombinant *Yersinia* protein tyrosine phosphatase. J Biol Chem 1992;267:23759–23766.

177. Cornelis GR. The Yersinia Ysc-Yop 'Type III' weaponry. Nature Rev Mol Cell Biol 2002;3:742–754.

178. Otto H, Tezcan-Merdol D, Girisch R et al. The spvB gene-product of the *Salmonella enterica* virulence plasmid is a mono(ADP-ribosyl)transferase. Mol Microbiol 2000;37:1106–1115.

179. Tezcan-Merdol D, Nyman T, Lindberg U et al. Actin is ADP-ribosylated by the *Salmonella enterica* virulence-associated protein SpvB. Mol Microbiol 2001;39:606–619.

180. Lesnick ML, Reiner NE, Fierer J et al. The *Salmonella* spvB virulence gene encodes an enzyme that ADP-ribosylates actin and destabilizes the cytoskeleton of eukaryotic cells. Mol Microbiol 2001;39:1464–1470.

181. Sansonetti PJ, Arondel J, Huerre M et al. Interleukin-8 controls bacterial transepithelial translocation at the cost of epithelial destruction in experimental shigellosis. Infect Immun 1999;67:1471–1480.

182. Ohtsuka Y, Lee J, Stamm DS et al. MIP-2 secreted by epithelial cells increases neutrophil and lymphocyte recruitment in the mouse intestine. Gut 2001;49:526–533.

183. Kolios G, Wright KL, Jordan NJ et al. C-X-C and C-C chemokine expression and secretion by the human colonic epithelial cell line, HT-29: differential effect of T lymphocyte-derived cytokines. Eur J Immunol 1999;29:530–536.

184. Kubens BS, Zanker KS. Differences in the migration capacity of primary human colon carcinoma cells (SW480) and their lymph node metastatic derivatives (SW620). Cancer Lett 1998;131:55–64.

185. Carethers JM, Hawn MT, Chauhan DP et al. Competency in mismatch repair prohibits clonal expansion of cancer cells treated with N-methyl-N'-nitro-N-nitrosoguanidine. J Clin Invest 1996;98:199–206.

186. Kleinert H, Wallerath T, Fritz G et al. Cytokine induction of NO synthase II in human DLD-1 cells: roles of the JAK-STAT, AP-1 and NFkB-signaling pathways. Br J Pharmacol 1998;125:193–201.

## CHAPTER 4

# Immune cell–epithelial cell interactions

Lloyd Mayer and Iris Dotan

## INTRODUCTION

Results from a number of animal models of inflammatory bowel diseases (IBD) indicate that several cellular elements contribute to the perpetuation of chronic inflammatory/immune responses[1-4] (see Chapter 9). Although most of the models focus on defects in immune regulation, many relate to the role of the barrier in controlling inflammation. The critical cell involved in barrier function is the intestinal epithelial cell (IEC). However, this cell is more than just a barrier, having incredibly pleiotropic activities. It functions in innate as well as adaptive immunity, acting as a facilitator of protective adaptive immune responses (transport of sIgA), a physical barrier (epithelial membrane, tight junctions, mucin and trefoil factor production) and a regulator of innate immunity (chemokine production following invasion by bacteria). Thus the epithelial cell stands as a critical mediator of intestinal homeostasis.

What has been less well explored is the role this cell has in regulating adaptive immunity directly through its interaction with mucosal T cells. There are three levels of this interaction:

1. Expression of cell surface molecules involved in T-cell activation (antigen presentation and co-stimulation);
2. Production of chemokines which attract T cells as well as professional antigen-presenting cells (APC);
3. Production of cytokines that can enhance or suppress mucosal inflammation and T-cell activation.

There may also be a symbiotic relationship between IEC and the T cells that they activate, with the potential for the latter to affect IEC growth and differentiation. In this chapter we will explore the nature of the interactions between IEC and T cells from the standpoint of cell–cell interactions (cognate interactions), antigen presentation and soluble mediator-regulated interactions (non-cognate interactions). At each step we will provide information regarding what is known about these processes in the normal state and contrast these with the findings in IBD.

## THE EPITHELIAL CELL AS AN ANTIGEN-PRESENTING CELL

### EXPRESSION OF RESTRICTION ELEMENTS

#### Major histocompatibility complex (MHC) class II expression

The first line of evidence to support the fact that IEC could interact with T cells came from the demonstration that cell surface molecules capable of mediating this interaction are expressed by IEC, the most important of these being classical restriction elements. These are antigen-presenting molecules that possess the capacity to bind peptides (processed antigens) and interact with the T-cell receptor. IEC express classical class I molecules (HLA-A, B, C in humans) and are the only non-professional APC to constitutively express MHC class II molecules (HLA-DR, DP in humans). This was first described by Mason et al.[5] in the rat and expanded to humans by Selby et al.[6] Selby went further to show, in immunohistochemical studies, that class II expression was increased on IEC derived from IBD tissues. The potential for these class II molecules to be functional (i.e. capable of activating CD4+ T cells) was realized with the description of invariant chain expression in normal IEC and IFN-γ stimulated IEC cell lines (see below).[7-9] The functional relevance of these findings came shortly thereafter, with the description that normal murine IEC that had been pulsed with ovalbumin (OVA) were capable of triggering an OVA-specific T-cell line to secrete IL-2.[10] Although the level of class II expressed by IEC is considerably less than that seen on a conventional APC, these molecules were sufficient to activate memory T cells. Later on, studies by Hershberg's group brought this into a human system.[11] A transfected T84 colon carcinoma line (transfected with HLA-DR4 as well as CIITA cDNA) could restore a tetanus-induced cytokine response in a T-cell hybridoma. Furthermore, this interaction was polarized, like the epithelium itself, such that apically introduced Ag could trigger a response basolaterally, but not vice versa. Further studies suggested a role for CD58 as well.[12] This molecule provided a needed co-stimulatory signal (see below). A number of groups have provided further indirect evidence for the integrity of the class II presentation pathway (Fig. 4.1). In the systemic immune system, Ags that gain access to the APC exogenously are processed through an endolysosomal pathway. Within the endosome and lysosome larger proteins are degraded (processed) by proteases (e.g. cathepsins) into smaller immunogenic peptides. Peptides generated in this fashion load into class II molecules in late endosomes and these traffic to the surface, fusing with the plasma membrane, resulting in the surface expression of an MHC II–peptide complex that can be recognized by specific T cells (through their T-cell antigen receptor). Using an ileal loop model, Gonnella et al.[13,14] showed that luminal administration of OVA led to uptake by the IEC and concentration of Ags within the endolysosomal pathway. These results were reproduced by Brandeis et al.,[15] who administered MHC peptides orally to a rat and traced them into endolysosomal structures in the upper small bowel epithelium. So et al.[16–18] analyzed this in vitro using three different cell line systems. She documented the uptake of soluble proteins by fluid phase endocytosis, followed by sequential trafficking to early and then late endosomes. The nature of the Ag appeared to be important in this process, as there appeared to be slow but selective uptake of all soluble protein Ags, with exclusion of insoluble proteins and carbohydrates. Hershberg's group[11,12] further showed that the late endosomes contained key elements involved in processing and presentation: endosomal cathepsins for processing, and HLA-DM for exchange of processed peptides with CLIP in

the class II pocket (Fig. 4.1). The presence of invariant chain confirmed that the class II molecules expressed by IEC were likely to be functional, but the ability of the engineered lines to take up intact tetanus toxoid and process it into a form (peptide) recognized by a peptide-specific DR4-restricted T-cell hybridoma (induction of IL-2 secretion by this hybridoma) was clear confirmation. Although these studies support the possibility of such an event occurring in vivo, direct evidence for a functional role of class II expression by IEC in vivo is still lacking.

The capability of IEC to function as APC and to stimulate CD4+ T cells was further supported by the demonstration[19] that, similar to professional APC, IEC secrete exosome-like particles (membrane blebs) that contain classical restriction elements. Interestingly, the phenotype of apically secreted exosomes differs significantly from that of basolaterally secreted exosomes in the polarized cell system model in which these experiments were conducted. Basolaterally secreted exosome-like particles had higher levels of MHC class II and CD63, and were able to cross 3 μM-pore filters, thus suggesting their potential to interact with cells in the lamina propria and activate the numerous CD4+ T cells residing in that environment. The possible functions of these exosome-like particles in vivo were demonstrated by Karlsson et al.,[20] who demonstrated in rats that exosome-like particles could be purified from the peripheral blood, and that transfer of these particles to naive animals after antigen feeding would result in antigen-specific tolerance in the recipients. The existence of exosomes/tolerosomes in the human intestinal mucosa has not been demonstrated, but their existence and potential function in both in vitro and in vivo animal models adds support to the notion that IEC are equipped and capable of functioning as APC in the GALT.

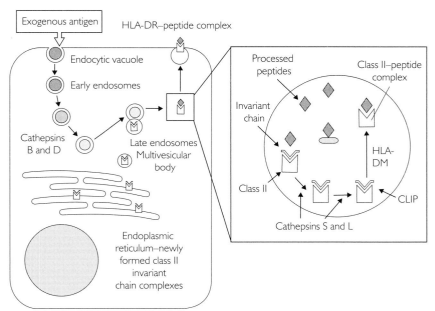

Fig. 4.1 Class II presentation pathway (exogenous antigen processing pathway). Antigens (mostly proteins) are taken up via many pathways into the cell (fluid phase endocytosis, receptor-mediated endocytosis) and targeted to the endosomal compartment. The early endosomes can recycle to the surface without processing of the antigen–transferrin receptor pathway), but most endosomes travel into the cytoplasm and activate H+ protopumps that lower the pH within the early endosome. At low pH, acid proteases (predominantly cathepsins B and D) present within the endosome are activated and cleave or 'process' the protein. The endoplasmic reticulum is producing new class II molecules. The antigen-binding groove of the class II molecule is complexed to a large glycoprotein, invariant chain (Ii), which prevents peptides within the ER from binding. From the ER to the Golgi, the class II/Ii complexes target the late endosome and fuse to its membrane. Cathepsins S and L (see inset) are activated and cleave the overhanging edges of Ii, leaving only the portion of the Ii within the groove. This peptide is called CLIP (class II associated invariant peptide). CLIP is removed from the groove with a peptide exchanger called HLA-DM and processed peptide within the late endosome is now able to bind in the groove of the class II molecule. This peptide class II complex is then transported to the cell surface, where the endosome fuses with the plasma membrane, and the complex is now present on the cell surface, where it can interact with the appropriate T-cell receptor.

# MHC CLASS I EXPRESSION

Like virtually all nucleated cells in the body, IEC also express class I MHC. This is the restriction element commonly used by CD8+ cytolytic T cells (CTL). Antigens recognized by these cells are typically the result of intracellular (endogenous) processing (proteasomal degradation and transport of the peptides to the endoplasmic reticulum (ER), a common scenario for viral infections (Fig. 4.2). Viral proteins produced in the cytoplasm of an infected cell are ubiquitinated and targeted for proteasomal degradation. Processed peptides are then transported to the endoplasmic reticulum using transporter (TAP) proteins.[18] Within the ER processed peptides can bind to newly synthesized class I molecules (empty peptide-binding groove). Binding of peptide to the class I molecule stabilizes the complex and allows for its transport to the cell surface. Once on the surface this complex can be recognized by a virus-specific CTL which becomes activated, releasing perforin and granzyme B, resulting in the lysis of the infected cell.

Does this happen to virally infected IEC? Although they express the full complement of proteasomes and transporters, interestingly, bulk lysis of the epithelium in a viral infection model is generally not seen. Early literature suggested that there was a dearth of cytolytic T cells in the lamina propria. The reason for the lack of lysis and cytolytic cells (providing a protective effect) is not yet known, but it speaks to mechanisms focused on maintaining epithelial integrity. Recent studies by

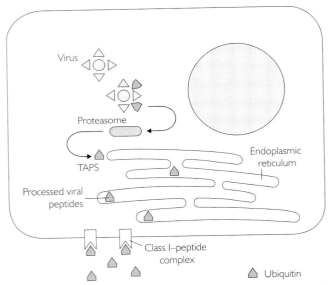

**Fig. 4.2** Class I presentation pathway (endogenous antigen processing pathway). Antigens in the form of intracellular infectious agents or mutated cells (malignant) utilize host protein synthetic machinery to generate required structural and replicative proteins. Some of these proteins are tagged with ubiquitin (ubiquitinated), which targets the molecule to the proteasome complex (made up of several subunits, its structure is similar to a barrel with enzymatic machinery inside). Proteins are processed by these proteasomal enzymes (e.g. LMP2, LMP7) and transported to the ER by cytoplasmic transporters (TAP). Within the ER, peptides load into the groove of newly synthesized class I molecules. This binding stabilizes the complex and allows it to go through the Golgi to the cell surface. On the surface these complexes can be recognized by antigen-specific MHC class I restricted CD8+ cytolytic T cells. Peptides are unable to bind to class II molecules in the ER because the groove is blanketed with invariant chain.

LeFrancois' group[21,22] support a failure of classic CTL to target IEC. This group generated a transgenic mouse that expressed a peptide of OVA on the surface of small bowel IEC that is known to be the Ag for a CD8+ cytolytic T-cell line. Transfer of this cytolytic line into these transgenic mice did not result in the killing of the IEC. Rather, it took an external viral infection (non-specific) to initiate the inflammatory process and promote IEC destruction. The T cells were in some manner inhibited from killing the IEC in the native state. Epithelial cells can be targets of cytolytic cells, as IEC lines can be lysed as targets for NK or LAK cells in in vitro assays.[23] Whether they can prime a CTL response remains to be clarified. The in vivo observations described above suggest that this may not be the case.

# NON-CLASSICAL CLASS I MOLECULES

Probably the most intriguing observation has been the identification of a number of non-classic class I molecules on the surface of IEC (Fig. 4.3). Non-classic class I or class Ib molecules comprise a family of class I-like molecules (structurally) that are generally non-polymorphic and less capable of binding conventional antigenic peptides. These include the CD1 family (CD1a-d in humans, CD1d in mice),[24,25] HLA-E, F and G in humans[26-35] MICA/B (mouse and human)[36,37] FcRn (mouse and human), and TL in the mouse.[38]

Data from several laboratories suggest that class Ib molecules might be important in T-cell recognition of the integrity of the epithelial cell and its response to stress. The receptors for some of the class Ib molecules are NK receptors that are expressed not only by NK cells but also by TCR $\gamma\delta$ and TCR $\alpha\beta$ CD8+ cells. Depending on the NK receptor, MHC class I molecules can either positively or negatively regulate NK and T-cell activity. Thus, class Ib molecules play a role in the regulation of the immune response and serve as a link between the innate and the adaptive immune systems.

## CD1d

CD1d is a class Ib molecule that is expressed in the thymus, placenta and intestine as well as on conventional APC such as B cells, monocytes and dendritic cells. It is encoded outside the MHC (on chromosome 1) and, although structurally similar to class I molecules, is non-polymporphic. Initial studies by Bleicher et al.[39] and Balk et al.[40] reported the expression of CD1d on both murine and human IEC. CD1d exists as two forms on normal IEC, a glycosylated $\beta_2$-microglobulin-associated form, expressed on the basolateral and apical membranes of the IEC, and a non-glycosylated non-$\beta_2$M-associated form expressed on the apical cell surface.[41] The expression of CD1d is TAP independent and is localized in late endosomes (similar to class II MHC molecules), supporting its ability to bind to Ag which are taken up via the exogenous pathway of Ag processing.[42,43] These features suggest that CD1d does not function like a classical class I molecule but may exhibit properties more in line with class II molecules. However, unlike class II molecules, CD1d binds unique antigenic forms. The crystal structure of CD1d has been resolved, demonstrating a deep hydrophobic pocket that would more likely bind lipid or glycolipid antigens rather than peptides.[44] In fact, the initial molecule shown to be capable of binding in the CD1d groove was a glycolipid derived from a marine sponge, $\alpha$-galactosyl ceramide.[24] Other members of the CD1 family bind lipids or carbohydrate antigens, suggesting that this entire family is involved in the immune response to bacterial antigens.

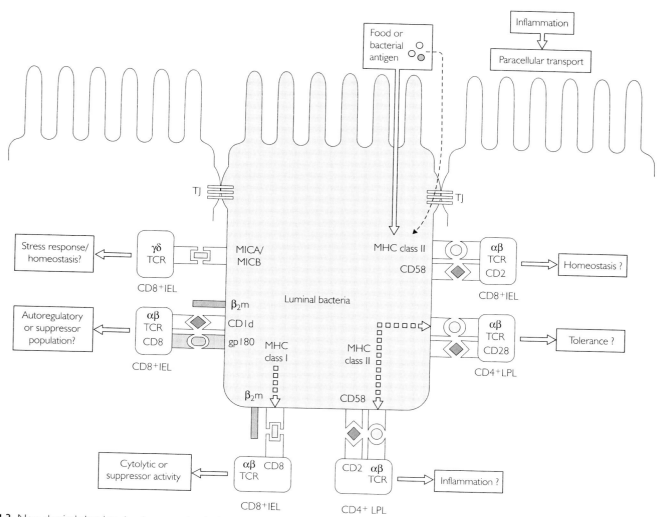

**Fig. 4.3** Non-classical class I molecule expression by intestinal epithelial cells. Intestinal epithelial cells express a normal complement of MHC class I molecules and are the only cell other than professional APC to constitutively express MHC class II molecules. In addition, IEC express a number of non-classic class I molecule which are class I-like in structure but are generally non-polymorphic. These restriction elements have been studied in a limited fashion but appear to be involved in the presentation of novel antigens (lipids, carbohydrates, and bacterial products) to distinct subpopulations of T cells. As will be discussed in the text, normal IEC activate CD8+ regulatory T cells via a CD1d-mediated interaction.

The first evidence that CD1d was involved in T cell–IEC interactions came from studies that demonstrated the capacity of IEC-induced T-cell proliferation to be inhibited by anti-CD1d mAbs.[45] Further studies suggested that some cytotoxic IEL lines were restricted by CD1d expressed on IEC.[46,47] There has been some recent controversy regarding the nature of CD1d expression on IEC, but a number of functional studies suggest that its expression is real and that it plays a regulatory role.[48] More recently, studies have shown that CD1d and a CD8 ligand, gp180 (see below), form a complex on the IEC surface which is recognized by regulatory CD8+ CD28- T cells.[49,50]

## HLA-E

HLA-E, another class Ib molecule, shares many functional features with MHC class I molecules. The most striking is the comparable structure composed of a heavy chain/$\beta_2$-microglobulin–peptide complex, a sequence homology that varies from 50 to 90%,[30] a ubiquitous tissue distribution (at the level of mRNA), and the requirement of TAP-1 for its function.[31,35] However,

there are some fundamental differences that indicate distinct biological functions. HLA-E has limited polymorphism[28,29] and a very restricted peptide-binding specificity imposed by the structure of the groove.[29,51] Furthermore, like its mouse homolog Qa-1, the leader peptide of HLA-E cannot bind HLA-E, whereas the majority (but not all) of MHC class I molecule-derived leader peptides, remarkably conserved, bind HLA-E with a high affinity. Interestingly, the leader peptide from the class Ib molecule HLA-G[33,52] can also bind HLA-E. Recently, the ligand of HLA-E has been identified:[26,27,32] CD94/NKG2 receptors. Among CD94/NKG2 receptors only NKG2A+ and NKG2C+ receptors have been shown to clearly recognize HLA-E. Interestingly, the only peptide recognized by the activating CD94/NKG2C receptor is the HLA-G-derived leader peptide present mainly in the placenta, suggesting a possible function for HLA-E in the protection against a maternal alloresponse or pathogens during the pregnancy. For the other CD94/NKG2 receptors it has not yet been determined whether the absence of staining by HLA-E tetramers with a conserved

MHC class I-derived leader peptide reflects a problem of sensitivity or an effective absence of binding. Cell surface expression of HLA-E, which broadly reflects the amount of class I within the cells, could be an indirect mechanism by which the immune system monitors the intracellular levels of MHC class I. Thus any modifications in the availability of MHC class I leader peptides directly influences the level of HLA-E expression and the recognition by CD94/NKG2A and C receptors. The downregulation of MHC-class I transcription by certain viruses may be indirectly responsible for the reduced expression of HLA-E, which then results in increased NK activity and cytotoxic activity in CD8+ T cells that express the inhibitory CD94/NKG2A receptor.

## MICA/B

MICA and B genes map to the MHC class I region and share a low level of homology (18–36%) with MHC class I molecules. Contrary to HLA-E and G, they display a relatively high level of polymorphism. MICA/B are highly glycosylated proteins that are unusual in their ability to be expressed and to function independently of $\beta_2$-microglobulin and TAP.[36] The distribution of these non-classical class I molecules is restricted to epithelial cells, mainly gastrointestinal epithelium and thymic cortical epithelium. MIC proteins are upregulated upon heat shock owing to a heat-shock response element in their promoters. They interact with V$\delta$1 $\gamma\delta$ IEL, probably (but not exclusively) via their TCR.[37] More recently, the NK-activating molecule NKG2D, broadly expressed on NK, TCR $\gamma\delta$ and CD8TCR $\alpha\beta$ cells, has also been found to recognize MICA and B and may be the main receptor for MICA/B proteins.[53] NKG2D is associated with the adaptor protein DAP10 in a activating receptor complex.[54] MIC glycoproteins appear to be crucial for maintaining the integrity of the gut epithelium by eliminating damaged epithelial cells.

The wide distribution of non-classical class I molecules on IEC suggests a unique role for these cells in the interface of innate and adaptive immunity in the GI tract. One hypothesis is that these molecules are involved in the activation of a series of regulatory T cells in the mucosal immune system. Alternatively, they may be involved in protective immune responses against luminal pathogens utilizing T cells with unique specificities. Regardless, the expression of all of the known restriction elements by IEC renders them capable of interacting with several T-cell subpopulations, potentially orchestrating mucosal homeostasis by activating or inhibiting mucosal immune responses.

Signals delivered via the restriction element–Ag complex involve the T-cell antigen receptor on the T-cell side (Fig. 4.1) and is only one part of a complex set of interactions between T cells and APCs. The TcR–restriction element–Ag complex interaction is described as signal 1 and is critical for specific T-cell activation. Alone, however, signal 1 is not optimal for priming and expansion of antigen-specific T cells. A second signal is required (cognate or cell contact dependent) for ultimate activation, with subsequent amplification dictated by non-cognate or cytokine factors. The following section describes the potential signal 2 interactions between T cells and IEC.

## CO-STIMULATORY MOLECULES

To generate a specific immune response, one needs to signal the T cell both through the TcR (MHC/peptide–signal 1) and through some form of co-stimulatory molecule (e.g. B7-1:CD28, CD40:CD40L – signal 2)[55-57] (Fig. 4.4). In the absence of signal 2, anergy ensues. There are several key co-stimulatory molecules that have been described in the systemic immune system. The initial co-stimulatory complex described involved two molecules (B7-1 and B7-2 – CD80/CD86) capable of interacting with CD28, a co-stimulatory molecule on T cells. Binding of CD28 promotes T-cell activation and cytokine production.[57] CD28 is constitutively expressed on all CD4+ T cells and roughly 50% of CD8+ T cells. A related CD28 family member, CTLA4, also binds to CD80 and CD86 but is induced after T-cell activation.[56] In contrast to CD28, CTLA4 inhibits T-cell activation by recruiting phosphatases into the TcR signaling complex, effectively shutting off critical kinase activity. CTLA4 has a higher affinity for CD80 and CD86, so in a cell expressing both molecules the inhibitory CTLA4-mediated response will be dominant. This may be the natural mechanism for downregulating a T-cell response after it has been activated. Although there appear to be differences between CD80 and CD86 in expression by different APC, differences in their function have been controversial (for example, it was thought for some time that CD80 was involved in the activation of Th1 responses, whereas CD86 was involved in the activation of Th2 responses; this is not absolute). However, it is clear that activation through the TcR results in anergy, in the absence of both CD80 and CD86. In the presence of either co-stimulatory molecule the T cell is 'rescued' from the anergic state. In normal IEC these co-stimulatory molecules are not expressed constitutively, raising further doubt as to the capacity of IEC to activate naive class II restricted CD4+ T cells. However, in memory T cells the absence of signal 2 may be less critical; these cells account for the majority of lymphocytes in the mucosal immune system away from lymphoid aggregates. In general, memory T cells are less rigorous in their requirement for activation. Induction of B7-2 (CD86) in UC suggests, at least in this disease, that IEC–CD4+ T-cell interactions might elicit an active immune response. Nakazawa et al.[58] demonstrated that this expression may be functionally significant, resulting in T-cell proliferation. In both UC and CD, CD80 and CD86 expression by professional APC in the lamina propria is increased, appearing to facilitate T-cell activation. However, these appear to be secondary events and may participate in disease perpetuation rather than induction.

More recently, additional members of the B7 family have been described (B7h[B7RP1, ICOS ligand] and B7H1 (PD1). These molecules bind to ligands on T cells similar to CD28 and CTLA4 (ICOS (inducible co-stimulator which, as the name implies, is activation dependent[59-61]) and PDL-1 and -2, respectively). Like CD28 and CTLA4, these ligands have stimulatory and inhibitory activities, respectively. The expression of B7h and B7H1 molecules on IEC had been studied in preliminary form only (Nakazawa et al., submitted) but they both appear to be expressed in normal and IBD epithelium. There is mRNA expression for the ligands of these co-stimulatory molecules (ICOS, PD1L) in IEL, but the level of protein expressed on the cell is modest. It is not clear whether these co-stimulatory molecules play a role in either normal IEC APC function or in IEC dysfunction in IBD.

Another potential co-stimulatory–adhesive interaction between the IEC and T cells can occur through CD58 (LFA-3 on the IEC) and CD2 (on the T cell). Hershberg's group reported that the CD58–CD2 interaction was critical for T-cell activation induced by the genetically engineered IEC line

A  Costimulatory signals are essential for T-cell activation

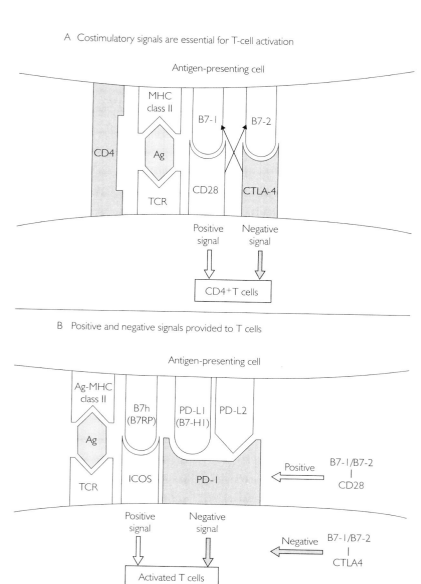

B  Positive and negative signals provided to T cells

**Fig. 4.4** Co-stimulatory molecule interactions between T cells and antigen-presenting cells. T cells are thought to be activated through a number of signals mediated by cell surface molecule interactions. Signal 1 has been used as the term indicating the interaction between the T-cell receptor and the MHC–peptide complex. Engagement of the antigen receptor alone leads to anergy. Amplifying or co-stimulatory signals are required to rescue the T cell from this anergic state. The most commonly described interaction involves CD28 on the T cell binding to either B7-1 (CD80) or B7-2 (CD86). CD28 binding allows for the optimal transcription of the IL-2 gene and cytokine synthesis (and T-cell proliferation and differentiation). A related molecule, CTLA4, is a CD28-regulated gene product that is transcribed several days after the initial T cell-activating event. Binding of CTLA4 by CD80 or CD86 results in an inhibition of TcR-mediated signaling by recruiting dephosphorylating enzymes (phosphatases) to the receptor and shutting off kinase activity important for the phosphorylation of DNA-binding proteins and transcription factors. CD40–CD40L is another important co-stimulatory complex. In the absence of CD40 ligand T-cell responses are defective and a poor antibody response ensues. CD40 is expressed on all professional APC but not on IEC. CD2–LFA-3 interactions may be particularly important for the activation of mucosal lymphocytes. Several groups have reported that CD2 ligation drives mucosal lymphocyte proliferation and cytokine production in the presence or absence of CD28 cross-linking. This may also allow for the non-specific expansion of mucosal lymphocytes. Newer B7 family members have recently been described. B7h (ICOS ligand) binds to ICOS on activated T cells and sends a positive signal to the nucleus (not unlike CD28 which, in contrast, is constitutively expressed). PDI (B7H1) on an APC binds to PD-L1 or PD-L2 that delivers a negative signal much like CTLA4. The functional significance of these newer co-stimulatory molecules has not been adequately addressed. It should be noted that other adhesive events (e.g. integrin interactions) probably deliver additional signals to T cells. It has been suggested that the combination of signals, as well as the strength of their interaction, dictates the nature of the T-cell response generated.

described earlier.[12] Others have shown that both IEL and LPL can proliferate in response to CD2 cross-linking (with or without concomitant CD28 cross-linking).[62–65] The CD2 signaling pathway has been noted to be dominant in mucosal lymphocytes, resulting in increased proliferation (these cells tend to be hyporesponsive) and cytokine secretion. This CD2-mediated signaling pathway can exist even in the absence of a TcR-mediated signal, although it is unclear whether such an event occurs in normal or diseased intestine. CD2 signaling is also associated with an increased susceptibility to Fas-mediated apoptosis, thus pointing to a possible regulatory role for IEC on the propensity for apoptosis of the lymphocytes that surround them. The decreased susceptibility of CD2-stimulated mucosal lymphocytes from IBD patients to undergo Fas-mediated apoptosis may be related to additional co-stimulatory signals that exist on IBD IEC, effects of other APC within the lamina propria or, as has already been demonstrated, to downstream signaling events (i.e. increased expression of anti-apoptotic proteins Bcl-2, an increased Bcl/Bax ratio in the mucosa, and decreased Bax expression in LPL).

The nature of signal 2 for IEC–T-cell interactions has not been clearly defined. Given the absence of CD80 and CD86, priming of naive CD4+ T cells is not likely to occur. The abundance of memory cells in the IEL and LPL compartments may render the expression of such molecules moot. The dominance of the CD2:CD58 pathway in mucosal T-cell activation is well described, and this fits well with the finding that CD58 is so abundantly expressed on IEC (as well as the data from Hershberg's group[66] documenting a requirement for a CD58–CD2 interaction in their CD4+ T-cell hybridoma activation system). Whether there is a defect in co-stimulatory pathways in mucosal lymphocytes in IBD that relates to IEC interactions has not been adequately explored. The limited data available at this time suggests that these pathways may amplify but do not initiate the inflammatory process in IBD.

## NON-COGNATE INTERACTIONS

The final component of the T-cell activation pathway is the recruitment and amplification step. This process generally involves the secretion of soluble mediators that augment the effects of signals 1 and 2. In general, the secretion of both IEC-derived chemokines and cytokines is increased in IBD, largely due to enhanced bacterial translocation and IFN-γ production. Enhancement of secretion of macrophage/dendritic cell and T-cell directed chemokines will increase mucosal inflammation. Altered production of suppressive cytokines, along with an upregulation of proinflammatory cytokines, may allow for the persistence of mucosal inflammation. It is evident that these events occur in IBD. How they play a role in T-cell–IEC interactions is another poorly explored area.

# CHEMOKINES PRODUCED BY IEC THAT ENHANCE T-CELL INTERACTIONS

One additional mechanism whereby the IEC can promote T-cell activation in the GALT is by producing factors that can attract T cells (directly or indirectly) into the local microenvironment (chemotaxis) and activate them once they get there. A list of such chemokines produced by IEC is given in Table 4.1. Many chemokines produced by IEC following bacterial infection are chemotactic for macrophages and dendritic cells. If these cells are recruited to the subepithelial layers they can then interact with T cells and promote inflammation. T cell-specific chemokines are limited in number. RANTES, secreted predominantly by macrophages, can be produced by human IEC as well.[67] RANTES may have a role in innate as well as adaptive mucosal immunity[68] and, interestingly, increased RANTES expression has been demonstrated in UC mucosa.[69] Other specific chemokines are seen at sites of high IFN-γ production. The CXC chemokines, monokine induced by interferon-γ (MIG), interferon-γ inducible protein 10 (IP-10) (this chemokine appears to promote Th1 responses and may therefore be relevant in CD tissues) and I-TAC are constitutively expressed by human colonic IEC. Their expression and polarized basolateral secretion increase after IFN-γ stimulation. Importantly, fresh human IEL, as well as CD4+ Th1 lymphocytes, express CXCR3, the common receptor for these chemokines. By attracting CD4+ Th1 cells that produce IFN-γ, upregulation of expression and secretion of CXC chemokines occurs, as IEC express IFN-γ receptors, thereby contributing to a positive feedback loop that may be relevant in inflammatory states, specifically IBD. In contrast to the 'inflammation-related' CXCR3 receptor, a 'tissue-specific' chemokine receptor, CCR9, is constitutively expressed on small bowel IEL and LPL.[70–72] Its ligand TECK (thymus-expressed chemokine – CCL25) is differentially expressed in the small bowel mucosa in the jejunal and ileal epithelium, especially in the crypts of Lieberkuhn, with decreasing levels of expression as one moves up the crypt/villus axis.[71–74] Svensson et al.[75] suggested that the function of CCL25/CCR9 expression in vivo might be the selective localization of MLN-activated CD8αβ+ lymphocytes, coexpressing $\alpha_E\beta_7$ to the small intestine, at least in a murine model. This demonstrated for the first time an in vivo function of a GALT-specific chemokine–chemokine receptor pair expressed on IEC and mucosal lymphocytes, respectively. These, as well as previous data, also suggested that the coordinated expression of chemokine receptors and mucosal homing molecules such as $\alpha_E\beta_7$ may serve as specific addresses

for mucosally activated lymphocytes, differentiating small intestinal from colonic immune responses. In inflamed small bowel of CD patients there is increased TECK expression on IEC, with decreased LPL CCR9 and increased PBL CCR9 expression.[71] These data support a potential role for this chemokine–chemokine receptor pair in the immunopathogenesis of IBD.

Another lymphocyte-attracting chemokine that is secreted by IEC is fractalkine. This unique chemokine, combining the properties of chemokines and adhesion molecules, attracts NK cells, monocytes and CD8+ T lymphocytes and, to a lesser extent, CD4+ T lymphocytes which express the specific receptor CX3CR1.[76] Fractalkine mRNA is expressed in small intestinal human IEC and its expression is significantly increased in CD. Interestingly, fractalkine staining of IEC parallels the mRNA expression pattern and shows polarization to the basolateral surface in active CD.[77] Muelhoefer et al.[77] also showed that activated human IEL were attracted to fractalkine in vitro, suggesting that this chemokine and its receptor may have a functional role in mucosal immunity and immunopathology. Pan et al.[78] described another chemokine produced by colonic IEC as well as its receptors MEC-CCR3/CC310. CD4+ memory lymphocytes and eosinophils are attracted in vitro by this chemokine, but its function in vivo has not yet been demonstrated. The existence of tissue-specific chemokines that are secreted by IEC suggests that this cell may play a key role in directing and segregating mucosal immune responses.

A CC chemokine, MDC/CCL2, which is constitutively expressed and secreted by colonic IEC, is unique in that it attracts CCR4+ Th2 cytokine-producing lymphocytes. Not surprisingly, polarized basolateral secretion of MDC/CCL2 from stimulated colonic IEC lines has been reported.[79] The specific recruitment of lymphocytes that preferentially secrete anti-inflammatory cytokines supports a role for the IEC in orchestrating normal mucosal homeostasis and adds to the accumulating data on these cells' ability to regulate mucosal immune responses.

Finally, a CC chemokine that attracts immature dendritic cells, MIP3α, is also expressed and produced by human small intestinal (mainly in the FAE)[80,81] and colonic IEC, and has been suggested to be the mediator of lymphocyte adhesion to the $\alpha_4\beta_7$ ligand MAdCAM-1. MIP3α expression and secretion are increased in colonic IBD IEC[82] and, as was shown for some of the previously mentioned chemokines, its stimulated secretion is polarized to the basolateral compartment. Mucosal memory T cells as well as IEC express CCR6, the cognate receptor for MIP3α. The interesting observation that CCR6 as well as CCR9 are coexpressed in T cells with the $\alpha_4\beta_7$ integrin, characteristic of mucosal lymphocytes, may suggest that in inflammatory states, and to some extent in the normal state, MIP3α and TECK expression by IEC attracts CCR9+ or CCR6+ lymphocytes that are activated in MLN, enter the peripheral blood, and then are recruited to the intestinal mucosa where they undergo activation-induced apoptosis or differentiation.

What has not been addressed here is the role of the IEC in regulating innate immune responses. The initial description of chemokine production by IEC involved the study of neutrophil chemokines IL-8, GROα and ENA-78.[83–85] These should be carefully considered when evaluating the role of the IEC in maintaining intestinal homeostasis rather than contributing to the immunopathology of IBD (see Chapter 3). Clearly there is a major interface between the innate and adaptive immune

## Table 4.1 Chemokines expressed/secreted by intestinal epithelial cells

| Chemokine | Expression/secretion | Comments/references |
|---|---|---|
| ENA 78 Epithelial–neutrophil activating protein 78 | Upregulated expression and basolateral secretion after bacterial stimulation-Caco2, HT29, Fresh normal colon IEC (Kim Clin Exp Immunol 2001 123:421–427) | Neutrophil chemoattraction |
| GRO Growth related oncogene | Upregulated expression and basolateral secretion after bacterial stimulation (Kim) | Neutrophil chemoattraction HT29 constitutively express GRO-a mRNA (Kim) |
| IL-8/CXCL8 | Low constitutive expression and secretion by fresh human colonic and small bowel IEC (Daig R, Gut 2000 46:350–58), Panja JI 1998;161:3675–3684) Upregulated expression and basolateral secretion after bacterial stimulation (Kim) | Neutrophil chemoattraction IEC cell lines – constitutive (HT29) and induced (HT29, Caco 2, T84) expression and basolateral secretion of IL-8 (Kim) (Eckmann Microbes and Infection 2001;3:1191–1200). |
| RANTES | Freshly isolated IEC, Caco2, HT29. Increased expression after S typhimurium and cytokine stimulation | Secreted also by IEL Gastro 1997;113:1214 Ligand CCR1/CCR5 |
| CCL25 (TECK) | Human and murine small intestinal IEC | CCR9 expressed on LPL and IEL, co-expression of mucosal homing molecules $\alpha_4\beta_7$, $\alpha_E\beta_7$. |
| MCP1 Monocyte Chemoattractant Protein 1 | mRNA expression induced in Caco2 by IL-1b and by non-pathogenic bacteria in the presence of PBMC (Haller Gut 2000 47:79–87), Secretion from Caco2 cells after IL-1$\beta$ and TNF-$\alpha$ stimulation, small amounts secreted from freshly isolated normal IEC, increased secretion after IL-1$\beta$ stimulation (Kucharzik Clin Exp Immunol 1998;111:152–157), | |
| CCL28 | Small intestinal IEC | CCR10 is the receptor for CCL28 (Wang JBC 2000:275;22313) |
| Fractalkine (Muelhoefer JI 2000 164 3368-3376) | Human small intestinal IEC and endothelial cells | The receptor is CX3CR1, expressed on activated IEL subset, NK, monocytes, CD8+ (CD4+low) Fractalkine mRNA is upregulated in active CD |
| MEC | Normal colon IEC – constitutive expression. Low & variable expression in small intestinal IEC | Receptors – CCR3, CCR10. MEC attracts memory lymphocytes and eosinophils. CCR10 is expressed in colon, Peyer's patches, stomach – Berin AJP 2001 280 G1217 |
| MDC/CCL22 | Normal human colon IEC | Receptor-CCR4 |
| MIP2 (GRO$\beta$) | When expressed in mice IEC attract neutrophils to small and large bowel, induce increased LPL/IEL | No constitutive/expression in normal human IEC, expressed in murine IEC after LPS/proinflammatory cytokine stimulation |
| MIP3a/CCL20/LARC | Human small bowel and colon IEC | Receptor-CCR6 on CD45RO lymphocytes and immature DCs. |
| IP10/CXCL10 | Human IEC. Induced by IFN-$\gamma$ | Receptor – CXCR3 – on Th1 cells and human IEL |
| MIG/CXCL9 | Human IEC. Induced by IFN -$\gamma$ | Receptor – CXCR3 – on Th1 cells and human IEL |
| ITAC/CCL11 | Human IEC. Induced by IFN -$\gamma$ | Receptor – CXCR3 – on Th1 cells and human IEL |

systems, and it is this that helps maintain controlled inflammation in the normal state but contributes to the uncontrolled inflammatory state that is IBD.

# CYTOKINES PRODUCED BY IEC THAT ENHANCE T-CELL INTERACTIONS

Equally as important as chemokines are the cytokines produced by IEC that may also play a role in the expansion or differentiation of mucosal lymphocytes. These include factors that promote (e.g. IL-6) as well as suppress (eg. IL-10, TGF-$\beta$) T-cell activation.[48,86–95] A full listing of cytokines produced by IEC is given in Table 4.2. In IBD the secretion of all these cytokines is generally increased.

## T CELL-ACTIVATING CYTOKINES

The accessory cytokine IL-6 is produced constitutively by freshly isolated human IEC[96] as well as by normal and malignant, non-stimulated and stimulated intestinal epithelial cell lines.[86–91] This cytokine promotes T-cell growth and B- and T-cell differentia-

tion. IL-6 levels are increased in the serum of IBD patients (CD, UC) and may contribute to the acute-phase response (i.e. CRP, increased fibrinogen, $\alpha_2$-macroglobulin), hypoalbuminemia, complement activation, hypergammaglobulinemia etc. seen in these diseases. Whether this multifunctional cytokine is secreted via the epithelial apical surface after neutrophil-derived stimulus, where it is capable of neutrophil activation, as has been demonstrated by Sitaraman et al.,[97] or may be secreted also basolaterally, remains to be determined. Preliminary studies suggest that interference with IL-6 activity (anti-IL-6 mAb therapy) ameliorates disease. Such studies are preliminary and are undergoing larger-scale trials. Whether the increased IL-6 levels seen in IBD patients are purely a reflection of IEC stores is unlikely. The major source of IL-6 is still macrophages, and such activated cells are plentiful in the lamina propria of IBD patients.

The common $\gamma c$ receptor cytokines IL-7 and IL-15 have also been reported to be produced by IEC.[98,99] Both cytokines have the capacity to promote the growth of mucosal lymphocytes. IL-7 was initially described as a pre-B cell growth factor, but its major role in thymocyte proliferation has become increasingly recognized. Interestingly, several groups have suggested that the GI tract, especially the intestinal epithelium, might be an

**Table 4.2 Cytokines expressed/secreted by intestinal epithelial cells**

| Cytokine | Expression/secretion | Comments/references |
|---|---|---|
| IL-1β | Induced in Caco2 by non-pathogenic bacteria in the presence of PBMCs (Haller Gut 2000 47:79–87) | No evidence that normal IEC produce IL-1. They do produce IL-1RA |
| IL-6 | IL-6 expression and secretion by fresh human IEC, upregulated by IL-1β (Panja Clin Exp Immunol 1995:100:298–305) expression in normal human enterocytes (Jones 1993 J Clin Pathol 46:1097–1110) and by stimulated IEC lines (McGee 1993 JI 151:970–978, Weinstein Infect Immun 1997 65:395–404) | |
| IL-7 | Expressed in fresh human IEC and cell lines (Madrigal Estebas Hum Immunol 1997;58:83–90) | Functional IL-7 receptor on fresh human IEC and colonic cell lines (Reinecker PNAS 1995;92:8353–8357) |
| IL-15 | Expressed in fresh human IEC cell lines (Reinecker Gastroenterology 1996;111:1706–1713) Important in CD8+ T cell expansion | Functional IL-15 receptors expressed by human IEC (Reinecker PNAS) |
| TNFα | Induced in Caco2 by non-pathogenic bacteria in the presence of PBMCs (Haller Gut 2000 47:79–87) | Little evidence for production of this cytokine by freshly isolated human or murine IEC |
| TGFβ | mRNA expression induced in Caco2 by bacteria (Haller Gut 2000 47:79–87 Produced by rat cell lines and upregulated by wounding of the monolayer | Little evidence for production of this cytokine by freshly isolated human or murine IEC |
| IL-10 | Produced following cross-linking of CD1d on the IEC surface in cell lines | |
| IL-18 | Produced by human and murine IEC. Increased in CD lesions. Absence of ICE prevents intracellular conversion to active form of cytokine | IL-18 binding protein- expressed by macrophages and upregulated in CD (Corbaz JI 2002;168:3608–16) |
| GMCSF | Produced by normal IEC and cell lines constitutively | |

extrathymic site of T-cell development. This was suggested after the presence of IEL (nearly 100% T cells) was noted in athymic mice, and genes encoding recombinases (RAG), critical for the generation of antigen receptors, were detected in the gut as well. IEL are notoriously difficult to activate, yet two groups simultaneously reported (in mouse and human) that these cells would proliferate in the presence of IL-7.[100,101] Consistent with these observations were the findings that there is a marked deficiency of IEL in either IL-7 or IL-7R knockout mice, and that IL-7 is a growth factor specifically for γδTCR CD8+ T cells, which are enriched among murine IEL.[102,103] The expression and secretion of IL-7 were detected in freshly isolated human small intestinal IEC as well as colonic tumor cell lines. The expression of functional IL-7R on colonic tumor epithelial cell lines, and on fresh human IEC, was demonstrated in earlier studies.

IL-15, in contrast, has been shown to be more selective, being involved mostly in CD8+ T-cell activation and NK T-cell differentiation.[104–106] IL-15 uses the IL-2Rβ and γ chains (the common γ chain used by IL-2, IL-4, IL-7, IL-9, IL-13 and IL-15Rs) but has a unique α chain. IL-15-deficient mice exhibit a defect in NK T-cell development and, like the IL-2 knockout, develop colitis (milder than in the IL-2–/– mouse).[107] Recent data suggest that IL-15 may be involved in the expansion of a population of CD8αα regulatory T cells. The absence of IL-15 may have repercussions in terms of regulatory T-cell activation, leading to a dysregulated immune response analogous to that seen in IBD. IL-15 expression was demonstrated in freshly isolated human IEC as well as in epithelial cell lines. Moreover, IEC also express functional receptors for IL-15 (common γc IL-2 receptor). IL-15 affects both T- and B-cell differentiation as well as IEC proliferation and migration (through TGF-β expression), and thus restitution.

IL-18 production by IEC has also been reported.[108] IL-18 possesses activities similar to those seen with IL-12 (enhances IFN-γ production). Interestingly, production of this cytokine

(IL-18) is increased in IBD. However, IL-18 is produced in a pro-form and requires processing by IL-1 converting enzyme (ICE), a factor that is not produced by IEC. The 24 kDa pro-form is inactive, and only upon cleavage to the 18 kDa form is the cytokine functionally active. Thus the role that IL-18 derived from IEC plays in either normal mucosal homeostasis or in IBD has not been clarified.

## T-CELL INHIBITORY CYTOKINES

Reports of cytokines secreted by IEC that inhibit T-cell activation, such as TGF-β, have been inconsistent.[93–95] TGF-β is the most potent immunosuppressive molecule known. In the GI tract it appears to serve several purposes:

1. Suppressing local immune responses to luminal antigens;
2. Promoting the production of the mucosal immunoglobulin secretory IgA (promotes an isotype switch from IgM to IgA);[109]
3. Enhancing barrier function.

In rat cell lines TGF-β is not only produced but is also critical to the maintenance of the epithelial barrier[94] (epithelial restitution). Malignant human IEC lines produce significant amounts of TGF-β as well, but there is little evidence that this cytokine is produced either in vivo or in vitro by normal IEC. Some groups have suggested that TGF-β may serve as a growth factor for some regulatory T cells, although the evidence for this is limited. Treatment of DC with TGF-β in the presence of antigen can enhance the activation of regulatory T cells after DC–T-cell interactions. Genetic deletion of TGF-β results in neonatal death, so the role that this cytokine plays in these processes is not easily explored.

IL-10, in contrast, can be produced by IEC (mRNA and protein).[48] Most recently one group reported that IL-10 secretion ensued following cross-linking of CD1d on the IEC surface.[48] This would occur during T-cell activation by IEC and may help to promote the generation of regulatory Tr1 cells (IL-10 secreting).[110] IL-10 inhibits APC function by inhibiting class II and co-stimulatory molecule expression. With its potential role in Treg activation this cytokine is well suited for mucosal sites. IL-10−/− mice develop colitis, and treatment of these mice with bacterially engineered (IL-10 expressing) normal luminal flora abrogates the intestinal inflammation.[3,111–113] Thus local IL-10 production may be critical for maintenance of intestinal homeostasis. As with IL-6 there are a large number of cell types that are able to produce IL-10. The actual contribution by IEC to the mucosal pool of IL-10 is unknown. However, it is intriguing to speculate on the potential of IEC-derived IL-10 to keep mucosal inflammation in check.

## NORMAL T CELL–IEC INTERACTIONS

We have focused on describing the molecules involved in the potential interaction of IEC with local T-cell populations, with a large number of cell surface molecules expressed by IEC that support this concept. However, most of the data regarding the actual interactions reflect in vitro findings, as it has been difficult to develop in vivo models to test the actual existence of a T-cell–IEC relationship.

The first studies to address this issue used freshly isolated cells from mouse, rat and human. These studies had in common the findings that IEC could present soluble Ag to T cells. However, the outcome of this interaction was different in each of the studies. In the mouse, Kaiserlian showed that IEC could present OVA peptides to Ag-specific CD4+ murine T-cell hybridomas (although the level of activation was less than that seen with conventional APC).[10,114] Bland et al.[115] in the rat and Mayer et al. in the human[116] showed that IEC could present Ag (OVA, tetanus, alloantigens) to T cells, but the proliferating cells in these experiments were CD8+. Functionally these cells were capable of suppressing immune responses; in the rat the suppression was Ag specific, whereas in humans it was Ag non-specific. The human studies were extended to show that the IEC–CD8+ T-cell interactions involved the CD8 molecule itself (activating the CD8-associated kinase p56 lck), a novel CD8 ligand, gp180, and the class Ib molecule CD1d.[45,49,50,117,118] CD1d and gp180 form a complex on the IEC surface which appears to be critical for CD8+ T-cell activation.[50] This serves an important purpose. As described above, normal T-cell activation involves the engagement of the TcR as well as a series of co-stimulatory molecules. To optimally provide signal 1 the MHC–peptide complex binds to the TcR as well as an accessory molecule CD4 (in the case of class II) or CD8 (in the case of class I), forming what has been termed the coreceptor complex. Engagement of the TcR/CD4 (or 8) complex on the T cell triggers the phosphorylation of key kinases that eventually deliver a signal into the nucleus stating that the appropriate Ag/MHC match has been made.[119] As with conventional co-stimulatory molecules (CD80/CD86), the absence of kinase (in the case of CD4 and CD8 it is p56lck) activation induced by the ligation of CD4 or 8 results in an aborted T-cell signal. These cells will then undergo apoptosis. CD1d can present novel Ag to the TcR, but alone does not appear to bind to CD8 and fails to establish a coreceptor complex formation on the T cell. The

CD1d–gp180 complex looks more class I-like, as CD1d can cross-link the TcR while gp180 cross-linksCD8 on the suppressor T-cell surface. gp180 binds to CD8 at sites that are distinct from those where MHC class I binds, so there is no competition between the two molecules.[118] The antigens presented by CD1d have not been elucidated, but studies from several groups suggest that this restriction element binds lipids or glycolipid Ag. There is recent evidence that the suppressor/regulatory T cells activated by IEC (via CD1d–gp180 interactions) are restricted in their repertoire and phenotypically distinct. IEC-activated T cells are CD8+, CD28−, CD101+ CD103+, and perforin and granzyme negative (non-cytolytic-terminal the cell).[49] They inhibit in an Ag non-specific manner, although they appear to be Ag driven with a limited TcR repertoire. This is consistent with the fact that CD1d is non-polymorphic and the Ag-binding groove is limited in its structure in terms of conventional Ag binding. It would be logical to assume that the source of the Ag would be luminal, quite possibly bacterial, in origin. CD1d expression is greater in the colon than in the small bowel, so bacterial products or bacteria themselves may have something to do with its expression.[39,40,120]

Normal IEC–T-cell interactions via surface molecules other than MHC class I or II, E-cadherin or CD1d was demonstrated in a mouse model by Yamamoto et al.[121] Here, IEC rendered IEL, but not splenic T cells, hypoproliferative and decreased cytokine secretion by IEL. This effect was contact dependent and was not demonstrated upon contact between thymocytes and IEC. An IEC regulatory effect specific to the GALT was therefore demonstrated. The inability to block this effect by antibodies to the restriction elements mentioned above or to TGF-β points to the possible existence of other surface molecules that may be responsible for this regulatory effect.

Thus in vitro data suggest that the cell surface and cytokine interactions proposed in the earlier sections may indeed be functional. However, there are no current data supporting a role of normal IEC in T-cell activation or regulation in vivo.

## IEC–T-CELL INTERACTIONS IN IBD

An indirect way to look for a role of the IEC in vivo would be to identify a disease with a notable defect in IEC function. As mentioned earlier, epithelial cells isolated from areas of active inflammation in patients with IBD express class II Ag at levels higher than that seen in normal control IEC.[6,122–127] Even at sites where inflammation is less apparent, class II molecule expression is greater than in normal controls. Furthermore, in UC, CD86 expression has been noted, suggesting that the class II-expressing IEC may be functionally capable of activating CD4+ T cells.[58] This was tested directly using the system described above (IEC–T-cell cocultures). In contrast to the activation of CD8+ regulatory T cells seen with normal IEC–T-cell cocultures, CD4+ T cell proliferation was noted.[128] This did not appear to relate solely to the increase in class II Ag expressed on these cells, as non-IBD inflammatory control IEC (expressing comparable levels of class II) activated CD8+ T cells comparably to normal IEC. Toy et al.[129] demonstrated that IBD IEC failed to express the CD8 ligand gp180 (Crohn's) or expressed it in an aberrant form (UC-apical expression only). Furthermore, IBD IEC fail to express CD1d both in areas of active inflammation as well as non-involved areas (Perera et al., submitted). Thus two key components involved in the activation of TrE cells are lacking in IBD IEC. Activation of CD4+ T cells by IBD IEC is class II restricted (mAbs to class II block proliferation and cytokine production) and results in the production of IFN-γ at levels that are comparable to those seen by T cells activated with conventional APC (monocytes/dendritic cells). Although this is not likely to be the only source of IFN-γ produced by mucosal T cells, it may contribute to the perpetuation of the inflammation in actively involved areas.

One key question that remains is why, if the defect in class II, gp180 and CD1d expression is global, do we see restricted patterns of disease in IBD (e.g. segmental colitis and skip lesions in CD, left sided vs. pancolitis in UC)? Clearly there are other factors involved in the initiation of disease activity. One possible mechanism may relate to the secretion of mediators that are localized to specific areas. As alluded to above, chemokines such as TECK may be secreted solely by small bowel IEC, whereas others such as MDC/CCL2 are secreted mainly by colonic IEC. This, combined with specific CD4+ T lymphocyte subsets that express the reciprocal receptors such as CCR9 (whose expression in IBD is increased),[72] may explain how local disease ensues. Another likely explanation is that luminal factors play a role. One need only look at the occurrence of pouchitis following ileoanal pullthrough in UC. Although the small bowel is rarely if ever involved in UC, pouchitis is a local inflammatory process that is bacterially mediated. A defect in epithelial cell presentation of the newly established anaerobic microbiota in the pouch may be sufficient to drive uncontrolled inflammation.

Does one need IEC-expressed class II to develop IBD? The answer to this question is unknown in humans, but a murine model suggests that this may not be the case. MHC class II–/– mice develop mild colitis,[3] which may reflect specific bacterial infections versus defects in the generation of T regulatory cells. However, in this case the absence of class II on IEC does not inhibit the development of colitis. Clearly, this is not a normal scenario and it is difficult to extrapolate it to human disease. Indeed, in an immunodeficiency syndrome, bare lymphocyte syndrome, where class II is absent owing to a defect in the gene encoding CIITA, no colitis is seen.[130]

## T-CELL FACTORS THAT AFFECT IEC

Thus far we have focused on the role of IEC in activating T cells. Clearly this interaction can be reciprocal, and there is strong evidence that T cells can influence epithelial cell phenotype and function. In the normal murine GI tract IEL have been shown to produce KGF1, a factor that promotes epithelial cell growth.[131,132] Epithelial cells express receptors for a number of cytokines. TGF-β is an immunosuppressive cytokine but also aids in epithelial restitution and repair.[94] Conversely, IFN-γ generally decreases barrier function, either alone or in combination with TNF.[133,134] IFN-γ increases the expression of class II molecules that may help promote CD4+ T-cell activation and inflammation in IBD. Studies by MacDonald's group, using fetal gut organ explants, have shown that activating T cells in the biopsies (by mitogen or αCD3) induce crypt hyperplasia and villus shortening.[135–138] In IL-10-deficient mice, one of the earliest histologic abnormalities noted is branching crypts, potential evidence that some of these cytokines have effects on epithelial cell differentiation (IEC express IL-10Rs). In the

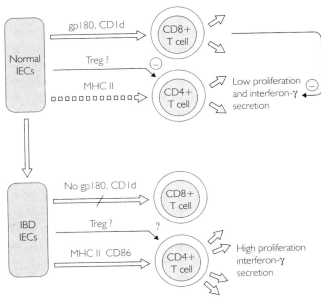

IEC:CD4+ T-cell interaction: suggested model

Fig. 4.5 Hypothetical model of the role of the IEC in the pathogenesis of IBD. Normal intestinal epithelial cells express many restriction elements that might be capable of activating a number of selected T-cell subpopulations. From in vitro studies, when normal IEC are used as an antigen-presenting cell there is a selective activation of CD8+ CD28– regulatory (suppressor) T cells. This activation is regulated by two cell surface molecules, the class Ib molecule CD1d and the novel CD8 ligand gp180. Normal IEC are capable of activating CD4+ T cells through their class II molecules, but the level of activation is much lower than a conventional APC. In IBD there is both a defect in the expression of gp180 (absent in Crohn's and an apically sorted form only in UC). CD1d expression is similarly depressed. In the absence of these signals regulatory CD8+ T cells are not generated and the increased expression of MHC class II on IEC that is seen in these diseases allows for vigorous activation of CD4+ T cells capable of secreting proinflammatory cytokines.

absence of critical T cell-derived cytokines normal IEC differentiation may fail to be achieved.

## SUMMARY

In many ways IEC may play a critical role in the initiation and perpetuation of IBD. Defects in barrier function are associated with colitis in mice (N cadherin dominant negative, ITF knockout, MDR1–/–),[139–141] and permeability defects in Crohn's disease have been described. The epithelial cell is also a bridge between innate and adaptive immunity, expressing molecules involved in NK-cell activation, possibly TLRs (innate immunity) as well as those involved in T-cell activation (e.g. MHC class II, class Ib, CD58). Thus one could propose a model where the IEC is the central regulator of mucosal inflammation. No testable model has been developed to date and we are left with a series of intriguing in vitro observations that point towards the central role that the IEC might play. In the normal state the IEC appear to promote more of a regulatory environment. In IBD either primary or secondary defects alter the ability of the IEC to promote suppression. Figure 4.5 depicts a hypothetical model as to how the IEC might function in IBD and the mechanisms involved in the dysfunction seen in IBD (e.g. absence of p180, lack of class Ib molecules). In the absence of controlled immune responses the IEC can participate in promoting active immunity to luminal antigens. This model needs to be explored in in vivo systems. If the in vitro data define an in vivo phenomenon, then novel approaches to therapy, targeting the IEC, will ensue.

# REFERENCES

1. Dieleman LA, Pena AS, Meuwissen SG, van Rees EP. Role of animal models for the pathogenesis and treatment of inflammatory bowel disease. Scand J Gastroenterol 1997;223( Suppl):99–104.

2. Louis E, Belaiche J. Experimental models of inflammatory bowel disease. Acta Gastroenterol Belg 1994;57:306–309.

3. Podolsky DK. Lessons from genetic models of inflammatory bowel disease. Acta Gastroenterol Belg 1997;60:163–165.

4. Sartor RB. Review article: How relevant to human inflammatory bowel disease are current animal models of intestinal inflammation? Aliment Pharmacol Ther 1997;11 (Suppl 3):89–96; discussion 96–87.

5. Mason DW, Dallman M, Barclay AN. Graft-versus-host disease induces expression of Ia antigen in rat epidermal cells and gut epithelium. Nature 1981;293:150–151.

6. Selby WS, Janossy G, Mason DY, Jewell DP. Expression of HLA-DR antigens by colonic epithelium in inflammatory bowel disease. Clin Exp Immunol 1983;53:614–618.

7. Momburg F, Moller P. Non-co-ordinate expression of HLA-DR antigens and invariant chain. Immunology 1988;63:551–553.

8. Ouellette AJ, Frederick D, Hagen SJ, Katz JD. Class II antigen-associated invariant chain mRNA in mouse small intestine. Biochem Biophys Res Commun 1991;179:1642–1648.

9. Sanderson IR, Ouellette AJ, Carter EA, Harmatz PR. Ontogeny of class II MHC mRNA in the mouse small intestinal epithelium. Mol Immunol 1992;29:1257–1263.

10. Kaiserlian D, Vidal K, Revillard JP. Murine enterocytes can present soluble antigen to specific class II-restricted CD4+ T cells. Eur J Immunol 1989;19:1513–1516.

11. Hershberg RM, Cho DH, Youakim A et al. Highly polarized HLA class II antigen processing and presentation by human intestinal epithelial cells. J Clin Invest 1998;102:792–803.

12. Hershberg RM, Blumberg RS. What's so (Co)stimulating about the intestinal epithelium? Gastroenterology 1999;117:726–728.

13. Gonnella PA, Neutra MR. Membrane-bound and fluid-phase macromolecules enter separate prelysosomal compartments in absorptive cells of suckling rat ileum. J Cell Biol 1984;99:909–917.

14. Gonnella PA, Wilmore DW. Co-localization of class II antigen and exogenous antigen in the rat enterocyte. J Cell Sci 1993;106:937–940.

15. Brandeis JM, Sayegh MH, Gallon L, Blumberg RS, Carpenter CB. Rat intestinal epithelial cells present major histocompatibility complex allopeptides to primed T cells. Gastroenterology 1994;107:1537–1542.

16. So AL, Small G, Sperber K et al. Factors affecting antigen uptake by human intestinal epithelial cell lines. Dig Dis Sci 2000;45:1130–1147.

17. Laiping So A, Pelton-Henrion K, Small G et al. Antigen uptake and trafficking in human intestinal epithelial cells. Dig Dis Sci 2000;45:1451–1461.

18. Lankat-Buttgereit B, Tampe R. The transporter associated with antigen processing: function and implications in human diseases. Physiol Rev 2002;82:187–204.

19. van Niel G, Raposo G, Candalh C et al. Intestinal epithelial cells secrete exosome-like vesicles. Gastroenterology 2001;121:337–349.

20. Karlsson M, Lundin S, Dahlgren U, Kahu H, Pettersson I, Telemo E. 'Tolerosomes' are produced by intestinal epithelial cells. Eur J Immunol 2001;31:2892–2900.

21. Vezys V, Olson S, Lefrancois L. Expression of intestine-specific antigen reveals novel pathways of CD8 T cell tolerance induction. Immunity 2000;12:505–514.

22. Kim SK, Reed DS, Heath WR, Carbone F, Lefrancois L. Activation and migration of CD8 T cells in the intestinal mucosa. J Immunol 1997;159:4295–4306.

23. Anelli R, Placido R, Sambuy Y, Bach S, Di Massimo A, Colizzi V. Cytotoxic activity of human lymphocytes against differentiated intestinal tumour cell lines. Immunology 1993;78:166–169.

24. Dutronc Y, Porcelli SA. The CD1 family and T cell recognition of lipid antigens. Tissue Antigens 2002;60:337–353.

25. Kronenberg M, Gapin L. The unconventional lifestyle of NKT cells. Nature Rev Immunol 2002;2:557–568.

26. Borrego F, Ulbrecht M, Weiss EH, Coligan JE, Brooks AG. Recognition of human histocompatibility leukocyte antigen (HLA)-E complexed with HLA class I signal sequence-derived peptides by CD94/NKG2 confers protection from natural killer cell-mediated lysis. J Exp Med 1998;187:813–818.

27. Braud VM, Allan DS, O'Callaghan CA et al. HLA-E binds to natural killer cell receptors CD94/NKG2A, B and C. Nature 1998;391:795–799.

28. Geraghty DE, Stockschleader M, Ishitani A, Hansen JA. Polymorphism at the HLA-E locus predates most HLA-A and -B polymorphism. Hum Immunol 1992;33:174–184.

29. Grimsley C, Ober C. Population genetic studies of HLA-E: evidence for selection. Hum Immunol 1997;52:33–40.

30. Koller BH, Geraghty DE, Shimizu Y, DeMars R, Orr HT. HLA-E. A novel HLA class I gene expressed in resting T lymphocytes. J Immunol 1988;141:897–904.

31. Lee N, Goodlett DR, Ishitani A, Marquardt H, Geraghty DE. HLA-E surface expression depends on binding of TAP-dependent peptides derived from certain HLA class I signal sequences. J Immunol 1998;160:4951–4960.

32. Lee N, Llano M, Carretero M et al. HLA-E is a major ligand for the natural killer inhibitory receptor CD94/NKG2A. Proc Natl Acad Sci USA 1998;95:5199–5204.

33. Llano M, Lee N, Navarro F et al. HLA-E-bound peptides influence recognition by inhibitory and triggering CD94/NKG2 receptors: preferential response to an HLA-G-derived nonamer. Eur J Immunol 1998;28:2854–2863.

34. Lopez-Botet M, Llano M, Navarro F, Bellon T. NK cell ecognition of non-classic HLA class I molecules. Semin Immunol 200;12:109–119.

35. Wei XH, Orr HT. Differential expression of HLA-E, HLA-F, and HLA-G transcripts in human tissue. Hum Immunol 1990;29:131–142.

36. Groh V, Bahram S, Bauer S, Herman A, Beauchamp M, Spies T. Cell stress-regulated human major histocompatibility complex class I gene expressed in gastrointestinal epithelium. Proc Natl Acad Sci USA 1996;93:12445–12450.

37. Groh V, Steinle A, Bauer S, Spies T. Recognition of stress-induced MHC molecules by intestinal epithelial gammadelta T cells. Science 1998;279:1737–1740.

38. Hershberg R, Eghtesady P, Sydora B et al. Expression of the thymus leukemia antigen in mouse intestinal epithelium. Proc Natl Acad Sci USA 1990;87:9727–9731.

39. Bleicher PA, Balk SP, Hagen SJ, Blumberg RS, Flotte TJ, Terhorst C. Expression of murine CD1 on gastrointestinal epithelium. Science 1990;250:679–682.

40. Balk SP, Burke S, Polischuk JE et al. Beta 2-microglobulin-independent MHC class Ib molecule expressed by human intestinal epithelium. Science 1994;265:259–262.

41. Somnay-Wadgaonkar K, Nusrat A, Kim HS et al. Immunolocalization of CD1d in human intestinal epithelial cells and identification of a beta2-microglobulin-associated form. Int Immunol 1999;11:383–392.

42. Rodionov DG, Nordeng TW, Kongsvik TL, Bakke O. The cytoplasmic tail of CD1d contains two overlapping basolateral sorting signals. J Biol Chem 2000;275:8279–8282.

43. Kim HS, Garcia J, Exley M, Johnson KW, Balk SP, Blumberg RS. Biochemical characterization of CD1d expression in the absence of beta2-microglobulin. J Biol Chem 1999;274:9289–9295.

44. Zeng Z, Castano AR, Segelke BW, Stura EA, Peterson PA, Wilson IA. Crystal structure of mouse CD1: An MHC-like fold with a large hydrophobic binding groove. Science 1997;277:339–345.

45. Panja A, Blumberg RS, Balk SP, Mayer L. CD1d is involved in T cell–intestinal epithelial cell interactions. J Exp Med 1993;178:1115–1119.

46. Roberts AI, Blumberg RS, Christ AD, Brolin RE, Ebert EC. Staphylococcal enterotoxin B induces potent cytotoxic activity by intraepithelial lymphocytes. Immunology 2000;101:185–190.

47. Balk SP, Ebert EC, Blumenthal RL et al. Oligoclonal expansion and CD1 recognition by human intestinal intraepithelial lymphocytes. Science 1991253:1411–1415.

48. Colgan SP, Hershberg RM, Furuta GT, Blumberg RS. Ligation of intestinal epithelial CD1d induces bioactive IL-10: critical role of the cytoplasmic tail in autocrine signaling. Proc Natl Acad Sci USA 1999;96:13938–13943.

49. Allez M, Brimnes J, Dotan I, Mayer L. Expansion of CD8+ T cells with regulatory function after interaction with intestinal epithelial cells. Gastroenterology 2002;123:1516–1526.

50. Campbell NA, Kim HS, Blumberg RS, Mayer L. The nonclassic class I molecule CD1d associates with the novel CD8 ligand gp180 on intestinal epithelial cells. J Biol Chem 1999;274:26259–26265.

51. Soloski MJ, DeCloux A, Aldrich CJ, Forman L. Structural and functional characteristics of the class IB molecule, Qa-1. Immunol Rev 1995;147:67–89.

52. Vales-Gomez M, Reyburn HT, Erskine RA, Lopez-Botet M, Strominger JL. Kinetics and peptide dependency of the binding of the inhibitory NK receptor CD94/NKG2-A and the activating receptor CD94/NKG2-C to HLA-E. EMBO J 1999;18:4250–4260.

53. Bauer S, Groh V, Wu J et al. Activation of NK cells and T cells by NKG2D, a receptor for stress-inducible MICA. Science 1999;285:727–729.

54. Wu J, Song Y, Bakker AB et al. An activating immunoreceptor complex formed by NKG2D and DAP10. Science 1999;285:730–732.

55. Norton SD, Zuckerman L, Urdahl KB, Shefner R, Miller J, Jenkins MK. The CD28 ligand, B7, enhances IL-2 production by providing a costimulatory signal to T cells. J Immunol 1992;149:1556–1561.

56. Noel PJ, Boise LH, Thompson CB. Regulation of T cell activation by CD28 and CTLA4. Adv Exp Med Biol 1996;406:209–217.

57. June CH, Bluestone JA, Nadler LM, Thompson CB. The B7 and CD28 receptor families. Immunol Today 1994;15:321–331.

58. Nakazawa A, Watanabe M, Kanai T et al. Functional expression of costimulatory molecule CD86 on epithelial cells in the inflamed colonic mucosa. Gastroenterology 1999;117:536–545.

59. Hutloff A, Dittrich AM, Beier KC et al. ICOS is an inducible T-cell co-stimulator structurally and functionally related to CD28. Nature 1999;397:263–266.

60. Coyle AJ, Lehar S, Lloyd C et al. The CD28-related molecule ICOS is required for effective T cell-dependent immune responses. Immunity 2000;13:95–105.

61. Kopf M, Coyle AJ, Schmitz N et al. Inducible costimulator protein (ICOS) controls T helper cell subset polarization after virus and parasite infection. J Exp Med 2000;192:53–61.

62. Boirivant M, Fuss I, Fiocchi C, Klein JS, Strong SA, Strober W. Hypoproliferative human lamina propria T cells retain the capacity to secrete lymphokines when stimulated via CD2/CD28 pathways. Proc Assoc Am Phys 1996;108:55–67.

63. Fuss IJ, Neurath M, Boirivant M et al. Disparate CD4+ lamina propria (LP) lymphokine secretion profiles in inflammatory bowel disease. Crohn's disease LP cells manifest increased secretion of IFN-gamma, whereas ulcerative colitis LP cells manifest increased secretion of IL-5. J Immunol 1996;157:1261–1270.

64. Qiao L, Schurmann G, Betzler M, Meuer SC. Activation and signaling status of human lamina propria T lymphocytes. Gastroenterology 1991;101:1529–1536.

65. Targan SR, Deem RL, Liu M, Wang S, Nel A. Definition of a lamina propria T cell responsive state. Enhanced cytokine responsiveness of T cells stimulated through the CD2 pathway. J Immunol 1995;154:664–675.

66. Framson PE, Cho DH, Lee LY, Hershberg RM. Polarized expression and function of the costimulatory molecule CD58 on human intestinal epithelial cells. Gastroenterology 1999;116:1054–1062.

67. Yang SK, Eckmann L, Panja A, Kagnoff MF. Differential and regulated expression of C-X-C, C-C, and C-chemokines by human colon epithelial cells. Gastroenterology 1997;113:1214–1223.

68. Lillard JW Jr, Boyaka PN, Taub DD, McGhee JR. RANTES potentiates antigen-specific mucosal immune responses. J Immunol 2001;166:162–169.

69. Yang SK, Choi MS, Kim OH et al. The increased expression of an array of C-X-C and C-C chemokines in the colonic mucosa of patients with ulcerative colitis: regulation by corticosteroids. Am J Gastroenterol 2002;97:126–132.

70. Zabel BA, Agace WW, Campbell JJ et al. Human G protein-coupled receptor GPR-9-6/CC chemokine receptor 9 is selectively expressed on intestinal homing T lymphocytes, mucosal lymphocytes, and thymocytes and is required for thymus-expressed chemokine-mediated chemotaxis. J Exp Med 1999;190:1241–1256.

71. Papadakis KA, Prehn J, Moreno ST et al. CCR9-positive lymphocytes and thymus-expressed chemokine distinguish small bowel from colonic Crohn's disease. Gastroenterology 2001;121:246–254.

72. Papadakis KA, Prehn J, Nelson V et al. The role of thymus-expressed chemokine and its receptor CCR9 on lymphocytes in the regional specialization of the mucosal immune system. J Immunol 2000;165:5069–5076.

73. Kunkel EJ, Campbell JJ, Haraldsen G et al. Lymphocyte CC chemokine receptor 9 and epithelial thymus-expressed chemokine (TECK) expression distinguish the small intestinal immune compartment: Epithelial expression of tissue-specific chemokines as an organizing principle in regional immunity. J Exp Med 2000;192:761–768.

74. Papadakis KA, Tung JK, Binder SW et al. Outcome of cytomegalovirus infections in patients with inflammatory bowel disease. Am J Gastroenterol 2001;96:2137–2142.

75. Svensson M, Marsal J, Ericsson A et al. CCL25 mediates the localization of recently activated CD8αβ(+) lymphocytes to the small-intestinal mucosa. J Clin Invest 2002;110:1113–1121.

76. Imai T, Hieshima K, Haskell C et al. Identification and molecular characterization of fractalkine receptor CX3CR1, which mediates both leukocyte migration and adhesion. Cell 1997;91:521–530.

77. Muehlhoefer A, Saubermann LJ, Gu X et al. Fractalkine is an epithelial and endothelial cell-derived chemoattractant for intraepithelial lymphocytes in the small intestinal mucosa. J Immunol 2000;164:3368–3376.

78. Pan J, Kunkel EJ, Gosslar U et al. A novel chemokine ligand for CCR10 and CCR3 expressed by epithelial cells in mucosal tissues. J Immunol 2000;165:2943–2949.

79. Kim JM, Cho SJ, Oh YK, Jung HY, Kim YJ, Kim N. Nuclear factor-kappa B activation pathway in intestinal epithelial cells is a major regulator of chemokine gene expression and neutrophil migration induced by Bacteroides fragilis enterotoxin. Clin Exp Immunol 2002;130:59–66.

80. Nakayama T, Fujisawa R, Yamada H et al. Inducible expression of a CC chemokine liver- and activation-regulated chemokine (LARC)/macrophage inflammatory protein (MIP)-3 alpha/CCL20 by epidermal keratinocytes and its role in atopic dermatitis. Int Immunol 2001;13:95–103.

81. Coulin F, Power CA, Alouani S et al. Characterisation of macrophage inflammatory protein-5/human CC cytokine-2, a member of the macrophage-inflammatory-protein family of chemokines. Eur J Biochem 1997;248:507–515.

82. Kwon JH, Keates S, Bassani L, Mayer LF, Keates AC. Colonic epithelial cells are a major site of macrophage inflammatory protein 3alpha (MIP-3alpha) production in normal colon and inflammatory bowel disease. Gut 2002;51:818–826.

83. Keates AC, Keates S, Kwon JH et al. ZBP-89, Sp1, and nuclear factor-kappa B regulate epithelial neutrophil-activating peptide-78 gene expression in Caco-2 human colonic epithelial cells. J Biol Chem 2001;276:43713–43722.

84. Eckmann L, Kagnoff MF, Fierer J. Epithelial cells secrete the chemokine interleukin-8 in response to bacterial entry. Infect Immun 1993;61:4569–4574.

85. Fierer J, Eckmann L, Kagnoff M. IL-8 secreted by epithelial cells invaded by bacteria. Infect Agents Dis 1993;2:255–258.

86. McGee DW, Beagley KW, Aicher WK, McGhee JR. Transforming growth factor-beta enhances interleukin-6 secretion by intestinal epithelial cells. Immunology 1992;77:7–12.

87. McGee DW, Beagley KW, Aicher WK, McGhee JR. Transforming growth factor-beta and IL-1 beta act in synergy to enhance IL-6 secretion by the intestinal epithelial cell line, IEC-6. J Immunol 1993;151:970–978.

88. Bao S, Goldstone S, Husband AJ. Localization of IFN-gamma and IL-6 mRNA in murine intestine by in situ hybridization. Immunology 1993;80:666–670.

89. Meyer TA, Noguchi Y, Ogle CK et al. Endotoxin stimulates interleukin-6 production in intestinal epithelial cells. A synergistic effect with prostaglandin E2. Arch Surg 1994;129:1290–1294; discussion 1294–1295.

90. Kontakou M, Przemioslo RT, Sturgess RP, Limb AG, Ciclitira PJ. Expression of tumour necrosis factor-alpha, interleukin-6, and interleukin-2 mRNA in the jejunum of patients with coeliac disease. Scand J Gastroenterol 1995;30:456–463.

91. Kusugami K, Fukatsu A, Tanimoto M et al. Elevation of interleukin-6 in inflammatory bowel disease is macrophage- and epithelial cell-dependent. Dig Dis Sci 1995;40:949–959.

92. Babyatsky MW, Rossiter G, Podolsky DK. Expression of transforming growth factors alpha and beta in colonic mucosa in inflammatory bowel disease. Gastroenterology 1996;110:975–984.

93. Scheiman JM, Meise KS, Greenson JK, Coffey RJ. Transforming growth factor-alpha (TGF-alpha) levels in human proximal gastrointestinal epithelium. Effect of mucosal injury and acid inhibition. Dig Dis Sci 1997;42:333–341.

94. Podolsky DK. Healing the epithelium: solving the problem from two sides. J Gastroenterol 1997;32:122–126.

95. Planchon S, Fiocchi C, Takafuji V, Roche JK. Transforming growth factor-beta1 preserves epithelial barrier function: identification of receptors, biochemical intermediates, and cytokine antagonists. J Cell Physiol 1999;181:55–66.

96. Panja A, Goldberg S, Eckmann L, Krishen P, Mayer L. The regulation and functional consequence of proinflammatory cytokine binding on human intestinal epithelial cells. J Immunol 1998;161:3675–3684.

97. Sitaraman SV, Merlin D, Wang L et al. Neutrophil–epithelial crosstalk at the intestinal lumenal surface mediated by reciprocal secretion of adenosine and IL-6. J Clin Invest 2001;107:861–869.

98. Madrigal-Estebas L, McManus R, Byrne B et al. Human small intestinal epithelial cells secrete interleukin-7 and differentially express two different interleukin-7 mRNA transcripts: implications for extrathymic T-cell differentiation. Hum Immunol 1997;58:83–90.

99. Meijssen MA, Brandwein SL, Reinecker HC, Bhan AK, Podolsky DK. Alteration of gene expression by intestinal epithelial cells precedes colitis in interleukin-2-deficient mice. Am J Physiol 1998;274:G472–479.

100. Bilenker M, Roberts AI, Brolin RE, Ebert EC. Interleukin-7 activates intestinal lymphocytes. Dig Dis Sci 1995;40:1744–1749.

101. Watanabe M, Ueno Y, Yajima T et al. Interleukin 7 is produced by human intestinal epithelial cells and regulates the proliferation of intestinal mucosal lymphocytes. J Clin Invest 1995;95:2945–2953.

102. Watanabe M, Ueno Y, Yajima T et al. Interleukin 7 transgenic mice develop chronic colitis with decreased interleukin 7 protein accumulation in the colonic mucosa. J Exp Med 1998;187:389–402.

103. Maeurer MJ, Lotze MT. Interleukin-7 (IL-7) knockout mice. Implications for lymphopoiesis and organ-specific immunity. Int Rev Immunol 1998;16:309–322.

104. Inagaki-Ohara K, Nishimura H, Mitani A, Yoshikai Y. Interleukin-15 preferentially promotes the growth of intestinal intraepithelial lymphocytes bearing gamma delta T cell receptor in mice. Eur J Immunol 1997;27:2885–2891.

105. Hirose K, Suzuki H, Nishimura H et al. Interleukin-15 may be responsible for early activation of intestinal intraepithelial lymphocytes after oral infection with Listeria monocytogenes in rats. Infect Immun 1998;66:5677–5683.

106. Lai YG, Gelfanov V, Gelfanova V et al. IL-15 promotes survival but not effector function differentiation of CD8+ TCRalphabeta+ intestinal intraepithelial lymphocytes. J Immunol 1999;163:5843–5850.

107. Ma A, Boone DL, Lodolce JP. The pleiotropic functions of interleukin 15: not so interleukin 2-like after all. J Exp Med 2000;191:753–756.

108. Pizarro TT, Michie MH, Bentz M et al. IL-18, a novel immunoregulatory cytokine, is up-regulated in Crohn's disease: expression and localization in intestinal mucosal cells. J Immunol 1999;162:6829–6835.

109. Coffman RL, Lebman DA, Shrader B. Transforming growth factor beta specifically enhances IgA production by lipopolysaccharide-stimulated murine B lymphocytes. J Exp Med 1989;170:1039–1044.

110. Roncarolo MG, Bacchetta R, Bordignon C et al. Type 1 T regulatory cells. Immunol Rev 2001;182:68–79.

111. Sellon RK, Tonkonogy S, Schultz M et al. Resident enteric bacteria are necessary for development of spontaneous colitis and immune system activation in interleukin-10-deficient mice. Infect Immun 1998;66:5224–5231.

112. Kuhn R, Lohler J, Rennick D et al. Interleukin-10-deficient mice develop chronic enterocolitis [see comments]. Cell 1993;75:263–274.

113. Davidson NJ, Leach MW, Fort MM et al. T helper cell 1-type CD4+ T cells, but not B cells, mediate colitis in interleukin 10-deficient mice. J Exp Med 1996;184:241–251.

114. Kaiserlian D, Vidal K. Antigen presentation by intestinal epithelial cells [letter]. Immunol Today 1993;14:144.

115. Bland PW, Warren LG. Antigen presentation by epithelial cells of the rat small intestine. II. Selective induction of suppressor T cells. Immunology 1986;58:9–14.

116. Mayer L, Shlien R. Evidence for function of Ia molecules on gut epithelial cells in man. J Exp Med 1987;166:1471–1483.

117. Yio XY, Mayer L. Characterization of a 180-kDa intestinal epithelial cell membrane glycoprotein, gp180. A candidate molecule mediating T cell–epithelial cell interactions. J Biol Chem 1997;272:12786–12792.

118. Campbell NA, Park MS, Toy LS et al. A non-class I MHC intestinal epithelial surface glycoprotein, gp180, binds to CD8. Clin Immunol 2002;102:267–274.

119. Li Y, Yio XY, Mayer L. Human intestinal epithelial cell-induced CD8+ T cell activation is mediated through CD8 and the activation of CD8-associated p56lck. J Exp Med 1995;182:1079–1088.

120. Kasai K, Matsuura A, Kikuchi K et al. Localization of rat CD1 transcripts and protein in rat tissues – an analysis of rat CD1 expression by in situ hybridization and immunohistochemistry. Clin Exp Immunol 1997;109:317–322.

121. Yamamoto M, Fujihashi K, Kawabata K et al. A mucosal intranet: intestinal epithelial cells down-regulate intraepithelial, but not peripheral, T lymphocytes. J Immunol 1998;160:2188–2196.

122. Mayer L, Eisenhardt D, Salomon P et al. Expression of class II molecules on intestinal epithelial cells in humans. Differences between normal and inflammatory bowel disease [see comments]. Gastroenterology 1991;100:3–12.

123. Fais S, Pallone F, Squarcia O et al. HLA-DR antigens on colonic epithelial cells in inflammatory bowel disease: I. Relation to the state of activation of lamina propria lymphocytes and to the epithelial expression of other surface markers. Clin Exp Immunol 1987;68:605–612.

124. McDonald GB, Jewell DP. Class II antigen (HLA-DR) expression by intestinal epithelial cells in inflammatory diseases of colon. J Clin Pathol 1987;40:312–317.

125. Chiba M, Iizuka M, Masamune O. Ubiquitous expression of HLA-DR antigens on human small intestinal epithelium. Gastroenterol Jpn 1988;23:109–116.

126. Geboes K, Rutgeerts P, Penninckx F et al. Changes in small intestinal epithelial expression of MHC class II antigen after terminal ileal resection for Crohn's disease. Int J Colorectal Dis 1988;3:102–108.

127. Chiba M, Iizuka M, Horie Y et al. HLA-DR antigen expression in macroscopically uninvolved areas of intestinal epithelia in Crohn's disease. Gastroenterol Jpn 1989;24:365–372.

128. Mayer L, Eisenhardt D. Lack of induction of suppressor T cells by intestinal epithelial cells from patients with inflammatory bowel disease. J Clin Invest 1990;86:1255–1260.

129. Toy LS, Yio XY, Lin A et al. Defective expression of gp180, a novel CD8 ligand on intestinal epithelial cells, in inflammatory bowel disease. J Clin Invest 1997;100:2062–2071.

130. Touraine JL, Betuel H. The bare lymphocyte syndrome: immunodeficiency resulting from the lack of expression of HLA antigens. Birth Defects Orig Artic Ser 1983;19:83–85.

131. Boismenu R, Havran WL. Modulation of epithelial cell growth by intraepithelial gamma delta T cells. Science 1994;266:1253–1255.

132. Chen Y, Chou K, Fuchs E et al. Protection of the intestinal mucosa by intraepithelial gamma delta T cells. Proc Natl Acad Sci USA 2002;99:14338–14343.

133. Adams RB, Planchon SM, Roche JK. IFN-gamma modulation of epithelial barrier function. Time course, reversibility, and site of cytokine binding. J Immunol 1993;150:2356–2363.

134. Madara JL, Stafford J. Interferon-gamma directly affects barrier function of cultured intestinal epithelial monolayers. J Clin Invest 1989;83:724–727.

135. Lionetti P, Breese E, Braegger CP et al. T-cell activation can induce either mucosal destruction or adaptation in cultured human fetal small intestine. Gastroenterology 1993;105:373–381.

136. MacDonald TT, Spencer J. Cell-mediated immune injury in the intestine. Gastroenterol Clin North Am 1992;21:367–386.

137. Pender SL, MacDonald TT. Regulation of matrix metalloproteinase production in human fetal intestinal mesenchymal cells by cytokines and the bacterial superantigen Staphylococcus aureus enterotoxin B. Ann NY Acad Sci 1998;859:188–191.

138. Salmela MT, MacDonald TT, Black D et al. Upregulation of matrix metalloproteinases in a model of T cell mediated tissue injury in the gut: analysis by gene array and in situ hybridisation. Gut 2002;51:540–547.

139. Panwala CM, Jones JC, Viney JL. A novel model of inflammatory bowel disease: mice deficient for the multiple drug resistance gene, mdr1a, spontaneously develop colitis. J Immunol 1998;161:5733–5744.

140. Hermiston ML, Gordon JI. Inflammatory bowel disease and adenomas in mice expressing a dominant negative N-cadherin. Science 1995;270:1203–1207.

141. Mashimo H, Wu DC, Podolsky DK et al. Impaired defense of intestinal mucosa in mice lacking intestinal trefoil factor. Science 1996;274:262–265.

## CHAPTER 5

# The regulation of mucosal homeostasis and its relation to inflammatory bowel diseases

Warren Strober and Ivan J Fuss

## INTRODUCTION

A consensus has emerged that the major cause of inflammatory bowel diseases (IBD) is the dysregulation of mucosal immune responses to antigens in the resident microbial (bacterial) microflora (or possibly to antigens in the food stream). This view derives its greatest support from the many rodent models of mucosal inflammation in which it has been shown that inflammation does not occur under germ-free conditions regardless of the underlying immune defect that is the root cause of the inflammation.[1] Thus, in these models and, by extension, in human IBD, antigens derived from non-pathogenic microflora to which the organism is ordinarily non-responsive (tolerant) provides the driving force for the inflammation[2] (see Chapter 10).

An understanding of the presumed dysregulation in IBD requires some knowledge of the factors that control mucosal immune responses in healthy animals. Mucosal responses result from the interplay of opposing mechanisms that lead on the one hand to immunogenic (effector cell) responses and on the other to tolerogenic (regulatory) cell responses. The former are necessary for host defense to pathogens, whereas the latter prevent responses to luminal antigens that would otherwise preoccupy the mucosal immune system with trivial responses and/or lead to excessive responses and autoimmunity. Antigens associated with the persistent commensal microflora are more or less equivalent to self-antigens. Thus, the need to not respond to such antigens is as compelling as the need to be non-responsive to 'true' self-antigens.

Mucosal immune dysregulation can be defined as either a heightened capacity to react to mucosal antigens with an abnormally increased effector cell response, or a diminished capacity to downregulate responses with an abnormally decreased regulatory cell response. Both of these possibilities are reflected in one or another of the animal models of intestinal inflammation and could be a cause of human IBD. In this chapter, however, we confine our discussion to the second or regulatory arm of the mucosal immune response, and to the possibility that IBD is due to inadequate regulation.

To this purpose, we consider the phenomenon of mucosal immune non-responsiveness to mucosal antigens, hereafter called oral tolerance, in some detail. Our focus is first on the antigens that do or do not induce oral tolerance, and second on the nature of the cellular mechanisms of such tolerance, most particularly the antigen-presenting cells (APC, dendritic cells) and the regulatory T cells mediating this phenomenon. Finally, we discuss the body of knowledge, mainly derived from animal models of mucosal inflammation, establishing that mucosal inflammation can indeed be derived from faulty regulation of the mucosal immune response. This allows us to turn to studies of immune regulation in patients with IBD, marshalling evidence that this type of abnormality may be a cause of these diseases.

## THE NATURE OF ANTIGENS THAT ELICIT EFFECTOR CELL OR SUPPRESSOR CELL RESPONSES IN THE MUCOSAL IMMUNE SYSTEM

Since the phenomenon of oral tolerance was first seriously studied some 40–50 years ago, the ability of a great number of potential antigens to elicit oral tolerance has been determined. It is now possible to describe a set of basic principles governing the types of antigens that induce responsiveness or unresponsiveness in the mucosal immune system. The first and foremost is that challenge of the mucosal immune system with the vast majority of soluble protein antigens (or peptides derived from such proteins) leads to oral tolerance if such challenge occurs in the absence of a mucosal adjuvant.[3] To some extent this rule is not different from that governing responses in the systemic immune system, although the mucosal response is more 'tilted' toward tolerance than is the systemic immune system, possibly because mucosal responses are governed by mucosa-specific active suppressor mechanisms that are not as evident in the systemic immune system. The activity of adjuvants necessary for mucosal effector responses may differ from that of adjuvants necessary for systemic responses, in that the former have the added role of neutralizing negative suppressor cell responses as well as the more conventional role of driving positive effector cell responses.

In accordance with the inherent tolerogenicity of protein antigens, oral administration of soluble proteins that are normally in the food stream, as well as most soluble proteins associated with commensal bacteria, are more likely to induce oral tolerance rather than oral immunization.[4] Even the oral administration of haptenating agents leading to the mucosal presentation of modified self-antigens induces oral tolerance,[5] even though the same agents applied to the skin induce immunity. Overall, it appears that the 'default' mucosal immune response to soluble proteins is tolerance, and a mucosal adjuvant has to be present to shift this response on to an immunogenic track. The mechanisms by which soluble proteins induce nonresponsiveness are the major focus of this chapter and are discussed in detail below.

A second principle of mucosal antigen immunogenicity/tolerogenicity is that particulate antigens are more likely to be immunogenic than soluble antigens when presented to the mucosal immune system. Such antigens often are compound materials that may include substances with inherent adjuvanticity. In addition, particulates have physical characteristics that influence their initial interactions with the antigen-presenting cells in the mucosal immune system and hence their ability to elicit effector cell responses. The difference between soluble and particulate antigens with respect to their ability to elicit mucosal responsiveness and non-responsiveness was noted quite early in the study of oral tolerance. Thus, whereas early studies of sheep red blood cells (SRBC) and later studies with killed or inactivated organisms showed that particulate antigens (or proteins released from the particulates during passage through the digestive tract) could be tolerogenic in the mucosal immune system,[6,7] the studies with SRBC showed that the appearance of tolerance was delayed owing to an initial (but transient) immune response.[8] This was the first indication that at least certain types of particulate antigens could be fundamentally different from soluble antigens in the induction of mucosal tolerance.

In further elaboration of mucosal immune responses to particulates, a difference was noted between dead and live organisms and between non-invasive and invasive organisms with regard to an antigen's tolerogenic potential. In particular, the same organisms that elicit tolerance in a non-invasive form can elicit immunity in an invasive form.[9] One possible explanation for this difference is that invasive organisms have a greater capacity to breach the mucosal surface barrier as an intact particle (or antigen) that is capable of addressing cells in an immunogenic form. A second and perhaps more important distinction is that the very properties that endow the organism with virulence and invasiveness are also the properties that favor immunogenicity; in essence, the molecules associated with the organism that allow virulence and invasiveness are built-in mucosal adjuvants. Support for this view comes from recent work which shows that

*Escherichia coli* that are genetically modified to express a normally tolerogenic antigen (ovalbumin, OVA) evoke immunogenic mucosal responses if they have the capacity to colonize and invade the mucosa, but not if they lack this property.[10,11] In addition, exposure of mice having transgenic T cells expressing a T-cell receptor (TCR) specific for OVA to colonizing *E. coli* organisms modified to produce OVA elicits a Th1 effector T-cell response that induces colitis, whereas exposure to OVA alone has no such effect.[12,13] The common theme is that antigen entering mucosal follicles in the presence of particulates with adjuvant properties have a more potent immunogenic effect than antigens alone, whether it is eliciting a de novo response among naive T cells or activating an established population of memory cells already capable of recognizing the antigen.

What, then, are the cellular and molecular factors that determine the adjuvant properties of some organisms? One such factor is almost certainly the ability of organisms to produce substances that interact with and stimulate cells in a way that leads to a positive immune response. For instance, the substance may act as an adjuvant because it interacts with cells via Toll-like receptors (TLR) on APC (including epithelial cells) that recognize 'dangerous' microbial antigens.[14] Such receptors lead to the activation of intracellular pathways that trigger cytokine responses, as well as other cell activation events that are necessary for innate immune responses. In turn, this innate response conditions the lymphoid milieu for the initiation of adaptive immune responses to many antigens associated with the organism. As discussed more fully below, there are a number of TLR and each TLR or combination of TLR is specialized in its ability to recognize and interact with various types of microbial products. A good example of such interaction in the mucosal immune system is the interaction between the *E. coli* virulence factor *P. fimbriae* with TLR4 on the surface of urinary epithelial cells, thus stimulating a chemokine response in the urinary tract that then 'calls in' cells capable of initiating an adaptive immune response.[15]

Other microbial substances, rather than (or in addition to) interacting with TLR, interact with other cell surface molecules such as CD91, a receptor for HSP(gp96),[16] or with various macrophage/antigen-presenting cell surface molecules such as CD14, and the $\beta_2$ integrin CD11b/CD18 (CR3).[17] This can also lead to adjuvant activity, as these receptors can influence antigen-presenting cell activation. The fact that such interactions can be specifically related to virulence is supported by recent work showing that the presence of specific adherence factors (intimin $\alpha$ or intimin $\beta$) intrinsic to the virulence of *E. coli* organisms led to a Th1 response, whereas *E. coli* organisms not expressing these factors or expressing alternative intimins did not have this effect.[18] Not surprisingly, these stimulatory effects correlate with the ability of the intimins to co-stimulate T cells in vitro.

One difficulty with the thesis that the ability of an organism to express components that interact with TLR and other cell activation molecules determines adjuvanticity is that enteric commensal organisms have this property, yet do not ordinarily induce an immune response. Thus, for example, the commensals express LPS, which reacts with TLR4 and peptidoglycans, which react with TLR2. One possibility is that even if bacteria express TLR-interactive components, they need to contain other proteins to stimulate the mucosal immune system. Thus, one can postulate that very early in life, i.e. at a time when the host does not have a fully developed immune system and exhibits neonatal tolerance, exposure to endogenous bacteria leads to non-responsiveness to all of their potentially immunogenic antigens, and thus no amount of adjuvant activity can reverse this primary tolerogenic response. Particulates without inherent adjuvant properties may induce an immunogenic mucosal response simply because of their physical properties. The most striking evidence in favor of this possibility is the capacity of normally tolerogenic soluble antigens when incorporated into biodegradable (polylactolol) microspheres, and to a lesser extent into microsomes (ISCOMS), to evoke mucosal and systemic responses when administered by the oral route.[19-22] Although the mechanism of action of such particulates is not completely understood, they require physical interaction with the antigen, so their adjuvanticity may be due to their function as an antigen delivery system. These microspheres protect mucosal antigens from proteolytic digestion as they pass through the gastrointestinal tract and then effectively deliver the antigens to Peyer's patch antigen-presenting cells capable of phagocytosis. This is consistent with the observation that the ability of microspheres to affect mucosal response is critically dependent on particle size and the ability of antigen-presenting cells to take up the particle within the mucosal lymphoid follicle.[22-24]

Size also helps determine whether the particle induces an immunogenic or a tolerogenic response. Thus, orally administered antigen-loaded particles that were 3–4 μm in diameter enhanced subsequent IgG responses to same antigen subsequently administered by a systemic route, whereas spheres twice as large, i.e. 7–10 μm in diameter, suppressed subsequent IgG and DTH responses but enhanced IgA responses.[24] These complex effects can be explained by postulating that the smaller particles are engulfed by specific dendritic cells in the Peyer's patches (PP) and spleen that favor IgG responses, whereas the larger particles are taken up by specific PP dendritic cells that facilitate the production of TGF-β, which favors IgA production and suppressor cell responses (see discussion below). However, this explanation does not correlate with the fact that the 7–10 μm particles induced high levels of IFN-γ, not TGF-β or IL-4, so that the cytokine pattern was not actually conducive to tolerance induction and IgA responses.

A third principle relating to the immunogenicity/tolerogenicity of mucosal antigens involves the T-cell dependence of the response to the antigen. Thus, whereas soluble protein antigens (i.e. T cell-dependent antigens) induce oral tolerance, soluble polysaccharides (i.e. T cell-independent antigens) have no such ability and instead evoke antibody responses. Stokes et al. nicely demonstrated this fact by showing that mice fed E. coli develop tolerance to the 'K' protein antigen but not to the 'O' polysaccharide antigen.[7] The distinction between T cell-dependent and -independent antigens point to an important feature of oral tolerance, namely that the latter is a T-cell tolerance not a B-cell tolerance. This was unequivocally demonstrated many years ago by Reese and Cebra, who showed that tolerance induction to a hapten on one carrier does not occur when the animal is challenged with the same hapten bound to a second carrier to which oral tolerance has been induced.[25] This lack of tolerance to T cell-independent antigens (with which the mucosa is replete) indicates that there is no need for unresponsiveness to this class of antigens, either because they are generally non-cross-reactive with host antigens or because the response induced is a non-pathogenic IgM/IgA antibody response which clears the circulation of the absorbed antigens.

A fourth principle of immunogenicity/tolerogenicity to mucosal antigens involves another physical property of antigens, i.e. the ability to bind to mucosal epithelial cells. Here the emphasis is on the adhesive properties rather than the adjuvanticity of the adhesin. Examples of immunogenic antigens with adherence properties are E. coli pilus antigens, heat-labile E.coli toxin B and certain bacterial lectins. Pilus administration elicited both mucosal (IgA and IgG) antibodies and systemic (mostly IgG, little or no IgA) antibodies, probably reflecting the capacity of these antigens to stimulate local (mucosal) immune cells as well as gain access to the circulation and thus stimulate the systemic immune system.[26] In contrast, various lectins elicited only systemic (IgG antibodies) and not mucosal IgA antibody responses.[26]

The importance of epithelial binding for the mucosal antigenicity of these types of antigen is shown by the fact that simple sugars that block binding also block immune responses.[26] Nevertheless, the relation of binding to mucosal immunogenicity is poorly understood. One possibility is that binding to colonic epithelial cells allows the antigen to bypass mucosal follicles and enter the lamina propria directly. Because the follicles are sites in the development of active suppressor cell-mediated tolerance, entering the lamina propria directly avoids at least one mechanism of tolerance induction. This view is supported by studies of mucosal responses to antigens incorporated into emulsions that enhance oral tolerance induction to the fed antigen even in TCR transgenic animals with a TCR specific for the antigen, presumably because the emulsion prevents binding to epithelial cells and delivers antigens into the Peyer's patches preferentially.[27]

A possible role for this avoidance of oral tolerance in the mucosal immune system may relate to the need for resident microflora or even transient pathogens to evoke low-level and/or early responses. This feature would help the animal regulate the mix and number of commensal organisms and provides a means of evoking responses to potential pathogens that are unimpeded by tolerogenic mechanisms. A fifth and somewhat unifying principle governing immunogenicity/tolerogenicity of mucosal antigens is the ability of some antigens to also act as mucosal adjuvants. For example, adhesins and other substances that interact with TLR or other pattern recognition receptors are possible adjuvants. The prototype antigens in this category are the various bacterial toxins such as cholera toxin (CT) and E. coli heat-labile toxin (LT), and are among the most potent mucosal adjuvants known. Thus, the study of how these antigens function as adjuvants is likely to provide detailed knowledge of the cellular mechanisms governing mucosal adjuvanticity.

Cholera (holo)toxin (CT), as well as E.coli heat-labile toxin (LT), is a heterodimeric molecule composed of one chain (subunit A) that influences G protein-coupled signaling function by affecting adenyl cyclase activity and ADP ribosylation, and another chain (subunit B) that binds to GM-1 ganglioside or (or in the case of LT, to other gangliosides) on the surface of many cells, and is thus responsible for the binding of toxin to the cell surface.[28] The A subunit of CT can function in the absence of the B subunit if it is bound by another binding moiety.[29] This was shown by Lycke et al., who demonstrated that the A subunit retains its adjuvant properties (at least with respect to IgA production) when combined with the Ig-binding domain of protein A, i.e. a substance that binds to the surface of B cells.[30,31] However, the B subunit, when bound to another antigen and administered in the absence of the A subunit, enhances oral tolerance to the bound antigen, whereas it retains adjuvanticity for unbound antigens.[32–37] These paradoxical affects of CT-B are discussed below.

The mechanism of action of CT and similar toxins is inherently complex. One factor clearly involved is their effect on G protein-coupled signaling. Recent evidence that mutant CT or LT retaining little or no enzymatic activity still retain adjuvanticity suggests that adjuvanticity may arise from the B subunit.[32–35,38] This is supported by the fact that mutant CT without enzymatic properties lacks adjuvanticity when linked to protein A as an alternative binding moiety.

These enzymatic properties of CT, LT and related toxins affect mucosal responses at several levels. First, it may affect epithelial cell cytokine secretion and epithelial layer barrier function, so as to increase access of antigen to antigen-presenting cells. Second, it may act on antigen-presenting cells to augment antigen adsorption and presentation, and to increase the expression of co-stimulatory molecules.[39] For example, CT increases the expression of MHC class II molecules as well as CD80 and CD86 co-stimulatory molecules on dendritic cells. Third, and perhaps most importantly, bacterial toxin signaling via G protein-coupled receptors has profound effects on cytokine secretion. Thus, CT and LT, substances that activate cells via Gs-protein-coupled signaling and lead to the induction of intracellular cAMP, suppress IL-12 p70 and TNF production and thus inhibit Th1 response and IFN-$\gamma$ production.[40] This finding explains the observation that CT and LT enhance Th2 responses (the former more than the latter) since, as discussed below, Th1 responses inhibit TGF-$\beta$ production.[41] In addition, it explains the positive effect of CT on IgA production, as Th1 cytokines inhibit the TGF-$\beta$ production necessary for IgA isotype switch differentiation. In contrast, activation of Gi-protein-coupled signaling (rather than Gs-protein-coupled signaling) by a variety of other substances, including certain chemokines, C5a and f-MetLeuPhi (fMLP), suppress IL-12 but not TNF production.[42] In addition, a bacterial toxin that inhibits Gi-protein-coupled signaling, such as pertussis toxin, causes increased IL-12 production and opposes the effect of C5a, certain chemokines and fMLP.[43] This explains the increased IL-12 responses and colitis that occur in certain strains of mice with Gi2$\alpha$ deficiency.[43]

CT may drive Th2 responses via effects that are independent of its ability to suppress IL-12 production. CT preferentially inhibits Th1 clonal proliferation via suppression of IL-2, but not IL-4 production and downregulation of IL-2 responsiveness.[44] In addition, CT causes the selective disappearance of IL-12-secreting CD8$\alpha$+ dendritic cells, the source of IL-12 (B. Kelsall, NIH, Bethesda, personal communication). These effects probably occur via the ability of CT to affect G protein-coupled signaling, but this remains to be proved.

Despite inhibiting Th1 cell development, CT is an adjuvant for CTL responses at mucosal surfaces. This paradoxical finding may be due to the fact that the (CD8+) CTL response requires far less IL-12 than does Th1 differentiation and thus is stimulated by CT via non-IL-12-related adjuvant functions in the presence of reduced amounts (but still sufficient) of IL-12. This is consistent with the finding that although CT augments the response to peptides of HIV gp120 given intrarectally, such augmentation does not occur in mice pretreated with anti-IL-12.[45] Finally, the possibility that CT directly augments the differentiation of CD8+ T cells into CTL is unlikely, however, as CT inhibits CD8+ T-cell activation in vitro.

The inhibitory effects of CT on IL-12 (and Th1 responses) are not as evident with LT. Indeed, LT induces a more balanced Ig subclass response, selecting both Th1 and Th2 helper activity for B cells.[41,46] The reason for this difference between the activity of the two toxins is currently unknown. However, because CT and LT bind to different gangliosides, it is possible that they address somewhat different antigen-presenting cell populations.

CT has an unparalleled ability to augment IgA responses, presumably because its 'general' adjuvant effects are coupled with the induction of cytokines favorable to IgA B-cell differentiation. Thus, it suppresses IL-12 production, a cytokine which inhibits TGF-$\beta$ production, and augments TGF-$\beta$, IL-10 and IL-6 production, cytokines that are necessary both for IgA B-cell switch differentiation and terminal differentiation. By promoting TGF-$\beta$ (and IL-10) production, CT is also acting as a tolerogenic agent (see discussion below). This apparently paradoxical state of affairs can be resolved by the fact that oral tolerance is a complex phenomenon, involving both cellular anergy/deletion and suppressor cell generation. Thus, whereas CT augments the suppressor cell mechanisms underlying oral tolerance by inducing TGF-$\beta$, it may have other, more important inhibitory effects, with the net effect of abrogating oral tolerance. In any case, these seemingly disparate effects of CT highlight the complexity of adjuvant activity of this substance and demonstrate that an adjuvant affects cells in multiple ways, and thus has variable effects under different conditions.

Finally, CT-B subunit has adjuvant properties in vivo and enhances antigen presentation and APC activation by an unbound or bound antigen. One mechanism to explain the latter is that antigen coupled to CT-B is targeted to APC via the binding of CT-B to cell surface GM-1 ganglioside. Under other circumstances, however, CT-B coupled to antigen leads to enhancement of oral tolerance to the linked antigen, and CT-B administered alone at high doses leads to inhibition of the Th1 response.[33,47] These tolerogenic effects of CT-B undoubtedly arise from the fact that CT-B tends to affect antigen-presenting cells in the same manner as the holotoxin, in that it induces a mixture of cytokines that favor certain forms of oral tolerance.

To summarize the antigenicity and tolerogencity of mucosal antigens, the development of oral tolerance appears to be a default response that occurs if the antigen lacks certain properties, such as the ability to bind to epithelial cells or other immune cells, lacks a particulate nature that ensures localization in cells that favor immunogenic mechanisms, and lacks the capacity to influence cell function via its adjuvant properties. Thus, although the default response of the mucosa is non-responsiveness, enteric pathogens manage to bypass such oral tolerance and elicit protective host defense responses.

## MECHANISMS OF ORAL TOLERANCE

Our understanding of oral tolerance has been recently expanded by the ability to study this phenomenon in animal models of mucosal inflammation and in transgenic mice bearing T-cell receptor (TCR) transgenes. These approaches provide a decisive advantage over previous studies that centered on mucosal responses to discrete antigens because in the case of either mice with inflammation or mice with transgenes, one is dealing with greatly amplified responses and more defined tolerance

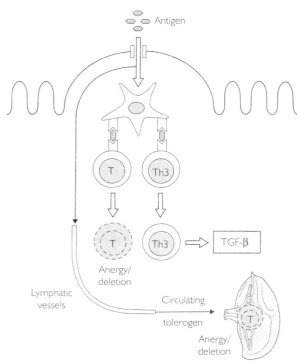

**Fig. 5.1** Mechanisms of oral tolerance. Oral tolerance is a complex phenomenon due to at least two major mechanisms: induction of cellular anergy and/or deletion and induction of suppressor T cells. The anergy/deletion mechanism can occur locally in the mucosal follicle or via mucosal antigen that gains access to the circulation via lymphatics. The suppression mechanism is mediated by 'Th3 cells' that produce TGF-β and (possibly) IL-10.

endpoints. These newer studies indicate that oral tolerance is a compound immunologic phenomenon mediated by at least two major mechanisms, an 'active' tolerance involving the induction of suppressor cells that regulate immune responses in an antigen non-specific fashion, and a passive tolerance due to the induction of cellular anergy and/or deletion (Fig. 5.1). This duality explains the many difficulties in understanding oral tolerance in the past and defines the challenge of future research in this area, which to a large extent now focuses on defining the factors affecting these mechanisms and how they interact.

## SUPPRESSOR T CELLS AS A CAUSE OF ORAL TOLERANCE

Suppressor T cells as a cause of oral tolerance was suggested and proved in the late 1970s with adoptive transfer studies showing that cells obtained from a mouse previously fed an antigen and transferred to a second mouse could render the latter tolerant (unresponsive) to the fed antigen given parenterally in an immunogenic form.[48] These suppressor cells were antigen specific in that they only suppressed responses to the fed antigen, not to an irrelevant antigen. Their existence was questioned in the 1980s and early 1990s when suppressor cells with antigen-specific suppressor–effector function were shown to be non-existent. However, whereas suppressor cells induced by antigen feeding are antigen specific in their induction, they exert antigen non-specific effector function by producing suppressive cytokines. These cells are now accepted among a number of known types of suppressor cells.

Several key characteristics of the suppressor cells of oral tolerance became evident. First, suppressor cells originate (or

undergo clonal expansion) in the mucosal follicles and only are noted in other tissues following migration from the latter site.[49,50] This relates to the important concept that mucosal sites may contain unique populations of cells that lead to suppressor cell development or proliferation, and that mucosal stimulation that bypasses this site does not lead to suppressor cell generation. Second, with regard to the phenotype of the suppressor cell, the cells were initially assumed to be CD8+ T cells (as were other suppressor cells), because in most adoptive transfer studies unresponsiveness could be abolished with antibodies generally associated with CD8+ T cells (rather than antibodies to CD8 itself). More recent evidence that CD8+ T cells mediate oral tolerance, at least under some conditions, has been confirmed with transfer studies using defined monoclonal anti-CD8+ antibodies.[51–53] This presents a dilemma, as oral tolerance occurs mainly after feeding soluble proteins that do not generally lead to antigen processing via the MHC class I pathway and the induction of CD8+ T cells. Two possible solutions to this dilemma need to be considered. The first is that antigen handling in mucosal and systemic lymphoid sites differs in that some of the antigen entering lymphoid follicles passes through epithelial cells and may thus assume a form that is processed by an endogenous APC pathway; this in turn results in presentation in the context of MHC class I molecules and the stimulation of CD8+ T cells. Such so-called 'cross-presentation' is now a well-recognized antigen processing pathway that applies to soluble antigen present in vesicular structures such as those formed around transported protein in cells.[51,54] A second possibility is that suppressor CD8+ T cells belong to a subpopulation of γδ T cells that are stimulated by antigen in the context on non-classic MHC antigens. Such cells are present in some forms of oral tolerance, particularly in the respiratory tract.[51,55,56] When CD8+ T cells function as suppressor cells, the mechanism of suppression may differ from that utilized by CD4+ T cells, for example by producing different suppressor cytokines. This is implied by the demonstration that whereas CD8–/– mice still manifest oral tolerance, they fail to downregulate mucosal IgA responses.[57] This can be explained by assuming that regulation of IgA responses and other responses by CD8+ T cells is not via the TGF-β-mediated mechanism exhibited by CD4+ cells.

In more recent studies of oral tolerance, the main suppressor T cell has been identified as a CD4+ T cell. This became evident when oral tolerance began to be studied in relation to experimental inflammatory states, such as EAE and various forms of colitis. The apparent primacy of a CD4+ rather than a CD8+ suppressor T cell in these contexts may be due to the fact that, whereas oral tolerance had largely been defined by its regulation of humoral responses, it was now being defined by its regulation of the Th1 T-cell response and, as alluded to above, CD8+ T cells may be more important for the former than the latter. The primacy of the CD4+ suppressor cell in oral tolerance has been formally shown by the fact that whereas oral tolerance is abolished in CD4–/– mice, it is retained in CD8–/– mice and β₂-microglobulin–/– mice (i.e. mice that lack MHC class I expression, necessary for stimulation of CD8+ cells).[58,59] This implies that even when CD8+ T cells are induced during oral tolerance they require the presence of a CD4+ T cell (as does the induction of CD8+ cytotoxic T cells).

A third key characteristic of oral antigen-induced suppressor T cells is that they are antigen-non-specific in their effector function and thus exhibit 'innocent-bystander' suppression. Weiner and colleagues[60–62] showed that oral administration of antigen is followed by the appearance of cells that subsequently downregulate responses to an irrelevant antigen if the latter is administered along with the original fed antigen (so that the suppressor cells are appropriately stimulated). These authors then showed that administration of a tolerogenic peptide derived from myelin basic protein inhibited EAE elicited by the systemic administration of an immunogenic (encephalogenic) peptide derive from the same molecule.[62] Thus, suppressor cells at lesional sites stimulated by tolerogenic peptides from endogenous myelin basic protein inhibited effector T cells of another specificity stimulated by immunogenic peptides.[60] Similarly, mice expressing a transgene encoding a CMV nucleoprotein under an insulin promoter (and thus expressing the CMV protein in pancreatic islet cells) develop diabetes when immunized with CMV, presumably because CMV-expressing islet cells elicit the development of CMV-specific CD8+ effector T cells, which then attack the CMV-expressing islet cells.[63–65] Feeding these mice insulin at the time of CMV immunization prevented diabetes because of the immunization. This can only be explained on the assumption that the feeding induces insulin-specific suppressor cells that are restimulated in the pancreas at sites of insulin production and then suppress the CMV-specific CD8+ cells capable of causing diabetes.

Establishing that suppressor cells elicited by antigen feeding manifest innocent bystander suppression has both theoretical and practical implications. It indicates that the suppressor cell of oral tolerance probably acts via the expression of an antigen-non-specific suppressor cytokine that operates at the level of either fully developed effector T cells or during stimulation of these cells during antigen presentation. In addition, feeding a limited number of antigens relevant to an autoimmune disease may influence the development of that disease, even if the latter is due to multiple antigens.[60–62,66] Therefore, tolerance induced by oral antigen administration could conceivably overcome the antigenic complexity of fully developed autoimmune responses.

## SUPPRESSOR CYTOKINES INVOLVED IN ORAL TOLERANCE

Having posited the existence of a suppressor cell of oral tolerance, we need to discuss the suppressor cytokines through which these cells can act. The first clues to the involvement of TGF-β in oral tolerance came from animal models of inflammation wherein antigen feeding was used to generate cells and cytokines that ameliorated inflammation.[3] These studies initially proceeded along two separate but parallel lines. First, it was established that T cells derived from rats undergoing induction of EAE (and thus encephalogenic T cells), when adoptively transferred to naive recipients, exhibit a greatly reduced capacity to confer EAE if they are exposed to TGF-β in vitro prior to transfer.[62,67–69] Further studies showed that production of IFN-γ by myelin basic protein (MBP)-stimulated encephalogenic T cells was inhibited if the latter were co-cultured with CD4+ T cells from rats that had recovered from EAE; this inhibition not only correlated with TGF-β production by the inhibiting CD4+ T cells, but was reversed by the presence of anti-TGF-β.[70] Meanwhile, an independent line of investigation showed that feeding MBP to rats prevented EAE, and that this prevention was mediated by CD8+ suppressor T cells.[71] Weiner et al. linked the two lines of investigation by showing that feeding MBP induced a cell producing TGF-β (ultimately called a Th3 T cell) that was responsible for both the development of oral tolerance and the

suppression of EAE. Furthermore, they showed that administration of anti-TGF-β prevented the inhibitory effect of feeding MBP and exacerbated EAE following systemic administration of MBP.[60–62,68,72] Finally, they showed that TGF-β could be identified in lesional tissues of resolving EAE.

Additional evidence supporting the role of TGF-β in oral tolerance has emerged from studies of experimental colitis models, which link oral tolerance and the secretion of TGF-β to maintaining mucosal homeostasis. SCID mice develop severe Th1 T cell-mediated colitis upon adoptive transfer of naive CD45RB(hi) T cells, but no colitis upon adoptive transfer of both naive and mature, CD45RB(lo) T cells, implying that the mature population of cells contains a regulatory (suppressor) T-cell subpopulation that prevents colitis.[73] Anti-TGF-β given at the time of mature T-cell co-administration abolished the suppressive effect of the latter, indicating that regulatory T cells in the CD45RB(lo) cell population act through TGF-β.[74] This observation was later refined by observing that a CD25+ subpopulation in the CD45RB(lo) cells population mediated regulatory activity through secretion of TGF-β.[75]

Parallel studies investigated Th1 T cell-mediated colitis obtained by the intrarectal administration of the haptenating agent trinitrol-benzene sulfonic acid (TNBS) to SJL/J or C57BL/10 mice. Feeding TNP-haptenated protein to mice prior to the induction of TNBS colitis by intrarectal TNBS administration prevented colitis.[76] Moreover, such feeding was associated with the appearance of TGF-β-producing cells in the lamina propria, and anti-TGF-β administered after feeding abolished the protective effect of the feeding. Finally, a recent study showed that although lamina propria T cells isolated from mice with TNBS colitis can transfer to naive recipient mice susceptibility to colitis elicited by low doses of TNBS, such susceptibility is abolished by co-administered lamina propria cells from mice fed TNP-haptenated protein.[77] Because the lamina propria cells from the recipient mice produced TGF-β, this co-transfer experiment is a formal demonstration that feeding of an antigen elicits a protective regulatory T-cell response mediated by TGF-β. Together, these studies directly link TGF-β-producing suppressor cells to oral tolerance, and link the development of such cells to mucosal homeostasis.

Whereas studies of oral tolerance analyzing mucosal immune responses to antigen feeding have consistently identified TGF-β as the major suppressor cytokine, some studies of experimental mucosal inflammation have identified IL-10 as a second mediator of oral tolerance. The involvement of IL-10 is evident from the facts that IL-10-deficient mice develop colitis, and that co-transfer of CD45RB(lo) cells from mice with IL-10 deficiency, or transfer of normal CD45RB(lo) cells with anti-IL10R, fails to prevent colitis in the SCID CD45RB(hi) transfer model.[78] In addition, in the spontaneous colitis that develops in LPS-non-responsive C3H/HeJ mice, T cells that produce IL-10 ultimately re-establish normal homeostasis and prevent colitis.[79] Finally, co-transfer of T-regulatory cell type 1, or Tr1, cells obtained by culturing cells in IL-10-containing media and which produce mainly IL-10 and only small amounts of TGF-β, prevents colitis in the SCID transfer model.[80] Such Tr1 cells represent an alternative regulatory cell type mediating oral tolerance that does not involve TGF-β.

Co-administration of either anti-TGF-β or anti-IL-10 more or less completely abolished the protective effect of the CD45RB(lo) cells in the SCID-transfer model of colitis. Thus it is apparent that TGF-β and IL-10 are not only co-equal, they have interrelated activities in suppressor cells that regulate mucosal homeostasis. Recently, the relation of TGF-β and IL-10 as regulatory cytokines was examined in their ability to suppress TNBS colitis. Administration of both anti-TGF-β and anti-IL-10 prevented the development of protection elicited by feeding TNP-haptenated protein, suggesting that both cytokines serve as regulatory elements.[77] However, studies of cytokines produced by lamina propria cells from mice treated with these antibodies revealed that whereas anti-IL-10 treatment inhibited both IL-10 and TGF-β secretion, anti-TGF-β treatment reduced TGF-β secretion but had no effect on IL-10 secretion. Thus, IL-10 production could not prevent colitis in the absence of TGF-β and so appeared to have a secondary role. The effect of anti-IL-10 was not on the initial induction of TGF-β-producing cells, but rather on their proliferation and/or expansion in the Th1 inflammatory milieu. This conclusion was solidified by studies of the ability of lamina propria T cells derived from fed mice to produce TGF-β ex vivo in the presence of Th1 cytokines, which was greatly hampered by the presence of both IL-12 and IL-18. Thus, the role of IL-10 as a regulatory cytokine lies mainly in its ability to act a facilitating factor for the expansion of TGF-β-producing cells. Although both of these cytokines are necessary for maintaining mucosal homeostasis, TGF-β has the more proximal role.

A functional relation between TGF-β and IL-10 is mirrored by the finding that TGF-β secretion can induce IL-10 production via activation of TGF-β-associated signaling molecules called Smads, followed by Smad-mediated transcriptional activation of the IL-10 gene (A Kitani, NIH, Bethesda, MD, personal communication). This supports the view that the co-secretion of TGF-β and IL-10 during the regulation of inflammation is not a mere redundancy, but a necessary interdependency. Thus, whereas IL-10 can downregulate Th1 responses, it cannot reverse established Th1-mediated inflammation unless it is present in extremely high, non-physiologic amounts. Conversely, TGF-β production is limited in the absence of IL-10- mediated downregulation of Th1 responses. In addition, IFN-γ and TNF block TGF-β function by upregulating Smad7, a Smad isoform that blocks TGF-β signaling via Smad2 and 3.[81]

## NATURE OF ORAL ANTIGEN-INDUCED SUPPRESSOR T CELLS PRODUCING TGF-β (TH3 CELLS) AND IL-10 (TR1 CELLS)

Th3 regulatory cells producing TGF-β appear to originate in organized mucosal lymphoid sites such as the Peyer's patches (PP) following antigen feeding. This leads naturally to the question as to whether these cells are preferentially produced in mucosal sites and are uniquely related to mucosal responses, or whether they are part of a larger population of regulatory cells that are simply more numerous or more easily detected in mucosal tissues. Two broad answers can be put forward. One is that conditions in mucosal follicles favor the induction and expansion of TGF-β-producing cells, and the other is that these cells are a subpopulation of regulatory cells that are specifically expanded in mucosal tissues simply because they encounter antigens intrinsic to the mucosal environment. To decide between these two possibilities we need to review the various types of suppressor cells described in recent years, emphasizing the origin of these cells and/or their unique sphere of function.

The first type of suppressor cell is the Th3 cell. Initial in vitro studies relating the origin of Th3 cells to Th1 and Th2 responses showed that the differentiation of naive CD4+ T cells into TGF-β-producing T cells is inhibited by Th1 cytokines and enhanced by Th2 cytokines.[82] This corresponds to in vivo studies showing that, following antigen feeding, the administration of anti-IL-12 or IL-4 increased TGF-β responses in PP.[83] Also, antigen-specific T-cell clones producing TGF-β (i.e. putative Th3 cells) derived from mesenteric lymph nodes of mice fed the stimulating antigen, can develop into cells also producing Th2 cytokines (although clearly clones producing TGF-β and not co-producing Th2 cytokines, or even co-producing Th1 cytokines, also develop).[61,84,85] This suggests that the Th3 cells developed under conditions that favor Th2 responses. However, although these data suggest that Th2 responses and IL-4 have a positive role in Th3 development, they do not indicate that Th2 cytokines are either necessary or sufficient for such development. On the contrary, feeding antigen can induce oral tolerance under conditions usually dependent on Th3 cells in IL-4 null mice, and oral antigen induction of Th3 responses is not necessarily accompanied by IL-4 responses.[82] Finally, in several models of mucosal inflammation, most notably in the SCID-transfer model and the IL-2-deficiency model, regulatory cells producing TGF-β can be induced with cells from IL-4-deficient mice in the presence of anti-IL-4 administration.[74,86]

In summary, although Th2 cytokines facilitate and Th1 cytokines inhibit Th3 T-cell development, neither is definitively involved in such development, either positively or negatively. In addition, the mucosal lymphoid follicles do not constitute a cellular milieu that is skewed exclusively to a Th2 response; thus, it is unlikely that the Th1/Th2 orientation of the mucosal lymphoid environment is responsible for the appearance of Th3 cells in mucosal tissues.

Dendritic cells in mucosal tissues, through preferential production of certain cytokines, could induce regulatory T cells. A subset of PP dendritic cells have been identified that have a unique cytokine profile in that they produce larger amounts of IL-10 than phenotypically similar cells in the spleen.[87] IL-10 produced by these cells could suppress IL-12 production and thus create conditions that allow the development of Th3 cells. Nevertheless, these dendritic cells do not produce substantial amounts TGF-β or induce T cells that produce this cytokine. Thus the concept that dendritic cells in mucosal follicles account for the development of Th3 cells is, at least as yet, poorly substantiated. However, recent evidence suggests that dendritic cells in the respiratory mucosa which preferentially secrete IL-10 induce regulatory T cells that produce IL-10.[88–90] Thus, although dendritic cells cannot be shown to induce Th3 cells they may induce an alternative regulatory cell, the Tr1 cell.

Another possibility regarding the origin of Th3 cells considers the fact that mucosal lymphoid follicles are juxtaposed to intestinal epithelial cells; thus they may be exposed to as yet undiscovered signaling molecules (e.g. cytokines) secreted by epithelial cells that induce Th3 T-cell generation. Yet another possibility is that Th3 T cells are a subset of regulatory T cells that develop centrally, i.e. in the thymus, and are preferentially expanded in the mucosal follicles after encountering mucosal antigens.

A second major type of suppressor T cell is the Tr1 cell (T-regulatory cell, type 1), which mediates suppression by the secretion of IL-10. Initially, this cell was identified in antigen-driven T-cell populations cultured in the presence of IL-10.[80] Thus, IL-10 emerged as the cytokine that defines these cells as well as being necessary for their development. More recently, a cell that is very similar to the Tr1 cell has been obtained by culturing antigen-driven cells in the presence of dexamethasone and vitamin $D_3$.[91] Induction could occur in the absence of APC, exogenous IL-10 acted as a positive proliferation factor, and exogenous IL-4, IL-12 or IFN-γ inhibited the development of these cells, suggesting that their development was independent of the Th1/Th2 axis. Finally, there is now evidence that IFN-α synergizes with IL-10 in support of human Tr1 cells.[92]

In the first description of Tr1 cells their suppressor function was inhibited by anti-TGF-β, suggesting that they also produced the latter cytokine.[80] In addition, Tr1 cells produced small amounts of other cytokines, particularly IL-5. However, Tr1 cells induced by dexamethasone and vitamin $D_3$ produce IL-10 in the absence of other cytokines, including TGF-β.[91] This suggests that under physiologic conditions 'hybrid' Tr1 cells produce cytokines other than IL-10.

The efficacy of Tr1 cells was initially shown to downregulate colitis in the SCID-transfer model, where Tr1 cells could substitute for CD45RB(lo) cells.[80] Recent studies show that *Helicobactor hepaticus* infection induced the formation of Tr1 cells (cells producing IL-10 but not TGF-β), which could then prevent colitis in the SCID-transfer model.[93] However, at least in the TNBS colitis model, IL-10 facilitates the suppression of inflammation by TGF-β, rather than mediating such suppression itself.[77] Thus, in both of these situations Tr1 cells could be serving as a source of IL-10 that allows the expansion of naturally occurring TGF-β-producing cells, rather than acting directly as suppressor cells. However, anti-TGF-β treatment of the SCID recipient mice did not affect the protective effect of the *H. hepaticus*-induced Tr1 cells. In addition, Tr1 cells induced by dexamethasone and vitamin $D_3$, which do not produce detectible TGF-β, prevent the development of EAE, particularly when given with antigen to activate the cells. Thus, in some cases, Tr1 cells seem to be the primary regulatory cells controlling inflammation, rather than merely facilitating TGF-β-producing regulatory cells.

Regulatory cells producing IL-10 have also been noted in a variety of other situations involving both mice and humans. They have been identified in mice following transplantation, after the administration of superantigens, and after intranasal immunization with soluble peptides.[94–96] In addition, they have been noted in SCID patients undergoing HLA-mismatched bone marrow transplantation, in patients tolerant to nematode infection, and in MS patients undergoing oral treatment with MBP to induce oral tolerance.[97] In some or all of these cases the IL-10 was being produced in association with TGF-β, so that it is not possible to say whether these cells are Tr1 or Th3. In reality, these regulatory cells exhibit considerable overlap, as illustrated by self-MHC-reactive T cells (i.e. cells reacting to self-antigens in the context of self-MHC antigens) which occur in normal individuals producing both TGF-β and IL-10 when appropriately stimulated.[98] Production of these cytokines is closely linked, and it may be artificial to define separate regulatory cell subsets producing one regulatory cytokine and not the other under physiologic conditions.

A third type of suppressor T cell is CD4+/CD25+. This cell has a long history in that human and mouse CD4+ cells with the capacity to downregulate B-cell function were identified over 20 years ago.[99] Nevertheless, it was not until the α chain of the IL-2 receptor (CD25) was identified as a marker that these cells became recognized as a defined regulatory T-cell subset. This marker is present on the surface of all activated T cells, not just this regulatory cell. This deficiency, however, is partially mitigated by the fact that the surface CD25 is not associated with other components of the IL-2 receptor, such as the β chain of the receptor, thereby distinguishing CD25+ regulatory cells from other activated cells. In addition, studies of gene expression differences between CD25+ regulatory cells and CD25+ non-regulatory activated cells using microarray technology reveal that the two cell populations are vastly different at the molecular level, and that the CD25+ cell is indeed unique.[100,101]

The existence of CD25+ regulatory cells were first inferred from studies showing that thymectomy in 2–3-day-old mice leads to multiple organ autoimmune disease, particularly gastritis and orchitis.[102,103] This observation, plus the fact that repletion of the thymectomized mice with thymocytes prevented the autoimmunity, whereas transfer of T cells from the thymectomized mice to athymic recipients led to autoimmunity, strongly suggested that a cell population developing in the thymus at an early age and then capable of sustaining itself in the periphery had important regulatory properties. Later, this regulatory cell was identified as a CD4+/CD25+ cell that was depleted in the thymectomized mice and was capable of preventing autoimmunity in such mice.[102,104] More recently, studies of various types of knockout mice and Rag-2-deficient mice have shown more or less definitively that CD25+ regulatory cells undergo positive selection in the thymus as a result of presentation of self-antigens in the context of self-MHC.[105] Whereas CD4+/CD25– cells selected in this way are deleted by negative selection (thus maintaining self-tolerance), CD4+/CD25+ cells are not so deleted and are thus released into the circulation. However, these self-reactive T cells do not cause autoimmunity themselves, probably because they are resistant to proliferation and because their activation leads to the suppression of responses. On the contrary, they prevent autoimmunity by responding to self-antigen at nascent sites of self-reactivity and then providing a negative regulatory (suppressor) response. CD25+ cells appear to mediate a silent immune surveillance that guards against autoimmunity. Finally, it is important to emphasize human self-MHC reactive T cells (formerly called autoreactive T cells) that belong to the Tr1 or Th3 category of suppressor cells. Because these cells have specificity for self-antigens they may also fit into the CD25+ cell category, although additional studies are necessary to determine their phenotype.

CD25+ cells comprise 5–10% of cells in the spleen of mice and a somewhat smaller percentage of human peripheral blood cells. They undergo proliferation only when stimulated under optimal conditions involving strong cross-linking of the T-cell receptor and the provision of co-stimulation and/or IL-2. However, activation of negative regulation does not require these stringent conditions and is instead triggered by antigen-loaded APC. There is some evidence that CTLA-4 co-stimulation delivers a positive signal for CD25+ cells, rather than the negative signal it delivers to CD25– cells.[46,106,107] The mechanism of suppression employed by CD25+ cells remains an enigma. Suppressor activity can be demonstrated in vitro simply by co-culturing of CD25+ and CD25– cells and then measuring proliferation of the CD25– cells. Under these conditions suppression requires cell–cell interaction without the secretion of a regulatory cytokine such as TGF-β or IL-10.[102,108] There is evidence, however, that CD25+ cells do not require cell–cell interaction. Recently, evidence has appeared showing that CD25+ cells secrete both TGF-β and IL-10 when stimulated under TCR-cross-linking conditions and in the presence of strong co-stimulation.[109] In addition, activated CD25+ cells express surface-inactive TGF-β associated with latency-associated protein (LAP), whereas CD25– cells express only marginal amounts of this protein. Such surface TGF-β is present both on mouse spleen cells and human peripheral blood cells, in which only the CD25+(hi) population is associated with suppressor cell activity.[109] Several groups have suggested that this surface TGF-β is responsible for cell contact-associated suppressor activity in vitro, as such surface TGF-β is upregulated under the relatively mild stimulation conditions of in vitro culture which does not elicit TGF-β secretion and, in addition, the latter is inhibited by high concentrations of anti-TGF-β.[106] Furthermore, unpublished work shows that in vitro suppression mediated by CD25+ cells can be inhibited by a component of latent TGF-β known as latency-associated protein in a dose-dependent fashion.

Although further verification is necessary, these results imply that CD25+ cells act as regulatory cells in one of two ways. When they are induced under strong activation conditions, such as those encountered in an inflammatory milieu, they secrete TGF-β and IL-10. In this functional form they act as conventional regulatory cells that are functionally indistinguishable from Th3 cells. However, relatively weak activation conditions upregulate surface TGF-β, which is activated upon cell–cell contact with a target (CD25–) cell without entering the fluid phase, and immediately commences signaling via its receptors on the target cell. This functional form of suppression may be more characteristic of the surveillance activity of the CD25+ cell, which acts to prevent inflammation.

## MISCELLANEOUS SUPPRESSOR CELLS

In addition to the regulatory cells described above, a number of other types of cell have been described which also mediate regulatory function. One cell in this category is the CD8+ suppressor cell elicited during oral tolerance induction in mice and rats, and which may be distinct from CD4+ suppressor cells on the basis of the cytokines they produce and the cellular events they influence. CD8+ suppressor cells occur both in humans undergoing transplantation and in patients with IBD. In IBD antigen presentation by epithelial cells involves unique interactions between CEA (gp180) on the epithelial cell surface, and CD8 on peripheral blood T cells leads to preferential stimulation of CD8+ cells with suppressor capability.[110–112] Induction of these cells is said to be impaired in IBD, possibly because of altered expression of CEA; however, it is not clear whether this is a primary or secondary disease factor. Finally, a particular subclass of dendritic cell, the DC2 plasmacytoid dendritic cells, induce CD8+T cells to undergo differentiation into regulatory T cells producing IL-10 (but not TGF-β) that resemble Tr1 cells.[113,114] γδ Intraepithelial T cells constitute yet another category that may display regulatory properties, particularly in the presence of oral tolerance. Cells of this type producing IL-10 and capable of mediating an antidiabetogenic effect were induced by oral insulin administration.[115] In addition, oral tolerance following low doses of antigen feeding cannot be induced or is severely impaired in mice lacking γδ T cells.[51] However, it is unclear how

or why γδ T cells play a significant role in oral tolerance, as they are limited to the intraepithelial cell compartment. One possibility is that these cells are necessary to support epithelial cell secretion of substances necessary for the development of Th3 cells and are thus only indirectly involved in oral tolerance. A final category of T cell with regulatory properties is the NK-T cell. Most of these cells manifest a specialized TCR that recognizes glycolipid antigens via an 'invariant TCR', characterized in humans by Vα24-JαQ (or in mice by a closely related TCR). NK-T cell-mediated regulation has been noted in NOD mice, where depletion of NK-T cells has been shown to lead to early-onset diabetes,[116–118] and in DSS-induced colitis where depletion led to more severe colitis, and the administration of an antigen that stimulates NK-T cells via the invariant TCR, α-galactosylceramide, improved disease.[119] Finally, NK-T cell number and function have been related to the severity of autoimmunity encountered in multiple sclerosis and diabetes.[120–122] The mechanism of action of NK-T cell regulation is completely unknown, although it undoubtedly relates to the cytokines produced by these cells. Different subsets of NK-T cells produce different cytokines, and so it may be possible to relate their regulatory function to the production of known suppressive cytokines.

The nature of the suppressor cell involved in oral tolerance is becoming better defined. The discovery that CD25+ regulatory T cells act through secreted or surface regulatory cytokines, particularly TGF-β, opens the question as to whether Th3 cells and CD25+ regulatory cells are identical. As mentioned, CD25+ cells are self-reactive T cells. If we assume that Th3 cells are, in general, specific for mucosal antigens, and further assume that commensal bacterial antigens are functionally equivalent to self-antigens because they are constantly present and have ready access to the internal milieu, then it is possible to say that Th3 cells are also self-reactive. Mucosal antigens that gain access to the circulation and enter the thymus may induce positive selection of CD25+ cells that are not materially different from other CD25+ cells. Furthermore, we speculate that the cells so induced ultimately re-enter the mucosal follicles, where they re-encounter mucosal antigens and undergo expansion. Thus, in this scenario Th3 cells are in fact CD25+ cells that appear to originate in mucosal tissues, but actually originate in the thymus and expand in mucosal tissues (Fig. 5.2).

Although the above hypothesis is not proven, it is nevertheless supported by certain observations. First, CD25+ cells with suppressor functions arise after both intravenous and oral administration of antigen to mice adoptively transferred with cells bearing a transgenic TCR specific for that antigen.[123] In these studies oral antigen administration is equivalent to systemic antigen administration in its ability to elicit an identical form of suppressor cell formation. Second, oral antigen administration to TCR-transgenic mice increased numbers of splenic CD25+ cell that secrete both TGF-β and IL-10 upon anti-CD3 stimulation, and when mixed in vitro with CD25– cells act as suppressor cells that are partially inhibited by anti-IL-10 and anti-TGF-β.[124] Third, there is good evidence that the regulatory cells that protect mice from colitis in the SCID-transfer model are CD25+ cells that act either directly or indirectly through the secretion of TGF-β, and there is emerging evidence that these cells are CD25+ cells with surface TGF-β[75] (K. Nakamura, NIH, Bethesda, MD, personal communication). If we assume that these cells are closely related to Th3 cells, as

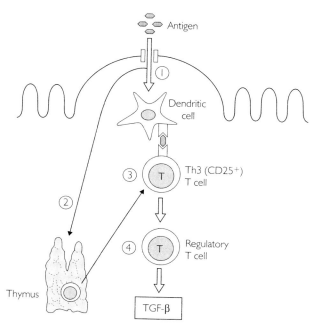

**Fig. 5.2** Hypothesis concerning the nature of suppressor cells mediating oral tolerance. As discussed in the text, recent work indicates that CD25+ T cells that develop in the thymus as a result of positive selection of self-antigens act via their production of TGF-β. This suggests that Th3 suppressor cells developing during the induction of oral tolerance enter mucosal follicles where they load dendritic cells (1). In addition, they enter the circulation and ultimately the thymus where they induce CD25+ regulatory cells by positive selection (2). Finally, the CD25+ cell migrates to the mucosal follicles, where it is restimulated by mucosal antigen (3) and then trafficks to the lamina propria where it mediates regulation (4).

suggested by induction of regulatory cells in the TNBS-colitis model by oral antigen administration, then these data also support the proposition that Th3 cells and CD25+ cells are the same. Finally, thymic abnormalities can lead to mucosal inflammation because of failure to generate regulatory cells. Thus, mice bearing a defective T-cell receptor (CD3ε) transgene manifest colitis when reconstituted with normal T cells. The colitis can be traced to thymic maldevelopment and the inability to generate regulatory T cells.[125] In a similar vein, IL-2-deficient mice have thymic abnormalities and colitis caused by the failure to generate regulatory T cells producing TGF-β.[86] Because the colitis developing in both of these models depends on a response to antigens in the microbial microflora, they can be considered to be due to a failure to develop oral tolerance and suppressor T cells. As such, they tie tolerance to a normal functioning thymus and so establish another link between Th3 and CD25+ T cells.

This evidence for the equivalence of the Th3 and CD25+ cells must be juxtaposed to evidence against this possibility. The most cogent argument is that it possible to induce oral tolerance to new antigens that cannot be considered self-antigens. However, oral tolerance is actually due to two competing immune processes, the induction of suppressor cells and the induction of clonal anergy and deletion. Thus, this objection is weakened by the fact that new antigen could be inducing oral tolerance via the second mechanism, having nothing to do with suppressor cells. Supporting this view is the fact that low-dose oral tolerance most frequently associated with suppressor cell-

mediated oral tolerance has been seen after oral administration of self-antigens such as MBP. In addition, it is seen after prolonged feeding of small doses of antigen dissolved in the drinking water, a form of antigen delivery that permits entry of antigens into the circulation and their subsequent induction of regulatory cells in the thymus. There remains the difficulty that oral tolerance due to suppressor cell formation, i.e. CD25+ T-cell induction, can presumably occur later in life when the thymus has involuted. Here we invoke the possibility that thymic involution is never complete, and there is always enough thymic tissue to allow positive selection and induction of suppressor cells.

Finally, it is important to consider the possible role of Tr1 cells (either CD4+ or perhaps CD8+ T cells) in oral tolerance. Because these cells are not specific for self-antigens, but rather for exogenous antigens, they may be induced by infectious agents and serve to limit inflammation induced by such agents without affecting the induction of immune responses that promote pathogen clearance. This would apply particularly well to protective antibodies, as IL-10 favors humoral responses while suppressing cellular responses. Exogenous agents confront the organism with a host of non-self antigens that have not been in the thymus and have not induced regulatory T cells that produce TGF-β. The recent study of *H. hepaticus* infection supports this possibility by showing that although colonic infection with *H. hepaticus* does not evoke an inflammatory response it does induce an IL-10-producing T cell that, when transferred to a SCID recipient, prevents SCID-transfer colitis that is not abrogated by systemic administration of TGF-β.[93] Therefore, Tr1 are not part of the oral tolerance response, but oral antigens can nevertheless elicit protective Tr1 cells under certain circumstances.

## ORAL TOLERANCE DUE TO INDUCTION OF T-CELL ANERGY OR DELETION

A second and perhaps more basic mechanism of oral tolerance involves the induction of clonal anergy or deletion. The first evidence in favor of this mechanism was the observation that unresponsiveness to fed antigens persists long after one can demonstrate by adoptive transfer the continued presence of oral antigen-induced suppressor cells.[48,49] In addition, although tolerance induced prior to systemic immunization can be attributed to the induction of suppressor cells, tolerance induced after immunization cannot. In retrospect, this is explainable by the fact that suppressor cells cannot easily expand in the face of an active Th1 response.

The first hard evidence that anergy/deletion accounted for oral tolerance was obtained by Ferguson and her colleagues in the 1980s, who demonstrated that oral antigen administration is followed by the appearance of a circulating form of antigen that could induce tolerance when transferred to naive recipient mice.[4] Such antigen was in fact equivalent to tolerogenic antigen existing in the circulation after the removal of immunogenic components by the RE system. These studies strongly suggested that oral antigen administration was similar to intravenous antigen administration in that both led to the 'production' of a tolerogenic form of antigen. In addition, as intravenous antigen administration is due to the induction of clonal anergy/deletion, it followed that oral antigen administration with systemic distribution was also due to this mechanism.

More recently, oral tolerance due to induction of clonal anergy/deletion has been investigated in the EAE model. Whitacre and colleagues[126,127] showed that feeding MBP led to unresponsiveness to MBP and the prevention of EAE. However, in contrast to other studies discussed above, tolerance to MBP was not accompanied by the development of suppressor cells acting through TGF-β. This apparent conflict was eventually resolved in further studies showing that whereas feeding relatively low doses of antigen leads to the induction of suppressor cells, feeding of high doses of antigen (as in the Whitacre studies) led to clonal anergy/deletion.

If anergy/deletion accounts for oral tolerance under some conditions it must necessarily involve the entire immune system. In studies of mice bearing TCR transgenes in whom the fate of cells bearing the transgene for a fed antigen can be readily determined, it was shown that although the induction of anergy/deletion that follows feeding is most evident in mucosal tissues, it also occurs in systemic tissues.[127] More deletion at mucosal than at systemic sites is reasonable, given the fact that mucosal lymphocytes comprise the cell population most exposed to mucosal antigens, and deletion of cells in systemic sites probably reflects either the export of cells about to be deleted or the induction of anergy/deletion by the tolerogenic circulating antigen that results from feeding.

Elucidation of anergy/deletion occurring in relation to oral antigen has come from studies of MBP-specific T cells in mice bearing a TCR transgene specific for MBP. These studies showed that feeding leads to the rapid appearance of activated cells that produce Th1 and Th2 cytokines, but which manifest transiently decreased expression of surface TCR due to TCR internalization.[128] When transgenic mice are challenged with antigens to induce EAE during this time, they do not develop disease, presumably reflecting the anergic state of the cells. Evidence that this is the case comes from mice that are thymectomized prior to feeding to prevent the generation of new, non-anergic cells.[128] In this situation, feeding is followed by a transient loss of TCR expression, but although such expression soon returns, the cells again gradually lose TCR expression and become unresponsive to stimulation. In addition, in situ TUNEL staining shows that after feeding the cells undergo apoptosis. These data agree with earlier results showing that mice transferred TCR-transgenic T cells and then fed antigen have TCR-positive cells in the spleen that are unresponsive to cognate antigen.[129] Collectively, these studies suggest that antigen feeding leads initially to short-lived cell activation, followed by a longer period of anergy and ultimately apoptotic deletion.

Feeding MBP to MBP-TCR transgenic mice results in a rapid loss of MBP-specific cells in the non-mucosal tissues: although such cells increased to near normal levels after 3 days, they again declined by 10 days, when the fed mice displayed protection from induction of EAE.[127,128] Interestingly, the number of MBP-specific cells in the lamina propria increased after feeding, whereas it declined in systemic tissues, reflecting the traffic of mucosal cells back to mucosal sites. These studies suggest that long-lived tolerance to fed antigen (and protection from EAE) results in the TCR-transgenic mouse from the depletion of cells reactive to antigen in the peripheral tissues. In normal mice (and presumably in normal humans), where the number of antigen specific cells are far less numerous than in transgenic mice, tolerance is probably not so much related to redistribution of cells as it is to deletion, particularly when antigen is fed repetitively.

The alacrity with which anergy and deletion is induced by feeding suggests that the mucosal microenvironment possesses unique characteristics that promote this outcome. One factor relates to the probability that high-dose oral antigen administration is equivalent to the administration of soluble antigen by an intravenous route, as tolerogenic antigen is found in the circulation after feeding. Another less well defined factor is the possibility that antigen presentation by epithelial cells favors tolerance over stimulation. Intestinal epithelial cells lack co-stimulatory molecules normally associated with strong stimulatory responses. However, this is probably not a major factor, as T-cell stimulation occurs primarily within the mucosal lymphoid follicles by dendritic cells. Support for the idea that Peyer's patch dendritic cells are 'tolerogenic' has recently emerged. Dendritic cells isolated from the mesenteric lymph node (which drain Peyer's patches) after feeding MBP and then adaptively transferred to recipient mice decreased induction of EAE in the recipients (C. Whitacre, Ohio State University, Columbus, OH, personal communication). Also, mice treated with Flt3 ligand, a substance that non-specifically induces dendritic cell expansion but not differentiation, manifest heightened oral tolerance, presumably because 'immature' cells are expanded which fail to express co-stimulatory molecules (CD80 and CD86).[130] In contrast, mice co-administered Flt-3 ligand and IL-1, an inflammatory cytokine that induces co-stimulatory molecules on the surface of DC, restored loss of tolerance.[131] These findings imply that the Peyer's patches normally contain immature DC that lead to tolerance rather than immunity. Finally, the idea that the mucosa contains tolerogenic APC is supported by unpublished studies showing that irradiated IL-10-deficient mice replete with bone marrow cells from OVA-TCR transgenic mice – i.e. transgenic mice lacking epithelial cells capable of producing IL-10 – are unable to manifest deletional tolerance following the feeding of OVA. This result suggests that IL-10 produced by mucosal epithelial cells conditions mucosal APC–T-cell interactions that lead to antigen unresponsiveness owing to anergy/deletion. Thus, it is possible that epithelial cell IL-10 acts to induce mucosal DC to act as tolerogenic rather than immunogenic presenting cells.

One of the remarkable aspects of oral tolerance due to cellular deletion is its persistence. Thus, even in mice bearing an MBP-specific TCR transgene, a single high dose of oral MBP prevents EAE for at least 40 days, despite the fact that new thymic immigrants are constantly being generated that were not present during the feeding period. A possible explanation is that feeding changes the trafficking of antigen-reactive cells by sequestering cells in the lamina propria or shunting cells to the liver, where they encounter conditions leading to apoptosis. These possibilities suggest that oral tolerance is due to redirection of cells away from sites where they can be sensed as antigen-reactive cells or cells that produce disease.

## THE INTERRELATION OF ACTIVE (SUPPRESSOR CELL-MEDIATED) AND PASSIVE (DELETIONAL) ORAL TOLERANCE

If oral tolerance depends on both active suppression and deletional mechanisms, it is important to determine which of these mechanisms predominates under various conditions. The most likely possibility is that both mechanisms are operative simultaneously but that one is more apparent than the other during low-

and high-dose oral antigen exposure. Feeding antigen to TCR-transgenic mice with cognate antigen induces early activation and Th1 cytokine response, which is followed by induction of clonal anergy/deletion. Because this Th1 response normally suppresses the TGF-β response, one would expect that feeding high doses of antigen suppresses the suppressor cell response by at least temporarily creating a non-permissive Th1 environment; hence high-dose feeding leads solely to anergic unresponsiveness. This view is nicely supported by the observation that the administration of anti-IL-12 to mice fed high doses of antigen is associated with the appearance of a suppressor cell response.[83]

In contrast, following low-dose antigen feeding the induced Th1 response is too weak to suppress the regulatory cell response, and the latter predominates. At the same time, the low-dose antigen feeding is unable to delete all of the antigen cells and, as a result, antigen-reactive cells (i.e. lack of anergy) and suppressor cells persist. A further question arises concerning different effects of a single low-dose antigen feed and multiple low-dose feedings. Multiple or continuous feedings (i.e. feeding regimens that more closely approximate the in vivo situation) are more likely to induce regulatory cells than are single feeds. This can be explained if we assume that suppressor cells arise primarily in the thymus as a result of exposure to mucosal antigens, so that feeding a new antigen can lead to the expansion of suppressor cells, first by initial induction by fed antigen that gains entry into the thymus, and second by the expansion of newly induced suppressor cells that recognize fed antigen in the mucosal tissues. Both processes are favored by low-dose continuous feeding, as this avoids the induction of high Th1 responses and allow for antigen entry and suppressor cell induction in the thymus. This sets the stage for unresponsiveness to ingested food antigens and antigens in the mucosal microflora.

A final consideration regarding low-dose suppressor T cell-mediated tolerance concerns Th2 responses, which favor suppressor T-cell development. As noted earlier, such responses are characteristic of adjuvant-induced responses such as cholera toxin, which leads to high IL-4 responses and low IL-12/IFN-γ responses. This raises a possible conundrum: how can the induction of high TGF-β suppressor cell responses be reconciled with high Th2 responses and mucosal IgA production? The answer may lie in the fact that TGF-β does not suppress Th2 responses unless present at very high concentrations, and on the other hand TGF-β is necessary for the isotype switching of B cells into IgA-producing B cells. Thus, low doses of oral antigen could induce TGF-β-producing T cells that suppress concomitant Th1 responses but not Th2 responses. The outcome is the differentiation of IgA B cells in the face of suppressor cell-mediated (Th1) unresponsiveness. Evidence in favor of this possibility comes from older studies showing that whereas Th1 responses are suppressed by antigen feeding, IgA responses are more resistant to such suppression.[5] This is not to say that humoral IgG and IgA responses are not suppressed by oral antigen feeding: this in fact does occur with high-dose antigen feeding, when helper T cells necessary to support humoral responses are deleted.

# THE ROLE OF MUCOSAL DENDRITIC CELLS IN THE REGULATION OF MUCOSAL RESPONSES

A key to the understanding of the positive and negative responses in the mucosal immune system is understanding the function of APC cells in the Peyer's patches and other mucosal lymphoid sites. Kelsall and Strober showed that dendritic cells form a dense layer of cells just below the epithelium overlying the Peyer's patches, and thus are in a perfect anatomic location to intercept incoming antigens at this major site of mucosal immune activity.[132] Other dendritic cells are either scattered through the patch or present in dense concentrations in the T cell-rich intrafollicular regions of the patch. Kelsall and colleagues showed that these mucosal dendritic cells are comprised of several subpopulations that occupy distinct positions within the follicle.[87,133] In the region beneath the epithelium (the subepithelial dome, SED) region, myeloid DC expressing CD11b but not CD8 are abundant, whereas in the intrafollicular regions lymphoid DC expressing CD8 but not CD11b are abundant. In addition, a third 'double-negative' DC population expressing neither CD11b nor CD8 is present in both the SED and intrafollicular regions; interestingly, this population is found between epithelial cells and thus is similar to a recently described mucosal CD11b DC subpopulation that is located in close apposition to epithelial cells and has processes that extend between epithelial cells allowing the direct sampling of luminal antigens. A final DC cell subpopulation is the so-called plasmacytic DC, which are distinguished by the expression of B220 and Ly6G/C markers and response to viral antigens with the production of type I interferons; in addition, when they mature they sometimes also express CD8, and may secrete IL-12 or IL-10 cytokines.[113] The location of these cells in the mucosal system has not yet been defined (see further discussion below).

The different DC subpopulations have been shown to produce different types of cytokine when stimulated by T cells or bacterial products (LPS). Lymphoid DC bearing CD8 (as well as plasmacytoid DC) usually produce large amounts of IL-12 but little or no IL-10, and thus support Th1 responses. In contrast, myeloid DC bearing CD11b usually produce large amounts of IL-10 and little or no IL-12, and thus support Th2 responses (Fig. 5.3). This has given rise to the notion that different subsets of DC induce different types of T-cell differentiation and that, by extension, cytokines that promote the differentiation of DC into one or the other subtypes ultimately affect the nature of the downstream T-cell response. However, DC exhibit a degree of 'plasticity' and can produce different cytokines under certain conditions despite their phenotype. Thus, such factors as antigen dose, tissue microenvironment and the presence of certain cytokines, chemokines and other factors may influence DC function in rather unpredictable ways. Finally, the above categorization of cytokine function of DC belonging to the gastrointestinal complement of DC may also apply to DC in the respiratory tract. Resident DC are immature cells that are skewed to the production of IL-10 and the induction of Th2 responses, thereby downregulating immune responses.[90] In addition, following stimulation they mature into a mixed population of cells that induce both Th1 and Th2 responses.

DC utilize separate receptors for antigen uptake and for activation. In the latter case, much attention has been focused on 'pattern recognition' receptors that include (but are not limited to) Toll-like receptors (TLR) that recognize evolutionarily conserved molecules on the surface of microbes. At least 10 different TLR have been described that, singly or in combination, recognize different microbial components. For example, LPS is recognized by TLR-4, peptidoglycans from *Staphylococcus aureus* are recognized by TLR-2, and CpG-containing oligonucleotides

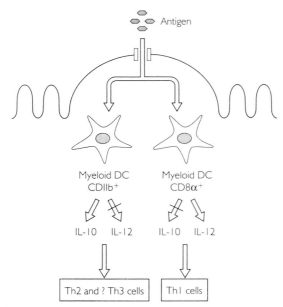

**Fig. 5.3** Dendritic cell subtypes and their relation to mucosal regulation. Antigen entering the mucosal follicle may encounter at least one of two types of dendritic cell (DC), myeloid DC producing cytokines that favor the development of Th2 and Th3 T cells (IL-10), or a lymphoid DC producing cytokines that favor the development of Th1 effector cells. The interrelation of these DC presentation pathways determines whether a given antigen will induce a tolerogenic or an immunogenic response.

are recognized by TLR-9.[16,134–137] These various TLR may be differentially expressed by DC subsets, suggesting that a particular microbe may address particular types of DC.

TLR signaling leads to the activation of intracellular adaptor molecules that, in turn, lead to NFκB activation and/or the activation of other cellular activation pathways. MyD88 is perhaps the most important of these adaptor molecules and is involved in all TLR signaling observed to date, although some TLR can manifest MyD88-independent signaling. Of interest, MyD88-deficient mice exhibit DC activation without the production of T-cell polarizing cytokines such as IL-12, IL-10 and IL-4. This has led to the notion that DC activation by a variety of stimuli in the absence of IL-12 production (e.g. schistosomal egg antigens and *P. gingivalis* LPS) leads to a default pathway and skewed Th2 responses.[138] Such stimulation could occur via suppression of MyD88 signaling, or signaling via a non-TLR pathway that results in selective IL-10 production and the consequent inhibition of IL-12 production. These include stimulation via the complement receptor CR3 and the chemokine receptor CCR5.

The knowledge that TLR are important in DC signaling has led to two as yet unresolved models of DC function. In an 'instructional' model, a DC with a particular phenotype can produce any set of cytokines depending on the type of stimulating microbe and the TLR(s) engaged by that microbe. In contrast, in a 'selectional model' different sets of DC, each with different expressed TLR and a genetically programmed cytokine production capability, determine the response; in this case, a given cytokine response is usually (but not always) associated with a particular DC phenotype based on selective expression of various TLR. Both of these models are compatible with the concept that phenotype of a DC does not absolutely specify a particular type of cytokine response, although the selectional

model is more consistent with this possibility than is the instructional model. In addition, although in both models DC control the type of cytokine production, other (exogenous) factors influence this as well. These include antigen dose, ratio of DC to T cells, duration of activation, and regulatory signals by cytokines, chemokines and products of arachidonic acid metabolism. In the latter regard, IFN-γ can stimulate DC to manifest a Th1-inducing capacity, whereas IL-10 and TGF-β may have the opposite effect.

An additional set of DC is the plasmacytoid DC, a type initially described in humans as a cell that arises from precursors circulating in the peripheral blood with plasma cell-like morphology. This cell is widely distributed in lymphoid tissues and occurs in both mice and humans. In humans, it is identified as a CD11b⁻ cell that only sometimes expresses CD8 (and then only following activation) and by the B220 and Ly6GC/C surface markers that are not found on other DC. Stimulation of this cell by viral antigens results in interferon α/β secretion, indicating that this cell was a component of 'innate immunity'.[113,139] Following their initial stimulation and consequent maturation, plasmacytoid DC cease production of interferon α/β and begin producing IL-12 or IL-10, depending on the mode of stimulation. However, the extent to which these cells induce Th1 or Th2 cells in adoptive immune responses remains to be defined. Human plasmacytoid DC may also induce regulatory T cells when stimulated by CD40L. The cells induced are anergic CD8+ cells that produce IL-10, but not TGF-β1 or the various Th1 or Th2 cytokines; in addition, they inhibit various T-cell responses through their production of IL-10, and thus appear to be a type of Tr1 regulatory cell.[53]

Considerable data support the concept that mucosal DC play a critical role in initiating the regulatory responses characteristic of this system. The first evidence of this kind is that dendritic cells in the respiratory tract tend to produce IL-10. Furthermore, mice exposed to ovalbumin by the intra-nasal route develop mature DC in the respiratory mucosa that transiently produce IL-10 and induce the development of Tr1 regulatory cells that produce IL-10 along with IL-4, but not TGF-β1. In addition, respiratory DC from IL-10+/+ mice, but not IL-10−/− mice, could transfer unresponsiveness to the stimulating antigen to naive mice. A similar series of observation were made in relation to respiratory exposure to a protein derived from a pathogen, *Bordetella pertussis*. The regulatory cells induced in this case produced high levels of IL-10 and IL-4, as well as low levels of TGF-β1.[90] However, the suppression was clearly due to the IL-10 secretion. As might be expected from this cytokine profile, they suppressed responses of Th1 cells but not Th2 cells in vitro. Of interest, the *B. pertussis* antigen used in these studies binds to CR3 on APC, a receptor that downregulates IL-12 production.[140] Thus, the mechanism of Tr1 cell induction may be preferential stimulation of IL-10-producing DC. Although these studies explain some aspects of the unresponsiveness of the respiratory mucosa, they do not explain all. This becomes evident from studies in which it has been shown that following exposure to aerosolized respiratory antigen, Th2 responses (IgE responses), but not Th1 responses, are suppressed; and the suppression in this case is not due to IFN-γ, i.e. not due to immune deviation.[141] If IL-10 were the sole mediator of respiratory unresponsiveness then Th2 responses should not be suppressed.

Studies of the capacity of gastrointestinal DC to induce regulatory cells is less extensive with respect to their cytokine profile but more extensive regarding how they function in inducing tolerance to the microbial microflora. Thus, in rats the intestinal lymphatics contain two populations of DC, a cell with strong antigen-presenting capability and bearing the OX41 antigen, and a cell with weak antigen-presenting capability and not bearing this antigen.[142] The OX41+ population is of particular interest because it contains apoptotic (TUNEL-positive) DNA and non-specific esterase inclusions probably derived from intestinal epithelial cells. This finding has led to the proposal that intestinal DC take up cellular remnants derived from dying epithelial cells and then migrate to draining nodes, where they induce regulatory cells specific for the antigens associated with the remnants. Such antigen uptake, migration and presentation are characteristic of DC in other sites and thus are unique only in the fact that the antigens being taken up are derived from dying epithelial cells. The latter include not only endogenous cellular antigens, but also antigens previously taken up by the epithelial cells from the intestinal lumen. In this way, oral antigens can induce tolerance in the intestinal tract as a whole, not only in the Peyer's patches. Still unanswered are questions regarding the types of T cell stimulated by migrating DC and the phenotype/cytokine profile of these cells. In addition, it is not clear why other OX41+ DC that are also migrating to draining nodes do not evoke effector responses to mucosal antigens. Nevertheless, it is tempting to speculate that such migrating DC are responsible for the restimulation of self-reactive regulatory T cells and, as such, are a major generator of TGF-β1-producing regulatory cells.

# EVIDENCE FOR DEFECTIVE ORAL TOLERANCE IN EXPERIMENTAL MUCOSAL INFLAMMATION AND IN HUMAN IBD

Having discussed the mechanisms of oral tolerance, we now address how these mechanisms apply to the pathogenesis of experimental inflammation and human IBD.

In recent years a great number of experimental models of mucosal inflammation have been described, and many of these have been intensively studied to determine the underlying pathogenesis. Such analyses have revealed the fact that the models can be placed in one of two broad categories: type 1 models are characterized by defects leading to the overactivity of effector mechanisms that overwhelm normal regulatory mechanisms, whereas type 2 models are characterized by the underactivity of regulatory mechanisms and thus unfettered activity of normal effector mechanisms (see Fig. 5.4 and Table 5.1 (reviewed in [1]). One example of a type 1 experimental inflammation is mice bearing a Stat4 transgene under a CMV promoter.[143] These mice have increased Th1 responses because of excessive responsiveness to IL-12 signaling. Thus, when unfractionated T cells from these mice are exposed to autologous commensal bacterial antigens and then transferred to a SCID recipient they induce colitis, whereas identical T cells from normal mice stimulated in the same way do not. Because unfractionated T cells contain populations of CD45RB(hi) naive T cells that are the source of effector T cells as well as populations of CD45RB(lo) memory T cells that are the source of regulatory T cells, this experiment indicates that

the Stat4 transgene leads to inflammation in the face of a normal regulatory population. Another example of a type I experimental inflammation is that seen in TNBS colitis. This colitis is induced in strains of mice that have a genetically determined hyperresponsiveness to LPS and thus greatly increased production of IL-12 when exposed to the microbial flora as a result of the disruption of the mucosal barrier by the ethanol vehicle used to deliver the TNBS.[144,145] It is believed that this initial (innate) IL-12 response sets the stage for the more prolonged Th1 response to TNBS-haptenated protein. In both of these examples (and presumably in other type 1 models), once a Th1 effector response is set in motion, the countervailing regulatory response is suppressed.

Corresponding examples of type II mucosal inflammations include the SCID-transfer model, in which colitis occurs after transferring cell populations lacking regulatory cells (CD45RB (lo) cells).[146] In addition, it occurs in models where there is an obvious lack of a regulatory cytokine, such as the IL-10-deficient mouse[147] or the TGF-β1-deficient mouse.[148] Other possible examples of type II inflammations include the C3H/HeJBir mouse, which develops spontaneous colitis that eventually resolves owing to the establishment of a regulatory cell response.[79] Because regulatory cells resolve the inflammation, it is reasonable to propose that the lack of these cells at an earlier stage causes disease.

Two other examples of type II inflammation, both associated with defects in thymic function, bear further discussion. The first of these is the IL-2-deficient mouse that either slowly develops colitis spontaneously, or rapidly develops colitis after injection with TNP-haptenated protein (in adjuvant).[86] These mice develop TNP-induced colitis because they lack regulatory T cells producing TGF-β1. In addition, upon injection of TNP-haptenated protein these mice generate thymic T cells that can induce colitis when transferred to naive recipients. One might presume that in the normal mouse, immunization with an antigen such as TNP-haptenated protein would result in the generation of effector T cells as well as regulatory T cells, but that in the absence of IL-2 the latter do not develop and one sees only effector cells. The second type II model associated with thymic abnormalities is the Tgε26, wherein a defect in the TCR complex due to overexpression of CDε leads to severe abnormalities of thymic development and colitis when the mice are replete with normal bone marrow cells, which give rise to precursor T cells that do not develop in a normal thymic microenvironment.[125] In this model repletion with normal bone marrow plus fetal thymus tissue does not lead to colitis, presumably because precursor T cells can develop in the thymus. However, because the cells passing through the normal thymus are inevitably mixed with cells passing through the abnormal thymus, the lack of disease indicates that the colitis developing in mice replete with bone marrow alone is because regulatory cells do not develop in these mice. These two models associated with thymic defects create a link between regulatory cell development and the thymus in experimental colitis, and provide indirect support for the concept that regulatory cells normally controlling mucosal responses and responding to antigens in the mucosal microflora are CD25+ regulatory cells.

Although the evidence supporting the existence of defective regulatory responses in a number of models of mucosal inflammation is quite extensive, very little evidence supports the existence of a similar defect in human IBD. IBD may be

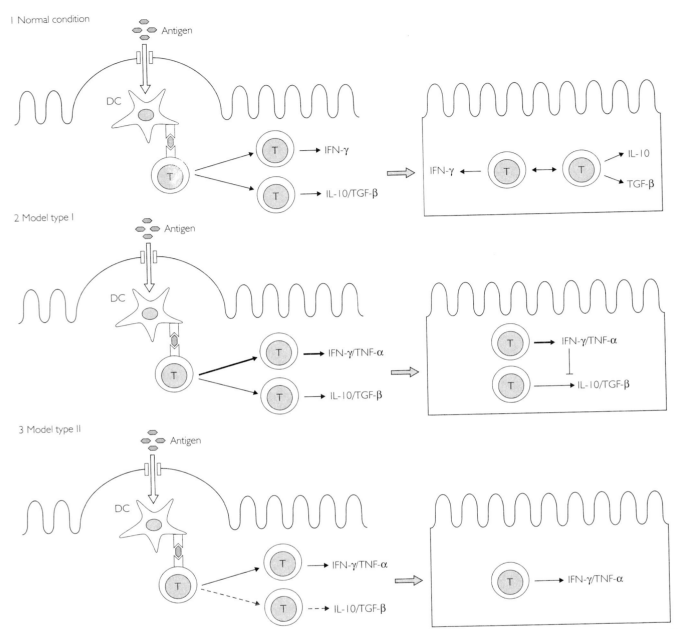

**Fig. 5.4** Type 1 and type 2 models of mucosal inflammation. As illustrated here and indicated in Table 5.1, models of mucosal inflammation can be classified as type 1, wherein the effector cell response to mucosal antigen is abnormally strong and overwhelms the regulatory response, and type 2, wherein the regulatory cell response to mucosal antigen is abnormal and cannot elicit a normal effector cell response. Type II models are therefore emblematic of IBD owing to definitive regulation.

characterized by a general regulatory defect to a large number of mucosal antigens, not just a few selected ones. Thus, although a defect in the regulatory response need not exist for all or even most antigens, impairment of the response to a substantial number of antigens needs to be present so that bystander suppression mediated by regulatory cells does not occur and responses are stimulated by a great number of antigens that do not ordinary elicit a regulatory response. This concept is consistent with the fact that various animal models of mucosal inflammation require the presence of a mucosal microflora and occur as a result of inappropriate responses to many bacterial antigens in the microflora, but to just a few selected antigens (reviewed in[1] and Chapter 10).

The best evidence of a regulatory defect in human IBD is the observation that normal individuals do not mount proliferative or cytokine T-cell responses to antigens derived from their own fecal extracts, whereas patients with Crohn's disease do mount such responses.[149] This coincides with the observation that normal mice do not react to antigens in autologous microflora but do react to those in the microflora of syngeneic littermates.[150] In addition, such self-tolerance is lost after the induction of TNBS colitis and restored when such colitis is successfully treated.[150] These data are compelling in their support of the loss of tolerance hypothesis, as it seems quite unlikely that patients would be hyperresponsive to mucosal microflora and not other antigens if they had a primary effector cell defect.

**Table 5.1 Classification of known models of mucosal inflammation based on whether the abnormality lies in the effector cell response (type I models) or the regulatory cell response (type II models)**

| Th1 models | Th2 models |
|---|---|
| TNBS colitis (SJL/J mice) | TCR-α chain deficiency |
| SCID-transfer colitis | TNBS colitis in BALB/c mice* |
| TCR Tg mice with lymphopenia | Oxazolone colitis |
| IL-10 deficiency colitis | WASP deficiency |
| IL-10 signaling defects (CRF2-4 deficiency) | |
| Tg.26 mice | |
| TNF$^{\Delta ARE}$ mice (TNF-α overproduction) | |
| C3H/HeJBir mice | |
| Gi2α-deficient mice | |
| Samp1/Yit mice | |
| T-bet Tg mice | |
| STAT4 Tg mice | |
| TGF-β RII dominant-negative Tg mice | |
| HLA-B27 Tg rats | |
| Mdr1a-deficient mice | |
| DSS colitis | |
| IL-7 Tg mice | |

SCID, severe combined immunodeficiency; TCR, T-cell receptor; CRF2-4, cyto receptor family 2-4; TNF, tumor necrosis factor; STAT-4, signal transduction and activators of transcription-4; TGF, transforming growth factor; DSS, dextran sulfate sodium; WASP, Wiskott–Aldrich syndrome protein.
* Mixed response but initially Th1, later Th2.

Additional evidence for the concept that IBD is due to a regulatory cell defect comes from the fact that IBD, especially ulcerative colitis, is usually accompanied by the presence of antibodies to a variety of mucosal constituents, including antigens associated with the normal flora, as well as antibodies to various gut constituents such as neutrophil cytoplasmic antigen and tropomyosin.[151] In fact, the discovery of these antibodies initially sparked the idea that IBD was due to an immune defect. Assuming that these antibodies are not secondary to abnormal effector cell responses to mucosal antigens presented in an immunogenic form as a result of the pathologic process, their existence is evidence of a selective loss of immunologic tolerance. However, as indicated above, such selective loss of tolerance can hardly explain the massive inflammation characteristic of IBD. A possible way of bridging this gap comes from a recent study that used representational difference analysis to identify an antigen associated with *Pseudomonas* organisms (termed I2): this is found in active Crohn's disease colonic lesions but not in adjacent non-lesional tissue. Crohn's disease patients respond to this antigen with the production of IgA antibodies.[152–154] This antigen does not require processing to evoke T-cell responses, but is nevertheless MHC restricted and thus has the characteristics of a superantigen. One additional characteristic of this antigen is that it induces T cells to produce IL-10 but not IFN-γ, and thus appears to selectively activate a type of regulatory cell. It was postulated that Crohn's disease may be caused by a defect in the development of B-cell tolerance to I2, and thus the production of antibodies to this molecule that block the ability of I2 to control/activate a large cohort of regulatory cells that are otherwise activated by I2 to control inflammation. This argument endows a molecule arising from a very small and minor population of bacteria to exert a global regulatory influence on mucosal immune responses, and is thus not very convincing.

Nevertheless, it establishes the fact that in order for a selective loss of tolerance to explain the non-selective or general loss of tolerance thought to underlie the occurrence of mucosal inflammation in murine models and, by extension, in human IBD, such selective loss must somehow affect regulatory function in general (reviewed in [1]).

A final body of information to consider in relation to whether or not human IBD is due to a defective regulatory response is the data relating to TGF-β expression in the lesional tissues of patients. TGF-β is a major (if not the major) regulatory cytokine in the control of mucosal immune responses, and thus the presence of a regulatory effect may be manifest as an abnormality in TGF-β expression. Evidence supporting this point, however, is inconclusive. TGF-β expression is, if anything, increased in both Crohn's disease and ulcerative colitis (compared to control tissues) as measured by mRNA expression.[155] In addition, the increased TGF-β expression was localized to inflammatory cells in the lamina propria, especially those situated near the luminal surface. In a more recent study of this point, ulcerative colitis and Crohn's disease differed with respect to TGF-β protein expression. In this study, lamina propria mononuclear cells stimulated in vitro produced increased amounts of TGF-β (compared to controls) if obtained from ulcerative colitis patients and decreased amounts of TGF-β if obtained from Crohn's disease patients. Similar finding were obtained with in vitro culture and stimulation of purified T cells (M. Boirivant, Istituto Superiore di Sanita, Rome, Italy, personal communication). Although it is possible that these changes represent primary defects and Crohn's disease is in fact associated with (and due to) decreased production of a key regulatory cytokine, it is also possible that the change observed is a secondary effect of the disease process, as Th1 responses inhibit TGF-β production. This view is favored by the fact that abnormalities of

TGF-β expression was not observed in cells obtained from non-lesional tissue. Increased TGF-β expression in ulcerative colitis also is probably a secondary effect, as this disease is most likely due to Th2-mediated inflammation, which facilitates TGF-β responses.

The concept that changes in TGF-β expression in IBD may be influenced by the inflammatory process itself also asserts itself in a recent study in which alterations in TGF-β activity was found. The concentration of Smad7, an inhibitor of TGF-β signaling, was increased in lesional cells of patients with Crohn's disease and, indeed, this was associated with defective TGF-β signaling and thus the ability of TGF-β to inhibit IFN-γ production.[156] It is known from previous studies, however, that Smad7 is induced by IFN-γ and/or TNF; thus, it is likely that this abnormality is also a result rather than a cause of the disease.[81]

## CONCLUSION

We have addressed the general question of mucosal responsiveness and non-responsiveness. In a number of mouse models of mucosal inflammation the basic defect leads directly or indirectly to faulty regulatory cell development or function and thus a problem in establishing appropriate unresponsiveness to commensal bacterial antigens, although the circle has not completed by clearly identifying a similar defect in patients with IBD. By and large, this awaits more probing studies of non-involved tissues of patients as well as tissues of disease-free family members who are at high risk for manifesting some of the underlying abnormalities causing IBD.

Although regulatory cell defects cannot yet be established as a cause of IBD, it is still possible that methods of enhancing regulatory cell activity can be a mode of treatment. In this regard, DNA encoding TGF-β delivered by an intranasal route can lead to the local generation of T cells and macrophages that produce TGF-β; such induced regulatory cells then migrate to intestinal lamina propria, where they prevent or even treat TNBS colitis.[157] Of interest, these induced TGF-β-producing cells do not lead to fibrosis despite the known fibrogenic role of TGF-β. This may be due to the fact that the cells producing TGF-β induce the co-production of IL-10 by other cells, and IL-10 then acts to prevent fibrosis. Thus, 'gene therapy' with intranasal TGF-β DNA appears to be both effective and safe. If methods can be devised to deliver TGF-β efficiently to patients, this could become a novel form of therapy for IBD.

## REFERENCES

1. Strober W, Fuss IJ, Blumberg RS. The immunology of mucosal models of inflammation. Annu Rev Immunol 2002;20:495–549.
2. Elson CO, Cong Y, Iqbal N, Weaver CT. Immuno-bacterial homeostasis in the gut: new insights into an old enigma. Semin Immunol 2001;13:187–194.
3. Strober W, Kelsall B, Marth T. Oral tolerance. J Clin Immunol 1998;18:1–30.
4. Mowat A, Weiner HL. Oral tolerance. Physiological basis and clinical applications. In: Ogra PL, Mestecky J, Lamm ME, Strober W, Bienenstock J, McGhee JR, eds. Mucosal immunology. New York: Academic Press; 1999:587–618.
5. Elson CO, Beagley KW, Sharmanov AT et al. Hapten-induced model of murine inflammatory bowel disease: mucosal immune response and protection by tolerance. J Immunol 1996;157:2174–2185.
6. Kagnoff MF. Effects of antigen-feeding on intestinal and systemic immune responses. II. Suppression of delayed-type hypersensitivity reactions. J Immunol 1978;120:1509–1513.
7. Stokes CR, Newby TJ, Huntley JH, Patel D, Bourne FJ. The immune response of mice to bacterial antigens given by mouth. Immunology 1979;38:497–502.
8. Kagnoff MF. Effects of antigen-feeding on intestinal and systemic immune responses. IV. Similarity between the suppressor factor in mice after erythrocyte-lysate injection and erythrocyte feeding. Gastroenterology 1980;79:54–61.
9. Rubin D, Weiner HL, Fields BN, Greene MI. Immunologic tolerance after oral administration of reovirus: requirement for two viral gene products for tolerance induction. J Immunol 1981;127:1697–1701.
10. Dahlgren UI, Wold AE, Hanson LA, Midtvedt T. Expression of a dietary protein in E. coli renders it strongly antigenic to gut lymphoid tissue. Immunology 1991;73:394–397.
11. Singh VK, Anand R, Sharma K, Agarwal SS. Suppression of experimental autoimmune uveitis in Lewis rats by oral administration of recombinant Escherichia coli expressing retinal S-antigen. Cell Immunol 1996;172:158–162.
12. Yoshida M, Watanabe T, Usui T et al. CD4 T cells monospecific to ovalbumin produced by Escherichia coli can induce colitis upon transfer to BALB/c and SCID mice. Int Immunol 2001;13:1561–1570.
13. Yoshida M, Shirai Y, Watanabe T et al. Differential localization of colitogenic Th1 and Th2 cells monospecific to a microflora-associated antigen in mice. Gastroenterology 2002;123:1949–1961.
14. Medzhitov R, Janeway C. The Toll receptor family and microbial recognition. Trends Microbiol 2000;8:452–456.
15. Fremdeus B, Wachtler C, Hedlund M et al. Escherichia coli P fimbriae utilize the Toll-like receptor 4 pathway for cell activation. Mol Microbiol 2001;40:37–51.
16. Wong SY. Innate immune trouble detectors. Trends Immunol 2001;22:235–236.
17. Perera PY, Mayadas TN, Takeuchi O et al. CD11b/CD18 acts in concert with CD14 and Toll-like receptor (TLR) 4 to elicit full lipopolysaccharide and taxol-inducible gene expression. J Immunol 2001;166:574–581.
18. Higgins LM, Frankel G, Connerton I, Goncalves N, Dougan G, MacDonald TT. Role of bacterial intimin in colonic hyperplasia and inflammation. Science 1999;285:588–591.
19. Eldridge JH, Meulborek JA, Staas JA, Tice TR, Gilley RM. Vaccine-containing biodegradable microspheres specifically enter the gut-associated lymphoid tissue following oral administration and induce a disseminated mucosal immune response. Adv Exp Med Biol 1989;251:191–202.
20. O'Hagan DT, McGhee JP, Holmgren J et al. Biodegradable microparticles for oral immunization. Vaccine 1993;11:149–154.
21. Maloy KJ, Donachie AM, Hagan DT, McIntosh Mowat A. Induction of mucosal and systemic immune response by immunization with ovalbumin entrapped in poly(lactide-co-glycolide) microparticles. Immunology 1994;81:661–667.
22. Tabata Y, Inoue Y, Ikada Y. Size effect on systemic and mucosal immune responses induced by oral administration of biodegradable microspheres. Vaccine 1996;14:1677–1685.
23. Barone KS, Reilly MR, Flanagan MP, Michael JG. Abrogation of oral tolerance by feeding encapsulated antigen. Cellular Antigen 2000;199:67–72.
24. Matsunaga Y, Wakatsuki Y, Tabata Y et al. Oral immunization with size-purified microsphere beads as a vehicle selectively induces systemic tolerance and sensitization. Vaccine 2001;19:579–588.
25. Reese RT, Cebra JJ. Anti-dinotrophenyl antibody production in strain 13 guinea pigs fed or sensitized with dinotrocholobenzene. J Immunol 1975;114:863–871.
26. Aizpura HJ, Russell-Jones GJ. Oral vaccination. Identification of classes of proteins that provoke an immune response upon oral feeding. J Exp Med 1988;167:440–451.
27. Elson CO, Tomasi M, Dertzbaugh MT, Thaggard G, Hunter R, Weaver C. Oral-antigen delivery by way of a multiple emulsion system enhances oral tolerance. Ann NY Acad Sci 1996;778:156–162.
28. Spangler BD. Structure and function of cholera toxin and the related Escherichia coli heat-labile enterotoxin. Microbiol Rev 1992;56:622–647.
29. Elson CO. Cholera toxin as a mucosal adjuvant. In: Kyono H, Ogra PL, McGhee J, eds. Mucosal vaccines. San Diego: Academic Press; 1996:59–72.
30. Lycke N, Schon K. The B cell targeted adjuvant, CTA1-DD, exhibits potent mucosal immunoenhancing activity despite pre-existing anti-toxin immunity. Vaccine 2001;19:2452–2458.
31. Mowat A, Donachie A, Jägewall S et al. CTA1-DD-immune stimulating complexes: a novel, rationally designed combined mucosal vaccine adjuvant effective with nanogram doses of antigen. J Immunol 2001;167:3398–3405.
32. Sun JB, Holmgren J, Czerkinsy C. Cholera-toxin B-subunit: an efficient transmural carrier-delivery system for induction of peripheral immunological tolerance. Proc Natl Acad Sci USA 1994;91:10795.
33. Sun JB, Xiao BG, Lindblad M et al. Oral administration of cholera toxin B subunit conjugated to myelin basic protein protects against experimental autoimmune encephaloymyelitis by inducing transforming growth factor-beta-secreting cells and suppressing chemokine expression. Int Immunol 2000;12:1449–1457.
34. Giuliani M, Del Guidice G, Giannelli V et al. Mucosal adjuvanticity and immunogenicity of LTR72, a novel mutant of Escherichia coli heat-labile enterotoxin with partial knockout of ADP-ribosyltransferase activity. J Exp Med 1998;187:1123–1132.
35. Park EJ, Chang JH, Kim JS, Chung I, Yum JS. Development of two novel nontoxic mutants of Escherichia coli heat-labile enterotoxin. Exp Mol Med 1999;31:101.

36. Sobel DO, Yankelovich D, Goyal D, Nelson D, Mazumder A. The B-subunit of cholera toxin induces immunoregulatory cells and prevents diabetes in the NOD mouse. Diabetes 1998;47:186–191.

37. Williams NA, Stasiuk LM, Nashar TO et al. Prevention of autoimmune diseases due to lymphocyte modulation by the B-subunit of Escherichia coli heat labile enterotoxin. Proc Natl Acad Sci USA 1997;94:5290.

38. George-Chandy A, Eriksson K, Lebens M, Nordstrom I, Schön E, Holmgren J. Cholera toxin B subunit as a carrier molecule promotes antigen presentation and increases CD40 and CD86 expression on antigen-presenting cells. Infect Immun 2001;69:5716–5725.

39. Cong Y, Weaver CT, Elson CO. The mucosal adjuvanticity of cholera toxin involves enhancement of costimulatory activity by selective upregulation of B7.2 expression. J Immunol 1997;159:5301–5308.

40. Braun MC, He J, Wu C, Kelsall BL. Cholera toxin suppresses interleukin (IL)-12 production and IL-12 receptor β1 and β2 chain expression. J Exp Med 1999;189:541–552.

41. Takashi T, Marinaro M, Kiyono H et al. Mechanisms for mucosal immunogenicity and adjuvancy of Escherichia coli labile enterotoxin. J Infect Dis 1996;173:627–635.

42. Braun MC, Lahey E, Kelsall BL. Selective suppression of IL-12 production by chemoattractants. J Immunol 2000;164:3009–3017.

43. He J, Gurunathan S, Iwasaki A, Ash-Shaheed B, Kelsall BL. Primary role for Gi protein signaling in the regulation of interleukin 12 production and the induction of T helper cell type 1 responses. J Exp Med 2000;191:1605–1610.

44. Anderson DL, Tsoukas CD. Cholera toxin inhibits resting human T cell activation via cAMP-independent pathway. J Immunol 1989;143:3647–3652.

45. Belyakov IM, Ahlers JD, Clements JD, Strober W, Berzofsky JA. Interplay of cytokines and adjuvants in the regulation of mucosal and systemic HIV-specific CTL. J Immunol 2000;165:6454–6462.

46. Takashi T, Tagami T, Yamazaki S et al. Immunologic self-tolerance maintained by CD25+CD4+ regulatory T cells constitutively expressing cytotoxic T lymphocyte-associated antigen 4. J Exp Med 2000;192:203–310.

47. Boirivant M, Fuss IJ, Ferroni L, De Pascale M, Strober W. Oral administration of recombinant cholera toxin subunit B inhibits IL-12-mediated murine experimental (trinitrobenzene sulfonic acid) colitis. J Immunol 2001;166:3522–3532.

48. Richman LK, Chiller JM, Brown WR, Hanson DG, Vaz NM. Enterically induced immunologic tolerance. I. Induction of suppressor T lymphocytes by intragastric administration of soluble proteins. J Immunol 1978;121:2429–2434.

49. Richman LK, Graeff AS, Yarchoan R, Strober W. Simultaneous induction of antigen-specific IgA helper T cells and IgG suppressor T cells in the murine Peyer's patch after protein feeding. J Immunol 1981;126:2079–2083.

50. Fujihashi K, Dohi T, Rennert PD et al. Peyer's patches are required for oral tolerance to poteins. Proc Natl Acad Sci USA 2001;98:3310–3315.

51. Ke Y, Pearce K, Lake JP, Ziegler HK, Kapp JA. γδ T lymphocytes regulate the induction and maintenance of oral tolerance. J Immunol 1997;158:3610–3618.

52. Miller A, Lider O, Roberts AB, Sporn MB, Weiner HL. Suppressor T cells generated by oral tolerization to myelin basic protein suppress both in vitro and in vivo immune responses by the release of transforming growth factor beta after antigen-specific triggering. Proc Natl Acad Sci USA 1992;89:421–425.

53. Gilliet M, Liu Y. Generation of human CD8 T regulatory cells by CD40 ligand- activated plasmacytoid dendritic cells. J Exp Med 2002;195:695–704.

54. Maecker HT, Ghanekar SA, Suni MA, He XS, Picker LJ, Maine VC. Factors affecting the efficiency of CD8+ T cell cross-priming with exogenous antigens. J Immunol 2001;166:7268–7275.

55. McMenamin C, McKersey M, Kuhnlein P, Hunig T, Holt PG. Gamma delta T cells downregulate primary IgE responses in rats to inhaled soluble protein antigens. J Immunol 1995;154:439–4394.

56. McNamin C, Holt PG. The natural immune response to inhaled soluble protein antigens involves major histocompatibility (MHC) class I-restricted CD8+ T cell- mediated but MHC class II-restricted CD4+ T cell-dependent immune deviation resulting in selective suppression of immunoglobulin E production. J Exp Med 1993;178:889-899.

57. Grdic D, Hornquist E, Kjerrulf M, Lycke N. Lack of local suppression in orally tolerant CD8-deficient mice reveals a critical regulatory role of CD8+ T cells in the normal gut mucosal. J Immunol 1998;160:754–762.

58. Vistica BP, Chanaud NP III, Felix N et al. CD8 T-cells are not essential for the induction of 'low dose' oral tolerance. Clin Immunol Immunopathol 1996;78:196–202.

59. Desvignes C, Bour H, Nicholas JF, Kaiserlian D. Lack of oral tolerance but oral priming for contact sensitivity to dinitrofluorobenzene in major histocompatibility complex case II-deficient mice and in CD4+ T cell-depleted mice. Eur J Immunol 1996;26:1756–1761.

60. Miller A, al-Sabbagh A, Santos LM, Das MP, Weiner HL. Epitopes of myelin basic protein that trigger TGF-beta release after oral tolerization are distinct from encephalitogenic epitopes and mediate epitope-driven bystander suppression. J Immunol 1993;151:7307–7315.

61. Santos LM, al-Sabbagh A, Londono A, Weiner HL. Oral tolerance to myelin basic protein induces regulatory TGF-beta-secreting T cells in Peyer's patches of SJL mice. Cell Immunol 1994;157:439–447.

62. Chen Y, Kuchroo VK, Inobe J, Hafler DA, Weiner HL. Regulatory T cell clones induced by oral tolerance: suppression of autoimmune encephalomyelitis. Science 1994;265:1237–1240.

63. Von Herrath MG, Dyrberg T, Oldstone M. Oral insulin treatment suppresses virus-induced antigen-specific destruction of beta cells and prevents autoimmune diabetes in transgenic mice. J Clin Invest 1996;98:1324–1331.

64. Von Herrath MG. Regulation of virally induced autoimmunity and immunopathology: contribution of LCMV transgenic models to understanding autoimmune insulin-dependent diabetes mellitus. Curr Top Microbiol Immunol 2002;263:145–175.

65. Laufer TM, von Herrath MG, Grusby MJ, Oldstone MB, Glimcher LH. Autoimmune diabetes can be induced in transgenic major histocompatibility complex class II-deficient mice. J Exp Med 1993;178:589–596.

66. Nagler Anderson C, Bober L, Robinson M, Siskind G, Thorbecke G. Suppression of type II collagen-induced arthritis by intragastric administration of soluble type II antigen. Proc Natl Acad Sci USA 1986;83:7443–7446.

67. Stevens DB, Gould KE, Swanborg RH. Transforming growth factor-beta 1 inhibits tumor necrosis factor-alpha/lymphotoxin production and adoptive transfer of disease by effector cells of autoimmune encephalomyelitis. J Neuroimmunol 1994;51:77–83.

68. Santambroglio L, Hochwald GM, Saxena B et al. Studies on the mechanisms by which transforming growth factor-beta (TGF-beta) protects against allergic encephalomyelitis. Antagonism between TGF-beta and tumor necrosis factor. J Immunol 1993;151:1116–1127.

69. Khoury SJ, Hancock WW, Weiner HL. Oral tolerance to myelin basic protein and natural recovery from experimental autoimmune encephalomyelitis are associated with downregulation of inflammatory cytokines and differential upregulation of transforming growth factor beta, interleukin 4, and prostaglandin E expression in the brain. J Exp Med 1992;176:1355–1364.

70. Schluesener H, Lider O. Transforming growth factors beta 1 and beta 2: cytokines with identical immunosuppressive effects and a potential role in the regulation of autoimmune T cell function. J Neuroimmunol 1989;24:249–258.

71. Karpus W, Swanborg R. CD4+ suppressor cells inhibit the function of effector cells of experimental autoimmune encephalomyelitis through a mechanism involving a transforming growth factor β. J Immunol 1991;146:1163–1169.

72. Higgins P, Weiner H. Suppression of experimental autoimmune encephalomyelitis by oral administration of myelin basic protein and its fragments. J Immunol 1998;140:440–445.

73. Powrie F, Correa-Oliveira R, Mauze S, Coffman RL. Regulatory interactions between CD45RBhigh and CD45RBlow CD4+ T cells are important for the balance between protective and pathogenic cell-mediated immunity. J Exp Med 1994;179:589–600.

74. Powrie F, Carlino J, Leach MW, Mauze S, Coffman RL. A critical role for transforming growth factor-beta but not interleukin 4 in the suppression of T helper type 1-mediated colitis by CD45RB(low) CD4+ T cells. J Exp Med 1996;183:2669–2774.

75. Read S, Malmstrom V, Powrie F. Cytotoxic T lymphocyte-associated antigen 4 plays an essential role in the function of CD25+CD4+ regulatory cells that control intestinal inflammation. J Exp Med 2000;192:295–302.

76. Neurath MF, Fuss I, Kelsall BL, Presky DH, Waegell W, Strober W. Experimental granulomatous colitis in mice is abrogated by induction of TGF-beta-mediated oral tolerance. J Exp Med 1996;183:2605–2616.

77. Fuss IJ, Boirivant M, Lacy B, Strober W. The interrelated roles of TGF-beta and IL-10 in the regulation of experimental colitis. J Immunol 2002;168:900–908.

78. Asseman C, Mauze S, Leach MW, Coffman RL, Powrie F. An essential role for interleukin 10 in the function of regulatory T cells that inhibit intestinal inflammation. J Exp Med 1999;190:995–1004.

79. Cong Y, Weaver CT, Lazenby A, Elson CO. Bacterial-reactive T regulatory cells inhibit pathogenic immune responses to the enteric flora. J Immunol 2002;169:6112–6119.

80. Groux H, O'Garra A, Bigler M et al. A CD4+ T-cell subset inhibits antigen-specific T-cell responses and prevents colitis. Nature 1997;389:737–742.

81. Ulloa L, Doody J, Massague J. Inhibition of transforming growth factor-beta/SMAD signaling by the interferon-gamma/STAT pathway. Nature 1999;397:710–713.

82. Seder RA, Marth T, Sieve MC et al. Factors involved in the differentiation of TGF-beta-producing cells from naïve CD4+ T cells: IL-4 and IFN-gamma have opposing effects, while TGF-beta positively regulates its own production. J Immunol 1998;160:5719–5728.

83. Marth T, Strober W, Kelsall BL. High dose oral tolerance in ovalbumin TCR- transgenic mice: systemic neutralization of IL-12 augments TGF-beta secretion and T cell apoptosis. J Immunol 1996;157:2348–2357.

84. Coffman RL, Mocci S, O'Garra A. The stability and reversibility of Th1 and Th2 populations. In: Coffman RL, Romagnani S, eds. Current topics in microbiology and immunology. London: Springer Verlag; 1999:1–29.

85. Fishman-Lobell J, Friedman A, Weiner H. Different kinetic patterns of cytokine gene expression in vivo in orally tolerant mice. Eur J Immunol 1994;24:2720–2724.

86. Ludviksson BR, Ehrhardt RO, Strober W. TGF-beta production regulates the development of the 2, 4, 6-trinitrophenol-conjugated keyhole limpet hemocyanin- induced colonic inflammation in IL-2-deficient mice. J Immunol 1997;159:3622–3628.

87. Iwasaki A, Kelsall BL. Freshly isolated Peyer's patch, but not spleen, dendritic cells produce interleukin 10 and induce the differentiation of T helper type 2 cells. J Exp Med 1999;190:229–239.

88. Akbari O, DeKruyff RH, Umetsu DT. Pulmonary dendritic cells producing IL-10 mediate tolerance induced by respiratory exposure to antigen. Nature Med 2001;7:725–731.

89. Stumbles PA, Thomas JA, Pimm CL et al. Rating respiratory tract dendritic cells preferentially stimulate T helper cell type 2 (Th2) responses and require obligatory cytokine signals for induction of Th1 immunity. J Exp Med 1998;188:2019–2031.

90. McGuirk P, McCann C, Mills KH. Pathogen-specific T regulatory 1 cells induced in the respiratory tract by a bacterial molecule that stimulates interleukin 10 production by dendritic cells: a novel strategy for evasion of protective T helper type 1 response by Bordetella pertussis. J Exp Med 2002;195:221–231.

91. Barrat FJ, Cua DJ, Boonstra A et al. In vitro generation of interleukin 10-producing regulatory CD4+ T cells is induced by immunosuppressive drugs and inhibited by T helper type 1 (Th1)- and Th2-inducing cytokines. J Exp Med 2001;195:603–616.

92. Levings MK, Sangregorio R, Galbiati F, Squadrone S, De Waal Malefyt R, Roncarolo MG. IFN-alpha and IL-10 induce the differentiation of human type 1 T regulatory cells. J Immunol 2001;166:5530–5539.

93. Kullberg MC, Jankovic D, Gorelick PL et al. Bacteria-triggered CD4+ T regulatory cells suppress Helicobacter hepaticus-induced colitis. J Exp Med 2002;196:505–515.

94. Roncarolo MG, Levings MK. The role of different subsets of T regulatory cells in controlling autoimmunity. Curr Opin Immunol 2000;12:676–683.

95. Mason D, Powrie F. Control of immune pathology by regulatory T cells. Curr Opin Immunol 1998;10:649–655.

96. Groux H, Powrie F. Regulatory T cells and inflammatory bowel disease. Immunol Today 1999;20:442–445.

97. Schevach EM. Regulatory T cells in autoimmunity. Annu Rev Immunol 2000;18:423–449.

98. Kitani A, Chua K, Nakamura K, Strober W. Activated self-MHC-reactive T cells have the cytokine phenotype of Th3/T regulatory cell 1 T cells. J Immunol 2000;165:691–702.

99. Kanof ME, Strober W, James SP. Induction of CD4 suppressor T cells with anti-Leau-8 antibody. J Immunol 1987;139:49–54.

100. McHugh RS, Whitters MJ, Piccirillo CA et al. CD4+CD25+ immunoregulatory T cells: gene expression analysis reveals a functional role for the glucocorticoid-induced TNF receptor. Immunity 2002;16:311–323.

101. Shimizu J, Yamazaki S, Takahashi T, Ishida Y, Sakaguchi S. Stimulation of CD25+CD4+ regulatory T cells through GITR breaks immunological self-tolerance. Nature Immunol 2002;3:135–142.

102. Thornton AM, Shevach EM. CD4+CD25+ immunoregulatory T cells suppress polyclonal T cell activation in vitro by inhibiting interleukin 2 production. J Exp Med 1998;188:287–296.

103. Asano M, Toda M, Sakaguchi N, Sakaguchi S. Autoimmune disease as a consequence of developmental abnormality of a T cell subpopulation. J Exp Med 1996;184:387–396.

104. McHugh RS, Shevach EM. Cutting edge: depletion of CD4+CD25+ regulatory T cells is necessary, but not sufficient, for induction of organ-specific autoimmune disease. J Immunol 2002;168:5979–5983.

105. Itoh M, Takahashi T, Sakaguchi N et al. Thymus and autoimmunity: production of CD25+CD4+ naturally anergic and suppressive T cells as a key function of the thymus in maintain immunologic self-tolerance. J Immunol 1999;162:5317–5326.

106. Annunziata F, Cosmi L, Liotta F et al. Phenotype, localization, and mechanism of suppression of CD4+CD25+ human thymocytes. J Exp Med 2002;196:379–387.

107. Sutmuller RP, van Duivenvoorde LM, val Elsas A et al. Synergism of cytotoxic T lymphocyte-associated antigen 4 blockade and depletion of CD25+ regulatory T cells in antitumor therapy reveals alternative pathways for suppression of autoreactive cytotoxic T lymphocyte response. J Exp Med 2001;194:823–832.

108. Piccirillo CA, Letterio JJ, Thornton AM et al. CD4+CD25+ regulatory T cells can mediate suppressor function in the absence of transforming growth factor beta1 production and responsiveness. J Exp Med 2002;196:237–246.

109. Nakamura K, Kitani A, Strober W. Cell contact-dependent immunosuppression by CD4+CD25+ regulatory T cells is mediated by cell surface-bound transforming growth factor beta. J Exp Med 2001;194:629–644.

110. Allez M, Brimnes J, Dotan I, Mayer L. Expansion of CD8+ T cells with regulatory function after interaction with intestinal epithelial cells. Gastroenterology 2002;123:1516–1526.

111. Campbell NA, Kim HS, Blumberg RS, Mayer L. The nonclassical class I molecule CD1d associates with the novel CD8 ligand gp180 on intestinal epithelial cells. J Biol Chem 1999;274:26259–26265.

112. Yio XY, Mayer L. Characterization of a 180-kDa intestinal epithelial cell membrane glycoprotein, gp180. A candidate molecule mediating T cell–epithelial cell interactions. J Biol Chem 1997;272:12786–12792.

113. Asselin-Paturel C, Boonstra A, Dalod M et al. Mouse type I IFN-producing cells are immature APCs with plasmacytoid morphology. Nature Immunol 2001;2:1144–1150.

114. Grouard G, Rissoan M, Filgueira L, Durand I, Banchereau J, Liu Y. The enigmatic plasmacytoid T cells develop into dendritic cells with interleukin (IL)-3 and CD40-ligand. J Exp Med 1997;185:1101–1111.

115. Hanninen A, Harrison LC. Gamma delta T cells as mediators of mucosal tolerance: the autoimmune diabetes model. Immunol Rev 2000;173:109–119.

116. Matsuda JL, Gapin L, Sidobre S et al. Homeostasis of V alpha 14i NK T cells. Nature Immunol 2002;3:966–974.

117. Laloux V, Beaudoin L, Jeske D, Carnaud C, Lehuen A. NK T cell-induced protection against diabetes in V alpha 14-J alpha transgenic nonobese diabetic mice is associated with a Th2 shift circumscribed regionally to the islets and functionally to islet autoantigens. J Immunol 2001;166:3749–3756.

118. Lehuen A, Lantz O, Beaudoin L et al. Overexpression of natural killer T cells protects V alpha-J alpha transgenic nonobese diabetic mice against diabetes. J Exp Med 1998;188:1831–1839.

119. Saubermann LJ, Beck P, De Jong YP et al. Activation of natural killer T cells by alpha-galacosylceramide in the presence of CD1d provides protection against colitis in mice. Gastroenterology 2000;19:119–28.

120. Jahng AW, Maricic I, Pedersen B et al. Activation of natural killer T cells potentiates or prevents experimental autoimmune encephalomyelitis. J Exp Med 2001;194:1789–1799.

121. Illes Z, Kondo T, Newcombe J, Oka N, Tabira T, Yammamura T. Differential expression of NK T cell V alpha 24J alpha Q invariant TCR chain in the lesions of multiple sclerosis and chronic inflammatory demyelinating polyneuropathy. J Immunol 2000;164:4375–4381.

122. Kukreja A, Cost G, Marker J et al. Multiple immuno-regulatory defects in type-1 diabetes. J Clin Invest 2002;109:131–140.

123. Thorsstenson KM, Khoruts A. Generation of anergic and potentially immunoregulatory CD25+CD4 T cells in vivo after induction of peripheral tolerance with intravenous or oral antigen. J Immunol 2001;167:188–195.

124. Zhang X, Izikson L, Liu L, Weiner HL. Activation of CD25+CD4+ regulatory T cells by oral antigenic administration. J Immunol 2001;167:425–453.

125. Hollander GA, Simpson SJ, Mizoguchi E et al. Severe colitis in mice with aberrant thymic selection. Immunity 1995;3:27–38.

126. Srinivasan M, Gienapp IE, Stuckman SS et al. Suppression of experimental autoimmune encephalomyelitis using peptide mimics of CD28. J Immunol 2002;169:2180–2188.

127. Meyer AL, Benson J, Song F et al. Rapid depletion of peripheral antigen-specific T cells in TCR-transgenic mice after oral administration of myelin basic protein. J Immunol 2001;166:5773–5781.

128. Benson JM, Campbell KA, Guan Z et al. T-cell activation and recpetor downmodulation precede deletion induced by mucosally administered antigen. J Clin Invest 2000;106:1031–1038.

129. Van Houten N, Blake SF. Direct measurement of anergy of antigen-specific T cells following oral tolerance induction. J Immunol 1996;157:1337–1341.

130. Viney JL, Mowat AM, O'Malley JM, Williamson E, Fanger NA. Expanding dendritic cells in vivo enhances the induction of oral tolerance. J Immunol 1998;160:5815–5825.

131. Williamson E, Westrich GM, Viney JL. Modulating dendritic cells to optimize mucosal immunization protocols. J Immunol 1999;163:3668–3675.

132. Kelsall BL, Strober W. Distinct populations of dendritic cells are present in the subepithelial dome and T cell regions of the murine Peyer's patch. J Exp Med 1996;183:237–247.

133. Iwasaki A, Kelsall B. Unique functions of CD11b+, CD8 alpha+ and double-negative Peyer's patch dendritic cells. J Immunol 2001;166:4884–4890.

134. Dziarski R, Wang Q, Miyake K, Kirschning CJ, Gupta D. MD-2 enables Toll-like receptor 2 (TLR2)-mediated responses to lipopolysaccharide and enhances TLR2- mediated responses to Gram-positive and Gram-negative bacteria and their cell wall components. J Immunol 2001;166:1938–1944.

135. Schilling JD, Mulvey MA, Vincent CD, Lorenz RG, Hultgren SJ. Bacterial invasion augments epithelial cytokine responses to Escherichia coli through a lipopolysaccharide-dependent mechanism. J Immunol 2001;166:1148–1155.

136. Krug A, Towarowski A, Britsch S et al. Toll-like receptor expression reveals CpG DNA as a unique microbial stimulus for plasmacytoid dendritic cells which synergizes with CD40 ligand to induce high amounts of IL-12. Eur J Immunol 2001;31:3026–3037.

137. Kadowaki N, Ho S, Antonenko S et al. Subsets of human dendritic cell precursors express different Toll-like receptors and respond to different microbial antigens. J Exp Med 2001;194:863–869.

138. Jankovic D, Kullberg MC, Hieny S, Caspar P, Callazo CM, Sher A. In the absence of IL-12, CD4+ T cell responses to intracellular pathogens fail to default to a Th2 pattern and are host protective in an IL-10–/– setting. Immunity 2002;16:429–439.

139. Nakano H, Yanagita M, Gunn MD. CD11c+B220+Gr-1+ cells in mouse lymph nodes and spleen display characteristics of plasmacytoid dendritic cells. J Exp Med 2001;194:1171–1178.

140. Marth T, Kelsall BL. Regulation of interleukin-12 by complement receptor 3 signaling. J Exp Med 1997;185:1987–1995.

141. Hurst SD, Seymour BW, Muchamuel T, Kurup VP, Coffman RL. Modulation of inhaled antigen-induced IgE tolerance by ongoing Th2 responses in the lung. J Immunol 2001;166:4922–4930.

142. Huang F, Platt N, Wykes M et al. A discrete subpopulation of dendritic cells transports apoptotic intestinal epithelial cells to T cell areas of mesenteric lymph nodes. J Exp Med 2000;191:435–443.

143. Wirtz S, Finotto S, Kanzler S et al. Cutting edge: chronic intestinal inflammation in STAT-4 transgenic mice: characterization of disease and adoptive transfer by TNF-plus IFN-gamma-producing CD4+ T cells that respond to bacterial antigens. J Immunol 1999;162:1884–1888.

144. Neurath MF, Fuss I, Kelsall BL, Stuber E, Strober W. Antibodies to interleukin 12 abrogate established experimental colitis in mice. J Exp Med 1995;182:1281–1290.

145. Bouma G, Kaushiva A, Strober W. Experimental murine colitis is regulated by two genetic loci, including one on chromosome 11 that regulates IL-12 responses. Gastroenterology 2002;123:554–565.

146. Powrie F, Leach MW, Mauze S, Caddle LB, Coffman RL. Phenotypically distinct subsets of CD4+ T cells induce or protect from chronic intestinal inflammation in C.B-17 scid mice. Int Immunol 1993;5:1461–1471.

147. Berg DJ, Davidson N, Kuhn R et al. Enterocolitis and colon cancer in interleukin-10-deficient mice are associated with aberrant cytokine production and CD4+ Th1-like responses. Clin Invest 1996;98:1010–1020.

148. Kulkarni AB, Karlsson S. Inflammation and TGF beta 1: lessons from the TGF beta 1 null mouse. Res Immunol 1997;148:453–456.

149. Duchmann R, Kaiser I, Hermann E, Mayet W, Ewe K, Meyer zum Buschenfelde KH. Tolerance exists towards resident intestinal flora in active inflammatory bowel disease (IBD). Clin Exp Immunol 1995;102:448–455.

150. Duchmann R, Schmitt E, Knolle P, Meyer zum Buschenfelde KH, Neurath M. Tolerance towards resident intestinal flora in mice is abrogated in experimental colitis and restored by treatment with interleukin-10 or antibodies to interleukin-12. Eur J Immunol 1996;26:934–938.

151. Podolsky DK. Inflammatory bowel disease. N Engl J Med 2002;347:417–429.

152. Dalwadi H, Wei B, Kronenberg M, Sutton CL, Braun J. The Crohn's disease-associated bacterial protein I2 is a novel enteric T cell superantigen. Immunity 2001;15:149–158.

153. Wei B, Huang T, Dalwadi H, Sutton CL, Bruckner D, Braun J. Pseudomonas fluorescence encodes the Crohn's disease-associated I2 sequence and T-cell superantigen. Infect Immunol 2002;70:6567–6575.

154. Sutton CL, Kim J, Yamane A et al. Identification of a novel bacterial sequence associated with Crohn's disease. Gastroenterology 2000;119:23–31.

155. Babyatsky MW, Rossiter G, Podolsky DK. Expression of transferring growth factors alpha and beta in colonic mucosa in inflammatory bowel disease. Gastroenterology 1996;110:975–984.

156. Monteleone G, Kumberova A, Croft NM, McKenzie C, Steer HW, MacDonald TT. Blocking Smad7 restores TGF-beta1 signaling in chronic inflammatory bowel disease. J Clin Invest 2001;108:601–609.

157. Kitani A, Fuss IJ, Nakamura K, Schwartz OM, Usui T, Strober W. Treatment of experimental (trinitrobenzene sulfonic acid) colitis by intranasal administration of transforming growth factor (TGF)-beta1 plasmid: TGF-beta1-mediated suppression of T helper type 1 response occurs by interleukin (IL)-10 induction and IL-12 receptor beta2 chain downregulation. J Exp Med 2000;192:41–52.

## CHAPTER 6

# T-lymphocyte trafficking

Terrence Barrett, Scott Snapper and Richard S Blumberg

## INTRODUCTION

Homing molecules expressed by circulating leukocytes allow the mucosal immune system to direct cells to locations where antigen recognition and effector responses are performed. Naive lymphocytes initiate immune responses to intestinal organisms, and therefore require access to sites within secondary lymphoid tissue where antigen derived from enteric organisms is presented. Naive T cells express a unique set of receptors that bind ligands only expressed on the specialized blood vessels of lymph nodes (LN) known as high endothelial venules (HEV).[1] Naive T cells are further restricted within secondary lymphoid organs to the T cell-rich paracortical areas in the LN and Peyer's patches (PP), and the pariarteriolar lymphoid sheath in the spleen.[2] In the intestinal immune network, naive T cells sample antigen (Ag) derived from enteric contents in several ways. In PP, Ag passes through specialized epithelial cells (M cells) before being delivered to dendritic cells (DC), which process and present the Ag to T cells. Antigen entry initiated in the intervening mucosa is taken up by immature DC that migrate through afferent lymphatics to sites of antigen presentation within draining LN such as the mesenteric lymph nodes (MLN).[3] The delivery of enteric Ag to T-cell zones within draining LN allows a relatively large pool of naive cells (in PP and MLN) to be exposed to peptides and lipids derived from luminal bacteria. Upon activation, naive T cells undergo clonal expansion (increase in numbers), functional differentiation (increase cytokine production) and modulation of surface phenotype. Modification of surface receptors facilitates cell movement between tissue compartments. For example, downregulation of surface ligands such as the chemokine receptor CCR7 releases (untethers) cells from T-cell areas, thereby allowing them to migrate to areas within the LN (e.g. germinal center) where they can provide B-cell help.[4] Upon activation, some T cells leave the LN and re-enter the circulation. Coincident with emigration from the LN, activated T cells

upregulate homing receptors that allow them to be selectively recruited by non-lymphoid tissues. The final step in lymphocyte recruitment allows activated cells to be delivered to sites within the mucosa where protective responses to enteric pathogen are delivered. Thus, mechanisms that control cell movement between tissues are critical for coordinating host responses to threats originating from the intestinal lumen. In this chapter we review the pathways involved in the recruitment of naive cells to 'inductive sites' within PP and MLN and those involved in the recruitment of activated cells to 'effector sites' within the non-lymphoid tissue of the intestinal lamina propria (iLP), and describe the implications for the pathogenesis and treatment of human inflammatory bowel diseases (IBD).

## THE MULTISTEP PARADIGM OF LYMPHOCYTE RECRUITMENT

The control of lymphocyte (and other leukocyte) recirculation is mediated by interactions that occur at the interface between circulating cells and the surface of vascular endothelium (Fig. 6.1; see Chapter 7). The current discussion will focus on lymphocyte recruitment; however, these processes are shared by several distinct leukocyte subsets (neutrophils, NK cells, macrophages etc.). Recruitment of cells to lymphoid and non-lymphoid tissue largely occurs in one region of the microvasculature, i.e. postcapillary venules (PCV, where free-flowing lymphocytes initially interact with endothelial cells in a transient and reversible interaction via adhesion receptors (usually selectins and selectin ligands, but also $\alpha_4$ integrins; Table 6.1).[5] This weak adhesive interaction results in a process called rolling (step 1). Rolling brings cells into contact with the surface of the endothelium, where they can sample for activating factors (typically chemokines; Tables 6.2 and 6.3). Signaling through G protein-coupled chemokine receptors activates surface integrins (step 2; see Table 6.1). Functionally competent integrins bind

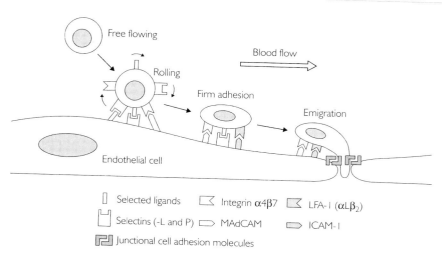

Fig. 6.1 Multistep model of lymphocyte recruitment. (Adapted from Refs. [1] and [23].)

## Table 6.1 Leukocyte–endothelial cell adhesion molecules and ligands (adapted from Panes and Granger[23])

| Adhesion molecule | Alternative designation | Localization | Expression Constitutive | Inducible | Ligand | Function |
|---|---|---|---|---|---|---|
| **Selectin family** | | | | | | |
| L-selectin | LAM-1, LECAM-1, MEL-14Ag, CD62L | All leukocytes | Yes | No: downregulation on activation | P-selectin, E-selectin, GlyCAM, CD14, MAdCAM | Rolling |
| P-selectin | PADGEM, GMP-140, CD62P | Endothelial cells, platelets | Yes | Yes | L-selectin, PSGL-1, 120 kDa PSL | Rolling |
| E-selectin | ELAM-1, CD62E | Endothelial cells | No | Yes | L-selectin, CLA, SSEA-1, 250 kDa ESL | Rolling |
| **Integrin family** | | | | | | |
| CD11a/CD18 | LFA-1, $\alpha_L\beta_2$ | All leukocytes | Yes | No | ICAM-1, ICAM-2 | Adherence/emigration |
| CD11b/CD18 | Mac-1, MO1, CR3, $\alpha_M\beta_2$ | Granulocytes, monocytes | Yes | Yes | ICAM-1, iC3b; Fb | Adherence/emigration |
| CD11c/CD18 | P150, 95, $\alpha_x\beta_2$ | Granulocytes, monocytes | Yes | Yes | Fb; iC3b? | ? |
| CD49d/CD29 | VLA-4, $\alpha_4\beta_2$ | Lymphocytes, monocytes, eosinophils, basophils | Yes | No | VCAM-1, extracellular matrix molecules | Adherence |
| CD49d/?$_7$ | $\alpha_4\beta_7$ | Lymphocytes | Yes | No | MAdCAM-1, VCAM-1, fibronectin | Adherence |
| **Ig supergene family** | | | | | | |
| ICAM-1 | CD54a | Endothelium, monocytes | Yes | No | LFA-1 Mac-1, CD43 | Adherence/emigration |
| ICAM-2 | CD102 | Endothelium | Yes | No | LFA-1 | Adherence/emigration |
| VCAM-1 | CD106 | Endothelium | No | Yes | VLA-4 | Adherenve |
| PECAM-1 | CD31 | Endothelium, leukocytes, platelets | Yes | No | PECAM-1 (homophilic) | Adherence/emigration |
| MAdCAM-1 | | Endothelium (intestine) | Yes | No | L-selectin, CD49d/?$_7$ | Adherence/emigration |

**Table 6.2 CXC, C and CX₃c family of chemokines and chemokine receptors (adapted from Ajuebor and Swain[55])**

| Systematic name | Human ligand | Mouse ligand | Chemokine receptors |
|---|---|---|---|
| **CXC family** | | | |
| CXCL1 | GRO-α/MGSA-α | GRO/KC | CXCR2 |
| CXCL2 | GRO-β/MGS-b/MIP-2α | GRO/KC | CXCR2 |
| CXCL3 | GRO-γ/MGSA-/MIP-2β | GRO/KC | CXCR2 |
| CXCL4 | PF₄ | PF₄ | Unknown |
| CXCL5 | ENA-78 | LIX | CXCR1; CXCR2 |
| CXCL6 | GCP-2 | C-3 | CXCR1 |
| CXCL7 | NAP-2 | Unknown | CXCR2 |
| CXCL8 | IL-8 | Unknown | CXCR1; CXCR2 |
| CXCL9 | Mig | MIG | CXCR3 |
| CXCL10 | IP-10 | IP-10 | CXCR3 |
| CXCL11 | I-TAC/H174 | Unknown | CXCR3 |
| CXCL12 | SDF-1α/β/PBSF | SDF-1 | CXCR4 |
| CXCL13 | BLC/BCA-1 | BLC/BCA-1 | CXCR5 |
| CXCL14 | BRAK/Bolekine | BRAK/BMAC | Unknown |
| CXCL15 | Unknown | Lungkine | Unknown |
| **C family** | | | |
| XCL1 | Lymphotactin/SCM-1α | Lyphotactin | XCR1 |
| XCL2 | SCM-1β/ATAC | Unknown | XCR2 |
| **CX₃C family** | | | |
| CX₃CL1 | Fractalkine | Fractalkine/neurotactin | CX₃CR1 |

ATAV, activation-induced, T cell-derived and chemokine-related; BCA-1, B-cell-attracting chemokine 1; BLC, B-lymphocyte chemoattractant; BMAC, B-cell and monocyte-activating chemokine; BRAK, breast and kidney derived chemokine; CXCL, CXC chemokine ligand; ENA-78, epithelial cell-derived neutrophil-activating peptide 78; GCP-2, granulocyte chemoattractant protein 2; GRO, growth-related oncogene; IL-8, interleukin 8; IP-10, interferon-inducible protein 10; I-TAC, interferon-inducible T-cell α chemoattractant; LIX, lipopolysaccharide-induced CXC chemokine; MGSA, melanocyte growth-stimulatory activity; Mig, monokine induced by interferon-γ; MIP, macrophage inflammatory protein; NAP-2, neutrophil-activating peptide 2; PF₄, platelet factor 4; SCM-1, single C motif-1; SDF-1, stromal cell-derived factor 1.

cellular adhesion molecules (CAM; Table 6.1), resulting in reversible arrest and firm adhesion of the lymphocyte (step 3).[1] Activation-dependent arrest allows cells to resist blood shear forces. Once arrested in endothelial surfaces, cells receive further signals derived from endothelia and tissue that induce transendothelial migration (step 4, diapedesis). Cells not induced to migrate into tissue resume rolling and return to the circulation.[1]

The complexity of the steps involved in lymphocyte migration allows tissue to selectively recruit cells with specific functional attributes. In the PP and MLN, HEV express ligands that facilitate migration of naive cells out of the circulation. As the pool of naive cells in the circulation expresses a broad repertoire of T-cell receptors, this population of cells is equipped to sample a wide range of enteric antigens. In contrast, immune cells in the iLP are preselected for enteric pathogens by encountering Ag-laden mucosal DC in lymphoid structures that drain the intestine (e.g. PP or MLN). Activation by antigen in draining lymphoid structures imprints cells with a specific profile of homing receptors needed for recruitment to the iLP. Preactivation permits the immune system to select cells that express high affinity TCR reactive for enteric Ag. Surface molecules expressed on gut-specific memory-like cells bind ligands on endothelial villous structures that facilitate recruitment to the iLP. Upon recruitment, lymphocyte populations respond rapidly and effectively to infectious agents. Thus, the selective recruitment of naive and activated cells to distinct compartments within the intestinal immune system allows the efficient induction of immune responses as well as the delivery of effector immune responses to sites within non-lymphoid tissues.

## ADHESION MOLECULES INVOLVED IN LYMPHOCYTE INTERACTIONS WITH PEYER'S PATCH VENULES

Homing of lymphocytes to the intestinal PP involves overlapping multimolecular adhesion events occurring on HEV. Data from Bargatze et al. indicate that arrest of naive cells in PP HEV requires the sequential engagement of L-selectin to initiate contact, α₄β₇ to slow rolling, and LFA-1 in conjunction with α₄β₇ to mediate activation-dependent arrest.[6] These studies demonstrate that the mucosal addressin, cellular adhesion molecule 1 (MAdCAM-1), is the predominant PP HEV ligand for both α₄β₇ and L-selectin. Once cells begin to roll, signaling through Gαi-coupled chemokine receptors triggers the adhesive arrest of rolling cells in PP venules. Fujimori et al.[7] examined PP homing by following the rolling and attachment of CFSE-labeled lymphocytes on intestinal microvessels by intravital fluorescence microscopy. Antibodies to L-selectin, α₄ integrin, β₇ integrin and MAdCAM-1 all reduced rolling of naive splenocytes within PP postcapillary venules (PCV). Furthermore, CD11a blockade detached >93% of cells from the venular walls. These results confirm that L-selectin and α₄β₇ are involved in rolling of lymphocytes in PP venules, whereas firm adhesion is mediated

## Table 6.3 CC family of chemokines and chemokine receptors (adapted from Ajuebor and Swain[55])

| Systematic name | Human ligand | Mouse ligand | Chemokine receptor |
|---|---|---|---|
| **CC family** | | | |
| CCL1 | I-309 | TCA-3/P500 | CCR8 |
| CCL2 | MCP-1/MCAF | JE/MCP-1 | CCR2 |
| CCL3 | MIP-1α/LD78 | MIP-1 | CCR1; CCR5 |
| CCL4 | MIP-1β/αT744.1/LAG-1 | MIP-1 | CCR5 |
| CCL5 | RANTES | RANTES | CCR1; CCR3; CCR5 |
| CCL6 | Unknown | C10/MRP-1 | Unknown |
| CCL7 | MCP-3 | MARC/FIC | CCR1-CCR3 |
| CCL8 | MCP-2/HC14 | MCP-2 | CCR1-CCR3; CCR5 |
| CCL9/10 | Unknown | MIP-1γ/MRP-2/CCF18 | Unknown |
| CCL11 | Eotaxin | Eotaxin | CCR3; CCR5 |
| CCL12 | Unknown | MCP-5 | ?CCR2 |
| CCL13 | MCP-4/CKβ-10/NCC-1 | Unknown | CCR1-CCR3; CCR5 |
| CCL14 | HCC-1-/NCC-2 | Unknown | CCR1; CCR3; CCR5 |
| CCL15 | HCC-2/MIP-5/Lkn-1/MIP-1δ | Unknown | CCR1; CCR3; CCR5 |
| CCL16 | HCC-4/LEC/NCC-3/4 | LCC-1 | CCR8 |
| CCL17 | TARC/dendrokine | TARC | CCR4 |
| CCL18 | DC-CK1/PARC/MIP-4/AMAC-1 | Unknown | Unknown |
| CCL19 | MIP-3β/ELC/exodus-3/CKb-11 | MIP-3 | CCR7 |
| CCL20 | MIP-3α/LARC/exodus-1 | MIP-3 | CCR6 |
| CCL21 | 6Ckine/TCA4/exodus-2/SLC | 6Ckine | CCR7 |
| CCL22 | MDC/STCP-1 | ABCD-1 | CCR4 |
| CCL23 | MPIF-1 | Unknown | CCR1 |
| CCL24 | MPIF-2/Eotaxin-2 | Unknown | CCR3 |
| CCL25 | TECK | TECK | CCR9 |
| CCL26 | Exotaxin-3 | Unknown | CCR3 |
| CCL27 | CTACK/ALP/ILC | Ctack/Eskine/ALP | CCR10 |

ABCD-1, activated B cells and dendritic cells-1; AMAC-1, alternative macrophage activation-associated CC-chemokine; CCL, CC chemokine ligand; CTACK, cutaneous T cell-attracting chemokine; DC-CK1, dendritic-cell-derived C-C chemokine; ELC, EBI1-ligand chemokine; FIC, fibroblast-induced cytokine; HCC, hemofiltrate CC chemokine; ILC interleukin-11 receptor α-locus chemokine; LARC, liver and activation-regulated chemokine; LCC 1, liver-specific CC chemokine 1; LEC, liver-expressed chemokine; Lkn 1, leukotactin 1; MCAF, monocyte chemotactic activating factor; MCP, monocyte chemoattractant protein; MDC, macrophage-derived chemokine; MIP, macrophage inflammatory protein; MPIF, myeloid progenitor inhibitory factor-1; MPR, multidrug resistance-associated protein; PARC, pulmonary and activation-regulated chemokine; RANTES, regulated upon activation normal T-cell expressed and secreted; TARC, thymus and activation-regulated chemokine; CA, T-cell activation gene; TECK, thymus-expressed chemokine; SLC, secondary lymphoid tissue chemokine; STCP-1, stimulated T-cell chemotactic protein.

by both MAdCAM-1/$\alpha_4\beta_7$ as well as ICAM-1/$\alpha L\beta_2$ integrin (LFA-1 (CD11a/CD18)) binding.[7,8] LFA-1 is expressed on the planar cell bodies of leukocytes rather than microvilli,[9] suggesting that this molecule functions in activation-triggered arrest and probably transendothelial migration.[6,10] MAdCAM-1 is also expressed on follicular DC and on DC in the 'buffer zone' between T- and B-cell regions.[11] Thus, the multistep cascade of events involved in lymphocyte recruitment to the PP may involve MAdCAM-1 interactions 1) at the initial rolling of cells (as a ligand for L-selectin), 2) at the point of firm adhesion (as a ligand for $\alpha_4\beta_7$ ), and 3) after diapedesis by enhancing activation of cells within DC-rich areas.[10]

Data from several groups suggest that PP recruitment of activated cells requires different adhesion events compared to naive cell migration. To examine this question, Ishii and colleagues followed the recruitment of iLP lymphocytes (iLPL) to PP HEV and microvessels in villus mucosa. iLPL are activated, memory-like populations (CD45RB[lo] and CD69[+]) that express high levels of $\alpha_4\beta_7$ and LFA-1.[7] Compared to splenic cells, iLPL were more

adherent to vessels in villous tips but failed to stick to PP venules. In other studies, Hokari et al. observed significantly reduced sticking of Con A-stimulated lymphocytes to PP PCV compared to naive cells.[8] These data differ from previous findings that TK1 cells, whose surface expression of adhesion molecules (L-selectin[lo-neg], $\alpha_4\beta_7^+$, LFA-1[+]) is similar to that of iLPL, bind avidly to PP HEV.[6,12] These data suggest that factors other than $\alpha_4\beta_7$ and LFA-1 mediate adhesion of activated lymphocytes to PP HEV[7] (see below).

## ADHESION MOLECULES INVOLVED IN LYMPHOCYTE INTERACTIONS WITH ILP VENULES

Recruitment of lymphocytes to non-lymphoid tissue in iLP is dominated by interactions between $\alpha_4\beta_7$ integrin and MAdCAM-1. MAdCAM-1 is expressed by postcapillary venules that traverse intestinal villi.[10] MAdCAM-1 is expressed throughout the small and large intestine and is upregulated during intestinal inflammation in ulcerative colitis, Crohn's disease[13] and celiac sprue.[10] MAdCAM-1 expressed in murine and human iLP contains two N-terminal immunoglobulin (Ig) domains that bind $\alpha_4\beta_7$.[14] The membrane-proximal mucin region serves to present the $\alpha_4\beta_7$-binding Ig domains ~20 nM from the cell membrane, thus facilitating interactions with lymphocyte homing receptors.[10] MAdCAM-1 detected in iLP lacks O-linked glycans that present L-selectin-binding carbohydrates which function to recruit naive cells to PP.[15] Thus, the distinct forms of MAdCAM-1 expressed in PP and iLP help to selectively recruit naive and activated effector cells to these separate sites.

$\alpha_4\beta_7$ is a heterodimeric integrin adhesion receptor expressed at low levels on resting lymphocytes in the circulation. The concentration of $\alpha_4\beta_7$ integrin on lymphocyte microvilli facilitates activation-independent tethering under shear and support lymphocyte rolling.[12] Activation mediated by T-cell receptor ligation, as well as signaling through chemoattractant receptors, increases expression and triggers functional activation of integrins, thereby promoting lymphocyte arrest.[16] $\alpha_4\beta_7$ integrin also binds fibronectin, the $\alpha_4$ integrin chain and VCAM-1.[10] However, these interactions are more likely involved in cell–cell and cell–matrix interactions within tissue.[10,17,18] The importance of $\alpha_4\beta_7$ integrin binding to MAdCAM-1-mediated recruitment of intestinal lymphocytes was first demonstrated by inhibition of in vivo lymphocyte recruitment using anti-$\alpha_4$ and anti-$\alpha_4\beta_7$ mAbs.[6,19] The requirement of $\alpha_4\beta_7$ to recruit intestinal lymphocytes was further highlighted by the severe depletion of cells in PP and iLP detected in $\beta_{7-/-}$ mice.[20] Thus, $\alpha_4\beta_7$–MAdCAM-1 interactions appear to be essential for the efficient recruitment of activated effector T cells to the iLP.

Whereas $\alpha_4\beta_7$–MAdCAM-1 interactions mediate recruitment of activated T cells under normal, uninflamed conditions in the colon, the data suggest that in colitis additional lymphocytes may be recruited to the intestine via alternative pathways. Specifically, L-selectin ligands may be aberrantly expressed in vessels of inflamed mucosa.[21,22] These data suggest that during intestinal inflammation, a wide array of lymphocytes, including naive T cells, are recruited to non-lymphoid intestinal compartments.

Data from Granger and colleagues[23] indicate that intestinal VCAM-1, as well as ICAM-1, levels are induced by injection of TNF.[24] Furthermore, Sans et al.[25] reported that both ICAM-1 and VCAM-1 are upregulated in colonic vessels in rats with TNBS colitis. These researchers found that immunoneutralization of ICAM-1 attenuated, and inhibition of VCAM-1 completely abrogated, leukocyte adhesion in colonic venules during colitis. Data from Fujimori et al.[7] suggest that these effects may be dependent on factors induced by tissue inflammation, as they found that blockade of LFA-1–ICAM-1 interactions had no effect on lymphocyte adhesion in normal (uninflamed) small intestine. Similarly, results from Butcher and colleagues[10] suggest that lymphocytes expressing the VCAM-1 ligand $\alpha_4\beta_1$ typically do not express $\alpha_4\beta_7$ and are therefore excluded from the intestine, even during states of inflammation. Taken together, these data suggest that under normal conditions ICAM-1 and VCAM-1 are probably not major determinants of lymphocyte recruitment to the iLP. However, as studies expand to include the effects of inflammation on tissue homing, the role of these molecules in intestinal leukocyte migration during IBD may become clear.

# THE ROLE OF P-SELECTIN IN LYMPHOCYTE RECRUITMENT TO PP AND ILP

Data from Austrup et al.[26] suggest that in vitro and in vivo differentiated Th1 cells express functional ligands for E- and P-selectin and migrate to acutely inflamed tissues. Data from Granger and colleagues suggest that P-selectin, but not E-selectin, is expressed constitutively on endothelial cells throughout the intestine.[27] In studies from Lee and colleagues[28] T-cell migration was followed to PP and LP tissue following a potent Th1-driven immune response in the abdominal cavity. To generate this model, transgenic T cells from OVA$_{323-339}$-specific DO11.10 x $RAG-1^{-/-}$ mice were transferred into BALB/c hosts prior to i.p. injections of antigen in complete Freund's adjuvant (CFA). Recruitment of activated cells to PP and iLP was detected in a MAdCAM-1-dependent pathway within 5–7 days of activation.[28] It was observed that P-selectin blockade inhibited the migration of in vivo-activated cells to the LP (–50%) without affecting the migration of cells to PP (T. Barrett, personal communication). In related studies we generated Th1 cells from transgenic mice and followed their recruitment to intestinal PP and LP. These studies revealed that Th1 cells were recruited in relatively high numbers by PP and LP tissue without requiring antigen to be present in vivo, and, as noted above, anti-P-selectin Ab completely abrogated Th1 iLP migration and reduced PP recruitment. Thus, P-selectin was found to play a significant role in the recruitment of differentiated effector cells to both PP and especially iLP. These findings differ from results published by Campbell et al.[29] In these studies P-selectin glycoprotein ligand-1 (PSGL-1) expression was detected on a subset of cells distinct from those expressing $\alpha_4\beta_7$. However, in these studies cells were examined 3 days after activation in vivo with antigen and LPS. Lee and colleagues[28] (and T. Barrett, personal observation), however, found that repeated activation in vivo with antigen in CFA effectively increased PSGL-1 on 'gut-homing' $\alpha_4\beta_7^+$ cells. The importance of P-selectin in mediating T-cell recruitment to the intestine is also supported by data from Salmi et al.[30] and Chu et al.,[31] who found that PSGL-1 was expressed by a substantial subset of LPL in colitic mice and in human IBD tissue, respectively. Taken together, these data indicate that P-selectin is an important mediator of both PP and iLP recruitment of activated Th1 effector cells.

# REGULATION OF HOMING MOLECULES AND ADDRESSINS

The major classes of molecules involved in leukocyte homing, the selectins,[32] immunoglobulin superfamily members[33] and integrins,[34] are highly regulated molecules. Presumably, this serves the purpose of both maintaining the recruitment of naive lymphocytes to the organized gut-associated lymphoid tissue (GALT) structures for education to relevant intestinal antigens, and to the effector compartments of the iLP and epithelium for the purposes of maintaining the basal immunologic defenses of these compartments. Moreover, during the course of pathologic insults that might be associated with the injurious events related to toxic exposures, infectious invasions or ischemia it would be beneficial to the host to increase the expression and function of these molecules to enhance mucosal defense through the recruitment of additional leukocyte populations. In the case of IBD, wherein the inflammation is presumed to be non-physiologic, such upregulation of expression and function of the molecules involved in leukocyte homing could be viewed as detrimental. Indeed, a wide variety of studies support increases in these classes of molecules both in humans with IBD and in chronic experimental intestinal inflammation. For example, the $\beta_2$ integrins $\alpha L\beta_2$ (LFA1) and CD11b/CD18 (MAC1) are increased on monocytes and neutrophils in IBD.[35] Similarly, ICAM-1 is increased on endothelial cells in human IBD, as are soluble ICAM-1 and VCAM-1 in the circulation of patients with ulcerative colitis in the former and Crohn's disease in the latter, consistent with the upregulation of these molecules in the inflammation associated with IBD.[36,37] Moreover, these molecules are hyperfunctional in that human intestinal mucosal endothelial cells (HIMEC) from patients with IBD exhibit increased adhesiveness for leukocyte populations.[38]

The proinflammatory environment that is present during these diseases regulates the molecules associated with leukocyte recruitment to the mucosal effector compartments. For example, IL-1$\beta$, TNF, IL-4 and IFN-$\gamma$ upregulate transcription of ICAM-1, VCAM-1, P-selectin, E-selectin and MAdCAM-1.[39] Whereas transcriptional activation of P-selectin and E-selectin occurs early after induction by these cytokines (3–5 hours), the Ig superfamily members VCAM-1 and ICAM-1 are transcriptionally activated somewhat later (6 and 12 hours, respectively) on endothelial cells.[40,41] Once expressed, the transcription of P-selectin, VCAM-1 and ICAM-1 tends to be persistent, in contrast to E-selectin expression, which is usually transient. Induction of these genes by cytokines and inflammatory mediators is integrated intracellularly through the induction of a number of transcription factors that ultimately determine expression of these molecules. Most important among these are NF$\kappa$B and AP1.[42] NF$\kappa$B binding sites can be detected in the E-selectin, VCAM-1, ICAM-1 and MAdCAM-1 genes. It is therefore not surprising that blockade of NF$\kappa$B pathways through antisense oligonucleotides ameliorated trinitrobenzene sulfonic acid-induced colitis.[43] AP1-binding sites, on the other hand, are found in ICAM-1, which also contains consensus sites for C/EBP.

The inflammatory milieu regulates function as well as expression of molecules involved in leukocyte homing. For example, the lipid mediators LTB4 and PAF activate the $\beta_2$ integrin CD11b/CD18, as do the chemokines IL-8 and MCP1.[44–46] Similarly, as noted above, homophilic interaction between the PECAM1 molecule on endothelial cells and leukocytes activates integrins. These interactions tend to promote leukocyte adhesion. In contrast, a number of soluble mediators, such as prostacyclin, NO, adenosine and TGF-$\beta$, are involved in decreasing leukocyte adhesion.[47,48] These immunosuppressive mediators provide tight regulation of leukocyte recruitment to mucosal tissues.

Consistent with the functional sequence of events involved in leukocyte homing into tissues, including the processes of rolling, adhesion, activation and transmigration, the various molecules involved in these processes are uniquely regulated in a manner consistent with supporting these functional events. The selectins, for example, are actively involved in both the early and late phases of leukocyte homing. Consistent with this, L-selectin is constitutively expressed by all leukocytes and shed from lymphocytes by the activity of sheddases during T-cell differentiation from the naive to the memory phenotype. Expression of L-selectin is regulated on leukocytes by IFN-$\alpha$. P- and E-selectin, on the other hand, are more involved in the recruitment of leukocytes into sites. Consistent with this, E-selectin, for example, is increased on the endothelium of active ulcerative colitis and Crohn's disease, but not inactive IBD.[35] Similarly, in rodents E-selectin is increased in several colitis models, including the CD45RB$^{hi}$ transfer model and IL-10-deficient mice.[49] E- and P-selectin are upregulated on endothelium when endothelial cells are stimulated by the inflammatory cytokines IFN-$\gamma$ and TNF, with maximal transcription by 3–6 hours and a return to baseline transcription by 12–24 hours.[50] P-selectin is uniquely activated by bacterial products such as LPS and reactive oxygen metabolites, consistent with an important role in inflammation.[51] In addition, P-selectin has a unique process of cell surface expression that involves rapid upregulation after activation that is transient owing to internalization as a result of endocytosis. This recycling presumably tightly regulates P-selectin on the cell surface after inflammatory stimuli. At the same time, bacterially stimulated P-selectin expression is associated with prolonged transcription, which maintains a large pool of this molecule during infection.[27]

The immunoglobulin superfamily members are also highly regulated by inflammatory mediators. Although ICAM-1 and ICAM-2 are expressed at low levels on endothelium in the absence of intestinal inflammation, ICAM-1 is expressed at high levels on the endothelium in patients with active IBD.[37,44,51] In contrast, ICAM-2 tends to be more constitutive, with little evidence of induction during the course of IBD in humans. Similar observations show that upregulation of ICAM-1 in endothelium and, interestingly, on epithelium, another site involved in recruitment of leukocytes (see Chapter 1), is increased during experimental colitis, including the CD45RB$^{hi}$ and IL-10–/– models.[49] Although VCAM-1 is increased in experimental colitis, upregulation in human IBD is less clear. MAdCAM-1, which mediates homing of both naive and memory cells, is highly expressed in the context of inflammation in both rodent models and human IBD at the sites of activity.[52] The major mechanisms of Ig superfamily regulation are transcriptional. Transcription of ICAM-1, for example, is dramatically increased by Th1 cytokines within 48 hours of stimulation. In general, regulation of the Ig superfamily members ICAM-1, VCAM-1 and MAdCAM-1 is through cytokine mediators that activate NF$\kappa$B.[53] Consistent with this, inhibition of NF$\kappa$B pathways leads to inhibition of these molecules, as shown by the inhibition of VCAM-1 expression in the peptidoglycan–polysaccharide rat model.[54]

The major integrins associated with leukocyte homing are the $\beta_2$ integrins ($\alpha_L\beta_2$ – LFA1 – and $\alpha_M\beta_2$ – Mac1) and $\alpha_4$ integrins ($\alpha_4\beta_1$-VLA4 and $\alpha_4\beta_7$ ). These molecules are regulated mainly through either the differentiation events associated with T-cell education to antigen or by leukocyte maturation and activation by other soluble mediators during the sequential events associated with leukocyte homing. For example, activation with chemokines at the site of homing causes conformational changes in the integrins that leads to increased adhesive function for either Ig superfamily members (ICAM-1, ICAM-2 or VCAM-1) or the connective tissue matrix.[34] For example, $\alpha_4\beta_1$ is involved in binding to fibronectins in the extracellular matrix.

# THE ROLE OF CHEMOKINES AND THEIR RECEPTORS IN LYMPHOID TRAFFICKING TO THE GI TRACT

The secretion and expression of chemoattractants (chemokines) and their receptors work in concert with adhesion molecules to orchestrate leukocyte trafficking to secondary lymphoid organs and specific tissue sites. Chemokines are small (7–15 kDa) structurally related heparin-binding proteins that are classified on the basis of the arrangement of their N-terminal cysteine residues (e.g. C, CC, CXC and $CX_3C$; see Tables 6.2 and 6.3) that mediate disulfide bonds. Chemokines mediate their effects through activation of G protein-coupled 7 transmembrane receptors that are classified based on the specific chemokines they bind (e.g. XCR1, CCR1-10, CXCR1-5 or CX3CR1; Tables 6.2 and 6.3). Following a chemokine-mediated signal (step 2 described above), surface integrins on rolling lymphocytes are activated and allow binding and firm adhesion to endothelial CAM (step 3). Although chemokines and chemokine receptors generally bind more than one ligand they bind to ligands only of the same class (e.g. CC chemokine bind to CCR receptors, CXC chemokines recognize CXCR chemokine receptors). Non-inflammatory chemokines are characterized by constitutive expression (e.g. SDF-1; MDC), whereas inflammatory chemokines are characterized by inducible expression (e.g. IL-8, MCP-1, RANTES, MIP-1). This latter class of chemokines has generated the most interest in IBD. Numerous studies in IBD patients and animal models have demonstrated that multiple inflammatory chemokines are upregulated in settings of active inflammation (e.g. IL-8, RANTES, MCP-1, MCP-3, IP-10, ENA-78, eotaxin).[55-70] Furthermore, increased chemokine receptor expression has also been associated with IBD (CXCR3, CCR1, CCR5).[55,67,71,72] In two murine models of IBD, chemical blockade or the absence of various chemokine receptors attenuated disease.[73,74] Human studies investigating the utility of chemokine – or chemokine receptor – blockade in IBD have not yet been reported.

One recently identified chemokine, Teck, and its ligand CCR9, plays a specific role in the trafficking of memory lymphocytes to the iLP. Teck is expressed by epithelial cells of the small intestine and CCR9 is expressed by most T lymphocytes found in the small intestine.[75-79] Teck and CCR9 are excluded from most other intestinal mucosal sites, suggesting that these molecules act specifically to drive the recruitment of cells to the small intestine. Interestingly, IgA-secreting B cells express CCR9 and migrate in response to Teck, suggesting a role for this receptor–ligand pair in the recruitment of B cells to the intestine.[80] The Teck/CCR9 interaction appears to have a complementary role to the $\alpha_4\beta_7$–MAdCAM-1 interactions that facilitate trafficking to the iLP.

A recent study by Targan and co-workers demonstrated that the Teck–CCR9 interactions may have relevance in IBD.[81] They demonstrated that CD patients with small intestinal disease, but not purely colonic involvement, had increased levels of Teck-reactive epithelium in the SI and elevated levels of CCR9+ lymphocytes in the peripheral blood. CCR9+ lymphocytes were reduced in inflamed versus uninflamed mucosa. They hypothesized that Teck may alter the partitioning of CCR9 lymphocytes to the small bowel in CD. The reduced levels of CCR9+ lymphocytes in the inflamed mucosa may result from increased activation-induced death of this cell type. Clearly there may be great therapeutic potential if the Teck–CCR9 interaction is necessary for the homing of intestinal lymphocytes in CD and required to initiate the inflammatory cascade. This has yet to be demonstrated. Trials investigating selective Teck inactivation or CCR9 blockade in the small intestine seem warranted. Moreover, if the combination of CCR9 and $\alpha_4\beta_7$ is the requisite 'address code' to lead to SI inflammation, dual modalities targeting these surface molecules may have promise.

# THERAPEUTIC IMPLICATIONS OF LEUKOCYTE HOMING MOLECULES FOR HUMAN IBD

The therapeutic importance of these molecular interactions involved in leukocyte homing has recently been appreciated as a potential target in the therapy of IBD. Significant insights for such a possibility have largely come from an examination of a variety of animal models. As a consequence of these observations, several classes of therapeutic targets have been identified among the leukocyte homing molecules on either the leukocyte or the endothelium. Thus far, the major classes of molecules that have been recognized to be potential targets include the Ig superfamily members and, in particular, ICAM-1, the integrins, in particular the $\alpha_4$ integrins, and the transcription molecules that regulate these molecules, in particular NF$\kappa$B.

ICAM-1 has been recognized as a potential target through an analysis of animal models. Either anti-ICAM-1 antibodies or anti-ICAM-1 antisense oligonucleotides that disrupt ICAM-1 have been shown to block the development of IBD in the SAMP-1/YIT model and the DSS colitis model.[82,83] Interestingly, in the SAMP-1/YIT model, blockade of VCAM-1 exhibits biologic activity nearly equivalent to that of ICAM-1, despite the fact that little VCAM-1 can be identified in inflammation in vivo. Similarly, blockade of the $\alpha_4$ integrins has been associated with amelioration of colitis in several animal models. Blockade of $\alpha_4$ with mAbs has shown efficacy in the cotton-top Tamarin model and the TNBS colitis model in rabbits.[84] Moreover, blockade of $\alpha_4\beta_7$ in particular, with a conformationally dependent antibody that recognizes this particular heterodimer, has activity in cotton-top Tamarins.[85] Interestingly, neither the selectins nor the $\beta_2$ integrins have so far been defined as potential targets in animal models. For example, blockade of E-selectin in cotton-top Tamarins has not ameliorated disease. Similarly, the absence of $\beta_2$ integrins in humans with leukocyte adhesion deficiency (LAD) is not associated with decreased chronic ileocolitis.[86] Whether this is due to redundancy of these molecular pathways or other factors is unknown, but more importantly, translates into the absence of potential efficacy of these molecules as potential therapeutic targets. As noted, many of these molecules involved in leukocyte adhesion are regulated by NF$\kappa$B. NF$\kappa$B is a common transcriptional pathway for a wide variety of cell surface and intracellular events, including a variety of cytokines and reactive oxygen metabolites. It is therefore interesting that NF$\kappa$B blockade ameliorates TNBS-induced colitis.[43] Clinical studies are now in progress. An equally appealing molecule based upon animal models is nitric oxide synthetase and its end product nitrous oxide (NO). This target, however, is likely to be quite complicated, as NO has been associated with both antiadhesive and proinflammatory processes. In terms of the former, NO, through its ability to decompose superoxide, can lead to decreased adhesion of leukocytes through the down-regulation of P-selectin expression. Regarding the latter, NO can promote TNF production by lymphocytes through the formation of peroxynitrate. Therefore, future interest in targeting this as a potential therapeutic pathway will probably be difficult. Thus, most interest has focused on the $\alpha_4$ integrins and the Ig superfamily member ICAM-1 as therapeutic targets for IBD patients.

There are two major approaches to blocking $\alpha_4$ integrins. These include a humanized $\alpha_4$ mAb capable of blocking $\alpha_4\beta_7$ and $\alpha_4\beta_1$, and hence interactions with MAdCAM-1 and VCAM-1, respectively. The other approach is conformational antibodies that recognize the $\alpha_4\beta_7$ integrin and are thus capable of specifically blocking $\alpha_4\beta_7$–MAdCAM-1 pathways. Two trials have investigated the utility of a humanized anti-$\alpha_4$ antibody in Crohn's disease. In the first study 30 patients with Crohn's disease with a CDAI between 150 and 450 were treated with 3 mg/kg of this mAb in comparison to a placebo group.[87,88] The $\alpha_4$ mAb antibody-treated group had a response rate of 39%, compared to an 8% remission rate in the placebo group at week 2. This response was short-lived, with a rebound of activity by 2 weeks. The relatively low efficacy rate may be related to the observed 50% decrease in the half-life of the antibody in the Crohn's disease patients compared to the controls. A larger study using the same antibody was recently published.[89] In this trial, 248 Crohn's disease patients with a CDAI between 220 and 450 were randomized to receive one of four treatments: two infusions of placebo; one infusion of 3 mg/kg humanized $\alpha_4$ mAb; two infusions of 3 mg/kg humanized $\alpha_4$ mAb; or two infusions of 6 mg/kg humanized $\alpha_4$ mAb. Notably, in the group that received two doses of 3 mg/kg of the humanized mAb, a 44% response rate at week 6, as defined by drop in the CDAI by 150, was noted, versus a 27% response rate in the placebo group. Although no significantly higher rate of clinical remission was found in the group receiving either two infusions of 6 mg/kg at 6 weeks (the primary endpoint) or one infusion of 3 mg/kg, there were higher remission rates in the former group at multiple other time points. Importantly, the response was maintained for up to 12 weeks. This monoclonal antibody therapy was observed to be safe, with mild infusion reactions seen in only two individuals. Taken together, these studies support targeting the $\alpha_4$ integrins as a means to treat IBD. It is unclear whether this response is due to decreased leukocyte homing, given the important co-stimulatory functions of the integrins and other classes of leukocyte homing molecules such as the Ig superfamily members, such that any significant effects observed could be related to modulating lymphocyte and leukocyte activity.

Significant attention has also been focused on blockade of the Ig superfamily member ICAM-1. As noted, blockade of $\beta_2$ integrins has not yet been supported by observations in either animal models or humans with deficiencies in these molecules. Two different strategies have thus far been utilized to attack ICAM-1 expression: antisense oligonucleotides and monoclonal antibodies. Four clinical trials have been published regarding the potential utility of antisense technology in the blockade of ICAM-1. In an initial preliminary study involving 20 Crohn's disease patients with a CDAI between 200 and 350, 15 patients received ISIS-2302 antisense compared to five placebo controls.[90] Groups received either 0.5 mg/kg, 1 mg/kg or 2 mg/kg, with an endpoint defined as either decreased CDAI, steroid use, or the Crohn's disease endoscopic index (CDEIS). When defined as a CDAI of less than 150, a clinical response was observed in seven of 15 ISIS-2302-treated patients versus one of five responses in the placebo control group. In addition, patients who received ISIS-2302 as a group exhibited decreased steroid use, improved IBDQ scores and increased circulating $\beta_7$ integrin-positive cells consistent with decreased leukocyte homing into the tissues. As a corollary, these investigators observed decreased tissue ICAM-1 expression following ISIS-2302 treatment. However, in three other studies ISIS-2302 did not exhibit significant efficacy.[91–93] In one of the largest studies, for example, 60 study subjects with a CDAI between 200 and 400, who had been steroid users for 6 months or more, received 0.5 mg/kg of ISIS-2302 subcutaneously. In this study, only two of 60 ISIS-2302-treated patients achieved a steroid-free remission, compared to none of 15 of the placebo-controlled subjects. Whether these latter results with ISIS-2302 reflect inadequate penetration into the tissues or inappropriate dose levels is not clear.

These studies emphasize the potential redundancy of these pathways, given the numerous molecular interactions involved in leukocyte homing. In this regard, simultaneous blockade of multiple pathways that are involved in the stepwise progression of leukocyte homing may be the appropriate strategy. In addition, focus on other potential therapeutic targets involved in leukocyte homing may make these types of approaches feasible, such as chemokine receptors including CCR9,[94] which is uniquely associated with small intestinal homing lymphocytes, and NF$\kappa$B pathways, as noted, which are broadly related to many of the molecules involved in leukocyte homing.

# REFERENCES

1. Butcher EC, Picker LJ. Lymphocyte homing and homeostasis. Science 1996;272:60.
2. Jenkins MK, Khoruts A, Ingulli E et al. In vivo activation of antigen-specific CD4 T cells. Annu Rev Immunol 2001;19:23.
3. Huang FP, Platt N, Wykes M et al. A discrete subpopulation of dendritic cells transports apoptotic intestinal epithelial cells to T cell areas of mesenteric lymph nodes. J Exp Med 2000;191:435.
4. Randolph DA, Huang G, Carruthers CJ et al. The role of CCR7 in TH1 and TH2 cell localization and delivery of B cell help in vivo. Science 1999;286:2159.
5. Kunkel EJ, Butcher EC. Chemokines and the tissue-specific migration of lymphocytes. Immunity 2002;16:1.
6. Bargatze R F, Jutila MA, Butcher EC. Distinct roles of L-selectin and integrins 47 and LFA-1 in lymphocyte homing to Peyer's patch-HEV in situ: the multistep model confirmed and refined. Immunity 1995;3:99.
7. Fujimori H, Miura S, Koseki S et al. Intravital observation of adhesion of lamina propria lymphocytes to microvessels of small intestine in mice. Gastroenterology 2002;122:734.
8. Hokari R, Miura S, Fujimori H et al. Altered migration of gut-derived T lymphocytes after activation with concanavalin A. Am J Physiol 1999;277:G763.
9. Erlandsen SL, Hasslen SR, Nelson RD. Detection and spatial distribution of the beta 2 integrin (Mac-1) and L-selectin (LECAM-1) adherence receptors on human neutrophils by high-resolution field emission SEM. J Histochem Cytochem 1993;41:327.
10. Butcher E, Williams CM, Youngman K et al. Lymphocyte trafficking and regional immunity. Adv Immunol 1999;72:209
11. Szabo MC, Butcher EC, McEvoy LM. Specialization of mucosal follicular dendritic cells revealed by mucosal addressin-cell adhesion molecule-1 display. J Immunol 1997;158:5584.
12. Berlin C, Bargatze RF, Campbell JJ et al. alpha 4 integrins mediate lymphocyte attachment and rolling under physiologic flow. Cell 1995;80:413.
13. Briskin M, Winsor-Hines D, Shyjan A et al. Human mucosal addressin cell adhesion molecule-1 is preferentially expressed in intestinal tract and associated lymphoid tissue. Am J Pathol 1997;151:97.
14. Briskin MJ, Rott L, Butcher EC. Structural requirements for mucosal vascular addressin binding to its lymphocyte receptor alpha 4 beta 7. Common themes among integrin-Ig family interactions. J Immunol 1996;156:719.

15. Berg EL, McEvoy LM, Berlin C et al. L-selectin-mediated lymphocyte rolling on MAdCAM-1. Nature 1993;366:695.

16. Takagi J, Springer TA. Integrin activation and structural rearrangement. Immunol Rev 2002;186:141.

17. Ruegg C, Postigo AA, Sikorski EE et al. Role of integrin alpha 4 beta 7/alpha 4 beta P in lymphocyte adherence to fibronectin and VCAM-1 and in homotypic cell clustering. J Cell Biol 1992;117:179.

18. Altevogt P, Hubbe M, Ruppert M et al. The alpha 4 integrin chain is a ligand for alpha 4 beta 7 and alpha 4 beta 1. J Exp Med 1995;182:345.

19. Hamann A, Andrew DP, Jablonski-Westrich D. Role of alpha 4 integrins in lymphocyte homing to mucosal tissues in vivo. J Immunol 1994;152:3282.

20. Wagner N, Lohler J, Kunkel EJ. Critical role for beta7 integrins in formation of the gut-associated lymphoid tissue. Nature 1996;382:366.

21. Michie SA, Streeter PR, Bolt PA. The human peripheral lymph node vascular addressin. An inducible endothelial antigen involved in lymphocyte homing. Am J Pathol 1993;143:1688.

22. Salmi M, Granfors K, MacDermott R et al. Aberrant binding of lamina propria lymphocytes to vascular endothelium in inflammatory bowel diseases. Gastroenterology 1994;106:596.

23. Panes J, Granger DN. Leukocyte-endothelial cell interactions: molecular mechanisms and implications in gastrointestinal disease. Gastroenterology 1998;114:1066.

24. Henninger DD, Panés J, Eppihimer M et al. Cytokine-induced VCAM-1 and ICAM-1 expression in different organs of the mouse. J Immunol 1997;158:1825.

25. Sans M, Salas A, Soriano A et al. Differential role of selectins in experimental colitis. Gastroenterology 2001;120;1162.

26. Austrup F, Vestweber D, Borges E et al. P- and E-selectin mediate recruitment of T-helper-1 but not T-helper-2 cells into inflamed tissues. Nature 1997; 385:81.

27. Eppihimer MJ, Wolitzky B, Anderson DC et al. Heterogeneity of expression of E- and P-selectins in vivo. Circ Res 1996;79:560.

28. Lee HO, Cooper CJ, Choi JH et al. The state of CD4+ T cell activation is a major factor for determining the kinetics and location of T cell responses to oral antigen. J Immunol 2002;168:3833.

29. Campbell DJ, Butcher EC. Rapid acquisition of tissue-specific homing phenotypes by CD4(+) T cells activated in cutaneous or mucosal lymphoid tissues. J Exp Med 2002;195:135.

30. Salmi M, Jalkanen S. Human leukocyte subpopulations from inflamed gut bind to joint vasculature using distinct sets of adhesion molecules. J Immunol 2001;166:4650.

31. Chu A, Hong K, Berg EL et al. Tissue specificity of E- and P-selectin ligands in Th1-mediated chronic inflammation. J Immunol 1999;163:5086.

32. Tedder TF, Steeber DA, Chen A et al. The selectins: vascular adhesion molecules. FASEB J 1995;9:866.

33. Granger DN. Cell adhesion and migration II: leukocyte-endothelial cell adhesion in the digestive system. Am J Physiol 1997;273:G982.

34. Springer TA. Traffic signals for lymphocyte recirculation and leukocyte emigration: the multistep paradigm. Cell 1994;76:301.

35. Nakamura S, Ohtani H, Watanabe Y et al. In situ expression of the cell adhesion molecules in inflammatory bowel disease: evidence of immunologic activation of vascular endothelial cells. Lab Invest 1993;69:77.

36. Nielsen OH, Langholz E, Hendel J et al. Circulating soluble intercellular adhesion molecule 1 (sICAM-1) in active inflammatory bowel disease. Dig Dis Sci 1994;39:1918.

37. Jones SC, Banks RE, Haidar A et al. Adhesion molecules in inflammatory bowel disease. Gut 1995;36:724.

38. Binion DG, West GA, Ina K et al. Enhanced leukocyte binding by intestinal microvascular endothelial cells in inflammatory bowel disease. Gastroenterology 1997;112:1895.

39. Silber A, Newman W, Reimann KA et al. Kinetic expression of endothelial adhesion molecules and relationship to leukocyte recruitment in two cutaneous models of inflammation. Lab Invest 1994;70:163.

40. Weller A, Isenmann S, Vestweber D. Cloning of the mouse endothelial selectins: expression of both E- and P-selectin is inducible by tumor necrosis factor alpha. J Biol Chem 1992;267:15176.

41. Fries JW, Williams AJ, Atkins RC et al. Expression of VCAM-1 and E-selectin in an in vivo model of endothelial activation. Am J Pathol 1993;143:725.

42. Baeuerele PA, Henkel T. Function and activation of NF-kB in the immune system. Annu Rev Immunol 1994;12:141.

43. Neurath MF, Petterson S, Buschenfelde KH et al. Local administration of antisense phosphorothioate oligonucleotides to the p65 subunit of NF-kB abrogates established experimental colitis in mice. Nature Med 1996;2:998.

44. Lefer AM. Significance of lipid mediators in shock states. Circ Shock 1989;27:3.

45. Bienvenu K, Russell J, Granger DN. Platelet-activating factor promotes shear rate-dependent leukocyte adhesion in postcapillary venules. J Lipid Mediat 1993;8:95.

46. Detmers PA, Powell DE, Walz A et al. Differential effects of neutrophil-activating peptide 1/IL-8 and its homologues on leukocyte adhesion and phagocytosis. J Immunol 1991;147:4211.

47. Kubes P, Suzuki M, Granger DN. Nitric oxide: an endogenous modulator of leukocyte adhesion. Proc Natl Acad Sci USA 1991;88:4561.

48. Gamble JR, Vadas MA. Endothelial adhesiveness for blood neutrophils is inhibited by transforming growth factor b. Science 1988;242:97.

49. Conner EM, Morise Z, Eppihimer MJ et al. Regional differences and magnitude of endothelial cell adhesion molecule expression in SCID mice reconstituted with CD45RBhigh T-lymphocytes. Gastroenterology 1998;114:A955.

50. Koizumi M, King N, Lobb R et al. Expression of vascular adhesion molecules in inflammatory bowel disease. Gastroenterology 1992;103:840–841.

51. Oshitani N, Campbell A, Bloom S et al. Adhesion molecule expression on vascular endothelium and nitroblue tetrazolium reducing activity in human colonic mucosa. Gastroenterology 1995;30:915.

52. Briskin M, Winsor-Hines D, Shyjan A et al. Human mucosal adressin cell adhesion molecule-1 is preferentially expressed in intestinal tract and associated lymphoid tissue. Am J Pathol 1997;151:97.

53. Read MA, Neish AS, Luscinskas FW et al. The proteasome pathway is required for cytokine-induced endothelial-leukocyte adhesion molecule expression. Immunity 1995;2:493.

54. Conner EM, Brand S, Davis JM et al. Proteosome inhibition attenuates nitric oxide synthase expression, VCAM-1 transcription and the development of chronic colitis. J Pharmacol Exp Ther 1997;282:1615–1622.

55. Ajuebor MN, Swain MG. Role of chemokines and chemokine receptors in the gastrointestinal tract. Immunology 2002;105:137–143.

56. Anezaki K, Asakura H, Honma T et al. Correlations between interleukin-8, and myeloperoxidase or luminol-dependent chemiluminescence in inflamed mucosa of ulcerative colitis. Intern Med 1998;37:253–258.

57. Daig R, Andus T, Aschenbrenner E, Falk W, Scholmerich J, Gross V. Increased interleukin 8 expression in the colon mucosa of patients with inflammatory bowel disease. Gut 1996;38:216–222.

58. Garcia-Zepeda EA, Rothenberg ME, Ownbey RT, Celestin J, Leder P, Luster AD. Human eotaxin is a specific chemoattractant for eosinophil cells and provides a new mechanism to explain tissue eosinophilia. Nature Med 1996;2: 449–456.

59. Grimm MC, Elsbury SK, Pavli P, Doe WF. Enhanced expression and production of monocyte chemoattractant protein-1 in inflammatory bowel disease mucosa. J Leukocyte Biol 1996;59:804–812.

60. Grimm MC, Elsbury SK, Pavli P, Doe WF. Interleukin 8: cells of origin in inflammatory bowel disease. Gut 1996;38:90–98.

61. Ina K, Kusugami K, Yamaguchi T et al. Mucosal interleukin-8 is involved in neutrophil migration and binding to extracellular matrix in inflammatory bowel disease. Am J Gastroenterol 1997;92:1342–1346.

62. Izzo RS, Witkon K, Chen AI, Hadjiyane C, Weinstein MI, Pellecchia C. Neutrophil-activating peptide (interleukin-8) in colonic mucosa from patients with Crohn's disease. Scand J Gastroenterol 1993;28:296–300.

63. Keshavarzian A, Fusunyan RD, Jacyno M, Winship D, MacDermott RP, Sanderson IR. Increased interleukin-8 (IL-8) in rectal dialysate from patients with ulcerative colitis: evidence for a biological role for IL-8 in inflammation of the colon. Am J Gastroenterol 1999;94:704–712.

64. Mahida YR, Ceska M, Effenberger F, Kurlak L, Lindley I, Hawkey CJ. Enhanced synthesis of neutrophil-activating peptide-1/interleukin-8 in active ulcerative colitis. Clin Sci (Lond) 1992;82:273–275.

65. Mazzucchelli L, Hauser C, Zgraggen K et al. Expression of interleukin-8 gene in inflammatory bowel disease is related to the histological grade of active inflammation. Am J Pathol 1994;144:997–1007.

66. Mazzucchelli L, Hauser C, Zgraggen K et al. Differential in situ expression of the genes encoding the chemokines MCP-1 and RANTES in human inflammatory bowel disease. J Pathol 1996;178:201–206.

67. Papadakis KA, Targan SR. The role of chemokines and chemokine receptors in mucosal inflammation. Inflamm Bowel Dis 2000;6:303–313.

68. Raab Y, Gerdin B, Ahlstedt S, Hallgren R. Neutrophil mucosal involvement is accompanied by enhanced local production of interleukin-8 in ulcerative colitis. Gut 1993;34:1203–1206.

69. Uguccioni M, Gionchetti P, Robbiani DF et al. Increased expression of IP-10, IL-8, MCP-1, and MCP-3 in ulcerative colitis. Am J Pathol 1999;155:331–336.

70. Z'Graggen K, Walz A, Mazzucchelli L, Strieter RM, Mueller C. The C-X-C chemokine ENA-78 is preferentially expressed in intestinal epithelium in inflammatory bowel disease. Gastroenterology 1997;113:808–816.

71. Qin S, Rottman JB. Myers P et al. The chemokine receptors CXCR3 and CCR5 mark subsets of T cells associated with certain inflammatory reactions. J Clin Invest 1998;101:746–754.

72. Williams EJ, Haque S, Banks C, Johnson P, Sarsfield P, Sheron N. Distribution of the interleukin-8 receptors, CXCR1 and CXCR2, in inflamed gut tissue. J Pathol 2000;192:533–539.

73. Ajuebor MN, Hogaboam CM, Kunkel SL, Proudfoot AE, Wallace JL. The chemokine RANTES is a crucial mediator of the progression from acute to chronic colitis in the rat. J Immunol 2001;166:552–558.

74. Andres PG, Beck PL, Mizoguchi E et al. Mice with a selective deletion of the CC chemokine receptors 5 or 2 are protected from dextran sodium sulfate-mediated colitis: lack of CC chemokine receptor 5 expression results in a NK1.1+ lymphocyte-associated Th2-type immune response in the intestine. J Immunol 2000;164:6303–6312.

75. Kunkel EJ, Campbell JJ, Haraldsen G et al. Lymphocyte CC chemokine receptor 9 and epithelial thymus-expressed chemokine (TECK) expression distinguish the small intestinal immune compartment: Epithelial expression of tissue-specific chemokines as an organizing principle in regional immunity. J Exp Med 2000;192:761–768.

76. Pan J, Kunkel EJ, Gosslar U et al. A novel chemokine ligand for CCR10 and CCR3 expressed by epithelial cells in mucosal tissues. J Immunol 2000;165:2943–2949.

77. Papadakis KA, Prehn J, Nelson V et al. The role of thymus-expressed chemokine and its receptor CCR9 on lymphocytes in the regional specialization of the mucosal immune system. J Immunol 2000;165:5069–5076.

78. Wurbel MA, Philippe JM, Nguyen C et al. The chemokine TECK is expressed by thymic and intestinal epithelial cells and attracts double- and single-positive thymocytes expressing the TECK receptor CCR9. Eur J Immunol 2000;30:262–271.

79. Zabel BA, Agace WW, Campbell JJ et al. Human G protein-coupled receptor GPR-9-6/CC chemokine receptor 9 is selectively expressed on intestinal homing T lymphocytes, mucosal lymphocytes, and thymocytes and is required for thymus-expressed chemokine-mediated chemotaxis. J Exp Med 1999;190:1241–1256.

80. Bowman EP, Kuklin NA, Youngman KR et al. The intestinal chemokine thymus-expressed chemokine (CCL25) attracts IgA antibody-secreting cells. J Exp Med 2002;195:269–275.

81. Papadakis KA, Prehn J, Moreno ST et al. CCR9-positive lymphocytes and thymus-expressed chemokine distinguish small bowel from colonic Crohn's disease. Gastroenterology 2001;121:246–254.

82. Sans M, Panes J, Ardite E et al. VCAM-1 and ICAM-1 mediate leukocyte-endothelial cell adhesion in rat experimental colitis. Gastroenterology 1999;116:874.

83. Burns RC, Rivera-Nieves J, Moskaluk CA et al. Antibody blockade of ICAM-1 and VCAM-1 ameliorates inflammation in the SAMP1/Yit adoptive transfer model of Crohn's disease in mice. Gastroenterology 2001;121:1428.

84. Podolsky DK, Lobb R, King N et al. Attenuation of colitis in the cotton-top tamarin by anti-alpha 4 integrin monoclonal antibody. J Clin Invest 1993;82:372.

85. Hesterberg PE, Winsor-Hines D, Briskin MJH et al. Rapid resolution of chronic colitis in the cotton-top tamarin with an antibody to a gut-homing integrin $\alpha 4\beta 7$. Gastroenterology 1996;111:173.

86. Uzel G, Kleiner DE, Kuhns DB et al. Dysfunctional LAD-1 neutrophils and colitis. Gastroenterology 2001;121:958.

87. Gordon FH, Clament WY, Lai Y et al. A randomized placebo controlled trial of a humanized monoclonal antibody to a4 integrin in active Crohn's disease. Gastroenterology 2001;121:268.

88. The Antegren Publication Committee. A randomized, double blind, placebo-controlled, pan European study of a recombinant humanized antibody to a4 integrin (Antegren TM) in moderate to severely active Crohn's disease. Gastroenterology 2001;120:A127.

89. Ghosh S, Goldin E, Gordon FH et al. Natalizumab for Crohn's disease. N Engl J Med 2003;348:24.

90. Yacyshyn BR, Bowen-Yacyshyn MB, Jewell L et al. A placebo-controlled trial of ICAM-1 antisense oligonucleotides in the treatment of Crohn's disease. Gastroenterology 1998;114:1133.

91. Yacyshyn BR, Cey WY, Goff J et al. A randomised, placebo-controlled trial of antisense ICAM-1 inhibitor (ISIS 2302) in steroid-dependent Crohn's disease showed clinical improvement at high serum levels. Gastroenterology 2001;120:A280.

92. Schreiber S, Nikolaus S, Malchow H et al. Absence of efficacy of subcutaneous antisense ICAM-1 treatment of chronic active Crohn's disease. Gastroenterology 2001;120:1339.

93. Yacyshyn BR, Chey W, Goff J et al. Double-blind, randomized, placebo-controlled trial of the remission induction and steroid sparing properties of two schedules of ISIS 2302 (ICAM-1 antisense) in active, steroid-dependent Crohn's disease. Gastroenterology 2000;118:A570.

94. Papadakis KA, Prehn J, Moreno ST et al. CCR9-positive lymphocytes and thymus-expressed chemokine distinguish small bowel from colonic Crohn's disease. Gastroenterology 2001;121:246.

## CHAPTER 7

# Leukocyte, platelet and endothelial cell interactions in the inflammatory bowel diseases

Matthew B Grisham and D Neil Granger

## INTRODUCTION

Active episodes of the inflammatory bowel diseases (IBD; e.g. Crohn's disease, ulcerative colitis) are characterized by the infiltration of large numbers of inflammatory cells, including neutrophils (polymorphonucleocytes, PMN), monocytes and lymphocytes into the intestinal interstitium. This inflammatory infiltrate is accompanied by extensive mucosal and/or transmural injury, including edema, loss of goblet cells, decreased mucus production, erosions and ulcerations, suggesting an important role for these leukocytes in the pathophysiology of IBD. Recent experimental and clinical investigations suggest that the enhanced leukocyte infiltrate and some of the pathophysiology observed in different models of colitis and in human IBD are mediated by the interaction between leukocytes and specific endothelial cell adhesion molecules (ECAM).[1-6] In addition to leukocyte–endothelial cell interactions there is a growing recognition that platelet–platelet, platelet–leukocyte and platelet–endothelial cell interactions may play important roles in the pathophysiology of IBD. Indeed, it is well known that platelet counts and their aggregation are enhanced in patients with active IBD.[7,8] The intestinal microvascular endothelium performs an important gatekeeper function by regulating the adhesion of leukocytes and platelets as well as the infiltration of protective and injurious immune cells into the gut interstitium.

Despite several decades of extensive investigation, the etiology and specific pathogenetic mechanisms responsible for IBD remain poorly defined. Recent experimental and clinical studies suggest that the initiation and pathogenesis of these diseases are multifactorial, involving interactions among genetic, environmental and immune factors.[9,10] Because the inflammation in IBD is localized primarily to the intestinal tract, investigators have focused on the intestinal lumen as the site for the antigenic trigger. Indeed, the chronic relapsing nature of IBD, coupled to the fact that a large percentage of patients with Crohn's disease

will experience recurrence following surgical resection of the diseased bowel, suggests that the antigen or antigens that initiate and perpetuate this disease are part of the normal gut flora[11] (see Chapter 10). Although several different etiologic theories have been proposed to account for this apparent immune activation, data obtained from multiple experimental studies suggest that the chronic gut inflammation may result from a dysregulated immune response to components of the normal gut flora.[12] This chapter presents a brief overview of the immunoregulatory mechanisms thought to contribute to and regulate the initiation of intestinal inflammation, and reviews the data implicating leukocyte, platelet and endothelial cell interactions as important determinants in the pathogenesis of IBD.

## FAILURE TO REGULATE INTESTINAL IMMUNE RESPONSES INDUCES CHRONIC GUT INFLAMMATION

The gastrointestinal (GI) mucosal interstitium is continuously exposed to large amounts of exogenous (i.e. dietary) and endogenous (e.g. commensal bacteria) antigens. Fortunately, the mucosal immune system has evolved efficient mechanisms to distinguish between potentially pathogenic bacterial, parasitic, viral and dietary antigens from non-pathologic antigens and resident gut microbiota. The gut mucosal immune system protects the body from invading pathogens via cell-mediated and humoral immunity. These protective immune responses involve not only activation of Th1 cells and the subsequent release of their cytokines, but also Th1 cytokine activation of innate immune cells, such as macrophages and other phagocytic leukocytes, to release additional proinflammatory cytokines such as tumor necrosis factor (TNF), IL-1β, IL-6, IL-8 and IL-12. Antigen-presenting cells (APC) endocytose, process and present

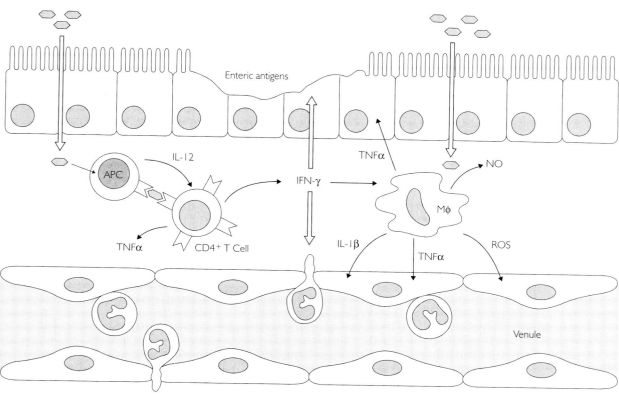

**Fig. 7.1** Cell-mediated immune responses in the gut interstitium. Antigen-presenting cells (APC) process and present enteric antigens that continuously gain access to the mucosal interstitium. T-cell–APC interactions activate previously polarized Th1 cells to produce IL-2 and IFN-γ, which activate tissue macrophages to release a variety of proinflammatory cytokines and mediators, including TNF-α, IL-1β, IL-12, nitric oxide (NO) and reactive oxygen species (ROS). IL-12 then further increases IFN-γ production by T cells. Both Th1- and macrophage-derived cytokines and mediators activate the microvascular endothelium to enhance expression of adhesion molecules, thereby promoting the recruitment of phagocytic leukocytes such as additional macrophages and PMN. The net result is the destruction of invading pathogens. Unregulated cell-mediated immunity may lead to epithelial injury, mucosal erosions and ulcerations.

luminal antigens that continuously gain access to the mucosal interstitium. T cell–APC interactions activate specific subsets of CD4+ T cells to produce IL-2 and IFN-γ, which in turn activate tissue macrophages to release a variety of proinflammatory cytokines and mediators, including TNF, IL-1β, IL-12, nitric oxide (NO) and reactive oxygen species (ROS) (Fig. 7.1). IL-12 feeds back on to the effector T cells to induce Th1 differentiation. Th1- and macrophage-derived cytokines, as well as ROS, activate the microvascular endothelium to enhance expression of adhesion molecules, thereby promoting the recruitment of phagocytic leukocytes (e.g. PMN, monocytes) into the extravascular space. The net result is the destruction of invading pathogens, but tissue damage can occur at the same time, which is intensified with protracted, dysregulated immune responses. The inability to regulate this normally protective response has been hypothesized to be importantly involved in the pathogenesis of IBD.

The potential for the immune system to lead to local and systemic injury suggests that healthy individuals possess mechanisms to appropriately downregulate immune responses after clearance of the inciting pathogen and to completely suppress pathogenic responses to ubiquitous antigens (see Chapter 5). This suppression is accomplished by additional subsets of CD4+ T cells collectively referred to as regulatory T (T_reg) cells

(Fig. 7.2).[13,14] This immunoregulatory group of T cells is composed of a naturally occurring CD4+CD25+ subset; T-regulatory-1 (Tr1) cells produced by repetitive antigenic stimulation of isolated CD4+ T cells (human or mouse) in the presence of IL-10 in vitro; and Th3 cells produced by oral exposure to antigen.[13,14] All three of these CD4+ T_reg subsets contain cells capable of inhibiting a variety of autoimmune disease models, including chronic colitis.[13–16] It is becoming increasingly appreciated that IL-10 and TGF-β are required for the regulatory function of T_reg cells in vivo, and that both of these regulatory cytokines play an important role in regulating tissue inflammation and injury in different models of IBD.[13,14,17–20] It has been proposed that interaction of T_reg cells with APC via their TCR–MHC interactions activates these leukocytes to release IL-10 and/or TGF-β. These cytokines inhibit Th1 activation as well as Th1-dependent activation of tissue macrophages. These regulatory cytokines also inhibit the activation of the venular endothelium within the mucosa, thereby downregulating the intestinal inflammatory response. These concepts are supported by the observations that virtually all of the genetically engineered or immune manipulated mouse models of IBD develop chronic colitis as a result of a lack of appropriate downregulation of normal cell-mediated immune responses to enteric antigens (see Chapter 9).

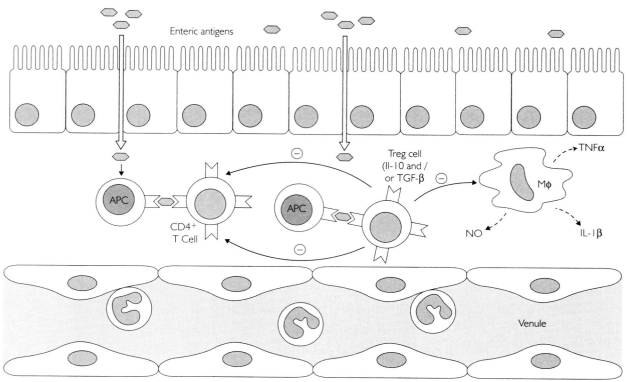

**Fig. 7.2** Regulation of intestinal immune responses to enteric antigens. Interaction of regulatory T cells ($T_{reg}$) with APC activates these leukocytes to release IL-10 and/or TGF-β. These regulatory cytokines inhibit effector T-cell activation as well as Th1-dependent activation of tissue macrophages. They also inhibit the activation of the venular endothelium within the mucosal interstitium, thereby downregulating the intestinal inflammatory response.

# SUSTAINED OVERPRODUCTION OF PROINFLAMMATORY CYTOKINES ACTIVATES THE MICROVASCULAR ENDOTHELIUM, THEREBY INITIATING CHRONIC INTESTINAL INFLAMMATION

## TRANSCRIPTIONAL REGULATION OF ENDOTHELIAL CELL ADHESION MOLECULES

The expression of Th1- and macrophage-derived cytokines such as TNF, IL-1β, IFN-γ, lymphotoxin or IL-12 is enhanced in both experimental and clinical colitis (Figs 7.1 and 7.3). Most of these cytokines promote leukocyte adhesion and extravasation in vitro and in vivo.[21] The mechanisms by which this diverse group of proinflammatory agents promote leukocyte recruitment in vivo are not entirely clear; however, recent data indicate that cytokine–receptor interactions transcriptionally activate the expression of certain ECAM (as well as many other inflammatory genes) via the activation of the nuclear transcription factor κB (NFκB). The remarkable effect of anti-TNF therapy in Crohn's disease attests to the importance of specific cytokines as important mediators of chronic gut inflammation. NFκB is a ubiquitous transcription factor and pleiotropic regulator of numerous inflammatory and immune responses.[22] Once activated, NFκB translocates from the cytosol to the nucleus of the cell, where it binds to its consensus sequence on the pro-

moter–enhancer region of multiple genes, thereby activating the transcription of a variety of inflammatory and protective genes (Fig. 7.4). For example, NFκB appears to regulate the transcription of several different ECAM, such as intercellular adhesion molecule-1 (ICAM-1), vascular cell adhesion molecule-1 (VCAM-1), E-selectin and mucosal addressin cell adhesion molecule-1 (MAdCAM-1), as well as NOS II and COX II and different cytokines (IL-1, IL-2, IL-6, IL-8, IL-12, TNF).[22-25] Thus, NFκB regulates the inflammatory response by enhancing surface expression of adhesion molecules and by inducing the synthesis of proinflammatory cytokines, thereby promoting leukocyte recruitment. NFκB belongs to the Rel family of transcription factors, in which members share a region of about 300 amino acids known as the Rel homology domain. The heterodimeric NFκB is composed of p50 and p65 subunits and is normally sequestered in the cytoplasm associated with its inhibitor IκB. In addition to proinflammatory cytokines, several different bacterial and viral products and lipid mediators also activate NFκB via pattern recognition receptors (see Chapter 10). Experimental data suggest that these stimuli activate multiple signaling pathways which converge to enhance intracellular reactive oxygen metabolism.[26-36]

These oxidants activate one or more redox-sensitive IκB kinases, which specifically phosphorylate IκB.[37,38] Once phosphorylated, IκB is selectively ubiquitinated and then degraded via the non-lysosomal, ATP-dependent 26S proteolytic complex (Fig. 7.4).[39-41] Inhibition of the proteasome pathway using selective yet structurally distinct inhibitors blocks cytokine synthesis and iNOS expression, as well as cytokine-mediated induction of ICAM-1, E-selectin and VCAM-1, with resultant alterations in adhesion of PMN and lymphocytes to endothelial

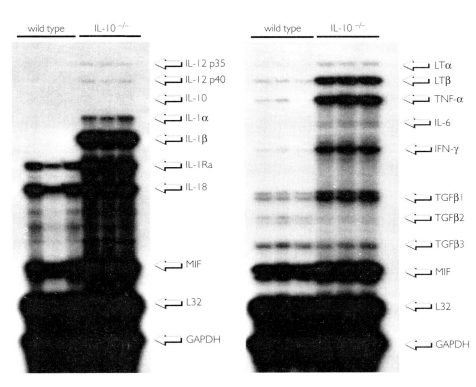

Fig. 7.3 Cytokine mRNA expression in healthy wildtype vs. IL-10-deficient (IL-10^-/-) mice with chronic colitis. RNase protection assay (RPA) analysis of colons from wildtype and colitic IL-10^-/- mice reveals marked increases in the mRNA for a variety of Th1- and macrophage-derived cytokines in diseased animals. Note the dramatic increases in lymphotoxin-β (LT-β), tumor necrosis factor (TNF), interleukin-1β (IL-1β), interferon-γ (IFN-γ) and IL-18. (Reproduced with permission from reference [119].)

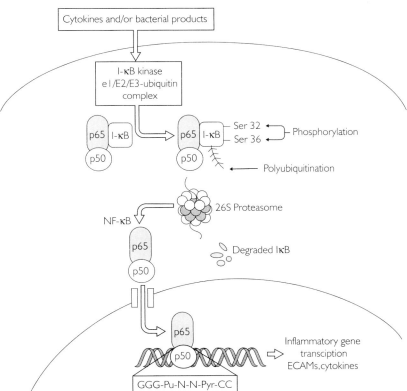

Fig. 7.4 Cytokine and/or bacterial product-induced activation of nuclear transcription factor-κB (NFκB). Cytokine–receptor interaction initiates multiple signaling pathways that activate one or more IκB kinases and ubiquitinating enzymes, resulting in the phosphorylation and polyubiquitination of IκB-α. The 26S proteasome complex selectively degrades the post-translationally modified IκB-α, thereby liberating the transcriptionally active p50/p65 heterodimer. This transcription factor is transported into the nucleus, where it binds to its consensus sequence in the promoter/enhancer region upstream of the different genes, where it activates the transcription of a variety of genes known to be important in the inflammatory response, such as endothelial cell adhesion molecules (ECAM) and proinflammatory cytokines.

monolayers.[42] Findings from our laboratory indicate that inhibition of NFκB using a selective proteasome inhibitor (PS-341) attenuates colonic as well as gastric mucosal and joint inflammation in models of chronic granulomatous colitis, non-steroidal anti-inflammatory drug (NSAID)-induced gastropathy and polyarthritis in rats, respectively.[43–46] In addition, Neurath and co-workers have demonstrated that antisense oligonucleotides specific for the p65 subunit of NFκB are also effective at inhibiting the colonic inflammation observed in two different models of colitis.[47] Of note, corticosteroids exert at least some of their potent anti-inflammatory activity in vivo by inhibiting the activation of NFκB.[48–55] Furthermore, sulfasalazine and possibly 5-ASA inhibit NFκB activation by inhibiting IKK activity in vitro.[56,57] The in vivo significance of these studies remains to be determined. Taken together, these data suggest that NFκB activation and its subsequent transcriptional activation of the

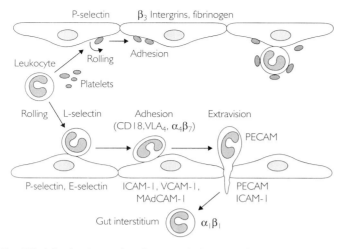

**Fig. 7.5** Adhesive interactions between leukocytes, platelets and the wall of postcapillary venules in inflamed intestine. Both leukocytes and platelets can roll and firmly adhere to the surface of activated endothelial cells through specific adhesion receptor–ligand interactions. Adherent leukocytes can also serve as a platform for platelet adhesion to the vessel wall.

microvascular endothelium, as well as cytokine expression, is crucial for the development of intestinal inflammation.

## LEUKOCYTE–ENDOTHELIAL-CELL INTERACTIONS

Leukocyte adhesion to microvascular endothelium involves a complex sequence of interactions between circulating leukocytes and vascular endothelial cells (Fig. 7.5).[58–60] The initial event involves a weak adhesive interaction which results in leukocytes 'rolling' along the endothelium. Subsequently, these adhesive forces strengthen, such that leukocytes become firmly attached to the endothelium and remain stationary. Finally, the leukocytes begin to change shape, send pseudopodia between endothelial cells, and extravasate into the interstitium. These adhesive interactions are regulated in an orderly, sequential activation of different families of membrane adherence receptors on leukocytes and endothelial cells. Although much of our current understanding of leukocyte–endothelial-cell interactions has come from studies describing PMN–endothelial-cell interactions, accumulating data suggest a very similar, multistep process for monocyte– or lymphocyte–endothelial-cell interactions, both of which involve the sequential rolling, activation, firm adhesion, and diapedesis of the leukocyte (Fig. 7.5). The following overview briefly outlines the general concepts involved in leukocyte–endothelial-cell interactions and their role in the pathophysiology of IBD.

## ROLLING

In vivo the initial adhesive interaction of leukocytes with vascular endothelium involves the movement of leukocytes from the central stream of circulating blood cells toward the vessel wall and subsequent rolling along the endothelium.[61,62] The movement of leukocytes toward the venular wall may be due to a hydrodynamic interaction between red blood cells and leukocytes as they pass from the smaller diameter capillaries to the larger diameter postcapillary venules, i.e. the faster-moving red blood cells displace the leukocytes from the axial stream

toward the venular endothelium.[62] The rolling of leukocytes along the endothelium is considered to be a result of weak adhesive interactions which are insufficient to overcome the effects of the shear stress along the vessel wall. L-selectin of leukocytes and the P- and E-selectins of endothelial cells have been implicated as the major ECAM involved in rolling of leukocytes along the endothelium (Table 7.1).[58–61] L-selectin is constitutively expressed on quiescent PMN and lymphocytes, whereas P- and E-selectins appear only on the surface of cytokine-activated endothelium. Mobilization of E-selectin to the surface of the endothelial cell is stimulated by certain Th1 and/or macrophage-derived cytokines (e.g. IFN-γ, lymphotoxin, TNF), and maximum surface levels are achieved several hours after activation, with a return to basal levels within 12–24 hours. Koizumi et al.[63] and Nakamura et al.[64] have demonstrated that E-selectin is significantly upregulated on the surface of endothelial cells in mucosa obtained from patients with active but not quiescent ulcerative or Crohn's colitis. We have demonstrated that colonic E-selectin expression is significantly enhanced with the onset of chronic colitis in SCID mice which have been reconstituted with CD45RB[high] T cells, or in the colons of IL-10-deficient (IL-10[−/−]) mice with colitis.[65–68] However, two different antibodies to E-selectin did not attenuate the spontaneous colitis that develops in cotton-top Tamarins, suggesting that E-selectin-dependent leukocyte adhesion may not represent an important interaction to sustain the inflammatory response in this model of colitis.[69] The authors suggested that if E-selectin is not necessary to promote leukocyte migration into the colonic mucosa, then other pathways for leukocyte adhesion must exist in the inflamed colon. P-selectin, on the other hand, is rapidly mobilized to the endothelial cell surface, reaching peak levels within 10–30 minutes. The expression of P-selectin is very transient, decreasing to negligible levels within minutes owing to internalization of the selectin via endocytosis. Interestingly, some stimuli (e.g. reactive oxygen species, bacterial products species) can activate endothelial cells in such a manner that P-selectin expression is prolonged for several hours.[70] Nakamura et al.[64] and Schurmann et al.[71] have shown that P-selectin is upregulated in venules of mucosa obtained from patients with active IBD. The ligands for the selectins have not been firmly established, but are thought to be Sialyl-Lewis X and other fucosylated carbohydrates.[58] A direct interaction between the selectins is also possible, i.e. PMN or lymphocyte L-selectin may interact with the P- or E-selectin on the endothelium. L-selectin is important for PMN or lymphocyte–endothelial rolling.[72] As with the earlier work using antibodies to E-selectin, studies addressing the importance of P- and E-selectin in experimental colitis using mice genetically deficient in these ECAM have also proved rather disappointing.[73] In these studies investigators found that colitis induced by acetic acid or TNBS in ethanol was not attenuated, and in some cases was actually enhanced in mice deficient in P- and/or E-selectin.[73] Interpretation of these studies in the context of human IBD is difficult, as neither the acetic acid nor the TNBS/ethanol model is immune based, and thus their clinical relevance is questionable.

## ADHESION

The rolling of leukocytes along the venular endothelium keeps these cells in close apposition to the endothelium, thereby facilitating their activation by inflammatory mediators generated

**TABLE 7.1 Adhesion glycoproteins involved in leukocyte-endothelial cell interactions**

| Adhesion molecule | Alternative designation | Localization | Constitutive expression | Inducible expression | Ligand | Function |
|---|---|---|---|---|---|---|
| *Immunoglobulin Supergene Family* | | | | | | |
| ICAM-1 | CD54a | Endothelium Monocytes | Yes | Yes | LFA-1; Mac-1 CD43 | Adherence Emigration |
| ICAM-2 | CD102 | Endothelium | Yes | No | LFA-1 | Adherence Emigration |
| VCAM-1 | CD106 | Endothelium | No | Yes | VLA-1($\alpha_4\beta_4$) | Adherence |
| PECAM-1 | CD31 | Endothelium Leukocytes | Yes | No (?) | PECAM-1 (homophilic) | Adherence Emigration |
| MAdCAM-1 | ———— | Endothelium (intestine) | Yes | Yes | VLA-4($\alpha_4\beta_1$) L-selectin CD49d/$\beta_7$ ($\alpha_4\beta_7$) | Adherence Emigration |
| *Selectin Family* | | | | | | |
| L-selectin | LAM-1 LECAM-1 MEL-14 Ag CD62L | All leukocytes | Yes | No; down-regulation on activation | P- selectin E-selectin GlyCAM CD14 MAdCAM | Rolling |
| P-selectin | PAGDEM GMP-140 CD62P | Endothelial cells Platelets | Yes | Yes | L- selectin PSGL-1 120 kDa PSL | Rolling |
| E- selectin | ELAM-1 CD62L | Endothelial cells | No | Yes | L- selectin CLA; SSEA-1 250 kDa ESL | Rolling |
| *Integrin Family* | | | | | | |
| CD11a/CD18 | LFA-1 $\alpha L\beta_2$ | All leukocytes | Yes | No | ICAM-1 ICAM-2 | Adherence Emigration |
| CD11b/CD18 | Mac-1, MO1 CR3, $\alpha M\beta_2$ | Granulocytes Monocytes | Yes | Yes | ICAM-1 iC3b; Fb | Adherence Emigration |
| CD11c/CD18 | p150, 95 $\alpha_x\beta_2$ | Granulocytes | Yes | Yes | Fb; iC3b? | ? |

by the endothelium or interstitial cells (e.g. lymphocytes, macrophages, mast cells). For example, activated PMN (or monocytes) and, to a lesser extent, lymphocytes adhere to venular endothelium (despite the shear stress of flowing blood) by virtue of the strong adhesive interactions between $\beta_2$ integrins (CD11/CD18) on these leukocytes and ICAM-1 on endothelial cells (Table 7.1). In vivo studies indicate that neutralization of L-selectin function or the removal of L-selectin from the PMN prevents firm adhesion to venules exposed to inflammatory mediators.[59] These latter observations support the contention that selectin-mediated rolling is a prerequisite for CD11/CD18-ICAM-1-mediated adhesion.

Upon activation, PMN and lymphocytes shed their L-selectin and upregulate and/or activate their integrins.[59,60] The $\beta_2$ integrins on PMN are heterodimers consisting of a common subunit (CD18) non-covalently linked to one of three immunologically distinct subunits designated CD11a, CD11b and CD11c (Table 7.1). CD11a/CD18 is basally expressed on the surface of PMN and lymphocytes, and interacts with ICAM-1 and ICAM-2 on endothelial cells to promote adhesive interactions.[74,75] The addition of unstimulated PMN to naive or cytokine-stimulated endothelial cell monolayers in vitro results in PMN adherence to the endothelial cells which is inhibited by monoclonal antibodies (MAb) directed against CD11a/CD18 or ICAM-1.[74] A variety of inflammatory mediators or cytokines are unable to increase the expression of CD11a/CD18 on the surface of PMN. By contrast, most of the CD11b/CD18 and CD11c/CD18 adherence glycoproteins are stored in PMN granules and can be rapidly (within minutes) mobilized to the surface of PMN by fusion of granule membranes with the cell membrane upon stimulation.[76] Stimulation of PMN with inflammatory mediators or cytokines results in a 3–10-fold increase in the expression of CD11b/CD18 and CD11c/CD18 on the PMN surface. Both anti-CD11a and anti-CD11b MAb can inhibit the adherence of activated PMN to cytokine-stimulated endothelial cell monolayers.

Although it has been generally assumed that CD11/CD18-dependent adhesion is essential for mediating much of the tissue injury and dysfunction during acute flares of colitis, recent reports by d'Agata et al.[77] and Uzel et al.[78] suggest that this concept may need to be re-examined. These authors report a case of CD11/CD18 deficiency characterized by chronic ileocolitis. Bone marrow transplantation completely resolved the

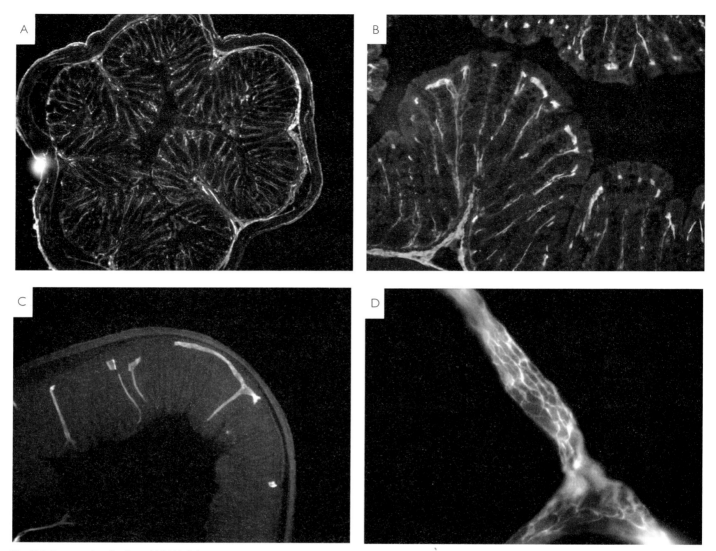

**Fig. 7.6** Immunolocalization of ICAM-2 (panels A and B) and MAdCAM-1 (panels C and D) in colons obtained from colitic IL-10[-/-] mice. At 3 months of age, rat antimouse monoclonal antibody specific for the two different ECAM was injected (IV), and tissues were processed as described elsewhere.[65] Frozen sections were stained with donkey antirat secondary antibody conjugated to Cy3 fluorochrome. Note the vascular immunolocalization of ICAM-2 demonstrating staining of the small and large vessels. Interestingly, MAdCAM-1 immunolocalizes to large vessels within the mucosa and submucosa and appears junctional in nature (magnification ×25 and ×100 for panels A and B, respectively; ×25 and ×200 for panels C and D, respectively).

intestinal inflammation, suggesting that marrow-derived leukocyte dysfunction may contribute to disease. These data are similar to those recently reported demonstrating that four of five Crohn's disease patients given allogenic marrow transplantation remained disease free for several years post transplantation[79] and support the concept that Crohn's disease may arise as a result of defective neutrophil function.

ICAM-1 and ICAM-2 are endothelial cell adhesion molecules which are members of the immunoglobulin supergene family.[72,76,80,81] ICAM-1 contains five Ig-like extracellular domains, of which the first $NH_2$-terminal Ig-like domain recognizes CD11a/CD18 and the third Ig-like domain recognizes CD11b/CD18 (Table 7.1).[80]

ICAM-1 is basally expressed on endothelial cells, and its expression is increased in response to activation of endothelial cells with certain Th1- and/or macrophage-derived cytokines. ICAM-2 is a truncated form of ICAM-1 and is also basally expressed on endothelial cells, but its level of expression is higher (10-fold) than that of ICAM-1.[81] In contrast to ICAM-

1, ICAM-2 expression is not increased on cytokine-activated endothelial cells. Indeed, ICAM-2 surface expression is useful for delineating vascular surface area. In our hands ICAM-2 expression does not appear to be localized exclusively to the postcapillary venules but rather is expressed on the capillaries as well (Fig.7.6). Several different reports have demonstrated enhanced staining for ICAM-1 on mucosal mononuclear or endothelial cells in biopsies obtained from patients with active ulcerative colitis and Crohn's disease.[64,82,83] We have shown that colonic ICAM-1 but not ICAM-2 expression is significantly enhanced in colitic SCID mice reconstituted with CD45RB[high] T cells or in colons from IL-10[-/-] mice with active enterocolitis.[65–68,84] Infusion of an antisense oligonucleotide or antibodies directed against ICAM-1 produces clinical improvement in mouse models of colitis or ileitis and in steroid-resistant Crohn's disease patients, respectively,[1,2,85] although larger controlled trials were negative.[86,87]

PMN–endothelial-cell interactions predominate in acute flares of IBD, whereas lymphocyte, monocyte, and in some cases eosinophil interactions with the microvascular endothelium are more prevalent during the chronic stages of gut inflammation. The mononuclear leukocytes possess a $\beta_1$ integrin called very-late activation antigen-4 (VLA-4; $\alpha_4\beta_1$), which binds to inducible VCAM-1 and MAdCAM-1 expressed on the surface of cytokine-activated endothelial cells (Table 7.1). Recent studies from our laboratory demonstrate a significant enhancement in colonic VCAM-1 expression with the onset of chronic colitis in the SCID/CD45RB[high] or IL-10[-/-] models of chronic colitis.[45,65–67,84] Although some recent studies have demonstrated that VCAM-1 blockade attenuates DSS-induced colitis,[88] several other laboratories have failed to consistently demonstrate enhanced expression of VCAM-1 in biopsies obtained from patients with active colitis.[63,64,82] These observations are somewhat surprising in view of two reports demonstrating that primary cultures of microvascular endothelial cells isolated from human intestine and colon respond to different proinflammatory cytokines with enhanced surface expression of VCAM-1.[89,90] The reasons for these differences between experimental and human IBD are not known, but may represent the inherent variability known to be associated with immunohistochemistry compared to the objective, more qualitative method to quantify ECAM expression in vivo.[65–67,84] Alternatively, the quality of the antibodies used for the immunolocalization studies may also represent an important determinant for accurate determination of VCAM-1.

Lymphocytes possess an additional ligand–counterreceptor pair, which is important in cell–cell adhesion, signaling, trafficking and regulation of the immune responses in mucosal tissues, especially in the gastrointestinal tract.[91,92] MAdCAM-1 is a member of the Ig supergene family that is expressed on gastrointestinal mucosal endothelial cells and high endothelial cells in lymph nodes and Peyer's patches, and is involved in the selective homing of lymphocytes to mucosal tissue (Table 7.1).[91,92] Surface expression of MAdCAM-1 is induced by certain Th1- or macrophage-derived cytokines and bacterial products and may last for several days.[30] Its lymphocyte-associated counterreceptor, $\alpha_4\beta_7$, is found primarily on a subpopulation of memory/ activated CD4+ T lymphocytes involved in mucosal immunity. Briskin et al.[93] reported that MAdCAM-1 surface expression on venular endothelial cells in the lamina propria of the gut is enhanced in inflammatory foci in biopsies obtained from patients with active UC or CD. Colonic and cecal but not ileal MAdCAM-1 expression increases dramatically (11-fold) with the onset of colitis in the SCID/CD45RB[high] and IL-10[-/-] models of colitis.[30,65–67,84] Several studies using low molecular weight antagonists or immunoneutralizing monoclonal antibodies to either $\alpha_4\beta_7$ or MAdCAM-1 demonstrate that the $\alpha_4\beta_7$– MAdCAM-1 interaction plays an important role in the pathophysiology in three different models of colitis.[3–5,94,95] MAdCAM-1 represents a potentially important therapeutic target for the treatment of IBD. There have been exciting reports using and Ab to $\alpha_4$ (Antegren; Elan Pharma, UK) which is directed against VLA-4 ($\alpha_4\beta_1$) and $\alpha_4\beta_7$ in patients with CD. In a large phase 2 clinical study natalizumab was significantly better than placebo.[96]

## TRANSENDOTHELIAL MIGRATION

Once leukocytes adhere to the endothelium, they send pseudopodia between endothelial cells and migrate into the interstitium. Based on studies using blocking antibodies, PMN transmigration across endothelial cell monolayers appears to require CD18–ICAM-1 interactions as well as platelet–endothelial-cell adhesion molecule-1 (PECAM-1).[97] PECAM-1 is preferentially distributed between endothelial cells (intercellular junctions), and the transmigration process appears to involve homotypic adhesive interactions between PECAM-1 on PMN and endothelial cells. A report by Shuermann et al. demonstrated a significant increase in PECAM expression on venules in mucosa obtained from patients with active UC.[98] Future work may elucidate the precise adhesive interactions involved in the transendothelial migration of PMN. Taken together, these studies suggest that the colonic and/or intestinal microvasculature regulates chronic gut inflammation by virtue of its ability to modulate the infiltration of different populations of leukocytes into the interstitium.

# PLATELETS AND INTESTINAL INFLAMMATION

## EVIDENCE IMPLICATING PLATELETS IN HUMAN AND EXPERIMENTAL IBD

There is growing recognition that platelets are not only involved in hemostasis and thrombosis, but can also modulate acute and chronic inflammatory responses. Platelets exhibit several proinflammatory properties, including the release of inflammatory mediators and the initiation of adhesion-dependent activation of other inflammatory cells (e.g. neutrophils). In human IBD there is an elevated platelet count, and this has been used as a marker of disease activity.[8] Furthermore, platelets isolated from patients with UC and Crohn's disease show that increased expression of P-selectin and other markers of cell activation (GP53, β-thromboglobulin, CD40 ligand) is associated with an increased aggregability both in vivo and in vitro.[99–101] Activated platelets not only express more P-selectin on the cell surface, but also shed this adhesion glycoprotein into blood plasma. Hence it is not surprising that some reports describe higher levels of circulating soluble P-selectin in both UC and CD patients than in healthy subjects.[102]

A reduced threshold for ADP, thrombin and collagen-induced platelet aggregation in vitro has also been demonstrated for IBD patients versus normal subjects.[103] 5-Aminosalicylate (5-ASA), which is widely used in the treatment of intestinal inflammation, has been shown to attenuate the platelet hyperreactivity seen in patients with IBD. Spontaneous ex vivo platelet activation is reduced by 50% in patients taking 5-ASA orally, compared to patients not receiving this treatment. 5-ASA was also shown to significantly reduce both spontaneous and thrombin-induced platelet activation following in vitro exposure of platelets to the drug.[104]

Intravascular platelet aggregates have been identified in mucosal biopsies of patients with UC, and there is an increased number of circulating platelet aggregates in the mesenteric venous circulation draining the inflamed bowel in UC.[7] These findings are consistent with evidence that patients with IBD are at increased risk of systemic thromboembolism.[105] This evidence has led to the proposal that multiple microvascular infarction contributes to the pathogenesis of CD.[106] A role for platelets and thromboembolism in the pathogenesis of IBD is supported by a study of 9000 patients with bleeding disorders, wherein a protective effect of inherited defects of coagulation, i.e. hemophilia and von Willebrand's disease, was shown against the occurrence of both CD and UC.[107]

There are a limited amount of data from experimental animal models that relate to the role of platelets in intestinal inflammation. Several models of acute intestinal inflammation, including ischemia/reperfusion and endotoxemia[108,109] are associated with the recruitment of adherent leukocytes and platelets in postcapillary venules. P-selectin-directed antibodies or antagonists appear to be effective in blunting both the thrombogenic and the inflammatory responses in these experimental models.[108] Inhibition of selectin function using the non-selective inhibitor fucoidan has been shown to confer protection against dextran sodium sulfate (DSS)-induced murine colitis.[110] Although this protective action was attributed to a reduction in leukocyte infiltration mediated by endothelial cell-associated P-selectin, another plausible explanation is that P-selectin expressed on the surface of platelets that are adherent to blood vessels participate in the leukocyte recruitment. Other experimental models of intestinal injury support this mechanism of platelet-associated, P-selectin-mediated leukocyte recruitment.[111]

## PLATELET–VESSEL WALL INTERACTIONS: MOLECULAR DETERMINANTS AND POTENTIAL THERAPEUTIC TARGETS

An important function of the normal microvasculature is to prevent the adhesion of platelets and the subsequent formation of microthrombi, which lead to impaired tissue perfusion. Endothelial cells help create this antithrombogenic surface by producing platelet inactivators (e.g. NO and $PGI_2$), by augmenting fibrinolysis (tPA) and by 'hiding' subendothelial matrix elements (e.g. collagen, fibronectin) from platelets and circulating coagulation factors (e.g. factor VIIa).[112] Hence, any endothelial denudation or injury will lead to immediate platelet adhesion and aggregation at the site of injury. The binding of platelets to exposed subendothelial matrix is mediated by specific adhesion glycoproteins expressed on platelets that bind to ligands or receptors embedded in the matrix, such as von Willebrand factor, collagen and fibronectin. These interactions mediate the initial binding, firm adhesion and spreading of platelets. Although much attention has been devoted to the adhesion of platelets to the subendothelial surface of damaged blood vessels, particularly as it relates to the genesis of thrombosis, there is a growing body of evidence that platelets can also bind to the surface of activated, undamaged vascular endothelial cells and to leukocytes that are already adherent to the vessel wall.[108,113]

The binding of activated platelets to endothelial cells and/or leukocytes appears to be important because it can influence the intensity of inflammatory responses by releasing different bioactive compounds. Many compounds released by activated neutrophils and endothelial cells may act as platelet agonists (e.g. superoxide, hydrogen peroxide) or antagonists (ADPases); conversely, platelets can release factors that may either inhibit (soluble P-selectin, NO) or activate (oxygen radicals, leukotrienes, thromboxane $A_2$) neutrophils.[114] Platelets can also facilitate the formation of inflammatory mediators by endothelial cells through transcellular exchange of precursor metabolites[112] and by upregulating the expression of endothelial VCAM, ICAM-1 and IL-8 through CD40 ligation and secretion of RANTES.[101] Platelets can also enhance the recruitment of leuko-

cytes into inflamed tissue by serving as a P-selectin-rich platform on endothelium for leukocyte adhesion, and by reducing shear rates in the microcirculation through the release of potent vasoconstrictors (e.g. TxA).

Adhesive interactions between platelets and endothelial cells can be mediated by a variety of glycoproteins expressed on the surface of activated platelets, including P-selectin, platelet–endothelial-cell adhesion molecule-1 (PECAM-1), von Willebrand factor (vWF) and $\beta_3$ integrins (GPIIb/IIIa). Some platelet glycoproteins, such as GPIIb/IIIa, can mediate the binding of platelets to subendothelial matrix proteins, the endothelial cell surface and other platelets (aggregation). Similarly, PECAM-1 can mediate both the homotypic aggregation of platelets as well as the heterotypic binding of platelets with endothelial cells and leukocytes. Integrin molecules (e.g. ICAM-1) that have been implicated as major molecular determinants of leukocyte–endothelial-cell adhesion also appear to contribute to platelet–endothelial-cell adhesion. For example, there is evidence that ICAM-1, which is constitutively expressed on the endothelial cells of most vascular beds,[115] mediates platelet–endothelial-cell adhesion by binding fibrinogen, to which the GPIIb/IIIa on activated platelets can attach.[116] Intravital microscopic analyses of platelet–endothelial-cell adhesion in acutely inflamed mesenteric venules of the mouse have capitalized on the availability of gene-targeted animals that are genetically deficient in either P-selectin, vWF or $\beta_3$ integrins, as well as blocking monoclonal antibodies to PECAM-1 and PSGL-1 (a ligand for P-selectin) to define the molecular determinants of P/E adhesion in vivo.[117] Most of these studies have focused on defining the P/E adhesion responses to exogenous stimuli (e.g. calcium ionophore, histamine or cytokines), whereas relatively little attention has been devoted to defining the molecular determinants of P/E adhesion in pathologic conditions such as IBD.

Preliminary results from our laboratory indicate that DSS-induced colitis in the mouse is associated with the recruitment of a large number of adherent platelets in venules of the inflamed colon. The magnitude of the platelet recruitment elicited in the DSS model far exceeds that observed in more acute models of inflammation.[108,109] P-selectin, expressed on platelets, appears to play a major role in mediating the platelet–vessel wall interactions in the DSS model of IBD. Because SCID mice with DSS colitis exhibit an attenuated platelet accumulation on the walls of colonic venules, it is possible that platelet-associated P-selectin may bind to its ligand, P-selectin glycoprotein ligand-1 (PSGL-1), which is constitutively expressed on the surface of lymphocytes.[111] These P-selectin-mediated platelet–leukocyte interactions may affect the intensity of the leukocyte activation responses that are elicited in the inflamed bowel. Platelets isolated from patients with UC enhance the production of reactive oxygen metabolites by isolated PMN; this effect was diminished by a P-selectin mAb, suggesting that the binding of activated platelets to PMN enhances the capacity of the latter to mediate tissue injury via ROM.[118]

## CONCLUSIONS

Our current understanding of the etiology and pathogenesis of IBD remains only speculative. A rapidly growing body of both experimental and clinical evidence suggests that a breakdown in the regulation of immune responses to ubiquitous luminal antigens may be a critical first step in activating the intestinal microvascular endothelium to enhance surface expression of ECAM. Leukocyte–endothelial-cell, as well as platelet–platelet, platelet–leukocyte and platelet–endothelial-cell, interactions appear to play important roles in the pathophysiology of IBD. Promising clinical studies suggest that interventions directed toward interfering with specific leukocyte, platelet and/or endothelial cell interactions may prove useful in the treatment of IBD.

# REFERENCES

1. Yacyshyn BR, Bowen-Yacyshyn MB, Jewell L et al. A placebo-controlled trial of ICAM-1 antisense oligonucleotide in the treatment of Crohn's disease. Gastroenterology 1998;114:1133–1142.
2. Bennett CF, Kornbrust D, Henry S et al. An ICAM-1 antisense oligonucleotide prevents and reverses dextran sulfate sodium-induced colitis in mice. J Pharmacol Exp Ther 1997;280:988–1000.
3. Picarella D, Hurlbut P, Rottman J, Shi X, Butcher E, Ringler DJ. Monoclonal antibodies specific for beta 7 integrin and mucosal addressin cell adhesion molecule-1 (MAdCAM-1) reduce inflammation in the colon of scid mice reconstituted with CD45RBhigh CD4+ T cells. J Immunol 1997;158:2099–2106.
4. Viney JL, Jones S, Chiu HH et al. Mucosal addressin cell adhesion molecule-1: a structural and functional analysis demarcates the integrin binding motif. J Immunol 1996;157:2488–2497.
5. Hesterberg PE, Winsor-Hines D, Briskin MJ et al. Rapid resolution of chronic colitis in the cotton-top tamarin with an antibody to a gut-homing integrin $\alpha 4\beta 7$. Gastroenterology 1996;111:1373–1380.
6. Viney JL, Fong S. Beta 7 integrins and their ligands in lymphocyte migration to the gut. Chem Immunol 1998;71:64–76.
7. Collins CE, Rampton DS, Rogers J, Williams NS. Platelet aggregation and neutrophil sequestration in the mesenteric circulation in inflammatory bowel disease. Eur J Gastroenterol Hepatol 1997;9:1213–1217.
8. Collins CE, Rampton DS. Review article: platelets in inflammatory bowel disease –pathogenetic role and therapeutic implications. Aliment Pharmacol Ther 1997;11:237–247.
9. Strober W, Fuss IJ, Ehrhardt RO, Neurath M, Boirivant M, Ludviksson BR. Mucosal immunoregulation and inflammatory bowel disease: new insights from murine models of inflammation. Scand J Immunol 1998;48:453–458.
10. Elson CO, Cong Y, Brandwein S et al. Experimental models to study molecular mechanisms underlying intestinal inflammation. Ann NY Acad Sci 1998; 859:85–95.
11. Sartor RB. The influence of normal microbial flora on the development of chronic mucosal inflammation. Res Immunol 1997;148:567–576.
12. Powrie F. T cells in inflammatory bowel disease: protective and pathogenic roles. Immunity 1995;3:171–174.
13. Singh B, Read S, Asseman C et al. Control of intestinal inflammation by regulatory T cells. Immunol Rev 2001;182:190–200.
14. Read S, Powrie F. CD4(+) regulatory T cells. Curr Opin Immunol 2001;13:644–649.
15. Groux H, Powrie F. Regulatory T cells and inflammatory bowel disease. Immunol Today 1999;20:442–445.
16. Groux H, O'Garra A, Bigler M et al. A CD4+ T cell subset inhibits antigen-specific T cell responses and prevents colitis. Nature 1997;389:737–742.
17. Lalani I, Bhol K, Ahmed AR. Interleukin-10: biology, role in inflammation and autoimmunity. Ann Allergy Asthma Immunol 1997;79:469–483. [published erratum appears in Ann Allergy Asthma Immunol 1998;80:A-6].
18. Strober W, Kelsall B, Fuss I et al. Reciprocal IFN-gamma and TGF-beta responses regulate the occurrence of mucosal inflammation. Immunol Today 1997;18:61–64.
19. Powrie F, Carlino J, Leach MW, Mauze S, Coffman RL. A critical role for transforming growth factor-beta but not interleukin 4 in the suppression of T helper type 1-mediated colitis by CD45RB(low) CD4+ T cells. J Exp Med 1996;183:2669–2674.
20. Chen Y, Kuchroo VK, Inobe J, Hafler DA, Weiner HL. Regulatory T cell clones induced by oral tolerance: suppression of autoimmune encephalomyelitis. Science 1994;265:1237–1240.
21. Winn R, Vedder N, Ramamoorthy C, Sharar S, Harlan J. Endothelial and leukocyte adhesion molecules in inflammation and disease. Blood Coag Fibrinol 1998;9 (Suppl 2):S17–S23.
22. Baeuerle PA, Baltimore D. NF-kappa B: ten years after. Cell 1996;87:13–20.
23. Read MA, Whitley MZ, Gupta S et al. Tumor necrosis factor $\alpha$-induced E-selectin expression is activated by the nuclear factor-$\kappa$B and c-JUN N-terminal kinase/p38 mitogen-activated protein kinase pathways. J Biol Chem 1997;272:2753–2761.
24. Collins T, Read MA, Neish AS, Whitley MZ, Thanos D, Maniatis T. Transcriptional regulation of endothelial cell adhesion molecules: NF-$\kappa$B and cytokine-inducible enhancers. FASEB J 1995;9:899–909.
25. Read MA, Whitley MZ, Williams AJ, Collins T. NF-$\kappa$B and I$\kappa$B$\alpha$: an inducible regulatory system in endothelial activation. J Exp Med 1994;179:503–512.
26. Schreck R, Baeuerle PA. Assessing oxygen radicals as mediators in activation of inducible eukaryotic transcription factor NF-$\kappa$B. Meth Enzymol 1994;234:151–163.
27. Sen CK, Packer L. Antioxidant and redox regulation of gene transcription [see comments]. FASEB J 1996;10:709–720.
28. Flohe L, Brigelius-Flohe R, Saliou C, Traber MG, Packer L. Redox regulation of NF-$\kappa$B activation. Free Radic Biol Med 1997;22:1115–1126.
29. Annacker O, Pimenta-Araujo R, Burlen-Defranoux O, Barbosa TC, Cumano A, Bandeira A. CD25+ CD4+ T cells regulate the expansion of peripheral CD4 T cells through the production of IL-10. J Immunol 2001;166:3008–3018.
30. Connor EM, Eppihimer MJ, Morise Z, Granger DN, Grisham MB. Expression of mucosal addressin cell adhesion molecule-1 (MAdCAM-1) in acute and chronic inflammation. J Leukocyte Biol 1999;65:349–355.
31. Munroe DG, Wang EY, MacIntyre JP et al. Novel intracellular signaling function of prostaglandin H synthase-1 in NF-$\kappa$B activation. J Inflamm 1995;45:260–268.
32. Suzuki Y, Wang W, Vu TH, Raffin TA. Effect of NADPH oxidase inhibition on endothelial cell ELAM-1 mRNA expression. Biochem Biophys Res Commun 1992;184:1339–1343.
33. Weber C, Erl W, Pietsch A, Strobel M, Ziegler-Heitbrock HW, Weber PC. Antioxidants inhibit monocyte adhesion by suppressing nuclear factor-$\kappa$B mobilization and induction of vascular cell adhesion molecule-1 in endothelial cells stimulated to generate radicals. Arterioscler Thromb 1994;14:1665–1673.
34. Blackwell TS, Blackwell TR, Holden EP, Christman BW, Christman JW. In vivo antioxidant treatment suppresses nuclear factor-$\kappa$B activation and neutrophilic lung inflammation. J Immunol 1996;157:1630–1637.
35. Liu SF, Ye X, Malik AB. Pyrrolidine dithiocarbamate prevents I$\kappa$B degradation and reduces microvascular injury induced by lipopolysaccharide in multiple organs. Mol Pharmacol 1999;55:658–667.
36. Liu SF, Ye X, Malik AB. In vivo inhibition of nuclear factor-$\kappa$B activation prevents inducible nitric oxide synthase expression and systemic hypotension in a rat model of septic shock. J Immunol 1997;159:3976–3983.
37. Mercurio F, Zhu H, Murray BW et al. IKK-1 and IKK-2: cytokine-activated I$\kappa$B kinases essential for NF-$\kappa$B activation [see comments]. Science 1997;278:860–866.
38. Woronicz JD, Gao X, Cao Z, Rothe M, Goeddel DV. I$\kappa$B kinase-$\beta$: NF-$\kappa$B activation and complex formation with I$\kappa$B kinase-$\alpha$ and NIK [see comments]. Science 1997;278:866–869.
39. Goldberg AL, Akopian TN, Kisselev AF, Lee DH, Rohrwild M. New insights into the mechanisms and importance of the proteasome in intracellular protein degradation. Biol Chem 1997;378:131–140.
40. Palombella VJ, Rando OJ, Goldberg AL, Maniatis T. The ubiquitin–proteasome pathway is required for processing the NF-$\kappa$B1 precursor protein and the activation of NF-$\kappa$B. Cell 1994;78:773–785.
41. Goldberg AL, Stein R, Adams J. New insights into proteasome function: from archaebacteria to drug development. Chem Biol 1995;2:503–508.
42. Read MA, Neish AS, Luscinskas FW, Palombella VJ, Maniatis T, Collins T. The proteasome pathway is required for cytokine-induced endothelial–leukocyte adhesion molecule expression. Immunity 1995;2:493–506.
43. Grisham MB, Palombella VJ, Elliott PJ et al. Inhibition of NF-$\kappa$B activation in vitro and in vivo: role of 26S proteasome. Meth Enzymol 1999;300:345–363.
44. Palombella VJ, Conner EM, Fuseler JW et al. Role of the proteasome and NF-$\kappa$B in streptococcal cell wall-induced polyarthritis. Proc Natl Acad Sci USA 1998;95:15671–15676.
45. Conner EM, Brand S, Davis JM et al. Proteasome inhibition attenuates nitric oxide synthase expression, VCAM-1 transcription and the development of chronic colitis. J Pharmacol Exp Ther 1997;282:1615–1622.
46. Brand SJ, Morise Z, Tagerud S, Mazzola L, Granger DN, Grisham MB. Role of the proteasome in rat indomethacin-induced gastropathy [see comments]. Gastroenterology 1999;116:865–873.
47. Neurath MF, Pettersson S, Meyer zum Buschenfelde KH, Strober W. Local administration of antisense phosphorothioate oligonucleotides to the p65 subunit of NF-$\kappa$B abrogates established experimental colitis in mice. Nature Med 1996;2:998–1004.
48. Auphan N, Didonato JA, Rosette C. Helmberg A, Karin M. Immunosuppression by glucocorticoids: inhibition of NF-$\kappa$B activity through induction of I$\kappa$B synthesis [see comments]. Science 1995;270:286–290.
49. Caldenhoven E, Liden J, Wissink S et al. Negative cross-talk between RelA and the glucocorticoid receptor: a possible mechanism for the antiinflammatory action of glucocorticoids. Mol Endocrinol 1995;9:401–412.
50. De Bosscher K, Schmitz ML, Vanden Berghe W, Plaisance S, Fiers W, Haegeman G. Glucocorticoid-mediated repression of nuclear factor-$\kappa$B-dependent transcription involves direct interference with transactivation. Proc Natl Acad Sci USA 1997;94:13504–13509.
51. Dumont A, Hehner SP, Schmitz ML et al. Cross-talk between steroids and NF-$\kappa$B: what language? Trends Biochem Sci 1998;23:233–235.
52. Ray A, Prefontaine KE. Physical association and functional antagonism between the p65 subunit of transcription factor NF-$\kappa$B and the glucocorticoid receptor. Proc Natl Acad Sci USA 1994;91:752–756.

53. Scheinman RI, Cogswell PC, Lofquist AK, Baldwin AS Jr. Role of transcriptional activation of IκBα in mediation of immunosuppression by glucocorticoids [see comments]. Science 1995;270:283–286.

54. Scheinman RI, Gualberto A, Jewell CM, Cidlowski JA, Baldwin AS Jr. Characterization of mechanisms involved in transrepression of NF-κB by activated glucocorticoid receptors. Mol Cell Biol 1995;15:943–953.

55. Wissink S, van Heerde EC, Schmitz ML et al. Distinct domains of the RelA NF-κB subunit are required for negative cross-talk and direct interaction with the glucocorticoid receptor. J Biol Chem 1997;272:22278–22284.

56. Kaiser GC, Yan F, Polk DB. Mesalamine blocks tumor necrosis factor growth inhibition and nuclear factor κB activation in mouse colonocytes. Gastroenterology 1999;116:602–609.

57. Wahl C, Liptay S, Adler G, Schmid RM. Sulfasalazine: a potent and specific inhibitor of nuclear factor κB. J Clin Invest 1998;101:1163–1174.

58. Granger DN. Cell adhesion and migration. II. Leukocyte–endothelial cell adhesion in the digestive system. Am J Physiol 1997;273:G982–G986.

59. Granger DN, Kubes P. The microcirculation and inflammation: modulation of leukocyte–endothelial cell adhesion. J Leukocyte Biol 1994;55:662–675.

60. Panes J, Granger DN. Leukocyte–endothelial cell interactions: molecular mechanisms and implications in gastrointestinal disease. Gastroenterology 1998;114:1066–1090.

61. Kishimoto TK, Rothlein R. Integrins, ICAMs, and selectins: role and regulation of adhesion molecules in neutrophil recruitment to inflammatory sites. Adv Pharmacol 1994;25:117–169.

62. Schmid-Schonbein GW, Usami S, Skalak R, Chien S. The interaction of leukocytes and erythrocytes in capillary and postcapillary vessels. Microvasc Res 1980;19:45–70.

63. Koizumi M, King N, Lobb R, Benjamin C, Podolsky DK. Expression of vascular adhesion molecules in inflammatory bowel disease. Gastroenterology 1992;103:840–847.

64. Nakamura S, Ohtani H, Watanabe Y et al. In situ expression of the cell adhesion molecules in inflammatory bowel disease. Evidence of immunologic activation of vascular endothelial cells. Lab Invest 1993;69:77–85.

65. Kawachi S, Jennings S, Panes J et al. Cytokine and endothelial cell adhesion molecule expression in interleukin-10-deficient mice. Am J Physiol Gastrointest Liver Physiol 2000;278:G734–G743.

66. Kawachi S, Morise Z, Conner E et al. E-Selectin expression in a murine model of chronic colitis. Biochem Biophys Res Commun 2000;268:547–552.

67. Kawachi S, Morise Z, Jennings SR et al. Cytokine and adhesion molecule expression in SCID mice reconstituted with CD4+ T cells. Inflamm Bowel Dis 2000;6:171–180.

68. Morise Z, Eppihimer M, Granger DN, Anderson DC, Grisham MB. Effects of lipopolysaccharide on endothelial cell adhesion molecule expression in interleukin-10 deficient mice. Inflammation 1999;23:99–110.

69. Podolsky DK, Lobb R, King N et al. Attenuation of colitis in the cotton-top tamarin by anti-alpha 4 integrin monoclonal antibody. J Clin Invest 1993;92:372–380.

70. Eppihimer MJ, Wolitzky B, Anderson DC, Labow MA, Granger DN. Heterogeneity of expression. Circ Res 1996;79:560–569.

71. Schurmann GM, Bishop AE, Facer P et al. Increased expression of cell adhesion molecule P-selectin in active inflammatory bowel disease. Gut 1995;36:411–418.

72. Springer TA. Traffic signals on endothelium for lymphocyte recirculation and leukocyte emigration. Annu Rev Physiol 1995;57:827–872.

73. McCafferty DM, Smith CW, Granger DN, Kubes P. Intestinal inflammation in adhesion molecule-deficient mice: an assessment of P-selectin alone and in combination with ICAM-1 or E-selectin. J Leukoc Biol 1999;66:67–74.

74. Smith CW, Marlin SD, Rothlein R, Toman C, Anderson DC. Cooperative interactions of LFA-1 and Mac-1 with intercellular adhesion molecule-1 in facilitating adherence and transendothelial migration of human neutrophils in vitro. J Clin Invest 1989;83:2008–2017.

75. Tsuchiya M, Miura S, Asakura H et al. Angiographic evaluation of vascular changes in ulcerative colitis. Angiology 1980;31:147–153.

76. Carlos TM, Harlan JM. Membrane proteins involved in phagocyte adherence to endothelium. Immunol Rev 1990;114:5–28.

77. D'Agata ID, Paradis K, Chad Z, Bonny Y, Seidman E. Leucocyte adhesion deficiency presenting as a chronic ileocolitis. Gut 1996;39:605–608.

78. Uzel G, Kleiner DE, Kuhns DB, Holland SM. Dysfunctional LAD-1 neutrophils and colitis. Gastroenterology 2001;121:958–964.

79. Lopez-Cubero SO, Sullivan KM, McDonald GB. Course of Crohn's disease after allogeneic marrow transplantation [see comments]. Gastroenterology 1998;114:433–440.

80. Diamond MS, Staunton DE, Marlin SD, Springer TA. Binding of the integrin Mac-1 (CD11b/CD18) to the third immunoglobulin-like domain of ICAM-1 (CD54) and its regulation by glycosylation. Cell 1991;65:961–971.

81. Staunton DE, Dustin ML, Springer TA. Functional cloning of ICAM-2, a cell adhesion ligand for LFA-1 homologous to ICAM-1. Nature 1989;339:61–64.

82. Jones SC, Banks RE, Haidar A et al. Adhesion molecules in inflammatory bowel disease. Gut 1995;36:724–730.

83. Oshitani N, Campbell A, Bloom S, Kitano A, Kobayashi K, Jewell DP. Adhesion molecule expression on vascular endothelium and nitroblue tetrazolium reducing activity in human colonic mucosa. Scand J Gastroenterol 1995;30:915–920.

84. Kawachi S, Cockrell A, Laroux FS et al. Role of inducible nitric oxide synthase in the regulation of VCAM-1 expression in gut inflammation. Am J Physiol 1999;277:G572–G576.

85. Burns RC, Rivera-Nieves J, Moskaluk CA, Matsumoto S, Cominelli F, Ley K. Antibody blockade of ICAM-1 and VCAM-1 ameliorates inflammation in the SAMP-1/Yit adoptive transfer model of Crohn's disease in mice. Gastroenterology 2001;121:1428–1436.

86. Yacyshyn BR, Chey WY, Goff J et al. Double blind, placebo controlled trial of the remission inducing and steroid sparing properties of an ICAM-1 antisense oligodeoxynucleotide, alicaforsen (ISIS 2302), in active steroid dependent Crohn's disease. Gut 2002;51:30–36.

87. Schreiber S, Nikolaus S, Malchow H et al. Absence of efficacy of subcutaneous antisense ICAM-1 treatment of chronic active Crohn's disease. Gastroenterology 2001;120:1339–1346.

88. Soriano A, Salas A, Salas A et al. VCAM-1, but not ICAM-1 or MAdCAM-1, immunoblockade ameliorates DSS-induced colitis in mice. Lab Invest 2000;80:1541–1551.

89. Binion DG, West GA, Ina K, Ziats NP, Emancipator SN, Fiocchi C. Enhanced leukocyte binding by intestinal microvascular endothelial cells in inflammatory bowel disease. Gastroenterology 1997;112:1895–1907.

90. Haraldsen G, Kvale D, Lien B, Farstad IN, Brandtzaeg P. Cytokine-regulated expression of E-selectin, intercellular adhesion molecule-1 (ICAM-1), and vascular cell adhesion molecule-1 (VCAM-1) in human microvascular endothelial cells. J Immunol 1996;156:2558–2565.

91. Butcher EC, Picker LJ. Lymphocyte homing and homeostasis. Science 1996;272:60–66.

92. Butcher EC, Williams M, Youngman K, Rott L, Briskin M. Lymphocyte trafficking and regional immunity. Adv Immunol 1999;72:209–253.

93. Briskin M, Winsor-Hines D, Shyjan A et al. Human mucosal addressin cell adhesion molecule-1 is preferentially expressed in intestinal tract and associated lymphoid tissue. Am J Pathol 1997;151:97–110.

94. Shigematsu T, Specian RD, Wolf RE, Grisham MB, Granger DN. MAdCAM mediates lymphocyte–endothelial cell adhesion in a murine model of chronic colitis. Am J Physiol Gastrointest Liver Physiol 2001;281:G1309–G1315.

95. Hokari R, Kato S, Matsuzaki K et al. Involvement of mucosal addressin cell adhesion molecule-1 (MAdCAM-1) in the pathogenesis of granulomatous colitis in rats. Clin Exp Immunol 2001;126:259–265.

96. Ghosh S, Goldin E, Gordon FH et al. Natalizumab for active Crohn's disease. N Engl J Med 2003;348:24–32.

97. Muller WA, Weigl SA, Deng X, Phillips DM. PECAM-1 is required for transendothelial migration of leukocytes. J Exp Med 1993; 178:449–460.

98. Schuermann GM, Aber-Bishop AE, Facer P et al. Altered expression of cell adhesion molecules in uninvolved gut in inflammatory bowel disease. Clin Exp Immunol 1993;94:341–347.

99. Collins CE, Cahill MR, Newland AC, Rampton DS. Platelets circulate in an activated state in inflammatory bowel disease. Gastroenterology 1994;106:840–845.

100. Stadnicki A, Gonciarz M, Niewiarowski TJ et al. Activation of plasma contact and coagulation systems and neutrophils in the active phase of ulcerative colitis. Dig Dis Sci 1997;42:2356–2366.

101. Danese S, la Motte, C, Sturm, A,West, G, Katz, J, Fiocchi, C. Platelets trigger a CD40-dependent inflammatory response in the microvasculature of IBD patients. Gastroenterology 2003 (in press).

102. Goke M, Hoffmann JC, Evers J, Kruger H, Manns MP. Elevated serum concentrations of soluble selectin and immunoglobulin type adhesion molecules in patients with inflammatory bowel disease. J Gastroenterol 1997;32:480–486.

103. van Wersch JW, Houben P, Rijken J. Platelet count, platelet function, coagulation activity and fibrinolysis in the acute phase of inflammatory bowel disease. J Clin Chem Clin Biochem 1990;28:513–517.

104. Carty E, MacEy M, Rampton DS. Inhibition of platelet activation by 5-aminosalicylic acid in inflammatory bowel disease. Aliment Pharmacol Ther 2000;14:1169–1179.

105. Talbot RW, Heppell J, Dozois RR, Beart RW Jr. Vascular complications of inflammatory bowel disease. Mayo Clin Proc 1986;61:140–145.

106. Wakefield AJ, Sawyerr AM, Dhillon AP et al. Pathogenesis of Crohn's disease: multifocal gastrointestinal infarction. Lancet 1989;2:1057–1062.

107. Thompson NP, Wakefield AJ, Pounder RE. Inherited disorders of coagulation appear to protect against inflammatory bowel disease. Gastroenterology 1995;108:1011–1015.

108. Massberg S, Enders G, Leiderer R et al. Platelet–endothelial cell interactions during ischemia/reperfusion: the role of P-selectin. Blood 1998;92:507–515.

109. Cerwinka WH, Cooper D, Krieglstein CF, Feelisch M, Granger DN. Nitric oxide modulates endotoxin-induced platelet–endothelial cell adhesion in intestinal venules. Am J Physiol Heart Circ Physiol 2002;282:H1111–H1117.

110. Zhang XW, Liu Q, Thorlacius H. Inhibition of selectin function and leukocyte rolling protects against dextran sodium sulfate-induced murine colitis. Scand J Gastroenterol 2001;36:270–275.

111. Salter JW, Krieglstein CF, Granger DN. DSS-induced colitis: a profile of P-selectin dependent platelet interactions and T cell involvement in the murine modlel, Gastroenterology 2003 (in press).

112. Body SC. Platelet activation and interactions with the microvasculature. J Cardiovasc Pharmacol 1996;27 Suppl 1:S13–S25.

113. Massberg S, Enders G, Matos FC et al. Fibrinogen deposition at the postischemic vessel wall promotes platelet adhesion during ischemia-reperfusion in vivo. Blood 1999;94:3829–3838.

114. Bazzoni G, Dejana E, Del Maschio A. Platelet–neutrophil interactions. Possible relevance in the pathogenesis of thrombosis and inflammation. Haematologica 1991;76:491–499.

115. Henninger DD, Panes J, Eppihimer M et al. Cytokine-induced VCAM-1 and ICAM-1 expression in different organs of the mouse. J Immunol 1997;158:1825–1832.

116. Bombeli T, Schwartz BR, Harlan JM. Adhesion of activated platelets to endothelial cells: evidence for a GPIIbIIIa-dependent bridging mechanism and novel roles for endothelial intercellular adhesion molecule 1 (ICAM-1), αvβ3 integrin, and GPIbα. J Exp Med 1998;187:329–339.

117. Andre P, Denis CV, Ware J et al. Platelets adhere to and translocate on von Willebrand factor presented by endothelium in stimulated veins. Blood 2000;96:3322–3328.

118. Suzuki K, Sugimura K, Hasegawa K et al. Activated platelets in ulcerative colitis enhance the production of reactive oxygen species by polymorphonuclear leukocytes. Scand J Gastroenterol 2001;36:1301–1306.

119. Laroux FS, Grisham MB. Immunological basis of inflammatory bowel disease: role of the microcirculation. Microcirculation 2001;8:283–301.

# ETIOLOGY AND PATHOGENESIS

## CHAPTER 8

# Genetics: molecular and chromosomal considerations

Judy Cho

## INTRODUCTION

Genetic approaches to the pathogenesis of the inflammatory bowel diseases (IBD) have been successful in identifying genetic associations with specific diseases and clinical phenotypes, particularly with respect to NOD2/CARD15 and Crohn's disease (CD). Genetic linkage studies suggest the presence of at least several additional contributing genes. The primary goal of genetic research is to identify genetic variants within specific genes that alter homeostatic mechanisms, thereby increasing disease susceptibility. The characterization of altered signaling pathways associated with specific genetic variants would potentially identify and prioritize novel therapeutic agents for CD and ulcerative colitis (UC). An additional goal of genetic research in IBD is to reclassify these disorders based on a more molecular basis of disease pathogenesis; CD and UC are probably each associated with a heterogeneous subset of susceptibility alleles and pathogenetic mechanisms, each with a discrete natural history and response to various treatments. A rational reclassification of disease on a genetic/molecular pathogenesis basis would potentially optimize prognostic information and allow the tailoring of specific therapies for individual patients. A third goal of IBD genetic research is to better understand the precise nature of gene–environment interactions, crucial to an understanding of the basic characteristics of chronic inflammatory disorders. In particular, for IBD the most important environmental contributions are the effects of tobacco and the complex microbial populations present within the intestine. Finally, the identification of specific disease genes highlights critical checkpoints in health and disease states, providing the potential to advance our knowledge of basic homeostatic mechanisms. The identification of HFE as the human hemachromatosis gene has fundamentally advanced our understanding of intestinal iron absorption, and the discovery of CFTR in cystic fibrosis has led to new mechanisms of epithelial secretion; similarly, the identification of IBD genes holds the potential of advancing our understanding of how the intestine limits the inflammatory response in an environment uniquely opposed to high concentrations of commensal and pathogenic microbes.

## EPIDEMIOLOGY OF IBD: RACIAL AND ETHNIC CONSIDERATIONS

CD and UC are common, chronic, relapsing inflammatory disorders of the intestines. The peak age of onset is between 15 and 30 years of age. Potentially reflecting changing environmental factors affecting the intraluminal microbial content, IBD has consistently been observed to occur at a higher frequency in cohorts with a higher standard of living and more pervasive public health measures, with prevalences changing in the second half of the 20th century in a number of populations. Observation of these changing prevalences provides evidence for the importance of environmental factors in disease pathogenesis. Epidemiologic studies demonstrate an increase in the incidence of Crohn's disease over the past three decades in almost all Western countries. Some places (Sweden, USA) have leveled off at a high incidence (6/100 000),[1] whereas others demonstrate continued increases.[2,3] In contrast, the incidence of UC in Western countries appears to have leveled off.[4] Among Caucasians, the prevalence of CD and UC among Jews in the US is significantly higher than in non-Jewish Caucasians.[5]

Prevalence rates among non-Caucasians in the US have consistently been reported as being lower than in Caucasian cohorts. In a health maintenance organization-based mail survey in the US the prevalence rates for CD per 100 000 were 43.6 among whites, 29.8 among African-Americans, 4.1 among Hispanics and 5.6 among Asians.[6] A recent 10-year retrospective study of African-American children living in Georgia reported a CD incidence rate of 7–12/100 000.[7] Although follow-up prospective studies are important, these data suggests that the incidence and prevalence rates among African-Americans are higher than previously reported, and the authors speculate that they may be increasing. This would be consistent with a cohort effect resulting from changing environmental exposures over time.

## FAMILY STUDIES

It has long been observed that cases of IBD cluster within families, suggesting the possibility that genetic factors may contribute to disease pathogenesis. In population-based studies[8–11] approximately 5–10% of all affected individuals with IBD report a positive family history (Table 8.1). Higher fractions of familial cases (as high as 20–30%) have been reported in some series, but these estimates may be biased by referral-based cohorts. Of the multiply affected families with IBD 75% are concordant for disease type (either all affected family members have either CD, or all have UC), with the remaining 25% being 'mixed' (having one member with CD and another with UC).[12] These data are consistent with a model of disease pathogenesis where some genetic variants contributing to disease are unique to either CD or UC, with some variants potentially being common to both, in which case the disease phenotype is influenced by environmental factors. Alternatively, familial disease could be explained by common environmental exposures.

The relative risk of developing disease in first-degree relatives of individuals affected by disease provides a general quantitative estimate of the extent to which genetic factors may contribute to disease pathogenesis. These data are useful both for assessing the overall feasibility of identifying disease genes for a particular disorder through genetic linkage approaches, as well as for providing counseling to unaffected relatives. The relative risk for IBD among first-degree relatives can be estimated using either a cohort or a case–control design. In a cohort study, Orholm[13] demonstrated a population relative risk of 10 for relatives of patients with UC and 14 for relatives of patients with CD. Similar relative risk estimates (14–15-fold increased risk) have been reported for first-degree relatives in two case–control studies.[14,15] These data from complementary epidemiologic approaches provide consistent estimates (10–15-fold increased risk) of the relative risk for IBD among first-degree relatives of an affected proband.

Familial aggregation reflects both shared genetic and environmental factors. Support for the contribution of genetic factors in IBD is provided by twin concordance studies, especially for CD.[16–18] If genetic factors contribute to disease pathogenesis, it would be predicted that concordance rates (given one twin affected by IBD, the fraction of the risk of the other twin also being affected) would be significantly higher among monozygotic than among dizygotic twins. In contrast, environmental influences would predict equal concordance rates in monozygotic and dizygotic twins. Monozygotic (MZ) twin concordance for CD is reported as 42–58%, whereas the dizygotic (DZ) twin concordance is not significantly different (<5%) from that for all siblings. The MZ and DZ concordances for UC have ranged between 6–17% and 0–5%, respectively. That MZ twin concordance has generally been reported to be higher for CD than for UC indicates that CD is likely to be a 'more genetic' disorder than UC, with UC having a greater environmental influence. That disease concordance is significantly less than 100% among MZ twins highlights the importance of developmental factors and environmental triggers in the pathogenesis of both CD and UC.

The contribution of environmental factors in the pathogenesis of IBD is suggested by the observation that more conjugal cases of IBD develop (especially *after* the onset of cohabitation) than would be expected by chance. This trend is most marked for couples where both members have CD.[19] Similarly, asymptomatic spouses of CD patients have an increased frequency of altered intestinal permeability, suggesting shared environmental exposure.[20,21] The prevalence of IBD among the offspring of couples where both are affected by IBD is extremely high, and has been reported to be between 10 and 36%,[14,19,22] representing (with the exception of risk to monozygotic twin pairs) the most significant risk factor for developing IBD. The most recent study from northern France and Belgium reported a 33% prevalence of IBD by age 28 among the offspring of parents both affected by IBD.[19] Taken together, these data are consistent with a model of IBD involving a complex combination of both genetic and environmental factors.

## FAMILIAL AND SPORADIC INFLAMMATORY BOWEL DISEASE

Only a minority of IBD patients have a positive family history; however, many of the genetic studies (especially genetic *linkage* studies; see below) are focused on 'familial' cases, where more than one member within a family has IBD. This raises the question of what the precise relationship is between familial and sporadic cases of IBD.[23] In particular, will genetic variants identified initially in familial cases of IBD also play a pathogenetic role to the same extent among the more common 'sporadic' cases? Furthermore, are there consistent clinical features that distinguish familial from sporadic cases?

Perhaps the most consistently observed finding between studies is an earlier age of onset for familial cases of IBD than in cases where no known family history exists. The average age of onset in familial CD is approximately 22 years, compared to 27 for sporadic cases.[24,25] Similarly, in UC, in a US-based study, the average age of diagnosis for familial compared to sporadic UC was 23.3 compared to 28.6 years.[26] This finding of earlier age of onset for familial cases has been a consistent theme in human genetics and provides some rationale in genetic studies for stratifying data based on age of diagnosis. For example, for two of the chromosomal regions (chromosomes 16 and 5) demonstrating evidence for a genetic linkage in IBD, greater evidence for linkage was observed by stratifying the analysis based on earlier age of onset.[27,28]

---

**Table 8.1 Genetic epidemiologic features of IBD**

- 5–10% of IBD patients have a positive family history
- Relative risk to first-degree relatives of an IBD proband: approximately 15-fold
- Monozygotic twin concordance is 42–58% (CD) and 6–17% (UC) compared to less than 5% (CD and UC) dizygotic twin concordance
- 10–36% prevalence of IBD if both parents are affected
- Familial cases with an average age of onset about 5 years earlier (22–23 vs. 27–28) than 'sporadic' cases

An intriguing finding in comparing familial and sporadic cases of IBD is the relative preponderance of female cases. The female:male ratio was between 1.23 and 1.68/1 in familial CD,[23] which is somewhat increased from sporadic cases, even given the slight female predominance found in all cases of CD. As opposed to CD, among all cases of UC there is a slight preponderance of male cases. Despite this, interestingly, a female preponderance among familial cases is observed for UC, with female:male ratios of 1.3–1.5/1 being observed in two separate series.[9,29] The underlying mechanisms for these findings are not yet established, but may provide an important clue for future genetic studies.

Numerous studies have examined the effect of family history on disease location. In the case of UC no consistent correlation has been observed between studies of disease extent (left-sided versus extensive colitis) and the presence or absence of a positive family history of UC.[29] In contrast, for CD a fairly consistent correlation has been found between age, family history and disease location, suggesting that the different locations observed in CD may reflect genetically distinct subsets. In a US cohort, earlier age of onset was associated with ileal involvement, with an increasing prevalence of colon-only disease among later-onset cases.[25] Consistent with this, the percentage of familial cases was lower in CD confined to the colon (2.4%) than in ileocolonic cases, where 9.7% had a positive family history.[30]

Disease severity is more difficult to evaluate, as there are no universally accepted standards of definition. Measuring disease severity by assessing therapeutic interventions, such as number of hospitalizations, surgical resections, or the institution of immunosuppressive therapies, may merely reflect differing clinical practices. Associating disease severity with the development of fistulous or stricturing complications is problematic, because these disease behaviors clearly change and accumulate over time. Furthermore, dissecting the effects of family history on disease location from the potentially independent effects that familiality may have on disease severity may be difficult; for example, ileal disease is associated with an increased number of surgical resections compared to colon-only CD. With these caveats, there is no evidence at present that family history is associated with a more severe course, a point of potential importance in counseling families with a strong history of IBD. Specifically, there were no differences in the need for either surgery or cyclosporin in familial compared to sporadic cases of IBD.[31,32]

# GENETIC APPROACHES TO IDENTIFY IBD GENES

Two broad, complementary approaches are typically utilized in genetic studies of IBD, namely genetic linkage and association studies.[33] *Genetic linkage* studies type families containing more than one affected member for the purposes of identifying general genomic regions shared in excess of statistical expectation (Fig. 8.1). During meiosis, recombination between homologous chromosomes occurs, so that a given proband receives genetic contributions from all four grandparents (Fig. 8.2). At any particular autosomal location two siblings might share no, one or two alleles. If a large cohort of random siblings were typed at a particular genetic marker, they would, on average, share 50%, or one of two possible alleles throughout the genome.

Genetic linkage studies type a large cohort of affected relative pairs (typically affected sibling pairs) with the same disease at genetic markers spaced throughout the genome. If a particular genetic marker is identified in which more than 50% allelic sharing is observed, this would imply that a disease-associated genes resides in that general area. Genetic linkage typically implicates broad genomic regions, encompassing scores of potential associated genes. Once linkage is identified by genome-wide searches, the identification of specific disease gene(s) requires the use of genetic association studies.

*Genetic association* studies test for differences in allelic frequencies in patients compared to control individuals. Whereas genetic linkage studies typically implicate broad genomic regions containing scores of potential genes, in outbred populations disease associations are typically observed over much more limited regions containing only one to several genes. The extent and functional characterization of human genetic variation is the fundamental current challenge of the Human Genome project. If DNA specimens from separate, unrelated individuals are sequenced at a particular genomic location, the sequence would be largely identical. As a rough estimate, at approximately every 500–1000 base pairs a genetic variant, or polymorphism, would be observed between individuals. This most commonly involves a simple nucleotide substitution known as an SNP (single nucleotide polymorphism). Undoubtedly, the large majority of SNP have no functional consequences, but an important subset

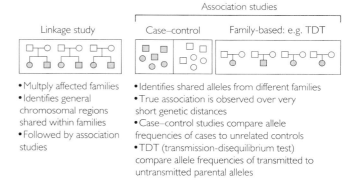

Fig. 8.1 Comparison between linkage and association studies.

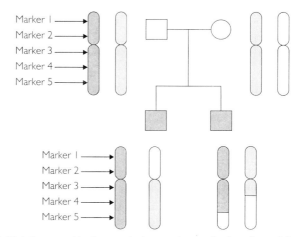

Fig. 8.2 Meiotic recombination results in genetic contributions from all four grandparents. If both parents are typed, haplotype patterns can be reconstructed with a high degree of certainty. At any particular autosomal location, two siblings might share no, one or two alleles.

of them will result in altered function of the gene product, which contributes to the continuum of normal phenotypic variation. A further subset of these functional SNP contribute to disease pathogenesis.[34,35]

An important concept which differentiates complex, multigenic disorders such as IBD from single-gene Mendelian disorders deals with the relative allelic frequency of the risk alleles. Typically, for single-gene disorders the risk allele, or associated allele, has a very low frequency in the general population. Mutations are genetic variants with an allele frequency of less than 1%; that is, if 100 chromosomes were tested, only one would carry the mutated allele. Polymorphisms are genetic variants with an allele frequency of greater than 1%. In contrast, for complex multigenic disorders, associated risk alleles might have a fairly high allelic frequency, with a reduced disease penetrance. For example, the CD-associated risk haplotype on chromosome 5q has an allelic frequency of 37%.[36] Such variants would have a very limited disease penetrance (that is, the fraction of individuals carrying a particular genotype who actually manifest disease). However, the epidemiologic significance of common risk alleles may be quite high. The population attributable risk (PAR) is one such measure and is defined by how much less frequent a disease would be if a particular risk allele did not exist in the population. PAR estimates are influenced in part by the allelic frequency of the risk allele in question.[37]

One of the biggest problems in dealing with complex diseases is heterogeneity.[33] Locus heterogeneity refers to the fact that different sets of genes at different genetic locations can contribute to produce a similar clinical/phenotypic picture. Allelic heterogeneity refers to the fact that multiple risk alleles or genetic variants within a gene might contribute to disease susceptibility. Allelic heterogeneity is a bigger problem for association studies than for linkage analyses, but locus heterogeneity affects the power of all stages of a gene-mapping project. One way to reduce the heterogeneity is to look at more homogeneous populations, for example Finnish or Ashkenazi Jewish groups, or to investigate subsets of the data at hand characterized by common ethnicity and/or geographical characteristics, in the hope that this strategy will reduce the genetic heterogeneity.

## GENETIC LINKAGE STUDIES IN IBD

Genetic linkage approaches were initially developed for monogenic disorders, where the extent of locus heterogeneity (i.e. different sets of genes contribute in different sets of patients) is relatively limited. The application of genetic linkage approaches for complex multigenic disorders such as IBD has been more challenging.[38] Ideally, the initial identification of linkage signals should be replicated in independent studies. However, because the signal to noise ratio for multigenic disorders is relatively modest, often linkage results have not been consistently replicated between studies. Furthermore, because it is anticipated that many of the risk alleles for complex disorders may be relatively common in allelic frequency,[34] the most pathophysiologically significant genes may not necessarily correspond to the most significant linkage signals.[39] Therefore, it is likely that significant disease associations will be established in IBD in chromosomal regions not implicated through the present linkage studies.

Table 8.2 lists some of the chromosomal regions implicated in IBD genetic linkage studies. The *IBD1* locus[40] in the pericentromeric region of chromosome 16 represents the best-

### Table 8.2 Chromosomal regions implicated in IBD

| Disease | Linkage region | | Putative association |
|---------|---------|---------|---------------------|
| IBD1 | CD | chr16cen | NOD2/CARD15 |
| IBD2 | UC, CD | chr12q | None reported |
| IBD3 | UC, CD | chr6p | MHC region, TNF |
| IBD4 | CD | chr14q | None reported |
| IBD5 | CD | chr5q | Cytokine 5q cluster |
| IBD6 | CD | chr19p | None reported |
| IBD7 | UC, CD | chr1p | None reported |

replicated region,[27,41–45] demonstrating positive evidence for linkage only in CD, and specifically not UC. Of particular interest is the extraordinarily high degree of evidence for linkage observed among Australian families at the *IBD1* locus.[44] It can be speculated that this linkage score may be due to environmental factors unique to the Australian cohort. The evidence for linkage in this region of chromosome 16 is now known to be accounted for largely by the association of three major, relatively uncommon, amino acid polymorphisms within the NOD2/CARD15 gene.[46,47] In a large, international IBD genetics consortium study including 613 nuclear families, definitive evidence for linkage at *IBD1* was established, with a lod score of 5.79.[41] In addition, because of the large number of families included in this analysis meaningful substratification of the families was achieved; it was determined that the increased allele sharing at the *IBD1* locus was equal in Jewish and non-Jewish cohorts. In addition, this analysis demonstrated the counterintuitive finding that increased allele sharing among affected siblings was only observed among those families with two affected siblings, but not greater numbers of siblings with Crohn's disease. Among those families with three or more affected siblings, no evidence of increased allele sharing was observed. This intriguing observation might be due to the presence of multiple rare risk alleles co-segregating in the densely affected families.

The levels of support for linkage for the *IBD2* locus on chromosome 12[48] for both CD and UC in the multicenter international consortium were weaker.[41] The mean allele sharing observed in this region was only 0.53 at D12S368, which corresponded to a maximum multipoint lod score of 1.2. However, within the small cohort of pure UC families the mean allele sharing was 0.59 at D12S85, suggesting that *IBD2* may be a predominantly UC locus. Because the current linkage studies have contained relatively more CD–CD-affected relative pairs, many of the linkage regions have demonstrated relatively greater evidence for linkage in CD than in UC. The *IBD2* locus is a notable exception to this, where the linkage evidence may be relatively greater in UC than in CD.[49]

The *IBD3* locus on chromosome 6p encompassing the MHC (major histocompatibility complex) has been implicated consistently for both CD and UC in a number of linkage studies.[50–53] One study demonstrated that the linkage at the *IBD3* locus on chromosome 6p was sex specific, being observed most notably among either CD- or UC-affected males, further demonstrating the likely complexity of disease pathogenesis.[54] A number of HLA associations have been reported in both CD and UC, with strong associations for UC and HLA-DR2 being observed in multiple studies (see below). Furthermore, this region contains the TNF gene, for which functional promoter polymorphisms affecting TNF expression have been reported.[55–57] Finally, the *IBD5* locus on chromosome 5q contains the cytokine gene cluster, which has been reported to be associated with CD.[36]

# NOD2/CARD15 AND CD

NOD2/CARD15 is located in the *IBD1* locus and is highly associated with CD, but not UC.[46,47] NOD2/CARD15 is expressed in peripheral blood monocytes[58] and dendritic cells, and can be upregulated in intestinal epithelial cells by TNF.[59] This intracellular receptor is structurally related to the well-described R proteins in plants,[60] which mediate host resistance to microbial pathogens. Figure 8.3 demonstrates the structural domains of NOD2/CARD15. The N-terminus portion of the gene contains two CARD (caspase-activation recruitment domains) motifs, which mediate protein–protein interactions. The central nucleotide-binding domain mediates self-oligomerization, required for activation. Of particular importance is the C-terminus leucine-rich repeat (LRR) domain.[58] This structural motif has been reported to function as a pattern recognition receptor for broad types of microbial components, such as bacterial lipopolysaccharide (LPS) and peptidoglycan.[61] Three major coding region polymorphisms (Arg702Trp, Gly908Arg, Leu1007fsinsC) within or near the LRR of NOD2/CARD15 have been highly associated with CD.[46,47,62–64] Table 8.3 lists the allelic frequencies reported in a variety of CD and control populations. The consistent presence of higher allelic frequencies for Arg702Trp, Gly908Arg and Leu1007fsinsC in Caucasian CD

patients compared to controls provides support for an association of NOD2/CARD15 with CD.

Carriage of one copy of the risk alleles increases the risk of developing CD two- to fourfold. Conferring a much greater risk is carriage of two copies of the risk alleles, which increases the risk of developing CD approximately 20–40-fold. The observation that homozygous or compound heterozygous risk alleles (i.e. double-dose carriers carrying two copies) confer such a greater risk than heterozygous, or single-dose, carriers indicates that NOD2/CARD15 functions to a large extent in an autosomal-recessive fashion. Approximately 8–17% of CD patients carry two copies of the major NOD2/CARD15 risk alleles (compared to less than 1% in Caucasian control populations). In contrast, approximately 27–32% of CD patients carry only one major risk allele (compared to about 20% of Caucasian controls). (Note that for uncommon polymorphisms, risk allele *carriage* is twice the allele *frequency*. If a variant has a 4% allele frequency, about 8% of individuals will carry that variant.) In addition to the three major risk alleles, a number of extremely rare amino acid polymorphisms, particularly within or near the LRR domain of NOD2/CARD15, have been defined,[65] which in aggregate appear to be similarly associated with disease pathogenesis. The precise genetic significance of individual rare LRR variants is difficult to establish, given the rarity of any single individual variant, but confirm the importance of this region of NOD2/CARD15 in the pathogenesis of a subset of CD patients.

For the frameshift variant Leu1007fsinsC, comparable allele frequencies were observed in Jewish (7.1%) and non-Jewish (8.4%) Caucasian CD patients. In contrast, the allele frequency of Gly908Arg was significantly higher among Jewish (10.2%) than non-Jewish (4.3%) CD patients ($P = 0.002$). The presence of higher allele frequencies observed for Gly908Arg in Jewish CD patients (10.2%) and controls (4.3%) than in non-Jewish patients (4.3%) and controls (1.7%), respectively,[66] is not unexpected for genuine risk alleles, given the higher prevalence of CD among Ashkenazi Jews.[5] It should be noted, however, that in both Jewish and non-Jewish CD patients the frequency of this

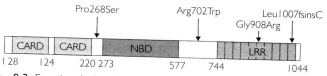

**Fig. 8.3** Functional domains of NOD2/CARD15. CARD, caspase-activation recruitment domain; NBD, nucleotide-binding domain; LRR, leucine-rich repeat domain.[58] The LRR domain contains a predominance of the CD-associated genetic variants. The NBD domain is responsible for oligomerization of NOD2/CARD15.

## Table 8.3 Genotype–phenotype correlations of NOD2/CARD15

|  | W. Europe[46, 65] | UK[62] | UK-G-D[80] | Quebec[64] | US [47, 123] |
|---|---|---|---|---|---|
| CD allele frequency | 0.33 | 0.26 | 0.22 | 0.31 | 0.26 |
| Control allele frequency | 0.10 | 0.08 | 0.07 | 0.10 | 0.10 |
| Age at diagnosis, all CD | 20.7 | 26.7 | — | 34 | 24.1 |
| Age at diagnosis, double-dose carriers | 18.4 | 23.5 | — | — | 21.4 |
| Any ileal disease, all CD | 74% | 82% | 76% | 67% | 79% |
| Any ileal disease, double-dose carriers | 77% | 100% | 87% | 80% | 97% |
| Colon only, all CD | — | 15% | 24% | 33% | 18% |
| Colon only, double-dose carriers | — | 0% | 13% | 20% | 3% |
| Any colon disease, all CD | 50% | 61% | 77% | 70% | 50% |
| Any colon disease, double-dose carriers | 38% | 55% | 60% | 66% | 39% |
| Fibrostenotic, all CD | 37% | 65% | — | 18% | 18% |
| Fibrostenotic double-dose carriers | 53% | 76% | — | 22% | 33% |

mutation is approximately 2.5 times the control frequency, suggesting that the apparent increase of this allele in Jewish CD patients merely reflects the higher frequency of this polymorphism in the Jewish population. In contrast, non-Jewish CD patients have a significantly higher allele frequency of Arg702Trp (10.8%) than Jewish CD patients (2.4%). The lack of association of Arg702Trp among Jewish CD patients does not merely reflect a genuine risk allele simply not present in the Jewish cohort: comparable allele frequencies for Arg702Trp were observed in Jewish (4.3%) and non-Jewish (4.0%) case controls.[66]

Because only a modest minority (approximately 10%) of CD patients have a positive family history of disease, and because genetic linkage studies by definition include only that subset, it was previously unclear whether risk alleles initially identified through genetic linkage studies would be observed at comparable frequencies in sporadic cases. Notably, in a population from Quebec[64] it was observed that the three major NOD2 risk alleles are observed at comparable frequencies in patients with sporadic IBD compared to familial cases of IBD.

To a large extent, NOD2/CARD15 Arg702Trp, Gly908Arg and Leu1007fsinsC confer an increased risk in primarily Caucasian CD patients. Among 350 Japanese patients with CD, 272 with UC and 292 case controls, none were carriers for any of the three major Caucasian risk alleles.[67] Among African-American CD patients, carriage of the three major risk alleles was considerably lower than in Caucasian CD cases or controls.[68] Furthermore, specific amino acid polymorphisms within or near the LRR of NOD2/CARD15, such as the Arg790Gln variant, are observed uniquely among the African-American population.[68] These data would indicate that the mechanisms of disease pathogenesis associated with Caucasian CD, namely amino acid polymorphisms within or near the LRR of NOD2/CARD15, are not observed in African or Asian populations. Whether other distinct variations within the NOD2/CARD15 gene, for example polymorphisms in the promoter region that alter regulation of expression, may play a role in CD pathogenesis, particularly in African or Asian populations, has yet to be fully determined and will require further study.

Interestingly, each of the three major risk alleles of NOD2/CARD15 occur on the same, relatively common, genetic background, observed primarily in Caucasian populations.[69] Evolutionarily rapid expansion of genetic variants, such as may have occurred for this background NOD2/CARD15 variant, may result from relatively random features of population history, or alternatively might reflect positive selective pressures.[70] Genes mediating host resistance to microbial pathogens represent an important class of genes exerting significant evolutionary selective pressures. The line between an effective versus an excessive immunologic response is probably fairly narrow and dependent on the stimulus. It can be speculated that genetic variants increasing susceptibility to chronic inflammatory disorders may have persisted and expanded in human populations owing to a beneficial effect in mediating host–microbial interactions.

## NOD2/CARD15 SIGNALING PATHWAYS

In addition to the statistical support for an association with CD, the function of NOD2/CARD15 supports a role for alterations of this molecule in the pathogenesis of CD. NOD2/CARD15 is known to interact with the serine threonine kinase RICK/RIP2, to activate NFκB (Fig. 8.4). With wild-type NOD2/CARD15, induction of NFκB is observed with treatment with either bacterial LPS or peptidoglycan.[58] The frameshift variant, Leu1007fsinsC, which truncates the last 3% of the NOD2/CARD15 protein, is associated with a marked hyporesponsiveness of NFκB activation in response to stimulation with certain types of LPS.[47] In contrast, the Arg702Trp and Gly908Arg variants responded to LPS to a greater extent than the frameshift variant, but overall exhibited a significantly diminished ability to activate NFκB with LPS stimulation.[66] Therefore, the three major variants Gly908Arg, Arg702Trp and Leu1007fsinsC exhibit a deficit in NFκB activation in response to bacterial components, providing a unifying mechanism for the major CD-associated NOD2/CARD15 variants.[66]

Several hypotheses can be developed whereby impaired NFκB activation in the innate immune system can result in an increased composite intestinal inflammatory/immune response. Decreased NFκB activation in the innate immune system might be associated with impaired killing of intracellular microbes, resulting in compensatory increases in other components of the innate and adaptive inflammatory/immune response. There is mounting evidence that activation of NFκB signaling pathways in response to bacterial components mediates protection of the host against invading pathogens. For example, mutant mice deficient in TNF or Toll-like receptor (TLR) signaling, which is associated with decreased NFκB activation, exhibit increased susceptibility to pathogen invasion.[71–73] In a similar fashion, decreased NOD-2/CARD15 activity could lead to defective clearance of intracellular pathogens. This hypothesis is supported by the observations of Hisamatsu et al., who demonstrated defective clearance of invasive Salmonella typhimurium in epithelial cells transfected with the Leu1007 fsinsC NOD2/CARD15 variant,[59] and detection of intracellular bacteria in the epithelial cells of some CD patients.[74] The innate immune system shapes the adaptive immune system response, through cytokine production and the expression of co-stimulatory proteins, thereby providing an essential function of context discrimination.[75] Decreased NFκB induction could result in decreased T-lymphocyte activity, including both effector and regulatory subsets. Of note, NFκB-deficient mice (p50–/–, p65–/+) are more susceptible to typhlocolitis in response to Helicobacter hepaticus infection.[76]

If a major function of NOD2/CARD15, a cytosolic protein, is to mediate host response to microbial components, a major unresolved issue is what the relationship is between the plasma membrane protein Toll-like receptors and the NOD family of proteins. Some insight into this issue is provided by RICK/RIP2-deficient mice. As the major known signaling partner for NOD2/CARD15, it is not surprising to observe that RICK/RIP2-deficient cells are deficient in NOD2/CARD15-induced NFκB activation. Interestingly, RICK/RIP2 deficiency results in impaired cellular responses to TLR2, TLR3 and TLR4, but not TLR9; consistent with this finding, RICK is transiently recruited to the TLR2 complex.[77] Defining the precise relationship between the TLR signaling pathway and the NOD family pathways will be important in advancing understanding of how specific NOD2/CARD15 mutations alter cellular signaling in response to various microbial components. IL-1 and

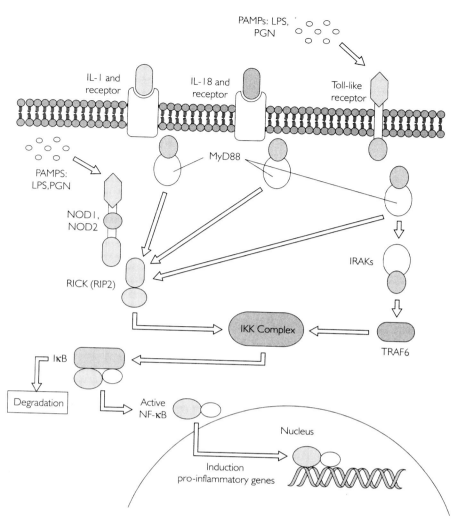

**Fig. 8.4** NOD2/CARD15 signaling. Activation of NOD2/CARD15 by PAMPs (pathogen-associated molecular patterns) such as LPS or PGN (peptidoglycan) results in oligomerization of NOD2, which results in the recruitment of the serine–threonine kinase RICK/RIP2.[58] This activates the IKK complex, resulting in NFκB activation. PAMPs are classically activated by the plasma membrane Toll-like receptors (TLR), which share components of the signaling pathway with IL-1 and IL-18, such as MyD88. RICK/RIP2-deficient cells have impaired signaling through the Toll-like receptors, as well as both IL-1 and IL-18 signaling.[77] This would imply some type of association between the plasma membrane (TLR) and cytoplasmic (NOD) PAMP receptors.

IL-18 receptors both have a TIR (Toll/IL1-receptor) domain within the cytoplasmic tail. Given this structural similarity, studies were performed which demonstrated that RICK-deficient Th1 and NK cells also demonstrate impaired responses to IL-1 and IL-18.[77] This finding suggests the possibility that, in addition to effects on NFκB activation, specific NOD2/CARD15 genetic variants may be associated through distinct pathways, with altered regulation of these proinflammatory cytokines and other yet to be defined inflammatory and protective pathways.

# GENOTYPE–PHENOTYPE CORRELATIONS OF NOD2/CARD15 IN CROHN'S DISEASE

The clinical cases currently classified as CD most likely encompass a heterogeneous subset of disorders, with differing pathogenic mechanisms. This pathogenic heterogeneity could include phenotypic differences, with altered clinical profiles possibly selectively responding to various therapeutic interventions. Numerous phenotypic classifications of Crohn's disease have been proposed,[78,79] encompassing many, often interacting, clinical variables.

The coding region polymorphisms within NOD2/CARD15 are associated with CD and not UC. Furthermore, ileal involvement in CD is associated with an earlier age of onset,[25] as well as a family history of CD. For these reasons, disease location would appear to be a reasonable clinical variable associated with NOD2/CARD15 genetic variants. The three most common disease location subtypes of CD are ileal-only disease, ileocolonic involvement, and isolated colonic disease. In particular, in several studies the 15–30% of CD patients with isolated colonic involvement are associated with a significantly lower carriage of major NOD2/CARD15 risk alleles.[62,64,65,80] These differences are most particularly observed for homozygous/compound heterozygous carriage of the risk alleles (double-dose carriers) (Table 8.3). Alternatively stated, NOD2/CARD15 carriage is positively associated with the presence of ileal disease. In one study the risk allele frequency of NOD2/CARD15 was observed to be highest in ileal-only disease, intermediate in ileocolonic disease, and lowest in colon-only disease.[80] The marked consistency across multiple studies clearly establishes the positive association of these NOD2/CARD15 risk alleles with ileal location; in particular, double-dose carriers are relatively uncommonly observed in colon-only CD (0–20% vs. 15–33% of all CD patients; Table 8.3). Because NOD2/CARD15 risk alleles are positively associated with ileal CD, with those individuals whose CD is confined to the colon having NOD2/CARD15 carriage rates more comparable to those of the control population, genotyping at NOD2/CARD15 would not be expected to have any prognostic value in characterizing cases of indeterminate colitis.

Less well established is the association of NOD2/CARD15 risk alleles with disease behavior (fistulizing, stricturing, inflammatory only). Part of the difficulty in classification resides in the use of different definitions, with some schemes including perianal fistulae in the fistulizing/perforating phenotype group, and others regarding perianal fistulae as being pathogenically distinct from primarily intra-abdominal fistulae. More problematic is the fact that disease behavior may change over time, with fistulous and stricturing complications increasing in prevalence with increasing disease duration.[81] Furthermore, distinctions between fistulous and stricturing behavior can often be difficult to differentiate, particularly in retrospective analyses. Given these caveats, some studies have demonstrated an association between NOD2/CARD15 risk allele carriage and stricturing disease,[62,65] but this has not been observed in all studies.[64] Finally, the age of disease onset among double-dose carriers of NOD2/CARD15 risk alleles is 2–3 years earlier than in all CD patients.[62,65]

## PROGNOSTIC VALUE OF NOD2/CARD15 IN CD

A critical issue is whether NOD2/CARD15 can provide prognostic information that will be useful in considering therapeutic interventions. If it could be established that carriers of NOD2/CARD15 risk alleles have a more severe clinical course, it would potentially justify the use of more potent therapeutic agents, such as immunosuppressive or biologic agents, earlier in the disease course. A retrospective analysis suggests that, once the effect of NOD2/CARD15 on disease location is considered, time to resectional surgery is not decreased among NOD2/CARD15 carriers.[62] Comprehensive assessment of the effect of NOD2/CARD15 carriage on disease course will benefit from additional, prospective analyses.

A separate but related issue is whether, with the identification of specific genes contributing to complex multigenic disorders, differences in response to specific therapeutic agents can be defined. If distinct pathogenic mechanisms resulting from genetic heterogeneity between different subsets of CD patients exist, it might be predicted that responses to specific medications may be different in carriers of different disease genes and risk alleles. One study demonstrated no difference in response to anti-TNF treatment (infliximab) among CD patients stratified by NOD2/CARD15 genotype.[82] However, given the pleiotropic effects exerted by TNF in the immune response, anti-TNF therapies may be too broad to exhibit genotype-specific differences in treatment response. As additional disease genes are identified, and the broad downstream functional consequences of genetic variants characterized, it is possible that a more individualized, rational approach to the medical treatment of IBD may be designed. Furthermore, given the plethora of potential therapeutic targets currently available in IBD, such considerations may be critical in prioritizing potential candidate drugs for further development, as well as defining molecular subsets of disease that will potentially respond more effectively to particular therapeutic approaches.

## ROLE OF NOD2/CARD15 IN OTHER CHRONIC INFLAMMATORY DISORDERS

A consistent theme in human genetics is that genes and specific risk alleles implicated in one disorder could potentially contribute to disease susceptibility in other, related disorders. NOD2/CARD15 is also involved in an extremely rare, monogenic dominant disorder characterized by skin rashes, uveitis and arthritis with granuloma formation known as Blau syndrome.[83] Interestingly, the mutations associated with Blau syndrome alter the central nucleotide-binding region of the protein, as opposed to CD mutations predominating in the LRR domain. This observation suggests that Blau syndrome is related to gain of function mutations, as opposed to Crohn's disease mutations, which appear to be recessive and characterized with respect to LPS and peptidoglycan signaling by a loss of function.[47,66]

Another related disorder that might be associated with genes overlapping those for IBD is psoriasis. CD patients have a sevenfold increased risk of developing psoriasis.[84] Furthermore, this linkage study implicated a psoriasis locus overlapping the IBD1 locus. However, in a large association study among psoriasis patients, no evidence for association was observed for the Leu1007fsinsC variant.[85] More extensive testing of variants throughout NOD2/CARD15 is required before a role for NOD2/CARD15 in psoriasis can definitively be eliminated.

## THE CHROMOSOME 5Q CYTOKINE CLUSTER

Significant evidence for association of a series of common genetic variants to CD was demonstrated over a 250 kb chromosomal region on chromosome 5q.[36] Heterozygous carriage of the risk alleles increases the risk of developing CD twofold, whereas homozygous carriage increases risk sixfold. This region contains a dense cluster of cytokine genes, including interleukins 3, 4, 5 and 13, as well as other potential candidate genes such as colony-stimulating factor isoform 2 (CSF2) and the transcription factor IRF1 (interferon regulatory factor, isoform 1). The associated genetic variants have a relatively high allelic frequency (37% among untransmitted parental alleles). However, the causative gene(s) and specific risk alleles are not currently established[36] and these observations have not yet been replicated. The disease association was tested for only in Caucasian families, with no correlative studies in African-American or Asian populations so far reported. A combination of genetic and expression studies may provide further insight into the precise gene(s) accounting for the observed association.

# LINKAGE AND ASSOCIATION STUDIES AT *IBD3*: COMPLEXITIES OF THE CHROMOSOME 6P REGION

Perhaps the most intensively studied genomic region for IBD has been the chromosome 6p region, which includes a broad array of genes mediating the host inflammatory response, including the MHC (major histocompatibility complex) region. This region is of particular interest in that it is highly polymorphic (that is, it exhibits significant genetic differences between individuals), in part reflecting marked selective evolutionary forces due to interindividual differences in proteins mediating host–environment interactions.

That this region significantly contributes to IBD pathogenesis has been clearly established through a number of linkage studies including cases of both CD and UC.[86] However, translating the replicated linkage studies into definitive disease associations has been extremely challenging, given the enormous genetic and immunologic complexity in this region. Furthermore, as opposed to the case for other disorders, such as type I diabetes mellitus[87] or celiac sprue,[88] where linkage findings at chromosome 6p dwarf the evidence for linkage observed elsewhere in the genome, the chromosome 6p region is only one of several equally important genetic linkage regions in IBD. This indicates that, as opposed to the case for type I diabetes mellitus, where disease pathogenesis can be to a large extent defined by specific HLA associations shaping host–environment interactions, IBD should not be thought of as an HLA-predominant disease. However, it is possible that subsets of UC or CD have an HLA-dependent pathogenesis, and it is well documented that HLA haplotypes are associated with complications of disease, especially extraintestinal manifestations.[89]

HLA proteins present peptides to T-cell receptors. Class I proteins are present in all cell types and consist of a single heavy chain encoded by three highly polymorphic genes (HLA-A, -B, -C). In contrast, class II molecules are normally only expressed on specialized immune cells and are comprised of α and β chains encoded by three genes (HLA-DP, -DQ, -DR). HLA-DP and -DQ are polymorphic for both chains, whereas HLA-DR is polymorphic for the β chain only. Many of the polymorphisms within these proteins are within or near the peptide-binding groove, suggesting interindividual differences in the capacity to bind peptide for presentation to the acquired arm of the immune system.[90]

In evaluating the various HLA studies reported in IBD over the years, it is important to distinguish studies utilizing the older serologic methods of HLA classification compared to the more recent methods of DNA-based typing, resulting in a larger number of HLA subtypes. Given the extensive polymorphism throughout this region, many of the individual reported association studies have been relatively underpowered to identify specific disease associations. Given these caveats, there is significant evidence that specific HLA associations contribute to overall disease pathogenesis, especially for UC. A meta-analysis combining results from 29 studies between 1966 and 1998 demonstrated significant positive associations in UC to DR2 (OR 2.00, CI 1.5–2.63), DRB1*1502 (serologically DR2) (OR 2.74, CI 2.20–6.38), DR9 (OR 1.54, CI 1.06–2.24), and

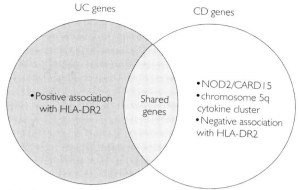

**Fig. 8.5** Relationship between UC- and CD-associated genes. NOD2/CARD15 and the cytokine 5q cluster are unique to CD, and not UC. It is anticipated that there will be risk alleles in shared genes common to CD and UC. Finally, there may be phenotype-modifying genes such as HLA-DR2, in which there appears to be an inverse relationship between CD and UC.[91]

DRB1*0103 (OR 3.42, CI 1.52–3.69), and a negative association with DR4 (OR 0.54, CI 0.43–0.68). Although the most significant associations between UC and HLA DR2 have been reported in Japanese populations (with an odds ratio of 4.92), a significant positive association with this locus was observed in pooled Caucasian population studies (odds ratio 1.51; 95% CI 1.20–1.90) as well.[91]

In contrast, significant positive associations in CD were found with DR7 (OR 1.42, CI 1.15–1.74), DRB3*0301 (OR 2.18, CI 1.25–3.80), and DQ4 (OR 1.88, CI 1.15–3.05) and negative associations with DR3 (OR 0.71, CI 0.56–0.90) and DR2 (OR 0.83, CI 0.70–0.98).[91] The very consistent observations of opposite associations of HLA-DR2 between CD and UC suggest that some disease associations at the class II genes represent phenotype-modifying factors rather than a primary pathogenic response to specific antigens required for disease expression[92] (Fig. 8.5).

There are a number of studies suggesting that HLA associations may be important in disease phenotype, most especially for disease location in UC, as well as extraintestinal manifestations. The rare variant HLA DRB1*0103, which demonstrates the highest odds ratio overall for UC, is present in 0.2–3.2% of the population, 6–10% of all UC cases, 15.8% of extensive UC, and 14.1–25% of severe UC requiring colectomy.[50,93-95]

The association between specific extraintestinal phenotypes and specific HLA associations has been examined. Orchard et al. demonstrated that non-erosive, seronegative peripheral arthropathies characterized by an acute, self-limited arthritis affecting fewer than five joints, lasting less than 5 weeks and associated with intestinal relapses, have associations with HLA-B27, HLA-B35 and HLA DR1*0103. More chronic peripheral arthropathies affecting five or more joints and associated with uveitis have been associated with HLA-B44.[89]

# TNF ASSOCIATIONS AND IBD

An important candidate gene contained within the *IBD3* linkage region on chromosome 6p is the TNF gene itself. The importance of TNF in the pathogenesis of intestinal inflammation, including CD, is clearly established through both clinical and animal studies. In murine studies, targeted deletion of an AU-rich region within the 3' untranslated region of TNF results in increased transcript stability and translational efficiency, thereby resulting in increased overall expression of TNF.[96] Ileitis and peripheral arthritis occur in this model of increased TNF expression, corresponding to the two major inflammatory conditions (CD and rheumatoid arthritis) for which anti-TNF therapies are effective.

A number of association studies of the TNF gene in CD have been reported. No identification of associated coding region polymorphisms changing protein structure or variants in the 3' untranslated region of the gene have been reported. Rather, a number of genetic variants in the promoter region (5' upstream of the transcriptional start site) of TNF exist, which could potentially affect the transcriptional regulation of TNF expression. Some functional studies demonstrate that some of these promoter variants (e.g. the –308, –863 and –238 variants) may result in differences in TNF transcriptional regulation.[55-57] However, in vitro studies examining altered TNF transcriptional activity can be difficult to interpret, given the complexity of the multiple promoter variants within the TNF gene. With respect to association studies, conflicting support for association to –308 have been reported.[90] A Japanese cohort demonstrated associations between CD and the less common variants at –1031, –863 and –857.[97] In contrast, a British cohort demonstrated association of the more common –857 variant within TNF in CD.[98] Furthermore, this study demonstrated allele-specific altered binding of a transcription factor, OCT-1, at the less common –857 variant. The apparent conflict between these two studies could reflect population differences in disease pathogenesis. Alternatively, these differences could reflect the possibility that the specific tested variants are not directly pathogenic. The reported association between the more common promoter variant at –857 with Caucasian CD could not entirely account for the observed evidence for linkage in this general region. This would indicate that the TNF gene by itself is unlikely to be the sole contributing factor within this important genomic region on chromosome 6p.

## ASSOCIATION OF TURNER'S SYNDROME AND INFLAMMATORY BOWEL DISEASES

Turner's syndrome has been consistently associated with both CD and UC. This association is with an altered, as opposed to a missing, X chromosome. Specifically, the karyotype XiXq, in pure or mosaic form, is most associated with IBD. This karyotype is associated with a relatively weak phenotypic form of Turner's syndrome.[99] This would suggest that genes on the X chromosome may be associated with the pathogenesis of several subsets of IBD. Along these lines, a detailed study of the X chromosome in a Belgian cohort of multiply affected families with IBD containing a predominance of CD cases demonstrated suggestive evidence for linkage near the genetic marker DXS1203.[100] Identification of associated genes on the X chromosome might provide insight into the modest female predominance observed in CD.

## IBD AND PRIMARY SCLEROSING CHOLANGITIS (PSC)

The unique epidemiologic relationship between IBD and PSC is well established, but the mechanistic basis for the observed findings remains incompletely defined. In a population-based Swedish cohort, 1500 patients with UC were identified and evaluations of liver function tests within the preceding 2 years were obtained from almost all (94%).[101] Within this cohort, 55 cases of ERCP-documented PSC were identified, which corresponds to a prevalence of 3.7%. Cases of PSC are strongly associated with male gender and extensive colitis: 95% of PSC cases had extensive colitis, compared with 62% of UC patients without PSC. Among cases of extensive colitis, the prevalence of PSC is 5.5%.[101] Conversely, the prevalence of IBD among diagnosed cases of PSC is as high as 70%.[102] Furthermore, this may be an underestimate, as the diagnosis of PSC may precede the diagnosis of IBD. For example, among those patients with PSC not carrying the diagnosis of IBD, a considerable fraction have endoscopic evidence of subclinical colitis.[103] Moreover, investigators at the Mayo Clinic have suggested that the phenotype of colitis associated with PSC is mild pancolitis, with a high incidence of ileal inflammation[104] that may account for the reported increased incidence of pouchitis.

Both UC and PSC are strongly associated with perinuclear antinuclear antibody (pANCA) positivity, suggesting the presence of shared antigenic epitopes. Along these lines, both disorders are associated with HLA class II risk alleles. The most commonly replicated HLA association in UC, DR2, has similarly been associated with PSC.[105] More recently, within the MHC region both positive and negative associations between PSC and specific alleles within the MICA gene have been reported.[106] Non-MHC associated candidate genes have also been reported in PSC; a functional polymorphism in the promoter region of stromelysin (matrix metalloproteinase-3), a gene which regulates tissue injury, repair and remodeling, has been associated with PSC.[107] The unique epidemiologic relationship between PSC and UC may represent an important means of understanding host–environment interactions with respect to response to intestinal antigens. Because of the relative rarity of PSC, efforts to increase the statistical power of genetic association studies by accruing larger PSC cohorts would be of considerable value.

## IBD AND PERIPHERAL SPONDYLOARTHROPATHIES

Spondyloarthropathies (SpA) are rheumatologic inflammations that involve other organ systems as well, most notably the gastrointestinal tract. Endoscopic evaluations have demonstrated the presence of intestinal inflammation in all SpA subtypes. Estimates of the prevalence of intestinal involvement in SpA have ranged between 20 and 70%.[108] HLA-B27 is strongly associated with SpA, particularly ankylosing spondylitis (AS), although this association decreases from more than 90% in sporadic AS to approximately 70% in AS associated with IBD. The direct role of HLA associations in the gut–joint inflammation axis is provided by HLA-B27 transgenic rat models, which develop chronic arthritis and colitis as well as gastroduodenitis, dermatitis and epididymitis. The presence of arthritis and intestinal inflammation is dependent on the presence of intraluminal commensal bacteria, as no inflammation in these organs was observed in rats raised in a germfree environment.[109]

The significance of non-HLA genes in contributing to AS is supported by a higher concordance of AS among monozygotic twins than in dizygotic twins concordant for HLA genotype. Candidate genes could include genes expressed in T cells mediating trafficking to both intestine and joints, such as $\beta_7$ integrins and VAP1.[110] Furthermore, the role of the innate immune system, such as TNF-associated processes, is provided both by the efficacy of anti-TNF therapies as well as by animal models of gut and joint inflammation associated with increased TNF expression.[96]

# DISEASE MARKERS UTILIZED IN IBD

The use of disease-specific antibodies, such as pANCA and anti-*Saccharomyces cerevisiae* (ASCA) to reclassify cases of IBD has been extensive and validated. The ASCA serologic response recognizes oligomannosidic epitopes in the *Saccharomyces cerevisiae* strain Su1.[111] Traditionally, neither pANCA nor ASCA antibody tests are sufficiently sensitive to be utilized as a screening test; however, a modified serodiagnostic assay with higher sensitivity (81%) and lower specificity has been reported.[112] Up to 64% of CD patients are positive for ASCA, with 42–83% of patients positive for UC.[113] However, the use of both tests concomitantly is fairly specific for either CD or UC. Although differences in the sensitivities and specificities of these tests between laboratories are observed, a commercially available test demonstrated a positive predictive value of 86% for CD, and 75% for UC.[113] Phenotypic studies based on the use of serologic markers suggest that pANCA and ASCA are serum markers for different mucosal inflammatory processes; for example, in CD the presence of pANCA is associated with a more 'UC-like' picture, i.e. left-sided colitis, more distal, continuous and superficial disease.[114]

Interestingly, the use of the pANCA and ASCA together has been proposed to be valuable in evaluating those 10% of colitis cases classified as indeterminate, although the use of these serologic markers is controversial. In a prospective study evaluating 97 cases of indeterminate colitis, 47 were seronegative, and 50 were positive for either pANCA or ASCA.[115] Only 14.9% of seronegative cases became CD or UC, compared to 48% of seropositive cases. However, the majority of the seropositive patients remained in the indeterminate category. Among the seropositive cases which developed into a definitive phenotype, 8 of 10 ASCA+/pANCA– cases developed CD, whereas 7 of 11 ASCA–/pANCA+ cases developed UC.[115] To date, expression of these serologic markers has not been linked to a specific gene or chromosomal region.

# EXPRESSION PROFILES IN INTESTINAL TISSUE SAMPLES OF IBD PATIENTS PROVIDE COMPREHENSIVE INSIGHT INTO GENE EXPRESSION

An additional impact of the completion of the Human Genome sequence is the capacity to comprehensively monitor tissue expression levels (mRNA, protein) in order to dissect pathogenetic mechanisms. In particular, cDNA or oligonucleotide microarrays containing large numbers of genes can be hybridized with mRNA from the tissue of interest. Comparisons of transcript expressions can then be performed to track relative expression levels, for example comparing diseased versus control tissues. These approaches have been utilized with great success in defining subsets of cases of breast cancers[116] and leukemias.[117] For example, the expression profiles of breast cancers from individuals harboring *BRCA1* rather than *BRCA2* mutations are different, implying differences in pathogenetic mechanisms. Recently, these DNA chip technologies have been applied to the study of mRNA expression levels in intestinal tissues taken from both UC and CD patients.[118,119] Reproducibility of hybridization from these sources has been established, and a number of differentially expressed transcripts have been identified. Studies in regions of active ulceration and inflammation will undoubtedly provide important insights into mechanisms of intestinal tissue regeneration and repair in the two diseases. For example, upregulated genes in UC patients included members of the metalloproteinase and collagen families. As expected, a number of the significantly upregulated genes were proinflammatory cytokines, as well as several HLA II transcripts.[119]

# GENES AND ENVIRONMENT: TOBACCO AND IBD

Although a number of environmental factors have been hypothesized and implicated in IBD, the best-established environmental modulator is the use of tobacco. It is quite clear that tobacco exerts a highly significant phenotype-modifying effect on chronic inflammatory disorders such as IBD. Tobacco use is protective against the development of UC; although less consistently observed, it has, however, been positively associated with CD. Specifically, active smokers were less likely to develop ulcerative colitis than were non-exposed non-smokers (OR 0.53, 95% CI 0.24–1.14). In addition, the risk was also decreased in individuals with passive smoke exposure, i.e. those whose parents had smoked (OR 0.50, 95% CI 0.25–1.00).[120] The protective effect of tobacco against the development of UC is similar to that observed with celiac disease, a chronic inflammatory disorder of the proximal intestine. The duration of the protective effect against UC in one study appears to be limited to 3 years. This would explain the frequently noted observation that UC is a disease of ex-smokers, with one study demonstrating a twofold increased risk of developing UC in recent ex-smokers. In contrast, the protective effect of tobacco use against developing celiac disease appears to be longer lived.[121]

The effect of tobacco on disease expression holds within multiply affected families with IBD as well.[29] Specifically, in a European cohort, within pure CD multiplex families the frequency of tobacco use was 64%, whereas within pure UC families 31% of affected individuals used tobacco. Interestingly, this trend held within those mixed families having one member with CD and another with UC; among CD members of mixed families the frequency of tobacco use was 64%, compared to 23% among individuals with UC.[29] These trends have subsequently been similarly observed in an additional cohort.[122]

There does not appear to be an association between NOD2/CARD15 risk allele carriage and tobacco status: that is, the frequency of tobacco use appears to be similar between NOD2/CARD15 carriers and non-carriers. Multivariate analysis suggests that both tobacco use and NOD2/CARD15 risk allele carriage independently increase the risk of developing ileal disease.[123]

# GENES AND ENVIRONMENT: THE INTESTINAL MICROBIAL MILIEU. TOWARD A COMPREHENSIVE MODEL OF IBD PATHOGENESIS

Although NOD2/CARD15 has been described as being constitutively expressed in peripheral blood monocytes and monocyte-derived cells, host responses to the intestinal microbial milieu involve the complex, coordinated function of epithelial cells, stromal cells, and acute and chronic inflammatory cells. Interindividual differences in epithelial barrier function, including the formation of an adequate mucus layer, may alter the subsequent exposure of intestinal microbes to the intestinal mucosal immune system. One study demonstrated an association between rare variants of the mucin 3 gene (MUC3) and UC in both a Japanese and a Caucasian cohort.[124]

Whether IBD represents primarily a dysfunctional immune response to commensal organisms, or rather a response to a pathogenic organism which remains within the intestine, resulting in chronic, remitting intestinal inflammation, is currently unknown (see Chapter 20). Intestinal tuberculosis can mimic CD, but so far there are no convincing data that a mycobacterial species is uniquely associated with CD. The possibility exists that, as was the case for peptic ulcer disease, currently unidentified organisms that are difficult to detect by current methods account for a large percentage of IBD cases. However, even if an infectious pathogen were involved, genetic factors are clearly important in determining whether IBD subsequently develops.[92]

Both the NOD2/CARD15 data, as well as data from animal models of IBD, have implicated the importance of commensal bacteria in disease pathogenesis (see Chapter 20). Although the intestine is normally colonized by large numbers of bacteria, normally the intestinal mucosa is relatively free of adherent bacteria. However, a number of studies have established that patients with IBD have increased numbers of different bacterial antigens within the intestinal mucosa.[92] One study suggested that increases in the populations of specific bacteria such as Escherichia coli, enterococci, bacteroides, and fusobacteria may be important in the postoperative recurrence of CD.[125] E. coli from the neoterminal ileum of patients with early reactivation of CD have adherent/invasive properties,[125] consistent with a separate study which demonstrated that some mucosa-associated E. coli strains are capable of altering the permeability of cultured intestinal cell monolayers.[126] Genetic factors may contribute both to the increased penetration of bacteria and bacterial products, as well as to an altered inflammatory response to those microbial products. A recent study demonstrated that adherent E. coli strains are able to survive and replicate within macrophages from IBD patients, but do not induce any cell death of the infected cells. These properties could be related to some features of CD, and particularly to granuloma formation, one of the hallmarks of CD lesions.[127] Whereas NOD2/CARD15 may be thought of as a cytosolic receptor of the innate immune system, providing a rapid response to broad groups of microbial patterns, marked differences in the capacity of wild-type NOD2/CARD15 to respond to different types of bacterial products are observed. The truncation mutant of NOD2/CARD15 is related to defective clearance of invasive bacteria.[59] The comprehensive elucidation of the pathogenesis of IBD will require the identification of multiple genes expressed in several intestinal cell types. Some of these genetic variants will probably affect specific aspects of the host response to the complex, intestinal microbial milieu. These discoveries may provide insights into how the intestine limits the inflammatory response in an environment uniquely apposed to high concentrations of commensal and pathogenic microbes in regard to immunologic tolerance, barrier function and bacterial killing.

# SUMMARY AND FUTURE PROSPECTS

The identification of specific, directly causative risk alleles within the NOD2/CARD15 gene with CD, combined with the reported associations in a number of additional chromosomal regions, notably the cytokine cluster on chromosome 5q with CD, has sparked a great deal of interest. These advances hold the potential to fundamentally change current concepts of IBD pathogenesis, prognosis and treatment. That the frameshift variant within NOD2/CARD15 is associated with decreased LPS-induced NFκB activation suggests that an important subset of genetic variants can be characterized which directly affect host responses to various environmental components, notably various microbial components. Double-dose carriage of NOD2/CARD15 risk alleles is associated with ileal CD, and specifically negatively associated with CD limited to the colon. For these reasons, genetic testing of NOD2/CARD15 will not be of diagnostic value in indeterminate colitis. Reports have suggested that NOD2/CARD15 is associated with CD complications, particularly fibrostenosing behavior. However, at present there is no evidence in retrospective analyses that NOD2/CARD15 carriage is associated with a more aggressive disease course warranting more aggressive therapeutic intervention. However, certain HLA genes have been associated with disease activity and extraintestinal complications. Genotyping of IBD risk alleles in the context of therapeutic trials and/or prospective natural history studies will provide important additional insights. The combination of genetic and expression studies may lead to the development of a molecular reclassification of IBD. This in turn may ultimately result in improved individualization of therapeutic approaches based on an improved understanding of pathophysiologic mechanisms. At present, testing unaffected family members for IBD risk alleles cannot be recommended, as no data are currently available on disease risk in these cohorts.

As will be the case generally for disease genes and risk alleles for complex disorders, none of the IBD susceptibility genes is either necessary or sufficient for disease expression. That the penetrance of disease (the fraction of individuals with a particular genotype manifesting disease) of NOD2/CARD15 double-dose carriers is less than 10% in the general population indicates the likely possibility that additional genetic risk factors and environmental triggers are required for disease expression. This prediction is supported by CD concordance rates of approximately 50% in identical twins. Identification of these interacting genes is of the highest priority, as potentially they could provide insight into the altered homeostasis of intracellular signaling pathways. Alternatively, genetically interacting genes could involve genes expressed in different cell types within the intestine, with multiple synergistic 'hits' required to pass a threshold of disease susceptibility.

# REFERENCES

1. Loftus EV Jr, Silverstein MD, Sandborn WJ, Tremaine WJ, Harmsen WS, Zinsmeister AR. Crohn's disease in Olmsted County, Minnesota, 1940–1993: incidence, prevalence, and survival. Gastroenterology 1998;114:1161–1168.

2. Thomas GA, Millar-Jones D, Rhodes J, Roberts GM, Williams GT, Mayberry JF. Incidence of Crohn's disease in Cardiff over 60 years: 1986–1990 an update. Eur J Gastroenterol Hepatol 1995;7:401–405.

3. Munkholm P, Langholz E, Nielsen OH, Kreiner S, Binder V. Incidence and prevalence of Crohn's disease in the county of Copenhagen, 1962–87: a sixfold increase in incidence. Scand J Gastroenterol 1992;27:609–614.

4. Langholz E, Munkholm P, Nielsen OH, Kreiner S, Binder V. Incidence and prevalence of ulcerative colitis in Copenhagen county from 1962 to 1987. Scand J Gastroenterol 1991;26:1247–1256.

5. Roth MP, Petersen GM, McElree C, Vadheim CM, Panish JF, Rotter JI. Familial empiric risk estimates of inflammatory bowel disease in Ashkenazi Jews. Gastroenterology 1989;96:1016–1020.

6. Kurata JH, Kantor-Fish S, Frankl H, Godby P, Vadheim CM. Crohn's disease among ethnic groups in a large health maintenance organization. Gastroenterology 1992;102:1940–1948.

7. Ogunbi SO, Ransom JA, Sullivan K, Schoen BT, Gold BD. Inflammatory bowel disease in African-American children living in Georgia. J Pediatr 1998;133:103–107.

8. Farmer RG, Michener WM, Mortimer EA. Studies of family history among patients with inflammatory bowel disease. Clin Gastroenterol 1980;9:271–277.

9. Monsen U, Brostrom O, Nordenvall B, Sorstad J, Hellers G. Prevalence of inflammatory bowel disease among relatives of patients with ulcerative colitis. Scand J Gastroenterol 1987;22:214–218.

10. Monsen U, Bernell O, Johansson C, Hellers G. Prevalence of inflammatory bowel disease among relatives of patients with Crohn's disease. Scand J Gastroenterol 1991;26:302–306.

11. Russel MG, Pastoor CJ, Janssen KM et al. Familial aggregation of inflammatory bowel disease: a population-based study in South Limburg, The Netherlands. The South Limburg IBD Study Group. Scand J Gastroenterol Suppl 1997;223:88–91.

12. Binder V. Genetic epidemiology in inflammatory bowel disease. Dig Dis 1998;16:351–355.

13. Orholm M, Munkholm P, Langholz E, Nielsen OH, Sorensen IA, Binder V. Familial occurrence of inflammatory bowel disease. N Engl J Med 1991;324:84–88.

14. Peeters M, Nevens H, Baert F et al. Familial aggregation in Crohn's disease: increased age-adjusted risk and concordance in clinical characteristics. Gastroenterology 1996;111:597–603.

15. Satsangi J, Jewell DP, Rosenberg WM, Bell JI. Genetics of inflammatory bowel disease. Gut 1994;35:696–700.

16. Subhani J MS, Ounder RE, Wakefield AJ. Concordance rates of twins and siblings in inflammatory bowel disease. Gut 1998;42 (Suppl I):A40.

17. Thompson NP, Driscoll R, Pounder RE, Wakefield AJ. Genetics versus environment in inflammatory bowel disease: results of a British twin study. Br Med J 1996;312:95–96.

18. Tysk C, Lindberg E, Jarnerot G, Floderus-Myrhed B. Ulcerative colitis and Crohn's disease in an unselected population of monozygotic and dizygotic twins. A study of heritability and the influence of smoking. Gut 1988;29:990–996.

19. Laharie D, Debeugny S, Peeters M, Van Gossum A, Gower-Rousseau C, Belaiche J, Fiasse R, Dupas JL, Lerebours E et al. Inflammatory bowel disease in spouses and their offspring. Gastroenterology 2001;120:816–819.

20. Breslin NP, Nash C, Hilsden RJ et al. Intestinal permeability is increased in a proportion of spouses of patients with Crohn's disease. Am J Gastroenterol 2001;96:2934–2938.

21. Soderholm JD, Olaison G, Lindberg E et al. Different intestinal permeability patterns in relatives and spouses of patients with Crohn's disease: an inherited defect in mucosal defence? Gut 1999;44:96–100.

22. Bennett RA, Rubin PH, Present DH. Frequency of inflammatory bowel disease in offspring of couples both presenting with inflammatory bowel disease. Gastroenterology 1991;100:1638–1643.

23. Peeters M, Cortot A, Vermeire S, Colombel JF. Familial and sporadic inflammatory bowel disease: different entities? Inflamm Bowel Dis 2000;6:314–320.

24. Colombel JF, Grandbastien B, Gower-Rousseau C et al. Clinical characteristics of Crohn's disease in 72 families. Gastroenterology 1996;111:604–607.

25. Polito JM II, Childs B, Mellits ED, Tokayer AZ, Harris ML, Bayless TM. Crohn's disease: influence of age at diagnosis on site and clinical type of disease. Gastroenterology 1996;111:580–586.

26. Yang H, McElree C, Roth MP, Shanahan F, Targan SR, Rotter JI. Familial empirical risks for inflammatory bowel disease: differences between Jews and non-Jews. Gut 1993;34:517–524.

27. Brant SR, Fu Y, Fields CT et al. American families with Crohn's disease have strong evidence for linkage to chromosome 16 but not chromosome 12. Gastroenterology 1998;115:1056–1061.

28. Rioux JD, Silverberg MS, Daly MJ et al. Genomewide search in Canadian families with inflammatory bowel disease reveals two novel susceptibility loci. Am J Hum Genet 2000;66:1863–1870.

29. Lee JC, Lennard-Jones JE. Inflammatory bowel disease in 67 families each with three or more affected first-degree relatives. Gastroenterology 1996;111:587–596.

30. Cottone M, Brignola C, Rosselli M et al. Relationship between site of disease and familial occurrence in Crohn's disease. Dig Dis Sci 1997;42:129–132.

31. Carbonnel F, Macaigne G, Beaugerie L, Gendre JP, Cosnes J. Crohn's disease severity in familial and sporadic cases. Gut 1999;44:91–95.

32. Lennon A, Keegan D, Grant D, Hyland J, O'Donoghue D. Severity of disease in familial inflammatory bowel disease. Gastroenterology 2000;188:A334.

33. Lander ES, Schork NJ. Genetic dissection of complex traits. Science 1994;265:2037–2048.

34. Chakravarti A. Population genetics – making sense out of sequence. Nature Genet 1999;21:56–60.

35. Chakravarti A. To a future of genetic medicine. Nature 2001;409:822–823.

36. Rioux JD, Daly MJ, Silverberg MS et al. Genetic variation in the 5q31 cytokine gene cluster confers susceptibility to Crohn disease. Nature Genet 2001;29:223–228.

37. Holtzman NA, Marteau TM. Will genetics revolutionize medicine? N Engl J Med 2000;343:141–144.

38. Risch NJ. Searching for genetic determinants in the new millennium. Nature 2000;405:847–856.

39. Risch N, Merikangas K. The future of genetic studies of complex human diseases. Science 1996;273:1516–1517.

40. Hugot JP, Laurent-Puig P, Gower-Rousseau C et al. Mapping of a susceptibility locus for Crohn's disease on chromosome 16. Nature 1996;379:821–823.

41. Cavanaugh J. International collaboration provides convincing linkage replication in complex disease through analysis of a large pooled data set: Crohn disease and chromosome 16. Am J Hum Genet 2001;68:1165–1171.

42. Ohmen JD, Yang HY, Yamamoto KK et al. Susceptibility locus for inflammatory bowel disease on chromosome 16 has a role in Crohn's disease, but not in ulcerative colitis. Hum Mol Genet 1996;5:1679–1683.

43. Curran ME, Lau KF, Hampe J et al. Genetic analysis of inflammatory bowel disease in a large European cohort supports linkage to chromosomes 12 and 16. Gastroenterology 1998;115:1066–1071.

44. Cavanaugh JA, Callen DF, Wilson SR et al. Analysis of Australian Crohn's disease pedigrees refines the localization for susceptibility to inflammatory bowel disease on chromosome 16. Ann Hum Genet 1998;62:291–298.

45. Annese V, Latiano A, Bovio P et al. Genetic analysis in Italian families with inflammatory bowel disease supports linkage to the IBD1 locus – a GISC study. Eur J Hum Genet 1999;7:567–573.

46. Hugot JP, Chamaillard M, Zouali H et al. Association of NOD2 leucine-rich repeat variants with susceptibility to Crohn's disease. Nature 2001;411:599–603.

47. Ogura Y, Bonen DK, Inohara N et al. A frameshift mutation in NOD2 associated with susceptibility to Crohn's disease. Nature 2001;411:603–606.

48. Satsangi J, Parkes M, Louis E et al. Two stage genome-wide search in inflammatory bowel disease provides evidence for susceptibility loci on chromosomes 3, 7 and 12. Nature Genet 1996;14:199–202.

49. Parkes M, Barmada MM, Satsangi J, Weeks DE, Jewell DP, Duerr RH. The IBD2 locus shows linkage heterogeneity between ulcerative colitis and Crohn disease. Am J Hum Genet 2000;67:1605–1610.

50. Bouma G, Crusius JB, Garcia-Gonzalez MA et al. Genetic markers in clinically well defined patients with ulcerative colitis (UC). Clin Exp Immunol 1999;115:294–300.

51. Ma Y, Ohmen JD, Li Z et al. A genome-wide search identifies potential new susceptibility loci for Crohn's disease. Inflamm Bowel Dis 1999;5:271–278.

52. Cho JH, Nicolae DL, Gold LH et al. Identification of novel susceptibility loci for inflammatory bowel disease on chromosomes 1p, 3q, and 4q: evidence for epistasis between 1p and IBD1. Proc Natl Acad Sci USA 1998;95:7502–7507.

53. Hampe J, Schreiber S, Shaw SH et al. A genomewide analysis provides evidence for novel linkages in inflammatory bowel disease in a large European cohort. Am J Hum Genet 1999;64:808–816.

54. Fisher SA, Hampe J, Macpherson AJ et al. Sex stratification of an inflammatory bowel disease genome search shows male-specific linkage to the HLA region of chromosome 6. Eur J Hum Genet 2002;10:259–265.

55. Skoog T, van't Hooft FM, Kallin B et al. A common functional polymorphism (C–>A substitution at position –863) in the promoter region of the tumour necrosis factor-alpha (TNF-alpha) gene associated with reduced circulating levels of TNF-alpha. Hum Mol Genet 1999;8:1443–1449.

56. McGuire W, Hill AV, Allsopp CE, Greenwood BM, Kwiatkowski D. Variation in the TNF-alpha promoter region associated with susceptibility to cerebral malaria. Nature 1994;371:508–510.

57. Knight JC, Udalova I, Hill AV et al. A polymorphism that affects OCT-1 binding to the TNF promoter region is associated with severe malaria. Nature Genet 1999;22:145–150.

58. Ogura Y, Inohara N, Benito A, Chen FF, Yamaoka S, Nunez G. Nod2, a Nod1/Apaf-1 family member that is restricted to monocytes and activates NF-kappaB. J Biol Chem 2001;276:4812–4818.

59. Hisamatsu T, Suzuki M, Reinecker HC et al. CARD15/NOD2 functions as an anti-bacterial factor in human intestinal epithelial cells. Gastroenterology 2003; 124:993–1000.

60. Holub EB. The arms race is ancient history in Arabidopsis, the wildflower. Nature Rev Genet 2001;2:516–527.

61. Inohara N, Ogura Y, Chen FF, Muto A, Nunez G. Human Nod1 confers responsiveness to bacterial lipopolysaccharides. J Biol Chem 2001;276:2551–2554.

62. Ahmad T, Armuzzi A, Bunce M et al. The molecular classification of the clinical manifestations of Crohn's disease. Gastroenterology 2002;122:854–866.

63. Hampe J, Cuthbert A, Croucher PJ et al. Association between insertion mutation in NOD2 gene and Crohn's disease in German and British populations. Lancet 2001;357:1925–1928.

64. Vermeire S, Wild G, Kocher K et al. CARD15 genetic variation in a Quebec population: prevalence, genotype–phenotype relationship, and haplotype structure. Am J Hum Genet 2002;71:74–83.

65. Lesage S, Zouali H, Cezard JP et al. CARD15/NOD2 mutational analysis and genotype–phenotype correlation in 612 patients with inflammatory bowel disease. Am J Hum Genet 2002;70:845–857.

66. Bonen DK, Ogura Y, Nicolae DL et al. Functional and genetic characterization of major CD-associated NOD2 variants [Abstract M1411]. Gastroenterology 2002;122(Suppl): A-296.

67. Inoue N, Tamura K, Kinouchi Y et al. Lack of common NOD2 variants in Japanese patients with Crohn's disease. Gastroenterology 2002;123:86–91.

68. Bonen DK, Nicolae DL, Moran T et al. Racial differences in NOD2 variation: characterization of NOD2 in African-Americans with Crohn's Disease [Abstract 248]. Gastroenterology 2002;122 (Suppl):A-29.

69. Cho JH. Update on the genetics of inflammatory bowel disease. Curr Gastroenterol Rep 2001;3:458–463.

70. Fay JC, Wyckoff GJ, Wu CI. Positive and negative selection on the human genome. Genetics 2001;158:1227–1234.

71. Pfeffer K, Matsuyama T, Kundig TM et al. Mice deficient for the 55 kd tumor necrosis factor receptor are resistant to endotoxic shock, yet succumb to L. monocytogenes infection. Cell 1993;73:457–467.

72. Takeuchi O, Hoshino K, Akira S. Cutting edge: TLR2-deficient and MyD88-deficient mice are highly susceptible to Staphylococcus aureus infection. J Immunol 2000;165:5392–5396.

73. Wang X, Moser C, Louboutin JP et al. Toll-like receptor 4 mediates innate immune responses to Haemophilus influenzae infection in mouse lung. J Immunol 2002;168:810–815.

74. Swidsinski A, Ladhoff A, Pernthaler A et al. Mucosal flora in inflammatory bowel disease. Gastroenterology 2002;122:44–54.

75. Lanzavecchia A, Sallusto F. Regulation of T cell immunity by dendritic cells. Cell 2001;106:263–266.

76. Erdman S, Fox JG, Dangler CA, Feldman D, Horwitz BH. Typhlocolitis in NF-kappa B-deficient mice. J Immunol 2001;166:1443–1447.

77. Kobayashi K, Inohara N, Hernandez LD et al. RICK/Rip2/CARDIAK mediates signalling for receptors of the innate and adaptive immune systems. Nature 2002;416:194–199.

78. Gasche C, Scholmerich J, Brynskov J et al. A simple classification of Crohn's disease: report of the Working Party for the World Congresses of Gastroenterology, Vienna 1998. Inflamm Bowel Dis 2000;6:8–15.

79. Sachar DB. Genomics and phenomics in Crohn's disease. Gastroenterology 2002;122:1161–1162.

80. Cuthbert AP, Fisher SA, Mirza MM et al. The contribution of NOD2 gene mutations to the risk and site of disease in inflammatory bowel disease. Gastroenterology 2002;122:867–874.

81. Louis E, Collard A, Oger AF et al. Behaviour of Crohn's disease according to the Vienna classification: changing pattern over the course of the disease. Gut 2001;49:777–782.

82. Vermeire S, Louis E, Rutgeerts P et al. NOD2/CARD15 does not influence response to infliximab in Crohn's disease. Gastroenterology 2002;123:106–111.

83. Miceli-Richard C, Lesage S, Rybojad M et al. CARD15 mutations in Blau syndrome. Nature Genet 2001;29:19–20.

84. Nair RP, Henseler T, Jenisch S et al. Evidence for two psoriasis susceptibility loci (HLA and 17q) and two novel candidate regions (16q and 20p) by genome-wide scan. Hum Mol Genet 1997;6:1349–1356.

85. Nair RP, Stuart P, Ogura Y et al. Lack of association between NOD2 3020InsC frameshift mutation and psoriasis. J Invest Dermatol 2001;117:1671–1672.

86. Yang H, Plevy SE, Taylor K et al. Linkage of Crohn's disease to the major histocompatibility complex region is detected by multiple non-parametric analyses. Gut 1999;44:519–526.

87. Concannon P, Gogolin-Ewens KJ, Hinds DA et al. A second-generation screen of the human genome for susceptibility to insulin-dependent diabetes mellitus. Nature Genet 1998;19:292–296.

88. Zhong F, McCombs CC, Olson JM et al. An autosomal screen for genes that predispose to celiac disease in the western counties of Ireland. Nature Genet 1996;14:329–333.

89. Orchard TR, Thiyagaraja S, Welsh KI et al. Clinical phenotype is related to HLA genotype in the peripheral arthropathies of inflammatory bowel disease. Gastroenterology 2000;118:274–278.

90. Ahmad T, Satsangi J, McGovern D, Bunce M, Jewell DP. The genetics of inflammatory bowel disease. Aliment Pharmacol Ther 2001;15:731–748.

91. Stokkers PC, Reitsma PH, Tytgat GN, van Deventer SJ. HLA-DR and -DQ phenotypes in inflammatory bowel disease: a meta-analysis. Gut 1999;45:395–401.

92. Hendrickson BA, Gokhale R, Cho JH. Clinical aspects and pathophysiology of inflammatory bowel disease. Clin Microbiol Rev 2002;15:79–94.

93. Roussomoustakaki M, Satsangi J, Welsh K et al. Genetic markers may predict disease behavior in patients with ulcerative colitis. Gastroenterology 1997;112:1845–1853.

94. Satsangi J, Welsh KI, Bunce M, Julier C, Farrant JM, Bell JI, Jewell DP. Contribution of genes of the major histocompatibility complex to susceptibility and disease phenotype in inflammatory bowel disease. Lancet 1996;347:1212–1217.

95. de la Concha EG, Fernandez-Arquero M, Martinez A et al. Amino acid polymorphism at residue 71 in HLA-DR beta chain plays a critical role in susceptibility to ulcerative colitis. Dig Dis Sci 1999;44:2324–2329.

96. Kontoyiannis D, Pasparakis M, Pizarro TT, Cominelli F, Kollias G. Impaired on/off regulation of TNF biosynthesis in mice lacking TNF AU-rich elements: implications for joint and gut-associated immunopathologies. Immunity 1999;10:387–398.

97. Negoro K, Kinouchi Y, Hiwatashi N et al. Crohn's disease is associated with novel polymorphisms in the 5'-flanking region of the tumor necrosis factor gene. Gastroenterology 1999;117:1062–1068.

98. Van Heel DA, Udalova IA, De Silva AP et al. Inflammatory bowel disease is associated with a TNF polymorphism that affects an interaction between the OCT1 and NF-kappaB transcription factors. Hum Mol Genet 2002;11:1281–1289.

99. Hayward PA, Satsangi J, Jewell DP. Inflammatory bowel disease and the X chromosome. Q J Med 1996;89:713–718.

100. Vermeire S, Satsangi J, Peeters M et al. Evidence for inflammatory bowel disease of a susceptibility locus on the X chromosome. Gastroenterology 2001;120:834–840.

101. Olsson R, Danielsson A, Jarnerot G et al. Prevalence of primary sclerosing cholangitis in patients with ulcerative colitis. Gastroenterology 1991;100:1319–1323.

102. Yang H, Taylor KD, Rotter JI. Inflammatory bowel disease. I. Genetic epidemiology. Mol Genet Metab 2001;74:1–21.

103. Broome U, Lofberg R, Lundqvist K, Veress B. Subclinical time span of inflammatory bowel disease in patients with primary sclerosing cholangitis. Dis Colon Rectum 1995;38:1301–1305.

104. Faubion WA Jr, Loftus EV, Sandborn WJ, Freese DK, Perrault J. Pediatric 'PSC-IBD': a descriptive report of associated inflammatory bowel disease among pediatric patients with PSC. J Pediatr Gastroenterol Nutr 2001;33:296–300.

105. Donaldson PT, Farrant JM, Wilkinson ML, Hayllar K, Portmann BC, Williams R. Dual association of HLA DR2 and DR3 with primary sclerosing cholangitis. Hepatology 1991;13:129–133.

106. Norris S, Kondeatis E, Collins R et al. Mapping MHC-encoded susceptibility and resistance in primary sclerosing cholangitis: the role of MICA polymorphism. Gastroenterology 2001;120:1475–1482.

107. Satsangi J, Chapman RW, Haldar N et al. A functional polymorphism of the stromelysin gene (MMP-3) influences susceptibility to primary sclerosing cholangitis. Gastroenterology 2001;121:124–130.

108. De Keyser F, Elewaut D, De Vos M et al. Bowel inflammation and the spondyloarthropathies. Rheum Dis Clin North Am 1998;24:785–813.

109. Rath HC, Herfarth HH, Ikeda JS et al. Normal luminal bacteria, especially Bacteroides species, mediate chronic colitis, gastritis, and arthritis in HLA-B27/human beta2 microglobulin transgenic rats. J Clin Invest 1996;98:945–953.

110. Baeten D, De Keyser F, Mielants H, Veys EM. Immune linkages between inflammatory bowel disease and spondyloarthropathies. Curr Opin Rheumatol 2002;14:342–347.

111. Sendid B, Colombel JF, Jacquinot PM et al. Specific antibody response to oligomannosidic epitopes in Crohn's disease. Clin Diagn Lab Immunol 1996;3:219–226.

112. Dubinsky MC, Ofman JJ, Urman M, Targan SR, Seidman EG. Clinical utility of serodiagnostic testing in suspected pediatric inflammatory bowel disease. Am J Gastroenterol 2001;96:758–765.

113. Sandborn WJ, Loftus EV Jr, Colombel JF et al. Evaluation of serologic disease markers in a population-based cohort of patients with ulcerative colitis and Crohn's disease. Inflamm Bowel Dis 2001;7:192–201.

114. Vasiliauskas EA, Kam LY, Karp LC, Gaiennie J, Yang H, Targan SR. Marker antibody expression stratifies Crohn's disease into immunologically homogeneous subgroups with distinct clinical characteristics. Gut 2000;47:487–496.

115. Joossens S, Reinisch W, Vermeire S et al. The value of serologic markers in indeterminate colitis: a prospective follow-up study. Gastroenterology 2002;122:1242–1247.

116. Hedenfalk I, Duggan D, Chen Y et al. Gene-expression profiles in hereditary breast cancer. N Engl J Med 2001;344:539–548.

117. Golub TR, Slonim DK, Tamayo P et al. Molecular classification of cancer: class discovery and class prediction by gene expression monitoring. Science 1999;286:531–537.

118. Dieckgraefe BK, Stenson WF, Korzenik JR, Swanson PE, Harrington CA. Analysis of mucosal gene expression in inflammatory bowel disease by parallel oligonucleotide arrays. Physiol Genomics 2000;4:1–11.

119. Lawrance IC, Fiocchi C, Chakravarti S. Ulcerative colitis and Crohn's disease: distinctive gene expression profiles and novel susceptibility candidate genes. Hum Mol Genet 2001;10:445–456.

120. Sandler RS, Sandler DP, McDonnell CW, Wurzelmann JI. Childhood exposure to environmental tobacco smoke and the risk of ulcerative colitis. Am J Epidemiol 1992;135:603–608.

121. Snook JA, Dwyer L, Lee-Elliott C, Khan S, Wheeler DW, Nicholas DS. Adult coeliac disease and cigarette smoking. Gut 1996;39:60–62.

122. Bridger S, Lee JC, Bjarnason I, Jones JE, Macpherson AJ. In siblings with similar genetic susceptibility for inflammatory bowel disease, smokers tend to develop Crohn's disease and non-smokers develop ulcerative colitis. Gut 2002;51:21–25.

123. Brant SR, Picco MF, Achkar JP et al. Crohn's disease: role of NOD2/CARD15 gene mutations in clinical heterogeneity. Am J Hum Genet 2002;(Abstract) In press.

124. Kyo K, Parkes M, Takei Y et al. Association of ulcerative colitis with rare VNTR alleles of the human intestinal mucin gene, MUC3. Hum Mol Genet 1999;8:307–311.

125. Neut C, Bulois P, Desreumaux P et al. Changes in the bacterial flora of the neoterminal ileum after ileocolonic resection for Crohn's disease. Am J Gastroenterol 2002;97:939–946.

126. Rocha F, Laughlin R, Musch MW, Hendrickson BA, Chang EB, Alverdy J. Surgical stress shifts the intestinal Escherichia coli population to that of a more adherent phenotype: role in barrier regulation. Surgery 2001;130:65–73.

127. Glasser AL, Boudeau J, Barnich N, Perruchot MH, Colombel JF, Darfeuille-Michaud A. Adherent invasive *Escherichia coli* strains from patients with Crohn's disease survive and replicate within macrophages without inducing host cell death. Infect Immun 2001;69:5529–5537.

## CHAPTER 9

# Animal models of intestinal inflammation

R Balfour Sartor

## INTRODUCTION

Animal models of intestinal inflammation have provided extremely important insights into the pathogenesis of the idiopathic inflammatory bowel diseases (IBD) and have been instrumental in attracting basic scientists to this discipline by providing a means to generate and test hypotheses.[1-5] In addition, these models, especially easily induced models, have been widely used in drug discovery and to explore in vivo mechanisms of action of various therapeutic agents. In the early 1960s Kraft and Kirsner[6] developed some of the first colitis models by inducing colonic hypersensitivity of ovalbumin combined with rectal formalin in rabbits. In the late 1970s Mee et al.[7] extended these studies by inducing more chronic distal colitis in rabbits immunized with *Escherichia coli*. The pace of discovery and applications of animal models of IBD accelerated in the 1980s and 1990s with chemically induced models,[8] and has dramatically intensified in the last decade by the advent of chronic models of T lymphocyte-mediated intestinal inflammation in genetically engineered mice and rats and T-lymphocyte transfer models.[1,3,4,9] These chronic, immune-mediated models are far more relevant to the pathogenesis of IBD than the more easily performed chemically induced models, although the latter are still useful to explore mechanisms of acute epithelial injury and repair and to screen therapeutic agents.

IBD models can be broadly characterized in several ways, ranging from the method of induction (Table 9.1) to the type of immune response that mediates inflammation (Table 9.2). Strober et al. have suggested a third category based on alterations of immunoregulation, where type I represents overaggressive effector cell function and type II is due to defective immunosuppression (regulation).[3] This chapter briefly discusses the clinical features, pathogenesis and unique features of the more frequently studied models, then outlines the insights these models have provided into the pathogenesis of IBD, and finally discusses their use in preclinical drug development. This chapter is designed to provide a conceptual overview with features of the more commonly used models, rather than attempting to present an exhaustive summary of all studies performed on each model.

## CLINICAL FEATURES/PATHOGENESIS/ ATTRIBUTES OF MAJOR MODELS

### INDUCED MODELS

#### Acetic acid colitis

*Clinical features*

Transient exposure of the distal colon (by enema) or ascending colon (by direct injection into a ligated colonic loop) to 4–5% acetic acid followed 20–30 seconds later by a buffer induces a bland epithelial necrosis that variably extends into the lamina propria, submucosa and external muscle layers, depending on the concentration of the acid and the duration of exposure.[10,11] This model has been used in rats, mice, guinea pigs and rabbits. Inflammation is acute, peaking between 1 and 3 days and healing over the ensuing 2–3 weeks in rats; in mice this response is accelerated, with resolution within 3 days.

*Pathogenesis*

Arachidonic acid pathways are activated in the acute phase of injury,[11] which can be prevented by leukotriene blockade, prostaglandin analogs, phospholipase A2 inhibitors, sulfasalazine, glucocorticoids, platelet-activating factor inhibitors, reactive oxygen metabolite scavengers, mast cell stabilizers, interleukin-1 receptor antagonist (IL-1RA) and somatostatin analogs.[1] Surprisingly, antineutrophil serum administered prior to acetic acid does not attenuate increased mucosal permeability or epithelial injury. This mucosal permeability enhances the uptake of luminal bacterial products, such as peptidoglycan-polysaccharide (PG-PS) polymers and bacterial chemotactic peptides; luminal PG-PS potentiates this injury.[12]

*Unique features, advantages/disadvantages*

Advantages of this model are its low cost, ease of administration (enema approach) and widespread availability. Disadvantages

**Table 9.1 Categories of animal models of intestinal inflammation based on method of induction**

| Induced | Spontaneous | Genetically engineered | T-cell transfer |
|---|---|---|---|
| Acetic acid | Cotton-top tamarin | HLA-B27/β2μ TG rat | |
| Immune complex/formalin | C3H/HeJ Bir | IL-2$^{-/-}$ | CD45RB$^{hi}$→SCID |
| Carageenan | Samp-1/Yit | IL-7$^{-/-}$ TG | BM→CD3ε TG |
| DSS | | IL-10$^{-/-}$, IL-10R$^{-/-}$ | |
| Indomethacin | | TCRα$^{-/-}$ | |
| TNBS/alcohol | | Giα2$^{-/-}$ | |
| PG-PS | | Mdr1$^{-/-}$ | |
| Oxazalone | | N-cadherin DN | |
| Methotrexate | | A20$^{-/-}$ | |
| | | TNF $^{\Delta ARE}$ | |
| | | STAT-3$^{-/-}$ | |
| | | STAT-4 TG | |
| | | T-bet TG | |
| | | WASP$^{-/-}$ | |

$-/-$, deficient, knockout; DN, dominant negative; TG, transgenic; BM, bone marrow.

**Table 9.2 Categories of animal models of intestinal inflammation based on type of immune response mediating inflammation**

| Innate | Th1 | Th2 |
|---|---|---|
| Acetic acid | IL-2$^{-/-}$ | TCRα$^{-/-}$ |
| DSS (acute) | IL-10$^{-/-}$ | Oxazalone |
| TNBS (acute) | TNBS (chronic) | WASP$^{-/-}$ |
| Carageenan | CD45RB$^{high}$→SCID | |
| Indomethacin | PG-PS | |
| Immune complex/formalin | Samp-1/Yit | |
| | Giα2$^{-/-}$ | |
| | HLA-B27 TG | |
| | Mdr-1$^{-/-}$ | |
| | BM→CD3ε TG | |
| | TNF $^{\Delta ARE}$ | |
| | T-bet TG | |
| | STAT-4 TG | |
| | IL-7 | |
| | A20$^{-/-}$ | |
| | TGF-β RII DN TG | |

include the variability in depth of injury induced by variable enema retention, the lack of chronicity, the non-specific nature of the initial mucosal injury, and lack of T-lymphocyte dependency. This absence of chronic, immune-mediated injury raises real questions regarding the relevancy of this model to human IBD, despite the ability of sulfasalazine and corticosteroids to prevent injury. However, it could be useful to explore mechanisms of mucosal repair and interactions with luminal bacteria.

## Indomethacin-induced enterocolitis
### Clinical features
Oral or subcutaneously administered indomethacin and other non-steroidal anti-inflammatory drugs (NSAID) induce dose-dependent mucosal ulcers in the mid and distal small intestine and cecum in rats, dogs and rabbits. Acute inflammation in rats, the most thoroughly studied species, peaks 2–3 days after injection,[13] with chronicity being dependent on genetic background.[14] Resistant Fischer rats undergo complete resolution of inflammation by 14 days after two subcutaneous injections of 7.5 mg/kg, whereas in outbred Sprague–Dawley rats active inflammation persists. In contrast, active small intestinal ulcerations are present at least 77 days after injection in highly susceptible Lewis rats.[14] The diffuse colonic ulcers resolve by 2 weeks, even in susceptible rat strains. Acute ulcers are small focal lesions in all regions of the mid to distal small intestine, whereas chronic lesions in Lewis rats are discrete, longitudinal ulcers on the mesenteric border associated with mesenteric 'fat wrapping' and adhesions. These intestinal features are associated with periportal hepatic inflammation, chronic anemia and leukocytosis.[14] Histologic features include discrete small intestinal ulcers with a neutrophilic exudate and adjacent crypt abscesses, but other areas appear entirely normal.[15]

### Pathogenesis
Inhibition of constitutive and inducible mucosal prostaglandins is important, as lesions can be prevented by the administration of prostaglandin analogs.[16] The protective role for prostaglandins is confirmed by the potentiation of DSS-induced colitis by deletion of COX-1 and COX-2,[17] exacerbation of TNBS-induced colitis by selective COX-2 inhibitors, and acceleration and potentiation of colitis in IL-10$^{-/-}$ mice on a resistant C57Bl/6 background.[18] Biliary secretion (enterohepatic circulation) of indomethacin is important, possibly through direct epithelial injury, as bile duct ligation dramatically attenuates disease and the combination of bile and indomethacin lyses intestinal epithelial cells in vitro.[13] Commensal bacteria are important as germ-free rats have minimal inflammation which resolves rapidly.[16,19] E. coli monoassociated rats develop ulcers[16] and tetracycline or metronidazole attenuate intestinal ulcers.[13,15] Inflammation can be prevented by sulfasalazine, thromboxane inhibitors, sucralfate and keratinocyte growth factor-2 (KGF-2); the latter appears to accelerate mucosal healing.[20]

### Advantages/disadvantages
This is an easily inducible model which uses a cheap, readily available and environmentally relevant agent which has been implicated in the reactivation of chronic, immune-mediated colitis[18] and human IBD.[21] It has the unique features of

mesenteric fat wrapping and chronic, longitudinal mucosal ulcers on the mesenteric border, which are characteristic of Crohn's disease. However, the location of chronic ulcers in the mid small intestine rather than the distal ileum is atypical, and there is no evidence that chronic inflammation in this model is T-cell mediated. In addition, confining this model to rats rather than mice limits mechanistic studies and increases costs for drug screening.

## Dextran sodium sulfate (DSS)-induced colitis
### Clinical features
Continuous administration of DSS (2.5–10%) in drinking water for 5–7 days induces pancolitis in mice, rats and hamsters, manifested by bloody diarrhea, weight loss, mucosal ulceration and colonic shortening.[22,23] The intensity of inflammation is dependent on concentration of DSS and the duration of administration. For example, 2.5% DSS induces mild colitis with no mortality, whereas 10% is associated with a high mortality rate.[17] A standard approach which induces reproducible colitis in most mouse strains is 5% DSS in drinking water for 7 days.[23] A modification of repeated cycles of DSS administration for 7 days followed by water alone for 7–21 days can induce chronic inflammation; three to four cycles of DSS are needed for optimal chronic inflammation.[23] The earliest histologic evidence of injury is shortening and dropout of crypts in the left colon, particularly over lymphoid aggregates. This progresses to focal ulceration, mononuclear cell and neutrophil infiltration, and rare crypt abscesses. DSS is concentrated within phagolysosomes in subepithelial macrophages. Chronic inflammation is associated with increased lymphoid aggregates in the lamina propria and submucosa, and focal inflammation. Chronic administration of DSS can lead to epithelial dysplasia and invasive adenocarcinoma.[10,23]

### Pathogenesis
This model bears a similarity to colitis induced in guinea pigs by chronic feeding of carrageenan, a heavily sulfated polymer extracted from red seaweed[24] deviated by anaerobic bacteria, especially *Bacteroides vulgatus*.[25] Similarly, *Bacteroides* species, especially *B. distasonis*, are increased[10] in DSS-induced colitis, and antibiotics, especially broad-spectrum combinations, attenuate disease,[26] but results in germ-free (sterile) mice are variable.[27–29] Treatment with bacterial DNA (CPG) oligonucleotide enhances disease.[30] Disease can be attenuated by α-galactosyl-ceramide, a bacterial glycolipid which binds to class I-like CD1d on innate immune cells and activates protective NK T cells.[31] Arachidonic acid metabolites and monokines (IL-1β, TNF, IL-6, IL-18) are increased in the acute phase and both Th1 (interferon-γ (IFN-γ), IL-12 and IL-18) and Th2 (IL-4 and IL-5) are elevated in chronic colitis.[32,33] Blockade of IL-18 inhibits disease.[32] Studies in COX-1- and COX-2-deficient mice indicate a protective role for constitutive and inducible mucosal prostaglandins.[17] However, it is clear that the standard acute colitis induced by 5–7 days of DSS is not T-lymphocyte dependent, as unabated disease occurs in SCID mice.[34,35] Inflammation can be attenuated by treatment with IL-1RA, luminal cyclosporin A, transforming growth factor-β (TGF-β) and several growth factors, including keratinocyte growth factor-2 (KGF-2) and fibroblast growth factor (FGF) 20.[1,36] These results suggest that acute inflammation is the result of epithelial cell injury, with subsequent activation of innate immune responses by luminal bacterial components and eventual activation of both Th1 and

Th2 responses. However, there is no indication that T lymphocytes are required for chronic inflammation, which may be related to the cumulative effects of repetitive injury without complete resolution between cycles of DSS administration, rather than the activation of pathogenic T-cell responses. Host genetic susceptibility is an important modifier of disease activity, based on variable intensity of disease in inbred murine strains. Mahler et al.[37] reported that NON/LtJ mice were relatively resistant, whereas C3H/HeJ and NOD/LtJ strains are highly susceptible to DSS-induced colitis.

### Advantages/disadvantages
This is a convenient model that generates reproducible pancolitis with an easily administered oral toxin which is widely available. A large number of studies have validated the timing of onset and resolution of acute inflammation in different mouse strains, and cyclical administration can produce chronic inflammation with dysplasia and adenocarcinoma. The well-validated clinical[23] and histologic[33] scoring systems provide a means to quantify responses to therapeutic interventions. Thus, this model is easily studied for drug discovery, and is quite useful to study consequences of targeted deletions or overexpression of intrinsic genes involved in the inflammatory process of knockout and transgenic mice.[17,38,39] The primary disadvantage of this model is that the inflammatory response is more related to direct epithelial injury than to T lymphocyte-mediated immune responses. Thus, DSS-induced colitis seems to be more applicable to the study of mechanisms of epithelial injury and resolution of acute injury than to exploring mechanisms of chronic inflammation. In addition, ulceration is quite focal, such that histologic scoring of inflammation must be performed on multiple sections, and even so does not correlate well with clinical scores. Therefore this model is most useful to investigate mechanisms of mucosal repair/healing in the resolution of inflammation and epithelial barrier function, to explore the consequences of deletion of endogenous genes in genetically engineered mice, and as a high-volume model for drug screening. However, any such results must be confirmed in a T lymphocyte-dependent model. The final caveat is that close attention must be paid to host genetic background when comparing separate studies, given the important differences in aggressiveness of disease in different inbred mouse strains. Furthermore, the onset of dysplasia and adenocarcinoma is quite variable and occurs late in the disease process, thereby complicating oncologic studies.

## Trinitrobenzene sulfonic acid (TNBS)/alcohol
### Clinical features
An enema of TNBS administered concomitantly with ethanol induces distal colitis in rats and mice, and a similar preparation has been adapted to produce ileitis in rabbits.[40–42] In the original rat model inflammation is acute, peaking 2–3 days after infusion and healing over 8 weeks, with focal distal colonic ulcers with transmural inflammation and local fibrosis. Acute pathologic features include focal necrosis and acute inflammation, followed by a chronic infiltration of mononuclear cells and rare granulomas. This response is different in mice, where host background is extremely important in the chronicity and intensity of lesions.[43] Most murine strains develop very short-lived, mild inflammation even with repeated administration. However, susceptible SJL/J mice develop very active chronic colitis, manifested by prominent mucosal hyperplasia, transmural

inflammation of mononuclear cells, and few ulcerations following a single rectal administration of TNBS/ETOH.[41]

## Pathogenesis

TNBS/ETOH-treated rats have increased tissue levels of $PGE_2$, leukotriene B4, IL-1, IL-6 and granulocyte–macrophage colony-stimulating factor (GM-CSF). Inflammation in rats can be inhibited by leukotriene inhibitors,[44] and rabbit ileitis is prevented by nitric oxide inhibitors,[42] but there is no compelling evidence of T-lymphocyte mediation of disease in either species. However, RANTES, a chemokine that stimulates T-lymphocyte migration, is required for the progression of acute to chronic colitis in rats.[45] In striking contrast, SJL/J mice treated with TNBS/ETOH have clear evidence of Th1-mediated inflammation[3,41] which is dependent on IL-12, TNF and CD40 ligand, as demonstrated by neutralizing antibody or knockout studies.[41,46,47] Moreover, STAT4, a transcription factor which mediates IFN-γ responses and is necessary for Th1 differentiation, appears important, as STAT4-transgenic mice develop colitis when stimulated with TNP-KLH in Freund's adjuvant.[48] An additional transcription factor, NFκB, is also involved, as antisense oligonucleotides to NFκB prevented and reversed established TNBS/ethanol-induced alcohol.[49] Of considerable interest, although the immune response is Th1-dominated, is the fact that colitis confined to the mucosa with crypt distortion and loss of goblet cells can occur in mice deficient in IFN-γ or IL-12.[50] The hapten trinitrophenol (TNP) appears to covalently bind either self-antigens, such as colonic proteins, or perhaps commensal enteric bacteria, although a direct T-cell response to TNBS is possible.[3] In support of an endogenous bacterial origin, Duchmann et al.[51] demonstrated T-cell proliferative responses to autologous enteric bacteria (loss of immunologic tolerance) in this model. Moreover, broad-spectrum antibiotics prevent TNBS/ETOH-induced colitis in rats.[52] Host genetic background is an essential determinant of chronicity and aggressiveness of disease. As mentioned earlier, many inbred mouse strains, including C57Bl/6, have mild, transient inflammation, whereas SJL/J mice have chronic aggressive disease with the same stimulant.[43] Studies in $F_2$ progeny of C57Bl/6 X SJL/J mice identified two susceptibility loci on murine chromosomes 9 and 11, respectively.[43] The chromosome 11 locus, which contains the IL-12 p40 gene, colocalizes with a genetic region regulating serum IL-12 responses to LPS. These results provide a potential mechanism for overly aggressive Th1 responses to TNBS.

Elegant studies have further addressed mechanisms of loss of immunologic tolerance to TNBS in this model. Independently, both Neurath et al.[53] and Elson et al.[54] showed that oral administration of TNBS (or TNP-haptenated colonic protein) prevented the subsequent induction of colitis by intrarectal TNBS/ETOH. This prevention was mediated by TGF-β-secreting regulatory T cells, based on enhanced production of lamina propria TGF-β after TNP-colonic protein feeding and blockade by anti-TGF-β antibody.[53] However, both IL-10 and TGF-β are involved with interactions between these two important immunosuppressive molecules.[55] The ability of TGF-β to inhibit inflammation is independently demonstrated by attenuation of TNBS/ETOH colitis by nasal plasmids encoding TGF-β,[56] and by adenoviral vectors encoding IL-10.[57]

## Advantages/disadvantages

This is an extremely well-validated murine model of Th1-mediated colitis induced with an exogenous agent.[58] TNBS, or its related hapten TNP, can be used for studies of oral tolerance. Disadvantages include the restricted genetic background of chronic inflammation, which does not include the common backgrounds (C57Bl/6, 129, Balb/c) used for most knockout and transgenic studies, and the high doses necessary to induce chronic inflammation, which results in high mortality rates. Furthermore, TNBS is a toxic compound whose use is becoming more restricted.

## Peptidoglycan-polysaccharide (PG-PS)-induced enterocolitis

PG-PS polymers, which are the primary structural component of both Gram-positive and Gram-negative bacteria, stimulate innate immune cells by binding to Toll-like receptor (TLR)-2 and NOD-2/CARD15, thereby activating NFκB[59-61] (see Chapter 10).

## Clinical features

Poorly biodegradable PG-PS polymers from group A streptococci injected intramurally (subserosally) into the cecum, distal ileum and distal ileal Peyer's patches induce biphasic granulomatous enterocolitis with extraintestinal inflammation in susceptible rat strains.[62] All rat strains studied develop acute inflammation in the subserosa and lamina propria at the site of injection that peaks 1–3 days after injection. This inflammation resolves over 10–14 days in resistant inbred Fischer F344 and Buffalo rats, but reactivates spontaneously after a brief quiescent phase in highly susceptible Lewis rats.[63,64] Chronic enterocolitis with distal cecal granulomas in Lewis rats appears between 10 and 18 days after injection and persists for at least 6 months after a single injection. Intestinal inflammation is accompanied by hepatic granulomas, erosive peripheral arthritis, anemia of chronic disease and protracted leukocytosis.[63,64] Histologic features include transmural acute and chronic inflammation with large non-caseating granulomas, focal fissuring ulcers, basilar lymphoid aggregates, hyperplasia and disorganization of the muscularis mucosa, increased myofibroblasts and prominent fibrosis.

## Pathogenesis

The acute phase is marked by macrophage activation and increased production of IL-1, TNF, IL-6, chemokines and nitric oxide.[65-68] The chronic granulomatous phase in Lewis rats is marked by increased expression of these same cytokines but is T-lymphocyte dependent, as determined by increased IFN-γ production, prevention and partial reversal by cyclosporin, and lack of development in nude (athymic) Lewis rats.[65,69] Acute and chronic intestinal and extraintestinal inflammation is attenuated by recombinant IL-1RA and IL-10, but IL-10 could not reverse established disease.[63,65] In contrast, corticosteroids completely prevent and reverse disease, but inflammation returns to pretreatment levels within 2 weeks of withdrawal,[70] consistent with continued stimulation by persistent antigen in a susceptible host and reminiscent of spontaneously relapsing human IBD. However, degradation of PG-PS by mutanolysin, an enzyme with the same specificity as lysozyme, eradicates chronic disease.[71] NFκB is an essential mediator of inflammation, as proteosome inhibitors which block IκBα degradation are quite effective in this model.[68] The fibrosis surrounding granulomas is associated with increased expression of insulin-like growth factor-1 (IGF-1) and TGF-β, the latter produced by myofibroblasts.[67,72]

### Unique features/advantages/disadvantages

This model has the unique features of a profile of extraintestinal manifestations which resemble those of human IBD, spontaneous reactivation of chronic inflammation, and induction by a purified bacterial adjuvant which has known receptors on innate immune cells. Although not unique, the frequency of granulomas and the degree of fibrosis are far greater than with other rodent models, and correspond more appropriately with these important features of Crohn's disease. However, applications of this model are limited by the requirement for laparotomy, tedious intramural injection requiring a skilled operator, lack of commercial availability of reproducible PG-PS, and lack of application to mice. Thus, this model, despite its attractive features, is not optimal as an initial screen for drug discovery, but can be highly useful to simultaneously investigate therapeutic responses in chronic enterocolitis, arthritis and hepatic granulomas and to investigate mechanisms of chronic granulomatous inflammation and intestinal/hepatic fibrosis.

## Oxazalone-induced colitis

### Clinical features

Rectal administration of a haptenating agent, oxazalone (3%), in 50% ETOH to SJL/J mice induces distal colitis which has an immediate onset and rapid (4–5 days) resolution in survivors, but a high mortality rate (up to 70%). This inflammation is concentrated in the mucosa and is characterized by infiltration of neutrophils and mononuclear cells, with luminal exudates, bowel wall edema and preservation of the crypt architecture.[73] Presensitization with 3% oxazalone skin painting before rectal administration of lower doses (1%) extends the duration of inflammation in C57Bl/10 mice to 7–10 days, but mortality remains in the 70% range.[74] Colitis in presensitized mice at 7 days after intrarectal administration is characterized by neutrophilic infiltration and focal necrotic ulcers with transmural inflammation.

### Pathogenesis

Th2 responses are dominant in both acute and presensitized models, with increased IL-4 and IL-5 produced by lamina propria T cells.[73,74] The acute model is mediated by IL-4, as anti-IL-4 antibodies prevent disease and colitis is potentiated by anti-IL-12.[73] The presensitized model is unique in that it is mediated by IL-13-producing NK T cells, based on blockade by neutralizing IL-13 or CD1, or by depleting NK T cells and lack of disease in $\beta_2$ microglobulin$^{-/-}$ mice.[74] Furthermore, IL-13 production is enhanced by non-specific anti-CD3/anti-CD28 stimulation of lamina propria mononuclear cells, or by incubation of NK T cells with $\alpha$-galactosylceramide, which selectively stimulates through CD1. Of considerable interest is that endogenous TGF-$\beta$, which is induced by oxazalone, particularly in the proximal colon of the acute (non-presensitized) model, appears to inhibit the progression of colitis and may be responsible for the rapid recovery of surviving mice. Anti-TGF-$\beta$ antibody administration induces severe pancolitis.[73]

### Unique features/advantages/disadvantages

The unique aspects of this model are its mediation by IL-13 and CD1-bearing NK T cells, which implicates a new class of effector cells. Its Th2 cytokine profile includes it in a relatively small group of IBD models. However, the very high mortality rate and the relatively short course of inflammation (even for the presensitization model) limit its usefulness in drug discovery, and

the toxic nature of this inducing agent may have limited relevancy to endogenous stimuli of human IBD. Furthermore, this model has not been validated in the most frequently used murine strains in published studies.

# GENETICALLY ENGINEERED MODELS

## Th1-dependent responses

### HLA B27/human $\beta_2$ microglobulin transgenic rats

*Clinical/pathologic features* Expression of human HLA-B27/β2 microglobulin in rats leads to pancolitis, gastroduodenal inflammation, peripheral and axial arthritis, psoriatic skin and nail lesions, and orchitis.[75] Colitis is evident by 10 weeks of age in conventional animal facilities, with diarrhea being the primary clinical manifestation. Histologic inflammation is characterized by crypt hyperplasia, mucosal thickening, infiltration of the lamina propria by predominantly mononuclear cells, and goblet cell depletion. Mucosal ulcers are not routinely seen. Gastritis is preferentially located in the antrum and extends into the duodenum. Colonic adenocarcinoma develops with chronic colitis. The onset and distribution of colitis are different when adult (8–12 weeks of age) germ-free HLA-B27 transgenic rats are colonized with specific pathogen-free (SPF) enteric bacteria. These rats develop predominantly cecal inflammation within 4 weeks of bacterial colonization.

*Pathogenesis* The exact mechanism of disease in this model is unclear, but appears to involve defective antigen-presenting cell (APC) processing of commensal enteric bacterial antigens.[76] HLA-B27 is not a risk factor for colitis in IBD patients, but is an important determinant of certain extraintestinal manifestations, including axial arthritis (sacroiliitis and ankylosing spondylitis) and uveitis (see Chapter 45). Expression of a human class I HLA molecule is not sufficient to induce disease, as HLA-A2 and HLA-B7 with $\beta_2$ microglobulin do not induce colitis.[75] Moreover, HLA-B27 TG mice do not develop disease. Mucosal expression of IL-1, TNF, IL-6, IL-10 and IFN-$\gamma$ is increased during active colitis, and mesenteric lymph node (MLN) cells secrete high concentrations of IL-12 and IFN-$\gamma$ upon stimulation with cecal bacterial lysates but relatively less IL-10 and TGF-$\beta$ compared to wildtype littermate MLN cells,[77–79] suggesting a Th1 cytokine profile. Colitis can be induced in nude HLA-B27 TG rats, which do not spontaneously develop disease, by transferring either CD4+ or CD8+ T cells from TG rats with colitis.[80] Furthermore, disease can be transferred by bone marrow transplant from HLA-B27 TG as well as HLA-B27 TG nude donors, and wildtype bone marrow transplantation can reverse disease.[81] These studies suggest that disease is mediated by a bone marrow-derived cell, so that HLA-B27 expression on intestinal epithelial cells is not necessary. Selected components of the endogenous bacterial population induce disease. Germ-free HLA-B27 TG rats fail to develop colitis, gastritis and arthritis, but exhibit orchitis and skin/nail lesions.[77,82] Of considerable importance is that only certain bacterial species induce disease. Gnotobiotic studies implicate *Bacteroides vulgatus*, with no disease being induced by *E. coli*.[77,83] Selectivity of inducing bacteria is seen even within the *Bacteroides* genus, with *B. vulgatus* and *B. thetaiotaomicron* monoassociation inducing disease, but no disease with *B. distasonis*; this disease induction corresponds with the presence of a 45 kDa protein recognized by sera from rats with colitis.[84] Colitis is attenuated, but not reversed, by antibiotics with selective spectra (metronidazole or ciprofloxacin), but is reversed by broad-spectrum antibiotics.[26] Importantly, disease recurs after transient antibiotic therapy, but this recurrence can be inhibited by probiotic administration.[85] In contrast to the PG-PS model, Fischer F344 vs. Lewis background rats do not exhibit different disease activities or phenotypes.[75]

*Unique features/advantages/disadvantages* This model is unique in its association of experimental colitis, gastritis and arthritis with a gene involved in human disease. The bacterial species inducing disease have been well characterized, and gnotobiotic rats can be selectively colonized to explore additional stimuli. However, the exact immunoregulatory defects have not yet been characterized, commercially available rats are quite expensive, and rats cannot be crossbred with various knockouts as can mice.

## IL-2$^{-/-}$ mice

*Clinical/pathologic features* Deletion of IL-2, which is a central activator of T and B lymphocytes, lymphokine-activated killer (LAK) and natural killer (NK) cells in mice on a mixed 129/C57Bl/6 background leads to severe hemolytic anemia, with a 50% mortality rate by 10 weeks of age.[86] Surviving mice develop pancolitis, characterized clinically by diarrhea, a wasting syndrome and rectal prolapse. This is a severe, progressive disease ending in death. Histologically, there is prominent mucosal hyperplasia, crypt abscesses, acute and chronic cellular infiltration in the lamina propria and submucosa, and goblet cell depletion. Antral and duodenal mucosal inflammation and periportal hepatitis are also present.[87] Amyloid deposition in the small bowel, liver and spleen is seen in some mice.[86]

*Pathogenesis* This model is quite confusing, as IL-2 was thought to generate clones of proinflammatory effector T cells. Early in life, IL-2$^{-/-}$ mice have increased numbers of activated T cells and increased circulating immunoglobulins, some with anti-colonic epithelial specificity, but as disease progresses B cells are depleted whereas polyclonal T cells expand.[88,89] Double knockout studies definitively indicate that T cells mediate disease, and that B lymphocytes are not required.[90] The effector cell is a CD4+ T cell with a Th1 cytokine profile[91] and defective Fas-mediated apoptosis,[92] perhaps accounting for the persistence and proliferation of these cells. Bone marrow reconstitution studies into Rag-2$^{-/-}$ mice[93] suggest defective regulatory cell function, which is confirmed by reports that IL-2$^{-/-}$ mice do not develop CD4+ CD25+ regulatory T cells,[94] which are required for suppression of colitis and induction of oral tolerance (see Chapter 5). Similar regulatory cell defects occur in IL-2R$\alpha^{-/-}$ mice, which develop a similar phenotype of colitis and systemic inflammation.[94,95] Another possibility is that depletion of regulatory B lymphocytes mediates colitis and systemic inflammatory processes. Commensal enteric bacteria clearly mediate colitis, but have less of a role in other organs. Germ-free IL-2$^{-/-}$ mice have very mild colitis but still have periportal hepatitis, gastritis and B-lymphocyte depletion.[87,89,96] Host genetic background alters phenotype, with C3H/HeJ and BALB/c being high responders and C57Bl/6 being low responders.[86]

*Advantages/disadvantages* This is a well-characterized murine model which has been very useful to investigate pathogenic mechanisms, i.e. T-cell/B-cell requirements and the genesis of

regulatory T cells, but the global inflammation and high mortality rate make pharmacologic studies difficult.

### Defective IL-10 function (IL-10$^{-/-}$, IL-10R$\beta^{-/-}$, conditional STAT-3$^{-/-}$ mice)

*Clinical/pathologic features* SPF IL-10$^{-/-}$ mice on a mixed 129/C57Bl/6 background develop progressive pancolitis, reproducibly beginning by 2 months of age.[97] Diarrhea and rectal prolapse are common, but weight loss is not. Histologic features include mucosal hyperplasia due to crypt elongation and mononuclear cell infiltration; crypt abscesses, focal mucosal ulcers and transmural inflammation occur in later phases. Inflammation is confined to the colon in SPF IL-10$^{-/-}$ mice,[97,98] but the phenotype of conventionally raised mice is far more aggressive, with perforating small intestinal disease and death.[97] Mice surviving for more than 6 months develop colonic adenocarcinomas.[99]

*Pathogenesis* IL-10 is an important immunosuppressive molecule which inhibits proinflammatory cytokine production by macrophages/monocytes and indirectly suppresses Th1 and Th2 lymphocyte activation by downregulating the expression of co-stimulatory molecules MHC II and IL-12 on APC, and potentiates TGF-$\beta$ activities[55] (see Chapter 5). Loss of this important inhibition leads to unrestrained activation of Th1 cells, APC, dendritic cells and macrophages/monocytes. For example, systemic injection of LPS leads to overwhelming TNF production in IL-10$^{-/-}$ mice,[100] whereas unfractionated splenocytes, MLN cells, APC and dendritic cells from IL-10$^{-/-}$ mice secrete significantly larger amounts of proinflammatory cytokines when stimulated in vitro with LPS or cecal bacterial lysates relative to cells from normal, congenic mice.[101,102] Thus, in the absence of endogenous IL-10 downregulation these mice display loss of immunologic tolerance to commensal bacterial stimuli. When activated in vivo by colonic bacteria, this loss of tolerance results in CD4+ Th1-dependent colitis. Double knockout studies show that T cells, but not B lymphocytes, are critical for colitis development,[103] despite the fact that systemic and mucosal immunoglobulins, including pANCA, are dramatically increased.[98,104] Transfer studies to Rag 2$^{-/-}$ recipients demonstrate the key role for CD4+ T cells.[103] Anti-IL-12 antibody blocks colitis, with less effect from anti-TNF and anti-IFN-$\gamma$.[105] Ex vivo studies show that IL-10$^{-/-}$ APC secrete large amounts of IL-12 in response to cecal bacterial lysates, whereas WT APC secrete no IL-12 but large amounts of IL-10.[102] Of considerable interest, IL-10$^{-/-}$ APC are more efficient in inducing Th1 responses than are wildtype APC, and can even induce IFN-$\gamma$ responses by wildtype MLN CD4+ T cells.[102] Surprisingly, recombinant IL-10 can prevent the onset of colitis in IL-10$^{-/-}$ mice, but does not reverse established disease.[103] This may be due to a selective role for IL-10 in preventing the activation of Th1 responses, but inability of this molecule to reverse an established Th1 response, which is consistent with observations in PG-PS-induced enterocolitis[65] and clinical trials of Crohn's disease.[106] Alternatively, it may be due to the change in the immunologic phenotype of IL-10$^{-/-}$ mice on a C57Bl/6 background as disease progresses.[107] In these studies, early stages of colitis of IL-10$^{-/-}$ mice have a Th1 cytokine profile and disease responds to anti-IL-12, but as disease progresses (>30 weeks) IFN-$\gamma$ secretion diminishes, IL-4 expression increases, and anti-IL-12 antibodies have no benefit.

Loss of immunologic tolerance to selected members of the colonic commensal bacterial population mediates colitis in

IL-10[-/-] mice. As mentioned, conventionally reared mice have aggressive, lethal enterocolitis, whereas SPF IL-10[-/-] mice have non-lethal disease confined to the colon.[97] Germ-free mice do not develop colitis nor exhibit immune activation.[98] Germ-free IL-10[-/-] mice develop cecal inflammation within 1 week of colonization with SPF bacteria; this progresses to a very aggressive disease by 5 weeks.[98] Induction of disease in gnotobiotic IL-10[-/-] mice is selective, with minimal effect from a group of six bacterial species, including *B. vulgatus*, that induce disease in HLA B27 TG rats,[98] *Helicobacter hepaticus*,[108] *Lactobacillus plantarum*,[109] *Clostridium* species and *Streptococci viridans*.[110] In contrast, monoassociation with *Enterococcus faecalis* and *E. coli* induces colitis with different clinical phenotypes.[111] *E. faecalis* causes delayed onset of distal colitis, whereas *E. coli* induces rapid onset, cecal-dominant disease. No inflammation is seen in identically colonized wildtype mice. In each situation, CD4+ T cells from the MLN of IL-10[-/-] mice secrete large amounts of IFN-γ in response to APC pulsed with the colonizing bacterial species, whereas wildtype mouse CD4+ T cells have negligible IFN-γ secretion. Preliminary studies demonstrate that transfer of in vitro *E. faecalis*-pulsed dendritic cells can accelerate the onset of colitis in *E. faecalis* monoassociated IL-10[-/-] mice.[112] Furthermore, broad-spectrum antibiotics can prevent and reverse colitis[113,114] and probiotics can attenuate disease.[109,115] In resistant SPF C57Bl/6 IL-10[-/-] mice, *H. hepaticus* can induce colitis and stimulate antigen-specific pathogenic as well as regulatory T cells.[116]

Genetic background is an important modifier of colitis and colonic adenocarcinoma. 129 SvEv IL-10[-/-] mice develop aggressive, rapid-onset disease and C57Bl/6 mice have slow-onset, mild colitis and limited cancer.[99] Subsequent studies demonstrate that BALB/c and C3H/HeJ Bir IL-10[-/-] mice have severe disease, which is a heritable trait.[117] Crossbreeding studies have identified a major susceptibility determinant on chromosome 3.[118] Interestingly, Berg et al.[18] demonstrated that 2-week exposure to piroxicam and other NSAIDs can accelerate the onset of disease in resistant C57Bl/6 IL-10[-/-] mice.

The importance of intrinsic IL-10 in suppressing pathologic immune responses is confirmed by similar phenotypes of colitis with deletion of components of the IL-10 signaling pathway. Deletion of the β chain of the IL-10 receptor (CRF-2), or selective deletion of STAT-3 in macrophages and neutrophils, leads to colitis.[119,120] The latter observation supports a primary role for innate immune cells in the genesis of this inflammation. Recent confirmation of a protective role for STAT-3 in innate immune responses is provided by a report of ileocolitis in conditional STAT-3[-/-] mice.[121] Deletion of STAT-3 in myeloid cells (but not T cells) leads to transmural ileocolitis with granulomas but no lymphocyte infiltration. Monocytes exhibit overly aggressive NFκB activation by LPS, but defective NADPH oxidase activity. These results suggest a predominant effect on innate immune cells.

*Advantages/disadvantages* This is a well-validated Th1-mediated murine model with a documented pathogenesis and response to various immunologic agents, antibiotics and probiotics. Unfortunately, commercial IL-10[-/-] mice are on a resistant (C57Bl/6) background, which slowly develops relatively mild colitis and has a low incidence of colon cancer. However, inflammation can be dramatically accelerated by briefly exposing C57BL/6 IL-10[-/-] mice[18] or by colonizing germ-free 129×C57Bl/6 IL-10[-/-] mice with SPF enteric bacteria.[98]

### Gi2α[-/-] mice

*Clinical/pathologic features* Deletion of the α subunit of Gi2, which regulates adenylate cyclose activity, leads to colitis and colonic adenocarcinoma associated with delayed growth, diarrhea, rectal prolapse and mortality.[122] Disease is evident between 8 and 12 weeks of age and is progressive; by 33 weeks approximately 1/3 of mice have developed colonic adenocarcinomas. Inflammation is confined to the colon, which is focally involved with mucosal ulcers, acute and chronic inflammatory cells, crypt abscesses and distortion, focal fibrosis and regenerative epithelial atypia.

*Pathogenesis* These mice exhibit mucosal Th1 responses with increased production of IL-12, IFN-γ, IL-1β and IgG2a and increased T-cell activation markers.[123] This immune activation precedes histologic evidence of disease.[124] It is unclear which antigens stimulate these Th1 responses and whether the primary defect is in epithelial cells, mucosal lymphocytes or APC, but the demonstration that dendritic cells from Gi2α[-/-] mice secrete high concentrations of IL-12 and TNF, and that inhibition of G1 signaling enhances IL-12, TNF and IL-10 secretion, suggests that defective APC function may drive this colitis.[125] As in many other models, the 129/Sv background is permissive, whereas Gi2α[-/-] mice on a C57Bl/6 background have less aggressive disease.[123]

*Advantages/disadvantages* This model is somewhat unique in that it involves a G-protein signaling defect, but the basic pathogenesis, including the role of commensal bacteria, remains unclear. However, the incidence of colonic adenocarcinoma is relatively high, providing a means to investigate mechanisms of carcinogenesis in inflammation.

### Multidrug resistance (Mdr)-1α[-/-] mice

*Clinical/pathologic features* Mdr genes express several transmembrane proteins which transport small amphiphilic and hydrophobic molecules, including drugs and potentially bacterial molecules, out of cells. Mdr-1α[-/-] mice develop diarrhea and anal mucus discharge at 20 weeks of age, with elongated crypts, crypt abscesses, focal mucosal ulcers, and infiltration of a mixed population of acute and chronic inflammatory cells, including CD4+ TCRα/β cells.[126] A Th1 profile of cytokines is present in the colon, with IFN-γ, TNF and IL-12 predominating.

*Pathogenesis* Bone marrow transplant experiments demonstrate that disease is *not* transferred by bone marrow-derived cells, suggesting that epithelial cells, which normally constitutively express large amounts of Mdr-1α, mediate this colitis.[126] The role of protective effects of Mdr-1α in colonic epithelial cells is demonstrated by enhanced susceptibility of Mdr-1[-/-] mice to DSS-induced colitis, but not TNBS/ETOH-induced disease.[127] Although LTB4 is increased in this model, blockade of this molecule did not affect disease.[127] Endogenous bacteria are involved, as broad-spectrum antibiotics treat colitis in this model and mucosal T cells proliferate in response to luminal bacteria.[126] Of note, *Helicobacter* species had variable effects, with *H. bilis* infection potentiating disease and *H. hepaticus* delaying the onset of colitis and attenuating disease.[128]

*Unique features/antibiotics/probiotics* A unique feature of this model is that the Mdr-1 gene has been implicated in human IBD[129,130] and as a factor mediating responses to drug treatment in IBD patients.[131] Thus, exploration of mechanisms of inflammation and responses to drugs relevant to human IBD in mice with defective mucosal expression of this molecule could have important implications for the pathogenesis and treatment of human IBD.

### TNF$^{\Delta ARE}$ mice overexpressing TNF

*Clinical/pathologic features*  Deletion of Au-rich regulatory elements in the 3' untranslated region of the murine TNF gene enhances mRNA stability, resulting in increased TNF production. These TNF$^{\Delta ARE}$ mice develop ileal inflammation, with some right colonic involvement in a dose-dependent fashion.[132] Homozygous mice have aggressive disease apparent by 1 month of age with early mortality (5–12 weeks of age) due to wasting, whereas heterozygous mice develop ileitis by 2 months of age. Disease is progressive and in later stages is transmural, associated with granulomas, loss of villi and increased lymphoid aggregates. Extraintestinal manifestations include erosive peripheral arthritis and focal stain lesions.

*Pathogenesis*  Interestingly, the pathogenesis of intestinal and joint inflammation is different.[132] TNFRII deletion attenuates intestinal inflammation but potentiates arthritis.[132] Similarly, ileal inflammation is T-lymphocyte dependent but arthritis is not.[132] Ileitis is Th1 dependent (increased IL-12 and IFN-γ), requires functional CD8+ T cells, and can be induced by both myeloid and T cell-derived cells as well as mesenchymal cells overexpressing TNF.[133] MAPK appears to inhibit disease, which is mediated by JNK-2 and COX/Tp12.

*Unique features/advantages/disadvantages*  TNF overexpression leading to transmural, granulomatous ileal inflammation is quite relevant to human Crohn's disease, in which TNF blockade has important therapeutic benefit and where ileal involvement is prominent. The lack of widespread availability of these mice limits large-scale studies.

### STAT-4 transgenic mice

*Clinical/pathologic features*  Overexpression of STAT-4, which is a transcription factor transmitting IL-12 signals to induce IFN-γ, does not lead to a spontaneous phenotype, but these mice develop colitis when stimulated with TNP-KLH in complete Freund's adjuvant.[48] They exhibit no disease when Freund's adjuvant is administered alone. Transmural inflammation in the ileum and colon begins 1–2 weeks after TNP/adjuvant administration.

*Pathogenesis*  This is a Th1-dominated response driven by commensal bacteria, as mucosal CD4+ T cells secrete IFN-γ and TNF in response to enteric bacterial stimulation.[48] Furthermore, colitis is transferred to T cell-deficient (SCID) mice by CD4+ T cells from transgenic mice stimulated in vitro by bacterial antigen. An important feature is the lack of spontaneous colitis, even with a potent adjuvant: inflammation requires a hapten that presumably sensitizes the susceptible host to commensal bacterial antigens. Transgenic expression depends on a triggering event.

*Advantages/disadvantages*  This model is an example of disease resulting from skewing signal transduction toward excessive (dysregulated) Th1 immune responses, and thus lends itself to investigating this signaling pathway. Furthermore, the ileum is involved, which is unusual in rodent colitis models. However, disease does not occur spontaneously and requires a triggering

event; it is unclear whether other, more environmentally relevant triggers, such as NSAIDs, might initiate similar processes.

### CD40 ligand transgenic mice

Engagement of the co-stimulatory molecule CD40, which is expressed on antigen-presenting cells (APC, dendritic cells, macrophages and B lymphocytes), and CD40 ligand (CD154) on T cells activates both APC and T lymphocytes. Overexpression of CD40L on T lymphocytes under the regulation of the lck promoter leads to multiorgan inflammation, manifested by wasting and diarrhea beginning soon after weaning (3 weeks of age).[134] Intestinal inflammation occurs primarily in the colon, but can involve the small intestine. This colitis consists of mucosal ulcers, focal transmural inflammation, occasional granulomas, and infiltration of the lamina propria and MLN with activated T and B lymphocytes. These findings and attenuation of experimental colitis by anti-CD40L antibody in a number of models are consistent with a key role for CD40/CD40L interactions in Th1 responses.[135,136]

### B7-related protein-1–IgG Fc fusion TG mice

Excessive production of a parallel co-stimulatory molecule similarly induces enterocolitis. B7-related protein-1 (B7RP-1) expressed on APC binds to inducible co-stimulator (ICOS) on activated T lymphocytes; this interaction activates both cell types. Overexpression of B7RP-1 fused to human IgG1 Fc by the liver (apolipoprotein E promoter) leads to transmural colitis with focal ulcers in less than 50% of mice over 6 months of age.[137] Disease can extend into the small intestine. Presumably the B7RP-1 fusion protein is secreted to activate T lymphocytes, which express ICOS. The concept that the B7RP-1/ICOS pathway contributes to chronic intestinal inflammation is supported by the ability of anti-ICOS antibodies to block CD45RB$^{high}$→SCID-induced colitis and increased ICOS expression in human IBD and experimental colitis.[138]

### IL-7 transgenic mice

*Clinical/pathologic features*  Overexpression of IL-7, an immunoregulatory molecule normally expressed by intestinal epithelial and stromal cells and recognized by T lymphocytes, leads to a variable induction of rectal predominant colitis with some ileal involvement.[138a] Histologic features include crypt abscesses, goblet cell depletion, Paneth cell metaplasia and infiltration of predominantly CD4+ T cells, macrophages and neutrophils with focal erosions.

*Pathogenesis*  The mechanisms of disease are unclear. Although IL-7 is normally expressed on non-lymphoid cells, transgenic mice had focal expression of IL-7 on activated lymphocytes but not epithelial cells. IFN-γ and IL-2 expression is increased following non-specific ex vivo stimulation, with decreased IL-4, suggesting that this is a Th1-mediated disease. IL-7R expression on lymphocytes is preserved.

*Advantages/disadvantages*  This model is not yet well characterized, so it is not well suited to preclinical pharmaceutical studies but could be explored to provide new mechanisms of inflammation through an understudied pathway.

### A20$^{-/-}$ mice

*Clinical/pathologic features*  In addition to activating proinflammatory pathways TNF induces the expression of protective molecules, including the zinc finger protein A20, which inhibits

TNF-activated NFκB. A20-deficient mice exhibit a wasting syndrome very early in life (pre-weaning) and die of multiorgan inflammation by 3–6 weeks of age.[139] Intestinal inflammation is characterized by infiltration of a mixed acute and chronic inflammatory response.

*Pathogenic mechanisms*  Inflammation is due to defective downregulation of inflammation selective for the TNF pathway, as TNF but not IL-1β induces exaggerated NFκB activation. This seems to be a selective defect in innate immune cells, as inflammation appears in T cell-deficient (RAG-1$^{-/-}$ X A20$^{-/-}$) mice.[140] Of interest, a similar pathology is seen for mice deficient in IκBα, which inhibits NFκB activity by complexing this transcription factor in the cytoplasm.[141] These similarities suggest that inhibitors of the NFκB pathway are central regulators of intestinal homeostasis.

### Disruption of TGF-β and the TGF-β signaling pathway (TGF-β1$^{-/-}$, TGF-βRII dn, Smad3$^{-/-}$ mice)

*Clinical and pathologic features*  TGF-β1$^{-/-}$ mice exhibit early-onset wasting, beginning soon after weaning (3–4 weeks of age) and which progresses to death by 5–6 weeks of age.[142,143] Inflammation is found in multiple organs, including the stomach and colon, with the location of gastrointestinal lesions dependent on genetic background. In most situations intestinal inflammation is a relatively minor manifestation of disease. Consistent with this model, similar multiorgan inflammation is seen with blockade of TGF-β signaling. A dominant negative (DN) TGF-βRII transgene expressed on a T lymphocyte-specific promoter leads to colitis and lung inflammation with autoantibodies, wasting and diarrhea.[144] The same transgene expressed in epithelial cells also leads to spontaneous colitis and enhanced susceptibility to DSS-induced colitis. Likewise, deletion of Smad3, a transcription factor phosphorylated by engagement of TGF-β to TGF-βRI/RII complex, leads to a wasting syndrome with the multiorgan inflammation and mucosal abscesses; a subset develop chronic intestinal inflammation.[145]

*Pathogenesis*  Multiorgan inflammation with deletion of any of three components of the TGF-β signaling pathway confirms a key role for TGF-β in downregulating T-cell responses. Regulatory T cells (Th3) producing TGF-β (secreted and possibly membrane bound) are integrally involved in the development of oral tolerance and suppression of Th1 pathogenic responses (see Chapter 5). Both Th1 and Th2 cytokines are increased in these models. CD4+ T cells mediate inflammation, as disease is absent when TGF-β1$^{-/-}$ mice are treated with anti-CD4 antibody or crossed with SCID or MHC II$^{-/-}$ mice.[146,147] Commensal bacteria have a secondary role, as disease persists, although perhaps mortality is delayed and colon cancer is absent in germ-free TGF-β1$^{-/-}$ mice.[148]

*Advantages/disadvantages*  Collectively, these genetically engineered mice provide an opportunity to dissect components of a key inhibitory pathway, as well as a means to determine the role of TGF-β in pathogenesis (see Chapter 5). However, the early mortality and the widespread non-specific inflammatory response limit use of these mice. The selective expression of DN TGF-βRII TG on epithelial and T cells allows studies of cell-specific signaling.

## Th2-mediated disease

### T-cell receptor α chain-deficient mice

*Clinical/pathologic features*  Deletion of TCRα, but not γ or δ, leads to predictable onset of colitis after 4 months of age; TCRβ$^{-/-}$ mice exhibit a far milder form.[149] Disease is progressive, confined to the colon, with diarrhea, weight loss and rectal prolapse. The colon, particularly the cecum, is thickened, contracted and edematous. Histologic inflammation is confined to the mucosa, consisting of crypt hyperplasia and branching, goblet cell depletion, occasional crypt abscesses, and prominent infiltration of the lamina propria with acute and chronic inflammatory cells. Ulceration and granulomas are not characteristic features.

*Pathogenesis*  This model has been extensively evaluated.[150] Although B lymphocytes are expanded and autoimmune responses relevant to human ulcerative colitis, such as antiepithelial, ANCA and antitropomysin antibodies,[151] are present, B lymphocytes are not required for disease expression, and in fact exert a protective role.[152] Whether B cells serve as regulatory cells or whether antibodies prevent inflammation remains to be determined. TNFRII and IL-6 appear to mediate the marked epithelial hyperplasia. The effector cells are TCRββ CD4+ T cells, which express unique ββ homodimeric TCR that are highly restricted and preferentially express the vβ8.2 chain.[153] The precise mechanism by which these pathogenic T cells develop is uncertain, but they may escape negative selection in the thymus.[3] Although TCRββ T cells expand in response to both autologous epithelial cells and bacterial stimulation, commensal bacteria are essential for disease induction, as germ-free TCRα$^{-/-}$ mice fail to develop colitis.[154] Organized cecal lymphoid aggregates (or, less probably, bacteria unique to the cecal tip) appear to be important in stimulating pathologic T cells, as cecal tip removal ('appendectomy') before the onset of colitis dramatically attenuates the development of disease; performing this procedure later in life does not substantially affect inflammation.[155] Host genetic background is an important determinant of disease expression.[149,150]

*Unique features/advantages/disadvantages*  This is one of the small number of Th2-mediated colitis models and the pathogenic mechanisms have been extensively studied. It has greater relevancy for ulcerative colitis than for Crohn's disease. A relative disadvantage is the slow onset of inflammation (4 months of age).

## Genetically engineered models with defective mucosal barrier function

### Dominant negative N-cadherin TG mice

*Clinical/pathologic features*  The creation of chimeric mice which focally express an N-cadherin DN on a fatty acid-binding protein promoter in the small intestine leads to focal areas of intestinal inflammation.[156] During the early phase of inflammation (1–2 months of age) mononuclear cells in the lamina propria and lymphoid aggregates expand, but by 3 months of age mucosal ulcers (aphthoid and longitudinal) form, with transmural inflammation, crypt abscesses, goblet cell depletion and lymphangiectasia. In the later phases (3–9 months) mucosal adenomas but no invasive cancers develop.

*Pathogenesis*  Inflammation is most likely due to defective epithelial cell–cell and cell–matrix contact, which is mediated by homophilic cadherin interactions. Expression in crypt cells is important for disease development, as TG expression in villous cells did not lead to disease. Presumably this defective cell–cell adhesion leads to enhanced uptake of luminal bacterial and/or dietary antigens and adjuvants that stimulate pathogenic innate and acquired immune responses. Although the cytokine profile has not been elucidated, the role of commensal bacteria has not been pursued by gnotobiotic, antibiotic or probiotic studies, and altered permeability has not been formally demonstrated.

*Unique features/advantages/disadvantages* The unique features of this chimera is the ability to study adjacent abnormal and normal epithelium in intact tissues. The disadvantages include the lack of documentation of immune responses and the lack of widespread availability of the model.

### Keratin 8-deficient mice
Keratin 8 and 18 filaments pair to form bonds that promote cell–cell junctions in epithelial cell monolayers. Although deletion of keratin 8 is a lethal mutation in most mouse strains, some FVB/N background mice survive. However, between 2 months and 1 year of age they eventually develop colitis, which is manifested by pancolonic inflammation and rectal prolapse.[157] Mucosal and submucosal inflammation is accompanied by crypt hyperplasia without ulcers, goblet cell depletion, or inflammation in other intestinal organs or extraintestinal sites. Of interest, targeted deletion of the reciprocal keratin fibril keratin 18 has no such phenotype, perhaps because of redundant function of these homologous molecules.

### Intestinal trefoil factor-deficient mice
Targeted deletion of ITF, a goblet cell glycoprotein which promotes epithelial restitution and enhances mucus viscosity, has no overt consequences unless the mucosa is injured by DSS.[38] After this trigger, DSS$^{-/-}$ mice develop more aggressive colitis and a higher mortality rate, which has been attributed to failure of appropriate mucosal healing.[38] Normal healing is restored by the exogenous administration of recombinant ITF in both the DSS and acetic acid models. Several growth factors, including KGF-2 and FGF20, stimulate expression of ITF in vitro and in vivo;[36,158] in preliminary data KGF-2 fails to accelerate healing of ITF$^{-/-}$ mice treated with DSS, suggesting that therapeutic effects of growth factors are mediated through upregulation of mucosal ITF.

### α1, 2-Fucosyltransferase transgenic mice
Overexpression of α1, 2-fucosyltransferase in transgenic mice leads to decreased sialic acid and galactose in colonic mucin.[159] These mice develop inflammation confined to the cecum and colon which consists of crypt abscesses and a mixed (acute and chronic) cellular infiltrate in the lamina propria. PNA lectin staining is increased in TG mice prior to the onset of inflammation. These results are consistent with the role of mucus as an integral component in mucosal barrier function, which is one mechanism by which ITF deficiency may affect colitis susceptibility. The role of bacteria in the pathogenesis of colitis is unknown in this model, but presumably defective mucous barrier function could lead to enhanced mucosal uptake of luminal bacteria.

## Genetically engineered mice with unknown pathogenesis

### Wiskott–Aldrich syndrome protein (WASP)-deficient mice
Humans with Wiskott–Aldrich syndrome have defective lymphocyte and megakaryocyte signaling and cytoskeletal function, resulting in X-linked immunodeficiency. Although colitis is not a feature of the human syndrome, WASP$^{-/-}$ mice develop an entirely different phenotype manifested by colitis beginning 4 months of age.[160] Numbers of circulating T cells and platelets are decreased and T-lymphocyte activation through the TCR is defective, although CD4+ T cells are increased in the colonic lamina propria. B-cell number and function remain normal.

### Antigen-specific TCR transgenic mice
T lymphocytes in most chronic rodent enterocolitis models respond to ubiquitous commensal enteric bacterial antigens or, possibly, self-antigens (see Chapter 10). Transgenes expressing TCR reactive to specific antigens permit investigation of defined exogenous and autoantigens. In one complex model, mice transgenic for mature (rearranged) α and β TCR recognizing cytochrome c were created.[161] When crossed with T cell-deficient mice (SCID or Rag$^{-/-}$), mice developed distal colitis with typical crypt hyperplasia and predominantly mononuclear cell infiltration. Infiltrating T cells were of an activated phenotype and expressed the TCRβ transgene, but not the TCRα transgene. Whether these cells are TCRββ, as in the TCRα$^{-/-}$ mice,[153] is unknown. Circulating CD4+ T cells were decreased. The pathogenesis and antigenic stimulation of this model are uncertain and could reflect defective regulatory cell function or inappropriate activation of self-reactive effector cells.

Transfer of DO11 TG T cells which specifically recognize ovalbumin (OVA) into T cell-deficient recipients has been a valuable tool to explore mechanisms of tolerance. Transfer of naive DO11 T lymphocytes into Rag-2$^{-/-}$ recipients colonized with *E. coli* expressing OVA did not cause disease.[162] However, transfer of polarized Th1 or Th2 cells induced disease with different phenotypes. No disease developed in the absence of luminal antigens. These results demonstrate the importance of early skewing of T-lymphocyte cytokine profiles and the presence of luminal bacterially derived antigen on disease induction and phenotype, and that a single antigen can drive different disease phenotypes in the same host. Yoshida et al.[163] confirmed these results and noted different migration patterns of Th1- and Th2 OVA-reactive cells.

## SPONTANEOUSLY OCCURRING MODELS

### Cotton-top Tamarins
#### Clinical/pathologic features
Cotton-top tamarins, marmosets from Colombia, in captivity spontaneously develop chronic progressive pancolitis with diarrhea and weight loss which begins at age 2–3 years.[164] This chronic inflammation persists throughout life, with episodic acute flares. Histologic features include infiltration of the lamina propria with mononuclear cells and mucin depletion, with superimposed acute colitis manifested by infiltrating neutrophils and crypt abscesses. Chronic inflammation is accompanied by epithelial dysplasia, which in a large percentage of animals evolves to chronic adenocarcinoma.

#### Pathogenesis
The profile of cytokines is unknown, but mucin abnormalities similar to those of human ulcerative colitis have been documented; whether these abnormalities precede colitis is unclear.[165] T cells are indirectly implicated by treatment of disease using anti-α$_4$ integrin antibody.[166] A role for luminal commensal bacteria is strongly suggested by studies in Thiry-Vella loops, in which inflammation does not occur in the absence of bacteria and is increased by perfusion with fecal matter.[167] Stress of captivity or changes in ambient temperature have been suggested as an etiologic function but remain speculative.[168] Colitis is presumably the result of a spontaneous genetic mutation, as yet unidentified. These animals have an unusual homogeneity in their HLA class I molecules which derives from HLA-G.

## Unique features/advantages/disadvantages

The well-documented spontaneous acute 'flares' of disease closely resemble human IBD, as does the chronic colitis/dysplasia/adenocarcinoma sequence. However, their endangered species status presents a major hurdle to studying these animals, as does the lack of defined immunologic reagents.

## C3H/HeJ Bir mice

### Clinical/pathologic features

The selective breeding of C3H/HeJ mice which sporadically developed colitis led to a substrain that develops ileal, right colonic and perianal ulcers at 3–6 weeks of age.[169] This relatively mild, focal inflammation resolves by 10–12 weeks of age. Histologic features of active lesions include acute and chronic inflammation, focal ulcers, crypt abscesses and epithelial regeneration. Crypt hyperplasia, granulomas and adenocarcinomas are not seen.

### Pathogenesis

Like the parental C3H/HeJ strain, these mice are LPS unresponsive owing to a point mutation in TLR4. Commensal bacteria are implicated by increased serum $IgG_1$ responses to multiple enteric bacterial antigens,[170] CD4 T cell IFN-$\gamma$ responses to cecal bacterial antigens, and the ability of Th1 cell lines expanded in vitro by cecal bacteria to induce colitis when transferred to SCID mice.[171] Cecal bacterial activation of Th1 responses in CD4+ T cells is dependent on CD4+–CD40 ligand interactions and is associated with an oligoclonal set of TCR chains.[135] Of considerable interest is that cecal bacteria stimulate regulatory Tr1 CD4+ T cells that secrete IL-10.[172] Co-transfer of the in vitro bacterially expanded IL-10-secreting CD4+ T cells with the CD1 CD4 T cells prevents the onset of colitis in recipient SCID mice.[172] Environmental influences, probably bacterial, are evident by a dramatic reduction in the frequency of colitis when mice are rederived into SPF conditions. Finally, although the gene(s) responsible for the increased frequency of spontaneous colitis in this substrain have not been identified, both the parental C3H/HeJ and C3H/HeJ Bir mice are highly susceptible to DSS- and TNBS-induced colitis, and IL-10$^{-/-}$ mice on the C3H/HeJ Bir background have extremely aggressive disease.[37,117]

### Unique features/advantages/disadvantages

This is the first model with documented counterbalancing bacterial antigen-specific Th1 and Tr1 immune responses, the balance of which probably account for the transient inflammation. These validated bacterial-responsive T-cell lines and their documented ability to induce and prevent colitis when transferred to SCID mice offer an opportunity to investigate mechanisms of effector and regulatory cell activation and function. Disadvantages include disappearance of the original disease phenotype in current SPF conditions, raising the possibility that *Helicobacter* species or other overt opportunistic pathogens could be causing the inflammatory response.

## SAMP-1/Yit mice

### Clinical/pathologic features

A substrain of the senescent accelerated mice (SAM), which exhibit accelerated aging and early death, was selectively bred based on the phenotype of skin lesions. A new inbred strain, SAMP-1/Yit, no longer had accelerated senescence, but developed ileal inflammation as early as 10–20 weeks of age and com-

plete penetrance by 30 weeks of age.[173,174] Inflammation was centered in the distal ileum, with lower degrees of inflammation in the mid to proximal ileum and in the right colon, with periportal inflammation occurring outside the intestine. Ileitis could be transferred by unfractionated MLN cells. Some mice developed ileal fibrosis and luminal narrowing, whereas occasional mice (~5%) developed perianal skin lesions and rare fistulae.[175] Histologic features include a mixed acute and chronic cell infiltration, influx of activated CD4+ and CD8$\alpha$+ TCR$\alpha$/$\beta$+ T cells, crypt abscesses, crypt hyperplasia and branching, with villous atrophy and occasional loose epithelial granulomas. The ratio of CD8$\alpha$+ TCR$\gamma\delta$/CD8$\alpha$+ TCR$\alpha$/$\beta$ CD4+ T cells is dramatically decreased.

### Pathogenesis

This is a Th1-mediated disorder, as MLN cells produce increased IFN-$\gamma$ and TNF but not increased IL-4, 5 and 10, and disease dramatically decreased following anti-TNF antibody treatment.[174] Commensal bacteria are involved, as germ-free SAMP-1/Yit mice have no disease and ileal inflammation occurs within 10 weeks of colonization with SPF bacteria,[173] and cipro/metronidazole attenuates disease in both preventive and therapeutic protocols and decreases TNF and IFN-$\gamma$.[176] It is important to determine whether the dominant antigens driving this response or bacteria specifically colonize the ileum. Finally, the genes regulating this spontaneous enterocolitis model are being studied. $F_2$ progeny of crosses with resistant mice implicate a region on murine chromosome 11.[177]

### Unique features/advantages/disadvantages

This is an important and unique model of spontaneously occurring ileocolitis with ileal fibrosis and perianal disease which is Th1 mediated. Identification of causative genes will help guide the search for genes causing Crohn's disease. Likewise, identifying which bacterial species preferentially induce disease will have considerable impact on the search for bacterial antigens causing Crohn's disease. Limited general access to this model, however, makes studying these important mice difficult.

# T-CELL OR BONE MARROW TRANSFER MODELS

## CD45RB$^{high}$ T-cell transfer to SCID mice

### Clinical/pathologic features

T cells can be divided into naive and effector/memory subsets based on expression of the surface marker CD45RB, which is expressed in high amounts in naive cells and decreases with T-cell activation. Adoptive transfer of CD45RB$^{high}$ CD4+ T cells from the spleens of normal mice to SCID mice, which lack TNB lymphocytes, induces pancolonic inflammation which appears 5–8 weeks after cell transfer.[178,179] This inflammation is progressive and leads to unrelenting non-bloody diarrhea, weight loss, and death within 4 weeks after the onset of symptoms. Histologic features include marked mucosal thickening, with crypt hyperplasia and infiltration of the lamina propria and, to a lesser extent, the submucosa with mononuclear cells. Neutrophils and crypt abscesses are occasionally seen, and granulomas are rarely visible. An extremely important observation in this model is that transfer of the reciprocal CD45RB$^{low}$ CD4+ T-cell population not only fails to induce disease, but actually *prevents* colitis when co-transferred with CD45RB$^{high}$ cells. These observations are not unique to mice, as they were first seen in rats with Ox22[high] naive T cells and activated Ox22[low] cells.[180]

### Pathogenesis of colitis and mechanisms of prevention

Colitis in this model is Th1 mediated, as demonstrated by increased IFN-γ, TNF, IL-1 and IL-6 expression and blockade by anti-IFN-γ, and to a lesser extent anti-TNF, as well as recombinant IL-10.[181] Colitis depends on CD40/CD40L (CD154) interactions as well as interaction with $\alpha_4\beta_7$ integrins.[136,182] T cells immigrate into both the small intestine and the colon, but inflammation is confined to the latter, presumably because of the antigenic bacterial species that preferentially reside in the colon. T-cell trafficking to the intestine is dependent on luminal bacteria:[183] these cells respond to fecal bacterial antigens[184] and disease is attenuated by 'simplified microflora' mice[183] and by antibiotics.[185] Furthermore, CD4+ T cells expansion in vivo is oligoclonal.[186] These results demonstrate that naive T cells from normal mice can be activated to become pathogenic competent Th1 cells by selected members of the commensal enteric bacterial population in the absence of proper thymic education.

The nature of the regulatory CD45RB[low] population promoting disease in normal hosts is being elucidated. Protection is due to the CD25+ subset of CD45RB[low] cells which express CTLA-4.[187] Prevention of colitis is dependent on both IL-10 and TGF-β, based on lack of prevention with anti-IL-10 receptor and anti-TGF-β antibody blockade and transfer of CD45RB[low] cells from IL-10[-/-] and TGF-β1[-/-] mice, lack of induction of colitis with CD45RB[high] CD4+ T cells from IL-10 TG mice, and prevention with IL-10 transfected T lymphocytes.[188-191] In contrast, IL-4 does not contribute to this protection.[188] The in vivo antigen(s) stimulating the development and regulatory function of CD45RB[low] CD4+ T cells are not yet determined, but preliminary data suggest that commensal bacterial antigens are involved, as CD45RB[low] CD4+ T cells from germ-free donors have decreased ability to prevent colitis.[192] Elegant experiments indicate that the antigens driving regulatory cells can be different from those stimulating disease. Groux et al.[193] showed that in vitro-expanded IL-10-secreting CD4+ T cells (Tr1) clones responding to OVA could prevent disease.

### Unique features/advantages/disadvantages

This model conclusively demonstrated a role for in vivo functional regulatory T cells. The convenient transfer of both effector and regulatory cell populations from normal murine splenocytes permits the investigator to obtain CD45RB[high] or [low] cells from an unlimited number of knockout or transgenic mouse strains. The same strategy could be used in gnotobiotic donors and recipient mice to determine key commensal bacterial species that induce and prevent disease. The disadvantage of this reductionist system is the absence of the normal mix of CD8+ and NK T cells and B lymphocytes, which themselves have regulatory activities.

## Bone marrow transplant → CD3εTG mice

### Clinical/pathologic features

Transgenic mice overexpressing human CD3ε (Tgε26 mice) have a blockade in early T-cell development leading to complete loss of T lymphocytes and NK cells, as well as a lack of thymic development.[194] T cell-depleted bone marrow reconstitution of adult Tgε26 mice from a normal mouse leads to progressive weight loss, diarrhea and pancolitis, which begins 4–6 weeks after bone marrow transplant. Disease is progressive, leading to death within 1–2 weeks after onset of symptoms. Histologic features of colitis include mucosal hyperplasia, goblet cell depletion, predominantly mononuclear cell infiltration of the lamina propria scattered crypt abscesses. Inflammation is confined to the colon. Transferred MLN CD4+ cells from Tgε26 mice with colitis induces a rapid onset of disease with a similar phenotype in non-bone marrow-reconstituted Tgε26 recipients, which is clinically evident within 2–4 weeks after transfer.

### Pathogenesis

Inflammation is Th1 mediated, with increased production of both IFN-γ and TNF by CD4 and CD8 T cells.[194] Inflammation is dependent on IL-12 and CD40/CD40L (CD154), based on attenuation of disease with neutralizing antibodies to these co-stimulatory factors and proinflammatory cytokines, as well as transplant of bone marrow from STAT-4-deficient mice.[136,195] Lymphotoxin and TNF are also involved,[196] but cytotoxic T cells and Fas-mediated apoptosis do not seem to be required.[195] Defective thymic education appears to be an important mechanism of disease, as transplant of a fetal thymus at the same time as the bone marrow transplant prevents disease. Regulatory cell function has not been thoroughly investigated, but it seems likely that the thymic defect prevents the development of thymic-dependent regulatory cells; whether this is the CD25+ Th3 population discussed in detail in Chapter 5 remains to be determined.

Commensal bacteria are required to both reduce and perpetuate disease.[197] CD4+ MLN T cells produce IFN-γ when stimulated by APC pulsed with cecal contents from SPF, but not germ-free mice; colonic epithelial cells from germ-free mice also induce no response. Germ-free recipients of normal T cell-depleted bone marrow, or even activated MLN CD4+ T cells from bone marrow transplanted Tgε26 mice with colitis, fail to develop colitis, although MLN cells from germ-free Tgε26 mice after bone marrow transplant induce disease in SPF recipients. Preliminary studies show specificity of induction by various bacterial species, as *Bacteroides vulgatus*, *Enterococcus faecalis* and *E. coli* do not induce disease in monoassociated recipients (Veltkamp, Kim and Sartor, unpublished results).

### Unique features/advantages/disadvantages

Various knockout and transgenic mouse strains can be used as the source of the bone marrow, and the microbial environment can be manipulated on both recipient and donor transfer sides with the MLN cell transfer. Furthermore, this model lends itself to the study of mechanisms of induction of thymic education of regulatory cells. Disadvantages include the global loss of thymic function.

# INSIGHTS INTO THE PATHOGENESIS OF IBD

Although no single model totally reproduces the clinical, pathogenic and immunoregulatory abnormalities of Crohn's disease and ulcerative colitis, numerous recurring themes that transcend several models are likely to be fundamental processes that are relevant to human disease (Table 9.3).

## Table 9.3 Recurring themes in animal models of chronic, immune intestinal inflammation

Chronic inflammation is T-lymphocyte mediated

Defective immunoregulatory or mucosal barrier function can induce chronic intestinal inflammation

Commensal enteric bacteria provide the constant antigenic and adjuvant stimulis driving chronic enterocolitis

Host genetic background modulates disease activity

## Table 9.4 Categories of animal models of IBD based on pathogenesis of inflammation

| Overly aggressive effector cell function | Defective regulatory cell activity | Defective epithelial barrier function |
|---|---|---|
| TNBS/ETOH | IL-10$^{-/-}$, IL-10R$^{-/-}$, STAT-3$^{-/-}$ | N-cadherin DN |
| TNF$^{\Delta ARE}$ | IL-2$^{-/-}$, IL-2R$^{-/-}$ | Mdr-1$\alpha^{-/-}$ |
| Gi$\alpha$2$^{-/-}$ | BM→CD3$\epsilon$ TG | Keratin 8$^{-/-}$ |
| STAT-4 TG | CD45RB$^{high}$→SCID | ITF$^{-/-}$ (inducible) |
| A20$^{-/-}$ | TGF-$\beta$ RII DN TG | IL-10$^{-/-}$ (?) |
| CD40 L TG | TGF-$\beta$1$^{-/-}$ | Gi$\alpha$2$^{-/-}$ (?) |

# CHRONIC INFLAMMATION IS T-LYMPHOCYTE MEDIATED

Every model studied to date that develops chronic inflammation in the absence of a pathogen is mediated by T lymphocytes. The effector T cells can have either Th1 (the majority of models) or Th2 (TCR$\alpha^{-/-}$ mice and oxazalone-induced colitis) cytokine profiles (see Table 9.2). Blockade of Th1-mediated colitis is most efficiently performed by inhibiting IL-12, pathways of IL-12 induction (CD40/CD40L/CD154) or signaling (STAT-4) rather than IFN-$\gamma$. Blockade of IL-4 abrogates Th2-mediated inflammation. IL-10 can inhibit induction of inflammation but not reverse established disease. Although most models show skewed Th1 or Th2 responses, this black and white picture is probably too simple; for example, IL-10$^{-/-}$ mice on a C57BL/6 background have a Th1 cytokine profile in the early phases of colitis which is lost in the chronic phase (>4 months of age).[107] Similarly, TNBS/ETOH normally induces Th1-mediated disease, but IFN-$\gamma$-deficient mice develop a Th2 profile, which has a different phenotype of superficial inflammation more consistent with ulcerative colitis.[50] Opportunistic pathogens such as *Helicobacter hepaticus* can induce chronic inflammation in T cell-deficient mice, raising a possible alternative mechanism of disease pathogenesis in immunosuppressed hosts or those with defective microbial clearance.

# DEFECTIVE IMMUNOREGULATION OR MUCOSAL BARRIER FUNCTION CAN INDUCE CHRONIC INFLAMMATION

Normal mice have redundant mechanisms of suppressing mucosal immune responses to ubiquitous antigens from the complex commensal enteric bacteria, dietary proteins and autologous proteins. This non-responsiveness, or immunologic tolerance, is mediated by IL-10, TGF-$\beta$ and prostaglandins (see Chapter 5) secreted by regulatory T cells (Tr1 lymphocytes secreting IL-10, Th3 secreting TGF-$\beta$, CD25+ T-regulatory cells) and perhaps intestinal epithelial cells. The CD25+ (IL-2 receptor) CD4+ T regulatory cells require thymic development and IL-2 stimulation, which perhaps explains the propensity for thymic-deficient mice (CD3$\epsilon$Tg) to develop disease after a bone marrow transplant from normal mice, or for IL-2$^{-/-}$ and IL-2Rd$^{-/-}$ mice to develop disease. There are two ways in which immunoregulatory defects induce disease: overly aggressive effector cells (i.e. TNF$^{\Delta ARE}$) or defective regulatory T cells (IL-10$^{-/-}$). The CD45RB$^{high}$ co-transfer model indicates that regulatory cells have dominance over effector cells. Results in IL-10$^{-/-}$, STAT3$^{-/-}$, A20$^{-/-}$ and Gi2$\alpha^{-/-}$ mice and HLA-B27 TG rats indicate that APC can be a primary determinant of dysregulated Th1 or Tr1 responses.

A second pathway to chronic enterocolitis is defective mucosal barrier function (Table 9.4). Defects in mucus production (MUC-2, possibly ITF$^{-/-}$), cell–cell and cell–matrix contact (N-cadherin and keratin-8 deficiency), and possibly epithelial restitution (ITF$^{-/-}$, COX-2$^{-/-}$), secretion of bacterial products or environmental toxins (Mdr-1$^{-/-}$) and epithelial function (Gi$\alpha$2$^{-/-}$) either lead to spontaneous inflammation or potentiation of disease, initiated by breaking the mucosal barrier (short-term DSS-induced colitis in ITF$^{-/-}$ or COX-2$^{-/-}$ mice).

# COMMENSAL ENTERIC BACTERIA PROVIDE THE CONSTANT ANTIGENIC AND ADJUVANT STIMULATION DRIVING CHRONIC INTESTINAL INFLAMMATION

As discussed in considerable detail in Chapter 10, commensal bacterial antigens and adjuvants regulate pathogenic innate and acquired effector immune responses which induce chronic intestinal inflammation. Despite systemic immunoregulatory defects, inflammation targets the colon and, in rare situations, the terminal ileum (SAMP-1/Yit and TNF$^{\Delta ARE}$ mice). A number of induced and genetically engineered models exhibit lack of inflammation in germ-free situations, attenuation with antibiotics, or surgical bypass and bacterial antigen-specific T-cell responses (see Table 4, Chapter 10). Recent studies in gnotobiotic rodents show both host- and bacterial-specific responses, with certain bacterial species causing disease in one, but not another host, and regional-specific responses in the same host (IL-10$^{-/-}$ mouse). Variable responses are seen within a single bacterial genus (*Bacteroides* species in HLA B27 transgenic rats), and may even be strain specific (*E. coli* virulence factors in Crohn's disease patients).[198] Intestinal inflammation responds to antibiotics or prebiotics that restore mucosal homeostasis. These studies have profound implications for the diagnosis and treatment of human IBD patients, particularly related to patient subsets.

# HOST GENETIC BACKGROUND MODULATES DISEASE INTENSITY AND PHENOTYPE

Background strain profoundly influences the aggressiveness of experimental colitis in both induced and genetically engineered models, with several consistent patterns appearing (Table 9.5). In murine models 129 and C3H are high responders, whereas C57Bl/6 mice are resistant, BALB/c intermediate or high responders, and 129 X C57Bl/6 F1 intermediate. LPS responsiveness does not seem to affect susceptibility to

**Table 9.5 Role of genetic background in experimental colitis: differential susceptibility in various inbred rodent strains**

| Model | Host strain | | |
|---|---|---|---|
| | Susceptible | Intermediate | Resistant |
| **A. Mouse models** | | | |
| DSS | C3H, NOD, BALB | C57Bl/6 | NON |
| TNBS/ETOH | SJL, C3H, BALB | | C57Bl/6, DBA/2 |
| IL-2$^{-/-}$ | C3H, BALB | | C57Bl/6 |
| IL-10$^{-/-}$ | 129, C3H | BALB, 129xC57Bl/6 | C57Bl/6 |
| TCRα$^{-/-}$ | 129, C3H | 129xC57Bl/6 | C57Bl/6 |
| Mdr-1α$^{-/-}$ | 129, C3H | 129xC57Bl/6 | C57Bl/6 |
| CD45RB$^{high}$→SCID | BALB | | C57Bl/6 |
| | | | |
| **B. Rat models** | | | |
| Indomethacin | Lewis | Sprague–Dawley | Fischer F344 |
| PG-PS | Lewis | Sprague–Dawley | Fischer F344, Buffalo |

disease, as C3H/HeJ, HeN and HeJ Bir have similar high susceptibility. Although no single gene has yet been identified, several common chromosomal regions (chromosome 11) have been implicated in at least three separate models which have obvious implications for the search for human IBD susceptibility genes.

# USE OF RODENT MODELS IN PHARMACOLOGIC STUDIES

In addition to the obligate toxicologic and pharmacokinetic studies performed in normal mice and rats, rodent models of intestinal inflammation are critically important in preclinical drug development to determine therapeutic efficacy and mechanisms of action. In addition, drug absorption, metabolism and distribution can be substantially different in the inflamed versus the normal intestine. Any of the available rodent models can be used for these studies, with the choice being dependent on the individual properties of the compounds under investigation. For example, a growth factor which is postulated to stimulate epithelial restitution should be investigated in the healing phase of a model which has self-limited mucosal ulceration (DSS, indomethacin, TNBS/ETOH), whereas an immunosuppressive molecule with systemic activities could simultaneously be used to block intestinal and extraintestinal inflammation in the PG-PS model of enterocolitis, erosive peripheral arthritis, hepatic granulomas and anemia of chronic disease; and a locally active compound or engineered T lymphocyte[191] will be tested in IL-10 knockout mice, CD45RB$^{high}$→SCID or any other T cell-mediated model.

In principle, an easily used, cheap, widely available model, such as DSS-induced murine colitis or perhaps TNBS/ETOH-induced colitis in mice or rats, should be used to screen high volumes of various pharmaceutical compounds. The more expensive, chronic immune-mediated models could then be used to determine whether an agent is effective in situations more relevant to human Crohn's disease or ulcerative colitis. Examples of the latter group of Th1-mediated models include IL-10$^{-/-}$, CD45RB$^{high}$→SCID transfer or chronic TNBS/ETOH (SJL/J background) mice, PG-PS enterocolitis in Lewis rats, or

possibly HLA B27 TG rats, although the latter is quite expensive. TCRα$^{-/-}$ mice present an excellent model for Th2-mediated disease. Logistically, the slow onset of mild disease in commercially available C57Bl/6 IL-10$^{-/-}$ mice limits their usefulness. This can be rectified in two ways: acceleration of disease by NSAID administration,[18] or the use of germ-free IL-10$^{-/-}$ mice on a 129 SvEv background colonized with SPF bacteria.[98]

Clinically relevant pharmacologic results should be generated in at least two independent models of chronic, T cell-mediated colitis or enterocolitis, and should demonstrate reversal of established disease rather than prevention of onset of inflammation, which is a relatively easily achieved endpoint. For example, both the IL-10$^{-/-}$ and PG-PS models predicted lack of therapeutic activity of recombinant IL-10 in IBD,[106] as experimental intestinal inflammation was prevented but not reversed.[65,99] A compound that possesses the characteristics of reversing established chronic T cell-mediated inflammation has a much higher likelihood of clinical success than an agent merely capable of preventing the onset of acute, specific mucosal injury.

# CONCLUSIONS

These overarching themes support the hypothesis that chronic intestinal inflammation is due to an overly aggressive cell-mediated immune response (loss of tolerance) to discrete components (adjuvants, antigens) of the complex commensal enteric bacterial population in genetically susceptible hosts. Mechanisms of genetic susceptibility include defective immunoregulation (APC–T-cell interactions) or altered barrier function/healing (restitution). Identifying the principal molecular mediators and genetic mechanisms of these defects can be best performed in animal models, thereby identifying precise targets for studies in human IBD patients.

# ACKNOWLEDGMENTS

The author thanks Susie May for diligent secretarial support. Original investigations were supported by NIH grants DK 40249, 53347 and 34987, Crohn's and Colitis Foundation of America and Broad Medical Research Foundation.

# REFERENCES

1. Elson CO, Sartor RB, Tennyson GS et al. Experimental models of inflammatory bowel disease. Gastroenterology 1995;109:1344–1367.

2. Sartor RB. Insights into the pathogenesis of inflammatory bowel diseases provided by new rodent models of spontaneous colitis. Inflammatory Bowel Diseases 1995;1:64–75.

3. Strober W, Fuss IJ, Blumberg RS. The immunology of mucosal models of inflammation. Annu Rev Immunol 2002;20:495–549.

4. Neurath MF, Finotto S, Glimcher LH. The role of Th1/Th2 polarization in mucosal immunity. Nature Med 2002;8:567–573.

5. Wirtz S, Neurath MF. Animal models of intestinal inflammation: new insights into the molecular pathogenesis and immunotherapy of inflammatory bowel disease. Int J Colorectal Dis 2000;15:144–160.

6. Kraft SC, Fitch FW, Kirsner JB. Histologic and immunohistochemical features of Auer 'colitis' in rabbits. Am J Pathol 1963;43:913–923.

7. Mee AS, Jewell DP. Factors inducing relapse in inflammatory bowel disease. Br Med J 1978;2:801–802.

8. Strober W. Animal models of inflammatory bowel disease – an overview. Dig Dis Sci 1985;30:3S–10S.

9. Powrie F. T cells in inflammatory bowel disease: protective and pathogenic roles. Immunity 1995;3:171–174.

10. Yamada Y, Marshall S, Specian RD et al. A comparative analysis of two models of colitis in rats. Gastroenterology 1992;102:1524–1534.

11. Sharon P, Stenson WF. Metabolism of arachidonic acid in acetic acid colitis in rats. Similarity to human inflammatory bowel disease. Gastroenterology 1985;88:55–63.

12. Sartor RB, Bond TM, Schwab JH. Systemic uptake and intestinal inflammatory effects of luminal bacterial cell wall polymers in rats with acute colonic injury. Infect Immun 1988;56:2101–2108.

13. Yamada T, Deitch E, Specian RD et al. Mechanisms of acute and chronic intestinal inflammation induced by indomethacin. Inflammation 1993;17:641–662.

14. Sartor RB, Bender DE, Holt LC. Susceptibility of inbred rat strains to intestinal and extraintestinal inflammation induced by indomethacin. Gastroenterology 1992;102:A690 (Abstract).

15. Banerjee AK, Peters TJ. Experimental non-steroidal anti-inflammatory drug-induced enteropathy in the rat: similarities to inflammatory bowel disease and effect of thromboxane synthetase inhibitors. Gut 31:1358–1364, 1990.

16. Robert A, Asano T. Resistance of germfree rats to indomethacin-induced intestinal lesions. Prostaglandins 1977;14:333–341.

17. Morteau O, Morham SG, Sellon R et al. Impaired mucosal defense to acute colonic injury in mice lacking cyclooxygenase-1 or cyclooxygenase-2. J Clin Invest 2000;105:469–478.

18. Berg DJ, Zhang J, Weinstock JV et al. Rapid development of colitis in NSAID-treated IL-10-deficient mice. Gastroenterology 2002;123:1527–1542.

19. Sartor RB, Bender DE, Grenther WB et al. Absolute requirement for ubiquitous luminal bacteria in the pathogenesis of chronic intestinal inflammation. Gastroenterology 1994;106:A767.

20. Han DS, Li F, Holt LC et al. Keratinocyte growth factor-2 (fibroblast growth factor-10) promotes healing of indomethacin-induced small intestinal ulceration in rats and stimulates epithelial cell restitution and protective molecules. Am J Physiol 2000;279:G1011–G1022.

21. Felder JB, Korelitz BI, Rajapakse R et al. Effects of nonsteroidal antiinflammatory drugs on inflammatory bowel disease: a case–control study. Am J Gastroenterol 2000;95:1949–1954.

22. Okayasu I, Hatakeyama S, Yamada M et al. A novel method in the induction of reliable experimental acute and chronic ulcerative colitis in mice. Gastroenterology 1990;98:694–702.

23. Cooper HS, Murthy SN, Shah RS et al. Clinicopathologic study of dextran sulfate sodium experimental murine colitis. Lab Invest 1993;69:238–249.

24. Watt J, Marcus R. Ulcerative colitis in the guinea-pig caused by seaweed extract. J Pharm Pharmacol 1969;21:187S.

25. Onderdonk AB, Franklin ML, Cisneros RL. Production of experimental ulcerative colitis in gnotobiotic guinea pigs with simplified microflora. Infect Immun 1981;32:225–231.

26. Rath HC, Schultz M, Freitag R et al. Different subsets of enteric bacteria induce and perpetuate experimental colitis in rats and mice. Infect Immun 2001;69:2277–2285.

27. Axelsson LG, Midtvedt T, Bylund-Fellenius AC. The role of intestinal bacteria, bacterial translocation and endotoxin in dextran sodium sulphate-induced colitis in the mouse. Microb Ecol Health Dis 1996;9:225–237.

28. Hudcovic T, Stepankova R, Cebra J et al. The role of microflora in the development of intestinal inflammation: acute and chronic colitis induced by dextran sulfate in germ-free and conventionally reared immunocompetent and immunodeficient mice. Folia Microbiol 2001;46:565–572.

29. Kitajima S, Morimoto M, Sagara E et al. Dextran sodium sulfate-induced colitis in germ-free IQI/Jic mice. Exp Anim 2001;50:387–395.

30. Obermeier F, Dunger N, Deml L et al. CpG motifs of bacterial DNA exacerbate colitis of dextran sulfate sodium-treated mice. Eur J Immunol 2002;32:2084–2092.

31. Saubermann LJ, Beck P, de Jong YP et al. Activation of natural killer T cells by alpha-galactosylceramide in the presence of CD1d provides protection against colitis in mice. Gastroenterology 2000;119:119–128.

32. Sivakumar PV, Westrich GM, Kanaly S et al. Interleukin 18 is a primary mediator of the inflammation associated with dextran sulphate sodium induced colitis: blocking interleukin 18 attenuates intestinal damage. Gut 2002;50:812–820.

33. Dieleman LA, Palmen MJ, Akol H et al. Chronic experimental colitis induced by dextran sulphate sodium (DSS) is characterized by Th1 and Th2 cytokines. Clin Exp Immunol 1998;114:385–391.

34. Axelsson LG, Landstrom E, Goldschmidt TJ et al. Dextran sulfate sodium (DSS) induced experimental colitis in immunodeficient mice: effects in CD4(+)-cell depleted, athymic and NK-cell depleted SCID mice. Inflammation Res 1996;45:181–191.

35. Dieleman LA, Ridwan BU, Tennyson GS et al. Dextran sulfate sodium-induced colitis occurs in severe combined immunodeficient mice. Gastroenterology 1994;107:1643–1652.

36. Jeffers M, McDonald WF, Chillakuru RA et al. A novel human fibroblast growth factor treats experimental intestinal inflammation. Gastroenterology 2002;123:1151–1162.

37. Mahler M, Bristol IJ, Leiter EH et al. Differential susceptibility of inbred mouse strains to dextran sulfate sodium-induced colitis. Am J Physiol 1998;274:G544–G551.

38. Mashimo H, Wu DC, Podolsky DK et al. Impaired defense of intestinal mucosa in mice lacking intestinal trefoil factor. Science 1996;274:262–265.

39. Williams KL, Fuller CR, Dieleman LA et al. Enhanced survival and mucosal repair after dextran sodium sulfate-induced colitis in transgenic mice that overexpress bovine growth hormone. Gastroenterology 2001;120:925–937.

40. Morris GP, Beck PL, Herridge MS et al. Hapten-induced model of chronic inflammation and ulceration in the rat colon. Gastroenterology 1989;96:795–803.

41. Neurath MF, Fuss I, Kelsall BL et al. Antibodies to interleukin 12 abrogate established experimental colitis in mice. J Exp Med 1995;182:1281–1290.

42. Miller MJ, Sadowski-Krowicka H, Chotinaruemol S et al. Amelioration of chronic ileitis by nitric oxide synthase inhibition. J Pharmacol Exp Ther 1993;264:11–16.

43. Bouma G, Kaushiva A, Strober W. Experimental murine colitis is regulated by two genetic loci, including one on chromosome 11 that regulates IL-12 responses. Gastroenterology 2002;123:554–565.

44. Wallace JL, Keenan CM. An orally active inhibitor of leukotriene synthesis accelerates healing in a rat model of colitis. Am J Physiol 1990;258:G527–G534.

45. Ajuebor MN, Hogaboam CM, Kunkel SL et al. The chemokine RANTES is a crucial mediator of the progression from acute to chronic colitis in the rat. J Immunol 2001;166:552–558.

46. Stuber E, Strober W, Neurath M. Blocking the CD40L–CD40 interaction in vivo specifically prevents the priming of T helper 1 cells through the inhibition of interleukin 12 secretion. J Exp Med 1996;183:693–698.

47. Neurath MF, Fuss I, Pasparakis M et al. Predominant pathogenic role of tumor necrosis factor in experimental colitis in mice. Eur J Immunol 1997;27:1743–1750.

48. Wirtz S, Finotto S, Kanzler S et al. Cutting edge: chronic intestinal inflammation in STAT-4 transgenic mice: characterization of disease and adoptive transfer by TNF- plus IFN-gamma-producing CD4+ T cells that respond to bacterial antigens. J Immunol 1999;162:1884–1888.

49. Neurath MF, Pettersson S, Meyer ZBK et al. Local administration of antisense phosphorothioate oligonucleotides to the p65 subunit of NF-kappa B abrogates established experimental colitis in mice. Nature Med 1996;2:998–1004.

50. Dohi T, Fujihashi K, Kiyono H et al. Mice deficient in Th1- and Th2-type cytokines develop distinct forms of hapten-induced colitis. Gastroenterology 2000;119:724–733.

51. Duchmann R, Schmitt E, Knolle P et al. Tolerance towards resident intestinal flora in mice is abrogated in experimental colitis and restored by treatment with interleukin-10 or antibodies to interleukin-12. Eur J Immunol 1996;26:934–938.

52. Videla S, Vilaseca J, Guarner F et al. Role of intestinal microflora in chronic inflammation and ulceration of the rat colon. Gut 1994;35:1090–1097.

53. Neurath MF, Fuss I, Kelsall BL et al. Experimental granulomatous colitis in mice is abrogated by induction of TGF-beta-mediated oral tolerance. J Exp Med 1996;183:2605–2616.

54. Elson CO, Beagley KW, Sharmanov AT et al. Hapten-induced model of murine inflammatory bowel disease: mucosa immune responses and protection by tolerance. J Immunol 1996;157:2174–2185.

55. Fuss IJ, Boirivant M, Lacy B et al. The interrelated roles of TGF-beta and IL-10 in the regulation of experimental colitis. J Immunol 2002;168:900–908.

56. Kitani A, Fuss IJ, Nakamura K et al. Treatment of experimental (trinitrobenzene sulfonic acid) colitis by intranasal administration of transforming growth factor (TGF-)-β1 plasmid: TGF-β1-mediated suppression of T helper cell type 1 response occurs by interleukin (IL)-10 induction and IL-12 receptor β2 chain downregulation. J Exp Med 2000;192:41–52.

57. Lindsay J, van Montfrans C, Brennan F et al. IL-10 gene therapy prevents TNBS-induced colitis. Gene Ther 2002;9:1715–1721.

58. Neurath M, Fuss I, Strober W: TNBS-colitis. Int Rev Immunol 2000;19:51–62.

59. Girardin SE, Travassos LH, Have M. Peptidoglycan molecular requirements allowing detection by NOD1 and NOD2. J Biol Chem 2003; (in press).

60. Beutler B. Toll-like receptors: how they work and what they do. Curr Opin Hematol 2002;9:2–10.

61. Jobin C. Intestinal epithelial cells and innate immunity in the intestine: Is CARD15/NOD2 another player? Gastroenterology 2003;124:1145–1149.

62. Sartor RB, Cromartie WJ, Powell DW et al. Granulomatous enterocolitis induced in rats by purified bacterial cell wall fragments. Gastroenterology 1985;89:587–595.

63. McCall RD, Haskill S, Zimmermann EM et al. Tissue interleukin 1 and interleukin-1 receptor antagonist expression in enterocolitis in resistant and susceptible rats. Gastroenterology 1994;106:960–972.

64. Sartor RB, De La Cadena RA, Green KD et al. Selective kallikrein–kinin system activation in inbred rats differentially susceptible to granulomatous enterocolitis. Gastroenterology 1996;110:1467–1481.

65. Herfarth HH, Mohanty SP, Rath HC et al. Interleukin 10 suppresses experimental chronic, granulomatous inflammation induced by bacterial cell wall polymers. Gut 1996;39:836–845.

66. Yamada T, Sartor RB, Marshall S et al. Mucosal injury and inflammation in a model of chronic granulomatous colitis in rats. Gastroenterology 1993;104:759–771.

67. Zimmermann EM, Sartor RB, McCall RD et al. Insulinlike growth factor I and interleukin 1 beta messenger RNA in a rat model of granulomatous enterocolitis and hepatitis. Gastroenterology 1993;105:399–409.

68. Conner EM, Brand S, Davis JM et al. Proteasome inhibition attenuates nitric oxide synthase expression, VCAM-1 transcription and the development of chronic colitis. J Pharmacol Exp Ther 1997;282:1615–1622.

69. Sartor RB, Bender DE, Allen JB et al. Chronic experimental enterocolitis and extraintestinal inflammation are T lymphocyte dependent. Gastroenterology 1993;104:775A (Abstract).

70. Herfarth HH, Bocker U, Janardhanam R et al. Subtherapeutic corticosteroids potentiate the ability of interleukin 10 to prevent chronic inflammation in rats. Gastroenterology 1998;115:856–865.

71. Sartor RB, Holt LC, Bender DE et al. Prevention and treatment of chronic relapsing enterocolitis in rats by in vivo degradation of bacterial cell wall polymers. Gastroenterology 1991;100:613A (Abstract).

72. van Tol EA, Holt L, Li FL et al. Bacterial cell wall polymers promote intestinal fibrosis by direct stimulation of myofibroblasts. Am J Physiol 1999;277:G245–G255.

73. Boirivant M, Fuss IJ, Chu A et al. Oxazolone colitis: A murine model of T helper cell type 2 colitis treatable with antibodies to interleukin 4. J Exp Med 1998;188:1929–1939.

74. Heller F, Fuss IJ, Nieuwenhuis EE et al. Oxazolone colitis, a Th2 colitis model resembling ulcerative colitis, is mediated by IL-13-producing NK-T cells. Immunity 2002;17:629–638.

75. Hammer RE, Maika SD, Richardson JA et al. Spontaneous inflammatory disease in transgenic rats expressing HLA-B27 and human beta 2m: an animal model of HLA-B27-associated human disorders. Cell 1990;63:1099–1112.

76. Sartor RB. Colitis in HLA-B27/beta 2 microglobulin transgenic rats. Int Rev Immunol 2000;19:39–50.

77. Rath HC, Herfarth HH, Ikeda JS et al. Normal luminal bacteria, especially Bacteroides species, mediate chronic colitis, gastritis, and arthritis in HLA-B27/human beta2 microglobulin transgenic rats. J Clin Invest 1996;98:945–953.

78. Dieleman LA, Hoentjen F, Williams R et al. B cells from mesenteric lymph nodes of resistant rats produce more interleukin-10 than those from B27 transgenic rats following in vitro stimulation with cecal bacterial lysate. Gastroenterology 2002;122:A261 (Abstract).

79. Hoentjen F, Tonkongy SL, Torrice C et al. B cells from mesenteric lymph nodes of resistant rats produce more TGF than those from B27 transgenic rats following in vitro stimulation with cecal bacterial lysate. Gastroenterology 2003;124: A487 (Abstract).

80. Breban M, Fernandez-Sueiro JL, Richardson JA et al. T cells, but not thymic exposure to HLA-B27, are required for the inflammatory disease of HLA-B27 transgenic rats. J Immunol 1996;156:794–803.

81. Breban M, Hammer RE, Richardson JA et al. Transfer of the inflammatory disease of HLA-B27 transgenic rats by bone marrow engraftment. J Exp Med 1993;178:1607–1616.

82. Taurog JD, Richardson JA, Croft JT et al. The germfree state prevents development of gut and joint inflammatory disease in HLA-B27 transgenic rats. J Exp Med 1994;180:2359–2364.

83. Rath HC, Wilson KH, Sartor RB. Differential induction of colitis and gastritis in HLA-B27 transgenic rats selectively colonized with Bacteroides vulgatus and Escherichia coli. Infect Immun 1999;67:2969–2974.

84. Mann BA, Kim SC, Sartor RB. Selective induction of experimental colitis by monoassociation of HLA-B27 transgenic rats with various enteric Bacteroides species. Gastroenterology 2003;124: A322 (Abstract).

85. Dieleman LA, Goerres M, Arends A et al. Lactobacillus GG prevents recurrence of colitis in HLA-B27 transgenic rats after antibiotic treatment. Gut 2003;52:370–376.

86. Sadlack B, Merz H, Schorle H et al. Ulcerative colitis-like disease in mice with a disrupted interleukin-2 gene. Cell 1993;75:253–261.

87. Schultz M, Tonkonogy SL, Sellon RK et al. IL-2-deficient mice raised under germfree conditions develop delayed mild focal intestinal inflammation. Am J Physiol 1999;276:G1461–G1472.

88. Kundig TM, Schorle H, Bachmann MF et al. Immune responses in interleukin-2-deficient mice. Science 1993;262:1059–1061.

89. Schultz M, Clarke SH, Arnold LW et al. Disrupted B-lymphocyte development and survival in interleukin-2-deficient mice. Immunology 2001;104:127–134.

90. Ma A, Datta M, Margosian E et al. T cells, but not B cells, are required for bowel inflammation in interleukin 2-deficient mice. J Exp Med 1995;182:1567–1572.

91. Ehrhardt RO, Ludviksson BR, Gray B et al. Induction and prevention of colonic inflammation in IL-2-deficient mice. J Immunol 1997;158:566–573.

92. Kneitz B, Herrmann T, Yonehara S et al. Normal clonal expansion but impaired Fas-mediated cell death and anergy induction in interleukin-2-deficient mice. Eur J Immunol 1995;25:2572–2577.

93. Kramer S, Schimpl A, Hunig T. Immunopathology of interleukin (IL) 2-deficient mice: thymus dependence and suppression by thymus-dependent cells with an intact IL-2 gene. J Exp Med 1995;182:1769–1776.

94. Almeida AR, Legrand N, Papiernik M et al. Homeostasis of peripheral CD4+ T cells: IL-2R alpha and IL-2 shape a population of regulatory cells that controls CD4+ T cell numbers. J Immunol 2002;169:4850–4860.

95. Papiernik M, de Moraes ML, Pontoux C et al. Regulatory CD4 T cells: expression of IL-2R alpha chain, resistance to clonal deletion and IL-2 dependency. Int Immunol 1998;10:371–378.

96. Contractor NV, Bassiri H, Reya T et al. Lymphoid hyperplasia, autoimmunity, and compromised intestinal intraepithelial lymphocyte development in colitis-free gnotobiotic IL-2-deficient mice. J Immunol 1998;160:385–394.

97. Kuhn R, Lohler J, Rennick D et al. Interleukin-10-deficient mice develop chronic enterocolitis. Cell 1993;75:263–274.

98. Sellon RK, Tonkonogy S, Schultz M et al. Resident enteric bacteria are necessary for development of spontaneous colitis and immune system activation in interleukin-10-deficient mice. Infect Immun 1998;66:5224–5231.

99. Berg DJ, Davidson N, Kuhn R et al. Enterocolitis and colon cancer in interleukin-10-deficient mice are associated with aberrant cytokine production and CD4(+) Th1-like responses. J Clin Invest 1996;98:1010–1020.

100. Berg DJ, Kuhn R, Rajewsky K et al. Interleukin-10 is a central regulator of the response to LPS in murine models of endotoxic shock and the Shwartzman reaction but not endotoxin tolerance. J Clin Invest 1995;96:2339–2347.

101. Kim SC, Tonkonogy SL, Sartor RB. Role of endogenous IL-10 in downregulating proinflammatory cytokine expression. Gastroenterology 2001;120:A183 (Abstract).

102. Albright C, Tonkonogy SL, Sartor RB. Endogenous IL-10 inhibits APC stimulation of T lymphocyte responses to luminal bacteria. Gastroenterology 2002;122:A270 (Abstract).

103. Davidson NJ, Leach MW, Fort MM et al. T helper cell 1-type CD4+ T cells, but not B cells, mediate colitis in interleukin 10-deficient mice. J Exp Med 1996;184:241–251.

104. Seibold F, Brandwein S, Simpson S et al. pANCA represents a cross-reactivity to enteric bacterial antigens. J Clin Immunol 1998;18:153–160.

105. Davidson NJ, Judak SA, Lesley RE et al. IL-12, but not IFN-gamma, plays a major role in sustaining the chronic phase of colitis in IL-10 deficient mice. J Immunol 1998;161:3143–3149.

106. Schreiber S, Fedorak RN, Nielsen OH et al. A safety and efficacy study of recombinant human interleukin-10 (rHuIL-10) treatment in 329 patients with chronic active Crohn's disease (CACD). Gastroenterology 1998;113:383–389.

107. Spencer DM, Veldman GM, Banerjee S et al. Distinct inflammatory mechanisms mediate early versus late colitis in mice. Gastroenterology 2002;122:94–105.

108. Dieleman LA, Arends A, Tonkonogy SL et al. Helicobacter hepaticus does not induce or potentiate colitis in interleukin-10-deficient mice. Infect Immun 2000;68:5107–5113.

109. Schultz M, Veltkamp C, Dieleman LA et al. Lactobacillus plantarum 299V in the treatment and prevention of spontaneous colitis in interleukin-10 deficient mice. Inflamm Bowel Dis 2002;8:71–80.

110. Sydora BC, Tavernini MM, Jewell LD et al. Effect of bacterial monoassociation on tolerance and intestinal inflammation in IL-10 gene-deficient mice. Gastroenterology 2001;120:A517 (Abstract).

111. Kim SC, Tonkonogy SL, Albright CA et al. Regional and host specificity of colitis in mice mono associated with different nonpathogenic bacteria. 2003;124: A485 (Abstract).

112. Albright C, Tonkonogy SL, Frelinger JA et al. Adoptive transfer of E. faecalis-pulsed dendritic cells accelerates colitis in IL-10 deficient mice. Gastroenterology 2003;124: A73 (Abstract).

113. Hoentjen F, Harmsen HJ, Bradt H et al. Antibodies with a selective aerobic on anaerobic spectrum have different therapeutic activities in various regions of the colon in IL-10 deficient mice. Gut 2003; (in press).

114. Madsen KL, Doyle JS, Tavernini MM et al. Antibiotic therapy attenuates colitis in interleukin 10 gene-deficient mice. Gastroenterology 2000;118:1094–1155.

115. Madsen K, Cornish A, Soper P et al. Probiotic bacteria enhance murine and human intestinal epithelial barrier function. Gastroenterology 2001;121:580–591.

116. Kullberg MC, Jankovic D, Gorelick PL et al. Bacteria-triggered CD4(+) T regulatory cells suppress Helicobacter hepaticus-induced colitis. J Exp Med 2003;196:505–515.

117. Bristol IJ, Farmer MA, Cong Y et al. Heritable susceptibility for colitis in mice induced by IL-10 deficiency. Inflamm Bowel Dis 2000;6:290–302.

118. Farmer MA, Sundberg JP, Bristol IJ et al. A major quantitative trait locus on chromosome 3 controls colitis severity in IL-10-deficient mice. Proc Natl Acad Sci USA 2001;98:13820–13825.

119. Spencer SD, Di Marco F, Hooley J et al. The orphan receptor CRF2-4 is an essential subunit of the interleukin 10 receptor. J Exp Med 1998;187:571–578.

120. Takeda K, Clausen BE, Kaisho T et al. Enhanced Th1 activity and development of chronic enterocolitis in mice devoid of Stat3 in macrophages and neutrophils. Immunity 1999;10:39–49.

121. Welte T, Zhang SSM, Wang T et al. STAT3 deletion during hematopoiesis causes Crohn's disease-like pathogenesis and lethality: A critical role of STAT3 in innate immunity. Proc Natl Acad Sci USA 2003;100:1879–1884.

122. Rudolph U, Finegold MJ, Rich SS et al. Ulcerative colitis and adenocarcinoma of the colon in G alpha i2-deficient mice. Nature Genet 1995;10:143–150.

123. Hornquist CE, Lu X, Rogers-Fani PM et al. G(alpha)i2-deficient mice with colitis exhibit a local increase in memory CD4+ T cells and proinflammatory Th1-type cytokines. J Immunol 1997;158:1068–1077.

124. Ohman L, Franzen L, Rudolph U et al. Immune activation in the intestinal mucosa before the onset of colitis in Gαi2-deficient mice. Scand J Immunol 2000;52:80–90.

125. He J, Gurunathan S, Iwasaki A et al. Primary role for Gi protein signaling in the regulation of interleukin 12 production and the induction of T helper cell type 1 responses. J Exp Med 2000;191:1605–1610.

126. Panwala CM, Jones JC, Viney JL. A novel model of inflammatory bowel disease: mice deficient for the multiple drug resistance gene, mdr1a, spontaneously develop colitis. J Immunol 1998;161:5733–5744.

127. ten Hove T, Drillenburg P, Wijnholds J et al. Differential susceptibility of multidrug resistance protein-1 deficient mice to DSS and TNBS-induced colitis. Dig Dis Sci 2002;47:2056–2063.

128. Maggio-Price L, Shows D, Waggie K et al. Helicobacter bilis infection accelerates and H. hepaticus infection delays the development of colitis in multiple drug resistance-deficient (mdr1a−/−) mice. Am J Pathol 2002;160:739–751.

129. Yacyshyn BR, Maksymowych W, Bowen-Yacyshyn MB. Differences in P-glycoprotein-170 expression and activity between Crohn's disease and ulcerative colitis. Hum Immunol 1999;60:677–687.

130. Schwab M, Schaeffeler E, Marx C et al. Association between the C3435T MDR1 gene polymorphism and susceptibility for ulcerative colitis. Gastroenterology 2003;124:26–33.

131. Farrell RJ, Murphy A, Long A et al. High multidrug resistance (P-glycoprotein 170) expression in inflammatory bowel disease patients who fail medical therapy. Gastroenterology 2000;118:279–288.

132. Kontoyiannis D, Pasparakis M, Pizarro TT et al. Impaired on/off regulation of TNF biosynthesis in mice lacking TNF AU-rich elements: implications for joint and gut-associated immunopathologies. Immunity 1999;10:387–398.

133. Kontoyannis D, Boulougouris G, Manoloukos M et al. Genetic dissection of the cellular pathways and signaling mechanisms in modeled tumor necrosis factor-induced Crohn's-like inflammatory bowel disease. J Exp Med 2002;196:1563–1574.

134. Clegg CH, Rulffes JT, Haugen HS et al. Thymus dysfunction and chronic inflammatory disease in gp39 transgenic mice. Int Immunol 1997;9:1111–1122.

135. Cong Y, Weaver CT, Lazenby A et al. Colitis induced by enteric bacterial antigen-specific CD4+ T cells requires CD40–CD40 ligand interactions for a sustained increase in mucosal IL-12. J Immunol 2000;165:2173–2182.

136. de Jong YP, Comiskey M, Kalled SL et al. Chronic murine colitis is dependent on the CD154/CD40 pathway and can be attenuated by anti-CD154 administration. Gastroenterology 2000;119:715–723.

137. Byrne RF, Whoriskey JS, Sarmiento U. Transgenic mice overexpressing the B7 related protein-1 (B7RP-1) develop an intestinal pathology similar to human Crohn's disease. A new mouse model of inflammatory bowel disease. Gastroenterology 2001;120:A47 (Abstract).

138. Totsuka T, Kanai T, Iiyama R et al. Ameliorating effect of anti-inducible co-stimulator monoclonal antibody in a murine model of chronic colitis. Gastroenterology 2003;124:410–421.

138a. Watanabe M, Ueno Y, Yajima T et al. Interleukin 7 transgenic mice develop chronic colitis with decreased IL-7 protein accumulation in colonic mucosa. J Exp Med 1998;187:389–402.

139. Lee EG, Boone DL, Chai S et al. Failure to regulate TNF-induced NF-kappaB and cell death responses in A20-deficient mice. Science 2000;289:2350–2354.

140. Boone DL, Lee EG, Libby S et al. Recent advances in understanding NF-κB regulation. Inflamm Bowel Dis 2002;8:201–212.

141. Jobin C, Sartor RB. The IκB/NF-κB system: a key determinant of mucosal inflammation and protection. Am J Physiol Cell Physiol 2000;278:C451–C462.

142. Shull MM, Ormsby I, Kier AB et al. Targeted disruption of the mouse transforming growth factor-beta 1 gene results in multifocal inflammatory disease. Nature 1992;359:693–699.

143. Kulkarni AB, Ward JM, Yaswen L et al. Transforming growth factor-beta 1 null mice. An animal model for inflammatory disorders. Am J Pathol 1995;146:264–275.

144. Flavell RA, Gorelik L, Flavell. Abrogation of TGF-beta signaling in T cells leads to spontaneous T cell differentiation and autoimmune disease. Immunity 2000;12:171–181.

145. Yang X, Letterio JJ, Lechleider RJ et al. Targeted disruption of SMAD3 results in impaired mucosal immunity and diminished T cell responsiveness to TGF-beta. EMBO J 1999;18:1280–1291.

146. Diebold RJ, Eis MJ, Yin M et al. Early-onset multifocal inflammation in the transforming growth factor beta 1-null mouse is lymphocyte mediated. Proc Natl Acad Sci USA 1995;92:12215–12219.

147. Letterio JJ, Geiser AG, Kulkarni AB et al. Autoimmunity associated with TGF-beta1-deficiency in mice is dependent on MHC class II antigen expression. J Clin Invest 1996;98:2109–2119.

148. Boivin GP, Ormsby I, Jones-Carson J et al. Germ-free and barrier-raised TGF-beta 1-deficient mice have similar inflammatory lesions. Transgenic Res 1997;6:197–202.

149. Mombaerts P, Mizoguchi E, Grusby MJ et al. Spontaneous development of inflammatory bowel disease in T cell receptor mutant mice. Cell 1993;75:274–282.

150. Bhan AK, Mizoguchi E, Smith RN et al. Spontaneous chronic colitis in TCR alpha-mutant mice; an experimental model of human ulcerative colitis. Int Rev Immunol 2000;29:123–138.

151. Das KM, Dasgupta A, Mandal A et al. Autoimmunity to cytoskeletal protein tropomyosin. A clue to the pathogenetic mechanism for ulcerative colitis. J Immunol 1993;150:2487–2493.

152. Mizoguchi A, Mizoguchi E, Smith RN et al. Suppressive role of B cells in chronic colitis of T cell receptor alpha mutant mice. J ExpMed 1997;186:1749–1756.

153. Mizoguchi A, Mizoguchi E, Saubermann LJ et al. Limited CD4 T-cell diversity associated with colitis in T-cell receptor alpha mutant mice requires a T helper 2 environment. Gastroenterology 2000;119:983–995.

154. Dianda L, Hanby AM, Wright NA et al. T cell receptor-αβ-deficient mice fail to develop colitis in the absence of a microbial environment. Am J Pathol 1997;150:91–97.

155. Mizoguchi A, Mizoguchi E, Chiba C et al. Role of appendix in the development of inflammatory bowel disease in TCR-alpha mutant mice. J Exp Med 1996;184:707–715.

156. Hermiston ML, Gordon JI. Inflammatory bowel disease and adenomas in mice expressing a dominant negative N-cadherin. Science 1995;270:1203–1207.

157. Baribault H, Penner J, Iozzo RV et al. Colorectal hyperplasia and inflammation in keratin 8-deficient FVB/N mice. Genes Dev 1994;8:2964–2973.

158. Iwakiri D, Podolsky DK. Keratinocyte growth factor promotes goblet cell differentiation through regulation of goblet cell silencer inhibitor. Gastroenterology 2001;120:1372–1380.

159. Miller AM, Elliot PR, Connell W et al. A novel model of ulcerative colitis based on genetic manipulation of the glycosylation of colonic mucins. Gastroenterology 2000;118:A687 (Abstract).

160. Snapper SB, Rosen FS, Mizoguchi E et al. Wiskott–Aldrich syndrome protein-deficient mice reveal a role for WASP in T but not B cell activation. Immunity 1998;9:81–91.

161. Koh WP, Chan E, Scott K et al. TCR-mediated involvement of CD4+ transgenic T cells in spontaneous inflammatory bowel disease in lymphopenic mice. J Immunol 1999;162:7208–7216.

162. Iqbal N, Oliver JR, Wagner FH et al. T helper 1 and T helper 2 cells are pathogenic in an antigen-specific model of colitis. J Exp Med 2002;195:71–84.

163. Yoshida M, Shirai Y, Watanabe T et al. Differential localization of colitogenic Th1 and Th2 cells monospecific to a micro flora-associated antigen in mice. Gastroenterology 2002;123:1949–1961.

164. Chalifoux LV, Bronson RT. Colonic adenocarcinoma associated with chronic colitis in cotton top marmosets, Saguinus oedipus. Gastroenterology 1981;80:942–946.

165. Podolsky DK, Madara JL, King N et al. Colonic mucin composition in primates. Selective alterations associated with spontaneous colitis in the cotton-top tamarin. Gastroenterology 1985;88:20–25.

166. Podolsky DK, Lobb R, King N et al. Attenuation of colitis in the cotton-top tamarin by anti-alpha 4 integrin monoclonal antibody. J Clin Invest 1993;92:372–380.

167. Wood JD, Peck OC, Tefend KS et al. Evidence that colitis is initiated by environmental stress and sustained by fecal factors in the cotton-top tamarin (Saguinus oedipus). Dig Dis Sci 2000;45:385–393.

168. Wood JD, Peck OC, Tefend KS et al. Colitis and colon cancer in cotton-top tamarins (Saguinus oedipus oedipus) living wild in their natural habitat. Dig Dis Sci 1998;3:1443–1453.

169. Sundberg JP, Elson CO, Bedigian H et al. Spontaneous, heritable colitis in a new substrain of C3H/HeJ mice. Gastroenterology 1994;107:1726–1735.

170. Brandwein SL, McCabe RP, Cong Y et al. Spontaneously colitic C3H/HeJBir mice demonstrate selective antibody reactivity to antigens of the enteric bacterial flora. J Immunol 1997;159:44–52.

171. Cong Y, Brandwein SL. McCabe RP et al. CD4+ T cells reactive to enteric bacterial antigens in spontaneously colitic C3H/HeJBir mice: increased T helper cell type 1 response and ability to transfer disease. J Exp Med 1998;187:855–864.

172. Cong Y, Weaver CT, Lazenby A et al. Bacterial-reactive T regulatory cells inhibit pathogenic immune responses to the enteric flora. J Immunol 2002;169:6112–6119.

173. Matsumoto S, Okabe Y, Setoyama H et al. Inflammatory bowel disease-like enteritis and caecitis in a senescence accelerated mouse P1/Yit strain. Gut 1998;43:71–78.

174. Kosiewicz MM, Nast CC, Krishnan A et al. Th1-type responses mediate spontaneous ileitis in a novel murine model of Crohn's disease. J Clin Invest 2001;107:695–702.

175. Rivera-Nieves J, Bamias G, Vidrich A et al. Emergence of perianal fistulizing disease in the SAMP1/YitFc mouse, a spontaneous model of chronic ileitis. Gastroenterology 2003;124:972–982.

176. Bamias G, Marini M, Moskaluk CA et al. Down-regulation of intestinal lymphocyte activation and Th1 cytokine production by antibiotic therapy in a murine model of Crohn's disease. J Immunol 2002;169:5308–5314.

177. Kozaiwa K, Sugawara K, Smith MF Jr et al. Identification of a quantitative trait for ileitis in a spontaneous mouse model of Crohn's disease: SAMP-1/Yit. Gastroenterology 2003;125:477–490.

178. Powrie F, Leach MW, Mauze S et al. Phenotypically distinct subsets of CD4+ T cells induce or protect from chronic intestinal inflammation in C. B-17 scid mice. Int Immunol 1993;5:1461–1471.

179. Morrissey PJ, Charrier K, Braddy S et al. CD4+ T cells that express high levels of CD45RB induce wasting disease when transferred into congenic severe combined

immunodeficient mice. Disease development is prevented by cotransfer of purified CD4+ T cells. J Exp Med 1993;178:237–244.

180. Powrie F, Mason D: OX-22high CD4+ T cells induce wasting disease with multiple organ pathology: prevention by the OX-22low subset. J Exp Med 1990;172:1701–1708.

181. Powrie F, Leach MW, Mauze S et al. Inhibition of Th1 responses prevents inflammatory bowel disease in scid mice reconstituted with CD45RBhi CD4+ T cells. Immunity 1994;1:553–562.

182. Picarella D, Hurlbut P, Rottman J et al. Monoclonal antibodies specific for beta 7 integrin and mucosal addressin cell adhesion molecule-1 (MAdCAM-1) reduce inflammation in the colon of scid mice reconstituted with CD45RBhigh CD4+ T cells. J Immunol 1997;158:2099–2106.

183. Aranda R, Sydora BC, McAllister PL et al. Analysis of intestinal lymphocytes in mouse colitis mediated by transfer of CD4+, CD45RBhigh T cells to SCID recipients. J Immunol 1997;158:3464–3473.

184. Brimnes J, Reimann J, Nissen M et al. Enteric bacterial antigens activate CD4(+) T cells from scid mice with inflammatory bowel disease. Eur J Immunol 2001;31:23–31.

185. Morrissey PJ, Charrier K. Induction of wasting disease in SCID mice by the transfer of normal CD4+/CD45RBhi T cells and the regulation of this autoreactivity by CD4+/CD45RBlo T cells. Res Immunol 1994;145:357–362.

186. Matsuda JL, Gapin L, Sydora BC et al. Systemic activation and antigen-driven oligoclonal expansion of T cells in a mouse model of colitis. J Immunol 2000;164:2797–2806.

187. Read S, Malmstrom V, Powrie F. Cytotoxic T lymphocyte-associated antigen 4 plays an essential role in the function of CD25(+)CD4(+) regulatory cells that control intestinal inflammation. J Exp Med 2000;192:295–302.

188. Powrie F, Carlino J, Leach MW et al. A critical role for transforming growth factor-beta but not interleukin 4 in the suppression of T helper type 1-mediated colitis by CD45RB(low) CD4+ T cells. J Exp Med 1996;183:2669–2674.

189. Hagenbaugh A, Sharma S, Dubinett SM et al. Altered immune responses in interleukin 10 transgenic mice. J Exp Med 1997;185:2101–2110.

190. Asseman C, Mauze S, Leach MW et al. An essential role for interleukin 10 in the function of regulatory T cells that inhibit intestinal inflammation. J Exp Med 1999;190:995–1004.

191. van Montfrans C, Rodriguez-Pena MS, Pronk I et al. Prevention of colitis by interleukin 10-transduced T lymphocytes in the SCID mice transfer model. Gastroenterology 2002;123:1865–1876.

192. Rietdijk ST, Faubion W, Albright C et al. CD4+ CD25+ regulatory T cells originating from germ free mice have impaired suppressive abilities. Gastroenterology 2002;122:A387 (Abstract).

193. Groux H, O'Garra A, Bigler M et al. A CD4+ T-cell subset inhibits antigen-specific T-cell responses and prevents colitis. Nature 1997;389:737–742.

194. Hollander GA, Simpson SJ, Mizoguchi E et al. Severe colitis in mice with aberrant thymic selection. Immunity 1995;3:27–38.

195. Simpson SJ, Shah S, Comiskey M et al. T cell-mediated pathology in two models of experimental colitis depends predominantly on the interleukin 12/Signal transducer and activator of transcription (Stat)-4 pathway, but is not conditional on interferon gamma expression by T cells. J Exp Med 1998;187:1225–1234.

196. Mackay F, Browning JL, Lawton P et al. Both the lymphotoxin and tumor necrosis factor pathways are involved in experimental murine models of colitis. Gastroenterology 1998;115:1464–1475.

197. Veltkamp C, Tonkonogy SL, de Jong YP et al. Continuous stimulation by normal luminal bacteria is essential for the development and perpetuation of colitis in Tg(epsilon26) mice. Gastroenterology 2001;120:900–913.

198. Darfeuille-Michaud A, Neut C, Barnich N et al. Presence of adherent *Escherichia coli* strains in ileal mucosa of patients with Crohn's disease. Gastroenterology 1998;115:1405–1413.

## CHAPTER 10

# Microbial influences in inflammatory bowel diseases: role in pathogenesis and clinical implications

R Balfour Sartor

## INTRODUCTION

Enteric microbial agents have a key role in the pathogenesis of chronic relapsing intestinal inflammation and its complications, as demonstrated by compelling results from experimental animal models (Chapter 9) and developing evidence in human inflammatory bowel diseases (IBD). These studies indicate that adjuvants and antigens from commensal bacteria are required to activate and sustain pathogenic cell-mediated immune responses, enteric pathogens can initiate and reactivate inflammation, and that secondarily invading bacteria induce septic complications. This chapter outlines current knowledge of intestinal microecology, provides data supporting or refuting the most widely accepted theories for the pathogenesis for IBD, discusses developing evidence for key genetic/environmental influences in IBD, and suggests potential therapeutic applications of these observations. The reader is referred to a recent review[1] describing the septic complications of IBD and the pathogens that reactivate or potentiate disease.

## INTESTINAL MICROECOLOGY

The mammalian gastrointestinal tract contains an extremely complex ecosystem composed of predominantly anaerobic bacteria, with marked regional differences in their concentration and composition (Table 10.1).[2,3] Moreover, the human and rodent microbiota are considerably different, with the human stomach and duodenum containing approximately $10^2$ bacteria/mL, in contrast to $10^5$/mL in rodents. Therefore, it is difficult to extrapolate results in the proximal intestine of rodent models to human IBD. The human small intestine contains a proximal to distal gradient of luminal bacteria, with a change from aerobic or microaerophilic to anaerobic. The distal ileum contains $10^5–10^6$ bacteria/mL, with *Clostridia*,

*Bacteroides* and coliforms predominating.[4,5] The composition of the small intestine can change dramatically with clinical interventions, including gastric acid suppression, partial obstruction, fistulization to the colon, loss of the ileocecal valve, and antibiotic or probiotic use.

The colonic bacterial ecology is extremely complex, with at least 200 different species in a given host and striking interindividual host variations, leading to 400–500 bacterial species in the study population.[4,6] However, an individual's bacterial population is remarkably stable over time. Older culture techniques detect only a relatively small fraction (35%) of colonic bacteria owing to the strict anaerobic nature of many components,[4] although this can be increased to 90% recovery by extremely thorough techniques.[6] Molecular techniques such as polymerase chain reaction (PCR), denaturing gradient gel electrophoresis (DGGE) and fluorescent-labeled in situ hybridization (FISH), which analyze variable sequences in the small subunit (16s) of ribosomal DNA (rDNA), have revolutionized the study of complex bacterial systems, including the colon.[2,3] Wilson et al.[7,8] developed a molecular taxonomic classification of the enteric microbiota and demonstrated that virtually all common colonic bacteria fall into four phylogenetic clusters: *Bacteroides* species, *Bifidobacterium*, *Clostridium coccoides* and *Clostridium leptum/Fusobacterium*. These genera contain species which were placed in different genera based on older, biochemical-based methods, for example the *Clostridium coccoides* group contains *Clostridium*, *Peptostreptococcus*, *Eubacterium* and *Ruminococcus* species.[7] Together, these four genera contain 90% of identifiable organisms and outnumber the more widely recognized Enterobacteriaceae (*Escherichia coli*, *Klebsiella*, *Pseudomonas*) and *Enterococcus* species by at least 1000:1. However, even with the molecular methods, many organisms cannot be identified. Recent studies using FISH demonstrated that most enteric organisms do not adhere to the mucosa in normal hosts.[9]

The enteric bacterial population within an individual is remarkably stable and resists colonization by introduced bacteria

**Table 10.1 Gastrointestinal luminal bacteria in normal humans**

| Location | Concentration | Composition (dominant organisms) |
|---|---|---|
| Stomach | $0-10^2$ | Lactobacillus, Candida, Streptococcus, Helicobacter pylori, Peptostreptococcus |
| Duodenum | $10^2$ | Streptococcus, Lactobacillus |
| Jejunum | $10^2$ | Streptococcus, Lactobacillus |
| Proximal ileum | $10^3$ | Streptococcus, Lactobacillus |
| Distal ileum | $10^5-10^6$ | Clostridium, Bacteroides sp.,coliforms |
| Colon | $10^{11}$ | Bacteroides, Bifidobacterium,Clostridium coccoides, Clostridium lepium/Fusobacterium |

by competing for energy substrates and mucosal binding sites. This property of 'colonization resistance' protects against invading pathogens, explaining why *Clostridium difficile* infection is far more likely following antibiotic clearance of commensals,[10] and accounts for the inability of ingested probiotic organisms to persist for more than 2 weeks after daily administration is stopped.[11] Furthermore, antibiotic therapy only transiently changes the enteric bacterial composition, which rapidly returns to its pretreatment state.[12] Factors accounting for individual variation of organisms are poorly understood, but genetic and dietary influences contribute to continuity of the intestinal microecology.[13] Although diet does not dramatically alter fecal bacterial composition in population studies, [14,15] obvious differences exist between breast- and bottle-fed infants[16] and before and after weaning.[17] *Bifidobacteria* predominate over *E. coli* by 100–1000:1 in breastfed infants, perhaps explaining some of the observed epidemiologic trends for IBD in developed versus underdeveloped countries (Sandler and Loftus, Chapter 17). In neonatal mice, *Lactobacillus* and *Streptococcus* species predominate during suckling and complex anaerobic bacteria proliferate after weaning, because of the altered dietary energy substrates.[17] Colonic bacteria metabolize non-absorbed plant polysaccharide such as cellulose, hemicelluloses, pectins and sugars into volatile fatty acids, including butyrate, propionic and acetic acids, as well as $CO_2$ and $H_2$.[18] Some commensal bacteria, particularly probiotic species such as *Lactobacillus* and *Bifidobacteria*, limit colonization by other species. Lactic acid bacteria alter the luminal microenvironment by changing the pH through the production of short-chain fatty acids (SCFA), altering the redox potential, or secreting bactericidal products (bacteriocins).[19] Furthermore, enteric bacteria rapidly and efficiently share DNA, including antibiotic resistance genes.[20]

Gut bacteria influence host epithelial metabolism, growth and differentiation and mucosal immune responses. Short-chain fatty acids (SCFA), particularly butyrate, are the primary energy source of colonocytes, particularly in the distal colon,[21] influence epithelial growth and differentiation[22] and regulate immune functions. Certain bacterial species produce sulfides from colonic mucins and dietary sulfates, particularly meat;[23] this sulfide production blocks epithelial butyrate utilization and has been postulated to cause ulcerative colitis.[24] *Bacteroides thetaiotaomicron* regulates host epithelial fucose metabolism with parallel derepression of fucose-metabolizing enzymes in luminal *B. thetaiotaomicron* by host-derived fucose.[25] Similarly, commensal enteric bacteria induce ileal mucosal expression of fucosyltransferase but inhibit epithelial sialyltransferase in mice.[26] It is likely that

a variety of similar microbial–host interactions profoundly influence host epithelial function. Commensal enteric bacteria also regulate mucosal immune responses. Germ-free (sterile) mice and rats have underdeveloped Peyer's patches, lamina propria and mesenteric lymph node (MLN) mononuclear cell populations, have defective B-cell responses, and fail to mount effective delayed-type hypersensitivity T-cell responses.[27] Of considerable potential importance to IBD is the fact that commensal bacteria, particularly Gram-negative organisms and LPS, induce certain forms of mucosal tolerance.[28,29]

Altered composition and functional activities of this exceedingly complex luminal microbiota could have profound implications for the pathogenesis, diagnosis and treatment of IBD. Abnormalities in the types and functions of bacteria colonizing the distal intestines of IBD patients are discussed in the section on dysbiosis.

# ROLE OF RESIDENT ENTERIC BACTERIA IN INTESTINAL AND SYSTEMIC INFLAMMATION

Adjuvants and antigens derived from commensal enteric bacteria stimulate cell-mediated immune responses, leading to chronic, relapsing enterocolitis (Table 10.2). The most obvious link is the consistent localization of intestinal inflammation to the colon, which is the site of highest luminal bacterial concentrations. These bacteria produce polymers (lipopolysaccharides (LPS), peptidoglycan and lipoteichoic acid) and DNA which activate innate immune cells (antigen-presenting and effector cells) through pattern recognition receptors (Toll-like receptors (TLR), NOD1, NOD2/CARD15) to secrete proinflammatory cytokines, inflammatory mediators and metalloproteases, as well as proteins and glycolipids that stimulate antigen-specific T-cell responses; Fig. 10.1A). Enhanced uptake of bacterial components occurs when environmental triggers (transient infections or toxic products) break the mucosal barrier or genetically mediated defects alter barrier function. Tissue damage and ulceration results from matrix destruction and cell death induced by products of bacterially activated macrophages, neutrophils, T lymphocytes, B cells, mesenchymal cells and biochemical cascades (complement, kallikrein–kinin). Secondary invasion of ulcerated tissues by viable bacteria perpetuate the local inflammatory response and cause septic complications (Fig. 10.1B).

**Table 10.2 Evidence that commensal luminal bacteria stimulate experimental and human chronic intestinal inflammation**

|  | Experimental enterocolitis | Crohn's disease | UC | Pouchitis |
|---|---|---|---|---|
| Location of ↑ bacterial concentrations | Colon | TI, colon | Colon | Ileal pouch |
| ↑ mucosal uptake of bacterial products | Yes | Yes | Yes | Yes |
| Response to anaerobic antibiotics | Yes | Yes | No | Yes |
| Response to aerobic antibiotics | +/– | Yes | +/– | Yes |
| ↓ inflammation with bypass | Yes | Yes | No | Yes |
| Disease in sterile environment | No | ? | ? | ? |
| Immune response to bacteria | Yes | Yes | Yes | ? |
| Exacerbation by pathogens | Yes | Yes | Yes | ? |
| Implicated commensal species | Bacteroides vulgatus E. coli Enterococcus faecium Helicobacter hepaticus | E. coli Bacteroides Enterococci Eubacteria Peptostrepto-coccus Fusobacterium | E. coli | Aerobic and anaerobic species |
| Protection with probiotics | Yes | ? | Yes | Yes |

# CLINICAL STUDIES

## Antibiotics

The results of clinical trials using antibiotics for the treatment of ulcerative colitis, Crohn's disease and pouchitis are detailed in Chapters 33, 34, 46, 47 and 49. In general, the results can be summarized as demonstrating no effect of antibiotics in active ulcerative colitis, a possible effect of metronidazole and/or ciprofloxacin for active Crohn's colitis, a possible effect of metronidazole and ornidazole for postoperative maintenance of remission in Crohn's disease, a possible effect of metronidazole and ciprofloxacin for perianal Crohn's disease, and a probable effect of metronidazole and ciprofloxacin for active pouchitis. Although the rationale for antibiotic use is clear from animal model studies, and many experienced clinicians use these agents extensively for Crohn's colitis, perianal fistulae and pouchitis, documentation by controlled clinical trials is meager.[30]

## Probiotics/prebiotics

The results of clinical trials using probiotics (a subset of commensal bacteria and species derived from fermented foods) to prevent or treat intestinal inflammation in patients with ulcerative colitis, Crohn's disease and pouchitis are detailed in Chapters 33, 34 and 46. In general, the results can be summarized as demonstrating definitive efficacy of an E. coli strain (E. coli Nissle 1917) for maintenance of remission in ulcerative colitis, and definite efficacy of a combination of four Lactobacillus species, three Bifidobacterium species and one Streptococcus salivarium species (VSL#3) for prophylaxis against pouchitis and maintenance of remission in patients with chronic pouchitis following colectomy with ileoanal pouch.[31-34] In patients with a history of chronic pouchitis, those treated with VSL#3 had increased tissue concentrations of IL-10 and decreased TNF levels.[35] Similarly, ex vivo exposure to certain Lactobacillus species decreased TNF secretion by active Crohn's disease mucosal tissues.[36]

Prebiotics are dietary substances, usually undigested carbohydrates, that foster the growth and metabolic activity of beneficial enteric bacteria, most notably Lactobacillus and Bifidobacteria.[37,38] These substances increase concentrations of commensal probiotic bacterial species, decrease luminal pH concentrations, enhance the production of short-chain fatty acids, especially butyrate, and improve the water-holding capacity of the stool. Although several prebiotics improve experimental colitis (see below), prebiotics have not been adequately tested in human IBD. Germinated barley extracts, a byproduct of beer production, decreased ulcerative colitis activity in a small uncontrolled study,[39] and psyllium fiber was superior to placebo in decreasing ulcerative colitis symptoms while increasing luminal Bifidobacterium concentrations and decreasing stool free water.[40]

## Bowel rest

Reducing concentrations of luminal bacteria, bacterial constituents and dietary antigens by surgical bypass, total parenteral nutrition (TPN) or elemental diets reproducibly diminishes symptoms and inflammation in Crohn's disease but has minimal benefit in ulcerative colitis.[41] Ninety-five per cent of patients with Crohn's colitis improve after surgical diversion of the fecal stream by a split ileostomy, but symptoms rapidly recur when bowel continuity is re-established.[42] Viable bacteria appear to mediate symptomatic recurrence rather than luminal antigens or toxic molecules, based on studies that introduced unfractionated or ultrafiltrates of ileal contents into the bypassed colon.[43] Similarly, proximal diverting ileostomy prevents recurrent inflammation in the bypassed neoterminal ileum after ileal resection, with rapid onset of distal ileitis following ileostomy takedown.[44] Infusion of ileostomy contents into the diverted ileum induced histologic and immunologic evidence of reactivation within 8 days.[45] Finally, Crohn's disease more frequently recurs following ileocolonic anastomosis than after standard ileostomy, despite identical exposure of the distal ileum to dietary antigens.

TPN or elemental diets improve two-thirds of patients with Crohn's disease, particularly those with small intestinal involvement.[46] In contrast, Crohn's colitis or ulcerative colitis symptoms do not consistently respond to nutritional therapy.

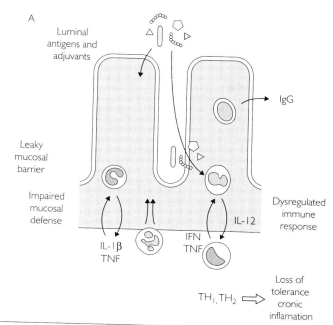

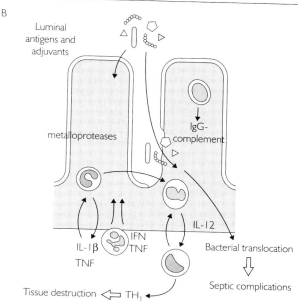

**Fig. 10.1** Induction and perpetuation of pathologic immune responses and tissue damage by commensal enteric bacteria in a susceptible host. (A) Initiation of inflammation. A complex mix of predominantly anaerobic bacteria populates the distal ileum and colon. Enhanced mucosal uptake of bacterial adjuvants and antigens due to an acquired (transient infection or ingested toxin) or intrinsic (host genetic) defect in mucosal barrier function activates resident innate immune responses. Genetically programmed immunoregulatory defects or continued antigenic stimulation (lack of mucosal healing or clearance of invading bacteria) lead to pathogenic (Th1 or Th2) immunologic responses to commensal bacterial antigens (loss of tolerance). (B) Perpetuation of inflammation, tissue damage and septic complications. Activation and recruitment of macrophages and neutrophils to the inflammatory focus and activation of the complement cascade stimulate production of cytokines and inflammatory mediators, such as reactive oxygen metabolites, nitric oxide etc., which cause tissue damage. Cytokine-induced metalloproteases damage matrix, leading to mucosal ulceration. Secondary bacterial translocation through these ulcers causes further tissue inflammation, local abscesses and regional and systemic distribution of bacterial products.

The beneficial mechanisms of these therapies remain obscure, as microbial concentrations are not altered, although total bacterial populations decrease with diminished fecal volume. Dietary antigens are probably not responsible, as TPN alone is not superior to TPN plus regular diet; elemental diets are not superior to polymeric diets; and exclusion diets have inconsistent results.[47] Roediger[48] suggests that lack of fat in enteral diets diminish the adjuvant activities of luminal bacteria, and Evans et al.[49] hypothesize that titanium dioxide and silica particles found in the Western diet induce disease. Further investigations are necessary to clarify the beneficial mechanisms of dietary manipulations in Crohn's ileitis.

## Secondary invasion by bacteria and uptake of bacterial components

Bacterial invasion of the inflamed mucosa of IBD patients and translocation to the lymphatic and portal circulations potentiate local tissue injury and cause local and systemic septic complica-

tions. Up to 27% of ulcerative colitis patients have portal vein bacteremia,[50] and IBD patients have an increased incidence of bacterial endocarditis and hepatic abscesses. The ulcerated mucosa and fistulae of Crohn's disease are particularly susceptible to bacterial invasion. Enteric bacteria were cultured from the serosa or MLN of 56% of Crohn's disease resected tissues but only 17% of those of controls.[51,52] E. coli and streptococcal antigen was present in two-thirds of inflamed Crohn's disease tissues, with immunohistochemical staining being particularly evident in areas of mucosal ulceration and fistulae, and bacterial antigen within granulomas.[52] E. coli antigen has been identified within lamina propria macrophages of ulcerative colitis patients.[53] Similarly, small rods and cocci invade the mucosa of 100% of ulcerative colitis patients, but not normal controls.[54] Similarly, intracellular bacteria-like structures have been reported within epithelial cells of IBD patients but not normal controls.[9] Bregman and Kirsner[55] reported biochemical evidence of bacterial invasion of ulcerative colitis tissues. Molecular techniques further document selective invasion of IBD tissues by

**Table 10.3 Serologic responses to specific microbial antigens by IBD patients and controls**

| Antigen | Frequency of positive serologic responses | | | |
| --- | --- | --- | --- | --- |
| | Ulcerative colitis, % | Crohn's disease, % | Inflammatory controls, % | Normal controls, % |
| pANCA[371,372] | 57–66 | 13–15 | 8 | 0–5 |
| ASCA[371,372] | 6–12 | 55–61 | 11 | 1–5 |
| Bacteroides vulgatus (26 kDa)[69] | 54 | NR[i] | NR | 9 |
| Pseudomonas fluorescens ($I_2$)[56] | 10 | 54 | 19 | 4 |
| Mycobacterium (HupB, 32 kDa)[81] | 10* | 90 | NR | 0 |
| Fusobacterium varium[80] | 61 | 13 | 13 | 3 |

*IgA antibody, $n = 10$/group. ASCA, anti-Saccharomyces cerevisiae antibody; NR, not reported; pANCA, perinuclear antineutrophil cytoplasmic antibody. Adapted from Sartor.[373]

commensal bacteria. Sutton et al.[56] identified a novel transcriptional regulation gene from *Pseudomonas fluorescens* within lamina propria mononuclear cells of 43% of Crohn's disease tissues compared with 9% ulcerative colitis and 5% control tissues. However, Chiba et al. were unable to document *Pseudomonas* 16s ribosomal RNA sequences in intestinal lymphoid follicles of Crohn's disease patients, although these investigators did find other commensal organisms in 28% of Crohn's tissues, 40% of ulcerative colitis samples, but only 2% of non-IBD control tissues.[57] Circulating bacterial products and immunologic responses to bacterial and dietary antigens further document enhanced uptake of luminal constituents in IBD patients. Circulating f-met-leu-phenylalanine (FMLP) is detectable in most patients with active Crohn's disease, ulcerative colitis and sclerosing cholangitis, but not in normal or inflammatory controls.[58] Approximately 10% of ambulatory and 94% of hospitalized patients with Crohn's disease have measurable plasma LPS; these levels correlate with disease activity.[59] Baldassano et al.[60] demonstrated enhanced reactivity of circulating monocytes from Crohn's disease patients. Serum from these patients contained increased LPS levels and could prime normal monocytes, a property reversed by removal of LPS. Similarly, Crohn's disease patients have increased serum antibodies to LPS and PG-PS, whereas patients with ulcerative colitis have intermediate levels.[61,62]

## Immune responses to commensal enteric bacteria

Antibody responses to multiple resident and pathogenic microbial and dietary antigens in IBD patients indicate either a generalized defect in mucosal permeability and/or enhanced immunologic responsiveness.[63–71] In addition, IBD patients have demonstrable T-lymphocyte responses to resident luminal bacteria.[72–75] These observations indicate a loss of immune tolerance in IBD patients.[76]

Selective serologic responses in IBD subpopulations to defined bacterial and yeast antigens raise the possibility that serologic markers can be used as diagnostic tools to differentiate Crohn's disease from ulcerative colitis and to identify homogeneous subpopulations of IBD patients which may selectively respond to different treatments[70] (see Chapter 29). Individual epitopes from *Bacteroides* species (*B. vulgatus*),[69] *B. ovatus*,[77] *B. caccae*,[78] *E. coli*,[79] *Pseudomonas fluorescens*,[56] *Fusobacterium varium*[80] and *Mycobacteria*[81] are selectively detected by sera from Crohn's disease or ulcerative colitis patients (Table 10.3).

Of potential clinical interest, Landers et al.[70] have identified IBD patient subsets with differing responses to defined microbial antigens. Cecal bacterial homogenates and several bacterial species react with perinuclear antineutrophilic cytoplasmic antibodies (pANCA), including *Bacteroides caccae*, *E. coli* and *Mycobacteria*.[79,81] Furthermore, the mycobacterial 32 kDa Hup B epitope exhibits homology with histone $H_1$, the putative mammalian epitope of pANCA.[81]

## Genetic regulation of immune responses to bacteria

Polymorphisms in the leucine-rich repeat (LRR) domain of intracellular NOD2/CARD15 are associated with Crohn's disease[82,83] (see Chapter 8). This domain binds to bacterial LPS and peptidoglycan (especially of Gram-negative organisms) to activate NFκB (Fig. 10.2).[84,85] The Crohn's disease-associated polymorphisms, particularly the 3020 insC mutation which truncates the C-terminal region of LRR, diminish NOD2 function.[83,85] NOD2/CARD15 is constitutively expressed in normal monocytes, macrophages and dendritic cells,[84] and in intestinal epithelial cells of IBD patients.[86,87] In vitro, TNF upregulates NOD2/CARD15 expression in intestinal epithelial cell lines, whereas epithelial expression is increased in active IBD.[86,87] NOD2/CARD15 expressed in intestinal epithelial cell lines mediate clearance of invasive *Salmonella* infection, whereas the 3020 insC truncation mutation of NOD2/CARD15 resulted in defective bacterial clearance,[86] suggesting that NOD2/CARD15 mutations associated with Crohn's disease may exert their biologic effects by defective clearance of invading intracellular pathogens, which is consistent with the recessive phenotype of this mutation.[82] An alternative mechanism is defective regulation of bacterially mediated induction of regulatory (suppressive) responses by mutated NOD2/CARD15. The observation that a polymorphism in the promoter region of CD14 is associated with Crohn's disease, but not ulcerative colitis,[88] provides independent support for defective innate immune responses to Gram-negative bacteria in Crohn's disease. CD14 is involved with LPS binding to Toll-like receptor-4 (TLR-4), which stimulates NFκB activation (Fig. 10.2). Thus, both intracellular and extracellular NFκB signaling by bacterial polymers are associated with Crohn's disease susceptibility. The NFκB signaling pathway is a key determinant of the inflammatory response and mucosal homeostasis.[89] The mechanism by which mdr1 polymorphisms mediate susceptibility to both chronically

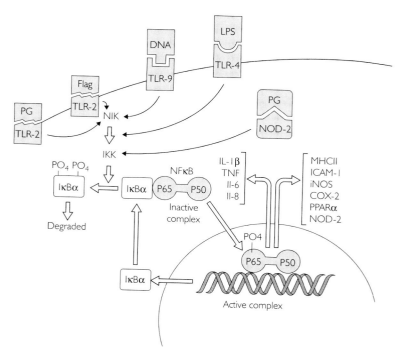

**Fig. 10.2** Activation of innate immune cells by bacterial adjuvants. Bacterial adjuvants (termed commensal associated molecular patterns) such as LPS, peptidoglycan (PG), flagellin (Flag) and unmethylated DNA (CpG) bind to pattern recognition receptors to activate NFκB. These receptors include membrane bound Toll-like receptors (TLR) and intracellular caspase activating receptor domain (CARD) family members, including NOD1 and NOD2/CARD15. These pathways converge on inhibitor of IκB kinase (IKK), which phosphorylates the inhibitor IκBα, releasing activated NFκB (p65/p50 heterodimer) to induce transcription of a number of proinflammatory and inhibitory gene products relevant to intestinal inflammation.

active, aggressive Crohn's disease and ulcerative colitis is unclear,[90] but this extracellular pump may excrete endogenous bacterial products, as mdr1a-deficient mice spontaneously develop colitis that can be prevented with antibiotics.[91]

## Induction and reactivation of IBD by transient infection with pathogens

In contrast to the controversy surrounding persistent infections as a cause of IBD (see below), there is abundant evidence that common pathogens can precipitate the onset of IBD, exacerbate inflammatory responses and reactivate quiescent disease.[1] Transient infection breaks the epithelial barrier and initiates mucosal inflammation, which we postulate can be perpetuated by specific immune responses in susceptible hosts (see Conclusions). Following epidemics of Shigella, Salmonella or Yersinia, a small percentage of patients develop typical ulcerative colitis or Crohn's disease after clearance of the inciting infection.[92] Patients not infrequently relate the onset of symptoms of IBD to foreign travel or a transient documented enteric infection. Furthermore, the unusual coexistence of IBD in close friends,[93] spouses[94] and large multiplex families[95] suggests common environmental exposures. These observations suggest that initiating (triggering) events may be entirely separate from factors perpetuating disease. Thus, the search for enteric pathogens in chronically inflamed tissue[96] may be negative despite an important role for these agents in initiation of disease. The rapid rise in incidence of IBD in developing countries and an altered frequency of IBD in the first generation of populations moving to a new country indicate important environmental influences. Moreover, the concordance rate of IBD in monozygotic (identical) twins is only 10% in ulcerative colitis and 50% in Crohn's disease,[97] confirming the importance of environmental factors in these disorders.

Symptomatic recurrence of both ulcerative colitis and Crohn's disease is associated with a number of viral, bacterial and parasitic infections.[1] Between 40% and 60% of relapses of IBD are associated with symptomatic respiratory infections.[98]

In a prospective study exacerbation of underlying IBD in children occurred contemporaneously with 43% of serologically diagnosed viral or Mycoplasma infections.[99] Conversely, 24% of clinical flares of IBD were associated with documented infections over the 21-month observation period. Exacerbation by respiratory infections may account for the seasonal variation in recurrence of IBD.[100]

Exacerbation of IBD by concurrent enteric pathogens is difficult to interpret, as symptoms could be caused by either the infection or a secondary reactivation of idiopathic IBD. Salmonella, Shigella, Campylobacter and Yersinia are detected in less than 2% of patients with relapsing IBD in industrialized countries[101] and only 4% of flaring cases in India,[102] suggesting that searching for enteric pathogens in uncomplicated flares of IBD is not cost effective. However, much higher rates of detection of Yersinia and toxigenic E. coli by PCR in resected tissues[103] indicate that cultures may understate the actual incidence of pathogens in refractory IBD.

C. difficile is the pathogen most frequently involved in relapsing IBD. Between 0 and 32% of active IBD patients have detectable C. difficile or its toxin.[104,105] Greenfield et al.[104] reported that 28% of IBD patients followed for 1 year had evidence of C. difficile infection on at least one occasion. In hospitalized patients, 13% of Crohn's disease patients, 14% of ulcerative colitis patients, 12% of diarrheal controls and 1% of healthy controls had positive toxin assays. Thirty-one per cent of patients taking antibiotics and 13% taking sulfasalazine had detectable C. difficile toxin, in contrast to only 6% of IBD patients taking no antimicrobial drugs. Most patients responded to therapy directed toward C. difficile infection. Weber et al.[101] demonstrated that 17% of IBD patients studied at the time of symptomatic recurrence had recoverable bacterial pathogens (9% had C. difficile and 5% had enteropathogenic E. coli). However, these authors did not attempt to isolate viruses.

Cytomegalovirus (CMV) infections can exacerbate IBD, particularly in immunosuppressed patients,[106,107] although this complication can rarely occur in steroid-naive patients;[108] 12% of resections had histological evidence of CMV infection, which occurred exclusively in patients with severe, steroid-treated disease,[109] and 36% of steroid-refractory IBD patients had CMV infection by biopsy and buffy coat analysis, with five of six patients responding to ganciclovir or foscarnet.[106] Clinical clues for CMV infection include worsening disease on steroids, fever, increased liver function studies and atypical circulating lymphocytes.

Less commonly, Epstein–Barr virus (EBV) and herpes virus 6 can potentiate IBD;[110,111] both intestinal and systemic symptoms can respond to IFN-$\alpha_{2a}$ treatment.[111] The presence of EBV DNA-positive lymphoma in IBD patients treated with immunosuppressive agents[112] raises the possibility of long-term neoplastic sequelae of these infections.

### Conclusions

The frequency of infectious exacerbation of IBD is probably understated, owing to the documented difficulty in detecting viral and enteric pathogens by culture and the much higher recovery rates by PCR. Whether viral and bacterial suprainfection of IBD is secondary to diminished host resistance (ulcerated mucosa, immunosuppression by drug therapy or malnutrition, or antibiotic therapy), increased exposure to nosocomial pathogens through hospitalization, or alternatively whether these infections influence the course of idiopathic IBD is difficult to determine. However, improved symptoms by specific treatment strongly suggest a pathogenic role in symptomatic flares. A role for transient infection in the initiation of chronic, relapsing disease in genetically susceptible hosts is supported by induction of persistent inflammation in susceptible rat strains[113] and IL-10$^{-/-}$ mice[114] by short-term NSAID administration.

## Extraintestinal inflammation induced by bacteria and bacterial components

Sclerosing cholangitis, reactive arthritis and uveitis are more common in patients with extensive colitis than in those with proctitis or isolated small intestinal disease, providing indirect evidence that enteric bacteria influence extraintestinal disease.[115] Proliferation of anaerobic bacteria in the bypassed small intestine induces systemic inflammation that mimics the extraintestinal manifestations of IBD.[115] Approximately 20% of morbidly obese patients who undergo jejunoileal bypass develop hepatic inflammation and steatosis, non-deforming migratory oligoarthritis and skin lesions that resemble those of Sweet's syndrome; the majority of patients improve with antibiotics active against anaerobes. Circulating immune complexes and cryoproteins contain antibodies recognizing *E. coli* and *Bacteroides* species.[116] A small number of patients with pouchitis after total colectomy for treatment of ulcerative colitis develop arthritis and erythema nodosum, which respond to metronidazole therapy.[117]

## EXPERIMENTAL ANIMAL MODELS

Studies in animal models of intestinal inflammation offer distinct advantages over clinical observations because the bacterial composition can be precisely manipulated in gnotobiotic rodents, commensal bacteria can be decreased or increased by antibiotics and experimental surgery, individual bacterial components can be administered or removed, and genetic background can be precisely controlled (see Chapter 9). Moreover, immune responses can be regulated in genetically engineered rodents and in lym-

phocyte and dendritic cell transfer studies. Therefore, it is not surprising that the most definitive evidence that subsets of commensal bacteria mediate chronic, immune-mediated inflammation is provided by rodent studies[118,119] (Table 10.4).

## GNOTOBIOTIC STUDIES

The luminal microenvironment can be manipulated by studying germ-free (sterile) rodents or ex-germ-free mice and rats colonized with a single (monoassociated) or a combination of bacterial species. In these studies the aggressiveness and location of intestinal inflammation correlates closely with the degree of microbial stimulation (Table 10.4). For example, IL-10-deficient (knockout) mice raised under conventional (dirty) conditions develop lethal small and colonic inflammation.[120] However, specific pathogen-free (SPF) mice have non-lethal inflammation restricted to the colon;[120] germ-free IL-10$^{-/-}$ mice exhibit no clinical, histologic or immunologic evidence of colitis.[121] A similar lack of colitis as well as gastritis and arthritis is found in germ-free HLA-B27/$\beta_2$-microglobulin transgenic rats, although skin and testicular lesions are unchanged.[122,123] Gnotobiotic B27 transgenic rats colonized with SPF bacteria develop progressively more aggressive colitis, which becomes statistically significant 4 weeks after colonization.[122] IL-10 knockout mice have a more aggressive course, with significant colitis 1 week after colonization with SPF bacteria and transmural cecal inflammation (typhlitis) within 5 weeks of exposure.[121] A consistent lack of colitis in all other germ-free knockout and transgenic murine colitis models studied to date and in most induced models indicates the near universal requirement for commensal bacteria to induce chronic immune-mediated enterocolitis (Table 10.4). The only known exceptions to this rule are IL-2$^{-/-}$ mice and dextran sodium sulfate (DSS)-induced colitis. IL-2 knockout mice develop aggressive, lethal gastritis, duodenitis and colitis in conventional and SPF conditions,[124,125] but continue to exhibit mild, focal, non-proliferative gastrointestinal inflammation with no mortality in the sterile state.[125] Interestingly, neither the periportal hepatic inflammation[125] nor the systemic immunologic abnormalities of autoimmune anemia, B-lymphocyte depletion and generalized lymphoid hyperplasia are altered by the germ-free state.[126,127] Standard germ-free technology excludes viable bacteria, viruses and parasites, but heat-killed bacteria with antigens and active cell wall polymers such as LPS and PG-PS are present in the autoclaved food, which could stimulate inflammation in highly susceptible hosts. The acute DSS model is the only experimental situation to date where the sterile environment does not strikingly diminish experimental colitis, although conflicting results have been reported.[128,129] Antibiotics active against enteric bacteria prevent and treat acute but not chronic DSS-induced colitis.[130,131] However, with these minor exceptions, the vast bulk of rodent models require resident enteric bacteria for the induction and perpetuation of intestinal inflammation.

Recent studies demonstrate that resident bacterial species have differential capacities to induce inflammation and that the dominant bacterial stimuli may depend on the host's immunologic (and perhaps genetic) background. *Bacteroides vulgatus* preferentially induces colitis in carrageenan-fed guinea pigs[132] and HLA-B27 transgenic rats;[122,133] *B. vulgatus* monoassociated B27 transgenic rats developed nearly as aggressive colitis as those colonized with six bacterial strains, including *B. vulgatus*, but *E. coli* monoassociated B27 transgenic rats failed to develop colitis.[133] Diversity was seen within the same genus, as *B. vul-*

**Table 10.4 The influence of the normal luminal bacterial environment on inflammation in animal models**

| Model | Species | SPF | Germ-free | Antibiotics | Intestinal bypass |
|---|---|---|---|---|---|
| **A. Induced disease** | | | | | |
| Indomethacin | Rat | Acute SB, colonic and gastric ulcers, chronic SB ulcers | Attenuated acute, absent chronic | ↓ by metronidazole, tetracycline | ND |
| Carrageenan | Guinea pig | Cecal inflammation | No colitis | ↓ by metronidazole, clindamycin | ND |
| DSS | Mouse | Colitis | ↑ or ↓ colitis | ↓ by cipro, imipenum/ vancomycin (acute phase) | |
| TNBS | Rat | Colitis | ND | ↓ by amoxicillin/ clavulanic acid | |
| **B. Genetically engineered** | | | | | |
| HLA-B27 transgenic | Rat | Gastritis, colitis, arthritis | No GI or joint inflammation | ↓ by metronidazole, vancomycin/ imipenum | ↓ bypass, ↑ blind loop |
| CD45 RB^hi → SCID | Mouse | Colitis | No colitis | ↓ by streptomycin and bacitracin | ND |
| IL-2−/− | Mouse | Colitis, gastritis, hepatitis | Absent-attenuated inflammation | ND | ND |
| IL-10−/− | Mouse | Colitis | No colitis | ↓ by metronidazole, cipro, vancomycin, imipenum | ND |
| TCRα−/− | Mouse | Colitis | No inflammation | ND | ↓ resection cecal tip |
| mdr1α−/− | Mouse | Colitis | ND | ↓ by streptomycin, neomycin, bacitracin, amphoteracin | ND |
| **C. Spontaneous mutations** | | | | | |
| Samp 1/Yit | Mouse | Ileitis | No ileitis | ↓ metronidazole/ cipro | ND |
| Cotton-top tamarin | Marmoset | Colitis | ND | ? | ↓ Thiry- Vella loop |

SB, small bowel; GI, gastrointestinal; ND, not done; ↓, attenuation of disease; ↑, potentiation of disease.

gatus and *B. thetaiotaomicron*, but not *B. distasonis*, monoassociation induced colitis.[134] However, IL-10-deficient mice, which develop aggressive cecal inflammation within 1 week of SPF bacterial colonization, have only very mild colonic inflammation when colonized with the same bacterial strains, including *B. vulgatus*, that cause active colitis in B27 transgenic rats.[121] *B. vulgatus*, *Helicobacter hepaticus*, *Clostridium sordelii* and *viridans*-type streptococci fail to induce colitis in monoassociated IL-10−/− mice.[135,136] However, IL-10−/− mice monoassociated with *Enterococcus faecalis*[137,138] or with a commensal murine *E. coli* strain[138] develop active colitis. Importantly, the phenotype of disease in the same host is different with these different bacterial species. *E. coli* induce a relatively rapid-onset cecal inflammation, whereas *E. faecalis* cause slow-onset distal colitis with dysplasia and duodenal obstruction.[138] Thus various hosts require different bacteria to induce chronic immune-mediated colitis, and illustrate the complexity of interpreting clinical investigations if ulcerative colitis and Crohn's disease are heterogeneous groups of genetically distinct disorders, each with different bacterial species preferentially stimulating immune responses, and with different bacteria causing variable phenotypes of disease in genetically distinct individuals.

## Probiotics/prebiotics

Not only do some luminal bacterial species preferentially induce inflammation, but other bacteria can prevent intestinal injury. *Lactobacillus* and *Bifidobacterium* species can attenuate colitis in IL-10 knockout mice. Serial feeding and rectal swabbing of native *Lactobacillus reuteri*[17] and daily administration of VSL#3[139], a combination of four *Lactobacillus*, three *Bifidobacterium* and one *Streptococcus* species, prevented colitis in IL-10 knockout mice. Probiotic bacterial species improved epithelial barrier function,[17,139] which was confirmed in rabbits, where *Lactobacillus GG* inhibited *E. coli* translocation.[140] Similarly, oral administration of an *L. plantarum* strain could partially reverse established colitis, prevent the onset of disease and decrease colonic IgG$_{2a}$ and IL-12 secretion.[141] Host background appears to determine which probiotic species is most effective, as *Lactobacillus GG* was more effective than *L. plantarum* in preventing recurrence of colitis in HLA-B27 transgenic rats.[142]

In these studies, neither *L. GG* nor *L. plantarum* alone was effective in reversing established colitis in SPF HLA-B27 transgenic rats, but *L. GG* decreased recurrent colitis after induction of remission by broad-spectrum antibiotics.[142] *L. plantarum* did not prevent relapse. These observations, together with the ability of VSL#3 to prevent relapse of chronic pouchitis after antibiotic-induced remission,[11] lay the foundation for additive effects of antibiotics and probiotics in the treatment of IBD. In innovative studies, colonizing the intestine with genetically engineered *Lactococcus lactis* that secrete recombinant IL-10 decreased colitis in two separate murine models.[143] Genetically engineered probiotic bacteria are now undergoing clinical trials in IBD patients.

Recent studies in experimental models demonstrate a potential therapeutic role for prebiotic substances in IBD. Madsen et al.[17] showed that feeding lactulose to IL-10−/− mice stimulated the growth of endogenous enteric *Lactobacillus* species and attenuated colitis. Similarly, oral administration of germinated barley extracts[144,145] or inulin[146] attenuated DSS-induced colitis in rats, increased SCFA production and augmented luminal concentrations of *Bifidobacterium* and *Lactobacillus* species. Fructo-oligosaccharides and inulin promote the growth of endogenous *Bifidobacterium* and *Lactobacillus* species, enhance the secretion of SCFA, especially butyrate, and decrease luminal pH.[37,147,148] Butyrate has numerous beneficial effects on epithelial function by serving as an energy source, enhancing barrier function and inducing protective molecules[22,149] (see next section).

## Antibiotics

Manipulating luminal bacteria by antibiotics, particularly combinations with broad-spectrum activity, further demonstrates the ability of ubiquitous microflora to perpetuate experimental colitis. A number of antibiotics can attenuate indomethacin-induced enterocolitis in rats. Metronidazole for 7 days significantly diminished mucosal permeability and almost totally inhibited small intestinal ulceration and inflammation, but had less impressive effects 3 days after indomethacin injection.[113] Ciprofloxacin and the combination of metronidazole and neomycin prevent colitis in IL-10−/− mice, but only the broad-spectrum combination could reverse established disease.[150] Similarly, metronidazole or ciprofloxacin prevented colitis in HLA-B27 transgenic rats, IL-10 knockout mice and DSS-fed mice.[130,151] However, broad-spectrum antibiotics (a combination of imipenum and vancomycin) not only prevented but also reversed established colitis in these studies. Luminal concentrations of bacteria were reduced further with the broad-spectrum combination than with metronidazole or ciprofloxacin alone.[130,151] Similarly, antibiotics with anaerobic and broad-spectrum activities prevented colitis in guinea pigs fed carrageenan,[152] reduced gross and histologic evidence of colitis induced by trinitrobenzene sulfonic acid (TNBS), and almost totally eliminated colonic fibrosis and granulomas.[153] Antibiotic decontamination or lactulose therapy decreased bacteremia, but this protocol had no apparent effect on colonic inflammation induced by TNBS.[59] However, broad-spectrum combination antibiotics are effective in almost all other models, including DSS-induced colitis,[131,144] colitis in mdr1a−/− mice[91] and ileitis in SAMP-1/Yit mice.[154]

These studies suggest that the complex commensal bacterial flora have synergistic activities in perpetuating colitis and that human IBD trials should explore combinations of antibiotics.

Results demonstrating that metronidazole preferentially decreases distal colitis, whereas ciprofloxacin selectively prevents cecal inflammation,[151] support the concept that different bacteria induce inflammation in different regions of the intestine[138] and that antibiotic treatment of Crohn's disease may need to be tailored to the region involved.

## Intestinal bypass and blind loops

Experimental colitis is affected by altering luminal bacterial concentrations by intestinal bypass or blind loops, further implicating commensal bacteria in the pathogenesis of intestinal inflammation. Cecal bypass in HLA-B27 transgenic rats decreased not only cecal inflammation, but also distal colitis and gastritis.[155] Cecal bypass dramatically decreased local concentrations of anaerobic bacteria, including *Bacteroides* species, but had no effect on bacterial populations in other gastrointestinal regions. In contrast, surgical creation of a self-filling blind loop of the cecum increased total anaerobic bacterial and *Bacteroides* species concentrations 1000-fold and enhanced cecal inflammation. Similar to Crohn's disease,[43,45] the exclusion of colonic loops from the fecal stream decreased colitis in cotton-top tamarins.[156] Upon infusion of fecal contents into the bypassed segment the inflammation rapidly returned. These studies demonstrate a consistent correlation between concentrations of luminal bacteria and intestinal inflammation.

## Induction of intestinal inflammation by purified bacterial products

### Non-viable bacterial constituents

Intestinal bacteria produce a number of constituents distinct from their innumerable surface antigens that can incite inflammation and activate innate immune cells.[157,158] Formylated oligopeptides, of which *n*-formyl-methionyl-leucyl-phenylalanine (FMLP) is the most active, are secreted by a number of intestinal bacteria, including *E. coli*. FMLP is synthesized as the N-terminal sequence of the UmuD protein of the *E. coli* SOS operon.[159] These proteins permit DNA repair in bacteria. Bacterial SOS genes are activated by exposure to oxygen free radicals, suggesting that enhanced production of FMLP by bacteria invading oxygenated tissues may signal host defense mechanisms.[159] LPS, a major component of the outer membrane of Gram-negative bacteria, consists of a hydrophobic lipid A moiety, which mediates the majority of LPS effects, a core oligosaccharide and a chain of repeating sugar units (O chain). LPS rapidly stimulates cytokine and procoagulant tissue factor synthesis, activates the complement cascade and is a polyclonal mitogen for B lymphocytes. Peptidoglycan–polysaccharide (PG–PS) complexes are the primary structural polymers of the cell walls of Gram-positive and Gram-negative bacteria.[158] These polymers are cross-linked by peptide chains which are inhibited by penicillin-class antibiotics. Like LPS, PG–PS is released by degradation of dead bacteria and can stimulate almost every limb of the inflammatory response, including activation of monocytes/macrophages to secrete cytokines, nitric oxide, lysosomal enzymes and eicosanoids, stimulation of neutrophil oxygen radical production, and has adjuvant activity, mitogenic and immunogenic responses in B cells, variable effects on T lymphocytes, and activates the complement and kallikrein–kinin cascades.[158,160,161] Bacterial DNA, which unlike mammalian DNA is not methylated and contains CpG motifs, serves as an adjuvant.[162]

Bacterial adjuvants such as LPS, PG–PS and CpG activate innate immune cells through pattern recognition receptors, most notably TLR[163-165] and intracellular CARD family receptors, including NOD1 and CARD15/NOD2[84,85] (Fig. 10.2). TLR-2 binds PG–PS polymers, mycobacterial components and teichoic acid; TLR-5 binds flagellins; TLR-4 binds LPS and bacterial heat-shock protein-60 (HSP-60); and TLR-9 binds bacterial DNA motifs (CpG). Optimal LPS binding to TLR-4 requires soluble LPS-binding protein and CD14, which is highly expressed on the membrane of activated monocytes, but decreases on mature intestinal macrophages. Ligation of TLR or NOD molecules by LPS, flagellin, PG–PS or CpG activates NFκB, which stimulates expression of proinflammatory cytokines, adhesion molecules, MHC class II molecules, iNOS and COX-2 in macrophages, monocytes, dendritic cells and neutrophils (Fig. 10.2). Similarly, *B. vulgatus* or *E. coli* lysates or purified LPS can activate NFκB and proinflammatory molecules in epithelial cells through TLR4[167]. NOD2/CARD15 is constitutively expressed in monocytes, macrophages and dendritic cells and Paneth cells, but not in resting intestinal epithelial cells.[84] However, this molecule is expressed in the inflamed epithelial cells of IBD patients and is upregulated by TNF and IFN8 in an NFκB-dependent manner.[86,87] Expression of Paneth cells in the distal ileum raises the possibility of defective regulation of anti-microbial defensins in Crohn's disease patients with NOD-2 polymorphisms.[167]

Purified components of normal luminal bacteria can cause experimental enterocolitis, demonstrating that tissue invasion by viable bacteria is not essential for the induction of intestinal inflammation. High luminal concentrations of FMLP cause acute colitis;[168] at more physiologic levels it increases mucosal permeability, particularly in the distal ileum.[169] Intravenous injection of LPS produces mid small bowel hemorrhagic injury that is mediated by platelet-activating factor[170] and induces diarrhea characterized by chloride secretion.[171]

In contrast to the acute experimental intestinal inflammation caused by FMLP and LPS, PG–PS can induce chronic, granulomatous enterocolitis with systemic inflammation in genetically susceptible hosts. Subserosal (intramural) ileocecal injection of poorly biodegradable PG–PS into Lewis rats induces biphasic enterocolitis which persists at least 6 months.[161,162] Acute inflammation confined to the injection site peaks at 1–2 days. After a quiescent phase, T lymphocyte-dependent diffuse granulomatous inflammation spontaneously reactivates.[172] Bacterial cell wall polymers can potentiate enterocolitis; these studies illustrate the proinflammatory potential of absorbed bacterial products. Gavage feeding of sterile PG–PS to germ-free rats treated with indomethacin increased acute small intestinal ulceration almost to levels observed in littermates conventionalized with specific pathogen-free flora,[173] and colonic instillation of PG–PS polymers modestly enhanced acetic acid-induced colitis in SPF rats.[174]

## Secondary mucosal invasion and uptake of bacterial products

Mucosal FMLP, LPS and PG–PS uptake is enhanced following experimental mucosal injury or intestinal bacterial overgrowth in rats.[175-177] Translocation of viable bacteria also occurs in experimental enterocolitis and small bowel bacterial overgrowth,[113,178,179] as well as in experimental small bowel bacterial overgrowth.[178]

## Immune responses to commensal bacteria

Mice and rats with experimental colitis mount humoral and cellular immune responses to ubiquitous enteric bacteria.[180-183] The Th1 immune responses found in most rodent models of chronic colitis are directed toward commensal intestinal bacteria.[91,138,181,182,184-186] Transfer of bacterial antigen-specific CD4+ T-cell lines from C3H/HeJ Bir mice with colitis induce colitis in SPF SCID recipients.[182] Studies in CD3e transgenic mice indicate lack of crossreaction of cecal bacterial-responsive CD4+ T cells to dietary and epithelial antigens in vitro or to self-antigens in vivo.[184] Monoassociated IL-10[-/-] mice exhibit antigen-specific responses to the bacterial species inducing colitis (*E. coli*, *Enterococcus faecalis*), but not to bacterial species incapable of inducing disease.[138] Bacterial-specific Th1 responses precede histologic or clinical evidence of inflammation.[138] However, Sydora et al.[136] reported that Th1-dominated immune responses to colonizing bacteria are not necessarily pathogenic. Similarly, cecal bacterial lysates activate pathogenic innate immune responses (increased IL-12, TNF, APC activity) in MLN cells, splenocytes or purified dendritic cells from IL-10[-/-] mice.[187,188] Although sera from rodents with experimental colitis react to numerous commensal bacterial species,[180] the core glycolipid region of LPS, and specific epitopes of *Bacteroides vulgatus*[134] B lymphocytes, do not mediate experimental colitis[189,190] and in fact are protective.[191] Therefore, serum and mucosal antibacterial antibodies are markers of enhanced permeability and/or heightened immunoresponsiveness rather than inducing disease. Cross-reactive bacterial/mammalian serologic responses exist, as pANCA serologic reactivity in IL-10-deficient mice can be blocked by preincubation with cecal bacteria.[192] Similarly, DSS-treated mice have crossreactive HSP-60 in enteric bacterial, epithelial and lamina propria mononuclear cells.[193]

Cecal lymphoid aggregates appear to be the preferential site of bacterial antigenic stimulation. 'Appendectomy' (actually removal of the cecal tip, which contains a large lymphoid aggregate) dramatically attenuates colitis in the remaining colon[194] and cecal bypass inhibited distal colitis as well as gastritis in HLA-B27 transgenic rats, even though luminal bacterial concentrations in the affected organs were not altered.[195] These results correspond to epidemiologic reports that appendectomy protects against the later onset of ulcerative colitis (see Chapter 17). Presumably naive T cells are activated by luminal bacteria in the appendiceal lymphoid aggregates, and then home to other colonic regions to mediate injury.

Commensal bacteria are also important in the induction of regulatory immune responses (tolerance) that prevent pathogenic immune responses to ubiquitous antigens. Antibiotics administered to neonatal mice enhanced in vitro expression of IL-4 but decreased IL-12 and IFN-γ,[196] consistent with more frequent atopy in children treated with antibiotics during infancy. Cong et al.[197] demonstrated that cecal bacterial-responsive Tr1 cells derived from C3H/HeJ Bir mice prevent colitis in SPF SCID recipients when co-transferred with Th1 cells. In vitro cecal lysate-stimulated Tr1 cells preferentially secrete IL-10, whereas Th1 cells secrete IFN-γ. In preliminary studies, CD4+RBlow T cells from germ-free mice were less able to prevent colitis in the CD45RB[high] co-transfer model than were similar cells from SPF controls.[198] Even potential pathogens can induce protective regulatory cells. Kullberg et al.[199] showed that CD4+ T cells from wildtype mice infected with *Helicobacter hepaticus* could prevent colitis in Rag[-/-] mice when co-transferred with CD4+ T cells from *H. hepaticus*-colonized IL-10[-/-] mice; this antigen-specific protection was dependent on IL-10 but not TGF-β. Cecal bacterial lysates or LPS induce the production of high concentrations of IL-10 by MLN cells or splenocytes; in murine cells the majority of IL-10 is produced by macrophages and dendritic cells,[187] but B lymphocytes account for the bulk of bacterial induced IL-10 and TGF-β production in rat MLN cells.[200,201] Commensal bacteria appear to regulate oral tolerance. Systemic antibody responses to oral sheep RBC are evident in germ-free mice but absent in SPF mice.[28] Similarly, tolerance to dietary ovalbumin is more easily broken in germ-free mice and more rapidly restored in SPF mice.[29,202] Selective bacterial stimulation may occur, with Gram-positive bacteria preferentially stimulating IL-12 production, whereas Gram-negative organisms induce IL-4[203] and Gram-negative bacteria and LPS were responsible for inducing oral tolerance.[28] In these studies oral tolerance was absent in germ-free mice, but was restored by colonization with Gram-negative bacteria (but not Gram-positive species) or by feeding LPS. Some reports indicate that selected probiotic bacterial species (*Lactobacillus* and *Bifidobacteria*), as well as DNA extracted from these species, preferentially induce IL-10 in vitro and in vivo.[204–207]

## Environmental triggers

Transient exposure to triggers that break the mucosal barrier can initiate chronic enterocolitis in genetically susceptible hosts. Chronic inflammation is then sustained by luminal bacterial adjuvants and antigens. For example, in SPF Lewis rats two injections of indomethacin induce chronic longitudinal small bowel ulcers with mesenteric fat wrapping, anemia of chronic disease and periportal inflammation which persists at least 77 days;[208] chronic ulceration does not occur in germ-free Lewis rats[209] and dramatically decreases with metronidazole therapy.[113] Similarly, piroxicam for 2 weeks dramatically accelerates and potentiates chronic colitis in SPF IL-10$^{-/-}$ mice on a relatively resistant C57Bl/6 background.[114] As in human IBD, bacterial infection can exacerbate colitis, as illustrated by TNF receptor-deficient mice infected with *Citrobacter rodentium*.[210] Finally, stress can initiate and reactivate experimental enterocolitis through mast cell[211] and T lymphocyte[212]-mediated mechanisms.

## Extraintestinal manifestations

Systemic distribution of luminal bacterial adjuvants and antigens, which are absorbed in higher amounts from the inflamed intestine, strongly influences the extraintestinal manifestations of intestinal inflammation.[115] For example, anaerobic bacterial overgrowth in jejunal self-filling blind loops induces hepatobiliary inflammation resembling sclerosing cholangitis[213] and reactivates quiescent peripheral arthritis in susceptible rat strains.[214] These systemic inflammatory events are prevented by metronidazole or tetracycline, but not gentamicin. Mechanistic studies indicate that luminal PG–PS polymers mediate this hepatobiliary inflammation, as mutanolysin, which selectively degrades PG–PS, inhibits hepatobiliary inflammation whereas polymyxin B, which binds and inactivates LPS, has no effect.[178,215] Furthermore, luminal PG–PS is absorbed and systematically distributed in the self-filling blind loop and acedic acid colitis models,[174,216] and intestinal intramural injection of PG–PS induces erosive arthritis, hepatic granulomas and chronic anemia in Lewis rats.[162] Additionally, repeated injections of emulsified muramyl dipeptide (MDP), the basic structure of PG, into the intestine[217] or heat-killed *E. coli* into the peripheral or portal veins[218] induce hepatobiliary inflammation. Finally, conventionally raised HLA-

B27 transgenic rats develop axial and peripheral arthritis; this arthritis is absent in the sterile state and decreased under SPF conditions.[122,123] In some models, however, extraintestinal manifestations are not totally dependent on luminal bacteria, as mild periportal inflammation persists in germ-free IL-2$^{-/-}$ mice.[125]

# ETIOLOGIC THEORIES

Crohn's disease and ulcerative colitis are chronic, relapsing, immunologically mediated conditions in genetically susceptible hosts. The persistent, relapsing nature of these disorders strongly suggests that the antigens and adjuvants driving the immune response are ubiquitous, derived from either exogenous (dietary products, commensal microflora or a persistent pathogen) or endogenous (host) sources. The presence of granulomas in Crohn's disease suggests that the inciting antigens are poorly biodegradable. Although the preponderance of data indicates that commensal luminal bacterial constituents provide the constant antigenic drive for chronic intestinal inflammation in the genetically susceptible host, other possibilities include dietary contributions, persistent pathogens and subtle alterations of the virulence factors in commensal organisms. This section discusses evidence to support or refute the most widely accepted etiologic hypotheses for IBD (Table 10.5), each of which involves microbial agents. The genetically determined host response to these microbial stimuli is integrally linked to the development of disease, so IBD must be considered a compendium of genetic/environmental interactions.

## PERSISTENT PATHOGENIC INFECTION

The causal role for *Helicobacter hepaticus* in peptic ulcer disease renewed credibility for an infectious etiology of IBD. Clinical observations have led a number of investigators to pursue the hypothesis that IBD is caused by a specific microbial pathogen. Crohn's disease is almost indistinguishable from ileocecal tuberculosis, *Yersinia enterocolitica* and anorectal chlamydial infections, whereas ulcerative colitis closely resembles chronic *Campylobacter*, *Shigella* and amebic colitis. Moreover, the onset of typical idiopathic IBD can follow epidemic or sporadic enteric infections, whereas respiratory tract or intestinal infections can precipitate exacerbations of long-standing ulcerative colitis or Crohn's disease. There is no evidence of transmission of Crohn's disease from patients to close contacts, including family members, spouses, or healthcare workers, but intriguing clusters of disease within close friends,[93] spouses[94] and families[95] suggest an infectious etiology. Chronic, recurrent inflammation could be due to ineffective clearance of a conventional enteric pathogen,

---

**Table 10.5 Etiologic theories for IBD**

Persistent pathogen: *Mycobacterium paratuberculosis*, virulent *E. coli*, *Pseudomonas* species, *Listeria monocytogenes*, non-*pylori* *Helicobacter* species, measles

Defective clearance of pathogenic and commensal bacteria

Defective mucosal barrier: enhanced permeability, ineffective healing

Dysbiosis: altered balance of protective/detrimental commensals

Dysregulated immune response: overly aggressive effectors, loss of tolerance

infection by an unusual intracellular or slowly replicating organism, or induction of an abnormal host immune response by a transient infection.

A number of microbial pathogens have been proposed as causes of ulcerative colitis or Crohn's disease,[1] although the majority of these have not been confirmed by blinded, controlled investigations. The availability of extremely sensitive molecular techniques to detect microbial agents has rekindled enthusiasm for the search for a specific pathogen.

## Mycobacterium paratuberculosis

In 1913, Dalziel[219] noted the similarity of the pathologic responses of ileocecal tuberculosis, Johne's disease and human idiopathic granulomatous enterocolitis. Johne's disease in ruminants is caused by Mycobacterium paratuberculosis, a fastidious and extremely slow-growing mycobactin-dependent organism.[220] Because M. paratuberculosis occurs in dairy herds around the world, and possibly within commercial milk and community water supplies,[221,222] a possible zoonotic infection has generated considerable debate.[221,223–225] It is unclear whether M. paratuberculosis DNA in Crohn's disease is due to passive uptake of non-viable dietary organisms into ulcerated tissues, or to pathogenic invasion of replicating bacteria which induce a cellular immune response, causing tissue destruction. Ongoing multicenter antibiotic and blinded molecular detection studies should help resolve this controversy.

Chiodini et al.[226] cultured slow-growing M. paratuberculosis from resected tissues of three patients with Crohn's disease, with confirmation by geographically dispersed investigators.[224] Although recovery of M. paratuberculosis from Crohn's disease tissues by culture is low (<15%) this method is specific, with very rare cultures from ulcerative colitis or normal control tissues. Detection of cultured spheroplasts (cell wall defective forms) by PCR is somewhat higher in both Crohn's disease (20–40%) and control (0–10%) tissues.[227,228] More widespread interest in this organism has been fostered by higher rates of detection by PCR and serologic methods. Sanderson et al.[229] detected IS-900, a multicopy DNA insertion element specific for M. paratuberculosis, in 65% of Crohn's disease tissues, 4% ulcerative colitis and 13% controls. However, other investigators report widely variable detection rates (0–100% for Crohn's disease),[222,230,231] lack of specificity[222,232] and lack of detection in tissues by 16s DNA technology.[57] Recent studies combining PCR with laser capture microdissection,[233] immunohistochemistry with confocal scanning laser microscopy,[234] and in situ hybridization[235] are more promising. M. paratuberculosis was detected by in situ hybridization in Crohn's disease tissues with granulomas (40%) more frequently than in those without (4.5%), which were no different from controls, although signals were within macrophages and myofibroblasts rather than within granulomas.[236] Disease-specific serologic responses to defined mycobacterial antigens have also been reported: 74–87% of Crohn's disease patients have positive IgM antibodies to M. paratuberculosis p35/p36 proteins, with 98% specificity for this disease.[237,238] In addition, Crohn's disease-specific IgA antibodies to a 32 kDa mycobacterial protein (HupB) homologous to human histone $H_1$ crossreact with ANCA.[81] However, these results must be interpreted cautiously because of the lack of replication, sensitivity and specificity are confined to single antibody classes, HupB is found in many mycobacterial species, pANCA is found in ulcerative colitis more than Crohn's disease,

and Crohn's disease patients have enhanced antibody responses to a number of pathogenic and commensal bacterial species. Lack of cell-mediated immune responses to M. paratuberculosis in Crohn's disease patients is a crucial weakness, because inflammation in a paucibacillary infection is immunologically mediated.

Crohn's disease is not more frequent in farm workers or veterinarians in close contact with M. paratuberculosis-infected ruminants: in fact, rural residents have a decreased prevalence of disease (see Chapter 17). Although M. paratuberculosis DNA has been detected in breast milk from mothers with Crohn's disease,[239] disease in offspring is not correlated with maternal rather than paternal Crohn's disease. However, some clinical observations support this theory. M. paratuberculosis was cultured from an enlarged cervical lymph node 5 years prior to the detection of distal ileal inflammation resembling Crohn's disease,[240] and BCG immunization decreased the detection rate of IS-900 fourfold.[232] The results of clinical trials of antibiotics directed against M. paratuberculosis are reviewed in Chapter 34. They can be summarized as not demonstrating efficacy for the treatment of active Crohn's disease or for maintenance of remission.

## Adherent/invasive E. coli

E. coli strains that adhere to epithelial cells in vitro by a mechanism distinct from that of enteropathogenic E. coli (EPEC) have been recovered from ulcerative colitis tissue,[241–243] although these findings were not universally replicated.[244,245] More recently, Darfeuille-Michaud and colleagues have described a novel adherent/invasive E. coli strain found in increased abundance in the postresection neoterminal ileum in recurrent Crohn's disease.[246] Eighty-five per cent of E. coli strains recovered from mucosal biopsies of chronic postoperative Crohn's disease patients adhere to differentiated Caco-2 cells, compared to 79% of strains from early recurrent disease and 33% of controls.[246] These E. coli invade macrophages by an actin monofilament and microtubule-dependent mechanism[247] and replicate within phagocytic cells without inducing apoptosis.[248] Adherence and invasion are mediated by type 1 pili.[249] These organisms replicate and persist within macrophages and induce protracted secretion of TNF.[248] 16s ribosomal DNA analysis demonstrates that these E. coli are not a single strain, but 79% belonged to a common genotype (cluster A). Although these recent observations have not been independently confirmed, other studies have demonstrated E. coli adherent to the epithelium,[9] invading ulcers and fistulae,[52,250] and within lamina propria macrophages[53] of IBD patients. It will be important to determine whether these clinical isolates preferentially invade and persist within CARD15/NOD2 defective phagocytes and epithelial cells, activate NFκB in epithelial cells and induce enterocolitis in genetically engineered rodents. These studies lay the foundation for postoperative prevention studies with ciprofloxacin or other antibiotics that target E. coli.

## Pseudomonas species

Spheroplast forms of Pseudomonas multiphilia have been recovered in increased frequency from Crohn's disease tissues,[251] but further analysis showed that the cell wall defective variants were due to the antibiotic bowel preparation used preoperatively. More recently a novel bacterial sequence, I2, was identified in the colonic lamina propria cells of 43% of Crohn's disease patients, but only 9% of ulcerative colitis patients and 5% of normal controls.[56] This sequence is a transcriptional regulation gene of *Pseudomonas fluorescens*.[252] This organism is a secondary invader, as it is found in approximately 50% of IBD and control ileal samples, although serologic responses are selectively increased in Crohn's disease patients.[56] However, *Pseudomonas* species were not found in Crohn's disease tissues by 16s ribosomal DNA methods. A potential role in disease is suggested by the finding that I2 is a superantigen that induces IFN-γ in CD4+ T cells from mice with colitis and IL-10 from normal mice by activating Vb5[253].

### Listeria monocytogenes

Listeria, a common environmental pathogen found in cheese and other foods, selectively invades M cells overlying lymphoid aggregates and persists within macrophages. Liu et al.[52] reported immunohistochemical detection of *L. monocytogenes* in 75% of Crohn's disease tissues and increased serologic responses in Crohn's disease versus controls (30% vs. 8%). However, subsequent investigators have reported either negative or non-specific results using immunohistochemical staining[250] or PCR,[57,254] although fulminant ulcerative colitis has been associated with *L. monocytogenes* superinfection.[255] It is likely that this common environmental pathogen secondarily invades the ulcers of Crohn's disease.

### Helicobacter species

Analogous to the role of *H. pylori* in peptic ulcer disease and gastric cancer, *Helicobacter* species have been sought as etiologic agents of IBD. Gastric *H. pylori* colonization is reduced in IBD patients, perhaps because of antibiotic use.[256] Moreover, *H. pylori* infection does not affect the incidence of focal active gastritis associated with Crohn's disease,[257,258] nor alter the phenotype of intestinal disease,[259] although some authors have suggested that *H. pylori* may be protective.[260] In contrast, intestinal *Helicobacter* species (*H. hepaticus, H. bilis, H. typhlonicus*, and a novel urease-negative species) cause typhlitis and hepatobiliary inflammation in immunodeficient mice.[261,262] *H. hepaticus* can potentiate experimental colitis, induce specific T cell-specific responses in IL-10$^{-/-}$ mice in the relatively resistant C57Bl/6 background,[199,263,264] and contribute to colitis and adenocarcinoma in TGFβ$^{-/-}$ mice.[265] *H. bilis* potentiated disease in IL-10$^{-/-}$, mdr1α$^{-/-}$ and TCRα$^{-/-}$ mice.[264,266] However, *H. hepaticus* does not stimulate colitis in IL-10$^{-/-}$ mice on a sensitive background[129,135] and inhibits the development of disease in mdr1a$^{-/-}$ mice.[266] Reports of novel intestinal *Helicobacter* species colonizing rhesus monkeys[267] and cotton-top tamarins[157] with colitis, and molecular detection of *Helicobacter* species in 3/11 Crohn's disease lymphoid tissues,[268] support a comprehensive search for this agent in IBD.

### Measles

Wakefield and colleagues[269]have suggested that Crohn's disease is caused by persistent measles infection of endothelial cells, leading to chronic granulomatous vasculitis. They postulate that infection occurs perinatally or in early infancy, or as a consequence of live viral vaccination. These investigators have detected paromyxo-like structures within endothelial cells, measles antigen by standard immunohistochemistry and immunogold labeling, and increased IgM antibody to measles in Crohn's disease patients, and in some studies, ulcerative colitis.[270] Moreover, they cite epidemiologic data showing an increased risk of Crohn's disease in children born to mothers with measles infection during pregnancy, in persons born during measles epidemics and in those receiving measles vaccination. These results evoked concern among parents of children approaching vaccination age. However, most experts downplay the association of Crohn's disease with measles vaccination,[271,272] based on the examination of large national vaccination databases.[273,274] No risk of Crohn's disease with maternal infection during pregnancy,[275] but a significant association of both ulcerative colitis and Crohn's disease with measles infection before age 9,[276] was found in the Mayo Clinic population-based database. Other investigators have not documented persistent infection by immunohistochemical, serologic or DNA analysis.[277–279] However, Israeli investigators reported more frequent exposure to measles during childhood in Crohn's disease patients, especially those with colonic involvement, although serologic studies were not supportive.[280]

### Conclusions

*M. paratuberculosis* is not responsible for the majority of cases of Crohn's disease, although there is an alarmingly high natural reservoir of this organism in the commercial food chain, nor are there convincing data for persistent measles, *Pseudomonas* or *Listeria* infection in Crohn's disease. However, adherent/invasive *E. coli* may contribute to postoperative recurrence of Crohn's disease. This organism needs to be further investigated in both new-onset and recurrent disease. *Helicobacter* species need to be adequately explored. Before discounting the notion that a specific infectious agent could cause IBD and attributing positive culture and nucleic acid hybridization results to environmental contaminants secondarily invading ulcerated mucosa, several considerations must be addressed. Crohn's disease and ulcerative colitis are almost certainly heterogeneous groups of disorders with different etiologies (see Chapters 8 and 29). Therefore, a specific pathogen would be expected to be recovered from a minority of patients in a randomly selected group. Immunological and therapeutic studies can only be properly interpreted if the presence of the organism is prospectively determined, so that patients harboring infection are selectively investigated. Second, new pathogens are continually being identified, as shown by relatively recent discoveries of C. *difficile* toxin, *Tropheryma whippelii*, *Legionella*, HIV, *Cryptosporidium*, *Microsporidia*, *Borrelia burgdorferi*, *E. coli* 0157:H7, hepatitis C and D viruses and *Helicobacter pylori* as human pathogens. The integral role for *H. pylori* in peptic ulcer disease is particularly instructive, as there was little clinical evidence of a transmissible agent in duodenal ulcers and the genetic and pathogenic factors of this syndrome were felt to be well understood. Finally, an environmental agent, probably infectious in nature, is the best explanation of sporadic reports of case clustering of Crohn's disease among family members[95] and close friends[93] following an apparent latency period.

## DEFECTIVE CLEARANCE OF PATHOGENIC AND COMMENSAL ORGANISMS

Defective killing of invading commensal bacteria, opportunistic microbial agents or traditional enteric pathogens may cause tissue destruction and induction of pathogenic immune responses. Korzenik and Dieckgraefe[281] postulate that defective neutrophil function can lead to Crohn's disease, based on the association of Crohn's disease-like lesions in genetic syndromes with defined neutrophil defects, such as chronic granulomatous disease, glycogen storage disease Ib and leukocyte adhesion deficiency. Furthermore, typhlitis frequently complicates chemotherapy-induced neutropenia, and defects in neutrophil migration, superoxide generation, phagocytosis and microbial killing have been reported in Crohn's disease.[282–284] Some *Bacteroides* species impair neutrophil phagocytosis and microbicidal activity, suggesting that enteric bacteria mediate these defects.[285] This hypothesis is supported by an open label trial of granulocyte–macrophage colony-stimulating factor (GM-CSF), which induced a remission in 8/15 Crohn's disease patients, with closure of fistulae[286] and by demonstration of *E. coli* within lamina propria macrophages in ulcerative colitis tissues.[53] Suppression of neutrophil function by nicotine[287] and NSAIDs could help explain several environmental risk factors for Crohn's disease.

This hypothesis would also explain the seemingly paradoxical observations that CARD15/NOD2 genetic variants in Crohn's disease are associated with defective activation of NFκB by LPS or PG–PS,[83,85] and that blockade of epithelial NFκB function is associated with enhanced DSS-induced colitis.[288,289] Furthermore, the 3020 insC truncation mutation of CARD15/NOD2 leads to defective intracellular bacterial killing.[86] NFκB activation accelerates killing of intracellular bacteria through the induction of bacteriocidal nitric oxide synthesis, β defensins and TNF expression. The importance of TNF signaling on clearance of enteric pathogens is documented by a dramatic worsening of colitis in TNF receptor[−/−] versus wildtype mice following *Citrobacter rodentium* infection.

Microbial products can also inhibit host defenses. *Bacteroides* species decrease neutrophil phagocytosis and bacterial killing,[285] and an Epstein–Barr virus protein (BCRF1) that shares structural homology with IL-10 can inhibit innate and cognate immune function.[290] Several bacterial products block NFκB activation, including *Yersinia* Yop proteins, which block IκBa phosphorylation,[291] and non-pathogenic *Salmonella* products, which block ubiquitination of IκBa.[292] A large toxin secreted by enteropathogenic *E. coli* inhibits lymphocyte activation by blocking IL-2, IL-4 and IL-5 expression.[293] Defective T-cell function fosters the growth of opportunistic pathogens, including intestinal *Helicobacter* species, which induce typhlitis and hepatobiliary disease in T cell-deficient mice.[262]

## DEFECTIVE MUCOSAL BARRIER FUNCTION OR EPITHELIAL RESTITUTION

Intrinsic (genetically determined) or acquired (environmental agent) defects in mucosal barrier function or healing can lead to continuous uptake of luminal antigens that overwhelm local protective mechanisms.[294] Endogenous luminal bacteria and their phlogistic products are transported across the inflamed mucosa in IBD, especially Crohn's disease, and experimental enterocolitis (see Fig. 10.1). The controversy concerns whether this permeability defect is a primary or a secondary event.[295,296] Intestinal inflammation increases mucosal permeability by numerous mechanisms, including epithelial cell loss and the effects of cytokines and neutrophil transmigration on epithelial tight junctions (see Chapter 1). The correlation between disease

activity and altered mucosal permeability in both Crohn's disease and ulcerative colitis, and enhanced permeability predicting flares of Crohn's disease, suggest an acquired defect.[297–300] Permeability defects in 'quiescent' Crohn's disease are difficult to interpret because of biochemical and immunologic evidence of occult inflammation despite normal gross, endoscopic and even histologic findings.[301] Mechanisms of acquired defects in mucosal permeability include stress, mediated by endogenous corticosteroids,[302] NSAIDs,[303,304] TNF,[305,306] secreted products of lamina propria mononuclear cells[307] and zinc deficiency.[308] Hollander et al.[297] postulated that susceptibility to Crohn's disease is caused by genetically determined defective barrier function, as patients with inactive Crohn's disease and two-thirds of their healthy relatives have increased permeability to inert markers. Thirty-five per cent of asymptomatic relatives of Crohn's disease patients have exaggerated permeability following aspirin challenge,[303] with similar findings after ibuprofen challenge.[304] Responsiveness to aspirin damage follows a familial pattern. However, other groups failed to show a significant increase in mucosal permeability to a number of markers in first-degree relatives of Crohn's disease patients,[309] even when the mucosa was stressed with hyperosmolar agents. However, a population-based study in Iceland demonstrated occult inflammation by fecal calprotectin levels in asymptomatic relatives of Crohn's disease probands.[310] May et al.[311] attempted to reconcile these differences by showing that only 10% of asymptomatic family members exhibit enhanced permeability, which is still greater than the number of family members who develop clinical disease. Further studies have indicated that spouses of Crohn's disease patients also have enhanced small bowel permeability, suggesting that familial aggregation of permeability defects is environmental rather than genetic.[312,313] Soderholm et al.[314] concluded that environmental factors contributed to baseline increased permeability, whereas response to aspirin challenge was genetically determined. The consequences of such defects are evident in experimental studies, where genetically susceptible Lewis rats or IL-10[−/−] mice develop chronic intestinal inflammation after brief exposure to NSAIDs;[114,208] gnotobiotic and antibiotic results indicate that this inflammation is mediated by commensal bacteria.[155,209]

Enhanced uptake of bacterial products and translocating bacteria owing to an intrinsic defect in mucosal barrier function can lead to intestinal inflammation. The mucous gel layer is depleted in ulcerative colitis with functionally abnormal mucus glycoproteins;[315] these mucous alterations are particularly evident in the distal colon.[316] Certain bacteria, including *Bacteroides* species, secrete mucolytic enzymes which could contribute to this thinned mucus layer.[317] In addition, both ulcerative colitis and experimental colitis are associated with goblet cell depletion due to increased secretion of mucus. The importance of an intact mucous gel layer in barrier function is illustrated by a 50-fold enhanced uptake of FMLP following dithiothreitol treatment, which removed mucus.[175] Mucosally associated bacterial concentrations are dramatically increased in IBD patients.[9] Animal studies elegantly illustrate the importance of an intact mucosal barrier. Several growth factors that prevent experimental colitis, including keratinocyte growth factor-2 and fibroblast growth factor 20, stimulate the expression of intestinal trefoil factor (ITF, TFF3),[318–320] which increases mucous viscosity and accelerates epithelial restitution after injury. ITF-deficient mice do not develop spontaneous inflammation, but have delayed healing and enhanced mortality following DSS challenge.[321] In contrast, defective N-cadherin function in the small intestine leads to spontaneous focal enteritis by targeting tight junctions.[322] Of considerable relevance is the fact that bacterial products can increase epithelial permeability, as shown by the effects of *Bacteroides fragilis* enterotoxin on HT-29 enterocytes.[323] Furthermore, IL-10 can prevent IFN-γ-mediated damage to HT-29 cell tight junctions,[324] IL-10[-/-] mice exhibit increased mucosal permeability prior to the onset of histologic colitis,[17] and IL-10[-/-] mice have defective MUC2 expression.[325] Thus, molecular defects in barrier function and/or restitution and healing could lead to chronic idiopathic IBD in humans, with enhanced uptake of luminal bacterial components driving a persistent mucosal immune response.

## ALTERED LUMINAL MICROBIAL COMPONENTS ('DYSBIOSIS')

Normal hosts could develop chronic intestinal inflammation as a result of the altered composition of commensal enteric bacteria or by harboring 'normal' fecal bacteria with subtle functional alterations that are extremely difficult to detect by standard culture or molecular genetic techniques. The extremely complex microbial ecology of the distal intestine is regulated by diet, pH, redox potential, motility, non-absorbed carbohydrates, anatomical variants such as loss of the ileocecal valve and fistulae, host genetics and antibiotic exposure.[13,145] Several of these parameters, notably pH, redox potential and SCFA production, are a function of the remarkably stable commensal bacteria population.

### Altered microbial composition

The balance of beneficial and detrimental enteric bacteria appears to be altered in patients with IBD and in the Western, industrialized population where IBD is most prevalent (Table 10.6). Fecal concentrations of certain anaerobic coccobacilli, including *Eubacteria*, *Peptostreptococci* and *Coprococci*, are increased in Crohn's disease patients and their asymptomatic relatives.[13,326] Prospective studies suggest that these bacterial profiles are genetically determined and precede (and perhaps predict) clinical symptoms.[13] *Bacteroides* species are increased in Crohn's disease,[9,327–329] and decreased fecal *Bacteroides vulgatus* concentrations correlate with response to metronidazole.[329] Similarly, mucosally associated *E. coli* are increased in Crohn's disease.[9,327] Neut and colleagues[327] found increased concentrations of mucosally associated *E. coli* and Enterococci in the neoterminal ileum of Crohn's disease patients after surgery; early disease recurrence was associated with increased concentrations of *E. coli*,

*Bacteroides* species and *Fusobacterium* species. In contrast, *Bifidobacteria* and Ruminococcus concentrations were decreased,[327] consistent with earlier reports of decreased fecal concentrations of *Bifidobacteria* and *Lactobacilli* in Crohn's disease.[330–332] Concentrations of Enterococci are increased in ulcerative colitis.[332,333] Mucosally associated aerobic and anaerobic bacteria, particularly *Bacteroides* species and Enterobacteriaceae, are significantly increased in IBD patients.[9] These increases are relatively non-specific, because mucosal bacteria were also increased in self-limited infectious colitis, although to a lesser extent than in IBD.[9] Other studies demonstrate increased mucosally associated bacteria in IBD[334] as well as a high frequency of small intestinal bacterial overgrowth in Crohn's disease, particularly with strictures and loss of the ileocecal valve.[335] Pouchitis appears to be due to an overgrowth of commensal enteric bacteria, but the abnormal components have not been thoroughly delineated.[336] Interestingly, increased fecal concentrations of *Bacteroides* and *Clostridia*, but decreased *Lactobacilli*, have been described in Westernized Swedish normals relative to Estonian subjects, who live in a less developed society.[337] Lack of childhood exposure to immunoregulatory microbial products (LPS, helminths) ubiquitously present in undeveloped countries has been postulated to account for the high rate of IBD and allergic disorders in Western countries (hygiene hypothesis).[338,339]

Similar observations in experimental models, which show the specific inflammatory potential of these bacterial species, provide additional support for the concept that altered composition of enteric commensal bacteria can influence disease. Madsen demonstrated early mucosal colonization of IL-10[-/-] mice with Streptococci and *Clostridium* species at 2 weeks of age (before onset of colitis) and decreased *Lactobacilli*.[17] *Bacteroides* species are increased in HLA-B27 transgenic rats with colitis[340] and in DSS-treated mice;[341] in the latter model *B. caccae* was particularly elevated and levels correlated with luminal concentrations of succinic acid, a *Bacteroides* metabolite which induced rectal ulceration upon enema administration. Furthermore, *B. vulgatus* induces experimental colitis in monoassociated HLA-B27 transgenic rats,[133] guinea pigs fed carrageenan[132] and T-cell receptor a[-/-] mice.[342] Moreover, *E. coli* or *Enterococcus faecalis* cause colitis in monoassociated IL-10[-/-] mice[137,138] and killed *Bacteroides* species induce fibrosis in TNBS-treated rats.[343] Finally, *Lactobacilli* and *Bifidobacteria* have protective roles in probiotic and prebiotic studies (see previous section).

### Altered function

Altered metabolic function or virulence properties in commensal bacteria isolated from IBD patients profoundly affect epithelial cell and mucosal barrier function, thereby inducing inflammation. As detailed above, *E. coli* strains isolated from ulcerative colitis patients exhibit increased epithelial adherence,[241] and those from the neoterminal ileum of postoperative Crohn's disease patients have an adherent/invasive phenotype and stimulate macrophage TNF production.[246,248] *E. coli* isolated from IBD patients produce cytotoxins,[243,246] whereas IBD-derived *B. vulgatus* and Enterococci secrete mucin-degrading enzymes,[344] Enterococci produce hyaluranidase[345] and *Pseudomonas fluorescence* I2 is a T-cell superantigen.[253]

Roediger[24] postulates that bacterial production of hydrogen sulfide, which blocks colonic epithelial cell metabolism of SCFA, causes ulcerative colitis through epithelial starvation. SCFA are

## Table 10.6 Balance of protective versus aggressive commensal bacterial species in the intestine

| Beneficial | Aggressive |
|---|---|
| *Lactobacillus* species | *Bacteroides* species |
| *Bifidobacterium* species | *Enterococcus faecalis* |
| Selected *E. coli* strains | Adherent/invasive or toxigenic *E. coli* strains |
| *Streptococcus salivarius* | *Eubacterium* and *Peptostreptococcus* species |
| | *Fusobacterium varium* |
| | *Helicobacter* species |

## Table 10.7 Therapeutic approaches to reversing inflammation induced by bacterial components

| Target | Strategy |
|---|---|
| Luminal antigens and adjuvants activating pathogenic responses | Antibiotics, probiotics, prebiotics (? combination) luminal binding agents (LPS), degrade PG–PS, LPS, FMLP |
| Bacterial adhesion to the mucosa | Block bacterial adhesins, epithelial binding sites |
| Adjuvant binding | Block TLR, NOD-1/2, CD14, LBP |
| Adjuvant signaling | Block NFκB, MAPK |
| Antigen binding | Selective blockade of MHC, TCR binding |
| Effector cell activation | Block macrophage, neutrophil, T-cell activation, cytokine expression |
| Regulatory cell function | Stimulate regulatory APC and T-cell activity |
| Mucosal barrier function | Stimulate healing, mucus, ITF, defensins, tight junctions, growth factor expression |
| Phagocytic cell killing of bacteria | Increase number and function of neutrophils and macrophages |

Strategies to selectively eliminate luminal antigens include antibiotics (narrow spectrum, broad spectrum and non-absorbable), probiotics and prebiotics. Based on current knowledge, antibiotic therapy should either be broad spectrum or selectively target *E. coli*, *Bacteroides* and Enterococci, and should be administered long term to eliminate chronic antigenic stimulation. Because this goal will be difficult to achieve owing to the emergence of resistant strains, short-term use of broad-spectrum antibiotics to eliminate targeted bacteria, followed by sustained administration of probiotic species, may be more effective.[142] Combining probiotics with prebiotics may sustain long-term colonization by beneficial organisms, as probiotic species disappear 2–4 weeks after cessation of probiotic administration[11] and are quite expensive. Elimination of luminal adjuvants by non-absorbed binding agents (soluble LPS-binding protein; soluble TLR 2, 3, 4, 9; polymyxin B; or LPS- and PG–PS-binding polymers) should decrease innate immune responses, including APC activation. Agents that degrade PG–PS (mutanolysin or lysosome) or FMLP (endopeptidases) should attenuate bacterial adjuvant and chemotactic signals. Because mucosally associated bacteria may provide greater antigenic stimulation than luminal bacteria, bacterial epithelial cell binding could be blocked. Antibodies or small molecules that bind without agonist activity or lactoferrin, which binds to soluble CD14[370], could block adjuvant binding to membrane or intracellular receptors. Obviously global blockade of APC and T-cell activation is hazardous because of infections. Finally, stimulation of defective phagocytic killing may be effective in selected cases.[286] Delivery of immunosuppressive molecules by genetically engineered enteric bacteria[143] establishes a precedent for delivering inhibitory proteins and growth factors to the site of disease activity, although the public health implications of using recombinant bacteria must be addressed.

## CONCLUSIONS

Adjuvants and antigens derived from the complex mix of commensal enteric bacteria constantly activate mucosal and systemic immune responses, culminating in chronic relapsing enterocolitis and associated extraintestinal inflammation in susceptible hosts. Microbial agents are strongly implicated in the pathogenesis of Crohn's disease, pouchitis and the septic complications of IBD, but evidence for their involvement in ulcerative colitis is more tangential and may relate to host defects in mucosal barrier function, healing or bacterial clearance, or perhaps subtle alterations in bacterial virulence factors. Pathogens (and environmental agents that break the mucosal barrier, such as NSAIDs) can initiate and reactivate chronic idiopathic IBD, but evidence for a persistent, specific pathogen causing disease is quite limited. However, a role for *M. paratuberculosis* in a subset of Crohn's disease patients, entero adherent/invasive *E. coli*, non-*pylori* *Helicobacter* species or yet to be defined pathogen(s) has not been excluded. Common environmental pathogens may perpetuate existing inflammation by secondarily invading the ulcerated mucosa in an immunosuppressed patient. Mechanisms by which bacterial adjuvants (pathogen-associated molecular patterns – LPS, PG–PS, CpG, flagellin HSP-60 etc.) interact with membrane-bound and intracellular receptors (pattern recognition receptors – TLR, CARD) to activate innate immune cells, including APC, phagocytes, intestinal epithelial cells and mesenchymal cells, through NFκB are rapidly being elucidated. A developing theme implicates deranged innate responses to these bacterial stimulants in the pathogenesis of Crohn's disease. These alterations in bacterial killing (defective NOD2/CARD15 or phagocytic/bacteriocidal function) and APC regulation could lead to persistence of pathogens and translocating commensal bacteria, excessive antigenic stimulation of T cells, and defective down-regulation of macrophage, Th1 and Th2 responses. Functional alterations of commensals can have pathologic consequences. For example, the acquisition of virulence factors, such as epithelial adhesion, invasion, secretion of cytokines, mucolytic enzymes or hydrogen sulfide, can damage the mucosal barrier and alter host immune responses. Finally, the relative balance of beneficial (*Lactobacilli*, *Bifidobacteria*) and aggressive (*Bacteroides*, *E. coli*, Enterococci) organisms in the lumen and at the mucosal surface may determine homeostatic versus inflammatory immune responses and help explain the predilection for developing IBD in the Westernized environment. Factors regulating the balance of bacterial populations include host genetics, diet, exposure to antibiotics and public health practices.

An overarching theme is host–microbial interactions and genetic regulation of host responses to commensal and pathogenic microbial agents (Fig. 10.4). The diversity of animal models indicates that multiple genetic defects in immunoregulation or barrier function/healing can lead to phenotypically similar immune and pathogenic responses. IBD patients exhibit loss of immunologic tolerance to autologous bacteria and have increased mucosally associated commensals. The first gene associated with Crohn's disease governs innate immune responses to bacterial adjuvants and clearance of intracellular pathogens. Provocative evidence suggests that a subset of asymptomatic relatives of Crohn's disease patients have defective mucosal barrier function and occult inflammation, with familial patterns of responses. Crohn's disease and ulcerative colitis almost certainly consist of heterogeneous groups of disorders, each with a defined genetic abnormality, immune response, natural history and response to treatment. Based on rodent model results, each host genetic background, and even each phenotype of IBD, may have a dominant bacterial stimulus, which has extremely important implications for designing optimal therapy for an individual patient.

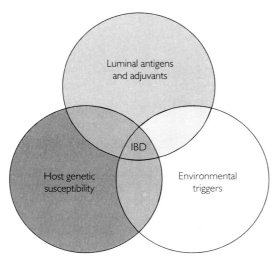

**Fig. 10.4** Host/microbial/environmental interactions. Induction of chronic inflammation requires the interaction of genetic, luminal (microbial or dietary) and environmental factors. Each of these components is necessary, but none alone is sufficient to induce disease. Microbial factors consist of adjuvants and antigens from the commensal enteric bacteria, or possibly a persistent pathogen, whereas environmental triggers include self-limited infections, microbial toxins and compounds that injure the mucosal barrier (NSAIDs).

We hypothesize that genetic susceptibility and luminal microbial composition govern host responses to environmental triggers (Fig. 10.5). Sporadic environmental insults are required to initiate disease, since the genetic defects of Crohn's disease and ulcerative colitis are subtle and are not sufficient to induce disease alone. It is more likely that genetically programmed defects in immunoregulation or mucosal defenses/healing determine whether the host promptly clears the inciting agent and heals the mucosa with return to immunologic tolerance (homeostasis) versus lapsing into a chronic inflammatory response perpetuated by antigenic stimulation and secondary invasion by commensal bacteria.

Many opportunities for improved clinical diagnosis and treatment emanate from our developing understanding of pathogenesis. Panels of bacteriologic antigens and 16s ribosomal DNA bacterial gene chips being developed and validated offer hope of identifying subsets of patients who will respond predictably to antibiotic, probiotic and prebiotic interventions. Biochemical or molecular identification of bacterial virulence factors will help identify subsets of bacteria upon which to target selective therapies. Understanding cellular receptors and signaling pathways used to activate innate and acquired immune responses to commensal bacteria will identify specific new therapeutic targets, and determining immunoregulatory mechanisms will allow the stimulation of tolerance. This approach, combined with manipulating the balance of beneficial and aggressive components of the commensal microbiota, offers a real prospect for long-term non-toxic means to maintain mucosal and immunologic homeostasis, thereby preventing relapse of these insidious diseases.

## ACKNOWLEDGMENTS

The author thanks Susie May for her expert secretarial assistance. Original research described in this review was supported by NIH grants DK 40249, DK 47700 and DK 34987, The Crohn's and Colitis Foundation of America, and the Broad Medical Research Foundation.

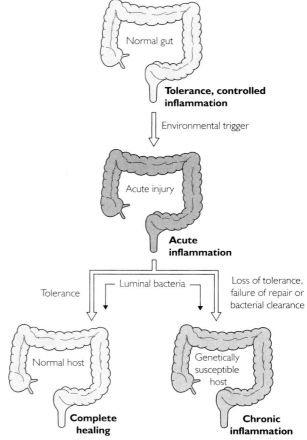

**Fig. 10.5** Variable responses to environmental triggers in genetically susceptible vs. normal hosts. Environmental triggers, including self-limiting infections or environmental agents such as NSAIDs, induce acute injury in all hosts. Normal hosts rapidly clear the inciting infection, heal the injured mucosa, and downregulate inflammation to return to the baseline state of immunologic non-responsiveness (tolerance) to commensal bacteria. However, genetically susceptible hosts with defective microbial clearance, mucosal healing or downregulation of inflammation develop chronic inflammation, which is driven by constant stimulation of pathogenic T lymphocytes by antigens from commensal bacteria (or persistent pathogens).

## REFERENCES

1. Sartor RB. Microbial agents in the pathogenesis, differential diagnosis, and complications of inflammatory bowel diseases. In: Blaser MJ, Smith PD, Ravdin JI et al, eds. Infections of the gastrointestinal tract, 2nd edn. Philadelphia: Lippincott Williams & Wilkins; 2002: 383–413.

2. Wilson KH. Natural biota of the human gastrointestinal tract. In: Blaser MJ, Smith PD, Ravdin JI et al., eds. Infections of the gastrointestinal tract, 2nd edn. Philadelphia: Lippincott Williams & Wilkins; 2002: 45–56.

3. Konstantinov SR, Fitzsimons N, Vaughan EE et al. From composition to functionality of the intestinal microbial communities. In: Tannock GW, ed. Probiotics and prebiotics: where are we going? Wymondham, UK: Caister Academic Press; 2002: 59–84.

4. Finegold SM, Sutter VL, Mathison GE. Normal indigenous intestinal flora. In: Hentges DJ, ed. Human intestinal microflora in health and disease. New York: Academic Press; 1983: 3–31.

5. Gorbach SL, Plaut AG, Nahas L et al. Studies of intestinal microflora. II. Microorganisms of the small intestine and their relations to oral and fecal flora. Gastroenterology 1967;53:856–867.

6. Moore WEC, Holdeman IV. Human fecal flora: The normal flora of 20 Japanese-Hawaiians. Appl Microbiol 1974;27:979.

7. Wilson KH, Blitchington RB. Human colonic biota studied by ribosomal DNA sequence analysis. Appl Environ Microbiol 1996;62:2273–2278.

8. Wilson KH, Ikeda JS, Blitchington RB. Phylogenetic placement of community members of human colonic biota. Clin Infect Dis 1997;25:S114–S116.

9. Swidsinski A, Ladhoff A, Pernthaler A et al. Mucosal flora in inflammatory bowel disease. Gastroenterology 2002;122:44–54.

10. Barza M, Guiliano M, Jacobus NV et al. Effect of broad-spectrum parenteral antibiotics on 'colonization resistance' of intestinal microflora of humans. Antimicrob Agents Chemother 1987;31:723–727.

11. Gionchetti P, Rizzello F, Venturi A et al. Oral bacteriotherapy as maintenance treatment in patients with chronic pouchitis: a double-blind, placebo-controlled trial. Gastroenterology 2000;119:305–309.

12. Buhling A, Radun D, Muller WA et al. Influence of anti-Helicobacter triple therapy with metronidazole, omeprazole and clarithromycin on intestinal microflora. Aliment Pharmacol Ther 2001;15:1445–1452.

13. van de Merwe JP, Schroder AM, Wensinck F et al. The obligate anaerobic faecal flora of patients with Crohn's disease and their first-degree relatives. Scand J Gastroenterol 1988;23:1125–1131.

14. Hentges DJ. Does diet influence human fecal microflora composition? Nutr Rev 1980;38:329–336.

15. Finegold SM, Attebery HR, Sutter VL. Effect of diet on human fecal flora: comparison of Japanese and American diets. Am J Clin Nutr 1974;27:1456–1469.

16. Lundequist B, Nord CE, Winberg J. The composition of the faecal microflora in breastfed and bottle fed infants from birth to eight weeks. Acta Paediatr Scand 1985;74:45–51.

17. Madsen KL, Doyle JS, Jewell LD et al. Lactobacillus species prevents colitis in interleukin 10 gene-deficient mice. Gastroenterology 1999;116:1107–1114.

18. Wolin MJ. Fermentation in the rumen and human large intestine. Science 1981;213:1463–1468.

19. Silva M, Jacobus NV, Deneke C et al. Antimicrobial substance from a human Lactobacillus strain. Antimicrob Agents Chemother 1987;31:1231–1233.

20. Salyers AA, Shoemaker NB, Stevens AM et al. Conjugative transposons: an unusual and diverse set of integrated gene transfer elements. Microbiol Rev 1995;59:579–590.

21. Roediger WE. Role of anaerobic bacteria in the metabolic welfare of the colonic mucosa in man. Gut 1980;21:793–798.

22. Bocker U, Nebe T, Herweck F et al. Butyrate modulates intestinal epithelial cell-mediated neutrophil migration. Clin Exp Immunol 2003;131:53–60.

23. Magee EA, Richardson CJ, Hughes R et al. Contribution of dietary protein to sulfide production in the large intestine: an in vitro and a controlled feeding study in humans. Am J Clin Nutr 2000;72:1488–1494.

24. Roediger WE, Duncan A, Kapaniris O et al. Reducing sulfur compounds of the colon impair colonocyte nutrition: implications for ulcerative colitis. Gastroenterology 1993;104:802–809.

25. Hooper LV, Gordon JI. Commensal host–bacterial relationships in the gut. Science 2001;292:1115–1118.

26. Narthakumar NN, Dai D, Newburg DS et al. The role of indigenous microflora in the development of murine intestinal fucosyl- and sialyltransferases. FASEB J 2003;17:44–46.

27. MacDonald TT, Carter PB. Requirement for a bacterial flora before mice generate cells capable of mediating the delayed hypersensitivity reaction to sheep red blood cells. J Immunol 1979;122:2624–2629.

28. Wannemuehler MJ, Kiyono H, Babb JL et al. Lipopolysacchairde (LPS) regulation of the immune responses: LPS converts germfree mice to sensitivity to oral tolerance induction. Clin Exp Immunol 1982;88:313–317.

29. Moreau MC, Gaboriau-Routhiau V. The absence of gut flora, the doses of antigen ingested and aging affect the long-term peripheral tolerance induced by ovalbumin feeding in mice. Res Immunol 1996;147:49–59.

30. Isaacs KL, Sartor RB. Antibodies in IBD. Gastroenterology Clin N Am 2003;(in press).

31. Madsen K. The use of probiotics in gastrointestinal disease. Can J Gastroenterol 2001;15:817–822.

32. Linskens RK, Huijsdens XW, Savelkoul PH et al. The bacterial flora in inflammatory bowel disease: current insights in pathogenesis and the influence of antibiotics and probiotics. Scand J Gastroenterol 2001; Suppl. 29–40.

33. Dunne C. Adaptation of bacteria to the intestinal niche: probiotics and gut disorder. Inflamm Bowel Dis 2001;7:136–145.

34. Gionchetti P, Rizzello F, Campieri M. Probiotics and antibiotics in inflammatory bowel diseases. Curr Opin Gastroenterol 2001;17:331–335.

35. Ulisse S, Gionchetti P, D'Alo S et al. Expression of cytokines, inducible nitric oxide synthase, and matrix metalloproteinases in pouchitis: effects of probiotic treatment. Am J Gastroenterol 2001;96:2691–2699.

36. Borruel N, Carol M, Casellas F et al. Increased mucosal tumour necrosis factor α production in Crohn's disease can be downregulated ex vivo by probiotic bacteria. Gut 2002;51:659–664.

37. Bird AR, Brown IL, Topping DL. Starches, resistant starches, the gut microflora and human health. Curr Issues Intest Microbiol 2000;1:25–37.

38. Jacobasch G, Schmiedl D, Kruschewski M et al. Dietary resistant starch and chronic inflammatory bowel diseases. Int J Colorectal Dis 1999;14:201–211.

39. Mitsuyama K, Saiki T, Kanauchi O et al. Treatment of ulcerative colitis with germinated barley foodstuff feeding: a pilot study. Aliment Pharmacol Ther 1998;12:1225–1230.

40. Hallert C, Kaldma M, Petersson BG. Ispaghula husk may relieve gastrointestinal symptoms in ulcerative colitis in remission. Scand J Gastroenterol 1991;26:747–750.

41. Sartor RB. Postoperative recurrence of Crohn's disease: the enemy is within the fecal stream. Gastroenterology 1998;114:398–400.

42. Harper PH, Truelove SC, Lee EC et al. Split ileostomy and ileocolostomy for Crohn's disease of the colon and ulcerative colitis: a 20 year survey. Gut 1983;24:106–113.

43. Harper PH, Lee EC, Kettlewell MG et al. Role of the faecal stream in the maintenance of Crohn's colitis. Gut 1985;26:279–284.

44. Rutgeerts P, Goboes K, Peeters M et al. Effect of faecal stream diversion on recurrence of Crohn's disease in the neoterminal ileum. Lancet 1991;338:771–774.

45. D'Haens GR, Geboes K, Peeters M et al. Early lesions of recurrent Crohn's disease caused by infusion of intestinal contents in excluded ileum. Gastroenterology 1998;114:262–267.

46. Dieleman LA, Heizer WD. Nutritional issues in inflammatory bowel disease. Gastroenterol Clin North Am 1998;27:435–451.

47. Greenberg GR, Fleming CR, Jeejeebhoy KN et al. Controlled trial of bowel rest and nutritional support in the management of Crohn's disease. Gut 1988;29:1309–1315.

48. Roediger WE. A new hypothesis for the etiology of Crohn's disease – evidence from lipid metabolism and intestinal tuberculosis. Postgrad Med J 1991;67:666–671.

49. Lomer MC, Harvey RS, Evans SM et al. Efficacy and tolerability of a low microparticle diet in a double blind, randomized, pilot study in Crohn's disease. Eur J Gastroenterol Hepatol 2001;13:101–106.

50. Brooke BN, Dykes PW, Walker FC. A study of liver disorder in ulcerative colitis. Postgrad Med J 1961;37:245–251.

51. Ambrose NS, Johnson M, Burdon DW et al. Incidence of pathogenic bacteria from mesenteric lymph nodes and ileal serosa during Crohn's disease surgery. Br J Surg 1984;71:623–625.

52. Liu Y, Van Kruiningen HJ, West AB et al. Immunocytochemical evidence of Listeria, Escherichia coli, and Streptococcus antigens in Crohn's disease. Gastroenterology 1995;108:1396–1404.

53. Rayment N, Mylonaki M, Rampton D et al. Co-localisation of E. coli with macrophages in lamina propria in patients with active inflammatory bowel disease (IBD). Gut 2003 (in press) (Abstract).

54. Ohkusa T, Okayasu I, Tokoi S et al. Bacterial invasion into the colonic mucosa in ulcerative colitis. J Gastroenterol Hepatol 1993;8:116–118.

55. Bregman E, Kirsner JB. Amino acids of colon and rectum. Possible involvement of diaminopimelic acid of intestinal bacteria in antigenicity of ulcerative colitis colon. Proc Soc Exp Biol Med 1965;118:7207.

56. Sutton CL, Kim J, Yamane A et al. Identification of a novel bacterial sequence associated with Crohn's disease. Gastroenterology 2000;119:23–31.

57. Chiba M, Kono M, Hoshina S et al. Presence of bacterial 16S ribosomal RNA gene segments in human intestinal lymph follicles. Scand J Gastroenterol 2000;35:824–831.

58. Anderson RP, Friend GM, Ferry DM et al. Formyl peptidemia in patients with inflammatory bowel disease and primary sclerosing cholangitis. Gastroenterology 1991;100:A557 (Abstract).

59. Gardiner KR, Halliday MI, Barclay GR et al. Significance of systemic endotoxaemia in inflammatory bowel disease. Gut 1995;36:897–901.

60. Baldassano RN, Schreiber S, Johnston RBJ et al. Crohn's disease monocytes are primed for accentuated release of toxic oxygen metabolites. Gastroenterology 1993;105:60–66.

61. Hazenberg MP, de Visser H, Bras MJ et al. Serum antibodies to peptidoglycan–polysaccharide complexes from the anaerobic intestinal flora in patients with Crohn's disease. Digestion 1990;47:172–180.

62. Currie CG, McCallum K, Poxton IR. Mucosal and systemic antibody responses to the lipopolysaccharide of Escherichia coli O157 in health and disease. J Med Microbiol 2001;50:345–354.

63. Auer IO, Roder A, Wensinck F et al. Selected bacterial antibodies in Crohn's disease and ulcerative colitis. Scand J Gastroenterol 1983;18:217–223.

64. Tabaqchali S, O'Donoghue DP, Bettelheim KA. Escherichia coli antibodies in patients with inflammatory bowel disease. Gut 1978;19:108–113.

65. Macpherson A, Khoo UY, Forgacs I et al. Mucosal antibodies in inflammatory bowel disease are directed against intestinal bacteria. Gut 1996;38:365–375.

66. Blaser MJ, Miller FA, Lacher J et al. Patients with active Crohn's disease have elevated serum antibodies to antigens of seven enteric bacterial pathogens. Gastroenterology 1984;87:888–894.

67. Lindberg E, Magnusson KE, Tysk C et al. Antibody (IgG, IgA, and IgM) to baker's yeast (Saccharomyces cerevisiae), yeast mannan, gliadin, ovalbumin and betalactoglobulin in monozygotic twins with inflammatory bowel disease. Gut 1992;33:909–913.

68. Linskens RK, Mallant-Hent RC, Groothuismink ZM et al. Evaluation of serological markers to differentiate between ulcerative colitis and Crohn's disease: pANCA, ASCA and agglutinating antibodies to anaerobic coccoid rods. Eur J Gastroenterol Hepatol 2002;14:1013–1018.

69. Matsuda H, Fujiyama Y, Andoh A et al. Characterization of antibody responses against rectal mucosa-associated bacterial flora in patients with ulcerative colitis. J Gastroenterol Hepatol 2000;15:61–68.

70. Landers CJ, Cohavy O, Misra R et al. Selected loss of tolerance evidenced by Crohn's disease-associated immune responses to auto- and microbial antigens. Gastroenterology 2002;123:689–699.

71. Elson CO. Commensal bacteria as targets in Crohn's disease. Gastroenterology 2000;119:254–257.

72. Duchmann R, Kaiser I, Hermann E et al. Tolerance exists towards resident intestinal flora but is broken in active inflammatory bowel disease (IBD). Clin Exp Immunol 1995;102:448–455.

73. Duchmann R, Marker-Hermann E, Meyer zum Buschenfelde KH. Bacteria-specific T-cell clones are selective in their reactivity towards different enterobacteria or H. pylori and increased in inflammatory bowel disease. Scand J Immunol 1996;44:71–79.

74. van den Bogaerde J, Kamm MA, Knight SC. Immune sensitization to food, yeast and bacteria in Crohn's disease. Aliment Pharmacol Ther 2001;15:1647–1653.

75. Pirzer U, Schonhaar A, Fleischer B et al. Reactivity of infiltrating T lymphocytes with microbial antigens in Crohn's disease. Lancet 1991;338:1238–1239.

76. Podolsky DK. Inflammatory bowel disease. N Engl J Med 2002;347:417–429.

77. Saitoh S, Noda S, Aiba Y et al. Bacteroides ovatus as the predominant commensal intestinal microbe causing a systemic antibody response in inflammatory bowel disease. Clin Diagn Lab Immunol 2002;9:54–59.

78. Wei B, Dalwadi H, Gordon LK et al. Molecular cloning of a Bacteroides caccae Ton B-linked outer membrane protein identified by an inflammatory bowel disease marker antibody. Infect Immun 2001;69:6044–6054.

79. Cohavy O, Bruckner D, Gordon LK et al. Colonic bacteria express an ulcerative colitis pANCA-related protein epitope. Infect Immun 2000;68:1542–1548.

80. Ohkusa T, Sato N, Ogihara T et al. Fusobacterium varium localized in the colonic mucosa of patients with ulcerative colitis stimulates species-specific antibody. J Gastroenterol Hepatol 2002;17:849–853.

81. Cohavy O, Harth G, Horwitz M et al. Identification of a novel mycobacterial histone H1 homologue (HupB) as an antigenic target of pANCA monoclonal antibody and serum immunoglobulin A from patients with Crohn's disease. Infect Immun 1999;67:6510–6517.

82. Hugot JP, Chamaillard M, Zouali H et al. Association of NOD2 leucine-rich repeat variants with susceptibility to Crohn's disease. Nature 2001;411:599–603.

83. Ogura Y, Bonen DK, Inohara N et al. A frameshift mutation in NOD2 associated with susceptibility to Crohn's disease. Nature 2001;411:603–606.

84. Givardin SE, Boneca IG, Viala J et al. NOD2 is a general sensor of peptidoglycan through MDP detection. J Biol Chem 2003;278:8869–8872.

85. Bonen DK, Ogura Y, Nicolae DL et al. NOD2 variants associated with Crohn's disease share a signaling defect in response to lipopolysaccharide and peptidoglycan. Gastroenterology 2002;124:140–146.

86. Hisamatsu T, Suzuki M, Reinecker HC et al. CARD15/NOD2 functions as an anti-bacterial factor in human intestinal epithelial cells. Gastroenterology 2003;(in press).

87. Rosenstiel P, Fantini M, Brautigam K et al. TNF-α and IFN-γ regulate the expression of NOD2 (CARD15) gene in human intestinal epithelial cells. Gastroenterology 2003;(in press).

88. Klein W, Tromm A, Griga T et al. A polymorphism in the CD14 gene is associated with Crohn disease. Scand J Gastroenterol 2002;37:189–191.

89. Jobin C, Sartor RB. The IκB/NFκB system: a key determinant of mucosal inflammation and protection. Am J Physiol Cell Physiol 2000;278:C451–C462.

90. Farrell RJ, Murphy A, Long A et al. High multidrug resistance (P-glycoprotein 170) expression in inflammatory bowel disease patients who fail medical therapy. Gastroenterology 2000;118:279–288.

91. Panwala CM, Jones JC, Viney JL. A novel model of inflammatory bowel disease: mice deficient for the multiple drug resistance gene, mdr1a, spontaneously develop colitis. J Immunol 1998;161:5733–5744.

92. Powell SJ, Wilmont AJ. Ulcerative postdysenteric colitis. Gut 1966;7:438–443.

93. Aisenberg J, Janowitz HD. Cluster of inflammatory bowel disease in three close college friends. J Clin Gastroenterol 1993;17:18–20.

94. Laharie D, Debeugny S, Peeters M et al. Inflammatory bowel disease in spouses and their offspring. Gastroenterology 2001;120:816–819.

95. Van Kruiningen HJ, Colombel JF, Cartun RW et al. An in-depth study of Crohn's disease in two French families. Gastroenterology 1993;104:351–360.

96. Cartun RW, Van Kruiningen HJ, Pedersen et al. An immunocytochemical search for infectious agents in Crohn's disease. Mod Pathol 1993;6:212–219.

97. Tysk C, Lindberg E, Jarnerot G et al. Ulcerative colitis and Crohn's disease in an unselected population of monozygotic and dizygotic twins. A study of heritability and the influence of smoking. Gut 1988;29:990–996.

98. Mee AS, Jewell DP. Factors inducing relapse in inflammatory bowel disease. Br Med J 1978;2:801–802.

99. Kangro HO, Chong SK, Hardiman A et al. A prospective study of viral and mycoplasma infections in chronic inflammatory bowel disease. Gastroenterology 1990;98:549–553.

100. Tysk C, Jarnerot G. Seasonal variation in exacerbations of ulcerative colitis. Scand J Gastroenterol 1993;28:95–96.

101. Weber P, Koch M, Heizmann WR et al. Microbic superinfection in relapse of inflammatory bowel disease. J Clin Gastroenterol 1992;14:302–308.

102. Kochhar R, Ayyagari A, Goenka MK et al. Role of infectious agents in exacerbations of ulcerative colitis in India. A study of Clostridium difficile. J Clin Gastroenterol 1993;16:26–30.

103. Kallinowski F, Wassmer A, Hofmann MA et al. Prevalence of enteropathogenic bacteria in surgically treated chronic inflammatory bowel disease. Hepatogastroenterology 1998;45:1552–1558.

104. Greenfield C, Aguilar-Ramirez JR, Pounder RE et al. Clostridium difficile and inflammatory bowel disease. Gut 1983;24:713–717.

105. Trnka YM, LaMont JT. Association of Clostridium difficile toxin with symptomatic relapse of chronic inflammatory bowel disease. Gastroenterology 1981;80:693–696.

106. Cottone M, Pietrosi G, Martorana G et al. Prevalence of cytomegalovirus infection in severe refractory ulcerative and Crohn's colitis. Am J Gastroenterol 2001;96:773–775.

107. Vega R, Bertran X, Menacho M et al. Cytomegalovirus infection in patients with inflammatory bowel disease. Am J Gastroenterol 1999;94:1053–1056.

108. Pfau P, Kochman ML, Furth EE et al. Cytomegalovirus colitis complicating ulcerative colitis in the steroid-naive patient. Am J Gastroenterol 2001;96:895–899.

109. Cooper HS, Raffensperger EC, Jonas L et al. Cytomegalovirus inclusions in patients with ulcerative colitis and toxic dilation requiring colonic resection. Gastroenterology 1977;72:1253–1256.

110. Ruther U, Nunnensiek C, Muller HA et al. Interferon α (IFN α$_{2a}$) therapy for herpes virus-associated inflammatory bowel disease (ulcerative colitis and Crohn's disease). Hepatogastroenterology 1998;45:691–699.

111. Bertalot G, Villanacci V, Gramegna M et al. Evidence of Epstein–Barr virus infection in ulcerative colitis. Dig Liver Dis 2001;33:551–558.

112. Dayharsh GA, Loftus EV, Sandborn WJ et al. Epstein–Barr virus-positive lymphoma in patients with inflammatory bowel disease treated with azathioprine or 6-mercaptopurine. Gastroenterology 2002;122:72–77.

113. Yamada T, Deitch E, Specian RD et al. Mechanisms of acute and chronic intestinal inflammation induced by indomethacin. Inflammation 1993;17:641–662.

114. Berg DJ, Zhang J, Weinstock JV et al. Rapid development of colitis in NSAID-treated IL-10-deficient mice. Gastroenterology 2002;123:1527–1542.

115. Sartor RB, Lichtman SN. Mechanisms of systemic inflammation associated with intestinal injury. In: Targan SR, Shanahan F, eds. Inflammatory bowel disease: From bench to bedside 2nd edn. Baltimore: Williams & Wilkins; 2003:305–335.

116. Wands JR, LaMont JT, Mann E et al. Arthritis associated with intestinal bypass procedure for morbid obesity. N Engl J Med 1976;294:121–124.

117. Balbir-Gurman A, Schapira D, Nahir M. Arthritis related to ileal pouchitis following total proctocolectomy for ulcerative colitis. Semin Arthritis Rheum 2001;30:242–248.

118. Sartor RB. Intestinal microflora in human and experimental inflammatory bowel disease. Curr Opin Gastroenterol 2001;17:555–561.

119. Elson CO, Cong Y, Iqbal N et al. Immuno-bacterial homeostasis in the gut: new insights into an old enigma. Semin Immunol 2001;13:187–194.

120. Kuhn R, Lohler J, Rennick D et al. Interleukin-10-deficient mice develop chronic enterocolitis. Cell 1993;75:263–274.

121. Sellon RK, Tonkonogy S, Schultz M et al. Resident enteric bacteria are necessary for development of spontaneous colitis and immune system activation in interleukin-10-deficient mice. Infect Immun 1998;66:5224–5231.

122. Rath HC, Herfarth HH, Ikeda JS et al. Normal luminal bacteria, especially Bacteroides species, mediate chronic colitis, gastritis, and arthritis in HLA-B27/human β$_2$ microglobulin transgenic rats. J Clin Invest 1996;98:945–953.

123. Taurog JD, Richardson JA, Croft JT et al. The germfree state prevents development of gut and joint inflammatory disease in HLA-B27 transgenic rats. J Exp Med 1994;180:2359–2364.

124. Sadlack B, Merz H, Schorle H et al. Ulcerative colitis-like disease in mice with a disrupted interleukin-2 gene. Cell 1993;75:253–261.

125. Schultz M, Tonkonogy SL, Sellon RK et al. IL-2-deficient mice raised under germfree conditions develop delayed mild focal intestinal inflammation. Am J Physiol 1999;276:G1461–G1472.

126. Contractor NV, Bassiri H, Reya T et al. Lymphoid hyperplasia, autoimmunity, and compromised intestinal intraepithelial lymphocyte development in colitis-free gnotobiotic IL-2-deficient mice. J Immunol 1998;160:385–394.

127. Schultz M, Clarke SH, Arnold LW et al. Disrupted B-lymphocyte development and survival in interleukin-2-deficient mice. Immunology 2001;104:127–134.

128. Axelsson LG, Midtvedt T, Bylund-Fellenius AC. The role of intestinal bacteria, bacterial translocation and endotoxin in dextran sodium sulphate-induced colitis in the mouse. Microb Ecol Health Dis 1996;9:225–237.

129. Hudcovic T, Stepankova R, Cebra J et al. The role of microflora in the development of intestinal inflammation: acute and chronic colitis induced by dextran sulfate in germ-free and conventionally reared immunocompetent and immunodeficient mice. Folia Microbiol 2001;46:565–572.

130. Rath HC, Schultz M, Freitag R et al. Different subsets of enteric bacteria induce and perpetuate experimental colitis in rats and mice. Infect Immun 2001;69:2277–2285.

131. Hans W, Scholmerich J, Gross V et al. The role of the resident intestinal flora in acute and chronic dextran sulfate sodium-induced colitis in mice. Eur J Gastroenterol Hepatol 2000;12:267–273.

132. Onderdonk AB, Franklin ML, Cisneros RL. Production of experimental ulcerative colitis in gnotobiotic guinea pigs with simplified microflora. Infect Immun 1981;32:225–231.

133. Rath HC, Wilson KH, Sartor RB. Differential induction of colitis and gastritis in HLA-B27 transgenic rats selectively colonized with Bacteroides vulgatus and Escherichia coli. Infect Immun 1999;67:2969–2974.

134. Mann BA, Kim SC, Sartor RB. Selective induction of experimental colitis by monoassociation of HLA-B27 transgenic rats with various enteric Bacteroides species. Gastroenterology 2003;124: A322 (Abstract).

135. Dieleman LA, Arends A, Tonkonogy SL et al. Helicobacter hepaticus does not induce or potentiate colitis in interleukin-10-deficient mice. Infect Immun 2000;68:5107–5113.

136. Sydora BC, Tavernini MM, Jewell LD et al. Effect of bacterial monoassociation on tolerance and intestinal inflammation in IL-10 gene-deficient mice. Gastroenterology 2001;120:A517 (Abstract).

137. Balish E, Warner T. *Enterococcus faecalis* induces inflammatory bowel disease in interleukin-10 knockout mice. Am J Pathol 2002;160:2253–2257.

138. Kim SC, Tonkongy SL, Albright CA et al. Regional and host specificity of colitis in mice monoassociated with different nonpathogenic bacteria. Gastroenterology 2003;124:(in press) (Abstract).

139. Madsen K, Cornish A, Soper P et al. Probiotic bacteria enhance murine and human intestinal epithelial barrier function. Gastroenterology 2001;121:580–591.

140. Mattar AF, Drongowski RA, Coran AG et al. Effect of probiotics on enterocyte bacterial translocation in vitro. Pediatr Surg Int 2001;17:265–268.

141. Schultz M, Veltkamp C, Dielman LA et al. Lactobacillus plantarum 299V in the treatment and prevention of spontaneous colitis in IL-10 deficient mice. Inflam Bowel Dis 2002;8:71–80.

142. Dieleman LA, Goerres M, Arends A et al. *Lactobacillus GG* prevents recurrence of colitis in HLA-B27 transgenic rats after antibiotic treatment. Gut 2002;52:370–376.

143. Steidler L, Hans W, Schotte L et al. Treatment of murine colitis by *Lactococcus lactis* secreting interleukin-10. Science 2000;289:1352–1355.

144. Fukuda M, Kanauchi O, Araki Y et al. Prebiotic treatment of experimental colitis with germinated barley foodstuff: a comparison with probiotic or antibiotic treatment. Int J Mol Med 2002;9:65–70.

145. Araki Y, Andoh A, Koyama S et al. Effects of germinated barley foodstuff on microflora and short chain fatty acid production in dextran sulfate sodium-induced colitis in rats. Biosci Biotech Biochem 2000;64:1794–1800.

146. Videla S, Vilaseca J, Antolin M et al. Dietary inulin improves distal colitis induced by dextran sodium sulfate in the rat. Am J Gastroenterol 2001;96:1486–1493.

147. Le Blay G, Michel C, Blottiere HM et al. Prolonged intake of fructo-oligosaccharides induces a short-term elevation of lactic acid-producing bacteria and a persistent increase in cecal butyrate in rats. J Nutr 1999;129:2231–2235.

148. Kleessen B, Hartmann L, Blaut M. Oligofructose and long-chain inulin: influence on the gut microbial ecology of rats associated with a human faecal flora. Br J Nutr 2001;86:291–300.

149. Roediger WE. The colonic epithelium in ulcerative colitis: an energy-deficiency disease? Lancet 1980;2:712–715.

150. Madsen KL, Doyle JS, Tavernini MM et al. Antibiotic therapy attenuates colitis in interleukin 10 gene-deficient mice. Gastroenterology 2000;118:1094–1155.

151. Hoentjen F, Harmstan HJ, Brant H et al. Antibodies with a selective aerobic or anaerobic spectrum have different therapeutic activities in various regions of the colon in IL-10 deficient mice. Gut 2003;(in press).

152. Onderdonk AB, Hermos JA, Dzink JL et al. Protective effect of metronidazole in experimental ulcerative colitis. Gastroenterology 1978;74:521–526.

153. Videla S, Vilaseca J, Guarner F et al. Role of intestinal microflora in chronic inflammation and ulceration of the rat colon. Gut 1994;35:1090–1097.

154. Bamias G, Marini M, Moskaluk CA et al. Down-regulation of intestinal lymphocyte activation and Th1 cytokine production by antibiotic therapy in a murine model of Crohn's disease. J Immunol 2002;169:5308–5314.

155. Rath HC, Ikeda JS, Linde HJ et al. Varying cecal bacterial loads influences colitis and gastritis in HLA-B27 transgenic rats. Gastroenterology 1999;116:310–319.

156. Wood JD, Peck OC, Tefend KS et al. Evidence that colitis is initiated by environmental stress and sustained by fecal factors in the cotton-top tamarin (*Saguinus oedipus*). Dig Dis Sci 2000;45:385–393.

157. Chadwick VS, Anderson RP. Microorganisms and their products in inflammatory bowel disease. In: MacDermott RP, Stenson WF, eds. Inflammatory bowel disease. New York: Elsevier; 1992: 241–248.

158. Schwab JH. Phlogistic properties of peptidoglycan–polysaccharide polymers from cell walls of pathogenic and normal-flora bacteria which colonize humans. Infect Immun 1993;61:4535–4539.

159. Broom MF, Scherriff RM, Ferry DM et al. Formylmethionylleucylphenylalanine and the SOS operon in *Escherichia coli*: a model of host bacterial interactions. Biochem J 1993;291:895–900.

160. McCall RD, Haskill S, Zimmermann EM et al. Tissue interleukin 1 and interleukin-1 receptor antagonist expression in enterocolitis in resistant and susceptible rats. Gastroenterology 1994;106:960–972.

161. Sartor RB, De La Cadena RA, Green KD et al. Selective kallikrein–kinin system activation in inbred rats differentially susceptible to granulomatous enterocolitis. Gastroenterology 1996;110:1467–1481.

162. Rachmilewitz D, Karmeli F, Takabayashi K et al. Immunostimulatory DNA ameliorates experimental and spontaneous murine colitis. Gastroenterology 2002;122:1428–1441.

163. Aderem A, Ulevitch RJ. Toll-like receptors in the induction of the innate immune response. Nature 2000;406:782–787.

164. Anderson KV. Toll signaling pathways in the innate immune response. Curr Opin Immunol 2000;12:13–19.

165. Krug A, Towarowski A, Britsch S et al. Toll-like receptor expression reveals CpG DNA as a unique microbial stimulus for plasmacytoid dendritic cells which synergizes with CD40 ligand to induce high amounts of IL-12. Eur J Immunol 2001;31:3026–3037.

166. Haller D, Russo MP, Sartor RB et al. IKKβ and phosphatidylinositol 3-kinase/Akt participate in non-pathogenic Gram-negative enteric bacteria-induced RelA

phosphorylation and NFκB activation in both primary and intestinal epithelial cell lines. J Biol Chem 2002;277:38168–38178.

167. Lalu S, Ogura Y, Osborne C et al. Crohn's disease and the NOD2 gene: a role for Paneth cells. Gastroenterology 2003;125:47–57.

168. Chester JF, Ross JS, Malt RA et al. Acute colitis produced by chemotactic peptides in rats and mice. Am J Pathol 1985;121:284–290.

169. Von Ritter C, Sekizuka E, Grisham MB et al. The chemotactic peptide N-formyl methionyl-leucyl-phenylalanine increases mucosal permeability in the distal ileum of the rat. Gastroenterology 1988;95:651–656.

170. Hsueh W, Gonzalez-Crussi F, Arroyave JL. Platelet-activating factor: an endogenous mediator for bowel necrosis in endotoxemia. FASEB J 1987;1:403–405.

171. Ciancio MJ, Vitiritti L, Dhar A et al. Endotoxin-induced alterations in rat colonic water and electrolyte transport. Gastroenterology 1992;103:1437–1443.

172. Sartor RB, Bender DE, Allen JB et al. Chronic experimental enterocolitis and extraintestinal inflammation are T lymphocyte dependent. Gastroenterology 1993;104:775A (Abstract).

173. Davis SW, Holt LC, Sartor RB. Luminal bacterial and bacterial polymers potentiate indomethacin induced intestinal injury in the rat. Gastroenterology 1990;98:444A (Abstract).

174. Sartor RB, Bond TM, Schwab JH. Systemic uptake and intestinal inflammatory effects of luminal bacterial cell wall polymers in rats with acute colonic injury. Infect Immun 1988;56:2101–2108.

175. Hobson CH, Butt TJ, Ferry DM et al. Enterohepatic circulation of bacterial chemotactic peptide in rats with experimental colitis. Gastroenterology 1988;94:1006–1013.

176. Gardiner KR, Anderson NH, Rowlands BJ et al. Colitis and colonic mucosal barrier dysfunction. Gut 1995;37:530–535.

177. Sartor RB, Anderle SK, Cromartie WJ et al. Localized gut-associated lymphoid tissue hemorrhage induced by intravenous peptidoglycan–polysaccharide polymers. Infect Immun 1986;51:521–528.

178. Lichtman SN, Keku J, Schwab JH et al. Hepatic injury associated with small bowel bacterial overgrowth in rats is prevented by metronidazole and tetracycline. Gastroenterology 1991;100:513–519.

179. Gardiner KR, Erwin PJ, Anderson NH et al. Colonic bacteria and bacterial translocation in experimental colitis. Br J Surg 1993;80:512–516.

180. Brandwein SL, McCabe RP, Cong Y et al. Spontaneous colitic C3H/HeJBir mice demonstrate selective antibody reactivity to antigens of the enteric bacterial flora. J Immunol 1997;159:44–52.

181. Duchmann R, Schmitt E, Knolle P et al. Tolerance towards resident intestinal flora in mice is abrogated in experimental colitis and restored by treatment with interleukin-10 or antibodies to interleukin-12. Eur J Immunol 1996;26:934–938.

182. Cong Y, Brandwein SL, McCabe RP et al. CD4+ T cells reactive to enteric bacterial antigens in spontaneously colitic C3H/HeJBir mice: increased T helper cell type 1 response and ability to transfer disease. J Exp Med 1998;187:855–864.

183. Sartor RB. Induction of mucosal immune responses by bacteria and bacterial components. Curr Opin Gastroenterol 2001;17:555–561.

184. Veltkamp C, Tonkonogy SL, de Jong YP et al. Continuous stimulation by normal luminal bacteria is essential for the development and perpetuation of colitis in Tg(ε26) mice. Gastroenterology 2001;120:900–913.

185. Higgins LM, Frankel G, Douce G et al. *Citrobacter rodentium* infection in mice elicits a mucosal Th1 cytokine response and lesions similar to those in murine inflammatory bowel disease. Infect Immun 1999;67:3031–3039.

186. Qian B-F, Hoentjen F, Dieleman LA et al. Dysregulated luminal bacterial antigen-specific T cell responses and antigen presenting cell function in HLA-B27 transgenic rats with chronic colitis. Gastroenterology 2003;124:A487 (Abstract).

187. Albright CA, Tonkongy SL, Sartor RB. Antigen presenting cells produce IL-10 in response to IFN gamma. Gastroenterology 2003;124:A332 (Abstract).

188. Albright C, Tonkongy SL, Frelinger JA et al. Adoptive transfer of *E. faecalis*-pulsed dendritic cells accelerates colitis in IL-10 deficient mice. Gastroenterology 2003;124:A73 (Abstract).

189. Ma A, Datta M, Margosian E et al. T cells, but not B cells, are required for bowel inflammation in interleukin 2-deficient mice. J Exp Med 1995;182:1567–1572.

190. Davidson NJ, Leach MW, Fort MM et al. T helper cell 1-type CD4+ T cells, but not B cells, mediate colitis in interleukin 10-deficient mice. J Exp Med 1996;184:241–251.

191. Mizoguchi A, Mizoguchi E, Smith RN et al. Suppressive role of B cells in chronic colitis of T cell receptor α mutant mice. J Exp Med 1997;186:1749–1756.

192. Seibold F, Brandwein S, Simpson S et al. pANCA represents a cross-reactivity to enteric bacterial antigens. J Clin Immunol 1998;18:153–160.

193. Leung FW, Heng MC, Allen S et al. Involvement of luminal bacteria, heat shock protein 60, macrophages and γδ T cells in dextran sulfate sodium-induced colitis in rats. Dig Dis Sci 2000;45:1472–1479.

194. Mizoguchi A, Mizoguchi E, Chiba C et al. Role of appendix in the development of inflammatory bowel disease in TCR-α mutant mice. J Exp Med 1996;184:707–715.

195. Rath HC, Ikeda JS, Wilson KH et al. Varying cecal bacterial loads influences colitis and gastritis in HLA-B27 transgenic rats. Gastroenterology 1998;112:A1068 (Abstract).

196. Oyama N, Sudo N, Sogawa H et al. Antibiotic use during infancy promotes a shift in the T(H)1/T(H)2 balance toward T(H)2-dominant immunity in mice. J Allergy Clin Immunol 2001;107:153–159.

197. Cong Y, Weaver CT. Lazenby A et al. Bacterial-reactive T regulatory cells inhibit pathogenic immune responses to the enteric flora. J Immunol 2002;169:6112–6119.

198. Rietdijk ST, Faubion W, Albright C et al. CD4+ CD25+ regulatory T cells originating from germ free mice have impaired suppressive abilities. Gastroenterology 2002;122:A387 (Abstract).

199. Kullberg MC, Jankovic D, Gorelick PL et al. Bacteria-triggered CD4(+) T regulatory cells suppress Helicobacter hepaticus-induced colitis. J Exp Med 2003;196:505–515.

200. Hoentjen F, Tonkongy SL, Torrice C et al. B cells from mesenteric lymph nodes of resistant rats produce more TGF than those from B27 transgenic rats following in vitro stimulation with cecal bacterial lysate. Gastroenterology 2003;124:A487 (Abstract).

201. Dieleman LA, Hoentjen F, Williams R et al. B cells from mesenteric lymph nodes of resistant rats produce more interleukin-10 than those from B27 transgenic rats following in vitro stimulation with cecal bacterial lysate. Gastroenterology 2002;122:A261 (Abstract).

202. Gaboriau-Routhiau V, Moreau MC. Gut flora allows recovery of oral tolerance to ovalbumin in mice after transient breakdown mediated by cholera toxin or Escherichia coli heat-labile enterotoxin. Pediatr Res 1996;39:625–629.

203. Hessle C, Hanson LA, Wold AE. Interleukin-10 produced by the innate immune system masks in vitro evidence of acquired T-cell immunity to E. coli. Scand J Immunol 2000;52:13–20.

204. Cender CJ, Haller D, Walters C et al. VSL #3 alters cytokine production of unfractionated splenocytes upon stimulation with cecal bacterial lysate: immunomodulation by this probiotic combination. Gastroenterology 2002;122:A145 (Abstract).

205. Nikolaus S, Bauditz J, Gionchetti P et al. Increased secretion of pro-inflammatory cytokines by circulating polymorphonuclear neutrophils and regulation by interleukin 10 during intestinal inflammation. Gut 1998;42:470–476.

206. Madsen K, Jijon H, Yeung H et al. DNA from probiotic bacteria exerts anti-inflammatory actions on intestinal epithelial cells by inhibition of NFκB. Gastroenterology 2002;122:A64 (Abstract).

207. Christensen HR, Frokiaer H, Pestka JJ. Lactobacilli differentially modulate expression of cytokines and maturation surface markers in murine dendritic cells. J Immunol 2002;168:171–178.

208. Sartor RB, Bender DE, Holt LC. Susceptibility of inbred rat strains to intestinal and extraintestinal inflammation induced by indomethacin. Gastroenterology 1992;102:A690 (Abstract).

209. Sartor RB, Bender DE, Grenther WB et al. Absolute requirement for ubiquitous luminal bacteria in the pathogenesis of chronic intestinal inflammation. Gastroenterology 1994;106:A767.

210. Goncalves NS, Ghaem-Maghami M, Monteleone G et al. Critical role for tumor necrosis factor α in controlling the number of lumenal pathogenic bacteria and immunopathology in infectious colitis. Infect Immun 2001;69:6651–6659.

211. Soderholm JD, Yang PC, Ceponis P et al. Chronic stress induces mast cell-dependent bacterial adherence and initiates mucosal inflammation in rat intestine. Gastroenterology 2002;123:1099–1108.

212. Qiu BS, Vallance BA, Blennerhassett PA et al. The role of CD4+ lymphocytes in the susceptibility of mice to stress-induced reactivation of experimental colitis. Nature Med 1999;5:1178–1182.

213. Lichtman SN, Sartor RB, Keku J et al. Hepatic inflammation in rats with experimental small intestinal bacterial overgrowth. Gastroenterology 1990;98:414–423.

214. Lichtman SN, Wang J, Sartor RB et al. Reactivation of arthritis induced by small bowel bacterial overgrowth in rats: role of cytokines, bacteria, and bacterial polymers. Infect Immun 1995;63:2295–2301.

215. Lichtman SN, Okoruwa EE, Keku J et al. Degradation of endogenous bacterial cell wall polymers by the muralytic enzyme mutanolysin prevents hepatobiliary injury in genetically susceptible rats with experimental intestinal bacterial overgrowth. J Clin Invest 1992;90:1313–1322.

216. Lichtman SN, Keku J, Schwab JH et al. Evidence for peptidoglycan absorption in rats with experimental small bowel bacterial overgrowth. Infect Immun 1991;59:555–562.

217. Kuroe K, Haga Y, Funakoshi O et al. Pericholangitis in a rabbit colitis model induced by injection of muramyl dipeptide emulsified with a long-chain fatty acid. J Gastroenterol 1996;31:347–352.

218. Kono K, Kunihiko O, Masao O. Experimental portal fibrosis produced by intraportal injection of killed nonpathogenic Escherichia coli in rabbits. Gastroenterology 1990;98:414–423.

219. Dalzeil TK. Chronic intestinal enteritis. Br Med J 1913;2:1068–1069.

220. Chiodini RJ. Crohn's disease and the mycobacterioses: a review and comparison of two disease entities. Clin Microbiol Rev 1989;2:90–117.

221. Lund BM, Gould GW, Rampling AM. Pasteurization of milk and the heat resistance of Mycobacterium avium subsp. paratuberculosis: a critical review of the data. Int J Food Microbiol 2002;77:135–145.

222. Mishina D, Katsel P, Brown ST et al. On the etiology of Crohn disease. Proc Natl Acad Sci USA 1996;93:9816–9820.

223. Hermon-Taylor J, Bull TJ, Sheridan JM et al. Causation of Crohn's disease by Mycobacterium avium subspecies paratuberculosis. Can J Gastroenterol 2000;14:521–539.

224. Hermon-Taylor J, Bull T. Crohn's disease caused by Mycobacterium avium subspecies paratuberculosis: a public health tragedy whose resolution is long overdue. J Med Microbiol 2002;51:3–6.

225. Van Kruiningen HJ. Lack of support for a common etiology in Johne's disease of animals and Crohn's disease in humans. Inflamm Bowel Dis 1999;5:183–191.

226. Chiodini RJ, Van Kruiningen HJ, Thayer WR et al. Possible role of mycobacteria in inflammatory bowel disease. I. An unclassified Mycobacterium species isolated from patients with Crohn's disease. Dig Dis Sci 1984;29:1073–1079.

227. Wall S, Kunze ZM, Saboor S. Identification of spheroplastlike agents isolated from tissues of patients with Crohn's disease and control tissues by polymerase chain reaction. J Clin Microbiol 1993;31:1241–1245.

228. Moss MT, Sanderson JD, Tizard ML et al. Polymerase chain reaction detection of Mycobacterium paratuberculosis and Mycobacterium avium subsp silvaticum in long term cultures from Crohn's disease and control tissues. Gut 1992;33:1209–1213.

229. Sanderson JD, Moss MT, Tizard ML et al. Mycobacterium paratuberculosis DNA in Crohn's disease tissue. Gut 1992;33:890–896.

230. Kanazawa K, Haga Y, Funakoshi O et al. Absence of Mycobacterium paratuberculosis DNA in intestinal tissues from Crohn's disease by nested polymerase chain reaction. J Gastroenterol 1999;34:200–206.

231. Fidler HM, Thurrel W, Johnson NM et al. Specific detection of Mycobacterium paratuberculosis DNA associated with granulomatous tissue in Crohn's disease. Gut 1994;35:506–510.

232. Collins MT, Lisby G, Moser C et al. Results of multiple diagnostic tests for Mycobacterium avium subsp. paratuberculosis in patients with inflammatory bowel disease and in controls. J Clin Microbiol 2000;38:4373–4381.

233. Ryan P, Bennett MW, Aarons S et al. PCR detection of Mycobacterium paratuberculosis in Crohn's disease granulomas isolated by laser capture microdissection. Gut 2002;51:665–670.

234. Naser SA, Shafran I, Schwartz D et al. In situ identification of mycobacteria in Crohn's disease patient tissue using confocal scanning laser microscopy. Mol Cell Probes 2002;16:41–48.

235. Sechi LA, Mura M, Tanda F et al. Identification of Mycobacterium avium subsp. paratuberculosis in biopsy specimens from patients with Crohn's disease identified by in situ hybridization. J Clin Microbiol 2001;39:4514–4517.

236. Hulten K, El-Zimaity HM, Karttunen TJ et al. Detection of Mycobacterium avium subspecies paratuberculosis in Crohn's diseased tissues by in situ hybridization. Am J Gastroenterol 2001;96:1529–1535.

237. Shafran I, Piromalli C, Decker JW et al. Seroreactivities against Saccharomyces cerevisiae and Mycobacterium avium subsp. paratuberculosis p35 and p36 antigens in Crohn's disease patients. Dig Dis Sci 2002;47:2079–2081.

238. Naser SA, Hulten K, Shafran I et al. Specific seroreactivity of Crohn's disease patients against p35 and p36 antigens of M. avium subsp. paratuberculosis. Vet Microbiol 2000;77:497–504.

239. Naser SA, Schwartz D, Shafran I. Isolation of Mycobacterium avium subsp paratuberculosis from breast milk of Crohn's disease patients. Am J Gastroenterol 2000;95:1094–1095.

240. Hermon-Taylor J, Barnes N, Clarke C et al. Mycobacterium paratuberculosis cervical lymphadenitis, followed five years later by terminal ileitis similar to Crohn's disease. Br Med J 1998;316:449–453.

241. Burke DA, Axon ATR. Adhesive Escherichia coli in inflammatory bowel disease and infective diarrhoea. Br Med J 1988;297:102–104.

242. Lobo AJ, Sagar PM, Rothwell J et al. Carriage of adhesive Escherichia coli after restorative proctocolectomy and pouch anal anastomosis: relation with functional outcome and inflammation. Gut 1993;34:1379–1383.

243. Giaffer MH, Holdsworth CD, Duerden BI. Virulence properties of Escherichia coli strains isolated from patients with inflammatory bowel disease. Gut 1992;33:646–650.

244. Hartley MG, Hudson MJ, Swarbrick ET et al. Adhesive and hydrophobic properties of Escherichia coli from the rectal mucosa of patients with ulcerative colitis. Gut 1993;34:63–67.

245. Schultsz C, Moussa M, van Ketel R et al. Frequency of pathogenic and enteroadherent Escherichia coli in patients with inflammatory bowel disease and controls. J Clin Pathol 1997;50:573–579.

246. Darfeuille-Michaud A, Neut C, Barnich N et al. Presence of adherent Escherichia coli strains in ileal mucosa of patients with Crohn's disease. Gastroenterology 1998;115:1405–1413.

247. Boudeau J, Glasser AL, Masseret E et al. Invasive ability of an Escherichia coli strain isolated from the ileal mucosa of a patient with Crohn's disease. Infect Immun 1999;67:4499–4509.

248. Glasser AL, Boudeau J, Barnich N et al. Adherent invasive Escherichia coli strains from patients with Crohn's disease survive and replicate within macrophages without inducing host cell death. Infect Immun 2001;69:5529–5537.

249. Boudeau J, Barnich N, Darfeuille-Michaud A. Type 1 pili-mediated adherence of Escherichia coli strain LF82 isolated from Crohn's disease is involved in bacterial invasion of intestinal epithelial cells. Mol Microbiol 2001;39:1272–1284.

250. Walmsley RS, Anthony A, Sim R et al. Absence of Escherichia coli, Listeria monocytogenes, and Klebsiella pneumoniae antigens within inflammatory bowel disease tissues. J Clin Pathol 1998;51:657–661.

251. Parent K, Mitchel P. Cell wall defective variants of Pseudomonas-like (group Va) bacteria in Crohn's disease. Gastroenterology 1978;75:368–372.

252. Wei B, Huang T, Dalwadi HN et al. Identification of Pseudomonas fluorescens as the microorganism expressing the Crohn's disease-associated I2 gene. Gastroenterology 2001;120:A82 (Abstract).

253. Dalwadi H, Wei B, Kronenberg M et al. The Crohn's disease-associated bacterial protein I2 is a novel enteric T cell superantigen. Immunity 2001;15:149–158.

254. Chen W, Li D, Paulus B et al. Detection of *Listeria monocytogenes* by polymerase chain reaction in intestinal mucosal biopsies from patients with inflammatory bowel disease and controls. J Gastroenterol Hepatol 2000;15:1145–1150.

255. Chiba M, Fukushima T, Horie Y et al. No *Mycobacterium paratuberculosis* detected in intestinal tissue, including Peyer's patches and lymph follicles, of Crohn's disease. J Gastroenterol 1998;33:482–487.

256. Feeney MA, Murphy F, Clegg AJ et al. A case–control study of childhood environmental risk factors for the development of inflammatory bowel disease. Eur J Gastroenterol Hepatol 2002;14:529–534.

257. Parente F, Cucino C, Bollani S et al. Focal gastric inflammatory infiltrates in inflammatory bowel diseases: prevalence, immunohistochemical characteristics, and diagnostic role. Am J Gastroenterol 2000;95:705–711.

258. Sharif F, McDermott M, Dillon M et al. Focally enhanced gastritis in children with Crohn's disease and ulcerative colitis. Am J Gastroenterol 2002;97:1415–1420.

259. Vare PO, Heikius B, Silvennoinen J et al. Seroprevalence of *Helicobacter pylori* infection in inflammatory bowel disease: is *Helicobacter pylori* infection a protective factor? Scand J Gastroenterol 2001;36:1295–1300.

260. Puspok A, Dejaco C, Oberhuber G et al. Influence of *Helicobacter pylori* infection on the phenotype of Crohn's disease. Am J Gastroenterol 1999;94:3239–3244.

261. Fox JG, Gorelick PL, Kullberg MC et al. A novel urease-negative *Helicobacter* species associated with colitis and typhlitis in IL-10-deficient mice. Infect Immun 1999;64:1757–1762.

262. Franklin CL, Riley LK, Livingston RS et al. Enteric lesions in SCID mice infected with 'Helicobacter typhlonicus,' a novel urease-negative *Helicobacter* species. Lab Anim Sci 1999;49:496–505.

263. Kullberg MC, Ward JM, Gorelick P et al. *Helicobacter hepaticus* triggers colitis in specific-pathogen-free interleukin-10 (IL-10)-deficient mice through an IL-12 and γ interferon-dependent mechanism. Infect Immun 1998;66:5157–5166.

264. Burich A, Hershberg R, Waggie K et al. *Helicobacter*-induced inflammatory bowel disease in IL-10 and T cell-deficient mice. Am J Physiol Gastrointest Liver Physiol 2001;281:G764–G778.

265. Engle SJ, Ormsby I, Pawlowski S et al. Elimination of colon cancer in germ-free transforming growth factor $\beta_1$-deficient mice. Cancer Res 2002;62:6362–6366.

266. Maggio-Price L, Shows D, Waggie K et al. *Helicobacter bilis* infection accelerates and *H. hepaticus* infection delays the development of colitis in multiple drug resistance-deficient (mdr1a−/−) mice. Am J Pathol 2002;160:739–751.

267. Fox JG, Handt L, Xu S et al. Novel *Helicobacter* species isolated from rhesus monkeys with chronic idiopathic colitis. J Med Microbiol 2001;50:421–429.

268. Tiveljung A, Soderholm JD, Olaison G et al. Presence of eubacteria in biopsies from Crohn's disease inflammatory lesions as determined by 16S rRNA gene-based PCR. J Med Microbiol 1999;48:263–268.

269. Wakefield AJ, Pittilo RM, Sim R et al. Evidence of persistent measles virus infection in Crohn's disease. J Med Virol 1993;39:345–353.

270. Wakefield AJ, Montgomery SM. Measles virus as a risk for inflammatory bowel disease: an unusually tolerant approach. Am J Gastroenterol 2000;95:1389–1392.

271. Robertson DJ, Sandler RS. Measles virus and Crohn's disease: a critical appraisal of the current literature. Inflamm Bowel Dis 2001;7:51–57.

272. Ghosh S, Armitage E, Wilson D et al. Detection of persistent measles virus infection in Crohn's disease: current status of experimental work. Gut 2001;48:748–752.

273. Morris CB, Cheng E, Thanawastien A et al. Effectiveness of intranasal immunization with HIV-gp160 and an HIV-1 env CTL epitope peptide (E7) in combination with the mucosal adjuvant LT(R192G). Vaccine 2000;18:1944–1951.

274. Davis RL, Kramarz P, Bohlke K et al. Measles–mumps–rubella and other measles-containing vaccines do not increase the risk for inflammatory bowel disease: a case–control study from the Vaccine Safety Datalink project. Arch Pediatr Adolesc Med 2001;155:354–359.

275. Pardi DS, Tremaine WJ, Sandborn WJ et al. Perinatal exposure to measles virus is not associated with the development of inflammatory bowel disease. Inflamm Bowel Dis 1999;5:104–106.

276. Pardi DS, Tremaine WJ, Sandborn WJ et al. Early measles virus infection is associated with the development of inflammatory bowel disease. Am J Gastroenterol 2000;95:1480–1485.

277. Van Kruiningen HJ, Mayo DR, Vanopdenbosch E et al. Virus serology in familial Crohn's disease. Scand J Gastroenterol 2000;35:403–407.

278. Afzal MA, Armitage E, Ghosh S et al. Further evidence of the absence of measles virus genome sequence in full thickness intestinal specimens from patients with Crohn's disease. J Med Virol 2000;62:377–382.

279. Kawashima H, Mori T, Kashiwagi Y et al. Detection and sequencing of measles virus from peripheral mononuclear cells from patients with inflammatory bowel disease and autism. Dig Dis Sci 2000;45:723–729.

280. Lavy A, Broide E, Reif S et al. Measles is more prevalent in Crohn's disease patients. A multicentre Israeli study. Dig Liver Dis 2001;33:472–476.

281. Korzenik JR, Dieckgraefe BK. Is Crohn's disease an immunodeficiency? A hypothesis suggesting possible early events in the pathogenesis of Crohn's disease. Dig Dis Sci 2000;45:1121–1129.

282. Segal AW, Loewi G. Neutrophil dysfunction in Crohn's disease. Lancet 1976;2:219–221.

283. Curran FT, Allan RN, Keighley MR. Superoxide production by Crohn's disease neutrophils. Gut 1991;32:399–402.

284. Uzel G, Kleiner DE, Kuhns DB et al. Dysfunctional LAD-1 neutrophils and colitis. Gastroenterology 2001;121:958–964.

285. Rotstein OD, Vittorini T, Kao J et al. A soluble *Bacteroides* by-product impairs phagocytic killing of *Escherichia coli* by neutrophils. Infect Immun 1989;57:745–753.

286. Dieckgraefe BK, Korzenik JR. Treatment of active Crohn's disease with recombinant human granulocyte–macrophage colony-stimulating factor. Lancet 2002;360:1478–1480.

287. Pabst MJ, Pabst KM, Collier JA et al. Inhibition of neutrophil and monocyte defensive functions by nicotine. J Periodontol 1995;66:1047–1055.

288. Russo MP, Boudreau F, Li F et al. NFκB blockade exacerbates experimental colitis in transgenic mice expressing an intestinal epithelial cells (IEC) specific IκB super-repressor. Gastroenterology 2001;120:A70 (Abstract).

289. Egan L, Eckmann L, Li Z-W et al. Systemic inflammation and decreased survival in conditional intestinal epithelial cell IKKβ knockout mice generated using a villin-cre transgenic mouse line. Gastroenterology 2002;122:A23 (Abstract).

290. Hsu DH, de Waal Malefyt R, Fiorentino DF. Expression of interleukin 10 activity by Epstein–Barr virus protein BCRF1. Science 1990;250:830–832.

291. Spiik AK, Meijer LK, Ridderstad A et al. Interference of eukaryotic signalling pathways by the bacteria *Yersinia* outer protein YopJ. Immunol Lett 1999;68:199–203.

292. Neish AS, Gewirtz AT, Zeng H et al. Prokaryotic regulation of epithelial responses by inhibition of IκBα ubiquitination. Science 2000;289:1560–1563.

293. Klapproth JM, Scaletsky IC, McNamara BP et al. A large toxin from pathogenic *Escherichia coli* strains that inhibits lymphocyte activation. Infect Immun 2000;68:2148–2155.

294. De Meo MT, Mutlu EA, Keshavarzian A et al. Intestinal permeation and gastrointestinal disease. J Clin Gastroenterol 2002;34:385–396.

295. Meddings JB. Intestinal permeability in Crohn's disease. Aliment Pharmacol Ther 1997;Suppl 11:47–53.

296. Hollander D. Intestinal permeability in patients with Crohn's disease and their relatives. Dig Liver Dis 2001;33:649–651.

297. Hollander D, Vadheim CM, Brettholz E et al. Increased intestinal permeability in patients with Crohn's disease and their relatives. A possible etiologic factor. Ann Intern Med 1986;105:883–885.

298. Gitter AH, Wullstein F, Fromm M et al. Epithelial barrier defects in ulcerative colitis: characterization and quantification by electrophysiological imaging. Gastroenterology 2001;121:1320–1328.

299. Irvine EJ, Marshall JK. Increased intestinal permeability precedes the onset of Crohn's disease in a subject with familial risk. Gastroenterology 2000;119:1740–1744.

300. Tibble JA, Sigthorsson G, Bridger S et al. Surrogate markers of intestinal inflammation are predictive of relapse in patients with inflammatory bowel disease. Gastroenterology 2000;119:15–22.

301. Isaacs KL, Sartor RB, Haskill S. Cytokine messenger RNA profiles in inflammatory bowel disease mucosa detected by polymerase chain reaction amplification. Gastroenterology 1992;103:1587–1595.

302. Meddings JB, Swain MG. Environmental stress-induced gastrointestinal permeability is mediated by endogenous glucocorticoids in the rat. Gastroenterology 2000;119:1019–1028.

303. Hilsden RJ, Meddings JB, Sutherland LR. Intestinal permeability changes in response to acetylsalicylic acid in relatives of patients with Crohn's disease. Gastroenterology 1996;110:1395–140.

304. Zamora SA, Hilsden RJ, Meddings JB et al. Intestinal permeability before and after ibuprofen in families of children with Crohn's disease. Can J Gastroenterol 1999;13:31–36.

305. Suenaert P, Bulteel V, Lemmens L et al. Anti-tumor necrosis factor treatment restores the gut barrier in Crohn's disease. Am J Gastroenterol 2002;97:2000–2004.

306. Colpaert S, Liu Z, De Greef B et al. Effects of anti-tumour necrosis factor, interleukin-10 and antibiotic therapy in the indometacin-induced bowel inflammation rat model. Aliment Pharmacol Ther 2001;15:1827–1836.

307. Willemsen LE, Schreurs CC, Kroes H et al. A coculture model mimicking the intestinal mucosa reveals a regulatory role for myofibroblasts in immune-mediated barrier disruption. Dig Dis Sci 2002;47:2316–2324.

308. Sturniolo GC, Di Leo V, Ferronato A et al. Zinc supplementation tightens 'leaky gut' in Crohn's disease. Inflamm Bowel Dis 2001;7:94–98.

309. Teahon K, Smethurst P, Levi AJ et al. Intestinal permeability in patients with Crohn's disease and their first degree relatives. Gut 1992;33:320–323.

310. Thjodleifsson B, Sigthorsson G, Cariglia N et al. Subclinical intestinal inflammation: An inherited abnormality in Crohn's disease relatives? Gastroenterology 2003;124:1728–1737.

311. May GR, Sutherland LR, Meddings JB. Is small intestinal permeability really increased in relatives of patients with Crohn's disease? Gastroenterology 1993;104:1627–1632.

312. Peeters M, Geypens B, Claus D et al. Clustering of increased small intestinal permeability in families with Crohn's disease. Gastroenterology 1997;113:802–807.

313. Breslin NP, Nash C, Hilsden RJ et al. Intestinal permeability is increased in a proportion of spouses of patients with Crohn's disease. Am J Gastroenterol 2001;96:2934–2938.

314. Soderholm JD, Olaison G, Lindberg E et al. Different intestinal permeability patterns in relatives and spouses of patients with Crohn's disease: an inherited defect in mucosal defence? Gut 1999;44:96–100.

315. Podolsky DK, Isselbacher KJ. Composition of human colonic mucin. Selective alteration in inflammatory bowel disease. J Clin Invest 1983;72:142–153.

316. Smithson JE, Campbell A, Andrews JM et al. Altered expression of mucins throughout the colon in ulcerative colitis. Gut 1997;40:234–240.

317. Cooke EM, Ewins SP, Hywel-Jones J et al. Properties of strains of Escherichia coli carried in different phases of ulcerative colitis. Gut 1974;15:143–146.

318. Iwakiri D, Podolsky DK. Keratinocyte growth factor promotes goblet cell differentiation through regulation of goblet cell silencer inhibitor. Gastroenterology 2001;120:1372–1380.

319. Jeffers M, McDonald WF, Chillakuru RA et al. A novel human fibroblast growth factor treats experimental intestinal inflammation. Gastroenterology 2002;123:1151–1162.

320. Nakase H, Peterson J, Benedele A et al. FGF-20 prevents and treats T-cell mediated colitis by promoting epithelial restitution and stimulating immunosuppressive pathways. Gastroenterology 2003;124:A491 (Abstract).

321. Mashimo H, Wu DC, Podolsky DK et al. Impaired defense of intestinal mucosa in mice lacking intestinal trefoil factor. Science 2003;274:262–265.

322. Hermiston ML, Gordon JI. Inflammatory bowel disease and adenomas in mice expressing a dominant negative N-cadherin. Science 1995; 270:1203–1207.

323. Wells CL, van de Westerlo EM, Jechorek RP et al. Bacteroides fragilis enterotoxin modulates epithelial permeability and bacterial internalization by HT-29 enterocytes. Gastroenterology 1996;110:1429–1437.

324. Madsen KL, Lewis SA, Tavernini MM et al. Interleukin 10 prevents cytokine-induced disruption of T84 monolayer barrier integrity and limits chloride secretion. Gastroenterology 1997;113:151–159.

325. Makkink MK, Schwerbrock NJ, van der Sluis M et al. Interleukin 10 deficient mice are defective in colonic MUC2 synthesis both before and after induction of colitis by commensal bacteria. Gastroenterology 2002;122:A30 (Abstract).

326. Ruseler-van Embden JG, Both-Patoir HC. Anaerobic gram-negative faecal flora in patients with Crohn's disease and healthy subjects. Antonie van Leeuwenhoek 1983;49:125–132.

327. Neut C, Bulois P, Desreumaux P et al. Changes in the bacterial flora of the neoterminal ileum after ileocolonic resection for Crohn's disease. Am J Gastroenterol 2002;97:939–946.

328. Keighley MR, Arabi Y, Dimock F et al. Influence of inflammatory bowel disease on intestinal microflora. Gut 1978;19:1099–1104.

329. Krook A, Lindstrom B, Kjellander J et al. Relation between concentrations of metronidazole and Bacteroides spp in faeces of patients with Crohn's disease and healthy individuals. J Clin Pathol 1978;34:645–650.

330. Giaffer MH, Holdsworth CD, Duerden BI. The assessment of faecal flora in patients with inflammatory bowel disease by a simplified bacteriological technique. J Med Microbiol 1991;35:238–243.

331. Favier C, Neut C, Mizon C et al. Fecal beta-D-galactosidase production and Bifidobacteria are decreased in Crohn's disease. Dig Dis Sci 1997;42:817–822.

332. Fabia R, Ar'Rajab A, Johansson ML et al. Impairment of bacterial flora in human ulcerative colitis and experimental colitis in the rat. Digestion 1993;54:248–255.

333. Hartley MG, Hudson MJ, Swarbrick ET et al. The rectal mucosa-associated microflora in patients with ulcerative colitis. J Med Microbiol 1992;36:96–103.

334. Schultsz C, Van Den Berg FM, Ten Kate FW et al. The intestinal mucus layer from patients with inflammatory bowel disease harbors high numbers of bacteria compared with controls. Gastroenterology 1999;117:1089–1097.

335. Mishkin D, Boston FM, Blank D et al. The glucose breath test: a diagnostic test for small bowel stricture(s) in Crohn's disease. Dig Dis Sci 2002;47:489–494.

336. Duffy M, O'Mahony L, Coffey JC et al. Sulfate-reducing bacteria colonize pouches formed for ulcerative colitis but not for familial adenomatous polyposis. Dis Colon Rectum 2002;45:384–388.

337. Sepp E, Julge K, Vasar M et al. Intestinal microflora of Estonian and Swedish infants. Acta Paediatr 1997;86:956–961.

338. Weiss ST. Eat dirt – the hygiene hypothesis and allergic diseases. N Engl J Med 1997;347:930–931.

339. Elliott DE, Urban JFJ, Argo CK et al. Does the failure to acquire helminthic parasites predispose to Crohn's disease? FASEB J 2000;14:1848–1855.

340. Hata K, Andoh A, Sato H et al. Sequential changes in luminal microflora and mucosal cytokine expression during developing of colitis in HLA-B27/$\beta_2$-microglobulin transgenic rats. Scand J Gastroenterol 2001;36:1185–1192.

341. Ariake K, Ohkusa T, Sakurazawa T et al. Roles of mucosal bacteria and succinic acid in colitis caused by dextran sulfate sodium in mice. J Med Dent Sci 2000;47:233–241.

342. Kishi D, Takahashi I, Kai Y et al. Alteration of V$\beta$ usage and cytokine production of CD4+ TCR$\beta$ $\beta$ homodimer T cells by elimination of Bacteroides vulgatus prevents colitis in TCR $\alpha$-chain-deficient mice. J Immunol 2000;165:5891–5899.

343. Mourelle M, Salas A, Guarner F et al. Stimulation of transforming growth factor $\beta$1 by enteric bacteria in the pathogenesis of rat intestinal fibrosis. Gastroenterology 1998;114:519–526.

344. Ruseler-van Embden JG, van Der Helm R, der HR et al. Degradation of intestinal glycoproteins by Bacteroides vulgatus. FEMS Microbiol Lett 1989;49:37–41.

345. van der Wiel-Korstanje JA, Winkler KC. The faecal flora in ulcerative colitis. J Med Microbiol 1975;8:491–501.

346. Harig JM, Soergel KH, Komorowski RA et al. Treatment of diversion colitis with short-chain-fatty acid irrigation. N Engl J Med 1989;320:23–28.

347. Segain JP, Raingeard dlB, Bourreille A et al. Butyrate inhibits inflammatory responses through NFκB inhibition: implications for Crohn's disease. Gut 2000;47:397–403.

348. Gibson GR, Cummings JH, Macfarlane GT. Growth and activities of sulphate-reducing bacteria in gut contents of healthy subjects and patients with ulcerative colitis. FEMS Microbiol Ecol 1991;86:103–111.

349. Levine J, Ellis CJ, Furne JK et al. Fecal hydrogen sulfide production in ulcerative colitis. Am J Gastroenterol 1998;93:83–87.

350. Roediger WE, Babidge WJ. Thiol methyltransferase activity in inflammatory bowel disease. Gut 2000;47:206–210.

351. Allan ES, Winter S, Light AM et al. Mucosal enzyme activity for butyrate oxidation: no defect in patients with ulcerative colitis. Gut 1996;38:886–893.

352. Den Hond E, Hiele M, Evenepoel P et al. In vivo butyrate metabolism and colonic permeability in extensive ulcerative colitis. Gastroenterology 1998;115:584–590.

353. Breuer RI, Soergel KH, Lashner BA et al. Short chain fatty acid rectal irrigation for left-sided ulcerative colitis: a randomised, placebo controlled trial. Gut 1997;40:485–491.

354. Furne JK, Suarez FL, Ewing SL et al. Binding of hydrogen sulfide by bismuth does not prevent dextran sulfate-induced colitis in rats. Dig Dis Sci 2000;45:1439–1443.

355. Porat R, Clark BD, Wolff SM et al. Enhancement of growth of virulent strains of Escherichia coli by interleukin1. Science 1991;254:430–432.

356. McCann ML, Abrams RS, Nelson RP Jr. Recolonization therapy with nonadhesive Escherichia coli for treatment of inflammatory bowel disease. Ann NY Acad Sci 1994;730:243–245.

357. Fuss IJ, Neurath M, Boirivant M et al. Disparate CD4+ lamina propria (LP) lymphokine secretion profiles in inflammatory bowel disease. Crohn's disease LP cells manifest increased secretion of IFN-γ, whereas ulcerative colitis LP cells manifest increased secretion of IL-5. J Immunol 1996;157:1261–1270.

358. Mizoguchi A, Mizoguchi E, Chiba C et al. Cytokine imbalance and autoantibody production in T cell receptor-α mutant mice with inflammatory bowel disease. J Exp Med 1996;183:847–856.

359. Duchmann R, May E, Heike M et al. T cell specificity and cross reactivity towards Enterobacteria, Bacteroides, Bifidobacterium, and antigens from resident intestinal flora in humans. Gut 1999;44:812–818.

360. Schreiber S, Heinig T, Thiele HG et al. Immunoregulatory role of interleukin 10 in patients with inflammatory bowel disease. Gastroenterology 1995;108:1434–1444.

361. Rioux JD, Daly M, Silverberg M et al. Genetic variation in the 5q31 cytokine gene cluster confers susceptibility to Crohn disease. Nature Genet 2001;29:223–228.

362. Berg DJ, Davidson N, Kuhn R et al. Enterocolitis and colon cancer in interleukin-10-deficient mice are associated with aberrant cytokine production and CD4(+) Th1-like responses. J Clin Invest 1996;98:1010–1020.

363. Mombaerts P, Mizoguchi E, Grusby MJ et al. Spontaneous development of inflammatory bowel disease in T cell receptor mutant mice. Cell 1993;75:274–282.

364. Sadlack B, Lohler J, Schorle H et al. Generalized autoimmune disease in interleukin-2-deficient mice is triggered by an uncontrolled activation and proliferation of CD4+ T cells. Eur J Immunol 1995;25:3053–3059.

365. Sundberg JP, Elson CO, Bedigian H et al. Spontaneous, heritable colitis in a new substrain of C3H/HeJ mice. Gastroenterology 1994;107:1726–1735.

366. Michalek SM, Kiyono H, Wannemuehler MJ et al. Lipopolysaccharide (LPS) regulation of the immune response: LPS influence on oral tolerance induction. J Immunol 1982;128:1992–1998.

367. Cong Y, Weaver CT, Lazenby A et al. T-regulatory-1 (Tr1) cells prevent colitis induced by enteric bacterial antigen-reactive pathogenic Th1 cells. Gastroenterology 2000;118:A683 (Abstract).

368. Kim SC, Tonkonogy SL, Sartor RB. Role of endogenous IL-10 in downregulating proinflammatory cytokine expression. Gastroenterology 2001;120:A183 (Abstract).

369. Albright C, Tonkonogy SL, Sartor RB. Endogenous IL-10 inhibits APC stimulation of T lymphocyte responses to luminal bacteria. Gastroenterology 2002;122:A270 (Abstract).

370. Baveye S, Elass E, Fernig DG et al. Human lactoferrin interacts with soluble CD14 and inhibits expression of endothelial adhesion molecules, E-selectin and ICAM-1, induced by the CD14-lipopolysaccharide complex. Infect Immun 2000;68:6519–6525.

371. Quinton JF, Sendid B, Reumaux D et al. Anti-Saccharomyces cerevisiae mannan antibodies combined with antineutrophil cytoplasmic autoantibodies in inflammatory bowel disease: prevalence and diagnostic role. Gut 1998;42:788–791.

372. Ruemmele FM, Targan SR, Levy G et al. Diagnostic accuracy of serological assays in pediatric inflammatory bowel disease. Gastroenterology 1998;115:822–829.

373. Sartor RB. Intestinal microflora in human and experimental inflammatory bowel disease. Curr Opin Gastroenterol 2001;17:324–330.

## CHAPTER 11

# Mechanisms of tissue injury

Thomas T MacDonald and Sylvia LF Pender

## INTRODUCTION

It is self-evident that the inflammatory bowel diseases (IBD) are caused by an excess of bloodborne inflammatory cells in the gut wall, superimposed upon and synergizing with the resident inflammatory cells present in normal intestine. However, once the excess inflammatory cells have migrated into the gut wall, they and their secreted and membrane-bound products have the ability to modulate the function of intestinal non-immune cells, such as lamina propria and submucosal fibroblasts, pericryptal myofibroblasts, structural smooth muscle cells and epithelial cells. These cells regulate the physiologic function of the gut as a digestive organ, such as the control of peristalsis, maintaining the epithelial barrier, and secreting the extracellular matrix that makes up the cores of the villi in the small intestine. In consequence, altered function of these structural cells has protean local manifestations, from changes in epithelial cells – e.g. secretion instead of absorption – to fibrosis and ulcer formation.

The intestinal mucosa is a soft tissue whose shape is controlled by the lamina propria. The highly vascular, loose connective tissue matrix contains structural collagens, glycoproteins such as laminin and fibronectin, chondroitin sulfate proteoglycans such as versican, hyaluronic acid, and ground substance.[1] These matrix constituents are secreted by lamina propria stromal cells (also known as myofibroblasts or mesenchymal cells). Where the stromal cells abut the epithelium and endothelium, the two cell types work in synergy to construct the basement membrane, which contains laminin, heparan sulfate proteoglycans, enactin and collagen IV.[2,3] The intestinal lamina propria is the most plastic tissue in the body and requires very tight control of extracellular matrix degradation and repair. For example, whereas matrix degradation in the rheumatoid joint causes pain, deformity and disability, matrix degradation in the gut leads to ulceration, diarrhea, malabsorption, protein-losing enteropathy and, in severe cases, death.

An extremely important component of tissue injury in the gut is the limited repertoire of responses. A flat mucosa can occur in nematode infection, giardiasis, celiac disease and other food-protein intolerances, Crohn's disease, small bowel allograft rejection, and intestinal graft-versus-host disease. Likewise, ulceration occurs in Crohn's disease and ulcerative colitis, amebiasis, campylobacter enteritis, T-cell lymphomas (ulcerative jejunitis) and in the stomach with *Helicobacter pylori* infection. The commonality in these responses suggests a stereotypic response of the intestine to injury, which in turn suggests that related biochemical and molecular events produce these changes.

A similar commonality in responses by inflammatory cells and cytokines occurs in end-stage inflammation. Although we now know that Crohn's disease is a T cell-mediated disorder and ulcerative colitis looks more like an antibody-mediated disease, in both conditions many end-stage effector pathways are shared. In both conditions vascular adhesion molecules are markedly increased,[4,5] resulting in increased migration of bloodborne inflammatory cells into the mucosa, which are easily visualized by reinfusing technetium- or indium-labeled blood neutrophils back into the patient.[6] UC is a more neutrophilic process, but in the gut tissues of both UC and Crohn's disease patients local concentrations of leukotrienes, prostaglandins, nitric oxide, free radicals, TNF, IL-1β, IL-6, IL-8, IL-10, IL-16 and numerous chemokines are markedly elevated (for details of cytokines in IBD mucosa, please refer to Chapter 12). An exception seems to be the Th1-inducing cytokines IL-12 and IL-18, which are preferentially upregulated in Crohn's disease.[7,8]

In this chapter we emphasize progress towards a better understanding of the interactions between inflammatory cells, cytokines and intestinal structural cells that lead to end-stage tissue injury in IBD. Mucosal ulceration is clearly severe tissue damage, but owing to the plasticity of the gut mucosa it is capable of undergoing extensive remodeling. Physiological remodeling during development occurs at about 20 weeks' gestation. Until this time, the colon has villi and is essentially identical to the ileum.[9] In long-standing ulcerative colitis, villous adenomas develop. In sprue, the villi in the upper small bowel disappear (villous atrophy). However, there is no evidence of actual villous atrophy in sprue: instead, the major structural change is a two- to threefold increase in the volume of the lamina propria.[10] Therefore, the flat mucosa in sprue should be viewed not as tissue damage, but as tissue growth. Although the intestine has only a limited repertoire of responses, many of the changes can be considered adaptive changes that alter function and provide the endogenous response of the mucosa to inflammation. We suggest that inflammatory cells and cytokines do not damage the gut per se, but instruct resident cells, primarily the lamina propria mesenchymal cell population,[11] to mediate the changes that compromise gut function. These mesenchymal cells comprise an extremely heterogeneous population made up of fibroblasts, smooth muscle cells and myofibroblasts,[12] but the distinction between these various types is not well defined in the gut, so we will not attempt to differentiate between them.

# THE ROLE OF PROTEASES IN INTESTINAL DAMAGE

## BACKGROUND

Degradation of the extracellular matrix and ulceration are the most serious consequences of intestinal inflammation. It is now realized that mucosal ulcers result from an ongoing host response and are not just due to necrotic injury. In this context, the most important mediators of ulceration are the various proteases produced by different cell types.

## THE MAJOR CLASSES OF PROTEASES AND THEIR INHIBITORS

### Background

In the past proteases were classified according to their substrate specificity or molecular size. Nowadays, a more rational system is based on their active sites, mechanisms of action and three-dimensional structures. Four classes of endoprotease (proteases that cleave at internal peptide bonds) are recognized by the International Union of Biochemistry: serine proteases, cysteine proteases, aspartic proteases and metalloproteinases (Table 11.1). These can be further grouped according to the mechanism by which they catalyse proteolysis: serine and cysteine proteases form covalent enzyme complexes with their substrates, whereas aspartic and metalloproteinases do not. This division has important consequences, as the two mechanisms by which catalysis occur are inhibited in completely different ways. Serine and cysteine proteases have strongly nucleophilic amino acids at their catalytic sites, at which hydrogen bond acceptors are aligned to promote the dissociation of the nucleophile in the approach to the transition state and thus increase the fraction in the hyperreactive state. However, the other two groups, aspartic and metalloproteinases, rely on general acid/general base catalysis of the attack of a water molecule, and therefore the catalytic residues lack the aggressive nucleophilicity of the serine and cysteine proteases. Otherwise, members of each class are believed to have descended from a common ancestor by divergent evolution.

The four classes of proteolytic enzyme, their substrate activities and specific inhibitors are summarized in Table 11.1. Proteolytic enzymes exist ubiquitously in all biological tissues and fluids; however, practical considerations have made some more amenable to study than others. Extracellular proteases such as pancreatic and gastric protease, mammary plasma protease and certain bacterial proteases are readily isolated and have therefore been widely studied. By comparison, much less is known about intracellular tissue proteases, their enzymatic specificity and physiological substrates. However, the overall enzymatic process (peptide bond scission) is identical in all cases and the differences between their catalytic mechanisms are rather subtle.

## The serine proteases

This is the most commonly studied class of enzymes in the protease field and is made up of two distinct families: the mammalian serine proteases such as plasminogen activators, chymotrypsin, trypsin, elastase, cathepsin G and kallikrein; and the bacterial serine proteases, for example subtitlisin. They differ from each other in amino acid sequence and three-dimensional structure, but share a common active site with the catalytic triad of Asp 102, His 57, Ser 195 (chymotrypsin numbering) and an enzymatic mechanism which proceeds via a tetrahedral transition state intermediate during both the acylation and deacylation steps of catalysis.[13]

The plasminogen activators are key regulators of connective tissue turnover, acting by specific catalysis of the generation of plasmin from its plasma zymogen, plasminogen.[14] Two major plasminogen activators have been described: tissue plasminogen activator (t-PA) and a urokinase-type plasminogen activator (u-PA). Both cleave plasminogen at an Arg–Val bond near the carboxy terminus, resulting in an autocatalytic cleavage near the amino terminus of the enzyme.

Considerable attention has been paid to another group of serine proteases which are expressed by granulocytes, leukocytes and mast cells.[15] These include leukocyte cathepsin G, neutrophil elastase and chymases, the chymotrypsin-like enzymes of mast cells. These enzymes are stored in granules as inactive precursors and are released in response to inflammatory or allergic reactions in an active form.[16] These enzymes lack a disulfide bond near the active serine site that is present in all other known mammalian serine proteases.

The serine protease inhibitors (serpins) include $\alpha_1$-antitrypsin, $\alpha_1$-antichymotrypsin, antithrombin III and protease-nexin. They are important regulators of neutrophil elastase activity and may also inhibit plasmin. Plasminogen activator inhibitors (PAI) are potential regulators of connective tissue degradation and inhibit both u-PA and t-PA. Synthetic inhibitors of serine proteases include di-isopropyl fluorophosphate (DPF) and phenylmethanesulphonyl fluoride (PMSF), which react with the serine in the active site; and chloromethyl ketone derivatives of amino acids and peptides which react with the histidine of the catalytic triad.

$\alpha_2$-Macroglobulin, the universal protease inhibitor, also inhibits proteases of this class. It is a 772 kDa protein which is confined to the blood, and is composed of four nearly identical, disulfide-bonding polypeptide chains. It displays very broad specificity, and traps the protease irreversibly in the so-called bait region.

## The cysteine proteases

This class of protease bears great similarity to the serine protease group because a covalent intermediate is formed and the attacking nucleophile is the sulfur atom of a cysteine side chain

**Table 11.1 Substrates and inhibitors of the four major classes of endoprotease**

| Protease class | Substrates[a] | Optimal pH | Inhibitors[a] |
|---|---|---|---|
| Aspartic | Hemoglobin<br>Amyloid<br>Invariant chain | 2–3 | Diazoacetyl compounds<br>Pepstatin A<br>$a_2$-Macroglobulin |
| Cysteine | Cartilage proteoglycan<br>Collagen<br>Connective tissue<br>protein | 3–5 | Cystatins<br>Iodoacetic acid<br>Leupeptin, E64<br>p-Hydroxymercuribenzoate<br>(PHMB)<br>$a_2$-Macroglobulin |
| Metalloproteinase | All extracellular matrix<br>(e.g. proteoglycans, collagen,<br>fibronectin, laminin, vitronectin)<br>Certain latent form of MMP<br>Fibroblast growth<br>factor-receptor-1<br>Insulin growth factor-binding<br>protein<br>L-selectin | 7–8 | 1,10-Phenanthroline<br>EDTA, EGTA<br>Hydroxamic acid<br>Phosphoramidon<br>TIMP<br>$a_2$-Macroglobulin |
| Serine | Certain MMP (e.g. interstitial<br>collagenase, stromelysin-1,<br>gelatinase B, MTI-MMP)<br>Fibronectin, laminin, tenascin<br>Hepatocyte growth factor<br>Latent form TGF-ß binding protein<br>Plasminogen<br>Proteoglycan (e.g. aggrecan,<br>syndecan) | 7 | Di-isopropyl fluorophospate<br>(DPF)<br>Phenylmethanesulphonyl<br>fluoride (PMSF)<br>Leupeptin, antipain, aprotinin<br>Plasminogen activator inhibitor<br>Serpins ($a_1$-antitrypsin, etc.)<br>$a_2$-Antiplasmin<br>$a_2$-Macroglobulin |

[a]Not all of the proteins noted in each group are cleaved by or inhibited by all the enzymes in the class.

(cysteine 25 in the papain numbering system, acting like serine 195 in chymotrypsin). This class of protease includes several mammalian lysosomal cathepsins, cytosolic calcium-activated proteases (calpains) and the plant proteases papain and actinidin. Cathepsins B, L, N and S are secreted by stimulated connective tissue cells and macrophages in liver and spleen. They have been shown to degrade connective tissue proteins in vitro.[17] Both cathepsins B and L are generally stored in lysosomal granules, often in a latent form requiring activation by proteolysis. They are stable at alkaline pH and are metabolically active at low pH values, and hence are often referred to as acidic proteases.[18,19] These proteinases have been directly implicated in bone resorption,[20] the degradation of cartilage proteoglycan and collagen, and experimentally induce kidney disease.[21–23]

Cystatins are a superfamily of cysteine proteinase inhibitors which have been divided into three families, type I (stefins), type 2 (cystatin C and S) and type 3 (kininogens), based on primary amino acid sequence homology and domain structure. The cystatins are tight-binding reversible inhibitors of many cysteine proteases and do not inhibit proteinases from other catalytic classes.

## The aspartic proteases

The aspartic proteases include bacterial penicillopepsin, mammalian pepsin, cathepsin D, renin, chymosin, and certain fungal proteases. This group of enzymes is believed to catalyze the cleavage of peptide bonds without the use of nucleophilic attack by a functional group of the enzyme.[24] The aspartic peptidases have two aspartic acid side chains (residues 32 and 215 of the porcine pepsin numbering system) in close proximity to each other. The enzymes are active in the pH range 2–3, and so fall into the generic grouping of acidic proteases and are found in lysosomes. Cathepsin D is involved in the enzymatic removal of invariant chain from the nascent class II MHC molecule during antigen processing, and is also involved in the production of antigenic peptides in the phagolysosome of antigen-presenting cells.[25] Mice deficient in cathepsin D exhibit progressive intestinal mucosal atrophy and extensive destruction of lymphoid cells, suggesting that apart from proteolytic functions this enzyme may regulate cell growth and tissue homeostasis.[26]

## The metalloproteinases

This group of enzymes catalyses the cleavage of peptide bonds without the use of nucleophilic attack by a functional group of the enzyme at neutral or near neutral pH. All matrix metalloproteinases (MMPs) have a $Zn^{2+}$-binding site HEXXH, and all require $Ca^{2+}$ for stability and exhibit a preferred cleavage specificity for the N-terminal side of hydrophobic residues.[27,28] MMPs are part of a larger superfamily of proteases, the metzincins, which also contains bone morphogenetic protein-1 (a serralysin) and the adamalysins.[29] The latter group contains a large family of transmembrane proteases which consist of a protease and a disintegrin domain, the best known of which is adamalysin 17, the TNF-α-converting enzyme that cleaves membrane TNF-α to generate soluble TNF, and which also is essential for the shedding of other cell surface proteins such as TGF-α and L-selectin.[30]

Twenty-five vertebrate MMPs have been identified so far, and 22 of them have human homologs (Table 11.2).[31–33] Together they have the capacity to degrade all components of the extracellular matrix, therefore their activity must be tightly controlled in vivo. They fall into four broad groups, the collagenases, the gelatinases, the stromelysins (all secreted) and membrane-type (MT-MMPs). They are secreted by various cell types, including mesenchymal cells, monocytes, macrophages, neutrophils, keratinocytes, tumor cells etc., nearly all as zymogens (latent enzyme).

MMPs can also be classified structurally (Fig. 11.1). They all have an N-terminal signal sequence (predomain) which directs them to the endoplasmic reticulum and is then removed. There is then a prodomain, which maintains latency by an unpaired cysteine sulfhydryl group near the C terminus of the propeptide.[34] This acts as a ligand for the zinc ion in the active site. Proteolytic cleavage of the propeptide by other enzymes such as plasmin allows the thiol group to be replaced by water to produce a smaller molecular weight active enzyme, which can then undergo autocatalytic activation. There is then a catalytic domain which determines substrate specificity, and finally a hemopexin/vitronectin-like domain which regulates binding of MMP inhibitors, substrate specificity and some proteolytic activities. The MT-MMPs have a transmembrane domain at their C terminus.

There is, however, considerable variation within family members. MMP-7 (matrilysin) lacks the hemopexin domain. The gelatinases have collagen-binding fibronectin type II domains within the catalytic domain. MMP-17 is GPI linked at its C terminus, and MMP-11 (stromelysin 3), MMP-28 (epilysin), and MMP-14, -15, -16, -17, -24 and -25 all contain a furin-like recognition motif within the catalytic domain. They can thus be activated by intracellular serine proteases, so that, when secreted or put on the cell surface, they are already activated.[35] However, one of the most studied MMPs, MMP-2 (gelatinase A), is not activated by serine proteases. Instead, MT1-MMP binds the N-terminus of its inhibitor TIMP-2. The C terminus of TIMP-2 then acts as a receptor for the hemopexin-like domain of MMP-2. The tethered MMP-2 is then activated by an adjacent MT1-MMP on the cell membrane.[36,37] MMPs can also activate each other – for example, stromelysin-1 is a potent activator of procollagenase[38] – and are activated by other proteases.[39,40]

Most MMPs are transcriptionally regulated, except for MMP-2, which is constitutively expressed by many cell types and whose activation is controlled by MT1-MMP. Once translated, most MMPs are secreted, with the exception of MMP-2 (neutrophil collagenase) and MMP-9 (gelatinase B) in granulocytes. These MMPs are made by granulocytes and then stored in granules and are released following neutrophil activation. MMP expression is regulated by many pathways, such as cytokines, growth factors and extracellular matrix. There is also cell-specific regulation and cell-specific expression. Even within the same cell a single factor can differentially regulate MMPs, such as TGF-β1, which suppresses MMP-1 and MMP-3 production but enhances MMP-13 (collagenase 3 expression).[41]

## ENDOGENOUS INHIBITORS OF MMPs

The proteolytic activity of MMP is regulated in the extracellular space by the tissue inhibitors of metalloproteinases (TIMPs), four of which have so far been identified.[42] TIMPs form high-affinity, 1:1 non-covalent complexes with the active forms of MMP. TIMPs are structurally similar, with a 37–51% homology, a conserved gene structure and a conserved six-loop two-domain structure owing to the pairing of 12 intrachain disulfide bridges. The inhibitory activity of TIMPs resides in the N-terminus of the molecule that binds to and blocks the catalytic site. TIMPs differ in their ability to inhibit different MMPs and, as stated above, TIMP-2 is required for the activation of MMP-2 by MT1-MMP. TIMP-2 and TIMP-3 inhibit MT1-MMP, but TIMP-1 does not. TIMP-3 binds to the extracellular matrix.

TIMPs have biological activity apart from MMP inhibition. TIMP-3 can induce apoptosis in various cell types.[43] TIMPs can also act as mitogens and, in fact, TIMP-1 was cloned as an erythroid-potentiating molecule. So far, however, no cell surface receptors for TIMPs have been identified.

The major inhibitor of MMPs is α2-microglobulin, abundant in serum and inflamed tissues. α2-Microglobulin is important for the removal of MMPs because the MMP/α2-microglubulin is removed from the circulation by scavenger receptor-mediated endocytosis.

## ARE PROTEASES INCREASED IN INTESTINAL ULCERATION?

There has only been recent recognition that proteolytic degradation is important in the development of ulcers in chronic IBD. The majority of studies have been descriptive. In 1994, Bailey et al.[44] used immunofluorescence to analyze MMP-1, -3 and -9 in IBD tissue. The most intense signal was detected with anti-MMP-9 in infiltrating neutrophils. MMP-1 staining was minimal. Interestingly, MMP-3 staining was seen in the matrix in IBD patients and was particularly strong around ulcers in patients with UC. Subsequent in situ hybridization studies extended these observations. Transcripts for MMP-1 and MMP-3 are abundant in the granulation tissue below and beside the ulcers of IBD patients, as well as in peptic and duodenal ulcers (Fig. 11.2).[45] Epithelium at the edge of ulcers was also strongly positive for matrilysin (MMP-7) and the basement membrane was disrupted below the matrilysin+ epithelium.[45] Further analysis revealed that the epithelium adjacent to IBD ulcers contained transcripts for stromelysin 2 (MMP-2).[46] Fibroblasts in ulcers also expressed collagenase 3 (MMP-13) and TIMP-3. Finally, macrophage metalloelastase (MMP-12)-positive cells were abundant in ulcers and below shedding epithelium.[46]

Zymography is a technique often used to analyze protease activity. This technique involves separating proteins on gelatin or casein gels, allowing the enzymes to degrade the substrates in the gel, and then staining the gel for protein with Coomassie blue. Clear bands appear where proteolysis has occurred. The class of protease can be identified by using appropriate inhibitors. The technique is very sensitive for gelatinases and, importantly, allows the identification of smaller molecular weight active enzyme as well as the latent enzyme, which itself is activated by SDS in the gel.

Homogenates of UC tissue analyzed by zymography show considerable gelatinolytic activity, which is mostly due to gelatinase B in neutrophils. In contrast, Crohn's disease does not show

## Table 11.2 The matrix metalloproteinases

| MMP | Name | Major activity |
|---|---|---|
| MMP-1 | Collagenase 1 | Aggrecan, collagen I, II, III, VII, VII, X, XI, fibronectin, laminin, link protein, tenascin, vitronectin, IL-1$\beta$, pro-TNF, CTGF |
| MMP-2 | Gelatinase A | Aggrecan, collagen I, III, IV, V, VII, X, XI, decorin, elastin fibronectin, gelatin, laminin, link protein, tenascin, vitronectin, IL-$\beta$, pro-TGFB, pro-TNF |
| MMP-3 | Stromelysin 1 | Aggrecan, collagen III, IV, V, VII, IX, X, XI, decorin, elastin, fibronectin. gelatin, laminin, link protein, tenascin, vitronectin, E-cadherin, IL-1$\beta$, pro-TNF, CTGF |
| MMP-7 | Matrilysin | Aggrecan, collagen I, IV, decorin, elastin, fibronectin, laminin, link protein, tenascin, vitronectin, E-cadherin, pro-TNF, $\alpha$-defensin, CTGF |
| MMP-8 | Collagenase 2 Neutrophil collagenase | Aggrecan, collagen I, II, III |
| MMP-9 | Gelatinase B | Aggrecan, collagen IV, V, XI, XIV, decorin, elastin, fibronectin, laminin link protein, vitronectin, IL-1$\beta$, pro-TGF$\beta$, pro-TNF |
| MMP-10 | Stromelysin 2 | Aggrecan, collagen III, IV, V, elastin, fibronectin, gelatin, link protein, fibrinogen |
| MMP-11 | Stromelysin 3 | |
| MMP-12 | Macrophage metalloelastase | Aggrecan, collagen I, IV, elastin, fibronectin, gelatin, laminin, vitronectin, pro-TNF |
| MMP-13 | Collagenase 3 | Aggrecan, collagen I, II, III, VI, IX, X, XI, XIV, fibronectin, gelatin, CTGF |
| MMP-14 | MT-1 MMP | Aggrecan, collagen I, II, III, fibronectin, gelatin, laminin, vitronectin, pro-MMP2, pro-TNF |
| MMP-15 | MT2-MMP | Collagen III, fibronectin |
| MMP-16 | MT3- MMP | |
| MMP-17 | MT4-MMP | |
| MMP-18 | Collagenase IV (Xenopus) | Collagen I |
| MMP-19 | RASI-1 | Collagen I, IV, fibronectin, gelatin, tenascin |
| MMP-20 | Enamelysin | |
| MMP-21 | XMMP (Xenopus) | |
| MMP-22 | CMMP chicken | |
| MMP-23 | | |
| MMP-24 | MT5-MMP | |
| MMP-25 | MT6-MMP | |
| MMP-26 | Endometase, matrilysin 2 | Collagen IV, fibronectin, gelatin, fibrinogen |
| MMP-27 | | |
| MMP-28 | Epilysin | |

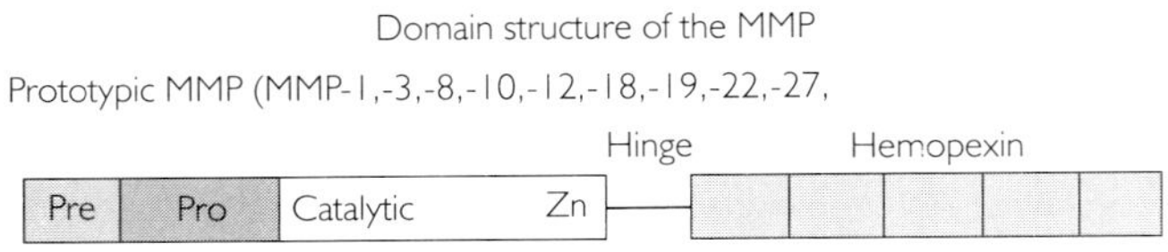

Domain structure of the MMP

Prototypic MMP (MMP-1,-3,-8,-10,-12,-18,-19,-22,-27,

Fig. 11.1 The modular nature of different MMP.

Structural modifications in the different MMPs
**MMP-7**, **MMP-26**, Minimal domain MMP– lacking domains
MMP-2,9, Gelatin-binding MMP–collagen-binding inserts between
catalytic and Zn regions
**MMP-11, 28** Furin-activated secreted MMPs–furin-susceptable
site in prodomain
**MMP-14-25-16-24** Transmembrane MMPs–transmembrane
domain at C terminus
**MMP-17-25** GPI-linked MMP–GPI anchoring domain at C terminus
**MMP-21**, XMMP Vitronectin-like insert-linker less MMPs–lack hinge,
vitronectin-like domain in prodomain
**MMP-23** Cysteine/proline-rich IL-1R-like domain MMP–replaces
hemopexin domains

activity.[47] Surprisingly, Western blotting for MMP-1 and MMP-3 has been expected as negative in most IBD samples.[47] However, these results have not been confirmed and it is now very clear that MMP-1 and -3 are highly overexpressed in IBD. Heuschkel et al. used quantitative RT-PCR and Western blotting to show marked overexpression of MMP-3 in the mucosa of children with IBD.[48] Importantly, lower molecular weight (active) enzyme was seen in most samples. Very similar results were obtained by von Lampe et al., who also showed increased transcripts for MMP-1 and MMP-3 in IBD mucosa, as well as an increase in MMP-14.[49] Louis et al. found markedly increased MMP-3 by immunoassay in supernatants from cultured biopsies from IBD patients, but not from controls.[50] Stallmach et al. showed that MMP-1 and -2 protein and RNA were markedly increased in pouchitis and ulcerative colitis.[51] Finally, Arihiro et al. reported that vascular smooth muscle cells and pericytes express MMP-1 and -9 in IBD mucosa.[52]

These results indicate rather conclusively that MMP are increased in IBD. Matrilysin and stromelysin 2 are overexpressed in epithelium adjacent to ulcers, MMP-12 is overexpressed in macrophages in the lamina propria of the inflamed gut, and MMP-1, -2, -3 and -13 are present adjacent to and below ulcers, almost certainly arising from stromal cells. However, information on other proteases is almost completely lacking. Stools and gut lavage fluid from IBD patients contain increased concentrations of neutrophil elastase,[53,54] but the role of any serine protease in intestinal injury has not been investigated in any detail. Neutrophils migrating across colon cancer cells in vitro cause death of the enterocytes, which is associated with loss of junctional complexes and can be inhibited with inhibitors of neutrophil elastase.[55]

## TIMP IN IBD

It is important to determine whether TIMPs are also increased in the mucosa in IBD, to counteract the demonstrated enhanced proteolytic activity during intestinal inflammation. TIMP-1 and TIMP-3 transcripts are abundant in ulcer bases in IBD.[45,46] However, it is not clear whether TIMP-1 is generally upregulated in IBD to counteract the increased MMP. Using quantitative RT-PCR, TIMP-1 transcripts are seen to be abundant in control and IBD tissues, and TIMP-1 protein is also equivalent by Western blotting.[48] However, others have reported that

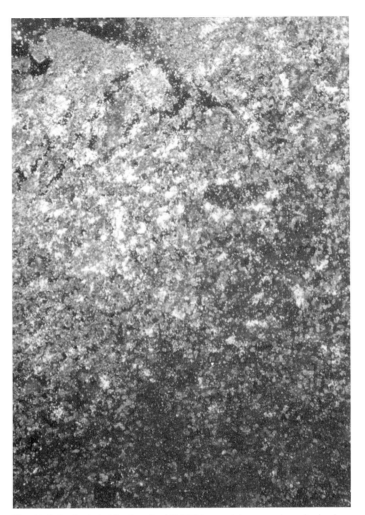

Fig. 11.2 In situ hybridization for MMP-3 transcripts around a colonic ulcer in a patient with Crohn's disease. Note the abundance of labeled cells around the ulcer margin, but their absence in the deeper layers of the mucosa.

TIMP-1 transcripts are moderately elevated in IBD, although TIMP-2 transcripts are abundant and not increased in all control and IBD tissues.[49] Mucosal TIMP-1 production is also increased in IBD, but was studied only in a few patients.[50] Overall, there is certainly no inhibition of TIMP production in IBD, and it may be moderately elevated.

## FUNCTIONAL STUDIES ON THE ROLE OF MMP IN MUCOSAL INJURY

It is crucial to show that the overexpression of various MMPs in IBD is functionally important, and that their inhibition can ameliorate tissue damage. Prior to treating patients this approach needs to be tested in model systems. Marimastat is a rather non-specific MMP inhibitor, but has greater specificity for gelatinase and collagenase than for stromelysin. Rats pretreated with marimastat, given TNBS intracolonically and then treated for a further 3 days show markedly reduced colitis scores on day 7.[56] TNF-α levels in tissue, however, remain elevated. Similar results have been obtained with batimastat, another broad MMP inhibitor, in rat TNBS colitis.[57] These experiments, however, do not demonstrate that MMP inhibitors directly heal intestinal

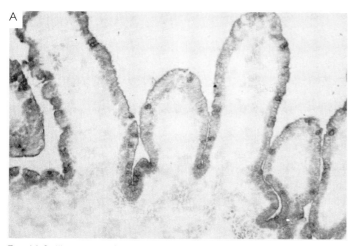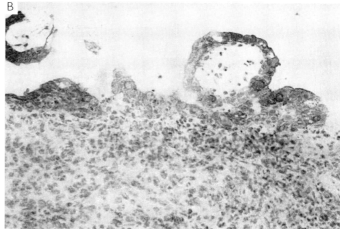

**Fig. 11.3** Illustration of the fetal gut explant organ culture system which was used to show that MMPs are important in immune-mediated damage in human intestine. Human gut contains T cells in the lamina propria and, when activated with anti-CD3 + IL-12, a massive Th1 immune response is initiated which results in degradation of the mucosa. This is associated with increased MMPs and is inhibited by MMP inhibitors and also by TNF inhibitors. (Immunoperoxidase histochemistry with anticytokeratin to highlight the epithelium; original magnification x20.)

ulcers, as the inhibitors were given prophylactically. It is now becoming clear that MMPs are involved in the immune response, and that gelatinases in particular are needed for the migration of dendritic cells and for T cells to cross basement membranes.[58,59] Because TNBS colitis is a T cell-dependent disease, the MMP inhibitors may function in an immunoregulatory or immunosuppressive fashion, rather than being antiulcerogenic. MMP inhibitors also prevent intestinal injury seen in acute graft-versus-host disease in mice.[60] However, again the MMP inhibitors were given throughout the experiment and the effect may be due to direct anti-inflammatory effects rather than preventing gut pathology. No studies have yet appeared in which MMP inhibitors have been used therapeutically to heal the gut in any of the numerous rodent models of IBD.

We have recently been investigating the biochemical and molecular basis for the mucosal degradation which is seen when the lectin, pokeweed mitogen (PWM), or anti-CD3 antibodies plus exogenous IL-12, are used to activate the resident T cells in the lamina propria of human fetal gut explants (Fig. 11.3).[11,16] This response is completely T-cell dependent, as injury is not seen if PWM is added to explants from younger specimens with few T cells, and is also inhibitable by cyclosporin A and FK506.[62] The first clue that proteases might be important in this system was that PWM-induced injury was associated with the loss of sulfated glycosaminoglycans (GAGs) from the lamina propria and their appearance in the organ culture supernatant.[63] These GAGs were identified as dermatan/chondroitin sulfate moieties, suggesting that they were associated with proteoglycans. Importantly, tissue injury was inhibited by $\alpha_2$-macroglobulin, suggesting that proteases were important. In further studies, injury was associated with markedly elevated interstitial collagenase and stromelysin-1 mRNA transcripts in the tissues, and increased inactive and active stromelysin and collagenase in the explant culture supernatants.[64] Gelatinase A concentration was not elevated, nor were TIMP-1 and TIMP-2.

Nanomolar amounts of stromelysin-1, but not interstitial collagenase or gelatinases, can cause rapid mucosal destruction and epithelial shedding when added directly to the explants. Further strong evidence for a major role for stromelysin in this system came from the observation that PWM-induced mucosal degra-

dation was inhibited by a stromelysin inhibitor and not a collagenase inhibitor. The stromelysin inhibitor was effective if added after the initiation of the T-cell response with PWM, and did not reduce the extent of the cell-mediated immune response in the tissue, implying that stromelysin-1-induced mucosal degradation was an end-stage event. Importantly, isolated stromal cells secreted large amounts of stromelysin and collagenase when activated with cytokines such as TNF-$\alpha$ or IL-1$\beta$, providing strong evidence that the injury was not caused by the T-cell and macrophage-derived cytokines directly, but was due to elevated production of stromelysin by mucosal myofibroblasts. Colocalization of MMP-3 and MMP-1 RNA-containing cells to smooth muscle actin-positive cells confirmed that the proteases were being made by myofibroblasts.

Mucosal degradation in this model is inhibited by a soluble p55 TNF receptor–human IgG$_1$ fusion protein.[65] Inhibition of the tissue injury is associated with a 95% reduction in the amount of stromelysin-1 detected in the organ culture supernatants, but not collagenase or gelatinases. This strongly suggests that TNF-$\alpha$ is driving tissue MMP production by stromal cells. Additional supporting data come from an analysis of the damage seen when explants are stimulated with anti-CD3 antibodies and Th1-inducing cytokines such as IL-12 or IL-18, where injury is T-cell mediated. In this situation anti-CD3, IL-12 and IL-18 have no effect on their own, but when anti-CD3 is added with IL-12 there is a massive Th1 response, with abundant TNF-$\alpha$ production, increased MMP and mucosal degradation.[61] Anti-CD3 plus IL-18 has no effect because there is no TNF-$\alpha$ produced. In this model, both TNFR-IgG and MMP inhibitors prevent injury.[61]

The evidence is therefore compelling that the overexpression of cytokines in inflamed gut is linked to the upregulation of matrix-degrading proteases by lamina propria myofibroblasts. Produced as zymogens into the extracellular space, activation into active enzyme can occur through a number of pathways, such as by free radicals, plasmin, mast cell proteases or other MMP-mediated cleavage of the MMP propeptide. However, there is only a very limited literature on the targets of MMP in the mucosa. Immediately below MMP-10+ epithelial cells in IBD there is loss of laminin staining, suggesting enzymatic degradation.[46] The loss of laminin staining has been confirmed by others,[66] although it is not possible to say that laminin protein has been lost; alternatively, the epitope recognized by the specific antibody may have been lost. In UC there is increased immunoreactivity for basement membrane type IV and type V collagen, suggesting a compensatory response.[66] Using an antibody specific for the denatured triple helix of collagen α1(IV), no staining is seen in active UC, suggesting the stability of type IV collagen in IBD.[67] However, using charge staining for the sulfated glycosaminoglycan side chains of lamina propria proteoglycans, we have demonstrated substantial loss of staining in active IBD,[68] presumably because of cleavage of the core protein. A thorough biochemical analysis of the matrix changes in IBD needs to be carried out.

Intestinal epithelial cells need to bind to extracellular matrix to survive. In ulcerative colitis there is extensive apoptosis of epithelial cells.[69] In addition, disruption of the interaction between epithelial cells and basement membrane in whole normal crypts with anti-integrin antibodies increases apoptosis.[70] These experiments indicate that MMP-mediated destruction of basement membrane, or, more subtly, the basement membrane ligands for epithelial cells, could lead to epithelial cell apoptosis in ulcerative colitis.

## COLLAGENOUS COLITIS

Although there are matrix changes in all forms of intestinal inflammation, the clearest case where changes in matrix are associated with the inflammatory response is in the rare condition collagenous colitis. In this condition there is increased deposition of extracellular matrix in the subepithelial space (Fig. 11.4). Patients have chronic watery diarrhea and, endoscopically, the colon is often normal. Mucosal biopsies show a lymphocytic infiltrate into the mucosa, loss and flattening of epithelial cells, and a band-like linear deposition of collagen I, II, VI and fibronectin below the epithelial basement membrane. Although no detailed immunological studies have been carried out, there

is increased HLA-DR expression on colonic epithelial cells suggestive of increased concentrations of inflammatory cytokines.[71] In situ hybridization reveals an increase in transcripts for procollagen I, VI and TIMP-1 in cells around the collagenous band, as well as increased immunostaining for tenascin, an extracellular matrix protein prominent in developing and remodeling intestine (Fig. 11.4). MMP-1 (interstitial collagenase) transcripts are sparse and MMP-13 (collagenase 3) transcripts absent.[72,73] Together these results suggest that the collagen band is due to increased collagen synthesis and reduced degradation. The dynamic nature of the band is illustrated by the fact that the band reduces in thickness when patients are treated with budesonide.[74] The relationship between the collagen band and the lymphocytic infiltrate is not understood, nor is the difference between collagenous colitis and a related condition, lymphocytic colitis, which does not develop the subepithelial collagen band.

## FIBROSIS AND STENOSIS IN IBD

One of the main features of Crohn's disease is the presence of fibrosis in the submucosa and external muscle layers, which can produce stenosis, strictures and complete luminal obstruction requiring surgical intervention. There is excess collagen deposition in lamina propria above strictures, expansion of the muscularis mucosa overlying the stricture, and collagen deposition in the submucosa and muscularis externa. These features are not seen in ulcerative colitis, where the inflammation is restricted to mucosa, suggesting that the cause of the fibrosis in the deeper layers is the transmural inflammation seen in Crohn's. There are differences in the collagen deposition in strictured bowel, with excess collagen V in deeper layers and collagen III in the lamina propria.[75] In situ hybridization reveals increased transcripts for procollagen types I, III, IV and V, especially in the deeper intestinal layers.[76] Functionally, smooth muscle cells isolated from the lamina propria of the strictured bowel secrete large amounts of collagen III when activated with TGF-β. In contrast, PDGF inhibits collagen III secretion.[77]

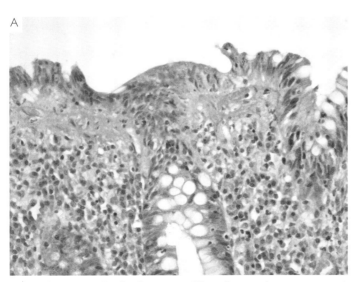
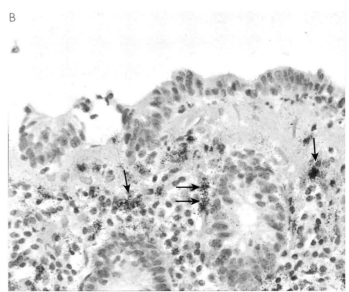

Fig. 11.4 An example of collagenous colitis, a disease where excess matrix deposition underlies the pathology and tissue injury. (A) The collagen band is highlighted by the red van Gieson stain. (B) In situ hybridization for procollagen I transcripts, which are abundant in fibroblasts around the area of collagen deposition (arrowed). Original magnification x40. Illustrations kindly supplied by Dr Adrian Bateman and Dr Ute Günther.

IL-1β is markedly overexpressed in Crohn's disease[78] and is a potent mitogen for human intestinal smooth muscle cells.[79] Interestingly, it also markedly increases the production of MMP-1 by these cells and decreases procollagen I and III mRNA.[79] This would suggest that IL-1β made by inflammatory cells in Crohn's is actually antifibrotic. Therefore, the excess extracellular matrix deposited in Crohn's strictures must reflect the overall balance of collagen production and collagen degradation by MMPs; after repeated insults, TGF-β₁-mediated collagen deposition predominates as an overzealous and final response to chronic injury and repair.

## COMPLEXITY OF THE ROLE OF MMPs IN INTESTINAL INFLAMMATION

MMPs play a much wider role than merely degrading extracellular matrix. Matrix plays a fundamental role in controlling cell survival, shape, growth and differentiation by sequestering growth factors and providing ligands for cell surface receptors.[80] Because MMPs alter the matrix, they must also alter all of these signals within the microenvironment. For example, latent TGF-β is sequestered in the matrix by decorin, a proteoglycan which is associated with collagen.[81] Degradation of decorin by MMPs produced by TNF-α-activated lamina propria myofibroblasts makes TGF-β bioavailable to drive collagen synthesis in fibroblasts.[81] But TGF-β is also a potent inhibitor of MMP-1 and MMP-3,[41] and so the release of TGF-β₁ feeds back and inhibits MMP production by the myofibroblasts. However, TGF-β itself activates a negative loop by inducing the expression of the inhibitory signaling molecule Smad7, which prevents signal transduction to the nucleus following TGF-β binding.[82] There is therefore a dampening of the TGF-β₁ inhibitory loop, allowing TNF-α to continue to drive MMP production (Fig. 11. 5). MMP-3 and MMP-7 can cleave the epithelial adherens junction protein E-cadherin, and the fragment produced disrupts other cells by acting as a competitive inhibitor of E-cadherin homotypic binding between cells.[83,84] Because E-cadherin is important not only in maintaining intestinal epithelial integrity, but also acts as a tumor suppressor,[85] MMP-3 in the gut wall may cause loss of barrier function and may even promote carcinogenesis. MMPs can cleave membrane-bound TNF-α, increasing local concentrations of this proinflammatory cytokine,[86] but can also degrade IL-1β, which will decrease inflammation.[87] MMP-7 cleaves the IL-2Rα chain, thereby making cells unresponsive to IL-2 and reducing T-cell proliferation.[88]

Importantly, MMPs may also be involved in healing. To reconstitute an ulcer, myofibroblasts have to migrate into granulation tissue, as do new endothelial cells, which are required for revascularization before the epithelium can restitute the barrier. We have shown that when gut myofibroblasts are activated through the α₄β₁ integrin (natural ligands fibronectin and VCAM-1), they upregulate MT1-MMP and active gelatinase A.[89] The cells then become capable of migrating through synthetic matrix. MT1-MMP mRNA+ cells are abundant around ulcers, which suggests that myofibroblasts are constantly attempting to migrate into the ulcer bed to heal the lesion.[89] Endothelial cells also use MT1-MMP to move through the matrix during revascularization.[90]

Epithelial cells at the edge of ulcers show strong expression of MMP-7.[45] In the airway, MMP-7 is needed for re-epithelialization after injury.[89] It is highly expressed in epithelium adjacent to damaged trachea in humans and mice. However, after wounding there is a complete failure of re-epithelialization in MMP-7 null mice.[89] Correspondingly, re-epithelialization of human tracheal epithelium is inhibited by MMP inhibitors. It is intriguing to speculate that MMP-7 null mice would be very susceptible to experimental colitis, and that the overexpression of matrilysin in human intestinal epithelium in IBD represents migrating epithelial cells remodeling the matrix as they crawl over granulation tissue.

A final important function of matrilysin in the gut is that it activates α-defensins produced by Paneth cells to mediate non-specific antimicrobial immunity.[92] This, however, is true only in mice; in humans this function is carried out by Paneth cell trypsin.[93]

MMP also play a very important role in cancer, but this topic is outside the scope of this chapter and readers are referred to recent excellent reviews.[94,95]

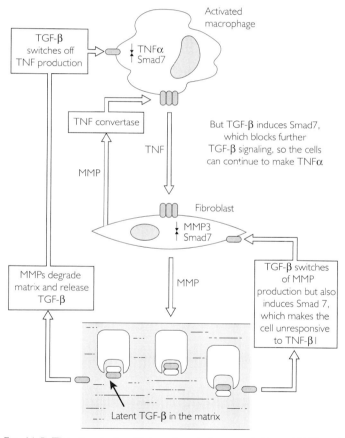

Fig. 11.5 The complexity of interactions between cytokines, MMPs and TGF-β in the inflammatory/pathological cascade. Activated macrophages in the mucosa secrete TNF, which is cleaved from the cell membrane by ADAM17. TNF then binds to the p55 receptor on fibroblasts and initiates transcription of MMPs. Secreted MMPs are activated extracellularly by molecules such as plasmin, which then degrades the matrix and releases and activates TGF-β. MMPs also function as TNF convertases. TGF-β can then negatively feed back on macrophages and fibroblasts and inhibit TNF and MMP production. However, TGF-β initiates its own inhibitory loop inside the cells and initiates synthesis of Smad7, which blocks TGF-β₁ signaling. The cells become refractory to TGF-β and the inflammatory cascade continues.

# MUCOSAL GROWTH AS A RESPONSE TO INFLAMMATION

## BACKGROUND

Although it may seem counterintuitive, inflammation often increases the size of a tissue. In psoriasis there is a marked thickening of the epidermis around the infiltrating T cells. In the colon in active ulcerative colitis and Crohn's disease there is also marked mucosal thickening, and crypt hyperplasia is a reproducible feature of T lymphocyte-mediated experimental colitis. In the upper small intestine of patients with celiac disease, detailed morphometric analysis has shown that the major feature of the transformation of the normal mucosa into the flat mucosa is a two- to threefold increase in the volume of the lamina propria, even although total mucosal thickness does not change.[10] Instead of villous atrophy, the villi in fact are swallowed up as the lamina propria grows upwards. Although most of this idea comes from the study of celiac disease it is applicable to Crohn's disease, where the small bowel mucosa is often flat and the colon obviously thickened.

In inflammation-induced mucosal growth considerable attention has been paid to the role of the hyperplastic epithelium and the lengthening of the glands in the colon or the crypts in the small bowel. In contrast, much less attention has been paid to the changes in the lamina propria, which forms the structure over which epithelial cells migrate. It is still contentious as to whether mucosal thickening is driven primarily by the epithelium or by the lamina propria, but in all likelihood mucosal remodeling and growth require a synergy between these two compartments.

## KERATINOCYTE GROWTH FACTORS

Growth factors made by TNF-α or IL-1β-activated stromal cells have the capacity to influence epithelial renewal. For example, TGF-β inhibits epithelial proliferation,[96] whereas glucagon-like peptide 2, IGF-1 and EGF enhance epithelial proliferation.[97–99] The keratinocyte growth factors (KGFs) are members of the fibroblast growth factor family, with FGF-7 also being known as KGF-1 and FGF-10 as KGF-2.

KGFs are important in controlling epithelial proliferation in the lungs and skin, especially following injury.[100–103] Expression of KGF and its receptor (a splice variant of the FGFRII) has been detected on epithelial cells throughout the GI tract, suggesting that KGF is an endogenous mediator of growth and differentiation in this tissue.[104]

Studies in animals have shown an important role for KGF in protection against injury. Pretreating mice with KGF-1 protects them from chemotherapy- and radiation-induced gut injury and mortality.[105] There is marked survival of crypts following these treatments in mice given KGF-1 systemically. Systemically administered KGF-1 or -2 also protects animals from dextran sulfate colitis or indomethacin-induced intestinal ulceration.[106–108] In cultured epithelial cells, KGF promotes goblet cell differentiation.[109] Together, these results show that KGF-1 and -2 function as gut epithelial mitogens in health and disease, and so KGF might play a role in driving the epithelial hyperplasia seen in all inflammatory diseases of the gut.

Like many growth factors KGF is held in the matrix, and it has been shown that it binds to perlecan core protein (a heparan sulfate proteoglycan) and collagens I, III and VI.[110,111]

In situ hybridization has shown clearly that KGF is overexpressed in the mucosa in active IBD, with abundant message in myofibroblasts (Fig. 11.6).[112–114] There is a report that in mice, intestinal epithelial γδ cells make KGF,[115] but in IBD and active celiac disease, where there are abundant γδ IEL, no KGF mRNA signal can be detected within the epithelium.[114,116]

Infusion of KGF into normal mice causes crypt hyperplasia, and so we determined whether KGF is involved in the crypt hyperplasia seen during immune reactions in the intestine. Using a modification of the human fetal gut organ system, where we activate a subpopulation of lamina propria T cells with the bacterial superantigen *Staphylococcus aureus* enterotoxin B (SEB), we can induce an immune-mediated crypt hyperplasia and an increase in the number of dividing crypt epithelial cells. In this system, T-cell activation leads to a large increase in KGF transcripts and protein; importantly, crypt cell hyperplasia is inhibited by anti-KGF antibody.[117] This suggests that KGF made by cytokine-activated stromal cells could be involved in the crypt hyperplasia seen in diseases such as IBD and celiac disease.

## LAMINA PROPRIA GROWTH

Concomitant with crypt lengthening in IBD there is increased volume of the lamina propria. As the crypts lengthen, the pericryptal myofibroblasts must also grow to underpin the increased epithelium. Likewise, the stromal cells between the glands must proliferate and lay down matrix as the tissue thickens. A number of cytokines and growth factors which are abundant in inflamed mucosa of IBD patients are mitogens for colonic subepithelial myofibroblasts.[118] These include PDGF, basic FGF, EGF, IL-1β and TNF-α. Another important mediator of fibroblast proliferation is connective tissue growth factor (CTGF),[119] the production of which is dramatically increased in fibroblasts by TGF-β₁.[120,121] CTGF promotes fibroblast migration, adhesion and extracellular matrix formation, as well as proliferation. Through its potent ability to induce extracellular matrix production[120,121] CTGF has been suggested to be an important mediator of fibrosis, and in fact the profibrogenic activity of TGF-β is probably through its induction of CTGF.

Studies on the role of CTGF in gut inflammation and fibrosis are only beginning, although it appears to play a role in pancreatic and hepatic fibrosis.[122,123] By in situ hybridization, CTGF is strongly expressed in the endothelial cells and fibroblasts (Fig. 11.7) of inflamed mucosa of patients with Crohn's or ulcerative colitis, and is also highly expressed in fibrotic areas of Crohn's disease tissue.[124] Although this is consistent with the fact that TGF-β₁ is also overexpressed in IBD,[125] a linear correlation between these two factors is unlikely. The only other publication on CTGF in gut inflammation shows that it is increased in indomethacin-induced gastric ulcers.[128] As with the relationship between MMPs and growth factors described above, MMPs can also modulate CTGF function. MMP-1, -3, -7 and -13 can all cleave CTGF into biologically inactive fragments.[127]

TGF-β₁ initiates signaling through the ligand-dependent activation of a complex of heterodimeric transmembrane serine/threonine kinases, consisting of type I (TGF-β₁ RI) and type II (TGF-β₁ RII) receptors.[126,127] Upon TGF-β₁ binding, the receptors rotate within the complex, resulting in phosphorylation and activation of TGF-β₁ RI by the constitutively active and autophosphorylated TGF-β₁ RII. TGF-β₁ signals from the receptor to the nucleus using a set of proteins, termed Smads, based on their high homology to the *Drosophila* Mad and the

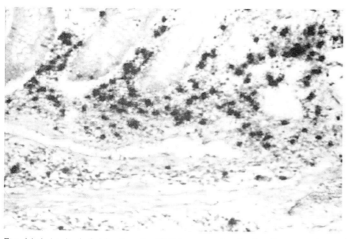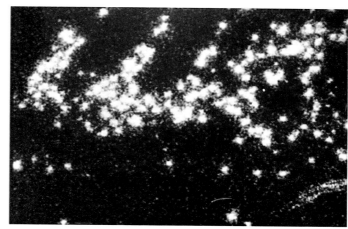

Fig. 11.6 In situ hybridization for KGF in a sample of colon from a patient with ulcerative colitis. The bright field image on the left shows that KGF mRNA-containing cells are situated next to the epithelium. The dark field shows the abundance of transcripts. No signal is seen in normal intestine. Original magnification x40. Illustration kindly supplied by Dr Richard Poulsom.

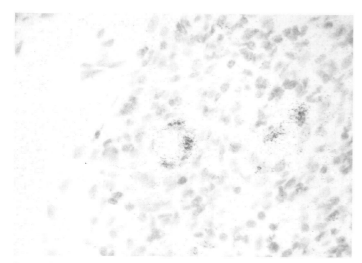

Fig. 11.7 In situ hybridization for CTGF in a colonic sample from a patient with UC. Transcripts are clearly visible in endothelial cells and fibroblasts. No signal is seen in normal intestine. Original magnification x40. Illustration kindly supplied by Dr Ute Günther.

*Caenorhabditis elegans* Sma proteins. To date, nine different Smad genes, which fall into three distinct functional sets, have been identified: signal-transducing receptor-activated Smads, which include Smad1, 2, 3, 5, 8 and 9; a single common mediator, Smad4, and inhibitory Smads 6 and 7. Activated TGF-$\beta_1$ RI directly phosphorylates Smad2 and Smad3 at serine residues in the carboxy-terminal SSXS sequence. Once activated, Smad2 and Smad3 associate with Smad4 and translocate to the nucleus, where Smad protein complexes participate in transcriptional control of target genes by binding to TGF-$\beta$ regulatory elements in the promoters of many genes. We have recently shown that the inhibitory Smad, Smad7, is highly overexpressed in inflammatory bowel disease mucosa, and that when lamina propria mononuclear cells (a mixture of T cells, plasma cells, stromal cells and macrophages) from Crohn's patients are stimulated with TGF-$\beta_1$ there is no phosphorylation of Smad2/3.[82] This raises the possibility that CTGF in IBD tissues is induced by factors other than TGF-$\beta_1$.

# THE MECHANISMS OF EPITHELIAL CELL DAMAGE IN IBD

## BACKGROUND

Epithelial damage is one of the most obvious markers of disease in the intestine and is especially obvious in ulcerative colitis. Damage may alter the function of the cells – for example chloride secretion as opposed to chloride absorption – with no obvious histologic change. In addition, epithelial damage may alter barrier integrity by compromising tight junctions, or it may lead to clear morphological changes to the cell and death by apoptosis or necrosis. In IBD all of these pathways occur.

## EPITHELIAL ABSORPTIVE FUNCTION IS COMPROMISED IN IBD

The primary function of the colonic epithelium is water and electrolyte absorption. In colitis these functions are impaired. In the left colon of healthy children, for example, there is net sodium and chloride absorption, but in children with IBD net chloride and sodium secretion is present.[130] Likewise, in collagenous colitis there is a net reduction in sodium and chloride ion absorption, coupled with electrogenic chloride secretion.[139] Epithelial transport is also compromised in pouchitis.[132]

Tight junctions between epithelial cells play a crucial role in the control of intestinal permeability. Their function can be measured by measuring transepithelial resistance as well as by the flux of macromolecules across the epithelium. In ulcerative colitis there is a 50% reduction in epithelial resistance, and tight junction strands are reduced by freeze fracture microscopy.[133] Western blotting and PCR reveals that in both active ulcerative colitis and Crohn's disease there is a marked reduction in occludin and ZO-1, both important tight junction proteins.[134]

## CYTOKINE-MEDIATED DAMAGE TO EPITHELIAL CELLS

Very little in vivo data exist on the role of cytokines in epithelial damage in IBD. Mouse models have shown biological effects, but their interpretation is difficult. The injection of LPS into mice causes widespread endothelial cell death by apoptosis, mediated by TNF-α.[135] TNF-α injection into animals induces apoptosis of intestinal endothelium, disrupts blood supply to the mucosa and induces local hypoxia and ischemia, which then induces apoptosis of epithelial cells.[136,137] IL-12 has similar effects, but works through an uncharacterized pathway which involves interferon-γ, but not TNF-α.[136] Injection of anti-CD3 antibody into mice also causes apoptosis of colonic crypt epithelial cells, which seems to depend on TNF-α, Fas and perforin.[139]

Control of epithelial structure and function has been extensively studied using polarized cancer cell lines in vitro. Interferon-γ increases tight junction permeability in T84 cells,[140] which is potentiated by hypoxia; this process involves an autocrine production of TNF-α by the T84 cells themselves.[141] The addition of TNF-α to IEC-18 cells (a rat gut epithelial cell line) causes direct cytotoxic and apoptotic damage, which is mediated through protein kinase C,[142] and TNF-α increases sodium and chloride conductance across CACO2 cells (a human colon carcinoma cell line).[143] Finally, TNF-α induces apoptosis and degradation of tight junctions in HT-29 cells in vitro, which vastly increases epithelial permeability.[144]

## OXIDANT DAMAGE TO EPITHELIAL CELLS

The large influx of neutrophils into IBD mucosa has tremendous potential to damage the epithelium, but this is covered extensively in Chapter 1. These cells are a rich source of free radicals which have the potential to directly damage many cell types in the intestine, including the epithelial cells, which have been most extensively studied. Normal epithelial cells are damaged by hydrogen peroxide,[144] nitric oxide and hypochlorous acid;[144] this damage is inhibited by 5-ASA.[147] Peroxynitrite induces apoptosis of T84 cells, which is also inhibited by mesalamine.[148] Epithelial cell glyceraldehyde-3-phosphate dehydrogenase (GAPDH) activity is markedly reduced in IBD owing to the oxidation of thiol groups.[146] Free radicals can also activate MMP proenzymes in the mucosa. Furthermore, it is well established that IBD tissues exhibit a loss of antioxidant capacity.[145]

## INFLAMMATION AND EPITHELIAL APOPTOSIS?

The intestinal epithelium is a highly dynamic tissue where epithelial cells are continually being produced in the stem cell compartment and being lost into the lumen. Epithelial proliferation increases in all gut inflammatory conditions, but the mechanism is not known. Above, we described a scenario where stromal cells stimulated epithelial renewal through the production of KGF. However, during inflammation the increased proliferation may be due to increased epithelial cell loss, although the lamina propria continues to be involved through enlargement of the pericryptal fibroblast sheath to support the increased crypt size. Any increase in apoptosis during inflammation must compromise epithelial function.

There is strong evidence for increased apoptosis in epithelial cells in IBD, especially in the crypts in ulcerative colitis. In contrast to the normal colon, where end-labeling of broken DNA strands is confined to surface epithelial cells, in colitis there is extensive end-labeling of crypt cells.[69] As apoptosis is an end-stage response to many different stimuli, there are probably many ways in which inflammation can increase epithelial apop-

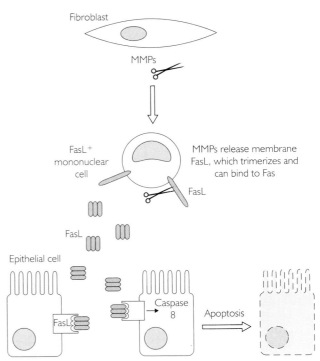

Fig. 11.8 Pathway by which elevated MMP concentrations in the lamina propria can induce epithelial cell death. MMP-3 can cleave FasL from the surface of mononuclear cells in the lamina propria. The FasL can then trimerize, diffuse into the epithelium and engage Fas, thereby inducing non-contact dependent Fas-mediated cell death.

tosis. CD95 (Fas) is a member of the TNF receptor superfamily whose ligand (FasL) is present on activated T cells.[149] Colonic epithelial cells constitutively express Fas[148] and so could be susceptible to Fas-mediated attack. Cross-linking Fas with antibodies substitutes for ligand binding and induces cell death in colonic epithelial cells.[150] In T84 cells this leads to the death of 50% of the cells by 24 hours.[151] High doses of anti-Fas antibody added to explants of colonic mucosa induce cell apoptosis, which is markedly increased if proinflammatory cytokines are also added.[152] Although these experiments show clearly that epithelial cells can die by Fas activation, it remains unclear whether this occurs in vivo, because FasL+ cells are abundant in the lamina propria of IBD patients but are not increased in the epithelium.[150,153] It has been proposed that soluble FasL from mononuclear cells in active colitis might be sufficient to trigger apoptosis in the epithelium.[150] Interestingly, MMP-3 and -7 can cleave FasL from the cell surface,[154,155] showing yet another way in which excess MMPs in the lamina propria can have activity beyond the degradation of extracellular matrix (Fig. 11.8). Neutrophils crossing model epithelium also trigger apoptosis, but the mechanism is unknown.[156] Finally, the epithelium in colitis appears to resist apoptosis to some extent, as the expression of the proapoptotic protein bax is dramatically decreased in colitis.[157]

## COMPLEMENT-MEDIATED DAMAGE

The flurry of interest in TNF-α and T cells in IBD has detracted from the important role played by humoral immunity in pathogenic mechanisms. One of the most striking features of Crohn's disease is the marked accumulation of IgG plasma cells adjacent to ulcers, and in chronic ulcerative colitis mucosal IgG plasma cells are increased.[158] Many of these plasma cells secrete $IgG_1$ antibodies, which are complement fixing. It has long been established that the complement system is activated in IBD.[159] The specificity of these $IgG_1$ antibodies is not known, but it is likely to be against antigens of the bacterial flora and/or self-antigens (especially in ulcerative colitis). There are two ways in which complement-mediated damage might affect the intestine in IBD. If the IgG antibodies are directed against bacterial antigens which are present in the lamina propria, then immune complex formation could initiate complement activation: the generation of C3a and C5a will provide chemoattractants for neutrophils. For example, rabbits given a non-specific rectal irritant and intravenous preformed immune complexes to bovine serum albumin develop a massive Arthus reaction as the immune complexes are deposited in the colon which is virtually identical to acute ulcerative colitis.[160] The influx of neutrophils then initiates the pathways of tissue damaged described above.

The second pathway involves complement-mediated lysis of target cells in the gut. In ulcerative colitis and Crohn's disease, $IgG_1$ antibodies can be visualised by immunofluorescence on the apical surface of epithelial cells.[161,162] The $IgG_1$ co-localizes with both C3b and the activated terminal complement complex of proteins, which mediate lysis. In addition, $IgG_1$ and activated complement components co-localize on the enterocyte membrane with the putative tropomysin autoantigen in ulcerative colitis, but not in Crohn's disease.[163]

# CONCLUSIONS

We have tried to illustrate how a synergistic interaction between inflammatory cells, cytokines, epithelial cells and gut mesenchymal cells can combine to produce pathological changes in the intestine. There is much we do not understand, but it is very clear that there is no linear path of damage. There is a complex interaction between MMPs, the matrix and growth factors; cells secrete molecules which feed back and switch off their own production in negative feedback loops; and there are changes in mucosal shape that represent tissue growth. Although an abundance of in vitro data is available, especially with transformed epithelial cell lines, it is impossible to rank the importance of the different mechanisms of damage that have been reported. Thus, is free radical damage of enterocytes more important than damage to the tight junctions, or is apoptosis of enterocytes the most important pathogenic event? Likewise, even though MMPs are certainly involved in intestinal ulceration, we do not know if the collagenases are more important than the stromelysins. Real insight into these pathways in IBD will only come from clinical studies where specific pathways can be targeted. Nevertheless, a more complete understanding of the various mechanisms of tissue damage offers the opportunity to therapeutically target key pathways of this complex system. In principal, these therapies could prevent and reverse the tissue damage of IBD that leads to the important complications of bleeding, stenosis, obstruction and mucosal ulceration, which contribute to secondary bacterial translocation, abscess formation and fistulae.

# REFERENCES

1. Pender SLF, MacDonald TT. Proteolytic enzymes in inflammatory bowel disease. Inflamm Bowel Dis 1998;4:157–164.
2. Simon-Assmann P, Kedinger M. Heterotypic cellular cooperation in gut morphogenesis and differentiation. Semin Cell Biol 1993;4:221–230.
3. Kedinger M, Lefebvre O, Duluc I et al. Cellular and molecular partners involved in gut morphogenesis and differentiation. Philos Trans Roy Soc Lond B Biol 1998;353:847–856.
4. Briskin M, Winsor-Hines D, Shyjan A et al. Human mucosal addressin cell adhesion molecule-1 is preferentially expressed in intestinal tract and associated lymphoid tissue. Am J Pathol 1997;151:97–110.
5. Souza HS, Elia CC, Spencer J et al. Expression of lymphocyte–endothelial receptor–ligand pairs, α4β7/MAdCAM-1 and OX40/OX40 ligand in the colon and jejunum of patients with inflammatory bowel disease. Gut 1999;45:856–863.
6. Saverymuttu SH, Camilleri M, Rees H et al. Indium 111-granulocyte scanning in the assessment of disease extent and disease activity in inflammatory bowel disease. A comparison with colonoscopy, histology, and fecal indium 111-granulocyte excretion. Gastroenterology. 1986;90:1121–1128.
7. Monteleone G, Biancone L, Marasco R et al. Interleukin 12 is expressed and actively released by Crohn's disease intestinal lamina propria mononuclear cells. Gastroenterology 1997;112:1169–1178.
8. Pizarro TT, Michie MH, Bentz M et al. IL-18, a novel immunoregulatory cytokine, is up-regulated in Crohn's disease: expression and localization in intestinal mucosal cells. J Immunol 1999;162:6829–6835.
9. Grand RJ, Watkins JB, Tarti F. Development of the human gastrointestinal tract. Gastroenterology 1976;70:790–810.
10. Marsh MN. Mucosal pathology in gluten sensitivity. In: Marsh MN, ed. Coeliac disease. Oxford: Blackwell Scientific; 1992:136–191.
11. MacDonald TT, Bajaj-Elliott M, Pender SL. T cells orchestrate intestinal mucosal shape and integrity. Immunol Today 1999;20:505–510.
12. Powell DW, Mifflin RC, Valentich JD et al. Myofibroblasts. I. Paracrine cells important in health and disease. Am J Physiol 1999;277:C1–9.
13. Kraut J. Serine proteases: structure and mechanism of catalysis. Annu Rev Biochem 1997;46:331–358.
14. Saksela O, Rifkin DB. Cell-associated plasminogen activation: Regulation and physiological functions. Annu Rev Cell Biol 1988;4:93–126.
15. Salvesen G, Farley D, Shuman J et al. Molecular cloning of human cathepsin G: structural similarity to mast cell and cytotoxic T lymphocytes proteinases. Biochemistry 1987;26:2289–2293.
16. Welle M. Development, significance, and heterogeneity of mast cells with particular regard to the mast cell-specific proteases chymase and tryptase. J Leukocyte Biol 1997;61:233–245.
17. Barrett AJ, Buttle DJ, Mason RW. Lysosomal cysteine proteinases. Biochemistry 1988;1:256–260.
18. Baron R, Neff L, Louvard D, Courtoy PJ. Cell-mediated extracellular acidification and bone resorption: Evidence for a low pH in resorbing lacunae and localization of a 100-kD lysosomal membrane protein at the osteoblast ruffled border. J Cell Biol 1985;101:2210–2222.
19. Silver IA, Murrills RJ, Etherington DJ. Microelectrode studies on the acid microenvironment beneath adherent macrophages and osteoclasts. Exp Cell Res 1988;175:266–276.
20. Delaisse JM, Boyde A, Maconnachie E et al. The effects of inhibitors of cysteine–proteinases and collagenase on the resorptive activity of isolated osteoclasts. Bone 1987;8:305–313.
21. Burleigh MC. Degradation of collagen by non-specific proteinases. In: Barrett AJ, ed. Proteinases in mammalian cells and tissues. Amsterdam: Elsevier/North-Holland; 1977:285–309.
22. Mason RW, Taylor MAJ, Etherington DJ. The purification and properties of cathepsin L from rabbit liver. Biochem J 1984;217:209–217.
23. Maciewicz RA, Wotton SF, Etherington DJ et al. Susceptibility of the cartilage collagens types II, IX and XI to degradation by the cysteine proteinases, cathepsins B and L. FEBS Lett 1990;269:189–193.
24. Hofmann T, Dunn BM, Fink AL. Cryoenzymology of penicillopepsin; with an appendix: mechanism of action of aspartyl proteinases. Biochemistry 1984;23:5241–5256.
25. Villadangos JA, Bryant RA, Reussing J et al. Proteases involved in MHC class II antigen presentation. Immunol Rev 1999;172:109–120.
26. Saftig P, Hetman M, Schmahl W et al. Mice deficient for the lysosomal proteinase cathepsin D exhibit progressive atrophy of the intestinal mucosa and profound destruction of lymphoid cells. EMBO J 1995;14:3599–3608.
27. Fields GB, Van Wart HE, Birkedal-Hansen H. Sequence specificity of human skin fibroblast collagenase. Evidence for the role of collagen structure in determining the collagenase cleavage site. J Biol Chem 1987;262:6221–6226.
28. Seltzer JL, Eisen AZ, Bauer EA, Morris NP, Glanville RW, Burgeson RE. Cleavage of type VII collagen by interstitial collagenase and type IV collagenase (gelatinase) derived from human skin. J Biol Chem 1989;264:3822–3826.

29. Stocker W, Grams F, Baumann U et al. The metzincins – topological and sequential relations between the astacins, adamalysins, serralysins, and matrixins (collagenases) define a superfamily of zinc-peptidases. Protein Sci 1995;4:823–840.

30. Peschon JJ, Slack JL, Reddy P et al. An essential role for ectodomain shedding in mammalian development. Science 1998; 282:1281–1284.

31. Nagase H, Woessner JF Jr. Matrix metalloproteinases. J Biol Chem 1999; 274:21491–21494.

32. Sternlicht MD, Werb Z. How matrix metalloproteinases regulate cell behaviour. Annu Rev Cell Dev Biol 2001;17:463–516.

33. Brinckerhoff CE, Matrisian LM. Matrix metalloproteinases: a tale of a frog that became a prince. Nat Rev Mol Cell Biol. 2002; 3:207–214.

34. Van Wart HE, Birkedal-Hansen H. The cysteine switch: a principle of regulation of metalloproteinase activity with potential applicability to the entire matrix metalloproteinase gene family. Proc Natl Acad Sci USA 1990;87:5578–5582.

35. Pei D, Weiss SJ. Furin-dependent intracellular activation of the human stromelysin-3 zymogen. Nature 1995;375:244–247.

36. Strongin AY, Collier I, Bannikov G et al. Mechanism of cell surface activation of 72-kDa type IV collagenase. Isolation of the activated form of the membrane metalloprotease. J Biol Chem 1995;270:5331–5338.

37. Butler GS, Butler MJ, Atkinson SJ et al. The TIMP2 membrane type I metalloproteinase "receptor" regulates the concentration and efficient activation of progelatinase A. A kinetic study. J Biol Chem 1998;273:870–880.

38. Murphy G, Cockett MI, Stephens PE et al. Stromelysin is an activator in procollagenase, a study with natural and recombinant enzymes. Biochem J 1987; 8:248–265.

39. Okada Y, Nakanishi I. Activation of matrix metalloproteinase 3 (stromelysin) and matrix metalloproteinase 2 (gelatinase) by human neutrophil elastase and cathepsin G. FEBS Lett 1989;249:353–356.

40. Suzuki K, Lees M, Newlands GF et al. Activation of precursors for matrix metalloproteinases 1 (interstitial collagenase) and 3 (stromelysin) by rat mast-cell proteinases I and II. Biochem J 1995;305:301–306.

41. Uria JA, Jimenez MG, Balbin M et al. Differential effects of transforming growth factor-beta on the expression of collagenase-1 and collagenase-3 in human fibroblasts. J Biol Chem 1998;273:9769–9777.

42. Gomez DE, Alonso DF, Yoshiji H et al. Tissue inhibitors of metalloproteinases: structure, regulation and biological functions. Eur J Cell Biol 1997;74:111–122.

43. Mannello F, Gazzanelli G. Tissue inhibitors of metalloproteinases and programmed cell death: conundrums, controversies and potential implications. Apoptosis 2001; 6:479–482.

44. Bailey CJ, Hembry RM, Alexander A et al. Distribution of the matrix metalloproteinases stromelysin, gelatinases A and B, and collagenase in Crohn's disease and normal intestine. J Clin Pathol 1994; 47:113–116.

45. Saarialho-Kere UK, Vaalamo M, Puolakkainen P et al. Enhanced expression of matrilysin, collagenase, and stromelysin-1 in gastrointestinal ulcers. Am J Pathol 1996; 148:519–526.

46. Vaalamo M, Karjalainen-Lindsberg ML, Puolakkainen P et al. Distinct expression profiles of stromelysin-2 (MMP-10), collagenase-3 (MMP-13), macrophage metalloelastase (MMP-12), and tissue inhibitor of metalloproteinases-3 (TIMP-3) in intestinal ulcerations. Am J Pathol 1998;152:1005–1014.

47. Baugh MD, Perry MJ, Hollander AP et al. Matrix metalloproteinase levels are elevated in inflammatory bowel disease. Gastroenterology 1999;117:814–822.

48. Heuschkel RB, MacDonald TT, Monteleone G et al. Imbalance of stromelysin-1 and TIMP-1 in the mucosal lesions of children with inflammatory bowel disease. Gut. 2000;47:57–62.

49. von Lampe B, Barthel B, Coupland SE et al. Differential expression of matrix metalloproteinases and their tissue inhibitors in colon mucosa of patients with inflammatory bowel disease. Gut 2000;47:63–73.

50. Louis E, Ribbens C, Godon A et al. Increased production of matrix metalloproteinase-3 and tissue inhibitor of metalloproteinase-1 by inflamed mucosa in inflammatory bowel disease. Clin Exp Immunol 2000;120:241–246.

51. Stallmach A, Chan CC, Ecker KW et al. Comparable expression of matrix metalloproteinases 1 and 2 in pouchitis and ulcerative colitis. Gut 2000;47:415–422.

52. Arihiro S, Ohtani H, Hiwatashi N et al. Vascular smooth muscle cells and pericytes express MMP-1, MMP-9, TIMP-1 and type I procollagen in inflammatory bowel disease. Histopathology 2001;39:50–59.

53. Adeyemi EO, Hodgson HJ. Faecal elastase reflects disease activity in active ulcerative colitis. Scand J Gastroenterol 1992;27:139–142.

54. Handy LM, Ghosh S, Ferguson A. Investigation of neutrophils in the gut lumen by assay of granulocyte elastase in whole-gut lavage fluid. Scand J Gastroenterol 1996;31:700–705.

55. Ginzberg HH, Cherapanov V, Dong Q et al. Neutrophil-mediated epithelial injury during transmigration: role of elastase. Am J Physiol Gastrointest Liver Physiol 2001;281:G705–717.

56. Sykes AP, Bhogal R, Brampton C et al. The effect of an inhibitor of matrix metalloproteinases on colonic inflammation in a trinitrobenzenesulphonic acid rat model of inflammatory bowel disease. Aliment Pharmacol Ther 1999;13:1535–1542.

57. Di Sebastiano P, di Mola FF, Artese L et al. Beneficial effects of Batimastat (BB-94), a matrix metalloproteinase inhibitor, in rat experimental colitis. Digestion 2001;63:234–239.

58. Leppert D, Waubant E, Galardy R et al. T cell gelatinases mediate basement membrane transmigration in vitro. Immunology 1995;154:4379–4389.

59. Ratzinger G, Stoitzner P, Ebner S et al. Matrix metalloproteinases 9 and 2 are necessary for the migration of Langerhans cells and dermal dendritic cells from human and murine skin. J Immunol 2002;168:4361–4371.

60. Hattori K, Hirano T, Ushiyama C et al. A metalloproteinase inhibitor prevents lethal acute graft-versus-host disease in mice. Blood 1997;90: 542–548.

61. Monteleone G, MacDonald TT, Wathen NC et al. Enhancing lamina propria Th1 cell responses with interleukin 12 produces severe tissue injury. Gastroenterology 1999;117:1069–1077.

62. Lionetti P, Breese E, Braegger CP et al. T-cell activation can induce either mucosal destruction or adaptation in cultured human fetal small intestine. Gastroenterology 1993;105:373–381.

63. Pender SLF, Lionetti P, Murch SH et al. Proteolytic degradation of intestinal mucosal extracellular matrix after lamina propria T cell activation. Gut 1996; 39: 284–290.

64. Pender SLF, Tickle SP, Docherty AJP et al. A major role for matrix metalloproteinases in T cell injury in the gut. J Immunol 1997;158:1582–1590.

65. Pender SLF, Fell JMC, Chamow SM et al. A p55 tumor necrosis factor (TNF) receptor immunoadhesin prevents T cell-mediated intestinal injury by inhibiting matrix metalloproteinase production. J Immunol 1998;160:4098–4103.

66. Schmehl K, Florian S, Jacobasch G et al. Deficiency of epithelial basement membrane laminin in ulcerative colitis affected human colonic mucosa. Int J Colorectal Dis 2000;15:39–48.

67. Wheatcroft AC, Hollander AP, Croucher LJ et al. Evidence of in situ stability of the type IV collagen triple helix in human inflammatory bowel disease using a denaturation specific epitope antibody. Matrix Biol 1999;18:361–372.

68. Murch SH, MacDonald TT, Walker-Smith JA et al. Disruption of sulphated glycosaminoglycans in intestinal inflammation. Lancet 1993;341:711–714.

69. Iwamoto M, Koji T, Makiyama K et al. Apoptosis of crypt epithelial cells in ulcerative colitis. J Pathol 1996;180:152–159.

70. Strater J, Wedding U, Barth TF et al. Rapid onset of apoptosis in vitro follows disruption of beta 1-integrin/matrix interactions in human colonic crypt cells. Gastroenterology 1996;110:1776–1784.

71. Mosnier JF, Larvol L, Barge J et al. Lymphocytic and collagenous colitis: an immunohistochemical study. Am J Gastroenterol 1996;91:709–713.

72. Aigner T, Neureiter D, Muller S et al. Extracellular matrix composition and gene expression in collagenous colitis. Gastroenterology 1997;113:136–143.

73. Gunther U, Schuppan D, Bauer M et al. Fibrogenesis and fibrolysis in collagenous colitis. Patterns of procollagen types I and IV, matrix-metalloproteinase-1 and -13, and TIMP-1 gene expression. Am J Pathol 1999;155:493–503.

74. Bonderup OK, Hansen JB, Birket-Smith L et al. Budesonide treatment of collagenous colitis: a randomized, double blind, placebo controlled study with morphometric analysis. Gut 2003;52:248–251.

75. Graham MF, Diegelmann RF, Elson CO et al. Collagen content and types in the intestinal strictures of Crohn's disease. Gastroenterology 1988;94:257–265.

76. Matthes H, Herbst H, Schuppan D et al. Cellular localization of procollagen gene transcripts in inflammatory bowel diseases. Gastroenterology 1992;102:431–442.

77. Stallmach A, Schuppan D, Riese HH et al. Increased collagen type III synthesis by fibroblasts isolated from strictures of patients with Crohn's disease. Gastroenterology 1992;102:1920–1929.

78. Mahida YR, Wu K, Jewell DP. Enhanced production of interleukin 1-beta by mononuclear cells isolated from mucosa with active ulcerative colitis of Crohn's disease. Gut 1989;30:835–838.

79. Graham MF, Willey A, Adams J et al. Interleukin 1 beta down-regulates collagen and augments collagenase expression in human intestinal smooth muscle cells. Gastroenterology 1996;110:344–350.

80. Lukashev ME, Werb Z. ECM signalling: orchestrating cell behaviour and misbehaviour. Trends Cell Biol 1998;:437–441.

81. Imai K, Hiramatsu A, Fukushima D et al. Degradation of decorin by matrix metalloproteinases: identification of the cleavage sites, kinetic analyses and transforming growth factor-beta1 release. Biochem J 1997;322:809–814.

82. Monteleone G, Kumberova A, Croft NM et al. Blocking Smad7 restores TGF-beta1 signaling in chronic inflammatory bowel disease. J Clin Invest 2001;108:601–609.

83. Lochter A, Galosy S, Muschler J et al. Matrix metalloproteinase stromelysin-1 triggers a cascade of molecular alterations that leads to stable epithelial-to-mesenchymal conversion and a premalignant phenotype in mammary epithelial cells. J Cell Biol 1997;139:1861–1872.

84. Noe V, Fingleton B, Jacobs K et al. Release of an invasion promoter E-cadherin fragment by matrilysin and stromelysin-1. J Cell Sci 2001;114:111–118.

85. Berx G, Cleton-Jansen AM, Nollet F et al. E-cadherin is a tumour/invasion suppressor gene mutated in human lobular breast cancers. EMBO J 1995;14:6107–6115.

86. Roghani M, Becherer JD, Moss ML et al. Metalloprotease-disintegrin MDC9: intracellular maturation and catalytic activity. J Biol Chem 1999;274:3531–3540.

87. Ito A, Mukaiyama A, Itoh Y et al. Degradation of interleukin 1β by matrix metalloproteinases. J Biol Chem 1996;271:14657–14660.

88. Sheu BC, Hsu SM, Ho HN et al. A novel role of metalloproteinase in cancer-mediated immunosuppression. Cancer Res 2001;61:237–242.

89. Pender SL, Salmela MT, Monteleone G et al. Ligation of a4β1 integrin on human intestinal mucosal mesenchymal cells selectively up-regulates membrane type-1 matrix metalloproteinase and confers a migratory phenotype. Am J Pathol 2000;157:1955–1962.

90. Hiraoka N, Allen E, Apel IJ et al.  Matrix metalloproteinases regulate neovascularization by acting as pericellular fibrinolysins. Cell 1998;95:365–377.

91. Parks WC, Lopez-Boado YS, Wilson CL. Matrilysin in epithelial repair and defense. Chest 2001;120: 36–41s.

92. Wilson CL, Ouellette AJ, Satchell DP et al. Regulation of intestinal alpha-defensin activation by the metalloproteinase matrilysin in innate host defense. Science 1999;286:113–117.

93. Ghosh D, Porter E, Shen B et al.  Paneth cell trypsin is the processing enzyme for human defensin-5. Nature Immunol 2002;3:583–590.

94. Coussens LM, Fingleton B, Matrisian LM . Matrix metalloproteinase inhibitors and cancer: trials and tribulations. Science 2002;295:2387–2392.

95. Egeblad M, Werb Z. New functions for the matrix metalloproteinases in cancer progression. Nat Rev Cancer 2002;2:161–174.

96. Kurokowa M, Lynch K, Podolsky DK. Effects of growth factors on intestinal epithelial cell line: transforming growth factor beta inhibits proliferation and stimulates differentiation. Biochem Biophys Res Commun 1987;142: 775–784.

97. Drucker DJ, Erlich P, Asa SL et al. Induction of intestinal epithelial proliferation by glucagon-like peptide 2. Proc Natl Acad Sci USA 1996;93:7911–7916.

98. Ohneda  K, Ulshen MH, Fuller CR et al. Enhanced growth of small bowel in transgenic mice expressing human insulin-like growth factor 1. Gastroenterology 1997;112: 444–454.

99. Playford RJ, Boulton R, Ghatei MA et al. Comparison of the effects of transforming growth factor alpha and the epidermal growth factor on gastrointestinal proliferation and hormone release. Digestion 1996;57:362–367.

100. Finch PW, Rubin JS, Miki T et al. Human KGF is FGF-related with properties of a paracrine effector of epithelial cell growth. Science 1989; 245:752–755.

101. Werner S, Peters KG, Longaker MT et al. Large induction of keratinocyte growth factor expression in the dermis during wound healing. Proc Natl Acad Sci USA 1992;89: 6896–6900.

102. Staiano-Coico L, Krueger JG, Rubin JS et al. Human keratinocyte growth factor effects in porcine model of epidermal wound healing. J Exp Med 1993;178:865–878.

103. Yi ES, Williams ST, Lee H. Keratinocyte growth factor ameliorates radiation and bleomycin-induced lung injury and mortality. Am J Pathol 1996;149:1963–1970.

104. Housley RM, Morris CF, Boyle W et al. Keratinocyte growth factor induces proliferation of hepatocytes and epithelial cells throughout the rat gastrointestinal tract. J Clin Invest 1994; 94:1764–1777.

105. Farrell CL, Bready JV, Rex KL et al. Keratinocyte growth factor protects mice from chemotherapy and radiation-induced gastrointestinal injury and mortality. Cancer Res 1998;58:933–939.

106. Egger B, Procaccino F, Sarosi I et al. Keratinocyte growth factor ameliorates dextran sodium sulfate colitis in mice. Dig Dis Sci 1999;44:836–844.

107. Han DS, Li F, Holt L et al. Keratinocyte growth factor-2 (FGF-10) promotes healing of experimental small intestinal ulceration in rats. Am J Physiol Gastrointest Liver Physiol 2000;279:G1011–1022.

108. Miceli R, Hubert M, Santiago G et al. Efficacy of keratinocyte growth factor-2 in dextran sulfate sodium-induced murine colitis. J Pharmacol Exp Ther 1999;290:464–471.

109. Iwakiri D, Podolsky DK. Keratinocyte growth factor promotes goblet cell differentiation through regulation of goblet cell silencer inhibitor. Gastroenterology 2001;120:1372–1380.

110. Ghiselli G, Eichstetter I, Iozzo RV. A role for the perlecan protein core in the activation of the keratinocyte growth factor receptor. Biochem J 2001;359:153–163.

111. Ruehl M, Somasundaram R, Schoenfelder I et al. The epithelial mitogen keratinocyte growth factor binds to collagens via the consensus sequence glycine–proline–hydroxyproline. J Biol Chem 2002;277:26872–26878.

112. Finch PW, Pricolo V, Wu A et al. Increased expression of keratinocyte growth factor messenger RNA associated with inflammatory bowel disease. Gastroenterology 1996; 110:441–451.

113. Brauchle M, Madlener M, Wagner AD et al. Keratinocyte growth factor is highly overexpressed in inflammatory bowel disease. Am J Pathol 1996;149:521–529.

114. Bajaj-Elliott M, Breese EJ, Poulsom R et al. Keratinocyte growth factor in inflammatory bowel disease – increased mRNA transcripts in ulcerative colitis compared with Crohn's disease in biopsies and isolated mucosal fibroblasts. Am J Pathol 1997;151:1469–1476.

115. Boismenu R, Havran WL. Modulation of epithelial cell growth by intraepithelial gamma delta T cells. Science 1994;226:1253–1255.

116. Salvati VM, Bajaj-Elliott M, Poulsom R et al. Keratinocyte growth factor and coeliac disease. Gut 2001;49:176–181.

117. Bajaj-Elliott M, Poulsom R, Pender SLF et al. Interactions between stromal cell-derived keratinocyte growth factor and epithelial transforming growth factor in immune-mediated crypt cell hyperplasia. J Clin Invest 1998;102:1473–1480.

118. Jobson TM, Billington CK, Hall IP. Regulation of proliferation of human colonic subepithelial myofibroblasts by mediators important in intestinal inflammation. J Clin Invest 1998;101:2650–2657.

119. Moussad EE, Brigstock DR. Connective tissue growth factor: what's in a name? Mol Genet Metab 2000;71:276–292.

120. Duncan MR, Frazier KS, Abramson S et al.  Connective tissue growth factor mediates transforming growth factor beta-induced collagen synthesis: down-regulation by cAMP. FASEB J 1999;13:1774–1786.

121. Leask A, Holmes A, Abraham DJ. Connective tissue growth factor: a new and important player in the pathogenesis of fibrosis. Curr Rheumatol Rep 2002;4:136–142.

122. di Mola FF, Friess H, Martignoni ME et al. Connective tissue growth factor is a regulator for fibrosis in human chronic pancreatitis. Ann Surg 1999;230:63–71.

123. Williams EJ, Gaca MD, Brigstock DR et al.  Increased expression of connective tissue growth factor in fibrotic human liver and in activated hepatic stellate cells. J Hepatol 2000;32:754–761.

124. Dammeier J, Brauchle M, Falk W et al. Connective tissue growth factor: a novel regulator of mucosal repair and fibrosis in inflammatory bowel disease? Int J Biochem Cell Biol 1998;30:909–922.

125. Babyatsky MW, Rossiter G, Podolsky DK. Expression of transforming growth factors alpha and beta in colonic mucosa in inflammatory bowel disease. Gastroenterology 1996;110:975–984.

126. Attisano L, Wrana JL. Signal transduction by the TGF-beta superfamily. Science 2002;296:1646–1647.

127. Moustakas A, Souchelnytskyi S, Heldin CH. Smad regulation in TGF-beta signal transduction. J Cell Sci 2001;114:4359–4369.

128. Lempinen M, Inkinen K, Wolff H, Ahonen J. Connective tissue growth factor in indomethacin-induced rat gastric ulcer. Eur Surg Res 2002;34:232–238.

129. Hashimoto G, Inoki I, Fujii Y et al. Matrix metalloproteinases cleave connective tissue growth factor and reactivate angiogenic activity of vascular endothelial growth factor 165. J Biol Chem 2002;277:36288–36295.

130. Jenkins HR, Milla PJ. The effect of colitis on large-intestinal electrolyte transport in early childhood. J Pediatr Gastroenterol Nutr 1993;16:402–405.

131. Burgel N, Bojarski C, Mankertz J et al.  Mechanisms of diarrhea in collagenous colitis. Gastroenterology 2002;123:433–443.

132. Kroesen AJ, Stockmann M, Ransco C et al.  Impairment of epithelial transport but not of barrier function in idiopathic pouchitis after ulcerative colitis. Gut 2002;50:821–826.

133. Schmitz H, Barmeyer C, Fromm M et al.  Altered tight junction structure contributes to the impaired epithelial barrier function in ulcerative colitis. Gastroenterology 1999;116:301–309.

134. Gassler N, Rohr C, Schneider A et al.  Inflammatory bowel disease is associated with changes of enterocytic junctions. Am J Physiol Gastrointest Liver Physiol 2001;281:G216–228.

135. Haimovitz-Friedman A, Cordon-Cardo C, Bayoumy S et al. Lipopolysaccharide induces disseminated endothelial apoptosis requiring ceramide generation. J Exp Med 1997;186:1831–1841.

136. Ikeda H, Suzuki Y, Suzuki M et al.  Apoptosis is a major mode of cell death caused by ischaemia and ischaemia/reperfusion injury to the rat intestinal epithelium. Gut 1998;42:530–537.

137. Kaufman HL, Swartout BG, Horig H et al.  Combination interleukin-2 and interleukin-12 induces severe gastrointestinal toxicity and epithelial cell apoptosis in mice. Cytokine 2002;17:43–52.

138. Guy-Grand D, DiSanto JP, Henchoz P et al.  Small bowel enteropathy: role of intraepithelial lymphocytes and of cytokines (IL-12, IFN-gamma, TNF) in the induction of epithelial cell death and renewal. Eur J Immunol 1998;28:730–744.

139. Merger M, Viney JL, Borojevic R et al.  Defining the roles of perforin, Fas/FasL, and tumour necrosis factor alpha in T cell induced mucosal damage in the mouse intestine. Gut 2002;51:155–163.

140. Madara JL, Stafford J. Interferon-gamma directly affects barrier function of cultured intestinal epithelial monolayers. J Clin Invest 1989;83:724–727.

141. Taylor CT, Dzus AL, Colgan SP. Autocrine regulation of epithelial permeability by hypoxia: role for polarized release of tumor necrosis factor alpha. Gastroenterology 1998;114:657–668.

142. Chang Q, Tepperman BL. The role of protein kinase C isozymes in TNF-alpha-induced cytotoxicity to a rat intestinal epithelial cell line. Am J Physiol Gastrointest Liver Physiol 2001;280:G572–583.

143. Marano CW, Lewis SA, Garulacan LA et al. Tumor necrosis factor-alpha increases sodium and chloride conductance across the tight junction of CACO-2 BBE, a human intestinal epithelial cell line. J Membrane Biol 1998;161:263–274.

144. Gitter AH, Bendfeldt K, Schulzke JD et al. Leaks in the epithelial barrier caused by spontaneous and TNF-alpha-induced single-cell apoptosis. FASEB J 2000;14:1749–1753.

145. Buffinton GD, Doe WF. Depleted mucosal antioxidant defences in inflammatory bowel disease. Free Radic Biol Med 1995;19:911–918.

146. McKenzie SJ, Baker MS, Buffinton GD et al. Evidence of oxidant-induced injury to epithelial cells during inflammatory bowel disease. J Clin Invest 1996;98:136–141.

147. McKenzie SM, Doe WF, Buffinton GD. 5-aminosalicylic acid prevents oxidant mediated damage of glyceraldehyde-3-phosphate dehydrogenase in colon epithelial cells. Gut 1999;44:180–185.

148. Sandoval M, Liu X, Mannick EE et al.  Peroxynitrite-induced apoptosis in human intestinal epithelial cells is attenuated by mesalamine. Gastroenterology 1997;113:1480–1488.

149. Strater J, Moller P. Expression and function of death receptors and their natural ligands in the intestine. Ann NY Acad Sci 2000;915:162–170.

150. Strater J, Wellisch I, Riedl S et al. CD95 (APO-1/Fas)-mediated apoptosis in colon epithelial cells: a possible role in ulcerative colitis. Gastroenterology 1997;113:160–167.

151. Abreu MT, Palladino AA, Arnold ET et al.  Modulation of barrier function during Fas-mediated apoptosis in human intestinal epithelial cells. Gastroenterology 2000;119:1524–1536.

152. Ruemmele FM, Russo P, Beaulieu J et al. Susceptibility to FAS-induced apoptosis in human nontumoral enterocytes: role of costimulatory factors. J Cell Physiol 1999;181:45–54.

153. Ueyama H, Kiyohara T, Sawada N et al. High Fas ligand expression on lymphocytes in lesions of ulcerative colitis. Gut 1998;43:48–55.

154. Mitsiades N, Yu WH, Poulaki V et al. Matrix metalloproteinase-7-mediated cleavage of Fas ligand protects tumor cells from chemotherapeutic drug cytotoxicity. Cancer Res 2001;61:577–581.

155. Matsuno H, Yudoh K, Watanabe Y et al. Stromelysin-1 (MMP-3) in synovial fluid of patients with rheumatoid arthritis has potential to cleave membrane bound Fas ligand. J Rheumatol 2001;28:22–28.

156. Le'Negrate G, Selva E, Auberger P et al. Sustained polymorphonuclear leukocyte transmigration induces apoptosis in T84 intestinal epithelial cells. J Cell Biol 2000;150:1479–1488.

157. Iimura M, Nakamura T, Shinozaki S et al. Bax is downregulated in inflamed colonic mucosa of ulcerative colitis. Gut 2000;47:228–235.

158. Brandtzaeg P. The B cell system. In: Brostoff J, Challacombe SJ, eds. Food allergy and intolerance. London; Baillière Tindall: 1987;7;118–155.

159. Hodgson HJ, Potter BJ, Jewell DP. C3 metabolism in ulcerative colitis and Crohn's disease. Clin Exp Immunol 1977;28:490–495.

160. Hodgson HJ, Potter BJ, Skinner J et al. Immune-complex mediated colitis in rabbits. An experimental model. Gut 1978;19:225–232.

161. Halstensen TS, Mollnes TE, Garred P et al. Epithelial deposition of immunoglobulin G1 and activated complement (C3b and terminal complement complex) in ulcerative colitis. Gastroenterology 1990;98:1264–1271.

162. Halstensen TS, Mollnes TE, Garred P et al. Surface epithelium related activation of complement differs in Crohn's disease and ulcerative colitis. Gut 1992;33:902–908.

163. Halstensen TS, Das KM, Brandtzaeg P. Epithelial deposits of immunoglobulin G1 and activated complement colocalise with the M(r) 40 kD putative autoantigen in ulcerative colitis. Gut 1993;34:650–657.

## CHAPTER 12

# Cytokines and inflammatory mediators

Fabio Cominelli, Kristen O Arseneau and Theresa T Pizarro

## INTRODUCTION

Cytokines and inflammatory mediators play a key pathogenic role in inflammatory bowel disease (IBD), as evidenced by the relative success of cytokine-targeted immunomodulatory therapy for the treatment of Crohn's disease, the most debilitating form of IBD. The precise cause of IBD remains elusive, but disease pathogenesis clearly involves genetic, immunologic and environmental risk factors. A current hypothesis for the etiology of IBD suggests that inflammation is initiated and perpetuated by a dysregulated immune response to an unknown environmental antigen in a genetically susceptible host.

In order to maintain gut homeostasis, the normal mucosal immune system must maintain a delicate balance between a network of inflammatory mediators, including proinflammatory, anti-inflammatory and regulatory cytokines (Fig. 12.1). During bacterial invasion, type 1 T-helper cell (Th1)-polarizing cytokines, including interleukin (IL)-12, IL-18, and tumor necrosis factor (TNF) are released from antigen-presenting cells (macrophages, dendritic cells etc.) and exert pleiotropic proinflammatory and inductive effects within the intestinal mucosa. Proinflammatory cytokines (i.e. IL-1, IL-6 and TNF) activate immune cells in the lamina propria and stimulate intestinal epithelial cells and macrophages to produce chemokines, which, when secreted, establish a chemotactic gradient across the intestinal mucosa, promoting leukocyte recruitment and extravasation across the intestinal endothelium. Meanwhile, Th1-polarizing cytokines released from antigen-presenting cells also induce activation of naive intraepithelial and lamina propria T lymphocytes and Th1 differentiation. These newly activated Th1 cells release Th1 cytokines (i.e. IL-2, interferon-gamma (IFN-$\gamma$), lymphotoxins (LT)), which further perpetuate inflammatory and delayed hypersensitivity immune responses in the gut.

In the normal gut mucosa this proinflammatory/inductive immune response is kept in balance by a network of anti-inflammatory and regulatory cytokines. Regulatory cytokines (i.e. IL-4, IL-5, IL-10, IL-13 and transforming growth factor-$\beta$ (TGF-$\beta$) are derived from many cellular sources within the intestine, including macrophages as well as type 2 T-helper (Th2) cells and Tr1-type (Tr1) T cells. Along with anti-inflammatory cytokines (i.e. IL-1 receptor antagonist (IL-1ra) and IL-11) derived primarily from intestinal epithelial cells and macrophages, these Th2 cytokines serve to counterbalance the proinflammatory effects of Th1-mediated immune responses.

For unknown reasons, patients with IBD cannot maintain normal gut homeostasis. An understanding of the cytokine network and its role in promoting IBD pathogenesis is a crucial step towards finding a cure for this devastating disease. This chapter provides an overview of the cytokines and other inflammatory mediators that have been implicated in IBD pathogenesis, with specific focus on what is known about targeted blockade of specific immune mediators.

## TH1-POLARIZING CYTOKINES (TNF, IL-12 AND IL-18)

Th1-polarizing cytokines are a group of inductive proinflammatory cytokines that mediate differentiation of CD4+ T cell to the Th1 phenotype (Fig. 12.2). These cytokines are derived primarily from stimulated antigen-presenting cells, especially macrophages, and include TNF, IL-12 and IL-18.

Because of their relatively early position in the inflammatory cascade, these cytokines are currently under investigation as promising targets for IBD therapy, at both the preclinical and the clinical levels. In particular, TNF has been clearly established as a key mediator of IBD pathogenesis, based on the dramatic efficacy of anti-TNF antibody therapy in the treatment of patients with refractory and fistulizing Crohn's disease.[1-3] Many biological properties of TNF in the intestine are relevant to mucosal inflammation; these include eliciting chemokine

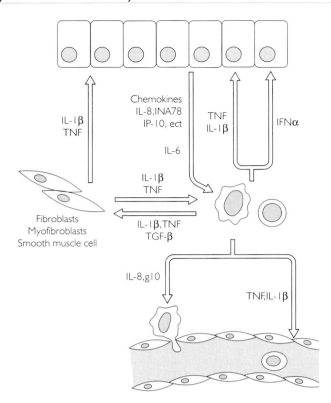

**Figure 12.1** Interaction of various types of intestinal cells, all of which secrete cytokines. Crosstalk between various cell lineages create the complex regulatory and inflammatory milieu of the intestine. Epithelial cells secrete chemokines which stimulate migration of neutrophils, monocytes/macrophages and T and B lymphocytes into the inflammatory focus. Activated lamina propria macrophages and T cells secrete IL-1β, TNF and IFNγ which stimulate cytokine production by epithelial, endothelial and mesenchymal cells. Activation of endothelial cells by proinflammatory cytokines (IL-1β, TNF and IFNγ) upregulate adhesion molecules on endothelial cells, leading to attachment of circulating effector cells, which migrate into the inflammatory focus under a chemokine gradient established by epithelial lamina propria cells. These inflammatory cytokines activate epithelial and mesenchymal cells, which in turn secrete their own cytokines. TGF-β induces collagen expression in mesenchymal cells, thus stimulating fibrogenesis.

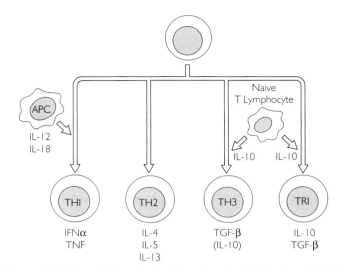

**Figure 12.2** Differentiation of naive T lymphocytes into T helper 1 (TH1), TH2, TH3 and T regulatory 1 (TR1) cells. Activated antigen presenting cells (APC) secreting cytokines determine the pathway of T cell differentiation.

secretion from intestinal epithelial cells, disrupting the epithelial barrier, and initiating apoptosis of villous epithelial cells.[4–6] In addition, TNF is capable of inducing cytokine and chemokine expression, as well as adhesion molecule production, in endothelial cells.[7,8] TNF exerts these effects by binding to two distinct receptors, TNFRI and TNFRII, which are expressed on a variety of cell types.[9] Together, these properties contribute to the initiation and perpetuation of mucosal immune responses, leading to the intestinal inflammation characteristic of IBD.

The initial evidence that TNF plays a critical role in mucosal immune responses came from blocking experiments in animal models of intestinal inflammation. Colitic mice treated with anti-TNF antibodies experience significant improvement in the clinical symptoms and histopathological signs of disease.[10] Similarly, when colitis is induced in mice that are deficient in TNF the severity of colitis is considerably attenuated. The most compelling evidence that TNF may directly initiate gut mucosal inflammation, in particular a Crohn's-like ileitis, comes from studies in which a deletion of AU-rich elements (ARE) in the

3' untranslated region of the TNF gene was introduced in mice.[11] Mice carrying this mutation in either a heterozygous or a homozygous state are normal at birth but soon develop two organ-specific pathologies, namely arthritis and a Crohn's-like enteritis. Another feature of these mice is high levels of circulating TNF, and the mice eventually succumb with a multiorgan failure syndrome. Interestingly, the main abnormality of TNF regulation in these mutant mice relates to the increased stability of TNF mRNA, which consequently results in an increased production of TNF protein. In a series of elegant studies with these mutant mice, Kontoyannis et al. demonstrated that Crohn's-like ileitis is dependent on T cells and requires the presence of both TNFRI and II. In recent studies, the same group has demonstrated that the development of intestinal inflammation in this model depends on Th1-like cytokines such as IL-12 and IFN-γ, and requires the function of CD8+ T lymphocytes.[12] Tissue-specific activation of the mutant TNF allele by CRE/loxP-mediated recombination demonstrated that either myeloid- or T cell-derived TNF can exhibit full pathogenic capacity. TNF also appears to mediate spontaneous ileitis in a recently described mouse model of Crohn's disease, the SAMP1/YitFc mouse. Administration of monoclonal antibodies against TNF to SCID mice adoptively transferred with CD4+ T cells from SAMP1/YitFc mice markedly diminishes disease severity in recipient animals.[13] The role of TNF in the SAMP1/YitFc model is of particular interest because of the spontaneous nature of intestinal lesions in these mice, and their resemblance to human disease. Thus, this model offers great promise for understanding the mechanism of anti-TNF treatment in patients with Crohn's disease.

Despite the beneficial effects of anti-TNF therapy in animal models of intestinal inflammation, clinical studies measuring TNF levels in the circulation and/or the gut lesions of IBD patients have generated controversial initial results, showing in some studies the absence of increased levels of TNF in intestinal lesions from IBD patients.[14–17] However, the demonstration that approximately two-thirds of patients with Crohn's disease experience a clinical response after treatment with a chimeric monoclonal antibody to TNF (infliximab) unquestionably proves the

## Table 12.1 Major activities of cytokines in the TH1 pathway

**A**

| Molecule | TH1 polarizing cytokines | | | |
|---|---|---|---|---|
| | Source | Receptors | Signaling | Biologic activity |
| TNF | Mφ, DC, TH1, mesenchymal cells | TNF RI, II | NFκB | Mediate experimental colitis, Crohn's disease, activation NFκB, activation of epithelial, mesenchymal, endothelial cells, monocytes, T cells |
| IL-12 | Mφ, DC | IL-12R β1, β2 | STAT-4 | ↑ production IFNγ, TNF, mediates experimental colitis, ? Crohn's disease |
| IL-18 | epithelial cells, Mφ, DC | IL-18R | NFκB IL-1Rrp | ↑ production IFNγ, TNF, IL-1β, C-C, C-X-C chemokines, Fas ligand, IL-8 |

**B**

| Molecule | TH1-derived cytokines | | | |
|---|---|---|---|---|
| | Source | Receptors | Signaling | Biologic activity |
| IFNγ | Th-1 | | STAT-1 | Activate APC, Mφ, epithelial cells, with TNF injure epithelial cells, mediate experimental colitis, ↑ in Crohn's disease |
| IL-2 | Th1, IEL | IL-2Rβ,γ | | Lymphocyte proliferation, activation of regulatory T cells (CD25) |
| LT | Th1 | TNFR, p55, p57 LTR | | Development Peyer's patches, LN, B cell follicles, ↑ expression adhesion molecules |

central role of TNF in Crohn's disease.[2,3] The role of TNF in ulcerative colitis is less clear, with an initial multicenter trial of infliximab showing inconclusive results owing to its small sample size.[18] However, two recent retrospective case series have reported dramatic improvements in patients with severe ulcerative colitis, with response rates ranging from 67 to 88%.[19,20] By comparison, a British study published in abstract form showed no clinical improvement in ulcerative colitis patients treated with infliximab compared to placebo.[21] A large, double-blind placebo-controlled multicenter trial in patients with moderate to severe ulcerative colitis is currently under way in the United States and Europe. A second monoclonal antibody to TNF, CDP571, has also been tested in patients with Crohn's disease, with encouraging but less dramatic results.[22] Because CDP571 is a humanized antibody consisting of the complementarity-determining regions of a mouse anti-human TNF antibody fused to human IgG$_4$, it is likely that fewer adverse reactions will be observed with this therapy.[23] Another potential biological therapy for patients with IBD is etanercept (Embril), which is a chimeric TNF inhibitory molecule consisting of the extracellular domain of the p75 TNFR spliced to an Ig heavy-chain molecule.[23,24] Although this compound is approved for the treatment for rheumatoid arthritis, an initial study showed no effect in patients with Crohn's disease using doses recommended for

the treatment of rheumatoid arthritis.[25] Interestingly, etanercept, unlike other anti-TNF therapies such as infliximab and CDP571, neutralizes lymphotoxin-α in addition to TNF, thereby preventing the activation of both TNF receptors. The reasons for these differences in efficacy are currently unknown; however, they may relate to their TNF-binding characteristics or the ability of infliximab to modulate intestinal mucosal cell apoptosis.[26,27] Finally, thalidomide, a synthetic TNF inhibitor tested for efficacy in Crohn's disease, has shown promising results for the treatment of mild to moderate disease.[28,29] Unfortunately, the well-known side effects of thalidomide represent a serious limitation to the widespread use of this drug in IBD. New and improved monoclonal antibodies against TNF are being developed, including fully humanized antibodies and PEGylated antibodies with increased half-lives. Altogether, these studies demonstrate the central role of TNF in the pathogenesis of Crohn's disease. The ability to generate safe, orally active compounds with TNF-inhibitory activity will represent a major advance in the treatment of IBD and allow better therapeutic options.

IL-12 is a second Th1-polarizing cytokine under investigation as a therapeutic target for Crohn's disease. IL-12 is secreted primarily by antigen-presenting cells in response to stimulation by bacterial antigens. Production is modulated by interactions between the surface marker CD40 on stimulated antigen-presenting cells and the CD40 ligand expressed on CD4+ T cells.[30–32] IL-12 induces the production of Th1 cytokines, such as IFN-γ and TNF, and initiates NK- and T-cell cytolytic activity through interactions with a high-affinity receptor complex composed of two subunits, designated $\beta_1$ and $\beta_2$.[33,34] The $\beta_2$ subunit is more tightly regulated than $\beta_1$ and may serve as a regulatory mechanism for IL-12 signaling.[35]

The therapeutic potential for agents directed at neutralizing IL-12 was initially realized from experiments in animal models of intestinal inflammation. Administration of recombinant IL-12 leads to severe exacerbation of colitis in mice, which is further aggravated by co-administration of both recombinant IL-12 and IL-18.[30,36,37] Meanwhile, administration of anti-IL-12 antibodies results in marked improvement in the clinical and histopathological features of disease, complete normalization of IFN-γ levels, and induction of Fas-mediated apoptosis of Th1 T cells in the lamina propria and spleen.[38–41] Interestingly, IL-12 neutralization ameliorates colitis in adult mice deficient in IL-10, but completely prevents colitis in younger mice. This differential effect appears to reflect distinct inflammatory mechanisms mediating the early versus the late phases of colitis in this model. The early phase is marked by a progressive increase in disease severity, with progressively greater production of IL-12 and interferon-γ; during the late phase IL-12 and interferon-γ levels fall drastically and return to prediesase levels, and the clinical phenotype resembles that of chronic colitis.[42] Thus, IL-12 appears to play an important role in the initiating steps of intestinal inflammation in this model.

Work by Neurath et al.[43] using mice with hapten-induced colitis reveals an important reciprocal relationship between IL-12 and the growth factor TGF-β. Hapten-induced colitis is characterized by a Th1-dominated distal colitis. However, mice fed hapten colonic proteins prior to the induction of colitis appear to develop oral tolerance to the disease, with elevated levels of TGF-β and Th2 cytokines and decreased levels of IL-12 and IFN-γ. The importance of IL-12 and TGF-β in this model is demonstrated by further experiments showing that these mice remain susceptible to colitis if treated with recombinant IL-12 or antibodies targeting TGF-β during oral tolerance. In addition, intranasal administration of a novel vector encoding TGF-β$_1$ has also been shown to prevent hapten-induced colitis through downregulation of IL-12, IL-12 receptor $\beta_2$ and IFN-γ, and upregulation of TGF-β and IL-10.[44] Thus, the balance of IL-12 and TGF-β may be an important mechanism for maintaining gut homeostasis.

To investigate the role of IL-12 in IBD in humans, Monteleone et al. studied the expression of IL-12 in lamina propria mononuclear cells isolated from patients with IBD and found increased expression associated with Crohn's disease, but not ulcerative colitis or healthy individuals.[45] In addition, they found that certain chemokines, as well as IFN-γ and prostaglandin E$_2$, modulate IL-12 production by activated lamina propria mononuclear cells.[46,47] Taken together, these findings indicate that IL-12, like TNF, may play a critical role in Th1-mediated intestinal inflammation and may have strong therapeutic potential for the treatment of Crohn's disease. However, preclinical data obtained in chemically induced or immunodeficient mice need to be confirmed in more relevant mouse models of IBD, and ultimately in patients with Crohn's disease. The results of an ongoing multicenter, double-blind placebo-controlled clinical trial using monoclonal antibodies against IL-12 will shed light on the efficacy of IL-12 neutralization in treating patients with Crohn's disease.

Unlike TNF and IL-12, investigations into the therapeutic potential of IL-18 neutralization remain at the preclinical level. IL-18, originally coined IFN-γ-inducing factor, was initially characterized as a novel IFN-γ stimulating factor in mice infected with *Propionibacterium acnes* and subsequently challenged with a sublethal dose of LPS.[48] Several similarities exist between IL-18 and the proinflammatory cytokine IL-1. Recombinant human IL-18 shares amino acid sequence homology with IL-1 (19% positional identity with hIL-1β and 12% with hIL-1α), but does not bind to the IL-1 receptor type I (IL-1RI), the signaling receptor for IL-1.[49] Like the precursor form of IL-1β (proIL-1β), the precursor form of IL-18 (proIL-18) does not contain a signal peptide required for the cellular secretion of the mature bioactive protein,[49] and both pro forms are cleaved by the IL-1β converting enzyme (ICE or caspase-1) to form mature, bioactive protein.[50] Finally, IL-18 binds to the IL-1R related protein (IL-1Rrp), a member of the IL-1 receptor family and an essential component of IL-1 and IL-18 signaling.[51] Thus, IL-18 may be considered a related member of the IL-1 family, including IL-1α, IL-1β and the IL-1 receptor antagonist.[52]

In addition to its ability to act as a co-stimulant for IFN-γ production, IL-18 possesses several other biological activities that highlight its potential role as a key proinflammatory cytokine.[52] IL-18 can induce the production of TNF, IL-1β and both C-C and C-X-C chemokines in peripheral blood mononuclear cells,[53] as well as Fas ligand and nuclear translocation of NFκB in activated T cells.[54,55] In addition, IL-18 may play a primary role in Th1-mediated immune responses,[56,57] as evidenced by its ability to directly stimulate TNF gene expression and synthesis from CD3+/CD4+ T cells and NK cells, which subsequently results in the production of IL-1β and IL-8 from the CD14+ population of peripheral blood mononuclear cells.[53] Based on these properties, IL-18 has become a promising target of preclinical investigation into the pathogenesis of Th1-mediated inflammatory disorders, including Crohn's disease.

Pizarro et al. were the first group to report that IL-18 is upregulated in patients with Crohn's disease, compared to ulcerative colitis and healthy individuals, and that IL-18 is primarily produced by three main cellular sources within the gut mucosa: intestinal epithelial cells, tissue macrophages (histiocytes) and dendritic cells.[58] In this study, more abundant IL-18 mRNA transcripts were found in intestinal epithelial cells than in lamina propria mononuclear cells, regardless of the patient source. However, increased IL-18 steady-state mRNA levels were observed in both intestinal epithelial cells and lamina propria mononuclear cells obtained from Crohn's disease compared to ulcerative colitis and control patients. Immunolocalization studies revealed that although Crohn's disease patients have an overall increase in gut IL-18 expression as disease severity increases, there is a dramatic shift in the cellular source of IL-18 from the epithelium to lamina propria mononuclear cells, with intestinal epithelial cells being the prevalent producer of IL-18 in non-involved areas, and macrophages and dendritic cells more severely involved lesions.[58] Work by Monteleone et al. supports these results and confirms that IL-18 produced in Crohn's disease tissues is functionally active. In this study, IL-18, as well as IFN-γ, production was decreased in lamina propria mononuclear cells derived from Crohn's disease patients following treatment with an antisense oligonucleotide specific for IL-18.[59] A recent study by Corbaz et al. shows that the neutralizing isoforms of IL-18-binding protein are present in intestinal tissue specimens for patients with active Crohn's disease, along with free, mature IL-18 protein, highlighting the complexity of the IL-18/IL-18-binding protein system.[60] Kanai et al. showed that lamina propria mononuclear cells possess IL-18 receptors, and in Crohn's disease this cell population expresses increased IL-2 receptors and proliferates more potently in response to IL-18 than those isolated from normal non-inflamed control patients.[61] These effects can be potentiated with the addition of IL-12 to Crohn's disease lamina propria mononuclear cells; however, proliferation of lamina propria mononuclear cells isolated from both ulcerative colitis and control patients also increase upon stimulation with IL-18 plus IL-12. Similarly, BALB/c mice given IL-18 and IL-12 experience more prominent intestinal mucosal inflammation when these Th1-polarizing cytokines are administered together than when given alone.[62]

Taken together, these data indicate that IL-18 may play a pivotal role in the pathogenesis of Crohn's disease. IL-18, in synergy with and independently of IL-12, promotes Th1-polarized immune response through IFN-γ production (inductive phase), and also stimulates TNF gene expression and secretion from activated T cells (effector phase).[53] In addition, IL-18 is capable of stimulating IL-1β and IL-8 secretion from activated macrophages, thus affecting the final common pathway of Crohn's disease immunopathogenesis.[53] Therefore, it is conceivable that IL-18 may, in fact, fulfill the specific requirements to be considered a primary initiating cytokine in Th1-mediated diseases such as Crohn's. Recent preclinical animal studies using neutralizing antibodies against IL-18 and recombinant IL-18-binding protein support this concept.[52,63–65] Based on the promising results from these animal studies, clinical trials focused on neutralization of IL-18 bioactivity are anticipated in the near future.

# TH1-DERIVED CYTOKINES (IFN-γ, IL-2 AND LYMPHOTOXIN)

Th1-derived cytokines, including IFN-γ, IL-2 and lymphotoxins (LT), are produced by Th1 CD4+ T cells in response to stimulation with TNF, IL-12 and IL-18, and promote chronic inflammation associated with a variety of disease states, includ-ing human Crohn's disease (Fig. 12.2). Owing to their important role in chronic gut inflammation, several of these cytokines have been or are being investigated at the clinical level as possible therapeutic targets for novel biological agents in patients with IBD.

Currently, the most promising of these therapeutic targets is IFN-γ, a pleiotropic cytokine with inductive effects on a variety of mucosal cell types, including intestinal epithelial cells, monocytes, endothelial cells and lymphocytes. Animal models of intestinal inflammation have provided several lines of evidence supporting a role for IFN-γ in the promotion of chronic intestinal inflammation. Studies by Bregenholt et al. demonstrate that SCID mice reconstituted with activated CD4+ T cells from IFN-γ-deficient mice develop a less severe colitis and have a two- to threefold increase in the number of IL-4-producing cells, compared to SCID mice reconstituted with cells from wildtype mice, suggesting that the absence of IFN-γ leads to an elevated Th2 response and hence a milder form of colitis.[66] Similarly, Powrie et al. showed that the administration of anti-IFN-γ antibodies to SCID mice adoptively transferred with pathogenic CD45Rb[hi] T cells prevents colitis for up to 12 weeks.[67]

Several studies in humans have shown elevated IFN-γ levels in the intestinal mucosa of Crohn's disease but not ulcerative colitis patients,[68–72] as well as from activated intestinal lamina propria lymphocytes isolated from patients with Crohn's disease, particularly when stimulated through the CD2/CD28 pathway.[73–75] However, work by Desreumaux et al. evaluating cytokine production from early (acute) and late (chronic) Crohn's disease lesions suggests that expression may depend on disease phase.[76] In this study, late Crohn's disease lesions displayed a characteristic Th1 immune response, but early lesions were in fact associated with Th2 responses, with increased IL-4 and decreased IFN-γ production. Thus, different cytokine profiles appear to be associated with acute and chronic phases of disease.

Phase II clinical trials are currently under way to study the efficacy of anti-IFN-γ monoclonal antibodies in treating patients with moderate to severe refractory Crohn's disease. Results from preclinical studies do not support IFN-γ as an especially strong target for immunomodulatory therapy. Although IFN-γ-deficient mice do display abnormalities in their immune system, they do not develop colitis resembling IBD. However, as mentioned above, neutralization studies in animal models have been successful at preventing intestinal inflammation. Ongoing randomized clinical trials should provide sufficient data to adequately assess the clinical utility of anti-IFN-γ therapy once and for all.

**Table 12.2 Major activities of TH2 cytokines**

| Cytokine | Source | Receptors | Signaling | Activity |
|---|---|---|---|---|
| IL-4 | Th2, MAST cells | | STAT-3 | ↑ expression IL-8, RANTES, MCP-1, iNOS, induce Th2-experimental colitis, suppress Th1-mediated colitis |
| IL-5 | Th2, MAST cells | | | Mediates parasitic, allergic diseases, ↑ IgE |
| IL-13 | Th2, NK T cells | IL-13 Rα2 | | Th2-mediated colitis |

IL-2 is a second Th1-derived cytokine involved primarily in lymphocyte proliferation and differentiation. In intraepithelial lymphocytes IL-2 is produced predominantly by cells expressing αβ+ T-cell receptors (TCRαβ+), and IL-2 receptors are localized on the surface of cells expressing γδ+ TCR (TCRγδ+). IL-2 signaling receptors are heterodimers composed of a β chain and a common γ chain. Through these receptors, IL-2 carefully regulates TCRγδ+ intestinal epithelial lymphocyte populations by promoting activation and differentiation, and inducing apoptosis after restimulation through the TCR.[77-79] IL-2 receptors are also found on intestinal epithelial cells.[80] In epithelial cells, IL-2 signaling leads to enhanced cellular restitution in vitro, suggesting a role for IL-2 in maintaining epithelial barrier function.[80-82] Taken together, these data may play an important role in mediating epithelial–lymphocyte interactions in the intestinal mucosa.

IL-2-deficient mice have been useful in understanding the functional role of IL-2 in IBD pathogenesis. These mice, when reared under conventional conditions or immunized with 2,4, 6-trinitrophenol (TNP)-conjugated keyhole limpet hemocyanin (KLH) and raised in a specific pathogen-free environment, develop a Th1-mediated colitis which is mediated by cytotoxic CD4+ TCRαβ+ lymphocytes that accumulate in the colon prior to the onset of macroscopic inflammation.[83,84] IL-2-deficient mice have enhanced expression of several important mediators of gut inflammation, including the proinflammatory cytokines IL-1, IL-6 and TNF, inducible nitric oxide synthase, the transcription factor NFκB, and IL-12-driven IFN-γ production, regulatory cytokines IL-15 and TGF-β, and the surface marker CD14.[85-88] One interesting aspect of this model involves the role of bacteria in initiating disease manifestations specific to the gut and characteristic of human IBD. Work by Schultz et al. demonstrates that IL-2-deficient mice raised under germ-free conditions develop only a mild focal colitis with delayed onset (compared to mice raised under specific pathogen-free conditions).[89] However, although their intestinal symptoms are greatly attenuated, germ-free mice still retain their extraintestinal pathologies, including anemia and extraintestinal lymphoid hyperplasia.[90] These studies clearly associate the presence of environmental antigens with the development of chronic inflammation specific to the intestine, but not other pathological conditions that occur in IL-2-deficient mice.

Although IL-2 production is increased in the intestines of patients with active Crohn's disease compared to ulcerative colitis or control patients,[68,70,71,91] a study by Fuss et al.[74] demonstrates that lamina propria T cells isolated from inflamed areas of intestinal tissue from Crohn's disease patients actually produce reduced levels of IL-2, compared to T cells taken from control patients and patients with ulcerative colitis. Interestingly, the mechanisms of action of several existing IBD drugs (i.e. corticosteroids and cyclosporin) may involve alterations of IL-2 production in the gut. In addition, variations in IL-2 and soluble IL-2 receptor plasma levels, as well as the percentage of IL-2-secreting cells, have been reported in Crohn's disease patients following treatment with cyclosporin and corticosteroids.[92,93] Reductions in IL-2 production have also been observed in ulcerative colitis and Crohn's disease patients treated with sulfasalazine, as well as in peripheral blood mononuclear cells isolated from healthy volunteers after treatment with transdermal nicotine, a possible therapeutic approach for ulcerative colitis.[94,95] Recent preclinical studies by Stallmach et al. have

shown possible therapeutic potential for an IL-2IgG2b fusion protein, which is capable of decreasing wasting and histopathological signs of colitis in TNBS-treated mice.[96] Van Assche et al.,[97] in an open-label pilot study, have recently reported the initial safety and efficacy of humanized anti-IL-2 receptor (CD25) antibodies (daclizumab) for refractory ulcerative colitis. Further controlled trials are being planned to confirm the therapeutic benefit of this biological therapy targeting IL-2.

Lymphotoxin (previously known as TNF-β) is the final Th1-derived cytokine and a member of the TNF family primarily involved in the early development of lymphoid tissue. It exists as both a membrane-bound heterotrimer composed of α and β subunits (LTαβ), and as a soluble homotrimer consisting of the α subunit (LTα3). LTαβ is expressed on the surface of activated CD4+ T cells, particularly Th1 cells; exposure to IL-4 or a Th2 environment leads to loss of LTαβ surface expression and down-regulation of soluble LTα3 and TNF.[98] Soluble LTα3 has the ability to bind to both the p55 and p57 TNF receptors, but surface LTαβ binds to an LTβ receptor. LTα may exert its effects on lymphoid organ development through the p55 TNF receptor, which is known to mediate TNF-induced Peyer's patch organogenesis.[99]

Animal models deficient in either LTα or β have provided useful information in understanding the role of these molecules in the intestinal immune system. LTα-deficient mice display splenic disorganization and non-segregating T/B-cell zones. These mice lack Peyer's patches, peripheral lymph nodes, B-cell follicles, germinal centers and follicular dendritic networks. In contrast, LTβ-deficient mice possess a similar phenotype but retain some ability to develop limited germinal centers and follicular dendritic networks, and have some segregation of T/B-cell zones.[100,101] LTβ receptor-deficient mice also lack Peyer's patches and colon-associated lymphoid tissue, as well as all lymph nodes.[102] Studies by Cuff et al.[103,104] in endothelial cell lines and LTα transgenic mice shed light on the role of LTα3 in promoting inflammation and lymphoid organ development. Results from these studies show that LTα3 induces cytotoxic activity, as well as expression of adhesion molecules (VCAM, ICAM, E-selectin, MAdCAM-1) and C-C chemokines (RANTES, IP-10, and MCP-1) both in vitro and in vivo.

Given the dramatic success of therapeutics targeting TNF, it is plausible that LT could be a strong candidate for immunomodulatory therapy in IBD. Evidence for this therapeutic potential can be seen in the CD45Rb[hi]/SCID adoptive transfer experiments as well as the tgε26 transgenic mouse model of colitis. In both of these models, fusion proteins, which bind to the LTβR and inhibit LTαβ signaling, are able to improve the clinical features of disease.[105] These findings suggest that LT may play an important role in IBD pathogenesis, similar to its close relative TNF. However, as mentioned earlier, blockade of LTα together with TNF by etanercept does not appear to have beneficial effects in a recently reported clinical trial.[25]

# TH2-DERIVED CYTOKINES (IL-4, IL-5, IL-13)

Th2-derived cytokines are a subset of immunoregulatory cytokines derived from Th2-type CD4+ T cells, and include IL-4, IL-5, IL-10 and IL-13 (Fig. 12.2). Th2 immune responses are associated with allergic reactions and atopic disorders, as well as intestinal nematode infections. Although it is well accepted that human IBD is associated with a dysregulated balance of Th1/Th2 immune responses, it is currently unclear whether up- or downregulation of Th2 responses plays a critical role in Crohn's disease or ulcerative colitis. However, as will be described below, there is substantial evidence that these cytokines are involved in regulating IBD pathogenesis.

IL-4 is a CD4+ T cell-derived Th2 cytokine that exhibits many regulatory functions within the intestinal mucosa, often in synergy with IL-10 and IL-13.[106] IL-4 and IL-13 mediate in vitro production of chemokines (i.e. IL-8, RANTES and MCP-1) and inducible nitric oxide synthase expression by intestinal epithelial cell lines,[107–111] and may play a role in mediating intestinal epithelial barrier function.[112] Both IL-4 and IL-13 are capable of synergizing with IL-10 to block the release of lysosomal enzymes from peripheral blood mononuclear cells and lamina propria mononuclear cells, thereby inhibiting mucosal cytotoxic activity.[113] IL-4, IL-10 and IL-13 also work together to inhibit the release of proinflammatory cytokines from intestinal monocytes.[114,115] However, monocytes isolated from IBD patients appear to be less responsive to IL-13 inhibition than those derived from healthy individuals.[113,114]

Different IL-4 secretion patterns are associated with ulcerative colitis and Crohn's disease. Overall, lamina propria mononuclear cells isolated from intestinal biopsies of patients with IBD produce reduced levels of IL-4 mRNA and protein than normal lamina propria mononuclear cells.[74,116,117] Likewise, reduced numbers of IL-4-secreting cells are found in diverted versus non-diverted areas of intestine from IBD patients who have undergone surgery.[118] In addition, peripheral monocytes and intestinal macrophages from IBD patients appear to be less responsive to the inhibitory effects of IL-4.[119] These differences are most likely attributable to Crohn's disease rather than ulcerative colitis, and may be dependent on the stage of disease.[73,120] In fact, increased levels of IL-4 can be detected in early Crohn's disease lesions along with decreased levels of IFN-γ, whereas chronic lesions display a Th1 cytokine profile, suggesting that Th2 responses are associated with acute inflammation in Crohn's disease, whereas Th1 responses are more predominant in chronic inflammation.[76]

Preclinical animal studies have evaluated the therapeutic potential of IL-4. Hogaboam et al.[121] found that two injections of retrovirally encoded IL-4 cause overexpression of IL-4 in TNBS-treated rats and significantly attenuates tissue damage, along with circulating and local levels of IFN-γ, inducible calcium-independent nitric oxide synthase gene expression, nitric oxide synthesis, and myeloperoxidase activity in the distal colon.

Comparatively less is known regarding the role of the Th2 cytokines IL-5 and IL-13 in IBD. IL-13 shares many similarities in structure and function to IL-4.[122] Genes encoding both cytokines are located in close proximity to each other on chromosome 5 and contain identical major transcriptional regulatory elements. They also share specific receptors and receptor subchains, as well as exhibit similar signal transduction pathways. As a result of these similarities, IL-4 and IL-13 appear to have overlapping functions and work in synergy as described above.

IL-5 has mainly been implicated in chronic parasitic and allergic diseases. However, increased levels of IL-5 have been detected in colonic patch T cells in hapten-induced colitis.[123] Elevated IL-5 production is also seen in stimulated T cells isolated from intestinal lesions in mice with oxazolone-induced colitis.[124] Finally, purified stimulated lamina propria CD4+ T cells from the inflamed intestinal mucosa of patients with ulcerative colitis produce increased concentrations of IL-5 than do those of normal controls.[74] In the oxazolone mouse model of intestinal inflammation, neutralization by IL-13Rα-2 Fc administration effectively prevents colitis. Interestingly, the source of IL-13 in this model was localized to NK T cells.[125] A possible role for IL-5 and IL-13 pharmacological modulation in the treatment of IBD has not yet been explored and may be a potential approach for targeted immunotherapy in the future. Studies in animal models have provided important evidence for the role of IL-13 in a Th2 colitis model.

# Tr1-DERIVED CYTOKINES (IL-10 AND TGF-β)

The Th1/Th2 paradigm is complicated in human IBD by the presence of a third subset of immunoregulatory CD4+ T cells, deemed type 1 T-regulatory (Tr1) cells, which are characterized by their ability to produce IL-10 (classically a Th2-derived cytokine) and TGF-β (Fig. 12.2). IL-10 is a potent anti-inflammatory cytokine implicated in the pathogenesis of IBD that promotes differentiation of both Th2 and Tr1 cells in the intestine. As evidence of the important role of Tr1-derived IL-10 in mediating intestinal inflammation, administration of recombinant IL-10 to SCID mice adoptively transferred with CD45Rb^hi T cells prevents the onset of colitis.[126] A similar protective effect is seen with co-transfer of Tr1 cells or CD45Rb^low T cells from IL-4-deficient mice, but not CD45Rb^low T cells from IL-10-deficient mice.[126,127] Thus, Tr1-derived IL-10 appears to be a critical mediator of gut homeostasis in this model.

Like other classic Th2 cytokines, IL-10 has the ability to suppress the production of proinflammatory cytokines secreted from macrophages, dendritic cells, T cells and NK cells within the inflamed intestinal mucosa.[128] This inhibitory effect is potentiated by synergy with IL-4 and IL-13 in monocytes and epithelial cells.[107,115] IL-10 also acts to counterbalance many of the proinflammatory functions of Th1-polarizing cytokines and suppresses proinflammatory cytokine and chemokine production by intestinal macrophages.[129] IL-10 regulates human intestinal T cells by blocking proliferation and activation of CD8+ T cells and inhibiting production of Th1 cytokines (i.e. IL-2, IFN-γ and TNF), while simultaneously enhancing IL-2-induced cytotoxicity, thus maintaining a basal level of host defense.[130]

Studies in IL-10-deficient mice clearly support this concept. These mice spontaneously develop colitis similar to human IBD when raised under conventional conditions.[131] Colitis first develops in the cecum and the ascending and transverse colon at around 3 weeks of age, and inflammation spreads through the entire colon and parts of the ileum as the mice age. A majority of IL-10-deficient mice develop colorectal adenocarcinomas by 60 weeks of age. The development of colitis in IL-10-deficient mice appears to be dependent on a combination of genetics, immunoregulatory and environmental factors. The intestinal inflammatory infiltrate in these mice is characterized by

## Table 12.3 Regulatory cytokines

| Cytokine | Source | Receptors | Signaling | Activity |
|---|---|---|---|---|
| IL-10 | TR1, TH3, DC, Mφ, B cells | | STAT-3 | Suppress APC activity, ↓ MHC II, IL-1β, TNF, IL-12, IFNγ expression |
| TGF-β | TH3, TR1, epithelial cells | TGF-βRI, II | Smad2, 3, 4 | Stimulates epithelial restitution, ↓ proliferation T cells, epithelial cells, ↑ collagen, ↑ IgA expression, mediates oral tolerance |

increased numbers of macrophages, B cells, plasma cells and CD4+ TCRαβ+ T cells, in addition to a dysregulated Th1 cytokine profile.[132] IL-1, IL-6, TNF, IFN-γ, LTβ and TGF-β mRNA levels are 10–35 times higher in the intestinal mucosa of IL-10-deficient mice than in wildtype controls, and adhesion molecules intracellular adhesion molecule-1, vascular cell adhesion molecule-1, and MAdCAM-1 mRNA and protein levels are also elevated 5–23-fold.[133] As noted earlier, treatment with anti-IL-12 antibodies completely abolishes colitis in young IL-10-deficient mice, and significantly improves disease in adult mice, suggesting that the inflammation in these mice is indeed Th1 mediated. Antibodies against IFN-γ can prevent colitis in young mice but, unlike anti-IL-12 antibodies, do not appear to be efficacious for treating established disease in adult mice.[40,132] The development of colitis in IL-10-deficient mice is believed to be mediated by pathogenic T-cell subsets. Intestinal epithelial and lamina propria lymphocytes from IL-10-deficient mice are capable of inducing colitis upon transfer to mice lacking B and T cells. The severity of the resulting colitis is dependent on the number of cells that are transferred.[134]

The normal enteric bacterial flora is also an important factor mediating the development of colitis in IL-10-deficient mice. IL-10-deficient mice raised under germ-free conditions do not develop colitis. However, when these mice are populated with specific bacterial strains found in the normal intestinal flora, they develop intestinal inflammation characteristic of IBD, indicating that the resident bacterial flora is necessary for the induction of colitis in this model.[135] Prior to the onset of colitis, IL-10-deficient mice display alterations in the appearance and number of mucosal adherent colonic bacteria, and antibiotic therapy is capable of attenuating the resulting intestinal inflammation.[136] Invasive bacteria may gain access to the intestinal mucosa through increased intestinal permeability, which can be detected in IL-10-deficient mice by 2 weeks of age.[137] Although it remains unclear which strains harbor pathogenic potential, studies have implicated novel *Helicobacter* species as well as *Bacteroides vulgates*.[135,138,139] On the other hand, some enteric bacteria may protect against colitis, including *Lactobacillus* species. In fact, IL-10-deficient neonates have reduced levels of colonic *Lactobacillus* species and elevated levels of mucosal adherent and translocated bacteria. When levels are normalized through rectal delivery of bacteria under specific-pathogen-free conditions, colitis is prevented.[140] Recent studies have also shown that the probiotic compound VSL#3 is effective in the treatment of colitis in IL-10-deficient mice.

These effects are associated with the ability of probiotic bacteria to enhance epithelial barrier function in this model.[141] Taken together, these observations support both pathogenic and protective roles for the bacterial flora in initiating and perpetuating colitis in IL-10-deficient mice.

In humans IL-10 is constitutively produced within the intestinal mucosa. Elevated levels of IL-10 mRNA and protein are seen in areas of active inflammation within the intestinal mucosa of IBD patients compared to non-inflamed areas as well as mucosa from healthy individuals.[68,70,72] IL-10 mRNA and protein expression by intestinal epithelial cells is similar in Crohn's disease, ulcerative colitis and healthy mucosa, but IBD samples have an increased number of IL-10-producing mononuclear cells (mainly macrophages) in the submucosa of inflamed tissues.[142] IL-10 production in the lamina propria of patients with active IBD is relatively low compared to that seen in the submucosa, suggesting that IBD patients may not be deficient in IL-10, but rather may have differential local distribution of IL-10 within the mucosa. Because IL-10 appears to be an important mediator of IBD pathogenesis, clinical studies have focused on its therapeutic potential in humans.

Human recombinant (hr) IL-10 has been tested in clinical trials as a new therapy for patients with Crohn's disease. Preclinical animal studies demonstrated that high doses of rIL-10 can ameliorate macroscopic formalin-induced colitis in rabbits and DSS-induced colitis in mice.[143,144] In recent work by De Winter et al.,[145] transgenic mice in which IL-10 is expressed by intestinal epithelial cells have elevated numbers of intraepithelial lymphocytes, as well as reduced Th1 immune responses and elevated levels of TGF-β. Experiments with these mice show that site-specific IL-10 expression can ameliorate both dextran sodium sulfate-induced colitis as well as colitis resulting from transfer of CD45Rb[hi] pathogenic splenocytes. Clinical trials in humans have shown hrIL-10 to be safe but not efficacious for the treatment of refractory Crohn's disease. Daily subcutaneous injections of hrIL-10 induced remission in up to 50% of steroid-refractory Crohn's disease patients after 3 weeks of treatment, compared to 23% of patients receiving placebo.[146] However, larger clinical trials to directly evaluate the efficacy of subcutaneous IL-10 administration in patients with Crohn's disease have shown a marginal beneficial effect.[147,148] The lack of efficacy of IL-10 has also been demonstrated in a subsequent large, double-blind placebo-controlled study yet to be published, as well as in a clinical trial for the prevention of postoperative recurrence of Crohn's disease.[149]

TGF-β is a second regulatory factor produced by intestinal Tr1 lymphocytes and plays a primary role in mediating intestinal immune responses. TGF-β is also produced by intestinal epithelial cells, and enhances epithelial restitution and inhibits growth and proliferation by downregulating cellular division in both intestinal epithelial cell lines and primary cultures.[150–153] TGF-β also enhances IL-1- and TNF-induced IL-6 secretion from intestinal epithelial cells in vitro, and maintains colonic epithelial barrier function in the presence of T cell-derived cytokines that promote intestinal permeability (i.e. IFN-γ, IL-4 and IL-10).[154,155] Certain bacterial strains contained within the normal intestinal flora stimulate TGF-β-induced collagen deposition, possibly supporting a role for TGF-β in the formation of intestinal strictures.[156] TGF-β may also be involved in regulating IgA production, as TGF-β-deficient mice lack IgA-committed B cells in the intestine.[157]

Animal models of intestinal inflammation have localized TGF-β to the surface epithelium of the murine small intestine, with expression predominantly in the villous tips, but not in the crypts.[158] Unstimulated cultured human intestinal endothelial cells also express TGF-β, and TGF-β receptors have been detected on the apical and basal colonic crypt surfaces.[154] The kinetics of TGF-β production appears to be different in intestinal epithelial cells versus lamina propria T cells. TGF-β mRNA is constitutively expressed by the colonic and small intestinal epithelium of IL-2-deficient mice, and increased concentrations can be detected in areas of active inflammation. Unlike in lamina propria T cells, elevated levels of TGF-β in the epithelium can be detected before the development of clinical symptoms, suggesting that TGF-β may play a role in the early phases of disease pathogenesis.[159]

As discussed earlier, TGF-β may share a reciprocal relationship with IFN-γ/IL-12.[160] Lamina propria T lymphocytes from TNP-KLH-immunized IL-2-deficient mice do not produce TGF-β during the early stages of colitis, compared to an eightfold increase in TGF-β protein production among wildtype mice. Induction of TGF-β in these mice inhibits IFN-γ production by lamina propria T cells and the development of colitis. Likewise, blocking TGF-β with neutralizing antibodies restores IFN-γ production and the resulting colitis, supporting a reciprocal relationship between these two cytokines.[161] One mechanism for this relationship in Crohn's disease may include expression of the transcription factor T-bet, which invokes production of Th1 immune responses through suppression of TGF-β signaling.[162]

Studies involving TGF-β have complicated the accepted Th1/Th2 paradigm in animal models of intestinal inflammation. As seen with IL-10-deficient mice, antibodies targeting TGF-β can reverse the protective effects of CD45Rb[low] T cells in the CD45Rb[hi]/*SCID* adoptive transfer model of colitis, suggesting that both IL-10 and TGF-β are essential in the regulation of pathogenic T cells.[163,164] Because this effect is independent of IL-4, these results suggest a more complicated relationship than the proposed Th1/Th2 paradigm, most likely involving Tr1 T-cell subsets.

TGF-β has shown therapeutic potential in preclinical studies using animal models of intestinal inflammation and appears to be a primary regulator of T-cell immune responses. In fact, recent work by Fuss et al. shows that TGF-β production is the primary mechanism for counterregulation of Th1-mediated intestinal inflammation, whereas the effects of IL-10 are only secondary and facilitate TGF-β production.[165] In gene therapy studies, 50% of rats administered TNBS and injected with an expression vector encoding the TGF-β gene developed minimal or no ulceration compared to controls, 83% of which had scores indicating maximal tissue damage.[166] Oral feeding of haptenized colonic proteins, which suppresses sensitivity to TNBS, is associated with a marked increase in TGF-β production.[43] This effect is abolished upon treatment with neutralizing antibodies against TGF-β. Taken together, these studies establish TGF-β as a primary regulator of immune responses in animal models of colitis.

TGF-β has been directly implicated in human IBD. In the inflamed mucosa of IBD patients, increased levels of TGF-β and increased numbers of TGF-β-producing T cells, neutrophils, monocytes and macrophages can be found in close proximity to luminal surfaces in the lamina propria, but expression in the epithelium is unchanged.[167,168] IBD patients also have abnormal expression patterns of TGF-β receptors type I and II, which are found on intestinal epithelial cells and fibroblasts during the early stages of fibrosis.[169] Increases in both TGF-β type I and II receptors can be seen in surgically resected intestinal specimens from Crohn's disease patients, along with striking increases in TGF-β, and both TGF-β and its signaling receptor are co-expressed in the intestinal mucosa of patients with Crohn's disease.[170] In contrast, mucosal samples from patients with ulcerative colitis have lower levels of TGF-β than normal mucosa, possibly reflecting differential mechanisms of disease pathogenesis for Crohn's disease and ulcerative colitis.[171] Perhaps some of the most compelling evidence for a role for TGF-β in IBD pathogenesis comes from a study by Monteleone et al.,[172] which demonstrates that TGF-β signaling is impaired in mucosal T cells isolated from patients with Crohn's disease due to over-expression of Smad7, an inhibitor of TGF-β signaling, resulting in the inability of TGF-β to inhibit proinflammatory cytokine production.

# THE IL-1–IL-1 RECEPTOR ANTAGONIST COMPLEX

Several other cytokines may be important in mediating the non-specific inflammatory phase of chronic intestinal inflammation. IL-1 is a pleiotropic proinflammatory cytokine produced in two forms, IL-1α and IL-1β, both of which bind to the same cell surface receptor and possess identical biological activities.[173] In contrast to IL-1α, which remains largely intracellular or membrane bound, the IL-1β precursor molecule is cleaved intracellularly by the IL-1β-converting enzyme to its mature form and is subsequently secreted. Two IL-1 receptors exist, IL-1 receptor type I and type II (IL-1RI and IL-1RII, respectively). The IL-1RI is present on intestinal epithelial cells, hepatocytes, fibroblasts, endothelial cells, T lymphocytes and keratinocytes, whereas the IL-1RII is found primarily on B lymphocytes, neutrophils and monocytes.[173] Several of the biological properties of IL-1, which is produced by activated monocytes, macrophages, fibroblasts, smooth muscle cells and endothelial cells, are relevant to IBD.[173] In the inflamed intestinal mucosa of IBD patients IL-1 expression is markedly increased, primarily in lamina propria mononuclear cells.[174] Locally, IL-1 amplifies gut inflammatory responses by inducing production of a variety of proinflammatory and immunoregulatory cytokines, as well as arachidonic acid metabolites by lamina propria immune and mesenchymal cells. As further evidence of its pleiotropic effects, IL-1 also increases expression of adhesion molecules on endothelial and immune cells, upregulates IL-2 receptors on T lymphocytes, stimulates proliferation of intestinal fibroblasts and smooth muscle cells, and enhances collagen synthesis by fibroblasts.[175] Thus, IL-1 appears to play a central role during gut inflammatory responses characteristic of IBD through recruitment of inflammatory cells to sites of injury and activation of classic and non-classic immune cells.

Three studies elucidate the primary role of IL-1 in the pathogenesis of intestinal inflammation. IL-1 has been shown to regulate the production of $PGE_2$, 6-keto-$PGI_2$ and $TXB_2$ in the normal and inflamed rabbit colon.[176] In this animal model of immune complex-induced colitis, IL-1 gene expression and synthesis occurs early in the course of disease and precedes the appearance of colonic $PGE_2$ and $LTB_4$; tissue levels of IL-1 correlate with the degree of tissue inflammation and necrosis.[177] Finally, specific blockade of IL-1 by recombinant IL-1 receptor antagonist dose-dependently suppresses the inflammatory response and production of $PGE_2$ and $LTB_2$ associated with experimental rabbit colitis.[178] The latter results have been confirmed in other animal models of intestinal inflammation and injury, suggesting that IL-1 may in fact play a role of paramount importance in gut inflammation.[179,180] Additional evidence that IL-1 may be an important inflammatory mediator in patients with IBD is also provided by the fact that compounds that are routinely used in the treatment of symptoms, such as sulfasalazine, corticosteroids and other immunosuppressive drugs, may exert some of their effects through the inhibition of IL-1 synthesis and/or activity.[181,182]

Expression of IL-1 in patients with IBD has been extensively investigated in different cell types. Satsangi et al. originally demonstrated that cultured peripheral blood mononuclear cells isolated from patients with Crohn's disease produced increased amounts of bioactive IL-1 than peripheral blood mononuclear cells isolated from controls.[183] These results have subsequently been confirmed using specific immunoassays in patients with active IBD.[173,184] Because peripheral blood mononuclear cells may not truly represent the lamina propria mononuclear cell population found in inflamed tissues of IBD patients, interest has focused more recently on measuring levels of IL-1 in freshly isolated lamina propria mononuclear cells. Elevated IL-1 levels in these cells have been reported in patients with IBD compared to controls.[185] Interestingly, freshly isolated intestinal epithelial cells do not express IL-1 mRNA transcripts or protein, supporting the hypothesis that production of IL-1 is localized to lamina propria mononuclear cells.[174]

The balance between IL-1 expression and its naturally occurring antagonist, deemed IL-1 receptor antagonist (IL-1ra), may be a potential mechanism of IBD pathogenesis. IL-1ra was originally isolated from human urine and partially purified as a 23 kDa protein that blocks the binding of IL-1 to T cells and fibroblasts, with a subsequent reduction in biological responses to IL-1.[186–188] This functional inhibitor comprises a homeostatic mechanism that has the ability to regulate IL-1 activity physiologically, thereby controlling inflammation. Because IBD is characterized by an inflammatory response that is not appropriately downregulated, an imbalance between the pro-

duction of IL-1 and its natural antagonist, IL-1ra, has been proposed as an important mechanism in perpetuating IBD immune responses. Casini-Raggi et al.[189] initially investigated the balance of IL-1 and IL-1ra in freshly isolated intestinal mucosal cells from patients with ulcerative colitis, Crohn's disease and surgical controls. IL-1 levels were markedly increased in freshly isolated mucosal cells from Crohn's disease and ulcerative colitis patients compared to controls, and IL-1ra levels were slightly elevated in Crohn's disease and significantly increased in ulcerative colitis compared to controls. Therefore, the ratio of IL-1ra to IL-1 was significantly decreased in intestinal mucosal cells from IBD patients compared to controls. These data suggest that an insufficient amount of intestinal IL-1ra may be produced during inflammation in IBD patients. The specificity of these findings was investigated by comparing the IL-1ra/IL-1 ratio in intestinal mucosal biopsies obtained from IBD patients with that in biopsies obtained from patients with self-limited acute colitis (inflammatory controls). The results of these studies showed that an imbalance of IL-1ra to IL-1 is present in inflamed tissues from IBD patients, whereas inflammatory controls have a ratio comparable with that present in intestinal tissues from normal surgical controls.[189] These data are in agreement with results from studies performed by other groups showing decreased intestinal IL-1ra mRNA transcripts or protein levels in IBD patients compared to inflammatory controls.[190,191] The discovery of IL-1ra genetic polymorphisms and the association of allele 2 of the IL-1ra gene with the incidence of ulcerative colitis in certain populations have suggested the interesting hypothesis that IL-1ra production may be genetically regulated.[192] Thus, a deficit of IL-1ra mucosal production may exist in patients carrying a specific IL-1ra polymorphism. Tountas et al. have demonstrated the association between allele 2 and ulcerative colitis in Hispanic and Jewish populations from the Los Angeles area, and that individuals carrying allele 2 produce decreased amounts of IL-1ra protein.[193] However, this association has not been detected in Caucasian northern European patients, although trends towards an association have been observed.[194,195] Two recent studies by Carter et al.[196,197] associate carriage of allele 2 with ulcerative colitis. The first study[196] reassessed the presence of a significant association in a large independent set of well-characterized Caucasian patients and performed a meta-analysis of reported patient series. Using this methodology, the association between IL-1ra allele 2 and ulcerative colitis was confirmed and shown to be weak, conferring only a small risk in this patient population. The second study[197] analyzed allele 2 carriage rates among ulcerative colitis patients who had undergone total colectomy and subsequent ileal pouch anal anastomosis, and found a significant association between carriage of IL-1ra allele 2 and the development of pouchitis.

Taken together, these findings strongly support the hypothesis that the imbalance of IL-1ra to IL-1 may be important in the pathophysiology of IBD. Based on this concept, providing exogenous IL-1ra or increasing the synthesis of endogenous IL-1ra has been proposed as a potential treatment for patients with IBD. Unfortunately, no reliable clinical trials have been performed to study the administration of either recombinant IL-1ra or monoclonal antibodies directly targeting IL-1 to patients with either Crohn's disease or ulcerative colitis.

# OTHER CYTOKINE MEDIATORS OF INTESTINAL INFLAMMATION (IL-6, IL-7, IL-11 AND IL-15)

Several other pro- and anti-inflammatory cytokines have been investigated in relation to intestinal inflammation and IBD pathogenesis. IL-6, along with IL-1 and TNF, is part of a group of classic macrophage-derived proinflammatory cytokines secreted into the intestinal mucosa in response to antigen stimulation or induction by Th1 cytokines. IL-6 has the ability to bind to both membrane-bound and soluble IL-6 receptors. Interestingly, IL-6 can interact with cells not expressing IL-6 receptors by a process known as trans-signaling in which IL-6 forms a complex with the soluble IL-6 receptor, which can then transduce signal to target cells.[198] In addition to macrophages, intestinal epithelial cells also secrete IL-6, and IL-6 receptors have been detected on both the apical and basal surfaces of intestinal epithelial cells in culture.[199,200] A variety of molecules are capable of inducing or potentiating IL-6 production from intestinal epithelial cells, including other proinflammatory and regulatory cytokines (i.e. IL-1, IFN-γ and TGF-β), heat-shock proteins, endotoxins and prostaglandins (PGE$_2$).[201–204] IL-6 has several biologic functions, including regulation of apoptosis and activation of mesenchymal cells.[205–207] IL-6 may also play a critical role in B-cell terminal differentiation, proliferation and immunoglobulin secretion, although conflicting reports using IL-6-deficient mice have made this finding somewhat controversial.[208–211]

Many studies have measured IL-6 production in patients with IBD. In the intestinal mucosa IL-6 has been detected in T and B lymphocytes, macrophages and intestinal epithelial cells.[212–214] IL-6 can be detected in normal mucosa, but levels are increased in areas of active inflammation; this local increase appears to correlate with the degree of inflammation.[215–218] However, it is unclear whether serum levels, which are also elevated in IBD patients, correlate with disease activity. Serum concentrations of IL-6 are elevated in patients with Crohn's disease compared to ulcerative colitis and normal controls, and ulcerative colitis patients have higher levels than healthy individuals.[219,220] Soluble IL-6 receptor levels are also elevated in patients with active IBD compared to inactive IBD, other types of intestinal inflammation or healthy individuals.[221]

The IL-6 system has been evaluated for therapeutic potential in several animal models of colitis. As in humans, IL-6 levels are elevated in the inflamed colons of IL-10-deficient mice and after acetic acid-induced tissue injury.[133,222] Furthermore, Yamamoto et al. have shown that blockade of IL-6 receptors ameliorates disease in the CD45Rb$^{hi}$/SCID adoptive transfer model of colitis, as evidenced by normal growth, decreased T-cell expansion, and a downregulation of adhesion molecules and proinflammatory cytokines.[223] This result has been confirmed in several models of Th1-mediated intestinal inflammation, and the mechanism of action for this improvement may involve induction of lamina propria T-cell apoptosis. As further support for this mechanism, recent work by Atreya et al. show evidence of trans-signaling through the IL-6/sIL-6 receptor complex in mucosal T cells isolated from patients with Crohn's disease. Specific blockade of this IL-6 trans-signaling

mechanisms induces T-cell apoptosis, suggesting that elevated mucosal levels of IL-6 and soluble IL-6 receptor in Crohn's disease may inhibit apoptosis of pathogenic T cells, leading to the development and perpetuation of IBD.[224] Novel therapeutic approaches neutralizing the IL-6/sIL-6 receptor trans-signaling system have been investigated at the preclinical level.[224]

IL-7 is another inductive cytokine that mediates B- and T-cell growth and differentiation and is produced by a variety of cell types, including bone marrow stromal cells, B cells, monocytes, macrophages, dendritic cells, keratinocytes and intestinal epithelial cells. IL-7 shares many biologic functions with IL-2 and preferentially targets proliferation of TCRγδ+ lymphocytes, as evidenced by IL-7 and IL-7 receptor-deficient mice, which have reduced numbers of B cells and retarded growth of TCRαβ+ T cells but few to no TCRγδ+ T cells.[225–227] Administration of IL-7 to IL-7-deficient mice results in restoration of TCRγδ+ T-cell populations, as well as the formation of Peyer's patches and crypt abscesses.[228] Work by von Freeden-Jeffry et al.[229] supports a role for IL-7 in colitis. Mice deficient in both T and B cells develop colitis when exposed to certain bacterial flora. However, these mice do not develop intestinal inflammation when crossed with IL-7-deficient mice and colonized with the same flora, suggesting that IL-7 may modulate the onset of colitis through a mechanism that is independent of B and T lymphocytes.[229] In support of this finding, genetically engineered mice that overexpress IL-7 develop chronic colitis similar to that observed in ulcerative colitis.[230] Therefore, IL-7 may play a role in intestinal inflammation, but it remains unclear whether or not this role is specific to IBD pathogenesis.

IL-15 is the final inductive cytokine and is derived mainly from non-lymphoid tissues, epithelial cells, fibroblasts, and activated monocytes and macrophages. IL-15 is produced in response to antigen and shares many biological activities with IL-2, including growth and differentiation of T and B lymphocytes, NK cells, epithelial cells, macrophages and monocytes within the intestinal mucosa. Most of these effects occur through interactions between IL-15 and a heterotrimeric receptor complex composed of the IL-2 receptor β chain, the IL-2 receptor common γ chain, and the IL-15 receptor α chain (IL-15 receptor α).[231]

Both IL-15 and IL-2 promote the growth of restimulated TCRγδ+ intraepithelial lymphocytes but have differential effects on survival. Intraepithelial lymphocytes expressing the γδ+ TCR constitutively express IL-15 and exhibit greater proliferation in response to IL-15 restimulation than do lymphocytes expressing the αβ+ TCR.[232] Restimulation of the TCR with IL-15 protects CD8+ TCRγδ+ lymphocytes against apoptosis, whereas restimulation with IL-2 causes increased programmed cell death.[78,233] In support of this concept, a study by Kennedy et al. found that mice deficient in IL-15 have marked reductions in CD8+ T cells, presumably due to apoptosis. Incidentally, these mice also completely lack NK cells, suggesting that IL-15 may also play a role in the development and maturation of NK cells.[234] Few studies have investigated the role of IL-15 in IBD pathogenesis. Elevated levels of IL-15 have been detected in the rectal mucosa of patients with active IBD and inactive ulcerative colitis.[16] Lamina propria T cells isolated from IBD patients, especially those with Crohn's disease, are hyperresponsive to IL-15 compared to controls, resulting in enhanced T-cell activation, proliferation and proinflammatory cytokine production.[235,236] However, more preclinical studies are needed before the medical potential of IL-15 targeting therapies can be established.

IL-11 is a stromal cell-derived growth factor with many functions, both extraintestinally and within the gut. As a hematopoietic agent, IL-11 stimulates peripheral platelet counts and is approved as a treatment for chemotherapy-induced thrombocytopenia. IL-11 is also involved in the induction of acute-phase reactants from the liver, and has a trophic effect for the damaged intestinal epithelium.[237] IL-11 plays an important role in gut tissue repair, especially with regard to small intestinal villi, and regulates normal growth control and proliferation of intestinal epithelial crypt cells, as well as partial suppression of apoptosis and extension of villous length.[238] These effects promote epithelial restitution in irradiated mice treated with rhIL-11, and may be mediated by TGF-β via the transcription factor-activating protein-1 (AP-1).[239,240] IL-11 also exhibits anti-inflammatory properties by blocking production of IL-1, IL-6, IL-12, TNF and nitric oxide by macrophages through inhibition of the transcription factor NFκB, as well as by downregulating Th1 cytokine production by CD4+ T cells and inducing Th2 cytokine production.[241,242]

Notably, these anti-inflammatory properties of rhIL-11 result in improvement of macroscopic and microscopic intestinal tissue damage in several animal models of IBD, including the acetic acid model of acute colitis, the TNBS-induced colitis, and HLA-B27 rats.[243–245] A similar effect is seen in rats that have undergone massive intestinal resections and subsequent treatment with rhIL-11. These animals have increased intestinal absorption and mucosal mass, indicating rhIL-11 as a potential therapy for patients with short-bowel syndrome.[246–248] These preclinical studies suggest a therapeutic potential for IL-11 in human IBD. Controlled clinical trials are currently under way to investigate the safety and efficacy of subcutaneous rhIL-11 injections in patients with Crohn's disease. In initial human trials, short-term treatment with rhIL-11 was well tolerated and mildly efficacious, with 42% of Crohn's disease patients experiencing a clinical response after five injections of rhIL-11 per week for 3 weeks, compared to 7% of patients treated with placebo.[249] A subsequent larger clinical trial of 148 patients with mild to moderately active Crohn's disease showed only a trend towards a decrease in mean percentage change of Crohn's disease activity index scores for patients treated twice weekly with rhIL-11 for 6 weeks versus placebo (–31.5% vs. –18.5%); however, a significantly greater number of IL-11-treated patients achieved remission during the study (36.7% vs. 16.3%).[250] In light of the more dramatic clinical responses seen with other biologic therapies for Crohn's disease, it is currently unclear whether rhIL-11 will find a niche in the arsenal of emerging treatments for IBD.

# C-X-C CHEMOKINES (IL-8, ENA-78, IP-10 AND FRACTALKINE)

Chemokines are chemotactic cytokines that play an important role in mucosal inflammation. These low molecular weight proteins consist of two subfamilies based primarily on their structure. The C-X-C chemokines (or α subfamily) have a single amino acid located between the first two of four cysteine residues; this amino acid is absent in the C-C chemokines (β subfamily). Chemokines, along with their abundant receptors, are expressed by a variety of cell types, including epithelial cells, macrophages, T and B lymphocytes, endothelial cells and neutrophils. Many of their effects are overlapping. In fact, one chemokine receptor can bind up to eight chemokines, and a single chemokine can bind up to four receptors. Chemokines have a variety of functions in the mucosal immune system. They activate immune cells and induce enzyme production and granule exocytosis. They also act as chemoattractants for infiltrating granulocytes, monocytes and lymphocytes. Chemokines regulate leukocyte cell trafficking to the gut, adherence to the endothelial lining of blood vessels, and migration into the intestinal mucosa. Upon stimulation they are secreted into the lamina propria and mucosa, where they establish a chemotactic gradient that attracts infiltrating leukocytes to sites of inflammation. This process normally leads to enhanced leukocyte extravasation and an increase in the number of infiltrating immune cells into the gut mucosa. However, similar to cytokine production during disease pathogenesis, dysregulated chemokine production may result in acute and chronic inflammation and tissue damage.

IL-8, the prototypic C-X-C chemokine, is a potent neutrophil chemoattractant and activator of polymorphonuclear cells. In vitro, IL-8 is secreted in a polarized fashion from the apical surface of intestinal epithelial cell lines in response to stimulation by bacteria and their products, as well as TNF and IL-1β.[251–253] In vivo studies have demonstrated that IL-8 is expressed primarily by macrophages, epithelial cells and neutrophils in areas of active inflammation within the intestinal mucosa of IBD patients.[254] IL-8 mRNA is consistently detected in macrophages and neutrophils in the inflamed lamina propria.[255–257] Transcripts have also been detected in intestinal epithelial cells located at the base of intestinal ulcers, in crypt abscesses, and along the border of fistulae and mucosal surfaces.[254] A differential distribution of IL-8 mRNA within the intestinal mucosa of patients with ulcerative colitis and Crohn's disease reflects characteristic histological differences between these two diseases. In ulcerative colitis, IL-8 mRNA is diffusely distributed throughout the entire affected mucosa, whereas IL-8 mRNA transcripts have a more focal distribution in inflamed tissue from Crohn's disease patients.[254]

Levels of IL-8 mRNA and protein concentrations are increased in inflamed tissue from IBD patients. Significantly higher levels of mRNA are found in involved versus uninvolved areas of intestinal mucosa from both Crohn's disease and ulcerative colitis patients.[258] Increased IL-8 protein concentrations are found in homogenates of colonic biopsies from patients with active Crohn's disease and ulcerative colitis, but not inactive disease, tissue from other inflammatory intestinal conditions, or normal mucosa. This increase correlates extremely well with the macroscopic grade of inflammation, the number of invading neutrophils in the mucosa, and tissue levels of TNF and IL-1β, all of which are associated with IL-8 activity.[259] Furthermore, the number of IL-8-producing cells in the colonic and small intestinal mucosa of patients with IBD also correlates well with the histological grade of disease severity.[254] These data strongly support an association between enhanced IL-8 production and disease pathogenesis in IBD.

Although IL-8 is implicated in the pathogenesis of both ulcerative colitis and Crohn's disease, evidence suggests a somewhat stronger association with ulcerative colitis. Enhanced production of IL-8 in the inflamed mucosa of patients with IBD is significantly greater in patients with ulcerative colitis than in those with Crohn's disease.[260–262] Similarly, although organ cultures of mucosal biopsies from IBD patients secrete higher levels of IL-8 than do normal biopsies, the effect is more pronounced in ulcerative colitis.[263] Increased IL-8 secretion in this culture system results in enhanced chemotactic activity and an increase in neutrophil-binding capacity, both of which are inhibited by pretreatment with anti-IL-8 antibodies, confirming the functional role of IL-8.[263] Taken together, these findings suggest that IL-8 may be a non-specific mediator of inflammation with a distinct role in IBD, particularly ulcerative colitis.

Epithelial cell-derived neutrophil-activating peptide-78 (ENA-78) is also a potent neutrophil chemoattractant and immune cell activator that shares 22% sequence homology with IL-8. Like IL-8, ENA-78 is a C-X-C chemokine produced by intestinal epithelial cell lines and monocytes in response to stimulation with bacteria and bacterial products (such as LPS), IL-1β and TNF.[264–268] ENA-78 and IL-8 secretion by human monocytes is drastically reduced by IFN-α and -γ, which also inhibit the function of ENA-78 and IL-8 in neutrophil activation, suggesting that IFN-α and -γ may regulate neutrophil chemotaxis.[268] Although these two chemokines share many common properties, differences in their kinetic profiles suggest that they are differentially regulated. After stimulation with IL-1β and TNF, intestinal epithelial cell lines produce IL-8 as early as 4 hours before ENA-78, with peak levels observed 12 hours before maximal levels of ENA-78.[267] Similar results are seen in freshly isolated colonic epithelial cells from patients with Crohn's disease and ulcerative colitis, with rapid and transient bursts of IL-8 secretion but delayed and steady production of ENA-78.[6] In monocytes stimulated with LPS, ENA-78 displays a biphasic kinetics profile after stimulation with IL-1β and TNF, with an initial peak between 8 and 12 hours post stimulation and a second peak between 20 and 28 hours.[266] This biphasic pattern may reflect differential regulation in acute and chronic inflammation. Of note, ENA-78 expression in both monocytes and epithelial cells does not begin until after IL-8 expression has ceased, further supporting differential regulation for these two neutrophil chemoattractants. Also, ENA-78 and IL-8 bind to chemokine receptors with different affinities. Both bind efficiently to CXCR2 but, unlike IL-8, higher concentrations of ENA-78 are needed for binding to CXCR1.[269] Thus, receptor-binding affinities may represent another layer of differential regulation for these two proteins.

ENA-78 production is enhanced in IBD. ENA-78 mRNA levels are 24 times higher in tissues from patients with ulcerative colitis than in normal mucosa, and protein levels are four times higher.[267] Immunoreactivity is primarily associated with the crypt epithelium. Similar levels of ENA-78 mRNA are expressed by intestinal epithelial cells from patients with either Crohn's disease or ulcerative colitis, and over 90% of epithelial cells from IBD patients stain positive for ENA-78 protein.[270] Little to no ENA-78 mRNA is detected in normal mucosa, and protein is produced by less than 30% of intestinal epithelial cells from patients not afflicted with IBD.[267,270] More preclinical studies need to be performed before we can understand whether or not ENA-78 holds any therapeutic potential as a target for IBD therapy.

Although IL-8 and ENA-78 are the primary C-X-C chemokines studied in relation to IBD pathogenesis, other C-X-C chemokines have also been associated with IBD. Interferon-inducible protein 10 (IP-10) is a potent chemoattractant for NK cells in vitro, and mediates NK-cell cytolytic responses by inducing degranulation.[271] Unlike other C-X-C chemokines, IP-10 can bind to receptors that are highly expressed on IL-2-activated T lymphocytes, but is incapable of inducing transendothelial migration among T-cell subsets.[272–274] However, recent studies have established IP-10 as a potent inducer of intestinal epithelial lymphocyte chemotaxis.[275] In addition, IP-10 is markedly expressed in normal intestinal mucosa, and the number of IP-10-expressing cells in colonic biopsies from patients with ulcerative colitis is significantly elevated compared to normal tissue.[276]

Fractalkine is a C-X-3C chemokine which also acts as an adhesion molecule on the surface of activated endothelial cells. Fractalkine induces adhesion between circulating monocytes and the intestinal endothelium through interactions with integrins and their ligands.[276,277] Intestinal epithelial and endothelial cells produce fractalkine in the normal mucosa, and fractalkine protein levels are upregulated in inflamed areas of mucosa obtained from patients with active Crohn's disease.[278] However, more recent studies have suggested the possibility that fractalkine is specifically expressed by intestinal epithelial cells.[278a] Intestinal epithelial cells express CX3CR1, a receptor for fractalkine, and respond to fractalkine activation by expressing both IL-8 and fractalkine mRNA, and neutrophil chemotaxis into but not through intestinal epithelial monolayers.[279] Subpopulations of intraepithelial lymphocytes also express CX3CR1, and migrate in response to a fractalkine chemotactic gradient following activation with IL-2, suggesting that fractalkine may also function as a lymphocyte chemoattractant.[278] Overall, the role of C-X-C chemokines in the pathogenesis of IBD and the potential role for their pharmacological modulation remain to be tested in patients with both Crohn's disease and ulcerative colitis.

## C-C CHEMOKINES (MCP-1 AND IL-16)

C-C chemokines (or α subfamily) lack a single amino acid located between the first two of four cysteine residues. Monocyte chemoattractant peptide (MCP)-1 is a C-C chemokine and important inducer of monocyte chemotaxis and transendothelial migration. Like other chemokines, MCP-1 elicits cellular migration by establishing a chemotactic gradient across the vascular endothelium that is inhibited by neutralizing antibodies against MCP-1 or disruption of the chemotactic gradient.[280] In addition to inducing monocytes chemotaxis, MCP-1 also promotes transmigration of specific T-cell subsets, including TCRαβ+ and TCRγδ+ T lymphocytes.[274] More recently, MCP-1 has been implicated as a key mediator of Th2 polarization, as MCP-1-deficient mice are incapable of mounting Th2 responses.[281] These mice express low levels of IL-4, IL-5 and IL-10 in their lymph nodes, but have normal levels of IFN-γ and IL-12. MCP-1-deficient mice also have normal trafficking of naive T cells, suggesting that defective polarization is a direct effect of MCP-1 rather than secondary to abnormal cell migration, and lack the ability to recruit monocytes.[282] Therefore, MCP-1 has dual functions, both as a monocyte chemoattractant in response to cytokine stimulation, and as a mediator of T-cell polarization.

MCP-1 gene expression and protein production are mediated by cytokines. In intestinal cell lines MCP-1 is secreted in response to stimulation with IL-1β or TNF.[283] IL-1β-induced MCP-1 mRNA expression and protein production is potentiated by co-stimulation with IFN-γ and IL-4, but with different kinetics.[284] IL-15 downregulates production of MCP-1 in both intestinal epithelial cell lines and freshly isolated human colonic epithelial cells.[285] However, IL-15 stimulation in monocytes induces monocyte chemotaxis, which in turn is blocked by neutralizing antibodies against MCP-1.[286] MCP-1 secretion can be detected in culture after IL-15 stimulation, and secretion is enhanced by co-stimulation with IFN-γ but inhibited by IL-4. Cytokines can also regulate expression of chemokine receptors on cell surfaces. The MCP-1 receptor CCR2 is expressed on the cell surface of monocyte cell lines, and expression is downregulated by incubation with either TNF or IL-1β.[287] As these two proinflammatory cytokines also stimulate MCP-1 expression and secretion from epithelial cells, chemokine receptors may function as an additional level of chemokine regulation for maintaining tissue homeostasis.

Elevated levels of MCP-1 have been associated with IBD. In the normal intestinal mucosa, MCP-1 mRNA is present in surface epithelial cells. However, in IBD many intestinal cell types have MCP-1 immunoreactivity, including spindle cells, mononuclear cells and endothelial cells. In addition, MCP-1 mRNA levels are elevated in IBD mucosa compared to normal tissue.[288] The number of MCP-1-expressing cells is also increased in the intestinal endothelium and lamina propria of tissues from IBD patients, but not in the intestinal epithelium.[276,288] Moreover, isolated intestinal epithelial cells from IBD patients are capable of inducing monocyte chemotaxis, which is inhibited by anti-MCP-1 antibodies. Facilitating its role as a potent mediator of chemotaxis, MCP-1 is produced by several cell types that surround the intestinal vasculature in IBD patients, including newly recruited infiltrating macrophages, medial smooth muscle cells, intraluminal cells and endothelial cells.[289,290] Based on these studies, it is evident that MCP-1 could represent a logical target for anti-inflammatory therapy and immunomodulation in patients with IBD.

IL-16 is a 56 kDa C-C chemokine originally identified as lymphocyte chemoattractant factor. The protein consists of four non-covalently linked monomers, which are initially synthesized as inactive precursor proteins (pro-IL-16) and cleaved by caspase-3 to form mature, biologically active IL-16 monomers.[291–293] IL-16 is produced primarily by CD8+ T lymphocytes, as well as eosinophils, mast cells and pulmonary epithelial cells.[294,295] With regard to function, IL-16 is a unique proinflammatory chemoattractant involved in T-cell recruitment, growth and proliferation. IL-16 binds to CD4 and subsequently induces migration in CD4+ immune cells, including T cells, macrophages and eosinophils.[296–298] In addition to its chemoattractant properties, IL-16 can also induce expression of IL-2 receptors and MHC class II molecules in target cells, thereby promoting T-cell growth and proliferation.[297,298]

IL-16 has recently been associated with intestinal inflammation in patients with Crohn's disease. In a study by Keates et al., colonic IL-16 protein levels were found to be significantly increased in patients with Crohn's disease, but not in ulcerative colitis.[299] These results were confirmed by Middel et al., who found elevated numbers of IL-16-producing CD4+ lymphocytes in the intestinal mucosa of Crohn's disease but not ulcerative colitis patients or normal controls.[300] A third study has reported elevated levels of IL-16 in the colonic mucosa of both Crohn's disease and ulcerative colitis patients compared to normal controls, but suggests that increased IL-16 production in ulcerative colitis may be limited to areas of active inflammation.[301] Preclinical experiments demonstrate that monoclonal antibody blockade of IL-16 in TNBS-treated mice attenuates colitis, resulting in decreased levels of mucosal ulceration, weight loss and myeloperoxidase activity, as well as reduced mucosal levels of IL-1β and TNF.[299] Thus, IL-16 may also represent a potential target for immunomodulatory therapy in Crohn's disease.

Although MCP-1 and IL-16 are the main C-C chemokines that have been evaluated in relation to IBD, there is some evidence that other C-C chemokines may have a role in IBD pathogenesis. These related C-C chemokines are chemotactic for monocyte, lymphocyte, NK cell, and possibly dendritic cell migration, and include eotaxin, RANTES (regulated on activation, normal T-cell expressed and secreted), MCP-2, MCP-3, macrophage inflammatory protein (MIP)-1α and MIP-1β. [271,273,274,302–304] Eotaxin is produced by epithelial and phagocytic cells and is a potent chemoattractant for eosinophils and basophils, and serum eotaxin concentrations are elevated in patients with Crohn's disease and ulcerative colitis compared to inactive disease and controls.[305,306] Elevated levels of RANTES expression are seen in intestinal epithelial cells and in the subepithelial lamina propria of intestinal mucosal samples obtained from IBD patients compared to normal controls.[289] Freshly isolated intestinal epithelial cells from patients with ulcerative colitis and Crohn's disease also secrete RANTES, MIP-1α and MIP-1β.[6] Finally, colonic biopsies from IBD patients contain an increased number of cells expressing MCP-3 compared to normal tissues. Taken together, these findings suggest a possible role for C-C chemokines in acute as well as chronic inflammation associated with IBD.

## NOVEL INTERLEUKINS

There are currently 29 interleukins officially reported and classified. Six of these – IL-19, IL-20, IL-21, IL-22, IL-24 and IL-26 – are recently described IL-10-related cytokines.[307] Although data indicate that these cytokines are involved in regulation of inflammatory and immune responses and may therefore have relevance to intestinal inflammation, their major functions remain to be elucidated. IL-23 and IL-27 are heterodimeric proinflammatory cytokines with similar activities to IL-12 and involvement with Th1 polarization, making them particularly relevant to IBD, and especially Crohn's disease – a prototypic Th1-mediated disease. Although there are currently no studies in animal models or humans, it is likely that these cytokines play an important role in the pathogenesis of IBD. In fact, an interesting recent paper suggests that IL-23, rather than IL-12, is the critical cytokine for autoimmune inflammation of the brain.[308] These data strongly suggest that IL-23 may be a critical Th1-polarizing cytokine and warrant careful investigation regarding its role in mediating chronic intestinal inflammation.

# REFERENCES

1. Rutgeerts P, D'Haens G et al. Efficacy and safety of retreatment with anti-tumor necrosis factor antibody (infliximab) to maintain remission in Crohn's disease. Gastroenterology 1999;117:761–769.

2. Present DH, Rutgeerts P et al. Infliximab for the treatment of fistulas in patients with Crohn's disease. N Engl J Med 1999;340:1398–1405.

3. Targan SR, Hanauer SB et al. A short-term study of chimeric monoclonal antibody cA2 to tumor necrosis factor α for Crohn's disease. Crohn's Disease cA2 Study Group. N Engl J Med 1997;337:1029–1035.

4. Guy-Grand D, DiSanto JP et al. Small bowel enteropathy: role of intraepithelial lymphocytes and of cytokines (IL-12, IFN-γ, TNF) in the induction of epithelial cell death and renewal. Eur J Immunol 1998;28:730–744.

5. Abreu-Martin MT, Vidrich A et al. Divergent induction of apoptosis and IL-8 secretion in HT-29 cells in response to TNF-a and ligation of Fas antigen. J Immunol 1995;155:4147–4154.

6. Yang SK, Eckmann L et al. Differential and regulated expression of C-X-C, C-C, and C-chemokines by human colon epithelial cells. Gastroenterology 1997;113:1214–1223.

7. Feldmann M, Elliott MJ et al. Anti-tumor necrosis factor–a therapy of rheumatoid arthritis. Adv Immunol 1997;61:283–350.

8. Nilsen EM, Johansen FE et al. Cytokine profiles of cultured microvascular endothelial cells from the human intestine. Gut 1998;42:635–642.

9. Bazzoni F, Beutler B. The tumor necrosis factor ligand and receptor families. N Engl J Med 1996;334:1717–1725.

10. Neurath MF, Fuss I et al. Predominant pathogenic role of tumor necrosis factor in experimental colitis in mice. Eur J Immunol 1997;27:1743–1750.

11. Kontoyiannis D, Pasparakis M et al. Impaired on/off regulation of TNF biosynthesis in mice lacking TNF AU-rich elements: implications for joint and gut-associated immunopathologies. Immunity 1999;10:387–398.

12. Kontoyiannis D, Boulougouris G et al. Genetic dissection of the cellular pathways and signaling mechanisms in modeled tumor necrosis factor-induced Crohn's-like inflammatory bowel disease. J Exp Med 2002;196:1563–1574.

13. Kosiewicz MM, Nast CC et al. Th1-type responses mediate spontaneous ileitis in a novel murine model of Crohn's disease [see comments]. J Clin Invest 2001;107:695–702.

14. Braegger CP, Nicholls S et al. Tumour necrosis factor α in stool as a marker of intestinal inflammation [see comments]. Lancet 1992;339:89–91.

15. Nicholls S, Stephens S et al. Cytokines in stools of children with inflammatory bowel disease or infective diarrhoea. J Clin Pathol 1993;46:757–760.

16. Saiki T, Mitsuyama K et al. Detection of pro- and anti-inflammatory cytokines in stools of patients with inflammatory bowel disease. Scand J Gastroenterol 1998;33:616–622.

17. Dionne S, Hiscott J et al. Quantitative PCR analysis of TNF-α and IL-1 β mRNA levels in pediatric IBD mucosal biopsies. Dig Dis Sci 1997;42:1557–1566.

18. Sands BE, Podolsky DK et al. Chimeric monoclonal anti-tumor necrosis factor antibody (cA2) in the treatment of severe, steroid refractory ulcerative colitis. Gastroenterology 1996;110:A1008.

19. Su C, Salzberg BA et al. Efficacy of anti-tumor necrosis factor therapy in patients with ulcerative colitis. Am J Gastroenterol 2002;97:2577–2584.

20. Chey WY, Hussain A et al. Infliximab for refractory ulcerative colitis. Am J Gastroenterol 2001;96:2373–2381.

21. Probert CJS, Hearing SD et al. Infliximab in steroid-resistant ulcerative colitis: a randomized controlled trial. Gastroenterology 2002;122:A-99.

22. Sandborn WJ, Feagan BG et al. An engineered human antibody to TNF (CDP571) for active Crohn's disease: a randomized double-blind placebo-controlled trial. Gastroenterology 2001;120:1330–1338.

23. Sandborn WJ, Hanauer SB. Antitumor necrosis factor therapy for inflammatory bowel disease: a review of agents, pharmacology, clinical results, and safety. Inflamm Bowel Dis 1999;5:119–133.

24. Kam LY, Targan SR. Cytokine-based therapies in inflammatory bowel disease. Curr Opin Gastroenterol 1999;15:302–307.

25. Sandborn WJ, Hanauer SB et al. Etanercept for active Crohn's disease: a randomized, double-blind, placebo-controlled trial. Gastroenterology 2001;121:1088–94.

26. Van Den Brande JM, Peppelenbosch MP et al. Treating Crohn's disease by inducing T lymphocyte apoptosis. Ann NY Acad Sci 2002;973:166–180.

27. Scallon B, Cai A et al. Binding and functional comparisons of two types of tumor necrosis factor antagonists. J Pharmacol Exp Ther 2002;301:418–426.

28. Ehrenpreis ED, Kane SVI et al. Thalidomide therapy for patients with refractory Crohn's disease: an open-label trial. Gastroenterology 1999;117:1271–1277.

29. Vasiliauskas EA, Kam LY et al. An open-label pilot study of low-dose thalidomide in chronically active, steroid-dependent Crohn's disease. Gastroenterology 1999;117:1278–1287.

30. Stuber E, Strober W et al. Blocking the CD40L–CD40 interaction in vivo specifically prevents the priming of T helper 1 cells through the inhibition of interleukin 12 secretion. J Exp Med 1996;183:693–698.

31. Cong Y, Weaver CT et al. Colitis induced by enteric bacterial antigen-specific CD4+ T cells requires CD40–CD40 ligand interactions for a sustained increase in mucosal IL-12. J Immunol 2000;165:2173–2182.

32. Liu Z, Colpaert S et al. Hyperexpression of CD40 ligand (CD154) in inflammatory bowel disease and its contribution to pathogenic cytokine production. J Immunol 1999;163:4049–4057.

33. Hessle C, Hanson LA et al. Lactobacilli from human gastrointestinal mucosa are strong stimulators of IL-12 production. Clin Exp Immunol 1999;116:276–282.

34. Monteleone G, MacDonald TT et al. Enhancing lamina propria Th1 cell responses with interleukin 12 produces severe tissue injury [see comments]. Gastroenterology 1999;117:1069–1077.

35. Gately MK, Renzetti LM et al. The interleukin-12/interleukin-12-receptor system: role in normal and pathologic immune responses. Annu Rev Immunol 1998;16:495–521.

36. Hans W, Scholmerich J et al. Interleukin-12 induced interferon-γ increases inflammation in acute dextran sulfate sodium induced colitis in mice. Eur Cytokine Netw 2000;11:67–74.

37. Nakamura S, Otani T et al. IFN-γ-dependent and -independent mechanisms in adverse effects caused by concomitant administration of IL-18 and IL-12. J Immunol 2000;164:3330–3336.

38. Neurath MF, Fuss I et al. Antibodies to interleukin 12 abrogate established experimental colitis in mice. J Exp Med 1995;182:1281–1290.

39. Fuss IJ, Marth T et al. Anti-interleukin 12 treatment regulates apoptosis of Th1 T cells in experimental colitis in mice [see comments]. Gastroenterology 1999;117:1078–1088.

40. Davidson NJ, Hudak SA et al. IL-12, but not IFN-γ, plays a major role in sustaining the chronic phase of colitis in IL-10-deficient mice. J Immunol 1998;161:3143–3149.

41. Simpson SJ, Shah S et al. T cell-mediated pathology in two models of experimental colitis depends predominantly on the interleukin 12/signal transducer and activator of transcription (Stat)-4 pathway, but is not conditional on interferon-γ expression by T cells. J Exp Med 1998;187:1225–1234.

42. Spencer DM, Veldman GM et al. Distinct inflammatory mechanisms mediate early versus late colitis in mice. Gastroenterology 2002;122:94–105.

43. Neurath MF, Fuss I et al. Experimental granulomatous colitis in mice is abrogated by induction of TGF-β-mediated oral tolerance. J Exp Med 1996;183:2605–2616.

44. Kitani A, Fuss IJ et al. Treatment of experimental (trinitrobenzene sulfonic acid) colitis by intranasal administration of transforming growth factor (TGF-)-β1 plasmid. TGF-β1-mediated suppression of T helper cell type 1 response occurs by interleukin (IL)-10 induction and IL-12 receptor β2 chain downregulation. J Exp Med 2000;192:41–52.

45. Monteleone G, Biancone L et al. Interleukin 12 is expressed and actively released by Crohn's disease intestinal lamina propria mononuclear cells. Gastroenterology 1997;112:1169–1178.

46. Braun MC, Lahey E et al. Selective suppression of IL-12 production by chemoattractants. J Immunol 2000;164:3009–3017.

47. Monteleone G, Parrello T et al. Interferon-γ (IFN-γ) and prostaglandin E₂ (PGE₂) regulate differently IL-12 production in human intestinal lamina propria mononuclear cells (LPMC). Clin Exp Immunol 1999;117:469-475.

48. Okamura H, Nagata K et al. A novel costimulatory factor for γ interferon induction found in the livers of mice causes endotoxic shock. Infect Immun 1995;63:3966–3972.

49. Bazan JF, Timans JC et al. A newly defined interleukin-1? [letter; comment]. Nature 1996;379:591.

50. Gu Y, Kuida K et al. Activation of interferon-γ inducing factor mediated by interleukin-1β converting enzyme. Science 1997;275:206–209.

51. Torigoe K, Ushio S et al. Purification and characterization of the human interleukin-18 receptor. J Biol Chem 1997;272:25737–25742.

52. Dinarello CA, Novick D et al. Overview of interleukin-18: more than an interferon-γ inducing factor. J Leukocyte Biol 1998;63:658–664.

53. Puren AJ, Fantuzzi G et al. Interleukin-18 (IFN-γ-inducing factor) induces IL-8 and IL-1β via TNFα production from non-CD14+ human blood mononuclear cells. J Clin Invest 1998;101:711–721.

54. Matsumoto S, Tsuji-Takayama K et al. Interleukin-18 activates NF-κB in murine T helper type 1 cells. Biochem Biophys Res Commun 1997;234:454–457.

55. Dao T, Ohashi K et al. Interferon-γ-inducing factor, a novel cytokine, enhances Fas ligand-mediated cytotoxicity of murine T helper 1 cells. Cell Immunol 1996;173:230–235.

56. Matsui K, Yoshimoto T et al. Propionibacterium acnes treatment diminishes CD4+ NK1.1 + T cells but induces type 1 T cells in the liver by induction of IL-12 and IL-18 production from Kupffer cells. J Immunol 1997;159:97–106.

57. Micallef MJ, Ohtsuki T et al. Interferon-γ-inducing factor enhances T helper 1 cytokine production by stimulated human T cells: synergism with interleukin-12 for interferon-γ production. Eur J Immunol 1996;26:1647–1651.

58. Pizarro TT, Michie MH et al. IL-18, a novel immunoregulatory cytokine, is upregulated in Crohn's disease: expression and localization in intestinal mucosal cells. J Immunol 1999;162:6829–6835.

59. Monteleone G, Trapasso F et al. Bioactive IL-18 expression is upregulated in Crohn's disease. J Immunol 1999;163:143–147.

60. Corbaz A, ten Hove T et al. IL-18-binding protein expression by endothelial cells and macrophages is upregulated during active Crohn's disease. J Immunol 2002;168:3608–3616.

61. Kanai T, Watanabe M et al. Interleukin-18 and Crohn's disease. Digestion 2001;63 Suppl 1:37–42.

62. Chikano S, Sawada K et al. IL-18 and IL-12 induce intestinal inflammation and fatty liver in mice in an IFN-γ dependent manner. Gut 2000;47:779–786.

63. Sivakumar PV, Westrich GM et al. Interleukin 18 is a primary mediator of the inflammation associated with dextran sulphate sodium induced colitis: blocking interleukin 18 attenuates intestinal damage. Gut 2002;50:812–820.

64. Siegmund B, Fantuzzi G et al. Neutralization of interleukin-18 reduces severity in murine colitis and intestinal IFN-γ and TNF-α production. Am J Physiol Regul Integr Comp Physiol 2001;281:R1264–1273.

65. Ten Hove T, Corbaz A et al. Blockade of endogenous IL-18 ameliorates TNBS-induced colitis by decreasing local TNF-α production in mice. Gastroenterology 2001;121:1372–1379.

66. Bregenholt S, Brimnes J et al. In vitro activated CD4+ T cells from interferon-γ (IFN-γ)-deficient mice induce intestinal inflammation in immunodeficient hosts. Clin Exp Immunol 1999;118:228–234.

67. Powrie F, Leach MW et al. Inhibition of Th1 responses prevents inflammatory bowel disease in scid mice reconstituted with CD45RBhi CD4+ T cells. Immunity 1994;1:553–562.

68. Niessner M, Volk BA. Altered Th1/Th2 cytokine profiles in the intestinal mucosa of patients with inflammatory bowel disease as assessed by quantitative reversed transcribed polymerase chain reaction (RT-PCR). Clin Exp Immunol 1995;101:428–435.

69. Noguchi M, Hiwatashi N et al. Enhanced interferon-γ production and B7-2 expression in isolated intestinal mononuclear cells from patients with Crohn's disease. J Gastroenterol 1995;30 Suppl 8:52–55.

70. Murata Y, Ishiguro Y et al. The role of proinflammatory and immunoregulatory cytokines in the pathogenesis of ulcerative colitis. J Gastroenterol 1995;30 (Suppl) 8:56–60.

71. Breese E, Braegger CP et al. Interleukin-2- and interferon-γ-secreting T cells in normal and diseased human intestinal mucosa. Immunology 1993;78:127–131.

72. Akagi S, Hiyama E et al. Interleukin-10 expression in intestine of Crohn disease. Int J Mol Med 2000;5:389–395.

73. Parronchi P, Romagnani P et al. Type 1 T-helper cell predominance and interleukin-12 expression in the gut of patients with Crohn's disease. Am J Pathol 1997;150:823–832.

74. Fuss IJ, Neurath M et al. Disparate CD4+ lamina propria (LP) lymphokine secretion profiles in inflammatory bowel disease. Crohn's disease LP cells manifest increased secretion of IFN-γ, whereas ulcerative colitis LP cells manifest increased secretion of IL-5. J Immunol 1996;157:1261–1270.

75. Fais S, Capobianchi MR et al. Interferon expression in Crohn's disease patients: increased interferon-γ and -α mRNA in the intestinal lamina propria mononuclear cells. J Interferon Res 1994;14:235–238.

76. Desreumaux P, Brandt E et al. Distinct cytokine patterns in early and chronic ileal lesions of Crohn's disease. Gastroenterology 1997;113:118–126.

77. Fujihashi K, Kawabata S et al. Interleukin 2 (IL-2) and interleukin 7 (IL-7) reciprocally induce IL-7 and IL-2 receptors on γ delta T-cell receptor-positive intraepithelial lymphocytes. Proc Natl Acad Sci USA 1996;93:3613–3618.

78. Chu CL, Chen SS et al. Differential effects of IL-2 and IL-15 on the death and survival of activated TCR γ delta+ intestinal intraepithelial lymphocytes. J Immunol 1999;162:1896–1903.

79. Porter BO, Malek TR. IL-2Rβ/IL-7Rα doubly deficient mice recapitulate the thymic and intraepithelial lymphocyte (IEL) developmental defects of γc-/- mice: roles for both IL-2 and IL-15 in CD8αα IEL development. J Immunol 1999;163:5906–5912.

80. Ciacci C, Mahida YR et al. Functional interleukin-2 receptors on intestinal epithelial cells. J Clin Invest 1993;92:527–532.

81. Reinecker HC, Podolsky DK. Human intestinal epithelial cells express functional cytokine receptors sharing the common γ c chain of the interleukin 2 receptor. Proc Natl Acad Sci USA 1995;92:8353–8357.

82. Dignass AU, Podolsky DK. Interleukin 2 modulates intestinal epithelial cell function in vitro. Exp Cell Res 1996;225:422–429.

83. Simpson SJ, Mizoguchi E et al. Evidence that CD4+, but not CD8+ T cells are responsible for murine interleukin-2-deficient colitis. Eur J Immunol 1995;25:2618–2625.

84. Ma A, Datta M et al. T cells, but not B cells, are required for bowel inflammation in interleukin 2-deficient mice. J Exp Med 1995;182:1567–1572.

85. Ehrhardt RO, Ludviksson BR et al. Induction and prevention of colonic inflammation in IL-2-deficient mice. J Immunol 1997;158:566–573.

86. Autenrieth IB, Bucheler N et al. Cytokine mRNA expression in intestinal tissue of interleukin-2 deficient mice with bowel inflammation. Gut 1997;41:793–800.

87. Yang F, de Villiers WJ et al. Increased nuclear factor-κB activation in colitis of interleukin-2-deficient mice. J Lab Clin Med 1999;134:378–385.

88. Harren M, Schonfelder G et al. High expression of inducible nitric oxide synthase correlates with intestinal inflammation of interleukin-2-deficient mice. Ann NY Acad Sci 1998;859:210–215.

89. Schultz M, Tonkonogy SL et al. IL-2-deficient mice raised under germfree conditions develop delayed mild focal intestinal inflammation. Am J Physiol 1999;276:G1461–1472.

90. Contractor NV, Bassiri H et al. Lymphoid hyperplasia, autoimmunity, and compromised intestinal intraepithelial lymphocyte development in colitis-free gnotobiotic IL-2-deficient mice. J Immunol 1998;160:385–394.

91. Mullin GE, Lazenby AJ et al. Increased interleukin-2 messenger RNA in the intestinal mucosal lesions of Crohn's disease but not ulcerative colitis. Gastroenterology 1992;102:1620–1627.

92. Brynskov J, Tvede N. Plasma interleukin-2 and a soluble/shed interleukin-2 receptor in serum of patients with Crohn's disease. Effect of cyclosporin. Gut 1990;31:795–799.

93. Breese EJ, Michie CA et al. The effect of treatment on lymphokine-secreting cells in the intestinal mucosa of children with Crohn's disease. Aliment Pharmacol Ther 1995;9:547–552.

94. van Dijk AP, Meijssen MA et al. Transdermal nicotine inhibits interleukin 2 synthesis by mononuclear cells derived from healthy volunteers. Eur J Clin Invest 1998;28:664–671.

95. Elsasser-Beile U, von Kleist S et al. Cytokine production in whole blood cell cultures of patients with Crohn's disease and ulcerative colitis. J Clin Lab Anal 1994;8:447–451.

96. Stallmach A, Wittig B et al. Protection of trinitrobenzene sulfonic acid-induced colitis by an interleukin 2-IgG2b fusion protein in mice. Gastroenterology 1999;117:866–876.

97. Van Assche G, Dalle I et al. A pilot study on the use of the humanized anti-interleukin-2 receptor antibody daclizumab in active ulcerative colitis. Am J Gastroenterol 2003;98:369–376.

98. Gramaglia I, Mauri DN et al. Lymphotoxin αβ is expressed on recently activated naive and Th1-like CD4 cells but is downregulated by IL-4 during Th2 differentiation. J Immunol 1999;162:1333–1338.

99. Neumann B, Luz A et al. Defective Peyer's patch organogenesis in mice lacking the 55-kD receptor for tumor necrosis factor. J Exp Med 1996;184:259–264.

100. Alexopoulou L, Pasparakis M et al. Complementation of lymphotoxin α knockout mice with tumor necrosis factor-expressing transgenes rectifies defective splenic structure and function. J Exp Med 1998;188:745–754.

101. Koni PA, Sacca R et al. Distinct roles in lymphoid organogenesis for lymphotoxins α and β revealed in lymphotoxin β-deficient mice. Immunity 1997;6:491–500.

102. Futterer A, Mink K et al. The lymphotoxin β receptor controls organogenesis and affinity maturation in peripheral lymphoid tissues. Immunity 1998;9:59–70.

103. Cuff CA, Schwartz J et al. Lymphotoxin α3 induces chemokines and adhesion molecules: insight into the role of LT α in inflammation and lymphoid organ development. J Immunol 1998;161:6853–6860.

104. Cuff CA, Sacca R et al. Differential induction of adhesion molecule and chemokine expression by LTα3 and LTαβ in inflammation elucidates potential mechanisms of mesenteric and peripheral lymph node development. J Immunol 1999;162:5965–5972.

105. Mackay F, Browning JL et al. Both the lymphotoxin and tumor necrosis factor pathways are involved in experimental murine models of colitis. Gastroenterology 1998;115:1464–1475.

106. Chang TL, Peng X et al. Interleukin-4 mediates cell growth inhibition through activation of Stat1. J Biol Chem 2000;275:10212–10217.

107. Kucharzik T, Lugering N et al. IL-4, IL-10 and IL-13 downregulate monocyte-chemoattracting protein-1 (MCP-1) production in activated intestinal epithelial cells. Clin Exp Immunol 1998;111:152–157.

108. Kolios G, Robertson DA et al. Interleukin-8 production by the human colon epithelial cell line HT-29: modulation by interleukin-13. Br J Pharmacol 1996;119:351–359.

109. Kolios G, Wright KL et al. C-X-C and C-C chemokine expression and secretion by the human colonic epithelial cell line, HT-29: differential effect of T lymphocyte-derived cytokines. Eur J Immunol 1999;29:530–536.

110. Kolios G, Rooney N et al. Expression of inducible nitric oxide synthase activity in human colon epithelial cells: modulation by T lymphocyte derived cytokines. Gut 1998;43:56–63.

111. Lugering N, Kucharzik T et al. Interleukin (IL)-13 and IL-4 are potent inhibitors of IL-8 secretion by human intestinal epithelial cells. Dig Dis Sci 1999;44:649–655.

112. Zund G, Madara JL et al. Interleukin-4 and interleukin-13 differentially regulate epithelial chloride secretion. J Biol Chem 1996;271:7460–7464.

113. Lugering N, Kucharzik T et al. IL-10 synergizes with IL-4 and IL-13 in inhibiting lysosomal enzyme secretion by human monocytes and lamina propria mononuclear cells from patients with inflammatory bowel disease. Dig Dis Sci 1998;43:706–714.

114. Kucharzik T, Lugering N et al. Immunoregulatory properties of IL-13 in patients with inflammatory bowel disease; comparison with IL-4 and IL-10. Clin Exp Immunol 1996;104:483–490.

115. Kucharzik T, Lugering N et al. Synergistic effect of immunoregulatory cytokines on peripheral blood monocytes from patients with inflammatory bowel disease. Dig Dis Sci 1997;42:805–812.

116. West GA, Matsuura T et al. Interleukin 4 in inflammatory bowel disease and mucosal immune reactivity. Gastroenterology 1996;110:1683–1695.

117. Karttunnen R, Breese EJ et al. Decreased mucosal interleukin-4 (IL-4) production in gut inflammation. J Clin Pathol 1994;47:1015–1018.

118. Schmit A, Van Gossum A et al. Diversion of intestinal flow decreases the numbers of interleukin 4 secreting and interferon γ secreting T lymphocytes in small bowel mucosa. Gut 2000;46:40–45.

119. Schreiber S, Heinig T et al. Impaired response of activated mononuclear phagocytes to interleukin 4 in inflammatory bowel disease [see comments]. Gastroenterology 1995;108:21–33.

120. Nielsen OH, Koppen T et al. Involvement of interleukin-4 and -10 in inflammatory bowel disease. Dig Dis Sci 1996;41:1786–1793.

121. Hogaboam CM, Vallance BA et al. Therapeutic effects of interleukin-4 gene transfer in experimental inflammatory bowel disease. J Clin Invest 1997;100:2766–2776.

122. Chomarat P, Banchereau J. Interleukin-4 and interleukin-13: their similarities and discrepancies. Int Rev Immunol 1998;17:1–52.

123. Dohi T, Fujihashi K et al. Hapten-induced colitis is associated with colonic patch hypertrophy and T helper cell 2-type responses. J Exp Med 1999;189:1169–1180.

124. Boirivant M, Fuss IJ et al. Oxazolone colitis: A murine model of T helper cell type 2 colitis treatable with antibodies to interleukin 4. J Exp Med 1998;188:1929–1939.

125. Heller F, Fuss IJ et al. Oxazolone colitis, a Th2 colitis model resembling ulcerative colitis, is mediated by IL-13-producing NK-T cells. Immunity 2002;17:629–638.

126. Groux H, O'Garra A et al. A CD4+ T-cell subset inhibits antigen-specific T-cell responses and prevents colitis. Nature 1997;389:737–742.

127. Asseman C, Powrie F. Interleukin 10 is a growth factor for a population of regulatory T cells. Gut 1998;42:157–158.

128. Moore KW, O'Garra A et al. Interleukin-10. Annu Rev Immunol 1993;11:165–190.

129. de Vries JE. Immunosuppressive and anti-inflammatory properties of interleukin 10. Ann Med 1995;27:537–541.

130. Ebert EC. IL-10 enhances IL-2-induced proliferation and cytotoxicity by human intestinal lymphocytes. Clin Exp Immunol 2000;119:426–432.

131. Kuhn R, Lohler J et al. Interleukin-10-deficient mice develop chronic enterocolitis [see comments]. Cell 1993;75:263–274.

132. Berg DJ, Davidson N et al. Enterocolitis and colon cancer in interleukin-10-deficient mice are associated with aberrant cytokine production and CD4(+) TH1-like responses. J Clin Invest 1996;98:1010–1020.

133. Kawachi S, Jennings S et al. Cytokine and endothelial cell adhesion molecule expression in interleukin-10-deficient mice. Am J Physiol Gastrointest Liver Physiol 2000;278:G734–743.

134. Davidson NJ, Leach MW et al. T helper cell 1-type CD4+ T cells, but not B cells, mediate colitis in interleukin 10-deficient mice. J Exp Med 1996;184:241–251.

135. Sellon RK, Tonkonogy S et al. Resident enteric bacteria are necessary for development of spontaneous colitis and immune system activation in interleukin-10-deficient mice. Infect Immun 1998;66:5224–5231.

136. Madsen KL, Doyle JS et al. Antibiotic therapy attenuates colitis in interleukin 10 gene-deficient mice. Gastroenterology 2000;118:1094–1105.

137. Madsen KL, Malfair D et al. Interleukin-10 gene-deficient mice develop a primary intestinal permeability defect in response to enteric microflora. Inflamm Bowel Dis 1999;5:262–270.

138. Kullberg MC, Ward JM et al. Helicobacter hepaticus triggers colitis in specific-pathogen-free interleukin-10 (IL-10)-deficient mice through an IL-12- and γ interferon-dependent mechanism. Infect Immun 1998;66:5157–5166.

139. Fox JG, Gorelick PL et al. A novel urease-negative Helicobacter species associated with colitis and typhlitis in IL-10-deficient mice. Infect Immun 1999;67:1757–1762.

140. Madsen KL, Doyle JS et al. Lactobacillus species prevents colitis in interleukin 10 gene-deficient mice [see comments]. Gastroenterology 1999;116:1107–1114.

141. Madsen KL. Inflammatory bowel disease: lessons from the IL-10 gene-deficient mouse. Clin Invest Med 2001;24:250–257.

142. Autschbach F, Braunstein J et al. In situ expression of interleukin-10 in noninflamed human gut and in inflammatory bowel disease. Am J Pathol 1998;153:121–130.

143. Grool TA, van Dullemen H et al. Anti-inflammatory effect of interleukin-10 in rabbit immune complex-induced colitis. Scand J Gastroenterol 1998;33:754–758.

144. Tomoyose M, Mitsuyama K et al. Role of interleukin-10 in a murine model of dextran sulfate sodium-induced colitis. Scand J Gastroenterol 1998;33:435–440.

145. De Winter H, Elewaut D et al. Regulation of mucosal immune responses by recombinant interleukin 10 produced by intestinal epithelial cells in mice. Gastroenterology 2002;122:1829–1841.

146. van Deventer SJ, Elson CO et al. Multiple doses of intravenous interleukin 10 in steroid-refractory Crohn's disease. Crohn's Disease Study Group. Gastroenterology 1997;113:383–389.

147. Schreiber S, Fedorak RN et al. Safety and efficacy of recombinant human interleukin 10 in chronic active Crohn's disease. Gastroenterology 2000;119:1461–1472.

148. Fedorak RN, Gangl A et al. Recombinant human interleukin 10 in the treatment of patients with mild to moderately active Crohn's disease. Gastroenterology 2000;119:1473–1482.

149. Bickston SJ, Cominelli F. Recombinant interleukin 10 for the treatment of active Crohn's disease: lessons in biologic therapy. Gastroenterology 2000;119:1781–1783.

150. Migdalska A, Molineux G et al. Growth inhibitory effects of transforming growth factor-β1 in vivo. Growth Factors 1991;4:239–245.

151. Dignass AU, Podolsky DK. Cytokine modulation of intestinal epithelial cell restitution: central role of transforming growth factor β. Gastroenterology 1993;105:1323–1332.

152. Booth C, Evans GS et al. Growth factor regulation of proliferation in primary cultures of small intestinal epithelium. In Vitro Cell Dev Biol Anim 1995;31:234–243.

153. Ebert EC. Inhibitory effects of transforming growth factor-β (TGF-β) on certain functions of intraepithelial lymphocytes. Clin Exp Immunol 1999;115:415–420.

154. Planchon S, Fiocchi C et al. Transforming growth factor-β1 preserves epithelial barrier function: identification of receptors, biochemical intermediates, and cytokine antagonists. J Cell Physiol 1999;181:55–66.

155. McGee DW, Bamberg T et al. A synergistic relationship between TNF-α, IL-1 β, and TGF-β 1 on IL-6 secretion by the IEC-6 intestinal epithelial cell line. Immunology 1995;86:6–11.

156. Mourelle M, Salas A et al. Stimulation of transforming growth factor β1 by enteric bacteria in the pathogenesis of rat intestinal fibrosis. Gastroenterology 1998;114:519–526.

157. van Ginkel FW, Wahl SM et al. Partial IgA-deficiency with increased Th2-type cytokines in TGF-β 1 knockout mice. J Immunol 1999;163:1951–1957.

158. Barnard JA, Warwick GJ et al. Localization of transforming growth factor β isoforms in the normal murine small intestine and colon. Gastroenterology 1993;105:67–73.

159. Meijssen MA, Brandwein SL et al. Alteration of gene expression by intestinal epithelial cells precedes colitis in interleukin-2-deficient mice. Am J Physiol 1998;274:G472–479.

160. Strober W, Kelsall B et al. Reciprocal IFN-γ and TGF-β responses regulate the occurrence of mucosal inflammation. Immunol Today 1997;18:61–64.

161. Ludviksson BR, Ehrhardt RO et al. TGF-β production regulates the development of the 2,4,6-trinitrophenol-conjugated keyhole limpet hemocyanin-induced colonic inflammation in IL-2-deficient mice. J Immunol 1997;159:3622–3628.

162. Neurath MF, Weigmann B et al. The transcription factor T-bet regulates mucosal T cell activation in experimental colitis and Crohn's disease. J Exp Med 2002;195:1129–1143.

163. Asseman C, Mauze S et al. An essential role for interleukin 10 in the function of regulatory T cells that inhibit intestinal inflammation. J Exp Med 1999;190:995–1004.

164. Powrie F, Carlino J et al. A critical role for transforming growth factor-β but not interleukin 4 in the suppression of T helper type 1-mediated colitis by CD45RB(low) CD4+ T cells. J Exp Med 1996;183:2669–2674.

165. Fuss IJ, Boirivant M et al. The interrelated roles of TGF-β and IL-10 in the regulation of experimental colitis. J Immunol 2002;168:900–908.

166. Giladi E, Raz E et al. Transforming growth factor-β gene therapy ameliorates experimental colitis in rats. Eur J Gastroenterol Hepatol 1995;7:341–347.

167. Babyatsky MW, Rossiter G et al. Expression of transforming growth factors α and β in colonic mucosa in inflammatory bowel disease. Gastroenterology 1996;110:975–984.

168. Xian CJ, Xu X et al. Site-specific changes in transforming growth factor-α and -β1 expression in colonic mucosa of adolescents with inflammatory bowel disease. Scand J Gastroenterol 1999;34:591–600.

169. Ohtani H, Kagaya H et al. Immunohistochemical localization of transforming growth factor-β receptors I and II in inflammatory bowel disease. J Gastroenterol 1995;30 (Suppl 8):76–77.

170. Friess H, di Mola FF et al. [Transforming growth factor-β controls pathogenesis of Crohn disease]. Langenbecks Arch Chir Suppl Kongressbd 1998;115:994–997.

171. Chowdhury A, Fukuda R et al. Growth factor mRNA expression in normal colorectal mucosa and in uninvolved mucosa from ulcerative colitis patients. J Gastroenterol 1996;31:353–360.

172. Monteleone G, Kumberova A et al. Blocking Smad7 restores TGF-β1 signaling in chronic inflammatory bowel disease. J Clin Invest 2001;108:601–609.

173. Dinarello CA. Interleukin-1 and interleukin-1 antagonism. Blood 1991;77:1627–1652.

174. Youngman KR, Simon PL et al. Localization of intestinal interleukin 1 activity and protein and gene expression to lamina propria cells. Gastroenterology 1993;104:749–758.

175. Dinarello CA, Wolff SM. The role of interleukin-1 in disease. N Engl J Med 1993;328:106–113.

176. Cominelli F, Nast CC et al. Regulation of eicosanoid production by interleukin-1 in normal rabbit colon. Gastroenterology 1989;97:1400–1405.

177. Cominelli F, Nast CC et al. Interleukin 1 (IL-1) gene expression, synthesis, and effect of specific IL-1 receptor blockade in rabbit immune complex colitis. J Clin Invest 1990;86:972–980.

178. Cominelli F, Nast CC et al. Recombinant interleukin-1 receptor antagonist blocks the proinflammatory activity of endogenous interleukin-1 in rabbit immune colitis. Gastroenterology 1992;103:65–71.

179. McCall RD, Haskill S et al. Tissue interleukin 1 and interleukin-1 receptor antagonist expression in enterocolitis in resistant and susceptible rats. Gastroenterology 1994;106:960–972.

180. Thomas TK, Will PC et al. Evaluation of an interleukin-1 receptor antagonist in the rat acetic acid-induced colitis model. Agents Actions 1991;34:187–190.

181. Ligumsky M, Simon PL et al. Role of interleukin 1 in inflammatory bowel disease-enhanced production during active disease. Gut 1990;31:686–689.

182. Kern JA, Lamb RJ et al. Dexamethasone inhibition of interleukin 1 β production by human monocytes. Posttranscriptional mechanisms. J Clin Invest 1988;81:237–244.

183. Satsangi J, Wolstencroft RA et al. Interleukin 1 in Crohn's disease. Clin Exp Immunol 1987;67:594–605.

184. Mazlam MZ, Hodgson HJ. Interrelations between interleukin-6, interleukin-1 β, plasma C-reactive protein values, and in vitro C-reactive protein generation in patients with inflammatory bowel disease. Gut 1994;35:77–83.

185. Mahida YR, Wu K et al. Enhanced production of interleukin 1-β by mononuclear cells isolated from mucosa with active ulcerative colitis of Crohn's disease. Gut 1989;30:835–838.

186. Arend WP. Interleukin-1 receptor antagonist. Adv Immunol 1993;54:167–227.

187. Arend WP, Malyak M et al. Binding of IL-1 α, IL-1 β, and IL-1 receptor antagonist by soluble IL-1 receptors and levels of soluble IL-1 receptors in synovial fluids. J Immunol 1994;153:4766–4774.

188. Balavoine JF, de Rochemonteix B et al. Prostaglandin E2 and collagenase production by fibroblasts and synovial cells is regulated by urine-derived human interleukin 1 and inhibitor(s). J Clin Invest 1986;78:1120–1124.

189. Casini-Raggi V, Kam L et al. Mucosal imbalance of IL-1 and IL-1 receptor antagonist in inflammatory bowel disease. A novel mechanism of chronic intestinal inflammation. J Immunol 1995;154:2434–2440.

190. Andus T, Daig R et al. Imbalance of the interleukin 1 system in colonic mucosa-association with intestinal inflammation and interleukin 1 receptor antagonist [corrected] genotype 2. Gut 1997;41:651–657.

191. Issacs KL, Sartor RB et al. Cytokine messenger RNA profiles in inflammatory bowel disease mucosa detected by polymerase chain reaction amplification. Gastroenterology 1992;103:1567–1595.

192. Mansfield JC, Holden H et al. Novel genetic association between ulcerative colitis and the anti-inflammatory cytokine interleukin-1 receptor antagonist. Gastroenterology 1994;106:637–642.

193. Tountas NA, Casini-Raggi V et al. Functional and ethnic association of allele 2 of the interleukin-1 receptor antagonist gene in ulcerative colitis. Gastroenterology 1999;117:806–813.

194. Hacker UT, Gomolka M et al. Lack of association between an interleukin-1 receptor antagonist gene polymorphism and ulcerative colitis. Gut 1997;40:623–627.

195. Gonzalez Sarmiento R, Araoz P et al. [Polymorphism of the IL1RN gene in Spanish patients with ulcerative colitis]. Med Clin (Barc) 1999;112:778–779.

196. Carter MJ, di Giovine FS et al. Association of the interleukin 1 receptor antagonist gene with ulcerative colitis in Northern European Caucasians. Gut 2001;48:461–467.

197. Carter MJ, Di Giovine FS et al. The interleukin 1 receptor antagonist gene allele 2 as a predictor of pouchitis following colectomy and IPAA in ulcerative colitis. Gastroenterology 2001;121:805–811.

198. Ward LD, Hammacher A et al. Influence of interleukin-6 (IL-6) dimerization on formation of the high affinity hexameric IL-6.receptor complex. J Biol Chem 1996;271:20138–20144.

199. Panja A, Goldberg S et al. The regulation and functional consequence of proinflammatory cytokine binding on human intestinal epithelial cells. J Immunol 1998;161:3675–3684.

200. Molmenti EP, Ziambaras T et al. Evidence for an acute phase response in human intestinal epithelial cells. J Biol Chem 1993;268:14116–14124.

201. McGee DW, Beagley KW et al. Transforming growth factor-β enhances interleukin-6 secretion by intestinal epithelial cells. Immunology 1992;77:7–12.

202. McGee DW, Beagley KW et al. Transforming growth factor-β and IL-1 β act in synergy to enhance IL-6 secretion by the intestinal epithelial cell line, IEC-6. J Immunol 1993;151:970–978.

203. Parikh AA, Moon MR et al. Interleukin-6 production in human intestinal epithelial cells increases in association with the heat shock response. J Surg Res 1998;77:40–44.

204. Parikh AA, Salzman AL et al. Interleukin-1 β and interferon-γ regulate interleukin-6 production in cultured human intestinal epithelial cells. Shock 1997;8:249–255.

205. Ishimura K, Tsubouchi T et al. Wound healing of intestinal anastomosis after digestive surgery under septic conditions: participation of local interleukin-6 expression [see comments]. World J Surg 1998;22:1069–1075; discussion 1076.

206. Strong SA, Pizarro TT et al. Proinflammatory cytokines differentially modulate their own expression in human intestinal mucosal mesenchymal cells. Gastroenterology 1998;114:1244–1256.

207. Swank GM, Lu Q et al. Effect of acute-phase and heat-shock stress on apoptosis in intestinal epithelial cells (Caco-2). Crit Care Med 1998;26:1213–1217.

208. Bromander AK, Ekman L et al. IL-6-deficient mice exhibit normal mucosal IgA responses to local immunizations and Helicobacter felis infection. J Immunol 1996;156:4290–4297.

209. Ramsay AJ, Husband AJ et al. The role of interleukin-6 in mucosal IgA antibody responses in vivo. Science 1994;264:561–563.

210. Bao S, Beagley KW et al. Exogenous IL-6 promotes enhanced intestinal antibody responses in vivo. Immunol Cell Biol 1998;76:560–562.

211. Bao S, Husband AJ et al. B1 B cell numbers and antibodies against phosphorylcholine and LPS are increased in IL-6 gene knockout mice. Cell Immunol 1999;198:139–142.

212. Jones SC, Trejdosiewicz LK et al. Expression of interleukin-6 by intestinal enterocytes. J Clin Pathol 1993;46:1097–1100.

213. Kusugami K, Fukatsu A et al. Elevation of interleukin-6 in inflammatory bowel disease is macrophage- and epithelial cell-dependent. Dig Dis Sci 1995;40:949–959.

214. Stevens C, Walz G et al. Tumor necrosis factor-α, interleukin-1 β, and interleukin-6 expression in inflammatory bowel disease. Dig Dis Sci 1992;37:818–826.

215. Reinecker HC, Steffen M et al. Enhanced secretion of tumour necrosis factor-α, IL-6, and IL-1β by isolated lamina propria mononuclear cells from patients with ulcerative colitis and Crohn's disease. Clin Exp Immunol 1993;94:174–181.

216. Daig R, Rogler G et al. Human intestinal epithelial cells secrete interleukin-1 receptor antagonist and interleukin-8 but not interleukin-1 or interleukin-6. Gut 2000;46:350–358.

217. Grottrup-Wolfers E, Moeller J et al. Elevated cell-associated levels of interleukin 1β and interleukin 6 in inflamed mucosa of inflammatory bowel disease. Eur J Clin Invest 1996;26:115–122.

218. Reimund JM, Wittersheim C et al. Increased production of tumour necrosis factor-α interleukin-1β, and interleukin-6 by morphologically normal intestinal biopsies from patients with Crohn's disease. Gut 1996;39:684–689.

219. Hyams JS, Fitzgerald JE et al. Relationship of functional and antigenic interleukin 6 to disease activity in inflammatory bowel disease. Gastroenterology 1993;104:1285–1292.

220. Gross V, Andus T et al. Evidence for continuous stimulation of interleukin-6 production in Crohn's disease [see comments]. Gastroenterology 1992;102:514–519.

221. Mitsuyama K, Toyonaga A et al. Soluble interleukin-6 receptors in inflammatory bowel disease: relation to circulating interleukin-6. Gut 1995;36:45–49.

222. Dieleman LA, Elson CO et al. Kinetics of cytokine expression during healing of acute colitis in mice. Am J Physiol 1996;271:G130–136.

223. Yamamoto M, Yoshizaki K et al. IL-6 is required for the development of Th1 cell-mediated murine colitis. J Immunol 2000;164:4878–4882.

224. Atreya R, Mudter J et al. Blockade of interleukin 6 trans signaling suppresses T-cell resistance against apoptosis in chronic intestinal inflammation: evidence in Crohn disease and experimental colitis in vivo. Nature Med 2000;6:583–588.

225. Maki K, Sunaga S et al. Interleukin 7 receptor-deficient mice lack γδ T cells. Proc Natl Acad Sci USA 1996;93:7172–7177.

226. Fujihashi K, McGhee JR et al. An interleukin-7 internet for intestinal intraepithelial T cell development: knockout of ligand or receptor reveal differences in the immunodeficient state. Eur J Immunol 1997;27:2133–2138.

227. Laky K, Lefrancois L et al. The role of IL-7 in thymic and extrathymic development of TCR γδ cells. J Immunol 1998;161:707–713.

228. Laky K, Lefrancois L et al. Enterocyte expression of interleukin 7 induces development of γδ T cells and Peyer's patches. J Exp Med 2000;191:1569–1580.

229. von Freeden-Jeffry U, Davidson N et al. IL-7 deficiency prevents development of a non-T cell non-B cell-mediated colitis. J Immunol 1998;161:5673–5680.

230. Watanabe M, Ueno Y et al. Interleukin 7 transgenic mice develop chronic colitis with decreased interleukin 7 protein accumulation in the colonic mucosa. J Exp Med 1998;187:389–402.

231. Kirman I, Vainer B et al. Interleukin-15 and its role in chronic inflammatory diseases. Inflamm Res 1998;47:285–289.

232. Inagaki-Ohara K, Nishimura H et al. Interleukin-15 preferentially promotes the growth of intestinal intraepithelial lymphocytes bearing γδ T cell receptor in mice. Eur J Immunol 1997;27:2885–2891.

233. Lai YG, Gelfanov V et al. IL-15 promotes survival but not effector function differentiation of CD8+ TCRαβ+ intestinal intraepithelial lymphocytes. J Immunol 1999;163:5843–5850.

234. Kennedy MK, Glaccum M et al. Reversible defects in natural killer and memory CD8 T cell lineages in interleukin 15-deficient mice [see comments]. J Exp Med 2000;191:771–780.

235. Sakai T, Kusugami K et al. Interleukin 15 activity in the rectal mucosa of inflammatory bowel disease. Gastroenterology 1998;114:1237–1243.

236. Liu Z, Geboes K et al. IL-15 is highly expressed in inflammatory bowel disease and regulates local T cell-dependent cytokine production. J Immunol 2000;164:3608–3615.

237. Schwertschlag US, Trepicchio WL et al. Hematopoietic, immunomodulatory and epithelial effects of interleukin-11. Leukemia 1999;13:1307–1315.

238. Leng SX, Elias JA. Interleukin-11. Int J Biochem Cell Biol 1997;29:1059–1062.

239. Orazi A, Du X et al. Interleukin-11 prevents apoptosis and accelerates recovery of small intestinal mucosa in mice treated with combined chemotherapy and radiation. Lab Invest 1996;75:33–42.

240. Tang W, Yang L et al. Transforming growth factor-β stimulates interleukin-11 transcription via complex activating protein-1-dependent pathways. J Biol Chem 1998;273:5506–5513.

241. Hill GR, Cooke KR et al. Interleukin-11 promotes T cell polarization and prevents acute graft-versus-host disease after allogeneic bone marrow transplantation. J Clin Invest 1998;102:115–123.

242. Trepicchio WL, Wang L et al. IL-11 regulates macrophage effector function through the inhibition of nuclear factor-κB. J Immunol 1997;159:5661–5670.

243. Qiu BS, Pfeiffer CJ et al. Protection by recombinant human interleukin-11 against experimental TNB-induced colitis in rats. Dig Dis Sci 1996;41:1625–1630.

244. Peterson RL, Wang L et al. Molecular effects of recombinant human interleukin-11 in the HLA-B27 rat model of inflammatory bowel disease. Lab Invest 1998;78:1503–1512.

245. Keith JC Jr., Albert L et al. IL-11, a pleiotropic cytokine: exciting new effects of IL-11 on gastrointestinal mucosal biology. Stem Cells 1994;12 (Suppl 1):79–89; discussion 89–90.

246. Alavi K, Prasad R et al. Interleukin-11 enhances small intestine absorptive function and mucosal mass after intestinal adaptation. J Pediatr Surg 2000;35:371–374.

247. Fiore NF, Ledniczky G et al. Comparison of interleukin-11 and epidermal growth factor on residual small intestine after massive small bowel resection. J Pediatr Surg 1998;33:24–29.

248. Liu Q, Du XX et al. Trophic effects of interleukin-11 in rats with experimental short bowel syndrome. J Pediatr Surg 1996;31:1047–1050; discussion 1050–1051.

249. Sands BE, Bank S et al. Preliminary evaluation of safety and activity of recombinant human interleukin 11 in patients with active Crohn's disease. Gastroenterology 1999;117:58–64.

250. Sands BE, Winston BD et al. Randomized, controlled trial of recombinant human interleukin-11 in patients with active Crohn's disease. Aliment Pharmacol Ther 2002;16:399–406.

251. Eckmann L, Kagnoff MF et al. Epithelial cells secrete the chemokine interleukin-8 in response to bacterial entry. Infect Immun 1993;61:4569–4574.

252. Schuerer-Maly CC, Eckmann L et al. Colonic epithelial cell lines as a source of interleukin-8: stimulation by inflammatory cytokines and bacterial lipopolysaccharide [see comments]. Immunology 1994;81:85–91.

253. McCormick BA, Colgan SP et al. Salmonella typhimurium attachment to human intestinal epithelial monolayers: transcellular signalling to subepithelial neutrophils. J Cell Biol 1993;123:895–907.

254. Mazzucchelli L, Hauser C et al. Expression of interleukin-8 gene in inflammatory bowel disease is related to the histological grade of active inflammation. Am J Pathol 1994;144:997–1007.

255. Daig R, Andus T et al. Increased interleukin 8 expression in the colon mucosa of patients with inflammatory bowel disease. Gut 1996;38:216–222.

256. Grimm MC, Elsbury SK et al. Interleukin 8: cells of origin in inflammatory bowel disease. Gut 1996;38:90–98.

257. Arai F, Takahashi T et al. Mucosal expression of interleukin-6 and interleukin-8 messenger RNA in ulcerative colitis and in Crohn's disease. Dig Dis Sci 1998;43:2071–2079.

258. Izutani R, Ohyanagi H et al. Quantitative PCR for detection of femtogram quantities of interleukin-8 mRNA expression. Microbiol Immunol 1994;38:233–237.

259. Mitsuyama K, Toyonaga A et al. IL-8 as an important chemoattractant for neutrophils in ulcerative colitis and Crohn's disease. Clin Exp Immunol 1994;96:432–436.

260. Mahida YR, Ceska M et al. Enhanced synthesis of neutrophil-activating peptide-1/interleukin-8 in active ulcerative colitis. Clin Sci 1992;82:273–275.

261. Izzo RS, Witkon K et al. Interleukin-8 and neutrophil markers in colonic mucosa from patients with ulcerative colitis. Am J Gastroenterol 1992;87:1447–1452.

262. Izzo RS, Witkon K et al. Neutrophil-activating peptide (interleukin-8) in colonic mucosa from patients with Crohn's disease. Scand J Gastroenterol 1993;28:296–300.

263. Ina K, Kusugami K et al. Mucosal interleukin-8 is involved in neutrophil migration and binding to extracellular matrix in inflammatory bowel disease. Am J Gastroenterol 1997;92:1342–1346.

264. Chang MS, McNinch J et al. Cloning and characterization of the human neutrophil-activating peptide (ENA-78) gene. J Biol Chem 1994;269:25277–25282.

265. Walz A, Burgener R et al. Structure and neutrophil-activating properties of a novel inflammatory peptide (ENA-78) with homology to interleukin 8. J Exp Med 1991;174:1355–1362.

266. Schnyder-Candrian S, Walz A. Neutrophil-activating protein ENA-78 and IL-8 exhibit different patterns of expression in lipopolysaccharide- and cytokine-stimulated human monocytes. J Immunol 1997;158:3888–3894.

267. Keates S, Keates AC et al. Enterocytes are the primary source of the chemokine ENA-78 in normal colon and ulcerative colitis. Am J Physiol 1997;273:G75–82.

268. Schnyder-Candrian S, Strieter RM et al. Interferon-α and interferon-γ downregulate the production of interleukin-8 and ENA-78 in human monocytes. J Leukocyte Biol 1995;57:929–935.

269. Wuyts A, Proost P et al. Differential usage of the CXC chemokine receptors 1 and 2 by interleukin-8, granulocyte chemotactic protein-2 and epithelial-cell-derived neutrophil attractant-78. Eur J Biochem 1998;255:67–73.

270. Z'Graggen K, Walz A et al. The C-X-C chemokine ENA-78 is preferentially expressed in intestinal epithelium in inflammatory bowel disease. Gastroenterology 1997;113:808–816.

271. Taub DD, Sayers TJ et al. α and β chemokines induce NK cell migration and enhance NK-mediated cytolysis. J Immunol 1995;155:3877–3888.

272. Loetscher M, Gerber B et al. Chemokine receptor specific for IP10 and mig: structure, function, and expression in activated T-lymphocytes [see comments]. J Exp Med 1996;184:963–969.

273. Roth SJ, Carr MW et al. C-C chemokines, but not the C-X-C chemokines interleukin-8 and interferon-γ inducible protein-10, stimulate transendothelial chemotaxis of T lymphocytes. Eur J Immunol 1995;25:3482–3488.

274. Roth SJ, Diacovo TG et al. Transendothelial chemotaxis of human α/β and γ/δ T lymphocytes to chemokines. Eur J Immunol 1998;28:104–113.

275. Shibahara T, Wilcox JN et al. Characterization of epithelial chemoattractants for human intestinal intraepithelial lymphocytes. Gastroenterology. 2001;120:60–70.

276. Uguccioni M, Gionchetti P et al. Increased expression of IP-10, IL-8, MCP-1, and MCP-3 in ulcerative colitis. Am J Pathol 1999;155:331–336.

277. Chapman GA, Moores KE et al. The role of fractalkine in the recruitment of monocytes to the endothelium. Eur J Pharmacol 2000;392:189–195.

278. Muehlhoefer A, Saubermann LJ et al. Fractalkine is an epithelial and endothelial cell-derived chemoattractant for intraepithelial lymphocytes in the small intestinal mucosa. J Immunol 2000;164:3368–3376.

278a. Lucas AD, Chadwick N, Warren BF et al. The transmembrane form of the CX3CL1 chemokine fractalkine is expressed predominantly by epithelial cells in vivo. Am J Pathol 2001;158:855–866.

279. Brand S, Sakaguchi T et al. Fractalkine-mediated signals regulate cell-survival and immune-modulatory responses in intestinal epithelial cells. Gastroenterology 2002;122:166–177.

280. Randolph GJ, Furie MB. A soluble gradient of endogenous monocyte chemoattractant protein-1 promotes the transendothelial migration of monocytes in vitro. J Immunol 1995;155:3610–3618.

281. Gu L, Tseng S et al. Control of TH2 polarization by the chemokine monocyte chemoattractant protein-1. Nature 2000;404:407–411.

282. Lu B, Rutledge BJ et al. Abnormalities in monocyte recruitment and cytokine expression in monocyte chemoattractant protein 1-deficient mice. J Exp Med 1998;187:601–608.

283. Warhurst AC, Hopkins SJ et al. Interferon γ induces differential upregulation of α and β chemokine secretion in colonic epithelial cell lines. Gut 1998;42:208–213.

284. Winsor GL, Waterhouse CC et al. Interleukin-4 and IFN-γ differentially stimulate macrophage chemoattractant protein-1 (MCP-1) and eotaxin production by intestinal epithelial cells. J Interferon Cytokine Res 2000;20:299–308.

285. Lugering N, Kucharzik T et al. Interleukin-15 strongly inhibits interleukin-8 and monocyte chemoattractant protein-1 production in human colonic epithelial cells. Immunology 1999;98:504–509.

286. Badolato R, Ponzi AN et al. Interleukin-15 (IL-15) induces IL-8 and monocyte chemotactic protein 1 production in human monocytes. Blood 1997;90:2804–2809.

287. Tangirala RK, Murao K et al. Regulation of expression of the human monocyte chemotactic protein-1 receptor (hCCR2) by cytokines. J Biol Chem 1997;272:8050–8056.

288. Reinecker HC, Loh EY et al. Monocyte-chemoattractant protein 1 gene expression in intestinal epithelial cells and inflammatory bowel disease mucosa. Gastroenterology 1995;108:40–50.

289. Mazzucchelli L, Hauser C et al. Differential in situ expression of the genes encoding the chemokines MCP-1 and RANTES in human inflammatory bowel disease. J Pathol 1996;178:201–206.

290. Grimm MC, Elsbury SK et al. Enhanced expression and production of monocyte chemoattractant protein-1 in inflammatory bowel disease mucosa. J Leukocyte Biol 1996;59:804–812.

291. Keane J, Nicoll J et al. Conservation of structure and function between human and murine IL-16. J Immunol 1998;160:5945–5954.

292. Zhang Y, Center DM et al. Processing and activation of pro-interleukin-16 by caspase-3. J Biol Chem 1998;273:1144–1149.

293. Baier M, Kurth R. Fighting HIV-1 with IL-16. Nature Med 1997;3:605–606.

294. Lim KG, Wan HC et al. Human eosinophils elaborate the lymphocyte chemoattractants. IL-16 (lymphocyte chemoattractant factor) and RANTES. J Immunol 1996;156:2566–2570.

295. Laberge S, Cruikshank WW et al. Histamine-induced secretion of lymphocyte chemoattractant factor from CD8+ T cells is independent of transcription and translation. Evidence for constitutive protein synthesis and storage. J Immunol 1995;155:2902–2910.

296. Rand TH, Cruikshank WW et al. CD4-mediated stimulation of human eosinophils: lymphocyte chemoattractant factor and other CD4-binding ligands elicit eosinophil migration. J Exp Med 1991;173:1521–1528.

297. Cruikshank WW, Berman JS et al. Lymphokine activation of T4+ T lymphocytes and monocytes. J Immunol 1987;138:3817–3823.

298. Cruikshank WW, Center DM et al. Molecular and functional analysis of a lymphocyte chemoattractant factor: association of biologic function with CD4 expression. Proc Natl Acad Sci USA 1994;91:5109–5113.

299. Keates AC, Castagliuolo I et al. Interleukin 16 is upregulated in Crohn's disease and participates in TNBS colitis in mice. Gastroenterology 2000;119:972–982.

300. Middel P, Reich K et al. Interleukin 16 expression and phenotype of interleukin 16 producing cells in Crohn's disease. Gut 2001;49:795–803.

301. Seegert D, Rosenstiel P et al. Increased expression of IL-16 in inflammatory bowel disease. Gut 2001;48:326–332.

302. Uguccioni M, D'Apuzzo M et al. Actions of the chemotactic cytokines MCP-1, MCP-2, MCP-3, RANTES, MIP-1 α and MIP-1 β on human monocytes. Eur J Immunol 1995;25:64–68.

303. Taub DD, Proost P et al. Monocyte chemotactic protein-1 (MCP-1), -2, and -3 are chemotactic for human T lymphocytes. J Clin Invest 1995;95:1370–1376.

304. Xu LL, Warren MK et al. Human recombinant monocyte chemotactic protein and other C-C chemokines bind and induce directional migration of dendritic cells in vitro. J Leukocyte Biol 1996;60:365–371.

305. Mir A, Minguez M et al. Elevated serum eotaxin levels in patients with inflammatory bowel disease. Am J Gastroenterol 2002;97:1452–1457.

306. Chen W, Paulus B et al. Increased serum levels of eotaxin in patients with inflammatory bowel disease. Scand J Gastroenterol 2001;36:515–520.

307. Kotenko SV. The family of IL-10-related cytokines and their receptors: related, but to what extent? Cytokine Growth Factor Rev 2002;13:223–240.

308. Trinchieri G. Interleukin-12 and the regulation of innate resistance and adaptive immunity. Nature Rev Immunol 2003;3:133–146.

## CHAPTER 13

# T-lymphocyte dysregulation

Markus F Neurath

The large mucosal surface of the intestine has many tasks, including absorption, macromolecule transport, barrier and secretory functions. However, the mucosal surface is continuously exposed to innumerable potentially harmful antigens (food and bacterial antigens). To deal with this, the gastrointestinal tract possesses a unique mucosal immune system that tightly controls the balance between mucosal responsiveness and non-responsiveness (tolerance) towards antigens. It consists of an integrated network of tissues, cells and effector molecules for host protection. Recent data suggest that T lymphocytes play a key role in regulating mucosal immune responses.[1–14] However, uncontrolled mucosal T-cell responses in response to bacterial antigens may lead to intestinal inflammation. Indeed, there is growing evidence that inflammatory bowel diseases (IBD: Crohn's disease (CD), ulcerative colitis (UC)) are due to a dysregulation of the mucosal immune system, with consecutive activation of mucosal T lymphocytes and production of proinflammatory cytokines such as tumor necrosis factor (TNF).[13,15] This chapter summarizes the data on T-lymphocyte dysregulation in IBD patients and discusses the implications of these findings for our understanding of the immunopathogenesis of IBD and for designing novel therapeutic approaches to treat these chronic inflammatory diseases.

## ROLE OF LYMPHOCYTES IN REGULATING MUCOSAL IMMUNE RESPONSES IN THE GUT

Various structural and functional unique properties separate the mucosal immune system from the peripheral immune system.[5,16–21] The mucosal immune system is highly regulated, so that the outcome of immune responses to foreign antigens and pathogens can range from local and systemic B- and T-cell responses to systemic anergy against a mucosally encountered antigen (oral tolerance). Intercellular and intertissue communication is crucial for an effective mucosal immune response, and

homing of lymphocytes via adhesion molecules is essential for the integration of immunologic responses in the diverse mucosal compartments located in the gastrointestinal, pulmonary and genitourinary tracts.[16,22] This homing highlights the communication between different mucosal sites, allowing specific antigen reactivity to extend quickly over mucosal tissues (common mucosal immune system). However, as a compensatory mechanism in response to the high antigen load at mucosal surfaces the mucosal immune system exhibits immunologic 'hyporesponsiveness' or unresponsiveness to commensal bacterial and dietary antigens; this is a key difference between the peripheral and the mucosal immune systems. On the other hand, the mucosal immune system must be capable of inducing effective cell- and antibody-mediated immune responses towards selected pathogenic microbial agents in local and peripheral lymphoid compartments.[17,23] It is evident that such a complex task requires tight structural and functional control elements, and that alterations to this system predispose to chronic inflammatory diseases such as IBD.

The mucosal immune system of the gut contains so-called inductive sites for antigen uptake and processing, as well as effector sites with lymphocytes, granulocytes and mast cells on the other hand.[16,17] The gut-associated lymphoreticular tissue (GALT) (e.g. Peyer's patches in the small bowel and colonic follicles in the large bowel) is an important inductive site and possesses both antigen-presenting cells (APC) and lymphocytes.[17] Following induction in the GALT, T and B lymphocytes migrate to the lamina propria, where they represent main effector cells of intestinal immune responses.[17] Immune responses generated in the GALT can lead to the development of B cells that produce antigen-specific immunoglobulins and to the differentiation of effector T cells. Such T cells can reach the lamina propria, where they secrete cytokines that are essential for the induction of suppressive T-cell responses, oral tolerance[17,24] and mucosal immunity. Furthermore, mucosal T-helper (Th) 1 and 2 T-cell subsets can produce proinflammatory cytokines (Fig. 13.1), as discussed below. Whereas Th1 cells secrete the cytokine IFN-γ, Th2 cells secrete the cytokines

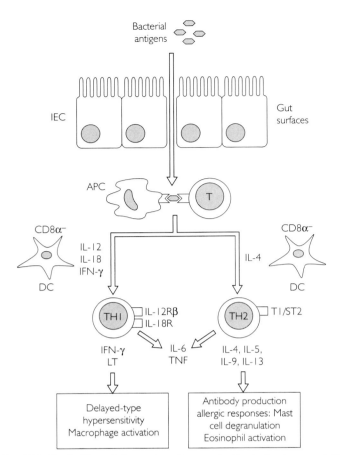

**Fig. 13.1** T-cell differentiation and cytokine production by lamina propria T cells in response to bacterial antigens (modified according to [14]). Bacterial antigens can be presented by antigen-presenting cells (APC) to mucosal T cells. In the presence of cytokines such as IL-12 and IFN-γ produced by APC, T cells can differentiate into Th1 effector cells, whereas IL-4 can induce Th2 T-cell differentiation.[67] IL-18 can augment IL-12-dependent Th1 T-cell differentiation. The Th2 T-cell subset produces cytokines such as IL-4, IL-5, IL-9 and IL-13, which are known to mediate B-cell isotype switching, antibody production and allergic responses. In contrast, the Th1 T-cell subset produces IFN-γ and mediates delayed-type hypersensitivity reactions and macrophage activation. IL-6 and TNF can be produced by both T-cell subsets, although Th1 cells produce larger amounts of TNF and Th2 cells larger amounts of IL-6.

IL-4, IL-5, IL-9 and IL-13. The functional differences between mucosal Th1 and Th2 cells can largely be explained by the activities of these subset-specific signature cytokines. Whereas cytokines produced by Th1 cells are known to mediate delayed-type hypersensitivity responses and macrophage activation, cytokines produced by Th2 cells regulate B-cell differentiation and activation, as well as allergic immune responses in the mucosal immune system (Fig. 13.1).

## A KEY ROLE FOR T LYMPHOCYTES IN THE PATHOGENESIS OF IBD

The gut is the largest reservoir for T lymphocytes and contains CD4+, CD8+ and NK T-cell populations. CD4+ T lymphocytes are recognized as key regulators of mucosal immune responses and can differentiate into functionally distinct subsets after receiving specific signals (processed antigen in the context of MHC class II molecules, co-stimulatory signals) from antigen-presenting cells, such as dendritic cells, macrophages and B lymphocytes. This maturation process is accompanied by changes in the expression of various surface molecules and cytokine production. Whereas naive human (or mouse) T cells express CD45RA (CD45RB high, CD62L+), memory T cells are known to express CD45RO (CD45RB low, CD62L–). With regard to cytokine production, naive T cells have been shown to produce low amounts of cytokines, whereas polarized effector T cells secrete larger amounts. Whereas Th1 cells secrete the signature cytokine IFN-γ, Th2 cells secrete IL-4, IL-5, IL-9 and IL-13 (Fig. 13.1).[25–27] Both Th1 and Th2 cells produce TNF, although Th1 cells tend to produce larger amounts. In addition, Th3 and regulatory CD25+ CD4+ T (TR) cells are present that produce membrane-bound TGF-β and soluble IL-10, respectively. Th3 cells appear to play a key role in regulating suppressive immune responses in oral tolerance, whereas CD25+ CD4+ T (TR) cells are important regulatory T cells that can antagonize the development of experimental models of IBD by producing IL-10.[23,24,28–30] The functional importance of these findings is supported by studies in knockout mice. In fact, mice in which the genes for the effector cytokines (IL-10 and TGF-β knockout mice) or signaling molecules (Smad3 for TGF-β) of CD25+ CD4+ T (TR) and Th3 cells have been inactivated by homologous recombination spontaneously develop chronic intestinal inflammation,[31–33] thereby highlighting the potential relevance of these T-cell subsets in suppressing intestinal immune responses. Although all T-cell subsets seem to occur in the normal gut, there is a predominance of anti-inflammatory and regulatory cytokine responses that is important for mucosal homeostasis (Fig. 13.2). It is currently assumed that immature dendritic cells in the gut are important in inducing such regulatory and suppressive immune responses, as these cells are known to induce differentiation of TR cells.[3,5,24]

T lymphocytes play an important role in regulating mucosal immune responses in IBD patients and animal models of chronic intestinal inflammation. In particular, an essential role for CD4+ T lymphocytes has been shown in many animal models of experimental colitis.[8,30,34,35] Of considerable importance is that both Th1 and Th2 cells have been shown to induce chronic intestinal inflammation in vivo,[30,35–40] and the action of these T-effector cells can be suppressed by cytokines produced by TR and Th3 cells, such as IL-10 and TGF-β.[29,41] Furthermore, CD4+ T cells seem to play a key pathogenic role in the pathogenesis of human IBD. This hypothesis is supported by the clinical effects of monoclonal anti-CD4+ antibodies in patients with Crohn's disease (CD)[42] and the observation that reduction of T-helper cell numbers by a concomitant HIV infection suppresses disease activity in CD.[43] Consistent with these observations, bone marrow transplantation because of concomitant leukemia can induce long-term remissions in CD, suggesting that the host immune dysregulation plays a role in the perpetuation of this disease that can be corrected by hematopoietic cell transplantation.[44,45] Finally, antibodies to TNF that are successfully used in treating Crohn's disease patients induce rapid mucosal T-cell apoptosis (programmed cell death) within 2 days, indicating that the therapeutic efficacy of these antibodies could be due to the elimination of T-effector cells in the gut.[46]

One possible reason for increased T-cell stimulation and activation in IBD is that bacterial antigens continuously activate these cells. Studies by Duchmann and co-workers suggest that

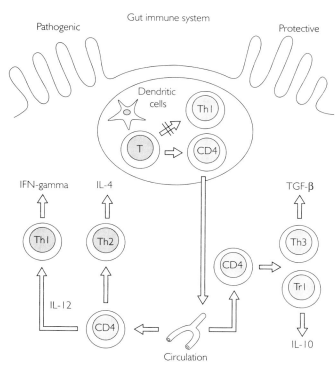

**Fig. 13.2** Pathogenic and protective cytokine responses in the lamina propria. Both Th1 and Th2 T cells have been shown to mediate chronic intestinal inflammation. In contrast, Th3 and regulatory Tr1 cells produce anti-inflammatory cytokines that can profoundly suppress intestinal inflammation. Whereas anti-inflammatory responses dominate in the uninflamed intestinal immune system, IBD are characterized by an activation of pathogenic T-cell responses and/or an insufficient counterregulation by regulatory T cells in the gut.

IBD T cells react to their autologous intestinal flora.[47] This concept is consistent with a study showing that infusion of intestinal contents into the excluded ileum induced early lesions of recurrent Crohn's disease with activated mucosal T cells.[48] A loss of T-cell tolerance to antigens from the normal intestinal flora has therefore been implicated as a key mechanism in the pathogenesis of IBD.[47,49-51] The hypothesis that intestinal T-cell responses in IBD are driven by bacterial antigens is also supported by studies showing that intestinal inflammation in various T cell-dependent animal models of IBD is suppressed when hosts are kept under germ-free (sterile) conditions, and that monoassociation with certain bacterial strains (e.g. *Bacteroides vulgatus* in HLA-B27 transgenic rats, *Enterococcus faecalis* in IL-10-/- mice) can cause disease development.[32,52,53] Furthermore, in some animal models colitis can by adoptively transferred by antigen-specific T cells that react with luminal bacterial antigens.[1,13,54,55] Finally, mutations in the *NOD2* gene, a gene that presumably controls innate immune responses to bacterial infections and commensal bacterial antigens in intestinal APC, have been associated with CD,[56-58] suggesting that dysregulated activation of the mucosal immune system in a genetically susceptible host is a key pathogenic factor at least in a subset of CD patients.[59,60]

In addition to signals provided by bacterial antigens, IBD T cells receive additional signals in the gut that appear to be important for their activation. For instance, it has been shown that lamina propria macrophages and intestinal epithelial cells produce various proinflammatory cytokines that can cause T-cell

activation.[61-63] Furthermore, co-stimulatory signals provided by these APC (e.g. via CD28/B7 or CD40/CD40 ligand interactions) may be important for the activation of IBD T cells. In addition, it has been shown that normal intestinal epithelial cells preferentially stimulate the proliferation of suppressor T cells in culture via the CD8 ligand gp180, whereas CD epithelial cells display defective gp180 expression and inappropriately induce activation of T-helper cells.[64]

# KEY PRINCIPLES OF T-HELPER CELL POLARIZATION AND THE ROLE OF ANTIGEN-PRESENTING CELLS

Because there is an increase in the number of cytokine-producing CD45RO CD4+ T cells in the lamina propria of IBD patients compared to controls, there has been a growing interest in understanding the principles of T-helper cell differentiation in IBD. Both Th1 and Th2 effector cells appear to play a fundamental role in regulating immune responses in the mucosal immune system, and it appears that various signals are required to induce such T-cell differentiation.[1,14,47,65] Although most of our knowledge on T-cell differentiation and activation has been derived from experiments using peripheral T lymphocytes, it appears that similar principles exist for mucosal T cells, although important exceptions exist, as discussed below. After differentiation and migration to the peripheral immune organs, CD4+ T-helper cells are termed naive T-helper precursor cells that are functionally immature. Much has been learned about the signals that drive these naive T cells to become Th1 or Th2 effector cells.[25,66,67] The activation and differentiation of T-helper precursor cells requires at least two separate signals. The first is delivered by the TCR/CD3 complex after its interaction with antigen/MHC on APC, such as DC and macrophages. Interestingly, this signal is known to induce stronger proliferation of T lymphocytes in the periphery than in the antigen-rich environment of the gut, as normal lamina propria T cells do not proliferate well on TCR/CD3 stimulation, in comparison to splenic lymphocytes.[68] This finding may contribute to the well-known 'hyporesponsiveness' of mucosal T cells in the normal gut. In patients with CD, however, T cells from the inflamed gut showed an increased proliferation comparable to that of peripheral blood-derived T cells.[68] Similarly, an increased proliferation of lamina propria T cells has been observed in UC patients.[69]

Several studies have analyzed the T-cell receptor repertoire in IBD in an attempt to identify responses to specific antigens or superantigens. CDR3 length analysis and sequencing of the TCR-Vβ regions demonstrated persistent oligoclonal CD4+ T-cell expansions within the peripheral blood and gut of IBD patients, suggesting the activation of a limited subset of antigen-specific T cells.[70,71] Recent studies have also addressed the potential role of superantigens, which can trigger large numbers of T cells without the requirement for prior antigen processing.[72] A recent study identified a DNA sequence, a homolog of a bacterial transcription family (tetR) denoted I2, in tissue from patients with active CD, but not control patients, as a potential superantigen relevant for CD pathogenesis. In mice, I2-induced immune responses resulted in the expansion of a Vβ5-restricted lymphocyte subset and the production of IL-10,[72] suggesting that I2 might play a role in limiting rather than promoting intestinal inflammation in CD.

The second signal necessary for T-cell polarization is produced by a number of co-stimulatory or accessory molecules on the APC that interact with their ligands on T cells (e.g. CD28/B7-1(CD 80), CD28/B7-2(CD 86), OX40/OX40L). Studies in mice in which the genes for these co-stimulatory molecules have been inactivated by homologous recombination show significantly reduced immune responses and defects in generating IL-4-producing effector cells, suggesting that these signals are key regulators of peripheral T-cell responses.[73-75] The co-stimulatory signal is also very important for mucosal T lymphocytes, as lamina propria T cells demonstrate normal or even enhanced proliferation and cytokine production in response to CD28-mediated co-stimulation.[76] Although CD28-dependent co-stimulation may induce very effective activation of mucosal T-cell responses, these co-stimulatory molecules are weakly expressed on most APC in the normal mucosal immune system, suggesting that co-stimulatory processes are tightly controlled in this antigen-rich environment. However, co-stimulatory signal activation is clearly important for the pathogenesis of T cell-mediated mucosal inflammation, as blockade of the CD28/B7 and OX40/OX40L systems has been shown to profoundly suppress chronic intestinal inflammation in mice.[77,78] Taken together, it appears that both co-stimulatory and TCR-derived signals exert important regulatory functions for peripheral and mucosal T lymphocytes.

Cytokines such as IL-12 and IL-4 play the most critical role in T-helper cell polarization.[25,26,66] In fact, both cytokines induce the generation of their own T-helper subset while simultaneously inhibiting the generation of the opposing subset. Their importance in T-helper differentiation has been demonstrated unequivocally by the phenotype of mice that lack these two cytokines or signaling molecules downstream of these cytokines.[66] Whereas mice lacking IL-12 p40 or the IL-12 receptor $\beta_2$ chain showed defective Th1 T-cell responses, mice that lack IL-4 or its receptor failed to develop Th2 cells in response to various stimuli.

Recent evidence suggests an important role for distinct subsets of dendritic cells as well as macrophages in orchestrating the lineage commitment of naive T-helper cells.[67,79-81] Two subsets of murine CD11c+ DC (CD8α+ versus CD8α− DC) and human DC (myeloid CD11c+ DC versus plasmacytoid CD1α− DC) have been identified that induce distinct classes of antigen-specific T-cell responses in vivo.[67] Whereas the former DC elicit Th1 responses, the latter favor Th2 responses.[82] Although both DC subsets can be found in murine Peyer's patches, Iwasaki et al.[79] showed that antigen-pulsed DC from the Peyer's patches induce Th2-type rather than Th1-type T-cell responses. Although the molecules produced by APC that induce Th2 responses are unknown, CD8α+ DC can be induced by bacterial antigens/products and IFN-γ to produce large amounts of IL-12 p35/p40 heterodimer, which appears to be essential for their potential to induce Th1 differentiation.[67] In addition to DC, macrophages and monocytes can be primed by IFN-γ to produce large amounts of IL-12 heterodimer upon LPS stimulation.[81,83] Although the role of DC in the pathogenesis of IBD has not yet been fully investigated, there appears to be an increase in DC numbers as well as an activation of these cells in patients with CD.[84] With regard to macrophages, however, recent data suggest that these cells may play an important role in controlling T-helper cell differentiation and augmenting gut inflammation in IBD,[62] as discussed below.

Taken together, substantial progress has been made in our understanding of Th1/Th2 polarization at the cellular level. The following paragraphs discuss the implications of these observations for the pathogenesis of IBD.

# CYTOKINE PRODUCTION BY LAMINA PROPRIA T CELLS IN IBD

Based on the above data it was important to understand the function of IBD T cells by determining their capacity to produce various regulatory lymphokines.[16,69,85-89] Fiocchi and co-workers found that lamina propria T cells from both CD and UC patients produce less IL-2 than do control lamina propria T cells.[69] Mullin et al.[87] used quantitative RT-PCR to measure messenger RNA levels of IL-2 and showed that IL-2 messenger RNA levels were increased in lesional tissues from patients with CD but not from patients with UC. Furthermore, Breese et al.[86] determined the numbers of lymphokine-secreting cells and showed that lesional CD tissues contained increased numbers of IL-2 secreting cells, whereas compared to control tissues UC tissues did not. These somewhat contradictory findings may indicate that basal production of IL-2 in T cells isolated from CD patients is elevated, but as a consequence their capacity to induce increased IL-2 production is reduced. However, IL-2 is an important growth and activation factor for regulatory T cells, as shown by the fact that IL-2-deficient mice develop gut inflammation owing to lack of regulatory T-cell responses.[53] One may therefore speculate that a reduced IL-2 production by IBD T cells may contribute to the recently observed decreased activity of TR cells in the lamina propria of patients with active IBD[90] and thus might contribute to disease pathogenesis.

Accessory pathway stimulation is important for T-cell activation in the mucosal immune response. Lamina propria T cells proliferate poorly in response to TCR/CD3 receptor stimulation compared with peripheral T cells,[47,76] but they manifest somewhat better proliferation in response to stimulation via the CD2/CD28 accessory pathway. Finally, with respect to lymphokine production, lamina propria T cells produce vastly more lymphokines in response to accessory pathway stimulation than do cells stimulated via the TCR/CD3 pathway. Based on these observations, it was of interest to determine cytokine production and T-cell proliferation in IBD under accessory pathway stimulation. It was found that whereas IBD lamina propria T cells both from UC and CD patients gave lower proliferative responses than did control lamina propria T cells via the TCR/CD3 signaling pathway, proliferative responses via the CD2/CD28 pathway were relatively preserved.[91] The production of IFN-γ, the signature cytokine of Th1 T cells, has also been measured in IBD lamina propria T cells after stimulation with anti-CD2 plus anti-CD28 antibodies. When purified lamina propria T cells from patients with CD were stimulated via accessory signaling pathways, IFN-γ production was significantly increased compared to T cells from control patients,[91] whereas IL-2 production was reduced. Thus in studies in which due consideration was made for how lamina propria T cells are stimulated, it was shown that CD T cells manifest an abnormal lymphokine profile characterized by increased IFN-γ and decreased IL-2 production. It should be noted that this is not a classic Th1 cytokine profile, however, as IL-2 production by CD

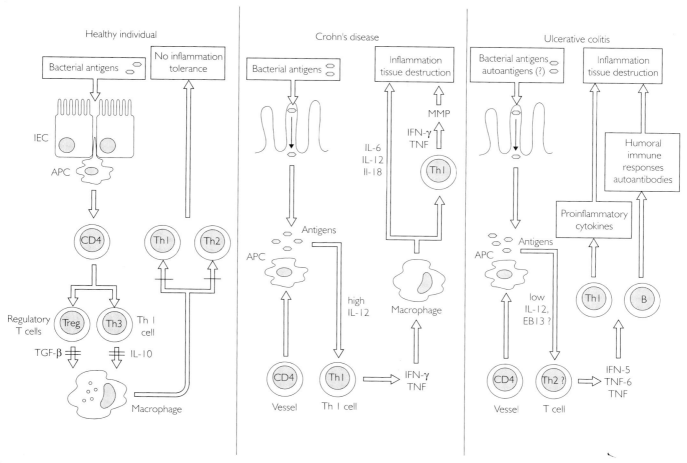

**Fig. 13.3** T-cell responses in the uninflamed and inflamed human gut. Immature dendritic cells appear to be important to induce suppressive T-cell responses in the normal gut by presenting bacterial antigens from the lumen to T cells.[164] In CD there is a predominance of Th1 responses, favored by increased production of IL-12 by APC. Th1 T cells produce large amounts of TNF and IFN-γ that activate macrophages to produce proinflammatory cytokines, leading to inflammation and tissue destruction. In contrast, there is a different cytokine production by T cells in patients with UC that may lead to B-cell activation and the production of autoantibodies in this disease.

lamina propria T cells was decreased. Thus this lymphokine profile may represent a modified Th1 cytokine profile present in patients with CD. Interestingly, TNF acts as a cofactor that strongly augments the production of Th1 cytokines by activated lamina propria T cells in CD, suggesting that TNF may play an important role in augmenting the effector functions of lamina propria T cells in this disease.[92]

In contrast to CD, few data are available on cytokine production by lamina propria T cells in patients with UC. However, Fuss et al. showed that upon stimulation with anti-CD2/CD28 antibodies purified lamina propria CD4+ T lymphocytes from UC patients produce equal amounts of the Th1 cytokine IFN-γ but large amounts of the Th2 cytokine IL-5 compared to T cells from control patients. Interestingly, the production of another Th2 cytokine, IL-4, was reduced by UC lamina propria T cells compared to T cells from control patients, suggesting the potential existence of a modified Th2 cytokine profile in UC patients.[91] This cytokine profile may at least partially account for the observed activation of B cells and the production of autoantibodies in UC patients, as Th2 cytokines are known to activate humoral immune responses.[15]

Taken together, the current data are consistent with a model in which anti-CD2/CD28 stimulated T cells from Crohn's disease patients produce a modified Th1 cytokine profile (high

IFN-γ, low IL-2), whereas T cells from UC patients exhibit a modified Th2 cytokine profile (high IL-5, low IL-4) (Fig. 13.3).

## CYTOKINE SIGNALING IN IBD T CELLS

Based on the above data on cytokine production and the therapeutic efficacy of several anticytokine strategies in IBD patients, there is a growing interest in understanding cytokine signaling events in IBD. In the case of Crohn's disease recent studies have focused on understanding the molecular pathways leading to Th1 T-cell differentiation in this disease. The cytokine IL-12 heterodimer (p35/p40) produced by DC or recently immigrated macrophages induces Th1 T-cell differentiation; this function requires the intracellular activation and nuclear translocation of the transcription factor Stat-4 (signal transducer and activator of transcription 4).[67,93–97] The IL-12/Stat-4 signaling pathway plays an important role in Th1-mediated intestinal inflammation. For instance, Th1-mediated models of chronic intestinal inflammation are associated with increased production of IL-12. In addition, neutralizing antibodies to IL-12 p40 or p70 prevent the development of Th1-mediated colitis, but they also suppress established Th1-mediated chronic intestinal inflammation. This remarkable effect is presumably mediated both by the prevention of Th1 T-cell development and the induction of Fas-mediated T-cell apoptosis in the inflamed gut.[39,98–102] Furthermore, Stat-4-deficient T cells fail to induce Th1-mediated colitis in an adoptive transfer system in *RAG* knockout mice, whereas Stat-4 transgenic mice (under control of the CMV promoter) develop Th1-mediated colitis upon immunization with DNP-KLH.[36,39] In addition to IL-12, however, the cytokine IL-23 (p19/p40) produced by APC has been recently shown to activate Stat-4 in T lymphocytes, raising the possibility that the observed Stat-4 activation in colitis could be at least partially due to IL-23.[103,104] Furthermore, the neutralizing antibodies to IL-12 used in the above studies on colitis activity appear to suppress the function of both IL-12 and IL-23, indicating that further studies are necessary to delineate the function of these cytokines individually. However, the importance of the IL-12/Stat-4 signaling pathway for CD pathogenesis has been highlighted by recent studies showing that IL-12 p35/p40 heterodimer secretion is increased in active CD, that T cells in this disease express large amounts of IL-12 receptor $\beta_2$ chain, and that Stat-4 is activated in mucosal T cells from active CD.[62,105] Finally, IL-12 has been suggested to cause intestinal tissue injury,[106] suggesting that it may play an active role in tissue destruction in CD patients.

In addition to Stat-4 the IFN-γ inducible transcription factor Stat-1 has been shown to be involved in Th1 T-cell differentiation.[107,108] IFN-γ signaling via Stat-1 leads to activation of the transcription factor T-bet,[109,110] a recently cloned member of the T-box protein family expressed in T lymphocytes.[111] High levels of T-bet have been found in IFN-γ-producing Th1 but not Th2 cells, suggesting a role for T-bet in controlling Th1 T-cell differentiation.[111,112] This is supported by recent studies showing profound suppression of IFN-γ production in CD4+ but not CD8+ T cells from T-bet deficient mice.[113] T-bet thus is an important factor for Th1 T-cell development and the regulation of T-cell effector function that acts independently of Stat-4 signaling and before IL-12-mediated selection of Th1 cells.[110,111,113,114] Therefore, it was of interest to determine the activation and expression of Stat-1 and T-bet in CD patients.[115] Stat-1 is overexpressed in CD patients, suggesting IFN-γ signaling in lamina propria T cells in this disease. Consistent with this idea, the IFN-γ inducible factor Smad7 was activated in CD, thereby suppressing TGF-β responsiveness and TGF-β signaling via Smad3 in mucosal CD T cells.[116–118] In addition, T-bet was overexpressed and activated in CD lamina propria T cells compared to control patients.[115] The potential relevance of this finding was highlighted by studies in murine models, where it was found that T-bet deficient T cells fail to induce Th1-mediated experimental colitis in an adoptive T-cell transfer system. This observation cannot be attributed to the effects of T-bet on IFN-γ production in CD4+ T cells, as CD4+ T cells from IFN-γ knockout mice are fully capable of inducing Th1-mediated colitis in an adoptive transfer system in *RAG* knockout mice.[39] Instead, these results suggest a more general role of T-bet in Th1 T-cell differentiation via regulation of IL-12 receptor $\beta_2$ chain expression.[109,114] Finally, overexpression of T-bet in T cells was found to augment Th1-mediated colitis, suggesting that T-bet controls Th1-mediated mucosal immune responses.[115] Taken together, these data suggest that CD lamina propria T cells display some characteristics of Th1 cells at the level of cytokine signaling.

In contrast to CD, few data are available on cytokine signaling and T-cell differentiation in patients with UC. However, it appears that there is no increase in IL-12 production by lamina propria cells in UC patients compared to control patients, whereas the expression of a potentially IL-12 antagonizing cytokine, denoted EBI3, is increased.[62,119,120] These data support the concept that T-cell differentiation is different between patients with CD and UC (Fig. 13.3). Whether UC lamina propria T cells exhibit some evidence for Th2 cytokine signaling remains to be seen, however. Interestingly, experimental colitis models support the notion that Th2 cytokines may play a key pathogenic role in regulating colitis activity in vivo.[35,37,40,121] In fact, transfer of Th2 cells has recently been shown to cause colitis in an antigen-specific colitis model.[40] Furthermore, antibodies to IL-4 attenuate T cell-mediated colitis induced by the hapten reagent oxazolone.[37] In addition, inactivation of the IL-4 but not the IFN-γ gene has been shown to suppress colitis activity in TCR knockout animals that normally display some features of human UC.[35] Furthermore, removal of the cecal tip early in life prevents colitis in TCR knockout mice,[122] suggesting that the immune system in this region initiates rather than perpetuates such colitis. This is reminiscent of the observed protective effect of early appendectomy on the development of colitis in UC patients.[123]

Administration of recombinant IL-4 prevents Th1-mediated colitis in an adoptive transfer model but can augment established Th1-mediated colitis,[30,124] suggesting that the effects of the Th2-type cytokine IL-4 may depend on the stage of the disease in T cell-mediated colitis. Consistently, Spencer and co-workers recently showed that colitis in young IL-10-deficient mice is mediated by IL-12-driven Th1 T cells, whereas later stages of disease appear to be mediated by the Th2-type cytokines IL-4 and IL-13.[125] These findings support the notion that T-cell cytokine production may differ during different phases of colitis in vivo. Additional data on this point are required for patients with early and late-stage IBD. Interestingly, a pilot study showed increased IL-4 mRNA levels in early but not late ileal lesions in CD, suggesting potential changes in cytokine production in T cells during the natural course of CD,[126] although the cellular source of the IL-4 was not determined in this study.

The above novel findings on transcriptional polarization of T cells not only give valuable new insights into the immunopathogenesis of IBD but also provide a rationale for selective targeting of transcription factors and signaling cascades in mucosal T cells in these diseases (Fig. 13.4).

# EFFECTOR CYTOKINES IN CHRONIC INTESTINAL INFLAMMATION

Various cytokines, such as IL-6, TNF and IL-18, have limited effects on Th1/Th2 polarization when given alone, but have important influences on the survival and activation of mucosal effector T cells. For instance, it has been shown that IL-18 alone cannot induce Th1 T-cell differentiation, although it strongly augments IL-12-dependent Th1 T-cell development and Th1 effector functions.[127–131] The latter effects are probably due to IL-18-induced upregulation of IL-12Rβ₂ chain expression on T cells and AP-1-(c-*fos*/c-*jun*) dependent *trans*-activation of the IFN-γ promoter.[131,132] The functional importance of IL-18 in colitis is underlined by very recent studies showing suppression

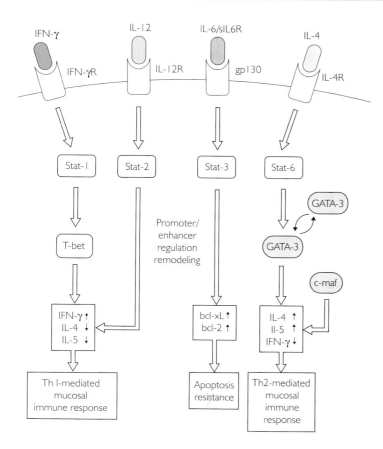

**Fig. 13.4** Cytokines and cytokine signaling in mucosal T lymphocytes via IFN-γ, IL-12, IL-6 and IL-4 (modified according to [14]). IFN-γ binds to its receptor on the T-cell surface, followed by activation of Stat-1 and consecutively of T-bet. T-bet induces Th1 cytokine production and IL-12 receptor $\beta_2$ chain expression. IL-12 then induces Th1 T-cell differentiation via activation of the transcription factor Stat-4 and consecutive induction of IFN-γ production via transactivation of the IFN-γ promoter.[95,111,113] Signaling via IL-6/sIL-6R complexes can augment mucosal Th1 effector functions by activation of the transcription factor Stat-3. IL-4 induces Th2 cytokine production in mucosal T cells by activation of the transcription factor Stat-6, followed by activation of the master transcription factor of Th2 cells GATA-3 165-169. GATA-3 exerts Stat-6-independent autoactivation, thus creating a feedback pathway stabilizing Th2 commitment (blue arrows). In addition to GATA-3, c-maf has been shown to regulate IL-4 production, at least in peripheral T cells. Various cytokine- or cytokine signaling-directed therapies for T cell-mediated mucosal diseases such as Crohn's disease have been performed using either recombinant anti-inflammatory cytokines such as IL-10 or IL-11 or anticytokine strategies.[170-172] The latter have been proven more beneficial in clinical trials so far, and include neutralizing antibodies against TNF in Crohn's disease.[170] However, specific targeting of signaling cascades in IBD could be a target for future therapies of IBD.

of Th1-mediated intestinal inflammation upon blockade of IL-18 expression or function by recombinant adenoviruses, neutralizing antibodies or IL-18 binding proteins.[133-136] Consistent with this observation, blockade of the enzyme ICE, which converts both IL-1 and IL-18 precursors into bioactive proteins, has been shown to suppress the activity of experimental colitis.[135] These data suggest that IL-18 plays an important role in chronic intestinal inflammation by stimulating cytokine production (IFN-γ, TNF) and augmenting the effector functions of lamina propria T cells.[133,137] The relevance of these studies for human IBD is supported by the observation that human intestinal cells such as epithelial cells and macrophages can produce IL-18, and that IL-18 production is increased in patients with CD but not UC.[61,63] Finally, IL-18 strongly enhances the proliferation of mucosal T cells in CD.[137] IL-18 may thus augment the effector functions of lamina propria T cells in patients with CD, and could be a potential target for future therapeutic approaches in this Th1- mediated disease.

The number of TNF-producing cells in the lamina propria of pediatric IBD patients is increased compared to control patients, with higher cell numbers noted in CD than in UC.[138] Soluble TNF augments cytokine production by mucosal effector cells and activates the production of tissue-degrading matrix metalloproteinases by intestinal mesenchymal cells (see Chapter 11), whereas membrane-bound TNF on APC provides an important antiapoptotic stimulus for T cells via interaction with TNF-R2[92,139,140] (Fig. 13.5). The relevance of these pathways for disease pathogenesis is further underlined by studies showing profound suppression of experimental, T cell-dependent colitis and Crohn's disease by the administration of anti-TNF antibodies[30] (see below).

# T-CELL RESISTANCE AGAINST APOPTOSIS: A NEW CONCEPT FOR UNDERSTANDING T-CELL DYSREGULATION IN IBD

Immune responses in the gut are frequently characterized by expansion of antigen-specific T cells which have potent effector functions.[19,47,88] On the one hand such T-cell expansion may be important for host defense against infections through the generation of pathogen-specific mucosal immune responses; on the other hand, however, this expansion might also lead to dysregulated effector cell populations with the capacity to cause gut inflammation. The mucosal immune system has therefore evolved strategies to control mucosal immune responses, such as the regulation of programmed T-cell death (apoptosis).[99,141-143] Such T-cell apoptosis can occur either via an active mechanism following T-cell receptor stimulation (so-called activation-induced cell death) or via a passive mechanism following lymphokine withdrawal. In contrast to the latter, the active mechanism involves death receptors such as Fas and its ligand (FasL).[144-146] Upon Fas/FasL interaction the adaptor molecule FADD (Fas-associated death domain-containing protein) and pro-caspase-8 are recruited to the Fas receptor, thereby forming a death-induced signaling complex (DISC). Recruitment of pro-caspase-8 to the DISC causes its autoproteolytic activation and the release of active caspase-8 (FLICE) into the cytosol. Active caspase-8 can then cleave the proapoptotic BID molecule, followed by the release of cytochrome c from mitochondria into the cytoplasm, resulting in cell death. Alternatively,

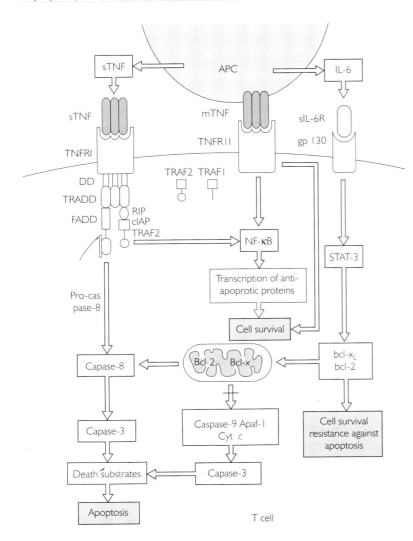

Fig. 13.5 IL-6 *trans*-signaling and TNF signaling events in IBD (modified according to [99]). Chronic intestinal inflammation in mice and humans is associated with increased production of both TNF and IL-6.[30,38, 173] IL-6 may bind to IBD lamina propria T cells lacking the membrane-bound IL-6R upon binding to its soluble receptor (sIL-6R; produced by shedding of the membrane-bound receptor from APC) and the gp130 molecule. Signaling via gp130 results in activation of Stat-3 and Stat-3 target molecules such bcl-2 and bcl-x_L.[151,156] This pathway contributes to T-cell resistance against apoptosis in IBD. Consistent with this idea, blockade of IL-6 *trans*-signaling causes suppression of intestinal inflammation by inhibiting T-cell resistance against apoptosis. TNF plays a dual role in T-cell apoptosis. Although it may induce reduced cell survival by signaling via TNFRI and activation of caspase-8, it may also provide anti-apoptotic signals via TNFR1/2 by activation of NFκB.[147] However, recent data indicate that antibodies to TNF appear to mediate their effects at least in part by rapid induction of T-cell apoptosis in the inflamed gut, suggesting an important function for TNF in promoting mucosal T-cell survival in IBD patients. This antiapoptotic effect is most likely mediated via interaction between mTNF on APC and TNFR2 on T cells. Cyt *c*, cytochrome *c*; DD, death domain; DISC, death-induced signaling complex; FADD, Fas-associated death domain; IL-6, interleukin-6; IL-6R, interleukin-6 receptor; TNF, tumor necrosis factor; TNFR, tumor necrosis factor receptor.

large amounts of caspase-8 can bypass mitochondria and activate other caspases, such as caspase-3, leading to apoptosis. Bcl-2 and bcl-x_L only inhibit apoptotic activities of mitochondria and thus can inhibit only the first but not the second pathway of caspase-8-mediated apoptosis. In contrast, Bcl-2 and bcl-x_L can inhibit passive forms of apoptosis involving activation of BID proteins that act exclusively via mitochondrial mechanisms.

Because most T cells in the lamina propria express memory cell markers such as CD45RO,[47] and because memory T cells are known to express high levels of Fas,[147] the Fas-mediated activation-induced cell death may be very important to downregulate effector cell function and cytokine production in the gut. Interestingly, Boirivant and co-workers showed that both resting and stimulated lamina propria T cells from normal subjects exhibit increased susceptibility to Fas-mediated apoptosis compared to peripheral blood T cells.[148] This is due to activation-induced apoptosis involving death receptors, as antibodies that block Fas extinguish it. Furthermore, they showed that lamina propria T cells exhibit increased spontaneous apoptosis compared to peripheral blood T cells. This finding is probably due to a passive apoptotic mechanism associated with IL-2 withdrawal, as spontaneous apoptosis was reduced when recombinant IL-2 was added.[148]

In contrast to lamina propria T cells from control patients, lamina propria T cells from patients with IBD (particularly CD) exhibit defective Fas-induced apoptosis upon stimulation via

CD2,[142,148] although they express the same amount of Fas on their surface. However, such resistance against apoptosis in Crohn's disease is not restricted to the Fas/FasL system, as CD lamina propria T cells are also more resistant to IL-2-deprivation-induced apoptosis and apoptosis mediated by nitric oxide.[142] This broad resistance to apoptosis could be due to the fact that T cells in inflamed tissue express increased levels of Bcl-2[142] and thus are resistant to various mitochondrial pathways of apoptosis.

In summary, lamina propria T cells in the non-inflamed gut exhibit increased spontaneous or activation-induced apoptosis mediated by the Fas pathway, which limits the expansion of antigen-specific T cells. In contrast, lamina propria T cells from IBD patients are resistant to multiple pathways of mitochondrial-mediated apoptosis, resulting in prolonged T-cell survival that might significantly aggravate the inflammation.

## TNF, IL-6 AND IL-12 REGULATE APOPTOSIS OF MUCOSAL T CELLS IN CHRONIC INTESTINAL INFLAMMATION

Recent data suggest that various proinflammatory cytokines such as IL-12, IL-6 and TNF contribute to T-cell resistance against apoptosis in IBD. In a Th1-mediated animal model of colitis the administration of a neutralizing anti-IL-12 antibody resulted in the rapid appearance of apoptotic CD4+ T cells in the colon.[100] This induction of T-cell apoptosis and elimination of mucosal effector T cells was followed by profound suppression of gut inflammation, and might explain the inhibition of intestinal inflammation in various Th1 models of colitis after treatment with anti-IL-12 antibodies.[39,98,101] Interestingly, the therapeutic effects of anti-IL-12 antibodies were greatly diminished in MRL/lpr mice, which exhibit defective apoptosis via the Fas pathway, as well as in mice administered Fas-Fc, an agent that blocks Fas signaling via FasL.[100] Therefore, it appears that activated mucosal Th1 cells producing inflammatory cytokines require the continued presence of IL-12 to avoid a Fas-mediated death.

Furthermore, administration of anti-IL-6R antibodies to mice with Th1-mediated colitis leads to a significant reduction in the severity of colitis and the rapid occurrence of apoptotic T cells in the inflamed tissues,[38] suggesting that IL-6 signaling provides an antiapoptotic stimulus. This antiapoptotic effect was mediated by complexes of soluble IL-6R (sIL-6R) and IL-6 that mediated their effects via the gp130 protein on the membrane of CD4+ T cells. Consistent with this idea, a gp130-Fc fusion protein that bound to sIL-6R but not to membrane-bound IL-6R also suppressed Th1-mediated colitis, presumably by blocking the interaction of the IL-6/sIL6R complex with membrane-bound gp.[130 149-152]

With regard to patients with IBD, it was shown that IL-6-specific signals appear to be transduced in vivo in lamina propria T cells, as these cells contain activated Stat-3,[38,153] although they also possess increased amounts of the Stat-3 inhibitor SOCS3 (possibly owing to insufficient endogenous counterregulation of Stat-3 activation). This idea is supported by the finding that anti-IL-6R antibodies blocked Stat-3 activation in cultured IBD T cells and resulted in T-cell apoptosis. Furthermore, IL-6-sIL-6R complexes were found in the serum of CD patients.[154] The antiapoptotic effect mediated by IL-6 trans-signaling via Stat-3, in contrast to the antiapoptotic effect mediated by IL-12, involves mitochondrial proteins such as Bcl-2 and bcl-$x_L$.[151,155-158] Indeed, Bcl-2 and bcl-$x_L$ are elevated in lamina propria cells from patients with CD, leading to an increase of the Bcl-2/Bax ratio,[142] and are known to be induced by Stat-3.

Additional complexity of this pathway is provided by the fact that TNF signaling via TNF receptor 1 (TNFR1) or TNFR2 can lead to pro- and antiapoptotic signals in T lymphocytes.[159,160] However, recent evidence suggests that administration of neutralizing anti-TNF antibodies to patients with Crohn's disease rapidly induces apoptosis of lamina propria T cells, suggesting that the overall effect provided by TNF signaling in IBD is an antiapoptotic signal.[46] This finding provides a possible explanation for the rapid and sustained beneficial effects of anti-TNF therapies. Furthermore, in an experimental animal model of colitis in SCID mice reconstituted with CD62L+ CD4+ T cells, overexpression of TNFR2 on T cells augments colitis activity by inducing T-cell resistance against apoptosis, suggesting that TNF signaling via TNFR2 is important for inducing or sustaining colitis activity.[140] Because TNFR2 on T cells is important for signaling via membrane-bound TNF (mTNF) on APC rather than for signaling via soluble TNF, these data suggest that the interaction between mTNF and TNFR2 is critical for the regulation of colitis activity (see Fig. 13.5). Consistent with this hypothesis, etanercept, a protein

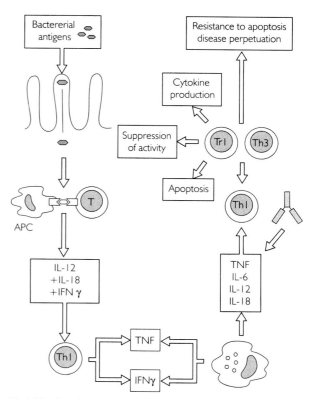

Fig. 13.6 T-cell resistance against apoptosis and novel therapeutic strategies in IBD (modified according to [99]). In CD, bacterial antigens in the gut induce mucosal T-cell activation and Th1 cell differentiation via IL-12.[47,49,62] Cytokines produced by Th1 cells such as TNF and IFN-γ can activate macrophages to produce large amounts of TNF, IL-18, IL-6, Fig.21.1 Pediatric IBD Consortium data and IL-12. Many proinflammatory cytokines, such as TNF and IL-6, in turn mediate T-cell resistance against apoptosis in the inflamed gut,[38,100] resulting in prolonged cytokine production by Th1 effector cells and, finally, tissue damage.[139] Such inflammation can be suppressed in experimental models of CD by suppressor cytokines such as IL-10 released by regulatory Tr1 cells or membrane-bound TGF-β on Th3 cells (blue arrows).[174,175] Alternatively, gut inflammation can be suppressed by neutralizing antibodies such as anti-IL-TNF and anti-IL-6R, which induce Th1-cell apoptosis (red arrows). Thus, these antibodies may provide attractive approaches to the therapy of CD. APC, antigen-presenting cell; IBD, inflammatory bowel disease; IFN, interferon; IL-6, interleukin-6; IL-6R, interleukin-6 receptor; TNF, tumor necrosis factor; Tr1, T regulatory cells 1.

that blocks soluble but not membrane-bound TNF, does not appear to be effective in the treatment of active Crohn's disease.[161,162]

Some very recent studies suggest that other regulatory molecules in addition to cytokines are important for the regulation of T-cell apoptosis in experimental colitis. For instance, leptin signaling via the leptin receptor on T cells has been identified as an important factor for mediating T-cell resistance against apoptosis. In fact, blocking leptin signaling in T cells prevents the development of colitis in an adoptive transfer model by suppressing T-cell resistance against apoptosis.[163] Similarly, anti-ICOS antibodies induce apoptosis in activated T cells and attenuate experimental colitis, demonstrating a contribution of co-stimulatory molecules to the regulation of apoptosis (Watanabe M, Gastroenterology, in press).

# CONCLUSIONS

In summary, it appears that T cells in experimental colitis and in IBD patients receive multiple different signals from the inflammatory environment that converge to induce T-cell resistance against apoptosis. Specific blocking of such resistance against apoptosis is a target mechanism for some drugs currently used for therapy of IBD, and will most likely be an important target for future specific therapies. For example, a recently described molecular mechanism of action of azathioprine is related to the induction of apoptosis in activated T lymphocytes by specific blockade of the Rac1/MEKK kinase signaling pathway (Tiede et al., unpublished data). These data suggest that both established and novel treatment modalities for IBD appear to mediate their rapid beneficial effects on colitis activity, at least in part by the suppression of T-cell resistance against apoptosis and the consecutive induction of mucosal T-cell death (Fig. 13.6). In Th1-mediated inflammation such as Crohn's disease[91,92] antibodies against proinflammatory cytokines such as TNF will not only result in suppression of disease by neutralization of the cytokines that augment the Th1 pathway of inflammation, but also by the death of activated CD4+ Th1 cells. It should also be noted that the T-cell death brought about by anti-TNF, anti-IL-12 and anti-IL-6R antibodies in intestinal inflammation is likely to occur via largely independent mechanisms. This introduces the possibility removing inflammatory CD4+ T cells in independent and possibly synergistic ways. Thus, the future of therapy for intestinal inflammation in IBD may lie in combined anticytokine therapies, rather than the use of a single agent.

# REFERENCES

1. Elson CO, Sartor RB, Tennyson GS, Riddell RH. Experimental models of inflammatory bowel disease. Gastroenterology 1995;109:1344–1367.
2. Wills-Karp M, Luyimbazi J, Xu X et al. Interleukin-13: central mediator of allergic asthma. Science 1998;282:2258–2261.
3. Strober W, Kelsall B, Fuss I et al. Reciprocal IFN-gamma and TGF-beta responses regulate the occurrence of mucosal inflammation. Immunol Today 1997;18:61–64.
4. Elias JA, Zhu Z, Chupp G, Homer RJ. Airway remodeling in asthma. J Clin Invest 1999;104:1001–1006.
5. Maloy KJ, Powrie F. Regulatory T cells in the control of immune pathology. Nature Immunol 2001;2:816–822.
6. Jong YPD, Abadia-Molina AC, Satoskar AR et al. Development of chronic colitis is dependent on the cytokine MIF. Nature Immunol 2001;2:1061–1066.
7. Podolsky DK. Mucosal immunity and inflammation. V. Innate mechanisms of mucosal defense and repair: the best offense is a good defense. Am J Physiol 1999;277:G495–499.
8. Blumberg RS, Saubermann LJ, Strober W. Animal models of mucosal inflammation and their relation to human inflammatory bowel disease. Curr Opin Immunol 1999;11:648–656.
9. Podolsky DK. Inflammatory bowel disease. N Engl J Med 1991;325:928–937.
10. Schölmerich J. Future developments in diagnosis and treatment of inflammatory bowel disease. Hepatogastroenterology 2000;47:101–114.
11. Abreu-Martin MT, Targan SR. Regulation of immune responses of the intestinal mucosa. Crit Rev Immunol 1996;16:277–309.
12. Alpan O, Rudomen G, Matzinger P. The role of dendritic cells, B cells, and M cells in gut-oriented immune responses. J Immunol 2001;166:4843–4852.
13. Elson CO. Genes, microbes, and T cells – new therapeutic targets in Crohn's disease. N Engl J Med 2002;346:614–616.
14. Neurath MF, Finotto S, Glimcher LH. The role of Th1/Th2 polarization in mucosal immunity. Nature Med 2002;8:567–573.
15. Friedman S, Blumberg RS. Inflammatory bowel disease. In: Ohta J, ed. Harrison's principles of internal medicine, 15th edn. San Diego: Wiley, 1999;1679–1691.
16. McGhee JR, Lamm ME, Strober W. Mucosal immune responses: an overview. In: Ogra P L, ed. Mucosal immunology. San Diego: Academic Press; 1999:485–506.
17. Kelsall B, Strober W. Gut-associated lymphoid tissue: antigen handling and T lymphocyte responses. In: Ogra PL. Mucosal immunology. San Diego: Academic Press; 1999:293–318.
18. Bienenstock J. T cells and the immune response: down-regulation via mucosal exposure. Can Respir J 1998; 5(Suppl. A):27–30.
19. Kagnoff MF. Immunology of the intestinal tract. Gastroenterology 1993;105:1275–1280.
20. Kyd JM, Foxwell AR, Cripps AW. Mucosal immunity in the lung and upper airway. Vaccine 2001;19:2527–2533.
21. MacDonald TT, Monteleone G, Pender SLF. Recent developments in the immunology of inflammatory bowel disease. Scand J Immunol 2000;51:2–9.
22. Butcher EC. Lymphocyte homing and intestinal immunity. In: Ogra PL. Mucosal immunology. San Diego: Academic Press; 1999:507–522.
23. Strober W, Kelsall B, Marth T. Oral tolerance. J Clin Immunol 1998;18:1–30.
24. Weiner HL. Oral tolerance: immune mechanisms and the generation of Th3-type TGF-beta-secreting regulatory cells. Microbes Infect 2001;3:947–954.
25. Mosmann TR, Sad S. The expanding universe of T-cell subsets: Th1, Th2 and more. Immunol Today 1996;17:138–146.
26. Romagnani S. The Th1/Th2 paradigm. Immunol Today 1997;18:263–266.
27. Paul WE, Seder RA. Lymphocyte responses and cytokines. Cell 1994;76:241–251.
28. Asseman C, Mauze S, Leach MW, Coffman RL, Powrie F. An essential role for interleukin-10 in the function of regulatory T cells that inhibit intestinal inflammation. J Exp Med 1999;190:995–1003.
29. Powrie F, Carlino J, Leach MW, Mauze S, Coffman RL. A critical role for transforming growth factor-beta but not interleukin-4 in the suppression of T-helper type 1-mediated colitis by CD45Rb(low) CD4+ T cells. J Exp Med 1996;183:2669–2674.
30. Powrie F, Leach MW, Mauze S, Menon S, Caddle LB, Coffman RL. Inhibition of Th1 responses prevents inflammatory bowel disease in scid mice reconstituted with CD45RBhi CD4+ T cells. Immunity 1994; 2:553–562.
31. Shull MM, Ormsby I, Kier AB et al. Targeted disruption of the mouse transforming growth factor beta-1 gene results in multifocal inflammatory disease. Nature 1992;359:693–699.
32. Kuhn R, Lohler J, Rennick D, Rajewsky K, Mueller W. Interleukin-10 deficient mice develop chronic enterocolitis. Cell 1993;75:263–274.
33. Yang X, Letterio JJ, Lechleider RJ et al. Targeted disruption of SMAD3 results in impaired mucosal immunity and diminished T cell responsiveness to TGF-beta. EMBO J 1999;18:1280–1291.
34. Mombaerts P, Mizoguchi E, Grusby MJ, Glimcher LH, Bahn AK, Tonegawa S. Spontaneous development of inflammatory bowel disease in T cell receptor mutant mice. Cell 1993;75:275–282.
35. Mizoguchi A, Mizoguchi E, Bhan AK. The critical role for interleukin-4 but not interferon-gamma in the pathogenesis of colitis in T-cell receptor alpha mutant mice. Gastroenterology 1999;116:320–326.
36. Wirtz S, Finotto S, Kanzler S et al. Cutting edge: chronic intestinal inflammation in STAT-4 transgenic mice: characterization of disease and adoptive transfer by TNF- plus IFN-gamma producing CD4+ T cells that respond to bacterial antigens. J Immunol 1999;162:1884–1888.
37. Boirivant M, Fuss IJ, Chu A, Strober W. Oxazolone colitis: a murine model of T-helper cell type 2 colitis treatable with antibodies to interleukin-4. J Exp Med 1998;188:1929–1939.
38. Atreya R, Mudter J, Finotto S et al. Blockade of IL-6 trans-signaling suppresses T cell resistance against apoptosis in chronic intestinal inflammation: Evidence in Crohn's disease and experimental colitis in vivo. Nature Med 2000;6:583–588.
39. Simpson SJ, Shah S, Comiskey M et al. T cell-mediated pathology in two models of experimental colitis depends predominantly on the interleukin 12/Signal transducer and activator of transcription (Stat)-4 pathway, but is not conditional on interferon gamma expression by T cells. J Exp Med 1998;187:1225–1234.
40. Iqbal N, Oliver JR, Wagner FH, Lazenby AS, Elson CO, Weaver CT. T-helper 1 and T-helper 2 cells are pathogenic in an antigen-specific model of colitis. J Exp Med 2002;195:71–84.
41. Neurath MF, Fuss I, Kelsall BL, Presky DH, Waegell W, Strober W. Experimental granulomatous colitis in mice is abrogated by induction of TGF-β-mediated oral tolerance. J Exp Med 1996;183:2515–2527.
42. Emmrich J, Seyfarth M, Fleig WE, Emmrich F. Treatment of inflammatory bowel disease with anti-CD4 monoclonal antibody. Lancet 1991;338:570–571.
43. Greenwald B, James SP. Long-term HIV infection with Crohn's disease. Am J Gastroenterol 1995;90:167–168.
44. Lopez-Cubero SO, Sullivan KM, McDonald GB. Course of Crohn's disease after allogeneic marrow transplantation. Gastroenterology 1998; 114:433–440.
45. Kashyap A, Forman SJ. Autologous bone marrow transplantation for non-Hodgkin's lymphoma resulting in long-term remission of coincidental Crohn's disease. Br J Haematol 1998;103:651–652.
46. Hove TT, Montfrans CV, Peppelenbosch MP, Deventer SJY. Infliximab treatment induces apoptosis of lamina propria T lymphocytes in Crohn's disease. Gut 2002;50:206–211.
47. Duchmann R, Zeitz M. Crohn's disease. In: Ogra P, Strober W, eds. Handbook of mucosal immunology. San Diego: Academic Press; 1998.

48. D'Haens GR, Geboes K, Peeters M, Baert F, Penninckx F, Rutgeerts P. Early lesions of recurrent Crohn's disease caused by infusion of intestinal contents in excluded ileum. Gastroenterology 1998;114:262–267.

49. Sartor R. Postoperative recurrence of Crohn's disease: the enemy is within the fecal stream. Gastroenterology 1998;114:398–400.

50. Brimnes J, Reimann J, Nissen M, Claesson M. Enteric bacterial antigens activate CD4(+) T cells from scid mice with inflammatory bowel disease. Eur J Immunol 2001;31:23–31.

51. Claesson MH, Bregenholt S, Bonhagen K et al. Colitis-inducing potency of CD4+ T cells in immunodeficient, adoptive hosts depends on their state of activation, IL-12 responsiveness, and CD45RB surface phenotype. J Immunol 1999;162:3702–3710.

52. Rath HC, Herfarth HH, Ikeda JS et al. Normal luminal bacteria, especially *Bacteroides* species, mediate chronic colitis, gastritis, and arthritis in HLA-B27/human beta2 microglobulin transgenic rats. J Clin Invest 1996;98:945–953.

53. Sadlack B, Merz H, Schorle H, Schimpl A, Feller AC, Horvak I. Ulcerative colitis-like disease in mice with a disrupted interleukin-2 gene. Cell 1993;75:253–261.

54. Cong Y, Brandwein SL, McCabe RP et al. CD4+ T cells reactive to enteric bacterial antigens in spontaneous colitic C3H/HeJBir mice: increased T-helper cell type 1 response and ability to transfer disease. J Exp Med 1998;187:855–864.

55. Wirtz S, Neurath MF. Animal models of intestinal inflammation: new insights into the molecular pathogenesis and immunotherapy of inflammatory bowel disease. Int J Colorectal Dis 2000;15:144–160.

56. Hugot JP, Chamaillard M, Zouali H et al. Association of NOD2 leucine-rich repeat variants with susceptibility to Crohn's disease. Nature 2001;411:599–603.

57. Ogura Y, Bonen DK, Inohara N et al. A frameshift mutation in NOD2 associated with susceptibility to Crohn's disease. Nature 2001;411:603–606.

58. Ogura Y, Inohara N, Benito N, Chen FF, Yamaoka S, Núñez G. Nod2, a Nod1/Apaf-1 family member that Is restricted to monocytes and activates NF-kappaB. J Biol Chem 2001;276:4812–4818.

59. Shanahan F. Inflammatory bowel disease: immunodiagnostics, immunotherapeutics, and ecotherapeutics. Gastroenterology 2001;120:622–635.

60. Shanahan F. Crohn's disease. Lancet 2002;359:62–69.

61. Pizarro TT, Michie MH, Bentz M et al. IL-18, a novel immunoregulatory cytokine, is upregulated in Crohn's disease: expression and localization in intestinal mucosal cells. J Immunol 1999;162:6829–6835.

62. Monteleone G, Biancone L, Marasco R et al. Interleukin-12 is expressed and actively released by Crohn's disease intestinal lamina propria mononuclear cells. Gastroenterology 1997;112:1169–1178.

63. Monteleone G, Trapasso F, Parello T et al. Bioactive IL-18 expression is upregulated in Crohn's disease. J Immunol 1999;163:143–147.

64. Toy LS, Yio XY, Lin A, Honig S, Mayer L. Defective expression of gp180, a novel CD8 ligand on intestinal epithelial cells, in inflammatory bowel disease. J Clin Invest 1997; 100:2062–2071.

65. Boismenu R, Chen Y. Insights from mouse models of colitis. J Leukocyte Biol 2000; 67:267–278.

66. Glimcher LH, Murphy KM. Lineage commitment in the immune system: the T-helper lymphocyte grows up. Genes Dev 2000;14:1693–1711.

67. Moser M, Murphy KM. Dendritic cell regulation of TH1–TH2 development. Nature Immunol 2000;1:199–205.

68. Pirzer U, Schonhaar A, Fleischer B, Hermann E, Buschenfelde KHMZ. Reactivity of infiltrating T lymphocytes with microbial antigens in Crohn's disease. Lancet 1991; 338:1238–1239.

69. Fiocchi C, Battisto JR, Farmer RG. Studies on isolated gut mucosal lymphocytes in inflammatory bowel disease. Dig Dis Sci 1981;26:728–736.

70. Probert CS, Chott A, Turner JR et al. Persistent clonal expansions of peripheral blood CD4+ lymphocytes in chronic inflammatory bowel disease. J Immunol 1996; 157:3183–3191.

71. Gulwani-Akolkar B, Akolkar PN, Minassian A et al. Selective expansion of specific T cell receptors in the inflamed colon of Crohn's disease. J Clin Invest 1996; 98:1344–1354.

72. Dalwadi H, Wei B, Kronenberg B et al. The Crohn's disease-associated bacterial protein I2 is a novel enteric T cell superantigen. Immunity 2001;15:149–158.

73. Kopf M, Ruedl C, Schmitz N et al. OX40-deficient mice are defective in Th cell proliferation but are competent in generating B cell and CTL responses after virus infection. Immunity 1999;11:699–708.

74. Dong C, Juedes AE, Temann UA et al. ICOS co-stimulatory receptor is essential for T-cell activation and function. Nature 2001;409:97–101.

75. Green JM, Noel PJ, Sperling AI et al. Absence of B7-dependent responses in CD28-deficient mice. Immunity 1994;1:501–508.

76. Targan SR, Deem RL, Liu M, Wang S, Nel A. Definition of a lamina propria T cell responsive state. Enhanced cytokine responsiveness of T cells stimulated through the CD2 pathway. J Immunol 1995;154:664–675.

77. Liu Z, Geboes K, Hellings P et al. B7 interactions with CD28 and CTLA-4 control tolerance or induction of mucosal inflammation in chronic experimental colitis. J Immunol 2001;167:1830–1838.

78. Higgins LM, McDonald SA, Whittle N, Crockett N, Shields JG, MacDonald TT. Regulation of T cell activation in vitro and in vivo by targeting the OX40–OX40 ligand interaction: amelioration of ongoing inflammatory bowel disease with an OX40–IgG fusion protein, but not with an OX40 ligand–IgG fusion protein. J Immunol 1999;162:486–493.

79. Iwasaki A, Kelsall BL. Freshly isolated Peyer's patch, but not spleen, dendritic cells produce interleukin 10 and induce the differentiation of T-helper type 2 cells. J Exp Med 1999;190:229–239.

80. Adorini L, Sinigaglia F. Pathogenesis and immunotherapy of autoimmune diseases. Immunol Today 1997;18:209–211.

81. Trinchieri G. Interleukin-12: a cytokine produced by antigen-presenting cells with immunoregulatory functions in the generation of T-helper cells type 1 and cytotoxic lymphocytes. Blood 1994; 84:4008–4027.

82. Pulendran B, Maraskovsky E, Banchereau J, Maliszewski C. Modulating the immune response with dendritic cells and their growth factors. Trends Immunol 2001; 22:41–47.

83. Ma X, Neurath MF, Gri G, Trinchieri G. Identification and characterization of a novel Ets-2-related nuclear complex implicated in the activation of the human interleukin-12 p40 gene promoter. J Biol Chem 1997; 272:10389–10394.

84. Bell SJ, Rigby R, English N et al. Migration and maturation of human colonic dendritic cells. J Immunol 2001;166:4958–4967.

85. Autschbach F, Schürmann G, Qiao L, Merz H, Wallich R, Meuer SC. Cytokine mRNA expression and proliferation status of intestinal mononuclear cells in noninflamed gut and Crohn's disease. Virchows Arch 1995;426:51–60.

86. Breese E, Braegger CP, Corrigan CJ, Walker-Smith JA, MacDonald TT. Interleukin-2 and interferon-gamma secreting T cells in normal and diseased human intestinal mucosa. Immunology 1993;78:127–131.

87. Mullin GE, Lazenby AJ, Harris ML, Bayless TM, James SP. Increased interleukin-2 messenger RNA in the intestinal mucosal lesions of Crohn's disease but not ulcerative colitis. Gastroenterology 1992;102:1620–1627.

88. Karp LC, Targan SR. Ulcerative colitis. In: Ogra PL, ed. Mucosal immunology, 2nd edn. San Diego: Academic Press; 1999:1047–1053.

89. Sher ME, d'Angelo AJ, Stein TA, Bruns G. Cytokines in Crohn's colitis. Am J Surg 1995;56:133–143.

90. Duchmann R. Downregulation of T reg cells in patients with active IBD. Gastroenterology/DDW A 2002; (in press).

91. Fuss I, Neurath MF, Boirivant M et al. Disparate CD4+ lamina propria (LP) lymphocyte secretion profiles in inflammatory bowel disease. J Immunol 1996; 157:1261–1270.

92. Plevy SE, Landers CJ, Prehn J et al. A role for TNF-alpha and mucosal T-helper-1 cytokines in the pathogenesis of Crohn's disease. J Immunol 1997;159:6276–6282.

93. Magram J, Connaughton SE, Warrier RR et al. IL-12-deficient mice are defective in IFN-gamma production and type 1 cytokine responses. Immunity 1996;4: 471–481.

94. Szabo SJ, Jacobson NG, Dighe AS, Gubler U, Murphy KM. Developmental commitment to the Th2 lineage by extinction of IL-12 signaling. Immunity 1995;2:665–675.

95. O'Shea JJ. Jaks, STATs, cytokine signal transduction, and immunoregulation: are we there yet? Immunity 1997;7:1–11.

96. Yoshimoto T, Takeda K, Tanaka T et al. IL-12 upregulates IL-18 receptor expression on T cells, Th1 cells and B cells: synergism with IL-18 for IFN-gamma production. J Immunol 1998;161:3400–3407.

97. Yamamoto K, Quelle FW, Thierfelder WE et al. Stat4, a novel gamma interferon activation site-binding protein expressed in early myeloid differentiation. Mol Cell Biol 1994;14:4342–4349.

98. Neurath MF, Fuss I, Kelsall BL, Stuber E, Strober W. Antibodies to IL-12 abrogate established experimental colitis in mice. J Exp Med 1995;182:1280–1289.

99. Neurath MF, Finotto S. Fuss I, Boirivant M, Galle PR, Strober W. Regulation of T-cell apoptosis in inflammatory bowel disease: to die or not to die, that is the mucosal question. Trends Immunol 2001;22:21–26.

100. Fuss IJ, Marth T, Neurath MF, Pearlstine GR, Jain A, Strober W. Anti-interleukin 12 treatment regulates apoptosis of Th1 T cells in experimental colitis in mice. Gastroenterology 1999;117:1078–1088.

101. Davidson NJ, Hudak SA, Lesley RE, Menon S, Leach MW, Rennick DM. IL-12, but not IFN-gamma, plays a major role in sustaining the chronic phase of colitis in IL-10-deficient mice. J Immunol 1998;161:3143–3149.

102. Marth T, Zeitz M, Ludviksson BR, Strober W, Kelsall BL. Extinction of IL-12 signaling promotes Fas-mediated apoptosis of antigen-specific T cells. J Immunol 1999; 162:7233–7240.

103. Oppmann B, Lesley R, Blom B et al. Novel p19 protein engages IL-12p40 to form a cytokine, IL-23, with biologic activities similar as well as distinct from IL-12. Immunity 2000;13:715–725.

104. Wiekowski MT, Leach MW, Evans EW et al. Ubiquitous transgenic expression of the IL-23 subunit p19 induces multiorgan inflammation, runting, infertility, and premature death. J Immunol 2001;166:7563–7570.

105. Parrello T, Monteleone G, Cucchiara S et al. Up-regulation of the IL-12 receptor beta 2 chain in Crohn's disease. J Immunol 2000;165:7234–7239.

106. Monteleone G, MacDonald TT, Wathen NC, Pallone F, Pender SL. Enhancing lamina propria Th1 cell responses with interleukin 12 produces severe tissue injury. Gastroenterology 1999;117:1069–1077.

107. Carter LL, Murphy KM. Lineage-specific requirement for signal transducer and activator of transcription Stat4 in interferon-gamma production from CD4(+) versus CD8(+) T cells. J Exp Med 1999;189:1355–1360.

108. Durbin JE, Hackenmiller R, Simon MC, Levy DE. Targeted disruption of the mouse Stat1 gene results in compromised innate immunity to viral disease. Cell 1996;84:443–450.

109. Afkarian M, Sedy JR, Yang J et al. T-bet is a STAT1-induced regulator of IL-12R expression in naive CD4(+) T cells. Nature Immunol 2002;3:361–369.

110. Lighvani AA, Frucht DM, Jankovic D et al. T-bet is rapidly induced by interferon-gamma in lymphoid and myeloid cells. Proc Natl Acad Sci USA 2001;98:15137–15142.

111. Szabo SJ, Kim ST, Costa GL, Zhang X, Fathman CG, Glimcher LH. A novel transcription factor, T-bet, directs Th1 lineage commitment. Cell 2000;100:655–669.

112. Grogan JL, Mohrs M, Harmon B, Lacy DA, Sedat JW, Locksley RM. Early transcription and silencing of cytokine genes underlie polarization of T-helper cell subsets. Immunity 2001;14:205–215.

113. Szabo SJ, Sullivan BM, Stemmann C, Satoskar AR, Sleckman BR, Glimcher LH. T-bet is essential for Th1 Lineage Commitment and IFN-gamma production in CD4 but not CD8 T Cells. Science 2002;295:338–342.

114. Mullen AC, High FA, Hutchins AS et al. Role of T-bet in commitment of TH1 cells before IL-12-dependent selection. Science 2001; 292:1907–1910.

115. Neurath MF, Weigmann B, Finotto S et al. The transcription factor T-bet regulates mucosal T cell activation in experimental colitis and Crohn's disease. J Exp Med 2002;195:1129–1143.

116. Monteleone G, Kumberova A, Croft NM, McKenzie C, Steer HW, MacDonald TT. Blocking Smad7 restores TGF-ß1 signaling in chronic inflammatory bowel disease. J Clin Invest 2001;108:601–609.

117. Nakao A, Afrakhte M, Moren A et al. Identification of Smad7, a TGF-beta-inducible antagonist of TGF-beta signalling. Nature 1997;389:631–635.

118. Piek E, Heldin CH, Dijke PT. Specificity, diversity, and regulation in TGF-beta superfamily signaling. FASEB J 1999;13:2105–2124.

119. Christ AD, Stevens AC, Koeppen H et al. An interleukin 12-related cytokine is up-regulated in ulcerative colitis but not in Crohn's disease. Gastroenterology 1998;115:307–313.

120. Omata F, Birkenbach M, Matsuzaki S, Christ AD, Blumberg RS. The expression of IL-12 p40 and its homologue, Epstein–Barr virus-induced gene 3, in inflammatory bowel disease. Inflamm Bowel Dis 2001;7:215–220.

121. Mizoguchi A, Mizoguchi E, Smith RN, Preffer FI, Bhan AK. The suppressive role of B cells in chronic colitis of T cell receptor alpha mutant mice. J Exp Med 1997;186:1749–1756.

122. Mizoguchi A, Mizoguchi E, Chiba C, Bhan AK. Role of appendix in the development of inflammatory bowel disease in TCR-alpha mutant mice. J Exp Med 1996; 184:707–715.

123. Russel MG, Dorant E, Brummer RJ et al. Appendectomy and the risk of developing ulcerative colitis or Crohn's disease: results of a large case–control study. South Limburg Inflammatory Bowel Disease Study Group. Gastroenterology 1997;113:377–382.

124. Fort M, Lesley R, Davidson N et al. IL-4 exacerbates disease in a Th1 cell transfer model of colitis. J Immunol 2001;166:2793–2800.

125. Spencer DM, Veldman GM, Banerjee S, Willis J, Levine AD. Distinct inflammatory mechanisms mediate early versus late colitis in mice. Gastroenterology 2002;122:94–105.

126. Desreumaux P, Brandt E, Gambiez L et al. Distinct cytokine patterns in early and chronic ileal lesions of Crohn's disease. Gastroenterology 1997;113:118–126.

127. Okamura H, Tsutsui H, Komatsu M et al. Cloning of a new cytokine that induces IFN-gamma production by T cells. Nature 1995;378:88–91.

128. Okamura H, Kashiwamura S, Tsutsui H, Yoshimoto T, Nakanishi K. Regulation of interferon-gamma production by IL-12 and IL-18. Curr Opin Immunol 1998;10:259–264.

129. Akira S. The role of IL-18 in innate immunity. Curr Opin Immunol 2000;12:59–63.

130. Dinarello CA. Interleukin-18. Methods 1999;19:121–132.

131. Dinarello CA. IL-18: a Th1-inducing proinflammatory cytokine and new member of the IL-1 family. J Allergy Clin Immunol 1999;103:11–19.

132. Barbulescu K, Becker C, Schlaak J, Schmitt E, Büschenfelde KHMz, Neurath MF. Cutting edge: Interleukin-12 and interleukin-18 differentially regulate the transcriptional activity of the human IFN-gamma promoter in primary CD4+ T lymphocytes. J Immunol 1998;160:3642–3647.

133. Hove TT, Corbaz A, Amitai H et al. Blockade of endogenous IL-18 ameliorates TNBS-induced colitis by decreasing local TNF-alpha production in mice. Gastroenterology 2001;121:1372–1379.

134. Kanai T, Watanabe M, Okazawa A et al. Macrophage-derived IL-18-mediated intestinal inflammation in the murine model of Crohn's disease. Gastroenterology 2001;121:875–888.

135. Siegmund B, Fantuzzi G, Rieder F et al. Neutralization of interleukin-18 reduces severity in murine colitis and intestinal IFN-gamma and TNF-alpha production. Am J Physiol Regul Integr Comp Physiol 2001;281:1264–1273.

136. Wirtz S, Becker C, Blumberg R, Galle PR, Neurath MF. Treatment of T cell-dependent experimental colitis in SCID mice by local administration of an adenovirus expressing IL-18 antisense mRNA. J Immunol 2002;168:411–420.

137. Kanai T, Watanabe M, Okazawa A et al. Interleukin-18 is a potent proliferative factor for intestinal mucosal lymphocytes in Crohn's disease. Gastroenterology 2000;119:1514–1523.

138. Breese EJ, Michie CA, Nicholls SW et al. Tumor necrosis factor alpha-producing cells in the intestinal mucosa of children with inflammatory bowel disease. Gastroenterology 1994;106:1455–1466.

139. Pender SL, Fell JM, Chamow SM, Ashkenazi A, MacDonald TT. A p55 TNF receptor immunoadhesin prevents T cell-mediated intestinal injury by inhibiting matrix metalloproteinase production. J Immunol 1998;160:4098–4103.

140. Holtmann MH, Douni E, Schütz M et al. Tumor necrosis factor-receptor 2 is upregulated on lamina propria T cells in Crohn's disease and promotes experimental colitis in vivo. Gastroenterology DDW issue 2002;156:A3102.

141. Shanahan F, Nally K, O'Sullivan GC. Turning on T-cell death and turning off Crohn's disease. Gastroenterology 2000;119:1166–1168.

142. Ina K, Itoh J, Fukushima K et al. Resistance of Crohn's disease T cells to multiple apoptotic signals is associated with a Bcl-2/Bax mucosal imbalance. J Immunol 1999;163:1081–1090.

143. Boirivant M, Marini M, Di-Felice G et al. Lamina propria T cells in Crohn's disease and other gastrointestinal inflammation show defective CD2 pathway-induced apoptosis. Gastroenterology 1999;116:557–565.

144. Scaffidi C, Fulda S, Srinivasan A et al. Two CD95 (APO-1/Fas) signaling pathways. EMBO J 1998;17:1675–1687.

145. Scaffidi C, Kirchhoff S, Krammer PH, Peter ME. Apoptosis signaling in lymphocytes. Curr Opin Immunol 1999;11:277–285.

146. Budd RC. Activation-induced cell death. Curr Opin Immunol 2001;13:356–362.

147. Lenardo M, Chan F, Hornung F et al. Mature T lymphocyte apoptosis – immune regulation in a dynamic and unpredictable antigenic environment. Annu Rev Immunol 1999;17:221–253.

148. Boirivant M, Pica R, DeMaria R, Testi R, Pallone F, Strober W. Stimulated human lamina propria T cells manifest enhanced Fas-mediated apoptosis. J Clin Invest 1996;98:2616–2622.

149. Rose-John S, Heinrich PC. Soluble receptors for cytokines and growth factors: generation and biological function. Biochem J 1994;300:281–290.

150. Hurst SM, Wilkinson TS, McLoughlin RM et al. IL-6 and its soluble receptor orchestrate a temporal switch in the pattern of leukocyte recruitment seen during acute inflammation. Immunity 2001;14:705–714.

151. Catlett-Falcone R, Landowski TH, Oshiro MM et al. Constitutive activation of Stat3 signaling confers resistance to apoptosis in human U266 myeloma cells. Immunity 1999;10:105–115.

152. Peters M, Müller A, Rose-John S. Interleukin-6 and soluble interleukin-6 receptor: direct stimulation of gp130 and hematopoiesis. Blood 1998;92:3295–3504.

153. Suzuki A, Hanada T, Mitsuyama K et al. CIS3/SOCS3/SSI3 plays a negative regulatory role in STAT3 activation and intestinal inflammation. J Exp Med 2001;193:471–481.

154. Mitsuyama K, Toyonaga A, Sasaki E et al. Soluble IL-6 receptors in inflammatory bowel disease: relation to circulating IL-6. Gut 1995;36:45–49.

155. Fukada T, Hibi M, Yamanaka Y et al. Two signals are necessary for cell proliferation induced by a cytokine receptor gp130: involvement of STAT3 in anti-apoptosis. Immunity 1996;5:449–460.

156. Shirogane T, Fukada T, Muller JMM, Shima DT, Hibi M, Hirano T. Synergistic roles for Pim-1 and c-myc in STAT3-mediated cell cycle progression and antiapoptosis. Immunity 1999;11:709–719.

157. Takeda K, Kaisho T, Yoshida N, Takeda J, Kishimoto T, Akira S. Stat3 activation is responsible for IL-6-dependent T cell proliferation through preventing apoptosis: generation and characterization of T cell-specific Stat3-deficient mice. J Immunol 1998;161:4652–4660.

158. Teague TK, Marrack P, Kappler JW, Vella AT. IL-6 rescues resting mouse T cells from apoptosis. J Immunol 1997;158:5791–5796.

159. Beutler B, Bazzoni F. TNF, apoptosis and autoimmunity: a common thread? Blood Cells Mol Dis 1998;24:216–230.

160. Beutler B. Autoimmunity and apoptosis: the Crohn's connection. Immunity 2001;15:5–14.

161. Sandborn WJ, Hanauer SB, Katz S et al. Etanercept for active Crohn's disease: a randomized, double-blind, placebo-controlled trial. Gastroenterology 2001;121:1088–1094.

162. Deventer SJV. Transmembrane TNF-alpha, induction of apoptosis, and the efficacy of TNF-targeting therapies in Crohn's disease. Gastroenterology 2001;121:1242–1246.

163. Siegmund B, Lehr HA, Fantuzzi G. Leptin: a pivotal mediator of intestinal inflammation in mice. Gastroenterology 2002;122:2011–25.

164. Rescigno M, Urbano M, Valzasina B et al. Dendritic cells express tight junction proteins and penetrate gut epithelial monolayers to sample bacteria. Nature Immunol 2001;2:362–367.

165. Ouyang W, Ranganath SH, Weindel K et al. Inhibition of Th1 development mediated by GATA-3 through an IL-4 independent mechanism. Immunity 1998;9:745–755.

166. Ouyang W, Löhning M, Gao Z et al. Stat-6 independent GATA-3 autoactivation directs IL-4 independent Th2 development and commitment. Immunity 2000;12:27–37.

167. Zheng W, Flavell RA. The transcription factor GATA-3 is necessary and sufficient for Th2 cytokine gene expression in CD4+ T cells. Cell 1997;89:587–596.

168. Zhang DH, Yang L, Cohn L et al. Inhibition of allergic inflammation in a murine model of asthma by expression of a dominant-negative mutant of GATA-3. Immunity 1999;11:473–482.

169. Finotto S, Sanctis GTD, Lehr HA et al. Treatment of allergic airway inflammation and hyperresponsiveness by local antisense-induced blockade of GATA-3 expression. J Exp Med 2001;193:1247–1260.

170. Targan SR, Hanauer SB, Deventer SJV et al. A short-term study of chimeric monoclonal antibody cA2 to tumor necrosis factor alpha for Crohn's disease. N Engl J Med 1997;337:1029–1035.

171. Deventer SJV, Elson CO, Fedorak RN. Multiple doses of intravenous interleukin 10 in steroid-refractory Crohn's disease. Gastroenterology 1997;113:383–389.

172. Schwertschlag US, Trepicchio WL, Dykstra KH, Keith JC, Turner KJ, Dorner AJ. Hematopoietic, immunomodulatory and epithelial effects of interleukin-11. Leukemia 1999;13:1307–1315.

173. Breese E, MacDonald TT. TNF-alpha secreting cells in normal and diseased human intestine. Adv Exp Med Biol 1996;371B:821–824.

174. Groux H, Powrie F. Regulatory T cells and inflammatory bowel disease. Immunol Today 1999;20:442–446.

175. Kitani A, Fuss IJ, Nakamura K, Schwartz OM, Usui T, Strober W. Treatment of experimental (TNBS)-colitis by intranasal administration of TGF-beta 1 plasmid: TGF-beta1-mediated suppression of Th1 response occurs by IL-10 induction and IL-12Rb2 chain down-regulation. J Exp Med 2000;192:41–52.

## CHAPTER 14

# Neuroimmune interactions in the inflamed intestine

Stephen M Collins

## HISTORICAL PERSPECTIVE

### NERVES AND IBD

The notion that the nervous system plays a role in the natural history of the idiopathic inflammatory bowel diseases (IBD) is not new. Indeed, ulcerative colitis was initially considered to be a psychosomatic disorder,[1] based in part on the perceived relationship between the activity of colitis and stress. This association was also based on a perceived relationship between behavior, functional bowel disorders (such as irritable bowel syndrome, IBS) and IBD; IBS was considered a prelude to IBD in some patients, and the linkage of these disorders was thought to be mediated via neural-induced changes in gut motility.[2] At the time, experiments demonstrated that induction of abnormal motility in dog colon produced changes in the organ that were indistinguishable from ulcerative colitis.[3] This colitis was initially considered to be ischemic, but further study showed that colitis induced by repeated administration of the parasympathomimetic drug methacholine could not be reproduced by injections of vasopressin.[4] In this early conceptual model of UC, a behavioral predisposition[5] led to abnormal motility and IBS, which in turn led to the development of UC. This concept influenced the early management of IBD, with the surgical interventions of truncal vagotomy and pelvic denervation offered to patients with refractory colitis.[6-8]

### IBS AS A RISK FACTOR FOR IBD

Although the psychosomatic model was subsequently discarded in favor of an exclusive organically based construct of IBD, it is interesting to note that a large cohort study suggested that IBS might be a risk factor for IBD.[9] In that study, 2956 patients with a recent diagnosis of IBS were followed for 3 years for a subsequent diagnosis of IBD, and results were compared with those from a cohort of healthy subjects. The authors found that patients with a diagnosis of IBS had a relative risk of 16.3 (95% confidence interval (CI) 6.6–40.7), which was constant throughout the 3-year follow-up period. The diagnosis of colorectal tumors (CRT) was used to detect a surveillance bias. Although the diagnosis of CRT increased predictably in the first year following a diagnosis of IBS, the relative risk was no different between IBS patients and controls over the duration of the study. The recent observations of a genetic susceptibility of IBS patients to inflammation,[10] increased inflammatory cell numbers in colonic biopsies of IBS patients, and evidence of immune activation in these tissues[11-16] support the notion, long held by this author, that low-grade inflammation is pathophysiologically relevant in at least a subset of IBS patients.[17,18]

### IBD AS A RISK FACTOR FOR IBS

The recognition that patients in remission from IBD exhibit a higher than expected incidence of IBS symptoms[19,20] and have abnormal motor-sensory function in the colon[21] has suggested that IBD may be a risk factor for IBS. This relationship is conceptually feasible in light of an increasing literature showing that previous inflammation leads to persistent changes in gastrointestinal motility.[22,23] Taken together, these data support a conceptual model in which IBD and at least a subset of the IBS population are interrelated (Fig. 14.1). This provocative model is offered to kindle interest not only in the hypothesis that a subset of IBS patients have an underlying predisposition to inflammation, but also to stimulate further investigation of the role of the nervous system in the pathogenesis of IBD.

## NERVES AND IBD: THE CONCEPTUAL FRAMEWORK

Investigation into the relationship of the nervous system and IBD is based on a bidirectional model in which the nervous system is altered by the presence of inflammation and the inflammatory process may be influenced by the nervous system

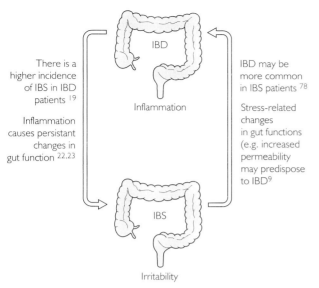

Fig. 14.1 A proposed relationship between idiopathic inflammatory bowel diseases (IBD) and irritable bowel syndrome (IBS).

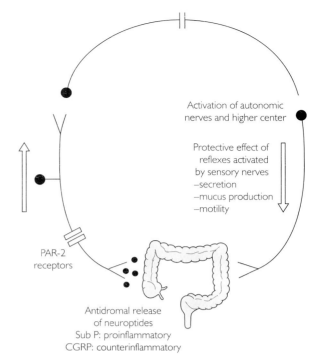

Fig. 14.2 The role of sensory pathways in intestinal inflammation. Neuropeptides are released from sensory nerve endings by inflammatory mediators. Substance P has proinflammatory properties, whereas calcitonin gene related peptide (CGRP) has counterinflammatory properties. Activation of sensory nerves also initiates reflex responses in the gut that contribute to host defense and which reduce inflammation. In addition, activation of sensory nerves may also alter higher circuits and autonomic outflow.

(Fig. 14.2). Products of inflammatory or immune cells can alter structure[24] and/or function[25] in enteric nerves, and biologically active receptors for neurotransmitters or growth factors are present on a variety of immune or inflammatory cells.[26,27] These observations, taken in conjunction with demonstrations of close proximity between nerves and immune or inflammatory cells,[28] form the basis for considering bidirectional neuroimmune interactions in IBD.

# THE EFFECT OF INFLAMMATION ON THE NERVOUS SYSTEM

## OBSERVATIONS IN IBD PATIENTS

Many studies show changes in neural number and structure, as well as changes in enteric neurotransmitter content in IBD.[29] The results of many of these studies have been compromised as a result of technical shortcomings and the profile of altered neurotransmitter content in IBD in these studies is variable. Nevertheless, it is evident that axonal degeneration occurs in both Crohn's disease and ulcerative colitis, and that such changes may occur early in the course of the disease and involve autonomic as well as enteric nerves.

A threefold increase in the number of ganglion cells has been observed in myenteric specimens from Crohn's disease[30] as well as ulcerative colitis.[31] In ulcerative colitis the changes were evident early in the course of the disease, whereas in Crohn's disease the neural changes became more evident with established inflammation. Interestingly, in both conditions changes in ganglion numbers were evident at adjacent non-involved sites. The significance of this is unclear, but similar findings have been associated with a higher risk of relapse in Crohn's patients. D'Haens and co-workers examined the proximal margin of ileal resections of patients undergoing surgery for Crohn's disease. Patients who subsequently relapsed 3 months after surgery had increased inflammatory cells around myenteric nerves in the sur-

gical specimen. In contrast, the presence of inflammatory cells in the mucosal compartment of the resected margin did not correlate with relapse.[32] This clinical observation suggests that enteric nerves may play an active role in the natural history of Crohn's disease.

The expression of MHC II on enteroglia in Crohn's disease suggests that changes in enteric nerves are immune mediated.[33] Interest has focused on tachykinins and their receptors because of their proinflammatory properties and their role in the sensation of pain. For example, a greater than 1000-fold increase in binding sites for substance P was reported in gut lymphoid tissue in both Crohn's disease and ulcerative colitis, suggesting that this neuropeptide may play a role in modulating inflammation in IBD.[34] Animal research supporting this concept is discussed below. In addition to neuropeptides and their receptors, changes also occur in neurotrophins in IBD.[35] Specifically, these investigators found increased expression of nerve growth factor (NGF), which possesses proinflammatory properties, and the high-affinity neurotrophin receptor A (TrkA) in tissues both from patients with ulcerative colitis and those with Crohn's disease. Increases in vasoactive intestinal peptide (VIP)-containing nerves have been reported in both inflamed and non-inflamed Crohn's disease tissues,[36,37] but later findings were not confirmatory.[38]

The involvement of nerves in IBD is not restricted to the gut. A chronic polyneuropathy has been associated with ulcerative colitis; electrophysiological studies have demonstrated a severe neuropathy with both axonal and demyelinating features. Biopsy of the sural nerve revealed perineuritis. These findings suggest that peripheral neuropathy may be an immunologically mediated extraintestinal manifestation of ulcerative colitis.[39]

Structural abnormalities have been identified in the brains of patients with IBD. Nuclear magnetic resonance studies showed the presence of focal lesions measuring 2–4 mm in the white matter of 10 of 28 patients with Crohn's disease and in 6 of 12 patients with ulcerative colitis; those with lesions tended to be older. The clinical significance of this finding remains unclear.[40,41] There is a small increase in the incidence of central neurological diseases in IBD patients whereby 3% had abnormalities compared to controls.[42] The most frequent abnormality was cerebrovascular disease, which might reflect hypercoagulability. Also found were myasthenia gravis, myelopathies, and an acute inflammatory demyelinating polyradicular neuropathy similar to that found in association with *Campylobacter jejuni* infection.

## FUNCTIONAL CHANGES

### Motor-sensory

Many studies show that motility is altered in IBD. As the enteric nervous system is an integral part of the motility apparatus, it is likely that these motility changes in IBD reflect primary alterations in neural function, although there is evidence that smooth muscle contraction[43] is altered in IBD.

### Autonomic imbalance

Studies of autonomic reflexes show abnormalities in patients with IBD. Thirty-five per cent of patients with ulcerative colitis had demonstrable autonomic neuropathy with parasympathetic impairment and hence sympathetic dominance;[44] almost 50% of patients with Crohn's disease also showed evidence of autonomic neuropathy, but without the sympathetic dominance seen in ulcerative colitis.[45] Studying cardiovascular and pupillary reflexes, Straub et al.[46] also found hyperreflexia in both Crohn's disease and ulcerative colitis patients. In the gastrointestinal tract, significant increases in catecholamine content have been identified in patients with ulcerative colitis, with the most marked changes being in the rectum.[47,48]

## INSIGHTS FROM ANIMAL MODELS

Studies in animal models have provided clear demonstrations that intestinal inflammation alters the structure and function of enteric nerves. Initial studies were performed in a model of intestinal inflammation due to primary infection with the nematode parasites *Trichinella spiralis* or *Nippostrongylus brasiliensis*. Subsequently studies have been extended to other models, such as hapten-induced colitis.

Initial studies in nematode-infected rats focused on changes in parasympathetic nerves. Acute infection with *Trichinella spiralis* produced mucosal inflammation in the jejunum, which was accompanied by a reduction in the release of the parasympathetic neurotransmitter acetylcholine from myenteric nerves.[49] The changes in cholinergic nerve function were attributed to the host inflammatory response, as they could be attenuated by steroid treatment. In contrast, these changes did not require T lymphocytes[50] and were therefore considered to reflect an innate immune response to the infection. Subsequent studies in mice showed that macrophages were required for the changes in cholinergic nerve function.[51] The critical subset of macrophages were macrophage colony-stimulating factor (M-CSF)

dependent.[52] These findings could be mimicked by the administration of interleukin-1β,[53] a known macrophage-derived cytokine, implicating IL-1β as a mediator in the suppression of cholinergic nerves in that model, particularly as there was increased expression of IL-1 and other proinflammatory cytokines in the myenteric plexus during inflammation.[54]

Suppression of adrenergic nerve function was also found in nematode-infected rats. Suppression of noradrenaline release was steroid sensitive, reflective of the inflammatory response rather than the presence of the parasite.[55] Studies were extended to other models, including colitis induced by trinitrobenzene sulfonic acid (TNBS), where decreased noradrenaline release was found not only at the site of inflammation in the distal colon but also at remote non-inflamed sites, including the small intestine. This provides a functional correlate of the observation in humans that changes exist in the enteric nervous system even in non-inflamed segments. Together these findings indicate that focal inflammation in the gastrointestinal tract could be a basis for widespread disruption of neurally mediated physiology that would include motility, secretion and epithelial function. This may be critical, for example, to intestinal permeability, as the integrity of the mucosal barrier is partly mediated by cholinergic nerves.[56]

There has been much interest in the effect of inflammation on substance P. The nematode-infected rat has a more than eightfold increase in substance P in the myenteric plexus. This increase was found in nerves, particularly primary afferents, as the increased substance P could be depleted using scorpion venom or capsaicin.[57] Interestingly, and in contrast to the mechanisms underlying the above-described changes in autonomic nerve function, increased substance P in this model was T lymphocyte dependent, as increases did not occur in infected athymic animals.[57] Thus, the changes in different types of enteric nerves reflect separate underlying immunological mechanisms and may involve components of the innate or adaptive immune systems.

Structural studies in rodent models of inflammation have provided evidence of remodeling and phenotypic change. The number of neuron-specific enolase (NSE)-staining nerves increased approximately 2.5-fold after infection of rats with *Nippostrongylus brasiliensis* and later returned to near control values. Immunoreactivity for the neural proteins B-50/GAP-43 was more extensive. B-50 immunoreactivity decreased minimally during infection but increased significantly after the peak inflammatory response to infection had subsided. These data demonstrate that early degenerative and later regenerative phases occur in the inflamed intestine. Regeneration of nerves was closely associated with mast cells.[58] Indeed, nerves are intimately associated with mucosal mast cells during intestinal inflammation.[59]

Functional studies show that intestinal inflammation results in functional changes in the brain. For example, inflammation-induced suppression of feeding seen in rats with experimental colitis[60] is mediated by both peripheral and central IL-1β.[61] Inflammation or immune activation in the gut produces rapid-onset extensive changes in neural activity. In a model of formalin-induced local colitis, Fos expression increased significantly in both myenteric neurons and enteric glia. Fos immunoreactive neuronal nuclei were significantly increased in the spinal cord, area postrema and nucleus of the solitary tract during inflammation. These changes were induced via sympathetic nerves, as they could be reversed by the $\alpha_2$ adrenoceptor antagonist yohimbine.[62] More restricted stimulation of the gut via antigen challenge in sensitized rats results in similar c-fos activation in the central nervous system via the involvement of primary afferents, the vagus nerve and 5-hydroxytryptamine.[63] Taken together, these observations indicate that inflammatory signals originating in the gut produce extensive changes in neural circuitry which involve the central nervous system.

The vagus nerve plays a critical role not only in transmitting information to the brain following immune activation in the gut, but also in mediating changes in CNS function, including temperature regulation and feeding behavior. Intravenously administered IL-1β activated the nucleus of the solitary tract (NTS), which is the primary pathway of sensory information from the vagus nerve. This effect was mediated by prostaglandins acting at the EP3 subtype of the prostaglandin $E_2$ receptor on neuronal cell bodies in the nodose ganglion.[64] IL-1β released during intestinal inflammation contributes to anorexia via both peripheral and central IL-1 receptors.[61,65] The febrile response to IL-1β is mediated via the vagus nerve, as this effect is blocked by truncal subdiaphragmatic vagotomy.[66]

# THE EFFECT OF NERVES ON INFLAMMATION

The notion that the nervous system influences inflammatory processes is not new. Chronic inflammatory conditions, including ulcerative colitis, were originally believed to represent 'psychosomatic' disorders.[67] Although a role for the nervous system in initiating IBD is no longer tenable, neural modulation of intestinal inflammation could influence the natural history of IBD.

The role of stress in IBD is controversial based on existing literature, and a full review of this is beyond the scope of this chapter (for review see[68,69] and Chapter 24). Although very good evidence indicates that stress increases or reactivates intestinal inflammatory responses in animals (see below), there are no controlled studies of the effect of antidepressants or anxiolytics in IBD; case reports suggest there may be a beneficial effect in selected patients.[70,71]

The relationship between smoking or nicotine treatment and IBD[72] may be construed as evidence of a neuromodulatory effect, although smoking may have nicotine-independent effects.[73] The evidence of autonomic imbalance in IBD does not apply to all patients. For example, in one study 35% of patients with ulcerative colitis had evidence of parasympathetic impairment.[44] As nicotine effects on inflammation are dose dependent and protection is seen only at low doses, it is likely that only those patients with parasympathetic impairment will respond beneficially to nicotine.

There are reports of therapeutic benefit from topical application of local anesthetics in ulcerative colitis.[74] Lidocaine not only produced symptomatic improvement but also reduced histologic inflammation. This suggests that sensory nerves modulate colitis, although the possibility of a systemic effect from absorbed lidocaine cannot be excluded. However, recent studies using ripivocaine have not demonstrated benefit in distal ulcerative colitis.[75]

Taken together, these clinical observations provide a basis for exploring mechanisms underlying the neuromodulation of intestinal inflammation.

# ANIMAL STUDIES: THE INTEGRITY OF THE NERVOUS SYSTEM AND REGULATION OF INFLAMMATION

## STRESS

Recent studies have elucidated underlying mechanisms of the proinflammatory potential of stress in experimental animals.[76] Stress applied prior to exposure to an inflammatory stimulus increases the severity of colitis in rats,[77] but this response is not mediated by either CRF or vasopressin pathways in the brain. Stress may facilitate the development of an inflammatory response via an increase in intestinal permeability;[78] in the rat this is mediated via cholinergic nerves.[56] Perhaps more relevant to clinical observations is the demonstration that mild restraint and acoustic stress reactivated colitis in mice that had fully recovered from colitis induced 6 weeks previously by the hapten dinitrobenzene sulfonic acid (DNBS).[79] This was accompanied by an increase in colonic permeability and was mediated by CD4+ lymphocytes. Indeed, the susceptibility to stress-induced reactivation could be adoptively transferred into naive mice by CD4+ cells from mice with previous colitis. This study provides an unambiguous demonstration of how stress can reactivate quiescent colitis, as has been suggested by clinical observation, and that control of immune activity in IBD patients may reduce the risk of relapse induced by stress.

## SENSORY NERVES

The role of sensory nerves in intestinal inflammatory processes is complex. Whereas the proinflammatory properties of the major sensory neurotransmitter substance P has long been recognized, the counterinflammatory properties of sensory nerves have been overlooked (Table 14.1). Stimulation of sensory nerves following tissue injury is accompanied by the antedromal release of substance P, which triggers plasma extravasation and initiates 'neurogenic inflammation'.[80] During inflammation, the activity of neutral endopeptidase (NEP EC 3.4.24.11), which degrades substance P, is markedly reduced, resulting in increased bioavailability of substance P and related ligands.[81] A role for endogenous NEP in intestinal inflammation was demonstrated by observations that hapten-induced colitis was more severe and prolonged in NEP-deficient mice.[82] Antagonism of substance P attenuates intestinal inflammation in some experimental models.[83] The therapeutic potential of inhibiting substance P via degradation (NEP) or via neurokinin (NK) receptor blockade is suggested by increased NK-binding sites in the intestine of patients with Crohn's disease.[34,84,85]

CGRP-containing nerves are prominent in Crohn's disease,[86] providing a structural basis for consideration of a role for this peptide in inflammation. Calcitonin gene-related peptide (CGRP)

### Table 14.1 Effects of neurotransmitters on inflammation

| Proinflammatory | Counterinflammatory |
| --- | --- |
| Nicotine (high dose)[94] | Nicotine (low dose)[94] |
| Substance P[80–85] | Calcitonin gene-related peptide (CGRP)[86–89] |
| Norepinephrine[98] | |

has anti-inflammatory properties and is protective in animal models of colitis.[87,88] It may also exert direct immunomodulatory effects on T lymphocytes as part of its protective action in colitis.[89]

G protein-coupled receptors activated by serine proteases, such as trypsin and tryptase, are present on sensory neurons and their activation has been implicated in the generation of inflammatory pain.[90,91] Protease concentrations are increased in the inflamed intestine of animals and humans, and are believed to contribute to the inflammatory process via PAR-2 activation; proteases fail to induce inflammation in PAR-2-deficient mice.[20] It has been proposed that PAR-2 activation produces inflammation via the release of substance P from sensory nerves.[20,92] However, this remains controversial, as recent evidence suggests that PAR-2 activation is protective in a model of experimental colitis, and that this effect is mediated in part via a direct effect on lymphocytes and the activation of sensory nerves. PAR-2 receptors were activated by the agonist peptide SLIGRL-NH2 in the hapten-induced model of colitis, which ameliorated the colitis.[20,89]

Thus, there are apparently conflicting data regarding the role of sensory nerve intestinal inflammation. Activation of sensory nerves causes the local release of neurotransmitters such as substance P and CGRP, which directly influence the inflammatory process. However, activation of these nerves also activates local and systemic reflexes, the efferent component of which influences blood flow, secretions and motility as well as immune and inflammatory cells. Ablation of sensory circuits by prior exposure to capsaicin markedly increased susceptibility to inflammatory stimuli in the gut, suggesting that the integrity of sensory nerves is an important component of host defense. The controversial therapeutic benefit of local anesthetics such as lidocaine is probably due to direct anti-inflammatory effects rather than via suppression of sensory input from the gut.[93] The therapeutic potential of this circuitry can only be harnessed via the selective activation of sensory nerves via receptors that are not shared on other cell types.

## THE AUTONOMIC NERVOUS SYSTEM

Autonomic imbalance occurs in IBD and persists in patients with ulcerative colitis following colectomy,[44] which raises the possibility that autonomic dysfunction contributes to the pathogenesis of this disorder. Studies in animals indicate that perturbation of autonomic function influences susceptibility to inflammatory stimuli in the gut. Cigarette smoke aggravated Th1-mediated colitis induced by TNBS, in keeping with its deleterious effect on Crohn's disease.[51] Studies using nicotine in animal models indicate a dose-dependent bivalent effect: low-dose nicotine protects against inflammation, whereas high-dose nicotine aggravates colitis.[94] There is also regional specificity[95] in the effect of nicotine on inflammatory processes in the gastrointestinal tract. Further evidence for a protective role for parasympathetic nerves comes from the observation that vagal stimulation protects against the inflammatory effects of endotoxin or salmonella infection in rats.[96,97]

The apparent benefit of smoking or nicotine in some patients with ulcerative colitis, taken in conjunction with the observation that there is vagal parasympathetic impairment in approximately 30% of ulcerative colitis patients, supports the notion that sympathetic nerves may be proinflammatory in colitis. This hypothesis is supported by experimental work. Chemical sympathectomy in the hapten model of colitis resulted in less colonic damage due to DNB in rats, indicating that sympathetic nerves contribute to the severity of colitis.[98] Taken together, these results support the hypothesis that autonomic balance is a determinant of the severity of intestinal inflammation, with parasympathetic nerves conferring protection and sympathetic nerves contributing to the inflammatory response.

## GLIA

Glial cells surround enteric nerves and extend into the mucosa. They are similar to astroglia, provide support for enteric nerves, and may engage in neuroimmune interactions via the expression of cytokines and MHC complexes.[99] Indeed, MHC II expression has been observed on glia in Crohn's disease.[33] Some reduction in glial cell number has been observed in Crohn's disease.[100] Studies involving genetic targeting of glia demonstrate that loss of this cell type is associated with a markedly increased susceptibility to inflammation.[101] The mechanism underlying the protective role of glia is unclear. It could be secondary to a loss of integrity of neural circuits or to a direct effect of glia on the inflammatory process, via either cytokine release or the production of trophic factors that possess anti-inflammatory properties.[102] Further investigation of glia and their products may yield novel approaches to the modulation of intestinal inflammation.

## REFERENCES

1. Aronowitz R, Spiro HM. The rise and fall of the psychosomatic hypothesis in ulcerative colitis. J Clin Gastroenterol 1999;10:298–301.
2. Hiatt RB. Abnormal intestinal motility as an etiological factor in inflammatory bowel disease J Clin Gastroenterol 1984;6:201–233.
3. Werner J, Hoff HE, Simon MA. Production of ulcerative colitis in dogs by prolonged administration of Mecholyl. Gastroenterology 1949;12:637–653.
4. Lium R. Etiology of ulcerative colitis II. Effects of induced muscular spasm on colonic explants in dogs with comment on relation of muscular spasm to ulcerative colitis. Arch Int Med 1939;63:210–225.
5. Murray CD. Psychogenic factors in the etiology of ulcerative colitis. Am J Dig Dis 1930;180:230–239.
6. Dennis C, Eddy FD, Frykman MH, McCarthy AM, Westover D. The response to vagotomy in idiopathic ulcerative colitis and regional enteritis. Ann Surg 1946;128:479–496.
7. Shafiroff GP, Hinton J. Denervation of the pelvic colon for ulcerative colitis. Surg Forum 1950;134–139.
8. Thorek P. Vagotomy for idiopathic ulcerative colitis and regional enteritis. JAMA 1951;145:140–146.
9. Garcia Rodriguez LA, Ruigomez A, Wallander MA, Johansson S, Olbe L. Detection of colorectal tumor and inflammatory bowel disease during follow-up of patients with initial diagnosis of irritable bowel syndrome. Scand J Gastroenterol 2000;35:306–311.
10. Chan J, Gonsalkorale W, Perrey M. CPVHAWPJ. IL-10 and TGF-β genotype in irritable bowel syndrome: evidence to support an inflammatory component? Gastroenterology 2000;118: A184.
11. Chadwick VS, Chen W, Shu D et al. Activation of the mucosal immune system in irritable bowel syndrome. Gastroenterology 2002;122:1778–1783.
12. Gwee KA, Leong YL, Graham C et al. The role of psychological and biological factors in postinfective gut dysfunction. Gut 1999;44:400–406.
13. O'Sullivan MA, Clayton N, Wong T, Bountra C, Buckley M, O'Morain C. Increased iNOS and nitrotyrosine expression in irritable bowel syndrome. Gastroenterology 2000;118:A702.
14. Salzmann JL, Peltier-Koch F, Bloch F, Petite JP, Camilleri JP. Methods in laboratory investigation: morphometric study of colonic biopsies: A new method of estimating inflammatory diseases. Lab Invest 1992;60:847–851.
15. Spiller RC, Jenkins D, Thornley JP et al. Increased rectal mucosal enteroendocrine cells, T lymphocytes and increased gut permeability following acute Campylobacter enteritis and in post-dysenteric irritable bowel syndrome. Gut 2000;47:804–811.
16. Weston AP, Biddle WL, Bhatia PS, Miner PB Jr. Terminal ileal mucosal mast cells in irritable bowel syndrome. Dig Dis Sci 1993;38:1590–1595.

17. Collins SM. Is the irritable gut an inflamed gut ? Scand J Gastroenterol 1992;27:192.

18. Hsueh CM, Chen SF, Lin RJ, Chao HJ. Cholinergic and serotonergic activities are required in triggering conditioned NK cell response. J Neuroimmunol 2002;123:102–111.

19. Isgar B, Harman M, Kaye MD, Whorwell PJ. Symptoms of irritable bowel syndrome in ulcerative colitis in remission. Gut 1983;24:190–192.

20. Cenac N, Coelho AM, Nguyen C et al. Induction of intestinal inflammation in mouse by activation of proteinase-activated receptor-2. Am J Pathol 2002;161:1903–1915.

21. Loening-Baucke V, Metcalf AM, Shirazi S. Rectosigmoid motility in patients with quiescent and active ulcerative colitis. Am J Gastroenterol 1989;84:34–39.

22. Barbara G, Vallance BA, Collins SM. Persistent intestinal neuromuscular dysfunction after acute nematode infection in mice. Gastroenterology. 1997;113:1224–32.

23. Barbara G, De Giorgio R, Deng Y, Vallance B, Blennerhassett P, Collins SM. Role of immunologic factors and cyclooxygenase 2 in persistent postinfective enteric muscle dysfunction in mice. Gastroenterology 2001;120:1729–1736.

24. Geboes K, Collins S. Structural abnormalities of the nervous system in Crohn's disease and ulcerative colitis. Neurogastroenterol Motil 1998;10:189–202.

25. Collins SM, Hurst SM, Main C et al. Effect of inflammation of enteric nerves. Cytokine-induced changes in neurotransmitter content and release. Ann NY Acad Sci 1992;664:415–424.

26. Ottaway CA, Greenberg GR. Interaction of VIP with mouse lymphocytes: Specific binding and the modulation of mitogen responses. J Immunol 1984;132:417–423.

27. Payan DG, Brewster DR, Goetzi EJ. Specific stimulation of human T lymphocytes by substance P. J Immunol 1983;131:1613–1615.

28. Stead RH. Innervation of mucosal immune cells in the gastrointestinal tract. Reg Immunol 1992;4:91–99.

29. Geboes K, Collins S. Structural abnormalities of the nervous system in Crohn's disease and ulcerative colitis. Neurogastroenterol Motil. 1998;10:189–202.

30. Davis DR, Dockerty MB, Mayo CB. The myenteric plexus in regional enteritis: A study of the number of ganglion cells in the ileum in 24 cases. Surg Gynecol Obstet 1953;101:208–216.

31. Storsteen KA, Kernohan JW, Bargen JA. The myenteric plexus in chronic ulcerative colis. Surg Gynecol Obstet 1953;97:335–343.

32. D'Haens G, Colpaert FC, Peeters F, Baert F, Penninckx F, Rutgeerts P. The presence and severity of neural inflammation predict severe post-operative recurrence of Crohn's disease. Gastroenterology 1998;114: A963.

33. Geboes K, Rutgeerts P, Ectors N et al. Major histocompatibility class II expression on the small intestinal nervous system in Crohn's disease. Gastroenterology 1992;103:439–447.

34. Mantyh CR, Gates TS, Zimmerman RP et al. Receptor binding sites for substance P, but not substance K or neuromedin K, are expressed in high concentrations by arterioles, venules, and lymph nodules in surgical specimens obtained from patients with ulcerative colitis and Crohn's disease. Proc Natl Acad Sci USA 1988;85:3235–3239.

35. di Mola FF, Friess H, Zhu ZW et al. Nerve growth factor and Trk high affinity receptor (TrkA) gene expression in inflammatory bowel disease. Gut 2000;46:670–679.

36. Bishop AE, Polack JM, Bryant MG, Bloom SR, Hamilton S. Abnormalities of vasoactive intestinal polypeptide containing nerves in Crohn's disease. Gastroenterology 1980;79:853–860.

37. O'Morain C, Bishop AE, McGregor GP et al. Vasoactive intestinal peptide concentrations and immunocytochemical studies in rectal biopsies from patients with inflammatory bowel disease. Gut 1984;25:56–61.

38. Sjolund K, Schaffalitzky OB, Muckadell DE et al. Peptide-containing nerve fibres in the gut wall in Crohn's disease. Gut 1983;24:724–733.

39. Chad DA, Smith TW, DeGirolami U, Hammer K. Perineuritis and ulcerative colitis. Neurology 1986;36:1377–1379.

40. Andus T, Geissler A, Roth M et al. Small focal white matter lesions in the brain of patients with inflammatory bowel disease – another extraintestinal manifestation? Gastroenterology 1994;106:A645.

41. Hart PE, Gould SR, MacSweeney JE, Clifton A, Schon F. Brain white-matter lesions in inflammatory bowel disease. Lancet 1998;351:1558.

42. Lossos A, River Y, Eliakim A, Steiner I. Neurological aspects of inflammatory bowel disease. Neurology 1995;45:416–421.

43. Snape WJ, Williams R, Hyman PE. Defect in colonic muscle contraction in patients with ulcerative colitis. Am J Physiol Gastrointest Liver Physiol 1991;261:G987–G991.

44. Lindgren S, Stewenius J, Sjolund K, Lilja B, Sundkvist G. Autonomic vagal nerve dysfunction in patients with ulcerative colitis. Scand J Gastroenterol 1993;28:638–422.

45. Lindgren S, Lilja B, Rosén I, Sundkvist G. Disturbed autonomic nerve function in patients with Crohn's disease. Scand J Gastroenterol 1991;26:361–366.

46. Straub RH, Antoniou E, Zeuner M, Gross V, Scholmerich J, Andus T. Association of autonomic nervous hyperreflexia and systemic inflammation in patients with Crohn's disease and ulcerative colitis. J Neuroimmunol 1997;80:149–157.

47. Kyosola K, Penttila O, Salaspuro M. Rectal mucosal adrenergic innervation and enterochromaffin cells in ulcerative colitis and irritable colon. Scand J Gastroenterol 1977;12:363–367.

48. Penttila O, Kyosola K, Klinge E, Ahonen A, Tallqvist G. Studies on rectal mucosal catecholamines in ulcerative colitis. Ann Clin Res 1975;7:32–36.

49. Collins SM, Blennerhassett PA, Blennerhassett MG, Vermillion DL. Impaired acetylcholine release from the myenteric plexus of Trichinella-infected rats. Am J Physiol 1989;257:G898–G903.

50. Blennerhassett MG, Vignjevic P, Vermillion DL, Ernst PB, Collins SM. Intestinal inflammation induces T-lymphocyte dependent hyperplasia of jejunal smooth muscle. Gastroenterology 1990;98:A328.

51. Galeazzi F, Haapala EM, van Rooijen N, Vallance BA, Collins SM. Inflammation-induced impairment of enteric nerve function in nematode-infected mice is macrophage dependent. Am J Physiol Gastrointest Liver Physiol 2000;278:G259–265.

52. Galeazzi F, Lovato P, Blennerhassett PA, Haapala EM, Vallance BA, Collins SM. Neural change in Trichinella-infected mice is MHC II independent and involves M-CSF-derived macrophages. Am J Physiol Gastrointest Liver Physiol 2001;281:G151–G158.

53. Main C, Blennerhassett P, Collins SM. Human recombinant interleukin 1 beta suppresses acetylcholine release from rat myenteric plexus. Gastroenterology 1993;104:1648–1654.

54. Khan I, Collins SM. Expression of cytokines in the longitudinal muscle myenteric plexus of the inflamed intestine of rat. Gastroenterology 1994;107:691–700.

55. Swain MG, Blennerhassett PA, Collins SM. Impaired sympathetic nerve function in the inflamed rat intestine. Gastroenterology 1991;100:675–682.

56. Saunders PR, Hanssen NP, Perdue MH. Cholinergic nerves mediate stress-induced intestinal transport abnormalities in Wistar-Kyoto rats. Am J Physiol 1997;273:G486–490.

57. Swain MG, Agro A, Blennerhassett PA, Stanisz A. Collins SM. Increased levels of substance P in the myenteric plexus of Trichinella-infected rats. Gastroenterology 1992;102:1913–1919.

58. Stead RH, Kosecka-Janiszewska U, Oestreicher AB, Dixon MF, Bienenstock J. Remodeling of B-50 (GAP-43)- and NSE-immunoreactive mucosal nerves in the intestines of rats infected with Nippostrongylus brasiliensis. J Neurosci 1991;11:3809–3821.

59. Stead RH, Tomioka M, Quinonez G, Simon GT, Felten SY, Bienenstock J. Intestinal mucosal mast cells in normal and nematode infected rat intestines are in intimate contact with peptidergic nerves. Proc Natl Acad Sci USA 1987;84:2975–2979.

60. McHugh K, Castonguay TW, Collins SM, Weingarten HP. Characterization of suppression of food intake following acute colon inflammation in the rat. Am J Physiol 1993;265:R1001–1005.

61. McHugh KJ, Collins SM, Weingarten HP. Central interleukin-1 receptors contribute to suppression of feeding after acute colitis in the rat. Am J Physiol 1994;266:R1659–1663.

62. Miampamba M, Sharkey KA. c-Fos expression in the myenteric plexus, spinal cord and brainstem following injection of formalin in the rat colonic wall. J Autonom Nerv Syst 1999;77:140–151.

63. Castex N, Fioramonti J, Fargeas MJ, Bueno L. c-fos expression in specific rat brain nuclei after intestinal anaphylaxis: involvement of 5-HT3 receptors and vagal afferent fibers. Brain Res 1995;688:149–160.

64. Ek M, Kurosawa M, Lundeberg T, Ericsson A. Activation of vagal afferents after intravenous injection of interleukin-1beta: role of endogenous prostaglandins. J Neurosci 1998;18:9471–9499.

65. McHugh K, Castonguay TW, Collins SM, Weingarten HP. Characterization of suppression of food intake following acute colon inflammation in the rat. Am J Physiol 1993;265:R1001–1005.

66. Gaykema RP, Goehler LE, Hansen MK, Maier SF, Watkins LR. Subdiaphragmatic vagotomy blocks interleukin-1beta-induced fever but does not reduce IL-1beta levels in the circulation. Autonom Neurosci 2000;85:72–77.

67. Engel GL. Psychological factors in ulcerative colitis in man and gibbon. Gastroenterology 1969;57:362–366.

68. Anton PA, Shanahan F. Neuroimmunomodulation in inflammatory bowel disease. How far from 'bench' to 'bedside'? Ann NY Acad Sci 1998l;840:723–734.

69. Talal AH, Drossman DA. Psychosocial factors in inflammatory bowel disease. Gastroenterol Clin North Am 1995;24:699–716.

70. Kast RE, Altschuler EL. Remission of Crohn's disease on bupropion. Gastroenterology 2001;121:1260–1261.

71. Kast RE. Crohn's disease remission with phenelzine treatment. Gastroenterology 1998;115:1034–1035.

72. Rubin DT, Hanauer SB. Smoking and inflammatory bowel disease. Eur J Gastroenterol Hepatol 2000;12:855–862.

73. Guo X, Shin VY, Cho CH. Modulation of heme oxygenase in tissue injury and its implication in protection against gastrointestinal diseases. Life Sci 2001;69:3113–3119.

74. Bjorck S, Dahlstrom A, Johansson L, Ahlman H. Treatment of the mucosa with local anaesthetics in ulcerative colitis. Agents Actions 1992;10:C61–C72.

75. Hillingso JG, Kjeldsen J, Schmidt PT et al. Effects of topical ropivacaine on eicosanoids and neurotransmitters in the rectum of patients with distal ulcerative colitis. Scand J Gastroenterol 2002;37:325–329.

76. Collins SM. Stress and the gastrointestinal tract IV. Modulation of intestinal inflammation by stress: basic mechanisms and clinical relevance. Am J Physiol Gastrointest Liver Physiol 2001;280:G315–G318.

77. Gue M, Bonbonne C, Fioramonti J et al. Stress-induced enhancement of colitis in rats: CRF and arginine vasopressin are not involved. Am J Physiol 1997;272:G84–91.

78. Kiliaan AJ, Saunders PR, Bijlsma PB et al. Stress stimulates transepithelial macromolecular uptake in rat jejunum. Am J Physiol 1998;275:G1037–1044.

79. Qiu B, Vallance B, Blennerhassett P, Collins SM. The role of CD4+ve lymphocytes in the susceptibility of the mice to stress-induced relapse of colitis. Nature Med 1999;5:1178–1182.

80. McDonald DM, Bowden JJ, Baluk P, Bunnett NW. Neurogenic inflammation. A model for studying efferent actions of sensory nerves. Adv Exp Med Biol 1996;410:453–462.

81. Hwang L, Leichter R, Okamoto A, Payan D, Collins SM, Bunnett NW. Downregulation of neutral endopeptidase (EC 3.4.24.11) in the inflamed rat intestine. Am J Physiol 1993;264:G735–743.

82. Sturiale S, Barbara G, Qiu B et al. Neutral endopeptidase (EC 3.4.24.11) terminates colitis by degrading substance P. Proc Natl Acad Sci USA 1999;96:11653–11688.

83. Agro A, Stanisz AM. Inhibition of murine intestinal inflammation by anti-substance P antibody. Reg Immunol 1993;5:120–126.

84. Renzi D, Pellegrini B, Tonelli F, Surrenti C, Calabro A. Substance P (neurokinin-1) and neurokinin A (neurokinin-2) receptor gene and protein expression in the healthy and inflamed human intestine. Am J Pathol 2000;157:1511–1522.

85. Stucchi AF, Shofer S, Leeman S et al. NK-1 antagonist reduces colonic inflammation and oxidative stress in dextran sulfate-induced colitis in rats. Am J Physiol Gastrointest Liver Physiol 2000;279:G1298–G1306.

86. Schneider J, Jehle EC, Starlinger MJ et al. Neurotransmitter coding of enteric neurones in the submucous plexus is changed in non-inflamed rectum of patients with Crohn's disease. Neurogastroenterol Motil 2001;13:255–264.

87. Eysselein VE, Reinshagen M, Patel A, Davis W, Nast C, Sternini C. Calcitonin gene related peptide in inflammatory bowel disease and experimentally induced colitis. Ann NY Acad Sci 1992;657:319–327.

88. Reinshagen M, Flaemig G, Ernst S, Geerling J, Eysselein V. Protective effect of calcitonin gene related peptide (CGRP) in chronic experimental colitis in the rat. Gastroenterology 1996;108: A676.

89. Fiorucci S, Mencarelli A, Palazzetti B et al. Proteinase-activated receptor 2 is an anti-inflammatory signal for colonic lamina propria lymphocytes in a mouse model of colitis. Proc Natl Acad Sci USA 2001;98:13936–13941.

90. Vergnolle N, Bunnett NW, Sharkey KA et al. Proteinase-activated receptor-2 and hyperalgesia: A novel pain pathway. Nature Med 2001;7:821–826.

91. Brain SD. New feelings about the role of sensory nerves in inflammation. Nature Med 2000;6:134–135.

92. Steinhoff M, Vergnolle N, Young SH et al. Agonists of proteinase-activated receptor 2 induce inflammation by a neurogenic mechanism. Nature Med 2000;6:151–158.

93. McCafferty DM, Sharkey KA, Wallace JL. Beneficial effects of local or systemic lidocaine in experimental colitis Am J Physiol 1994;266:G560–577.

94. Eliakim R, Karmeli F, Rachmilewitz D, Cohen P, Fich A. Effect of chronic nicotine administration on trinitrobenzene sulphonic acid-induced colitis. Eur J Gastroenterol Hepatol 1998;10:1013–1019.

95. Eliakim R, Fan QX, Babyatsky MW. Chronic nicotine administration differentially alters jejunal and colonic inflammation in interleukin-10 deficient mice. Eur J Gastroenterol Hepatol 2002;14:607–614.

96. Borovikova LV, Ivanova S, Zhang M et al. Vagus nerve stimulation attenuates the systemic inflammatory response to endotoxin. Nature 2000;405:458–462.

97. Wang X, Wang BR, Zhang XJ, Xu Z, Ding YQ, Ju G. Evidences for vagus nerve in maintenance of immune balance and transmission of immune information from gut to brain in STM-infected rats. World J Gastroenterol 2002;8:540–545.

98. McCafferty DM, Wallace JL, Sharkey KA. Effects of chemical sympathectomy and sensory nerve ablation on experimental colitis in the rat. Am J Physiol 1997;272:G272–800.

99. Bannerman PG, Mirsky R, Jessen KR. Analysis of enteric neurons, glia and their interactions using explant cultures of the myenteric plexus. Dev Neurosci 1987;9:201–227.

100. Cornet A, Savidge TC, Cabarrocas J et al. Enterocolitis induced by autoimmune targeting of enteric glial cells: a possible mechanism in Crohn's disease? Proc Natl Acad Sci USA 2001;98:13306–13311.

101. Bush TG, Savidge TC, Freeman TC et al. Fulminant jejuno-ileitis following ablation of enteric glia in adult transgenic mice. Cell 1998;93:189–201.

102. Reinshagen M, von Boyen G, Adler G, Steinkamp M. Role of neurotrophins in inflammation of the gut. Curr Opin Invest Drugs 2002;3:565–568.

## CHAPTER 15

# Fibrogenesis

Ellen Zimmermann and P Kay Lund

## INTRODUCTION

In the idiopathic inflammatory bowel diseases (IBD), particularly Crohn's disease, intestinal fibrosis is a consequence of long-standing chronic inflammation. Fibrosis is variable in presentation, but extensive transmural collagen deposition and muscular hyperplasia frequently lead to critical luminal narrowing (termed stenosis or stricture) and obstruction. In less severe cases, luminal narrowing and loss of wall compliance probably contribute to symptoms such as pain, early satiety, anorexia, diarrhea and constipation due to partial obstruction and bacterial overgrowth in proximal segments. Despite recent advances, current therapies do little to interrupt the seemingly relentless progression from inflammation to fibrosis that occurs in some patients, perhaps on a genetic basis. Available medical therapies do little to change well-established strictures which may present years after the active inflammation has subsided. Indeed, fibrogenic complications are the most common cause of surgical intervention in Crohn's disease.[1] A better understanding of the early phases of inflammation and the initiators of fibrosis is essential to the development of therapeutic strategies that will prevent fibrogenesis before strictures develop. The cellular and molecular mechanisms that lead to fibrosis in Crohn's disease have been much less extensively studied than the immunologic basis of this disease. This chapter addresses several key questions relevant to the clinical features, molecular pathogenesis and therapeutic implications of intestinal fibrogenesis.

## WHAT ARE THE CLINICAL FEATURES OF FIBROSIS IN IBD?

### CLINICAL PRESENTATION

Abdominal pain is a common clinical symptom of an intestinal stricture and fibrosis but there are many other causes of pain in IBD. Stricture and luminal narrowing may be due to inflamma-

tion (edema), fibrosis or both. Pain associated with systemic inflammatory signs or symptoms, including increased peripheral WBC count, increased erythrocyte sedimentation rate, C-reactive protein, or platelet count, rash, fever, joint symptoms or bloody diarrhea, favors an inflammatory component. A bland fibrotic stricture may present with episodic pain but no associated systemic inflammatory signs. Typically, inflammatory signs are not clear-cut owing to concomitant disease or anti-inflammatory therapy creating a confusing picture. Pain typical of critical luminal narrowing is usually postprandial cramping, with bloating that lasts from minutes to hours. Longer-lasting symptoms of pain and bloating associated with vomiting and decreased stool output are more ominous and suggest intermittent or chronic obstruction. Symptoms may be precipitated by a large meal or eating food with significant indigestible fiber components. The stricture acts like a funnel that is unnoticed when meals are small or the fiber content of ingested food is low, but may prevent the passage of an increased load of larger particulate matter. Pain is the result of increased pressure and distension in the upstream bowel segment, with activation of the local stretch receptors. If this segment of bowel is inflamed, cytokines and neuromediators may further activate pain receptors. The situation of increased luminal pressure in an ulcerated segment of bowel can create conditions appropriate for fistula formation. Sudden improvement in obstructive symptoms may occur as a fistula forms. Interestingly, even tight strictures may be completely asymptomatic and symptoms do not correlate well with radiographic or endoscopic findings.

## DIFFERENTIAL DIAGNOSIS AND EVALUATION

The differential diagnosis of luminal narrowing/stricture with or without fibrosis is broad. The timing of pain in relation to a flare of disease is important. For example, pain occurring in the setting of a flare is probably related to inflammation, whereas pain remote from a typical flare may signify a critical fibrotic stricture or a malignancy. The possibility of malignancy may be difficult to eliminate, particularly if the stricture is inaccessible to endoscopic examination. Strictures in the terminal ileum may mimic appendicitis. Strictures in the small or large intestine may mimic strictures from other causes, such as malignant and non-malignant tumors, infections or ischemia, and duodenal or pyloric strictures mimic peptic or neoplastic gastric outlet obstruction.

The choice of imaging modality to evaluate a potential intestinal stricture depends on the most likely site of the stricture. Colonic, anastomotic or distal ileal strictures are usually best evaluated by colonoscopy. Colonoscopy allows visualization of the stricture to assess associated intestinal inflammation, biopsy of the lesion to rule out malignancy, and the performance of balloon dilation if indicated. Suspected terminal ileal strictures may not be accessible colonoscopically because of the stricture itself, anatomic factors, or inflammation that prevent intubation of the ileocecal valve. A CT scan is indicated if an abscess or tumor is suspected. A radiographic small bowel study is currently the test of choice to evaluate the degree of functional blockage, the length of the stricture and the extent of inflammation of the small intestine. Choices include a dedicated small bowel follow-through (SBFT), combined upper GI (UGI) study and small bowel examination, or enteroclysis. A dedicated SBFT is preferred to a combined procedure because of the compromised small bowel detail caused by the thick barium used for the upper examination. The choice between SBFT and enteroclysis depends largely on local expertise. In either examination, distinguishing between luminal narrowing caused by active inflammatory disease versus a fixed fibrotic stricture is based largely on indirect data and is not always possible, although dilation of the proximal intestine strongly suggests a fixed, chronic obstruction. Improvement following an empiric trial of steroids or infliximab indicates an inflammatory component to the stricture. Clearly, improved non-invasive means to distinguish between luminal narrowing due to inflammation and fibrosis are needed. Abdominal ultrasound has been employed in an attempt to distinguish between active disease and fibrosis. Ultrasonographic bowel wall thickening correlates with fibrosis, but only in quiescent disease, limiting its usefulness.[2] High-resolution CT enterography may, in the future, distinguish fibrotic strictures from inflammation as new generations of scanners are able to generate three-dimensional reconstructions, and venous and arterial phase contrast enhances inflamed areas. Emerging technologies, including magnetic resonance imaging (MRI) may further refine the available images, but video capsules are contraindicated because of the possible obstruction.

Limited data on blood tests for monitoring fibrosis are available in IBD patients, but additional markers are needed. Fibronectin appears to have limited value in assessing disease activity but may be useful for detecting fibrostenosing disease.[3]

## RISK FACTORS

Intestinal fibrosis with bowel wall thickening and loss of wall compliance is considered a long-standing consequence of chronic intestinal inflammation. Patients with Crohn's disease are more likely to develop symptomatic strictures than patients with ulcerative colitis because of the full-thickness bowel wall inflammation and the typical occurrence of disease in the narrow-caliber small intestine. Fibrosis, which is a more common complication of Crohn's disease than of ulcerative colitis, is typified by excessive deposition of fibrillar collagen and other extracellular matrix (ECM) components, and by the overgrowth of smooth muscle layers. Increased collagen expression or deposition can occur in ulcerative colitis but is generally limited to regions of inflammation within the mucosa and submucosa.[4,5] One challenge to defining the etiology and pathophysiology of fibrosis in IBD is that it is variable not only between patients but also in different regions of involved intestine within a given patient.[1]

Disease subtypes exist in Crohn's disease such that certain patients tend to develop intestinal fibrosis and strictures whereas others develop a fistulizing phenotype. Exciting new data indicate a genetic basis for particular IBD phenotypes. Several groups have reported that the first Crohn's susceptibility gene, a mutation in NOD2, is more common in patients with fibrostenosing ileal disease than are other phenotypes.[6,7] The mechanism whereby NOD2 mutation predisposes to fibrosis is not clear and may not correlate with fibrosis directly but with disease in the terminal ileum. NOD2 is an intracellular receptor for bacterial peptidoglycan-polysaccharide and lipopolysaccharide.[8] NOD2 mutations results in defective activation of nuclear factor-$\kappa$B (NF$\kappa$B), leading to abnormal macrophage/dendritic cell maturation and cytokine synthesis and defective clearance of invasive bacterial pathogens by epithelial cells. The downstream mechanisms linking this mutation to excessive fibrosis are unclear.

It has been hypothesized that rapid tissue healing resulting from treatment with potent immunosuppressive medications may predispose to scarring and fibrotic strictures. Several cases of patients who developed symptomatic strictures, and even obstruction requiring surgery, have been reported after infliximab infusion.[9] Most of these patients had known strictures prior to infusion, but the infusion was temporally related to the development of a symptomatic critical stricture. Although the data are too limited for firm recommendations, caution has been advised in using infliximab therapy in patients with known intestinal strictures. It will be important to establish whether the NOD2 mutation predisposes to accelerated stricture associated with infliximab.

# WHAT CELL TYPES MEDIATE THE ONSET, PROGRESSION AND PERPETUATION OF FIBROSIS IN CROHN'S DISEASE?

## A WORKING MODEL OF THE CELLULAR BASIS OF FIBROSIS

Fibrosis in Crohn's disease can be considered an overzealous healing response to chronic injury and inflammation. Figure 15.1 depicts a simple working model comparing normal healing and fibrosis in the intestine in response to acute or chronic inflammation and injury. In this model injury causes initial activation of normal intestinal mesenchymal cells to a 'fibrogenic' phenotype, with an increased capability for extracellular matrix (ECM) synthesis and deposition. Following acute injury, fibrogenic mesenchymal cells mediate normal wound healing and restore normal intestinal architecture. During normal wound healing, post-transcriptional and post-translational mechanisms prevent the net accumulation of ECM and the activated fibrogenic cells revert to normal phenotype or are eliminated. In contrast, fibrosis occurs when the intestine is subject to chronic inflammation

**Model of normal tissue repair and fibrosis**

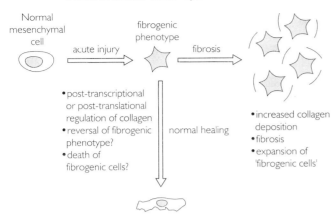

Fig. 15.1 Hypothetical model of normal tissue repair and fibrosis. Acute injury activates normal mesenchymal cells to develop a fibrogenic phenotype with increased ECM synthesis. Normal healing or fibrosis may follow activation. During normal healing, excess ECM deposition is prevented by post-transcriptional or post-translation regulation of collagen, reversal of the fibrogenic phenotype, or selective death of fibrogenic cells. Fibrosis results if these events do not occur, are not sufficiently active, or if the fibrogenic cell population expands.

and injury because mechanisms to degrade ECM are not operative at appropriate levels, and fibrogenic mesenchymal cells are not only maintained but are expanded in number. This model has parallels with models of fibrosis in other organs, notably the liver.[10] In the liver, acute injury causes normal, quiescent hepatic mesenchymal cells (stellate cells) to transform to an activated phenotype typified by the expression of $\alpha$ smooth muscle (SM)-actin, organization of $\alpha$SM-actin into stress fibers, and increased collagen synthesis. However, persistence and expansion of the activated stellate cells, net deposition of collagen and fibrosis only occur if inflammation and injury persist.

Some challenges exist to testing whether the model proposed in Figure 15.1 describes the etiology of fibrosis in Crohn's disease. First, apart from their ability to synthesize and deposit large amounts of ECM, we do not yet have a useful definition of an 'activated' or 'fibrogenic' phenotype of intestinal mesenchymal cells. In the liver, the induction of $\alpha$SM-actin has proved very useful to identify and functionally characterize activated, fibrogenic, hepatic stellate cells. The intestine is more complicated because the normal intestine has a large, heterogeneous population of mesenchymal cells, some of which synthesize significant amounts of collagen in the normal setting. These cells could therefore be considered to have a constitutive fibrogenic phenotype. A second point is that hyperproliferation of normal mesenchymal cells may be of equal or greater importance than ECM synthesis in the development of stenosis, stricture and irreversible fibrosis, yet we know little about the temporal or functional relationship between mesenchymal cell proliferation and the initiation or progression of fibrosis in Crohn's disease or experimental models. Third, our ability to study cellular events associated with fibrosis in humans is limited to studies on mucosal biopsies or resected intestine. Mucosal biopsies fail to provide information about submucosal layers, where fibrosis is most prevalent and severe in Crohn's disease. Resected tissues necessarily provide insights into end-stage disease and are of limited value in analyzing the etiology and pathophysiology of the onset and progression of fibrosis. None

the less, subsequent sections of this chapter review current information about the cellular mediators of fibrosis.

## MESENCHYMAL CELLS IN NORMAL INTESTINE

Mesenchymal cells in the normal intestine consist of fibroblasts, smooth muscle cells, myofibroblasts and interstitial cells of Cajal (ICC), which have been categorized by their immunostaining properties with antibodies to vimentin (V) and $\alpha$SM-actin (A) or other markers.[11,12] Typically, V+/A- fibroblasts are present in the submucosa and serosa of the normal intestine.[13] V-A+ smooth muscle cells predominate in the normal muscularis mucosa and muscularis propria.[13] Subepithelial myofibroblasts (SEMF) with V+/A+ phenotype are found adjacent to epithelial cells.[11-13] In the normal intestine, SEMF and fibroblasts found in submucosa, serosa and intermuscular connective tissue are the primary sites of expression of collagen mRNA and protein.[4,13] ICC, a myofibroblast-related subtype specific to the gastrointestinal tract, are located between enteric smooth muscle layers, where they regulate gut motility.[11,12] The c-kit receptor, which binds the proto-oncogene stem cell or steel factor, is a marker of ICC.[11-13] ICC in normal human intestine also express vimentin, but not $\alpha$SM-actin or desmin.[13] The categorization of mesenchymal cell subtypes in normal intestine based on these phenotypic markers is useful but an oversimplifcation.[11,12] Some cells that share common features with V+/A+ myofibroblasts do not express $\alpha$SM-actin.[11,12] Desmin, an intermediate filament protein typically found in normal smooth muscle, represents a marker of myofibroblasts in some tissues,[11,12] even though it is expressed only in enteric smooth muscle in normal intestine.[13] The c-kit receptor is expressed in mast cells as well as ICC,[14] complicating the identification of ICC in inflamed intestine.

## IS THERE AN ACTIVATED, FIBROGENIC PHENOTYPE OF MESENCHYMAL CELLS IN INTESTINAL INFLAMMATION?

In both ulcerative colitis and Crohn's disease the expression of mRNA encoding multiple collagen subtypes is upregulated in lamina propria mesenchymal cells, probably SEMF and mucosal fibroblasts, suggesting that chronic inflammation further increases the constitutive fibrogenic activity of these cells.[4,15] In ulcerative colitis, however, one report suggests that this increased collagen mRNA is not associated with as pronounced an increase in deposition of collagen protein as in Crohn's disease.[4,15] This raises the possibility that SEMF or mucosal fibroblasts in Crohn's and ulcerative colitis differ in their post-transcriptional or post-translational mechanisms, or perhaps degradation, which lead to net collagen accumulation.[4,15] Fibroblasts isolated from fibrotic bowel from Crohn's disease demonstrate increased type III collagen synthesis in response to TGF-$\beta$ compared to cells derived from inflamed but not fibrotic intestine from the same patient.[15] Fibroblasts from patients with Crohn's disease or ulcerative colitis were found to proliferate faster in response to TGF-$\beta$1, PDGF and bFGF.[5] These findings suggest that inflammation alters the phenotype of intestinal fibroblasts or myofibroblasts, which may predispose to fibrosis.

Myofibroblasts are expanded in number in the mucosa of Crohn's disease patients and may mediate or contribute to mucosal fibrosis.[13] In Crohn's disease activated SEMF or mucosal fibroblasts may migrate to submucosal layers to mediate fibrosis in deeper tissue layers. Evidence in other diseases, however, suggests that increased collagen synthesis by SEMF does not necessarily lead to irreversible fibrosis. Patients with collagenous colitis, for example, exhibit a microscopic, regionally limited fibrosis associated with a chronic inflammatory infiltrate in the mucosa that is thought to be mediated by SEMF.[16,17] In this disease, fibrosis is limited to a subepithelial collagen band composed primarily of the non-fibrillar collagen subtype, collagen VI.[16,17] Importantly, this collagen band may completely resolve after inflammation resolves.[17] Therefore, collagen VI may serve as a useful marker of normal, reversible SEMF responses to injury compared with SEMF responses, which lead to irreversible fibrosis. More extensive analysis of the expression of collagen VI in IBD tissues and animal models is required to test this possibility. Intriguingly, recent gene microarray studies indicate that collagen VI gene expression is selectively increased in ulcerative colitis.[18]

Loss of integrity of the muscularis mucosa is a hallmark of Crohn's disease and could expose SEMF or submucosal fibroblasts to the chemotactic, proliferative or profibrogenic activities of cytokines associated with inflammation. An unexplored possibility is that breaching of the muscularis mucosa could facilitate the invasion of fibrogenic submucosal fibroblasts into the mucosa. Alternatively, activated SEMF could migrate from the disorganized muscularis mucosa to the submucosa and muscularis propria and, if expanded in number, could mediate transmural fibrosis. Regulation of intestinal mesenchymal cell motility and migration is not well defined. Recent studies indicate that cultured colonic mucosal myofibroblasts secrete heat-sensitive factors which stimulate migration, and that platelet-derived growth factors (PDGFA or B) and insulin-like growth factor-1 (IGF-1) potently enhance migration, whereas epidermal growth factor (EGF) and transforming growth factor-β1 (TGF-β1) are less potent, and basic fibroblast growth factor (bFGF) has no effect.[19]

Graham[20] proposed that smooth muscle cells may be the cellular mediators of fibrosis in Crohn's disease. Cells that retain phenotypic characteristics of smooth muscle cells in culture, including αSM-actin and tropomyosin expression, can synthesize collagen.[20,21] However, whether or not cells with a 'normal' smooth muscle phenotype are the same cells that synthesize excessive collagen in Crohn's disease in vivo is uncertain. Cells with a V+/A− or V+/A+ phenotype, typically associated with fibroblasts and myofibroblasts, predominate at sites of increased type I collagen mRNA expression and collagen deposition in the muscularis layers of fibrotic intestines from Crohn's disease patients.[13] These collagen-producing cells do not express desmin, a typical marker of smooth muscle cells.[13] It is possible that the V+/A− or V+/A+ cells are modified smooth muscle cells activated to a collagen-overexpressing phenotype, but currently we have no useful markers to trace the lineage of these cells conclusively. The cells could also derive from activated or expanded local fibroblasts or myofibroblasts that reside in connective tissue between smooth muscle bundles, or from the migration of 'activated' fibroblasts and myofibroblasts from the mucosa or submucosa to the muscularis layers.

ICC could represent other cellular mediators of fibrosis by transforming to a collagen-expressing fibroblast or myofibroblast phenotype.[11,12] Our studies of involved Crohn's disease tissues failed to reveal c-kit positive ICC even though such cells were evident in uninvolved segments from the same patients and from non-inflammatory controls.[13] However, V+/A− positive cells and increased collagen mRNA and protein were commonly observed in involved Crohn's intestine at sites normally populated by ICC, indicating that phenotypically modified ICC could indeed be cellular sources of collagen in fibrotic intestine. In vitro studies with isolated strips of muscularis propria indicate that ICC are altered by inflammatory stimuli.[22] Another possibility is that ICC are destroyed during fibrosis and replaced by collagen-expressing V+/A− fibroblasts.

Defining the lineage of the collagen-expressing V+/A− or V+/A+ cells at sites of fibrosis in Crohn's disease requires additional studies. Analyses at the onset of fibrosis would be especially useful but cannot easily be done in humans, although animal models of inflammation represent an obvious alternate approach. Strategies to permanently label or identify particular mesenchymal cell lineages in normal intestine of mice using cell-specific promoters linked to reporter genes could be particularly useful. Gene expression profiling on homogeneous, phenotypically characterized intestinal mesenchymal cell subtypes would also be of great value.

## TRANSCRIPTIONAL ACTIVATION OF COLLAGEN SYNTHESIS AS A POSSIBLE MARKER OF FIBROGENIC PHENOTYPE

Transcriptional activation of collagen genes could provide an early biochemical or histological marker of conversion of normal cells to a fibrogenic phenotype. Our prediction that intestinal mesenchymal cells have activated collagen genes during both normal tissue healing and fibrosis (Fig. 15.1) has not been examined directly. A transgenic mouse with a green fluorescent protein (GFP) reporter gene linked to a procollagen α1 (I) promoter[23] potentially provides a simple, highly sensitive and readily quantifiable measure of transcriptional activation of the procollagen α1 (I) gene in vivo. Detection of GFP combined with immunostaining for markers of particular cell phenotypes could identify cell types that exhibit type I collagen gene activation at different stages of intestinal inflammation, injury, normal wound healing or fibrosis. Preliminary data indicate that the procollagen α1 (I)-GFP reporter gene is specifically induced in intestinal mesenchymal cells in vivo during mucosal injury and inflammation, and is induced in vitro by fibrogenic cytokines such as TGF-β.[24] Procollagen α1 (I) promoter-GFP mice may therefore provide a novel model to help define the phenotype of fibrogenic intestinal mesenchymal cells.

## MUSCULARIS OVERGROWTH DURING INTESTINAL INFLAMMATION AND FIBROSIS

In Crohn's disease overgrowth of the muscularis mucosa and muscularis propria is frequently observed in regions of fibrosis but can occur in its absence.[1] Muscularis overgrowth also occurs in some animal models of chronic intestinal inflammation.[21,25–27] The contributions of increased cell size, increased cell proliferation or reduced cell death to muscularis overgrowth during Crohn's disease and the significance of muscularis overgrowth for the initiation, progression or severity of fibrosis are not well understood. Figure 15.2 illustrates two hypothetical models describing the development of muscularis overgrowth and its relationship to fibrosis. In one model, acute injury activates fibrogenic cells, followed by expansion of this fibrogenic cell population during chronic inflammation. In the second, proliferation of normal smooth muscle cells precedes activation or transformation to the fibrogenic phenotype. Either model results

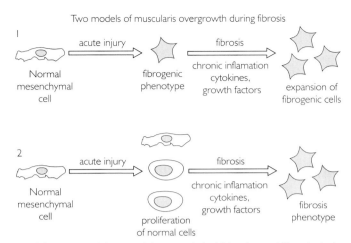

Two models of muscularis overgrowth during fibrosis

**Fig. 15.2** Two models to explain muscularis thickening and fibrosis during inflammation of the intestine.

in expanded numbers of fibrogenic mesenchymal cells within the muscularis layers. The possibility that normal intestinal smooth muscle cells might transiently expand in number during injury has not, to our knowledge, been addressed. If such an event precedes conversion to fibrogenic phenotype, strategies to control smooth muscle cell proliferation or hypertrophy could prove useful as prophylactic or therapeutic measures to control or limit fibrosis. Quantitative analyses of muscularis overgrowth over the course of inflammation and fibrosis in animal models, using either morphometric measurements or quantitative assays of cytoskeletal antigens in conjunction with assays of cell phenotype and levels of collagen synthesis, will determine which of these models is correct. Direct evaluation of smooth muscle cell proliferation would also be valuable. Recent studies reported a high prevalence (approximately 30%) of obliterative muscularization of the submucosa (OMUS) in ileal resections that significantly correlated with luminal narrowing but not fibrosis. OMUS is similar, if not identical, to the neuromuscular and vascular hamartoma reported by Shepherd and Jass,[28] and may represent an earlier pathophysiologic manifestation of disease than luminal narrowing with fibrosis.[29] Whatever its etiology, OMUS suggests that aberrant hyperplasia of smooth muscle within the submucosa is a mesenchymal response to inflammation in a significant number of Crohn's disease patients.

## MAST CELLS AND FIBROSIS

Mast cells are new putative mediators of fibrosis in Crohn's disease.[14,30–33] Mast cells express the c-kit receptor and are chemotactic to mesenchymal cells and lymphocytes. These long-lived cells can be stimulated by bacterial products to release pre-stored or newly synthesized cytokines, including TNF.[14,30–33] Major increases in TNF-producing mast cells occur in the intestine of patients with Crohn's disease relative to those with ulcerative colitis, particularly in the submucosa and muscularis propria of strictured bowel.[31,32] Increased urinary excretion of methylhistamine, a mast cell product, correlates positively with disease activity.[34] Fibrosing colonopathy, an inflammatory and fibrosing disorder in children with cystic fibrosis given particular pancreatic enzyme supplements, is characterized by increased numbers of submucosal and muscularis propria mast cells.[35,36] Co-culture of mast cells and mesenchymal cells stimulates mesenchymal cell proliferation and collagen synthesis.[37,38] Mast cells expressing tryptase (MC$_T$) predominate in the mucosa, whereas those expressing chymase and tryptase (MC$_{TC}$) predominate in the submucosal layers, particularly the muscularis propria.[14,30–32] Tryptase stimulates the proliferation of lung-derived fibroblasts via protease-activated receptor-2.[39] Chymase increases the formation of collagen fibrils.[40] Enzymes expressed by mast cells may therefore contribute to fibrosis. TGF-β is a potent chemoattractant for mast cells, which can produce TGF-β, prolong its half-life and cause its release from ECM.[33,38] Rats deficient in c-kit show reduced radiation-induced intestinal fibrosis, which has been attributed to mast cell deficiency[38] but could reflect a deficiency in ICC.[14] The c-kit-deficient rats show reduced mucosal inflammation with sodium dextran sulfate[41] but enhanced radiation-induced mucosal injury;[38] therefore the role of mucosal mast cells in mucosal inflammation is not clear. Rat and mouse models deficient in c-kit or stem cell factor none the less represent powerful models to study the role of mast cells and ICC in IBD.[14] It would also be of interest to develop methods to transfer activated mucosal or submucosal mast cells to animal models of IBD and test the impact on ECM synthesis or development of fibrosis.

# MOLECULAR MEDIATORS OF FIBROSIS

## ECM COMPONENTS

Although excessive net deposition of collagens and ECM defines fibrosis in Crohn's disease, precisely which ECM components are involved and the biosynthetic mechanisms that dictate excessive synthesis and deposition are unclear. Common collagen types have been quantified in normal intestine, inflamed non-strictured intestine, and strictured intestine resected from patents with Crohn's disease.[42] Type I is the major collagen in normal ileum, accounting for 68% of total collagen. Types III and V account for 20% and 12%, respectively, of total collagen in normal ileum. In strictured ileum, type V collagen is enriched approximately 40% over control tissue.[42] Types I and III collagen are reportedly increased in ulcerated areas, especially around capillaries, and types IV and V are increased in perivascular regions in the muscularis propria and around ganglia.[43] Consistent with smooth muscle cells as possible sources of collagen during fibrosis, intestinal smooth muscle cells isolated from normal human jejunum synthesize the same predominant collagen types, types I, III and V, as found in normal and strictured intestine.[42,44] Other studies suggest that increased laminin associated with infiltration of mast cells into submucosa and muscularis propria may be a distinguishing feature of Crohn's disease.[31] Intriguingly, a recent microarray analysis found that numerous ECM genes, including fibronectin, collagen IV and collagen VI, were selectively upregulated in ulcerative colitis and not Crohn's disease.[18]

## MATRIX METALLOPROTEINASES (MMP) AND TISSUE INHIBITORS OF METALLOPROTEINASES (TIMP)

Increasing evidence indicates a central role for MMP and TIMP in dictating the balance between ECM synthesis and degradation and normal wound healing or fibrosis. MMP are an expanding family of structurally related zinc-dependent matrix-degrading proteinases.[45,46] As shown in Table 15.1, MMP can be classified based on specificity for particular substrates, such as fibrillar collagens (collagenases), denatured collagens (gelatinases) and non-collagen ECM components (stromelysins), and can be secreted (MMP) or exist as transmembrane proteins (MT-MMP). Secreted MMP are initially released as inactive precursors and must be proteolytically cleaved to be activated. Some MT-MMP activate other MMP family members and act on ECM.[45] Active MMP form stable complexes with TIMP (TIMP-1, TIMP-2 or TIMP-3); the balance between active MMP and their TIMP inhibitors exerts a complex control over net ECM degradation. Although initially studied for their role in dictating the balance between ECM synthesis and degradation during tissue injury and healing, MMP/TIMP have major effects on organ growth and development, disease and tumorigenesis.[45,46] MMP/TIMP play a major role in the liberation of active cytokines or growth factors from the cell surface or ECM, and in processing growth factor/cytokine precursors from an inactive to an active form (Table 15.1). Thus, in addition to their direct actions on ECM, MMP/TIMP may influence fibrosis by dictating the local milieu of active fibrogenic cytokines or growth factors that control mesenchymal cell proliferation or ECM deposition or degradation. At present there is no clear evidence to correlate fibrosis in IBD with increased levels of particular MMP or TIMP within the mucosa. Mucosal biopsies from patients with ulcerative colitis and Crohn's disease show both elevated mRNA and elevated protein levels of mesenchymal cell-derived MMP, including MMP-1, -2, -3 and -14.[47,48] It will be important to assay MMP/TIMP activity directly to determine whether they correlate with fibrosis, and to examine them in submucosal layers. Mice with targeted deletion of specific MMP or TIMP[49,50] provide useful models to address the role of MMP in normal mucosal repair and fibrosis.

## CYTOKINES AND GROWTH FACTORS

Direct effects on ECM synthesis or proliferative effects on intestinal mesenchymal cells implicate a large number of cytokines and growth factors as mediators of fibrosis. Insulin-like growth factor-1 (IGF-1) and TGF-β are among the most intensively studied. Both show increased expression in the intestine of Crohn's disease patients.[13,51]

Increased local expression of IGF-1 mRNA occurs in all layers of inflamed or fibrotic intestine of patients with Crohn's disease,[52] but is only focally increased in ulcerative colitis tissues.[5,53] Local expression of IGF-1 mRNA is increased in every animal model of enterocolitis examined to date.[27,54–56] Increased IGF-1 expression occurs primarily in myofibroblasts and smooth muscle cells at sites of increased collagen mRNA expression and fibrosis in Crohn's disease and chronic experimental intestinal inflammation.[21,27,52,56] IGF-1 is mitogenic for enteric smooth muscle cells,[21,57] intestinal myofibroblasts or fibroblasts in vitro[58] and in vivo,[59,60] and stimulates collagen synthesis in these cells.[21,61,62] Together, these data indicate that locally expressed, mesenchymal cell-derived IGF-1 is probably a key mediator of fibrosis during chronic intestinal inflammation. The IGF-binding protein (IGFBP) family has complex effects on IGF bioavailability and action and can inhibit or potentiate IGF-1 action. In Crohn's disease and animal models IGFBP5 shows increased expression at similar sites as IGF-1.[21,63] IGFBP5 potentiates IGF action and may contribute to fibrosis. Other IGFBP, such as IGFBP3 and IGFBP4, which can inhibit IGF

### Table 15.1 MMP and growth factor action

| Type | MMP | Cytokine/growth factor release |
|---|---|---|
| Matrilysin | MMP-7 | TGF-β, TNF |
| | MMP-26 | |
| Collagenase | MMP-1 | FGF, IGF, TNF, IGFBP2, |
| | MMP-8 | IGFBP3, IGFBP5 |
| | MMP-13 | |
| Stromelysin | MMP-3 | TGF-β, TNF, IL-1β, IGF, |
| | MMP-10 | TNF, FGFRI, IGFBP2, |
| | MMP-11 | IGFBP3, VEGF, TGF-β2, |
| Gelatinase | MMP-2 | TGF-β, TNF-α, IL-1β, IGF, |
| | MMP-9 | TNF, FGFRI, IGFBP2, IGFBP3, VEGF, TGF-β2, IGF-1, IGFBP3, IGFBP5 |
| Membrane associated | | IGF, FGF |
| MT-1-MMP | MMP-14 | IGF |
| MT-2-MMP | MMP-15 | IGF |
| MT-3-MMP | MMP-16 | IGF, TNF |
| MT-4-MMP | MMP-17 | |
| MT-5-MMP | MMP-24 | |
| MT-6-MMP | MMP-25 | |
| | MMP-23 | |
| Metalloelastase | MMP-12 | |
| RASI | MMP-19 | |
| Enamelysin | MMP-20 | |
| Epilysin | MMP-28 | |
| TACE/ADAM 17 | | TNF |

Data compiled from references[46,121,122]

action by limiting bioavailability, are expressed in intestinal mesenchymal cells.[64] Specific MMP are known to cleave IGFBP[46] and thus may influence fibrosis by affecting the actions or bioavailability of IGF-1.

TGF-β has a complex role in IBD through immunoregulatory, immunosuppressive and profibrogenic functions.[65] Considerable evidence supports a profibrogenic role of TGF-β in fibrosis in many organ systems, including the intestine.[66–68] TGF-β directly stimulates collagen production in all intestinal mesenchymal cell subtypes.[67–69] Bacterial cell wall polymers induce increased collagen synthesis in intestinal myofibroblasts by TGF-β-dependent mechanisms.[68] Adenovirus-mediated gene transfer studies provide powerful support for an in vivo role of TGF-β to promote fibrosis within many organs.[70–72] TGF-β stimulates quiescent mesenchymal cells to become activated myofibroblasts, typified by the expression of αSM-actin, organization of αSM-actin into stress fibers, and increased

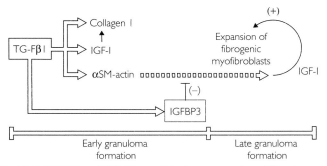

**Fig. 15.3** TGF-β1 and IGF-1 interact during progression of fibrosis associated with early and late granulomas and determine their role in early wound healing versus prolonged, excessive fibrosis.

collagen expression.[11,12,67] Although profibrogenic, TGF-β inhibits cell proliferation and so does not account for the expansion of fibrogenic mesenchymal cells in IBD. In the liver TGF-β acts in concert with other mitogenic cytokines, such as platelet-derived growth factor (PDGF) or basic fibroblast growth factor (bFGF), to elicit proliferation of activated, fibrogenic mesenchymal cells.[10] TGF-β and IGF-1 show partially overlapping sites of expression in an animal model of granulomatous enterocolitis and fibrosis, but IGF-1 is expressed in a larger number of mesenchymal cells.[67] These findings and recent in vitro studies support an interaction of TGF-β and IGF-1 during normal wound healing or fibrosis[67] (Fig. 15.3). This model proposes that TGF-β expressed in immune cells recruits fibroblasts, converts them to activated fibrogenic phenotype, and induces IGF-1 expression in these or neighboring fibroblasts/myofibroblasts. Combined actions of TGF-β and IGF-1 stimulate collagen expression and normal wound healing. Inappropriate expansion of fibrogenic mesenchymal cells is, however, limited by the antagonistic actions of TGF-β on IGF-1-induced proliferation and the fact that TGF-β induces IGFBP3, an inhibitor of the proliferative actions of IGF-1. However, in an experimental model,[67] and probably in Crohn's disease fibrosis,[13,51,73] increased IGF-1 expression persists in mesenchymal cells at sites distant from TGF-β which permits IGF-1 to chronically expand the population of TGF-β-activated fibrogenic mesenchymal cells[67] (Fig. 15.3). Crohn's disease myofibroblasts show increased release of TGF-β2 and reduced expression of TGF-β3,[74] indicating that changes in patterns of TGF-β expression may contribute to the pathophysiology of Crohn's disease. In hepatic stellate cells TGF-β-mediated induction of myofibroblast phenotype is obligatorily linked to increased collagen production. Recent studies[75] question this concept. Pan et al.[75] show that a novel protein, P311, is expressed specifically in smooth muscle cells and myofibroblasts but not fibroblasts at sites of wound healing in a number of organs. P311 induces myofibroblast phenotype in embryonic mesenchymal cells, but downregulates TGF-β and collagen. P311 may therefore be a useful phenotypic marker of smooth muscle and myofibroblasts in IBD and may have a critical role in the balance between normal wound healing or TGF-β-mediated fibrosis. Analyses of this protein in IBD tissues and animal models will be of great interest.

Emerging information suggests that TNF, which plays a central role in the pathophysiology of CD, may be a mediator of fibrosis.[76–79] TNF is expressed in myofibroblasts derived from the intestine of patients with IBD.[82] In other organ systems TNF contributes to inflammation-induced fibrosis.[83–86] TNF stimulates proliferation and type I collagen transcription in lung-derived fibroblasts.[84] Mice deficient in either the 55 or the 75 kDa TNF receptor show greatly diminished experimentally induced pulmonary fibrosis[84] or renal fibrosis,[87] even though they still exhibit inflammation and tissue damage. Intriguingly, in silica-induced pulmonary fibrosis TNF receptor-null mice show similar increases in type I collagen gene expression as wildtype mice, but impaired induction of TIMP-1, an inhibitor of collagen degradation.[84] NFκB activation is also normal in P55- or P75-null mice, but activation of AP-1, a key mediator of TIMP-1 gene expression,[88] is impaired.[84] TIMP-1 expression is increased in the intestine of patients with CD.[89] Preliminary data indicate that TNF directly increases type I collagen accumulation and TIMP-1 expression in intestinal myofibroblasts, and that IGF-1 and TNF have additive or synergistic actions on myofibroblast proliferation (Lund, Simmons and Goodrich, unpublished observations). The role of TNF in fibrosis in Crohn's disease warrants further study. It is clear that the story will be complex, given the conflicting effects of TNF on collagen synthesis in different systems[83–85] and the difficulty of distinguishing direct effects of TNF on fibrosis from secondary effects due to its proinflammatory actions.

This section has emphasized the most thoroughly studied candidate mediators or modulators of fibrosis. However, many other cytokines, including connective tissue growth factor (CTGF),[90] VEGF[91] and angiotensin II are emerging as potential mediators. Angiotensin II is particularly interesting as it mediates mesenchymal cell expansion in vascular, hepatic and renal injury or fibrosis,[92–96] and in other systems induces TGF-β and IGF-1.[92,97,98] Findings in experimentally induced fibrosis of other organs[99–101] suggest that angiotensin-converting enzyme (ACE) inhibitors or angiotensin receptor antagonists could be promising antifibrosis therapies in IBD. Furthermore, interleukin-10 (IL-10) may contributes to fibrosis in chronic inflammation. IL-10 attenuates fibrosis in the liver and pancreas,[50,102] suggesting that analysis of the antifibrogenic actions of IL-10 is warranted in IBD.

## WHICH ANIMAL MODELS MAY PROVE USEFUL TO STUDY FIBROSIS?

Well-characterized animal models of inflammation-induced intestinal fibrosis with features in common with Crohn's disease are desirable to better define the cellular and molecular mediators of the onset and perpetuation of fibrosis. Comparisons in models where the same stimulus administered in different paradigms can cause acute mucosal inflammation followed by normal wound healing or chronic transmural inflammation associated with fibrosis would be particularly valuable. Animal models are essential to test therapies that may limit fibrosis without compromising the desired tissue healing responses.

Table 15.2 reviews some existing animal models that may prove useful for analysis of normal mucosal healing and fibrosis (see Chapter 9). None of these models has been well characterized for disease-related changes in expression of ECM proteins or phenotype of intestinal mesenchymal cells. Inflammation occurs predominantly in the mucosa of IL-10-null mice, suggesting that this model could be useful to study the role of mucosal mesenchymal cells in inflammation-induced fibrosis.[103] The TNF$^{\Delta ARE}$ mouse overexpresses TNF mRNA in

## Table 15.2 Animal models of fibrosis and IBD

| | IL-10 null | TNF$^{\Delta\,ARE}$ | SAMP1/ Yit | PG-PS | TNBS | DSS | γ IRR |
|---|---|---|---|---|---|---|---|
| Mucosal inflammation | + | + | + | + | + | + | + |
| **Transmural inflammation** | | | | | | | |
| Ileum | + | + | + | + | ? | +/– | + |
| Colon | + | + | – | + | + | + | + |
| Bowel wall thickening | + | + | + | + | + | + | + |
| Muscle hyperplasia | (+) | + | + | + | (+) | (+) | + |
| **Collagen gene activation** | | | | | | | |
| Mucosa | ? | ? | ? | + | ? | + | + |
| Submucosa | ? | ? | ? | + | ? | + | + |
| Muscularis propria | ? | ? | ? | + | ? | + | + |
| **Increased collagen deposition** | | | | | | | |
| Mucosa | + | ? | + | + | + | + | + |
| Submucosa | +/– | ? | + | + | + | + | + |
| Muscularis propria | +/– | ? | + | + | + | + | + |
| **Mucosal healing** | | | | | | | |
| Chronic mucosal damage | – | – | – | + | + | + | + |
| Genetic background | + | + | + | + | + | + | + |
| Dependence | + | ? | ? | + | + | + | ? |

+ feature of the model; (+) not verified; +/– observed in some strains or conditions;- not observed; ? not established; Data are modified from [123].

ileal and colonic macrophages or other cells of hemopoietic origin,[80,81] making this a potentially very attractive mouse model to study the role of TNF-mediated transmural inflammation in fibrosis. It would be of interest to establish whether mast cells are sources of TNF overexpression in TNF$^{\Delta\,ARE}$ mice. Cross-bred models with TNF$^{\Delta\,ARE}$ mutation in conjunction with absolute deficiency of TNFR1 and TNFRII[80,81] could provide insights into the role of the different TNF-α receptors in inflammation and fibrosis. Some disadvantages of the TNF$^{\Delta\,ARE}$ model are that disease onset begins prior to puberty, leading to significant growth retardation and mortality which may indirectly affect fibrosis. The SAMP1/Yit model generated from the senescence accelerated mouse (SAM) line shares many features with the TNF$^{\Delta\,ARE}$ model and may overcome this disadvantage, as disease develops later in life.[81] Adoptive transfer of CD4+ cells from SAMP1/Yit mice into SCID mice also provides a useful model of ileitis in Crohn's disease which will be very valuable for studies of fibrosis.[104]

Inflammation induced by peptidoglycan-polysaccharide (PG-PS) or ethanol trinitrobenzensulfonic acid (TNBS) in rats definitively demonstrates transmural inflammation associated with transmural fibrosis and overexpression of TGF-β and/or IGF-1, as occurs in Crohn's disease.[27,68,105] The acute, quiescent and reactivation phases in PG-PS-induced enterocolitis, together with dramatic transmural, granulomatous fibrosis, permit analysis of collagen subtypes, mesenchymal phenotypes and cytokines, growth factors, and consequences of interventions at different stages in inflammation-induced fibrosis. Disadvantages of the model are the limited availability of PG-PS, its technically demanding nature, and its unsuccessful adaptation to mice (Lund and Sartor, unpublished data). Fibrosis has been less well characterized in the rat TNBS model. However, repeated treat-ments of CD-1 mice with progressively increasing doses of TNBS over a 6–8-week period cause increased ECM deposition and a high occurrence of fibrosis.[106] The TNBS model may therefore prove useful for studying fibrosis in other mouse strains.

An inducible mouse model of fibrosis that can be easily applied to transgenic or gene knockout mice and their wildtype littermates on different genetic backgrounds is particularly desirable. Acute colitis induced by DSS in drinking water has been extensively used in genetically manipulated mice to study the genes involved in mucosal protection or repair.[26,52,55] Most studies have analyzed animals given a single treatment with 3–10% DSS for 5–7 days, which induces acute inflammation of the colonic mucosa and mucosal damage that probably results from direct toxicity of DSS to epithelial cells.[26] Acute colitis is followed by restoration of mucosal architecture once DSS is withdrawn,[26,55,107] making this an ideal model to study normal mucosal healing. Low doses of DSS (3–3.5%) should be used if animals are to be studied subsequent to DSS treatment, as higher doses lead to unacceptably high morbidity in several mouse strains[55] (Lund, unpublished data). A single treatment with 3–5% DSS does not lead to significant fibrosis at the end of DSS or during recovery (Lund and Williams, unpublished observations). Preliminary data indicate that two cycles of DSS cause chronic transmural inflammation and transmural fibrosis in several mouse strains (Lund, unpublished observations).[24] Advantages of the DSS model include technical ease and the potential to compare mechanisms of normal mucosal healing and fibrosis in response to the same injurious agent. Disadvantages are that the immunological features of mucosal healing and chronic inflammation have not yet been well characterized, generating considerable debate about the relevance of this model to IBD.

Irradiation of the small intestine or colon leads to early fibrosis underlying mucosal ulcers, attributed to induction of mucosal repair mechanisms.[38,108–110] Submucosal and muscularis propria fibrosis develops later and is attributed to direct damage or death of mesenchymal cells in these layers. Differences in induction of collagens I and III have been noted in mucosal and submucosal fibrosis, although fibroblasts appear to mediate fibrosis in both locations.[108,109] The relevance of irradiation-induced intestinal fibrosis to IBD is uncertain, but this model may be very useful to study differences in molecular or cellular mediators of mucosal and submucosal fibrosis and, by comparison with immune-mediated models, to delineate those features of fibrosis specific to IBD. Recent studies implicate c-kit-expressing cells and TGF-β as mediators of irradiation-induced fibrosis,[110] indicating common features with fibrosis in CD.

As indicated previously, procollagen α1 (I) promoter-GFP transgenic mice provide a model to easily and sensitively assess collagen gene activation in vivo and in vitro.[23] Mice with different portions of the procollagen α1 (I) promoter linked to GFP[23] will permit dissection of the *cis*-acting genetic elements that regulate collagen gene activation in the intestine in vivo. The GFP reporter provides an early histological marker of cell types that exhibit type I collagen gene activation, which should facilitate the identification of 'activated' mesenchymal cell phenotypes early in the course of intestinal inflammation or fibrosis. The procollagen α1 (I)-GFP reporter gene is induced in intestinal mesenchymal cells in vivo by DSS and in vitro by TGF-β and IGF-1.[24] Procollagen α1 (I) promoter-GFP transgenics serve as a prototype for similar approaches linking GFP to promoters that regulate the expression of other collagen types or other ECM components, and could provide a rapid and easy model system to test the effects of interventions aimed at controlling collagen synthesis in vivo.

## WHAT ARE THE PROSPECTS FOR THE DEVELOPMENT OF NEW ANTIFIBROSIS THERAPIES?

Surgical resection and stricturoplasty are the only current therapies for fibrosis and strictures. Stricturoplasty preserves bowel integrity and mucosal surface area[11,111] and is most effectively employed in patients with multiple short strictures that have quiescent disease. Endoscopic balloon dilation can be effective for short anastomotic strictures.

No specific medical therapy is available for the treatment of intestinal fibrosis in IBD. Medical therapies for other fibrotic diseases, such as idiopathic pulmonary fibrosis, cirrhosis and retroperitoneal fibrosis, are primarily experimental. Experimental therapies include a wide variety of agents that have shown promise in vivo and in vitro, and include TGF-β-soluble receptor,[113] p38 MAPK inhibitors,[114] colchicine,[115] mycophenolate mofetil,[116] ACE inhibitors or angiotensin II type 1 receptor blockade,[94,99–101] tamoxifen, thalidomide,[117] and D-penicillamine. Studies of these therapies for fibrosis associated with IBD have been hampered by the lack of suitable tests to monitor intestinal fibrosis. Other experimental therapies, such as tranilast or batimastat, inhibit MMP.[118,119] Findings that COX-2-null mice show prolonged inflammation and fibrosis in a model of lung injury[120] have implications for the profibrogenic actions of COX-2 inhibitors.

Recent studies establishing the safety and efficacy of potent immunosuppressives such as infliximab and azathioprine/6-mercaptopurine have changed the approach to patients with complicated IBD. The effect of these therapies to modify disease progression, specifically their effect on stricture formation, is unknown. This is largely due to the inherent difficulty in monitoring bowel strictures and the slow progression of the disease. The lack of a reproducible, non-invasive, widely available test for following strictures over time is a serious handicap in our ability to study potential disease-modifying agents. The rapid development of stricture and obstruction in a subset of patients given infliximab[9] is a concern and somewhat paradoxical, given the evidence described above that TNF may be a causative agent in fibrosis. The problem may relate to indirect rapid anti-inflammatory effects of infliximab on wound healing. If these immunosuppressive agents or other experimental therapies are shown to prevent or delay stricture formation, then their use earlier in the disease process, after resection, and in children with IBD, may be warranted, although they will be expensive and potentially toxic.

## CONCLUSIONS

Our understanding of the etiology and pathophysiology of fibrosis in IBD is much more limited than our knowledge of immune mechanisms, even though fibrosis is a major cause of surgery and morbidity in IBD patients, particularly those with Crohn's disease. It is increasingly apparent that fibrosis is not simply a single wound healing response that shares similar cellular and molecular mediators and mechanisms across all organs. Animal models and new tools and approaches to further our understanding of intestinal fibrosis should facilitate the testing of potential therapies and determine whether fibrosis is an obligatory end-stage response to chronic inflammation in Crohn's disease or may be attenuated, cured or prevented.

## ACKNOWLEDGMENTS

This work was supported by NIH grant DK DK56750 to Ellen Zimmermann and DK-47769 and DK-40247 to P. K. Lund. Prior funding from the Crohn's and Colitis Foundation of America for research into fibrosis and IBD is also acknowledged. The authors thank Drs David Brenner, Leo Dieleman, Shira Fruchtman, Arianne Goodrich, Martin Graham, Jolanta Pucilowska, Balfour Sartor, Jim Simmons and Kristen Williams for useful discussions about IBD and fibrosis. The authors also thank Katherine Kershaw and Eileen Hoyt for assistance with graphics, and Natasha Waglow and Heidi Karp for secretarial assistance.

## REFERENCES

1. Becker JM. Surgical therapy for ulcerative colitis and Crohn's disease. Gastroenterol Clin North Am 1999;28:371–390.
2. Maconi G, Parente F, Bollani S, Cesana B, Bianchi Porro G. Abdominal ultrasound in the assessment of extent and activity of Crohn's disease: clinical significance and implication of bowel wall thickening. Am J Gastroenterol 1996;91:1604–1609.
3. Verspaget HW, Biemond I, Allaart CF et al. Assessment of plasma fibronectin in Crohn's disease. Hepatogastroenterology 1991;38:231–234.
4. Matthes H, Herbst H, Suchuppan D, Stallmach A, Milani S, Stein H. Cellular localization of procollagen gene transcripts in inflammatory bowel disease. Gastroenterology 1992;102:431–442.
5. Lawrance IC, Maxwell L, Doe W. Altered response of intestinal mucosal fibroblasts to profibrogenic cytokines in inflammatory bowel disease. Inflamm Bowel Dis 2001;7:226–236.

6. Abreu MT, Taylor KD, Lin YC et al. Mutations in NOD2 are associated with fibrostenosing disease in patients with Crohn's disease. Gastroenterology 2002;123:679–688.

7. Radlmayr M, Torok HP, Martin K, Folwaczny C. The c-insertion mutation of the NOD2 gene is associated with fistulizing and fibrostenotic phenotypes in Crohn's disease. Gastroenterology 2002;122:2091–2092.

8. Inohara N, Ogura Y, Nunez G. Nods: a family of cytosolic proteins that regulate the host response to pathogens. Curr Opin Microbiol 2002;5:76–80.

9. Toy L, Scheri E, Kornbluth A et al. Complete bowel obstruction following initial response to infliximab therapy for Crohn's disease: a series of a newly described complication. Gastroenterology 2000;118:G2974.

10. Li D, Friedman SL. Liver fibrogenesis and the role of hepatic stellate cells: new insights and prospects for therapy. J Gastroenterol Hepatol 1999;14:618–633.

11. Powell DW, Mifflin RC, Valentich JD, Crowe SE, Saada JI, West AB. Myofibroblasts. I. Paracrine cells important in health and disease. Am J Physiol 1999;277:C1–C9.

12. Powell DW, Mifflin RC, Valentich JD, Crowe SE, Saada JI, West AB. Myofibroblasts. II. Intestinal subepithelial myofibroblasts. Am J Physiol 1999;277:C183–201.

13. Pucilowska JB, McNaughton KK, Mohapatra NK et al. IGF-1 and procollagen α1(I) are coexpressed in a subset of mesenchymal cells in active Crohn's disease. Am J Physiol Gastrointest Liver Physiol 2000;279:G1307–1322.

14. Wershil BK. IX. Mast cell-deficient mice and intestinal biology. Am J Physiol Gastrointest Liver Physiol 2000;278:G343–348.

15. Stallmach A, Schuppan D, Riese HH, Matthes H, Riecken EO. Increased collagen type III synthesis by fibroblasts isolated from strictures of patients with Crohn's disease. Gastroenterology 1992;102:1920–1929.

16. Aigner T, Neureiter D, Muller S, Kuspert G, Belke J, Kirchner T. Extracellular matrix composition and gene expression in collagenous colitis. Gastroenterology 1997;113:136–143.

17. Tremaine WJ. Collagenous colitis and lymphocytic colitis. J Clin Gastroenterol 2000;30:245–249.

18. Lawrance IC, Fiocchi C, Chakravarti S. Ulcerative colitis and Crohn's disease: distinctive gene expression profiles and novel susceptibility candidate genes. Hum Mol Genet 2001;10:445–456.

19. Leeb SN, Vogl D, Falk W, Scholmerich J, Rogler G, Gelbmann CM. Regulation of migration of human colonic myofibroblasts. Growth Factors 2002;20:81–91.

20. Graham MF. Pathogenesis of intestinal strictures in CD–an update. Inflamm Bowel Dis 1995;1:220–227.

21. Zimmermann EM, Li L, Hou YT, Cannon M, Christman GM, Bitar KN. IGF-1 induces collagen and IGFBP-5 mRNA in rat intestinal smooth muscle. Am J Physiol 1997;273:G875–882.

22. Lu G, Qian X, Berezin I, Telford GL, Huizinga JD, Sarna SK. Inflammation modulates in vitro colonic myoelectric and contractile activity and interstitial cells of Cajal. Am J Physiol 1997;273:G1233–1245.

23. Krempen K, Grotkopp D, Hall K et al. Far upstream regulatory elements enhance position-independent and uterus-specific expression of the murine α1(I) collagen promoter in transgenic mice. Gene Expression 1999;8:151–163.

24. Dacosta CM, Simmons JG, Fuller CR et al. Collagen promoter-GFP transgenic mice provide a model to study collagen gene expression during experimental intestinal inflammation and injury in vivo and in vitro. Gastroenterology 2001;120:A135.

25. Blennerhassett MG, Bovell FM, Lourenssen S, McHugh KM. Characteristics of inflammation-induced hypertrophy of rat intestinal smooth muscle cell. Dig Dis Sci 1999;44:1265–1272.

26. Elson CO, Cony Y, Brandwein S et al. Experimental models to study molecular mechanisms underlying intestinal inflammation. Ann NY Acad Sci 1998;3859:85–95.

27. Zeeh JM, Mohapatra N, Lund PK, Eysselein VE, McRoberts JA. Differential expression and localization of IGF-1 and IGF binding proteins in inflamed rat colon. J Receptor Signal Trans Res 1998;18:265–280.

28. Shepherd NA, Jass JR. Neuromuscular and vascular hamartoma of the small intestine: is it Crohn's disease? Gut 1987;28:1663–1668.

29. Koukoulis G, Ke Y, Henley JD, Cummings OW. Obliterative muscularization of the small bowel submucosa in Crohn disease: a possible mechanism of small bowel obstruction. Arch Pathol Lab Med 2001;125:1331–1334.

30. Bischoff SC, Lorentz A, Schwengberg S, Weier G, Raab R, Manns MP. Mast cells are an important cellular source of tumour necrosis factor α in human intestinal tissue. Gut 1999;44:643–652.

31. Gelbmann CM, Mestermann S, Gross V, Kollinger M, Scholmerich J, Falk W. Strictures in Crohn's disease are characterised by an accumulation of mast cells colocalised with laminin but not with fibronectin or vitronectin. Gut 1999;45:210–217.

32. Lilja I, Gustafson-Svard C, Franzen L, Sjodahl R. Tumor necrosis factor-α in ileal mast cells in patients with Crohn's disease. Digestion 2000;61:68–76.

33. Malaviya R, Abraham SN. Clinical implications of mast cell–bacteria interaction. J Mol Med 1998;76:617–623.

34. Weidenhiller M, Raithel M, Winterkamp S, Otte P, Stolper J, Hahn EG. Methylhistamine in Crohn's disease (CD): increased production and elevated urine excretion correlates with disease activity. Inflamm Res 2000;49:S35–36.

35. Dodge JA. Fibrosing colonopathy. Gut 2000;46:152–153.

36. Pawel BR, de Chadarevian JP, Franco ME. The pathology of fibrosing colonopathy of cystic fibrosis: a study of 12 cases and review of the literature. Hum Pathol 1997;28:395–399.

37. Berton A, Levi-Schaffer F, Emonard H, Garbuzenko E, Gillery P, Maquart FX. Activation of fibroblasts in collagen lattices by mast cell extract: a model of fibrosis. Clin Exp Allergy 2000;30:485–492.

38. Zheng H, Wang J, Hauer-Jensen M. Role of mast cells in early and delayed radiation injury in rat intestine. Radiat Res 2000;153:533–539.

39. Akers IA, Parsons M, Hill MR et al. Mast cell tryptase stimulates human lung fibroblast proliferation via protease-activated receptor-2. Am J Physiol Lung Cell Mol Physiol 2000;278:L193–201.

40. Kofford MW, Schwartz LB, Schechter NM, Yager DR, Diegelmann RF, Graham MF. Cleavage of type I procollagen by human mast cell chymase initiates collagen fibril formation and generates a unique carboxyl-terminal propeptide. J Biol Chem 1997;272:7127–7131.

41. Araki Y, Andoh A, Fujiyama Y, Bamba T. Development of dextran sulphate sodium-induced experimental colitis is suppressed in genetically mast cell-deficient Ws/Ws rats. Clin Exp Immunol 2000;119:264–269.

42. Graham MF, Diegelmann RF, Elson CO et al. Collagen content and types in the intestinal strictures of Crohn's disease. Gastroenterology 1988;94:257–265.

43. Geboes KP, Cabooter L, Geboes K. Contribution of morphology for the comprehension of mechanisms of fibrosis in inflammatory enterocolitis. Acta Gastroenterol Belg 2000;63:371–376.

44. Graham MF, Drucker DE, Diegelmann RF, Elson CO. Collagen synthesis by human intestinal smooth muscle cells in culture. Gastroenterology 1987;92:400–405.

45. Nagase H, Woessner JF Jr. Matrix metalloproteinases. J Biol Chem 1999;274:21491–21494.

46. Winkler MK, Fowlkes JL. Metalloproteinase and growth factor interactions: do they play a role in pulmonary fibrosis? Am J Physiol Lung Cell Mol Physiol 2002;283:L1–11.

47. Schuppan D, Hahn EG. MMP in the gut: inflammation hits the matrix. Gut 2000;47:12–14.

48. von Lampe B, Barthel B, Coupland SE, Riecken EO, Rosewicz S. Differential expression of matrix metalloproteinases and their tissue inhibitors in colon mucosa of patients with inflammatory bowel disease. Gut 2000;47:63–73.

49. Garcia-Gonzalez MA, Crusius JB, Strunk MH et al. TGF-B1 gene polymorphisms and inflammatory bowel disease. Immunogenetics 2000;51:869–872.

50. Vaillant B, Chiaramonte MG, Cheever AW, Soloway PD, Wynn TA. Regulation of hepatic fibrosis and extracellular matrix genes by the th response: new insight into the role of tissue inhibitors of matrix metalloproteinases. J Immunol 2001;167:7017–7026.

51. Babyatsky MW, Rossiter G, Podolsky DK. Expression of transforming growth factors α and β in colonic mucosa in inflammatory bowel disease. Gastroenterology 1996;110:975–984.

52. Pucilowska JB, Williams KL, Lund PK. Fibrogenesis. IV. Fibrosis and inflammatory bowel disease: cellular mediators and animal models. Am J Physiol Gastrointest Liver Physiol 2000;279:G653–659.

53. Lawrance IC, Maxwell L, Doe W. Inflammation location, but not type, determines the increase in TGF-β1 and IGF-1 expression and collagen deposition in IBD intestine. Inflamm Bowel Dis 2001;7:16–26.

54. Savendahl L, Underwood LE, Haldeman KM, Ulshen MH, Lund PK. Fasting prevents experimental murine colitis produced by dextran sulfate sodium and decreases interleukin-1-β and insulin-like growth factor I messenger ribonucleic acid. Endocrinology 1997;138:734–740.

55. Williams KL, Fuller CR, Dieleman LA et al. Enhanced survival and mucosal repair after dextran sodium sulfate-induced colitis in transgenic mice that overexpress growth hormone. Gastroenterology 2001;120:925–937.

56. Zimmermann EM, McNaughton K, Sartor RB, Lund PK. IGF-1 is overexpressed in cells with a smooth muscle phenotype in peptidoglycan-poly saccharide induced chronic enterocolitis in the rat. Gastroenterology 1993;104:A808.

57. Kuemmerle JF. Endogenous IGF-1 regulates IGF binding protein production in human intestinal smooth muscle cells. Am J Physiol Gastrointest Liver Physiol 2000;278:G710–717.

58. Simmons JG, Pucilowska JB, Lund PK. Autocrine and paracrine actions of intestinal fibroblast-derived insulin-like growth factors. Am J Physiol 1999;276:G817–827.

59. Wang J, Niu W, Nikiforov Y et al. Targeted overexpression of IGF-1 evokes distinct patterns of organ remodeling in smooth muscle cell tissue beds of transgenic mice. J Clin Invest 1997;100:1425–1439.

60. Williams KL, Fuller CR, Dieleman LA et al. Enhanced survival and mucosal repair after dextran sodium sulfate-induced colitis in transgenic mice that overexpress growth hormone. Gastroenterology 2001;120:925–937.

61. Simmons JG, Hoyt EC, Westwick JK, Brenner DA, Pucilowska JB, Lund PK. Insulin-like growth factor-1 and epidermal growth factor interact to regulate growth and gene expression in IEC-6 intestinal epithelial cells. Mol Endocrinol 1995;9:1157–1165.

62. Simmons JG, Pucilowska JB, Keku TO, Lund PK. IGF-I and TGF-beta1 have distinct effects on phenotype and proliferation of intestinal fibroblasts. Am J Physiol Gastrointest Liver Physiol. 2002;283:G809–818.

63. Zimmermann EM, Li L, Hou YT, Mohapatra NK, Pucilowska JB. Insulin-like growth factor I and insulin-like growth factor binding protein 5 in Crohn's disease. Am J Physiol Gastrointest Liver Physiol 2001;280:G1022–1029.

64. Williams KL, Fuller CR, Fagin J, Lund PK. Mesenchymal IGF-1 overexpression: paracrine effects in the intestine, distinct from endocrine actions. Am J Physiol Gastrointest Liver Physiol 2002;283:G875–885.

65. Fiocchi C. TGF-β/Smad signaling defects in inflammatory bowel disease: mechanisms and possible novel therapies for chronic inflammation. J Clin Invest 2001;108:523–526.

66. Friedman SL. Molecular regulation of hepatic fibrosis, an integrated cellular response to tissue injury. J Biol Chem 2000;275:2247–2250.

67. Simmons JG, Pucilowska JB, Keku TO, Lund PK. IGF-1 and TGF-β1 have distinct effects on phenotype and proliferation of intestinal fibroblasts. Am J Physiol Gastrointest Liver Physiol 2002;283:G809–818.

68. van Tol EA, Holt L, Li FL et al. Bacterial cell wall polymers promote intestinal fibrosis by direct stimulation of myofibroblasts. Am J Physiol 1999;277:G245–255.

69. Graham MF, Bryson GR, Diegelmann RF. Transforming growth factor β1 selectively augments collagen synthesis by human intestinal smooth muscle cells. Gastroenterology 1990;99:447–453.

70. Hellerbrand C, Stefanovic B, Giordano F, Burchardt ER, Brenner DA. The role of TGF-β1 in initiating hepatic stellate cell activation in vivo. J Hepatol 1999;30:77–87.

71. Kolb M, Bonniaud P, Galt T et al. Differences in the fibrogenic response after transfer of active transforming growth factor-β1 gene to lungs of "fibrosis-prone" and "fibrosis-resistant" mouse strains. Am J Respir Cell Mol Biol 2002;27:141–150.

72. Liu JY, Sime PJ, Wu T et al. Transforming growth factor-β(1) overexpression in tumor necrosis factor-α receptor knockout mice induces fibroproliferative lung disease. Am J Respir Cell Mol Biol 2001;25:3–7.

73. di Mola FF, Friess H, Scheuren A et al. Transforming growth factor-βs and their signaling receptors are coexpressed in Crohn's disease. Ann Surg 1999;229:67–75.

74. McKaig BC, Hughes K, Tighe PJ, Mahida YR. Differential expression of TGF-β isoforms by normal and inflammatory bowel disease intestinal myofibroblasts. Am J Physiol Cell Physiol 2002;282:C172–182.

75. Pan D, Zhe X, Jakkaraju S, Taylor GA, Schuger L. P311 induces a TGF-β1-independent, nonfibrogenic myofibroblast phenotype. J Clin Invest 2002;110:1349–1358.

76. Fiocchi C. Inflammatory bowel disease: etiology and pathogenesis. Gastroenterology 1998;115:182–205.

77. Sandborn WJ, Hanauer SB. Antitumor necrosis factor therapy for inflammatory bowel disease: a review of agents, pharmacology, clinical results, and safety. Inflamm Bowel Dis 1999;5:119–133.

78. Stack WA, Mann SD, Roy AJ et al. Randomised controlled trial of CDP571 antibody to tumour necrosis factor-α in Crohn's disease. Lancet 1997;349:521–524.

79. Targan SR, Hanauer SB, van Deventer SJ et al. A short-term study of chimeric monoclonal antibody cA2 to tumor necrosis factor α for Crohn's disease. Crohn's Disease cA2 Study Group. N Engl J Med 1997;337:1029–1035.

80. Kontoyiannis D, Pasparakis M, Pizarro TT, Cominelli F, Kollias G. Impaired on/off regulation of TNF biosynthesis in mice lacking TNF Au-rich elements: implications for joint and gut-associated immunopathologies. Immunity 1999;10:387–398.

81. Pizarro TT, Arseneau KO, Cominelli F. Lessons from genetically engineered animal models. XI. Novel mouse models to study pathogenic mechanisms of Crohn's disease. Am J Physiol 2000;278:G665–G669.

82. Strong SA, Pizarro TT, Klein JS, Cominelli F, Fiocchi C. Proinflammatory cytokines differentially modulate their own expression in human intestinal mucosal mesenchymal cells. Gastroenterology 1998;114:1244–1256.

83. Liu JY, Brody AR. Increased TGF-β1 in the lungs of asbestos-exposed rats and mice: reduced expression in TNF-α receptor knockout mice. J Environ Pathol Toxicol Oncol 2001;20:97–108.

84. Ortiz LA, Lasky J, Gozal E et al. Tumor necrosis factor receptor deficiency alters matrix metalloproteinase 13/tissue inhibitor of metalloproteinase 1 expression in murine silicosis. Am J Respir Crit Care Med 2001;163:244–252.

85. Ortiz LA, Lasky J, Lungarella G et al. Upregulation of the p75 but not the p55 TNF-α receptor mRNA after silica and bleomycin exposure and protection from lung injury in double receptor knockout mice. Am J Respir Cell Mol Biol 1999;20:825–833.

86. Sime PJ, Marr RA, Gauldie D et al. Transfer of tumor necrosis factor-α to rat lung induces severe pulmonary inflammation and patchy interstitial fibrogenesis with induction of transforming growth factor-β1 and myofibroblasts. Am J Pathol 1998;153:825–832.

87. Guo G, Morrissey J, McCracken R, Tolley T, Liapis H, Klahr S. Contributions of angiotensin II and tumor necrosis factor-α to the development of renal fibrosis. Am J Physiol Renal Physiol 2001;280:F777–785.

88. Phillips BW, Sharma R, Leco PA, Edwards DR. A sequence-selective single-strand DNA-binding protein regulates basal transcription of the murine tissue inhibitor of metalloproteinases-1 (Timp-1) gene. J Biol Chem 1999;274:22197–22207.

89. Lawrance IC, Fiocchi C, Chakravarti S. Differential expression of metalloproteinases (MMPS), tissue inhibitor of metaloproteinase (TIMP)-1 and extracellular matrix (ECM) components in fibrosed, inflamed and normal intestine. Gastroenterology 1999;116:G3291.

90. Gore-Hyer E, Shegogue D, Markiewicz M et al. TGF-β and CTGF- have overlapping and distinct fibrogenic effects on human renal cells. Am J Physiol Renal Physiol 2002;283:F707–716.

91. Griga T, Voigt E, Gretzer B, Brasch F, May B. Increased production of vascular endothelial growth factor by intestinal mucosa of patients with inflammatory bowel disease. Hepatogastroenterology 1999;46:920–923.

92. Border WA, Noble NA. Interactions of transforming growth factor-β and angiotensin II in renal fibrosis. Hypertension 1998;31:181–188.

93. Datta PK, Moulder JE, Fish BL, Cohen EP, Lianos EA. TGF-β 1 production in radiation nephropathy: role of angiotensin II. Int J Radiat Biol 1999;75:473–479.

94. Fukuda N, Hu WY, Kubo A et al. Angiotensin II upregulates transforming growth factor-β type I receptor on rat vascular smooth muscle cells. Am J Hypertens 2000;13:191–198.

95. Lim DS, Lutucuta S, Bachireddy P et al. Angiotensin II blockade reverses myocardial fibrosis in a transgenic mouse model of human hypertrophic cardiomyopathy. Circulation 2001;103:789–791.

96. Molteni A, Moulder JE, Cohen EF et al. Control of radiation-induced pneumopathy and lung fibrosis by angiotensin-converting enzyme inhibitors and an angiotensin II type I receptor blocker. Int J Radiat Biol 2000;76:523–532.

97. Peeters AC, Netea MG, Kullberg BJ, Thien T, van der Meer JW. The effect of renin–angiotensin system inhibitors on pro- and anti-inflammatory cytokine production. Immunology 1998;94:376–379.

98. Schultz Jel J, Witt SA, Glascock BJ et al. TGF-β1 mediates the hypertrophic cardiomyocyte growth induced by angiotensin II. J Clin Invest 2002;109:787–796.

99. Jonsson JR, Clouston AD, Ando Y et al. Angiotensin-converting enzyme inhibition attenuates the progression of rat hepatic fibrosis. Gastroenterology 2001;121:148–155.

100. Tzanidis A, Lim S, Hannan RD, See F, Ugoni AM, Krum H. Combined angiotensin and endothelin receptor blockade attenuates adverse cardiac remodeling post-myocardial infarction in the rat: possible role of transforming growth factor β(1). J Mol Cell Cardiol 2001;33:969–981.

101. Yoshiji H, Kuriyama S, Yoshii J et al. Angiotensin-II type I receptor interaction is a major regulator for liver fibrosis development in rats. Hepatology 2001;34:745–750.

102. Demols A, Van Laethem JL, Quertinmont E et al. Endogenous interleukin-10 modulates fibrosis and regeneration in experimental chronic pancreatitis. Am J Physiol Gastrointest Liver Physiol 2002;282:G1105–1112.

103. McCafferty DM, Sihota E, Muscara M, Wallace JL, Sharkey KA, Kubes P. Spontaneously developing chronic colitis in IL-10/iNOS double-deficient mice. Am J Physiol Gastrointest Liver Physiol 2000;279:G90–99.

104. Burns RC, Rivera-Nieves J, Moskaluk CA, Matsumoto S, Cominelli F, Ley K. Antibody blockade of ICAM-1 and VCAM-1 ameliorates inflammation in the SAMP-1/Yit adoptive transfer model of Crohn's disease in mice. Gastroenterology 2001;121:1428–1436.

105. Zimmermann EM, Sartor RB, McCall RD, Pardo M, Bender D, K. LP. Insulin-like growth factor-1 and interleukin 1 β messenger RNA in a rat model of granulomatous enterocolitis and hepatitis. Gastroenterology 1993;105:399–409.

106. Lawrance IC, Fiocchi C, Chakravarti S. TNBS-induced intestinal inflammation in CD-1 mice: A model for Crohn's disease-associated fibrosis. Gastroenterology 1999;116:G3292.

107. Dieleman LA, Elson CO, Tennyson GS, Beagley KW. Kinetics of cytokine expression during healing of acute colitis in mice. Am J Physiol 1996;271:G130–136.

108. Followill DS, Travis EL. Differential expression of collagen types I and III in consequential and primary fibrosis in irradiated mouse colon. Radiat Res 1995;144:318–328.

109. Langberg CW, Hauer-Jensen M. Influence of fraction size on the development of late radiation enteropathy. An experimental study in the rat. Acta Oncol 1996;35:89–94.

110. Zheng H, Wang J, Koteliansky VE, Gotwals PJ, Hauer-Jensen M. Recombinant soluble transforming growth factor β type II receptor ameliorates radiation enteropathy in mice. Gastroenterology 2000;119:1286–1296.

111. Pritchard TJ, Schoetz DJ Jr, Caushaj FP et al. Strictureplasty of the small bowel in patients with Crohn's disease. An effective surgical option. Arch Surg 1990;125:715–717.

112. Canin-Endres J, Salky B, Gattorno F, Edye M. Laparoscopically assisted intestinal resection in 88 patients with Crohn's disease. Surg Endosc 1999;13:595–599.

113. Wang Q, Hyde DM, Gotwals PJ, Giri SN. Effects of delayed treatment with transforming growth factor-β soluble receptor in a three-dose bleomycin model of lung fibrosis in hamsters. Exp Lung Res 2002;28:405–417.

114. Matsuoka H, Arai T, Mori M et al. A p38 MAPK inhibitor, FR-167653, ameliorates murine bleomycin-induced pulmonary fibrosis. Am J Physiol Lung Cell Mol Physiol 2002;283:L103–112.

115. Addrizzo-Harris DJ, Harkin TJ, Tchou-Wong KM et al. Mechanisms of colchicine effect in the treatment of asbestosis and idiopathic pulmonary fibrosis. Lung 2002;180:61–72.

116. Grotz W, von Zedtwitz I, Andre M, Schollmeyer P. Treatment of retroperitoneal fibrosis by mycophenolate mofetil and corticosteroids. Lancet 1998;352:1195.

117. Tsirigotis P, Venetis E, Rontogianni D, Dervenoulas J, Kontopidou F, Apostolidis P. Thalidomide in the treatment of myelodysplastic syndrome with fibrosis. Leuk Res 2002;26:965–966.

118. Corbel M, Lanchou J, Germain N, Malledant Y, Boichot E, Lagente V. Modulation of airway remodeling-associated mediators by the antifibrotic compound, pirfenidone, and the matrix metalloproteinase inhibitor, batimastat, during acute lung injury in mice. Eur J Pharmacol 2001;426:113–121.

119. Platten M, Wild-Bode C, Wick W, Leitlein J, Dichgans J, Weller M. N-[3,4-dimethoxycinnamoyl]-anthranilic acid (tranilast) inhibits transforming growth factor-β release and reduces migration and invasiveness of human malignant glioma cells. Int J Cancer 2001;93:53–61.

120. Bonner JC, Rice AB, Ingram JL et al. Susceptibility of cyclooxygenase-2-deficient mice to pulmonary fibrogenesis. Am J Pathol 2002;161:459–470.

121. Blobel CP. Remarkable roles of proteolysis on and beyond the cell surface. Curr Opin Cell Biol 2000;12:606–612.

122. McCawley LJ, Matrisian LM. Matrix metalloproteinases: they're not just for matrix anymore! Curr Opin Cell Biol 2001;13:534–540.

123. Lund PK, Zuniga C. Fibrosis in inflammatory bowel disease: animal models. Curr Concepts Gastroenterol 2001:318–323.

## CHAPTER 16

# Colorectal cancer in inflammatory bowel disease: molecular considerations

Steven H Itzkowitz

## INTRODUCTION

Colorectal cancer (CRC) develops from a dysplastic precursor lesion. This is true regardless of whether the cancer arises sporadically, in the setting of high-risk hereditary conditions such as familial adenomatous polyposis (FAP) and hereditary non-polyposis colorectal cancer (HNPCC), or in the setting of chronic inflammation such as inflammatory bowel diseases (IBD). Although the dysplastic lesion in most of these clinical settings is an adenomatous polyp, in IBD the premalignant histologic change is often flat dysplasia, rather than polypoid. Indeed, the uniqueness of the macroscopic appearance and biological behavior of dysplasia in IBD has stimulated a considerable amount of research into the natural history and molecular pathogenesis of CRC in patients with IBD. This chapter focuses on the molecular alterations that accompany CRC pathogenesis in IBD. Although none of the molecular alterations discussed has yet been integrated into clinical practice, examples are provided which highlight the potential for molecular diagnostics to one day enhance the management of patients with long-standing IBD. Most of our current understanding of the molecular alterations involved in colitis-associated carcinogenesis has come from studies of patients with ulcerative colitis (UC), not Crohn's disease (CD). Because Crohn's colitis carries essentially the same CRC risk as UC of similar disease duration and anatomic extent,[1] it is possible that the molecular changes discussed below will apply to both types of IBD, but formal testing of this hypothesis in patients with CD will be necessary.

## GENETIC CONTRIBUTION TO COLORECTAL CANCER

The genesis of CRC involves an interplay between genetic and environmental factors. Studies concerning the autosomal dom-

inant syndromes FAP and HNPCC have elucidated the important role of heredity. Inheritance of a mutated *adenomatous polyposis coli* (*APC*) gene causes FAP, whereas patients with HNPCC inherit a mutation in one of the genes responsible for DNA repair. In both circumstances, affected individuals demonstrate a very high genetic predisposition to colorectal and other cancers. Together, FAP and HNPCC account for fewer than 5% of all colorectal cancers. Another 25–30% of CRC cases are considered familial, occurring in individuals who have a family history of CRC but do not clearly fit into one of the hereditary syndromes.[2] Fully two-thirds of CRC cases, therefore, arise in individuals who have no demonstrable family history; these are considered sporadic CRC. To what extent genetics contributes to familial and sporadic CRC is not clear, but a variety of predisposing genetic polymorphisms have been suggested.[2]

Colon cancers arising in patients with IBD account for well under 1% of all CRC cases, but patients with IBD represent one of the highest risk groups for developing CRC. It is assumed that the increased risk of CRC in patients with IBD relates to the many years of colonic inflammation. This is certainly the most likely explanation, but how much of their predisposition might be genetic as opposed to environmental is not known. A potential role for hereditable factors is suggested by the observation that patients with IBD who have a family history of CRC have an approximate twofold greater risk of developing CRC than an IBD patient with no such family history.[3,4] A similar degree of familial risk for CRC has been observed in cotton-top tamarins – marmosets that develop CRC in a setting of chronic inflammation.[5] It is not yet clear which hereditable genes, if any, may contribute to increased CRC risk in IBD.

Environmental factors can modify colon cancer risk. For example, aspirin and non-steroidal anti-inflammatory drugs (NSAIDs) have been shown to decrease the risk of sporadic CRC[6] and rectal adenomatous polyps in patients with FAP.[7] Indeed, evidence is emerging that the use of the anti-inflammatory agent 5-aminosalicylic acid appears to lower the risk of CRC in IBD patients.[8] Although the mechanisms underlying the chemopreventative effect of anti-inflammatory agents remain to be elucidated, a partial explanation in the case of some NSAIDs relates to their inhibition of cyclooxygenase-2 (COX-2), a protein that is not expressed in normal colonic mucosa but is induced in premalignant and malignant lesions of the colon,[9] including those from IBD patients.[10] In a rat model of colon cancer, folate deficiency induced progressive DNA strand breaks within exons 5–8 of the *p53* gene (but did not affect the *APC* gene), and folate supplementation increased the steady-state levels of *p53* transcript.[11] Likewise, in a handful of UC patients who demonstrated microsatellite instability (MSI; see below) in non-neoplastic colonic mucosa, serum and colonic tissue folate levels tended to be lower than those without MSI, and in one patient folate supplementation for 6 months resulted in an altered pattern of some microsatellite markers.[12] Thus, it seems that environmental factors such as medications, diet and vitamins can interact with certain genes responsible for colon carcinogenesis, but research into gene–environment interaction is still in its infancy. Much more is known about the molecular genetic events involved in the development of colon carcinogenesis, as described in the sections that follow.

# MOLECULAR PATHWAYS OF SPORADIC COLON CARCINOGENESIS

To place the molecular pathogenesis of colitis-associated neoplasia in its proper perspective, it is first helpful to appreciate the molecular events involved in the development of sporadic colorectal neoplasia, which in many cases has drawn lessons from the molecular alterations that contribute to carcinogenesis in FAP and HNPCC patients.[13,14] CRC arises as a result of genomic instability. It is currently believed that there are two main types of genomic instability that contribute to colon carcinogenesis: chromosomal instability (CIN) and microsatellite instability (MSI) (Fig. 16.1). The vast majority (80–85%) of sporadic CRC appear to arise via the chromosomal instability pathway. This results in abnormal segregation of chromosomes and abnormal DNA content (aneuploidy). As a result, loss of chromosomal material (so-called loss of heterozygosity, or LOH) often occurs, and this contributes to the loss of function of key tumor suppressor genes such as *APC* and *p53*. Besides undergoing LOH, these genes can also be rendered non-functional by mutations of the genes themselves. In either event, it is the accumulation of molecular disturbances – mainly in tumor suppressor genes – that drives the sporadic adenoma-to-carcinoma progression, and therefore this pathway has sometimes been referred to as the 'suppressor pathway'. Colon cancers arising in patients with FAP tend to proceed via the suppressor pathway.

In the development of sporadic CRC, loss of *APC* function is typically an early event. Indeed, it is often considered the initiating event that allows subsequent molecular alterations to give rise to an adenoma (Fig. 16.2). For this reason, the *APC* gene has been termed the 'gatekeeper' of the colon. Some have argued that *APC* mutation may not be the universal initiating event, but may instead occur at somewhat later stages of adenoma progression.[15] However, *APC* may still contribute to the process of CIN.[16] Normally in the colonocyte, the APC protein forms a complex with other proteins in the cytoplasm, all of which act to phosphorylate β-catenin, a protein involved

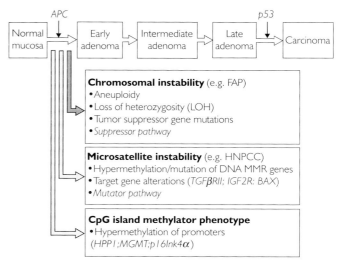

**Fig. 16.1** Schematic diagram of the major pathways of sporadic colon carcinogenesis.

in normal cell adhesion. Under normal physiological circumstances, the APC protein complex maintains the balance of β-catenin levels by phosphorylating β-catenin, a process that destines β-catenin for degradation in the cytoplasm, preventing it from entering the nucleus. If APC protein is mutated or lost, the protein complex that engages β-catenin does not function correctly, so β-catenin is not properly phosphorylated or degraded. This allows β-catenin to gain access to the cell nucleus, where it complexes with specific transcription factors to turn on genes which in turn contribute to adenoma formation by altering critical cellular functions, such as proliferation, apoptosis (programmed cell death) and cell–cell adhesion. Thus, nuclear β-catenin expression can be considered a surrogate indicator of abnormal APC function.

Once small adenomas form, some of them progress in size, villous histology and degree of dysplasia, and this is associated with conversion to malignancy. During this process other changes in genetic regulation occur, such as induction of *k-ras* oncogene and loss of function of tumor suppressor genes on chromosome 18q in the region of the *DCC* (*d*eleted in *c*olon *c*ancer) and *DPC4* genes. Loss of *p53* gene function occurs late, and is believed to be the defining event that drives the adenoma to carcinoma (Fig.16.2).

Tumors that arise via the CIN/tumor suppressor gene pathway are typically microsatellite stable (MSS). The remaining 15% of sporadic CRC arise through the MSI pathway (Fig. 16.1). This pathway also seems to explain the majority of CRC that occur in patients with HNPCC. The MSI pathway involves loss of function of genes that normally repair mismatches between DNA base pairs that occur during the normal process of DNA replication in dividing cells. Several DNA mismatch repair (MMR) genes cooperate to repair DNA base mismatches. Two of these, *hMLH1* and *hMSH2*, are most commonly affected by loss of function in CRC, but mutation or loss of other members of the DNA MMR system can also result in DNA replication errors throughout the genome, and this so-called replication error characteristic is what is detected as the MSI phenotype. In MSI colon cancers, instead of tumor suppressor genes such as *APC*, *p53* and candidate loci on chromosome 18q being lost, different genes are affected, notably

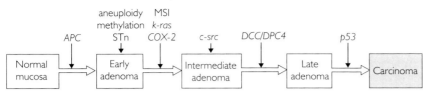

**Sporadic colon cancer**

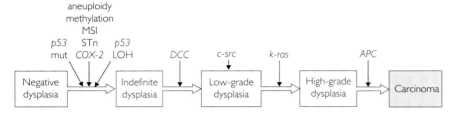

**Colitis-associated colon cancer**

Fig. 16.2 Comparison of molecular alterations in sporadic colon cancer and colitis-associated colon cancer.

*TGFβRII, IGF2R*, and *BAX*. These genes contain in their coding regions short nucleotide repeats which are intrinsically unstable and therefore prone to be copied incorrectly during DNA replication. The incorrect replica of these genes becomes the template strand for the next round of cell division, generating daughter cells with a permanent mutation in these genes. This pathway of colon carcinogenesis has been referred to as the 'mutator' pathway because of the many mutations in key genes involved in colonocyte homeostasis. Compared with MSS sporadic colon cancers, MSI sporadic colon cancers are more likely to be diploid (normal DNA content), located in the proximal colon, mucinous, poorly differentiated, show lymphocytic infiltration, and associated with a more favorable prognosis.[15]

The MSI phenotype is detected in tissues using a panel of markers that recognize microsatellite sequences in various parts of the genome. Soon after the discovery of MSI it became clear that some colon cancers manifest high degrees of MSI (termed MSI-H), whereas others demonstrate low levels of MSI (MSI-L). The MSI-H phenotype in HNPCC-associated CRC is usually caused by mutations of DNA MMR genes, whereas the same phenotype in sporadic CRC is usually due to hypermethylation of *hMLH1* gene promoter (see below). Because investigators had been using different microsatellite markers and applied different criteria to classify a tumor as MSI positive, an NIH consensus conference resolved that a panel of five standard markers should be employed.[17] The panel includes two mononucleotide (BAT25 and BAT26) and three dinucleotide (D5S346, D2S123, D17S250) markers. Cancers are classified as MSI-H if two or more markers are unstable, as MSI-L if only one marker is unstable, and as MSS if no marker demonstrates instability.

In addition to genetic events such as mutations or LOH of key genes, epigenetic alterations also contribute to altered gene expression in colon carcinogenesis. A recently recognized molecular alteration is the CpG island methylator phenotype (CIMP) (Fig. 16.1).[18] CpG islands are dense aggregates of cytosine–guanine dinucleotide sequences that may occur in the promoter region of genes. Extensive methylation of the cytosine bases is associated with promoter silencing and hence loss of gene expression. Many genes involved in cell cycle control, cell adhesion and DNA repair can be methylated in colon cancer (Table 16.1). So-called type A methylation, as for example the

### Table 16.1 Genes methylated in colorectal cancer

| Gene | Function |
|------|----------|
| hMLH1 | DNA mismatch repair |
| ER (estrogen receptor) | Growth and differentiation |
| p16INK4a | Cell cycle control |
| p14ARF | p53 regulation |
| HPP1/TPEF (hyperplastic polyposis protein) | apoptosis |
| MGMT (O-6-methylguanine-DNA methyltransferase) | DNA repair |
| APC | 'Gatekeeper' |
| COX-2 | Growth regulation |
| CDH1 (E-cadherin) | Cell adhesion |

Modified from Jass 2002.[15]

estrogen receptor (*ER*), occurs as a function of age, and is found in both normal colon and colon cancer. Type C methylation, however, is cancer associated, leading to pathogenic silencing of genes such as *hMLH1, MGMT, p16, p14* and *HPP1/TPEF.*

In general there is little overlap between CIN and MSI: tumors manifest either one phenotype or the other. However, there can be overlap between CIMP phenotype and MSI. For example, hypermethylation of *hMLH1* can produce the MSI-H cancer phenotype. By the same token, methylation of *MGMT* rather than *hMLH1* underlies MSI-L cancers.[15] The process of methylation is an area of intense investigation and it is anticipated that this line of research will help to further define the molecular pathways involved in CRC in a variety of clinical settings.

## GENOMIC INSTABILITY AND CLONAL EXPANSION IN IBD

Like sporadic CRC, colon carcinogenesis in IBD is a consequence of sequential episodes of somatic genetic mutation and clonal expansion. However, unlike sporadic colonic neoplasia, where only one or two dysplastic lesions arise in very focal areas of the colon, in colitic mucosa it is not unusual for dysplasia or cancer to be multifocal, reflecting a broader 'field change'. This is perhaps best exemplified by careful mapping studies that used DNA aneuploidy as a molecular marker to gain insights into temporal and topographical molecular changes in patients with UC. On the basis of DNA indices, individual cell populations were observed in the same locations of the colon on repeated examinations, and became more widely distributed over time, occupying larger areas of the mucosa.[19,20] Moreover, within an aneuploid area additional subclones of aneuploidy seemed to emerge from their predecessors.[19] Indeed, whereas only a handful of different aneuploid cell populations have been detected in aneuploid areas without dysplasia, up to 46 different aneuploid populations may be found in areas of aneuploidy that show dysplastic changes.[19] These observations highlight two crucial features of tumor development: genomic instability of increasingly dysregulated subclones of cells, and clonal expansion of mutant cell populations at the expense of the normal surrounding tissues. It is not known whether the re-epithelialization of large patches of colonic mucosa by abnormal clones is simply a consequence of the healing response to ulceration caused by chronic inflammation, or whether the epithelial cells of IBD patients have an innate ability to replace surrounding epithelium. Regardless, because aneuploidy is often more widespread than dysplasia, this indicates that substantial genomic alterations can occur in colonic mucosa without disturbing morphology. The fact that genetically abnormal cells have been observed in histologically non-dysplastic mucosa adjacent to or even remote from dysplasia suggests that the dysplastic cells arise from the pre-existing mutant clones.[19–21]

## ROLE OF CHRONIC INFLAMMATION IN IBD NEOPLASIA

The colonic mucosa of patients with IBD demonstrates enhanced epithelial cell turnover. Compared to normal colonic biopsies taken from patients with sporadic adenomas, mucosal biopsies from patients with UC demonstrate higher rates of mitosis and apoptosis, especially in areas of active, as opposed to quiescent, inflammation.[22] In addition, inflammation-associated genes such as cyclooxygenase-2,[10] nitric oxide synthase-2[23] and the interferon-inducible gene 1-8U[24] are increased not only in the inflamed mucosa of UC patients but also in their neoplastic tissues. Animal models suggest that inflammation predisposes to colorectal cancer. For example, dysplasia and cancer can be induced in healthy mice with colitis induced by repeated cycles[25,26] or even a single cycle[26] of dextran sulfate sodium (DSS). In this model, longer disease duration was associated with an increased rate of neoplasia, even in mice given the identical initial colitis insult and in the setting of clinical remission.[26] Similarly, dysplasia and adenocarcinoma occur in the chronic phase of T lymphocyte-mediated colitis in multiple knockout mice (see Chapter 9).

Because colitis-associated cancers arise in the setting of chronic inflammation, it is logical to assume that factors associated with inflammation, such as oxidative stress, contribute to the molecular alterations seen in IBD tissues. Support for this theory comes from a study showing a high frequency of *p53* mutations in inflamed tissue – more so than in uninflamed

tissues of UC patients.[23] This study also revealed that reactive oxygen species, which are common byproducts of inflammation, contributed to the *p53* mutations. Others have observed increased p53 expression in actively inflamed UC tissues compared to mucosa in histological remission, not only in patients with long-standing UC, but even in those with shorter disease duration.[22] Additional support for how inflammation might affect molecular pathways of colon carcinogenesis comes from in vitro studies demonstrating that oxidative stress can interfere with the function of the DNA mismatch repair enzymes, thereby contributing to the development of MSI.[27] Even in vivo, the induction of chronic inflammation by DSS results in more frequent development of LGD and HGD in *Msh2* knockout mice compared to wildtype controls, and colonic mucosa remote from dysplastic lesions in the DNA mismatch repair-deficient animals also demonstrates MSI.[28]

Thus, chronic inflammation appears to predispose to colon carcinogenesis, but it remains unknown which aspects of the inflammatory response are responsible for instigating neoplastic progression. Colonic dysplasia and adenocarcinoma develop in interleukin-10 (IL-10) knockout mice, suggesting that Th1 responses may be important.[29] In addition, $\beta_2$-microglobulin/IL-2 double knockout mice also develop colonic neoplasia, suggesting that a lack of MHC class I expression by the tumors allows them to escape detection by the host immune system.[30] Of relevance to human colitis-associated colon cancers is the fact that neoplastic lesions in both of these models develop only after 6–12 months of chronic colitis. The double knockout model demonstrates mutations in *APC* and *p53*, confirming the role of these important tumor suppressor genes in colon carcinogenesis.[31]

An intriguing observation in animal models of colitis-associated CRC is that bacterial flora appear to contribute to carcinogenesis. For example, TGF-$\beta$1-deficient mice on an immunodeficient background develop colon adenocarcinoma in association with inflammation.[32] When these mice are raised under germ-free conditions neoplasia does not develop, but when the animals are recolonized with enteric flora neoplasms occur in association with colitis, and *Helicobacter* species may contribute to the carcinogenesis process.[33] In this model, colitis is required but is not sufficient for cancer formation: a genetic predisposition to cancer appears to contribute. Whether the enteric bacteria directly affect carcinogenesis or induce inflammation which results in neoplastic events is unclear. These animal models highlight the complex interaction between genetic predisposition, inflammation and bacterial flora in colitis-associated neoplasia.

## MOLECULAR PATHWAYS OF COLITIS-ASSOCIATED COLON CARCINOGENESIS

To help decipher the molecular events involved in colitis-associated colon carcinogenesis, investigators have applied the lessons learned from studies of sporadic CRC. Perhaps not surprisingly, many of the molecular alterations that are responsible for sporadic CRC development also play a role in colitis-associated colon carcinogenesis (Table 16.2). In fact, the emerging evidence suggests that the two major pathways of CIN

## Table 16.2 Genetic alterations in colitis-associated and sporadic colorectal cancer

| | Colitis-associated CRC (%) | Sporadic CRC (%) | References |
|---|---|---|---|
| **CHROMOSOMAL INSTABILITY** | | | |
| Overall CIN | 85 | 85 | 34,45 |
| APC-related alterations: | | | |
| 5q loss | 56 | 26 | 45 |
| APC LOH | 0–33 | 31 | 61–63 |
| APC mutation | 6 | 74 | 36 |
| β-catenin LOH | 7 | 34 | 62 |
| p53-related alterations: | | | |
| 17p loss | 44 | 57 | 45 |
| P53 LOH | 47–85 | 50 | 39,63 |
| P53 mutation | 33–100 | 75–80 | 40,58,66 |
| Chromosome 18q genes: | | | |
| 18q loss | 78 | 69 | 45 |
| DCC LOH | 54 | 38 | 62 |
| DPC4 mutation | 0 (1 case) | – | 70 (69) |
| E-cadherin: | | | |
| LOH | 0 | 17 | 62 |
| Protein decrease | 43 | 37 | 95 |
| CDH1 methylation | 57 | 36 | 96 |
| | | | |
| **MICROSATELLITE INSTABILITY** | | | |
| Overall MSI-positive | 15–40 | 15–20 | 15,35,77,80,81 |
| MSI-H / MSI-L | 10/12 | – | 35 |
| MSI-H / MSI-L | 40/ 40 | – | 77 |
| MSI-H / MSI-L | 14/7 | – | 34 |
| MSI-H / MSI-L | 13/38 | – | 61 |
| MSI-H / MSI-L | 9/11 | – | 82 |
| MSI-H / MSI-L | 1/30 | – | 80 |
| MSI-H / MSI-L | 2/12 | – | 81 |
| HMLH1 methylation* | 46 | 76 | 82,86 |
| TGFbRII mutation* | 17 | 81 | 87 |
| | | | |
| **HYPERMETHYLATION** | | | |
| P16INK4a | 100 | 40 | 91 |
| P14ARF | 50 | 28–33 | 89,90,92 |
| HPP1 | 50 | 84 | 93,94 |

*in MSI tumors only.

and MSI also apply to colitis-associated CRC, and with roughly the same frequency (CIN 85%, MSI 15%).[34,35] However, as discussed in the following sections, the timing of these genomic alterations appears to differ between colitis-associated and sporadic neoplasms (Fig. 16.2). For example, loss of *APC* function, considered to be a very common early event in sporadic colon carcinogenesis, is much less frequent and usually occurs late in the colitis-associated dysplasia–carcinoma sequence.[36-38] Conversely, *p53* mutations in sporadic neoplasia usually occur late in the adenoma–carcinoma sequence, whereas in colitis patients *p53* mutations occur early and are often detected in mucosa that is non-dysplastic or indefinite for dysplasia.[39-42] Indeed, the fact that non-dysplastic mucosa from patients with UC demonstrates abnormalities in p53 and DNA mismatch repair function strongly suggests that genomic instability occurs quite early in carcinogenesis (see below).

The model presented in Figure 16.2 suggests that colitic mucosa progresses in a systematic fashion in the following way:

no dysplasia–indefinite dysplasia–low-grade dysplasia (LGD)–high-grade dysplasia (HGD)–carcinoma. This is a useful paradigm which facilitates the study of cancer risk markers in IBD and allows comparisons with the progression of molecular changes in sporadic colon neoplasia. However, it is important to realize that the natural history of dysplasia in IBD is often unpredictable. For example, LGD may progress to cancer without demonstrating HGD, and cancers can arise in colitic colons without any apparent prior dysplasia.[43,44] These caveats should be borne in mind when interpreting the results of studies describing the predictive value of dysplasia or molecular markers in IBD.

## CHROMOSOMAL INSTABILITY

Just as with sporadic CRC, chromosomal instability represents the major pathway by which cancers seem to arise in IBD patients. This pathway is marked by DNA aneuploidy, mutations and LOH of tumor suppressor genes, and activation of proto-oncogenes. The technique of comparative genomic hybridization demonstrates that a similar number of chromosomal alterations occur in UC-associated and sporadic CRC, and the frequency of losses and gains of various chromosomal arms is quite similar between the two types of neoplasm.[45] Using probes specific for chromosomes 8, 11, 17 and 18, studies employing fluorescent in situ hybridization noted that patients with UC who had a neoplasm (HGD or cancer) in their colon demonstrated abnormalities in these chromosomal arms, not only in the neoplastic lesions themselves, but even in non-dysplastic rectal mucosa remote from the neoplastic areas.[21] Normal mucosa from control subjects without UC, and non-dysplastic mucosa of UC patients who did not harbor a neoplasm in their colon, did not exhibit chromosomal instability. This observation was reinforced by studies in which DNA fingerprinting demonstrated substantial genomic instability in both the dysplastic as well as the non-dysplastic mucosa of UC patients harboring a neoplasm.[46] This instability, which was not present in organs outside the colon or in the colons of normal controls, remained at a steady state in precancerous and cancerous biopsies from the same patient, suggesting that genomic instability had reached the maximum level early in neoplastic progression. These findings suggest that widespread genomic instability occurs in patients with UC who develop colonic neoplasia, but not in patients with UC who have not yet developed neoplasia despite comparable disease duration. Thus, genomic instability may be a marker of cancer risk in UC.

A possible mechanism to explain the chromosomal instability associated with UC is telomere shortening. Telomeres are the protective ends of chromosomes that shorten with age and inflammation. Shorter telomeres become sticky, predisposing chromosomal ends to fuse together indiscriminately, forming bridges that subsequently cause the chromosomal arms to break.[46] Indeed, in biopsies of non-dysplastic mucosa from UC patients with dysplasia or cancer, chromosomal losses were greater and telomeres were shorter than in similar biopsies from UC patients without neoplasia or from non-UC controls.[47] Support for this comes from a limited study in which telomerase activity was detected in neoplastic as well as non-dysplastic colonic mucosa of UC patients.[48]

## ANEUPLOIDY

Diploidy refers to the normal complement of DNA in a cell. Aneuploidy, or abnormal DNA content, occurs as a consequence of chromosomal instability. Of all of the molecular markers in IBD colon carcinogenesis aneuploidy has been the most extensively studied, with observations dating back almost two decades. Usually measured by flow cytometry on fresh biopsies, aneuploidy occurs in approximately 14–33% of patients with long-standing UC,[20,49–51] and its presence has been associated with longer duration of colitis.[52,53] This molecular change correlates directly with histological dysplasia in that approximately 20–50% of dysplastic lesions and 50–90% of cancers will demonstrate aneuploidy.[39,50,53–56] Some studies suggest that aneuploidy is more frequent in HGD than in LGD lesions,[54,57] but others have not confirmed this finding.[39,52,58] Importantly, anywhere from 2 to 35% of histologically non-dysplastic mucosal biopsies already demonstrate aneuploidy.[39,50,52,53,55,56,58] Thus, aneuploidy is a relatively early event. Curiously, there are examples where

a diploid colon cancer occurs on a background of aneuploid mucosa.[52] Moreover, despite intensive repeated surveillance biopsies, colon cancers may arise without preceding dysplasia or aneuploidy.[59] Thus, although aneuploidy as a surrogate measure of CIN appears to be a useful marker of the high-risk colon, it may not be universally present nor required for progression to the malignant phenotype. This suggests that other pathways, such as MSI, also contribute.

## LOSS OF TUMOR SUPPRESSOR GENES

Tumor suppressor genes are normal cellular genes that control cell proliferation, death and differentiation. Loss of function of both copies of tumor suppressor genes impairs their function and predisposes to cancer. Inactivation occurs typically by two separate mechanisms: allelic deletion (LOH) of one allele, and mutation of the other. New insights suggest that promoter hypermethylation is another important mechanism of gene inactivation. The classic tumor suppressor genes *APC*, *p53* and *DCC/DPC4*, which are important for sporadic colon carcinogenesis, have also been implicated in colitis-associated CRC.

### *APC* tumor suppressor gene

Unlike sporadic colon carcinogenesis, where *APC* mutations are common and early events, in UC neoplasms *APC* mutations are rare and occur late in the dysplasia–carcinoma progression (Fig. 16.2). Mutations in *APC* are rarely if ever encountered in colitic mucosa that is negative or indefinite for dysplasia,[37] and fewer than 14% of tissues manifesting LGD harbor *APC* mutations.[37,60] Indeed, fewer than 14% of UC cancers demonstrate *APC* mutations.[37,38,61] The frequency of *APC* mutations in HGD lesions has been reported to be as high as 50–100%,[37,60] but this is based on very few cases. With respect to allelic deletion of *APC*, two studies observed a 33% rate of *APC* LOH,[62,63] whereas a third study found no *APC* LOH.[61] Because LOH and mutational analyses are often considered rather accurate for assessing genetic alterations in cancer, the literature to date suggests that *APC* gene aberrations in UC neoplasia are rare. It is worth noting, however, that the APC protein was reported to be abnormally expressed in 76% of UC cancers by immunohistochemistry.[64]

### *p53* tumor suppressor gene

Mutations of the *p53* gene occur in about 50% of all human cancers. The normal p53 protein, considered an important guardian of the genome, is thought to prevent clonal expansion of mutant cells by preventing cells that have acquired damaged DNA from progressing through the cell cycle. Allelic deletion of *p53* occurs in approximately 47–85% of UC-associated CRC (see Table 16.2).[39,42,63] Burmer et al.[39] found that *p53* LOH correlated with malignant progression, finding this molecular change in 6% of biopsies without dysplasia, 9% with indefinite dysplasia, 33% with LGD, 63% with HGD and 85% with cancer. They also noted that *p53* LOH was restricted to biopsies that were aneuploid, suggesting that aneuploidy precedes *p53* LOH. Further studies from these investigators indicated that *p53* mutations were distributed more extensively than *p53* LOH in carefully mapped colectomy specimens, and that mutation but not LOH of *p53* was found in diploid, non-dysplastic mucosa, suggesting that *p53* mutation was an early molecular change that occurred prior to aneuploidy, which in turn preceded *p53* LOH[40]

(Fig. 16.2). Other investigators found a more variable association between *p53* mutation and aneuploidy, but confirmed that *p53* mutations occurred in 19% of biopsies without dysplasia, with a steady increase in frequency among biopsies that showed progressive degrees of dysplasia.[58] In fact, using tissues from UC patients who did not have cancer, Hussain et al.[23] demonstrated a high frequency of *p53* mutations in inflamed mucosa, suggesting that chronic inflammation itself may predispose to these early mutations. Additional evidence from immunohistochemical studies links altered p53 expression with dysplasia in UC; with this technique, biopsies that are negative for dysplasia do not often demonstrate p53 staining.[41,65–67] Thus, considerable evidence implicates p53 as playing an instrumental role in UC carcinogenesis, and apparently at an earlier stage than in sporadic cancer.

## Tumor suppressor genes on 18q (*DCC/DPC4*)

Allelic losses of 18q, in particular 18q21.1, are common in both sporadic and colitis-associated CRC. Allelic loss of 18q has been reported to occur in 78% of UC-associated CRC compared to 69% of sporadic CRC (see Table 16.2).[45] Moreover, 3/5 (60%) dysplastic lesions and 1/5 (20%) non-dysplastic samples manifested 18q allelic deletion.[68] A similar trend, but with lower rates of 18q loss, has been reported by others.[29] Candidate tumor suppressor genes that reside in this location include *DCC* and *DPC4*. LOH at *DCC* has been reported to occur in 54% of colitis-associated CRC compared to 38% of sporadic CRC.[62] One study of 10 colitis-associated CRC found 18q LOH in three cases, one of which also demonstrated mutation in *DPC4*.[69] Others were unable to detect any DPC4 mutations among 10 colitis-associated CRC.[70]

## ACTIVATION OF PROTO-ONCOGENES

Proto-oncogenes are normal cellular genes which, when activated by mutation of one allele, can disrupt normal cell growth and differentiation and enhance the progression to neoplastic transformation. With regard to colitis-associated CRC, two proto-oncogenes have received the most attention: *K-ras* and *c-src*.

### *K-ras* oncogene

Mutations of the *k-ras* oncogene result in a permanently activated gene product that enhances cell proliferation and alters differentiation pathways. *K-ras* mutations typically are not found in UC mucosa that is negative for dysplasia. In fact, most studies also indicate that *k-ras* mutations are rare even in LGD,[58,61,71–73] although one study using a highly sensitive assay detected *k-ras* mutations in 36% and 14% of lesions that were indefinite for dysplasia and LGD, respectively.[37] When *k-ras* mutations occur, they tend to be found in HGD or cancerous lesions. Early studies suggested that the 8–24% frequency of *k-ras* mutations in UC cancers was lower than the approximate 40–50% rate in sporadic CRC,[61,66,71–73] but more recent studies suggest that 40–50% of UC-associated CRC demonstrate *k-ras* mutations.[37,58,60,74]

### *Src* oncogene

The cellular oncogene *c-src* is a tyrosine kinase that is associated with malignant transformation in a variety of tumors. Elevated *c-src* levels have been reported in sporadic colon adenomas and carcinomas.[75] In UC patients *c-src* activity was low in areas of inflammation but demonstrated a progressive increase in activity in LGD, HGD, DALM and cancer lesions.[76]

## MICROSATELLITE INSTABILITY

Microsatellite instability is not found in normal colonic mucosa from healthy controls or from patients with other types of benign inflammatory colitis.[77,78] It is also quite rare in colonic mucosa from patients with Crohn's colitis.[79] However, as many as 15–40% of patients with UC demonstrate MSI in cancer tissues (see Table 16.2). In some studies UC-associated cancers were more likely to express MSI-L than MSI-H,[61,80,81] but other studies indicate that the two types of instability can occur with similar frequency.[34,35,77,82] Some of this difference may relate to the fact that not all studies applied the NIH consensus microsatellite marker panel. Curiously, MSI has been detected as an early event, occurring in non-dysplastic mucosa even from patients with disease of rather short duration.[77,78] The DNA mismatch repair system is important for repairing frameshift mutations that can be induced by the oxidative stress that accompanies chronic inflammation. Cells that are deficient in MMR, and even cells that are MMR proficient, accumulate frameshift mutations, suggesting that oxidative stress acts as a mutagen.[83] Also, oxidative stress can functionally impair the protein components of the MMR system without necessarily causing genetic mutations.[27] This may contribute to the MSI-L phenotype seen in both non-neoplastic and neoplastic mucosa of IBD patients. A germline *hMSH2* mutation was reported to be more frequent in UC patients who developed HGD and cancer than in those who did not,[84] but this finding was not substantiated by other investigators.[85] In sporadic CRC hypermethylation of *hMLH1* is an important mechanism for silencing the function of this gene, resulting in MSI-H tumors.[15,86] Likewise, in UC-associated neoplasms hypermethylation of *hMLH1* was detected in almost half of MSI-H cancers and dysplasias.[82]

## IMPAIRMENT OF *TGFβRII*

Responsiveness to TGF-β1 is important for maintaining normal colonocyte growth and differentiation. Consequently, mutations of the TGF-β1 receptor permit colonic cells to escape growth control. The type II TGF-β1 receptor (TGFβRII) has two microsatellites within its coding region that predispose this gene to replication errors in cells which have abnormal DNA mismatch repair. Thus, as a target gene for MSI, TGFβRII instability has been demonstrated in as many as 81% of MSI sporadic CRC.[87] By contrast, among 18 UC neoplasms that demonstrated MSI, only three (17%) demonstrated instability of TGFβRII,[87] indicating that this same phenomenon occurs in colitis-associated colon carcinogenesis but with a lesser frequency.

## PROMOTER METHYLATION

Methylation is being increasingly recognized as an important mechanism contributing to the genetic alterations in colitis-associated CRC (Fig. 16.2, Table 16.2). Indeed, methylation of CpG islands in several genes seems to precede dysplasia and is more widespread throughout the mucosa.[88] In colitis-associated neoplasms *hMLH1* hypermethylation was observed in 6/13 (46%) MSI-H, 1/6 (16%) MSI-L and 4/27 (15%) MSS specimens, implicating this epigenetic change as a cause of microsatellite instability.[82] The cell cycle inhibitor $p16^{INK4\alpha}$, loss of which has been implicated in sporadic CRC,[89,90] is commonly hypermethylated in UC neoplasms.[91] Approximately 10% of biopsies without dysplasia already demonstrate *p16* promoter hypermethylation, the rate increasing with higher grades of dysplasia and reaching 100% in cancer specimens. Curiously, almost all specimens with *p16* promoter hypermethylation are also aneuploid. *p14^ARF* is an indirect regulator of p53 and resides at the same locus as *p16^INK4α*. Loss of *p14^ARF* function by promoter hypermethylation has been reported in 50% of adenocarcinomas, 33% of dysplastic lesions, and even in 60% of non-dysplastic mucosal samples in patients with UC.[92] Another gene, *HPP1*, recently implicated in the hyperplastic polyp–serrated adenoma–carcinoma pathway of colorectal cancer,[93] undergoes methylation silencing in 50% and 40% of colitis-associated cancers and dysplasias, respectively.[94] The significance of this latter observation remains to be elucidated.

E-cadherin (*CDH1*), a member of the calcium-dependent cell adhesion molecule family, plays an important role in cell–cell contacts, thereby functioning as a tumor suppressor gene. Loss of E-cadherin function has been implicated in various cancers, including diffuse gastric cancer, breast cancer and prostate cancer. Loss of E-cadherin expression has been reported in approximately 57% of colitis-associated CRC, as a result of hypermethylation of the E-cadherin promoter rather than allelic loss.[95,96] In fact, *CDH1* promoter hypermethylation was detected in 13/14 (93%) colonoscopies where dysplasia was present, compared to only 1/17 (6%) of colonoscopies without detectable dysplasia, and it is typically the dysplastic lesion itself that manifests reduced E-cadherin protein expression.[97] Methylation of *CDH1* was seen in 75% of aneuploid tissue samples compared to 26% of diploid samples.[97]

## OTHER PHENOTYPIC MARKERS IN IBD NEOPLASMS

### MUCINS

Changes in mucin glycoproteins in patients with IBD have been observed in studies dating back more than two decades. These studies used primarily histochemical or immunohistochemical methods to analyze glycoconjugates, and as such the changes described represent post-translational modifications rather than genetic mutations. None the less, one repeated observation was that upon neoplastic transformation colonic mucosa from patients with UC frequently demonstrated a conversion from predominantly sulfomucin to sialomucin.[98] In some cases sialomucin expression was detected several years before the advanced dysplasia.[59,99] Others noted an increase in sialomucin expression as well as in binding of peanut agglutinin, a lectin that recognizes a cancer-associated carbohydrate antigen, in dysplastic mucosa of UC patients, but similar changes were also noted in non-dysplastic, actively inflamed tissues.[100] Using a combination of lectins to stain rectal biopsies, another study reported that dysplasia developed over a 4-year follow-up period in six of 13 patients who initially manifested abnormal lectin-binding patterns, but in only one of five patients with normal lectin binding.[101]

More detailed studies have been performed using a monoclonal antibody that recognizes a particular sialomucin epitope, sialyl-Tn (STn) antigen. This disaccharide antigen resides on mucin glycoproteins, but the functional significance of this epitope is not yet known. STn is found only rarely in normal colonic mucosa, but it is expressed in half of sporadic adenocarcinomas.[102] In sporadic CRC STn is expressed in the tumors of 85–90% of patients and is associated with a poor prognosis.[103] Expression of STn has been evaluated in UC tissues both at a single point in time and chronologically. In UC, STn was expressed in 49% of tissue samples taken from cancer-bearing colons compared to only 13% in cancer-free colons.[104] As shown in Figure 16.3, STn antigen can be detected rather diffusely throughout the colon, even in biopsies that do not demonstrate dysplasia.[105] In addition, STn expression was independent of aneuploidy.[106] Furthermore, in many instances STn antigen was detected several years before the initial finding of dysplasia. In two case–control studies, patients who underwent colectomy for cancer or dysplasia had considerably more STn expression in their prior serial colonoscopic biopsies than those who did not progress to dysplasia, despite comparable durations of colitis and intensity of surveillance.[105,106] STn expression was occasionally found in patients who never manifested dysplasia, but its expression was weak, limited to only one to two biopsies per colonoscopy, and was usually not sustained over time.

## POTENTIAL CLINICAL APPLICATION OF MOLECULAR MARKERS

### MARKERS OF CANCER PROGRESSION

So far, histologic evidence of dysplasia on colonic biopsies is the gold-standard marker for determining cancer risk and deciding upon clinical management. However, there are many limitations of dysplasia, such as variations in pathological interpretation (particularly in the setting of active inflammation), the focality of dysplasia making random biopsy detection often difficult, and the fact that cancers can arise without any apparent preceding detectable dysplasia. This has raised the question of whether newer molecular markers could be complementary to dysplasia for assigning cancer risk. The studies defining molecular alterations that accompany colitis-associated colon carcinogenesis are not only important for helping to understand how these neoplasms arise, but they also provide an opportunity to learn whether these same molecular changes might be useful clinical markers of colon cancer progression.

To date, most of our knowledge about the types of molecular alterations in colitis-associated neoplasia has come from studies that took a particular marker of interest and analyzed its expression in pathological lesions at a single time point from several patients, representing the pathological spectrum of no dysplasia, indefinite dysplasia, LGD, HGD and cancer. In this type of horizontal, cross-sectional study design, any particular genetic alteration that demonstrates a preferential or increased expression in neoplastic (dysplasia and/or cancer) tissues is considered potentially useful, and might be thought of as a marker of cancer progression. Many such markers have been evaluated in this way, as listed in Table 16.2.

This type of horizontal, one-time analysis is important for several reasons. First, it establishes whether a given marker correlates with dysplasia, and if so, at what stage in the dysplasia–carcinoma sequence it is associated. Second, it is the most feasible type of study design and therefore readily accomplished. Third, it provides an assessment of the anatomical distribution of the marker compared to dysplasia (which is often focal in nature). Often in these studies, when a marker is expressed in non-dysplastic tissue from a patient who also has

**A**

| | CE | AC | HF | TR | SF | DC | SIG | RECT |
|---|---|---|---|---|---|---|---|---|
| CASE | | | | | | | | |
| Colectomy: | | | HGD | LGD | | | | |
| 1989 | ++ | + | +++ (LGD) | +++ | +++ | ++ | | +++ |
| 1984 | ++ | +++ | | +++ | +++ | +++ | +++ | +++ |
| 1983 | ++ | | ++ | +++ | +++ | +++ | +++ | ++ |
| Control: | | | | | | | | |
| 1993 | – | – | – | – | – | +++ | – | – |
| 1990 | – | – | – | – | – | ++ | – | – |
| 1987 | – | | – | | | – | + | – |
| 1985 | – | – | – | | – | + | – | – |

**B**

| | CE | AC | HF | TR | SF | DC | SIG | RECT |
|---|---|---|---|---|---|---|---|---|
| CASE | | | | | | | | |
| Colectomy: | | | | HGD | HGD | HGD | | HGD |
| 1990 | – | – | – | – | – | + | + | +++ |
| 1987 | – | – | – | – | – | – | – | |
| 1986 | – | – | – | – | – | +++ | +++ | +++ |
| 1984 | – | – | – | – | – | – | – | +++ |
| 1983 | – | – | – | – | | | | |
| 1981 | – | – | ++ | – | | | | |
| Control: | | | | | | | | |
| 1991 | – | – | – | – | – | – | – | – |
| 1989 | – | – | – | – | – | – | + | + |
| 1984 | – | – | – | – | – | ++ | ++ | ++ |
| 1982 | – | – | – | – | – | – | – | – |
| 1979 | – | | – | – | | – | – | – |

Fig. 16.3 Example of how a molecular marker can be applied to clinical specimens. Shown is the expression of STn mucin-associated antigen in serial colonoscopic biopsies. STn expression is indicated as strong (+++), moderate (++), weak (+) or absent (–). Biopsies were examined from the cecum (CE), ascending colon (AC), hepatic flexure (HF), transverse colon (TR), splenic flexure (SF), descending colon (DC), sigmoid (SIG) and rectum (RECT). 'Cases' represent individuals who underwent colectomy because of dysplasia or a suspicion of cancer. 'Controls', who did not manifest dysplasia and did not undergo colectomy, were matched to each case on the basis of comparable disease duration and intensity of surveillance. (A) The case developed LGD of the hepatic flexure which prompted colectomy, revealing HGD and LGD in the hepatic flexure and transverse colon, respectively. The case demonstrated strong expression of STn in essentially every surveillance biopsy for several years prior to the detection of dysplasia. The control had minimal STn expression in only an occasional biopsy. (B) The case developed a tubulovillous adenoma of the rectum in 1990, prompting colectomy. Multifocal HGD was detected in the colectomy specimen. In hindsight, the rectal mucosa had demonstrated strong STn expression for 7 years prior to the detection of the adenoma. The control had some STn expression on one colonoscopy which disappeared on subsequent examinations. (Modified from Itzkowitz et al. Gastroenterology 1996;110:694–704.)

dysplasia or cancer elsewhere in the colon, the marker is considered to be expressed 'earlier' than dysplasia. Although this concept may be plausible, it is not biologically or clinically accurate to assign a chronological sequence to marker expression when the tissue derives from one time point (see next section).

## MOLECULAR MARKERS OF FUTURE CANCER RISK

An advantage to studying patients with IBD is that they typically undergo periodic surveillance colonoscopies with repeated tissue sampling. In colon cancer research, IBD is essentially the only clinical setting in which multiple repetitive sampling of colonic tissue is routinely performed, and provides a unique opportunity to study histological and molecular changes chronologically. A marker that correlates with subsequent development of dysplasia or cancer can be thought of as a marker of cancer risk. To date, few studies describing a promising new marker in IBD tissues have tested the marker in using a chronological study design. The reasons for this are multifactorial, but include difficulty in obtaining these tissues (which are often more plentiful in tertiary referral centers), interest of the investigator to study the marker chronologically, and definition of what a 'marker-positive' patient is. The latter issue is not trivial. Does one classify a patient as high risk if only one biopsy from one colonoscopy is positive? Do we insist that more than one biopsy from a given colonoscopy be marker positive? Should we require more than one colonoscopy to be 'marker positive', and if so, do they have to be consecutive examinations? The answers to these questions are not readily apparent from the existing literature.

To date, only three molecular markers, aneuploidy, p53, and the mucin-associated sialyl-Tn antigen, have been evaluated in a chronological context, and each has been demonstrated to be a harbinger of subsequent risk of developing dysplasia or cancer. Longitudinal, prospective studies have demonstrated that aneuploidy is a marker of subsequent progression to neoplasia in patients with long-standing UC who have not yet demonstrated dysplasia. Among 25 high-risk UC patients without dysplasia, all five who showed aneuploidy progressed to dysplasia within 1–2.5 years, whereas 19/20 (95%) without aneuploidy did not progress to either dysplasia or aneuploidy over a 2–9-year period.[19] Likewise, among 34 UC patients without dysplasia, 3/4 (75%) with aneuploidy progressed to LGD, whereas only 2/30 (7%) without aneuploidy progressed to LGD over a 10-year period.[49] These and other studies indicate that when aneuploidy is detected it is usually found either before or at the same time as dysplasia.[19,20,49,51] In the largest study with the longest follow-up, all of the 10 patients who developed HGD or cancer had aneuploidy detected either before or simultaneously with these histologically more advanced neoplastic lesions, whereas five of 12 (42%) patients with LGD had aneuploidy detected after LGD.[51] Aneuploidy following dysplasia has also been reported by others.[20] Thus, it appears that finding aneuploidy may be a useful marker of cancer risk, but not finding it does not offer reassurance.

Sialyl-Tn antigen expression has been studied in both cross-sectional and longitudinal study designs, and it fulfills the criteria of being both more widespread and chronologically earlier than dysplasia (Fig. 16.3).[105,106] In fact, STn expression was noted as early as 2–9 years before the first detection of dysplasia. Importantly, STn expression does not just overlap with dysplasia, but is complementary to it. Moreover, STn expression is also independent of aneuploidy, thereby adding information beyond what dysplasia or aneuploidy provide.[106]

Little is known about whether p53 expression in surveillance biopsies predicts the future development of dysplasia or cancer. One study suggested that abnormal p53 immunostaining may precede LGD, HGD and cancer by 8 months, 26 months and 38 months, respectively.[107] Other reports in a handful of patients also suggest that p53 expression may precede cancer by 2–4 years.[108,109]

Another study retrospectively analyzed biopsy specimens for MSI and k-ras mutations prior to surgical resection.[80] The presence of MSI in the biopsies did not predict the presence of MSI in the resection specimens. There were three cases in which k-ras mutations were detected in dysplastic presurgical biopsies, and two of them demonstrated the identical mutation in the resection specimen.

There is no consensus as to how, or even whether, these markers of cancer risk should be incorporated into clinical management of patients with long-standing IBD. In part, this field suffers from the same dilemmas as prognostic marker research in other areas of cancer research. For example, what does it take for a prognostic marker to become accepted for use in clinical practice? Do we insist on a prospective randomized controlled trial? More than one? Would data from one or more good retrospective case–control studies suffice? Given our current knowledge, no-one is likely to recommend colectomy to a patient solely on the basis of marker positivity without some evidence of dysplasia, even if the patient's tissue demonstrated marker positivity on several colonoscopies. Perhaps more intensive surveillance should be offered to such patients. These issues should be considered as more research is conducted in this field.

## THE PROBLEM OF POLYPOID DYSPLASIA IN IBD

One dilemma that plagues clinicians is the finding of dysplasia in a polypoid lesion of a patient with long-standing IBD. If the lesion is considered a sporadic adenoma, it can be removed endoscopically and the patient continued under surveillance. However, if it is a more ominous dysplasia-associated lesion or mass (DALM), this usually prompts a recommendation for total proctocolectomy because of the very high synchronous and metachronous rate of CRC. The difficulty is that histology alone cannot distinguish between these two types of dysplastic lesions, and even clinical considerations such as patient age or duration of colitis offer little help. Two recent studies have suggested that if the polypoid lesion can be confidently removed in its entirety by endoscopic polypectomy, and if numerous biopsies of mucosa adjacent to the polyp base and throughout the rest of colon are negative for dysplasia, the polypectomy alone may be sufficient, and colectomy can be deferred while the patient continues to undergo surveillance.[110,111]

Apparent 'sporadic adenomas' in UC patients differ somewhat from more ominous polypoid dysplastic lesions (DALM) in that the adenomas tend to occur in somewhat older patients who have shorter disease duration and less frequent pancolitis (Table 16.3). Moreover, the sporadic adenomas in UC patients are more likely to be simple tubular adenomas and are less likely

to demonstrate HGD or cancer than are polypoid dysplastic lesions. It would be helpful if molecular markers could help distinguish between a sporadic adenoma and a polypoid dysplastic lesion in a UC patient. As shown in Table 16.3, LOH for certain genetic loci are somewhat more common in PDL/DALM than in sporadic adenomas from either UC patients or those without UC.[112] Unfortunately, although these studies suggest a difference between sporadic adenomas and PDL, none of these markers, alone or in combination, has high enough sensitivity or specificity to be clinically practical. A more promising approach might be to study global gene expression profiles using cDNA microarray technology. Indeed, this has been performed in the context of using an artificial neural network to interpret the results.[113] It appears that once the network is trained to recognize patterns of gene expression between the two types of dysplastic lesions on a training set, it was able to distinguish between sporadic adenomas and colitis-associated neoplasms on a validation set. This technology therefore holds great promise for the future of molecular diagnostics in IBD.

## NEW MOLECULAR SCREENING APPROACHES

Most efforts to date have understandably focused on studying tissues from IBD patients to identify molecular markers that might be helpful for understanding cancer pathogenesis or possibly assigning risk. Given the limitations of finding and interpreting dysplasia as a tissue marker, additional studies using IBD tissues are important and should continue to be pursued. At the same time, it is worth considering alternative approaches to identifying cancer risk in this disease.

One approach is single-nucleotide polymorphism (SNP) analysis. Performed on DNA from peripheral blood leukocytes, this technique can detect subtle germline alterations in key genes that might be implicated in the carcinogenesis process. A preliminary report suggests that a polymorphism in human *disheveled 1* gene, a member of the β-catenin signaling pathway, may correlate with dysplasia risk in UC.[114] Using DNA extracted from serum, k-ras mutations have been detected in two of four patients with UC but not in any of three patients with Crohn's disease or in healthy controls.[115]

Another approach worth considering is to examine the stool of patients with IBD for molecular alterations. This technology, which uses markers associated with the more common molecular alterations associated with CIN, MSI and abnormal apoptosis, has already been shown to have reasonable sensitivity and rather high specificity for sporadic CRC and adenomas.[116] As the DNA shed into stool should theoretically provide a more comprehensive sampling of abnormal cells than random pinch biopsies, stool DNA testing could significantly contribute to the management of patients with long-standing IBD who are at risk for developing CRC.

Molecular markers have also been studied in colonic lavage fluid taken at the time of colonoscopy. One such study analyzed p53 and k-ras mutations in colonic effluent and noted mutations in either gene in up to 19% of UC patients, particularly those with longer disease duration.[117] In addition, 15% of patients with Crohn's colitis, but not ileitis, had a positive mutation. Mutations were also found in 2% of non-inflammatory controls

**Table 16.3 Features of sporadic adenomas versus DALM in UC**

| Feature | CUC polypoid dysplacia (DALM) | CUC 'sporadic' adenoma | Non-CUC sporadic adenoma |
|---|---|---|---|
| **Clinical setting** | | | |
| Age | 53 | 60 | 66 |
| Duration >10 years | 60% | 29% | NA |
| Pancolitis | 100% | 24% | NA |
| | | | |
| **Histology** | | | |
| Lesion manifests HGD | 63% | 38% | 30% |
| Lesion manifests CA | 63% | 0 | 9% |
| Tubular | 45% | 81% | 87% |
| Tubulovillous | 55% | 19% | 9% |
| Villous | 0 | 0 | 4% |
| | | | |
| **Molecular markers** | | | |
| LOH for APC (5q) | 43% | 33% | 33% |
| LOH for VHL (3p) | 50% | 28% | 5% |
| LOH for p16 (9p) | 56% | 5% | 4% |

Modified from Odze. Am J Surg Pathol 2000;24:1209–1216.
NA – not applicable

and in only 50% of sporadic colon cancer patients. In several patients the molecular alteration could not be confirmed on subsequent lavage samples, and only one patient who repeatedly had a *p53* mutation in the fluid had the same mutation discovered in biopsy tissues. The appealing concept behind stool- or lavage-based molecular diagnostics is the potential to sample a much larger surface area of the colon than the multiple random pinch biopsies currently performed. As this technology becomes further developed and newer, more specific molecular markers become available, this approach may assume greater importance.

# REFERENCES

1. Sachar DB. Cancer in Crohn's disease: dispelling the myths. Gut 1994;35:1507–1508.
2. Burt RW. Colon cancer screening. Gastroenterology 2000;119:837–853.
3. Askling J, Dickman PW, Karlen P et al. Family history as a risk factor for colorectal cancer in inflammatory bowel disease. Gastroenterology 2001;120:1356–1362.
4. Nuako KW, Ahlquist DA, Mahoney DW et al. Familial predisposition for colorectal cancer in chronic ulcerative colitis: a case–control study. Gastroenterology 1998;115;1079–1983.
5. Bertone ER, Giovannucci EL, King NW Jr et al. Family history as a risk factor for ulcerative colitis-associated colon cancer in cotton-top tamarin. Gastroenterology 1998;114:669–674.
6. Janne PA, Mayer RJ. Chemoprevention of colorectal cancer. N Engl J Med 2000;342:1960–1968.
7. Cruz-Correa M, Hylind LM, Romans KE et al. Long-term treatment with sulindac in familial adenomatous polyposis: a prospective cohort study. Gastroenterology. 2002;122:641–645.
8. Itzkowitz SH. Cancer prevention in patients with inflammatory bowel disease. Gastroenterol Clin North Am 2002;31:1133–1144.
9. Gupta RA, DuBois RN, Wallace MC. New avenues for the prevention of colorectal cancer: targeting cyclo-oxygenase-2 activity. Best Practice Res Clin Gastroenterol 2002;16:945–956.
10. Agoff SN, Brentnall TA, Crispin DA et al. The role of cyclooxygenase 2 in ulcerative colitis-associated neoplasia. Am J Pathol 2000;157:737–745.
11. Kim YI, Shirwadkar S, Choi SW et al. Effects of dietary folate on DNA strand breaks within mutation-prone exons of the p53 gene in rat colon. Gastroenterology 2000;119:151–161.
12. Cravo ML, Albuquerque CM, de Sousa S et al. Microsatellite instability in non-neoplastic mucosa of patients with ulcerative colitis: effect of folate supplementation. Am J Gastroenterol 1998;93:2060–2064.
13. Chung DC. The genetic basis of colorectal cancer: Insights into critical pathways of tumorigenesis. Gastroenterology 2000;119:854–865.
14. Calvert PM, Frucht H. The genetics of colorectal cancer. Ann Intern Med 2002;137;603–612.
15. Jass JR, Whitehall VLJ, Young J et al. Emerging concepts in colorectal neoplasia. Gastroenterology 2002;123:862–876, 3370–3374.
16. Fodde R, Kuipers J, Rosenberg C et al. Mutations in the APC tumor suppressor gene cause chromosomal instability. Nature Cell Biol 2001;3:433–438.
17. Boland CR, Thibodeau SN, Hamilton SR et al. A National Cancer Institute Workshop on microsatellite instability for cancer detection and familial predisposition: development of international criteria for the determination of microsatellite instability in colorectal cancer. Cancer Res 1998;58:5248–5257.
18. Ahuja N, Mohan AL, Li Q et al. Association between CpG island methylation and microsatellite instability in colorectal cancer. Cancer Res 1997;57:3370–3374
19. Rubin CE, Haggitt RC, Burmer GC et al. DNA aneuploidy in colonic biopsies predicts future development of dysplasia in ulcerative colitis. Gastroenterology 1992;103:1611–1620.
20. Lofberg R, Brostrom O, Karlen P et al. DNA aneuploidy in ulcerative colitis: reproducibility, topographic distribution, and relation to dysplasia. Gastroenterology 1992;102:1149–1154.
21. Rabinovitch PS, Dziadon S, Brentnall TA et al. Pancolonic chromosomal instability precedes dysplasia and cancer in ulcerative colitis. Cancer Res 1999;59:5148–5153.
22. Arai N, Mitomi H, Ohtani Y et al. Enhanced epithelial cell turnover associated with p53 accumulation and high p21WAF1/CIP1 expression in ulcerative colitis. Mod Pathol 1999;12:604–611.
23. Hussain SP, Amstad P, Raja K et al. Increased p53 mutation load in noncancerous colon tissue from ulcerative colitis: a cancer-prone chronic inflammatory bowel disease. Cancer Res 2000;60:3333–3337.
24. Hisamatsu T, Watanabe M, Ogata H et al. Interferon-inducible gene family 1-8U expression in colitis-associated colon cancer and severely inflamed mucosa in ulcerative colitis. Cancer Res 1999;59:5927–5931.
25. Okayasu I, Yamada M, Mikami T et al. Dysplasia and carcinoma development in experimental colitis. J Gastroenterol Hepatol 2002;17:1078–1083.
26. Cooper HS, Murthy S, Kido K et al. Dysplasia and cancer in the dextran sulfate sodium mouse colitis model. Relevance to colitis-associated neoplasia in the human. Carcinogenesis 2000;21:757–768.
27. Chang CL, Marra G, Chauhan DP et al. Oxidative stress inactivates the human DNA mismatch repair system. Am J Physiol Cell Physiol 2002;283:C148–154.
28. Kohonen-Corish MRJ, Daniel JJ, Riele H et al. Susceptibility of Msh2-deficient mice to inflammation-associated colorectal tumors. Cancer Res. 2002;62:2092–2097.
29. Berg DJ, Davidson N, Kuhn R et al. Enterocolitis in colon cancer in interleukin-10-deficient mice are associated with aberrant cytokine production and CD(+) Th1-like responses. J Clin Invest 1995;98:1010–1020.
30. Shah SA, Simpson SJ, Brown LF et al. Development of colonic adenocarcinomas in a mouse model of ulcerative colitis. Inflamm Bowel Dis 1998;4:196–202.

31. Sohn KJ, Shah SA, Reid S et al. Molecular genetics of ulcerative colitis-associated colon cancer in the interleukin 2- and b(2)microglobulin-deficient mouse. Cancer Res 2001;61:6912–6917.

32. Engle SJ, Hoying JB, Boivin GP et al. Transforming growth factor β1 suppresses nonmetastatic colon cancer at an early stage of tumorigenesis. Cancer Res 1999;59:3379–3386.

33. Engle SJ, Ormsby I, Pawlowski S et al. Elimination of colon cancer in germ-free transforming growth factor β1-deficient mice. Cancer Res 2002;62:6362–6366.

34. Willenbucher RF, Aust DE, Chang CG et al. Genomic instability is an early event during the progression pathway of ulcerative colitis-related neoplasia. Am J Pathol 1999;154:1825–1830.

35. Suzuki H, Harpaz N, Tarmin L et al. Microsatellite instability in ulcerative colitis-associated colorectal dysplasias and cancers. Cancer Res 1994;54:4841–4844.

36. Tarmin L, Yin J, Harpaz N et al. Adenomatous polyposis coli gene mutations in ulcerative colitis-associated dysplasias and cancers versus sporadic colon neoplasms. Cancer Res 1995;55:2035–2038.

37. Redston MS, Papadopoulos N, Caldas C et al. Common occurrence of APC and K-ras gene mutations in the spectrum of colitis-associated neoplasias. Gastroenterology 1995;108:383–392.

38. Aust DE, Terdiman JP, Willenbucher RF et al. The APC/β-catenin pathway in ulcerative colitis-related colorectal carcinomas. Cancer 2002;94:1421–1427.

39. Burmer GC, Rabinovitch PS, Haggitt RC et al. Neoplastic progression in ulcerative colitis: histology, DNA content, and loss of a p53 allele. Gastroenterology 1992;103:1602–1610.

40. Brentnall TA, Crispin DA, Rabinovitch PS et al. Mutations of the p53 gene: an early marker of neoplastic progression in ulcerative colitis. Gastroenterology 1994;107:369–378.

41. Klump B, Holzmann K, Kuhn A et al. Distribution of cell populations with DNA aneuploidy and p53 protein expression in ulcerative colitis. Eur J Gastro Hepatol 1997;9:789–794.

42. Yin J, Harpaz N, Tong Y et al. p53 mutations in dysplastic and cancerous ulcerative colitis lesions. Gastroenterology 1993;104:1633–1639.

43. Lennard-Jones JE, Morson BC, Ritchie JK, Williams CB. Cancer surveillance in ulcerative colitis. Experience over 15 years. Lancet 1983;ii:149–152.

44. Rosenstock E, Farmer RG, Petras R et al. Surveillance for colonic carcinoma in ulcerative colitis. Gastroenterology 1985;89:1342–1346.

45. Aust DE, Willenbucher RF, Terdiman JP et al. Chromosomal alterations in ulcerative colitis-related and sporadic colorectal cancers by comparative genomic hybridization. Hum Pathol 2000;31:109–114.

46. Brentnall TA. Molecular underpinnings of cancer in ulcerative colitis. Curr Opin Gastroenterol 2003;19:64–68.

47. O'Sullivan JN, Bronner MP, Brentnall TA et al. Chromosomal instability in ulcerative colitis is related to telomere shortening. Nature Genet 2002;32:280–284.

48. Holzmann K, Klump B, Weis-Klemm M et al. Telomerase activity in long-standing ulcerative colitis. Anticancer Res 2000;20:3951–3956.

49. Befrits R, Hammarberg C, Rubio C et al. DNA aneuploidy and histologic dysplasia in long-standing ulcerative colitis: a 10-year follow-up study. Dis Colon Rectum 1994;37:313–320.

50. Melville DM, Jass JR, Shepherd NA et al. Dysplasia and deoxyribonucleic acid aneuploidy in the assessment of precancerous changes in chronic ulcerative colitis. Gastroenterology 1988;95:668–675.

51. Lindberg JO, Stenling RB, Rutegard JN. DNA aneuploidy as a marker of premalignancy in surveillance of patients with ulcerative colitis. Br J Surg 1999;86:947–950.

52. Fozard JBJ, Quirke P, Dixon MF et al. DNA aneuploidy in ulcerative colitis. Gut 1986;27:1414–1418.

53. Hammarberg C, Slezak P, Tribukait B. Early detection of malignancy in ulcerative colitis; a flow cytometric DNA study. Cancer 1984;53:291–295.

54. Cuvelier CA, Morson BC, Roels HJ. The DNA content in cancer and dysplasia in chronic ulcerative colitis. Histopathology 1987;11:927–939.

55. Lofberg R, Tribukait B, Ost A et al. Flow cytometric DNA analysis in longstanding ulcerative colitis: a method of prediction of dysplasia and carcinoma development? Gut 1987;28:1100–1106.

56. Meling GI, Clausen OPF, Bergan A et al. Flow cytometric DNA ploidy pattern in dysplastic mucosa, and in primary and metastatic carcinomas in patients with longstanding ulcerative colitis. Br J Cancer 1991;64:339–344.

57. Suzuki K, Muto T, Masaki T, and Morioka Y. Microspectrophotometric DNA analysis in ulcerative colitis with special reference to its application in diagnosis of carcinoma and dysplasia. Gut 1990;31:1266–1270

58. Holzmann K, Klump B, Borchard F et al. Comparative analysis of histology, DNA content, p53, and Ki-ras mutations in colectomy specimens with long-standing ulcerative colitis. Int J Cancer 1998;76:1–6.

59. Lofberg R, Lindquist K, Veress B, Tribukait B. Highly malignant carcinoma in chronic ulcerative colitis without preceding dysplasia or DNA aneuploidy. Dis Colon Rectum 1992;35:82–86.

60. Kern SE, Redston M, Seymour AB et al. Molecular genetic profiles of colitis associated neoplasms. Gastroenterology 1994;107:420–428.

61. Umetani N, Sasaki S, Watanabe T et al. Genetic alterations in ulcerative colitis-associated neoplasia focusing on APC, K-ras gene and microsatellite instability. Jpn J Cancer Res 1999;90:1081–1987.

62. Tomlinson I, Ilyas M, Johnson V et al. A comparison of the genetic pathways involved in the pathogenesis of three types of colorectal cancer. J Pathol 1998;184:148–152.

63. Greenwald BD, Harpaz N, Yin J et al. Loss of heterozygosity affecting the p53, Rb, and mcc/apc tumor suppressor gene loci in dysplastic and cancerous ulcerative colitis. Cancer Res 1992;52:741–745.

64. Aust DE, Terdiman JP, Willenbucher RF et al. Altered distribution of β-catenin, and its binding proteins E-cadherin and APC, in ulcerative colitis-related colorectal cancers. Mod Pathol 2001;14:29–39.

65. Harpaz N, Peck AL, Yin J et al. P53 protein expression in ulcerative colitis-associated colorectal dysplasia and carcinoma. Hum Pathol 1994;25:1069–1074.

66. Chaubert P, Benhattar J, Saraga E et al. K-ras mutations and p53 alterations in neoplastic and nonneoplastic lesions associated with longstanding ulcerative colitis. Am J Pathol 1994;144:767.

67. Wong NACS, Mayer NJ, MacKell S et al. Immunohistochemical assessment of Ki67 and p53 expression assists the diagnosis and grading of ulcerative colitis-related dysplasia. Histopathology 2000;37:108–114.

68. Willenbucher RF, Zelman SJ, Ferrell LD et al. Chromosomal alterations in ulcerative colitis-related neoplastic progression. Gastroenterology 1997;113:791–801.

69. Hoque ATMS, Hahn SA, Schutte M et al. DPC4 gene mutation in colitis associated neoplasia. Gut 1997;40:120–122.

70. Lei J, Zou TT, Shi YQ et al. Infrequent DPC4 gene mutation in esophageal cancer, gastric cancer and ulcerative colitis-associated neoplasms. Oncogene 1996;13:2459–2462.

71. Burmer GC, Levine DS, Kulander BG et al. c-Ki-ras mutations in chronic ulcerative colitis and sporadic colon carcinoma. Gastroenterology 1990;99:416–420.

72. Meltzer SJ, Mane SM, Wood PK et al. Activation of c-Ki-ras in human gastrointestinal dysplasias determined by direct sequencing of polymerase chain reaction products. Cancer Res 1990;50:3627–3630.

73. Bell SM, Kelly SA, Hoyle JA et al. c-Ki-ras gene mutations in dysplasia and carcinomas complicating ulcerative colitis. Br J Cancer 1991;64:174–178.

74. Chen J, Compton C, Cheng B et al. c-Ki-ras mutations in dysplastic fields and cancer in ulcerative colitis. Gastroenterology 1992;102:1983–1987.

75. Cartwright CA, Meisler AI, Eckhart W. Activation of the pp60c-src protein kinase is an early event in colonic carcinogenesis. Proc Natl Acad Sci USA 1990;87:558–562.

76. Cartwright CA, Coad CA, Egbert BM. Elevated c-src tyrosine kinase activity in premalignant epithelia of ulcerative colitis. J Clin Invest 1994;93:509–515.

77. Brentnall TA, Crispin DA, Bronner MP et al. Microsatellite instability in nonneoplastic mucosa from patients with chronic ulcerative colitis. Cancer Res 1996;56:1237–1240.

78. Heinen CD, Noffsinger AE, Belli J et al. Regenerative lesions in ulcerative colitis are characterized by microsatellite mutation. Genes Chromosom Cancer 1997;19:170–175.

79. Noffsinger A, Kretschmer S, Belli J et al. Microsatellite instability is uncommon in intestinal mucosa of patients with Crohn's disease. Dig Dis Sciences 2000;45:378–384.

80. Lyda MH, Noffsinger A, Belli J et al. Microsatellite instability and K-ras mutations in patients with ulcerative colitis. Hum Pathol 2000;31:665–671.

81. Cawkwell L, Sutherland F, Murgatroyd H et al. Defective hMSH2/hMLH1 protein expression is seen infrequently in ulcerative colitis associated colorectal cancers. Gut 2000;46:367–369.

82. Fleisher AS, Esteller M, Harpaz N et al. Microsatellite instability in inflammatory bowel disease-associated neoplastic lesions is associated with hypermethylation and diminished expression of the DNA mismatch repair gene, hMLH1. Cancer Res 2000;60:4864–4868.

83. Gasche C, Chang CL, Rhees J et al. Oxidative stress increases frameshift mutations in human colorectal cancer cells. Cancer Res 2001;61:7444–7448.

84. Brentnall TA, Rubin CE. Crispin DA et al. A germline substitution in the human MSH2 gene is associated with high-grade dysplasia and cancer in ulcerative colitis. Gastroenterology 1995;109:151–155.

85. Noffsinger AE, Belli J, Fogt F et al. A germline hMSH2 alteration is unrelated to colonic microsatellite instability in patients with ulcerative colitis. Hum Pathol 1999;30:8–12.

86. Cunningham JM, Christensen ER, Tester DJ et al. Hypermethylation of the hMLH1 promoter in colon cancer with microsatellite instability. Cancer Res 1998;58:3455–3460.

87. Souza RF, Lei J, Yin J et al. A transforming growth factor b1 receptor type II mutation in ulcerative colitis-associated neoplasms. Gastroenterology 1997;112:40–45.

88. Issa JPJ, Ahuja N, Toyota M et al. Accelerated age-related CpG island methylation in ulcerative colitis. Cancer Res 2001;61:3573–3577.

89. Esteller M, Tortola S, Toyota M et al. Hypermethylation-associated inactivation of p14ARF is independent of p16INK4a methylation and p53 mutational status. Cancer Res 2000;60:129–133.

90. Burri N, Shaw P, Bouzourene H et al. Methylation silencing and mutations of the p14ARF and p16INK4? genes in colon cancer. Lab Invest 2001;81:217–229.

91. Hsieh CJ, Klump B, Holzmann K et al. Hypermethylation of the p16INK4a promoter in colectomy specimens of patients with long-standing and extensive ulcerative colitis. Cancer Res 1998;58:3942–3945.

92. Sato F, Harpaz N, Shibata D et al. Hypermethylation of the p14ARF gene in ulcerative colitis-associated colorectal carcinogenesis. Cancer Res 2002;62:1148–1151.

93. Young J, Biden KG, Simms LA et al. HPP1: a transmembrane protein-encoding gene commonly methylated in colorectal polyps and cancers. Proc Natl Acad Sci USA 2001;98:265–270.

94. Sato F, Shibata D, Harpaz N et al. Aberrant methylation of the HPP1 gene in ulcerative colitis-associated colorectal carcinoma. Cancer Res 2002;62:6820–6822.

95. Ilyas M, Tomlinson IP, Hanby A et al. Allele loss, replication errors and loss of expression of E-cadherin in colorectal cancers. Gut 1997;40:654–659.

96. Wheeler JMD, Kim HC, Efstathiou JA et al. Hypermethylation of the promoter region of the E-cadherin gene (CDH1) in sporadic and ulcerative colitis associated colorectal cancer. Gut 2001;48:367–371.

97. Azarschab P, Porschen R, Gregor M et al. Epigenetic control of the E-cadherin gene (CDH1) by CpG methylation in colectomy samples of patients with ulcerative colitis. Genes Chrom Cancer 2002;35:121–126.

98. Ehsanullah M, Filipe MI, Gazzard B. Mucin secretion in inflammatory bowel disease: correlation with disease activity and dysplasia. Gut 1982;23:385–489.

99. Fozard JBJ, Dixon MF, Axon ATR et al. Lectin and mucin histochemistry as an aid to cancer surveillance in ulcerative colitis. Histopathology 1987;11:385–394.

100. Ahnen DJ, Warren GH, Greene LJ et al. Search for a specific marker of mucosal dysplasia in chronic ulcerative colitis. Gastroenterology 1987;93:1346–1355.

101. Boland CR, Lance P, Levin B et al. Abnormal goblet cell glycoconjugates in rectal biopsies associated with an increased risk of neoplasia in patients with ulcerative colitis: early results of a prospective study. Gut 1984;25:1364–1371.

102. Itzkowitz SH, Bloom EJ, Lau TS et al. Mucin-associated Tn and sialosyl-Tn antigen expression in colorectal polyps. Gut 1992;33:518–523.

103. Itzkowitz SH, Bloom EJ, Kokal WA et al. Sialosyl-Tn: a novel mucin antigen associated with prognosis in colorectal cancer patients. Cancer 1990;66:1960–1966.

104. Itzkowitz SH, Marshall A, Kornbluth A et al. Sialosyl-Tn antigen: initial report of a new marker of malignant progression in long-standing ulcerative colitis. Gastroenterology 1995;109:490–497.

105. Itzkowitz SH, Young E, Dubois D et al. Sialosyl-Tn antigen is prevalent and precede dysplasia in ulcerative colitis: a retrospective case–control study. Gastroenterology 1996;110:694–704.

106. Karlen P, Young E, Brostrom O et al. Sialyl-Tn antigen as a marker of colon cancer risk in ulcerative colitis: relation to dysplasia and DNA aneuploidy. Gastroenterology 1998;115:1395–1404.

107. Lashner BA, Shapiro BD, Husain A et al. Evaluation of the usefulness of testing for p53 mutations in colorectal cancer surveillance for ulcerative colitis. Am J Gastroenterol 1999;94:456–462.

108. Sato A, Machinami R. p53 immunohistochemistry of ulcerative colitis associated with dysplasia and carcinoma. Pathol Int 1999;49:858–868.

109. Ilyas M, Talbot IC. p53 expression in ulcerative colitis: a longitudinal study. Gut 1995;37:802–804.

110. Rubin PH, Friedman S, Harpaz S et al. Colonoscopic polypectomy in chronic colitis: conservative management after endoscopic resection of dysplastic polyps. Gastroenterology 1999;117:1295–1300.

111. Engelsgjerd M, Farraye FA, Odze RD. Polypectomy may be adequate treatment for adenoma-like dysplastic lesions in chronic ulcerative colitis. Gastroenterology 1999;117:1288–1294.

112. Odze RD, Brown CA, Hartmann CJ et al. Genetic alterations in chronic ulcerative colitis-associated adenoma-like DALMs are similar to non-colitic sporadic adenomas. Am J Surg Pathol 2000;24:1209–1216.

113. Selaru FM, Xu Y, Yin J et al. Artificial neural networks distinguish among subtypes of neoplastic colorectal lesions. Gastroenterology 2002:122:606–613.

114. Uthoff SMS, Hilliard D, Eichenberger M et al. Significance of the wnt-pathway for cancer risk in inflammatory bowel disease: association of a genetic polymorphism in human disheveled 1 with dysplasia in ulcerative colitis. Gastroenterology 2002;122:A104.

115. Borchers R, Heinzlmann M, Zahn R et al. K-ras mutations in sera of patients with colorectal neoplasia and long-standing inflammatory bowel disease. Scand J Gastroenterol 2002;37:715–718.

116. Ahlquist DA, Skoletsky JE, Boynton KA et al. Colorectal cancer screening by detection of altered human DNA in stool: feasibility of a multitarget assay panel. Gastroenterology 2000;119:1219–1227.

117. Heinzlmann M, Lang SM, Neynaber S et al. Screening for p53 and k-ras mutations in whole-gut lavage in chronic inflammatory bowel disease. Eur J Gastroenterol Hepatol 2002;14:1061–1066.

# EPIDEMIOLOGY, CLINICAL FEATURES AND NATURAL HISTORY

## CHAPTER 17

# Epidemiology of inflammatory bowel diseases

Robert S Sandler and Edward V Loftus Jr

## INTRODUCTION

Epidemiologists have made important contributions to our understanding of a number of chronic diseases. The inflammatory bowel diseases (IBD), however, pose a number of problems for epidemiologists, and their contributions to our understanding of IBD have been modest. None the less, the large body of epidemiological data on the distribution of ulcerative colitis and Crohn's disease in diverse populations over time has laid important groundwork. The descriptive data serve as a benchmark against which to measure potential etiologic factors. Credible hypotheses must fit with geographic and temporal trends. This chapter summarizes current knowledge about the epidemiology of IBD.

## DESCRIPTIVE EPIDEMIOLOGY

### INCIDENCE

Incidence is the number of new cases of disease that develop in a specific time interval, generally 1 year. Comparing the incidence of disease across different geographic regions could provide clues to etiology. Studying changes in incidence within an area over time may also provide valuable information.

### Ulcerative colitis

The incidence rates for ulcerative colitis have remained relatively constant in areas such as northern Europe and North America, where data have been available for several years (Fig. 17.1). In areas that previously had a low incidence, such as southern Europe and East Asia, the incidence appears to be increasing. It may be difficult to directly compare rates of disease in different areas, however, because disease definitions vary. Because most investigators do not have access to true population-based registries, surrogates (including hospitalization) are sometimes used to estimate incidence. Finally, the age structure of populations

may differ. IBD is diagnosed preferentially in young people, so areas with a younger population will appear to have higher incidence rates unless standardization procedures are employed.

Table 17.1 summarizes more recent incidence data from a number of investigators.[1-17] Rates tend to be generally higher in the Scandinavian countries, Great Britain and North America. Rates in southern and central Europe are somewhat lower. Ulcerative colitis is being increasingly reported in Asia,[18] Africa and Latin America. Rates in some of the underdeveloped countries, which tend to be lower, may be less reliable. Data from India are limited. Chuttani et al.[19] found that the number of hospital admissions for ulcerative colitis in India was not significantly different from that in the United Kingdom, but the conclusions are suspect because there was no population denominator.

Ulcerative proctitis significantly complicates the published literature on ulcerative colitis. Several authors have excluded cases with ulcerative proctitis,[20] some have included them with the ulcerative colitis group,[2] and others have grouped them with colitis affecting the sigmoid colon as an entity denoted 'distal colitis'.[1] The variation in proportion of patients with ulcerative proctitis ranges from 17 and 49% of all ulcerative colitis patients.[21-23]

### Crohn's disease

Crohn's disease is a relatively new condition. The initial description is generally attributed to Crohn, Ginzburg and Oppenheimer[24] in 1932, although isolated cases were described much earlier.[25] We have witnessed a remarkable rise in disease incidence. Figure 17.2 demonstrates the changes in incidence over time in selected registries. All of these registries demonstrate a rise in incidence followed by a plateau. The explanation for these trends is unknown. Some increase in incidence could be secondary to shortening of the time interval between symptom onset and disease diagnosis,[26] or to better appreciation of the disease, but these explanations cannot explain the profound changes in incidence. Diagnostic transfer from ulcerative colitis to Crohn's is also not an adequate explanation for the

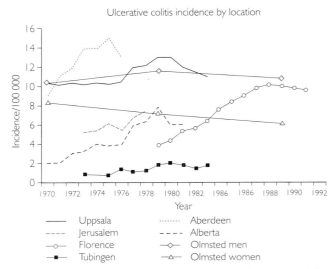

Fig. 17.1  Incidence rates of ulcerative colitis (per 100 000 population) from Aberdeen, Scotland,[1] Uppsala, Sweden,[39] Jerusalem, Israel,[94] and Tubingen, Germany,[37] Alberta, Canada[14] and Florence, Italy,[12] 1970–1992.

trends over time, given the relatively stable or increasing rates for ulcerative colitis. The inescapable conclusion is that most of the increase in incidence of Crohn's disease is real. One must also conclude that some environmental factors are partially responsible – genetic factors do not change this quickly.

Table 17.1 summarizes published data about Crohn's disease incidence from a selected group of studies. These studies are all relatively recent. Calkins and Mendeloff[27] provide an excellent review of incidence data from earlier studies. The incidence rates in Table 17.2 vary considerably. There is a greater than 10-fold difference between the registries with the highest and lowest incidence rates. Although part of this variation must be due to differences in disease definition, recognition and coding, there is little doubt that disease incidence varies with geography. As a general rule, areas of high incidence for Crohn's disease are also high incidence areas for ulcerative colitis.

Although the data are somewhat limited for certain regions, the disease appears most common in Scandinavia, Great Britain and North America, with lower rates from southern Europe,[28] Africa and Asia.[29,30] Estimates from Australia suggest that the rates may be intermediate.[31] The incidence of Crohn's disease has now exceeded that for ulcerative colitis in many parts of the world, including Stockholm,[32,33] Rochester, NY,[34] Cardiff, Wales,[35,36] Tubingen, Germany,[37] northwestern France[38] and Scotland.[1] In Uppsala, Sweden, Crohn's disease is more common than extensive colitis, but less common when extensive colitis and ulcerative proctitis are combined.[39]

## PREVALENCE

Prevalence is the number of individuals with a specific condition at a given time. As a rule of thumb, prevalence is approximately equal to the incidence of a disease multiplied by its duration. For self-limited conditions with short duration (e.g. influenza or appendicitis), the prevalence is equal to the incidence. Chronic conditions, on the other hand, have a prevalence that considerably exceeds incidence. Although prevalence figures are hard to come by, they are very important. Prevalence of disease represents the healthcare burden in a population. Policy makers need to know the number affected so that they can allocate appropriate healthcare funding. Research agencies may wish to know

prevalence so that they can prioritize funds for investigation. Pharmaceutical companies need prevalence information to project sales.

Selected studies that present both incidence and prevalence for both Crohn's disease and ulcerative colitis are shown in Table 17.2.[12,14,16,23,28,37,40–55] The highest reported prevalence of ulcerative colitis is from Olmsted County, Minnesota (229 cases per 100 000 persons). The highest reported prevalence rates of Crohn's disease are from Manitoba, Canada (198 per 10[5]) and from a survey in Great Britain (214 per 10[5]). If one applied the 1991 prevalence rates in Olmsted County to the United States population in 2000 (281 million), there would be approximately 1 000 000 individuals with inflammatory bowel disease in the US. Rates in Olmsted County may be somewhat higher than most of the US, however, thereby inflating the national prevalence figures. Using 1994 Manitoba prevalence data and 2001 Census data (30 million), the estimated IBD population in Canada is approximately 110 000 persons. If the highest prevalence figures from European studies are extrapolated to the combined population of Europe (approximately 400 million), there may be as many as 1.8 million persons with IBD.

The variability of data shown in Table 17.2 is hard to explain. If one assumes that prevalence is equal to incidence multiplied by duration, and if the duration of disease is presumed to be roughly the same everywhere, it is surprising that the prevalence/incidence ratio in published studies has such a wide range. The prevalence/incidence ratio for Crohn's disease ranges from 15 in Rochester, Minnesota, to 6.6 in North Tees, England. The prevalence/incidence ratio for ulcerative colitis also varies between registries. Because asymptomatic persons and patients in remission are probably undercounted in prevalence studies, the prevalence figures are more likely to be incorrect than the incidence figures. Based on the data in Table 17.3, one might estimate that prevalence is approximately 10–15 times incidence for ulcerative colitis and Crohn's disease.

## MORTALITY

IBD mortality statistics present several problems for epidemiologists. First, IBD is an uncommon cause of death and small errors in classification can have major effects on death rates. Moreover, although IBD may be a contributing cause of death, death certificate data on underlying causes of death may be unreliable. A Rochester, NY, study compared death certificates with physician chart review and found only 80% concordance over a 16-year period.[56] Second, International Classification of Disease (ICD) codes for IBD have changed over time.[57] This makes it difficult to plot trends over time. Finally, it is difficult to compare mortality rates between different areas. Differences in the age structure of different populations make crude comparison of mortality rates potentially erroneous, and age-standardized mortality data have not been available.

As a general rule, mortality rates for UC have declined over time. Although some population-based studies of mortality for UC in Scandinavia have demonstrated a significantly elevated standardized mortality ratio (SMR) ranging from 1.4 to 1.6,[58,59] other studies from the United Kingdom or Scandinavia have not.[60–62] Two studies of mortality rates in ulcerative colitis from Italy found no increased mortality.[63,64] Survival among ulcerative colitis patients residing in Olmsted County, Minnesota, has not been significantly different from that expected in the general population.[23,65] In the few recent studies that have demonstrated increased mortality in UC, gastrointestinal events were the

## Table 17.1 Incidence of ulcerative colitis and Crohn's disease from selected registries since 1980

| Author(s) (reference) | Setting | Case ascertainment | Incidence dates | Incidence of UC* | Incidence of CD* |
|---|---|---|---|---|---|
| **NORTH AMERICA** | | | | | |
| Pinchbeck et al.[14] | Northern Alberta | Population | 1981 | 6 | 10 |
| Hiatt et al.[83] | Northern California | HMO | 1980–81 | 10.9 | 7.0 |
| Stowe et al.[34] | Monroe County, NY | Hospital | 1980–89 | 2.3 | 3.9 |
| Kurata et al.[40] | Southern California | HMO, outpatient | 1987–88 | NA | 3.6 |
| | | HMO, hospital | 1988 | NA | 5.4 |
| Loftus et al.[23,41] | Olmsted County, MN | Population | 1984–93 | 8.3 | 6.9 |
| Bernstein et al.[16] | Manitoba | Population | 1989–94 | 14.3 | 14.6 |
| Blanchard et al.[86] | Manitoba | Population | 1987–96 | 15.6 | 15.6 |
| **EUROPE** | | | | | |
| Shivananda et al.[17] | 8 N. European cities | Population | 1991–93 | 11.8 | 7.0 |
| Shivananda et al.[17] | 12 S. European cities | Population | 1991–93 | 8.7 | 3.9 |
| **SCANDINAVIA** | | | | | |
| Bjornsson et al.[286] | Iceland | Population | 1990–94 | 16.5 | 5.5 |
| Munkholm et al.[287] | Copenhagen County | Population | 1980–87 | 9.2 | 4.1 |
| Langholz et al.[42] | | | | | |
| Moum et al.[13] | S.E. Norway | Population | 1990–93 | 13.6 | 5.8 |
| Roin et al.[288] | Faroe Isles, Denmark | Population | 1981–99 | 20.3 | 3.6 |
| Lapidus et al.[104] | Stockholm County | Population | 1985–89 | NA | 4.9 |
| **UNITED KINGDOM** | | | | | |
| Rubin et al.[289] | North Tees, UK | Population | 1985–94 | 13.9 | 8.3 |
| Yapp et al.[290] | Cardiff, Wales, UK | Population | 1991–95 | NA | 5.6 |
| Kyle[291] | N.E. Scotland, UK | Population | 1985–87 | NA | 9.8 |
| **NORTHERN EUROPE** | | | | | |
| Russel et al.[292] | S. Limburg, Netherlands | Population | 1991–94 | 10.0 | 6.9 |
| Gower-Rousseau et al.[293] | N.W. France | Population | 1988–90 | 3.2 | 4.9 |
| **SOUTHERN/CENTRAL EUROPE** | | | | | |
| Maté-Jiminez et al.[45] | 2 Spanish regions | Hospital | 1981–88 | 3.2 | 1.6 |
| Manousos et al.[294] | Heraklion, Crete | Population | 1990–94 | 9.4 | 3.3 |
| Vucelic et al.[46] | Zagreb, Croatia | Population | 1980–89 | 1.5 | 0.7 |
| Trallori et al.[295] | Florence, Italy | Population | 1990–92 | 9.6 | 3.4 |
| Tragnone et al.[11] | 8 Italian cities | Population | 1989–92 | 5.2 | 2.3 |
| **ASIA AND OCEANIA** | | | | | |
| Odes et al.[296] | Southern Israel | Population | 1987–92 | NA | 4.2 |
| Yang et al.[55] | Seoul, Korea | Population | 1992–94 | 1.2 | NA |
| Morita et al.[53] | Japan | Survey | 1991 | 1.9 | 0.5 |
| **AFRICA** | | | | | |
| Wright et al.[88] | Cape Town, South Africa | Population, white | 1980–84 | 5.0 | 2.6 |
| | | Population, coloured | 1980–84 | 1.9 | 1.8 |
| | | Population, black | 1980–84 | 0.6 | 0.3 |
| **LATIN AMERICA** | | | | | |
| Linares de la Cal et al.[297] | Colon, Panama | Hospital | 1987–93 | 1.2 | 0 |
| Linares de la Cal et al.[297] | Partido General de Pueyrredon, Argentina | Hospital | 1987–93 | 2.2 | 0.03 |

* Cases per 100 000 person-years.

primary reason for the higher rates, but UC patients also had higher rates of death from colorectal cancer, respiratory disease and hepatobiliary disease than the general population.[58,66,67] Several studies that did not find an increased mortality overall found that mortality was increased in the first year after diagnosis,[60,62,63] probably reflecting the higher mortality associated with acute fulminant colitis.

Similarly, although most studies have noted higher mortality rates and lower survival among patients with Crohn's disease,[41,58,64,64,68–70] other reports show mortality in Crohn's disease to be similar to that in the general population.[18,67,71–74]

A well-characterized cohort from Copenhagen was initially noted to have no increased mortality,[43] but extension of follow-up revealed an excess mortality restricted to women who had been diagnosed before the age of 50 years and who had disease duration greater than 20 years.[71] The results of other subgroup analyses in these studies are conflicting; whereas some have suggested that patients with ileal or jejunal disease are at increased mortality risk,[48,64] others have suggested that patients with colonic or perianal involvement are more at risk.[62,62,72]

Looking at trends over time, the mortality from Crohn's disease increased in England and Wales and the United States

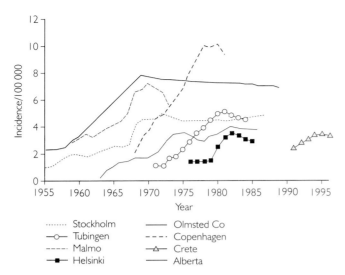

Fig. 17.2 Incidence rates of Crohn's disease (per 100 000 population) from Malmo, Sweden,[306] Stockholm, Sweden,[104] Olmsted County, Minnesota,[41] Tubingen, Germany,[37] Copenhagen, Denmark,[287] Helsinki, Finland[106] and Heraklion, Crete,[15] 1955–1995. Interval data from published reports were interpolated.

during the period between 1950 and the early 1970s, and then decreased.[73] The death rate for ulcerative colitis decreased throughout the entire observation period for both men and women. Mortality rates for whites were twice those for non-whites, although the non-white rates may not be completely reliable. During the period from 1980 to 1982, mortality rates in the US were approximately 1 per million population for both men and women for both Crohn's and ulcerative colitis. In England and Wales during 1980–1983 the mortality rates for Crohn's disease for men were 2.19 per million and 4.13 for

women. Corresponding rates for ulcerative colitis were 2.80 and 4.30 per million population for men and women, respectively. It is safer to compare mortality rates between sexes and over time within countries than between countries, because coding and classification are likely to be relatively similar within a country.

## MORBIDITY

Although the mortality from IBD is low, the disease confers considerable morbidity. Morbidity is particularly difficult to study because there are no standard measures. Not surprisingly, there have been few epidemiological studies of IBD-related morbidity.

IBD can have serious socioeconomic implications because it often affects young people and can last a lifetime. Using statistics from the German social security system to assess the impact of IBD on disability, Sonnenberg[74] identified 1321 employees who were granted disability from 1982 to 1986 because of Crohn's disease and 766 for ulcerative colitis. The age distribution was younger than that for other conditions. Disability for both Crohn's disease and ulcerative colitis was more common in white-collar workers. The study is a good example of the creative use of data collected for other purposes (administrative data sets) to provide valuable information about IBD epidemiology. Among 2700 survey responders representing 60% of a population-based cohort of IBD patients from Manitoba, Canada, self-reported unemployment was twice as high as that expected in the general population.[75] Crohn's disease patients were more likely to report unemployment or disability than ulcerative colitis patients.

Hospitalization can be viewed as another measure of IBD morbidity. In England during the period 1982–1985 2530 men with Crohn's disease and 2750 with ulcerative colitis were discharged annually from hospital.[76] Figures for women were 3400 and 3020. Data from the US National Hospital Discharge

## Table 17.2 Prevalence of IBD from selected registries after 1980

| Author (s) (ref) | Setting | Case ascertainment | Prevalence date | Prevalence of UC | Prevalence of CD |
|---|---|---|---|---|---|
| **NORTH AMERICA** | | | | | |
| Pinchbeck et al.[14] | Northern Alberta | Population | 12/31/81 | 37.5 | 44.4 |
| Kurata et al.[40] | Southern California | HMO | 1988 | NA | 26.0 |
| Loftus et al.[23,41] | Olmsted County, MN | Population | 1/1/91 | 229 | 144.1 |
| Bernstein et al.[16] | Manitoba | Population | 12/31/94 | 169.7 | 198.5 |
| **EUROPE** | | | | | |
| Langholz et al.[42] Munkholm et al.[43] | Copenhagen | Population | 12/31/87 | 161.2 | 4 |
| Kyle et al.[44] | N.E. Scotland, UK | Population | 12/31/88 | NA | 147 |
| Maté-Jiminez et al.[45] | 2 Spanish regions | Hospital | 12/31/88 | 43.4 | 19.8 |
| Vucelic et al.[28,46] | Zagreb, Croatia | Population | 12/31/89 | 21.4 | 8.3 |
| Trallori et al.[12] | Florence, Italy | Population | 12/31/92 | 121 | 40 |
| Rubin et al.[47] | North Tees, UK | Population | 1/1/95 | 243 | 144 |
| Daiss et al.[37] | Tubingen, Germany | Population | 12/31/84 | 24.8 | 54.6 |
| Montgomery et al.[48] | United Kingdom | Survey | 1996 | 122 | 214 |
| **ASIA** | | | | | |
| Fireman et al.[49] Grossman et al.[50] | Central Israel | Population | 1980 | 55.2 | 19.5 |
| Odes et al.[51] | Southern Israel | Population | 12/31/85 | 70.6 | NA |
| Odes et al.[52] | Southern Israel | Population | 12/31/92 | NA | 50.6 |
| Morita et al.[53] | Japan | Survey | 1991 | 18.1 | 5.8 |
| Lee et al.[54] | Singapore | Hospital | 1985–96 | 6.0 | 3.6 |
| Yang et al.[55] | Seoul, Korea | Population | 12/31/97 | 7.6 | NA |

**Table 17.3 Prevalence of ulcerative colitis (per 100 000 population) in Israel by place of birth**

| | | Place of birth | | | |
|---|---|---|---|---|---|
| Location (ref) | Year | Europe/America | Asia/Africa | Israel | Total |
| Tel Aviv[98] [a] | 1970 | 37.3 | 18.7 | 25.7 | 37.4 |
| Tel Aviv[50] [c] | 1980 | 52.7 | 48.5 | 45.8 | 55.2 |
| Jerusalem[94] | 1978 | 92.9 | 31.3 | 64.7 | 56.9 |
| Galilee[298] | 1986 | 61.5 | 40.8 | 138.2 | 64.2 |
| Beer Sheva[299] [b] | 1987 | 145 | 81 | 74 | 89 |
| Kinneret[96] | 1994 | NA | NA | NA | 86.7 |
| Kibbutzes[300] | 1987 | 78.3 | 139.2 | 220.5 | 121 |
| | 1997 | 265.3 | 71.1 | 116.5 | 167.2 |

[a] age standardized to Tel Aviv.
[b] age standardized to world standard population.
[c] age standardized to Jerusalem population.
Prevalence refers to the last date during the interval.

Survey from 1984 to 1987 show an average of 26 630 men discharged annually from US hospitals with Crohn's disease and 19 040 with ulcerative colitis.[76] For women the corresponding numbers were 39 330 and 20 690. Temporal trends for hospital discharges parallel those for mortality rates.

## GEOGRAPHY

The variation in IBD rates with geography may serve as a valuable clue to etiology. There appears to be a distinct north–south gradient in risk. As noted previously, the highest rates in Europe come from the Scandinavian countries and the United Kingdom. Rates in southern Europe had historically been much lower than in Scandinavia and the UK, but more recent studies have shown rapid increases in incidence in Italy, Greece and Spain.[17] A prospective multicenter study in Europe, the EC-IBD study, assessed incidence over a 2-year period.[17] The investigators found the highest incidence of ulcerative colitis in Iceland, and the lowest in southern Portugal. For Crohn's disease the highest incidence was in The Netherlands and northwest France, with the lowest incidence in Greece. The overall adjusted rate for ulcerative colitis in all northern centers was 40% higher than in all of the southern centers and 80% higher for Crohn's disease. The study confirmed the presence of a north–south gradient in incidence, but the differences were smaller than expected.

Sonnenberg et al.[77] used data on 17.5 million hospital discharges of Medicare beneficiaries over a 2-year period in the mid-1980s to examine geographic variation in IBD in the United States. In general, hospitalization for IBD was significantly more common in northern states. This pattern was seen for men and women and for blacks and whites. Crohn's disease and ulcerative colitis had similar geographic variations that were not shared by other gastrointestinal diseases.[77] Hospital discharge data from Veterans Affairs hospitals showed a similar north–south gradient.[78]

The explanation for this gradient in IBD risk is unknown. People in southern climates presumably spend less time in buildings. Perhaps their lower rates are related to sunlight, indoor air pollution, and either lack of transmissible agents or increased exposure to protective microbial agents (hygiene hypothesis).

Several reports from East and Southeast Asia have documented the emergence of IBD, especially UC, in recent decades.[29,53,54,79] The epidemiology of IBD in Asia has recently been reviewed.[80] The incidence of UC increased 10-fold in a district of Seoul, Korea, between 1986 and 1997,[55] and the prevalence of IBD in Japan in 1991[81] was comparable to that of IBD in Croatia in 1989.[28,46] Such rapid changes in incidence and prevalence may point to environmental changes associated with a so-called 'westernization' of lifestyle (e.g. dietary changes, cigarette smoking etc.) as potential risk factors.

## RACE AND ETHNICITY

In the past, IBD was thought to be much more common in Caucasians than African-Americans. This impression probably arose because most of the studies were conducted in areas where non-white minorities are underrepresented. In data from Baltimore, the age-adjusted rates for white men were about twice those of non-whites, whereas the rates for non-white women were higher than those for white women.[82] Although hospital-based studies of US military veterans and Medicare beneficiaries showed that blacks were about half as likely to have IBD as whites,[77,78] these data are now 12–15 years old. In addition, the Medicare rates are based on patients over the age of 65 and may not be generalizable.

Data on hospitalization among members of the Kaiser Permanente Medical Care Program in northern California showed no differences between whites and blacks.[83] A study from a southern California HMO found that hospitalization rates for Crohn's disease were similar for whites and blacks, and that the overall prevalence of Crohn's disease in blacks was approximately two-thirds that of whites.[40] Afro-Caribbean children in the UK have a risk of IBD similar to that of Caucasian children[84] and the incidence of Crohn's disease is similar among Afro-Caribbean and Caucasian adults residing in Derby, UK.[85]

Other US minority groups appear to develop ulcerative colitis and Crohn's disease much less commonly. Among US Medicare beneficiaries, Hispanics, Asian-Americans and native Americans were infrequently admitted to hospital with IBD.[77] Hospitalizations for IBD were uncommon among Asians in a northern California HMO.[83] The prevalence of Crohn's disease among Hispanics and Asian-Americans was one-tenth that of whites in a southern California HMO in the 1980s.[40] Native

Americans from Manitoba, Canada, are half as likely as Caucasians residing in that province to develop ulcerative colitis and one-tenth as likely to develop Crohn's disease.[86]

In Johannesburg, ulcerative colitis is infrequently seen among blacks,[87] and black IBD patients tend to be urbanized and belong to upper social and educational strata with a western or partially westernized diet. In Cape Town, incidence rates between 1980 and 1984 were eight times higher for whites than blacks and about two and a half times higher than for mixed ethnic backgrounds for both ulcerative colitis and Crohn's.[88]

South Asian migrants to the UK are at increased risk of UC and at nearly equal risk of Crohn's disease compared to Caucasians.[89–92] Within the South Asian population in the UK, Sikhs may be at higher risk than Hindus or Muslims.[89] Second-generation South Asians residing in the UK also appear to be at increased risk of UC (but not Crohn's) compared to Caucasians.[84,91] In Singapore, South Asians are at increased risk of UC relative to ethnic Chinese residents, although their absolute risk appears to be much lower than that of South Asian migrants to the UK.[54] In New Zealand, ulcerative colitis is rare among Maoris.[93]

Reports from Israel demonstrate a higher prevalence of ulcerative colitis in European- and American-born Jews than in Jews from Asia and Africa[50,94–98] (Table 17.3). Because these prevalent cases may have developed their ulcerative colitis before emigrating to Israel, the results may simply reflect disease risk in parent countries. In fact, a study from Jerusalem showed that 29% of the European/American group developed ulcerative colitis prior to immigration to Israel.[94] Incidence figures demonstrate the same trend, however. In Beer Sheva, over a 20-year period, the incidence rates were greater among those born in Europe/America than among those born in Asia/Africa or Israel. Ulcerative colitis is uncommon among Israeli Arabs.[99]

Crohn's disease is more common in Jews than non-Jews. A population-based study conducted in southeast Wales demonstrated that the risk of developing Crohn's disease among Jews was increased between five- and eightfold compared to non-Jews.[100] Crohn's disease is uncommon among Israeli, Kuwaiti and Bedouin Arabs.[99]

In 1970, the prevalence rates of Crohn's disease among immigrants from Europe and America to Tel Aviv were seven times those of Jews born in Asia/Africa.[49] By 1980 this had decreased to about twofold. A more recent study from southern Israel assessed outpatient cases of Crohn's disease for the period 1968–1992.[101] The prevalence rates were $55.0/10^5$ for Asian/African-born Jews and $58.7/10^5$ for Europe/America-born Jews.

Although the prevalence of IBD is generally higher in Jews than in non-Jews, there is considerable variation in disease rates among Jews in different countries. In general, the rates for Jews parallel those of the general population. In areas where Crohn's disease is common in the general population, the rates of Crohn's disease among Jews are higher than they are in areas where the disease is less common. The same holds true for ulcerative colitis.[102]

The experience of Jews points to gene–environment interaction with respect to IBD etiology. The higher rates among Jews in a number of areas supports a genetic predisposition. The fact that rates among Jews vary by country suggests that environmental factors can influence this inherited predisposition in important ways. Although IBD rates appear to vary by country,

some of the differences could be due to differences in disease definition and case ascertainment.

## SEX

Epidemiologists commonly examine sex ratios for insights into disease etiology. Differences in disease risk by sex could indicate that hormonal, occupational or lifestyle factors were responsible.

In the case of IBD, men and women are generally at similar risk. Studies using somewhat different methods and definitions conducted at different times show that women are at 20–30% greater risk of developing Crohn's disease than men. In 10 studies of Crohn's disease incidence performed in North America, the female proportion ranged from 48% to 66%, with most studies ranging from 50% to 60%.[103] The situation is reversed for ulcerative colitis. Although the male to female ratio is close to unity, men are slightly more likely to develop ulcerative colitis. The findings suggest that susceptibility factors for the two diseases may be different. On the other hand, the fact that the ratios for both diseases are close to unity further suggests no major sex-related risk.

## AGE

IBD is more common in young people. Crohn's disease is most frequently diagnosed in late adolescence or early adulthood, with a median age of diagnosis in the third decade.[43] The average age at diagnosis of ulcerative colitis is in the fourth decade. A 'bimodal' age distribution of incidence[104] refers to a large peak in incidence seen in the second or third decades, followed by a second smaller peak in incidence later in life. Although some studies show a bimodal age distribution for Crohn's disease,[2,34,35,39,85,105–108] others do not.[16,17,41] It is not clear whether these variations in age distribution represent real differences in the age of onset of Crohn's disease or whether they are due to differences in classification of various entities that might be confused with Crohn's disease (e.g. diverticulitis, infectious colitis or ischemic colitis). In general, studies of Crohn's disease incidence performed within the past decade have not observed the second peak. In contrast, the existence of a bimodal distribution of incidence in ulcerative colitis seems to be consistent across many studies.[2,3,9,16,17,34,39,41] Interestingly, in some of these studies there is a gender divergence later in life.[16,17,41] In men, new cases of ulcerative colitis continue to be diagnosed later in life, whereas in women the incidence of this disease decreases dramatically after a peak seen in the third or fourth decades.

Some investigators have suggested that the late onset of IBD is due to exposure to an environmental agent that manifests itself later in life, but no such agent has been identified. The second peak might be secondary to greater susceptibility to disease with increasing age, or to mesenteric vascular disease that is confused with IBD. The second peak might be partially explained by the fact that the elderly are more likely to be hospitalized and carefully evaluated. It has been hypothesized that the gender-related differences in ulcerative colitis incidence could be due to varying rates of current or previous smoking, but this has not been confirmed.

Other diseases that have demonstrated a bimodal age distribution include aplastic anemia,[109] multiple sclerosis[110–113] and Hodgkin's disease.[114] Perhaps each of these conditions involves inherited genetic susceptibility that becomes manifest during periods of life that produce immunologic susceptibility or an increased exposure to infection. For each of these conditions there might be two different ages that satisfy this requirement.

## URBAN/RURAL RESIDENCE

Studies of urban/rural differences might provide clues to etiology. Urban exposures include industrial chemicals, pollutants of air and water, and infections that are spread more easily with close human contact. Risk factors in rural areas could be related to zoonoses or agricultural chemicals.

Crohn's disease has been reported to be more common in urban areas from Northern Ireland,[115] Aberdeen,[44] Minnesota,[116] Baltimore,[117] Alberta,[14] The Netherlands[118] and Manitoba.[86] Ulcerative colitis appears more common in urban areas based on studies from Scotland,[1] Minnesota [23] and Manitoba.[86] Not all studies confirm these findings.[21,108] In interpreting these results one should consider whether residents of rural areas have similar availability and/or access to health care, or whether cases of IBD might be misclassified as other conditions. Definitions of rural and urban may vary from study to study.

Sweden provides unique opportunities for studying IBD because the medical system provides all citizens equal access to high-quality, free medical care.[39] This should limit biased ascertainment as an explanation of urban/rural differences. Studies from Sweden show that both Crohn's disease and ulcerative colitis are more common in urban areas.[39] Incidence rates in urban Copenhagen have also been found to be higher than in the Faroe Islands, despite similar medical systems.[20,22]

# RISK FACTORS

## DIET

The marked geographic differences in IBD incidence and the experience of migrants could be explained by differences in diet. For example, contact of dietary factors or metabolites with the intestine, or alterations in bacterial profiles, could influence IBD development or persistence. Although there have been a number of studies of diet and IBD, the results have not been definitive. There are plausible biological mechanisms that could explain an association between IBD and diet. Dietary antigens represent the majority of non-bacterial and non-self antigens presented to the gut. Antibodies to dietary wheat and maize have been reported in both ulcerative colitis and Crohn's disease.[119] Glassman et al.[120] noted cow's milk protein sensitivity during infancy in patients with IBD. Although milk is not generally thought to be causative, it may exacerbate the symptoms of ulcerative colitis.[121] Furthermore, food additives could provide toxic products that affect vascular or immune functions, and dietary fiber can affect luminal microecology. Whether dietary factors are etiologic, consequent or coincident to IBD remains to be determined.

## CARBOHYDRATES

A number of investigators have examined the association between carbohydrate consumption, particularly refined sugar, and Crohn's disease.[122-129] These studies generally show a higher consumption of sugar in Crohn's patients. Reif et al.[130] compared IBD patients to clinic and population controls and found that high sucrose intake was a risk factor. Other investigators have suggested that increased sugar intake was a consequence of disease rather than a cause.[126,127] Thornton et al.[124] interviewed newly diagnosed Crohn's patients and concluded that a diet high in refined sugar and low in raw fruits and vegetables preceded and might favor the development of Crohn's disease. They did not find differences in intake between those with recent and those with longer-lasting symptoms. A study from Cardiff also found no difference in sugar consumption by Crohn's patients over time.[131] Sonnenberg used available data on per capita consumption of sugar from a number of countries and correlated it with geographic and temporal trends in the incidence and mortality of Crohn's disease.[132] The study failed to show a close relationship.

## MARGARINE

There are marked geographic differences in margarine consumption. Intake has also increased markedly over time in parallel with increases in incidence in Crohn's disease. Consumption is low in some Western countries with low incidence of Crohn's. Sonnenberg, however, found no significant correlation between margarine consumption and Crohn's disease.[132]

## FRUITS AND VEGETABLES

Fruit and vegetable consumption may be lower in IBD patients.[124] In Israel, the diet of the high-risk Ashkenazi Jews in Tel Aviv includes more meat, milk and eggs than that of the low-risk non-Ashkenazi population who eat more non-meat protein.[133] These finding must be accepted cautiously. Patients with strictures due to Crohn's disease may have difficulty tolerating fiber-containing foods.

## BEVERAGES

Coffee does not appear to be associated with ulcerative colitis.[134] Alcohol consumption has been found to decrease UC in one study.[134] The mechanism for this effect is not known.

## FAT

Omega-3 fatty acids, found in higher concentrations in fish oil, have received attention. These fatty acids can alter arachidonic acid metabolism and may be anti-inflammatory. It has been noted that IBD rates are low in Japan, where fish consumption is high.[135] There have been no studies that have tried to assess fish consumption in IBD patients. It is difficult to obtain accurate information on omega-3 fatty acid consumption from questionnaires. Unsaturated fatty acids may have a suppressive effect on cell-mediated immunity via eicosanoid release, receptor affinity changes or interactions with intracellular signal transduction. Fat absorption has also been thought to lead to cytokine release from intestinal epithelial cells following long-chain fatty acid absorption.[136] In a study from The Netherlands polyunsaturated fat was also reported to be associated with an increased risk of ulcerative colitis.[137]

## FOOD ADDITIVES

Powell et al.[137a] have postulated that non-degradeable microparticles, such as silica dioxide, can induce lymphangitis, lymphatic obstruction, focal injury and granulomas, resulting in intestinal inflammation. These microparticles are used as stabilizers in powdered sugar, refined flour, and even as fillers in medications. The presence of microparticles in toothpaste has been suggested as a cause of Crohn's disease. A crude ecological comparison showed some parallels between toothpaste use and Crohn's.[138] Toothpaste contains abrasives, foaming agents, flavoring mixtures, and thickening agents or binders that might be responsible. Toothpaste is swallowed, especially by children. Particulate material such as talc can produce lesions reminiscent of Crohn's.

## BREASTFEEDING AND PERINATAL EVENTS

Because IBD affects young people, early life events may be important in the etiology. Breastfeeding and perinatal events have been investigated. In one of the best studies, Koletzko et al.[139] found that children with Crohn's disease were more than three times less likely to have been breastfed and nearly three times more likely to have had a diarrheal illness during infancy. Similar results were obtained by some,[140] but not other authors.[141,142]

Koletzko et al.[144] found ulcerative colitis cases three times more likely to have had diarrheal diseases during infancy than their unaffected siblings, but breastfeeding was not associated with ulcerative colitis risk. There was no association with breastfeeding in two other studies of children with ulcerative colitis,[141,142] but not in two studies of adults with ulcerative colitis.[142,145] Additional studies of children focused on early life events are needed.

Infectious diseases during the early years of life could influence IBD rates. A meticulous population-based study in Sweden found higher incidence rates for IBD among individuals born in the first half of certain years.[39] During the years in question there were small, annual influenza epidemics lasting 1 or more months from December to May. The authors have proposed that early life or perinatal infectious events might influence the subsequent risks of IBD.[39]

Ekbom et al.[142] compared perinatal health events in 257 IBD patients born in one Swedish hospital from 1924 to 1957 with 514 controls delivered at the hospital during the same interval. The risk for IBD was increased fourfold for those with infectious events in mothers and children. Febrile viral infections other than upper respiratory infections were particularly strong risk factors. Low socioeconomic status was also an independent risk factor for IBD, possibly due to overcrowded conditions leading to more frequent but unrecognized infections. Whorwell et al.[143] found a higher frequency of gastroenteritis during the first 6 months of life of infants who subsequently developed IBD.

In contrast, others have suggested that absence of infections might be a risk factor. One study found that Crohn's disease (but not ulcerative colitis) was more common in individuals whose first houses had a hot water tap (odds ratio 5.9, 95% CI 1.4–17.3) and a separate bathroom (OR 3.3, 95%CI 1.3–8.3) than in age- and gender-matched controls.[146] The authors speculated that the increased incidence of Crohn's disease over the past 50 years could be due to delayed exposure to enteric infections.

## MARITAL STATUS

Patients with IBD have been reported as being less likely to be married.[117,147] Given the early age of onset of IBD, this difference may be a consequence of steroid-induced cosmetic changes, growth retardation, ostomy, psychological effects on confidence,

body image and social skills, or the long-term effects of a serious chronic disorder that might reduce the probability of getting married. Not all studies show IBD to be more common in single individuals.[148] A survey of 2700 Manitobans with IBD showed that more were married than in the general population (66% versus 55%); however, IBD patients were also more likely to be separated or divorced (7.6% vs. 6.5%).[75] Among those married at the time of diagnosis and whose disease duration was at least 5 years, 10% of men and nearly 20% of women were no longer married.[75]

Married people share potential infectious risk factors, and husband–wife pairs would be likely to develop IBD if the disease had an infectious etiology. There are numerous reported series of husband–wife pairs both of whom have IBD.[149–153] In a report from northwestern France and Belgium where both spouses had IBD, 22 of 30 couples both developed the disease after the marriage, and this was significantly more frequent than would be expected by chance.[154] The data on couples could be attributed to shared environmental exposures, but the role of chance cannot be dismissed. Increased intestinal permeability, thought to be a risk marker for Crohn's disease, has been noted in 13–36% of spouses of Crohn's disease patients.[155–157] These studies suggest that abnormal permeability, and by extension Crohn's disease, may arise from a shared environmental exposure.

## OCCUPATION AND SOCIAL CLASS

IBD is generally more common among those of higher socioeconomic status in most[104,167,168,178,179, 89] but not all studies.[75] A study of IBD incidence by postal area in Manitoba showed that the postal codes associated with the highest tertile of family income had IBD incidence rates that were on average 20% higher than those in postal codes associated with the lowest tertile of family income.[86] On the other hand, a study of Canadian Census information from individuals with IBD from the same region showed no significant differences in income or education between IBD patients and the general population.[75]

There have been attempts to link IBD with specific occupations, but most studies simply classify job types rather than looking at specific occupations. There may be a deficit among farmers.[147] Sonnenberg[158] used data from the German social security system to examine the distribution of IBD by individual occupations. For men, bricklayers, road construction workers, unskilled workers in brick and stone, unskilled laborers and security personnel had a lower prevalence of IBD. Lower rates were found for women employed in cleaning and maintenance and in those without occupation. Higher rates for men were found for instrument makers, electricians, bakers and technical assistants. For women higher rates were found for sales representatives, office workers, health workers and hairdressers. There was a good correlation between the occupational distributions for Crohn's disease and ulcerative colitis for both genders. A Danish prospective cohort study from 1981 to 1990 found no consistent pattern of occupations at increased risk for IBD, except that predominantly sedentary work appeared to be a risk factor.[159]

Occupational mortality statistics from England and Wales show elevations of IBD-related mortality in managerial, clerical and selling occupations.[160] Mortality from Crohn's disease was low in security and protective services, occupations involving catering, cleaning and personal services, and farming. Mortality from ulcerative colitis was low in occupations of security and protective services and construction work. A study of occupational mortality due to IBD in the United States showed reduced mortality among those employed in the livestock production, mining and grocery store industries.[161] Specific occupations associated with reduced IBD-related mortality included farming, mining machine operation, and unskilled labor. There were no industries or occupations associated with increased IBD-related mortality, although non-significant trends were noted in food products, investments/insurance, military and administration.[161]

IBD mortality appears lower in occupations associated with physically demanding work and lower social status. Higher mortality is associated with sedentary occupations and types of work that are done indoors.[160] Sonnenberg[158] has hypothesized that occupations involving work in the open air and physical activity could be protective, whereas work in air-conditioned, artificial conditions, with extended or irregular shift work could increase the risk of developing IBD. This hypothesis fits with the geographic distribution: IBD is more common in northern climates, where people spend more time indoors. It is also consistent with recent trends in IBD incidence, where rates have increased in developed countries and among migrants to developed countries. An alternative explanation, however, is that patients with recurrent symptoms seek less physically active occupations, and those with active disease and recurrent symptoms gravitate toward less demanding jobs or become disabled.

## ORAL CONTRACEPTIVES

Several cohort studies have shown an increased risk of IBD in users of oral contraceptives. Vessey et al.[162] conducted a prospective study of 17 032 white married women aged 25–39 using data from the Oxford Family Planning Association contraceptive study. For women who used oral contraceptives at the start of the study, the risk of developing ulcerative colitis was increased 2.5 times (95% CI 1.06–5.81). The risk for Crohn's disease was increased 1.7 times, with the greatest risk among women who used oral contraceptives for more than 2 years. Another cohort study using data from the Royal College of General Practitioners Oral Contraceptive Study[163] found a statistically non-significant increase in risk for both ulcerative colitis (relative risk 1.3; 95% CI 0.82–2.0) and Crohn's disease (RR 1.7; 95% CI 0.88–3.2). The Walnut Creek Contraceptive Study followed 17 939 women for an average of 6.5 years between 1968 and 1972.[164] The risk of developing IBD among current oral contraceptive users was increased 3.4-fold.

Results from several case–control studies are not as consistent as those from cohort studies. Lesko et al.,[165] in a hospital-based study of 57 women admitted with Crohn's disease and 2189 controls admitted with other conditions, found that users of oral contraceptives were at nearly twice the risk for Crohn's. The risk was greatest for those who had taken oral contraceptives for more than 5 years. Risk declined when oral contraceptives were discontinued.

Lashner et al.,[166] in another small case–control study, found no excess risk for current, former or ever-users of oral contraceptives. There was no interaction with cigarette smoking, no dose response, and no variation with location of disease. A similar study in ulcerative colitis patients by the same authors was also negative.[167] Data from North Carolina showed an increased risk for Crohn's disease in oral contraceptive users who also smoked cigarettes.[168] There was no risk attributed to oral contraceptives for non-smokers or for ulcerative colitis.

The thrombogenic properties of oral contraceptives have been proposed as a possible mechanism to explain the association with IBD. Morphologic studies have suggested that multifocal, microvascular gastrointestinal infarction may be involved in Crohn's disease,[169] and contraceptives might contribute to this. A form of ischemic colitis has been reported in young adults taking estrogen-containing drugs, presumably as a consequence of occlusion of small blood vessels,[170] but a similar evanescent condition has occurred in young people not taking contraceptives.[171] A number of features of this transient, self-limited colitis resemble Crohn's disease, specifically rectal sparing, segmental involvement of the colon, and discrete ulcers with normal adjacent mucosa.[172] Alternatively, transient ischemia caused by oral contraceptives could alter mucosal integrity to permit the absorption of luminal antigens.

## CIGARETTE SMOKING

Epidemiologists have studied the association between cigarette smoking and a number of diseases. Compared to most environmental exposures, it is relatively simple to determine smoking status. Information about cigarette smoking is often collected in general health surveys, making it possible to examine information on smoking and IBD. There have been a large number of studies on the association between cigarette smoking and IBD.[162,173–183]

### Ulcerative colitis

The inverse association between cigarette smoking and ulcerative colitis was first described as part of a comprehensive epidemiological investigation of ulcerative colitis in central Sweden in 1976.[183] However, this finding was not widely disseminated. The observation that smoking protects against ulcerative colitis was again discovered serendipitously during a study of cigarette smoking and nutrition.[175] Since that initial report, numerous studies, using different case groups in vastly different geographic areas, have shown remarkably consistent results. Virtually all of them indicate a decreased risk of ulcerative colitis for current smokers (Table 17.4). One notable exception is a lack of an association between smoking and ulcerative colitis in an Israeli Jewish population, a group thought to be at higher risk for ulcerative colitis.[184] The study suggests that genetic factors could mediate the effect of smoking.

Several meta-analyses have been published that pool the estimates from the methodologically sound studies.[185–188] As is often the case with meta-analyses, different authors have pooled slightly different studies. Fortunately they have each reached similar conclusions: the risk of developing ulcerative colitis among current smokers is 40% that of non-smokers. The findings are generally similar in men and women.[180] The risk of developing primary sclerosing cholangitis (PSC) may also be reduced among current smokers.[189,190] The protective effect against PSC suggests a systemic protective effect rather than a local effect in the colon.

The findings for *former* smokers are also quite consistent, but opposite to those for current smokers (Table 17.4). Former smokers are at increased risk for ulcerative colitis. Some studies have shown this increased risk to be statistically significant, but others have not. However, the meta-analyses suggest that former smokers are approximately 1.7 times more likely to develop ulcerative colitis than never-smokers. If cigarette smoking is

**Table 17.4 Selected case–control studies of cigarette smoking and ulcerative colitis**

| Author (ref) | Current smokers | | Former smokers | |
|---|---|---|---|---|
| | Relative risk* | 95% CI | Relative risk* | 95% CI |
| Harries[175] | 0.1 | 0.1–0.3 | 1.5 | 0.9–2.4 |
| Gyde[301] | 0.2 | 0.1–0.5 | 0.7 | 0.3–1.5 |
| Tobin[180] | 0.2 | 0.1–0.3 | 1.5 | 0.8–2.8 |
| Jick[176] | 0.3 | 0.2–0.4 | 1.1 | 0.8–1.8 |
| Logan[177] | 0.3 | 0.2–0.6 | 2.8 | 1.5–5.0 |
| Lorusso[182] | 0.3 | 0.1–0.9 | 1.4 | 0.5–4.1 |
| Thornton[207] | 0.3 | 0.1–1.1 | 12.2 | 2.1–89.9 |
| Nakamura[194] | 0.3 | 0.2–0.5 | 1.5 | 0.9–2.6 |
| Sandler[218] | 0.5 | 0.2–1.1 | 1.3 | 0.7–2.5 |
| Boyko[173] | 0.6 | 0.4–1.0 | 2.0 | 1.1–3.7 |
| Lindberg[178] | 0.6 | 0.4–0.9 | 2.2 | 1.4–3.5 |
| Franceschi[174] | 0.6 | 0.3–1.0 | 2.6 | 1.4–4.6 |
| Vessey[162] | 0.8 | 0.4–1.4 | 1.2 | 0.6–2.6 |
| Persson[179] | 0.8 | 0.5–1.3 | 1.5 | 0.8–2.6 |

*Relative risks for current and former smokers compared to non-smokers.

'protective' against ulcerative colitis, it is not unexpected that ex-smokers lose this protection, but it is hard to explain why the risk becomes higher. Some have suggested that early symptoms of ulcerative colitis might have led to smoking cessation, which would explain the apparent increased risk. However, when Boyko et al.[173] stratified their data by interval between smoking cessation and onset of ulcerative colitis they found that even remote cessation was associated with increased risk. Although other studies have suggested clustering of cessation shortly before onset,[191,192] this may have been coincident with disease onset and not causally related.

Dose response is one of the features of an exposure–disease association that epidemiologists use to evaluate cause and effect.[193] Several studies have explored dose response, and although some demonstrate a lower risk of ulcerative colitis with heavier smoking than lighter smoking,[174,176,178,180,194] others do not.[173,195] Although the presence of a consistent dose response would support causality, its absence may simply indicate a threshold, rather than dose response.

Investigators have also examined the effect of cigarette smoking on the course of ulcerative colitis. Boyko et al.[196] reported that current smokers were half as likely to be hospitalized for ulcerative colitis than non-smokers, whereas former smokers were 50% more likely to be hospitalized. Ex-smokers were twice as likely to require colectomy as current or never-smokers. Rudra et al.[197] found that 14 of 30 patients with ulcerative colitis who resumed smoking had an improvement in their symptoms over a median period of 6 weeks. Interestingly, the responders smoked twice as many cigarettes daily as the non-responders. The study was not controlled and may be subject to significant bias. A study of smokers with ulcerative colitis who stopped smoking demonstrated increased severity of disease, more hospitalizations, and more need for corticosteroids or azathioprine than patients who were non-smokers or who continued to smoke.[198]

The results of the observational studies have led to treatment with nicotine, although the effects of smoking could be due to any one of the thousands of chemicals present in tobacco smoke.

Roberts and Diggle[199] described a woman who repeatedly induced remission with nicotine gum. Lashner et al.[200] formally tested the effect of nicotine gum in a double-blind randomized crossover trial with individual patients (single-patient trial, or *n* of 1 clinical trial). Three of seven patients (all former smokers) improved when nicotine gum was added to their regimens. However, not all studies confirm benefit from nicotine gum.[201]

Several clinical trials have evaluated the potential beneficial effects of nicotine on ulcerative colitis utilizing a transdermal route. Two randomized, double-blind placebo-controlled trials of transdermal nicotine (11–25 mg/day) for active disease demonstrated clinical improvement in 40–50% of patients receiving nicotine versus 9–24% of those receiving placebo;[202,203] however, neither study demonstrated significantly higher remission rates with nicotine. A randomized trial of transdermal nicotine versus placebo patches for maintenance of remission showed no benefit of nicotine over placebo.[204] Another randomized clinical trial compared transdermal nicotine against 15 mg of oral prednisolone for active disease.[205] The nicotine group had fewer remissions and more side effects than the prednisolone group. Only one in five patients in the nicotine group reached full sigmoidoscopic remission in the 6-week trial. The plateau nicotine levels achieved with transdermal patches are lower than the peaks seen in smokers.[206] Perhaps the benefit of smoking on ulcerative colitis depends on these peaks, or perhaps other components of cigarette smoke contribute to the protective effects.

## Crohn's disease

In stark contrast to the protective effect of cigarette smoking on ulcerative colitis, several studies have demonstrated that smoking increases the risk for Crohn's disease[174,180,207,208] (Table 17.5). Meta-analyses pooling results from methodologically sound studies have concluded that smokers are more than twice as likely to develop Crohn's disease.[185–187] Interestingly, the association appears to be stronger in women. Ex-smokers also appear to be at increased risk, although the level of risk is somewhat less than that for current smokers. There is no apparent dose response.[174,178,180] The association between

**Table 17.5 Selected case–control studies of cigarette smoking and Crohn's disease**

| Author (ref) | Current smokers | | Former smokers | |
|---|---|---|---|---|
| | Relative risk* | 95% CI | Relative risk* | 95% CI |
| Franceschi[174] | 3.9 | 2.2–7.0 | 3.2 | 1.3–8.1 |
| Silverstein[208] | 3.7 | 1.9–7.1 | N/A | N/A |
| Somerville[181] | 3.5 | 1.8–6.6 | N/A | N/A |
| Sicilia[302] | 3.1 | 1.6–6.1 | N/A | N/A |
| Lindberg[178] | 2.0 | 1.3–3.1 | 1.9 | 0.8–4.3 |
| Tobin[180] | 1.9 | 1.1–3.1 | 1.6 | 0.6–4.1 |
| Vessey[162] | 1.8 | 1.3–2.6 | 0.8 | 0.1–5.0 |
| Harries[303] | 1.2 | 0.7–1.9 | 1.7 | 1.0–2.8 |

*Relative risk for current and former smokers compared to non-smokers.

smoking and Crohn's disease may not apply to all ethnic groups or geographic regions. Three Israeli studies did not demonstrate an elevated risk of Crohn's disease among current or former smokers.[209,210]

Smoking may modify the clinical course of Crohn's disease. Several studies suggest that Crohn's disease patients who smoke are more likely to have ileal than colonic or ileocolonic involvement.[211,212] Continued cigarette smoking following surgical resection increases the risk of recurrent disease. Sutherland et al.[213] found that women smokers were more than four times more likely to require another operation for recurrent Crohn's disease than were non-smokers (odds ratio 4.1, 95% CI 2.0–4.2). A dose–response effect of smoking on the risk of requiring a second surgery in women was noted. The risk was slightly increased in men as well (odds ratio 1.5, 95% CI 0.8–6.0). This finding has been replicated by a number of researchers.[214,215] Crohn's disease patients who smoke are more likely to require immunosuppressive agents.[214] The health-related quality of life of female patients who smoke is significantly lower than that of those who do not.[216] Conversely, patients who quit smoking noted fewer exacerbations and required less corticosteroid or immunosuppressive therapy than patients who continued to smoke.[217]

## Passive smoking

Passive smoking has also been linked to IBD risk, but results have been conflicting. One case–control study conducted in North Carolina found that adult subjects exposed as children to environmental tobacco smoke in the home were half as likely to develop ulcerative colitis as those not so exposed.[218] The effect of passive smoking in childhood was comparable to that of active smoking in adulthood. However, another study[219] found that passive smoking exposure at birth was significantly associated with the development of both Crohn's disease (OR 5.3) and ulcerative colitis (OR 2.2). The association for Crohn's disease demonstrated a dose–response relationship. In a Swedish study exposure to secondhand cigarette smoke in childhood increased the risk of CD but not ulcerative colitis.[211] An Israeli study of passive smoking among adults with IBD showed no overall differences in exposure among patients or controls, although ulcerative colitis patients may have had less exposure to secondhand smoke when a quantitative index was employed.[220]

## Non-steroidal anti-inflammatory drugs

Non-steroidal anti-inflammatory drugs (NSAIDs) have a variety of effects on the intestinal tract, ranging from asymptomatic mucosal inflammation to strictures, obstruction, perforation and major hemorrhage.[221,222] NSAIDs block the cyclooxygenase pathway of arachidonic acid metabolism.[223] Given the possible role of prostaglandins in intestinal inflammation and immuno-regulation, it is not surprising that these drugs might influence IBD. The specific effects have been somewhat unexpected, however. Although prostaglandin inhibitors might be anticipated to be beneficial in the treatment of IBD, studies of indomethacin have found the opposite: they caused an exacerbation of disease in some patients.[223,224]

These results are supported by the induction of mid small intestinal ulcers in susceptible rat strains by short-term injection of indomethacin,[225,226] activation of chronic aggressive colitis in IL-10$^{-/-}$ mice on a low susceptibility genetic background by NSAIDs,[227] and more aggressive induced colitis in COX-1 and -2 knockout mice.[228] Prostaglandins mediate secretory diarrhea but have important immunosuppressive properties. Oral administration of indomethacin can produce an ulcerative enterocolitis in dogs which resembles features of Crohn's disease, including ulceration of the terminal ileum or colonic skip lesions, and transmural inflammation.[229] The intestinal lesions resemble those of inflammatory bowel disease in particular.

Orally administered NSAIDs have been reported to precipitate relapse in patients with inactive ulcerative proctocolitis.[230,231] The effect is not confined to those with an established diagnosis of IBD. Hall et al.[232] reported two patients who developed colitis while on mefenamic acid who had rapid and permanent improvement in symptoms when NSAID treatment was stopped. The patients had a recurrence on re-exposure. There have been a number of similar reports.[233–236] There are also isolated reports of salicylates exacerbating proctocolitis.[237,238] Sulfasalazine, a mainstay in the therapy of ulcerative colitis, has been rarely reported to exacerbate ulcerative colitis,[239] possibly owing to the salicylate component of the sulfasalazine.

Using the indium-111 ($^{111}$In) leukocyte technique, NSAIDs have been shown to cause small intestinal inflammation in two-thirds of patients on long-term treatment for rheumatoid arthritis.[240] Patients with rheumatoid arthritis who had not received NSAIDs showed no evidence of intestinal inflammation. Some of the patients had radiographic evidence of ileal mucosal irregularity, ulceration and strictures that resembled Crohn's disease. In other patients NSAIDs have been shown to produce an unusual form of intestinal stricture characterized by a bland external appearance of the small bowel at surgery, but a striking mucosal appearance with multiple concentric circumferential diaphragmatic strictures that caused luminal stenosis to a pinhole.[241] The septa were due to submucosal fibrosis.

NSAID use is widespread. Some individuals would be expected to develop intestinal inflammation simply by chance. Because the literature on the association between NSAIDs and IBD consists largely of case reports it is difficult to estimate the magnitude of the problem. As a rough approximation, Tanner and Raghunath[242] have estimated that NSAID use increased the risk of Crohn's colitis fivefold.

## APPENDECTOMY

Appendectomy has been reported to be a potential protective factor for ulcerative colitis. The association was first reported by Gilat et al.[141] in an international study of childhood IBD. The inverse relationship between appendectomy and ulcerative colitis has been confirmed in numerous studies[243–251] (Table 17.6). A meta-analysis of 13 case–control studies involving over 2700 cases and 3300 controls yielded a pooled odds ratio of 0.31 (95% CI 0.25–0.38).[243] Stated another way, appendectomy was associated with a 69% reduction in the subsequent risk of ulcerative colitis.[243] Some (but not all) of these case–control studies adjusted for other important factors, such as age, gender, socioeconomic factors and cigarette smoking. In virtually all studies where such factors were taken into account, the apparent protective effect of appendectomy remained significant. Table 17.6 summarizes the studies of ulcerative colitis and appendectomy.

Two large population-based cohort studies of appendectomy and subsequent risk of ulcerative colitis have recently been published, with conflicting results.[244,246] Andersson et al.[244,245] utilized a national inpatient register in Sweden to assemble a cohort of over 212 000 patients who had undergone appendectomy over a 30-year period and a cohort of age-, gender- and location-matched controls. These cohorts were followed for over 5 million person-years for a subsequent hospital diagnosis of ulcerative colitis. Those undergoing appendectomy had a lower subsequent incidence of ulcerative colitis (incidence rate ratio 0.74; 95% CI 0.64–0.86). When indication for appendectomy was examined, those who underwent operation for appendicitis and mesenteric lymphadenitis had a significantly lower incidence rate of ulcerative colitis, whereas those who underwent appendectomy for non-specific abdominal pain did not.[244] The cumulative incidence of ulcerative colitis among those undergoing appendectomy for appendicitis before the age of 20 was significantly lower than that of the cohort of matched controls, but this difference was not seen in those undergoing surgery after the age of 20. Using similar methodology in Denmark, Frisch et al.[246] developed a cohort of 154 000 patients who had undergone appendectomy over a 13-year period. They were followed for over 1 million person-years for a subsequent hospital diagnosis of IBD. Expected numbers of hospitalizations for IBD were derived from previously published national rates.[8] Although fewer hospital diagnoses of UC than expected were observed (RR 0.87), this was not statistically significant (95% CI 0.69–1.07). The reasons for these disparate results remain unclear. The Swedish study excluded UC diagnosed within 1 year of appendectomy, whereas the Danish study did not; however, even if these UC diagnoses are included, the results are little changed.[244,245] Overall, the bulk of the evidence from both case–control and cohort studies suggests that appendectomy is a protective factor for ulcerative colitis.

As with smoking, there has been an opposite positive association between appendectomy and Crohn's disease.[150,298,300–303] However, the association has been smaller than for ulcerative colitis. In the case of Crohn's disease, appendectomies are frequently performed near the time of the diagnosis, suggesting that surgery may have been a function of undiagnosed Crohn's disease.[251]

The mechanisms whereby appendectomy might protect against ulcerative colitis but not Crohn's disease are unknown. It is postulated that chronic intestinal inflammation is due to defective mucosal immunoregulation. Removal of the appendix, with its large lymphoid aggregates, might alter the balance of regulatory and effector T cells. This concept is supported by decreased experimental colitis when the tip of the cecum is resected or bypassed in genetically engineered rodents.[252,253] Alternatively, individuals who are predisposed to ulcerative colitis might be less likely to develop appendicitis. Finally, the finding may be spurious, the result of incomplete control for some confounding factor. The rates of appendicitis have declined. If appendectomies had an important protective role in ulcerative colitis, then the incidence of ulcerative colitis should be increasing. There has been no such increase.

## MEASLES

During the past decade there has been considerable interest in a possible association between exposure to measles virus and the subsequent development of IBD.[254–256] Although wildtype measles virus has been the focus of most investigations, the attenuated live-virus measles vaccine has also been implicated.[257]

## Table 17.6 Appendectomy and ulcerative colitis

| Author (ref) | Cases | | Controls | | Odds Ratio | 95% CI |
|---|---|---|---|---|---|---|
| | No. | % | No. | % | | |
| Rutgeerts[304] | 1/174 | 0.6 | 41/161 | 26.0 | 0.02 | 0.002–0.89 |
| Duggan[249] | 9/213 | 4.5 | 57/337 | 16.9 | 0.20 | 0.1–0.4 |
| Gilat[141] | 4/133 | 3.0 | 27/266 | 10.2 | 0.20 | 0.1–0.8 |
| Gent[146] | 9/220 | 4.1 | 32/220 | 14.5 | 0.30 | 0.1–0.6 |
| Smithson[305] | 7/197 | 3.6 | 26/243 | 10.7 | 0.30 | 0.1–0.7 |
| Russel[251] | 21/423 | 5.0 | 44/423 | 9.7 | 0.36 | 0.2–0.8 |

Investigators have looked for serologic evidence of measles infection in patients with Crohn's disease and their families.[258,259] These studies have not supported an association. Four separate groups have tried to isolate measles virus RNA from intestinal tissue of patients with Crohn's disease.[260–263] Attempts have been uniformly unsuccessful.

Hermon-Taylor and colleagues[264] examined the number of reported measles cases in England and Wales over the period from 1940 to 1990 and found a dramatic reduction in measles cases after 1968, corresponding to the introduction of the measles vaccine. Despite a substantial decline in wildtype measles infection, the incidence of Crohn's disease continued to rise. Although one might argue that measles vaccine (rather than wildtype measles) was responsible for this trend, the incidence of Crohn's disease was already rising before the vaccine was introduced.

Feeney and colleagues[265] performed a case–control study in 140 patients with IBD (83 with Crohn's) and 280 controls matched for age, sex and general practitioner area. They found essentially no difference in the crude rates of measles vaccination between IBD cases (56.4%) and controls (57.1%). Matched odds ratios for measles vaccination were 1.08 (95% CI 0.62–1.88) in patients with CD and 0.84 (0.44–1.58) in patients with ulcerative colitis.

Longitudinal data from several British cohort studies have been used to examine the association between measles or measles vaccination and IBD. Morris and colleagues[266] found no significant association between measles vaccination and subsequent development of Crohn's disease (RR 1.21, 95% CI 0.5–2.89) or ulcerative colitis (RR 1.31, 95% CI 0.47–3.65). Montgomery and colleagues[267] examined data on individuals participating in a 1970 British Cohort study. Measles infection alone was not a risk factor for the subsequent development of either CD or ulcerative colitis. Thompson et al.[268] found that measles infection was not associated with an increased risk for Crohn's disease (OR 1.09, 95% CI 0.36–3.52) or for ulcerative colitis (OR 1.52, 95% CI 0.47–5.46).

Several groups have investigated whether the offspring of women exposed to measles in utero might be at increased risk.[269–272] The studies do not support the hypothesis that antenatal exposure to measles is a risk factor for the subsequent development of Crohn's disease.

It would be a mistake to avoid vaccinating children against measles because of fear of Crohn's disease. The risk of death and disability from measles virus infection has been unequivocally demonstrated, whereas the association between measles virus and Crohn's disease remains a poorly supported conjecture.[256,273]

## MISCELLANEOUS

Thrombotic mesenteric microvascular occlusion has been postulated to be a cause of IBD. A national survey in the UK evaluating the prevalence of IBD among patients with inherited disorders of coagulation showed that IBD occurred less frequently than expected in patients with hemophilia or von Willebrand's disease (standardized morbidity ratios 0.33–0.24, 95% CI 0.90–0.01).[274] These results were not explained by age- or sex-related differences from the general population, mortality or HIV infection. They support the theory that thrombotic events may be crucial in the development of IBD and may help explain associations with cigarette smoking and oral contraceptives.

Lichen planus is a relatively common inflammatory disease affecting the skin, nails and mucous membranes that may be due to defects in cell-mediated immunity. A large multicenter case–control study in Italy has shown an association between lichen planus and ulcerative colitis.[275] Eczema and psoriasis are more common in patients with IBD and their first-degree relatives.[276,277]

IBD might be due to an allergy.[278] Like IBD, allergy and asthma have dramatically increased in frequency in industrialized societies in the second half of the 20th century, possibly as a result of public health measures and medical practices that have created a cleaner environment (hygiene hypothesis).[279] A survey of IBD patients found a high proportion with allergic diatheses. Immunoregulation is important in the development and course of both IBD and allergies/asthma, but the role of allergy in IBD has not been properly tested in an epidemiological study.

There has been a suggestion of a familial concurrence of multiple sclerosis and IBD, perhaps owing to shared genetic factors.[280,281] A report from Vancouver found a striking concordance between multiple sclerosis and IBD.[282] The authors speculated that one or more loci contributing to IBD might determine susceptibility to multiple sclerosis. Alternatively, a generalized problem of immune control could result in familial occurrence of both diseases. Similarly, psoriasis and IBD have been linked in families.[277]

## CONCLUSIONS

Despite genuine uncertainty about the etiology of IBD, there are certain epidemiologic facts that are incontrovertible. Both Crohn's disease and ulcerative colitis are more common in the developed countries of Scandinavia, Europe and North America, and uncommon in Asia, Africa and South America. However, the incidence of IBD is increasing in these less developed countries as they become more industrialized and adopt Western dietary and cultural practices. There also appears to be a distinct north–south gradient in incidence. The incidence of ulcerative colitis has remained relatively stable, but the incidence of Crohn's has increased precipitously since its description in 1932. This rising incidence has plateaued and may be decreasing in most areas. Ulcerative colitis has been more common than Crohn's disease, but now Crohn's disease is more common than ulcerative colitis in many areas. IBD typically affects young people, but may have a bimodal incidence with a second peak in later life. The explanation for the second peak is not known. Men are slightly more likely to be affected with ulcerative colitis and women with Crohn's disease. The incidence of IBD among blacks in Africa is low, but in the United States there is evidence from Baltimore to suggest that the rates in blacks are similar to those in whites. The rates among Jews are high relative to the non-Jewish population in every country studied, but rates among Jews in different countries vary considerably and mirror the overall incidence and prevalence rates. IBD is more common in urban than in rural areas, and among those with sedentary indoor occupations. Early life events (possibly infectious) may alter adult susceptibility. Exposure to tobacco smoke, oral contraceptives, non-steroidal anti-inflammatory agents and possibly diet also influences disease expression.

Great strides have been made in our understanding of the genetic basis for many diseases. There is now indisputable evidence of heritable factors in the genesis of IBD, but it is clear that genetic factors interact with environmental influences. The most obvious evidence of an environmental influence is the discordance rates in identical twins of 85–90% in ulcerative colitis and 50–55% in Crohn's disease.[283, 284] Similarly, smoking may influence the phenotype of disease. In multiplex families with both ulcerative colitis and Crohn's disease, smoking is highly associated with Crohn's disease and non-smoking with ulcerative colitis.[285] The rapid changes in rates over time for Crohn's disease are due to environmental, not genetic, factors. Changes in disease rates with geography and population migrations further support non-genetic factors. Evidence of higher rates of IBD in urban areas and among those with indoor occupations raises the possibility of a transmissible agent or public health measures that may be responsible for disease expression or increased susceptibility.

The evidence in support of important environmental causes for IBD does not imply that genes are unimportant. The observations outlined in this chapter strongly support the necessity for genetic–environmental interactions in the pathogenesis of IBD, with important contributions by dietary influences on enteric commensal bacteria and environmental triggers such as infections or NSAIDs.

# REFERENCES

1. Sinclair TS, Brunt PW, Mowat NA. Nonspecific proctocolitis in northeastern Scotland: a community study. Gastroenterology 1983;85:1–11.

2. Haug K, Schrumpf E, Barstad S et al. Epidemiology of ulcerative colitis in western Norway. Scand J Gastroenterol 1988;23:517–522.

3. Kildebo S, Nordgaard K, Aronsen O et al. The incidence of ulcerative colitis in Northern Norway from 1983 to 1986. The Northern Norwegian Gastroenterology Society. Scand J Gastroenterol 1990;25:890–896.

4. Shivananda S, Weterman IT, Pena AS. Epidemiology of inflammatory bowel disease in the Netherlands. Front Gastrointest Res 1986;11:54–57.

5. Odes HS, Fraser D, Krawiec J. Incidence of idiopathic ulcerative colitis in Jewish population subgroups in the Beer Sheva region of Israel. Am J Gastroenterol 1987;82:854–858.

6. Niv Y, Torten D, Tamir A et al. Incidence and prevalence of ulcerative colitis in the upper Galilee, Northern Israel, 1967–1986. Am J Gastroenterol 1990;85:1580–1583.

7. Desai Y, Seebaran AR, Pillay CN. Crohn's disease in the Indian population of Durban. S Africa J Surg 1987;25:144–145.

8. Fonager K, Sorensen HT, Olsen J. Change in incidence of Crohn's disease and ulcerative colitis in Denmark. A study based on the National Registry of Patients, 1981–1992. Int J Epidemiol 1997;26:1003–1008.

9. Flamenbaum M, Zenut M, Aublet-Cuvelier B et al. Incidence of inflammatory bowel diseases in the department of Puy-de-Dome in 1993 and 1994. EPIMICI. Epidémiologie des Maladies Inflammatoires Cryptogénétiques de l'Intestin group. Gastroenterol Clin Biol 1997;21:491–496.

10. Pagenault M, Tron I, Alexandre JL et al. Incidence of inflammatory bowel diseases in Bretagne (1994–1995). ABERMAD. Association Bertonne d'Etude et de Recherche des Maladies de l'Appareil Digestif. Gastroenterol Clin Biol 1997;21:483–490.

11. Tragnone A, Corrao G, Miglio F et al. Incidence of inflammatory bowel disease in Italy: a nationwide population-based study. Gruppo Italiano per lo Studio del Colon e del Retto (GISC). Int J Epidemiol 1996;25:1044–1052.

12. Trallori G, Palli D, Saieva C et al. A population-based study of inflammatory bowel disease in Florence over 15 years (1978–92). Scand J Gastroenterol 1996;31:892–899.

13. Moum B, Vatn MH, Ekbom A et al. Incidence of Crohn's disease in four counties in southeastern Norway, 1990–93. A prospective population-based study. The Inflammatory Bowel South-Eastern Norway (IBSEN) Study Group of Gastroenterologists. Scand J Gastroenterol 1996;31:355–361.

14. Pinchbeck BR, Kirdeikis J, Thomson AB. Inflammatory bowel disease in northern Alberta. An epidemiologic study. J Clin Gastroenterol 1988;10:505–515.

15. Manousos ON, Koutroubakis I, Potamianos S et al. A prospective epidemiologic study of Crohn's disease in Heraklion, Crete. Incidence over a 5-year period. Scand J Gastroenterol 1996;31:599–603.

16. Bernstein CN, Blanchard JF, Rawsthorne P et al. Epidemiology of Crohn's disease and ulcerative colitis in a central Canadian province: a population-based study. Am J Epidemiol 1999;149:916–924.

17. Shivananda S, Lennard-Jones J, Logan R et al. Incidence of inflammatory bowel disease across Europe: is there a difference between north and south? Results of the European Collaborative Study on Inflammatory Bowel Disease (EC-IBD). Gut 1996;39:690–697.

18. Law NM, Lim CC, Chong R et al. Crohn's disease in the Singapore Chinese population. J Clin Gastroenterol 1998;26:27–29.

19. Chuttani HK, Nigam SP, Sama SK et al. Ulcerative colitis in the tropics. Br Med J 1967;4:204–207.

20. Binder V, Both H, Hansen PK et al. Incidence and prevalence of ulcerative colitis and Crohn's disease in the County of Copenhagen, 1962 to 1978. Gastroenterology 1982;83:563–568.

21. Evans JG, Acheson ED. An epidemiological study of ulcerative colitis and regional enteritis in the Oxford area. Gut 1965;6:311–324.

22. Berner J, Kiaer T. Ulcerative colitis and Crohn's disease on the Faroe Islands 1964–83. A retrospective epidemiological survey. Scand J Gastroenterol 1986;21:188–192.

23. Loftus EV Jr, Silverstein MD, Sandborn WJ et al. Ulcerative colitis in Olmsted County, Minnesota, 1940–1993: incidence, prevalence, and survival. Gut 2000;46:336–343.

24. Crohn BB, Ginzburg L, Oppenheimer GD. Regional ileitis: a pathologic and clinical entity. JAMA 1932;99:1323–1329.

25. Kirsner JB. Origins and directions of inflammatory bowel disease. Dordrecht: Kluwer Academic Publishers; 2001.

26. Gilat T, Langman MJS, Rozen P. Environmental factors in inflammatory bowel disease. Front Gastrointest Res 1986;11:158–176.

27. Calkins BM, Mendeloff AI. Epidemiology of inflammatory bowel disease. Epidemiol Rev 1986;8:60–91.

28. Vucelic B, Korac B, Sentic M et al. Epidemiology of Crohn's disease in Zagreb, Yugoslavia: a ten-year prospective study. Int J Epidemiol 1991;20:216–220.

29. Teh LB, Ng HS, Ho MS et al. Crohn's disease – a diagnostic rarity in Singapore. Ann Acad Med Singapore 1987;16:480–487.

30. Tandon BN, Mathur AK, Mohapatra LN et al. A study of the prevalence and clinical pattern of non-specific ulcerative colitis in northern India. Gut 1965;6:448–453.

31. McDermott FT, Whelan G, St John DJ et al. Relative incidence of Crohn's disease and ulcerative colitis in six Melbourne hospitals. Med J Aust 1987;146:525, 528–529.

32. Monsen U. Inflammatory bowel disease. An epidemiological and genetic study. Acta Chir Scand 1990;559(Suppl):1–42.

33. Hellers G. Crohn's disease in Stockholm County 1955–1974. A study of epidemiology, results of surgical treatment and long-term prognosis. Acta Chir Scand Suppl 1979;490:1–84.

34. Stowe SP, Redmond SR, Stormont JM et al. An epidemiologic study of inflammatory bowel disease in Rochester, New York. Hospital incidence. Gastroenterology 1990;98:104–110.

35. Thomas GA, Millar-Jones D, Rhodes J et al. Incidence of Crohn's disease in Cardiff over 60 years: 1986–1990 an update. Eur J Gastroenterol Hepatol 1995;7:401–405.

36. Morris T, Rhodes J. Incidence of ulcerative colitis in the Cardiff region 1968–1977. Gut 1984;25:846–848.

37. Daiss W, Scheurlen M, Malchow H. Epidemiology of inflammatory bowel disease in the county of Tubingen (West Germany). Scand J Gastroenterol Suppl 1989;170:39–43.

38. Colombel JF, Cortot A et al. Incidence of inflammatory bowel disease in northwestern France. Preliminary results in region Nord-Pas-de-Calais. Scand J Gastroenterol 1989;170(Suppl):22–24.

39. Ekbom A, Helmick C, Zack M et al. The epidemiology of inflammatory bowel disease: a large, population-based study in Sweden. Gastroenterology 1991;100:350–358.

40. Kurata JH, Kantor-Fish S, Frankl H et al. Crohn's disease among ethnic groups in a large health maintenance organization. Gastroenterology 1992;102:1940–1948.

41. Loftus EV, Silverstein MD, Sandborn WJ et al. Crohn's disease in Olmsted County, Minnesota, 1940–1993: incidence, prevalence, and survival. Gastroenterology 1998;114:1161–1168.

42. Langholz E, Munkholm P, Nielsen OH et al. Incidence and prevalence of ulcerative colitis in Copenhagen county from 1962 to 1987. Scand J Gastroenterol 1991;26:1247–1256.

43. Munkholm P, Langholz E, Nielsen OH et al. Incidence and prevalence of Crohn's disease in the county of Copenhagen, 1962–87: a sixfold increase in incidence. Scand J Gastroenterol 1992;27:609–614.

44. Kyle J. An epidemiological study of Crohn's disease in Northeast Scotland. Gastroenterology 1971;61:826–833.

45. Mate-Jimenez J, Munoz S, Vicent D et al. Incidence and prevalence of ulcerative colitis and Crohn's disease in urban and rural areas of Spain from 1981 to 1988. J Clin Gastroenterol 1994;18:27–31.

46. Vucelic B, Korac B, Sentic M et al. Ulcerative colitis in Zagreb, Yugoslavia: incidence and prevalence 1980–1989. Int J Epidemiol 1991;20:1043–1047.

47. Rubin DT, Hanauer SB. Smoking and inflammatory bowel disease. Eur J Gastroenterol Hepatol 2000;12:855–862.

48. Montgomery SM, Morris DL, Thompson NP et al. Prevalence of inflammatory bowel disease in British 26 year olds: national longitudinal birth cohort. Br Med J 1998;316:1058–1059.

49. Fireman Z, Grossman A, Lilos P et al. Epidemiology of Crohn's disease in the Jewish population of central Israel, 1970–1980. Am J Gastroenterol 1989;84:255–258.

50. Grossman A, Fireman Z, Lilos P et al. Epidemiology of ulcerative colitis in the Jewish population of central Israel 1970–1980. Hepatogastroenterology 1989;36:193–197.

51. Odes HS, Fraser D, Krawiec J. Incidence of idiopathic ulcerative colitis in Jewish population subgroups in the Beer Sheva region of Israel. Am J Gastroenterol 1987;82:854–858.

52. Odes HS, Locker C, Neumann L et al. Epidemiology of Crohn's disease in southern Israel. Am J Gastroenterol 1994;89:1859–1862.

53. Morita N, Toki S, Hirohashi T et al. Incidence and prevalence of inflammatory bowel disease in Japan: nationwide epidemiological survey during the year 1991. J Gastroenterol 1995;30(Suppl 8):1–4.

54. Lee YM, Fock KM, See SJ et al. Racial differences in the prevalence of ulcerative colitis and Crohn's disease in Singapore. J Gastroenterol Hepatol 2000;15:622–625.

55. Yang SK, Hong WS, Min YI et al. Incidence and prevalence of ulcerative colitis in the Songpa-Kangdong District, Seoul, Korea, 1986–1997. J Gastroenterol Hepatol 2000;15:1037–1042.

56. Nordenholtz KE, Stowe SP, Stormont JM et al. The cause of death in inflammatory bowel disease: a comparison of death certificates and hospital charts in Rochester, New York. Am J Gastroenterol 1995;90:927–932.

57. Sonnenberg A, Koch TR. Period and generation effects on mortality from idiopathic inflammatory bowel disease. Dig Dis Sci 1989;34:1720–1729.

58. Persson PG, Bernell O, Leijonmarck CE et al. Survival and cause-specific mortality in inflammatory bowel disease: a population-based cohort study. Gastroenterology 1996;110:1339–1345.

59. Ekbom A, Helmick C, Zack M et al. Ulcerative proctitis in central Sweden 1965–1983. A population-based epidemiological study. Dig Dis Sci 1991;6:97–102.

60. Langholz E, Munkholm P, Davidsen M et al. Colorectal cancer risk and mortality in patients with ulcerative colitis. Gastroenterology 1992;103:1444–1451.

61. Probert CS, Jayanthi V, Wicks AC et al. Mortality in patients with ulcerative colitis in Leicestershire, 1972–1989. An epidemiological study. Dig Dis Sci 1993;38:538–541.

62. Farrokhyar F, Swarbrick ET, Grace RH et al. Low mortality in ulcerative colitis and Crohn's disease in three regional centers in England. Am J Gastroenterol 2001;96:501–507.

63. Davoli M, Prantera C, Berto E et al. Mortality among patients with ulcerative colitis: Rome 1970–1989. Eur J Epidemiol 1997;13:189–194.

64. Palli D, Trallori G, Saieva C et al. General and cancer specific mortality of a population based cohort of patients with inflammatory bowel disease: the Florence Study. Gut 1998;42:175–179.

65. Stonnington CM, Phillips SF, Melton LJD et al. Chronic ulcerative colitis: incidence and prevalence in a community. Gut 1987; 28:402–409.

66. Ekbom A, Helmick CG, Zack M et al. Survival and causes of death in patients with inflammatory bowel disease: a population-based study. Gastroenterology 1992;103:954–960.

67. Ekbom A, Helmick CG, Zack M et al. Survival and causes of death in patients with inflammatory bowel disease: a population-based study. Gastroenterology 1992;103:954–960.

68. Ekbom A, Helmick CG, Zack M et al. Survival and causes of death in patients with inflammatory bowel disease: a population-based study. Gastroenterology 1992;103:954–960.

69. Mayberry JF, Newcombe RG, Rhodes J. Mortality in Crohn's disease. QJ Med 1980;49:63–68.

70. Ekbom A, Helmick CG, Zack M et al. Survival and causes of death in patients with inflammatory bowel disease: a population-based study. Gastroenterology 1992;103:954–960.

71. Jess T, Winther KV, Munkholm P et al. Mortality and causes of death in Crohn's disease: follow-up of a population-based cohort in Copenhagen County, Denmark. Gastroenterology 2002; 122:1808–1814.

72. Probert CS, Jayanthi V, Wicks AC et al. Mortality from Crohn's disease in Leicestershire, 1972–1989: an epidemiological community based study. Gut 1992;33:1226–1228.

73. Sonnenberg A. Mortality from Crohn's disease and ulcerative colitis in England–Wales and the US from 1950 to 1983. Dis Colon Rectum 1986;29:624–629.

74. Sonnenberg A. Disability from inflammatory bowel disease among employees in West Germany. Gut 1989;30:367–370.

75. Bernstein CN, Kraut A, Blanchard JF et al. The relationship between inflammatory bowel disease and socioeconomic variables. Am J Gastroenterol 2001;96:2117–2125.

76. Sonnenberg A. Hospital discharges for inflammatory bowel disease. Time trends from England and the United States. Dig Dis Sci 1990;35:375–381.

77. Sonnenberg A, McCarty DJ, Jacobsen SJ. Geographic variation of inflammatory bowel disease within the United States. Gastroenterology 1991;100:143–149.

78. Sonnenberg A, Wasserman IH. Epidemiology of inflammatory bowel disease among US military veterans. Gastroenterology 1991;101:122–130.

79. Yang S, Loftus EV, Sandborn WJ. Epidemiology of inflammatory bowel disease in Asia. Inflamm Bowel Dis 2001;7:260–270.

80. Yang HY, Taylor KD, Rotter JI. Inflammatory bowel disease – I. Genetic epidemiology. Mol Genet Metab 2001;74:1–21.

81. Yao T, Matsui T, Hiwatashi N. Crohn's disease in Japan – Diagnostic criteria and epidemiology. Dis Colon Rectum 2000;43:S85–S93.

82. Calkins BM, Lilienfeld AM, Garland CF et al. Trends in incidence rates of ulcerative colitis and Crohn's disease. Dig Dis Sci 1984;29:913–920.

83. Hiatt RA, Kaufman L. Epidemiology of inflammatory bowel disease in a defined northern California population. West J Med 1988;149:541–546.

84. Sawczenko A, Sandhu BK, Logan RFA et al. Prospective survey of childhood inflammatory bowel disease in the British Isles. Lancet 2001;357:1093–1094.

85. Fellows IW, Freeman JG, Holmes GK. Crohn's disease in the city of Derby, 1951–85. Gut 1990;31:1262–1265.

86. Blanchard JF, Bernstein CN, Wajda A et al. Small-area variations and sociodemographic correlates for the incidence of Crohn's disease and ulcerative colitis. Am J Epidemiol 2001;154:328–335.

87. Segal I, Tim LO, Hamilton DG et al. The rarity of ulcerative colitis in South African blacks. Am J Gastroenterol 1980;74:332–336.

88. Wright JP, Froggatt J, O'Keefe EA et al. The epidemiology of inflammatory bowel disease in Cape Town 1980–1984. S Africa Med J 1986;70:10–15.

89. Probert CS, Jayanthi V, Pinder D et al. Epidemiological study of ulcerative proctocolitis in Indian migrants and the indigenous population of Leicestershire. Gut 1992;33:687–693.

90. Jayanthi V, Probert CS, Pinder D et al. Epidemiology of Crohn's disease in Indian migrants and the indigenous population in Leicestershire. Q J Med 1992;82:125–138.

91. Montgomery SM, Morris DL, Pounder RE et al. Asian ethnic origin and the risk of inflammatory bowel disease. Eur J Gastroenterol Hepatol 1999;11:543–546.

92. Carr I, Mayberry JF. The effects of migration on ulcerative colitis: A three-year prospective study among Europeans and first- and second-generation South Asians in Leicester (1991–1994). Am J Gastroenterol 1999;94:2918–2922.

93. Wigley RD, Maclaurin BP. A study of ulcerative colitis in New Zealand, showing a low incidence in Maoris. Br Med J 1962;2:228–231.

94. Jacobsohn WZ, Levine Y. Incidence and prevalence of ulcerative colitis in the Jewish population of Jerusalem. Israel J Med Sci 1986;22:559–563.

95. Odes HS, Fraser D, Krawiec J. Incidence of idiopathic ulcerative colitis in Jewish population subgroups in the Beer Sheva region of Israel. Am J Gastroenterol 1987;82:854–858.

96. Shapira M, Tamir A. Ulcerative colitis in the Kinneret sub district, Israel 1965–1994: incidence and prevalence in different subgroups. J Clin Gastroenterol 1998;27:134–137.

97. Niv Y, Abuksis G, Fraser GM. Epidemiology of ulcerative colitis in Israel: A survey of Israeli kibbutz settlements. Am J Gastroenterol 2000;95:693–698.

98. Gilat T, Ribak J, Benaroya Y et al. Ulcerative colitis in the Jewish population of Tel-Aviv Jafo. I. Epidemiology. Gastroenterology 1974; 66:335–342.

99. Odes HS, Fraser D. Ulcerative colitis in Israel: epidemiology, morbidity, and genetics. Public Health Rev 1989;17:297–319.

100. Mayberry JF, Judd D, Smart H et al. Crohn's disease in Jewish people – an epidemiological study in south-east Wales. Digestion 1986; 5:237–240.

101. Odes HS, Locker C, Neumann L et al. Epidemiology of Crohn's disease in southern Israel. Am J Gastroenterol 1994;89:1859–1862.

102. Gilat T, Grossman A, Fireman Z et al. Inflammatory bowel disease in Jews. Front Gastrointest Res 1986;11:135–140.

103. Loftus EV Jr., Schoenfeld P, Sandborn WJ. The epidemiology and natural history of Crohn's disease in population-based patient cohorts from North America: a systematic review. Aliment Pharmacol Ther 2002;16:51–60.

104. Lapidus A, Bernell O, Hellers G et al. Incidence of Crohn's disease in Stockholm County 1955–1989. Gut 1997;41:480–486.

105. Lee FI, Costello FT. Crohn's disease in Blackpool – incidence and prevalence 1968–80. Gut 1985;26:274–278.

106. Halme L, von Smitten K, Husa A. The incidence of Crohn's disease in the Helsinki metropolitan area during 1975–1985. Ann Chir Gynaecol 1989;78:115–119.

107. Fahrlander H, Baerlocher C. Clinical features and epidemiological data on Crohn's disease in the Basle area. Scand J Gastroenterol 1971;6:657–662.

108. Norlen BJ, Krause U, Bergman L. An epidemiological study of Crohn's disease. Scand J Gastroenterol 1970;5:385–390.

109. Szklo M, Sensenbrenner L, Markowitz J et al. Incidence of aplastic anemia in metropolitan Baltimore: a population-based study. Blood 1985;66:115–119.

110. Dean G, Kurtzke JF. On the risk of multiple sclerosis according to age at immigration to South Africa. Br Med J 1971;3:725–729.

111. Poskanzer D, Schapira K, Miller H. Epidemiology of multiple sclerosis in the counties of Northumberland and Durham. Acta Neurol Scand 1966;42:Suppl–6.

112. Morariu MA, Linden M. Multiple sclerosis in American blacks. Acta Neurol Scand 1980;62:180–187.

113. Fischman HR. Multiple sclerosis: a new perspective on epidemiologic patterns. Neurology 1982;32:864–870.

114. Paffenbarger RS Jr, Wing AL, Hyde RT. Characteristics in youth predictive of adult-onset malignant lymphomas, melanomas, and leukemias: brief communication. J Natl Cancer Inst 1978;60:89–92.

115. Humphreys WG, Parks TG. Crohn's disease in Northern Ireland – a retrospective survey of 159 cases. Ir J Med Sci 1975;144:437–446.

116. Gollop JH, Phillips SF, Melton LJ III et al. Epidemiologic aspects of Crohn's disease: a population based study in Olmsted County, Minnesota, 1943–1982. Gut 1988;29:49–56.

117. Monk M, Mendeloff AI, Siegel CI et al. An epidemiological study of ulcerative colitis and regional enteritis among adults in Baltimore. II. Social and demographic factors. Gastroenterology 1969; 6:847–857.

118. Shivananda S, Hordijk ML, Pena AS et al. Inflammatory bowel disease: one condition or two? Digestion 1987;38:187–192.

119. Elson CO. The immunology of inflammatory bowel disease. In: Kirsner JB, Shorter RG, eds. Inflammatory bowel disease. Philadelphia: Lea & Febiger; 1988:97–174.

120. Glassman MS, Newman LJ, Berezin S et al. Cow's milk protein sensitivity during infancy in patients with inflammatory bowel disease. Am J Gastroenterol 1990;85:838–840.

121. Truelove SC. Ulcerative colitis provoked by milk. Br Med J 1961;1:161.

122. Martini GA, Brandes JW. Increased consumption of refined carbohydrates in patients with Crohn's disease. Klin Wochenschr 1976;54:367–371.

123. Graham WB, Torrance B, Taylor TV. Breakfast and Crohn's disease. Br Med J 1978;2:768.

124. Thornton JR, Emmett PM, Heaton KW. Diet and Crohn's disease: characteristics of the pre-illness habit. Br Med J 1979;2:762–764.

125. Mayberry JF, Rhodes J, Allan R et al. Diet in Crohn's disease two studies of current and previous habits in newly diagnosed patients. Dig Dis Sci 1981;26:444–448.

126. Silkoff K, Hallak A, Yegena L et al. Consumption of refined carbohydrate by patients with Crohn's disease in Tel-Aviv-Yafo. Postgrad Med J 1980;56:842–846.

127. Jarnerot G, Jarnmark I, Nilsson K. Consumption of refined sugar by patients with Crohn's disease, ulcerative colitis, or irritable bowel syndrome. Scand J Gastroenterol 1983;18:999–1002.

128. Katschinski B, Logan RF, Edmond M et al. Smoking and sugar intake are separate but interactive risk factors in Crohn's disease. Gut 1988;29:1202–1206.

129. Probert CS, Bhakta P, Bhamra B et al. Diet of South Asians with inflammatory bowel disease. Arq Gastroenterol 1996;33:132–135.

130. Reif S, Klein I, Lubin F et al. Pre-illness dietary factors in inflammatory bowel disease. Gut 1997;40:754–760.

131. Mayberry JF, Rhodes J, Newcombe RG. Increased sugar consumption in Crohn's disease. Digestion 1980;20:323–326.

132. Sonnenberg A. Geographic and temporal variations of sugar and margarine consumption in relation to Crohn's disease. Digestion 1988;41:161–171.

133. Rozen P, Zonis J, Yekutiel P et al. Crohn's disease in the Jewish population of Tel-Aviv-Yafo. Epidemiologic and clinical aspects. Gastroenterology 1979;76:25–30.

134. Boyko EJ, Perera DR, Koepsell TD et al. Coffee and alcohol use and the risk of ulcerative colitis. Am J Gastroenterol 1989;84:530–534.

135. O'Morain C, Tobin A, Suzuki Y et al. Risk factors in inflammatory bowel disease. Scand J Gastroenterol 1989;170(Suppl):58–60.

136. Miura S, Tsuzuki Y, Hokari R et al. Modulation of intestinal immune system by dietary fat intake: relevance to Crohn's disease. J Gastroenterol Hepatol 1998;13:1183–1190.

137. Geerling BJ, Dagnelie PC, Badart-Smook A et al. Diet as a risk factor for the development of ulcerative colitis. Am J Gastroenterol 2000;95:1008–1013.

137a. Powell JJ, Harvey RS, Thompson RP. Microparticles in Crohn's disease – has the dust settled? Gut 1996;9:340–341.

138. Sullivan SN. Hypothesis revisited: toothpaste and the cause of Crohn's disease. Lancet 1990;336:1096–1097.

139. Koletzko S, Sherman P, Corey M et al. Role of infant feeding practices in development of Crohn's disease in childhood. Br Med J 1989;298:1617–1618.

140. Bergstrand O, Hellers G. Breast-feeding during infancy in patients who later develop Crohn's disease. Scand J Gastroenterol 1983;18:903–906.

141. Gilat T, Hacohen D, Lilos P et al. Childhood factors in ulcerative colitis and Crohn's disease. An international cooperative study. Scand J Gastroenterol 1987;22:1009–1024.

142. Ekbom A, Adami HO, Helmick CG et al. Perinatal risk factors for inflammatory bowel disease: a case–control study. Am J Epidemiol 1990;132:1111–1119.

143. Whorwell PJ, Holdstock G, Whorwell GM et al. Bottle feeding, early gastroenteritis, and inflammatory bowel disease. Br Med J 1979;1:382.

144. Koletzko S, Griffiths A, Corey M et al. Infant feeding practices and ulcerative colitis in childhood. Br Med J 1991;302:1580–1581.

145. Acheson ED, Truelove SC. Early weaning in the aetiology of ulcerative colitis: a study of feeding in infancy in cases and controls. Br Med J 1981;2:929–933.

146. Gent AE, Hellier MD, Grace RH et al. Inflammatory bowel disease and domestic hygiene in infancy. Lancet 1994;343:766–767.

147. Rogers BH, Clark LM, Kirsner JB. The epidemiologic and demographic characteristics of inflammatory bowel disease: an analysis of a computerized file of 1400 patients. J Chronic Dis 1971;24:743–773.

148. Keighley A, Miller DS, Hughes AO et al. The demographic and social characteristics of patients with Crohn's disease in the Nottingham area. Scand J Gastroenterol 1976;11:293–296.

149. Almy T, Sherlock P. Genetic aspects of ulcerative colitis and regional enteritis. Gastroenterology 1966;51:757–761.

150. Rosenberg JL, Kraft SC, Kirsner JB. Inflammatory bowel disease in all three members of one family. Gastroenterology 1976;70:759–760.

151. Whorwell PJ, Eade OE, Hossenbocus A et al. Crohn's disease in a husband and wife. Lancet 1978;2:186–187.

152. Bennett RA, Rubin PH, Present DH. Frequency of inflammatory bowel disease in offspring of couples both presenting with inflammatory bowel disease. Gastroenterology 1991;100:1638–1643.

153. Murray CJ, Thomson AB. Marital idiopathic inflammatory bowel disease. Crohn's disease in a husband and wife. J Clin Gastroenterol 1988;10:95–97.

154. Laharie D, Debeugny S, Peeters M et al. Inflammatory bowel disease in spouses and their offspring. Gastroenterology 2001;120:816–819.

155. Peeters M, Geypens B, Claus D et al. Clustering of increased small intestinal permeability in families with Crohn's disease. Gastroenterology 1997;113:802–807.

156. Soderholm JD, Olaison G, Lindberg E et al. Different intestinal permeability patterns in relatives and spouses of patients with Crohn's disease: an inherited defect in mucosal defence? Gut 1999;44:96–100.

157. Breslin NP, Nash C, Hilsden RJ et al. Intestinal permeability is increased in a proportion of spouses of patients with Crohn's disease. Am J Gastroenterol 2001;96:2934–2938.

158. Sonnenberg A. Occupational distribution of inflammatory bowel disease among German employees. Gut 1990;31:1037–1040.

159. Boggild H, Tuchsen F, Orhede E. Occupation, employment status and chronic inflammatory bowel disease in Denmark. Int J Epidemiol 1996;25:630–637.

160. Sonnenberg A. Occupational mortality of inflammatory bowel disease. Digestion 1990;46:10–18.

161. Cucino C, Sonnenberg A. Occupational mortality from inflammatory bowel disease in the United States 1991–1996. Am J Gastroenterol 2001;96:1101–1105.

162. Vessey M, Jewell D, Smith A et al. Chronic inflammatory bowel disease, cigarette smoking, and use of oral contraceptives: findings in a large cohort study of women of childbearing age. Br Med J (Clin Res Ed) 1986;292:1101–1103.

163. Logan RF, Kay CR. Oral contraception, smoking and inflammatory bowel disease – findings in the Royal College of General Practitioners Oral Contraception Study. Int J Epidemiol 1989;18:105–107.

164. Ramcharan S. The Walnut Creek Contraceptive Drug Study: a prospective study of the side effects of oral contraceptives. Bethesda, MD: US Department of Health, Education, and Welfare, Public Health Service, National Institutes of Health, National Institute of Child Health and Human Development, Center for Population Research, 1981.

165. Lesko SM, Kaufman DW, Rosenberg L et al. Evidence for an increased risk of Crohn's disease in oral contraceptive users. Gastroenterology 1985;89:1046–1049.

166. Lashner BA, Kane SV, Hanauer SB. Lack of association between oral contraceptive use and Crohn's disease: a community-based matched case–control study. Gastroenterology 1989;97:1442–1447.

167. Lashner BA, Kane SV, Hanauer SB. Lack of association between oral contraceptive use and ulcerative colitis. Gastroenterology 1990;99:1032–1036.

168. Sandler RS, Wurzelmann JI, Lyles CM. Oral contraceptive use and the risk of inflammatory bowel disease. Epidemiology 1992;3:374–378.

169. Wakefield AJ, Sawyerr AM, Dhillon AP et al. Pathogenesis of Crohn's disease: multifocal gastrointestinal infarction. Lancet 1989;2:1057–1062.

170. Barcewicz PA, Welch JP. Ischemic colitis in young adult patients. Dis Colon Rectum 1980;23:109–114.

171. Heron HC, Khubchandani IT, Trimpi HD et al. Evanescent colitis. Dis Colon Rectum 1981;24:555–561.

172. Tedesco FJ, Volpicelli NA, Moore FS. Estrogen- and progesterone-associated colitis: a disorder with clinical and endoscopic features mimicking Crohn's colitis. Gastrointest Endosc 1982;28:247–249.

173. Boyko EJ, Koepsell TD, Perera DR et al. Risk of ulcerative colitis among former and current cigarette smokers. N Engl J Med 1987;316:707–710.

174. Franceschi S, Panza E, La Vecchia C et al. Nonspecific inflammatory bowel disease and smoking. Am J Epidemiol 1987;125:445–452.

175. Harries AD, Baird A, Rhodes J. Non-smoking: a feature of ulcerative colitis. Br Med J (Clin Res Ed) 1982;284:706.

176. Jick H, Walker AM. Cigarette smoking and ulcerative colitis. N Engl J Med 1983;308:261–263.

177. Logan RF, Edmond M, Somerville KW et al. Smoking and ulcerative colitis. Br Med J (Clin Res Ed) 1984;288:751–753.

178. Lindberg E, Tysk C, Andersson K et al. Smoking and inflammatory bowel disease. A case control study. Gut 1988;29:352–357.

179. Persson PG, Ahlbom A, Hellers G. Inflammatory bowel disease and tobacco smoke – a case–control study. Gut 1990; 31:1377–1381.

180. Tobin MV, Logan RF, Langman MJ et al. Cigarette smoking and inflammatory bowel disease. Gastroenterology 1987; 93:316–321.

181. Somerville KW, Logan RF, Edmond M et al. Smoking and Crohn's disease. Br Med J (Clin Res Ed) 1984;289:954–956.

182. Lorusso D, Leo S, Misciagna G et al. Cigarette smoking and ulcerative colitis. A case control study. Hepatogastroenterology 1989;36:202–204.

183. Samuelsson SM. Ulceros colit och proctit. Uppsala: Department of Social Medicine, University of Uppsala, 2002.

184. Reif S, Klein I, Arber N et al. Lack of association between smoking and inflammatory bowel disease in Jewish patients in Israel. Gastroenterology 1995;108:1683–1687.

185. Boyko EJ. A critical appraisal of the association between cigarette smoking and risk of ulcerative colitis. In: MacDermott RP, ed. Inflammatory bowel disease: current status and future approach. New York: Elsevier Science; 1988:671–676.

186. Calkins BM. A meta-analysis of the role of smoking in inflammatory bowel disease. Dig Dis Sci 1989;34:1841–1854.

187. Logan R. Smoking and inflammatory bowel disease – an overview of recent studies. In: MacDermott RP, ed. Inflammatory bowel disease: current status and future approach. New York: Elsevier Science; 1988:663–669.

188. Cope GF, Heatley RV, Kelleher J et al. Cigarette smoking and inflammatory bowel disease: a review. Hum Toxicol 1987;6:189–193.

189. Loftus EV Jr., Sandborn WJ, Tremaine WJ et al. Primary sclerosing cholangitis is associated with nonsmoking: a case–control study. Gastroenterology 1996;110:1496–1502.

190. Van Erpecum KJ, Smits SJ, van de Meeberg PC et al. Risk of primary sclerosing cholangitis is associated with nonsmoking behavior. Gastroenterology 1996;110:1503–1506.

191. Benoni C, Nilsson A. Smoking habits in patients with inflammatory bowel disease. A case–control study. Scand J Gastroenterol 1987;22:1130–1136.

192. Motley RJ, Rhodes J, Ford GA et al. Time relationships between cessation of smoking and onset of ulcerative colitis. Digestion 1987;37:125–127.

193. Bradford-Hill AB. The environment and disease: association or causation? Proc Roy Soc Med 1965;58:295–300.

194. Nakamura Y, Labarthe DR. A case–control study of ulcerative colitis with relation to smoking habits and alcohol consumption in Japan. Am J Epidemiol 1994;140:902–911.

195. Silverstein MD, Lashner BA, Hanauer SB. Cigarette smoking and ulcerative colitis: a case–control study. Mayo Clin Proc 1994;69:425–429.

196. Boyko EJ, Perera DR, Koepsell TD et al. Effects of cigarette smoking on the clinical course of ulcerative colitis. Scand J Gastroenterol 1988;23:1147–1152.

197. Rudra T, Motley R, Rhodes J. Does smoking improve colitis? Scand J Gastroenterol Suppl 1989;170:61–63.

198. Beaugerie L, Massot N, Carbonnel F et al. Impact of cessation of smoking on the course of ulcerative colitis. Am J Gastroenterol 2001;96:2113–2116.

199. Roberts CJ, Diggle R. Non-smoking a feature of ulcerative colitis. Br Med J 1982;285:440.

200. Lashner BA, Hanauer SB, Silverstein MD. Testing nicotine gum for ulcerative colitis patients. Experience with single-patient trials. Dig Dis Sci 1990;35:827–832.

201. Perera DR, Janeway CM, Feld A et al. Smoking and ulcerative colitis. Br Med J (Clin Res Ed) 1984;288:1533.

202. Pullan RD, Rhodes J, Ganesh S et al. Transdermal nicotine for active ulcerative colitis. N Engl J Med 1994;330:811–815.

203. Sandborn WJ, Tremaine WJ, Offord KP et al. Transdermal nicotine for mildly to moderately active ulcerative colitis – a randomized, double-blind, placebo-controlled trial. Ann Intern Med 1997;126:364.

204. Thomas GA, Rhodes J, Mani V et al. Transdermal nicotine as maintenance therapy for ulcerative colitis. N Engl J Med 1995;332:988–992.

205. Thomas GA, Rhodes J, Ragunath K et al. Transdermal nicotine compared with oral prednisolone therapy for active ulcerative colitis. Eur J Gastroenterol Hepatol 1996;8:769–776.

206. Thomas GA, Rhodes J, Green JT. Inflammatory bowel disease and smoking – a review. Am J Gastroenterol 1998;93:144–149.

207. Thornton JR, Emmett PM, Heaton KW. Smoking, sugar, and inflammatory bowel disease. Br Med J (Clin Res Ed) 1985; 290:1786–1787.

208. Silverstein MD, Lashner BA, Hanauer SB et al. Cigarette smoking in Crohn's disease. Am J Gastroenterol 1989;84:31–33.

209. Fich A, Eliakim R, Sperber AD et al. The association between smoking and inflammatory bowel disease among Israeli Jewish patients. Inflamm Bowel Dis 1997;3:6–9.

210. Reif S, Lavy A, Keter D et al. Lack of association between smoking and Crohn's disease but the usual association with ulcerative colitis in Jewish patients in Israel: A multicenter study. Am J Gastroenterol 2000;95:474–478.

211. Lindberg E, Jarnerot G, Huitfeldt B. Smoking in Crohn's disease: effect on localisation and clinical course. Gut 1992;33:779–782.

212. Russel MG, Volovics A, Schoon EJ et al. Inflammatory bowel disease: is there any relation between smoking status and disease presentation? European Collaborative IBD Study Group. Inflamm Bowel Dis 1998;4:182–186.

213. Sutherland LR, Ramcharan S, Bryant H et al. Effect of cigarette smoking on recurrence of Crohn's disease. Gastroenterology 1990;98:1123–1128.

214. Cosnes J, Carbonnel F, Carrat F et al. Effects of current and former cigarette smoking on the clinical course of Crohn's disease. Aliment Pharmacol Ther 1999;13:1403–1411.

215. Breuer-Katschinski BD, Hollander N, Goebell H. Effect of cigarette smoking on the course of Crohn's disease. Eur J Gastroenterol Hepatol 1996;8:225–228.

216. Russel MG, Nieman FH, Bergers JM et al. Cigarette smoking and quality of life in patients with inflammatory bowel disease. South Limburg IBD Study Group. Eur J Gastroenterol Hepatol 1996;8:1075–1081.

217. Cosnes J, Beaugerie L, Carbonnel F et al. Smoking cessation and the course of Crohn's disease: An intervention study. Gastroenterology 2001;120:1093–1099.

218. Sandler RS, Sandler DP, McDonnell CW et al. Childhood exposure to environmental tobacco smoke and the risk of ulcerative colitis. Am J Epidemiol 1992;135:603–608.

219. Lashner BA, Shaheen NJ, Hanauer SB et al. Passive smoking is associated with an increased risk of developing inflammatory bowel disease in children. Am J Gastroenterol 1993;88:356–359.

220. Eliakim R, Reif S, Lavy A et al. Passive smoking in patients with inflammatory bowel disease: an Israeli multicentre case–control study. Eur J Gastroenterol Hepatol 2000;12:975–979.

221. Aabakken L, Osnes M. Non-steroidal anti-inflammatory drug-induced disease in the distal ileum and large bowel. Scand J Gastroenterol Suppl 1989;163:48–55.

222. Bjarnason I, Hayllar J, Macpherson AJ et al. Side effects of nonsteroidal anti-inflammatory drugs on the small and large intestine in humans. Gastroenterology 1993;104:1832–1847.

223. Donowitz M. Arachidonic acid metabolites and their role in inflammatory bowel disease. An update requiring addition of a pathway. Gastroenterology 1985;88:580–587.

224. Gould SR, Brash AR, Conolly ME et al. Studies of prostaglandins and sulphasalazine in ulcerative colitis. Prostaglandins Med 1981;6:165–182.

225. Fang WF, Broughton A, Jacobson ED. Indomethacin-induced intestinal inflammation. Am J Dig Dis 1977;22:749–760.

226. Yamada T, Deitch E, Specian RD et al. Mechanisms of acute and chronic intestinal inflammation induced by indomethacin. Inflammation 1993;17:641–662.

227. Berg DJ, Zhang J, Weinstock JV et al. Rapid development of colitis in NSAID-treated IL-10-deficient mice. Gastroenterology 2002;123:1527–1542.

228. Morteau O, Morham SG, Sellon R et al. Impaired mucosal defense to acute colonic injury in mice lacking cyclooxygenase-1 or cyclooxygenase-2. J Clin Invest 2000;105:469–478.

229. Stewart TH, Hetenyi C, Rowsell H et al. Ulcerative enterocolitis in dogs induced by drugs. J Pathol 1980;131:363–378.

230. Rampton DS, Sladen GE. Relapse of ulcerative proctocolitis during treatment with non-steriodal anti-inflammatory drugs. Postgrad Med J 1981;57:297–299.

231. Kaufmann HJ, Taubin HL. Nonsteroidal anti-inflammatory drugs activate quiescent inflammatory bowel disease. Ann Intern Med 1987;107:513–516.

232. Hall RI, Petty AH, Cobden I et al. Enteritis and colitis associated with mefenamic acid. Br Med J (Clin Res Ed) 1983;287:1182.

233. Phillips MS, Fehilly B, Stewart S et al. Enteritis and colitis associated with mefenamic acid. Br Med J 1983;287:1626.

234. Edwards AL, Heagerty AM, Bing RF. Enteritis and colitis associated with mefenamic acid. Br Med J 1983;287:1626–1627.

235. Rampton DS, Tapping PJ. Enteritis and colitis associated with mefenamic acid. Br Med J 1983;287:1627.

236. Williams R, Glazer G. Enteritis and colitis associated with mefenamic acid. Br Med J 1983;287:1627.

237. Pearson DJ, Stones NA, Bentley SJ. Proctocolitis induced by salicylate and associated with asthma and recurrent nasal polyps. Br Med J (Clin Res Ed) 1983;287:1675.

238. Rutherford D, Stockdill G, Hamer-Hodges DW et al. Proctocolitis induced by salicylate. Br Med J (Clin Res Ed) 1984;288:794.

239. Schwartz AG, Targan SR, Saxon A et al. Sulfasalazine-induced exacerbation of ulcerative colitis. N Engl J Med 1982;306:409–412.

240. Bjarnason I, Zanelli G, Smith T et al. Nonsteroidal antiinflammatory drug-induced intestinal inflammation in humans. Gastroenterology 1987;93:480–489.

241. Bjarnason I, Price AB, Zanelli G et al. Clinicopathological features of nonsteroidal antiinflammatory drug-induced small intestinal strictures. Gastroenterology 1988;94:1070–1074.

242. Tanner AR, Raghunath AS. Colonic inflammation and nonsteroidal anti-inflammatory drug administration. An assessment of the frequency of the problem. Digestion 1988;41:116–120.

243. Koutroubakis IE, Vlachonikolis IG. Appendectomy and the development of ulcerative colitis: results of a metaanalysis of published case–control studies. Am J Gastroenterol 2000;95:171–176.

244. Andersson RE, Olaison G, Tysk C et al. Appendectomy and protection against ulcerative colitis. N Engl J Med 2001;344:808–814.

245. Andersson RE, Ekbom A. Appendectomy and protection against ulcerative colitis. N Engl J Med 2001;345:223–224.

246. Frisch M, Johansen C, Mellemkjaer L et al. Appendectomy and subsequent risk of inflammatory bowel diseases. Surgery 2001;130:36–43.

247. Wurzelmann JI, Lyles CM, Sandler RS. Childhood infections and the risk of inflammatory bowel disease. Dig Dis Sci 1994;39:555–560.

248. Breslin NP, McDonnell C, O'Morain.C. Surgical and smoking history in inflammatory bowel disease: a case–control study. Inflamm Bowel Dis 1997;3:1–5.

249. Duggan AE, Usmani I, Neal KR et al. Appendicectomy, childhood hygiene, *Helicobacter pylori* status, and risk of inflammatory bowel disease: a case control study. Gut 1998;43:494–498.

250. Reif S, Lavy A, Keter D et al. Appendectomy is more frequent but not a risk factor in Crohn's disease while being protective in ulcerative colitis: A comparison of surgical procedures in inflammatory bowel disease. Am J Gastroenterol 2001;96:829–832.

251. Russel MG, Dorant E, Brummer RJ et al. Appendectomy and the risk of developing ulcerative colitis or Crohn's disease: results of a large case–control study. South Limburg Inflammatory Bowel Disease Study Group. Gastroenterology 1997;113:377–382.

252. Mizoguchi A, Mizoguchi E, Chiba C et al. Role of appendix in the development of inflammatory bowel disease in TCR-alpha mutant mice. J Exp Med 1996;184:707–715.

253. Rath HC, Ikeda JS, Linde HJ et al. Varying cecal bacterial loads influences colitis and gastritis in HLA-B27 transgenic rats. Gastroenterology 1999;116:310–319.

254. Wakefield AJ, Ekbom A, Dhillon AP et al. Crohn's disease: pathogenesis and persistent measles virus infection. Gastroenterology 1995;108:911–916.

255. Wakefield AJ, Pittilo RM, Sim R et al. Evidence of persistent measles virus infection in Crohn's disease. J Med Virol 1993;39:345–353.

256. Robertson DJ, Sandler RS. Measles virus and Crohn's disease: a critical appraisal of the current literature. Inflamm Bowel Dis 2001;7:51–57.

257. Thompson NP, Montgomery SM, Pounder RE et al. Is measles vaccination a risk factor for inflammatory bowel disease? Lancet 1995;345:1071–1074.

258. Fisher NC, Yee L, Nightingale P et al. Measles virus serology in Crohn's disease. Gut 1997;41:66–69.

259. Touze I, Dubucquoi S, Cortot A et al. IgM-specific measles-virus antibody in families with a high frequency of Crohn's disease . Lancet 1995;346:967.

260. Chadwick N, Bruce IJ, Schepelmann S et al. Measles virus RNA is not detected in inflammatory bowel disease using hybrid capture and reverse transcription followed by the polymerase chain reaction. J Med Virol 1998;55:305–311.

261. Iizuka M, Saito H, Yukawa M et al. No evidence of persistent mumps virus infection in inflammatory bowel disease. Gut 2001;48:637–641.

262. Afzal MA, Armitage E, Begley J et al. Absence of detectable measles virus genome sequence in inflammatory bowel disease tissues and peripheral blood lymphocytes. J Med Virol 1998;55:243–249.

263. Haga Y, Funakoshi O, Kuroe K et al. Absence of measles viral genomic sequence in intestinal tissues from Crohn's disease by nested polymerase chain reaction. Gut 1996;38:211–215.

264. Hermon-Taylor J, Ford J, Sumar N et al. Measles virus and Crohn's disease. Lancet 1995;345:922–923.

265. Feeney M, Ciegg A, Winwood P et al. A case–control study of measles vaccination and inflammatory bowel disease. The East Dorset Gastroenterology Group. Lancet 1997;350:764–766.

266. Morris DL, Montgomery SM, Thompson NP et al. Measles vaccination and inflammatory bowel disease: a national British Cohort Study. Am J Gastroenterol 2000;95:3507–3512.

267. Montgomery SM, Morris DL, Pounder RE et al. Paramyxovirus infections in childhood and subsequent inflammatory bowel disease. Gastroenterology 1999;116:796–803.

268. Thompson NP, Montgomery SM, Wadsworth ME et al. Early determinants of inflammatory bowel disease: use of two national longitudinal birth cohorts. Eur J Gastroenterol Hepatol 2000;12:25–30.

269. Jones P, Fine P, Piracha S. Crohn's disease and measles. Lancet 1997;349:473.

270. Fine PE, Adelstein AM, Snowman J et al. Long term effects of exposure to viral infections in utero. Br Med J (Clin Res Ed) 1985;290:509–511.

271. Nielsen LL, Nielsen NM, Melbye M et al. Exposure to measles in utero and Crohn's disease: Danish register study. Br Med J 1998;316:196–197.

272. Pardi DS, Tremaine WJ, Sandborn WJ et al. Perinatal exposure to measles virus is not associated with the development of inflammatory bowel disease. Inflamm Bowel Dis 1999;5:104–106.

273. Davis RL, Bohlke K. Measles vaccination and inflammatory bowel disease: controversy laid to rest? Drug Safety 2001;24:939–946.

274. Thompson NP, Wakefield AJ, Pounder RE. Inherited disorders of coagulation appear to protect against inflammatory bowel disease. Gastroenterology 1995;108:1011–1015.

275. Epidemiological evidence of the association between lichen planus and two immune-related diseases. Alopecia areata and ulcerative colitis. Gruppo Italiano Studi Epidemiologici in Dermatologia. Arch Dermatol 1991;127:688–691.

276. Pugh SM, Rhodes J, Mayberry JF et al. Atopic disease in ulcerative colitis and Crohn's disease. Clin Allergy 1979;9:221–223.

277. Lee FI, Bellary SV, Francis C. Increased occurrence of psoriasis in patients with Crohn's disease and their relatives. Am J Gastroenterol 1990; 85:962–963.

278. Siege J. Inflammatory bowel disease: another possible facet of allergic diathesis. Ann Allergy 1981;47:92–94.

279. Weiss ST. Eat dirt – the hygiene hypothesis and allergic diseases. N Engl J Med 2002;347:930–931.

280. Minuk GY, Lewkonia RM. Possible familial association of multiple sclerosis and inflammatory bowel disease. N Engl J Med 1986;314:586.

281. Rang EH, Brooke BN, Hermon-Taylor J. Association of ulcerative colitis with multiple sclerosis. Lancet 1982;2:555.

282. Sadovnick AD, Paty DW, Yannakoulias G. Concurrence of multiple sclerosis and inflammatory bowel disease. N Engl J Med 1989;321:762–763.

283. Tysk C, Lindberg E, Jarnerot G et al. Ulcerative colitis and Crohn's disease in an unselected population of monozygotic and dizygotic twins. A study of heritability and the influence of smoking. Gut 1988;29:990–996.

284. Orholm M, Binder V, Sorensen TI et al. Concordance of inflammatory bowel disease among Danish twins. Results of a nationwide study. Scand J Gastroenterol 2000;35:1075–1081.

285. Bridger S, Lee JC, Bjarnason I et al. In siblings with similar genetic susceptibility for inflammatory bowel disease, smokers tend to develop Crohn's disease and non-smokers develop ulcerative colitis. Gut 2002;51:21–25.

286. Bjornsson S, Johannsson JH. Inflammatory bowel disease in Iceland, 1990–1994: a prospective, nationwide, epidemiological study. Eur J Gastroenterol Hepatol 2000;12:31–38.

287. Munkholm P, Langholz E, Nielsen OH et al. Incidence and prevalence of Crohn's disease in the county of Copenhagen, 1962–87: a sixfold increase in incidence. Scand J Gastroenterol 1992;27:609–614.

288. Roin F, Roin J. Inflammatory bowel disease of the Faroe Islands, 1981–1988. A prospective epidemiologic study: primary report. Scand J Gastroenterol 1989;170(Suppl):44–46.

289. Rubin GP, Hungin APS, Kelly PJ et al. Inflammatory bowel disease: epidemiology and management in an English general practice population. Aliment Pharmacol Ther 2000;14:1553–1559.

290. Yapp TR, Stenson R, Thomas GAO et al. Crohn's disease incidence in Cardiff from 1930: an update for 1991–1995. Eur J Gastroenterol Hepatol 2000;12:907–911.

291. Kyle J. Crohn's disease in the northeastern and northern Isles of Scotland: an epidemiological review. Gastroenterology 1992;103:392–399.

292. Russel MG, Dorant E, Volovics A et al. High incidence of inflammatory bowel disease in The Netherlands: results of a prospective study. The South Limburg IBD Study Group. Dis Colon Rectum 1998;41:33–40.

293. Gower-Rousseau C, Salomez JL, Dupas JL et al. Incidence of inflammatory bowel disease in northern France (1988–1990). Gut 1994;35:1433–1438.

294. Manousos ON, Giannadaki E, Mouzas IA et al. Ulcerative colitis is as common in Crete as in northern Europe: a 5-year prospective study. Eur J Gastroenterol Hepatol 1996;8:893–898.

295. Trallori G, Palli D, Saieva C et al. A population-based study of inflammatory bowel disease in Florence over 15 years (1978–92). Scand J Gastroenterol 1996;31:892–899.

296. Odes HS, Locker C, Neumann L et al. Epidemiology of Crohn's disease in southern Israel. Am J Gastroenterol 1994;89:1859–1862.

297. Linares de la Cal JA, Canton C, Pajares JM et al. Inflammatory bowel disease in Argentina and Panama (1987–1993). Eur J Gastroenterol Hepatol 1997;9:1129.

298. Niv Y, Torten D, Tamir A et al. Incidence and prevalence of ulcerative colitis in the upper Galilee, Northern Israel, 1967–1986. Am J Gastroenterol 1990;85:1580–1583.

299. Odes HS, Fraser D, Krawiec J. Incidence of idiopathic ulcerative colitis in Jewish population subgroups in the Beer Sheva region of Israel. Am J Gastroenterol 1987;82(9):854–858.

300. Niv Y, Abuksis G, Fraser GM. Epidemiology of ulcerative colitis in Israel: a survey of Israeli kibbutz settlements. Am J Gastroenterol 2000;95:693–698.

301. Gyde SN, Prior P, Alexander F et al. Ulcerative colitis: why is the mortality from cardiovascular disease reduced? QJ Med 1984;53:351–357.

302. Sicilia B, Miguel CL, Arribas F et al. Environmental risk factors and Crohn's disease: a population-based, case–control study in Spain. Dig Liver Dis 2001;33:762–767.

303. Harries AD, Jones L, Heatley RV et al. Smoking habits and inflammatory bowel disease: effect on nutrition. Br Med J 1982;284:1161.

304. Rutgeerts P, D'Haens G, Hiele M et al. Appendectomy protects against ulcerative colitis. Gastroenterology 1994;106:1251–1253.

305. Smithson JE, Radford-Smith G, Jewell GP. Appendectomy and tonsillectomy in patients with inflammatory bowel disease. J Clin Gastroenterol 1995;21:283–286.

306. Brahme F, Lindstrom C, Wenckert A. Crohn's disease in a defined population. An epidemiological study of incidence, prevalence, mortality, and secular trends in the city of Malmo, Sweden. Gastroenterology 1975;69:342–351.

## CHAPTER 18

# Clinical genetics of inflammatory bowel diseases: genetic epidemiology, genotype–phenotype correlations and pharmacogenetics

Jean-Frédéric Colombel, Cyrus Pesi Tamboli and Jean-Pierre Hugot

The pathophysiology of inflammatory bowel diseases (IBD) is still unknown, but epidemiological studies show clear evidence of genetic susceptibility.[1] This evidence has been supplemented by molecular genetic data from genome-wide linkage scans and candidate gene studies. Identification of the first IBD susceptibility gene, *NOD2/CARD15*, has been a major breakthrough in genetic research and may provide a key step to unravelling the etiology of Crohn's disease (CD).[2] The clinical impact of genetic studies is becoming more apparent in understanding disease heterogeneity and responses to treatment. It also promises to expand the opportunities for genetic counselling regarding IBD.

## GENETIC EPIDEMIOLOGY

The role of genetics in IBD susceptibility is suggested by epidemiological data, including twin studies, ethnic differences in disease prevalence, studies of familial aggregation, and by association with recognized genetic syndromes.[3]

## TWIN STUDIES

Twin studies provide a powerful tool to evaluate the respective roles of environmental and genetic factors in the pathophysiology of IBD. In theory, greater concordance for a disease in monozygotic twin pairs compared to dizygotic twin pairs suggests that genetic factors are responsible for this difference. Three twin studies performed in Sweden,[4] the United Kingdom[5] and Denmark[6] have examined the concordance for IBD. The two Scandinavian studies were based on nationwide twin registries, whereas the British study was based on questionnaires to

the National Association for Colitis and Crohn's disease. Tysk[4] and Orholm[6] showed remarkably consistent disease concordance rates of 44% and 50%, respectively, among monozygotic twin pairs with CD. This contrasts with ulcerative colitis (UC) concordance rates of 6.3%[4] and 18.2%.[6] Subhani[6] found a CD concordance rate of 42.4% and a UC concordance rate of 16.5% among monozygotic twins. All studies showed higher concordance (i.e. more genetic influence) in CD than in UC. The concordance rates in dizygotic twins ranged from 0 to 12% in CD and from 0 to 5.3% in UC, suggesting a greater influence of genetic factors in CD, but environmental influences in UC. Concordance rates in IBD twins compared with other complex diseases are given in Table 18.1. From these concordance rates, an estimation of the relative contribution of genetics to disease etiology can be calculated (coefficient of heritability).[7] The coefficient for CD is of the same magnitude as that for asthma or type I diabetes mellitus. Only one case has been described of monozygotic twins in whom one had CD and the other UC,[8] suggesting that the net genetic susceptibility factors causing CD and UC are different. Ongoing Scandinavian studies on environmental factors in childhood and adolescence in discordant monozygotic twins may give important clues to which external factors are worth studying in IBD.

## ETHNIC DIFFERENCES

There are large differences in IBD frequency between various ethnic groups. It is of particular interest that the prevalence in the Jewish population is two to nine times higher than in other ethnic groups.[7] This difference is maintained irrespective of time period or geographical location, which strongly suggests the

**Table 18.1 Concordance rate (%) for various diseases in monozygotic and dizygotic twins**

| Disease | Monozygotic twins | Dizygotic twins |
|---|---|---|
| Cancer, same site | 7 | 3 |
| Cancer, different site | 16 | 14 |
| **Ulcerative colitis** | **6.3–18.2** | **0–5.3** |
| Myocardial infarction | 19 | 9 |
| Harelip | 30 | 5 |
| **Crohn's disease** | **42–58.5** | **0–12** |
| Type I diabetes | 56 | 11 |
| Asthma | 50 | 4 |
| Schizophrenia | 65 | 12 |

existence of a genetic predisposition. The Jewish population is comprised of two major genetically distinct subgroups: Ashkenazi Jews of European descent, and non-Ashkenazi primarily of Asian–African extraction. In Israel, most studies reported higher rates of CD in the Ashkenazi than in the non-Ashkenazi Jewish population,[9,10] and a study from California showed a significant excess of IBD in the Ashkenazi Jewish population that originated in middle Europe relative to those from Poland and Russia.[11] It has been suggested that these higher prevalence rates result from a stronger genetic predisposition.[12] However, the prevalence of IBD in Israel is rather low, suggesting that environmental factors also play an important role.

Epidemiological studies have reported the highest prevalence rates of IBD in whites, lower rates in black Americans, and the lowest rates in Asians.[13,14] These data should be interpreted with caution: studies have shown that young Asians who were born in Britain were at a significantly higher risk of developing IBD than was the indigenous European population.[15] This may in fact reflect a greater genetic predisposition to IBD in Asians that is uncovered by exposure to relevant environmental factors not present in the region of lower incidence.

## FAMILY STUDIES

### Estimation of risk

Epidemiologic studies on the familial prevalence of IBD have shown strong and significant associations. In families with a positive family history, the prevalence varies between 5.5 and 22.5 %.[16–21] The population relative risk of IBD among relatives of patients with IBD has been estimated by cohort studies and case–control studies. Orholm et al.[22] studied a regional group of 637 patients with IBD. Standardized for age and sex, a population relative risk of 10 was found for relatives of patients for both UC and CD. The prevalence of IBD in first-degree relatives was 1.6% and 1.3% for UC and CD, respectively. Peeters et al.[21] using a case–control study design, found that 14.5% of 640 patients with CD had at least one first-degree relative with IBD, compared to 1.1% of the controls. The prevalence of IBD among first-degree relatives was 2.8%, compared to 0.2% among relatives of controls. The population relative risk was 14, almost exactly the same as found by Orholm et al. The crude prevalence rates were 3.3% for siblings, 1.6% for parents and 2.0% for offspring. Calculated as lifetime risk of IBD, based on age-adjusted incidence rates and assuming a life expectancy of 70 years, the risk was reported to be 7.4 for offspring, 1.9 for parents and 4.9 for siblings. Satsangi et al.[20] studied 433 patients with CD, by

postal questionnaire. Seventy-eight respondents (18%) reported having at least one first- or second-degree relative with IBD. The prevalence of IBD among first-degree relatives was found to be 2.6%, and was estimated to be 15 times higher than in the general population. Thus, the population relative risk for first-degree relatives is almost identical in the three studies, as is the prevalence values of IBD for parents of patients with CD. The relative risk to a sibling (λs ratio) has been estimated to be somewhere between 15 and 35 for CD, and between 7 and 17 for UC.[7] This compares with λs ratios of 3 for hypertension, 7 for schizophrenia, 10–20 for type I diabetes mellitus and 450 for cystic fibrosis, which is a monogenic disease. Familial risks appear to show ethnic differences, with the highest risk in Ashkenazi Jews and the lowest in Asians.[12,14] However, these latter estimates may reflect the low prevalence of IBD in Asian countries. Even though a rare circumstance, the risk of IBD to a child of parents who both have IBD may be very high: in a study from New York City involving 19 couples, 52% of the children who were aged 20 years or older developed IBD.[23] In our own experience involving 25 couples with IBD, the probability of their children developing IBD was estimated to be 33% at age 28.[24]

## Familial phenotype

Many studies of familial IBD have shown a high degree of concordance for CD or UC within families.[21,25,26] However, the cross-occurrence of CD and UC is also significant. In a Danish study,[22] first-degree relatives of patients with CD had a 3.85-fold greater risk than the general population for developing UC. Similarly, the risk for UC patients with CD relatives was 1.72.

Most data concerning the clinical similarities of IBD within families are also convincing. Bayless et al.[27] studied a group of 133 patients with CD from 60 families. Concordance for disease location among at least two family members was found in 88% of families. Concordance for disease type – either UC or CD – was found in 82% of families. In Oxford, Satsangi et al. reported a crude concordance rate of 80.3% for disease extent and 80.3% for extraintestinal manifestations among 82 CD–CD sibling pairs.[25] Lower concordance rates were observed in 31 parent–child pairs (75% and 68%, respectively). A French familial CD study was comprised of 72 families.[28] There were 176 patients with CD, 82% being siblings, 29% parent–child and 13% second-degree relatives. Among relatives of families with two affected members, 56% were concordant for disease location and 49% for disease type. These percentages reached 83% and 76%, respectively, in 17 families with more than two affected members. Similarities were particularly striking in two families that have been reported in detail.[29] In a Belgian series[21] the overall concordance rate in 51 families with two affected members was 58% for location, 44% for type and 42% for number of bowel resections. Using the κ value a significant agreement was found for disease location (ileal, ileocolonic and perianal). The strongest agreement was detected in sibling–sibling and parent–child pairs. Familiality for disease type could only be shown in multiplex families. These combined observations suggest that the familial IBD subgroup is more homogeneous than expected, and they support a role for familiality in both disease site and disease behavior. On the other hand, no significant similarities have been found for disease location and type in CD couples.[24] This suggests that genetic rather than environmental factors significantly shape the expression of the disease. However, it should be mentioned that not all studies regarding clinical similarities within CD families are in agreement. Lee and Lennard-Jones observed no significant similarities in clinical behavior (including extent, type and extraintestinal manifestations) or course in 67 families, each with three or more members affected with IBD.[30] In the Danish twin registry, no homogeneous pattern regarding the clinical characteristics was observed within the concordant CD pairs.[6]

Far fewer data exist for familial UC. Concordance rates for disease extent were 53% in 17 parent–child pairs and 69% in 35 sibling pairs in Satsangi's study.[25] In an Italian study involving 64 families, concordance rates of 33%, 47% and 34% were found for disease extension, need for steroids and relapse rate, respectively.[31] These figures are lower than for CD–CD pairs. This is in accordance with the hypothesis that CD depends more heavily on genetic influences.

Association between familial IBD and early age at onset or diagnosis has been documented in some, but not all, family studies. In our series[28] the median age at onset in 176 patients with familial CD was 22 years. This was significantly younger than in 1377 sporadic cases: 26.5 years ($P<0.01$). These results were strengthened by the early onset of disease in multicase families (median age 20 years). Among 552 consecutive patients followed at Johns Hopkins Hospital, 95 (17%) had a family history of CD.[32] These 95 patients were significantly younger at the time of diagnosis than the 432 with a negative family history: 21.8 years versus 26.8 years, respectively ($P<0.005$). Additionally, it has been reported that CD patients with early age at onset have an increased positive family history compared with patient populations with a more varied age of onset. Thirty-five per cent of CD patients with an onset of disease before the age of 21 followed at the Cleveland Clinic had a positive family history of IBD.[33] Fewer data are available in UC: in a series from Los Angeles[12] the age at onset of disease was significantly lower in patients with a positive family history than in those with sporadic cases (23.3 vs. 28.6 years). In the study by Lee and Lennard-Jones[30] no control sporadic cases were available. The median age at UC diagnosis in 20 families with three or more affected first-degree relatives was 27 years. Although this was 6 years younger than the 33 years observed in a large Swedish epidemiological study,[34] the authors did not consider this difference to be significant.

A preponderance of women has been observed in familial IBD, with a female to male ratio ranging from 1.23:1 to 1.68:1 in familial CD[19,28,30] and from 1.3:1 to 1.5:1 in familial UC.[18,30] In the majority of large clinical series, women with CD usually outnumber men, but the opposite trend is frequent in UC. In a series of 135 families in which both a parent and a child had IBD, 93 families involved transmission of susceptibility to disease from mother to child, versus 42 examples of transmission from father to child ($P=0.0001$), suggesting either genomic imprinting or a maternally associated environmental factor.[35] Imprinting is observed when affected offspring show different phenotypic effects of genes carried on maternally derived as opposed to paternally derived chromosomes.[36] It may induce differences in age of onset, disease type or severity. However, this distortion of transmission was observed only among non-Jewish pairs with CD and has not been confirmed in other series.

Several series suggest that CD location and type may be different in familial and sporadic cases. More patients with both small bowel and colonic involvement and fewer with pure colonic disease have been reported in familial series from France and Belgium.[28,37] Cottone et al.[38] found that familial occurrence in CD was less frequent when the disease was located in the colon (2.4%) than in the ileum and the colon (9.7%) ($P<0.006$). In our familial cases[28] the type of disease was fistulizing in 14%, fibrostenotic in 48% and inflammatory in 38%. There was a significant statistical link between the fibrostenotic type and the presence of small bowel involvement, with an odds ratio of 1.3 ($P<10^{-4}$). It is quite possible that these features are secondary to the early age at onset. The literature strongly supports the concept of higher rates of small bowel disease in childhood and adolescent patients, and more colonic disease in older-onset populations. In the large series from Johns Hopkins[32] the age at diagnosis was associated with the site of involvement of CD, regardless of the presence or absence of a positive family history. As age at diagnosis increased, the proportion of patients having small bowel involvement decreased and, conversely, colonic involvement was significantly more common in the group aged 40 and older. Data in UC are less available. In the families studied by Monsen et al.[18] pancolitis tended to be more common among familial than among non-familial cases, whereas Lee and Lennard-Jones found approximately equal proportions of patients with pancolitis and distal or left-sided colitis.[30] This is in accordance with large epidemiological series.

Although so far there is no accepted index of severity in IBD, requirements for medical or surgical therapy may be a useful surrogate. In the series from Baltimore,[32] a positive family history for CD was significantly associated with surgery for abscess or perforation (26.3% vs. 16.6%; $P<0.05$; odds ratio 1.79). In contrast, Carbonnel et al.[39] found no differences in medical therapy or the incidence and extent of excisional surgery between 152 patients with a positive familial history of CD and 1164 sporadic cases. Kaplan–Meier-estimated times for prescription of immunosuppressive drugs and first intestinal resection were similar in familial and sporadic cases (Figs 18.1, 18.2). In the families with UC studied by Lee and Lennard-Jones,[30] 24 of the 93 patients (26%) had been treated surgically, a similar figure to those observed in large epidemiological studies.[40,41]

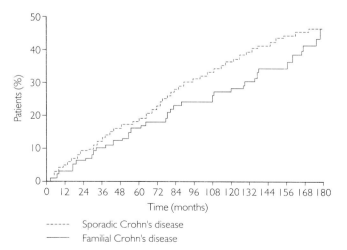

**Fig. 18.1** Kaplan–Meier estimated time to first prescription of immunosuppressive drugs in familial and sporadic Crohn's disease. __, familial Crohn's disease ($n=152$).---, sporadic Crohn's disease ($n=1164$). (From [39], with permission.)

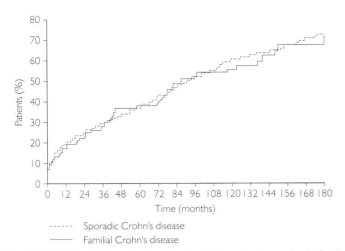

**Fig. 18.2** Kaplan–Meier estimated time to first intestinal resection in familial and sporadic Crohn's disease. ___, familial Crohn's disease (n = 152); ---, sporadic Crohn's disease (n = 1164). (From [39], with permission.)

Although these series were retrospective and mostly hospital based, they suggest that having a positive family history does not significantly influence the course of IBD in affected members. Finally, a Scandinavian study demonstrated that first-degree relatives of patients with IBD are not at increased risk of colorectal cancer relative to sporadic cases.[42]

In conclusion, based on the available literature, there are few phenotypic differences between the familial and sporadic forms of IBD.[43] No particular phenotype has been associated with familial cases. An earlier age at onset or diagnosis is the most significant familial characteristic that has been observed in population-based studies, which may account for the higher rates of ileal Crohn's disease in some familial series.

## Genetic anticipation

Because an earlier age at onset (which could influence disease site and type) may be the single most important difference between familial and sporadic IBD, a proper interpretation of early onset in families is critical. Genetic anticipation has been suggested as a possible explanation. This term denotes a decrease in the age at onset and an increase in severity as a disease is passed through generations. Genetic anticipation has been described in monogenic neurologic illnesses such as Huntington's disease, myotonic dystrophy and, more recently, Friedreich's ataxia.[44–46] In these diseases there is strong evidence that anticipation reflects the influence of genetic factors and has a true molecular basis. Amplification of DNA triplet repeats within or adjacent to the disease gene occurs in successive generations, and this instability of DNA is associated with increasing disease severity and earlier age at onset.[45–47] The consistent finding in CD familial series of an earlier age at diagnosis in affected children than in affected parents, with an average difference of 15 years, has led to speculation about genetic anticipation.[48] However, this interpretation has been challenged because of possible methodological biases.[49–51] An increased awareness and diagnostic acuity may influence age at diagnosis in later generations. For example, in our series there was a shorter time interval between symptoms and age at diagnosis in children than in parents. However, the difference only accounted for 2 years.[50] Another complicating factor, inherent in retrospective studies

of familial IBD, is the differential age at interview. This results in a greater chance of finding a later age at diagnosis in the older generation (recall bias).[49] A third potential bias is the preferential ascertainment of parents with late age at diagnosis. The median age at IBD diagnosis in the affected parents was higher in all published familial series than the one observed in sporadic cases. This might well reflect a selection bias (also called truncation bias), with lower recruitment of parents with an early onset and reduced fertility. This bias was displayed in two studies in which parent–child pairs were stratified according to age at diagnosis in the parents. No anticipation persisted in the parent–child pairs who had a relatively early diagnosis, except in a Jewish subset.[50,52] Finally, the main confounder in assessing anticipation in IBD is probably the inadequate follow-up time of the entire younger generation cohort which is at risk. In this situation, some members of the younger generation who are eventually destined to develop disease may not be recognized because they have not yet lived through their later years of disease susceptibility.[51] Additional evidence against genetic anticipation was provided by the observation that there was no difference between disease extent and type (a marker of disease severity) in parent–child pairs.[50,51] In summary, apparent genetic anticipation can be explained by observational biases without invoking any additional genetic influence.[53] In addition, there is no molecular evidence of triplet repeats in the NOD2 gene.

Alternative explanations for earlier disease onset in IBD families have been proposed. As in other polygenic diseases, it could merely reflect a heavier genetic load in families compared with sporadic cases. The genetic contribution to disease is greater in patients with an early onset. This is supported by studies that have demonstrated stronger evidence for linkage to markers on chromosomes 1, 3, 16 and 12 in families with at least one member less than 20 years old at diagnosis.[54,55] A study by Akolkar et al. reported strong linkage to the IBD1 gene locus in Ashkenazi Jewish CD patients with early-onset disease, whereas the group of Ashkenazi Jewish patients as a whole showed only a weak association.[56] Increased and/or earlier exposure to causal environmental factors may also explain younger age at onset in families.[57,58]

## Smoking habit in families

Cigarette smoking is the most established environmental risk factor to date in the development of IBD.[59] It has been well described that there is a relationship between smoking and the risk of developing the various forms of IBD. Interestingly, this risk extends in opposite directions for UC (decreased risk) and CD (increased risk). Although these observations have been noted for the past 40 years, the reasons for this discrepancy are completely unclear. Relatively few investigations have been performed to define the relationship between smoking and genetic factors in familial IBD.

A Swedish twin registry study could not explain discordance for IBD between twin pairs on the basis of smoking habits.[4] This study demonstrated similar smoking patterns at the time of diagnosis in each of monozygotic twin pair members who were discordant for UC or CD. The smoking patterns were similar for the disease-concordant and -discordant twin pairs. It was concluded that identical heredity and similar smoking habits are by themselves insufficient to cause CD. More recently, the Danish twin registry study did find discordant smoking habits to be significantly associated with discordance for UC, but this did not reach statistical significance for CD.[6] Both studies confirmed significant overall correlations between smoking and CD and negative associations for UC. Similarly, Smith et al. found a high concordance rate for smoking habits and for IBD type between 62 IBD probands and affected family members (first-, second- or third-degree relatives) from the University of Chicago IBD registry.[60] In this small study, the contribution of genetic factors, as measured by concordance of IBD type, was not statistically different from the concordance of smoking habit. A larger Italian study has focused on familial IBD and the relationship of smoking to CD in several groups, including healthy controls. The authors found no significant difference in the percentage of affected smokers from CD families versus sporadic cases of CD.[61] However, in families with at least one sibling affected with CD, the second affected CD family member had a significantly higher chance of being a smoker than did healthy siblings (OR 3.46, CI 1.03–11.65, $P<0.04$). This result suggests an influence of smoking on the development of familial cases of CD, and perhaps even its differentiation into a CD phenotype. Smoking habits were analysed in 242 IBD pedigrees in a recent study from London.[62] Of 89 sibling pairs discordant for smoking at diagnosis, 23 were also discordant for disease type: in 21 of these CD occurred in the smoker and UC in the non-smoker (OR 10.5; 2.6–92; $P<0.0001$), suggesting that in those cases tobacco acts on IBD genetic predisposition to displace the phenotype from UC to CD.

Overall, comparisons between these studies are difficult because of different methodologies, but the results have suggested that smoking may be a more important determinant for CD development in those instances where genetic factors are less powerful, i.e. CD expression in non-twin siblings or family members, rather than in twins.

## Subclinical markers

In recent years there has been a great interest in searching for subclinical markers of IBD in families.[63] Their presence in clinically unaffected members may provide insights into the genetic and/or environmental factors predisposing to a disease, or identify those in an earlier phase of subclinical disease (Table 18.2). The three most studied markers have been intestinal permeability, antineutrophil cytoplasmic autoantibodies (ANCA) and anti-*Saccharomyces cerevisiae* mannan antibodies (ASCA).

Intestinal permeability is increased in patients with CD and a fraction of their healthy relatives. Hollander et al.[64] first reported an increased permeability in 78% of healthy relatives of patients with CD. Additional results were controversial, mainly due to a lack of methodologic standardization.[65,66] More recent studies detected an increased permeability index in a fraction of 10–25% of healthy relatives.[67,68] There have been interesting reports regarding increased sensitivity to NSAID challenge in healthy first-degree relatives of IBD patients. A significantly higher fraction of relatives showed an increased intestinal permeability compared to controls.[69] One might speculate that this represents a genetically determined hypersensitivity of the bowel mucosa to environmental factors, particularly as this trait seemed to be conserved among families. However, this hypothesis conflicts with the finding that permeability is also increased in 30% of spouses of CD patients.[68,70] Söderhölm et al. suggested that baseline permeability (increased in a subset of both spouses and relatives) may be determined by environmental factors, whereas permeability provoked by acetylsalicylic

**Table 18.2 Potential subclinical markers in IBD**

| Antibodies | Increased frequency in healthy relatives | IBD | Reference |
|---|---|---|---|
| Intestinal permeability | + | CD | 64–70 |
| ANCA | + (not consistently) | UC | 73–79 |
| ASCA | + | CD | 81–84, 86 |
| Antigoblet cells | + | CD/UC | 181 |
| Antipancreas | – | CD | 182 |
| Lymphocytotoxic | + | CD | 183 |
| Antitropomyosin | – | UC | 184 |

ASCA, anti-*Saccharomyces cerevisiae* mannan antibodies; ANCA, antineutrophil cytoplasmic antibodies; CD, Crohn's disease; UC, ulcerative colitis.

acid (only increased in relatives) may be a function of the genetically determined state of the mucosal barrier.[70]

Antineutrophil cytoplasmic autoantibodies (ANCA) were first described in sera from patients with systemic vasculitides such as Wegener's granulomatosis, but were subsequently found in many inflammatory disorders.[71] In 1990, Saxon et al. reported that ANCA were present in patients with IBD, particularly in UC.[72] UC-associated ANCA are characterized by perinuclear highlighting on indirect immunofluorescence microscopy and have been described commonly as pANCA. In 1992, Shanahan et al. found an increased frequency of pANCA in healthy relatives (16%) of UC patients compared to controls (3%), with higher titers in relatives from ANCA-positive patients.[73] Another family study reported ANCA positivity in 30% of the first-degree relatives of UC patients.[74] However, these results have not been replicated.[75–79] Moreover, the frequency of pANCA was not significantly increased in the healthy marker of monozygotic twin pairs discordant for UC compared with healthy controls.[80] Overall, these studies have not supported the hypothesis that pANCA are a subclinical marker for susceptibility to UC.

ASCA, an antibody against oligomannosidic epitopes of the yeast *Saccharomyces cerevisiae*, has been associated with CD but not with UC. The reported prevalence is 60–70% in patients with CD, 10–15% in patients with UC, and 0–5% in control subjects.[63] In a first set of CD families, ASCA were detected in 35/51 (69%) patients with CD and in 13/66 (20%) healthy relatives versus 1/163 in the control group ($P < 0.001$).[81] The presence of ASCA in healthy relatives was observed in 12 of 20 families and was not restricted to a few particular multiplex families. The prevalence of ASCA in relatives did not depend on the ASCA status of affected family members. In 15 families in this series, children with CD were born to healthy parents; in eight of these families at least one of the parents was ASCA positive. This has led to the suggestion that ASCA positivity in parents is at least as potent a risk factor for children to develop CD as parental CD itself. Seibold et al.[82] confirmed these findings: ASCA was found in 48 (25%) of 193 healthy first-degree relatives. Despite the fact that 20–25% of relatives are ASCA positive, the generation of ASCA does not seem to be due to an autosomally dominantly inherited trait, as there are families composed of ASCA-positive children with ASCA-

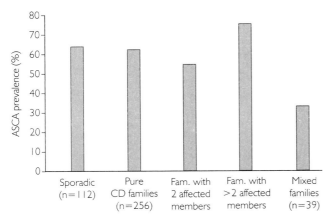

**Fig. 18.3** Prevalence of ASCA in sporadic CD, CD patients from pure CD families and mixed families, and in healthy relatives from pure CD families. ASCA prevalence in large families with more than two affected members was significantly higher than in families with two affected members ($P = 0.002$). (Modified from[84].)

negative parents.[81] Conversely, Sutton et al.[80] did not find a significantly increased frequency of ASCA in unaffected relatives of CD patients (9.3%) compared to healthy controls (4%).[83] However, they demonstrated a high concordance for ASCA seropositivity rates (defined as either ASCA positive or ASCA negative, based on an arbitrary cutoff value) in family members, in two separately analysed seronegative and seropositive proband subgroups. In addition, these authors performed an intraclass correlation of quantitative ASCA levels in both affected and unaffected family members, and found a significant familial aggregation of ASCA titers within families. This latter association was strongest among siblings. The authors concluded that these observations support the concept of both ASCA occurrence and ASCA titer levels as distinctly familial traits in CD families. Familial aspects of ASCA were further investigated in a large series of Belgian families having one, two or more affected members.[84] Overall, ASCA prevalence was the same in both sporadic (63.4%) and familial (62.1%) CD. Interestingly, CD patients from mixed families (UC plus CD) showed a significantly lower ASCA prevalence (33.3%) than sporadic cases and pure familial CD, suggesting that these families represent a distinct entity with a different immunologic response. Within pure CD families, ASCA were present in 54.2% of CD patients with two members affected, versus 74.7% in CD patients with three or more members affected ($P = 0.002$). The presence of ASCA was confirmed in 21% of healthy relatives in CD families (Fig. 18.3). These data provide convincing arguments for the hypothesis that ASCA is an expression of familiality of CD. The lack of concordance for the marker in marital pairs[84] may indicate that their presence in families is due in part to a genetic factor or childhood environmental exposure. However, the claim that ASCA may represent a specific marker of susceptibility for CD was challenged by Annese et al., who found that the frequency of ASCA in healthy relatives of UC and mixed families did not differ from that of CD families.[85] In support of this observation Poulain et al. showed that familiality of ASCA might occur in control families independent of CD, with evidence for a vertical transmission of the marker from mother to child.[86]

Thjodleifsson et al. have reported in a large Icelandic population that fecal calprotection, a product of neutrophils, was

increased in 49% of asymptomatic first-degree relatives of patients with Crohn's disease; spouses had no such increase. These authors suggested that the prevalence of subclinical inflammation in their relatives conformed to a dominant or additive inheritance pattern.[86a]

The presence of subclinical markers in healthy relatives of IBD does not yet have practical clinical implications, but intestinal permeability has been identified as possibly useful in this regard. Irvine and Marshall measured intestinal permeabilities in a small cohort of CD families. They described an initially asymptomatic 13-year-old girl with an elevated permeability to $^{51}$Cr-EDTA. Her mother and an older brother both had CD requiring multiple surgical resections. She subsequently developed symptoms of IBD at age 21, and repeat investigations revealed ileocolonic CD. In that case, a permeability defect was clearly identified to precede the onset of CD in a subject at increased risk.[87] It is clear that the majority of asymptomatic relatives do not develop overt clinical symptoms.

## Associated diseases

IBD is associated with well-defined genetic syndromes, including Turner's syndrome,[88] Hermansky–Pudlak syndrome,[89] glycogen storage disease IB,[90] cystic fibrosis[91] and pachydermoperiostosis.[92] Patients with these syndromes could potentially increase our understanding of IBD genetics, as they may carry genes that are also important in IBD susceptibility. For instance, the association of CD with Turner's syndrome has prompted the tentative localization of a CD susceptibility gene on the X chromosome.[93] IBD is also more common in patients with ankylosing spondylitis,[94] psoriasis,[95] multiple sclerosis[96] and celiac disease.[97] These are all multifactorial diseases for which there is strong evidence for genetic susceptibility and involvement of the immune system. Interestingly, clustering of non-MHC susceptibility loci between different autoimmune diseases, including CD, has been observed.[98] This supports the hypothesis that distinct chronic inflammatory disorders may have some common susceptibility genes.[99] However, the reported associations between CD and other autoimmune diseases need to be confirmed in population-based studies.

# CLINICAL IMPACT OF GENETIC STUDIES

The major focus of genetic research in IBD has been on disease susceptibility genes. It is almost certain that IBD encompasses a spectrum of heterogeneous diseases with great variations in disease presentation. Increasing data suggest that disease heterogeneity and variable responses to treatment are both genetically determined.

## SUSCEPTIBILITY GENES

Hugot and colleagues reported the first genome-wide screen for CD in 1996.[100] Since then, other genome scans for IBD have become available.[101–117] Collectively, these genome scans confirm that inflammatory bowel diseases are complex genetic disorders with several predisposing genes, and that no major gene locus carries an attributable relative risk higher than 2. At least 16 susceptibility loci have been identified (Fig. 18.4). Seven of them, on chromosomes 1, 5, 6, 12, 14, 16 and 19, have been deemed

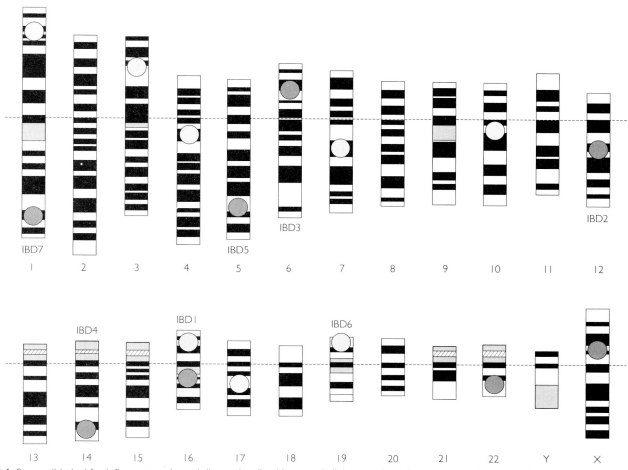

**Fig. 18.4** Susceptible loci for inflammatory bowel disease localized by genetic linkage analyses in genome-wide scan studies. *Red:* loci that have been localized with high statistical significance and replicated by several independent groups; *blue:* other proposed loci.

important in IBD susceptibility, considering their statistical threshold of significance for linkage or replication studies. Of these, only *IBD1* (chromosome 16) has been universally replicated and three others – *IBD2* (chromosome 12), *IBD3* (chromosome 6) and *IBD4* (chromosome 14) – have been widely, although not universally, replicated. The International IBD Genetics Consortium is a collaboration of 12 investigator groups involved in the positional cloning approach of identifying IBD gene loci. They have pooled large amounts of genetic data from 603 affected sibling pairs for these proposed localizations, and have undisputedly confirmed a positive linkage for chromosome 16 (*IBD1*), but not for chromosome 12 (*IBD2*).[118] For *IBD2*, LOD scores have only been 1.8 for IBD, 1.2 for UC and 1.1 for CD. This contrasts with a LOD score of 5.8 for the *IBD1* locus. However, the legitimacy of the *IBD2* locus is still likely, especially as it might pertain to UC. This is based on the observation that linkage with *IBD2* is stronger in studies with a higher number (and statistical power) of UC-relative pairs.[105] In that study, *IBD2* had a LOD score of 3.91 when analyzed for UC-only pairs, compared with LOD scores of 1.66 for CD-only family pairs. Gene identification will probably occur in the near future for *IBD2*, thus having the potential to advance our understanding of UC genetics, which so far has lagged behind advances made in CD genetics.

Out of the seven recognized IBD susceptibility loci, so far only the *IBD1* gene locus has progressed from simple localization to

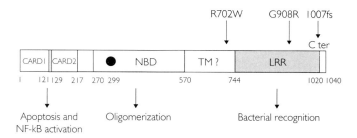

**Fig. 18.5** Structure of the NOD2/CARD15 gene and location of the Crohn's disease associated variants. The numbers represent the amino acid position. The C insertion at nucleotide 3020 causes a Leu1007Pro amino acid change followed by a stop codon. CARD, caspase recruitment domain; NBD, nucleotide binding domain; LRR, leucine-rich repeat.

actual identification: NOD2/CARD15.[119-121] Originally called NOD2, it has been re-named CARD15 by the International Nomenclature Committee. CARD15 is an intracellular protein expressed in monocytes and macrophages and has high binding affinities for bacterial peptidoglycan through its leucine-rich repeat (LRR) domain. The latter is located in the carboxy-terminal region of CARD15 (Fig. 18. 5). Binding of peptidoglycan to CARD15 leads to nuclear factor-κB (NFκB) activation under normal circumstances. Further details regarding the structure and proposed function(s) of CARD15 can be found elsewhere in this

**Table 18.3 Risk of developing Crohn's disease (CD) according to inheritance of a combination of the three CARD15 mutations based on the data of Hugot et al.[119]**

| Genotype | Relative risk of CD | Absolute risk of CD |
|---|---|---|
| No mutation | 1 | 0.007 |
| Simple heterozygous | 3 | 0.002 |
| Compound heterozygous | 44 | 0.03 |
| Homozygous | 38 | 0.03 |

Reprinted with permission from Nature (Hugot et al. Association of NOD2 leucine-rich repeat variants with susceptibilty to Crohn's disease) 2001. Macmillan Magazines Limited.

book (see Chapter 8). Mutation screening in more than 450 CD subjects has revealed 67 sequence variations, of which 31 non-conservative mutations could have a potential functional effect, based on their locations in encoding portions of the gene.[119,122] More than 90% of these mutations observed in CD patients are located in the distal, LRR portion of the protein, suggesting that this region plays a crucial role in CD susceptibility. Out of the 31 identified genetic variants, only three are frequently encountered in CD patients, but not UC: one frameshift mutation (3020insC) and two missense mutations (Arg702Trp and Gly908Arg) (Fig. 18.5). Altogether, the three main mutations are present in 10–30% of CD patients at a single dose (heterozygotes) and 3–15% at double dose (homozygotes and compound heterozygotes). By comparison, heterozygotes and mutated homozygotes are respectively 8–15% and 0–1% in healthy controls.[3,119–121,123,124] Thus, CD patients often carry a mutation on both chromosomes, suggesting some recessive properties of CARD15. On this basis, the relative risk to develop CD can be roughly estimated to be in the range of 1.5–3 in people carrying one mutation and in the range of 10–40 in people carrying two mutations. Assuming a prevalence of 1/1000 for CD inhabitants in Western countries, the probability to develop the disease is no more than 0.04 for mutated homozygotes[119] (Table 18.3). Other CARD15 allelic variants were identified in Lesage's study,[122] but owing to their rarity statistical correlation with disease susceptibility was not possible; functional analyses of these gene products are needed before their role in disease susceptibility can be confirmed.

Based on previously referenced studies, it has been proposed that less than 30% of overall susceptibility to CD may be attributable to the effect of CARD15.[3,123] This contribution to disease susceptibility may be variable in selected subpopulations owing to the association with specific gene–gene or gene– environment interactions. Similar rates of mutation have been observed in Jewish and non-Jewish patients and in Ashkenazi and non-Ashkenazi Jewish patients, although their susceptibility to CD is different.[120,124,125] The frequency of CARD15 mutations is lower in African-American than in Caucasian cohorts,[126] and it is noteworthy that CARD15 mutations are not associated with Crohn's disease in the Japanese population.[127] These data suggest that CARD15 mutations may neither be sufficient nor necessary for the development of CD, and confirm the long-held point of view that CD represents a complex genetic trait with important environmental influences.

## Genotype–phenotype relationships

Sachar has suggested that the process of identifying specific (CD) phenotypes associated with specific genotypes be called phenomics.[128] This is felt to be an essential exercise for determining the role of various 'disease-causing' mutations. CD is a clinically heterogeneous disorder, and many authors have asserted that this could be related to genetic heterogeneity. This point of view is supported by the observation that within CD families affected members show some clinical resemblance between cases (see Section 1; Genetic Epidemiology). However, this clinical concordance is limited and it was never expected to be easy to classify CD by familial risk factors, including genes. The Vienna Classification of Crohn's disease[129] attempts to standardize the clinical description of CD based on parameters such as age, disease location and behavior. However, it has been suggested that this scheme is too simplistic to account for all of the observed CD variations. As yet, there is no universally applicable CD phenotypic classification scheme. This becomes obvious when comparing the published studies on CD phenomics, and caution is required when making conclusions from such studies. Despite these qualifications, obvious phenotypic patterns are associated with discrete genotypes.

## CARD15

Since the identification of the CARD15 mutations in CD, several investigators have turned their attention to defining genotype–phenotype relationships.[3,122–124,130–133] In clinical practice, the CARD15 genotypes do not solely define specific phenotypic entities. All of the clinically recognized forms of CD can be found in both mutated and non-mutated patients.[122] Nevertheless, the main pattern emerging from these studies is that CARD15 variants are strongly associated with younger age at onset, ileal (versus non-ileal) disease, and a tendency to develop strictures (Table 18.4). Both Lesage and Ahmad's studies have shown that double-dose variants, either compound heterozygotes or homozygotes, were associated with significantly earlier age at disease presentation than patients with no variant allele.[3,122] All of the published studies have shown a propensity for ileal involvement in mutants, although it is here that the phenotypic definitions start to diverge considerably. For example, Lesage found that 'the involvement of the transverse colon, left colon, or rectum was significantly less common at the onset of disease' in double-dose mutants than in no mutants (43% vs. 62%, $P = 0.003$) for the three main mutations. In that study, left-sided colonic involvement was defined at the *onset* of disease and included the transverse colon. Similarly, ileocolonic disease was defined by involvement of the terminal ileum and/or the appendix and/or the right colon.[122] Ahmad found a significant association between ileal disease and the possession of one or more variant CARD15 alleles (43% vs. 16% controls, $P<0.0001$; RR = 23.1 for >1 variant), where ileal disease included patchy inflammation of the cecum.[3] Colonic involvement was not specifically defined. The point in the course of the disease at which evaluation occurred was also not specified. The Leu1007fsinsC frameshift mutation was identified as conferring the single highest relative risk for ileal involvement. Cuthbert and Hampe have also found a statistically significant association for ileum-specific disease and ileocolonic disease with the three mutant CARD15 haplotypes, compared with non-ileal cases.[123,130] Once again, the definitions of location remain open to interpretation. Despite the limitations of these studies, the main message is as follows: CARD15 variants are associated with ileal but not colonic CD. As an explanation for these phenotypic differences, it has been suggested that the association of

## Table 18.4 Comparison of genotype–phenotype observations for *NOD2/CARD15* mutations in the literature

| Reference | Mean age at onset | Disease location | Disease behavior |
|---|---|---|---|
| Lesage[122] | Younger, for double-dose mutations (16.9 yr) versus one mutation (20.0 yrs) or no mutation (19.8 yr) | Less frequent involvement of the transverse colon, left colon, or rectum at onset of disease | Stenosis development during evolution of disease (53% for double-dose mutations, versus 28% for no mutation) |
| Ahmad[3] | Carriage of Leu1007fsinsC – 23.1 yr<br>Homozygote or compound heterozygote – 23.5 yr<br>Carriage of any 1 of the 3 variants – 26.4 yr<br>Simple heterozygote – 27.7 yr<br>None of the 3 variants – 29.0 yr | Ileal disease associated with possession of one or more *NOD2/CARD15* variant alleles | All-stenosis and surgical-stenosing disease not significantly associated with mutations alone (logistical regression analysis showed association only with ileal disease)<br>Carriage of 1 or more variant alleles protective against fistulizing disease |
| Cuthbert[123] | Not specified | Increased frequency of mutant haplotypes in ileum-specific disease versus colon-specific disease | Not specified |
| Hampe[130] | No association | Association between mutant haplotypes and ileal and right-colonic disease | Not specified |
| Radlmayr[131] | Not specified | Not specified | Positive association between 1007fs mutation and fistulizing and fibrostenotic type – negative association with inflammatory type |
| Vermeire[132] | No association | Patients with ileal disease had a 2.3–2.9 increased risk of carrying CARD15 variants compared with solely colonic involvement | No association |
| Murillo[133] | No association | No association | No association |
| Abreu[124] | No association | Association with small bowel disease but not significant | Patients with fibrostenosing disease had a 2.8 increased risk of carrying CARD15 variants compared with patients without fibrostenosing disease – multivariate and conditioning analyses showed that the association was independent of small bowel involvement |

CARD15 mutations with ileal disease represents an important difference between the immune tolerance mechanisms of the ileum and of the colon. The colon, which is exposed to much higher bacterial concentrations than the ileum, may invoke immune mechanisms that do not depend on intact CARD15 function as much as the ileum does. This theory has not been well examined. An alternative explanation is selective colonization of the ileum by bacterial species that are suppressed by normal CARD15 function. Furthermore, there has been no association found in the existing studies between CARD15 variants and perianal disease or extraintestinal manifestations, including eye, skin, joint or liver involvement.[122]

Of all the phenotypes studied in association with CARD15 mutations so far, disease behavior (i.e. stricturing or fistulizing phenotype) is the most difficult to reproduce. It has been shown that these phenotypes are dependent upon the duration of disease,[134,135] with an ever-increasing likelihood of stricturing or penetrating behavior over the course of years. The published results are not directly comparable to the extent that they have not standardized the duration of disease in their cohorts. Such studies may show stronger associations with CARD15 variants if the mean duration of disease is sufficiently long. Lesage et al.[122] have associated the development of stenosis with double-dose mutants (OR 2.92 vs. no mutation subjects). However, stricturing behavior is more likely to occur in patients with ileal CD. Indeed, Ahmad's logistic regression showed no association between any CARD15 variant and the stricturing phenotype, independent of ileal disease.[3] These authors also found the Leu1007fsinsC frameshift mutation to be protective against fistulizing disease. In the study by Abreu et al. 46% of CD patients with fibrostenosing disease had at least one CARD15 mutation, compared to 23% of CD patients without fibrostenosing disease (OR 2.8; 95% CI 1.56–5.18).[124] Contrary to Ahmad's study, multivariate analysis suggested a primary association of CARD15 variants and fibrostenosing disease independent of small bowel involvement. Further carefully designed studies will be required to accurately determine real associations of variant alleles with disease behavior based on clear duration of disease.

Some studies have suggested that familial and sporadic CD are two distinct entities, based on differences in disease location and natural history (see Section 1); however, no difference in the frequency of CARD15 variants was found in familial and non-familial cases.[122,132] No significant association has been found between CARD15 variants and ASCA.[124] Finally, smoking habits were similar between mutation carriers and non-carriers, suggesting that additional, independent factors may interact with this well-characterized environmental risk factor.[122]

## HLA region

The major histocompatibility complex (MHC)/HLA genes and/or genes in the HLA region on chromosome 6 may have a greater role in modifying IBD phenotype than on overall disease susceptibility. In UC, genetic markers within the MHC have been associated with the development of severe steroid-resistant disease: notably, allelic variations of HLA class II genes and polymorphisms of the IκBL gene. The genetic association of the HLA-DRB1*0103 allele with severe disease has been replicated widely in the Caucasian population. Studies from Oxford first identified the HLA-DRB1*0103 allele as a potential determinant of need for colectomy in ulcerative colitis.[136] Of 99 patients with ulcerative colitis requiring colectomy, 14.1% carried the HLA-DRB1*0103 allele, compared to 3.2% of controls ($P<10^{-5}$, OR 5.5). These data were confirmed by an independent study in Amsterdam.[137] Meta-analysis has also supported these initial observations.[138] HLA associations have also been reported for subtypes of peripheral arthropathy, based on their natural history and articular distribution.[139,140] Type I peripheral arthropathy (defined as acute, self-limiting inflammation affecting fewer than five joints, lasting less than 5 weeks, associated with IBD relapses and the presence of other extraintestinal manifestations) had associations with HLA-B*27, HLA-B*35 and the strongest association to date with HLA-DRB1*0103 (40% vs. 3%). Type II arthropathy (affecting five or more joints, median duration of symptoms of 3 years, and associated with uveitis but not erythema nodosum) was associated with HLA-B*44 and MICA*008. A recent report from the same group that uveitis was strongly associated with HLA-B*27, B*58 and HLA-DRB1*0103 further supports the hypothesis that genes in the HLA region play an important role in determining the presence of extraintestinal manifestations in IBD.[141]

Several other HLA-phenotypic associations in patients with CD have been reported.[3] These include the association of HLA-DRB1*0701 with ileal disease only in the absence of variant CARD15 alleles, and the association of HLA haplotypes A1-B8-DR3 with colonic disease. Fistulizing CD has been significantly associated with HLA-DRB1*0103. A novel HLA haplotype, MICA*010, is associated with an increased risk of perianal disease, as is HLA-DRB*0103 and Cw*0802. Age at diagnosis has not been associated with any HLA haplotype or allele.

## Other genes

Other examples of reported associations between genotypes and phenotypes include the following:

- In patients with UC, carriage of allele 2 of the IL-1ra gene was highest in extensive colitis and in patients who have undergone colectomy,[142] and predicts pouchitis after ileal-pouch anastomosis.[143]
- The IκBL gene lies telomeric to the TNF cluster and carries a structural polymorphism at position 738. In a Spanish Caucasian population of patients with UC, the IκBL +

738(c) allele marked a propensity to extensive and intractable disease.[138]
- A –308 single base pair polymorphism is located in the promoter region of the TNF gene. In CD, the frequency of the allele TNF2 was significantly higher in patients with steroid-dependent than with non-steroid-dependent disease. It tended to be higher in colonic than in small bowel disease, and in fistulizing versus stricturing disease.[144]
- The CD-associated TNF haplotype a2b1c2d4e1 has been associated with a subgroup of medically unresponsive UC patients who are predisposed to a higher incidence of pouchitis after ileoanal anastomosis.[145]
- Bone loss and osteoporosis are well-known sequelae of IBD, but the risk factors for increased bone loss have not been identified. IL-1 and IL-6 have a central role in the stimulation of osteoclast development and regulation of bone resorption. A prospective study over more than 1 year in 83 IBD patients showed that genetic variations in the IL-6 and IL-1ra genes identified IBD patients at risk for increased bone loss.[146]
- A 250 kb haplotype on chromosome 5q31 (IBD5 locus) has been linked with CD.[146a] In a study from Oxford, IBD5 was specifically associated with perineal CD, and ileal disease in patients not carrying the Leu1007fsinsC CARD15 variant.[147]

In conclusion, studies defining the genotype–phenotype relationships are promising. However, there are significant difficulties in interpreting the current literature because of suboptimal standardization of clinical criteria, the lack of prospective studies with sufficient long-term follow-up, and variable data sources introducing potential investigation and referral biases.

## Molecular classification of IBD

With the increasing number of observed genotype–phenotype relationships, it is hoped that a molecular classification scheme can be created for IBD in which various disease subtypes are categorized according to their specific molecular defects. Such a classification scheme is beginning to emerge already, in which the genotype–phenotype relationships can be depicted graphically (Fig. 18.6).[3] Such a scheme could hold the possibility of tailoring 'customized' IBD therapies for the specific disease phenotype, something that has not yet been possible. At present, clinical responses to various pharmacologic agents have been largely a determination of trial and error. Molecular classifications are also felt to hold an explanation for the observed individual differences in response to treatments such as infliximab, although initial studies have not demonstrated a relationship of response to this drug with mutations in CARD15 (see below).

## PHARMACOGENETICS

Interindividual variability in drug response is a major problem in clinical practice and drug development. The main causes for the variation in drug metabolism are genetic polymorphisms, enzyme induction, and inhibition due to concomitant drug therapies, environmental factors, physiologic status and various coexisting disease states. Pharmacogenetics is the study of how genetic differences influence the variability in the responses of patients to drugs. Such variability can be manifested as a lack of response or by the occurrence of adverse drug reactions.

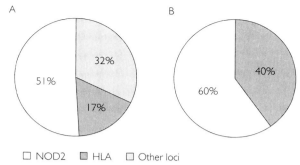

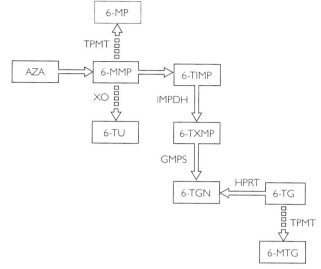

**Fig. 18.6** Population attributable risk (PAR) (%) of the NOD2/CARD15 variants, the HLA region and other loci in patients with CD and ileal disease (A) and colonic and/or perianal disease (B). PAR% were defined as the excess rate of disease in individuals with a NOD2/CARD15 variant or HLA haplotype compared with those without and are reported separately for patients with ileal disease and those with colonic and/or perianal disease. To estimate the PAR% of the NOD2/CARD15 variants the RR associated with carriage of one or more of the NOD2/CARD15 variants was calculated. To estimate the PAR% of the HLA region for ileal disease the RR associated with possession of either the DRB1*0701 or Cw*0802 haplotypes was calculated, and for colonic and/or perianal disease the RR associated with possession of either the DRB1*0701, Cw*0802, MICA*010, or BAT 1 in 10 NcoI C haplotypes was calculated. (From [3], with permission.)

## Azathioprine/6-mercaptopurine

The immunosuppressive properties of azathioprine (AZA) and 6-mercaptopurine (6-MP) are mediated through their interference with protein synthesis and nucleic acid metabolism, as well as induction of apoptosis of activated lymphocytes. After absorption, AZA is rapidly converted to 6-MP by a non-enzymatic reaction. Three enzymes then compete to metabolize 6-MP: xanthine oxidase, hypoxanthine–guanine phosphorybosyltransferase (HPRT) and thiopurine S-methyltransferase (TPMT). HPRT initiates the production of 6-thioinosine monophosphate (6-TIMP) and the 6-thioguanine nucleotides (6-TGN), the putative active metabolites. TPMT catalyzes S-methylation of 6-MP, 6-TIMP and 6-thioguanosine monophosphate (Fig. 18.7).[148] AZA/6-MP myelotoxicity has been attributed to the low activity of TPMT, which in vivo is subject to interindividual and interethnic variability owing to TPMT gene polymorphisms. Three major phenotypes have been described: high, intermediate and low methylators. Less efficient methylation leads to increasing levels of 6-TGN and thereby to an increased risk of hematopoietic toxicity.[149–151] In the past 5 years the genetic basis of the TPMT polymorphism has been largely unraveled. A substantial number of point mutations have been identified in various populations, occurring alone or in combination on different alleles of the TPMT gene. In vitro and in vivo studies have allowed clarification of the functional consequences of mutations on TPMT activity.[152–155] Several non-functional variants of the gene have been characterized and major mutations causing 'loss of function' of alleles have been recognized. Identification of these mutations has provided a molecular basis for TPMT polymorphisms and has led to the development of simple DNA-based assays to predict TPMT phenotype.[83,152–158]

Colombel et al. performed a genotypic analysis of TPMT in 41 patients with Crohn's disease and severe myelosuppression during AZA treatment.[159] Four patients (10%) had two mutant alleles associated with TPMT deficiency, seven (17%) had one mutant allele and 30 (73%) had no known TPMT mutations. An

**Fig. 18.7** Azathioprine (AZA) metabolism. Oral AZA is rapidly converted to 6-mercaptopurine (6-MP) by a non-enzymatic process. Initial 6-MP transformation occurs along competing pathways: XO, xanthine oxidase; TPMT, thiopurine S-methyltransferase; HGPRT, hypoxanthine–guanine phosphoribosyltransferase. Once formed, 6 thio-inosine monophosphate (6-TIMP) may be transformed in active 6-thioguanine nucleotides by the rate-limiting inosine monophosphate dehydrogenase (IMPDH) or methylated into 6-methyl-mercaptopurine ribonucleotides (6-MMPR). (From [162], with permission.)

important finding of this study was the relationship between the duration of AZA/6-MP treatment, the occurrence of myelotoxicity and TPMT genotype: in the four patients homozygous for an inactivating mutation, myelosuppression occurred within 1.5 months after azathioprine was started. On the other hand, myelosuppression occurred over a much wider range of time in heterozygous patients or patients having no mutation (Fig. 18.8). This study suggested that delayed neutropenia in patients receiving AZA/6MP was most likely to be due to factors other than TPMT deficiency, possibly associated treatments or environmental factors.

Several studies have suggested that 6-TGN levels are significantly associated with clinical remission in IBD.[160–162] In a series of 92 pediatric patients, the frequency of therapeutic response significantly increased at 6-TGN levels higher than 235 pmol/$8 \times 10^8$ erythrocytes and leukopenia was associated with higher 6-TGN levels.[160] Conversely, increased methylation with elevated 6-methylmercaptopurine (6-MMP) levels correlated with hepatotoxicity. 6-TGN levels have also been used to optimize AZA/6-MP therapy in a group of 82 adult patients with IBD. 6-TGN levels >250pmol/$8 \times 10^8$ erythrocytes correlated with clinical response in patients with fistulizing and colonic CD, but not in those with ileocolonic disease.[161] More recently, serial metabolite measurement in 51 IBD patients identified a subgroup of patients resistant to AZA/6-MP therapy and characterized by preferential 6-MMP production upon dose escalation.[163] Monitoring 6-MP metabolite levels may thus assist clinicians in optimizing therapeutic response to AZA/6-MP. Nevertheless, reported results have been controversial regarding the prediction of responsiveness to AZA/6-MP based on 6-TGN levels,[164,165] and no prospective study is yet available. In a series of 170 patients with IBD treated with AZA or 6-MP,

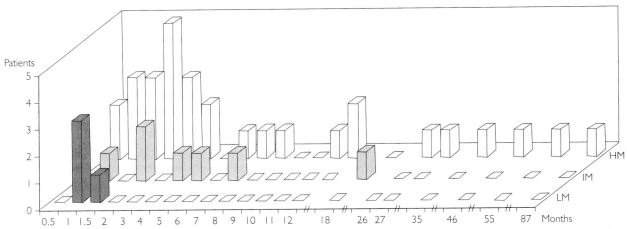

**Fig. 18.8** Delay (months) between the first administration of AZA/6-MP and the occurrence of bone marrow toxicity in 41 patients having had severe myelosuppression during AZA therapy. Patients classified as low methylators (LM) (n = 4) were homozygous for one non-functional mutation or heterozygous for two non-functional mutations; patients classified as intermediate methylators (IM) (n = 7) were heterozygous for one non-functional mutation; patients classified as high methylators (HM) (n = 29) were homozygous for the wildtype or heterozygous for two functional alleles. One patient not represented was heterozygous for a previously unknown mutation. (From [159], with permission.)

there was no correlation between disease activity as measured by the Inflammatory Bowel Disease Questionnaire and 6-TGN concentrations. The median 6-TGN concentrations in 56 patients with active disease and 114 patients in remission were similar.[165]

In summary, the utility of TPMT genotyping and 6-TGN concentrations measurement in clinical practice remains unclear[166] (see Chapter 32, Clinical Pharmacology). Testing for TPMT activity or genotype is recommended prior to initiating AZA or 6-MP therapy, in order to avoid using the drug in the rare instance of absent TPMT activity (1/300 patients). Alternatively, starting at lower doses (1 mg/kg 6MP or 1.5–2 mg/kg AZA) with blood counts at 2 weeks can identify patients at risk for early neutropenia. It is also recommended to adjust the dose in those with intermediate TPMT activity. Myelosuppression is more often due to other factors than TPMT deficiency. Continued monitoring of blood cell counts remains mandatory in patients treated with AZA/6-MP. Monitoring of 6-TGN is not necessary but should be considered in patients suspected of non-adherence and those failing to respond to standard doses of the drugs. Failure to respond is likely due to as yet unexplained mechanisms, rather than merely an inadequate systemic exposure to 6-TGN.[167] If confirmed by independent studies, measuring 6-TGN/6-MMP in non-responding patients may be helpful to identify which may respond to increased dosages.[163]

## Sulfasalazine and 5-aminosalicylate

Colonic bacterial metabolism of sulfasalazine leads to the formation of sulfapyridine and 5-aminosalicylate. Acetylation of 5-aminosalicylate is catalyzed by arylamine-N-acetyltransferase 1 (NAT1), which is expressed in the human intestine. Several alleles of the *NAT1* gene have been described.[168] A significant interindividual variation in NAT1 activity correlating with its genotype has been demonstrated in the colon and small bowel of four organ donors.[169] One subject with the NAT1*14 allele had a strongly reduced level of activity. The sulfapyridine moiety of sulfasalazine, which is associated with toxicity, is degraded by NAT2 within the liver. Intuitively, a relationship between clinical efficacy and various NAT1 and 2 polymorphisms would be

expected, but a study from the Mayo Clinic has shown that there is no such relationship. NAT1 and NAT2 genotypes did not predict response to mesalamine or sulfasalazine, or toxicity to sulfasalazine in patients with UC.[170]

## CORTICOSTEROIDS

Considerable progress has been made in understanding the complex molecular mechanisms that underlie the anti-inflammatory effects of glucocorticoids, and a number of key regulatory points have been identified. IBD studies have strongly implicated two further potential markers of drug responsiveness: the multidrug resistance (MDR) gene[171] and the glucocorticoid receptor gene.[172] The MDR1 genotype encodes a 170 kDa cell membrane-based drug efflux pump, P-glycoprotein 170 (PGP170). This protein actively transports MDR substrates out of cells, thereby lowering their intracellular concentrations. In vitro studies have demonstrated that corticosteroids and cyclosporin concentrations are significantly affected by PGP170 activity. Farrell and colleagues have demonstrated that peripheral blood lymphocyte MDR expression is increased in patients with medically refractory UC.[171] Glucocorticoids bind to glucocorticoid cytoplasmic receptors (GCR), which dimerize and translocate to the cell nucleus. The β-splice variant of the glucocorticoid receptor (hGRß), which encodes a truncated protein of amino acid #742, does not bind glucocorticoid and lacks transrepression activity. Data in UC suggest that overexpression of hGRß may be associated with steroid-refractory disease. Among corticosteroid-resistant UC patients, hGRß was found in 83%, compared to 9% in corticosteroid-sensitive patients and 10% in controls.[172]

## Infliximab

Twenty-five to fifty per cent of patients do not clinically respond to infliximab, and the presence or absence of response appears stable over time. This suggests that some biological characteristics, possibly genetically determined, may be involved. Several polymorphisms in the gene encoding TNF and the TNF receptor have been examined, but most have proved without success.

In a Belgian cohort of 226 patients with CD treated with infliximab a clinical response was associated with a higher CRP level before treatment, but there was no relevant association with –308 TNF polymorphism.[173] A study in a small number of treated Crohn's patients showed that homozygosity for the lymphocytotoxin LTA Nco1-TNFc-aa13L-aa26 haplotype and a pANCA fluorescence pattern are associated with a poor response to infliximab.[174] Further confirmation is awaited.

Targeted deletion of the LRR region of CARD15 is associated with increased NFκB activity, but the truncation mutation in the region leads to decreased activation of NFκB by bacterial components[175] Therefore, mutations in CARD15 could well be involved in the differences in response seen with infliximab, based on dysregulated NFκB activation and TNF production. Vermeire et al. studied the identified mutations in CARD15 in a large cohort of infliximab-treated CD patients, to assess whether these mutations are predictive of clinical response.[176] There was no relationship between the overall presence of a mutation in CARD15, nor of any of the mutations separately, and short-term infliximab response or median response duration. Multivariate analysis could not identify any clinical characteristics that were associated with response to infliximab in combination with CARD15 mutations.[176]

## GENETIC COUNSELING

Historically, genetic counseling has been addressed by medical geneticists and involves detailed case preparation.[177] This includes obtaining family history information and pedigree construction, obtaining information on the genetic condition, performing risk assessments, genetic testing, and providing support group contacts. Traditionally, this has pertained to diseases of simple Mendelian inheritance, or single-gene disorders, which manifest at birth or soon thereafter. This formed the basis for prenatal genetic testing for disorders such as trisomy 21 (Down's syndrome), cystic fibrosis, and inherited disorders of metabolism. Other examples include Huntington's disease. These services are provided by only a few tertiary medical centers. Over the past several years advances have been made in understanding the genetic basis of common diseases, including prostate, breast, ovarian and colorectal cancers, Alzheimer's disease, diabetes mellitus, and also IBD. Widespread genetic testing would generate a demand for technical resources and counseling that exceeded current availability, requiring that many more professionals be trained in genetic counseling. Primary care and medical specialty providers would require training in the fundamentals of the genetic basis of disease, genetic testing and counseling.

Also challenging is the question of how genetic testing and counseling may be applied to susceptibility genes, which are not found in many afflicted persons and yet may also be found in persons who never manifest the disease. Such is the case for the CARD15 gene polymorphism of CD. Thus, a specific genetic factor is neither necessary nor sufficient to develop the disease. This point of view is supported by genome-wide scan analyses which have failed to localize any gene with an attributable relative risk higher than 2. In addition, our knowledge of the interaction between the various environmental and genetic risk factors is quite limited. Currently, there is no comprehensive model of CD development. Thus, questions which patients will have on risk estimates, severity estimates and familial risk are currently uncertain. None the less, new observations from clinical studies may be useful for genetic counseling. The main message is that the relative risk of IBD in first-degree relatives is increased by a factor of 10–15 compared to general populations. Based on the available literature, no genetic counseling information should be given to families about age at onset and disease severity.

Considering that IBD relatives are at higher risk to develop the disease, families frequently ask for presymptomatic screening or diagnosis. Subclinical markers such as ASCA, ANCA or intestinal permeability tests have been proposed, but currently their predictive value is too limited to use in clinical practice. From the genetic markers, the most convincing argument could be made for CARD15 screening. However, even for the three main CD-associated mutations the relative risk to develop CD is too low to provide useful information for populations at risk. Indeed, the probability of developing CD for the highest risk genotype is in the range of only a few per cent. Even if it were possible to provide more useful information, it would be questionable to perform presymptomatic diagnosis for IBD. Such an approach is usually proposed only for very severe diseases in the fetus, or when a presymptomatic preventive therapy exists. This is not the case for either CD or UC. Thus, in our opinion (and currently is the state of the art) it is not recommended to screen healthy at-risk people such as CD relatives for the CARD15 polymorphism. However, it is useful to inform them to avoid cigarette smoking.

The presence of CARD15 polymorphisms may be an argument to consider its use in patients presenting with clinical symptoms suggestive of CD. However, because CARD15 polymorphisms are present in only a small proportion of CD patients, the sensitivity of the genotyping test is too low for this purpose. Thus, it is not possible to consider CARD15 screening as a stand-alone tool in the clinical diagnosis of CD. IBD diagnosis still requires the necessary art of due consideration of all clinical, laboratory, radiological, endoscopic and histological data. In this context, CARD15 testing may be considered as one of the parameters.

Because CARD15 is not involved in UC predisposition, it could be attractive to use this test in cases of indeterminate colitis. However, results of genotype/phenotype analyses suggest that CARD15 may have only a limited role in this clinical situation. Indeed, CARD15 polymorphisms are infrequent in colitis without ileal involvement.

Genotyping methods may also be useful for the clinician in order to establish a prognosis. The first results on CARD15 suggest that stenoses are more frequent in patients carrying two mutations. This information may become useful in clinical practice, for example to avoid therapeutic agents that could worsen bowel strictures. HLA genotypes may also be useful to predict the severity of the disease or extraintestinal manifestations. However, additional studies are needed before the impact of genotyping on clinical practice can be understood.

Even though pharmacogenetics carries the promise of improving rational dosing of IBD treatments, the current enthusiasm should be tempered in view of the available data. The patient's response to a drug is multifactorial and is similar to complex diseases in that there are primary genes, modifier genes and environmental factors that all interact. Evans and Relling have provided an illustration of such complexity.[178] They considered the hypothetical effects of two polymorphic genes: one that determines the extent of drug inactivation and another that determines the sensitivity of the drug receptor. These two genetic polymorphisms yielded nine different theoretical patterns of drug effects. The therapeutic ratio ranged from a favorable 75 in the patient with wt/wt genotypes for drug metabolism and receptors, to less than 0.13 in the patient with an m/m genotype. This situation might be found, for instance, in patients with IBD treated with AZA/6-MP.[179] Somatic mutations may arise in T cells, including those affecting the gene encoding HPRT. Therefore, clinical AZA/6-MP efficacy or resistance and toxicity may depend both on TPMT and HPRT polymorphisms. In general, it will probably be very difficult, if not impossible, to characterize all of the genetically determined variability in drug response.

In conclusion, genetic testing in patients and their relatives seems premature because of the low penetrance of disease and our current lack of effective intervention at a preclinical stage.[180] As each new IBD gene is discovered, it will need to be investigated further in many clinical situations. Therefore, it would be useful to widely genotype all IBD patients involved in clinical research studies. It is expected that this resource will help to better define the place of genotyping in clinical practice, and pave the way for meaningful genetic counseling and eventual therapeutic intervention to prevent disease onset.

# REFERENCES

1. Podolsky D. Inflammatory bowel disease. N Engl J Med 2002;347:417–429.
2. Cho JH. The Nod2 gene in Crohn's disease: implications for future research into the genetics and immunology of Crohn's disease. Inflamm Bowel Dis 2001;7:271–275.
3. Ahmad T, Armuzzi A, Bunce M et al. The molecular classification of the clinical manifestations of Crohn's disease. Gastroenterology 2002;122:854–866.
4. Tysk C, Lindberg E, Jarnerot G, Floderus-Myrhed B. Ulcerative colitis and Crohn's disease in an unselected population of monozygotic and dizygotic twins. A study of heritability and the influence of smoking. Gut 1988;29:990–996.
5. Subhani J, Montgomery S, Pounder R, Wakefield A. Concordance rates of twins and siblings in inflammatory bowel diseases. Gut 1998;42 (Suppl 1):A40.
6. Orholm M, Binder V, Sorensen TI, Rasmussen LP, Kyvik KO. Concordance of inflammatory bowel disease among Danish twins. Results of a nationwide study. Scand J Gastroenterol 2000;35:1075–1081.
7. Ahmad T, Satsangi J, McGovern D, Bunce M, Jewell DP. Review article: the genetics of inflammatory bowel disease. Aliment Pharmacol Ther 2001;15:731–748.
8. Breslin NP, Todd A, Kilgallen C, O'Morain C. Monozygotic twins with Crohn's disease and ulcerative colitis: a unique case report. Gut 1997;41:557–560.
9. Odes HS, Fraser D, Hollander L. Epidemiological data of Crohn's disease in Israel: etiological implications. Public Health Rev 1989;17:321–335.
10. Niv Y, Abuksis G, Fraser GM. Epidemiology of Crohn's disease in Israel: a survey of Israeli kibbutz settlements. Am J Gastroenterol 1999;94:2691–2695.
11. Roth MP, Petersen GM, McElree C, Feldman E, Rotter JI. Geographic origins of Jewish patients with inflammatory bowel disease. Gastroenterology 1989;97:900–904.
12. Yang H, McElree C, Roth MP, Shanahan F, Targan SR, Rotter JI. Familial empirical risks for inflammatory bowel disease: differences between Jews and non-Jews. Gut 1993;34:517–524.
13. Sonnenberg A, Wasserman IH. Epidemiology of inflammatory bowel disease among US military veterans. Gastroenterology 1991;101:122–130.
14. Yang SK, Loftus EV Jr, Sandborn WJ. Epidemiology of inflammatory bowel disease in Asia. Inflamm Bowel Dis 2001;7:260–270.
15. Montgomery SM, Morris DL, Pounder RE, Wakefield AJ. Asian ethnic origin and the risk of inflammatory bowel disease. Eur J Gastroenterol Hepatol 1999;11:543–546.
16. Weterman IT, Pena AS. Familial incidence of Crohn's disease in The Netherlands and a review of the literature. Gastroenterology 1984;86:449–452.
17. Farmer RG. Study of family history among patients with inflammatory bowel disease. Scand J Gastroenterol 1989;170(Suppl):64–65.
18. Monsen U, Brostrom O, Nordenvall B, Sorstad J, Hellers G. Prevalence of inflammatory bowel disease among relatives of patients with ulcerative colitis. Scand J Gastroenterol 1987;22:214–218.
19. Monsen U, Bernell O, Johansson C, Hellers G. Prevalence of inflammatory bowel disease among relatives of patients with Crohn's disease. Scand J Gastroenterol 1991;26:302–306.
20. Satsangi J, Rosenberg WMC, Jewell DP. The prevalence of inflammatory bowel disease in relatives of patients with Crohn's disease. Eur J Gastroenterol Hepatol 1994;6:413–416.
21. Peeters M, Nevens H, Baert F et al. Familial aggregation in Crohn's disease: increased age-adjusted risk and concordance in clinical characteristics. Gastroenterology 1996;111:597–603.
22. Orholm M, Munkholm P, Langholz E, Nielsen OH, Sorensen IA, Binder V. Familial occurrence of inflammatory bowel disease. N Engl J Med 1991;324:84–88.
23. Bennett RA, Rubin PH, Present DH. Frequency of inflammatory bowel disease in offspring of couples both presenting with inflammatory bowel disease. Gastroenterology 1991;100:1638–1643.
24. Laharie D, Debeugny S, Peeters M et al. Inflammatory bowel disease in spouses and their offspring. Gastroenterology 2001;120:816–819.
25. Satsangi J, Grootscholten C, Holt H, Jewell DP. Clinical patterns of familial inflammatory bowel disease. Gut 1996;38:738–741.
26. Orholm M, Fonager K, Sorensen HT. Risk of ulcerative colitis and Crohn's disease among offspring of patients with chronic inflammatory bowel disease. Am J Gastroenterol 1999;94:3236–3238.
27. Bayless TM, Tokayer AZ, Polito JM II, Quaskey SA, Mellits ED, Harris ML. Crohn's disease: concordance for site and clinical type in affected family members – potential hereditary influences. Gastroenterology 1996;111:573–579.
28. Colombel JF, Grandbastien B, Gower-Rousseau C et al. Clinical characteristics of Crohn's disease in 72 families. Gastroenterology 1996;111:604–607.
29. Van Kruiningen HJ, Colombel JF, Cartun RW et al. An in-depth study of Crohn's disease in two French families. Gastroenterology 1993;104:351–360.
30. Lee JC, Lennard-Jones JE. Inflammatory bowel disease in 67 families each with three or more affected first-degree relatives. Gastroenterology 1996;111:587–596.
31. Annese V, Andreoli A, Astegiano M et al. Clinical features in familial cases of Crohn's disease and ulcerative colitis in Italy: a GISC study. Italian Study Group for the Disease of Colon and Rectum. Am J Gastroenterol 2001;96:2939–2945.
32. Polito JM II, Childs B, Mellits ED, Tokayer AZ, Harris ML, Bayless TM. Crohn's disease: influence of age at diagnosis on site and clinical type of disease. Gastroenterology 1996;111:580–586.
33. Farmer RG, Michener WM, Mortimer EA. Studies of family history among patients with inflammatory bowel disease. Clin Gastroenterol 1980;9:271–277.
34. Ekbom A, Helmick C, Zack M, Adami HO. The epidemiology of inflammatory bowel disease: a large, population-based study in Sweden. Gastroenterology 1991;100:350–358.
35. Akolkar PN, Gulwani-Akolkar B, Heresbach D et al. Differences in risk of Crohn's disease in offspring of mothers and fathers with inflammatory bowel disease. Am J Gastroenterol 1997;92:2241–2244.
36. Hall J. Genomic imprinting: nature and clinical relevance. Annu Rev Med 1997;48:35–44.
37. Franchimont D, Belaiche J, Louis E et al. Familial Crohn's disease: a study of 18 families. Acta Gastroenterol Belg 1997;60:134–137.
38. Cottone M, Brignola C, Rosselli M et al. Relationship between site of disease and familial occurrence in Crohn's disease. Dig Dis Sci 1997;42:129–132.
39. Carbonnel F, Macaigne G, Beaugerie L, Gendre JP, Cosnes J. Crohn's disease severity in familial and sporadic cases. Gut 1999;44:91–95.
40. Leijonmarck CE, Persson PG, Hellers G. Factors affecting colectomy rate in ulcerative colitis: an epidemiologic study. Gut 1990;31:329–333.
41. Langholz E, Munkholm P, Davidsen M, Binder V. Colorectal cancer risk and mortality in patients with ulcerative colitis. Gastroenterology 1992;103:1444–1451.
42. Askling J, Dickman PW, Karlen P et al. Colorectal cancer rates among first-degree relatives of patients with inflammatory bowel disease: a population-based cohort study. Lancet 2001;357:262–266.
43. Peeters M, Cortot A, Vermeire S, Colombel JF. Familial and sporadic inflammatory bowel disease: different entities? Inflamm Bowel Dis 2000;6:314–320.
44. Harper PS, Harley HG, Reardon W, Shaw DJ. Anticipation in myotonic dystrophy: new light on an old problem. Am J Hum Genet 1992;51:10–16.
45. Durr A, Cossee M, Agid Y et al. Clinical and genetic abnormalities in patients with Friedreich's ataxia. N Engl J Med 1996;335:1169–1175.
46. Ranen NG, Stine OC, Abbott MH et al. Anticipation and instability of IT–15 (CAG)n repeats in parent–offspring pairs with Huntington disease. Am J Hum Genet 1995;57:593–602.
47. Tsilfidis C, MacKenzie AE, Mettler G, Barcelo J, Korneluk RG. Correlation between CTG trinucleotide repeat length and frequency of severe congenital myotonic dystrophy. Nature Genet 1992;1:192–195.
48. Polito JM II, Rees RC, Childs B, Mendeloff AI, Harris ML, Bayless TM. Preliminary evidence for genetic anticipation in Crohn's disease. Lancet 1996;347:798–800.
49. Bayless TM, Picco MF, LaBuda MC. Genetic anticipation in Crohn's disease. Am J Gastroenterol 1998;93:2322–2325.
50. Grandbastien B, Peeters M, Franchimont D et al. Anticipation in familial Crohn's disease. Gut 1998;42:170–174.
51. Lee JC, Bridger S, McGregor C, Macpherson AJ, Jones JE. Why children with inflammatory bowel disease are diagnosed at a younger age than their affected parent. Gut 1999;44:808–811.
52. Heresbach D, Gulwani-Akolkar B, Lesser M et al. Anticipation in Crohn's disease may be influenced by gender and ethnicity of the transmitting parent. Am J Gastroenterol 1998;93:2368–2372.

53. Picco MF, Goodman S, Reed J, Bayless TM. Methodologic pitfalls in the determination of genetic anticipation: the case of Crohn disease. Ann Intern Med 2001;134:1124–1129.

54. Brant SR, Panhuysen CI, Bailey-Wilson JE et al. Linkage heterogeneity for the IBD1 locus in Crohn's disease pedigrees by disease onset and severity. Gastroenterology 2000;119:1483–1490.

55. Van Heel D, Satsangi J, Carey A, Jewell D. Chromosome 12 linkage for inflammatory bowel disease is greater in families identified by early age at diagonosis. Gut 2000;46 (Suppl 11):A6.

56. Akolkar PN, Gulwani-Akolkar B, Lin XY et al. The IBD1 locus for susceptibility to Crohn's disease has a greater impact in Ashkenazi Jews with early onset disease. Am J Gastroenterol 2001;96:1127–1132.

57. Sachar DB. Crohn's disease: a family affair. Gastroenterology 1996;111:813–815.

58. Van Kruiningen HJ, Cortot A, Colombel JF. The importance of familial clusterings in Crohn's disease. Inflamm Bowel Dis 2001;7:170–173; discussion 174.

59. Calkins BM. A meta-analysis of the role of smoking in inflammatory bowel disease. Dig Dis Sci 1989;34:1841–1854.

60. Smith MB, Lashner BA, Hanauer SB. Smoking and inflammatory bowel disease in families. Am J Gastroenterol 1988;83:407–409.

61. Brignola C, Belloli C, Ardizzone S, Astegiano M, Cottone M, Trallori G. The relationship between heritability and smoking habits in Crohn's disease. Italian Cooperative Study Group. Am J Gastroenterol 2000;95:3171–3175.

62. Bridger S, Lee JCW, Bjarnason I, Lennard Jones J, MacPherson AJ. In siblings with similar genetic susceptibility for inflammatory bowel disease, smokers tend to develop Crohn's disease and non-smokers develop ulcerative colitis. Gut 2002;51:21–25.

63. Reumaux D, Sendid B, Dewit O, Poulain D, Duthilleul P, Colombel JF. Serological markers in inflammatory bowel diseases. Best Prac Res Clin Gastroenterol 2002;17.

64. Hollander D, Vadheim CM, Brettholz E, Petersen GM, Delahunty T, Rotter JI. Increased intestinal permeability in patients with Crohn's disease and their relatives. A possible etiologic factor. Ann Intern Med 1986;105:883–885.

65. Ainsworth M, Eriksen J, Rasmussen JW, Schaffalitzky de Muckadell OB. Intestinal permeability of 51Cr-labelled ethylenediaminetetraacetic acid in patients with Crohn's disease and their healthy relatives. Scand J Gastroenterol 1989;24:993–998.

66. Teahon K, Smethurst P, Levi AJ, Menzies IS, Bjarnason I. Intestinal permeability in patients with Crohn's disease and their first degree relatives. Gut 1992;33:320–323.

67. May GR, Sutherland LR, Meddings JB. Is small intestinal permeability really increased in relatives of patients with Crohn's disease? Gastroenterology 1993;104:1627–1632.

68. Peeters M, Geypens B, Claus D et al. Clustering of increased small intestinal permeability in families with Crohn's disease. Gastroenterology 1997;113:802–807.

69. Hilsden RJ, Meddings JB, Sutherland LR. Intestinal permeability changes in response to acetylsalicylic acid in relatives of patients with Crohn's disease. Gastroenterology 1996;110:1395–1403.

70. Soderholm JD, Olaison G, Lindberg E et al. Different intestinal permeability patterns in relatives and spouses of patients with Crohn's disease: an inherited defect in mucosal defence? Gut 1999;44:96–100.

71. Hoffman GS, Specks U. Antineutrophil cytoplasmic antibodies. Arthritis Rheum 1998;41:1521–1537.

72. Saxon A, Shanahan F, Landers C, Ganz T, Targan S. A distinct subset of antineutrophil cytoplasmic antibodies is associated with inflammatory bowel disease. J Allergy Clin Immunol 1990;86:202–210.

73. Shanahan F, Duerr RH, Rotter JI et al. Neutrophil autoantibodies in ulcerative colitis: familial aggregation and genetic heterogeneity. Gastroenterology 1992;103:456–461.

74. Seibold F, Slametschka D, Gregor M, Weber P. Neutrophil autoantibodies: a genetic marker in primary sclerosing cholangitis and ulcerative colitis. Gastroenterology 1994;107:532–536.

75. Reumaux D, Colombel JF, Duclos B et al. Antineutrophil cytoplasmic auto-antibodies in sera from patients with ulcerative colitis after proctocolectomy with ileo-anal anastomosis. Adv Exp Med Biol 1993;336:523–525.

76. Lee JC, Lennard-Jones JE, Cambridge G. Antineutrophil antibodies in familial inflammatory bowel disease. Gastroenterology 1995;108:428–433.

77. Bansi DS, Lo S, Chapman RW, Fleming KA. Absence of antineutrophil cytoplasmic antibodies in relatives of UK patients with primary sclerosing cholangitis and ulcerative colitis. Eur J Gastroenterol Hepatol 1996;8:111–116.

78. Folwaczny C, Noehl N, Endres SP, Loeschke K, Fricke H. Antineutrophil and pancreatic autoantibodies in first-degree relatives of patients with inflammatory bowel disease. Scand J Gastroenterol 1998;33:523–528.

79. Papo M, Quer JC, Pastor RM et al. Antineutrophil cytoplasmic antibodies in relatives of patients with inflammatory bowel disease. Am J Gastroenterol 1996;91:1512–1515.

80. Yang P, Jarnerot G, Danielsson D, Tysk C, Lindberg E. P-ANCA in monozygotic twins with inflammatory bowel disease. Gut 1995;36:887–890.

81. Sendid B, Quinton JF, Charrier G et al. Anti-Saccharomyces cerevisiae mannan antibodies in familial Crohn's disease. Am J Gastroenterol 1998;93:1306–1310.

82. Seibold F, Stich O, Hufnagl R, Kamil S, Scheurlen M. Anti-Saccharomyces cerevisiae antibodies in inflammatory bowel disease: a family study. Scand J Gastroenterol 2001;36:196–201.

83. Sutton CL, Yang H, Li Z, Rotter JI, Targan SR, Braun J. Familial expression of anti-Saccharomyces cerevisiae mannan antibodies in affected and unaffected relatives of patients with Crohn's disease. Gut 2000;46:58–63.

84. Vermeire S, Peeters M, Vlietinck R et al. Anti-Saccharomyces cerevisiae antibodies (ASCA), phenotypes of IBD, and intestinal permeability: a study in IBD families. Inflamm Bowel Dis 2001;7:8–15.

85. Annese V, Andreoli A, Andriulli A et al. Familial expression of anti-Saccharomyces cerevisiae mannan antibodies in Crohn's disease and ulcerative colitis: a GISC study. Am J Gastroenterol 2001;96:2407–2412.

86. Poulain D, Sendid B, Fajardy I, Danze PM, Colombel JF. Mother to child transmission of anti-S. cerevisiae mannan antibodies (ASCA) in non-IBD families. Gut 2000;47:870–871.

86a. Thjodleifsson B, Sigthorsson C, Cariglia N et al. Subclinical intestinal inflammation: an inherited abnormality in Crohn's disease relatives. Gastroenterology 2003;124:1728–1737.

87. Irvine EJ, Marshall JK. Increased intestinal permeability precedes the onset of Crohn's disease in a subject with familial risk. Gastroenterology 2000;119:1740–1744.

88. Hayward PA, Satsangi J, Jewell DP. Inflammatory bowel disease and the X chromosome. Q J Med 1996;89:713–718.

89. Schinella RA, Greco MA, Cobert BL, Denmark LW, Cox RP. Hermansky–Pudlak syndrome with granulomatous colitis. Ann Intern Med 1980;92:20–23.

90. Couper R, Kapelushnik J, Griffiths AM. Neutrophil dysfunction in glycogen storage disease Ib: association with Crohn's-like colitis. Gastroenterology 1991;100:549–554.

91. Lloyd-Still J. Crohn's disease and cystic fibrosis. Dig Dis Sci 1994;39:880–885.

92. Compton RF, Sandborn WJ, Yang H et al. A new syndrome of Crohn's disease and pachydermoperiostosis in a family. Gastroenterology 1997;112:241–249.

93. Vermeire S, Satsangi J, Peeters M et al. Evidence for inflammatory bowel disease of a susceptibility locus on the X chromosome. Gastroenterology 2001;120:834–840.

94. Purrmann J, Zeidler H, Bertrams J et al. HLA antigens in ankylosing spondylitis associated with Crohn's disease. Increased frequency of the HLA phenotype B27,B44. J Rheumatol 1988;15:1658–1661.

95. Lee FI, Bellary SV, Francis C. Increased occurrence of psoriasis in patients with Crohn's disease and their relatives. Am J Gastroenterol 1990;85:962–963.

96. Minuk GY, Lewkonia RM. Possible familial association of multiple sclerosis and inflammatory bowel disease. N Engl J Med 1986;314:586.

97. Cottone M, Cappello M, Puleo A, Cipolla C, Filippazzo MG. Familial association of Crohn's and coeliac diseases. Lancet 1989;2:338.

98. Becker KG, Simon RM, Bailey-Wilson JE et al. Clustering of non-major histocompatibility complex susceptibility candidate loci in human autoimmune diseases. Proc Natl Acad Sci USA 1998;95:9979–9984.

99. Cho JH. Update on the genetics of inflammatory bowel disease. Curr Gastroenterol Rep 2001;3:458–463.

100. Hugot JP, Laurent-Puig P, Gower-Rousseau C et al. Mapping of a susceptibility locus for Crohn's disease on chromosome 16. Nature 1996;379:821–823.

101. Satsangi J, Parkes M, Louis E et al. Two stage genome-wide search in inflammatory bowel disease provides evidence for susceptibility loci on chromosomes 3, 7 and 12. Nature Genet 1996;14:199–202.

102. Ohmen JD, Yang HY, Yamamoto KK et al. Susceptibility locus for inflammatory bowel disease on chromosome 16 has a role in Crohn's disease, but not in ulcerative colitis. Hum Mol Genet 1996;5:1679–1683.

103. Parkes M, Satsangi J, Lathrop GM, Bell JI, Jewell DP. Susceptibility loci in inflammatory bowel disease. Lancet 1996;348:1588.

104. Brant SR, Fu Y, Fields CT et al. American families with Crohn's disease have strong evidence for linkage to chromosome 16 but not chromosome 12. Gastroenterology 1998;115:1056–1061.

105. Curran ME, Lau KF, Hampe J et al. Genetic analysis of inflammatory bowel disease in a large European cohort supports linkage to chromosomes 12 and 16. Gastroenterology 1998;115:1066–1071.

106. Cavanaugh JA, Callen DF, Wilson SR et al. Analysis of Australian Crohn's disease pedigrees refines the localization for susceptibility to inflammatory bowel disease on chromosome 16. Ann Hum Genet 1998;62:291–298.

107. Duerr RH, Barmada MM, Zhang L et al. Linkage and association between inflammatory bowel disease and a locus on chromosome 12. Am J Hum Genet 1998;63:95–100.

108. Cho JH, Nicolae DL, Gold LH et al. Identification of novel susceptibility loci for inflammatory bowel disease on chromosomes 1p, 3q, and 4q: evidence for epistasis between 1p and IBD1. Proc Natl Acad Sci USA 1998;95:7502–7507.

109. Annese V, Latiano A, Bovio P et al. Genetic analysis in Italian families with inflammatory bowel disease supports linkage to the IBD1 locus – a GISC study. Eur J Hum Genet 1999;7:567–573.

110. Hampe J, Schreiber S, Shaw SH et al. A genomewide analysis provides evidence for novel linkages in inflammatory bowel disease in a large European cohort. Am J Hum Genet 1999;64:808–816.

111. Hampe J, Shaw SH, Saiz R et al. Linkage of inflammatory bowel disease to human chromosome 6p. Am J Hum Genet 1999;65:1647–1655.

112. Yang H, Plevy SE, Taylor K et al. Linkage of Crohn's disease to the major histocompatibility complex region is detected by multiple non-parametric analyses. Gut 1999;44:519–526.

113. Ma Y, Ohmen JD, Li Z et al. A genome-wide search identifies potential new susceptibility loci for Crohn's disease. Inflamm Bowel Dis 1999;5:271–278.

114. Mirza MM, Lee J, Teare D et al. Evidence of linkage of the inflammatory bowel disease susceptibility locus on chromosome 16 (IBD1) to ulcerative colitis. J Med Genet 1998;35:218–221.

115. Duerr RH, Barmada MM, Zhang L, Pfutzer R, Weeks DE. High-density genome scan in Crohn disease shows confirmed linkage to chromosome 14q11-12. Am J Hum Genet 2000;66:1857–1862.

116. Rioux JD, Silverberg MS, Daly MJ et al. Genomewide search in Canadian families with inflammatory bowel disease reveals two novel susceptibility loci. Am J Hum Genet 2000;66:1863–1870.

117. Cho JH, Nicolae DL, Ramos R et al. Linkage and linkage disequilibrium in chromosome band 1p36 in American Chaldeans with inflammatory bowel disease. Hum Mol Genet 2000;9:1425–1432.

118. Cavanaugh J. International collaboration provides convincing linkage replication in complex disease through analysis of a large pooled data set: Crohn disease and chromosome 16. Am J Hum Genet 2001;68:1165–1171.

119. Hugot JP, Chamaillard M, Zouali H et al. Association of NOD2 leucine-rich repeat variants with susceptibility to Crohn's disease. Nature 2001;411:599–603.

120. Ogura Y, Bonen DK, Inohara N et al. A frameshift mutation in NOD2 associated with susceptibility to Crohn's disease. Nature 2001;411:603–606.

121. Hampe J, Cuthbert A, Croucher PJ et al. Association between insertion mutation in NOD2 gene and Crohn's disease in German and British populations. Lancet 2001;357:1925–1928.

122. Lesage S, Zouali H, Cezard JP et al. CARD15/NOD2 mutational analysis and genotype–phenotype correlation in 612 patients with inflammatory bowel disease. Am J Hum Genet 2002;70:845–857.

123. Cuthbert AP, Fisher SA, Mirza MM et al. The contribution of NOD2 gene mutations to the risk and site of disease in inflammatory bowel disease. Gastroenterology 2002;122:867–874.

124. Abreu MT, Taylor KD, Lin YC et al. Mutations in NOD2 are associated with fibrostenosing disease in patients with Crohn's disease. Gastroenterology 2002;123:679–688.

125. Fidder HH, Olschwang S, Avidan B et al. Association between mutations in the CARD15 (NOD2) gene and Crohn's disease in Israeli Jewish patients. Submitted 2002.

126. Bonen DK, Nicolae DL, Moran T et al. Racial differences in Nod2 variation: characterization of Nod2 in African-Americans with Crohn's disease. Gastroenterology 2002;122:A29 (abstract).

127. Inoue N, Tamura K, Kinouchi Y et al. Lack of common Nod2 variants in Japanese patients with Crohn's disease. Gastroenterology 2002;123:86–91.

128. Sachar D. Genomics and phenomics in Crohn's disease. Gastroenterology 2002;122:1161–1162.

129. Gasche C, Scholmerich J, Brynskov J et al. A simple classification of Crohn's disease: report of the Working Party for the World Congress of Gastroenterology, Vienna 1998. Inflamm Bowel Dis 1998;6:8–15.

130. Hampe J, Grebe J, Nikolaus S et al. Association of NOD2 (CARD15) genotype with clinical course of Crohn's disease: a cohort study. Lancet 2002;359:1661–1665.

131. Radlmayr M, Torok HP, Martin K, Folwaczny C. The c-insertion mutation of the NOD2 gene is associated with fistulizing and fibrostenotic phenotypes in Crohn's disease (letter). Gastroenterology 2002;122:2091–2092.

132. Vermeire S, Wild G, Kocher K et al. CARD15 genetic variation in a Quebec population: prevalence, genotype–phenotype relationship, and haplotype structure. Am J Hum Genet 2002;71:74–83.

133. Murillo L, Crusius B, van Bodegraven AA, Alizadeh BZ, Pena AS. CARD15 gene and the classification of Crohn's disease. Immunogenetics 2002;54:59–61.

134. Louis E, Collard A, Oger AF, Degroote E, Aboul Nasr El Yafi FA, Belaiche J. Behaviour of Crohn's disease according to the Vienna classification: changing pattern over the course of the disease. Gut 2001;49:777–782.

135. Cosnes J, Cattan S, Blain A et al. Long-term evolution of disease behavior of Crohn's disease. Inflamm Bowel Dis 2002;8:244–250.

136. Roussomoustakaki M, Satsangi J, Welsh K et al. Genetic markers may predict disease behavior in patients with ulcerative colitis. Gastroenterology 1997;112:1845–1853.

137. Bouma G, Crusius JB, Garcia-Gonzalez MA et al. Genetic markers in clinically well defined patients with ulcerative colitis (UC). Clin Exp Immunol 1999;115:294–300.

138. De la Concha EG, Fernandez-Arquero M, Lopez-Nava G et al. Susceptibility to severe ulcerative colitis is associated with polymorphism in the central MHC gene IKBL. Gastroenterology 2000;119:1491–1495.

139. Orchard TR, Thiyagaraja S, Welsh KI, Wordsworth BP, Hill Gaston JS, Jewell DP. Clinical phenotype is related to HLA genotype in the peripheral arthropathies of inflammatory bowel disease. Gastroenterology 2000;118:274–278.

140. Orchard TR, Dhar A, Simmons JD, Vaughan R, Welsh KI, Jewell DP. MHC class I chain-like gene A (MICA) and its associations with inflammatory bowel disease and peripheral arthropathy. Clin Exp Immunol 2001;126:437–440.

141. Orchard TR, Chua CN, Ahmad T, Cheng H, Welsh KI, Jewell DP. Uveitis and erythema nodosum in inflammatory bowel disease: clinical features and the role of HLA genes. Gastroenterology 2002;123:714–718.

142. Carter MJ, di Giovine FS, Jones S et al. Association of the interleukin 1 receptor antagonist gene with ulcerative colitis in Northern European Caucasians. Gut 2001;48:461–467.

143. Carter MJ, Di Giovine FS, Cox A, Goodfellow P, Jones S, Shorthouse AJ, Duff GW, Lobo AJ. The interleukin 1 receptor antagonist gene allele 2 as a predictor of pouchitis following colectomy and IPAA in ulcerative colitis. Gastroenterology 2001;121:805–811.

144. Louis E, Peeters M, Franchimont D et al. Tumour necrosis factor (TNF) gene polymorphism in Crohn's disease (CD): influence on disease behaviour? Clin Exp Immunol 2000;119:64–68.

145. Facklis K, Plevy SE, Vasiliauskas EA et al. Crohn's disease-associated genetic marker is seen in medically unresponsive ulcerative colitis patients and may be associated with pouch-specific complications. Dis Colon Rectum 1999;42:601–605; discussion 605–606.

146. Schulte CM, Dignass AU, Goebell H, Roher HD, Schulte KM. Genetic factors determine extent of bone loss in inflammatory bowel disease. Gastroenterology 2000;119:909–920.

146a. Rioux JD, Daly M, Silverberg M et al. Genetic variation in the 5q31 cytokine gene cluster confers susceptibility to Crohn disease. Nature Genet 2001;29:223–228.

147. Armuzzi A, Ahmad T, De Silva AP et al. The 5q31/IBD5 risk haplotype determines perianal phenotype in Crohn's disease. Gastroenterology 2002;122:A229.

148. Krynetski EY, Krynetskaia NF, Yanishevski Y, Evans WE. Methylation of mercaptopurine, thioguanine, and their nucleotide metabolites by heterologously expressed human thiopurine S-methyltransferase. Mol Pharmacol 1995;47:1141–1147.

149. Weinshilboum RM, Sladek SL. Mercaptopurine pharmacogenetics: monogenic inheritance of erythrocyte thiopurine methyltransferase activity. Am J Hum Genet 1980;32:651–662.

150. Lennard L, Van Loon JA, Lilleyman JS, Weinshilboum RM. Thiopurine pharmacogenetics in leukemia: correlation of erythrocyte thiopurine methyltransferase activity and 6-thioguanine nucleotide concentrations. Clin Pharmacol Ther 1987;41:18–25.

151. Lennard L, Lilleyman JS, Van Loon J, Weinshilboum RM. Genetic variation in response to 6-mercaptopurine for childhood acute lymphoblastic leukaemia. Lancet 1990;336:225–229.

152. Otterness D, Szumlanski C, Lennard L et al. Human thiopurine methyltransferase pharmacogenetics: gene sequence polymorphisms. Clin Pharmacol Ther 1997;62:60–73.

153. Otterness DM, Szumlanski CL, Wood TC, Weinshilboum RM. Human thiopurine methyltransferase pharmacogenetics. Kindred with a terminal exon splice junction mutation that results in loss of activity. J Clin Invest 1998;101:1036–1044.

154. Szumlanski C, Otterness D, Her C et al. Thiopurine methyltransferase pharmacogenetics: human gene cloning and characterization of a common polymorphism. DNA Cell Biol 1996;15:17–30.

155. Tai HL, Krynetski EY, Yates CR et al. Thiopurine S-methyltransferase deficiency: two nucleotide transitions define the most prevalent mutant allele associated with loss of catalytic activity in Caucasians. Am J Hum Genet 1996;58:694–702.

156. Strik WO, Strik W. [Familial occurrence of Crohn's regional enteritis in binovular twins and 2 other siblings]. Munch Med Wochenschr 1972;114:1852–1856.

157. Sung JY, Chan FK, Lawton J et al. Anti-neutrophil cytoplasmic antibodies (ANCA) and inflammatory bowel diseases in Chinese. Dig Dis Sci 1994;39:886–892.

158. Yates CR, Krynetski EY, Loennechen T et al. Molecular diagnosis of thiopurine S-methyltransferase deficiency: genetic basis for azathioprine and mercaptopurine intolerance. Ann Intern Med 1997;126:608–614.

159. Colombel JF, Ferrari N, Debuysere H et al. Genotypic analysis of thiopurine S-methyltransferase in patients with Crohn's disease and severe myelosuppression during azathioprine therapy. Gastroenterology 2000;118:1025–1030.

160. Cuffari C, Theoret Y, Latour S, Seidman G. 6-Mercaptopurine metabolism in Crohn's disease: correlation with efficacy and toxicity. Gut 1996;39:401–406.

161. Cuffari C, Hunt S, Bayless T. Utilisation of erythrocyte 6-thioguanine metabolite levels to optimise azathioprine therapy in patients with inflammatory bowel disease. Gut 2001;48:642–646.

162. Dubinsky MC, Lamothe S, Yang HY et al. Pharmacogenomics and metabolite measurement for 6-mercaptopurine therapy in inflammatory bowel disease. Gastroenterology 2000;118:705–713.

163. Dubinsky MC, Yang H, Hassard PV et al. 6-MP metabolite profiles provide a biochemical explanation for 6-MP resistance in patients with inflammatory bowel disease. Gastroenterology 2002;122:904–915.

164. Belaiche J, Desager JP, Horsmans Y, Louis E. Therapeutic drug monitoring of azathioprine and 6-mercaptopurine metabolites in Crohn disease. Scand J Gastroenterol 2001;36:71–76.

165. Lowry PW, Franklin CL, Weaver AL et al. Measurement of thiopurine methyltransferase activity and azathioprine metabolites in patients with inflammatory bowel disease. Gut 2001;49:665–670.

166. Sandborn WJ. Rational dosing of azathioprine and 6-mercaptopurine. Gut 2001;48:591–592.

167. Tremaine WJ. Failure to yield: drug resistance in inflammatory bowel disease. Gastroenterology 2002;122:1165–1167.

168. Meyer UA, Zanger UM. Molecular mechanisms of genetic polymorphisms of drug metabolism. Annu Rev Pharmacol Toxicol 1997;37:269–296.

169. Hickman D, Pope J, Patil SD et al. Expression of arylamine N-acetyltransferase in human intestine. Gut 1998;42:402–409.

170. Ricard E, Taylor W, Loftus E et al. N-acetyl transferase 1 and 2 genotypes do not predict response or toxicity to treatment with mesalamine and sulfasalazine in patients with ulcerative colitis. Am J Gastroenterol 2002;97:1763–1768.

171. Farrell RJ, Murphy A, Long A et al. High multidrug resistance (P-glycoprotein 170) expression in inflammatory bowel disease patients who fail medical therapy. Gastroenterology 2000;118:279–288.

172. Honda M, Orii F, Ayabe T et al. Expression of glucocorticoid receptor beta in lymphocytes of patients with glucocorticoid-resistant ulcerative colitis. Gastroenterology 2000;118:859–866.

173. Louis E, Vermeire S, Rutgeerts P et al. A positive response to infliximab in Crohn's disease: aasociation with a higher systemic inflammation before treatment but not with −308 TNF polymorphism. Scand J Gastroenterol 2002;37:818–824.

174. Taylor KD, Plevy SE, Yang H et al. ANCA pattern and LTA haplotype relationship to clinical responses to anti-TNF antibody treatment in Crohn's disease. Gastroenterology 2001;120:1347–1355.

175. Ogura Y, Inohara N, Benito A, Chen FF, Yamaoka S, Nunez G. Nod2, a Nod1/Apaf-1 family member that is restricted to monocytes and activates NF-kB. J Biol Chem 2001;276:4812–4818.

176. Vermeire S, Louis E, Rutgeerts P et al. NOD2/CARD15 does not influence response to Infliximab in Crohn's disease. Gastroenterology 2002;123:106–111.

177. Guttmacher AE, Jenkins J, Uhlmann WR. Genomic medicine: Who will practice it? A call to open arms. Am J Med Genet 2001;106:216–222.

178. Evans WE, Relling MV. Pharmacogenomics: translating functional genomics into rational therapeutics. Science 1999;286:487–491.

179. Danesi R, Mosca M, Boggi U, Mosca F, Del Tacca M. Genetics of drug response to immunosuppressive treatment and prospects for personalized therapy. Mol Med Today 2000;6:475–482.

180. Colombel JF. The CARD15 gene in Crohn's disease: are there implications for current clinical practice ? Clin Gastroenterol Hepatol 2003;(in press).

181. Folwaczny C, Noehl N, Tschop K et al. Goblet cell autoantibodies in patients with inflammatory bowel disease and their first-degree relatives. Gastroenterology 1997;113:101–106.

182. Seibold F, Mork H, Tanza S et al. Pancreatic autoantibodies in Crohn's disease: a family study. Gut 1997;40:481–484.

183. Korsmeyer SJ WR, Wilson ID, Strickland RG. Lymphocytotoxic antibody in inflammatory bowel disease. A family study. N Engl J Med 1975;293:1117–1120.

184. Biancone L, Monteleone G, Marasco R, Pallone F. Autoimmunity to tropomyosin isoforms in ulcerative colitis (UC) patients and unaffected relatives. Clin Exp Immunol 1998;113:198–205.

## CHAPTER 19

# Clinical course and natural history of ulcerative colitis

Michael Cantor and Charles N Bernstein

## INTRODUCTION

Ulcerative colitis (UC) is a disease with no known etiology and an unpredictable course. However, there are sufficient longitudinal studies published that give some guidance as to expected outcomes. Five clinical outcomes are encountered: chronic relapsing disease, chronic unremitting disease, a single episode with no recurrence of symptoms (most uncommon in bona fide UC), colectomy and death.[1] In this chapter, the course and outcomes of UC are reviewed.

## OUTCOME AFTER THE INITIAL ATTACK

As illustrated in Table 19.1, most patients with ulcerative colitis have a chronic relapsing course. A Danish study[2] examined the natural history of ulcerative colitis in 1161 patients over a 25-year period. Overall, 77% of patients experienced a chronic relapsing course, with a cumulative probability of 90% at 25 years. In contrast, chronic continuous disease was exceedingly rare, with a cumulative probability of 1% after 5 years and 0.1% after 25 years. Surprisingly, 23% of patients had only one episode of disease with no subsequent symptomatic recurrence. However, the median follow-up in this group was limited to 3 years.[3] It is also conceivable that some of these cases may have been due to undiagnosed bacterial-mediated colonic infections.[3]

Placebo groups from clinical trials may also define the natural history of ulcerative colitis. It is controversial whether taking placebo allows for any insight into the natural history of a disease or whether it simply reflects a different form of active intervention. Unfortunately, most placebo-controlled trials are heterogeneous with respect to disease severity, selection criteria and follow-up, thereby limiting the applicability of any one trial to standard clinical practice.[4] To overcome these deficiencies, a synthesis analysis of 38 placebo-controlled treatment trials for active UC was undertaken.[5] Placebo remission and benefit rates were assessed using clinical, endoscopic and histological criteria. The results are summarized in Table 19.2. Overall, the authors concluded that remission occurs in 10% and significant symptomatic improvement occurs in 30% of patients with active UC treated with placebo. The one variable that most significantly influenced the placebo response was the number of visits to the healthcare provider: subjects who had three or more visits exhibited the highest placebo response rates. Because placebo may represent an active intervention, it may be that placebo response rates reflect outcomes from active intervention of any type, as opposed to a true natural history of simply expectant management without healthcare visits.

## THE NEED FOR SURGERY

Several factors affect the reported surgical rates for ulcerative colitis. These include: (a) patient population (whether the sample is referral-based, community-based, or population-based); (b) heterogeneity in disease extent (proctitis versus pancolitis); and (c) the period during which the study was conducted, as medical management has changed over time.

Most studies indicate that the need for surgery in ulcerative colitis is highest within the first few years of diagnosis.[6] Population-based data from Denmark revealed a colectomy rate of 9% in the first year of disease and 3% per year during the next 4 years.[2] Thereafter, the rate diminished to 1% per year. Overall, 20% of patients underwent colectomy during the study period. A Swedish study of 1586 patients between 1955 and 1984 with a mean follow-up of 13 years reported similar results.[7] During the first year after diagnosis, 10% of patients underwent colectomy. The colectomy rate in the second year after diagnosis was 4% and over the following 20 years was 1% per year. In total, 32% of patients underwent colectomy. Table 19.3 summarizes the colectomy rates from several large studies.

There have been two risk factors consistently identified with increased colectomy rates for patients with ulcerative colitis. These include extent of disease at diagnosis,[2,6-9] and disease

**Table 19.1 Disease course of ulcerative colitis. Adapted with modification from Kirsner JB. Inflammatory bowel disease, 5th edn. Philadelphia: WB Saunders; 2000.**

|  | Langholz et al.[2] | Stonnington et al.[42] | Sinclair et al.[8]* |
|---|---|---|---|
| Number of patients | 1161 | 182 | 537 |
| Setting | Community Denmark | Community Rochester, MN | Community Scotland |
| Period of study | 1962–1987 | 1935–1979 | 1967–1976 |
| Median length of follow-up (years) | 12 | 14 | N/A |
| Disease activity relapsing | 77% | 65% | 40% at 2 years |
| Single episode | 23% | 28% | 28% at 5 years |
| Continuous | 0.1% at 25 years | 6% | 8% |

\* The data do not add up to 100% because they are reported for different points in time.

**Table 19.2 Placebo response in ulcerative colitis by assessment end points. Reproduced with permission from Ilnyckyj et al. Gastroenterology 1997; 112:1855.**

| End point | Percent remission rate (CI) | Percent benefit rate (CI) |
|---|---|---|
| Clinical | 9.1 (6.6–11.6) | 26.7 (24.1–29.2) |
| Endoscopic | 13.5 (10.0–17.1) | 30.3 (26.6–34.0) |
| Histological | 8.6 (5.0–12.0) | 25.2 (20.8–29.6) |

activity at diagnosis.[2,6,8] Among patients who presented with pancolitis, left-sided colitis and proctitis, the 5-year cumulative colectomy rates were 32%, 14% and 14%, respectively.[7] It is not surprising that Sinclair et al.[8] reported an overall low colectomy rate of 3%, as most of the patients in this study had proctitis. This compares to other studies that included more patients with extensive disease and reported colectomy rates that exceeded 20%.[2,7,10] Similarly, the risk of colectomy is increased in patients who present with a severe first attack; in this group, up to 30% of patients require surgical intervention.[2,8] Although younger age has been reported as a risk factor,[8] other studies have not confirmed this finding.[2,7]

## RISK OF RELAPSE

The course of UC is usually marked by intermittent relapses and remissions. Langholz et al.[2] identified three risk factors for UC relapse:

(1) *Preceding disease activity.* In patients who experienced disease activity during the preceding year, the risk of relapse in the following year was 70%. In contrast, for

**Table 19.3 Colectomy rates for ulcerative colitis**

|  | Langholz et al.[2] | Hendriksen et al.[9] | Farmer et al.[10] | Leijonmarck et al.[7] |
|---|---|---|---|---|
| Number of patients | 1161 | 783 | 1116 | 1586 |
| Setting | Community Denmark | Community Denmark | Referral USA | Community Sweden |
| Colectomy rate |  |  |  |  |
|  Total | 20% | 19% | 38% | 32% |
|  First year | 9% | 10% | Not reported | 10% |
|  10-year cumulative | 24% | 23% | 34% | 28% |

patients who were in remission during the preceding year, only 20% relapsed the following year.

(2) *Systemic symptoms at diagnosis.* Surprisingly, the presence of fever and weight loss at diagnosis predicted a less active disease course so long as the patients responded to medical treatment and did not undergo colectomy during that episode.

(3) *The point in time of the study in which the diagnosis of ulcerative colitis was established.* Relapse rates were lower among patients diagnosed with ulcerative colitis during the latter years of the study than in those diagnosed earlier. Disease severity was not a factor. The authors postulated that physician experience and improved medical treatments might have played a role.

In the literature, much attention has been focused on the specific infectious and environmental influences that contribute to relapse in ulcerative colitis. Clinically, it is imperative to identify these factors in order to achieve optimal relapse prevention and treatment (see Chapter 10).

## CYTOMEGALOVIRUS (CMV) INFECTION AND UC

Population-based data from the United States indicate that 16% of patients with ulcerative colitis are refractory to corticosteroid treatment.[11] It has been postulated that CMV infections may contribute to flares that develop in corticosteroid refractory colitis.[12–15] Although the precise mechanism remains unclear, CMV may selectively inhabit the injured proliferating colonic mucosa present in ulcerative colitis.[12] Indeed, increased rates of relapse and toxic megacolon have been observed in UC patients infected with CMV.[15] Until recently, most evidence linking CMV to corticosteroid-refractory colitis was limited to case reports and case series.[12,15,16] Cottone et al.[13] carried out the first prospective study to evaluate the prevalence of CMV in acute, corticosteroid-refractory IBD. They identified 62 patients with severe colitis (55 UC and seven Crohn's colitis), all of whom were initially treated with intravenous corticosteroids for 5–10 days. Thirty per cent of patients were refractory to corticosteroids. All corticosteroid-refractory patients underwent rectal biopsy to detect underlying CMV infection. The prevalence of CMV within the group with corticosteroid-refractory colitis was 36% (five ulcerative colitis and two Crohn's disease patients). Six of the seven patients with CMV and corticosteroid-refractory colitis were using corticosteroids or azathioprine prior to presenting with the acute flare. Although not specifically studied, the effect of antiviral therapy (ganciclovir) has been suggested to be favorable.[12,14] The most recent study reported that of 14 CMV IgG-positive hospitalized UC patients, 100% had CMV DNA in their stool. Eight had CMV DNA in their blood. However, antiviral therapy did not change the course of the disease.[17]

## NSAIDS

Data regarding non-steroidal anti-inflammatory drug (NSAID) use and its effect on IBD are limited.[17] A recent case–control study determined NSAID use in 60 patients with IBD (36 Crohn's disease, 24 UC) requiring hospitalization and 62 age-/sex-matched patients with irritable bowel syndrome.[18] In 31% of IBD cases, but only 2% of IBS controls, there was a correlation between NSAID use and disease activity. Among patients with ulcerative colitis, 35% reported NSAID use within 1 month of exacerbation or onset of symptoms.

The best evidence linking NSAIDs to IBD relapse comes from a recent study evaluating three groups of patients with quiescent Crohn's disease and UC before and after the administration of paracetamol 1 g tid, naproxen 500 mg bid and nabumetone 1 g bid.[19] The aim of this study was to delineate the mechanism and frequency of NSAID-related exacerbations in IBD. Although naproxen and nabumetone both exhibit non-selective COX inhibition, naproxen causes topical mucosal injury whereas nabumetone does not. Paracetamol (acetaminophen) served as the control. Fecal calprotectin was used as a marker of active inflammation. At 1 and 4 weeks of treatment paracetamol had no effect on disease activity, whereas the naproxen and nabumetone groups had significantly increased disease activity. Approximately 25% of patients in the NSAID groups had clinical relapses. The authors concluded that NSAIDs are associated with increased intestinal inflammation mediated mostly by their effects on COX inhibition rather than a topical effect. Leading theories to explain the mechanism by which NSAIDs provoke inflammatory bowel disease include: inhibition of protective prostaglandin synthesis (via COX inhibition), uncoupling of oxidative phosphorylation in enterocyte mitochondria, and increased intestinal permeability.[20] In humans, the effects of COX-2 inhibitors on ulcerative colitis activity is controversial.[16,21] However, in an interleukin-10 knockout mouse model of colitis, celecoxib and rofecoxib both exacerbated disease activity.[22] In addition, dextran sodium sulfate-induced colitis is potentiated in COX-2-deficient mice.[23]

## SMOKING

Epidemiological data strongly support the notion that ulcerative colitis occurs more commonly in non-smokers than in smokers[23] (see Chapter 17). A meta-analysis from nine case–control studies of ulcerative colitis revealed a pooled odds ratio of 0.41 (CI 0.34–0.48) for current smokers compared to lifetime non-smokers.[24] The effect of smoking on UC disease activity has also been evaluated. Several studies have linked smoking with reduced rates of relapse, improved symptoms and lower colectomy rates.[25–28] UC patients who stop smoking during the course of their disease tend to have increased disease activity, higher rates of hospitalization and a need for major medical therapy (corticosteroids or immunomodulators).[28] Individuals who stop smoking just prior to diagnosis may be at higher risk for a complicated course.[27]

## MISCELLANEOUS

There are other variables, albeit less well studied, that may affect the disease activity of ulcerative colitis. Elevated levels of long-term psychological stress were recently found to triple the baseline risk of UC exacerbation.[29] There appears to be a seasonal variability in UC exacerbations, with peak relapse rates occurring in the autumn.[31,32] It is possible that virally mediated acute upper respiratory tract infections contribute to this variability.[33] Although the precise mechanism is unknown, a generalized heightened immune response aimed at clearing the viral infection, with inadvertent hyperactivity within the gastrointestinal mucosal immune system, may be responsible.[20] Bacterial colonic infections such as *Campylobacter jejuni*, *Salmonella*, *Shigella*, *Yersinia*, *Escherichia coli* and *Clostridium* may also be associated with flares of ulcerative colitis.[20] Perhaps the triggering of leukocyte trafficking to the gut to neutralize the infection fails to downregulate once the infection is cleared (see Chapter 10). Interestingly, appendectomy in patients with acute appendicitis appears to be inversely correlated to the subsequent development of ulcerative colitis.[30,34] A recent multicenter case–control study from Japan demonstrated reduced UC recurrence rates in patients who underwent appendectomy.[31] The explanation to account for these findings remains elusive, but alterations within the T-lymphocyte population and a reduction in intestinal microbes and antigens are thought to be relevant.[31] Preliminary results from an open study of appendectomy as therapy for refractory UC have been reported.[35]

## ASSESSMENT OF DISEASE ACTIVITY

To date, the assessment of disease activity in ulcerative colitis has an unclear role in ongoing patient management (see Chapter 33). It is as yet uncertain whether endoscopic or histologic remission should be the goal of therapy (as opposed to clinical remission). It is plausible to postulate that an endoscopic remission will be more durable, or alternatively that patients with clinical remission but active endoscopic inflammation will be more likely to relapse. However, this remains unproven.

Unfortunately, a single 'gold standard' UC activity index does not currently exist (see Chapter 30). Over 45 years have passed since Truelove and Witts described the first UC severity index (Table 19.4).[36] Utilizing clinical parameters and basic laboratory investigations, this index classifies patients as having mild, moderate or severe disease. There are, however, several shortcomings. The index utilizes only three simple categories (mild, moderate and severe) to define disease activity, but because of overlapping symptoms not all patients match to a single category.[37] None the less, retrospective data indicate a correlation between these three grades of severity and the outcome of an attack.[38] For clinical trials, the Powell-Tuck[39] and Rachmilewitz[40] indices have been used but their value in day-to-day clinical management is limited.

Approximately 10% of UC patients present with severe disease.[8,42,43] In this select group, it is important to identify the parameters that predict treatment outcome as the prolonged ineffectual use of corticosteroids and subsequent delay of surgery may have adverse consequences.[44] There are several

## Table 19.4 Truelove and Witts' classification of disease severity in ulcerative colitis

| Mild | Moderate | Severe |
|---|---|---|
| ≤ 4 bowel movements/day | Intermediate between mild and severe | ≥ 6 bowel movements/day |
| Small amounts of blood in stool | | Large amounts of blood in stool |
| Fever absent | | Temperature > 99.5°F (37.5° C) |
| Tachycardia absent | | Heart rate > 90 bpm |
| Hemoglobin > 75% of normal | | Hemoglobin ≤ 75% of normal |
| ESR < 30 | | ESR > 30 |

## Table 19.5 Factors with the highest predictive value for steroid-refractory severe ulcerative colitis. (Adapted with modification from Gelbmann CM. Inflammatory bowel diseases 2000;6:2.)

| Day after start of treatment | Number of bowel movements/day | C-reactive protein concentration | Risk of colectomy (%) |
|---|---|---|---|
| 3 | >8 | – | 85 |
| | 3–8 | > 45 mg/dL | 85 |

variables that may predict which patients with severe UC will be refractory to high-dose corticosteroid treatment and require colectomy.[45] One such variable is persistent bloody diarrhea. In patients who fail corticosteroid treatment and require surgery, the stool frequency tends to decrease at a significantly slower rate than in those who achieve either partial or complete remission.[45] Patients who do not have a significant reduction in bowel movement frequency by day 3 appear to have increased rates of medical treatment failure and higher rates of colectomy. Determining C-reactive protein levels may also add to the predictive power that identifies those patients who will fail medical treatment and require surgery (Table 19.5).[45] Serum prealbumin concentrations usually rise in patients who respond to medical therapy but remain depressed or continue to decline in those who fail.[46] Serum albumin levels may also predict treatment outcome but, given the significantly shorter half-life of prealbumin compared to albumin, it is not surprising that prealbumin correlates more closely to treatment outcome.[46] Recently, much interest has focused on a fecal measure of a neutrophil protein, calprotectin. Current evidence suggests that fecal calprotectin predicts clinical relapse of disease activity in both adults and children with UC.[47,48]

Although endoscopy can be performed safely in severe flares of ulcerative colitis,[49,50] concern regarding the risk of perforation and toxic megacolon continues to remain an issue.[45] In one retrospective study, colonoscopic findings of extensive deep ulcerations, mucosal detachment on the edge of these ulcerations, well-like ulcerations and large mucosal ulcerations defined patients with severe endoscopic colitis.[49] Forty-three of the 46 patients (93%) with severe endoscopic colitis were refractory to intensive medical treatment and underwent colectomy. In contrast, 29 of 36 patients (74%) with less extensive colonic ulceration (moderate endoscopic colitis) responded to medical treatment and entered clinical remission.[49]

## Table 19.6 Risk of macroscopic extension in ulcerative proctitis

| | Meucci et al.[53] | Ayres et al.[54*] | Ritchie et al.[110] |
|---|---|---|---|
| Number of patients | 341 | 145 | 269 |
| Study period | 1989–1994 | 1953–1993 | 1966–1975 |
| Overall risk of extension: | | | |
|   Absolute percent | 27 | 37 | 7 |
|   5-year cumulative probability | 20 | 27 | 5 |
|   10-year cumulative probability | 54 | 49 | |

*Result includes patients with proctitis and/or proctosigmoiditis.

## EXTENT OF DISEASE

Because of the considerable heterogeneity among studies, it is difficult to clearly define the true rate of proximal extension of ulcerative colitis. Differences in disease evaluation (endoscopy versus barium enema), definitions of extent (proctitis versus proctosigmoiditis), statistical methods (cumulative probability versus absolute percent) and the lack of use of histological parameters all contribute to the problem. Of particular clinical interest is the potential for progression of ulcerative proctitis. Individuals with proctitis have a similar colorectal cancer (CRC) risk as the general population.[51] However, this risk may be increased if disease extension occurs.[52] Table 19.6 summarizes the studies outlining the risk of disease progression in ulcerative proctitis.

In a recent retrospective study from Italy, 273 patients with ulcerative proctitis were followed for a mean of 52 months.[53] Disease extension occurred in 74 (27%), with 5- and 10-year cumulative probabilities of 20% and 54%, respectively. In 41% of these patients, mucosal inflammation progressed beyond the sigmoid colon. As stated previously, the extension of proctitis has implications for colon cancer surveillance but its implications for prognosis are unclear.

Among studies that assess the rate of disease extension of ulcerative proctitis, a common problem continues to be the lack of uniformity regarding the definition of proctitis. In the strictest sense, ulcerative proctitis should only be diagnosed if biopsies from above the rectum (15–20 cm from the anal verge) are proved to be normal. It may be that a patient has endoscopic proctitis but on biopsy the inflammation extends more proximally; thus, the diagnosis of ulcerative proctitis may not be completely accurate.

The risk of disease progression in ulcerative proctosigmoiditis has also been evaluated. Rates vary among studies, with disease extension occurring in 12–27% at 5 years and 30–41% at 10 years.[8,54,55]

Of the reported risk factors associated with proximal disease extension, the most important is poorly controlled, severe disease.[10,53,55] This may consist simply of a history of severe disease[10] or active symptoms.[53,56] In those with active symptoms, the most relevant features are persistent abdominal pain and diarrhea,[55] the presence of refractory disease as defined by more than three relapses per year, or the need for corticosteroids or immunosuppressives.[53] It is important to note that both macroscopic and microscopic disease extension may occur in the setting of quiescent disease.

# CLINICAL FEATURES

## SYMPTOMS

UC is characterized by chronic mucosal inflammation that typically starts in the rectum and proceeds proximally. The small intestine is not involved except in cases of backwash ileitis. The disease is divided into four major categories based on the length of involved colon: (a) ulcerative proctitis refers to inflammation that is confined to the rectum; (b) proctosigmoiditis is inflammation that extends to the sigmoid colon; (c) left-sided colitis refers to inflammation that extends to the splenic flexure; and (d) pancolitis defines patients with inflammation beyond the splenic flexure that may extend to the cecum.

Patients with active proctitis typically complain of the insidious onset of increased stool frequency, hematochezia (the presence of visible blood in the stool) and tenesmus (continuous proclivity to eliminate the bowels accompanied by painful straining ('dry heaves of the rectum')).[56] Bowel movements are generally liquid and patients may experience nocturnal diarrhea and fecal incontinence. Interestingly, approximately one-quarter of patients with active proctitis complain of constipation and the passage of hard stools.[56] Under these circumstances, blood, mucus, tenesmus and incomplete evacuation are almost always present.[56] Systemic symptoms are usually absent. Patients with proctosigmoiditis and left-sided colitis have similar symptoms to those with proctitis but are more apt to complain of left lower quadrant abdominal pain. In cases of increasingly severe disease, nausea, vomiting and weight loss may also be present. Because most patients have rectal involvement, and because inflamma-tion of the rectum leads to urgency, frequency and tenesmus, rectal therapy may benefit even patients with extensive disease.

## SIGNS

With mild to moderate disease the physical examination is usually normal. In a patient with chronic symptoms, pallor and signs of malnutrition may be evident. With more severe acute disease, systemic manifestations, including fever, postural hypotension and tachycardia, may be present. In the setting of toxic megacolon delirium may occur. The abdomen may be distended and diffusely tender, with rebound tenderness. Rebound tenderness should alert the examiner to the possibility of microperforations and frank perforation. This sign, together with an increasing need for narcotic analgesia, should particularly heighten the concern regarding perforation. During this stage, hypoactive bowel sounds may also be noted.

Extraintestinal manifestations such as peripheral arthritis and erythema nodosum may flare only during disease activity. Other extraintestinal manifestations, such as ankylosing spondylitis, pyoderma gangrenosum and primary sclerosing cholangitis (PSC), may run courses independent of the underlying bowel disease activity.

## LABORATORY INVESTIGATIONS

With mild disease there are usually no abnormal laboratory values detected, although iron deficiency or mild anemia may exist. With moderate to severe disease laboratory abnormalities may be noted, but none is specific for ulcerative colitis. None the less, these deviations may be helpful in distinguishing UC from irritable bowel syndrome, a condition characterized by normal laboratory investigations. Examples of abnormal laboratory tests in active UC include anemia, thrombocytosis, iron deficiency, hypoalbuminemia and electrolyte abnormalities. Stool tests for bacteria, *Clostridium difficile* toxin and ova and parasites should be submitted in cases of newly diagnosed or newly flaring disease.

## ENDOSCOPIC FEATURES OF ULCERATIVE COLITIS

Under normal conditions the colonic mucosa is smooth and glistening. The underlying vascular pattern is branching and clearly visible. Although not specific for ulcerative colitis, there are several endoscopic changes that result from colonic inflammation. These include edema with subsequent loss of the fine vascular pattern, and mucosal friability (bleeding that occurs spontaneously or upon contact with the endoscope). Mucosal granularity imparts a 'wet sandpaper' appearance as the mucosa scatters the light reflection from the endoscope into multiple small points.[57] Ulcers, exudates and pseudopolyps may also be evident. In more long-standing disease the colon may become tubular and featureless.[58]

Traditionally, the endoscopic distribution of inflammation in UC is described as continuous, starting and being most severe in the rectum and then spreading in a proximal fashion without skip lesions.[58] However, there is a growing body of evidence that describes a high prevalence of endoscopic patchiness with or without rectal sparing in patients with treated ulcerative colitis.[59-62] D'Haens et al.[62] prospectively followed 20 patients with proctitis or left-sided colitis for a minimum of 8 years. In 15 patients (75%) the periappendiceal orifice was macroscopically inflamed and separated from the distal colitis by normal-appearing mucosa. Bernstein et al.[63] conducted the first prospective study to evaluate the prevalence of endoscopic patchiness and rectal sparing in 39 patients with long-standing treated ulcerative colitis. The mean duration of disease was 12 years. In all, 17 patients (44%) were determined to have patchiness by endoscopic criteria and five(13%) were found to have rectal sparing. Kim et al.[61] recently assessed the prevalence of endoscopic patchiness and rectal sparing in treated ulcerative colitis over time. They examined 32 patients with a median duration of disease of 15 years. A median of five endoscopies per patient were performed over a maximum of 13 years. Seven patients (22%) were found to have endoscopic patchiness and 10 (31%) had rectal sparing. Interestingly, in the studies by Bernstein et al. and Kim et al. the presence of endoscopic patchiness and rectal sparing were not related to specific therapy. To date, reports of patchy inflammation and rectal sparing in untreated ulcerative colitis are limited to the pediatric population.[59,63] It is currently unknown whether the presence of endoscopic patchiness has an influence on the course of ulcerative colitis.

In addition to endoscopic patchiness, the pathology literature is replete with reports of histologic patchiness in UC.[64,65] Thus, the finding of patchiness or even rectal sparing in treated UC should not mandate a change in diagnosis to Crohn's disease. However, it should be recognized that bona fide segmental colitis – for example disease limited to the rectum and the hepatic flexure with completely normal mucosa in between – is not patchy UC but more likely the segmental colitis of Crohn's disease.

# COMPLICATIONS OF ULCERATIVE COLITIS

Both intestinal and extraintestinal complications can occur in ulcerative colitis. These can be further divided into non-neoplastic and neoplastic manifestations.

## NON-NEOPLASTIC INTESTINAL COMPLICATIONS

### Toxic megacolon, perforation, hemorrhage and stricture

Toxic megacolon is a potentially life-threatening condition that is defined by non-obstructive colonic dilatation of at least 6 cm in conjunction with systemic toxicity.[66] Earlier reports suggested that 1–5% of all UC patients develop toxic megacolon during their lifetime. However, because of heightened awareness and improved medical management of severe colitis, the risk of toxic megacolon continues to decline.[66] The risk appears greatest during the first few months following diagnosis. Approximately 30% of patients who develop toxic megacolon do so within 3 months of receiving the diagnosis of UC, and 60% within the first 3 years.[66] Toxic megacolon is mostly a disease of patients with pancolitis, but cases involving left-sided colitis have been reported.[67] Precipitants include *Clostridium difficile*, *Campylobacter*, *Shigella*, *Salmonella* and amebic infections.[66] More recent attention has focused on CMV as a potential inciting agent.[68,69]

Most cases of perforation in ulcerative colitis occur in the setting of toxic megacolon.[70] In fact, perforation is 28 times more frequent in patients with toxic megacolon than in those without.[70] The mortality rate following perforation in the setting of toxic megacolon can be as high as 40–50%.[71,70]

Acute gastrointestinal hemorrhage is relatively rare in UC, occurring in less than 5% of all patients.[72,73] Despite this, acute hemorrhage comprises approximately 10% of all urgent colectomies for UC.[73] Severe bleeding tends to occur early on in the disease, with a mean onset of 2.6 years after the initial diagnosis.[73] Patients with pancolitis appear to be at higher risk than those with left-sided colitis.[72,73]

Both benign and malignant strictures develop in UC, with an overall frequency that ranges from 3% to 10%.[74] Because strictures are associated with malignancy in up to 30% of cases, the old dogma that 'all strictures are malignant until proven otherwise' may be overstated, but should nevertheless be heeded. Several factors are known to increase the likelihood that a stricture is malignant.[74] Disease duration is an important factor, as 60% of malignant strictures are found in patients with at least 20 years of disease. In terms of location, benign strictures occur predominantly in the left side of the colon; malignant strictures, on the other hand, are more likely to locate proximal to the splenic flexure.[74] Interestingly, most UC patients with malignant strictures present with obstructive symptoms (constipation, bowel obstruction), compared to those with benign strictures, who rarely express these same complaints.[74]

## NEOPLASTIC INTESTINAL COMPLICATIONS
*(see Chapter 43)*

A recent population-based study from Manitoba, Canada, evaluated 2672 UC patients over a 14-year period.[76] Compared to the non-IBD population, increased rates of rectal cancer and colon cancer were found in UC patients with incidence rate ratios of 1.9 (CI 1.05–3.43) and 2.8 (CI 1.91–3.97), respectively. The risk of cancer has been estimated to be approximately 1/400 person-years in a population-based Canadian study[75] and 1/333 person-years in a meta-analysis.[76]

Several risk factors for CRC in UC have been identified. Ekbom et al.[78] found that the relative risk of colon cancer in UC was directly related to disease extent, with incidence ratios of 2.8 (CI 1.6–4.4) for left-sided colitis and 14.8 (CI 11.4–18.9) for pancolitis. As stated previously, patients with proctitis are probably not at increased risk of colorectal cancer.[51] Duration of disease is also an import factor. In patients with pancolitis the risk of CRC begins to increase after 8–10 years of disease.[78] It is estimated that the risk of CRC 10 years after the diagnosis of UC is 2%, by 20 years is 8%, and by 30 years is as high as 18%.[76] The presence of PSC also increases the risk of CRC: patients with PSC and UC are five times more likely to develop colon cancer than control patients with UC.[79–82] Other recently described risk factors include a family history of sporadic colorectal cancer[83,84] and the presence of backwash ileitis.[85]

A recent case–control study suggested that the chronic use of 5-aminosalicylates may reduce the incidence of colorectal cancer in UC.[86] The risk of colorectal cancer was reduced by 81% in patients who used mesalamine at a daily dosage of 1.2 g or more.[86] It is possible, however, that this reduced risk of CRC may be a function of patient compliance: patients compliant with their 5-aminosalicylate use might also be more compliant in general and seek more thorough medical care. A recent cross-sectional study suggested a possible reduction in colonic dysplasia in UC patients with PSC using ursodeoxycholic acid compared to those who were not (OR 0.18 (0.05–0.61)).[87]

There does not appear to be an increased risk of lymphoma in patients with ulcerative colitis. There is, however, an increased risk of cholangiocarcinoma in patients with PSC and UC.[75]

# EXTRAINTESTINAL COMPLICATIONS

Population-based data from Canada and data from a large European inception cohort suggest that approximately 6–11% of UC patients will develop at least one of the extraintestinal manifestations listed below.[88,89] It is important to note that most of the major extraintestinal manifestations occur with similar frequencies in both UC and Crohn's disease, thereby limiting their usefulness in distinguishing between these two disorders.

## Osteopenia and osteoporosis

Both osteopenia and osteoporosis, diagnosed by dual-energy X-ray absorptiometry, are common in IBD, with estimated rates of prevalence that range from 40 to 50% and 15%, respectively.[90] IBD patients are at an increased risk for fracture of the hip, spine and forearm, with an overall fracture incidence that is 40% higher than in the general population. Overall, however, the magnitude of this increased risk is quite modest.[90] The increased fracture rates appear to be similar in both Crohn's disease and ulcerative colitis, irrespective of gender. The fracture rate is approximately 1 per 100 patient-years.[90]

## Venous thrombosis

Patients with UC are at increased risk of thrombotic complications. Recently published population-based data indicate an incidence rate ratio of 2.8 (CI 2.1–3.7) for deep venous thrombosis and 3.6 (CI 2.5–5.2) for pulmonary embolism.[91] The incidence rate is approximately 1 per 200 patient-years. The highest incidence rate ratios were noted for patients under the age of 40. The underlying mechanisms accounting for this increased risk remains unknown. Although plausible, increased rates of hospitalization and surgery do not seem to account for this increased risk.[91]

## Hepatobiliary

PSC is the most common hepatobiliary manifestation associated with IBD. The prevalence of PSC in UC is approximately 3%.[89] PSC is more often associated with extensive UC than with Crohn's disease, although in a subset of Crohn's colitis patients the prevalence rates of PSC appear similar to that of ulcerative colitis.[92] In addition, PSC tends to affect men (70%) more often than women.[89,92] Other less commonly encountered hepatic disorders associated with ulcerative colitis include hepatic steatosis, drug-induced hepatotoxicity, hepatic amyloidosis and chronic autoimmune hepatitis.[92]

## Musculoskeletal

The most common extraintestinal manifestations of IBD are musculoskeletal,[88,93] the most common complaint being arthralgias in the absence of any signs of arthritis. Regarding specific joint inflammation two classic patterns occur: peripheral arthritis and axial disease. It is estimated that 5–20% of all IBD patients experience peripheral arthritis.[94] Peripheral arthritis usually manifests as an acute, asymmetric, large joint arthritis or a polyarticular small joint arthritis.[95] It is typically self-limiting and non-deforming and is distributed equally between the sexes.[95] Flares of peripheral arthritis tend to parallel the underlying bowel disease activity, such that symptomatic relief is generally achieved with successful treatment of the colitis.[95]

The prevalence of axial involvement (ankylosing spondylitis) in IBD ranges from 2% to 7%, with most data suggesting an equal distribution between Crohn's disease and UC.[89,96] Males are affected more than females.[95] The course of ankylosing spondylitis is typically unrelated to the underling IBD activity and is usually indistinguishable from non-IBD-associated ankylosing spondylitis.[93] Interestingly, up to 52% of UC patients may have asymptomatic sacroiliitis.[89,95] At present, it is not clear how many of these patients progress to clinically active disease.

# CUTANEOUS AND OPHTHALMOLOGIC MANIFESTATIONS

The reported prevalence of pyoderma gangrenosum in UC ranges from 0.5 to 5%.[89] Although classic teaching indicates a stronger association between pyoderma gangrenosum and UC than Crohn's disease, not all studies support this contention.[89] The activity of pyoderma gangrenosum appears to be associated with the underlying bowel disease activity, although the courses of the two diseases may be unrelated.[97]

The prevalence of erythema nodosum in ulcerative colitis ranges from 0.9 to 4% and it occurs more often in females.[89] Whether erythema nodosum is more frequent in Crohn's disease than UC is controversial.[89,98] The activity of erythema nodosum usually parallels that of the underlying bowel disease.[98]

Oral lesions occur more frequently in Crohn's disease than in UC.[99] The oral manifestations associated with ulcerative colitis include aphthous ulcers, pyostomatitis vegetans and major ulcers.[99] Aphthous ulcers commonly occur during disease flares. These lesions are identical to the frequently encountered canker sores that afflict healthy individuals and are usually painless.[98]

Both iritis and uveitis have similar rates of prevalence in Crohn's disease and UC of approximately 2%, and afflict men more often than women.[89] The course of iritis and uveitis is generally unrelated to the underlying enteral disease activity.[100] Episcleritis occurs in 5–8% of patients with IBD and its activity tends to be related to the underlying UC activity.[100,101] Ophthalmologic manifestations may also result from medications used to treat ulcerative colitis. For example, corticosteroid use is associated with posterior subcapsular cataracts and increased intraocular pressure.[100]

# RESPIRATORY MANIFESTATIONS

Up to 42% of patients with IBD demonstrate asymptomatic abnormal pulmonary function tests, as manifested by reduced $FEV_1$, IVC and $D_{LCO}$.[102] Some studies indicate a predilection for UC,[103] whereas others indicate an equal distribution for Crohn's disease and UC.[102] Lung disease associated with UC can be divided into four main categories, including airway disease (tracheal inflammation/stenosis, bronchitis, bronchiectasis), pulmonary parenchymal disease (interstitial lung disease, bronchiolitis obliterans with organizing pneumonia), serositis and drug related.[104,106] It is unknown whether these respiratory complications are truly increased in patients with UC, as population-based studies addressing this issue have not been conducted. Drug-induced pulmonary complications occur most frequently with sulfasalazine and mesalamine, although these reactions are quite rare.[105]

# MORTALITY

Most studies indicate that long-term survival rates for patients with UC are equivalent to that of the general population.[41,89,106]

However, within the first few years of diagnosis the mortality rate does appear to be increased.[106,107] In fact, Langholz et al.[107] found the relative risk of death to be 2.4 within the first few years of establishing the diagnosis of UC. The two most commonly reported risk factors associated with an increased mortality are pancolitis and severe disease at diagnosis.[9,106,107]

Some studies, however, show overall higher mortality rates for UC. In a Swedish population-based study the mortality rate was slightly increased, with a 10-year relative survival rate of 96% (95% CI 94.3–97.5).[107] Disease extent was an important determinant of mortality; the relative survival rate was not reduced for proctitis but was increased for left-sided colitis and pancolitis. Another population-based study from Sweden revealed a 15-year relative UC survival rate of 94% (95% CI 92–96%) and a mortality ratio of 1.37.[108] Most deaths were related to the underlying UC, but colorectal cancer, asthma and non-alcohol-related fatty liver disease also contributed.

## CONCLUSIONS

The majority of patients with UC have a chronic relapsing course, but very few (1%) have continuously active disease. Inflammation initially confined to the rectum (proctitis) extends proximally in approximately 25% of patients. The risk of colectomy at 10 years after diagnosis is approximately 25%, with almost half of the colectomies occurring in the first year after diagnosis. Mortality rate is only minimally increased over control values, with most UC-associated mortality occurring in the first year of disease activity. The rate of colorectal cancer is increased. Factors that are associated with an increased risk of colorectal cancer in UC include duration of disease, extensive colitis, family history of colorectal cancer (particularly in relatives that develop colorectal cancer below the age of 50), PSC, and perhaps backwash ileitis. Frequent complications include peripheral arthritis, which is associated with underlying disease activity, whereas toxic megacolon, PSC and colorectal cancer are relatively unusual but severe complications. Protective environmental factors include smoking and appendectomy, whereas NSAID ingestion, cessation of smoking, and respiratory and enteric infections can precipitate onset and flares of disease.

## REFERENCES

1. Selby W. The natural history of ulcerative colitis. Gastroenterology 1997;11:53–64.
2. Langholz E, Munkholm P, Davidsen M, Binder V. Course of ulcerative colitis: analysis of changes in disease activity over years. Gastroenterology 1994;107:3–11.
3. Hodgson HJ. The natural history of treated ulcerative colitis. Gastroenterology 1994;107:300–302.
4. Meyers S, Janowitz HD. The 'natural history' of ulcerative colitis: an analysis of the placebo response. J Clin Gastroenterol 1989;11:33–37.
5. Ilnyckyj A, Shanahan F, Anton PA, Cheang M, Bernstein CN. Quantification of the placebo response in ulcerative colitis. Gastroenterology 1997;112:1854–1858.
6. Brostrom O. Prognosis in ulcerative colitis. Med Clin North Am 1990;74:201–218.
7. Leijonmarck CE, Persson PG, Hellers G. Factors affecting colectomy rate in ulcerative colitis: an epidemiologic study. Gut 1990;31:329–333.
8. Sinclair TS, Brunt PW, Mowat NA. Nonspecific proctocolitis in northeastern Scotland: a community study. Gastroenterology 1983;85:1–11.
9. Hendriksen C, Kreiner S, Binder V. Long term prognosis in ulcerative colitis – based on results from a regional patient group from the county of Copenhagen. Gut 1985;26:158–163.
10. Farmer RG, Easley KA, Rankin GB. Clinical patterns, natural history, and progression of ulcerative colitis. A long-term follow-up of 1116 patients. Dig Dis Sci 1993;38:1137–1146.
11. Faubion WA Jr, Loftus EV Jr, Harmsen WS, Zinsmeister AR, Sandborn WJ. The natural history of corticosteroid therapy for inflammatory bowel disease: a population-based study. Gastroenterology 2001;121:255–260.
12. Pfau P, Kochman ML, Furth EE, Lichtenstein GR. Cytomegalovirus colitis complicating ulcerative colitis in the steroid-naive patient. Am J Gastroenterol 2001;96:895–899.
13. Cottone M, Pietrosi G, Martorana G et al. Prevalence of cytomegalovirus infection in severe refractory ulcerative and Crohn's colitis. Am J Gastroenterol 2001;96:773–775.
14. Papadakis KA, Tung JK, Binder SW et al. Outcome of cytomegalovirus infections in patients with inflammatory bowel disease. Am J Gastroenterol 2001;96:2137–2142.
15. Vega R, Bertran X, Menacho M et al. Cytomegalovirus infection in patients with inflammatory bowel disease. Am J Gastroenterol 1999;94:1053–1056.
16. Hommes D, Sterringa G, Boom R, Bartelsman J, Van Deventer S, Weel J. Incidence and outcome of cytomegalovirus infecton in patients with inflammatory bowel disease. Gastroenterology 2002;122:4.
17. Mahadevan U, Loftus E, Tremaine WJ, Sandborn WJ. Safety of selective cyclooxygenase-2 inhbitors in inflammatory bowel disease. Am J Gastroenterol 2002;97:910–914.
18. Felder JB, Korelitz BI, Rajapakse R, Schwarz S, Horatagis AP, Gleim G. Effects of nonsteroidal antiinflammatory drugs on inflammatory bowel disease: a case–control study. Am J Gastroenterol 2000;95:1949–1954.
19. Smale S, Sighorsson G, Foster R, Forgacs I, Bjarnason I. NSAIDs and relapse of IBD. Gastroenterology 2002;122:4.
20. Miner PB Jr. Factors influencing the relapse of patients with inflammatory bowel disease. Am J Gastroenterol 1997;92:1S–4S.
21. Meyer A, Ramzan N, Heigh R, Hernandez JL, Leighton J. NSAID use (including aspirin and selective COX II inhibitors) is associated with relapses of inflammatory bowel disease (IBD). Gastroenterology 2002;122:4.
22. Hegazi R, Mady H, Melhem M, Mohy MHH. Celecoxib and rofecoxib exacerbate chronic colitis and pre-malignant changes in IL-10 knockout mice. Gastroenterology 2002;122:4.
23. Morteau O, Morham SG, Sellon R et al. Impaired mucosal defense to acute colonic injury in mice lacking cyclooxygenase-1 or cyclooxygenase-2. J Clin Invest 2000;105:469–478.
24. Thomas GA, Rhodes J, Green JT. Inflammatory bowel disease and smoking – a review. Am J Gastroenterol 1998;93:144–149.
25. Calkins BM. A meta-analysis of the role of smoking in inflammatory bowel disease. Dig Dis Sci 1989;4:1841–1854.
26. Odes HS, Fich A, Reif S et al. Effects of current cigarette smoking on clinical course of Crohn's disease and ulcerative colitis. Dig Dis Sci 2001;46:1717–1721.
27. Green JT, Rhodes J, Ragunath K et al. Clinical status of ulcerative colitis in patients who smoke. Am J Gastroenterol 1998;93:1463–1467.
28. Boyko EJ, Perera DR, Koepsell TD, Keane EM, Inui TS. Effects of cigarette smoking on the clinical course of ulcerative colitis. Scand J Gastroenterol 1988;23:1147–1152.
29. Beaugerie L, Massot N, Carbonnel F, Cattan S, Gendre JP, Cosnes J. Impact of cessation of smoking on the course of ulcerative colitis. Am J Gastroenterol 2001;96:2113–2116.
30. Levenstein S, Prantera C, Varvo V et al. Stress and exacerbation in ulcerative colitis: a prospective study of patients enrolled in remission. Am J Gastroenterol 2000;95:1213–1220.
31. Jowett SL, Barton SJ, Welfare MR. Factors predictive of relapse in ulcerative colitis. Gastroenterology 2002;122:4.
32. Karamanolis DG, Delis KC, Papatheodoridis GV, Kalafatis E, Paspatis G, Xourgias VC. Seasonal variation in exacerbations of ulcerative colitis. Hepatogastroenterology 1997;44:1334–1338.
33. Russel MG, Dorant E, Brummer RJ et al. Appendectomy and the risk of developing ulcerative colitis or Crohn's disease: results of a large case–control study. South Limburg Inflammatory Bowel Disease Study Group. Gastroenterology 1997;113:377–382.
34. Andersson RE, Olaison G, Tysk C, Ekbom A. Appendectomy and protection against ulcerative colitis. N Engl J Med 2001;344:808–814.
35. Naganuma M, Iizuka B, Torii A et al. Appendectomy protects against the development of ulcerative colitis and reduces its recurrence: results of a multicenter case–controlled study in Japan. Am J Gastroenterol 2001;96:1123–1126.
36. Eri R, Cross S, Misko I et al. Appendectomy for refractory ulcerative colitis: targeting the right patient. Gastroenterology 2000;122:4; A–61.
37. Truelove S, Witts LJ. Cortisone in ulcerative colitis; final report on a therapeutic trial. Br Med J 1955;2:1041–1048.
38. Kjeldsen J, Schaffalitzky de Muckadell OB. Assessment of disease severity and activity in inflammatory bowel disease. Scand J Gastroenterol 1993;28:1–9.
39. Lennard-Jones JE, Ritchie JK, Hilder W, Spicer CC. Assessment of severity in colitis: a preliminary study. Gut 1975;16:579–584.
40. Powell-Tuck J, Day DW, Buckell NA, Wadsworth J, Lennard-Jones JE. Correlations between defined sigmoidoscopic appearances and other measures of disease activity in ulcerative colitis. Dig Dis Sci 1982;27:533–537.
41. Rachmilewitz D. Coated mesalazine (5-aminosalicylic acid) versus sulphasalazine in the treatment of active ulcerative colitis: a randomised trial. Br Med J 1989;298:82–86.
42. Stonnington CM, Phillips SF, Zinsmeister AR, Melton LJ III. Prognosis of chronic ulcerative colitis in a community. Gut 1987;28:1261–1266.
43. Langholz E, Munkholm P, Nielsen OH, Kreiner S, Binder V. Incidence and prevalence of ulcerative colitis in Copenhagen county from 1962 to 1987. Scand J Gastroenterol 1991;26:1247–1256.
44. Edwards F, Truelove SC. The course and prognosis of ulcerative colitis. Gut 1965;5:15–22.

45. Travis SP, Farrant JM, Ricketts C et al. Predicting outcome in severe ulcerative colitis. Gut 1996;38:905–910.

46. Gelbmann CM. Prediction of treatment refractoriness in ulcerative colitis and Crohn's disease – do we have reliable markers? Inflamm Bowel Dis 2000;6:123–131.

47. Buckell NA, Lennard-Jones JE, Hernandez MA, Kohn J, Riches PG, Wadsworth J. Measurement of serum proteins during attacks of ulcerative colitis as a guide to patient management. Gut 1979;20:22–27.

48. Bunn SK, Bisset WM, Main MJ, Gray ES, Olson S, Golden BE. Fecal calprotectin: validation as a noninvasive measure of bowel inflammation in childhood inflammatory bowel disease. J Pediatr Gastroenterol Nutr 2001;33:14–22.

49. Tibble JA, Sigthorsson G, Bridger S, Fagerhol MK, Bjarnason I. Surrogate markers of intestinal inflammation are predictive of relapse in patients with inflammatory bowel disease. Gastroenterology 2000;119:15–22.

50. Carbonnel F, Lavergne A, Lemann M et al. Colonoscopy of acute colitis. A safe and reliable tool for assessment of severity. Dig Dis Sci 1994;39:1550–1557.

51. Alemayehu G, Jarnerot G. Colonoscopy during an attack of severe ulcerative colitis is a safe procedure and of great value in clinical decision making. Am J Gastroenterol 1991;86:187–190.

52. Levin B. Inflammatory bowel disease and colon cancer. Cancer 1992;70:1313–1316.

53. Connell WR, Lennard-Jones JE, Williams CB, Talbot IC, Price AB, Wilkinson KH. Factors affecting the outcome of endoscopic surveillance for cancer in ulcerative colitis. Gastroenterology 1994;107:934–944.

54. Meucci G, Vecchi M, Astegiano M et al. The natural history of ulcerative proctitis: a multicenter, retrospective study. Gruppo di Studio per le Malattie Infiammatorie Intestinali (GSMII). Am J Gastroenterol 2000;95:469–473.

55. Ayres RC, Gillen CD, Walmsley RS, Allan RN. Progression of ulcerative proctosigmoiditis: incidence and factors influencing progression. Eur J Gastroenterol Hepatol 1996;8:555–558.

56. Langholz E, Munkholm P, Davidsen M, Nielsen OH, Binder V. Changes in extent of ulcerative colitis: a study on the course and prognostic factors. Scand J Gastroenterol 1996;31:260–266.

57. Rao SS, Holdsworth CD, Read NW. Symptoms and stool patterns in patients with ulcerative colitis. Gut 1988;29:342–345.

58. Waye JD. The role of colonoscopy in the differential diagnosis of inflammatory bowel disease. Gastrointest Endosc 1977;23:150–154.

59. Bernstein CN. On making the diagnosis of ulcerative colitis. Am J Gastroenterol 1997;92:1247–1252.

60. Markowitz J, Kahn E, Grancher K, Hyams J, Treem W, Daum F. Atypical rectosigmoid histology in children with newly diagnosed ulcerative colitis. Am J Gastroenterol 1993;88:2034–2037.

61. Kim B, Barnett JL, Kleer CG, Appelman HD. Endoscopic and histological patchiness in treated ulcerative colitis. Am J Gastroenterol 1999;94:3258–3262.

62. D'Haens G, Geboes K, Peeters M, Baert F, Ectors N, Rutgeerts P. Patchy cecal inflammation associated with distal ulcerative colitis: a prospective endoscopic study. Am J Gastroenterol 1997;92:1275–1279.

63. Bernstein CN, Shanahan F, Anton PA, Weinstein WM. Patchiness of mucosal inflammation in treated ulcerative colitis: a prospective study. Gastrointest Endosc 1995;42:232–237.

64. Glickman A, Bousvaros A, Farraye FA et al. Relative rectal sparing and skip lesions are not uncommon at initial presentation in pediatric patients with chronic ulcerative colitis (CUC). United States and Canadian Academy of Pathology Annual Meeting, 2002.

65. Levine TS, Tzardi M, Mitchell S, Sowter C, Price AB. Diagnostic difficulty arising from rectal recovery in ulcerative colitis. J Clin Pathol 1996;49:319–323.

66. Kleer CG, Appelman HD. Ulcerative colitis: patterns of involvement in colorectal biopsies and changes with time. Am J Surg Pathol 1998;22:983–989.

67. Sheth SG, LaMont JT. Toxic megacolon. Lancet 1998;351:509–513.

68. Binder SC, Patterson JF, Glotzer DJ. Toxic megacolon in ulcerative colitis. Gastroenterology 1974;66:909–915.

69. Kotanagi H, Fukuoka T, Shibata Y et al. A case of toxic megacolon in ulcerative colitis associated with cytomegalovirus infection. J Gastroenterol 1994;29:501–505.

70. Berk T, Gordon SJ, Choi HY, Cooper HS. Cytomegalovirus infection of the colon: a possible role in exacerbations of inflammatory bowel disease. Am J Gastroenterol 1985;80:355–360.

71. Greenstein AJ, Aufses AH Jr. Differences in pathogenesis, incidence and outcome of perforation in inflammatory bowel disease. Surg Gynecol Obstet 1985; 160:63–69.

72. Danovitch SH. Fulminant colitis and toxic megacolon. Gastroenterol Clin North Am 1989;18:73–82.

73. Pardi DS, Loftus EV Jr, Tremaine WJ et al. Acute major gastrointestinal hemorrhage in inflammatory bowel disease. Gastrointest Endosc 1999;49:153–157.

74. Robert JH, Sachar DB, Aufses AH Jr, Greenstein AJ. Management of severe hemorrhage in ulcerative colitis. Am J Surg 1990;159:550–555.

75. Gumaste V, Sachar DB, Greenstein AJ. Benign and malignant colorectal strictures in ulcerative colitis. Gut 1992;33:938–941.

76. Bernstein CN, Blanchard JF, Kliewer E, Wajda A. Cancer risk in patients with inflammatory bowel disease: a population-based study. Cancer 2001;91:854–862.

77. Eaden JA, Abrams KR, Mayberry JF. The risk of colorectal cancer in ulcerative colitis: a meta-analysis. Gut 2001;48:526–535.

78. Ekbom A, Helmick C, Zack M, Adami HO. Ulcerative colitis and colorectal cancer. A population-based study. N Engl J Med 1990;323:1228–1233.

79. Nugent FW, Haggitt RC, Gilpin PA. Cancer surveillance in ulcerative colitis. Gastroenterology 1991;100:1241–1248.

80. Shetty K, Rybicki L, Brzezinski A, Carey WD, Lashner BA. The risk for cancer or dysplasia in ulcerative colitis patients with primary sclerosing cholangitis. Am J Gastroenterol 1999;94:1643–1649.

81. Kornfeld D, Ekbom A, Ihre T. Is there an excess risk for colorectal cancer in patients with ulcerative colitis and concomitant primary sclerosing cholangitis? A population based study. Gut 1997;41:522–525.

82. Broome U, Lofberg R, Veress B, Eriksson LS. Primary sclerosing cholangitis and ulcerative colitis: evidence for increased neoplastic potential. Hepatology 1995;22:1404–1408.

83. Brentnall TA, Haggitt RC, Rabinovitch PS et al. Risk and natural history of colonic neoplasia in patients with primary sclerosing cholangitis and ulcerative colitis. Gastroenterology 1996;110:331–338.

84. Nuako KW, Ahlquist DA, Mahoney DW, Schaid DJ, Siems DM, Lindor NM. Familial predisposition for colorectal cancer in chronic ulcerative colitis: a case–control study. Gastroenterology 1998;115:1079–1083.

85. Askling J, Dickman PW, Karlen P et al. Family history as a risk factor for colorectal cancer in inflammatory bowel disease. Gastroenterology 2001;120:1356–1362.

86. Heuschen UA, Hinz U, Allemeyer EH et al. Backwash ileitis is strongly associated with colorectal carcinoma in ulcerative colitis. Gastroenterology 2001;120:841–847.

87. Eaden J, Abrams K, Ekbom A, Jackson E, Mayberry J. Colorectal cancer prevention in ulcerative colitis: a case–control study. Aliment Pharmacol Ther 2000;14:145–153.

88. Tung BY, Emond MJ, Haggitt RC et al. Ursodiol use is associated with lower prevalence of colonic neoplasia in patients with ulcerative colitis and primary sclerosing cholangitis. Ann Intern Med 2001;134:89–95.

89. Ryan BM, Van der Eijk I, Fornaciari G, Mouzas I, Stockbrugger R, Russel GR. Extraintestinal manifestations of IBD significantly adversely affect quality of life: results from the population-based European collaborative study group for IBD. Gastroenterology 2002;122:4.

90. Bernstein CN, Blanchard JF, Rawsthorne P, Yu N. The prevalence of extraintestinal diseases in inflammatory bowel disease: a population-based study. Am J Gastroenterol 2001;96:1116–1122.

91. Bernstein CN, Blanchard JF, Leslie W, Wajda A, Yu BN. The incidence of fracture among patients with inflammatory bowel disease. A population-based cohort study. Ann Intern Med 2000;133:795–799.

92. Bernstein CN, Blanchard JF, Houston DS, Wajda A. The incidence of deep venous thrombosis and pulmonary embolism among patients with inflammatory bowel disease: a population-based cohort study. Thromb Haemost 2001;85:430–434.

93. Raj V, Lichtenstein DR. Hepatobiliary manifestations of inflammatory bowel disease. Gastroenterol Clin North Am 1999;28:491–513.

94. Fornaciari G, Salvarani C, Beltrami M, Macchioni P, Stockbrugger RW, Russel MG. Muscoloskeletal manifestations in inflammatory bowel disease. Can J Gastroenterol 2001;15:399–403.

95. Orchard TR, Wordsworth BP, Jewell DP. Peripheral arthropathies in inflammatory bowel disease: their articular distribution and natural history. Gut 1998;42:387–391.

96. Katz JP, Lichtenstein GR. Rheumatologic manifestations of gastrointestinal diseases. Gastroenterol Clin North Am 1998;27:533–562.

97. Greenstein AJ, Janowitz HD, Sachar DB. The extra-intestinal complications of Crohn's disease and ulcerative colitis: a study of 700 patients. Medicine (Baltimore) 1976;55:401–412.

98. Ward SK, Roenigk HH, Gordon KB. Dermatologic manifestations of gastrointestinal disorders. Gastroenterol Clin North Am 1998;27:615–636.

99. Lebwohl M, Lebwohl O. Cutaneous manifestations of inflammatory bowel disease. Inflamm Bowel Dis 1998;4:142–148.

100. Lisciandrano D, Ranzi T, Carrassi A et al. Prevalence of oral lesions in inflammatory bowel disease. Am J Gastroenterol 1996;91:7–10.

101. Hendrickson BA, Gokhale R, Cho JH. Clinical aspects and pathophysiology of inflammatory bowel disease. Clin Microbiol Rev 2002;15:79–94.

102. Petrelli EA, McKinley M, Troncale FJ. Ocular manifestations of inflammatory bowel disease. Ann Ophthalmol 1982;14:356–360.

103. Herrlinger KR, Noftz MK, Dalhoff K, Ludwig D, Stange EF, Fellermann K. Alterations in pulmonary function in inflammatory bowel disease are frequent and persist during remission. Am J Gastroenterol 2002;97:377–381.

104. Camus P, Piard F, Ashcroft T, Gal AA, Colby TV. The lung in inflammatory bowel disease. Medicine (Baltimore) 1993;72:151–183.

105. Mahadeva R, Walsh G, Flower CD, Shneerson JM. Clinical and radiological characteristics of lung disease in inflammatory bowel disease. Eur Respir J 2000;15:41–48.

106. Parry SD, Barbatzas C, Peel ET, Barton JR. Sulphasalazine and lung toxicity. Eur Respir J 2002;19:756–764.

107. Langholz E, Munkholm P, Davidsen M, Binder V. Colorectal cancer risk and mortality in patients with ulcerative colitis. Gastroenterology 1992;103:1444–1451.

108. Ekbom A, Helmick CG, Zack M, Holmberg L, Adami HO. Survival and causes of death in patients with inflammatory bowel disease: a population-based study. Gastroenterology 1992;103:954–960.

109. Persson PG, Bernell O, Leijonmarck CE, Farahmand BY, Hellers G, Ahlbom A. Survival and cause-specific mortality in inflammatory bowel disease: a population-based cohort study. Gastroenterology 1996;110:1339–1345.

110. Ritchie JK, Powell-Tuck J, Lennard-Jones JE. Clinical outcome of the first ten years of ulcerative colitis and proctitis. Lancet 1978;1:1140–1143.

## CHAPTER 20

# Clinical features and natural history of Crohn's disease

## Pia Munkholm and Vibeke Binder

Crohn's disease is a pan-enteric disease with focal exacerbations and with intermittent activity throughout the patient's life. Therefore it is not possible to cure Crohn's disease by medical therapy or by surgical excision, it can only be managed.

*J Alexander-Williams, Professor of gastrointestinal surgery, Birmingham, 1990*

## INTRODUCTION

A natural course of Crohn's disease and ulcerative colitis does not exist, as almost no patient with IBD remains untreated for an extended period either by current drugs or surgery. Older studies with long-term follow-up of large but selected patient groups from tertiary referral centers revealed the worst possible prognosis as, for instance, the study by Devroede et al.,[1] who found a very high mortality and cancer incidence in ulcerative colitis. Similarly, the study by Weedon et al.[2] reported a very high incidence of cancer in Crohn's disease. These studies have become a burden for patients, as they have been considered to depict the true prognosis. These studies have been read by, among others, insurance companies, and have made it difficult for patients to obtain insurance at reasonable rates.

The clinical presentation of Crohn's disease is often insidious, and although the interval between the initial symptom and the final diagnosis of the disease may be quite long, the retrospective description of this initial disease course is rather non-specific, as regards bowel symptoms, systemic symptoms and extraintestinal symptoms and signs. Combined delays by both patients and physicians contribute to the interval from onset to diagnosis, which tends to become longer the milder the symptoms are.[3] The early untreated course of disease is thus neither representative nor accurate enough to form the basis for a description of the natural course of Crohn's disease.

The closest we get to a natural course of these diseases is probably the outcome of patients receiving placebo in controlled therapeutic trials. Even then, clinicians have learned that the mere act of participating in a study, with frequent outpatient interactions with doctors and members of the healthcare team, may change the disease course. Furthermore, placebo-treated patients are to some degree selected, as for ethical reasons patients with severe and threatening symptoms will not be included in a placebo-controlled study and are eliminated from such a study if their disease worsens. As stated by Meyers and Janowitz,[4] valuable information can nevertheless be obtained, if the following questions can be answered: 'Can a patient, sick enough to need treatment get better by himself?', and 'Can a patient in remission stay in remission without medical therapy?' Large placebo-controlled studies of Crohn's disease[5,6] have shown that within 3 months, between one out of four and one out of two patients in active disease went into remission spontaneously, but after 12 months only 15–18% of the patients were still in remission (Table 20.1).

Patients who were brought into remission, either by medical or by surgical treatment, remained in remission in the placebo arm of controlled studies in over 50% of cases after 1 year and between 35 and 46% after 2 years,[7,8] as shown in Table 20.2.

These trials indicate that even without treatment, the course of Crohn's disease in a substantial proportion of patients is mild, with spontaneous clinical remission.

In today's environment of widespread access to medical care, a legitimate question is whether a *natural* history of disease is particularly important, as evidence-based medical and surgical treatments are available for most patients. A more relevant issue is the long-term prognosis and disease course in regional, population-based patient groups that are treated with widely accepted medical and surgical approaches. Such studies have been performed in Europe and North America during recent years, and provide a basis for information about prognosis and risk factors in response to modern medical and surgical

**Table 20.1 Patients with active Crohn's disease treated in the placebo arm of controlled studies obtaining spontaneous remission (% of total)**

|  | 3 months (%) | 12 months (%) | 24 months (%) |
|---|---|---|---|
| Summers et al. 1979[5] (n=77) | 26 | 18 | 12 |
| Malchow et al. 1984[6] (n=58) | 42 | 15 | 8 |

**Table 20.2 Patients in remission continuing placebo treatment in controlled study**

|  | 1 year (%) | 1½ year (%) | 2 years (%) |
|---|---|---|---|
| Summers et al. 1979[5] (n=101) | 64 |  | 40 |
| Malchow et al. 1984[6] (n=52) | 52 |  | 35 |
| Gendre et al. 1993[7] (n=81) | 57 |  | 46 |
| Lochs et al. 2000[8] (n=166) |  | 69 |  |

treatment. This information provides an important resource for evaluating newly introduced treatment modalities and a mechanism to estimate the long-term risk of new medications relative to existing treatments. This chapter is based principally on these types of population-based outcome studies.

## CLINICAL APPEARANCE

Because of the lack of a known etiology, Crohn's disease is diagnosed as a syndrome of chronic inflammation in the absence of infection within one or more segments of the gastrointestinal tract. Four clinically relevant diagnostic criteria have been described regarding clinical symptoms, radiological, endoscopical and histological signs. At least two of these four criteria must be fulfilled to establish the diagnosis, after excluding infectious, ischemic and neoplastic diseases.[9,10] These diagnostic criteria have been generally accepted internationally for epidemiological and clinical studies.

The clinical appearance of Crohn's disease can differ considerably, according to the location of disease, the inflammatory activity, the degree of fibrosis and the degree of penetration through the intestinal wall.

A comprehensive survey of the disease manifestations is possible through the clinical epidemiological studies of unselected, regional patient populations that have been published during recent years. However, it has not yet been possible to actively predict the subsequent course of disease based on the phenotype at diagnosis. It is the hope of ongoing large studies to define phenotypes of patients based on the clinical appearance at diagnosis, the course of disease during the first several years, and the genotype.

## LOCATION OF CROHN'S DISEASE

Although the disease can be localized throughout the gastrointestinal tract from mouth to anus, and although chronic inflammation histologically can be evident in endoscopically uninvolved areas, more than 90% of new cases of grossly detectable Crohn's disease is located in three main sites: isolated small intestinal involvement, restricted to the colon, and combined small and large bowel involvement. The single most often affected segment is the terminal ileum, which is clinically inflamed in two-thirds of patients. The distribution of patients within these three different disease locations at diagnosis is shown in Table 20.3, based on population studies.[11–19]

In an attempt to specify further the different localization of Crohn's disease, in 1998 an international group of IBD specialists worked out a clinical classification.[20] According to this Vienna classification, Crohn's disease can be divided into several distinct locations:

● *Terminal ileum* – less than one-third of the small bowel, with or without spillover into the cecum;

**Table 20.3 Localization of Crohn's disease at diagnosis in population-based studies**

|  | Small and large intestine (%) | Small intestine only (%) | Colon only (%) |
|---|---|---|---|
| Munkholm et al. 1992[11] | 33 | 29 | 30 |
| Lapidus et al. 1997[12] | 41 | 27 | 32 |
| Nyhlin et al. 1986[13] | 32 | 48 | 20 |
| Ekbom et al. 1991[14] | 26 | 39 | 25 |
| Loftus et al. 1998[15] | 45 | 22 | 32 |
| Gower-Rousseau 1994[16] | 48 | 11 | 19 |
| Moum et al. 1996[17] | 29 | 27 | 44 |
| Bjørnsson et al. 2000[18] | 31 | 18 | 51 |
| Witte 2000 EC-IBD[19] | 31 | 29 | 38 |
| Overall (range) | 35 (26–48) | 28 (11–48) | 32 (19–51) |

- *Colon* – any colonic location between cecum and rectum, with no small bowel or upper gastrointestinal involvement;
- *Ileocolon* – disease of the terminal ileum and any location between ascending colon and rectum;
- *Upper gastrointestinal* – any disease location proximal to the terminal ileum, regardless of additional involvement of the terminal ileum or colon.

The maximum extent is defined as disease involvement at any time before the first resection. Minimum involvement for a location is defined as any aphthous lesion or ulceration, whereas the appearance of only mucosal erythema and edema is not adequate. For classification, examination of both the small and large bowel is required.

An internal validation was initially carried out, based on three existing population-based Crohn's disease patient groups from Denmark, Norway and North America, and further patient data from a surgical and a medical referral center from Canada and New York were included. Some differences were found, indicating regional differences, but all disease locations were recognized in all five databases.[20]

A prospective evaluation of this classification in a large regional group of unselected patients has not so far been carried out, but Louis et al.[21] retrospectively classified 297 patients with Crohn's disease, followed in a Belgian university clinic, for a median of 9 years. This analysis revealed that over a course of 10 years, 16% of the patients changed from one location to another. This is in concordance with other studies showing that the localization of disease in an individual patient may change over time. Lapidus[22] found that 24% of patients with Crohn's colitis subsequently developed inflammation in the small bowel. An ongoing study of disease course in a European multicenter epidemiological study is including the Vienna classification during a follow-up over 10 years.[23]

Esophageal, gastric and duodenal ulcerations, oral ulcers and lip lesions are less typical presentations of Crohn's disease and are rare primary manifestations of the disease, as they seldom occur without Crohn's disease in small and/or large bowel simultaneously.

Crohn's disease of the esophagus was reported during the disease course in only 20 of approximately 9900 patients (0.2%) with Crohn's disease treated in the Mayo Clinic between 1976 and 1998. All patients with esophageal involvement had associated small intestinal or large colonic involvement.[24] The endoscopic appearances of the esophageal lesions were similar to the findings in the bowel: aphthous ulcers (40%), larger and deeper ulcerations (85%), stenosis (20%) and pseudopolyps (5%). All patients had esophageal symptoms, including dysphagia (55%), odynophagia (40%), heartburn (30%) and chest pain (10%).

Gastric and duodenal involvement has an estimated incidence of 1–4% of adult patients with Crohn's disease described in two series.[25,26] Gastroduodenal Crohn's disease occurred in association with Crohn's disease elsewhere in 96% of these patients, most often in the small bowel (69%). The endoscopic and histological findings were not different from the spectrum of findings in other locations of Crohn's disease. Fistulization to the transverse colon, other parts of the GI tract or the skin are rare and serious complications, as are duodenal and enteral obstruction. However, in general gastroduodenal Crohn's disease generated less morbidity than did more distal Crohn's disease. In contrast, gastroduodenal Crohn's disease is more common in children, being reported in 30–40 % of patients.[26a] Perianal localization of the disease is often connected to simultaneous rectoanal localization, but may occur as the initial lesion, without intestinal involvement, in about 5%.[3]

Fistulizing Crohn's disease at diagnosis has been reported in 14–20% of patients in different population-based studies,[11,17,27] most frequently in patients with colorectal disease, of whom 37% have been reported with fistulae.[22] Schwartz et al.[27] reported that 34% of 169 patients from a population-based study, followed for a median of 9 years, developed at least one fistula during the course of disease. The fistula sites were perianal (54%), enteroenteric (24%), rectovaginal (9%), enterocutaneous (6%), enterovesical (3%) and enterointra-abdominal (3%). Sixty-six per cent of patients experiencing fistula had only one episode, whereas 22 % had two and 12% had three or more episodes during the follow-up period. The frequency of recurrence periods was similar when patients with perianal fistula were analyzed separately.

## CLINICAL SYMPTOMS

The dominant symptoms in Crohn's disease are abdominal pain and diarrhea, which are present in more than 70% of all patients at diagnosis. Although present at all localizations, a positive correlation has been found between ileal disease and abdominal pain, and between diarrhea, bloody stools and colonic disease.[11] Weight loss and fever are present at diagnosis in 38–69% of patients at diagnosis, independent of disease localization. Figure 20.1 shows the symptoms from the Danish population-based cohort of patients with Crohn's disease.

The chronic transmural inflammatory process of Crohn's disease may lead to stricture of the gut lumen by the formation of fibrosis in the bowel wall and also, with or without stenosis, to penetration through the bowel wall, with fistulae connecting to adjacent organs or to the skin. The Vienna classification[20] has defined three different types of behavior of Crohn's disease: inflammatory, stricturing and penetrating. It is important, however, to realize that the behavior of the disease may change during its course. For example, inflammatory presentation at diagnosis can become stricturing within few years and penetrating later on. Louis et al.[21] found that after 10 years with the disease, almost half of the patients exhibited a change in disease

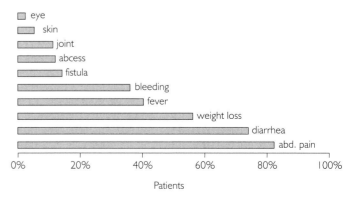

Fig. 20.1 Frequency of symptoms at diagnosis among 373 Danish patients with Crohn's disease. (Modified from Munkholm P et al. Incidence and prevalence of Crohn's disease in the County of Copenhagen, 1962–87: A sixfold increase in incidence. Scand J Gastroenterol 1992;27:609.)

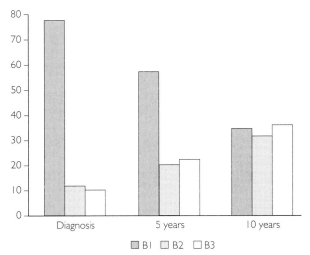

**Fig. 20.2** Evolution of disease behaviour according to the Vienna classification system over 10 years in 125 patients with Crohn's disease. The proportion of patients with non-stricturing non-penetrating (B1), stricturing (B2) and penetrating (B3) disease are shown at diagnosis and after 5 and 10 years of evolution. The proportion of patients with a change in disease behavior was highly significant over 10 years ($P<0.0001$) and was already significantly different from baseline after 1 year ($P=0.04$). (From Louis E et al. Behavior of Crohn's disease according to the Vienna classification: changing pattern over the course of the disease. Gut 2001;49:777.)

behavior, predominantly from inflammatory to stricturing and penetrating. At diagnosis 74% of patients were classified as B1: inflammatory behavior, 11% as B2: stricturing behavior, and 15% as B3: penetrating behavior. Ten years later, only 30% could be classified as B1, whereas 32% were B2 and 37% B3, as shown in Figure 20.2.

These results indicate that disease behavior must be compared in patients with similar disease durations, as the characteristics of the inflammatory process evolve during the course of disease. Future studies may reveal individual characteristics that predict the evolution of the inflammatory process in a given patient.

## EXTRAINTESTINAL MANIFESTATIONS

Extraintestinal manifestations may be temporally related to a clinical flare of symptoms of Crohn's disease, appear independently of intestinal activity, or may even be present before diagnosis.

### Joints

The most frequent extraintestinal manifestations of Crohn's disease are associated with the joints, in the form of either arthralgias or acute peripheral arthritis types 1 and 2, as described by Orchard et al.[28] Type 1 is characterized by being pauciarticular, i.e. fewer than five and especially large joints affected, short duration, and usually in relation to flares in disease activity. This type is clinically and genetically connected to reactive arthritis and is associated with HLA class I genes, like the axial forms of arthropathy, including ankylosing spondylitis. Type 2 arthritis affects multiple small joints, with no correlation to flares in CD. This type is not closely associated with HLA

class I genes and may have a different etiology. In a large group of patients with Crohn's disease in Oxford[29] 32.9% of 483 patients currently or previously had arthropathy, including 14.3% with arthralgia without swelling, 6% with type 1 arthritis, 4% with type 2 and 9.9% with axial arthropathy. Eleven per cent of the patients in the Danish cohort had clinical joint manifestations, not further specified, at diagnosis.[11]

### Skin

Erythema nodosum, Sweet's syndrome and pyoderma gangrenosum are all reported to have an increased frequency in patients with Crohn's disease. A large German study revealed retrospectively a prevalence of 2.1% of cutaneous manifestations among 1043 patients with ulcerative colitis and Crohn's disease,[30] similar to the findings of Bernstein et al. in a large Canadian study.[31] Erythema nodosum was found three times more frequently than pyoderma. Both were more frequent in Crohn's disease than in ulcerative colitis. Sweet's syndrome, defined as acute febrile neutrophilic dermatosis, has been described in only 30 patients with inflammatory bowel diseases.[32]

Non-specific eczema has been reported with a greater frequency in patients with Crohn's disease than in healthy controls – unrelated to relapse of bowel disease[33-] and an increased occurrence of psoriasis has similarly been shown in patients with Crohn's disease and their relatives.[34] Psoriasis may be genetically linked to Crohn's disease in that these Th1-mediated disorders can occur in the same families, and familial psoriasis has been linked to a region on chromosome 16.[35]

### Eyes

Iridocyclitis/uveitis and episcleritis were reported in 1–2% of patients with IBD in a large population-based database from Canada,[31] most frequently among patients with ulcerative colitis and among women, where a percentage of 3.8 was found.

### Primary sclerosing cholangitis (PSC)

This is often classified as an extraintestinal manifestation, but may be a coincidental disease to both ulcerative colitis and Crohn's disease. PSC has been reported in between 1 and 3% of patients with Crohn's disease, less than in patients with ulcerative colitis, and may precede the bowel disease by several years or present after total colectomy in ulcerative colitis patients.[31,36,37]

## CLINICAL COURSE

The chronic, relapsing nature of Crohn's disease imparts physical, psychological and social strains on the patient, and although these are not mutually independent it has become recognized that they are each important and deserve attention in patient management. This thus comprises three cornerstones: treatment, information and support. A long-term strategy includes the goals of improving survival, decreasing morbidity, avoiding complications, and maintaining a daily life as close to normal as possible.

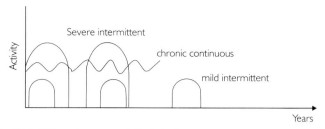

**Fig. 20.3** Different courses of Crohn's disease.

## CLINICAL INFLAMMATORY ACTIVITY COURSE

Different disease patterns are described, which include chronic intermittent disease, with remission periods of more than 1 month without glucocorticoid treatment, and chronic continuous symptoms, without such remission periods. In response to current medical and surgical treatment, most cases of Crohn's disease follow a chronic intermittent course, with clinical remission lasting from a few months to several years. Different patterns of disease are shown in Figure 20.3.

Although the individual courses are unpredictable and the provoking factors for relapse are unknown, statistical analyses in cohorts of patients give us some understanding of the long-term course of Crohn's disease. In a population-based incidence cohort of patients, Munkholm et al.[38] found that about half of the patients at any time appeared to be in clinical remission. During the course of the individual patient, however, considerable changes in the state of activity were found. The relapse rate was influenced by the length of the foregoing remission. Experiencing one full year in clinical remission increases the chance of remaining in remission in the following year to 80%. For a patient with active Crohn's disease, the probability of having active disease the following year is 70%. Within 3 years however, the chance of obtaining a full year in remission is 50%.

For further analysis, the 5-year course from the third to the eighth year after diagnosis was characterized as remission all years – 22%; relapse every year – 25%; and years with alternating remission and relapse – 53%. The only predictor for the 5-year course was the course of disease in the preceding 2 years, whereas other clinical characteristics, such as age, gender, location of disease and familial occurrence, do not seem to correlate with the course of activity during the subsequent years (Fig. 20.4).

Expressed in another way, as shown in Figure 20.5, 13% of the patients have had a relapse-free course, 20% have had relapses every year, and 67% have experienced both years in relapse and years in remission within the first 8 years with the disease.

A chronic continuous course over years, without even short remissions, is rare: 4% after 5 years and 1% after 10 years.

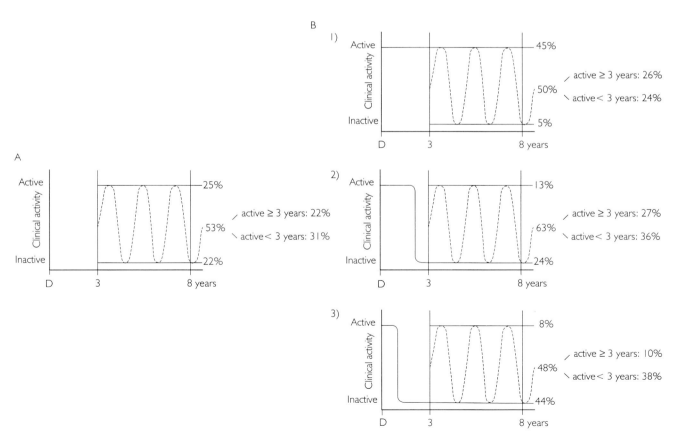

**Fig. 20.4** Distribution of Crohn's disease patients according to years in remission and years with relapse during a 5-year period from the third to the eighth year after diagnosis. (A) Total patient group. (B) 1. Active disease every year before the 5-year period; 2. 1 year in remission; 3. 2 years in remission after the year of diagnosis. (From Munkholm P et al. Disease activity courses in a regional cohort of Crohn's disease patients. Scand J Gastroenterol 1995;30:699.)

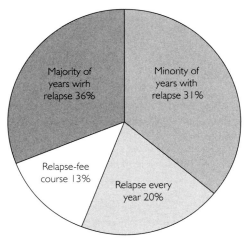

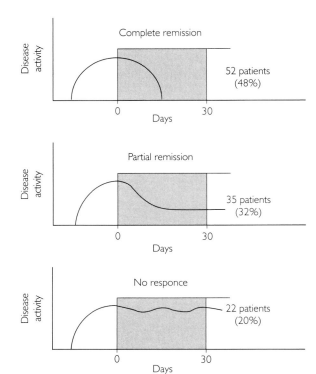

**Fig. 20.5** Frequency of relapse during the first 8 years from diagnosis of Crohn's disease in 171 patients. (Modified from Munkholm P et al. Disease activity courses in a regional cohort of Crohn's disease patients. Scand J Gastroenterol 1995;30:699.)

**Fig. 20.6** Initial outcome of the first steroid treatment course after 1 month of prednisolone (1mg/kg) administration in 109 patients with Crohn's disease. (From Munkholm P et al. Frequency of glucocorticoid resistance and dependency in Crohn's disease. Gut 1994;35:360.)

Using a slightly different approach with Markov chain analysis, in a Mayo Clinic study Silverstein et al.[39] found in a population-based inception cohort of patients that the future 'disease expectancy' for a representative Crohn's disease patient consisted of 24% of time spent in medical remission (no medication), 41% in postsurgical remission (no medications), and 27% in medical treatment with a 5-ASA preparation only, whereas only 7% of the years would be expected to have a severity of disease requiring glucucorticoid treatment or immunosuppressives.

The short- and long-term responses to steroid treatment in Crohn's disease have been analysed in two studies by Munkholm et al.[40] and Faubion et al.[41] showing very concordant results. A flare-up of Crohn's disease responded to medical treatment with glucocorticoids within 1 month, with complete remission in 48–58% of patients, and with improvement in an additional 26–32% of patients. No response at all was found in 16–20% (Fig. 20.6). Furthermore, close to 30% of the patients became steroid dependent, with immediate flare-ups after cessation of treatment.

## SURGICAL INTERVENTIONS IN THE DISEASE COURSE

Most of the patients who do not respond to glucocorticoids will need surgery, with either resection of the inflamed/stenosed segment of small intestine or large bowel or a colectomy. The indication for an intestinal resection may be acute, caused by a complication such as an intra-abdominal fistula, abscess or even frank perforation. Elective operation, which carries a much better prognosis, is indicated in case of stenosis of a segment of the bowel or persisting, severe inflammation in a short segment, refractory to intensive medical treatment. The cumulative rate of surgical intervention in Crohn's disease has been reported from two Scandinavian population-based follow-up studies, as shown in Table 20.4. Patients with ileal or ileocecal location at diagnosis have a 3.2 times higher frequency of operation than patients with colonic inflammation only. Age, but not gender, influenced the rate of primary surgery, being low in childhood (RR 0.8 (0.6–0.96), $P=0.02$) and high in the 45–59-year age

group (RR 1.2 (1.00–1.4), $P=0.04$).[42] Patients with fistula/perianal disease had an independantly higher operation rate than patients without fistulizing disease (RR 1.2 (1.03–1.3), $P= 0.006$).

The cumulative probability of colectomy for Crohn's colitis, based on the Danish population-based study,[3] was of the same order of magnitude as in patients with ulcerative colitis, as shown in Figure 20.7.

## RECURRENCE AFTER SURGICAL INTERVENTION

The cumulative clinical relapse rate for patients who had undergone an intestinal resection for Crohn's disease was found by Bernell et al.[42,43] to be 33% after 5 years, 44% after 10 years and 50% after 15 years, higher for women (RR 1.2) and higher in patients with small bowel or continuous ileocolonic disease (RR:1.8) compared to colorectal Crohn's disease (Fig. 20.8). No influence of age on the rate of recurrence was found.

The frequency of recurrence depends on the definition of recurrence, as it was reported by Rutgeerts et al.[44] that 73% of patients, 1 year after ileal resection, showed endoscopic signs of recurrence at anastomosis or in the neoterminal ileum, although only 20% had clinical symptoms. These surprising results have been confirmed by Olaison et al.[45] However, McLeod et al.,[46] by studying the placebo arm of a large controlled study of postoperative course, reported an endoscopic or radiographic recurrence rate of 28% after 1 year, 61% after 2 years and 77% after 3 years. Also in this study, a discrepancy between endoscopic/radiographic and clinical recurrence was found, as seen in Figure 20.9.

## Table 20.4 Cumulative probability of resective surgery in Crohn's disease during the course of disease

|  | 1 year (%) | 5 years (%) | 10 years (%) | 15 years (%) |
|---|---|---|---|---|
| Bernell et al.[41] All patients CD | 44 | 61 | 71 | |
| Munkholm et al.[3] All patients CD | 31 | 44 | 61 | 70 |
| Bernell et al.[42] Ileocaecal CD | 61 | 77 | 83 | |
| Munkholm et al.[3] Ileocaecal CD | 60 | 78 | 78 | 78 |
| Lapidus et al.[22] Colorectal CD | 18 | 33 | 47 | |

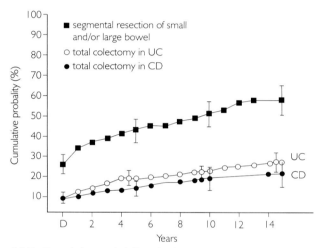

**Fig. 20.7** Cumulative probability of colectomy and segmental small and large bowel resection, respectively, in Crohn's disease patients compared to colectomy in patients with ulcerative colitis in Copenhagen County. (From Munkholm P. Crohn's disease – occurrence, course and prognosis. An epidemilogic cohort-study. Dan Med Bull 1997;44(3):287.)

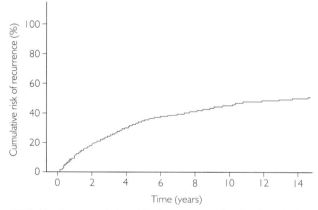

**Fig. 20.8** Absolute cumulative risk of recurrence after first intestinal resection in patients diagnosed with CD, Stockholm County, Sweden, 1956–89. (From Bernell O, Lapidus A, Hellers G. Risk factors for surgery and postoperative recurrence in Crohn's disease. Ann Surg 2000;231:38.)

The apparent discrepancy between endoscopic severity and clinical symptoms has been further revealed in a prospective French study of 121 CD patients with colonic or ileocolonic disease.[47] The correlation between clinical disease activity, endoscopic severity and biochemical parameters was found to be remarkably weak.

The cumulative operation rates for first and second operations for Crohn's disease, from Munkholm et al.[3] are shown in Figure 20.10. Within the first 15 years with Crohn's disease, slightly less than one-third of all patients will remain on medical treatment without surgical resection, one-third will have had only one resection and one-third will have had two or more operations.

The recurrence rate of Crohn's disease has been studied based on the hypothesis of the existence of an aggressive subtype of the disease characterized by early recurrence after operation. Borley et al.[48,49] analyzed 482 operations in 280 patients with Crohn's disease in Oxford. No difference was found between recurrence in patients with penetrating, stenosing or inflamma-

tory phenotypes. The recurrence rate was significantly higher for ileal disease than for ileocolonic and colonic disease. Furthermore, they found that patients treated with stricturoplasty, either alone or combined with resection, had a shorter reoperation-free survival than patients treated by resection alone. Moskovitz et al.[50] found that, after ileocecal resection for Crohn's disease, smoking affected both symptomatic and operative recurrence rates (RR 2.38 and 3.13, respectively, $P=0.03$). For unclear reasons, smoking has a greater influence on postoperative recurrence in women than in men.

## QUALITY OF LIFE WITH CROHN'S DISEASE

There is no doubt that having a chronic inflammatory bowel disease is a burden to the patient, but the impact of the disease is highly variable. This influence on daily life depends on the severity of the inflammation, the presence of complications, the personality of the patient, and the psychological and social support offered by the medical profession and the community. An early case–control study[51] demonstrated that most patients with Crohn's disease are able to lead a near normal social and family life. However, after 15 years with the disease up to 20% of the patients were unable to maintain employment.[3]

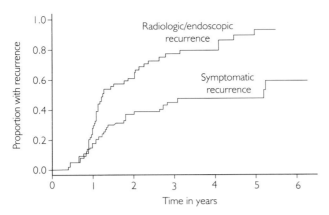

**Fig. 20.9** Endoscopic/radiological and symptomatic recurrence rates in all patients after resection. (Reprinted from Gastroenterology, 113, McLeod et al, Risk and significance of endoscopic/radiologic evidence of recurrent Crohn's disease, 1823, 1997, with permission from the American Gastroenterological Association).

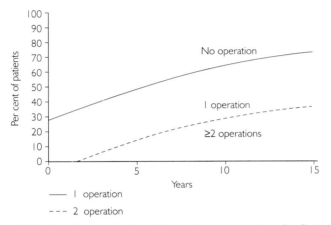

**Fig. 20.10** Cumulative probability of first and second operations for Crohn's disease within 15 years, based on follow-up of 373 Crohn's disease patients in Copenhagen County. (From Munkholm P. Crohn's disease – occurrence, course and prognosis. An epidemiologic cohort study. Dan Med Bull 1997;44(3):287.)

Using the general, so-called short-form-36 (SF-36) questionnaire and the specific RFIPC (Rating Form of Inflammatory Bowel Disease Patient Concerns), described by Drossman et al.,[52] a prospective French multicenter study of 231 Crohn's disease patients was carried out over 1 year, with follow-up every 3 months. Clinical variables found to have significant negative impact on quality of life were active disease, hospitalization, corticosteroid treatment and surgery, whereas patients on immunosuppressive treatment experienced a better quality of life.[53]

A subjective measurement for Health-Related IBD Quality of life (HRIBDQ) has been developed and validated.[54] This was tested in a large controlled study in Canada by Irvine et al.[55] in 1994 and found to correlate well with the CDAI (Crohn's Disease Activity Index), traditionally used as a quantitative measurement for severity of disease. In contrast to the CDAI, the IBDQ can be completed relatively easily by the patient, and has been proposed as a marker for efficiency of a certain treatment modality. A slightly modified version of the McMaster questionnaire, in which bowel dimension questions were removed, was used by Guassora et al.[56] to study a regional group

**Table 20.5 IBDQ values validated in 94 CD patients in remission and in relapse respectively. (Modified from Guassora et al. Quality of life in a regional group of patients with Crohn's disease. A structured interview study. Scand J Gastroenterol 2000;35(10):1068.)**

| IBDQ[1] | Crohn's disease | | Healthy controls |
| | Relapse | Remission | |
|---|---|---|---|
| Overall | 5.1*** | 5.8 | 6.1 |
| Systemic | 3.8*** | 5.6 | 5.8 |
| Emotional | 5.5* | 6.0 | 6.0 |
| Social | 5.6** | 6.4 | 7.0 |

[1]Score 7 best *** P<0.001 **P<0.01 *P<0.05 vs. healthy controls

of patients with Crohn's disease and an age- and sex-matched group of healthy controls. A significant, but modest, reduction in score was found in patients with Crohn's disease who were consecutively recruited from the outpatient clinic. The quality of life score in patients in relapse was significantly lower than among those in remission, with the most pronounced change in the systemic dimension of the questionnaire, and less but still significant alterations in emotional and social dimensions, as shown in Table 20.5.

## COMPLICATIONS

A complication is defined as an unexpected, serious development related to the disease, which could be an adverse response to a treatment or a consequence of the disease itself.

### FISTULATION AND ABSCESS FORMATION

Long-standing inflammation may lead to local penetration, abscess (microscopic or macroscopic) and fistula formation from the diseased intestinal segment to a neighboring organ, for example the urinary bladder, the vagina, another bowel segment, or to retroperitoneum, forming a psoas abscess. Surgical treatment in due time before fistula formation is the best protection and may save bowel length, as once fistulation is present surgery tends to be extensive.

### OSTEOPOROSIS

In recent years it has been shown that patients with Crohn's disease have an increased risk of fractures,[57,58] and several population-based studies have shown decreased bone mineral content in a substantial proportion of patients with Crohn's disease.[59] Risk factors are a high cumulative dose of glucocorticoids, low body weight, malabsorption of calcium and lipid-soluble vitamins, and the inflammatory process.

### LEUKOPENIA

Myelosuppression is an important and potentially lethal complication of immunosuppressive treatment with azathioprine or 6-MP. In a large retrospective study of 739 patients with inflammatory bowel disease, treated in St. Mark's hospital in London, 5% of those treated with these agents developed bone marrow toxicity, from which two patients died. Myelotoxicity developed both early and late during drug treatment, ranging from 2 weeks to 11 years after starting the drug, and the majority of the patients were asymptomatic. It is therefore recommended that hematologic parameters be regularly monitored during treatment.[60]

## INFECTIONS

Patients with Crohn's disease do not generally have an increased frequency of non-gut-related infections. However, immunosuppressive therapy, especially with powerful agents, such as infliximab, cyclosporin etc., may give rise to reactivation of tuberculosis, viral infections such as cytomegalovirus, herpes virus, and opportunistic infections such as *Pneumocystis carinii*, because of the depressed immune defense. In a recent large, randomized multicenter trial of effect and safety of infliximab in Crohn's disease, serious infections occurred in 4% of the 573 patients, independent of whether the drug was given once or several times.[61] Another recent American study reported 70 patients with active tuberculosis after treatment with infliximab, significantly more than could be expected by chance.[62]

## NEPHROPATHY

There is no direct connection between Crohn's disease and nephropathy, but medical therapy may imply a risk of renal complications. 5-Aminosalicylic acid preparations have been reported to cause interstitial nephritis in rare cases, and therefore treatment with this drug necessitates periodic analysis of renal function.[63] Nephrolithiasis is a well-recognized complication of extensive small bowel resection, where oxylate stones form as a consequence of luminal calcium complexing with fat, leading to heightened urate absorption. In addition, uric acid stones form as a result of chronic dehydration due to ileostomy or chronic diarrhea.[64]

## THROMBOEMBOLIC DISEASE

Bernstein et al.[65] have recently quantified previous sporadic reports of deep venous thrombosis in patients with inflammatory bowel diseases. The age-adjusted incidence ratio for patients with Crohn's disease versus the normal population was found to be 4.7 for venous thrombosis and 2.9 for pulmonary embolism, compared to background population of similar age, gender and postal area of residence. Whether these complications are directly related to Crohn's disease or represent non-specific reactions to the inflammatory response, with or without surgery, is unclear.

## LYMPHOMA

There does not seem to be an increased risk of lymphoma among patients with Crohn's disease, compared to the population in general,[66–70] although previous reports from referral centers have found such a possible correlation.[71] The increasing use of immunosuppressant drugs, and especially the new, potent biologic therapies, makes it necessary to monitor cautiously for lymphoma development. An increased frequency of Epstein–Barr virus-related lymphomas at the Mayo Clinic in the past decade, since the increased use of azathioprine, raises concerns about this treatment causing viral-induced lymphomas.[72]

## COLORECTAL CANCER

As in ulcerative colitis, Crohn's disease carries an increased risk of colorectal cancer. The magnitude of the risk, however, differs in population-based studies. Ekbom et al.[73] found a relative risk of 5.6 for colorectal cancer among patients with Crohn's disease, whereas Persson et al., in another Swedish patient cohort study,[74] did not find an increased population relative risk. Similarly, Fireman et al. from Israel[75] and Jess et al. in the Danish cohort,[69] did not find an increased risk of colorectal cancer among their patients with Crohn's disease. However, these studies did not individually assess risk based on disease location. From the study of Gillen et al.[76] it appears that the malignant potential in Crohn's disease and ulcerative colitis is of the same order of magnitude. They directly compared the colorectal cancer risk in patients with extensive ulcerative colitis ($n=486$) and patients with extensive Crohn's colitis ($n=125$), extracted from their previously published series from Birmingham. The cumulative risk for developing colorectal cancer was 7% after 20 years for ulcerative colitis and 8% for Crohn's colitis, increased 18- and 19-fold compared to the background population of similar age and gender. Further, Choi and Zelig[77] compared 80 patients with concomitant colorectal cancer, out of 3124 patients with Crohn's disease and 3093 with ulcerative colitis. During the same period 5266 patients with colorectal cancer but without inflammatory bowel disease were seen in the clinic. The cancers in ulcerative colitis and Crohn's disease occurred 15 and 18 years, respectively, after onset of inflammatory bowel disease. The tumors were multiple in 11 and 12%, respectively, and occurred in connection with dysplasia in 73 and 79%. The histological picture was very similar in the two diseases. Five-year survival rates were 46 and 50%, respectively. Cancers developed in inflamed areas in both diseases and were thus located in the right colon in 49% in patients with Crohn's disease, compared to 36% in ulcerative colitis, reflecting the difference in inflammatory sites in the two diseases. On this background the low incidence of colorectal cancer in the population-based studies presented is remarkable, and possible explanations must be determined.

Many patients with extensive Crohn's disease have had resections of their entire colon or the inflamed portion, thereby eliminating the risk for colonic adenocarcinoma. The cumulative probability for having an ileostomy was 16, 25 and 38% after 5, 10 and 25 years in the Swedish study of Lapidus et al.[22] which comprised 507 patients with colorectal Crohn's disease. Similar percentages were found in the Danish material by Munkholm et al.[3] (see Fig. 20.7). Another possible cancer-protective factor could be treatment with 5-aminosalicylic acid (5-ASA) preparations. These drugs have been used as maintenance, relapse-preventing therapy in patients with Crohn's disease, similar to ulcerative colitis, for many years, despite controlled studies and meta-analyses which have thrown doubt upon its efficacy as a maintenance treatment for Crohn's disease.[8,78]

5-ASA may have benefit in the chemoprevention of colorectal cancer in inflammatory bowel diseases.[79] 5-ASA maintenance therapy of IBD may protect against dysplasia and carcinoma by reducing inflammation, thereby altering the increased epithelial cell turnover and proliferation, or by altering mucosal cytokine and adhesion molecule profiles.[80] Reducing mucosal inflammation may also modify intestinal bacterial flora, either by a direct effect of bacteria on colonic mucosa or by altering the production of short-chain fatty acids, which may be anticarcinogenic. There may also be a direct effect of treatment with 5-ASA on mucosal neoplasia. Among the mechanisms that have been suggested are the antioxidant, antiproliferative and proapoptotic effects of 5-ASA.[81–84] It is of great importance that the possible effect of 5-ASA treatment on colorectal cancer risk is tested and considered in the future.

## SMALL INTESTINAL CANCER

In contrast to adenocarcinoma of the large bowel adenocarcinoma of the small intestine is extremely rare. Although only relatively few small bowel cancers have been reported in Crohn's disease, their frequency is significantly increased in relation to the expected number, and relative risks have been found to be 16, 40 and 50 times normal values in studies from Sweden,[74] the UK[85] and Denmark.[86] Adenocarcinomas develop only in affected segments of the small intestine, and are difficult to diagnose at an early stage because the radiological appearance is similar to that of stricturing Crohn's disease. Proper surveillance is thus difficult or impossible, but this diagnosis should be borne in mind when surgery for a Crohn's-affected small bowel segment is considered.

## SURVIVAL

Unlike ulcerative colitis, which has been shown to carry a slightly increased mortality at onset but a normal survival after 1 year,[87] Crohn's disease seems to become more dangerous with increasing disease duration. Long-term follow-up studies of population-based cohorts of patients have shown slightly increased mortality in patients with Crohn's disease late in the disease course.[15,66–68,88] Jess et al.[88] found an excess mortality among women only, and especially among women under 50 years of age at diagnosis. In contrast, Loftus et al.[15] found that older age at diagnosis was associated with diminished survival. None of these population studies showed a correlation between localization of Crohn's disease and survival. The difference in survival among men and women in the Danish study was surprising, and was not present in the other population-based studies. Weterman et al.,[89] however, in their study from Leiden, reviewing 50 years' experience with Crohn's disease, found a similar excess mortality among women. The possibility that women exhibit a more aggressive course of Crohn's disease has been considered, and in fact significantly more women than men underwent surgery during the first 5 years after diagnosis.[86] Thirty-one per cent of the deaths among women in this cohort were connected to Crohn's disease, similar to the 35% rate found in the study from Olmsted county.[15] Twenty-one per cent of the deaths among men in the Danish cohort were connected directly to Crohn's disease. Figure 20.11 shows the survival curves for men and women, compared to the expected survival and to constructed survival curves for the patient group, where the Crohn's disease related deaths are subtracted.

Probert et al.,[90] and later, in a relatively small study, Farrokhyar et al.,[91] found no excess mortality in CD but found that, although the standard mortality rate (SMR) did not vary significantly with the age at diagnosis, the highest SMR was found in the patient group aged 25–34 years. The SMR was not

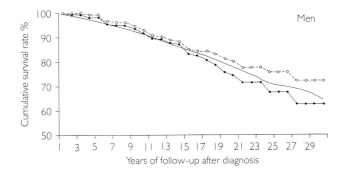

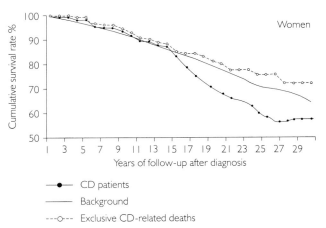

Fig. 20.11 Cumulative probability of survival among men and women in the Danish inception cohort of 374 CD patients diagnosed 1962–87 and followed up to 35 years, median 17 years. The only significant difference from survival of the background population was in women with 21–25 years of disease duration. SMR for this group was 2.85 (1.30–5.41). (Reprinted from Gastroenterology, 122, Jess et al, Mortality and causes of death in Crohn's disease: follow-up of a population-based cohort in Copenhagen County, Denmark, 1808-1814, 2002, with permission from the American Gastroenterological Association).

influenced by gender. Patients who had perianal disease or Crohn's colitis did have a higher SMR than expected values.

## CONCLUSION

More than three decades of clinical epidemiological research in inflammatory bowel diseases have revealed Crohn's disease as a condition with a broad spectrum of clinical courses, ranging from mild disease with multiyear remission periods to severe, life-threatening disease. At any time, however, half of the patients will be in clinical remission, and only 20% will have relapse of their disease every year. This corresponds to the fact that patients with Crohn's disease are generally able to lead a normal family and social life. These generally positive prognostic features are based on studies where patients are in regular treatment, with easy access to outpatient medical care and early onset of treatment at the time of relapse by a specialized team composed of a gastroenterologist, surgeon, stoma care nurse and dietitian. It is likely that a better understanding of clinical, genetic and pathophysiologic disease subsets will permit a more precise prediction of the natural history of the course of disease for an individual, and the prevention of complications by more rapid initiation of individualized treatment with a high likelihood of suppressing inflammation.

# REFERENCES

1. Devroede GJ, Taylor WF, Sauer WG, Jackman RJ, Stickler GB. Cancer risk and life expectancy of children with ulcerative colitis. N Engl J Med 1971;285:17–21.

2. Weedon DD, Shorter RG, Duane M, Ilstrup MS, Huizenga KA, Taylor WF. Crohn's disease and cancer. N Engl J Med 1973;289:1099–1103.

3. Munkholm P. Crohn's disease – occurrence, course and prognosis. An epidemiologic cohort study. Dan Med Bull 1997;44(3):287–302. (Thesis review).

4. Meyers S, Janowitz HD. 'Natural history' of Crohn's disease. An analytic review of the placebo lesson. Gastroenterology 1984;87:1189–1192.

5. Summers RW, Switz DM, Sessions JT et al. National cooperative Crohn's disease study: Results of drug treatment. Gastroenterology 1979;77:847–869.

6. Malchow H, Ewe K, Brandes JW et al. European cooperative Crohn's disease study (ECCDS): Results of drug treatment. Gastroenterology 1984;86:249–266.

7. Gendre J-P, Mary J-Y, Florent C et al. and the Groupe d'Etudes Thérapeutiques des Affections Inflammatoires Digestifs (GETAID). Gastroenterology 1993;104:435–439.

8. Lochs H, Mayer M, Fleig WE et al. Prophylaxis of postoperative relapse in Crohn's disease with mesalamine: European cooperative Crohn's disease study VI. Gastroenterology 2000;118:264–273.

9. Binder V, Both H, Hansen PK, Hendriksen C, Kreiner S, Torp-Pedersen K. Incidence and prevalence of ulcerative colitis and Crohn's disease in the county of Copenhagen 1962–1978. Gastroenterology 1982;83:563–568.

10. Lennard-Jones JE. Classification of inflammatory bowel disease. Scand J Gastroenterol 1989;24(Suppl 170):2–6.

11. Munkholm P, Langholz E, Nielsen OH, Kreiner S, Binder V. Incidence and prevalence of Crohn's disease in the county of Copenhagen 1962–87: a sixfold increase in incidence. Scand J Gastroenterol 1992;27:609–614.

12. Lapidus A, Bernell O, Hellers G, Person P-G, Löfberg R. Incidence of Crohn's disease in Stockholm County 1955–1989. Gut 1997;41:480–486.

13. Nyhlin H, Danielsson Å. Incidence of Crohn's disease in a defined population in Northern Sweden, 1974–81. Scand J Gatroenterol 1986;21:1185–1192.

14. Ekbom A, Helmick C, Zack M, Adami H-O. The epidemiology of inflammatory bowel disease: a large, population-based study in Sweden. Gastroenterology 1991;100:350–358.

15. Loftus EV Jr, Silverstein MD, Sandborn WJ, Tremaine WJ, Harmsen WS, Zinsmeister AR. Crohn's disease in Olmsted County, Minnesota, 1940–1993. Incidence, prevalence and survival. Gastroenterology 1998;114:1161–1168.

16. Gower-Rousseau C, Salomez J-L, Dupas J-L et al. Incidence of inflammatory bowel disease in northern France (1988–1990). Gut 1994;35:1433–1438.

17. Moum B, Vatn MH, Ekbom A et al. Incidence of Crohn's disease in four counties in Southeastern Norway, 1990–93. Scand J Gastroenterol 1996;31:355–361.

18. Bjørnsson S, Jóhannsson JH. Inflammatory bowel disease in Iceland, 1990–1994: a prospective, nationwide, epidemiological study. Eur J Gastroenterol Hepatol 2000;12:31–38.

19. Witte J, Shivananda S, Lennard-Jones JE et al. Disease outcome in inflammatory bowel disease. Scand J Gastroenterol 2000;35:1272–1277.

20. Gasche C, Schölmerich J, Brynskov J et al. A simple classification of Crohn's disease: report of the working party for the world congresses of gastroenterology Vienna 1998. Inflamm Bowel Dis 2000;6:8–15.

21. Louis E, Collard A, Oger AF, Degroote E, El Yafi FAN, Belaiche J. Behaviour of Crohn's disease according to the Vienna classification: changing pattern over the course of the disease. Gut 2001;49:777–782.

22. Lapidus A, Bernell O, Hellers G, Löfberg R. Clinical course of colorectal Crohn's disease: a 35 year follow-up study of 507 patients. Gastroenterology 1998;114:1151–1160.

23. Shivananda S, Lennard-Jones J, Logan R et al. and the EC-IBD study group. Incidence of inflammatory bowel disease across Europe: is there a difference between north and south? Results of the European collaborative study on inflammatory bowel disease (EC-IBD). Gut 1996;39:690–697.

24. Anton G, Decker G, Loftus EV, Pasha TM, Tremaine WJ, Sandborn WJ. Crohn's disease in the esophagus: clinical features and outcomes. Inflamm Bowel Dis 2001;7:113–119.

25. Yamamoto T, Allan RN, Keighley MR. An audit of gastroduodenal Crohn's disease: clinicopathologic features and management. Scand J Gastroenterol 1999;34:1019–1024.

26. Nugent FW, Roy MA. Duodenal Crohn's disease: an analysis of 89 cases. Am J Gastroenterol 1989;84:249–254.

26a. Ruuska T, Vaajalahti P, Arajarvi P, Maki M. Prospective evaluation of upper gastrointestinal mucosal lesions in children with ulcerative colitis and Crohn's disease. J Pediatr Gastroenterol Nutr. 1994;19:181–186.

27. Schwartz DA, Loftus EV, Tremaine WJ et al. The natural history of fistulizing Crohn´s disease in Olmstead County, Minnesota. Gastroenterology 2002;122:875–880.

28. Orchard TR, Wordsworth B, Jewell DP. Peripheral arthropathies in inflammatory bowel disease: their articular distribution and natural history. Gut 1998;42:387–391.

29. Orchard TR, Thiyagaraja S, Welsh KI, Wordsworth BP, Hill GJS, Jewell DP. Clinical phenotype is related to HLA genotype in the peripheral arthropathies of inflammatory bowel disease. Gastroenterology 2000;118:274–278.

30. Tromm A, May D, Almus E, Voigt E, Greving I, Schwegler U, Griga T. Cutaneous manifestations in inflammatory bowel disease. Zeitschr Gastroenterol 2001;39:137–144.

31. Bernstein CN, Blanchard JF, Rawsthorne P, Yu N. The prevalence of extraintestinal diseases in inflammatory bowel disease: a population-based study. Am J Gastroenterol 2001;96:1116–1122.

32. Travis S, Innes N, Davies MG, Tawfique D, Hughes S. Sweets syndrome: an unusual cutaneous feature of Crohn's disease or ulcerative colitis. Eur J Gastroenterol Hepatol 1997;9:715–720.

33. Gilat T, Hacohen D, Lilos P, Langman MJS. Childhood factors in ulcerative colitis and Crohn's disease. An international cooperative study. Scand J Gastroenterol 1987;22:1009–1024.

34. Lee FI, Bellary SV, Francis C. Increased occurrence of psoriasis in patients with Crohn's disease and their relatives. Am J Gastroenterol 1990;85:962–963.

35. Bhalerao J, Bowcock AM. The genetics of psoriasis: a complex disorder of the skin and immune system. Hum Mol Genet 1998;7:1537–1545.

36. Wewer V, Gluud C, Schlichting P, Burchardt F, Binder V. Prevalence of hepatobiliary dysfunction in a regional group of patients with chronic inflammatory bowel disease. Scand J Gastroenterol 1991;26:97–102.

37. Rasmussen HH, Fallingborg JF, Mortensen PB, Vyberg M, Tage-Jensen U, Rasmussen SN. Hepatobiliary dysfunction and primary sclerosing cholangitis in patients with inflammatory disease. Scand J Gastroenterol 1997;32:604–610.

38. Munkholm P, Langholz E, Davidsen M, Binder V. Disease activity courses in a regional cohort of Crohn's disease patients. Scand J Gastroenterol 1995;30:699–706.

39. Silverstein MD, Loftus EV, Sandborn WJ et al. Clinical course and costs of care for Crohn's disease: Markov model analysis of a population-based cohort. Gastroenterology 1999;117:49–57.

40. Munkholm P, Langholz E, Davidsen M, Binder V. Frequency of glucocorticoid resistance and dependency in Crohn's disease. Gut 1994;35:360–362.

41. Faubion WA, Loftus EV, Harmsen WS, Zinsmeister AR, Sandborn WJ. The natural history of corticoid therapy for inflammatory bowel disease: A population-based study. Gastroenterology 2001;121:255–260.

42. Bernell O, Lapidus A, Hellers G. Risk factors for surgery and postoperative recurrence in Crohn's disease. Ann Surg 2000;231:38–45.

43. Bernell O, Lapidus A, Hellers G. Risk factors for surgery and recurrence in 907 patients with primary ileocaecal Crohn's disease. Br J Surg 2000;87:1697–1701.

44. Rutgeerts P, Geboes K, Vantrappen G, Kerremans R, Coenegrachts JL, Coremans G. Natural history of recurrent Crohn's disease at the ileocolonic anastomosis after curative surgery. Gut 1984;25:665–672.

45. Olaison G, Smedh K, Sjödahl R. Natural course of Crohn's disease after ileocolic resection: endoscopically visualized ileal ulcers preceeding symptoms. Gut 1992;33:331–335.

46. McLeod RS, Wolff BG, Steinhardt AH et al. Risk and significance of endoscopic/radiological evidence of recurrent Crohn's disease. Gastroenterology 1997;113:1823–1827.

47. Cellier C, Sahmoud T, Froguel E et al. and the Groupe d'Etudes Thérapeutiques des Affections Inflammatoires Digestifs. Correlations between clinical activity, endoscopic severity and biologic parameters in colonic or ileocolonic Crohn's disease. A prospective multicenter study of 121 cases. Gut 1994;35:231–235.

48. Borley NR, Mortensen NJMcC, Chaudry MA et al. Recurrence after abdominal surgery for Crohn's disease. Dis Colon Rectum 2002;45:377–383.

49. Borley NR, Mortensen NJMcC, Chaudry MA, Mohammed S, Clarke T, Jewell DP. Evidence for separate disease phenotypes in intestinal Crohn's disease. Br J Surg 2002;89:201–205.

50. Moskovitz D, McLeod RS, Greenberg GR, Cohen Z. Operative and environmental risk factors for recurrence of Crohn's disease. Int J Colorectal Dis 1999;14:224–226.

51. Sørensen VZ, Olsen BG, Binder V. Life prospects and quality of life in patients with Crohn's disease. Gut 1987;28:382–385.

52. Drossman DA, Patrick DL, Mitchell CM, Zagami EA, Appelbaum MI. Health-related quality of life in inflammatory bowel disease. Functional status and patient worries and concerns. Dig Dis Sci 1989;34:1379–1386.

53. Blondel-Kucharski F, Chircop C, Marquis P et al. Health-related quality of life in Crohn's disease. A prospective, longitudinal study in 231 patients. Am J Gastroenterol 2001;96:2915–2920.

54. Guyatt G, Mitchell A, Irvine EJ et al. A new measure of health status for clinical trials in inflammatory bowel disease. Gastroenterology 1989;96:804–810.

55. Irvine EJ, Feagan B, Rochon J et al. Quality of life: a valid and reliable measure of therapeutic efficacy in the treatment of inflammatory bowel disease. Canadian Crohn's relapse prevention study group. Gastroenterology 1994;106:287–296.

56. Guassora AD, Kruuse C, Thomsen OØ, Binder V. Quality of life study in a regional group of patients with Crohn's disease. A structured interview study. Scand J Gastroenterol 2000;35:1068–1074.

57. Vestergaard P, Krogh K, Rejnmark L, Laurberg S, Mosekilde L. Fracture risk is increased in Crohn's disease, but not in ulcerative colitis. Gut 2000;46:176–181.

58. Bernstein CN, Blanchard JF, Leslie W, Wajda A, Yu N. The incidence of fracture among patients with inflammatory bowel disease – a population-based cohort study. Ann Intern Med 2000;133:795–799.

59. Jahnsen J, Falch JA, Aadland E, Mowinckel P. Bone mineral density is reduced in patients with Crohn's disease, but not in patients with ulcerative colitis: a population-based study. Gut 1997;40:313–319.

60. Connell WR, Kamm MA, Ritchie JK, Lennard-Jones JE. Bone marrow toxicity by azathioprine in inflammatory bowel disease: 27 years of experience. Gut 1993;34:1081–1085.

61. Hanauer SB, Feagan BG, Lichtenstein GR et al. Maintenance infliximab for Crohn's disease: the ACCENT I randomised trial. Lancet. 2002;359:1541–1549.

62. Keane J, Gershon S, Wise RP et al. Tuberculosis associated with infliximab, a tumor necrosis factor -neutralizing agent. N Engl J Med 2001;345:1098–1104.

63. Corrigan G, Stevens PE. Review article: interstitial nephritis associated with the use of mesalazine in inflammatory bowel disease. Aliment Pharmacol Ther 2000;14:1–6.

64. Buno Soto A, Torres Jimenez R, Olveira A et al. Lithogenic risk factors for renal stones in patients with Crohn's disease. Arch Esp Urol 2001;54:282–292.

65. Bernstein CN, Blanchard JF, Houston DS, Wajda A. The incidence of deep venous trombosis and pulmonary embolism among patients with inflammatory bowel disease. Thromb Haemost 2001;85:430–434.

66. Ekbom A, Helmick CG, Zack M, Holmberg L, Adami HO. Survival and causes of death in patients with inflammatory bowel disease: a population-based study. Gastroenterology 1992;103:954–960.

67. Persson P-G, Bernell O, Leijonmarck C-E, Farahmand BY, Hellers G, Ahlbom A. Survival and cause-specific mortality in inflammatory bowel disease: a population-based cohort study. Gastroenterology 1996;110:1339–1345.

68. Palli D, Trallori G, Saieva C et al. General and cancer specific mortality of a population based cohort of patients with inflammatory bowel disease: the Florence Study. Gut 1998;42:175–179.

69. Jess T, Winther K, Munkholm P, Langholz E, Binder V. Is there an increased risk of intestinal and extra intestinal cancer in patients with Crohn's disease? A population-based cohort followed from 1962 to 1997. Gastroenterology 2000;118(Suppl 2):1472.

70. Loftus EV, Tremaine WJ, Habermann TM, Harmsen WS, Zinsmeister AR, Sandborn WJ. Risk of lymphoma in inflammatory bowel disease. Am J Gastroenterol 2000;95:2308–2312.

71. Greenstein AJ, Mullin GE, Strauchen JA et al. Lymphoma in inflammatory bowel disease. Cancer 1992;69(5):1119–1123.

72. Dayharsh GA, Loftus EV, Sandborn WJ et al. Epstein–Barr virus-positive lymphoma in patients with inflammatory bowel disease treated with azathioprine or 6-mercaptopurine. Gastroenterology 2002;122:72–77.

73. Ekbom A, Helmick C, Zack M, Adami H-O. Increased risk of large bowel cancer in Crohn's disease with colonic involvement. Lancet 1990;336:357–359.

74. Persson PG, Karlén P, Leijonmarck CE, Broström O, Ahlbom A, Hellers G. Crohn's disease and cancer: a population-based cohort study. Gastroenterology 1994;107:1675–1679.

75. Fireman Z, Grossman A, Lilos P et al. Intestinal cancer in patients with Crohn's disease. Scand J Gastroenterol 1989;24:346–350.

76. Gillen CD, Walmsley RS, Prior P, Andrews HA, Allan RN. Ulcerative colitis and Crohn's disease: a comparison of the colorectal cancer risk in extensive colitis. Gut 1994;35:1507–1508.

77. Choi PM, Zelig MP. Similarity of colorectal cancer in Crohn's disease and ulcerative colitis: implications for carcinogenesis and prevention. Gut 1994;35:950–954.

78. Camma C, Giunta M, Rosselli M, Cottone M. Mesalamine in the maintenance treatment of Crohn's disease: a meta-analysis adjusted for confounding variables. Gastroenterology 2001;113:1465–1473.

79. Bernstein CN, Eaden J, Steinhart H, Munkholm P, Gordon P. Cancer prevention in IBD and the chemoprophylactic potential of 5-aminosalicylic acid. Inflamm Bowel Dis 2002;8:356–361.

80. Greenfield SM, Punchard NA, Teare JP, Thompson RP. Review article: the mode of action of the aminosalicylates in inflammatory bowel disease. Aliment Pharmacol Ther 1993;7:369–383.

81. Bus PJ, Nagtegaal ID, Verspaget HW et al. Mesalazine-induced apoptosis of colorectal cancer: on the verge of a new chemopreventative era? Aliment Pharmacol Ther 1999;13:1397–1402.

82. Allgayer H, Kruis W. Aminosalycylates: Potential antineoplastic actions in colon cancer prevention. Scand J Gastroenterol 2002;37:125–131.

83. Brown WA, Farmer KC, Skinner SA, Malcontenti-Wilson C, Misajon A, O'Brien PE. Aminosalicylic acid and olsalazine inhibit tumor growth in a rodent model of colorectal cancer. Dig Dis Sci 2000;45:1578–1584.

84. MacGregor DJ, Kim YS, Sleisenger MH, Johnson LK. Chemoprevention of colon cancer carcinogenesis by balsalazide: Inhibition of azoxymethane-induced aberrant crypt formation in the rat colon and intestinal tumor formation in the B6-Min/+ mouse. Int J Oncol 2000;17:173–179.

85. Gillen CD, Andrews HA, Prior P, Allan RN. Crohn's disease and colorectal cancer. Gut 1994;35:651–655.

86. Munkholm P, Langholz E, Davidsen M, Binder V. Intestinal cancer risk and mortality in patients with Crohn's disease. Gastroenterology 1993;105:1716–1723.

87. Langholz E, Munkholm P, Davidsen M, Binder V. Colorectal cancer risk and mortality in patients with ulcerative colitis. Gastroenterology 1992;103:1444–1451.

88. Jess T, Winther KV, Munkholm P, Langholz E, Binder V. Mortality and causes of death in Crohn's disease: follow-up of a population-based cohort in Copenhagen county, Denmark. Gastroenterology 2002;122:1808–1814.

89. Weterman IT, Biemond I, Pena AS. Mortality and causes of death in Crohn's disease. Review of 50 years' experience in Leiden University Hospital. Gut 1990;31:1387–1390.

90. Probert CS, Jayanthi V, Wicks AC, Mayberry JF. Mortality from Crohn's disease in Leicestershire, 1972–89: an epidemiological community based study. Gut 1992;33:1226–1228.

91. Farrokhyar F, Swarbrick ET, Grace RH, Hellier MD, Gent AE, Irvine EJ. Low mortality in ulcerative colitis and Crohn's disease in three regional centers in England. Am J Gastroenterol 2001;96:501–507.

## CHAPTER 21

# Clinical features and natural history of pediatric inflammatory bowel diseases

Petar Mamula, Jonathan E Markowitz and Robert N Baldassano

'Are children just small adults?'

In the minds of pediatricians the answer to this question is often negative. We believe it is important to point out significant physiologic differences between children and adults, and to emphasize the importance of unique characteristics of the pediatric population. As in many other disorders, these differences have important clinical consequences for inflammatory bowel diseases (IBD). Although the similarities between adult and pediatric patients diagnosed with IBD are numerous, several important differences should be emphasized. The diagnosis of IBD in children comes often at a vulnerable time of growth and development. Despite the increased nutritional needs related to the rapid periods of growth during childhood and adolescence, many pediatric patients afflicted with IBD will paradoxically demonstrate decreased appetite, increased metabolism and decreased absorptive capacity. Clinical presentation is often uncharacteristic, and environmental and genetic factors have a strong potential to influence the natural history of disease.[1,2] As a result, IBD may have profound effects on weight gain, linear growth and bone mineralization, some of which may not be reversible. Additionally, delayed sexual development may have significant adverse effects on self-esteem and socialization. Beyond treating the overt symptoms of disease, therapy in children with IBD must be directed towards overcoming nutritional deficiencies to allow the maximal potential for growth. These issues add a level of complexity to the management of a child or adolescent with IBD. This chapter reviews aspects of IBD diagnosis and management unique to the pediatric population.

## EPIDEMIOLOGY

IBD is recognized as one of the most significant chronic diseases to affect children and adolescents.[3] Pediatric IBD population-based epidemiological studies are sparse. They are difficult to perform because of the large number of patients needed, the high cost and the potential for surveillance error, and difficult to compare because of different criteria and designs.[4,5] In the United States most of the data come from large tertiary care centers, with a potential for a bias owing to referral practice. Because demographic data are important factors allowing for a better understanding of IBD there is an urgent need for a nationwide pediatric IBD registry, which would allow centralized data collection and simplify the execution of true epidemiological studies. A long-term analysis of a large cohort of patients is necessary to identify the risk factors associated with IBD, true epidemiologic distribution and trends, clinical features, and natural history.[6] In addition, a multicenter database would serve as a tool for the design and execution of pediatric pharmaceutical clinical trials and the development of disease severity and quality of life indices. Most importantly, it would enhance development of a standard of care for the management of children and adolescents with IBD based on clinical outcomes research.

The demographic data usually describe the sex, age and racial distribution of a particular disease. The sex distribution of IBD among children indicates a slightly increased preponderance of Crohn's disease (CD) in boys,[7] whereas ulcerative colitis (UC) affects both sexes equally. The age distribution follows a bimodal pattern of incidence, with the first peak in the second and third decades and a smaller peak in the sixth decade.[8-10] Up to 30% of all patients with IBD are diagnosed during childhood.[3] At the Center for Pediatric IBD at The Children's Hospital of Philadelphia we follow 1100 children with IBD. The demographic data on a sample of 425 children seen at the main hospital site during the last 12 months are presented in Table 21.1.

During the last several decades the incidence of IBD has increased, more so for CD than UC.[9,11] Analysis of time trends indicates a rapid rise in the incidence of Crohn's disease from the 1960s to the 1980s, with subsequent stabilization,[12] although some studies indicate a continuing rise in recent years.[4,9,13] The incidence of ulcerative colitis showed a more

**Table 21.1 Demographic data on a sample of 425 children with inflammatory bowel disease seen 06/2001–05/2002 at The Children's Hospital of Philadelphia**

| Demographic characteristics | Crohn's disease and indeterminant Colitis (%) | Ulcerative colitis (%) |
|---|---|---|
| Male | 204 (48) | 42 (10) |
| Female | 123 (29) | 56 (13) |
| 0–5 years old | 12 (3) | 3 (1) |
| 6–9 years old | 26 (6) | 8 (2) |
| 10–13 years old | 69 (16) | 32 (7) |
| 14–17 years old | 136 (32) | 35 (8) |
| 18–23 years old | 84 (20) | 20 (5) |
| Caucasian | 268 (63) | 80 (19) |
| African-American | 43 (10) | 14 (3) |
| Hispanic | 3 (1) | 0 |
| Asian | 1 (<1) | 1 (<1) |
| Other | 11 (3) | 4 (1) |
| Total number | 327 (73) | 98 (27) |

high rate of concordance between monozygotic twins (44.4%) compared to dizygotic twins (3.8%),[27] and frequent multiple family members.[28] Increased genetic influence in early-onset CD, or perhaps genetic anticipation, may account for the fact that patients with CD below 20 years of age have a family history of this disorder in 30% of cases, whereas only 13% of patients diagnosed later have a family history. The newly discovered NOD2 gene in CD supports the interaction between genetic predisposition and the environment, as this gene regulates immune responses to bacterial products.[29,30] Other studies evaluated environmental factors: housing with hot tap-water and a separate bathroom, and low infant mortality rate coincide with the higher incidence of CD. These results may suggest that clean environments delay exposure to enteric infections, resulting in failure of the normal immunologic maturation process necessary to develop oral tolerance later in life.[31–33] It is imperative that large, prospective genetic studies, as well as studies of environmental exposures to infections and living conditions, are performed in children. The pediatric population is ideal for this type of research, for various reasons: environmental factors potentially leading to IBD may occur early in life; modification of early environment may be attempted; patients with early-onset disease tend to show more aggressive disease with a stronger genetic influence; and access to patients' relatives is easier than in the adult population.[6]

stable pattern, although again with a tendency for an increase over the years.[9,13] Pediatric incidence studies from Europe indicate similar patterns of increased incidence for both types of IBD, although lower than in adults (Table 21.2).[5,14–26] The incidence rates for pediatric IBD range from 0.2 to 8.5 per 100 000 for CD and 0.5 to 4.3 per 100 000 for UC.

A recent hypothesis regarding the etiology of IBD supports the multifactorial theory, encompassing genetic predisposition, internal and external environmental influences, and immune system disorder.[6] Genetic factors are well recognized, with a

## CLINICAL PRESENTATION

The presentation of IBD in children and adults depends on the location and extent of inflammation.[34] The most commonly encountered gastrointestinal symptoms are abdominal pain and diarrhea. The list of presenting clinical features compiled from several studies is presented in Table 21.3.[3,14,35–42] Abdominal pain can be located anywhere in the abdomen, although in

**Table 21.2 Epidemiologic studies in pediatric Crohn's disease (CD) and ulcerative colitis (UC)**

| Author | Country | Time period | Incidence CD | Incidence UC |
|---|---|---|---|---|
| Langholz et al.[16] | Denmark | 1962-1987 | 0.2 | 2 |
| Barton et al.[18] | Scotland | 1968-1983 | 2.3 | 1.6 |
| Armitage et al.[21] | Scotland | 1981-1995 | 2.5 | 1.3 |
| Olafsdottir et al.[27] | Norway | 1984-1985 | 2.5 | 4.3 |
| Lindberg et al.[4] | Sweden | 1984-1986 | 1.2 | 1.4 |
|  |  | 1993-1995 | 1.3 | 3.2 |
| Hildebrand et al.[19] | Sweden | 1984-1985 | 1.7 | 1.7 |
| Askling et al.[17] | Sweden | 1990-1998 | 3.8 | 2.1 |
| Cosgrove et al.[20] | United Kingdom (Wales) | 1983-1988 | 1.3 | 0.7 |
|  |  | 1989-1993 | 3.1 | 0.7 |
| Hassan et al.[24] | United Kingdom (Wales) | 1995-1997 | 1.4 | 0.8 |
| RCPHC[28] | United Kingdom |  | 5.3 |  |
| Sawczenko et al.[23] | United Kingdom/ R. of Ireland | 1998-1999 | 5.2 |  |
| Tourtelier et al.[22] | France | 1994-1997 | 1.6 | 0.6 |
| Gottrand et al.[25] | France | 1984-1989 | 2.1 | 0.5 |
| Bjornsson et al.[26] | Iceland | 1990-1994 | 8.5 |  |

## Table 21.3 Frequency of common presenting symptoms

| Symptom | Crohn's disease (%) | Ulcerative colitis (%) |
|---|---|---|
| Abdominal pain | 62–95 | 54–76 |
| Diarrhea | 52–78 | 67–93 |
| Hematochezia | 14–60 | 52–97 |
| Weight loss | 43–92 | 22–55 |
| Fever | 11–48 | 4–34 |

patients with CD it occurs frequently in the right mid quadrant, whereas in patients with UC it is located in the lower abdomen. Diarrhea may be associated with blood in the stool, more so in UC. Other gastrointestinal symptoms include loss of appetite, weight loss, nausea, vomiting, and perianal disease, which are more common in CD than in UC. Features such as growth and pubertal delay may cause confusion during the diagnostic process, especially if they are predominant. These will be discussed separately.

Delay in the diagnosis of pediatric IBD continues to be a concern, even with the increasing incidence and heightened awareness of the disease. Mean delay for CD in children is reported to be between 7 and 11 months, in UC between 5 and 8 months, and in indeterminate colitis (IC) 14 months.[20,36,43] At the same time the delay in the adult population is even longer and is measured in years.[44] The time lag between the onset of symptoms and correct diagnosis of Crohn's disease appears to be prolonged if the disease affects more proximal bowel, and if presenting symptoms do not include diarrhea. The diagnosis is particularly difficult when the presenting symptoms are uncharacteristic and consist mainly of extraintestinal manifestations.

## EXTRAINTESTINAL MANIFESTATIONS

Up to 35% of pediatric IBD patients in some series have at least one extraintestinal manifestation as a presenting sign.[45,46] Common symptoms in a series of pediatric IBD patients from Israel included anorexia, joint complaints and anemia.[47] Table 21.4 lists extraintestinal manifestations commonly seen in children with IBD. These manifestations may also be noted concurrently with, or after the diagnosis of IBD is made.[45]

Skin manifestations include erythema nodosum and pyoderma gangrenosum. Erythema nodosum is more common in CD and affects 3% of pediatric patients with CD.[48] It is estimated that 75% of the patients with erythema nodosum ultimately develop arthritis.[49] Pyoderma gangrenosum, on the other hand, is more common in patients with UC and affects less than 1% of patients.

Mouth ulceration is the most common oral manifestation of IBD. It is more common in CD, frequently associated with skin and joint lesions, and together with skin and eye manifestations often parallels the disease activity.[35]

Ophthalmologic manifestations occur in about 4% of the adult population with IBD, but less frequently in children and adolescents with UC and CD.[50] The most common ocular findings are episcleritis and anterior uveitis.

Arthritis is the most common extraintestinal manifestation in children and adolescents, occurring in 7–25% of pediatric IBD patients.[51] The arthritis is usually transient non-deforming

## Table 21.4 Extraintestinal manifestations of inflammatory bowel disease

**SKIN**
Erythema nodosum
Pyoderma gangrenosum
Perianal disease
Metastatic Crohn's disease

**MOUTH**
Cheilitis
Stomatitis
Aphtae

**LIVER**
Primary sclerosing cholangitis
Hepatitis
Cholelithiasis

**PANCREAS**
Pancreatitis

**KIDNEY**
Nephrolithiasis
Obstructive hydronephrosis
Enterovesical fistula
Urinary tract infection
Amyloidosis

**GROWTH**
Delayed growth
Delayed puberty

**BONE**
Osteoporosis
Osteopenia

**EYE**
Uveitis
Episcleritis
Conjunctivitis

**LUNGS**
Pulmonary vasculitis
Fibrosing alveolitis

**VASCULAR**
Vasculitis
Thrombosis (pulmonary, limb, cerebrovascular)

**JOINTS**
Arthralgia
Arthritis
Ankylosing spondylitis

**BLOOD**
Iron deficiency anemia
Anemia of chronic disease
Thrombocytosis
Autoimmune hemolytic anemia
Vitamin B12 deficiency

**GENERAL**
Fever
Fatigue
Weight loss
Anorexia

synovitis, asymmetric in distribution, and involves the large joints of the lower extremities. In adults the arthritis occurs when the disease is active, but in children it may occur years before any gastrointestinal symptoms develop.[52]

Hepatobiliary manifestations in children may precede the onset of IBD, accompany active disease, or develop after surgical resection of all diseased bowel.[53] Hepatic manifestations include elevation of aminotransferases, chronic active hepatitis, granulomatous hepatitis, amyloidosis, fatty liver and sclerosing cholangitis. Abnormal serum aminotransferases are commonly transient and appear to relate to medications or disease activity. If elevation persists patients should be evaluated for the etiology of viral hepatitis. Chronic active hepatitis develops in less than 1% of children with IBD.[54] Colitis at the time may be relatively asymptomatic, although the hepatitis may proceed to cirrhosis. Sclerosing cholangitis develops in 3.5% of pediatric patients with UC, usually extensive disease, and less than 1% of pediatric patients with CD.[54] It is not related to disease activity and may appear years before any gastrointestinal disease develops, or even years after a colectomy for UC. In a series of 36 pediatric patients with IBD who developed sclerosing cholangitis only four had CD and 32 had UC.[55] The authors suggested heightened endoscopic surveillance once the diagnosis of IBD is made in the setting of sclerosing cholangitis, as the time to dysplasia may be accelerated, as noted in three pediatric patients who underwent proctocolectomy for dysplasia. Endoscopic retrograde cholangiopancreatography and magnetic resonance cholangiopancreatography have significantly improved the ability to diagnose this disease in the pediatric population. Cholelithiasis has been described in both UC and CD, but more frequently in CD, especially after ileal resection.

The urologic manifestations of IBD include nephrolithiasis, hydronephrosis and enterovesical fistulae. Nephrolithiasis is a common renal complication in pediatrics, and occurs in approximately 5% of children with IBD.[3] It is usually the result of the fat malabsorption that occurs with small bowel CD. Dietary calcium binds to malabsorbed fatty acids in the colonic lumen and free oxalate is absorbed. This results in hyperoxaluria and oxalate stones.[56] In patients with an ileostomy, increased fluid and electrolyte losses may lead to a concentrated acidic urine and the formation of uric acid stones. External compression of the ureter by an inflammatory mass or abscess may lead to hydronephrosis. Enterovesical fistulae, which are more common in males, may present with recurrent urinary tract infections or pneumaturia.

Thromboembolic disease is a rare but severe complication of IBD. Both UC and CD are thought to be associated with a prothrombotic state with enhanced parameters of coagulation.[57] Several different coagulation abnormalities have been reported in patients with IBD, imparting an increased risk of thrombotic vascular disease over the general population: increased fibrinogen, thrombocytosis and abnormal platelet activation, accelerated thromboplastin generation, elevation of factors V and VIII, decreased antithrombin III, protein S and C deficiency, elevated anticardiolipin antibodies, high plasma factor VII coagulant activity, resistance to activated protein C, and prothrombin gene mutation (G20210).[58-60] Thromboembolic complications are reported in 1.3–6.4% of pediatric patients with IBD.[57,59] In the adult population, pulmonary, abdominal and peripheral veins and arteries are more commonly involved than cerebral or retinal vessels. In pediatric IBD patients' cerebral and retinal vessels

seem to be affected more frequently than others, and thrombosis in these sites carries a better prognosis than in adults.[59,61] The majority of patients have active disease at the time of the thromboembolic event, more so in children than in the adult population.

Other extraintestinal manifestations may develop as side effects of treatment. These include pancreatitis, pericarditis, alopecia, osteoporosis, cataracts, acne, hepatitis, anemia, neutropenia, fibrosing alveolitis, interstitial pneumonitis and peripheral neuropathy. For example, pancreatitis may result from therapy with 5-aminosalicylic acid, 6-mercaptopurine, corticosteroids and methotrexate, and peripheral neuropathy may occur with metronidazole therapy; corticosteroid therapy is associated with acne, cataracts and osteoporosis.

# DISEASE DISTRIBUTION AND NATURAL HISTORY OF IBD IN CHILDREN VERSUS ADULTS

The anatomic distribution of IBD is an important clinical feature which, when thoroughly documented and described, allows for improved comparisons of response to therapy and natural history among reported studies.

## CROHN'S DISEASE

In 139 adult patients with CD at the time of diagnosis 27% had small bowel, 28% large bowel and 43% ileocolonic disease.[61] The extent of disease progressed with time: eventually 75% of patients had ileocolonic disease and 88% underwent at least one operation. Pooled data of 14 pediatric studies with a total of 1153 children with CD revealed isolated small bowel disease in 38%, small bowel and large bowel in 38%, and large bowel alone in 20% of cases.[62] In children 10 years of age and younger 40% had ileocolonic disease, which over time increased to 60%, and 43% of patients required surgery.[38] In our series of children 5 years of age and younger, isolated small bowel disease was seen in 11%, small bowel and large bowel in 59%, and isolated large bowel disease in 30% of cases.[63] Perianal disease is seen in 11–18% of children with CD,[7,64] whereas in children less than 5 years of age the documented rate was significantly higher at 34%, similar to the adult rate of 36–46%.[63,65–70] Upper gastrointestinal CD is seen in 30–40% of children, and endoscopic studies have shown even higher rates of up to 80%.[3,71,72]

Studies of the natural course of CD in adults probably indicate a benign course if patients stay in remission in the year after diagnosis.[73] However, predicting the course is difficult until 2 years into the course of disease.[74] Early age at diagnosis was shown to be associated with more complicated disease in adults,[10] although a more recent study indicated that age had no influence on change of location or behavior of the disease.[75] Studies on the natural course of disease in children with CD are lacking. In one study children with ileal disease had a better prognosis than those with ileocolonic disease.[48] In a series of 100 consecutively diagnosed prepubertal patients from Toronto, one-third had mild disease never requiring corticosteroid therapy, and one-third had at least one exacerbation requiring corticosteroids.[76] An additional 19% of patients had chronically active disease, but achieved sustained remission with the use of immunomodulatory or surgical therapy, and 10% of patients had chronically active steroid-dependent or steroid-refractory disease. In the same series, 36% of patients required surgical therapy, which is significantly less than reported in earlier studies.[77,78] The proportion of pediatric patients with CD requiring surgery was 28% in a recent study, and this was shown to decrease over time, which was mainly attributed to advances in medical therapy.[5] After the year of diagnosis about 50% of patients with CD will be in a remission during any given year,[14] and less than 1% of patients have only a single episode of disease activity.[41]

In the series of 639 Swedish children with IBD, 8% of patients were 5 years old or younger, and almost half carried a diagnosis of indeterminate colitis (IC).[5] The number of children diagnosed with IC is higher than that seen in the adult population. In a large multicenter adult study in Europe 5% of adult patients were diagnosed with IC and a similar proportion of 6% was seen in a series of 475 patients newly diagnosed with IBD in The Netherlands.[79] In pediatric series of older children, 14–23% were diagnosed with IC.[15,17,80] In our experience of 82 children diagnosed with IBD at 5 years of age and younger, 23% were diagnosed with IC.[63] Reasons for this difference are unclear, but one possible explanation is a longer duration of disease in adults with a better chance of establishing a specific diagnosis of CD or UC. Also, pediatric gastroenterologists have in the past exhibited a less aggressive approach to colonoscopy. During the period from 1984 to 1995 in the study of pediatric IBD by Lindberg et al.[5] the percentage of diagnoses made by colonoscopy as opposed to rectosigmoidoscopy increased significantly, from 50% during 1984–1986 to 90% in 1995. With recent more extensive colonoscopy and histologic sampling of the terminal ileum, the proportion of children diagnosed with IC is likely to decrease.

## ULCERATIVE COLITIS

In UC, the distribution of disease is categorized as distal (disease involving the rectum, or rectum and sigmoid colon), left-sided (disease extending beyond the rectosigmoid region) and pancolitis (disease involving the whole large intestine). In a large cohort of 1116 adult patients the disease distribution was 63% with distal and left-sided colitis, and 37% with pancolitis.[81] Data compiled from several studies indicated that 14–37% of adult patients have pancolitis, 36–41% left-sided colitis, and 44–49% involve the rectum/sigmoid colon.[8] Barton et al.[62] found that the distribution of disease in a group of 37 Scottish children with UC corresponded with seven additional studies in 357 aggregate patients. Proctitis was present in 22% of patients, left-sided colitis in 35%, and extensive disease or pancolitis in 43%. The course and prognosis of idiopathic ulcerative proctosigmoiditis was studied in 85 young patients whose symptoms had begun before the age of 21 and the results were compared with those with a similar onset of disease as adults. The natural history of proctosigmoiditis in young patients was found to be somewhat different from that in adults, being characterized by a greater tendency to proximal extension (38% vs. 10%). When the disease remained confined to the rectosigmoid region, the course and prognosis were no different than in adults. Extension of the disease was unpredictable in individual patients, but occurred in 73% of patients within 5 years from the onset of symptoms;[82] in contrast, proximal extension was noted in 27% of adult patients in a separate study.[83]

In a study by Langholz et al. comparing clinical features and natural history of UC in Swedish children and adults, abdominal pain was more frequently found in children.[14] The distribution of the disease was pancolitis in 29% and proctitis in 25% of children, compared to 14% and 46%, respectively, in adults. The cumulative colectomy rate after 20 years in childhood onset UC was 29%, which was the same as in adults. Extension of the disease was noted in 65% of the pediatric patients, and 70% of patients were in remission during 1 year. In a study at the Cleveland Clinic, pancolitis was seen in 63% of patients, left-sided colitis in 22%, and proctitis in 15%.[84] In the largest reported series of 171 children with UC, 22% had proctosigmoiditis, 36% left-sided colitis, and 43% pancolitis.[85] Mild disease was initially seen in 43%, and moderate to severe in 57% of patients. Ninety per cent of patients in the mild group had cessation of symptoms within 6 months, compared to 81% in the moderate to severe group. The response was independent of disease distribution and the overall 5-year risk of surgery was 19%. During any subsequent year of follow-up 55% of patients were symptom free, 38% had chronic intermittent symptoms, and 7% had continuous symptoms. In their review, Hofley and Piccoli reported that 10% of children had only a single episode, 20% had intermittent symptoms, 50% had chronic symptoms but were not incapacitated, and 20% had incapacitating disease.[41] Ten per cent of patients had fulminant colitis, defined as more than six bloody bowel movements, abdominal tenderness, fever, weight loss, anemia, leukocytosis and low albumin.

Disease in patients with early onset of UC has been reported to have variable courses. In young children (<10 years of age) with UC 11% of patients had severe, 37% moderate and 53% mild disease.[86] Eventually 89% had total colonic disease within 2–10 years of the disease, from 75% at the presentation. An early study indicated that mild disease at presentation was usually followed by a mild course.[87] In our series of 36 children with UC less than 5 years of age, 60% had proctitis and left-sided disease, whereas 40% had pancolitis.[63] Four patients (11%) required colectomy. In a series of patients diagnosed with UC before the age of 20, 22% required surgery after a mean follow-up of 18 years[88], and up to 73% of steroid-dependent patients with pancolitis required the same.[89]

## GROWTH AND NUTRITIONAL ISSUES

Abnormal nutritional status in IBD is now universally acknowledged. Poor growth in IBD is often attributed to chronic malnutrition related to decreased intake, as well as increased intestinal losses and metabolic demands which, if present, concurrently produce a situation almost impossible to compensate for by oral intake alone.[90–92]

Growth failure may be the earliest sign of IBD in children and adolescents. Up to 85% of children with CD, and as many as 65% of those with UC, will demonstrate growth failure at the time of diagnosis.[93] A decreased rate of height accrual may also precede diagnosis. In a review of 50 children and prepubescent adolescents with CD, 88% showed a decrease in height velocity before diagnosis.[94] Perhaps more importantly, 46% revealed evidence of decreased height velocity prior to the development of symptoms attributable to CD. Surprisingly, 34 of the 44 patients with decreased linear growth were still above the fifth percentile for height based on age. This fact may have contributed to a further delay in diagnosis, as the duration between onset of growth failure and diagnosis was more than twice as long in the group with heights above the fifth percentile. Accordingly, growth velocity (rather than height for age percentile) has been incorporated into the scoring system of the Pediatric Crohn's Disease Activity Index (PCDAI) (Fig. 21.1). This index was developed and validated by a group of senior pediatric gastroenterologists in 1991[95] and correlates well with the original Crohn's Disease Activity Index (CDAI) developed for adult patients.[96] An activity index for use in pediatric UC is currently being developed.

Because decreasing height velocity is evident in the majority of CD patients several months or years before they develop symptoms attributable to the disease, there is a high likelihood they already demonstrate signs of chronic malnutrition at the time of diagnosis. Therefore, management of these patients should incorporate a plan for nutritional rehabilitation.

Poor intake is commonly felt to be the most important etiology of malnutrition in IBD.[3,97,98] Several studies have documented that dietary intake is chronically deficient in the majority of growth-retarded children with Crohn's disease.[92,99,100] The causes of decreased food intake are multifactorial. Children and adolescents with IBD may limit their diet because eating exacerbates abdominal symptoms, including pain, nausea and bloating from partial obstruction, or diarrhea. Additionally, they may suffer from anorexia related to depression, increased inflammatory mediators such as tumor necrosis factor (TNF-α) and interleukin-1 (IL-1).[103] These repeated symptoms after eating lead to behavioral conditioning.[101]

Several studies of patients with IBD demonstrate significant weight gain when calories are supplemented by a variety of means. Intravenous nutrition administered during acute exacer-

bations has been demonstrated to maintain fluid and electrolyte status and to arrest some of the early catabolism of protein stores.[102,103] Kirschner et al., in a small series of children with CD, demonstrated that growth retardation responded to enterally administered calories, as measured by height velocity and height percentile.[104] To achieve these results, caloric intake was increased from 56% to 91% of the recommended goal for a period of 12 months. Improved linear growth rates and percentiles were seen in all patients. This study was among the first to show that nutritional therapy was a useful adjunct to medical therapy of CD, and suggested that enteral nutrition should be employed before more invasive therapies such as surgery or parenteral nutrition. The ability of enteral feeding to reverse malnutrition was also demonstrated by Motil et al.[99] In a series of six adolescents with active CD, caloric intake was increased by over 40% (from 67 to 96 kcal/kg/day), with protein intake increasing from 2.3 to 3.2 g/kg/day for a period of 3 weeks. Patients gained an average of 3.3 kg over the study period, with a resultant increase in newly synthesized body protein stores as measured by radiolabeled leucine metabolism. The authors concluded that significant weight gain is achievable with short-term enteral nutritional supplementation, and that the gain resulted largely from lean body mass accretion.

Despite the ability to induce both weight and height acquisition through calorie and nutrient supplementation, it is also clear that some effects of malnutrition are irreversible. When adjusting height for genetic potential based on parental height, many patients with CD never achieve expected levels,[98] as was demonstrated by measuring body composition in 132 subjects with CD and 66 controls aged 5 to 25 years. In this population, adjusted height Z scores were significantly lower than predicted heights. These findings were most pronounced in male patients, in whom the average adjusted height Z score was a full standard deviation below expected.

## ASSESSING GROWTH AND NUTRITIONAL STATUS

Accurately assessing growth and nutritional status is the first step in successfully addressing these issues in IBD. Growth irregularities in children with IBD have been measured in various ways, including weight for age, height for age, height- and weight-adjusted Z score, height velocity, and various anthropometric measures such as head circumference, midarm circumference, and triceps skinfold thickness.[93,105] When assessing a patient with IBD for growth failure, one must first use accurate measurements. Weight measurement should be performed on the same scale, with the patient wearing similar amounts of clothing each time. Height measurement should be obtained using a stadiometer, and the patient should be measured without shoes.

Accurate assessment of nutritional status, however, relies on more than just height and weight at a given time. Genetic height potential, determined by midparental height, should be calculated.[106] Previous height and weight points should be considered, with calculation of growth velocity. Height and weight deficit calculations, expressed as a ratio of the actual height or weight divided by the expected value based on the 50th percentile for age, can give insight into the duration of malnutrition. In cases

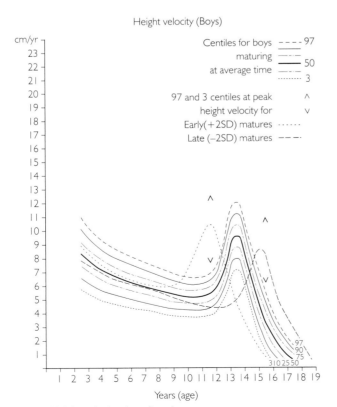

**Fig. 21.1** Height velocity chart (boys).

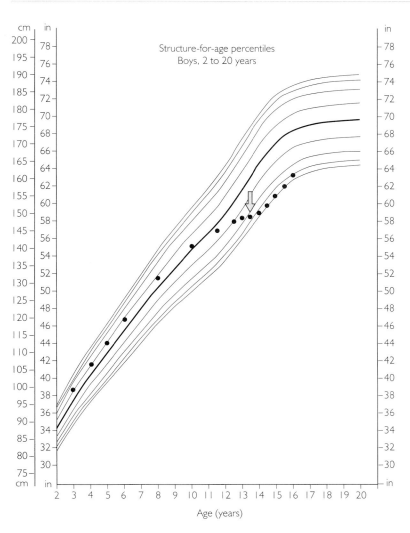

cm in — Structure-for-age percentiles
Boys, 2 to 20 years

Age (years)

**Fig.21.2** Growth chart of a 16-year-old boy diagnosed with Crohn's disease at the age of $3\frac{1}{2}$ years (arrow).

of short-term deficiency one can expect weight deficit (wasting), whereas long-term malnutrition often results in height deficit (stunting).[105]

Stage of sexual maturation is an important reflection of nutritional status, with significant implications for the patient. Adolescents with CD often have delay in the onset of pubertal development, and active disease could potentially delay the onset of puberty indefinitely, with a deleterious effect on growth.[107] Duration of puberty can also be affected in children with IBD, as active or relapsing disease during the years after puberty may slow down or even arrest the progression of puberty.

Patients who are in remission by the time they reach puberty may experience good catch-up growth, with improved height velocity.[108] However, the persistence of growth deficits after the development of secondary sexual characteristics may signify irreversible loss of growth potential (Fig. 21.2). Therefore, accurate staging of sexual development, using the parameters described by Tanner,[109] should be a routine component of the ongoing evaluation and care of any young patient with IBD.

Nutritional assessment should also include evaluation for macro- and micronutrient deficiencies. Overall caloric intake should be assessed using diet diaries, recorded for at least 3 consecutive days. This type of assessment allows accurate calculation of not just overall calories, but the breakdown of fat, protein and carbohydrate intake, as well as the amount of various micronutrients in the diet.

Iron intake is important in the diet of all children and adolescents, especially in IBD, with over 70% of patients manifesting iron deficiency.[110] Small bowel disease, a history of small bowel resection, and increased intestinal transit rate may result in poor absorption of iron. Iron supplementation may cause frequent adverse side effects, including indigestion and diarrhea, resulting in poor patient compliance.[111] Diet diaries may suggest that one is at risk of iron deficiency, with confirmation from objective measures such as hemoglobin, mean corpuscular volume, reticulocyte count, and levels of iron, ferritin and transferrin saturation. Absorption of other micronutrients, in particular vitamin $B_{12}$, folic acid, vitamin D and calcium, may also be impaired under various conditions in IBD. For example, extensive ileal disease or resection may result in $B_{12}$ deficiency, whereas sulfasalazine administration can interfere with folate metabolism, resulting in megaloblastic anemia. Of all the micronutrients, calcium and vitamin D have received the greatest attention because of their role in bone disease.

## BONE DISEASE IN PEDIATRIC IBD

Calcium homeostasis and bone growth are among the most important aspects of malnutrition in pediatric IBD. Bone disease suffered by patients with IBD can be a combination of osteomalacia, defined as abnormal bone mineralization, and osteoporosis, defined as reduced bone mass.[112] Osteopenia is the general term used for any abnormality of bone density and may occur in the context of either osteomalacia or osteoporosis.

Osteoporosis can be reliably detected by measurement of bone mineral density, of which dual energy X-ray absorptiometry (DEXA) is the favored approach.[113] When measured by DEXA, bone mineral density is expressed as the number of standard deviations above or below the mean for age-matched controls (Z score). One must be careful in interpreting bone density under circumstances of abnormal growth, however. For example, a patient with significant stunting may exhibit an abnormal Z score for age, but may in turn have a normal Z score for height. Under these circumstances, the bone density changes over time have more clinical significance than any individual Z score. One should also be aware of the use of T scores in the expression of bone density. These scores express bone density as compared to other young adults, and have little interpretive value for pediatric patients with IBD.

It is now believed that osteoporosis in the elderly has its roots in childhood. Adult levels of bone mineralization are achieved mainly during childhood and adolescence,[114] and there remains no definitive treatment for significant osteoporosis. Therefore, derangements in calcium intake and bone growth early in life, such as occur with early-onset IBD, may have profound permanent results on bone density. One of the serious consequences of osteoporosis is bone fracture, with vertebral compression fracture representing a frequent complication.[115] The healthcare costs of disability due to osteoporosis-related fractures are considerable.[116] As a result, childhood prevention of adult bone disease takes on a high level of significance. Effective prevention of osteoporosis and its consequences must occur during childhood, and identifying those patients at risk is the cornerstone of successful prevention.

Rates of bone turnover are higher in children and adolescents than in adults. In a study of bone mass and biochemical markers of bone turnover in children at various stages of sexual development, bone formation markers were found to be highest at midpuberty, with a reduction in late puberty.[117] Measures of bone formation correlated most highly with bone density, emphasizing the importance of this period of development on final bone composition.

The skeletal complications of IBD are largely related to poor nutrition. Vitamin D deficiency is common among patients with IBD, and CD in particular, with over 50% of patients demonstrating abnormal levels.[118] This deficiency could relate to decreased intake of dairy products, which may exacerbate abdominal symptoms in patients with lactose intolerance. Alternatively, patients with a history of ileal resection or active ileal disease may undergo treatment with cholestyramine, which binds vitamin D in addition to binding bile acids. Other disordered mechanisms of vitamin D homeostasis may be present in IBD patients, such as changes in the metabolic clearance of vitamin D related to calcium deficiency,[119,120] and could explain why ultraviolet light is not adequate to overcome dietary deficiencies. This would be of particular importance in IBD as, once established, a derangement in vitamin D or calcium homeostasis could become a self-perpetuating problem.[112]

Calcium homeostasis is another important factor in bone mineralization and density in IBD patients. As with vitamin D, decreased intake coupled with avoidance of dairy products may lead to inadequate dietary calcium. In contrast to vitamin D, however, calcium cannot be synthesized de novo. Furthermore, calcium deficiency may be exacerbated by fat malabsorption, present in patients with CD-related small bowel disease. The most important effects on calcium homeostasis may be secondary to the use of corticosteroids, as long-term corticosteroid therapy has been shown to inhibit intestinal calcium absorption and tubular resorption of calcium in the kidney.[121,122]

Beyond calcium malabsorption, corticosteroids may have a negative impact on bone remodeling in IBD patients. This includes the inhibition of osteoblastic activity, which limits bone formation, while osteoblastic activity continues unabated.[123,124] Corticosteroids also depress calcitonin levels, resulting in further bone resorption.[125] The clinician treating IBD is often faced with a 'double-edged sword' when considering treatment with corticosteroids. Disease activity may be improved by treatment with corticosteroids, resulting in improved intake and absorption of vital nutrients. However, the use of corticosteroids may also undermine the development of adequate linear growth and bone density. It is unclear which situation is less desirable, but neither is optimal. It is still debated whether the short-term benefits that corticosteroids offer for control of symptoms offset the long-term effects on bones. This dilemma may be resolved by rapidly metabolized corticosteroids such as budesonide, or the avoidance of corticosteroids by using alternatives such as anti-TNF agents.

Various inflammatory cytokines also affect calcium homeostasis. IBD patients who have increased secretion of the proinflammatory cytokine IL-1β on a genetic basis are at increased risk of developing osteopenia.[126] Seventy-five IBD patients expressing a polymorphism associated with increased secretion of IL-1β had significantly lower bone density of the femoral neck and lumbar spine than IBD patients who did not have increased expression. In healthy controls, these polymorphisms did not affect bone density. The authors suggested that these findings may help to predict which IBD patients are at the greatest risk of developing bone abnormalities. Further evidence as to the role of IL-1β in osteopenia of IBD relates to the negative association between the IL-1 receptor antagonist (IL-1ra), which helps to mediate the proinflammatory effects of IL-1β, and the development of bone disease. In a study of 83 patients with IBD it was shown that non-carriage of the allele for normal IL-1ra expression was independently associated with the development of increased bone loss.[127] In this same study, carrying an allele for increased expression of IL-6 was correlated with bone loss. Bone loss in this study was not, however, related to disease severity or use of corticosteroids. Based on these results, it was felt that genetic variation in the genes responsible for cytokine expression has a significant role in whether patients with IBD develop metabolic bone disease.

Just as there are a number of mechanisms responsible for the development of osteopenia in IBD, there are a number of potential treatments directed at its prevention (Table 21.5). Intuitively, supplementation of the nutrients most directly responsible for normal bone development is reasonable. Indeed, calcium supplementation is a useful way to improve bone mineralization. In a study of normal twin children[128] one twin of each set was randomized to receive 1000 mg of calcium citrate in excess of their normal dietary intake. The other twin received placebo and calcium through dietary intake alone. At the end of a 3-year period the twins who received calcium supplementation were found to have higher bone mineral density in the

| Disease severity | Therapy |
|---|---|
| Mild | Calcium supplementation |
| ↓ | Exercise |
| | Vitamin D |
| | Tube feeding |
| | Fluoride |
| | Hormone therapy |
| Severe | Bisphosphonates |

radius and lumbar spine than their twins who had received placebo. Of note, the average dietary calcium intake of both groups of twins approximated the recommended dietary allowance before calcium supplementation, implying that supplementation imparts benefits even when the diet contains appropriate amounts of calcium. This argues that patients with IBD, regardless of dietary calcium intake, should receive calcium supplementation. Those patients with IBD whose dietary calcium intake is inadequate may have more to gain. To address this possibility, Chinese children with habitually low calcium intake were randomized to receive supplementation with 300 mg of calcium for 18 months or placebo.[129] The supplemented group had higher bone mineral content and bone mineral density than the placebo group at the end of the study period.[129] However, a follow-up study revealed that these improvements were reversible, and that any benefits imparted by calcium supplementation disappeared after 18 months without further supplementation.[130]

It appears that calcium supplementation has its greatest utility early in development, and that the window of opportunity to affect bone density may close with puberty. Several studies have demonstrated improved bone mineral density when supplementation is started in premenarchal girls.[131,132] However, in the twin study mentioned above, the benefits of calcium supplementation were not evident when comparing twins who had already entered or completed puberty.[128]

Calcium supplementation may also be more effective when combined with vitamin D. In a meta-analysis of combination therapy with vitamin D and calcium supplementation for patients receiving corticosteroids, there was a statistically and clinically significant difference in lumbar spine and radial bone density after 2 years of therapy.[133] A reduction in fracture risk was not definitively demonstrated, however. Vitamin D has also been shown to reduce the risk of bone mineral loss, when supplemented alone. In a study of 75 patients with CD, 1000 IU/day of vitamin D for 1 year resulted in significantly less bone loss compared with controls who received placebo.[134] Further benefit may be imparted by the addition of sodium fluoride, which resulted in increased bone density in IBD patients compared to calcium and vitamin D alone.[135]

Another important factor for minimizing bone loss is exercise. Weight bearing against gravity and the forces of muscle pull on bones produce strain on the axial skeleton, which stimulates bone formation.[136] However, increased disease activity and hospitalization are associated with decreased exercise. Accordingly, low-impact exercise programs may have a role in the prevention of bone disease in IBD patients.[137]

Bisphosphonates are newer compounds that have been used in osteoporosis because of their ability to suppress bone resorption and reduce bone turnover. These compounds increase bone mass and reduce the frequency of vertebral compression fractures in menopausal women[138-140] and in patients receiving corticosteroids for various conditions.[141,142] Subsequently, one of these compounds (alendronate) was shown to improve bone mineral density in adult patients with CD also supplemented with calcium and vitamin D, compared with a group receiving placebo for 12 months.[143] In the alendronate group, bone mineral density was increased by over 4% as measured in the lumbar spine, whereas bone mineral density dropped by 0.9% in the placebo group. Additionally, biochemical markers of bone turnover decreased significantly in the alendronate group; however, no difference was found in fracture rate between treatment groups.

Although these results are encouraging, potential effects on bone remodeling raise some concern over the use of bisphosphonates in pediatric patients. However, long-term adverse effects of these medications on bone remodeling have yet to be demonstrated in pediatric patients.[144] There have also been studies showing normal vertebral remodeling in children receiving bisphosphonates for other bone disorders.[145] Because of the relative lack of data specific to pediatric IBD, use of these medications should be limited to those with severe osteoporosis unresponsive to the proven, better-studied modalities. Controlled trials of these medications are needed in the pediatric IBD population, and it is likely that more information on the long-term effects of bisphosphonates will be available soon.

# NUTRITION AND INFLAMMATORY BOWEL DISEASES

Nutritional therapy in IBD is still underused, although it is gaining wider acceptance. One of the most appealing aspects of nutritional therapy is that it addresses the well-known effects of malnutrition while providing a therapeutic option as well. There are several hypotheses for the mechanisms by which nutritional therapy works for IBD.

Elimination of detrimental dietary antigens is one proposed theory to explain the utility of nutritional therapy for IBD, and forms the basis for the use of either elemental or polymeric diets. Elemental diets provide a protein source in the form of non-antigenic peptides or amino acids. The protein in polymeric diets is antigenic, but is generally derived from only one source. The belief that providing a limited antigenic diet may help with disease activity makes intuitive sense, as the gastrointestinal tract is routinely exposed to uncounted numbers of antigens from many sources, including the food ingested and the endogenous bacterial flora. Immunologic tolerance to these antigens is necessary to maintain a state of mucosal homeostasis, and disordered immune responses may be exacerbated by continued exposure to complex intestinal antigens through an inflamed mucosa.[146,147] Therefore, limited antigenic exposure may result in decreased pathogenic immune responses. Normalization of the cytokine profile, with downregulation of inflammatory cytokines and stimulation of anti-inflammatory cytokines may also result from nutritional therapy in IBD. In a study of children with Crohn's disease, enteral nutrition reduced the proinflammatory cytokines IL-2 and interferon-γ comparably to the effects of cyclosporin.[148] Furthermore, intestinal permeability may also improve with nutritional therapy,[149–151] resulting in less antigenic stimulation of the GI tract.

Changes in dietary components may also have profound effects on the antigenically active bacterial flora.[152–154] Elemental diets were initially developed for use in space travel, as a low-residue, nutritionally complete food. Not surprisingly, there are changes in the colonic flora following a journey to space.[155] Nutritional therapy may therefore affect the inflammatory response through its modulation of the bacterial flora.

In the early 1970s elemental diets were employed in IBD patients awaiting surgery, to maximize nutritional status prior to operation. It was serendipitously discovered that the patients not only improved nutritionally, but also had improved disease activity.[156] Subsequently, nutritional therapies have received increasing attention as an alternative to medical therapy. Because of the numerous nutritional issues associated with IBD in pediatric patients, nutritional therapy has been extensively studied in this population.

Perhaps the most basic form of nutritional therapy in IBD is the use of bowel rest and parenteral nutrition. In 1977, it was suggested that home total parenteral nutrition (TPN) be employed for the treatment of severe small bowel CD in children.[102] This study demonstrated that home TPN was safe and effective at promoting growth, while allowing the slow reintroduction of oral alimentation. Subsequently, trials of TPN and bowel rest have resulted in clinical remission of CD in both adolescents and adults. Response rates as high as 90% have been reported with the use of exclusive TPN, even in steroid-refractory disease.[157] A study comparing TPN with a specified liquid diet and combined oral and parenteral nutrition showed that 71% of patients receiving solely TPN achieved remission after 21 days.[158] The other forms of nutritional support resulted in remission rates of 58% and 60%, respectively, with 1-year remission rates decreasing to 42% in the TPN group and 55% in the other groups. A subsequent study similarly demonstrated superior response rates in a group receiving TPN, compared to elemental and polymeric diets.[159]

Despite the reported success with TPN, enteral nutrition represents a more physiologic and safer delivery system, and therefore would be preferable if similar results could be achieved. In 1995, Griffiths et al.[160] reviewed 37 pediatric and adult trials of enteral nutrition as primary therapy for active Crohn's disease. Thirteen trials met the inclusion criteria for meta-analysis, with eight trials comprising 413 patients comparing liquid diet and corticosteroids. In this analysis, the pooled odds ratio for the likelihood of clinical remission with liquid diet therapy versus corticosteroids was 0.35, demonstrating that diet therapy alone was inferior to corticosteroid therapy for the induction of remission. Various sensitivity analyses did not significantly change the results. Approximately 20% of patients randomized to receive nutritional therapy failed to complete the trials owing to intolerance of the formulas. The likelihood of intolerance was lower (8%) when the formula was administered strictly via nasogastric tube. The remaining five studies in the meta-analysis compared the efficacies of polymeric and elemental diets. In 134 patients tolerance for the liquid diets was quite high, with 94% completing the trials. In this analysis there was no demonstrable difference in efficacy between the two types of diet. A subsequent meta-analysis demonstrated similar

findings.[161] When including 10 studies comparing elemental diet with polymeric diet, no significant difference in efficacy of inducing remission was found. It should be noted that both TPN and enteral feeding are more effective for CD than for UC, where these interventions should be reserved for repletion of malnutrition rather than treatment of active disease.

Although the data in favor of corticosteroid therapy for the induction of remission seem compelling, the importance of nutritional therapy as an adjuvant to other therapies for IBD should not be underestimated. It remains to be determined whether the added benefits of nutritional therapy beyond effects on disease activity outweigh the increased efficacy of corticosteroids in inducing remission. For instance, a lower efficacy would be compensated if other disease complications such as growth failure and osteoporosis were successfully treated by nutritional therapy. This is particularly applicable to pediatric and adolescent patients, where growth issues take on paramount importance. Furthermore, the increased efficacy of corticosteroids may be counterbalanced by their negative effects on growth and bone development. Chronic corticosteroid therapy carries other undesirable side effects, including cosmetic and behavioral, that may make nutritional therapy more desirable in the pediatric and adolescent population.

# QUALITY OF LIFE AND COPING STRATEGIES

Childhood and adolescence is a period of intense physical, emotional, social and intellectual growth and change. The transition into adulthood is a turbulent time when adolescents are finding their identity, improving their social skills and cognitive abilities, and when their belief systems are being shaped. To a great extent this development affects how they will respond to events as adults later in life. This may explain why various psychological and social issues may be more pronounced in children and adolescents than adults with IBD. Adults may be better equipped to express their wants, needs and feelings in a social situation or with their family. Furthermore, adults may have developed problem-solving skills that allow them to adjust to these situations better than children, who have yet to develop these skills.

Physicians are becoming increasingly aware that traditional methods of evaluating the clinical status of patients with IBD may not accurately reflect how patients feel about their illness, how they function on a day-to-day basis, and their worries and concerns.[162] This is why health-related quality of life (HRQOL), defined as 'a global measure of the patient's perceptions, illness experience, and functional status that incorporates social, cultural, psychological, and disease-related factors',[163] becomes an important aspect of care. Questionnaires have been developed which attempt to quantify the patient's subjective evaluation of various aspects of their experience with IBD. These questionnaires incorporate physical, emotional and social functioning, including social activity, sexual functioning, ability to attend school or work, participation in sports and recreation, and body image. HRQOL questionnaires have been studied extensively in adult populations, but similar child and adolescent studies are lacking.[164–169] This may be because of a lack of uniform pediatric measures, as physical, intellectual and emotional functioning is constantly changing with normal development.[170] A disease-specific quality of life measure that encompasses the issues unique to the pediatric population is currently being developed and validated.

The concerns of children and adolescents diagnosed with IBD mostly overlap with those of adults, but some are unique to the pediatric population. It has been reported that children initially deny that IBD interferes with their lives, but with further probing many admit frustration and anger about their physical symptoms, unpleasant treatments, and the lack of understanding of the illness by others.[171] Major concerns of children are also energy level and body image.[170,172] Children often feel a lack of control with their choices regarding a variety of activities, ranging from leisure and sports to school and employment. They believe they are missing opportunities because of lack of energy, exacerbation of the disease, and feelings of isolation. In a meta-analysis of different chronic diseases in children, IBD had the most profound effect on mental health of all the medical diseases reviewed.[173] In a study that compared mental health and psychological functioning in 20 children with IBD against children with chronic headaches, diabetes mellitus, and healthy children, the rates of psychiatric disorders, assessed by the Child Assessment Schedule Interview, were 60% in children with IBD, 30% in children with chronic headaches, 20% in children with diabetes mellitus, and in 15% of healthy controls.[174] In a separate study, the prevalence of psychiatric disorders was noted to be 56% in children with IBD compared to 18% in a control group.[175]

When a child or adolescent is diagnosed with IBD, he/she is not the only person affected. Parents and siblings also have to learn how to cope with the illness.[176] The dynamics of the family may change by bringing more attention to the child with the illness, which may cause jealous feelings in siblings. Parents may have worries and fears about how the disease will affect the child's future, potential problems at school, side effects of medications, and feelings of guilt. The most common concerns of siblings of IBD patients are that they are being kept in the dark about the disease, fear about the disease and treatment, and feeling jealous of parents' overprotection of the ill child. Children with IBD experience a multitude of stressors, including altered physical appearance, decreased physical functioning, diarrhea and fecal incontinence, demanding treatment regimens, pain, and school absences. Some of the variability in children's adjustment to illness may be due to differences in the degree of disease severity, and the age and sex of the child. However, psychosocial factors also influence adjustment to IBD.[177] Thus, the way a child responds to illness-specific stressors must be considered, as this will affect the course of the illness as well as the child's overall adjustment.[178] Understanding the role of coping strategies is thus essential to facilitating maximal adjustment to a chronic illness.

Coping strategies are commonly classified as either problem focused or emotion focused. Problem-focused strategies attempt to alter the situation by changing the way an individual manages the disease, or by making a change in the environment. Children who utilize problem-focused strategies cope by gathering information.[179] They then make educated decisions about how to manage the situation most effectively through direct action. Emotion-focused strategies seek to manage somatic, subjective and affective responses to the stressor.[180] In this case, typical coping mechanisms include denial and distraction. One study suggested that patients who less frequently utilize maladaptive coping have more adaptive responses to hospitalization and surgery.[181] Similarly, social support has been found to positively influence the quality of life of adolescents with IBD.[182]

A child's perception of her/his ability to modify a stressor or its impact may influence their choice of coping strategy. Problem-focused strategies are most often used when one perceives a certain degree of control over a stressor; emotion-focused strategies are often associated with internal cues of emotional arousal, and when one perceives little control over the stressor.[183] Children with inflammatory bowel disease are typically affected by the stressors previously discussed. Gillman[184] notes that these children may have difficulty recognizing or acknowledging such stressors, and may therefore continually use ineffective coping strategies. In addition, the strategies they employ most often tend to be passive, and they make less effort to initiate problem solving.

A positive approach style includes problem-focused strategies of cognitive restructuring and problem solving, emotional regulation and social support. A negative/avoidance style includes emotion-focused strategies of distraction, denial, wishful thinking and resignation, as well as social withdrawal, blaming others and self-criticism. An additional factor determining adjustment to illness is the presence of mental health issues such as anxiety and depression. In adults with IBD, Turnbull and Vallis found that coping significantly correlated with psychological distress.[185] Underlying mental disorders may affect the way a child responds to her/his stressors, and hence the illness. Future research examining the effect of underlying mental disorders on adjustment to illness would be a valuable addition to our knowledge.

Multidisciplinary teams treating patients with IBD and their families need to recognize the aforementioned concepts, and use this information accordingly. Psychological treatment may be used to teach patients ways to facilitate their adjustment and maintain their typical daily lives. For example, these patients may be guided to utilize family and peer support to adjust to changes in their appearance caused by medications. They may learn to schedule activities when they feel most energetic, and to rest at other times. They may get through episodes of pain by performing learned techniques such as muscle relaxation and deep breathing, and by becoming attuned to the specific techniques that are most helpful to their personal illness experience. Harbeck-Weber et al.[179] suggest that children who engage in these proactive, problem-focused strategies are able to learn that information changes the way they manage a situation. In doing so they gain control over their lives at a time when their symptoms may cause them to feel somewhat out of control.

Casati and Toner recognized communication as a component of positive coping.[186] By expressing concerns to physicians, these issues may be alleviated and quality of life improved. Educational intervention is crucial, to inform children and adolescents about their medical condition so that they can use appropriate coping strategies. Education may be achieved through informal conversation with their parents and professional staff, as well as through formal educational programs and literature. Developmental differences in comprehension must be considered when educating children of various ages.

Parents will also benefit from intensive education about their children's conditions and learning strategies to help them gain control and adapt to living with a child with a chronic illness. Teaching parents strategies to facilitate appropriate systemic involvement, such as school participation with medications and special arrangements, will help them gain their own sense of competence and control while simultaneously helping to improve their children's quality of life.

# TRANSITION OF THE PATIENT WITH IBD FROM PEDIATRIC TO ADULT CARE

Children with IBD should be cared for by a physician trained to manage issues unique to pediatric patients.[187] Pediatric gastroenterologists have the expertise to address a multitude of important problems that occur uniquely during childhood, particularly growth and development. Internist gastroenterologists have a different set of skills that are necessary to provide optimal care to adult patients with IBD.

The passage from adolescence to adulthood is a time of internal turmoil and intense examination of personal goals and wishes. Being ill during this time of growth and change may cause frustration about the present and anxiety about the future. The growing adolescent must be able to progressively shed the sheltered environment of childhood and achieve self-reliance and independent living as a decision-maker. Under normal circumstances this process is painful for the healthiest of individuals. For the chronically ill adolescent this period of transition can be stressful not only for the patient, but also for their families and their healthcare providers.[188-192]

During the transition to an internist gastroenterologist, patients, parents and other family members may feel threatened by changes in the pattern of care, and resentful of the effort required to adjust to a new setting and different staff. They have weathered many crises and made vital decisions with the support of the pediatric team, and frequently regard this strong source of advocacy as a permanent arrangement. In contrast, they may perceive the internist who expects to care for an independent individual as less involved or less sensitive to the developmental and social aspects of their medical conditions.

Healthcare providers may also feel ambivalent during this period of change. The pediatrician may view the maturation of the child as a professional and personal achievement, and find difficulty in relinquishing the patient to others whose style of practice he or she may not know well.

Why transition? The goal of a transition program is to achieve for each chronically ill individual a continuum of care that includes normalization of social and emotional development and the development of independent living skills. A successful program should result in improved compliance with therapy and effective planning of long-term life needs. The successful transition from pediatric to adult healthcare systems is a part of this process.

The process of transition should begin when a patient enters early to mid adolescence. The pediatric gastroenterologist should begin seeing adolescent patients without their parents in order to build a relationship that promotes independence and self-reliance. It is important to discuss with the patient and the family that in the future they will need to transfer to a gastroenterologist who is also trained in internal medicine, with expertise in dealing with medical problems that occur during adulthood, including pregnancy, fertility and cancer surveillance.

Once the decision to pursue a transition program has been made, the next step is to identify a skilled gastroenterologist who cares for young adults. This individual must realize that a young adult with childhood-onset IBD may have a different set of expectations from young adults with recent-onset disease. These young adults also have a heightened risk of developing cancer and will require an increased need for cancer surveillance. The pediatrician needs to provide all of the necessary medical records and medical summaries so that all providers work together to deliver excellent care.

The timing of transition will require some flexibility, as many patients have 'special circumstances'. Any adolescent who has additional growth potential as a result of delayed puberty should be followed by a pediatric gastroenterologist. Also, children with neurologic delay should be transferred to an adult gastroenterologist who has the expertise and the support necessary to provide comprehensive care.

## TEAM APPROACH

Because of the complex nature of issues surrounding the care of a child or adolescent with IBD it is necessary to adopt a multidisciplinary approach, and devise an individual plan for therapy. In addition to parents, siblings and family members, teachers and school nurses should also be part of the team. They should be informed about important aspects of IBD, especially symptoms. The medical support team ideally should include physician, nurses and nurse practitioners, nutritionist, social worker and psychologist (Fig. 21.3). We believe that a team effort is necessary to ensure comprehensive, state-of-the-art care, which will allow IBD patients to achieve appropriate levels of physical, mental and social wellbeing.

The authors would like to thank Melissa Shepanski for her help during the preparation of the manuscript.

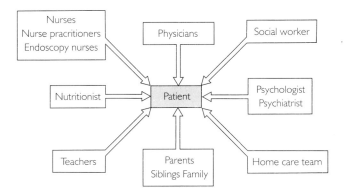

**Fig. 21.3** Inflammatory bowel disease support team.

# REFERENCES

1. Cohen MB, Seidman E, Winter H et al. Controversies in pediatric inflammatory bowel disease. Inflamm Bowel Dis 1998;4:203–227.
2. Kim S, Ferry G. Inflammatory bowel diseases in children. Curr Probl Pediatr Adolesc Health Care 2002;32:108–132.
3. Baldassano RN, Piccoli DA. Inflammatory bowel disease in pediatric and adolescent patients. Gastroenterol Clin North Am 1999;28:445–458.
4. Fonager K, Sorensen HT, Olsen J. Change in incidence of Crohn's disease and ulcerative colitis in Denmark. A study based on the National Registry of Patients, 1981–1992. Int J Epidemiol 1997;26:1003–1008.
5. Lindberg E, Lindquist B, Holmquist L et al. Inflammatory bowel disease in children and adolescents in Sweden, 1984–1995. J Pediatr Gastroenterol Nutr 2000;30:259–264.
6. Oliva-Hemker M, Fiocchi C. Etiopathogenesis of inflammatory bowel disease: the importance of the pediatric perspective. Inflamm Bowel Dis 2002;8:112–128.
7. Farmer RG, Michener WM. Prognosis of Crohn's disease with onset in childhood or adolescence. Dig Dis Sci 1979;24:752–757.
8. Andres PG, Friedman LS. Epidemiology and the natural course of inflammatory bowel disease. Gastroenterol Clin North Am 1999;28:255–281.
9. Logan RF. Inflammatory bowel disease incidence: up, down or unchanged? Gut 1998;42:309–311.
10. Polito JM II, Childs B, Mellits ED et al. Crohn's disease: influence of age at diagnosis on site and clinical type of disease. Gastroenterology 1996;111:580–586.
11. Kirschner BS, Heyman M, Ferry G et al. The pediatric IBD Consortium Database – Initial Demographic Data. Gastroenterology 2002;122:A611.
12. Russel MG, Stockbrugger RW. Epidemiology of inflammatory bowel disease: an update. Scand J Gastroenterol 1996;31:417–427.
13. Bjornsson S, Johannsson JH, Oddsson E. Inflammatory bowel disease in Iceland, 1980–89. A retrospective nationwide epidemiologic study. Scand J Gastroenterol 1998;33:71–77.
14. Langholz E, Munkholm P, Krasilnikoff PA et al. Inflammatory bowel diseases with onset in childhood. Clinical features, morbidity, and mortality in a regional cohort. Scand J Gastroenterol 1997;32:139–147.
15. Askling J, Grahnquist L, Ekbom A et al. Incidence of paediatric Crohn's disease in Stockholm, Sweden. Lancet 1999;354:1179.
16. Barton JR, Gillon S, Ferguson A. Incidence of inflammatory bowel disease in Scottish children between 1968 and 1983; marginal fall in ulcerative colitis, threefold rise in Crohn's disease. Gut 1989;30:618–622.
17. Hildebrand H, Fredrikzon B, Holmquist L et al. Chronic inflammatory bowel disease in children and adolescents in Sweden. J Pediatr Gastroenterol Nutr 1991;13:293–297.
18. Cosgrove M, Al-Atia RF, Jenkins HR. The epidemiology of paediatric inflammatory bowel disease. Arch Dis Child 1996;74:460–461.
19. Armitage E, Drummond HE, Wilson DC et al. Increasing incidence of both juvenile-onset Crohn's disease and ulcerative colitis in Scotland. Eur J Gastroenterol Hepatol 2001;13:1439–1447.
20. Tourtelier Y, Dabadie A, Tron I et al. Incidence of inflammatory bowel disease in children in Brittany (1994–1997). Breton association of study and research on digestive system diseases (Abermad). Arch Pediatr 2000;7:377–384.
21. Sawczenko A, Sandhu BK, Logan RF et al. Prospective survey of childhood inflammatory bowel disease in the British Isles. Lancet 2001;357:1093–1094.
22. Hassan K, Cowan FJ, Jenkins HR. The incidence of childhood inflammatory bowel disease in Wales. Eur J Pediatr 2000;159:261–263.
23. Gottrand F, Colombel JF, Moreno L et al. Incidence of inflammatory bowel diseases in children in the Nord–Pas-de-Calais region. Arch Fr Pediatr 1991;48:25–28.
24. Bjornsson S, Johannsson JH. Inflammatory bowel disease in Iceland, 1990–1994: a prospective, nationwide, epidemiological study. Eur J Gastroenterol Hepatol 2000;12:31–38.
25. Olafsdottir EJ, Fluge G, Haug K. Chronic inflammatory bowel disease in children in western Norway. J Pediatr Gastroenterol Nutr 1989;8:454–458.
26. RCPCH. Inflammatory bowel disease in under 20 year olds. RCPCH British Surveillance Unit 14th Annual report. London, 1999–2000:25–27.
27. Tysk C, Lindberg E, Jarnerot G et al. Ulcerative colitis and Crohn's disease in an unselected population of monozygotic and dizygotic twins. A study of heritability and the influence of smoking. Gut 1988;29:990–996.
28. Cohen Z, Weizman Z, Kurtzbart E et al. Infantile colonic Crohn's disease: a report of four cases in one family. J Pediatr Gastroenterol Nutr 2000;30:461–463.
29. Hugot J-P, Chamaillard M, Zouali H et al. Association of NOD2 leucine-rich repeat variants with susceptibility to Crohn's disease. Nature 2001;411:599–603.
30. Ogura Y, Bonen DK, Inohara N et al. A frameshift mutation in NOD2 associated with susceptibility to Crohn's disease. Nature 2001;411:603–606.
31. Montgomery SM, Pounder RE, Wakefield AJ. Infant mortality and the incidence of inflammatory bowel disease. Lancet 1997;349:472–473.
32. Gent AE, Hellier MD, Grace RH et al. Inflammatory bowel disease and domestic hygiene in infancy. Lancet 1994;343:766–767.
33. Duggan AE, Usmani I, Neal KR et al. Appendicectomy, childhood hygiene, Helicobacter pylori status, and risk of inflammatory bowel disease: a case control study. Gut 1998;43:494–498.
34. Statter MB, Hirschl RB, Coran AC. Inflammatory bowel disease. Pediatr Clin North Am 1993;40:1213–1231.
35. Hyams JS. Extraintestinal manifestations of inflammatory bowel disease in children. J Pediatr Gastroenterol Nutr 1994;19:7–21.
36. Heikenen JB, Werlin SL, Brown CW et al. Presenting symptoms and diagnostic lag in children with inflammatory bowel disease. Inflamm Bowel Dis 1999;5:158–160.
37. Kirschner BS. Inflammatory bowel disease in children. Pediatr Clin North Am 1988;35:189–208.
38. Gryboski JD. Crohn's disease in children 10 years old and younger: comparison with ulcerative colitis. J Pediatr Gastroenterol Nutr 1994;18:174–182.
39. Langholz E, Munkholm P, Krasilnikoff PA et al. Inflammatory bowel diseases in children. Ugeskr Laeger 1998;160:5648–5654.
40. O'Donoghue DP, Dawson AM. Crohn's disease in childhood. Arch Dis Child 1977;52:627–632.
41. Hofley PM, Piccoli DA. Inflammatory bowel disease in children. Med Clin North Am 1994;78:1281–1302.
42. Griffiths A, Buller HB. Inflammatory bowel disease. In: Walker-Smith J, Durie PB, Hamilton MI, Walker A, Watkins JB, eds. Pediatric gastrointestinal disease, 3rd edn. Hamilton, Ontario: BC Decker; 2000:613–652.
43. Spray C, Debelle GD, Murphy MS. Current diagnosis, management and morbidity in paediatric inflammatory bowel disease. Acta Paediatr 2001;90:400–405.
44. Wagtmans MJ, Verspaget HW, Lamers CB et al. Crohn's disease in the elderly: a comparison with young adults. J Clin Gastroenterol 1998;27:129–133.
45. Danzi JT. Extraintestinal manifestations of idiopathic inflammatory bowel disease. Arch Intern Med 1988;148:297–302.
46. Hyams JS. Crohn's disease in children. Pediatr Clin North Am 1996;43:255–277.
47. Menachem Y, Weizman Z, Locker C et al. Clinical characteristics of Crohn's disease in children and adults. Harefuah 1998;134:173–175, 247.
48. Gryboski JD, Spiro HM. Prognosis in children with Crohn's disease. Gastroenterology 1978;74:807–817.
49. Winesett M. Inflammatory bowel disease in children and adolescents. Pediatr Ann 1997;26:227–234.
50. Hofley P, Roarty J, McGinnity G et al. Asymptomatic uveitis in children with chronic inflammatory bowel diseases. J Pediatr Gastroenterol Nutr 1993;17:397–400.
51. Burbige EJ, Huang SH, Bayless TM. Clinical manifestations of Crohn's disease in children and adolescents. Pediatrics 1975;55:866–871.
52. Lindsley C, Schaller JG. Arthritis associated with inflammatory bowel disease in children. J Pediatr 1974;86:76.
53. Kane W, Miller K, Sharp HL. Inflammatory bowel disease presenting as liver disease during childhood. J Pediatr 1980; 97:775–778.
54. Hyams J, Markowitz J, Treem W et al. Characterization of hepatic abnormalities in children with inflammatory bowel disease. Inflamm Bowel Dis 1995;1:27–33.
55. Faubion WA Jr, Loftus EV, Sandborn WJ et al. Pediatric 'PSC-IBD': a descriptive report of associated inflammatory bowel disease among pediatric patients with PSC. J Pediatr Gastroenterol Nutr 2001;33:296–300.
56. McLeod RS, Churchill DN. Urolithiasis complicating inflammatory bowel disease. J Urol 1992;148:974–978.
57. Lloyd-Still JD, Tomasi L. Neurovascular and thromboembolic complications of inflammatory bowel disease in childhood. J Pediatr Gastroenterol Nutr 1989;9:461–466.
58. Hudson M, Chitolie A, Hutton RA et al. Thrombotic vascular risk factors in inflammatory bowel disease. Gut 1996;38:733–737.
59. Markowitz RL, Ment LR, Gryboski JD. Cerebral thromboembolic disease in pediatric and adult inflammatory bowel disease: case report and review of the literature. J Pediatr Gastroenterol Nutr 1989;8:413–420.
60. Reuner KH, Ruf A, Grau A et al. Prothrombin gene G20210->A transition is a risk factor for cerebral venous thrombosis. Stroke 1998;29:1765–1769.
61. Harper PH, Fazio VW, Lavery IC et al. The long-term outcome in Crohn's disease. Dis Colon Rectum 1987;30:174–179.
62. Barton JR, Ferguson A. Clinical features, morbidity and mortality of Scottish children with inflammatory bowel disease. Q J Med 1990;75:423–439.
63. Mamula P, Telega GW, Markowitz JE et al. Inflammatory bowel disease in children 5 years of age and younger. Am J Gastroenterol 2002;97:2005–2110.
64. Markowitz J, Daum F, Aiges H et al. Perianal disease in children and adolescents with Crohn's disease. Gastroenterology 1984;86:829–833.
65. Winter AM, Hanauer SB. Medical management of perianal Crohn's disease. Semin Gastrointest Dis 1998;9:10–14.
66. Rankin GB, Watts HD, Melnyk CS et al. National Cooperative Crohn's Disease Study: extraintestinal manifestations and perianal complications. Gastroenterology 1979;77:914–920.
67. Homan WP, Tang C, Thorgjarnarson B. Anal lesions complicating Crohn disease. Arch Surg 1976;111:1333–1335.
68. Gray BK, Lockhartmummery HE, Morson BC. Crohn's disease of the anal region. Gut 1965;6:515–524.
69. Farmer RG, Hawk WA, Turnbull RB Jr. Clinical patterns in Crohn's disease: a statistical study of 615 cases. Gastroenterology 1975;68:627–635.
70. Schwartz DA, Pemberton JH, Sandborn WJ. Diagnosis and treatment of perianal fistulas in Crohn disease. Ann Intern Med 2001;135:906–918.

71. Ruuska T, Vaajalahti P, Arajarvi P et al. Prospective evaluation of upper gastrointestinal mucosal lesions in children with ulcerative colitis and Crohn's disease. J Pediatr Gastroenterol Nutr 1994;19:181–186.

72. Cameron DJ. Upper and lower gastrointestinal endoscopy in children and adolescents with Crohn's disease: a prospective study. J Gastroenterol Hepatol 1991;6:355–358.

73. Veloso FT, Ferreira JT, Barros L et al. Clinical outcome of Crohn's disease: analysis according to the Vienna classification and clinical activity. Inflamm Bowel Dis 2001;7:306–313.

74. Beaugerie L, Le Quintrec Y, Paris JC et al. Testing for course patterns in Crohn's disease using clustering analysis. Gastroenterol Clin Biol 1989;13:1036–1041.

75. Louis E, Collard A, Oger AF et al. Behaviour of Crohn's disease according to the Vienna classification: changing pattern over the course of the disease. Gut 2001;49:777–782.

76. Griffiths AM, Nguyen P, Smith C et al. Growth and clinical course of children with Crohn's disease. Gut 1993;34:939–943.

77. Puntis J, McNeish AS, Allan RN. Long term prognosis of Crohn's disease with onset in childhood and adolescence. Gut 1984;25:329–336.

78. Michener WM, Whelan G, Greenstreet RL et al. Comparison of the clinical features of Crohn's disease and ulcerative colitis with onset in childhood or adolescence. Cleveland Clin Q 1982;49:13–16.

79. Shivananda S, Lennard-Jones J, Logan R et al. Incidence of inflammatory bowel disease across Europe: is there a difference between north and south? Results of the European Collaborative Study on Inflammatory Bowel Disease (EC-IBD). Gut 1996;39:690–697.

80. Holmquist L, Rudic N, Ahren C et al. The diagnostic value of colonoscopy compared with rectosigmoidoscopy in children and adolescents with symptoms of chronic inflammatory bowel disease of the colon. Scand J Gastroenterol 1988;23:577–584.

81. Farmer RG, Easley KA, Rankin GB. Clinical patterns, natural history, and progression of ulcerative colitis. A long-term follow-up of 1116 patients. Dig Dis Sci 1993;38:1137–1146.

82. Mir-Madjlessi SH, Michener WM, Farmer RG. Course and prognosis of idiopathic ulcerative proctosigmoiditis in young patients. J Pediatr Gastroenterol Nutr 1986;5:571–575.

83. Meucci G, Vecchi M, Astegiano M et al. The natural history of ulcerative proctitis: a multicenter, retrospective study. Gruppo di Studio per le Malattie Infiammatorie Intestinali (GSMII). Am J Gastroenterol 2000;95:469–473.

84. Michener WM, Farmer RG, Mortimer EA. Long-term prognosis of ulcerative colitis with onset in childhood or adolescence. J Clin Gastroenterol 1979;1:301–305.

85. Hyams JS, Davis P, Grancher K et al. Clinical outcome of ulcerative colitis in children. J Pediatr 1996;129:81–88.

86. Gryboski JD. Ulcerative colitis in children 10 years old or younger. J Pediatr Gastroenterol Nutr 1993;17:24–31.

87. Werlin SL, Grand RJ. Severe colitis in children and adolescents: diagnosis, course, and treatment. Gastroenterology 1977;73:828–832.

88. Ahsgren L, Jonsson B, Stenling R et al. Prognosis after early onset of ulcerative colitis. A study from an unselected patient population. Hepatogastroenterology 1993;40:467–470.

89. Falcone RA Jr, Lewis LG, Warner BW. Predicting the need for colectomy in pediatric patients with ulcerative colitis. J Gastrointest Surg 2000;4:201–206.

90. Motil KJ, Grand RJ, Maletskos CJ et al. The effect of disease, drug, and diet on whole body protein metabolism in adolescents with Crohn disease and growth failure. J Pediatr 1982;101:345–351.

91. Grill BB, Hillemeier AC, Gryboski JD. Fecal alpha 1-antitrypsin clearance in patients with inflammatory bowel disease. J Pediatr Gastroenterol Nutr 1984;3:56–61.

92. Kelts D, Grand R, Shen G et al. Nutritional basis of growth failure in children and adolescents with Crohn's disease. Gastroenterology 1979;76:720–727.

93. Seidman E, LeLeiko N, Ament M et al. Nutritional issues in pediatric inflammatory bowel disease. J Pediatr Gastroenterol Nutr 1991;12:424–438.

94. Kanof ME, Lake AM, Bayless TM. Decreased height velocity in children and adolescents before the diagnosis of Crohn's disease. Gastroenterology 1988;95:1523–1527.

95. Hyams JS, Ferry GD, Mandel FS et al. Development and validation of pediatric Crohn's Disease Activity Index. J Pediatr Gastroenterol Nutr 1991;12:439–447.

96. Otley A, Loonen H, Parekh N et al. Assessing activity of pediatric Crohn's disease: which index to use? Gastroenterology 1999;116:527–531.

97. Rigaud D, Cosnes J, Le Quintrec Y et al. Controlled trial comparing two types of enteral nutrition in treatment of active Crohn's disease: elemental vs. polymeric diet. Gut 1991;32:1492–1497.

98. Sentongo T, Semeao E, Piccoli D et al. Growth, body composition, and nutritional status in children and adolescents with Crohn's disease. J Pediatr Gastroenterol Nutr 2000;31:33–40.

99. Motil K, Grand R, Matthews D et al. Whole body leucine metabolism in adolescents with Crohn's disease and growth failure during nutritional supplementation. Gastroenterology 1982;82:1361–1368.

100. Layden T, Rosenberg F, Nemchausky G et al. Reversal of growth arrest in adolescents with Crohn's disease after parenteral alimentation. Gastroenterology 1976;70:1017–1021.

101. Ferguson A, Glen M, Ghosh S. Crohn's disease: nutrition and nutritional therapy. Baillière's Clin Gastroenterol 1998;12:93–114.

102. Byrne W, Halpin T, Asch M et al. Home total parenteral nutrition: an alternative approach to the management of children with severe chronic small bowel disease. J Pediatr Surg 1977;12:359–366.

103. Christie P, Hill G. Effect of intravenous nutrition on nutrition and function in acute attacks of inflammatory bowel disease. Gastroenterology 1990;99:730–736.

104. Kirschner B, Klich J, Kalman S et al. Reversal of growth retardation in Crohn's disease with therapy emphasizing oral nutritional restitution. Gastroenterology 1980;80:10–15.

105. Motil K. Aggressive nutritional therapy in growth retardation. Clin Nutr 1985;4:75–84.

106. Himes JH, Roche AF, Thissen D et al. Parent-specific adjustments for evaluation of recumbent length and stature of children. Pediatrics 1985;75:304–313.

107. Rosen DS. Pubertal growth and sexual maturation for adolescents with chronic illness or disability. Pediatrician 1991;18:105–120.

108. Brain CE, Savage MO. Growth and puberty in chronic inflammatory bowel disease. Baillière's Clin Gastroenterol 1994;8:83–100.

109. Tanner JM. Growth at adolescence. Oxford: Blackwell Scientific; 1972.

110. de Vizia B, Poggi V, Conenna R et al. Iron absorption and iron deficiency in infants and children with gastrointestinal diseases. J Pediatr Gastroenterol Nutr 1992;14:21–26.

111. Galloway R, McGuire J. Determinants of compliance with iron supplementation: supplies, side effects, or psychology? Soc Sci Med 1994;39:381–390.

112. Mailloux R, Sitrin M. The skeletal complications of inflammatory bowel disease and their treatment. Prog Inflamm Bowel Dis 1994;15:1–21.

113. Scott EM, Gaywood I, Scott BB. Guidelines for osteoporosis in coeliac disease and inflammatory bowel disease. British Society of Gastroenterology. Gut 2000;46(Suppl 1):1–8.

114. Caulfield L, Himes J, Rivera J. Nutritional supplementation during early childhood and bone mineralization during adolescence. J Nutr 1995;125:1104–1110.

115. Kanis JA, Pitt FA. Epidemiology of osteoporosis. Bone 1992;13(Suppl 1):S7–15.

116. Kanis JA, McCloskey EV. Epidemiology of vertebral osteoporosis. Bone 1992;(13 Suppl):2:S1–10.

117. Mora S, Pitukcheewanont P, Kaufman F et al. Biochemical markers of bone turnover and the volume and the density of bone in children at different stages of sexual development. J Bone Miner Res 1999;14:1664–1671.

118. Compston JE, Creamer B. Plasma levels and intestinal absorption of 25–hydroxyvitamin D in patients with small bowel resection. Gut1977;18:171–175.

119. Bell NH, Shaw S, Turner RT. Evidence that calcium modulates circulating 25-hydroxyvitamin D in man. J Bone Miner Res 1987;2:211–214.

120. Clements MR, Johnson L, Fraser DR. A new mechanism for induced vitamin D deficiency in calcium deprivation. Nature 1987;325:62–65.

121. Caniggia A, Nuti R, Lore F et al. Pathophysiology of the adverse effects of glucoactive corticosteroids on calcium metabolism in man. J Steroid Biochem 1981;15:153–161.

122. Suzuki Y, Ichikawa Y, Saito E et al. Importance of increased urinary calcium excretion in the development of secondary hyperparathyroidism of patients under glucocorticoid therapy. Metabolism 1983;32:151–156.

123. Lukert BP, Raisz LG. Glucocorticoid-induced osteoporosis: pathogenesis and management. Ann Intern Med 1990;112:352–364.

124. Schoon EJ, Geerling BG, Van Dooren IM et al. Abnormal bone turnover in long-standing Crohn's disease in remission. Aliment Pharmacol Ther 2001;15:783–792.

125. LoCascio V, Adami S, Avioli LV et al. Suppressive effect of chronic glucocorticoid treatment on circulating calcitonin in man. Calcif Tissue Int 1982;34:309–310.

126. Nemetz A, Toth M, Garcia-Gonzalez MA et al. Allelic variation at the interleukin 1beta gene is associated with decreased bone mass in patients with inflammatory bowel diseases. Gut 2001;49:644–649.

127. Schulte CM, Dignass AU, Goebell H et al. Genetic factors determine extent of bone loss in inflammatory bowel disease. Gastroenterology 2000;119:909–920.

128. Johnston C, Miller J, Slemenda C et al. Calcium supplementation and increases in bone mineral density in children. N Engl J Med 1992;327:82–87.

129. Lee W, Leung S, Wang S-H et al. Double-blind, controlled calcium supplementation and bone mineral accretion in children accustomed to a low-calcium diet. Am J Clin Nutr 1994;60:744–750.

130. Lee W, Leung S, Leung D et al. A follow-up study on the effects of calcium-supplement withdrawal and puberty on bone acquisition of children. Am J Clin Nutr 1996;64:71–77.

131. Chan G, Hoffman K, McMurry M. Effects of dairy products on bone and body composition in pubertal girls. J Pediatr 1995;126:551–556.

132. Lloyd T, Andon M, Rollings N et al. Calcium supplementation and bone mineral density in adolescent girls. JAMA 1993;270:841–844.

133. Homik J, Suarez-Almazor ME, Shea B et al. Calcium and vitamin D for corticosteroid-induced osteoporosis. Cochrane Database Syst Rev 2000:CD000952.

134. Vogelsang H, Ferenci P, Resch H et al. Prevention of bone mineral loss in patients with Crohn's disease by long-term oral vitamin D supplementation. Eur J Gastroenterol Hepatol 1995;7:609–614.

135. von Tirpitz C, Klaus J, Bruckel J et al. Increase of bone mineral density with sodium fluoride in patients with Crohn's disease. Eur J Gastroenterol Hepatol 2000;12:19–24.

136. Frost HM. Suggested fundamental concepts in skeletal physiology. Calcif Tissue Int 1993;52:1–4.

137. Robinson RJ, Iqbal SJ, Abrams K et al. Increased bone resorption in patients with Crohn's disease. Aliment Pharmacol Ther 1998;12:699–705.

138. Adami S, Passeri M, Ortolani S et al. Effects of oral alendronate and intranasal salmon calcitonin on bone mass and biochemical markers of bone turnover in postmenopausal women with osteoporosis. Bone 1995;17:383–390.

139. Harris ST, Gertz BJ, Genant HK et al. The effect of short term treatment with alendronate on vertebral density and biochemical markers of bone remodeling in early postmenopausal women. J Clin Endocrinol Metab 1993;76:1399–1406.

140. Harris ST, Watts NB, Jackson RD et al. Four-year study of intermittent cyclic etidronate treatment of postmenopausal osteoporosis: three years of blinded therapy followed by one year of open therapy. Am J Med 1993;95:557–567.

141. Saag KG, Emkey R, Schnitzer TJ et al. Alendronate for the prevention and treatment of glucocorticoid-induced osteoporosis. Glucocorticoid-Induced Osteoporosis Intervention Study Group. N Engl J Med 1998;339:292–299.

142. Adachi JD, Bensen WG, Brown J et al. Intermittent etidronate therapy to prevent corticosteroid-induced osteoporosis. N Engl J Med 1997;337:382–387.

143. Haderslev KV, Tjellesen L, Sorensen HA et al. Alendronate increases lumbar spine bone mineral density in patients with Crohn's disease. Gastroenterology 2000;119:639–646.

144. Brumsen C, Hamdy N, Papapoulos S. Long-term effects of bisphosphonates on the growing skeleton: studies of young patients with severe osteoporosis. Medicine (Baltimore) 1997;76:266–283.

145. Astrom E, Soderhall S. Beneficial effect of long term intravenous bisphosphonate treatment of osteogenesis imperfecta. Arch Dis Child 2002;86:356–364.

146. Linskens RK, Huijsdens XW, Savelkoul PH et al. The bacterial flora in inflammatory bowel disease: current insights in pathogenesis and the influence of antibiotics and probiotics. Scand J Gastroenterol Suppl 2001:29–40.

147. Murch S, Walker-Smith J. Nutrition in inflammatory bowel disease. Baillière's Clin Gastroenterol 1998;12:719–739.

148. Breese EJ, Michie CA, Nicholls SW et al. The effect of treatment on lymphokine-secreting cells in the intestinal mucosa of children with Crohn's disease. Aliment Pharmacol Ther 1995;9:547–552.

149. Zoli G, Care M, Parazza M et al. A randomized controlled study comparing elemental diet and steroid treatment in Crohn's disease. Aliment Pharmacol Ther 1997;11:735–740.

150. Sanderson IR, Boulton P, Menzies I et al. Improvement of abnormal lactulose/rhamnose permeability in active Crohn's disease of the small bowel by an elemental diet. Gut 1987;28:1073–1076.

151. Teahon K, Smethurst P, Pearson M et al. The effect of elemental diet on intestinal permeability and inflammation in Crohn's disease. Gastroenterology 1991;101:84–89.

152. Bengmark S. Ecological control of the gastrointestinal tract. The role of probiotic flora. Gut 1998;42:2–7.

153. Gibson GR, Roberfroid MB. Dietary modulation of the human colonic microbiota: introducing the concept of prebiotics. J Nutr 1995;125:1401–1412.

154. Roberfroid MB. Prebiotics and synbiotics: concepts and nutritional properties. Br J Nutr 1998;80:S197–202.

155. Lencner AA, Lencner CP, Mikelsaar ME et al. The quantitative composition of the intestinal lactoflora before and after space flights of different lengths. Nahrung 1984;28:607–613.

156. Voitk AJ, Echave V, Feller JH et al. Experience with elemental diet in the treatment of inflammatory bowel disease. Is this primary therapy? Arch Surg 1973;107:329–333.

157. Forbes A. Crohn's disease – the role of nutritional therapy. Aliment Pharmacol Ther 2002;16(Suppl 4):48–52.

158. Greenberg G, Fleming C, Jeejeebhoy K et al. Controlled trial of bowel rest and nutritional support in the management of Crohn's disease. Gut 1988;29:1309–1315.

159. Kobayashi K, Katsumata T, Yokoyama K et al. A randomized controlled study of total parenteral nutrition and enteral nutrition by elemental and polymeric diet as primary therapy in active phase of Crohn's disease. Nippon Shokakibyo Gakkai Zasshi 1998;95:1212–1221.

160. Griffiths AM, Ohlsson A, Sherman PM et al. Meta-analysis of enteral nutrition as a primary treatment of active Crohn's disease. Gastroenterology 1995;108:1056–1067.

161. Zachos M, Tondeur M, Griffiths AM. Enteral nutritional therapy for inducing remission of Crohn's disease. Cochrane Database Syst Rev 2001:CD000542.

162. Ferry GD. Quality of life in inflammatory bowel disease: background and definitions. J Pediatr Gastroenterol Nutr 1999;28:S15–18.

163. Maunder RG, Cohen Z, McLeod RS et al. Effect of intervention in inflammatory bowel disease on health-related quality of life: a critical review. Dis Colon Rectum 1995;38:1147–1161.

164. Yacavone RF, Locke GR 3rd, Provenzale DT et al. Quality of life measurement in gastroenterology: what is available? Am J Gastroenterol 2001; 96:285–297.

165. Pallis AG, Mouzas IA. Instruments for quality of life assessment in patients with inflammatory bowel disease. Dig Liver Dis 2000;32:682–688.

166. Casellas F, Lopez-Vivancos J, Vergara M et al. Impact of inflammatory bowel disease on health-related quality of life. Dig Dis 1999;17:208–218.

167. Koot HM, Bouman NH. Potential uses for quality-of-life measures in childhood inflammatory bowel disease. J Pediatr Gastroenterol Nutr 1999;28:S56–61.

168. Irvine EJ. Quality of life issues in patients with inflammatory bowel disease. Am J Gastroenterol 1997;92:18S–24S.

169. Sandborn WJ, Feagan BG, Hanauer SB et al. A review of activity indices and efficacy endpoints for clinical trials of medical therapy in adults with Crohn's disease. Gastroenterology 2002;122:512–530.

170. Griffiths AM, Nicholas D, Smith C et al. Development of a quality-of-life index for pediatric inflammatory bowel-disease: dealing with differences related to age and IBD type. J Pediatr Gastroenterol Nutr 1999;28:S46–52.

171. Akobeng AK, Suresh-Babu MV, Firth D et al. Quality of life in children with Crohn's disease: a pilot study. J Pediatr Gastroenterol Nutr 1999;28:S37–39.

172. Rabbett H, Elbadri A, Thwaites R et al. Quality of life in children with Crohn's disease. J Pediatr Gastroenterol Nutr 1996;23:528–533.

173. Lavigne JV, Faier-Routman J. Psychological adjustment to pediatric physical disorders: a meta-analytic review. J Pediatr Psychol 1992;17:133–157.

174. Engstrom I, Lindquist BL. Inflammatory bowel disease in children and adolescents: a somatic and psychiatric investigation. Acta Paediatr Scand 1991;80:640–647.

175. Burke P, Meyer V, Kocoshis S et al. Depression and anxiety in pediatric inflammatory bowel disease and cystic fibrosis. J Am Acad Child Adolesc Psychiatry 1989;28:948–951.

176. Akobeng AK, Miller V, Firth D et al. Quality of life of parents and siblings of children with inflammatory bowel disease. J Pediatr Gastroenterol Nutr 1999;28:S40–42.

177. Ringel Y, Drossman DA. Psychosocial aspects of Crohn's disease. Surg Clin North Am 2001;81:231–252.

178. Spirito A, Stark LJ, Williams C. Development of a brief coping checklist for use with pediatric populations. J Pediatr Psychol 1988;13:555–574.

179. Harbeck-Weber C, McKee DH. Prevention of emotional and behavioral distress in children experiencing hospitalization and chronic illness. In: Roberts MC, ed. Handbook of pediatric psychology. New York: Guilford Publications; 1995:167–184.

180. Tobin DL, Holroyd KA, Reynolds RV et al. The hierarchical factor structure of the coping strategies inventory. Cognitive Ther Res 1989;13:343–361.

181. Moskovitz DN, Maunder RG, Cohen Z et al. Coping behavior and social support contribute independently to quality of life after surgery for inflammatory bowel disease. Dis Colon Rectum 2000;43:517–521.

182. MacPhee M, Hoffenberg EJ, Feranchak A. Quality-of-life factors in adolescent inflammatory bowel disease. Inflamm Bowel Dis; 1998:4:6–11.

183. Compas BE, Worsham NL, Ey S. Conceptual and developmental issues in children's coping with stress. In: La Greca AM, Siegel LJ, Wallander JL, Walker CE, eds. Stress and coping in child health. New York: Guilford Publications; 1991:7–24.

184. Gillman JB. Inflammatory bowel diseases: psychological issues. In: Olson RA, Mullins LL, Gillman JB, Chaney JM, eds. The sourcebook of pediatric psychology. Boston: Allyn & Bacon; 1994:135–144.

185. Turnbull GK, Vallis TM. Quality of life in inflammatory bowel disease: the interaction of disease activity with psychosocial function. Am J Gastroenterol 1995;90:1450–1454.

186. Casati J, Toner BB. Psychosocial aspects of inflammatory bowel disease. Biomed Pharmacother 2000;54:388–393.

187. Baldassano R, Ferry G, Griffiths A et al. Transition of the patient with inflammatory bowel disease from pediatric to adult care: recommendations of the North American Society for Pediatric Gastroenterology, Hepatology and Nutrition. J Pediatr Gastroenterol Nutr 2002;34:245–248.

188. Betz CL. Facilitating the transition of adolescents with chronic conditions from pediatric to adult health care and community settings. Issues Compr Pediatr Nurs 1998;21:97–115.

189. Blum RW, Garell D, Hodgman CH et al. Transition from child-centered to adult health-care systems for adolescents with chronic conditions. A position paper of the Society for Adolescent Medicine. J Adolesc Health 1993;14:570–576.

190. Rosen D. Between two worlds: bridging the cultures of child health and adult medicine. J Adolesc Health 1995;17:10–16.

191. Sawyer SM, Blair S, Bowes G. Chronic illness in adolescents: transfer or transition to adult services? J Paediatr Child Health 1997;33:88–90.

192. Transition of care provided for adolescents with special health care needs. American Academy of Pediatrics Committee on Children with Disabilities and Committee on Adolescence. Pediatrics 1996;98:1203–1206.

## CHAPTER 22

# Physiologic consequences of surgical treatment for inflammatory bowel disease

Ishaan S Kalha and Joseph H Sellin

The normal intestinal tract has several major functions, including nutrient absorption, fluid and electrolyte conservation, and maintenance of an appropriate barrier against the potentially hostile environment of bacteria, antigens and toxins within the intestinal lumen. This function is always challenged and usually compromised by inflammatory bowel disease (IBD) itself. Although surgery can ameliorate (or eliminate) the symptoms of IBD, it may at the same time either exacerbate pre-existing problems with intestinal function or superimpose a new set of challenges for the gut. This chapter describes the consequences of IBD surgery on the intestine and colon and the adaptive responses of the gut to maintain homeostasis. In this era of molecular biology, we have the opportunity to understand in far greater detail the adaptive responses of the intestine and, perhaps, provide innovative therapeutic interventions.

## SPATIAL HETEROGENEITY OF THE GASTROINTESTINAL TRACT

There is a very specific spatial heterogeneity in the gut along two different axes. The duodenal–colonic axis has long been appreciated: there are major differences when comparing the upper small bowel and rectum in regard to both structure and function. Either IBD itself or surgical intervention may have a significant impact along this axis, removing or eliminating a specific transporter, for example. Changes along the second axis, the crypt:villus (small intestine) or crypt:surface (colon) axis, may be more subtle but are no less important. As epithelial cells move along this axis there are major changes in protein expression and function. Increased rates of proliferation may occur either with injury, inflammation and cytokine modulation of IBD, or alternatively with adaptation following surgical resection. This change in proliferation may alter the balance between immature (secretory) cells of the crypt and the mature (absorptive) cells of the villus (surface). This change in the gradient

may modify the overall absorptive, digestive and specific transport function of the epithelium.

## DIARRHEA AND MALABSORPTION IN INFLAMMATORY BOWEL DISEASE

Before focusing in detail on the alterations in gut function caused by surgery, it is important to consider the baseline changes induced by IBD. Diarrhea is, perhaps, the most common symptom in both ulcerative colitis and Crohn's disease. Although it may seem obvious that an inflamed intestine or colon would lead to diarrhea, current understanding of the underlying pathophysiology is limited. The colonic epithelial cells do have an increased turnover when an inflammatory process is active. Even when there is no inflammatory infiltrate, IBD patients may have an intrinsic abnormality in their colonic epithelium making them more susceptible to the effects of IBD.

Numerous factors contribute to the diarrhea in IBD: active ion secretion stimulated by inflammatory mediators; changes in permeability; alterations in motility; malabsorption of nutrients, ions and water; and 'sick cell syndrome'. Although it is clear that there is a significant increase in inflammatory mediators within the IBD epithelium and that these mediators can stimulate electrogenic ion secretion in the normal intestine in vitro, it is less apparent that this is the dominant mechanism of diarrhea in IBD. Several studies have suggested that the inflamed epithelium is less responsive to secretory stimuli than its healthy counterpart. This has led to the concept of the sick cell syndrome, in which the epithelium is unable to perform its normal (absorptive) functions. For each patient there probably is an individual mix of these multiple factors that leads to diarrhea.

Although weight loss is common in IBD, it is relatively unusual for this to be due to an extensive malabsorption of nutrients. The exception is Crohn's disease involving most of the small intestine. Weight loss of more than 20% of body weight is uncommon but may occur. In contrast to global malabsorption, nutrient-specific malabsorption is common. Ileal dysfunction impairs both bile salt and vitamin $B_{12}$ absorption. The colon's role in fluid and electrolyte absorption is well recognized, but it is not generally thought of as a site for absorption of calories and nutrients. Nevertheless, colonic dysfunction may have important nutritional consequences related to mineral metabolism and absorption of short-chain fatty acids (SCFA).

# COMMON SURGICAL PROCEDURES FOR INFLAMMATORY BOWEL DISEASE

The most common surgical procedures performed for IBD patients are limited segmental resection of the small intestine, most commonly the ileum; total proctocolectomy with ileostomy; proctocolectomy with ileal pouch–anal anastomosis; proctocolectomy with ileorectal anastomosis; segmental colonic resection in Crohn's disease; and major or successive resections of the small intestine, resulting in short bowel syndrome in Crohn's disease. The development of strictureplasty in Crohn's disease surgery has resulted in intestine-sparing operations that maintain a sufficient absorptive area to prevent short bowel syndrome. Each type of operation will have characteristic consequences and predictable effects on the gastrointestinal (GI) tract. The ileal pouch–anal anastomosis is being used more commonly, with better outcomes. This procedure has created a whole new understanding of ileal physiology and its ability to adapt to a distinctly different environment. It has yielded new terms such as pouchitis and has led to a greater appreciation of the physiological changes that surgery induces.

Even though there are different surgical techniques for patients with ulcerative colitis and Crohn's disease any of these operations results in four distinct outcomes. These are:

- Ileal resection
- Short bowel syndrome
- Colectomy
- Formation of an ileal pouch.

The chapter will now focus on each of these surgical outcomes in terms of the physiological changes, clinical presentation and therapeutic interventions.

# PHYSIOLOGICAL EFFECTS OF ILEAL RESECTION

The ileum is up to 6 m long in the adult. The small intestinal epithelium is characterized by the formation of crypts and villi. There are receptors for growth factors, hormones, peptides and neurotransmitters. Activation of these receptors will affect enterocyte permeability, solute transport, migration and differentiation. In addition to its generalized capacity to absorb fluid and nutrients the ileum has some very specialized functions. It has the unique ability to absorb bile salts and vitamin $B_{12}$. The ileum is a critical component of the enterohepatic circulation. The ileum is also central to the concept of the 'ileal brake', the primary inhibitory feedback mechanism to control transit of a meal through the gastrointestinal tract so that nutrient digestion and absorption are optimized. Neurohormonal factors are felt to mediate this response.[1] Ileal resection can therefore lead to significant alterations in intestinal function affecting bile salts, $B_{12}$ absorption and nutrient absorption.

## ENTEROHEPATIC CIRCULATION

Organic anions, drugs and hormone metabolites are conserved by a recycling process that involves biliary secretion, ileal absorption and hepatic uptake: the enterohepatic circulation. Bile salts are the most important participant in the enterohepatic circulation; they stimulate hepatic bile flow, micellularize dietary lipids, solubilize biliary cholesterol, and stimulate intestinal fluid secretion. Ileal resection disrupts bile salt metabolism and therefore will have an impact on these functions. The bile acid pool remains constant as a result of a balance between hepatic bile acid synthesis and intestinal absorption. The rate-limiting step is usually intestinal absorption; however, in the short bowel syndrome the limiting step is hepatic synthesis.

There are two different mechanisms of intestinal absorption of bile acids: (1) passive permeation, which occurs throughout the length of the gut, and (2) active absorption, which is restricted to the terminal ileum. The more polar (conjugated) bile acids are well absorbed by the active transport mechanism of the ileum. This absorption is dependent on $Na^+$ and is similar to other $Na^+$-coupled transport systems in the small bowel that link the intracellular accumulation of a solute to the downhill movement of $Na^+$ across the apical membrane. This transporter recently has been cloned and its transport properties characterized.[2]

In contrast, passive absorption is greater for the less polar bile salts and depends on the concentration of the bile salt within the intestinal lumen and its permeability coefficient (lipid solubility). Passive absorption is affected by the functional surface area of the small intestine, the type of bile salts within the lumen, and other factors in the luminal environment (pH, calcium), but is not strictly dependent on the terminal ileum. The ileal absorptive mechanism is highly efficient, whereas the passive absorptive mechanism, which may account for up to half the bile acids absorbed in the normal gut, demonstrates relatively low efficiency.

Ileal resection obviously blocks the active component of bile acid absorption. With relatively small resections of the ileum (<100 cm) there is mild malabsorption of the bile acids, particularly chenodeoxycholate. The dihydroxy bile acids are potent cathartics. In the colon they alter intestinal permeability and stimulate active electrolyte secretion in colonocytes. Bile salts increase both intracellular cyclic AMP (c-AMP) and calcium, causing a cascade of events that results in the opening of apical membrane chloride channels and hence chloride secretion. Clinically, this results in watery diarrhea, generally worse in the morning when the bile salt pool is higher after an overnight fast. The diarrhea responds to cholestyramine. With small ileal resections there is minimal nutrient malabsorption.

With small ileal resections, increased hepatic synthesis of bile salts compensates for intestinal losses. The bile salt pool and intestinal micelle formation are maintained at near-normal levels. However, with larger ileal resections (>100 cm) the magnitude of losses from the enterohepatic circulation may be profound and can no longer be matched by increased production in the liver. Overall bile acid synthesis increases but the luminal concentration in the jejunum falls. At this point the concentration of bile salts in the upper GI tract drops sufficiently to impair micelle formation and fat absorption (Fig. 22.1). Secretory diarrhea persists, but the stimulus is different. Long-chain fatty acids entering the colonic lumen as a result of the steatorrhea, such as dihydroxy bile acids, can serve as a potent stimulus for electrogenic anion secretion. The severity of the diarrhea can be reduced to some extent by severe restriction of dietary fat.

Bile salts solubilize cholesterol in the bile. As the bile salt pool is depleted by ileal resection the concentration of bile salts in the bile decreases, leading to cholesterol supersaturation and an increased probability of cholesterol gallstone formation. Although this is the textbook explanation of the increased incidence of gallstones in patients with ileal resections, the clinical realities are less clear. A significant proportion of stones are pigment, rather than cholesterol. The reasons for this are unknown.[3] Whether they may be precipitated by total parenteral nutrition and prolonged periods of gallbladder stasis has not been determined (see later discussion).

## VITAMIN $B_{12}$

Vitamin $B_{12}$ (cobalamin), an essential cofactor in the conversion of homocysteine to methionine, is necessary for folic acid metabolism and DNA synthesis. Cobalamin deficiency leads to a megaloblastic maturation pattern well recognized in hematopoietic cells but also occurring in epithelial cells. The body's cobalamin stores are dependent on intake, absorption, and conservation. Vitamin $B_{12}$ is found only in animal products, and thus strict vegetarians are at risk for developing a deficiency. About 10–20 μg/day are ingested in an average diet, and of this about 1–2 μg/day are needed to provide for normal requirements. Absorption is complex, depending on salivary and gastric R proteins, gastric intrinsic factor and pancreatic secretions. In contrast to bile salts, which have alternative absorptive pathways, cobalamin's sole mechanism of absorption depends on specific receptors on the ileal brush border, which recognize and bind the intrinsic factor: cobalamin complex and allow intracellular entry into the enterocyte and subsequent export into the portal circulation bound to transcobalamin II. Cobalamin is taken up by the liver; this is its major storage site in the body. There also is an enterohepatic circulation of vitamin $B_{12}$. In the context of IBD surgical resection of the terminal ileum, obviously, vitamin $B_{12}$ absorption is eliminated. The extent of the surgical resection resulting in cobalamin malabsorption is not known, but usually requires more than 60 cm to be removed for absorption to become impaired. Simply assessing circulating vitamin $B_{12}$ levels may provide an inaccurate picture. The hepatic stores of cobalamin can meet the physiologic requirements for several years, and serum levels may be normal even though there is inadequate intestinal absorption. Interruption of the enterohepatic circulation of vitamin $B_{12}$ may hasten the onset of a deficiency state. These possibilities can be distinguished by a multistep Schilling test (Table 22.1). Patients with documented vitamin $B_{12}$ malabsorption will require parenteral vitamin $B_{12}$ administration for life.

## ILEAL AND COLONIC BRAKE

A negative feedback loop has been described that inhibits duodenal motility when nutrients are infused into the ileum and colon of experimental animals. This has been termed the ileal

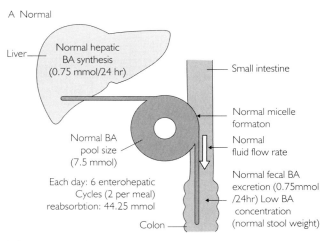

A  Normal

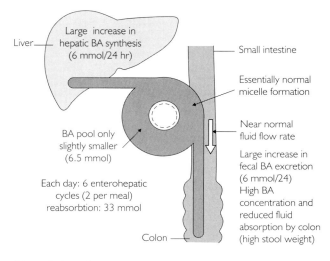

B  Small ileal resection

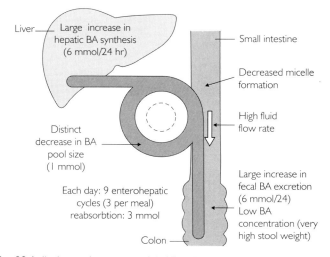

C  Large ileal resection

Fig. 22.1  Ileal resections can result in bile acid malabsorption and will cause secretory diarrhea if bile acid (BA) concentration in the colon becomes high enough. (A) Normal enterohepatic circulation of bile acids. (B) Effect of small (<100 cm) ileal resection, which results in BA malabsorption without interruption of fat digestion or fluid absorption by the small intestine. (C) More substantial ileal resection results in malabsorption of fluid, bile salt, and fat. In this instance, the steatorrhea may overshadow any secretory diarrhea caused by BA malabsorption. (From Schiller LR. Secretory diarrhea. In: Feldman M, ed. Gastroenterology and hepatology: the comprehensive visual reference, Vol 7. Philadelphia: Churchill Livingstone; 1997:4.10, with permission.)

**Table 22.1 Results of Schilling test in different clinical conditions**

| Stage | Normal | Pernicious anemia | Ileal abnormality | Bacterial overgrowth | Pancreatic insufficiency |
|---|---|---|---|---|---|
| Stage I: radioactive vitamin $B_{12}$ | Normal | Decreased | Decreased | Decreased | Decreased |
| Stage II: radioactive vitamin $B_{12}$; IF | NA | Normal | Decreased | Decreased | Decreased |
| Stage III: radioactive vitamin $B_{12}$; pancreatic enzymes | NA | NA | Decreased | Decreased | Normal |
| Stage IV: antibiotics; radioactive vitamin $B_{12}$ | NA | NA | Decreased | Normal | Decreased |

NA, not applicable; IF, = intrinsic factor.

(colonic) brake and may serve as an adaptive response to slow intestinal transit in clinical situations in which there is significant malabsorption, and thus unabsorbed nutrients in the ileum. Recent studies have suggested that there are at least two components to the brake phenomenon, volume-induced and nutrient-induced. Volume-induced effects are mediated via extrinsic nerves.[4] The effect of extrinsic innervation may be mediated through intestinal $5HT_3$ receptors and adrenoreceptors. Nutrient-induced slowing of transit is related to humoral factors, specifically plasma levels of peptide YY, enteroglucagon and the glucagon-like peptides and luminal factors such as short-chain fatty acids.[4] The 'ileal brake' has been shown to continue to function following ileal pouch–anal anastomosis. Fatty acids placed into the ileal pouch slowed gastrointestinal transit and delayed defecation. These effects have clinical applications which will be addressed later.[5] The small intestine has also been shown to have distal and proximal components to the braking mechanism. Fat in the proximal and distal gut inhibits intestinal transit as, respectively, the 'jejunal brake' and the 'ileal brake'. It is known that surgical removal of the distal small intestine induces faster transit times and greater steatorrhea than removal of the proximal small intestine. Studies have shown that intestinal transit was inhibited more potently by fat in the distal than in the proximal half of the gut. Intestinal transit is therefore more potently inhibited by the fat-induced 'ileal brake' than the 'jejunal brake'.[6] These concepts have important clinical application in those patients with short bowels and those who have ileoanal anastomoses.

## LOSS OF ILEOCECAL VALVE

Loss of the ileocecal valve putatively leads to both decreased small bowel transit time and, probably, an increase in anaerobic bacteria in the remaining small intestine, with the development of a bacterial overgrowth syndrome. Bacterial overgrowth may have several significant consequences that potentiate the deleterious effects of ileal resection. Anaerobic bacteria, primarily *Bacteroides*, may compete very successfully with the ileal receptors for cobalamin absorption, decreasing the intraluminal availability of vitamin $B_{12}$. Bacteria will deconjugate bile salts, resulting in physicochemical changes that decrease their bioavailability and efficacy in fat malabsorption. Thus, small bowel

bacterial overgrowth can impair the two ileal-specific absorptive pathways that may already be marginal secondary to resection. Small intestinal bacteria may compete with the host organism for luminal nutrients, metabolizing proteins and carbohydrates before they can be absorbed. When this occurs in the colon it is an integral component of the luminal ecology, providing a mechanism for absorption of SCFA. However, when it occurs in the small intestine the effects are less beneficial. Whether the more rapid small bowel transit associated with loss of the ileal brake and the ileocecal valve overrides the tendency to bacterial contamination of the ileum has not been carefully investigated.

In general, breath tests are the best way to diagnose bacterial overgrowth. A radiolabeled cholylglycine breath test can detect deconjugation of bile salts. A glucose hydrogen breath test will be positive in the presence of significant bacterial metabolism of the test sugar. Unfortunately, the specificity of these tests in Crohn's disease is limited by other complicating factors of intestinal physiology.[7]

# PHYSIOLOGICAL EFFECTS OF THE SHORT BOWEL SYNDROME

The small intestine has a considerable reserve capacity for absorption of nutrients and fluids. In addition it exhibits major anatomic and functional adaptive responses (see following discussion) that compensate for loss of absorptive area. However, there is some point beyond which adaptation can no longer suffice, and significant losses of nutrients and fluid occur. The short bowel syndrome (SBS) can be defined as a malabsorption syndrome that results from extensive small intestinal resection. There is a process of adaptation, which involves crypt dilatation, hypertrophy and mucosal hyperplasia, primarily in the region distal to the area of bowel loss. The response of the remaining bowel is mediated by several factors, including luminal nutrition, pancreaticobiliary secretions, luminal growth factors and humoral factors. Generally it occurs when more than 75% of the small intestine is resected or there is less than 120 cm of intestine remaining (Table 22.2). In most patients the duodenum is intact and there is a variable length of jejunum. Specific cases may be affected by the health of the remaining small bowel, the

## Table 22.2 Predicted outcomes after small bowel resection

| Remaining jejunal length | Outcome | |
| --- | --- | --- |
| | Colon present | S/P colectomy |
| 0–50 cm | Total parenteral nutrition | Total parenteral nutrition |
| 50–100 cm | Modified oral diet | IV fluids/minerals or TPN |
| 100–150 cm | Regular diet | Modified oral/regular diet |
| >200 cm | Regular diet | Regular diet |

Source: Adapted from Lennard-Jones JE. Practical management of the short bowel. Aliment Pharmacol Ther 1994;8:563.

adaptive response of the intestine, adherence to specific diets, and the age of the patient. The leading cause of SBS in adults is Crohn's disease. Crohn's disease can account for up to 70% of cases of SBS. Short bowel syndrome in Crohn's disease is similar to that occurring in other diseases.[8] This chapter focuses on several aspects of the SBS that are particularly germane to the IBD patient.

## WATER AND ELECTROLYTE MALABSORPTION

The most clinically disabling problem of the short bowel syndrome is fluid and electrolyte loss, causing diarrhea. Whereas the diarrhea associated with ileal resection tends to be secretory, short bowel syndrome is more commonly due to a predominantly osmotic diarrhea. The proximal small bowel receives about 9 L of fluid per day, of which about 8 L are absorbed. On an unrestricted diet patients with SBS cannot deal with such volumes, leading to torrential diarrhea, hypovolemia, hyponatremia and hypokalemia. The conventional American diet contains many hyperosmolar items: colas, for example, are approximately 700 mmol. Therefore, in the normal course of digestive events the jejunal lumen is exposed to hypertonic fluids from dietary intake that may be exacerbated by digestion into simpler sugars. This results in substantial fluid entry across the epithelium into the intestinal lumen. As the fluid progresses downstream into the more distal jejunum and ileum, this fluid shift normally is reversed. Absorption of sugars, amino acids and sodium 'pulls' water out of the lumen across the epithelium (solvent drag), resulting in net fluid absorption. Of course, if there is significant loss of intestinal surface and length, this reversal cannot occur. Thus, there is generally a large osmotic component to the diarrhea of short bowel syndrome.

The clinical consequences depend to a certain degree on whether ileum or jejunum has been resected; the presence of a colon; and volume depletion-induced hormonal stimulation of sodium absorption. In response to volume depletion there is an increase in circulating mineralocorticoids. Aldosterone stimulates electrogenic sodium absorption, primarily in the rectum and distal colon. There is an ileal adaptive response, with more efficient fluid absorption, but the specific transport mechanisms involved are less clearly defined. The colon can increase its absorption of fluid from a normal 1.5 L/day to 4–6 L/day. Short-chain fatty acids stimulate colonic fluid absorption, and may also play an important role in colonic adaptation. Therefore, preservation of the colon can have significant effects on water and electrolyte loss in patients with SBS. When patients with

## Table 22.3 Causes of ileostomy diarrhea

Stenosis of ileostomy
Osmotic diarrhea (partial small bowel resection)
Recurrence of disease
Loss of ileal brake mechanism
Bacterial overgrowth

Source: Adapted from Schiller LR. Secretory diarrhea. In: Feldman M, ed. Gastroenterology and hepatology. The comprehensive visual reference, Vol 7. Philadelphia: Churchill Livingstone; 1997:4.7.

similar jejunal length are compared, those who have a jejunostomy will have higher requirements of oral or intravenous supplementation than those in whom the colon is intact. The colon also has a role in salvaging unabsorbed/malabsorbed carbohydrates (see below). Persistence of high-output ostomy diarrhea may be a troubling clinical problem (Table 22.3).

## MALABSORPTION

### Carbohydrate, protein and fat

Carbohydrates are absorbed across the enterocytes in the form of monosaccharides after the terminal action of hydrolases located in the brush border of the duodenum and jejunum. Intestinal resection may affect carbohydrate absorption by decreased brush border carbohydrases and by decreased action of available enzymes, owing to shortened intestinal transit time. However, after intestinal adaptation has occurred, adequate mean net carbohydrate absorption of approximately two-thirds of ingested calories occurs as long as there is residual small bowel up to the midjejunum.[9] Large jejunal resections may be associated with lactose malabsorption because lactase is predominantly localized in the jejunum.

Carbohydrates that escape small intestinal absorption are converted to short-chain fatty acids (SCFA) in the colon by bacterial fermentation. In normal individuals this provides 5–10% of dietary sources of energy and is important in maintaining colonic cell viability. This assumes clinical significance in patients with intestinal resection who retain part or all of their colon, and may account for the slightly higher carbohydrate absorption in patients with SBS and residual colon.[10] This process of salvaging carbohydrates can provide an additional 500 kcal/day.

Protein is absorbed primarily as amino acids and peptides through different transport systems and after sequential action by luminal enzymes and brush border enzymes and cytoplasmic peptidases. Amino acids mainly are absorbed in the jejunum, and dipeptides and tripeptides are absorbed in the more distal jejunum and proximal ileum. Patients with 50 cm or less of residual small intestine have net protein absorption that is more than 40% of their dietary intake.[10] Mean net protein absorption after intestinal adaptation in SBS ranges from 60 to 80%.[8,9] Protein absorption is not affected by the presence/absence of the colon in patients with SBS.

Fat absorption occurs mainly in the upper two-thirds of the jejunum. Normal fat absorption not only requires adequate absorptive surface but presupposes optimal pancreatic function, the right intraluminal pH, presence of bile salts, and diffusion of mixed micelles across the unstirred water layer into the microvilli.[11] Fat absorption in SBS patients may exceed 50%.[9,10] Steatorrhea may be observed in patients with more than 100 cm of ileal resection. This occurs because of decreased enterohepatic circulation of bile salts. In the presence of residual colon, excess fatty acids may decrease sodium and water absorption and contribute to diarrhea.

## Calcium

Calcium metabolism is problematic in IBD without the added insult of intestinal resection. Dietary calcium intake often is restricted, whether justified or not. Chronic steroid therapy also impairs calcium absorption. Prolonged restriction of physical activity or bed rest may lead to loss of bone mass. Vitamin D and its metabolites are critical for intestinal calcium absorption. Restricted diets, with avoidance of milk products, and steatorrhea may limit intestinal absorption of vitamin D, and lack of exposure to sunlight may reduce the non-dietary source of vitamin D. Surgical resection, by reducing the absorptive surface area, will have a deleterious effect on calcium absorption. The major impact of marginal deficient calcium absorption is chronic and subtle loss of bone mass, and therefore the full impact of calcium malabsorption may not be fully appreciated until several years after surgery.

Active calcium absorption is restricted primarily to the duodenum and is responsive to changes in calcium balance and modulated by vitamin D. Unlike cobalamin, but similar to bile salts, a large component of calcium absorption is passive and not site specific. Passive calcium absorption occurs throughout the small intestine and, in normal physiology, may be responsible for the majority of calcium absorption. Therefore, although the duodenum is rarely affected by Crohn's disease and is even more rarely the target of surgery, small bowel resection can have a considerable impact on calcium balance. Prospective studies on intestinal calcium absorption in patients undergoing jejunoileal bypass demonstrate a significant decrease in calcium absorption with no functional or surgical changes in the duodenum, emphasizing the importance of the distal reaches of the small intestine in calcium absorption.[12] Additionally, adequate vitamin D intake and levels are critical to maintaining as efficient an absorptive process as possible.

## Iron

The duodenum is the primary site for active iron absorption. Although there is increasing recognition that iron deficiency can result from malabsorption in adults, especially with celiac sprue, iron deficiency in IBD occurs more frequently as a result of

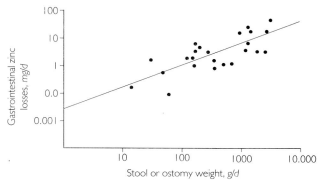

**Fig. 22.2** Relationship between zinc losses and stool output. The gastrointestinal tract is the major route for zinc excretion. Normally, 2–3 mg are excreted in the feces each day. This figure shows the results from a study performed in patients receiving only parenteral feeding, which demonstrated that the amount of zinc lost was proportional to stool or ostomy volume. Patients with massive small bowel resection lost approximately 15 mg of zinc per liter or kilogram of stool or ostomy output. (From Klein S. Nutrient malabsorption. In: Feldman M, ed. Gastroenterology and hepatology: the comprehensive visual reference, Vol 7. Philadelphia: Churchill Livingstone; 1997:5.14, with permission.)

chronic gastrointestinal blood loss. However, iron replacement in patients with IBD is problematic because of the difficulties in tolerating oral iron. Not infrequently such patients may require intravenous iron therapy and/or treatment with erythropoietin.

## Zinc

The potential role of zinc in IBD is twofold: first, the development of zinc deficiency may be secondary to inadequate absorption and loss in diarrheal fluids; second, the zinc deficiency state has a negative impact on intestinal function, perhaps exacerbating the zinc deficiency. In this way, it is much like the megaloblastic anemias that develop with cobalamin and folate deficiency, i.e. the deficiency state develops because of some primary intestinal pathologic change, but once developed it further impairs intestinal function, thereby creating a vicious circle.

Dietary zinc is found in meat, cereals and legumes. In global malabsorption, complexed dietary zinc fails to be released into its soluble form and may therefore be unavailable for absorption. Zinc appears to be absorbed primarily in the distal small intestine. There is an enterohepatic circulation of zinc.[13] Both of these characteristics of zinc absorption put the patient with ileal Crohn's disease at risk. The normal gut responds to zinc deficiency with increased absorption; whether this occurs after ileal resection in Crohn's disease is unclear. Because fecal zinc losses in patients with SBS parallel the volume of diarrhea, this may be the most important factor in creating a negative zinc balance[14] (Fig. 22.2). Assessment of nutritional zinc status is not straightforward: the serum zinc level is affected by inflammatory mediators and serum albumin, among other factors that may be important in Crohn's disease.[15] Although a fully developed clinical presentation of zinc deficiency with acral dermatitis and dysgeusia is uncommon in patients with Crohn's disease, marginal zinc status is probably not a rare finding.[16]

Recent observations have demonstrated structural and functional intestinal abnormalities associated with zinc deficiency that may either cause or exacerbate diarrhea. Zinc may modulate apical ion channels and mucosal permeability in the gut.[17,18] Zinc deficiency appears to increase an endogenous secretory stimulus, uroguanylin, that may increase the severity of diarrhea.[19] Zinc deficiency also may alter intestinal metalloproteinases. The clinical relevance of these findings is emphasized by reports that zinc supplementation reduces the duration and severity of acute diarrheas in young children in India.[20,21] There may be an interplay between inflammatory mediators and zinc deficiency in promoting diarrhea.[22]

## LOSS OF GASTROINTESTINAL HORMONES

Hormones are produced in the intestinal mucosa throughout the GI tract. Gastrin, cholecystokinin, secretin, gastric inhibitory polypeptide and motilin are produced in the proximal tract and regulate secretion and gut motility. The regions of the gut where these hormones are made are not typically affected in SBS patients, and their profiles are normal. However, in those who have undergone massive small bowel resection there have been documented incidences of transient gastric hypersecretion and peptic ulceration. Also, impaired digestion and absorption,[23–25] with high-output jejunostomy, with or without severe metabolic alkalosis,[26] may occur in the immediate postoperative period in patients with SBS. This gastric hypersecretory state has been correlated with increased serum gastrin.[23,27–31] Although several mechanisms have been proposed to explain this transient hypergastrinemia, none is firmly established as the cause. The situation improves with intestinal adaptation, and generally is well controlled with $H_2$-blockers.[24–27] Enteroglucagon, neurotensin and peptide YY are gut hormones produced in the ileum in response to intraluminal fats or carbohydrates, and are lost when the ileum and proximal colon are resected. Both enteroglucagon and peptide YY are involved in the 'ileal brake' phenomenon and cause delay in gastric emptying. Therefore, loss of these hormones may explain the altered motility, rapid intestinal transit time and rapid gastric emptying seen in patients with SBS.

## KIDNEY STONES: OXALATE AND URATE

Patients with IBD have an increased incidence of renal stone formation (oxalate and uric acid). The incidence is further increased by intestinal resections or ileostomy.[32–34] The risk of forming stones depends on the saturation of urine with the various stone-forming salts and the effect of inhibiting versus promoting factors for stone growth. Uric acid stones constitute 60% of the stones found in patients with ileostomy. The intestinal loss of water, sodium and bicarbonate in these patients causes reduced pH and urine volume, which results in relative supersaturation of uric acid.[35,36] Actually, the 24-hour uric acid secretion from these patients is not high, but because the urinary pH is lower than the pKa for uric acid, uric acid crystallization can readily occur. Compared with control subjects, patients with either an ileostomy or a J pouch had significantly lowered urine volumes and pH, higher concentrations of calcium and oxalate, and an increased risk of forming uric acid stones.[37] In contrast to J-pouch patients, ileostomy patients had an increased risk of forming calcium stones. This may be related to a significantly decreased concentration of glycosaminoglycans (GAG) in these patients.[37] GAG are high molecular weight anions that form part of the connective tissue matrix and may be important because they inhibit stone formation by retarding crystal growth.

Calcium oxalate stone formation is related to both increased urinary concentrations of oxalate and decreased concentration of inhibitors of crystal growth, such as citrate[38] and magnesium.[33,38,39] Fat malabsorption secondary to bile acid deficiency in SBS patients leads to an increased risk of oxalate stone formation when the colon is preserved. The presence of bile salts and fatty acids in the colon may also increase the permeability to oxalate. In the presence of fat malabsorption calcium binds preferentially to fatty acids, leaving oxalate in a more soluble form, sodium oxalate, which is absorbed.[40] Enteric hyperoxaluria is at maximum level after ileal resection of 50 cm or more.[39] About a quarter of patients with SBS and a preserved colon will develop symptomatic kidney stones within 2 years of surgery.[41,42]

## GALLSTONES

Gallstones occur in as many as 30–40% of patients with SBS. In patients with IBD undergoing ileal resection or ileostomy, the enterohepatic circulation of bile acids is disturbed. When hepatic synthesis of bile acids cannot compensate for the increased losses, the bile acid pool decreases, leading to precipitation of cholesterol crystals and subsequent stone formation. Another factor that can contribute to decreased bile acids in these patients is bacterial colonization, which causes deconjugation of bile acids. Similar to findings in the general population, Kurchin et al.,[43] in their retrospective study of 152 ileostomates with inflammatory disease, found age (over 50 years) and female sex to be significant risk factors for cholelithiasis. They did not demonstrate the significance of other factors, perhaps owing to the small sample size, difficulty in measuring residual small bowel, and misdiagnosis of Crohn's colitis as chronic ulcerative colitis.

Contrary to most preconceptions, there also is an increased risk of pigment stone formation in these patients.[44–47] Experimental studies have provided some insight into the mechanisms involved. Pitt et al. studied adult male prairie dogs subjected to ileal resection or sham surgery and showed that the cholesterol saturation index in gallbladder bile was no different in these two groups.[47] However, calcium and total bilirubin concentrations in gallbladder bile were significantly greater in dogs with ileal resection than in those with sham surgery, putting them at increased risk for pigment stone formation.[47]

## PHYSIOLOGICAL EFFECTS OF COLECTOMY

Colectomy is performed in inflammatory bowel disease. The surgical variants include ileostomy with or without pouch, ileorectal anastomosis or ileal pouch–anal anastomosis (IPAA). In patients with Crohn's colitis the continent ileostomy and IPAA operations are contraindicated. For patients with ulcerative colitis a proctocolectomy with ileostomy, or IPAA can return the majority to good health and remove the risk of subsequent malignancy.

The colon is often thought of as a simple reservoir, but it has several complex functions that can be more fully appreciated after surgical intervention. Patients undergoing both small and large intestine resections fare worse than those who only have a small bowel resection.[48] A major function of the intact large intestine is to absorb water and electrolytes. After colectomy almost a liter of nearly isotonic ileostomy fluid may be excreted, resulting in a chronic salt and water loss. This is compensated to some extent by activation of the renin–angiotensin–aldosterone system, which increases sodium absorption in the ileum.

## SHORT-CHAIN FATTY ACIDS

Colonic bacteria metabolize unabsorbed carbohydrate, protein and fiber, forming short-chain fatty acids (SCFA), hydrogen and carbon dioxide. This is an important function of the large bowel. The SCFA, primarily acetate, proprionate and butyrate, are weak electrolytes that constitute approximately two-thirds of the colonic anion concentration (70–130 mmol/L). SCFA are important in the colonic ecology and in various systemic metabolic functions. The recognition that luminal SCFA concentrations are significantly decreased in severe ulcerative colitis has led to an increased interest in the potential role of these compounds in IBD.

SCFA, particularly butyrate, are the preferred metabolic substrate for colonocytes. Roediger[49] has hypothesized that colitis is a relative nutritional deficiency state resulting from impaired butyrate utilization.

SCFA are critical in the understanding of the physiological properties of dietary fiber and its possible role in colorectal cancer. SCFA production and absorption are related to the nourishment of the colonocytes, sodium and water absorption, and potential mechanisms of diarrhea. It was once assumed that SCFA contributed to or exacerbated the diarrhea of carbohydrate malabsorption, but this is not the case. SCFA are rapidly absorbed in vivo, enhancing sodium and water absorption while stimulating bicarbonate secretion. The specific in vitro transport mechanisms have not been fully defined, but probably involve either $Na^+$–$H^+$ exchangers or anion transport linked to bicarbonate. SCFA cause an increase in the expression of sodium/hydrogen membrane exchangers in the apical membrane of the epithelial cells.[50] SCFA exert this effect only on colonic epithelial cells, and not in the ileum. Therefore this adaptive mechanism is restricted to the colon. SCFA are integral to fluid absorption in the colon; changes in SCFA production, utilization, and concentration may alter the propensity to diarrhea in colitis.

Patients with an intact colon and severe carbohydrate malabsorption compensate by metabolizing osmotically active saccharides to SCFA, which are readily absorbed and used as a source of energy. SCFA production from dietary carbohydrates is a mechanism that can produce considerable amounts of calories. Given a typical Western diet approximately 10% of total caloric value may be supplied when fiber, carbohydrate and protein are converted to SCFA and are absorbed in the colon. For high-fiber diets the proportion may be greater. This salvage pathway provides the physiologic basis for the high-carbohydrate low-fat diets prescribed for SBS. SCFA formation depends on the colon. For ileostomy patients bacterial metabolism of carbohydrates is negligible, which leads to a significant loss of potential calories in the ileostomy fluid. Thus removal of the colon will prevent the salvage mechanism from occurring and will lead to loss of calories and significant diarrhea in SBS and ileoanal anastomosis patients. Diminished production of SCFA is also associated with antibiotic-associated diarrhea, diversion colitis, and possibly pouchitis.

SCFA have been shown to be a differentiating agent in cancer cell lines but a proliferative and an antiapoptotic factor

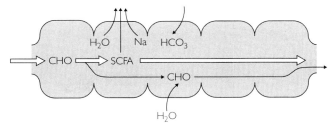

**Fig. 22.3** Short-chain fatty acids (SCFA) arise from carbohydrate (CHO) not absorbed in the small intestine that is then converted by colonic bacteria to acetate, propionate, butyrate, $H_2$ and $CO_2$. SCFA are rapidly absorbed by the normal colon and also stimulate Na and $H_2O$ absorption along with bicarbonate ($HCO_3$) secretion. This process may be disrupted by (1) insufficient bacterial conversion of CHO to SCFA, due to either massive small bowel CHO malabsorption or inefficient bacterial metabolism (e.g. antibiotics), or (2) epithelial dysfunction or loss of surface area. This may result in diarrhea, due either to an osmolar driving force (CHO malabsorption) or to failure to adequately absorb Na in the colon.

in normal epithelium. SCFA have been postulated to be the link between fiber and decreased colon cancer risk. SCFA also stimulate motor activity in the terminal ileum and the colon.[51] The motility effects may be modulated by release of peptide YY[52] (Fig. 22.3). SCFA are clearly trophic factors for the colon, and in all probability for the small bowel as well. This has clinical importance when considering 'bowel rest' as a management option in IBD.[53] In the course of complex surgery for Crohn's disease, a colonic pouch diverted from the fecal stream may be created during the formation of an ileostomy or colostomy. This segment becomes at risk for diversion colitis, a clinical syndrome of abdominal pain and bloody diarrhea. SCFA may be an effective therapy for diversion colitis, suggesting that the presence of luminal SCFA is necessary for epithelial integrity.[54] However, several studies have also shown no benefit for this form of therapy.[55,56]

## MINERAL METABOLISM

Although not generally considered as a site for mineral absorption, the colon absorbs significant amounts of calcium, primarily in the cecum and proximal colon.[57] Colonic calcium absorption plays a minor role in the normal gut but assumes greater importance in malabsorption and short bowel syndrome.[58]

# PHYSIOLOGICAL EFFECTS OF ILEAL POUCH–ANAL ANASTOMOSIS

Ileal pouch–anal anastomosis (IPAA) has become the operation of choice following proctocolectomy for ulcerative colitis and familial adenomatous polyposis. The aim of this surgical technique is to preserve anal sphincter function and thus maintain continence. The adaptive changes in the pouch mucosa are due to either an altered luminal environment or the onset of acute/chronic inflammation known as pouchitis. The concept and etiology of ileal adaptation, with further examples, is discussed below. The IPAA may in part substitute for the functions of the removed colon. Pouches are colonized by bacterial flora similar to colonic bacteria. Both dehydration and renal sodium retention are seen to a lesser extent in patients with IPAA than in those with ileorectal anastomosis. In those patients with an IPAA, conservation of energy from malabsorbed substrate may be similar to that in healthy subjects.[59]

## MORPHOLOGIC CHANGES IN IPAA

The physiologic and anatomic consequences of the construction of an ileal pouch are intriguing, from both a basic science and a clinical perspective. The creation of a pouch results in stasis of fecal material and colonization with fecal flora, thereby forming a new ileal environment. The process of adaptation of the terminal ileum to its neorectal function is accompanied by a gradual transformation to colonic-type mucosa, with progressive flattening of ileal villi and an increase in crypt size and number. Three basic patterns of mucosal adaptation have been observed and are given in Table 22.4.[60] These reflect chronic changes in the pouch mucosa over a period of several years. Although ileal pouches acquire certain colonic characteristics, complete colonic metaplasia does not occur.[61] The degree of colonic metaplasia in ileoanal pouches is variable. Goblet cells and enlarged Paneth's cells with atypical granules are seen. Goblet cells will acquire colon characteristics even in the absence of inflammation. Villous atrophy, mucin changes and chronic inflammation occur to varying degrees in all patients with IPAA, whereas pouchitis tends to affect those with a history of ulcerative colitis.

In some patients with ulcerative colitis the mucosa of the pouch adapts with constant severe villous atrophy accompanied by long-standing pouchitis. The combination of chronic inflammation and colonic metaplasia over time may lead to cell atypia and dysplasia. The incidence of dysplasia in a pouch remains to be determined. Low-grade dysplasia has occurred in a small number of patients with the type C response.[62] A recent study portrayed the risk as minimal even after 15–20 years from the time the pouch was formed.[63,64] It is difficult to delineate whether villous atrophy is a direct result of pouchitis, or whether, because of the altered luminal environment, villous atrophy leads to pouchitis through bacterial interaction with the mucosa and/or malabsorption and malutilization of luminal nutrients.[65] There is an increase in the number of peptide YY-positive cells in pouch mucosa. Peptide YY is known to inhibit gastrointestinal motility and transit. Delayed transit time and crypt elongation are manifestations of intestinal adaptation that assist in optimizing the absorption of luminal contents.[66] Despite

the presence of chronic inflammation in the majority of patients with IPAA, the functional adaptation with reduced permeability occurs primarily in conjunction with colonic metaplasia.[65]

## METABOLIC CHANGES IN IPAA

The degree of mucosal adaptation that may occur in response to changes in nutrient supply and fecal stasis, after the formation of an ileoanal pouch, is variable and still being studied.

The major nutrients for the colon and small bowel mucosa are butyrate and glutamine, respectively. Ileoanal pouch construction, with subsequent bacterial colonization and fecal stasis, results in a significant reduction in the ability to oxidize glutamine, whereas there is no difference in the rate of butyrate oxidation.[67] SCFA concentrations in the pouch are similar to those in the normal fecal stream. Pouch adaptation gradually increases SCFA production and concentration severalfold, and reaches concentrations normally found in non-colectomized individuals after approximately 1 year.[68] There is also major adaptation in the form of increased water and electrolyte absorption.[69] The ability to increase absorption is related to the increased SCFA production. The bacterial production of SCFA is low in non-adapted pouches, resulting in low concentrations of SCFA comparable to concentrations found in conventional ileostomies.

Within the pouch there are alterations in bile acid absorption, resulting from its mucosa adapting to assume the functional characteristics of normal colon, thereby making it less able to participate in enterohepatic circulation. The absorption of bile acids decreases by up to 83% in some patients, consistent with the progressive transformation of ileal to colonic function.[70] The relative reduction in bile acid absorption is lower after IPAA than after ileostomy.[71] Forty per cent of patients will have increased fecal bile acid excretion. Although there is moderate bile acid deconjugation within the pouch, malabsorption will still occur in about one-third to half of patients because the loss of bile acids may be greater than the hepatic compensatory response.[72] These changes are not as frequent in those patients with less severe villous abnormalities. Moderate steatorrhea is present in 30% of the patients by 3 months postoperatively, but fecal fat excretion will normalize with time. Calcium absorption remains normal in all patients regardless of time after operation, but substitution therapy with vitamin $B_{12}$ is necessary in about one-third of patients.

## FUNCTIONAL CHANGES IN IPAA

Stool studies on patients with IPAA have shown an increase in stool mass (median 609 g/24 h) which is found in nearly all patients and does not change with time. Stool frequency after IPAA adaptation is about 5/day during the first year. Stool frequency depends on stool volume and pouch capacity and not on the design of the pouch.[73] For the majority of patients evacuation is spontaneous and as complete as in healthy persons. Two-thirds of patients are perfectly continent, but 19% have to wear incontinence pads because of intermittent leakage. Complete incontinence is reported in only 0–4% of patients. Despite altered reflex activity, stool discrimination is preserved in most patients.

The ileal mucosa within the pouch must change its role from an absorptive surface to a unit with storage capacity. There are limited observations concerning the functional consequences of

| Table 22.4 Patterns of mucosal adaptation in an ileal pouch | |
|---|---|
| **Type of metaplasia** | **Description** |
| A | Normal ileal mucosa or mild villous atrophy and no or mild inflammation |
| B | Transient atrophy with moderate or severe villous atrophy followed by some degree of normalization |
| C | Persistent atrophy with permanent subtotal or total villous atrophy accompanied by crypt hyperplasia and severe pouchitis |

Source: Adapted from Veress B et al. Long-term histomorphological surveillance of the pelvic ileal pouch: dysplasia develops in a subgroup of patients. Gastroenterology 1995;109(4):1090–1097.

the pouch.[68,74] Lerch et al., in 1989,[70] reported their experience regarding morphologic and functional changes in the residual small bowel and ileal pouch 3 years after total colectomy. They noted decreased frequency of bowel movements with time and showed that the size of the pouch inversely correlated with the number of bowel movements per 24 hours. There is some difference in pouch emptying time between patients with and without pouchitis. Patients with acute pouchitis that responded to metronidazole therapy were found to have a trend toward a prolonged pouch emptying time compared with those without pouchitis. Ileal pouch anastomosis for ulcerative colitis results in increased stool mass in all patients. This suggests that there is a link between the development of mucosal inflammation and delayed pouch emptying.[75]

## POUCHITIS: PATHOPHYSIOLOGY AND METABOLIC CONSEQUENCES

Inflammation is expected as a consequence of the transformation of the normal ileum to a reservoir with uncleared bacterial flora. The question is, when does the expected increase in inflammatory cells become abnormal? In a subset of patients with colectomy and creation of a surgical pouch a clinical syndrome of diarrhea, rectal bleeding and abdominal cramping develops, designated as pouchitis. This is described in detail in Chapter 44. Pouchitis is strongly associated with villous atrophy. Similar atrophy, however, is seen in the mucosa of the pouch without inflammation, representing colonic metaplasia and adaptation to a new luminal environment. The underlying causes are unknown. The histological picture in pouchitis is highly variable.

There is a lower SCFA concentration in pouchitis patients. The 24-hour production of total SCFA in patients with pouchitis can be increased by the addition of saccharides to the local environment. Pouch concentrations of saccharides are normally reduced in pouchitis owing to dilution, because of increased water and electrolyte output, and therefore whether this is a cause or effect of the pouchitis is unclear.[76] Metabolic consequences after IPAA are closely associated with the degree of pouchitis, the grade of villous atrophy and the extent of inflammation in the remaining ileum. Pouchitis will lead to decreased vitamin $B_{12}$, bile acid and cholesterol absorption. In IPAA patients with subtotal or total villous atrophy secondary to pouchitis, serum levels of albumin, calcium, triglycerides and vitamin E are reduced. Vitamin D deficiency is seen in 10%, and vitamin A and $B_{12}$ deficiency in approximately 5%. Bile acid and vitamin $B_{12}$ absorption rates are lowest in those patients with inflammation in the proximal limb of the pouch.[77]

Risk factors identified for pouchitis include the presence of extraintestinal manifestations, primary sclerosing cholangitis, cessation of smoking, and previous course of the disease. Several pathophysiological pathways have been identified as potential mechanisms of pouchitis, but the topic is still controversial. These mechanisms include inflammatory mediators, adhesion molecules, oxygen radical species, pANCA, and SCFA. The microflora in the pouch is also an important factor in causing inflammation.[78] Mucosal lesions of pouchitis are characterized by a neutrophil infiltrate. Interleukin (IL)-8 is a key mediator in neutrophil recruitment and is downregulated by IL-10. Histologic lesions of pouchitis are associated with a mucosal imbalance between IL-8 and IL-10. IL-10 could be proposed as a new treatment for pouchitis to restore this balance.[79] Induction of nitric oxide synthase-2 (NOS-2) correlates with both the clinical degree of pouchitis and the severity of acute inflammation. NOS-3 activity is increased in all pouchitis groups.[80] Prostaglandins are synthesized by cyclooxygenase-2 (COX-2) and are also involved in the inflammatory process. COX-2 and NOS-2 are both increased in normal IPAA and in pouchitis, compared with healthy subjects.[81]

## INTESTINAL ADAPTATION

Intestinal adaptation is the process by which the gut undergoes significant changes to maintain nutritional and fluid balance in the most economical manner. Although intestinal adaptation is more commonly thought of in terms of modified function after surgical resections, the normal gut exhibits adaptation in response to changes in the luminal environment. Unlike bacteria, vertebrate cells are exposed to an almost constant external medium; the exception, of course, is the intestinal epithelium, which is routinely challenged by dramatic changes in its extracellular environment. Thus, in a broader sense, the gut is constantly adapting.

Adaptation can take many directions. It generally is assumed that the gut has a huge reserve capacity to absorb nutrients; however, Diamond has argued that this is an overestimation, and that such an overcapacity would be evolutionarily inefficient.[82] In response to either an isolated deficiency state or low luminal concentrations, the gut can upregulate transporters to increase the efficiency of intestinal absorption. This occurs most notably with iron deficiency.

In contrast, the gut will respond to changes in diet composition with changes in brush border enzymes critical to digestion. The most striking examples of this are during weaning and hibernation.[83] During the postnatal period in sheep, as the diet changes from milk to grass, there is a decrease in the in vitro glucose uptake and a decline in the lamb's intestinal $Na^+$-glucose co-transporter. However, this decline can be prevented by maintaining the post-weanling sheep on a milk diet.[84] This suggests that luminal nutrient supply and composition will modify the absorptive machinery in the intestinal epithelium to appropriately accommodate (i.e. adapt to) changes in the diet. With intestinal hypertrophy, there is global adaptation with a generalized upregulation of epithelial digestive enzymes and transporters.

Surgical resection of the small intestine entrains a series of adaptive responses to maintain adequate absorption of nutrients and fluids. Although this adaptation usually is effective in general absorptive processes, it does not occur with specialized, geographically discrete functions, such as cobalamin or calcium absorption. The occurrence of an adaptive response in 'enterohormones' after surgical resection is less clear. For example, what is the impact of jejunal resection on cholecystokinin or secretin function?

The different surgical techniques mentioned so far all lead to changes in the small bowel in terms of remaining length or in terms of asking it to perform a 'new role', as seen in IPAA. There is strong evidence that humoral factors play an important role in intestinal adaptation; characterization of the nature of the humoral factors and their relationship with other influences such as luminal nutrition and pancreaticobiliary secretions may facilitate the development of new therapeutic strategies for the short bowel syndromes. The following sections will summarize the adaptive changes seen in the small bowel after resection and will detail the numerous regulatory factors that allow such changes to occur.

## MORPHOLOGIC CHANGES IN ADAPTATION

After extensive small bowel resections morphologic changes consist of an increase in crypt cellularity without an increase in the total number of crypts, resulting in increased villus height and crypt depth.[85] This change is associated with an increased rate of mitosis, with increased DNA, RNA and protein content in the intestinal mucosa per unit length.[85] What happens may be likened to remodeling of the epithelium, because no corresponding increase in apoptosis or exfoliation of mucosal cells occurs to accommodate the increased proliferation. The muscle layer of the intestine is likewise affected with hyperplasia, which is most prominent in the longitudinal muscle layer. These changes lead to increased circumference and length of the residual small bowel (Fig. 22.4). The end result is a compensatory adaptation to maintain absorptive capacity. The absorptive surface area may increase by as much as 70%. The level of increase will depend on the remaining length of intestine and the time course. Interestingly, there is a lag between the increase in cell numbers and the expected corresponding increase in cellular transport proteins. When normalized to the increase in ileal surface area, the flux of $Na^+$ and $Cl^-$ is seen to be generally lower. Therefore, following intestinal resection the upregulation of intestinal cell transports for $Na^+$, $Cl^-$ and glucose absorption are relatively diminished.

The role of apoptosis in adaptation is still controversial. Recent studies have shown that adaptation is essentially a balance of intestinal cell proliferation and apoptosis, and that after small bowel resection the influence of both is important.[86–88]

## MOTILITY CHANGES IN ADAPTATION

Unlike morphologic changes, the motility changes after extensive small bowel resection are not as well defined, but there are adaptive responses. Studies on motility after small bowel resection have utilized either the transit time of radioactive markers or electromyographic (EMG) studies. Animal studies demonstrate that, in general, proximal resections are better tolerated than distal ones in terms of recovery of functional motility.[89–92]

Similar studies performed in humans emphasize the role of intestinal motility in the development of adaptation after small bowel resection. Schmidt et al.[93] described 24-hour manometry findings in 13 patients with limited ileal resections, followed for a mean of 15 months after surgery, and compared this with findings in 50 healthy subjects. They made use of changes observed in the migrating motor complex (MMC), i.e. a band of regular contractions that migrate periodically from the stomach to the distal small intestine during fasting.[94] Persons with extensive ileal resection demonstrate a shorter MMC cycle and a shorter duration but normal frequency and amplitude of postprandial response. The early postprandial return of phase III

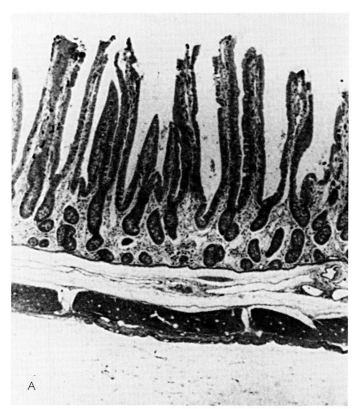
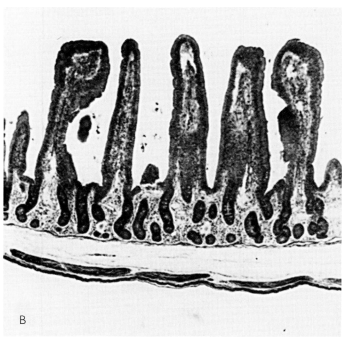

**Fig. 22.4** (A) Photomicrograph of the ileum of a pig 5 weeks after 75% small bowel resection. (B) Photomicrograph of the ileum of a normal pig. Note the taller, thinner, and more numerous villi, slightly deeper crypts, and thicker muscle layers in A that occur with adaptation. (From Collins JB et al. Short bowel syndrome. Semin Pediatr Surg 1995; 4:61, with permission.)

activity of the MMC may account for decreased intestinal transit time, which may contribute to malabsorption and diarrhea in patients with extensive resections and SBS. In dogs with massive proximal small bowel resection the major adaptive response was markedly delayed gastroduodenal emptying with subsequent decreases in intestinal flow rates, suggesting that SBS may elicit a feedback mechanism to control gastric function. The modifications in postprandial motor activity of the small bowel appear more rapidly and are more pronounced after jejunal resection than after ileal resection.

## REGULATION OF INTESTINAL ADAPTATION

Several factors may modify the process of intestinal adaptation (Table 22.5). The length of resection – or expressed as the inverse, the length of remaining small bowel – is clearly a factor. The age of the patient may play a role: younger patients may exhibit more of an adaptive response. The portion of bowel removed (jejunum versus ileum) may affect how well the patient does. Time after resection may be important. In experimental animals the adaptive response begins within 24–48 hours, with crypt hyperplasia and villus lengthening. The

adaptive response may continue for several months, but after a certain length of time the process plateaus. This becomes a critical factor to consider when contemplating therapeutic interventions in patients with short bowel syndrome. The effect of a particular intervention may be quite different early or late in the course of the adaptive process. Finally, the role of luminal nutrients is critical.

## NUTRIENTS

The presence of nutrients in the small intestinal lumen is necessary for adaptation. The quantity of nutrients may be a factor. It also appears that the type of nutrient may be important. The intestine seems to have adopted a Puritan ethic in the process of adaptation: work is good. Complex nutrients that require more digestion are more potent stimuli for adaptation. Disaccharides are more effective in stimulating adaptation than their component monosaccharides.[95] In a comparison of the relative stimulatory effects of carbohydrate, protein and fat in jejunectomized rats, fat provided the most potent stimulus to mucosal growth.[96] Intravenous SCFA have been shown to enhance intestinal adaptation after 80% small bowel resections

**Table 22.5 Endocrine/paracrine/autocrine factors in intestinal adaptation**

| Factors | Observed effects |
|---|---|
| Cholecystokinin (CCK) | CCK levels rise with increasing percentage gut resection, stimulate pancreaticobiliary secretions |
| Corticosteroids | Impair mucosal hyperplasia |
| Epidermal growth factor (EGF) | Increased cell proliferation, increased disaccharidase, increased ornithine decarboxylase expression |
| Enteroglucagon | Parallel between adaptive response and enteroglucagon levels |
| Gastrin | Increase in colonic epithelial proliferation (?) |
| Growth hormone | Mucosal weight, DNA, protein, and sucrase activity increase |
| Insulin-like growth factor | Body weight gain; hyperplasia of duodenojejunum; increased ileal activity of sucrase, maltase, and leucine aminopeptidase leucine aminopeptidase |
| Neurotensin | Postprandial elevations; 'pharmacologic' effects on proximal small intestinal proliferation |
| Prostaglandin $E_2$ | Increase in mucosal weight protein, DNA, and disaccharidase levels in distal ileum |
| Somatostatin | Inhibits postresectional hyperplasia |
| Testosterone | Enhance weight gain, increase in hyperplasia |
| Transforming growth factor-α | Effects through EGF receptor |
| Vasoactive intestinal polypeptide | Reduced by about 50% after small bowel resection. VIP is an inhibitory transmitter[110] |
| Neurotensin | Potentiates the growth of intestinal villi and accelerates the trophic response after bowel resection[115] |
| Secretin and cholecystokinin | Trophic effect on intestinal adaptation[116,117] |

Source: Adapted from Wolvekamp MIC, Heineman E, Taylor RG et al. Towards understanding the process of intestinal adaptation. Dig Dis 1996;14:59.

in rats. Even though the delivery was not luminal, the ileal RNA/DNA concentration and ileal proglucagon were elevated within 24 hours of starting the infusion. Glucose transporter-2 (GLUT-2) mRNA was significantly higher. Sodium-glucose cotransporter (SGLT-1) and uptake of D-glucose did not differ.[97] Delivery of SCFA may have some therapeutic advantage.

## GLUTAMINE

Much of the recent advance in our understanding of intestinal adaptation after surgery has been based on delineating specific factors – luminal, hormonal or paracrine – that are critical to the ability of the gut to respond in an appropriate adaptive manner (Fig. 22.5). Several intraluminal substances have been implicated in promoting intestinal adaptation.[98] Glutamine deserves special mention because it is the principal metabolic fuel for the small bowel. Experimentally, glutamine has been shown to stimulate electrogenic and electroneutral NaCl absorption. It has been shown to have beneficial effects on mucosal function and repair, especially in conditions associated with gut stress.[98] Glutamine enhances intestinal blood flow, and this may be another mechanism favoring intestinal adaptation.[99]

Intestinal adaptation after extensive small bowel resection is augmented by the provision of diets supplemented with glutamine, which may significantly enhance adaptive ileal hyperplasia. Synergistic effects have been shown with insulin-like growth factors (IGF-1) and/or growth hormone, supporting the concept that specific gut-trophic nutrients and growth factors work together to enhance intestinal adaptation via an enteral axis.[100,101] In rat models, growth hormone treatment significantly increased the plasma insulin-like growth factor 1 (IGF-1) level, body weight, jejunal and ileal villous height and mucosal thickness. Glutamine supplementation alone did not produce a significant difference. When combined with GH treatment, glutamine supplementation did lead to increased body weight,

plasma IGF-1 level, jejunal and ileal villous height and mucosal thickness. Therefore, after massive small bowel resection in rats, enteral glutamine supplementation alone has a marginal adaptive effect on the bowel remnant. However, in combination with GH there was the predicted gut-trophic effect.[102]

The clinical data on glutamine as a therapeutic modality in SBS are not definitive. Byrne et al. showed improved nutrient absorption, decreased stool output and reduced total parental nutrition (TPN) requirements in patients with severe SBS treated with a combination of growth hormone (GH), glutamine and a modified high-fiber, high-carbohydrate diet.[103,104] It was difficult to distinguish the individual effects of these three factors. However, Scolapio et al., in a randomized, double-blind placebo-controlled crossover study of eight patients with SBS similarly treated with GH, glutamine and a high-carbohydrate, low-fat diet, found no significant effects on small bowel morphology, stool losses or macronutrient absorption.[105] Several critical and confounding variables preclude definitive assessment: the length of small bowel remaining, underlying disease, the presence or absence of colon, and duration of the SBS. Each of these may alter the results of a potential therapeutic intervention. For example, in the Scolapio study patients were studied more than 10 years from their surgery. Would intervention in the first year make a difference in intestinal adaptation? It is unclear whether glutamine, GH or other stimulants would increase the intestinal adaptation that occurs normally after resection.[106]

## HORMONE-MEDIATED ADAPTATION

Strong evidence for a humoral or hormonal component to intestinal adaptation is based on the observation that there is increased crypt cell production in Thiry–Vella fistulae when additional resection of a segment of the bowel in continuity is performed.[107,108] Likewise, parabiotic vascular studies in rats show increased mucosal proliferation and DNA synthesis in the recipient small bowel after small bowel resection in the donor rat.[109] Different hormones have attracted interest, in the hope of explaining and understanding the changes associated with intestinal adaptation.

As mentioned earlier, following small bowel resection the adaptation of intestinal digestive and absorptive function does not parallel the degree of mucosal hyperplasia. Administration of epidermal growth factor to rats, however, can substantially increase glucose absorption by increasing membrane transport.[110] This hormone is among several others that are implicated in enhancing ileal adaptation. Increased basal and postprandial levels of gastrin, cholecystokinin (CCK), glucose-dependent insulinotropic peptide (GIP), peptide YY and enteroglucagon are seen at 1 month after small bowel resection. In contrast, no significant changes are seen in concentrations of secretin, motilin, neurotensin, somatostatin or glucagon. Enteroglucagon, GIP and peptide YY will remain high, whereas gastrin and CCK levels are usually normal by 3 months.

### Enteroglucagon

Recognition of the importance of enteroglucagon in adaptation was somewhat serendipitous. A patient with an enteroglucagon-secreting tumor presented with small bowel dilatation and villous hyperplasia, which normalized with removal of the

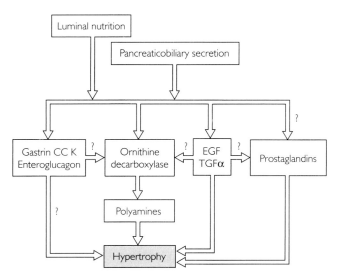

**Fig. 22.5** Intestinal adaptation. Interrelationships between the major factors concerned with inducing mucosal hypertrophy, such as may follow intestinal resection. (From Marsh IVIN, Riley SA. Digestion and absorption of nutrients and vitamins. In: Feldman M et al., eds. Gastrointestinal and liver disease, 6th edn, Vol. II. Philadelphia: WB Saunders; 1998: 1493, with permission.)

tumor.[111] The enteroglucagon family represents a group of prohormones and hormones. Enteroglucagon, which is synthesized in the L cells of the intestinal mucosa, is thought to be an important humoral factor. The increase in peptide YY and enteroglucagon in portal blood supports their role in postresectional adaptation. There is an excellent correlation between states of hyperproliferation in the small intestine (e.g. resection, sprue) and circulating enteroglucagon levels. Enteroglucagon appears to be elevated in proportion to the degree of adaptation. In rats after gut resection, enteroglucagon was elevated and the degree of elevation correlated closely with the crypt cell production rate. Thus, enteroglucagon is the most attractive candidate for hormonal regulation of adaptation, but whether it is a stimulatory factor, a secondary response factor, or simply an epiphenomenon needs to be determined. In addition to enteroglucagon, families of proglucagon-like peptides may be involved.[112] Glucagon-like peptides-1 (GLP-1) and -2 are a part of the enteroglucagon family. GLP-1 and GLP-2 are insulinotropic hormones which are secreted from endocrine cells of the intestinal mucosa in relation to meal ingestion. They are potent inhibitors of gastrointestinal secretion and motility, and assist in mediation of the 'ileal brake'. This slowing down of ileal transit time is an adaptive effect on the remnant small bowel.[113] GLP-2 has a more trophic effect than GLP-1, and will induce mucosal hyperplasia as well as enhancing the rate and magnitude of the proximal intestinal adaptive response following bowel resection. This has been reproduced in studies where the action of native GLP-2 has been prolonged, resulting in significant intestinotrophic effects, such as increases in cell numbers, crypt/villus architecture and RNA concentration.[114]

## Peptide YY

Peptide YY is a gastrointestinal hormone secreted from intestinal L cells.[115] It is released in response to intraluminal nutrients from the distal intestine, and via a neurohormonal pathway in the proximal intestine. Its major function is inhibition of small bowel motility. After small bowel resection, basal and postprandial peptide YY concentrations are greatly elevated. This occurs as a result of an increased amount of peptide YY per L cell and an increased postprandial response.[116] Peptide YY release from the distal intestine does not have an adaptive trophic response but suppresses gastric acid secretion and gastric motility,[117] and stimulates pancreatic secretion. After proctocolectomy, peptide YY levels are initially reduced, as the colon also contains peptide YY-producing cells.[116] The levels gradually increase with time, contributing to adaptation of the digestive organs to the new condition. Moderately elevated peptide YY levels are seen in patients with inflammatory bowel disease and those recovering from acute infective diarrhea. These changes highlight the adaptive response peptide YY has in other digestive disorders. There are several forms of circulating peptide YY, each with different bioactivity but with the same overall effect.[118]

## Somatostatin

Somatostatin is a peptide with diverse inhibitory functions from which various clinical uses are derived. Although it may be tempting to use this agent in the immediate postoperative period to decrease excessive fluid losses in patients with extensive small bowel resection, this may be ill-advised because of observed interference with morphologic changes of intestinal adaptation.[119] The intestinal adaptation seen after colectomy is associated with lower somatostatin and higher growth hormone plasma levels. Hodin et al.[120] tried to elucidate the mechanism by which somatostatin exerts its antiproliferative effect. Somatostatin inhibits epidermal growth factor (EGF)-induced proliferation of rat crypt cells (IEC-6) by decreased production of c-*fos*, c-*jun*, and *jun-B* gene expression. Inhibition of other gut hormones or secretions (e.g. pancreaticobiliary secretion) may be possible.

## Growth hormone

Growth hormone (GH) will increase the number of proliferating cells and crypt and villus length. GH can markedly increase the trophic response of intestinal mucosa after bowel resection, and will enhance morphologic and proliferative adaptation.[121] After small bowel resection, absorption depends on how fast the mucosal adaptation takes place. Morphologic changes include mucosal thickness, villus height, crypt depth, and the villous surface area of the residual bowel. The underlying mechanisms involve increased proliferation and decreased apoptosis.[102] Wheeler and Challacombe also demonstrated increased crypt cell proliferation in human duodenal mucosa cultured in vitro with recombinant human growth hormone (GH), insulin-like growth factor-1, and insulin.[122] IGF-1 has a potent mitogenic action on the bowel. The increase in IGF-2 in the ileal mucosa, without changes in plasma, implies autocrine or paracrine growth stimulation at this stage after resection.[123] Vanderhoof et al. also showed a positive effect of both IGF-1 (native IGF-1) and des-IGF-1 (truncated IGF-1) on intestinal adaptation.[124] Growth hormone has been a component of several clinical trials to increase adaptation. For example, in one study growth hormone was found to have a beneficial therapeutic role in the treatment of inflammatory bowel disease.[125,126] Other hormones have been studied but have not played a major role in intestinal adaptation.

## Polyamines

The cellular mechanisms controlling intestinal adaptation are dependent on the activity of the key enzymes controlling polyamine synthesis, ornithine decarboxylase (ODC), and degradation, diamine oxidase (DAO). Luminal factors may interact with hormones and function sequentially to produce changes of intestinal maturation and adaptation.[127,128]

Ornithine decarboyxlase increases polyamine synthesis and subsequent stimulation of DNA, RNA and protein synthesis that produces adaptive tissue growth.[129] Similar positive effects of dietary polyamines in the maturation of villus and crypt cell functions in the rat small intestine can occur even after complete inhibition of ornithine decarboxylase activity by α-difluromethyorithine (DFMO).[130] There are significant changes in polyamines associated with fasting and refeeding. Mucosal polyamines drop rapidly in response to a 24-hour fast in experimental animals but increase rapidly after refeeding; this suggests a constitutive role for polyamines in the maintenance of the normal epithelium. In terms of adaptation, ODC levels increase after resection, and pharmacologic inhibition of ODC prevents the expected adaptive response. Both enteroglucagon and ODC increase early after resection, suggesting but certainly not proving a linkage.[131] The increases in ODC activity and polyamine biosynthesis are critical for ileal adaptation, as manifested by crypt cell proliferation, and that the critical and limiting step performed by polyamines in this adaptive process is the onset of new DNA synthesis.[132,133]

Suppression of ODC activity is associated with a very significant absence of DNA synthesis, and results in a complete abolition of intestinal adaptation, as manifested by marginal intestinal weight gain with no increase in mucosal thickness, or in crypt cell production. The expected adaptive intestinal changes from pancreaticobiliary diversion are inhibited when polyamine synthesis is blocked by DFMO, an inhibitor of ODC. This clearly suggests a trophic role for polyamines (putrescine, spermidine and spermine).[129]

## GROWTH FACTORS

There is strong evidence that humoral factors play an important role in intestinal adaptation. Identifying the nature of the humoral factors and their complex relationship with other influences, such as luminal nutrition and pancreatic secretions, may facilitate the development of new therapeutic strategies for the sequelae of small bowel resection. The identification of specific peptide families that modulate the growth of the intestine through autocrine and paracrine processes has provided an opportunity to reassess the regulation of adaptation and ponder the possibility of therapeutic intervention. Most of these growth factors, unfortunately, have become burdened by names, given at the time of their discovery, that may not reflect their recognized spectrum of activities. Growth factors generally exert their effect through specific receptors linked to tyrosine kinases. Epidermal growth factor, fibroblast growth factor, transforming growth factor P and trefoil peptides have all been implicated in the regulation of epithelial growth, proliferation and adaptation. Trefoil peptides are a group of small peptides produced in significant amounts at mucosal surfaces, which define mechanisms of mucosal differentiation and preservation of mucosal integrity.[134] The peptides form a secondary structure that leads to intrinsic resistance to protease digestion. Induction of these peptides has been associated with response to injury in the gastrointestinal tract. Intestinal trefoil peptides are secreted on to the intestinal surface by goblet cells, suggesting that this may be an important component of an intrinsic mechanism for maintaining mucosal integrity.[135]

## SUMMARY

Surgical intervention is an integral part of the therapy of IBD. Surgery clearly benefits the patient but, at the same time, can exacerbate existing problems or create new ones. For the most part, a firm grasp of the physiology of the GI tract makes these problems predictable and points to the appropriate therapy (e.g. vitamin $B_{12}$ replacement after ileal resection). Occasionally, surgery creates a 'new' disease, such as pouchitis, which highlights our current limited understanding of the relationship between the luminal environment and mucosal inflammation. Intestinal adaptation after surgery represents a homeostatic response to maintain intestinal function. The molecular and physiologic mechanisms that underlie these processes may provide important clues for possible therapeutic interventions to optimize adaptation and, in the future, minimize the consequences of surgery.

## REFERENCES

1. Van Citters GW, Lin HC. The ileal brake: a fifteen-year progress report. Curr Gastroenterol Rep 1999;1(5):404–409.
2. VCraddock AL, Love MW, Daniel RW et al. Expression and transport properties of the human ileal and renal sodiurndependent bile acid transporter. Am J Physiol 1998;274:G157.
3. VBrink MA, Mendez-Sanchez N, Carey MC. Bilirubin cycles enterohepatically after ileal resection in the rat. Gastroenterology 1996;110(6):1945–1957.
4. VWen J, Luque-de Leon E, Kost Q et al. Duodenal motility in fasting dogs: Human and neural pathways mediating the colonic brake. Am J Physiol 1998;274:G192.
5. Soper NJ, Chapman NJ, Kelly KA, Brown ML, Phillips SF, Go VL. The 'ileal brake' after ileal pouch–anal anastomosis. Gastroenterology 1990;98(1):111–116.
6. Lin HC, Zhao XT, Wang L. Intestinal transit is more potently inhibited by fat in the distal (ileal brake) than in the proximal (jejunal brake) gut. Dig Dis Sci 1997;42(1):19–25.
7. Sellin JH, Hart R. Glucose malabsorption associated with rapid intestinal transport. Am J Gastroenterol 1992;87:584.
8. Vanderhoof JA, Langnas AN. Short bowel syndrome in children and adults. Gastroenterology 1997;113:1767.
9. Woolf GM, Miller C, Kurian R et al. Nutritional absorption in short bowel syndrome. Dig Dis Sci 1987;320:8.
10. Messing I, Pigot F, Rongier M et al. Intestinal absorption of free oral hyperalimentation in the very short bowel syndrome. Gastroenterology 1991;100:1502.
11. Nord-aard I, Hansen BS, Mortensen P. Colon as a digestive organ in patients with short bowel. Lancet 1994;343:373.
12. Sellin JH, Meredith SC, Kelly S et al. Prospective evaluation of metabolic bone disease after jejunoileal bypass. Gastroenterology 1984;87:123.
13. Taylor CM, Bacon JR, Agett PJ et al. The homeostatic regulation of zinc absorption and endogenous zinc losses in zinc deprived man. Am J Clin Nutr 1991;53:755.
14. Woman SL, Anderson GH, Marliss EB et al. Zinc in total parenteral nutrition: Requirements and metabolic effects. Gastroenterology 1979;76:458.
15. Ainby CC, Cason J, Carlsson LK et al. Zinc status in inflammatory bowel disease. Clin Sci 1988;75:277.
16. McClain C, Soutor C, Zieve L. Zinc deficiency: A complication of Crohn's disease. Gastroenterology 1980;78:272.
17. Ghishan FK. Transport of electrolytes, water, and glucose in zinc deficiency. J Pediatr Gastroenterol Nutr 1984;3:608.
18. Rodriguez P, Darmon N, Chappuis C et al. Intestinal paracellular permeability during malnutrition in guinea pigs: Effect of high dietary zinc. Gut 1996;39:416.
19. Blanchard RK, Cousins RJ. Upregulation of rat intestinal uroguanylin mRNA by dietary zinc restriction. Am J Physiol 1997;272:G972.
20. Sazawal S, Black RE, Bhan MJ et al. Zinc supplementation in young children with acute diarrhea in India. N Engl J Med 1995;333:839.
21. Rosado JL, Lopez P, Munoz E et al. Zinc supplementation reduced morbidity but neither zinc nor iron supplementation affected growth or body composition of Mexican preschoolers. Am J Clin Nutr 1997;65:13.
22. Cui L, Takagi Y, Wasa M et al. Induction of nitric oxide synthase in rat intestine by interleukin 1 alpha may explain diarrhea associated with zinc deficiency. J Nutr 1997;127:1729.
23. Thompson JS, Harty RF. Postresection hypergastrinemia correlates with malabsorption but not adaptation. J Invest Surg 1994;7:469.
24. Cortot A, Fleming CR, Malagelada JR. Improved nutrient absorption after cimetidine in short-bowel syndrome with gastric hypersecretion. N Engl J Med 1979;300(2):79.
25. Jacobsen O, Lodefoged K, Stage JG et al. Effects of cimetidine in jejunostomy effluents in patients with severe short bowel syndrome. Scand J Gastroenterol 1986;21:828.
26. Doherty NJ, Sufian S, Pavlides CA et al. Cimetidine in the treatment of severe metabolic alkalosis secondary to short bowel syndrome. Int Surg 1978;63(3):140.
27. Murphy JP, King DR, Dubois A. Treatment of gastric hypersecretion with cimetidine in the short-bowel syndrome. N Engl J Med 1979;300(2):80.
28. Wickbom G, McGuigan JE, Landor JH. Role of gastrin in short-bowel hypersecretion. Surg Forum 1973;24:353.
29. Windsor CWO, Fejfar J, Woodward DAK. Gastric secretion after massive small bowel resection. Gut 1969;10:779.
30. Wickbom G, Landor JH, Bushkin FL et al. Changes in canine gastric acid output and serum gastrin levels following massive small intestinal resection. Gastroenterology 1975;69:448.
31. Strauss E, Gerson CD, Yalow RS. Hypersecretion of gastrin associated with short bowel syndrome. Gastroenterology 1974;66(2):175.
32. Gelzayd EA, Breuer RI, Kirsner JB. Nephrolithiasis in inflammatory bowel disease. Am J Dig Dis 1968;13:1027.

33. Caudarella R, Rizzoli E, Pironi L et al. Renal stone formation in patients with inflammatory bowel disease. Scanning Microsc 1993;7:371.

34. Shield DE, Lytton B, Weiss RH et al. Urologic complications of inflammatory bowel disease. J Urol 1976;115:701.

35. Clarke AM, Mckenzie RG. Ileostomy and the risk of urinary uric acid stones. Lancet 1969;2:395.

36. Christie PM, Knight GS, Hill GL. Metabolism of body water and electrolytes after surgery for ulcerative colitis: Conventional ileostomy vs J-pouch. Br J Surg 1990;77:149.

37. Christie PM, Knight GS, Hill GL. Comparison of relative risks of urinary stone formation after surgery for ulcerative colitis: Conventional ileostomy vs J-pouch – a comparative study. Dis Colon Rectum 1996;39:50.

38. Fleming R, George L, Stoner G et al. The importance of urinary magnesium values in persons with gut failure. Mayo Clin Proc 1996;71:21.

39. Farmer RG, Mir-Madjlessi SH. Urinary excretion of oxalate, calcium, magnesium, and uric acid in inflammatory bowel disease-Relationship to urolithiasis. Cleveland Clin Q 1974;41:109.

40. Stauffer JQ, Humpreys MH, Weir GJ. Acquired hyperoxaluria with regional enteritis after ileal resection. Role of dietary oxalate. Ann Intern Med 1973;79:383.

41. Hoffman AF, Laker MF, Dharmsathaphorn K et al. Complex pathogenesis of hyperoxaluria after jejunoileal bypass surgery: Oxalogenic substances in diet contribute to urinary oxalate. Gastroenterology 1983;84:2930.

42. Earnest DL. Perspectives on incidence, etiology and treatment of enteric hyperoxaluria. Am J Clin Nutr 1997;30:72.

43. Kurchin A, Ray JE, Bluth EL et al. Cholelithiasis in ileostomy patients. Dis Colon Rectum 1984;27(9):585.

44. Pitt HA, King W III, Mann LL et al. Increased risk of cholelithiasis with prolonged total parenteral nutrition. Am J Surg 1983;45:106.

45. Bickerstaff KI, Moossa AR. Effects of resection or bypass of the distal ileum on the lithogenicity of bile. Am J Surg 1983;145:34.

46. Coyle JJ, Hoyt DB, Sedaghat A. Relationship of intestinal bypass operations and cholelithiasis. Surg Forum 1980;21:139.

47. Pitt HA, Lewinski MA, Muller EL. Ileal-resection induced gallstones: Altered bilirubin or cholesterol metabolism. Surgery 1984;96:154.

48. Kusunoki M, Shoji Y, Yanagi H et al. Function after anoabdominal rectal resection and colonic J pouch–anal anastomosis. Br J Surg 1991;78(12):1434–1438.

49. Roediger WEW. The starved colon – diminished mucosal nutrition, diminished absorption, and colitis. Dis Colon Rectum 1990;33:858.

50. Musch MW, Bookstein C, Xie Y, Sellin JH, Chang EB. SCFA increase intestinal Na absorption by induction of NHE3 in rat colon and human intestinal C2/bbe cells. Am J Physiol Gastrointest Liver Physiol 2001;280: G687–G693.

51. Richardson A, Delbridge AT, Brown NJ et al. Short chain fatty acids in the terminal ileum accelerate stomach to caecum transit time in the rat. Gut 1991;32:269.

52. Longo E, Ballantyne GH, Savoca PE. Short chain fatty acid release of peptideYY in the isolated rabbit distal colon. Scand J Gastroenterol 1991;26:442.

53. Tappenden KA, Thomson ABR, Wild GE et al. Short chain fatty acid-supplemented total parenteral nutrition enhances functional adaptation to intestinal resection in rats. Gastroenterology 1997;112:792.

54. Harig JM, Soergel KH, Komorowski RA et al. Treatment of diversion colitis with short chain-fatty acid irrigation. N Engl J Med 1989;320:23.

55. Neut C, Guillemot F, Gower-Rousseau C et al. Treatment of diversion colitis with short chain fatty acids. Bacteriological study. Gastroenterol Clin Biol 1995;11:871–875.

56. Guillemot F, Colombel JF, Neut C et al. Treatment of diversion colitis by short chain fatty acids. Prospective and double blind study. Dis Col Rectum 1991;10:861–864.

57. Favus MJ, Kathpalia SC, Coe FL. Kinetic characteristics of calcium absorption and secretion by rat colon. Am J Physiol 1981;240:G350.

58. Hylander E, Ladefoged K, Jarnum S. Calcium absorption after intestinal resection. The importance of a preserved colon. Scand J Gastroenterol 1990;25:705.

59. Christl SU, Scheppach W. Metabolic consequences of total colectomy. Scand J Gastroenterol 1997;222(Suppl):20–24.

60. Kuisma J, Nuutinen H, Luukkonen P, Jarvinen H, Kahri A, Farkkila M. Long term metabolic consequences of ileal pouch–anal anastomosis for ulcerative colitis. Am J Gastroenterol 2001;96(11):3110–3116.

61. de Silva HJ, Millard PR, Kettlewell M, Mortensen NJ, Prince C, Jewell DP. Mucosal characteristics of pelvic ileal pouches. Gut 1991;32(1):61–65.

62. Heuschen UA, Heuschen G, Autschbach F, Allemeyer EH, Herfarth C. Adenocarcinoma in the ileal pouch: late risk of cancer after restorative proctocolectomy. Int J Colorectal Dis 2001;16(2):126–130.

63. Veress B, Reinholt FP, Lindquist K, Lofberg R, Liljeqvist L. Long-term histomorphological surveillance of the pelvic ileal pouch: dysplasia develops in a subgroup of patients. Gastroenterology 1995;109(4):1090–1097.

64. Marciniak R, Majewski P, Drews M et al. Endoscopical and histological aspects of inflammatory changes in J-pouch mucosa. Pol J Pathol 2000;51(1):25–30.

65. Merrett MN, Soper N, Mortensen N, Jewell DP. Intestinal permeability in the ileal pouch. Gut 1996;39(2):226–230.

66. Tsukamoto Y, Koh K. [Adaptation and effects of ileal reservoir on ileo-proctostomy following total colectomy in dogs]. J Smooth Muscle Res 1994;30(1):35–50.

67. Chapman MA, Hutton M, Grahn MF, Williams NS. Metabolic adaptation of terminal ileal mucosa after construction of an ileoanal pouch. Br J Surg 1997;84(1):71–73.

68. Hove H, Mortensen PB. Short-chain fatty acids in the non-adapted and adapted pelvic ileal pouch. Scand J Gastroenterol 1996;31(6):568–574.

69. Mibu R, Itoh H, Nakayama F. Effect of total colectomy and mucosal proctectomy on intestinal absorptive capacity in dogs. Dis Colon Rectum 1987; 30:47.

70. Lerch MM, Braun J, Harder M et al. Post-operative adaptation of the small intestine after total colectomy and J-pouch–anal anastomosis. Dis Colon Rectum 1989;32:600.

71. Schumpelick V, Willis S, Schippers E. [Ulcerative colitis – late functional results of ileoanal pouch anastomosis]. Chirurg 1998;69(10):1013–1019.

72. Hylander E, Rannem T, Hegnhoj J, Kirkegaard P, Thale M, Jarnum S. Absorption studies after ileal J-pouch anastomosis for ulcerative colitis. A prospective study. Scand J Gastroenterol 1991;26(1):65–72.

73. de Silva HJ, Millard PR, Soper N, Kettlewell M, Mortensen N, Jewell DP. Effects of the faecal stream and stasis on the ileal pouch mucosa. Gut 1991;32(10):1166–1169.

74. Ambroze WL, Pemberton JH, Phillips SF et al. Fecal short fatty acids concentrations and effect on ileal pouch function. Dis Col Rectum 1993;36:235.

75. Takesue Y, Sakashita Y, Akagi S et al. Gut transit time after ileal pouch–anal anastomosis using a radiopaque marker. Dis Colon Rectum 2001;44(12):1808–1813.

76. Clausen MR, Tvede M, Mortensen PB. Short-chain fatty acids in pouch contents from patients with and without pouchitis after ileal pouch–anal anastomosis. Gastroenterology 1992;103:1144.

77. Kuisma J, Nuutinen H, Luukkonen P, Jarvinen H, Kahri A, Farkkila M. Long term metabolic consequences of ileal pouch–anal anastomosis for ulcerative colitis. Am J Gastroenterol 2001;96(11):3110–3116.

78. Kuhbacher T, Schreiber S, Runkel N. Pouchitis: pathophysiology and treatment. Int J Colorectal Dis 1998;13(5–6):196–207.

79. Bulois P, Tremaine WJ, Maunoury V et al. Pouchitis is associated with mucosal imbalance between interleukin-8 and interleukin-10. Inflamm Bowel Dis 2000;6(3):157–164.

80. Vento P, Kiviluoto T, Jarvinen HJ, Karkkainen P, Kivilaakso E, Soinila S. Expression of inducible and endothelial nitric oxide synthases in pouchitis. Inflamm Bowel Dis 2001;7(2):120–127.

81. Leplingard A, Brung-Lefebvre M, Guedon C et al. Increase in cyclooxygenase-2 and nitric oxide-synthase-2 mRNAs in pouchitis without modification of inducible isoenzyme heme-oxygenase-1. Am J Gastroenterol 2001;96(7):2129–2136.

82. Diamond J. Evolutionary design of intestinal nutrient absorption: Enough but not too much. NIPS 1991;6:92.

83. Carey HV. Gut feelings about hibernation. NIPS 1995;10:55.

84. Shiraz-Beechy SP, Hirayam BA, Wang Y et al. Ontogenetic development of lamb intestinal sodium glucose cotransporter is regulated by diet. J Physiol 1991; 437:699.

85. Williamson RCN. Intestinal adaptation. Structural, functional and cytokinetic changes. N Engl J Med 1978;298(25):1393.

86. Thompson JS. Somatostatin analogue predisposes enterocytes to apoptosis. J Gastrointest Surg 1998;2(2):167–173.

87. Welters CF, Piersma FE, Hockenbery DM, Heineman E. The role of apoptosis during intestinal adaptation after small bowel resection. J Pediatr Surg 2000;35(1):20–24.

88. Stern LE, Huang F, Kemp CJ, Falcone RA, Jr, Erwin CR, Warner BW. Bax is required for increased enterocyte apoptosis after massive small bowel resection. Surgery 2000;128(2):165–170.

89. Nygaard K. Resection of the small intestine in rats: Adaptation of astrointestinal motility. Acta Chir Scand 1967;133:407.

90. Quigley EMM, Thompson JS. Clustered motor activity – the dominant motor pattern in short bowel syndrome: An analysis of regional and temporal distribution. Transplant Proc 1994;26:1451.

91. Quigley EMM, Thompson JS. The motor response to intestinal resection: Motor activity in canine small intestine following distal resection. Gastroenterology 1993;105:791.

92. Thompson JS, Quigley EM, Adrian TE. Smooth muscle adaptation after intestinal transection and resection. Dig Dis Sci 1996;41:1760.

93. Schmidt T, Pfeiffer A, Hackelsberger N et al. Effect of intestinal resection on human small bowel motility. Gut 1996;38:859.

94. Wingate DL. Backwards and forwards with the migrating complex. Dig Dis Sci 1981;26:641.

95. Weser E, Babbit J, Hoban M et al. Intestinal adaptation. Different growth responses to disaccharides compared with monosaccharides in rat small bowel. Gastroenterology 1986;91:1521.

96. Dowling RH. Small bowel adaptation and its regulation. Scand J Gastroenterol 1982;74(Suppl):53.

97. Tappenden KA, Drozdowski LA, Thomson AB, McBurney MI. Short-chain fatty acid-supplemented total parenteral nutrition alters intestinal structure, glucose transporter 2 (GLUT2) mRNA and protein, and proglucagon mRNA abundance in normal rats. Am J Clin Nutr 1998;68(1):118–125.

98. LeLeiko NS, Walsh MJ. The role of glutamine, short-chain fatty acids, and nucleotides in intestinal adaptation to gastrointestinal disease. Pediatr Gastroenterol 1996;43(2):451.

99. Houdijk AP, Van Leeuwen PA, Boermeester MA et al. Glutamine-enriched enteral diet increases splanchnic blood flow in the rat. Am J Physiol 1994;267:G1035.

100. Ziegler TR, Mantell MP, Chow JC, Rombeau JL, Smith RJ. Gut adaptation and the insulin-like growth factor system: regulation by glutamine and IGF-I administration. Am J Physiol 1996;271(5 Pt I):G866–875.

101. Gu Y, Wu ZH, Xie JX, Jin DY, Zhuo HC. Effects of growth hormone (rhGH) and glutamine supplemented parenteral nutrition on intestinal adaptation in short bowel rats. Clin Nutr 2001;20(2):159–166.

102. Zhou X, Li YX, Li N, Li JS. Glutamine enhances the gut-trophic effect of growth hormone in rat after massive small bowel resection. J Surg Res 2001;99(1):47–52.

103. Byrne TA, Morrissey T, Naltakom T et al. Growth hormone, glutamine and modified diet enhance nutrient absorption in persons with severe short bowel syndrome. JPEN 1995;19:296.

104. Byrne TA, Persinger RL, Young LS et al. A new treatment for patients with short bowel syndrome. Ann Surg 1995;222:243.

105. Scolapio JS, Camilleri M, Fleming CR et al. Effect of growth hormone, glutamine and diet on adaptation in short bowel syndrome: A randomized, controlled study. Gastroenterology 1997;113:1074.

106. Thompson JS. Can the intestine adapt to a changing environment? (Editorial). Gastroenterology 1997;113:1402.

107. Bloom SR. Gut hormones in adaptation. Gut 1987;28 (Suppl):31.

108. Appleton GVN, Bristol JB, Williamson RCN. Proximal enterectomy provides stronger systemic stimulus to intestinal adaptation than distal enterectomy. Gut 1987;28(Suppl):165.

109. Dowling RH. Small bowel adaptation and its regulation. Scand J Gastroenterol 1982;74(Suppl):53.

110. O'Loughlin E, Winter M, Shun A, Hardin JA, Gall DG. Structural and functional adaptation following jejunal resection in rabbits: effect of epidermal growth factor. Gastroenterology 1994;107(1):87–93.

111. Gleeson MH, Bloom SR, Polak JM et al. Endocrine tumor of kidney affecting small bowel structure, motility and absorptive function. Gut 1971;12:773.

112. Drucker DJ, DeForest L, Brubaker PL. Intestinal response to growth factors administered alone or in combination with human [Gly-2] glucagon-like peptide. Am J Physiol 1997;273:G1252.

113. Holst JJ. Enteroglucagon. Annu Rev Physiol 1997;59:257–271.

114. Tappenden KA, Bartholome AL. ALX-0600, a glucagon-like peptide (GLP-2) analog, enhances intestinal structure and function in patients with short bowel syndrome. Abstract presentation. Digestive Disease Week 2002.

115. Armstrong DN, Ballantyne GH, Adrian TE, Bilchik AJ, McMillen MA, Modlin IM. Adaptive increase in peptide YY and enteroglucagon after proctocolectomy and pelvic ileal reservoir construction. Dis Colon Rectum 1991;34(2):119–125.

116. Imamura M, Nakajima H, Mikami Y, Yamauchi H. Morphological and immunohistochemical changes in intestinal mucosa and PYY release following total colectomy with ileal pouch–anal anastomosis in dogs. Dig Dis Sci 1999;44(5):1000–1007.

117. Olesen M, Gudmand-Hoyer E, Holst JJ, Jorgensen S. Importance of colonic bacterial fermentation in short bowel patients: small intestinal malabsorption of easily digestible carbohydrate. Dig Dis Sci 1999;44(9):1914–1923.

118. Imamura M. Effects of surgical manipulation of the intestine on peptide YY and its physiology. Peptides 2002;23(2):403–407.

119. Bloom SR, Polak JM. The hormonal pattern of intestinal adaptation. A major role for enteroglucagon. Scand J Gastroenterol 1982;74(Suppl):93.

120. Hodin RA, Saldinger P, Meng S. Small bowel adaptation: Counterregulatory effects of epidermal growth factor and somatostatin on the program of early gene expression. Surgery 1995;118:206.

121. Gomez de Segura IA, Aguilera MJ, Codesal J, De Miguel E. [Administration of growth hormone enhances the intestinal adaptive response after resection of small intestine in rats]. Rev Esp Enferm Dig 1995;87(4):288–293.

122. Wheeler EE, Challacombe DN. The trophic action of growth hormone, insulin-like GF-I and insulin on human duodenal mucosa cultured in vitro. Gut 1997;40(l):57.

123. Wiren M, Adrian TE, Arnelo U, Permert J, Staab P, Larsson J. An increase in mucosal insulin-like growth factor II content in postresectional rat intestine suggests autocrine or paracrine growth stimulation. Scand J Gastroenterol 1998;33(10):1080–1086.

124. Vanderhoof JA, McCusker RH, Clark R et al. Truncated and native insulin like growth factor-I enhance mucosal adaptation after jejunoileal resection. Gastroenterology 1992;102:1949.

125. Sandborn WJ, Targan SR. Biologic therapy of inflammatory bowel disease. Gastroenterology 2002;122(6):1592–1608.

126. Slonim AE, Bulone L, Damore MB, Goldberg T, Wingertzahn MA, McKinley MJ. A preliminary study of growth hormone therapy for Crohn's disease. N Engl J Med 2000;342(22):1633–1637.

127. Jonas A, Diver-Haber A, Yahav J. Adaptive response of ileal mucosa to malnutrition in the rat: role of polyamines. Acta Physiol Scand 1991;142(3):387–395.

128. Luk GD, Baylin SB. Polyamines and intestinal growth-increased polyamine biosynthesis after jejunectomy. Am J Physiol 1983;245(5 Pt 1):G656–660.

129. Dowling RH, Hosomi M, Stace NH et al. Hormones and polyamines in intestinal and pancreatic adaptation. Scand J Gastroenterol 1985;112(Suppl):84.

130. Buts JP, De Keyser N, Kotanowski J et al. Maturation of villus and crypt cell functions in rat small intestine. Role of dietary polyamines. Dig Dis Sci 1993;38:1091.

131. Bamba T, Vaja S, Murphy GM, Dowling RH. Role of polyamines in the early adaptive response to jejunectomy in the rat: effect of DFMO on the ileal villus:crypt axis. Digestion 1990;46 (Suppl 2):410–423.

132. Hosomi M, Stace NH, Lirussi F, Smith SM, Murphy GM, Dowling RH. Role of polyamines in intestinal adaptation in the rat. Eur J Clin Invest 1987;17(5):375–385.

133. Johnson LR, McCormack SA. Regulation of mucosal growth. In: Johnson LR, ed. Physiology of the gastrointestinal tract, 3rd edn., Vol 1. New York: Raven Press; 1994:611.

134. Podolsky DK, Lynch-Devaney K, Stow JL et al. Identification of human intestinal trefoil factor. Goblet cell-specific expression of a peptide targeted for apical secretion. J Biol Chem 1993;268(9):6694–6702.

135. Amorim MJ, Ferreira JP. Microparticles for delivering therapeutic peptides and proteins to the lumen of the small intestine. Eur J Pharm Biopharm 2001;52(1):39–44.

*Additional References*

1. Brink MA, Slors JFM, Keulerrians YCA et al. Enterohepatic cycling of bilirubin: A putative mechanism for pigment gallstone formation in ileal Crohn's disease. Gastroenterology 1999;116:1420.

2. Lapidus A, Einarsson C. Bile composition in patients with ileal resection due to Crohn's disease. Inflamm Bowel Dis 1998;4(2):89.

## CHAPTER 23

# Fertility and pregnancy

Sunanda Kane and Stephen Hanauer

The incidence of one form of chronic inflammatory bowel disease (IBD), ulcerative colitis, has remained stable whereas the incidence of the other form, Crohn's disease, has increased over the past few decades. The consequence of this trend is a growing population of patients in their childbearing years with concerns about fertility and pregnancy. Issues of importance to the female patient with IBD who is pregnant or contemplating pregnancy include: 1) inheritance in the offspring; 2) fertility; 3) the effect of the IBD on the pregnancy; 4) initial onset and new diagnosis during pregnancy; 5) the effect of the pregnancy on the IBD; and 6) the safety of drugs used to treat IBD on the developing fetus and nursing newborn. Issues of importance to male patients with IBD whose partner is pregnant or contemplating pregnancy include: 1) fertility; and 2) the potential teratogenicity of medications used to treat IBD.

## INHERITANCE

Current data suggest that a child of affected parents has a 5% risk when the proband has CD and 1.6% when the proband has UC.[1] However, the risk of IBD increases as high as 37% if both parents have the disease. The risk of inheriting IBD is higher in Jewish (7.8%) than in non-Jewish (5.8%) families.[2] It is important to emphasize to patients that although their offspring may have an increased risk of developing IBD relative to the general population, the absolute risk is small. Thus, a decision to remain childless for fear of disease transmission to offspring seems unfounded.

## FERTILITY

Overall, the fertility rates for women with ulcerative colitis are similar to those of the general population.[3] Early studies suggesting lower fertility rates in women with IBD had not taken into account an important confounding factor, an increased rate of voluntary childlessness.

The systemic effects of Crohn's disease, including fever, pain, diarrhea, and suboptimal nutrition, have been implicated in decreased fertility. In patients with active Crohn's disease, inflammation involving either the colon or terminal ileum can reduce fertility, presumably due to scarring of the fallopian tubes.[4,5] Similarly, women who have undergone surgical resection for either Crohn's disease or ulcerative colitis[6–8] are at risk for pelvic adhesions, which can also impair tubal function. Women with perianal disease may have secondary dyspareunia and decreased libido, which also contribute to lower fertility rates. The overall reproductive capacity of men with IBD has not been found to be decreased, although male patients with CD have been noted to have small families.[9]

Finally, fear of pregnancy may also play a role in the reported reduced fertility seen in women with CD. The obstetrician or gastroenterologist, who may overemphasize the potential fetal toxicity of drug therapy or adverse outcome, can contribute to these fears. None of the medications used to treat IBD have an adverse effect on female fertility, but it is important to remember that sulfasalazine therapy reduces sperm motility and count in male patients.[10–13] These effects on sperm are dose related and do not respond to supplemental folic acid. A recent study of sperm analysis in patients with IBD taking azathioprine did not show significant differences in sperm count or morphology as determined by WHO criteria.[14]

## EFFECT OF IBD ON PREGNANCY

Women with inactive IBD appear no more likely than controls to experience spontaneous abortion, stillbirth, or children born with a congenital abnormality.[15] Some studies have suggested that babies born to women with IBD, regardless of disease activity, are of smaller birthweight.[16] This appears to be particularly true in women with Crohn's disease.[5,16] Thus, if a woman is in symptomatic remission, there is every reason to expect the pregnancy will proceed smoothly. Although there is no evidence-based minimum required time period for quiescent disease prior to a planned conception, some experts recommend at least 3 months.

In contrast, women with active disease run a greater risk for premature birth.[17] One study in patients with UC showed an increased rate of premature birth when the first hospitalization for UC occurred during pregnancy.[18] Others have shown an increased rate for preterm births[19] and small size for gestational age.[20] In a recent study by Dominitz et al.[21] babies born to mothers with Crohn's disease were 3.5 times more likely to have a low birthweight and twice as likely to be small for gestational age than babies born to mothers without IBD. Thus, if active disease is present, it is likely to continue through pregnancy and will place the pregnancy at greater risk for a complication.[5] This risk appears to be higher in CD than in UC.

The presence of IBD does not appear to have an impact on maternal complications related to pregnancy, including hypertension or proteinuria.[22]

## MODE OF DELIVERY

The mode of delivery is often an obstetric decision. The indications for cesarean section for obstetric reasons are not different in women with IBD. The presence of UC does not have a significant impact on the method of delivery, nor is it an indication for a C-section per se. However, active perianal disease in Crohn's disease may worsen after a vaginal delivery. One retrospective a study of women with CD found that 18% of those without previous perianal disease developed such disease after delivery, usually involving an extensive episiotomy.[23] General guidelines include a planned C-section for any woman with known perianal or rectal Crohn's disease, or if the birth appears to be more complicated than initially presumed.

## INITIAL ONSET AND NEW DIAGNOSIS DURING PREGNANCY

An early clinical series suggested that the prognosis was poor for women diagnosed with ulcerative colitis during pregnancy.[24] Subsequently, epidemiologic and natural history studies have failed to confirm that these patients have a worse disease course than those diagnosed with ulcerative colitis at other times.[25] There has been no large study involving the initial diagnosis of Crohn's disease during pregnancy; thus, no conclusions about the severity and natural history of these patients can be reached.

## EFFECT OF PREGNANCY ON IBD

The activity of IBD at conception is the primary predictor of the disease course during pregnancy. For women with quiescent UC at the time of conception, the rate of relapse is approximately the same in pregnant versus non-pregnant patients.[5] This is in contrast to the presence of active disease at the time of conception, which is associated with continued or worsening disease activity in approximately 70% of women. Comparable observations are seen in Crohn's disease.[26] The older literature suggested a trend for disease to flare in the first trimester, but this was

documented prior to the accepted practice of maintenance therapy, continued even during pregnancy. Occasionally, pregnancy will induce an improvement in disease activity or clinical remission, usually in the first trimester.[19] In addition, some patients will have symptomatic disease only when pregnant, with quiescence between pregnancies and exacerbations during subsequent pregnancies. A single study suggested that psychological factors play a role in disease course during pregnancy.[27] Investigators found that 38% of unwanted pregnancies were associated with an increased activity of the disease during pregnancy, compared with only 12% among women with planned pregnancies. The clinical course or outcome of previous pregnancies cannot predict either the clinical course of IBD or the outcome of a subsequent pregnancy.

One study has suggested that the course of both UC and CD correlates with HLA maternal–fetal disparity.[28] Over 50 mother–child pairs were studied for maternal disease course in relation to the amount of shared HLA alleles. In those pregnancies where the mother and fetus had disparity at both the DR and DQ alleles, the mother tended to experience an improvement in disease scores over time, compared to those pregnant women who shared more alleles with the fetus. Subsequent pregnancies in the same women showed the same effect.

There are data suggesting that a history of childbearing changes the natural history of Crohn's disease.[29] Women with a history of pregnancy had fewer resections and/or longer intervals between resections than women who had not had children but who had otherwise similar disease. One theory proposed by the authors is the inhibition of macrophage function by relaxin. Relaxin is a hormone produced exclusively during pregnancy that may decrease fibrosis and stricture formation through inhibition of macrophages.

## MANAGEMENT OF IBD DURING PREGNANCY

### CLINICAL EVALUATION

Many pregnant women will have intermittent abdominal discomfort related to changes in bowel habits or gastroesophageal reflux, which commonly occur during pregnancy. In addition, it is important to remember that abdominal pain in the pregnant IBD patient could be related to cholelithiasis, pancreatitis, toxemia, or a problem with the pregnancy itself. Clinically, these processes can be distinguished from a flare of IBD by a careful history, physical examination, laboratory evaluation, and judicious use of radiographic and endoscopic studies.

During pregnancy hemoglobin and albumin levels decrease by 1 g/dL, sedimentation rate increases two- to threefold, and there is a 1.5-fold rise in serum alkaline phosphatase. Because of these normal physiologic changes, disease assessment during pregnancy should rely more on clinical symptoms than laboratory parameters. It is also important to bear in mind that a growing uterus changes normal anatomy, with the terminal ileum and appendix being higher in the right upper quadrant.

With respect to radiographic testing, ultrasound examination is safe, as is magnetic resonance imaging (MRI),[30] but these are rarely used for clinical assessment of IBD during pregnancy. Clearly, it is best to avoid exposure of the fetus to radiation from abdominal X-rays, especially early in the pregnancy. However, the absolute risk to the fetus of abdominal radiography is minimal, and clinical necessity should guide the decision making.[31]

With respect to endoscopy, sigmoidoscopy will provide sufficient information for clinical management in most patients. There is no evidence that sigmoidoscopy will induce premature labor.[32,33] Full colonoscopy can be performed when needed to establish the diagnosis or to determine the extent and severity of disease. Fetal monitoring can be considered when patients require colonoscopy.

## MEDICAL THERAPIES

The guiding principle to medical management of IBD during pregnancy is to remember that the greatest risk is active disease, not active therapy.[34] The two fundamental issues regarding medical therapy in the pregnant IBD patient are the beneficial effect of maintaining IBD remission during pregnancy on the outcome of the pregnancy; and the safety and efficacy of the medications used to induce and maintain remission. The focus should be on establishing remission before conception and maintaining it during pregnancy.

Early studies suggested that the rates of prematurity, spontaneous abortions and fetal malformations among mothers with IBD undergoing medical treatment were increased.[18,35] However, most investigators have shown that medical therapy, when analyzed as an independent variable, has no effect on pregnancy outcome.[20,21,35,36] As previously discussed, it is evident that disease activity, not medication, most strongly affects the outcome of pregnancy. Reported adverse birth outcomes tend to occur more often in the setting of active disease. Table 23.1 outlines the relative safety profiles of those medications used in IBD.

## Antidiarrheals

Symptomatic therapies used in IBD include the antidiarrheals and antispasmodics, as well as pain medications. Loperamide use has not been associated with an increased rate of first trimester fetal malformations, spontaneous abortion, low birthweight or premature delivery,[37] and is considered safe. However, increased stool frequency may be a sign of increased activity, and loperamide use should be monitored. Diphenoxylate with atropine is teratogenic in animals, and fetal malformations have been

observed in infants exposed during the first trimester.[38] Antispasmodics and anticholinergics have been associated with non-life-threatening fetal malformations and are probably best avoided during pregnancy.[38] Codeine has been used for many years during pregnancy without reports of associated fetal abnormalities. Drug dependence and withdrawal in the newborn can occur, but is rare.

## Sulfasalazine

Sulfasalazine has been used for over 50 years in the treatment of IBD. Although there have been a few case reports of congenital abnormalities associated with its use during pregnancy,[39,40] several large studies have shown it to be safe.[3,20,22,25,26] One study of 1400 patients reports that the rate of congenital malformations among the offspring of male IBD patients taking sulfasalazine was greater than that in the offspring of untreated IBD patients, but nearly identical to that in the general population.[41]

Because sulfasalazine interferes with normal folate metabolism through competitive inhibition of the enzyme folate conjugase, it is recommended that pregnant women take 2 mg of supplemental folate daily. Both sulfasalazine and its metabolite sulfapyridine cross the placenta with fetal serum levels equivalent to maternal levels.[42] However, numerous studies have shown that there is no increased incidence of abnormal birth outcomes.[20,22,25,41]

## 5-Aminosalicylic acid

The safety of treatment with 5-aminosalicylic acid (5-ASA) during pregnancy has been demonstrated in a number of trials.[43–46] In a postmarketing study of controlled-release mesalamine capsules, 55 women were treated with 1.5–4 g/day during 76 pregnancies. Three fetal malformations occurred, a frequency similar to that in the general population.

Diav-Citrin and colleagues[44] conducted a prospective controlled cohort study of 165 women exposed to 5-ASA during pregnancy, 146 of them having exposure in the first trimester. Pregnancy outcomes were matched with a control group. The mean daily 5-ASA dose was 2 g, with 20% of women taking between 2.4 and 3.2 g/day and another 20% taking more than 3.2 g/day. There was no increase in major malformations in the infants of 5-ASA-treated women compared with controls. There was a statistically significant increase in preterm deliveries (13% vs. 5%) and a decrease in mean birthweight (3.2 kg vs. 3.4 kg). Women with active IBD during pregnancy had significantly lower birthweight than women with inactive disease. No significant differences in the rates of live births, miscarriages, terminations or fetal distress were detected between the two groups. There is a single case report of renal interstitial damage in a child born to a woman taking mesalamine.[47] To date, this finding has not been confirmed by other investigators.

The single study looking at topical (rectal) administration of 5-ASA agents during pregnancy did not demonstrate an increase in adverse birth outcomes.[43] 5-Aminosalicylic acid and its metabolite N-acetyl-5-aminosalicylic acid are found in the maternal plasma of women taking mesalamine as well as in the fetal plasma.

## Antibiotics

The most frequently used antibiotics in IBD include metronidazole and ciprofloxacin. Animal studies have shown no evidence

### Table 23.1 Safety of IBD medications during pregnancy

| Safe to use when indicated | Contraindicated |
| --- | --- |
| Oral, topical mesalamine | Methotrexate |
| Sulfasalazine | Thalidomide |
| Corticosteroids | Diphenoxylate |
| Loperamide | |
| Azathioprine/6-mercaptopurine | |
| Total parenteral nutrition | |
| Cyclosporin | |
| Infliximab | |
| Metronidazole* | |
| Ciprofloxacin* | |

* Probably safe after first trimester.

of teratogenicity or increased fetal loss with metronidazole.[48] Although there have been a few reports of cleft lip with metronidazole use in early pregnancy in humans,[49,50] two separate meta-analyses have failed to show any relationship between metronidazole exposure and birth defects.[51,52] The most recent study of 228 women exposed to metronidazole during pregnancy followed the subjects prospectively through their pregnancies.[53] Eighty-six per cent of women were exposed during the first trimester. The malformation rate was 1.6% in the treatment group, and 1.4% in the control group.

In animal studies, no teratogenicity has been seen with ciprofloxacin, although cartilage abnormalities have been identified in immature animals.[54] This initially led to restricted use of ciprofloxacin during pregnancy, but a report of 35 women who received ciprofloxacin during the first trimester for treatment of infection showed no association with fetal malformations or arthropathies.[55] A larger prospective controlled trial showed similar results.[54] Although these data are reassuring, it should be emphasized that this information comes from the non-IBD population, where antibiotics are used in the short term. In IBD, where medications are often used for prolonged periods, there are insufficient safety data to advocate the long-term use of antibiotics during pregnancy, particularly as alternative agents that are at least as effective, with more long-term safety data, are available. Thus, the use of metronidazole and ciprofloxacin during pregnancy should currently be restricted to short-term courses of treatment.

## Corticosteroids

Studies of women with IBD treated with corticosteroids have not demonstrated harmful effects to the fetus.[16,35] In a study by Mogadam, 168 of 531 pregnant women received steroids for an extended period, mostly during the second and third trimesters. No increased incidence of prematurity, spontaneous abortion, stillbirth or developmental defects was noted. Corticosteroids cross the placenta and are transferred into breast milk, but the ratio of maternal to fetal serum concentration depends on the choice of corticosteroid used. Prednisolone is more efficiently metabolized than dexamethasone or betamethasone, and fetal concentrations are approximately 10% of maternal levels.[56] Although there is theoretically some concern regarding possible adrenal suppression among neonates born to mothers taking corticosteroids, in practice this has rarely been seen.[57] When therapy with corticosteroids is required during pregnancy, it makes sense to use one of the steroids that undergoes more extensive metabolism by the placenta, such as prednisone.

## Immunomodulators

The largest experience with use of azathioprine/6-mercaptopurine during pregnancy comes from the renal transplant literature. Among 238 pregnancies in renal transplant patients, 93% were receiving azathioprine, most often in combination with steroids and/or cyclosporin.[58] In this cohort there was a 7% rate of spontaneous abortion, 3% had stillbirths, and of the remaining pregnancies 52% of the births were premature (before 37 weeks' gestation). The neonatal death rate was 2.4%. Neonatal complications occurred in 50% of infants, but this figure includes apnea and jaundice, as well as other unspecified congenital abnormalities.

The data regarding use of azathioprine and 6-mercaptopurine for IBD during pregnancy come from small retrospective series.[59–61] In a study of short- and long-term toxicity of 6-MP, Present et al. reported on 13 children born to patients who had been taking 6-MP, although only three of them were taking the drug at the time of conception. No congenital anomalies were found in any of the children.[61] Subsequently these same investigators reported on a larger group of 72 patients who conceived while taking 6-MP, although only eight continued to do so during the pregnancy. The rate of spontaneous abortion was 18%, prematurity 3%, and congenital abnormalities 4%.[60] Compared with a group of patients who conceived after stopping 6-MP, or prior to ever taking 6-MP, there were no significant differences. The authors concluded that 6-MP is safe in pregnancy but recommended further study.

Another small retrospective study of 16 pregnancies in 14 women with IBD treated with azathioprine found no increased rate of spontaneous abortion, fetal anomalies, prematurity or lower birthweight.[59] Seven women continued azathioprine throughout the pregnancy, five stopped before week 16, and two had elective terminations. All pregnancies went to term except for the voluntary terminations and an elective cesarean section at 32 weeks' gestation. No congenital anomalies or subsequent health problems occurred among 15 children. All neonates weighed 2.5 kg or more. The authors recommended continuing azathioprine therapy throughout pregnancy if the drug is considered to help control disease symptoms. Based on these data, and evidence from other conditions as outlined above, clinicians experienced in the management of IBD generally believe that 6-MP and azathioprine can be used safely during pregnancy if the mother's health mandates therapy.

Recent interest has focused on the safety of these medications in the father. In a retrospective review of pregnancy outcome among fathers treated with 6-MP compared with fathers who had never been treated with 6-MP, the incidence of pregnancy-related complications was significantly increased when fathers used 6-MP within 3 months of conception.[62] Specifically, there were two spontaneous abortions (first trimester) and two congenital anomalies among 13 pregnancies where the father took 6-MP within 3 months of conception. This resulted in a highly statistically significant difference when compared with men who had never taken 6-MP ($P < 0.002$) or men who had conceived at least 3 months after stopping 6-MP ($P < 0.013$). However, the validity of this observation is limited by the retrospective nature of the data collection, the small sample size, the lack of a true normal control group, and the lack of information regarding disease activity in the fathers and comorbid conditions in the mothers.[63]

Azathioprine and 6-MP have been shown to be teratogenic in mice and rabbits, but not in rats.[59] This species difference suggests that variable metabolism may play a role in potential drug toxicity. Azathioprine crosses the placenta, but the fetal liver lacks the enzyme inosinate pyrophosphorylase, which converts azathioprine to its active metabolites.

Methotrexate (MTX), another immunomodulatory medication, has been used on an increasing basis for refractory Crohn's disease.[64] In a variety of animals, including mice, rats and chicks, embryonic exposure to MTX has been associated with fetal loss and congenital anomalies, including neural tube and craniofacial defects.[65] In addition, a spontaneous abortion rate as high as 40% has been reported after MTX exposure, along with a variety of neural tube defects, including spina bifida.[66] In humans, high doses of MTX are an abortifacient.[67] For these reasons, MTX use is contraindicated prior to and during pregnancy. There is, however, a single study of women exposed to low doses of MTX who carried successfully to term.[68] When trying to counsel women with the risk to benefit ratio, it is probably best to discuss the issue of pregnancy termination carefully with each individual couple. Whereas certain congenital abnormalities, such as spina bifida, can be screened for with blood tests and ultrasound, others are undetectable. The optimum management includes careful counseling and effective contraception prior to any initiation with MTX therapy.

## Biologic agents

Infliximab is the first biologic agent approved by the FDA for the treatment of inflammatory and fistulizing Crohn's disease. The safety of infliximab prior to and during pregnancy has not yet been adequately defined. The only published literature for Crohn's disease and infliximab use is in the form of a letter.[69] A woman with active perianal disease treated with a combination of medications including a single dose of infliximab gave birth to an infant at 23 weeks which subsequently died from intracranial hemorrhage after 3 days. Katz et al. reported in abstract form data from the Med-Watch program, a self-reporting mechanism for adverse events.[70] In 34 women followed after infliximab infusions for either CD or rheumatoid arthritis, 26 live births occurred. There was one tetralogy of Fallot that was surgically corrected. Although the early data are encouraging, clearly more information is needed before broad recommendations can be made.

## OTHER IMMUNOMODULATING AGENTS

The experience in pregnancy with CsA comes from the transplant population. In a review of 75 pregnancies in 70 women, renal and liver function tests were normal in exposed infants.[71] Other larger series have reported increased rates of low birthweight and prematurity.[58,72] Despite these increases, Armenti et al. have found lower neonatal complications among CsA-treated patients and no congenital malformations. Follow-up studies have also found no persistent nephrotoxicity among the children of mothers treated with CsA.

In the IBD literature there are only case reports and case series of CsA use during pregnancy.[73] One patient was treated for steroid-resistant colitis in the 29th week. A healthy baby was delivered at 36 weeks following induction of remission with CsA. In a series of five women treated with first oral and then IV CsA, Marion and colleagues reported four live births and one spontaneous abortion at 8 weeks.[74] No congenital abnormalities were observed and no renal toxicity was noted in the neonates. Two infants were premature. The use of cyclosporin should be considered in cases of severe colitis as a means of avoiding urgent surgery and reaching a gestational age when the fetus can be delivered safely.

At 10 mg/kg/day, CsA showed no fetal toxicity in rats.[65] Cyclosporin does cross the placenta, but the concentration of the drug in the newborn falls rapidly within days.

Thalidomide has been found to have some clinical benefit in the treatment of Crohn's disease.[75,76] Thalidomide, however, is a potent teratogen and should not be given to women of childbearing age except those who have undergone careful counseling and adhere strictly to contraceptive use. Its use is restricted and it is only available to those women with negative serum pregnancy tests done on a monthly basis.

Some of the newer immunomodulators used in refractory Crohn's disease include tacrolimus and mycophenolate mofetil. Again, the safety data during pregnancy come from the transplant populations. The experience with tacrolimus has been favorable overall, with no evident increase in adverse outcomes based on case reports and National Transplant Registry data.[68,77,78] The National Registry followed 100 women's status post solid organ transplant and reported four neonatal malformations in 68 live births.

The use of mycophenolate in CD has been recent, and to date there are no data regarding any pregnancies occurring with its use.

## NUTRITIONAL THERAPIES

Both total parenteral (TPN) and enteral supplementation have been used to support the pregnant IBD patient.[79–81] Despite the theoretical concern about fat embolization to the placenta, pregnant patients have tolerated TPN with intravenous lipids well. The infants born to these mothers have been healthy, and examination of the placenta has failed to show any signs of fat emboli. Elemental diets have also been used safely during pregnancy, both as primary therapy for active CD as well as a source of supplemental nutrition.

## BREASTFEEDING

Table 23.2 summarizes the safety data regarding medications and their use during breastfeeding. The medications known to be safe for breastfeeding (i.e. acceptable milk:serum ratios) include sulfasalazine, the 5-ASA formulations (Asacol, Pentasa, Rowasa) and steroids. Mothers planning on breastfeeding should discontinue the use of cyclosporin, metronidazole, ciprofloxacin and methotrexate. In addition, the antidiarrheals loperamide and diphenoxylate should be discontinued. No data are available regarding the thiopurines, and these should be discussed on a case-by-case basis.

## SURGERY AND PREGNANCY

In the pregnant IBD patient elective surgical procedures are uncommon, but those that are performed in the second trimester do not appear to carry a significant increase in perinatal mortality over those in women without IBD.[82]

### Table 23.2 Safety of IBD medications during breastfeeding

| Safe to use when indicated | Very limited data | Contraindicated |
| --- | --- | --- |
| Oral mesalamine | Olsalazine | Methotrexate |
| Topical mesalamine | Azathioprine | Thalidomide |
| Sulfasalazine | 6-MP | Cyclosporin |
| Corticosteroids | Infliximab | Ciprofloxacin |
| | | Metronidazole |
| | | Loperamide |
| | | Diphenoxylate |

The indications for surgery during pregnancy are identical to those of non-pregnant patients. They include obstruction, perforation, abscess and hemorrhage. In the ill pregnant IBD patient, the greater risk to the child is continued maternal illness rather than surgical intervention.[81,83] In general, what is best for the mother is ultimately best for the fetus.

Numerous case reports and one small case series make up the literature documenting successful surgical intervention for treatment of severe colitis in the pregnant patient.[83-87] Anderson[84] reported on the outcomes of four pregnant women who experienced disease activity between the 28th and 37th weeks of gestation. Three patients were treated medically and allowed to progress to labor. Two babies were stillborn and one child was healthy. All three mothers required colectomy in the weeks after delivery. The fourth patient relapsed at 28 weeks' gestation, had surgery for toxic megacolon at 31 weeks, and delivered at 34 weeks.

In patients with Crohn's disease, Hill and colleagues described three pregnant patients with intraperitoneal sepsis requiring surgery.[88] All three women recovered and delivered healthy infants. Most reports suggest proceeding to surgery when indicated. A variety of procedures have been performed, including proctocolectomy, subtotal colectomy with ileostomy, hemicolectomy or segmental resection, and combined subtotal colectomy and cesarean section. Two general points should be made: 1) primary anastomosis carries a greater risk of postoperative complication rate, and thus a temporary ileostomy is generally preferred; and 2) if the fetus is significantly mature, then cesarean section along with bowel resection is indicated.

In women who have a total proctocolectomy with ileal pouch–anal anastomosis (IPAA) prior to pregnancy, there is controversy regarding postoperative fertility and sexual function. One study suggests that these are maintained,[89] but the most recent study[90] suggests a significant decrease in fertility following this type of surgery. There has been debate about whether women who have had IPAA should be allowed to deliver vaginally, or whether cesarean section should be planned. One study suggests normal delivery is possible.[89] In another study of 43 pregnancies in women post IPAA, pregnancy was well tolerated, with a complication rate lower than in women who had had an ileostomy.[91] Although more cesarean sections were performed in women with IPAA, the explanation was probably due to the uncertainty about the pouch function. An extended follow-up of women with an IPAA who delivered vaginally showed no adverse long-term effects on pouch function. During actual pregnancy, however, women with IPAA did note an increase in stool frequency, incontinence and pad use, with symptoms resolving after delivery. The authors suggest that the type of delivery in patients with an IPAA be dictated by obstetric considerations. Other surgeons feel that the risk to permanent pouch failure is higher with a vaginal delivery, and recommend that any patient with surgery for UC undergo cesarean section.

Pregnancy has not been shown to complicate stoma function. Women may experience some prolapse due to abdominal pressure, but no increased risk to the pregnancy is encountered.

# REFERENCES

1. Orholm M, Fonager K, Sorensen HT. Risk of ulcerative colitis and Crohn's disease among offspring of patients with chronic inflammatory bowel disease. Am J Gastroenterol 1999;94:3236–3238.

2. Yang H, McElree C, Roth MP et al. Familial empirical risks for inflammatory bowel disease: differences between Jews and non-Jews. Gut 1993;34:517–524.

3. Woolfson K, Cohen Z, McLeod RS. Crohn's disease and pregnancy. Dis Colon Rectum 1990;33:869–873.

4. Mayberry JF, Weterman IT. European survey of fertility and pregnancy in women with Crohn's disease: a case control study by European collaborative group. Gut 1986;27:821–825.

5. Fonager K, Sorensen HT, Olsen J et al. Pregnancy outcome for women with Crohn's disease: a follow-up study based on linkage between national registries. Am J Gastroenterol 1998;93:2426–2430.

6. Arkuran C. Crohn's disease and tubal infertility: the effect of adhesion formation. Clin Exp Obstet Gynecol 2000;27:12–13.

7. Olsen KO. Fertility after ileal pouch–anal anastomosis in women with ulcerative colitis. Br J Surg 1999;86:493–495.

8. Olsen KO. Ulcerative colitis: female fecundity before diagnosis, during disease, and after surgery compared with a population sample. Gastroenterology 2002;122:15–19.

9. Burnell D, Mayberry J, Calcraft BJ et al. Male fertility in Crohn's disease. Postgrad Med J 1986;62:269–272.

10. Birnie GG, McLeod TI, Watkinson G. Incidence of sulphasalazine-induced male infertility. Gut 1981;22:452–455.

11. Levi AJ, Fisher AM, Hughes L et al. Male infertility due to sulphasalazine. Lancet 1979;2:276–278.

12. O'Morain C, Smethurst P, Dore CHG et al. Reversible male infertility due to sulphasalazine: studies in man and rat. Gut 1984;25:1078–1084.

13. Toth A. Reversible toxic effect of salicylazosulfapyridine on semen quality. Fertil Steril 1979;31:538–540.

14. Dejaco C, Mittermaier C, Rejnisch W et al. Azathioprine treatment and male fertility in inflammatory bowel disease. Gastroenterology 2001;121:1048–1053.

15. Miller JP. Inflammatory bowel disease in pregnancy: a review. J Roy Soc Med 1986;79:221–225.

16. Moser MA, Okun NB, Mayes DC et al. Crohn's disease, pregnancy, and birth weight. Am J Gastroenterol 2000;95:1021–1026.

17. Baiocco PJ, Korelitz BI. The influence of inflammatory bowel disease and its treatment on pregnancy and fetal outcome. J Clin Gastroenterol 1984;6:211–216.

18. Nielsen O, Andreasson B, Bondesen S et al. Pregnancy in ulcerative colitis. Scand J Gastroenterol 1983;18:735–742.

19. Kornfeld D, Cnattingius S, Ekbom A. Pregnancy outcomes in women with inflammatory bowel disease – a population-based cohort study. Am J Obstet Gynecol 1997;177:942–946.

20. Schade RR, Van Thiel DH, Gavaler JS. Chronic idiopathic ulcerative colitis. Pregnancy and fetal outcome. Dig Dis Sci 1984;29:614–619.

21. Dominitz J, Young, JCC, Boyko, EJ. Outcomes of infants born to mothers with inflammatory bowel disease: a population-based study. Am J Gastroenterol 2002;97:641–648.

22. Porter RJ, Stirrat GM. The effects of inflammatory bowel disease on pregnancy: a case-controlled retrospective analysis. Br J Obstet Gynaecol 1986;93:1124–1131.

23. Ilnyckyj A, Blanchard JF, Rawsthorne P et al. Perianal Crohn's disease and pregnancy: role of the mode of delivery. Am J Gastroenterol 1999;94:3274–3278.

24. Banks B, Korelitz BI, Zetzel L. The course of non-specific ulcerative colitis: a review of twenty years of experience and late results. Gastroenterology 1957;32:983–1012.

25. Willoughby CP, Truelove SC. Ulcerative colitis and pregnancy. Gut 1980;21:469–74.

26. Mogadam M, Korelitz BI, Ahmed SW et al. The course of inflammatory bowel disease during pregnancy and postpartum. Am J Gastroenterol 1981;75:265–269.

27. Levy N, Roisman I, Teodor I. Ulcerative colitis in pregnancy in Israel. Dis Colon Rectum 1981;24:351–354.

28. Kane S, Hanauer, SB, Kiesel J et al. HLA disparity determines disease activity through pregnancy in women with IBD. Gastroenterology 1998;114:A1006.

29. Nwokolo C, Tan WC, Andrews HA et al. Surgical resections in parous patients with distal ileal and colonic Crohn's disease. Gut 1994;35:220–223.

30. Shoenut JP, Semelka RC, Silverman R et al. MRI in the diagnosis of Crohn's disease in two pregnant women. J Clin Gastroenterol 1993;17:244–247.

31. Brent RL. The effect of embryonic and fetal exposure to x-ray, microwaves, and ultrasound: counseling the pregnant and nonpregnant patient about these risks. Semin Oncol 1989;16:347–368.

32. Cappell MS, Sidhom O. Multicenter, multiyear study of safety and efficacy of flexible sigmoidoscopy during pregnancy in 24 females with follow-up of fetal outcome. Dig Dis Sci 1995;40:472–479.

33. Cappell MS, Colon VJ, Sidhom OA. A study at 10 medical centers of the safety and efficacy of 48 flexible sigmoidoscopies and 8 colonoscopies during pregnancy with follow-up of fetal outcome and with comparison to control groups. Dig Dis Sci 1996;41:2353–2361.

34. Sachar D. Exposure to mesalamine during pregnancy increased preterm deliveries (but not birth defects) and decreased birth weight. Gut 1998;43:316.

35. Warrell D, Taylor R. Outcome for the foetus of mothers receiving prednisolone during pregnancy. Lancet 1968;1:117–118.

36. Norgard B, Fonager K, Sorensen HT et al. Birth outcomes of women with ulcerative colitis: a nationwide Danish cohort study. Am J Gastroenterol 2000;95:3165–3170.

37. Einarson A, Mastroiacovo P, Arnon J et al. Prospective, controlled multicenter study of loperamide in pregnancy. Can J Gastroenterol 2000;4:185–187.

38. Bonapace E, Fisher RS. Constipation and diarrhea in pregnancy. Gastroenterol Clin North Am 1998;27:197–211.

39. Hoo JJ, Hadro TA, Von Behren P. Possible teratogenicity of sulfasalazine. N Engl J Med 1988;318:1128.

40. Newman NM, Correy JF. Possible teratogenicity of sulphasalazine. Med J Aust 1983;1:528–529.

41. Moody GA, Probert C, Jayanthi V et al. The effects of chronic ill health and treatment with sulphasalazine on fertility amongst men and women with inflammatory bowel disease in Leicestershire. Int J Colorectal Dis 1997;12:220–224.

42. Esbjorner E, Jarnerot G, Wranne L. Sulphasalazine and sulphapyridine levels in children to mothers treated with sulphasalazine during pregnancy and lactation. Acta Paediatr Scand 1987;76:137–142.

43. Bell CM, Habal FM. Safety of topical 5-aminosalicylic acid in pregnancy. Am J Gastroenterol 1997;92:2201–2202.

44. Diav-Citrin O, Park YH, Veeruntharam G et al. The safety of mesalamine in human pregnancy: a prospective controlled cohort study. Gastroenterology 1998;114:23–28.

45. Habal FM, Hui G, Greenberg GR. Oral 5-aminosalicylic acid for inflammatory bowel disease in pregnancy: safety and clinical course. Gastroenterology 1993;105:1057–1060.

46. Marteau P, Tennenbaum R, Elefant E et al. Foetal outcome in women with inflammatory bowel disease treated during pregnancy with oral mesalazine microgranules. Aliment Pharmacol Ther 1998;12:1101–1108.

47. Colombel JF, Brabant G, Gubler MC et al. Renal insufficiency in infant: side-effect of prenatal exposure to mesalazine? Lancet 1994;344:620–621.

48. Roe F. Toxicologic evaluation of metronidazole with particular reference to carcinogenic, mutagenic, and teratogenic potential. Surgery 1983;93:158–164.

49. Czeizel AE, Rockenbauer M. A population based case–control teratologic study of oral metronidazole treatment during pregnancy. Br J Obstet Gynaecol 1998;105:322–327.

50. Greenberg F. Possible metronidazole teratogenicity and clefting. Am J Med Genet 1985;22:825.

51. Burtin P, Taddio A, Ariburnu O et al. Safety of metronidaozle in pregnancy: a meta-analysis. Am J Obstet Gynecol 1995;172:525–529.

52. Caro-Paton T, Carvajal A, Diego IM et al. Is metronidazole teratogenic? A meta-analysis. Br J Clin Pharmacol 1997;44:179–183.

53. Diav-Citrin O, Shechtman S, Gotteiner T et al. Pregnancy outcome after gestational exposure to metronidazole: a prospective controlled cohort study. Teratology 2001;63:186–192.

54. Linseman DA, Hampton LA, Branstetter DG. Quinolone-induced arthropathy in the neonatal mouse. Morphological analysis of articular lesions produced by pipemidic acid and ciprofloxacin. Fundam Appl Toxicol 1995;28:59–64.

55. Berkovitch M, Pastuszak A, Gasrzarian M et al. Safety of the new quinolones in pregnancy. Obstet Gynecol 1994;84:535–538.

56. Beitens I, Bayard, F, Ances IG et al. The transplacental passage of prednisone and prednisolone in pregnancy near term. J Pediatr 1972;81:936–945.

57. Fraser FSA. Teratogenic potential of corticosteroids in humans. Teratology 1995;51:45–46.

58. Armenti V, Ahlswede KM, Ahlswede RA et al. National transplant pregnancy registry-outcomes of 154 pregnancies in cyclosporine-treated female kidney transplant recipients. Transplantation 1994;57:502–506.

59. Alstead EM, Ritchie JK, Lennard-Jones JE et al. Safety of azathioprine in pregnancy in inflammatory bowel disease. Gastroenterology 1990;99:443–446.

60. Francella A, Dayan, A, Rubin, P et al. 6-Mercaptopurine is a safe therapy for child bearing patients with inflammatory bowel disease: a case controlled study. Gastroenterology 1996;110:A909.

61. Present D, Meltzer S, Krumholz M et al. 6-Mercaptopurine in the management of inflammatory bowel disease: short- and long-term toxicity. Ann Intern Med 1989;111:641–649.

62. Rajapakse RO, Korelitz BI, Zlatanic J et al. Outcome of pregnancies when fathers are treated with 6-mercaptopurine for inflammatory bowel disease. Am J Gastroenterol 2000;95:684–688.

63. Kane SV. What's good for the goose should be good for the gander—6-MP use in fathers with inflammatory bowel disease. Am J Gastroenterol 2000;95:581–582.

64. Feagan BG, Rochon J, Fedorak RN et al. Methotrexate for the treatment of Crohn's disease. The North American Crohn's Study Group Investigators. N Engl J Med 1995;332:292–297.

65. Ramsey-Goldman R SE. Immunosuppressive drug use during pregnancy. Rheum Clin North Am 1997;23:149–167.

66. Donnenfield A, Pastuszak A, Noah JS et al. Methotrexate exposure prior to and during pregnancy. Teratology 1994;49:79-81.

67. Goldenberg M, Bider D, Admon D et al. Methotrexate therapy of tubal pregnancy. Hum Reprod 1993;8:660–666.

68. Kozlowski RD, Steinbrunner JV, MacKenzie AH et al. Outcome of first-trimester exposure to low-dose methotrexate in eight patients with rheumatic disease. Am J Med 1990;88:589–592.

69. Srinivasan R. Infliximab treatment and pregnancy outcome in active Crohn's disease. Am J Gastroenterol 2001;96:2274–2275.

70. Katz J, Lichtenstein, GR, Keenan, GF, et al. Outcome of pregnancy in women receiving Remicade (infliximab) for the treatment of Crohn's disease or rheumatoid arthritis. Gastroenterology 2001;120:A69.

71. Ostensen M. Treatment with immunosuppressive and disease modifying drugs during pregnancy and lactation. Am J Reprod Immunol 1992;28:148–152.

72. Haugen G, Fauchald P, Sodal G et al. Pregnancy outcome in renal allograft recipients in Norway. The importance of immunosuppressive drug regimen and health status before pregnancy. Acta Obstet Gynecol Scand 1994;73:541–546.

73. Bertschinger P, Himmelmann A, Risti B et al. Cyclosporine treatment of severe ulcerative colitis during pregnancy. Am J Gastroenterol 1995;90:330.

74. Marion JRP, Lichtiger S et al. Cyclosporine is safe for severe colitis complicating pregnancy. Am J Gastroenoterol 1996;91:A1975.

75. Ehrenpreis ED, Kane SV, Cohen LB et al. Thalidomide therapy for patients with refractory Crohn's disease: an open-label trial. Gastroenterology 1999;117:1271–1277.

76. Vasiliauskas EA, Kam LY, Abreu-Martin MT et al. An open-label pilot study of low-dose thalidomide in chronically active, steroid-dependent Crohn's disease. Gastroenterology 1999;117:1278–1287.

77. Kainz A, Harabacz I, Cowlrick IS et al. Analysis of 100 pregnancy outcomes in women treated systemically with tacrolimus. Transpl Int 2000;13:S299–300.

78. Pergola PE, Kancharla A, Riley DJ. Kidney transplantation during the first trimester of pregnancy: immunosuppression with mycophenolate mofetil, tacrolimus, and prednisone. Transplantation 2001;71:994–997.

79. Jacobson L, Clapp, DH. Total parenetal nutrition in pregacy complicated by Crohn's disease. JPEN 1987;11:93–96.

80. Nugent F, Rajala, M, O'Shea, RA et al. Total parenteral nutrition in pregnancy: conception to delivery. JPEN 1987;11:424–427.

81. Subhani JM, Hamiliton MI. Review article: The management of inflammatory bowel disease during pregnancy. Aliment Pharmacol Ther 1998;12:1039–1053.

82. Levine W, Diamond B. Surgical procedures during pregnancy. Am J Obstet Gynecol 1961;81:1046–1052.

83. Kelly M, Hunt TM, Wicks ACB et al. Fulminant ulcerative colitis and parturition: a need to alter current management? Br J Obstet Gynaecol 1994;101:166–167.

84. Anderson JB, Turner GM, Williamson RC. Fulminant ulcerative colitis in late pregnancy and the puerperium. J Roy Soc Med 1987;80:492–494.

85. Bohe M, Ekelund GR, Genell SN et al. Surgery for fulminating colitis during pregnancy. Dis Colon Rectum 1983;26:119–122.

86. Boulton R, Hamilton M, Lewis A et al. Fulminant ulcerative colitis in pregnancy. Am J Gastroenterol 1994;89:931–933.

87. Greenfield C, Pounder RE, Craft IL et al. Severe ulcerative colitis during successful pregnancy. Postgrad Med J 1983;59:459–461.

88. Hill J, Clark A, Scott NA. Surgical treatment of acute manifestations of Crohn's disease during pregnancy. J Roy Soc Med 1997;90:64–66.

89. Metcalf A, Dozois RR, Baert RW et al. Pregnancy following ileal pouch–anal anastomosis. Dis Colon Rectum 1985;28:859–861.

90. Olsen K, Juul S, Berndtsson I et al. Ulcerative colitis: female fecundity before diagnosis, during disease, and after surgery compared with a population sample. Gastroenterology 2002;122:15–19.

91. Juhasz ES, Fozard B, Dozois RR et al. Ileal pouch–anal anastomosis function following childbirth. An extended evaluation. Dis Colon Rectum 1995;38:159–165.

## CHAPTER 24

# Psychosocial factors in ulcerative colitis and Crohn's disease

Douglas A Drossman and Yehuda Ringel

## INTRODUCTION

Although our understanding of inflammatory bowel disease (IBD) (ulcerative colitis and Crohn's disease) has advanced significantly over the last decade, knowledge of the etiology, natural history, and even the clinical expression of these disorders is still developing. Although physicians have considered psychosocial factors to be important in chronic ulcerative colitis (CUC) and Crohn's disease (CD), confusion and controversy still exists as to their precise role. Often, this relates to forming opinions from anecdotal observations or limited scientific data. Clinical experience indicates that psychosocial factors can play a prominent role in the experience and clinical expression of IBD. Recent advances in the investigation of the relationships between psychological and neural, endocrine and immune systems help to 'close the gap' between clinical observations and the scientific understanding of this contention.

This chapter addresses several issues that will assist in understanding the role of psychosocial factors in IBD:

1. The need for an integrated model of illness and disease.
2. The influence of stress on GI function, intestinal inflammation and IBD.
3. Mechanisms mediating stress, neuroendocrine immune function and IBD.
4. The psychosocial concomitants and consequences of IBD.
5. Methods to integrate the relevant psychosocial factors in diagnosis and treatment.

## THE NEED FOR AN INTEGRATED MODEL OF ILLNESS AND DISEASE

The traditional – and for these conditions less effective – model for understanding illness and disease in Western civilization has been the biomedical model.[1,2] (For the purpose of this discussion, disease is defined as abnormalities in the structure and function of organs and tissues, and illness as the experience of ill health or bodily dysfunction. Illness is a broader concept that is determined by disease activity and its psychosocial influences.) This proposes that any illness can be reduced to a single etiology (reductionism). So, finding and treating this etiology is considered sufficient to explain the illness and ultimately lead to cure. Furthermore, illness is dichotomized either to an 'organic' disorder having objectively defined pathophysiology, or a 'functional' disorder with no specific etiology or pathophysiology (dualism). This categorization also presumes that organic and functional illnesses are separate.

However, this understanding leads to inconsistencies in clinical practice. First, over 80% of medical illnesses (e.g. fatigue, abdominal pain) seen in primary care have no structural etiology, and yet they are not necessarily psychologically based.[3] Second, psychiatric diagnoses such as anxiety disorder and major depression also have a biologic basis. Third, 'organic' (e.g. IBD) and functional (e.g. irritable bowel syndrome) or psychiatric disorders (e.g. depression) may coexist in the same patient.[4–6] When this occurs, it is important to understand that IBD can vary not only in the extent and severity of the intestinal and extraintestinal involvement, but also in its clinical presentation. It is now recognized that disease activity is not sufficient to explain the variability in symptoms or behavior (i.e. the illness) in IBD.[7] For example, with an 8 cm segment of ileitis one patient may be disabled from severe symptoms, whereas another reports no complaints and functions normally.[7] It is also not rare for physicians to care for a patient in whom there are discrepancies between the 'disease' activity and the severity of the illness, the symptom experience, and the patient's behavior. Here, psychological factors and environmental modulators must be considered to allow for a complete understanding of the patient's health status.

The biopsychosocial model[2,8,9] embodies the complex biological and psychosocial interactions that explain human illness and its effects. It presumes that illness is the product of

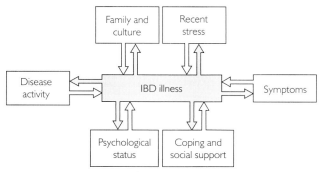

**Fig. 24.1** Relationship between IBD illness, disease activity and psychosocial factors. It can be seen that illness – the patient's experience of ill health – is determined by multiple factors. Furthermore, this association is reciprocal, so that the severity of the illness will also affect its determinants.

subsystems interacting at multiple levels, from the organ system to the patient, the family, the healthcare system and society. As shown in Figure 24.1, biological and psychosocial factors simultaneously define the illness, and the illness reciprocates with its determinants. So increased disease activity has varying effects on individuals, depending on the status of the other subsystems. A recent stress, such as a death or other traumatic experience, could affect the severity of symptoms, the psychological state and, consistent with recent studies, even the nature of the inflammatory process. These effects also depend on pre-existing psychiatric status, social support networks or coping style. Finally, chronic illness itself is a stressful event, and this will adversely affect psychologic status leading, for example, to clinical depression.

The existence of mutually interacting systems to explain illness and disease is an advantage over the proposed separation of mind and body implicit in the biomedical model. It provides an operating framework for emerging studies in psycho-neuroimmunology, neuroendocrinology and brain–gut interactions where environmental factors (e.g. psychosocial stress) are shown to have direct effects on the development and expression of inflammatory conditions. Taken from this perspective, attention to the psychosocial factors associated with IBD may have consequences not only for psychosocial wellbeing and quality of life, but also for the activity of the disease itself.

# THE INFLUENCE OF STRESS ON GI FUNCTION, INTESTINAL INFLAMMATION AND IBD

## CURRENT MEDICAL THINKING

Research relating psychologic stress to IBD is evolving from clinical opinion to scientific investigation. (Stress is difficult to understand and even harder to study; no definition is satisfactory. Humans function in constantly changing environments, and any influence on one's steady state requiring adjustment or adaptation can, in its broadest sense, be considered stress. The term encompasses both the stimulus (e.g. a biologic event such as infection, a social event such as a change of residence, or merely a disturbing thought) and its effects, from no effect to a psychological response (anxiety, depression), physiologic change (diarrhea, diaphoresis), possibly disease activation, or any

combination. Individuals may interpret a stressor as desirable or undesirable; pain, sex or threat of injury, usually elicit predictable responses. In contrast, life events and other psychologic processes have more varied effects: a change of job may be of little concern to one person, yet lead to crisis in another who views the event as a personal failure. Both a person's interpretation of events as stressful or not, and his or her response, depend on prior experience, attitudes, coping, personality, culture and biological factors including susceptibility to disease.) In a random sample of 1000 members of the American Gastroenterological Association (53% clinical practice, 33% academic practice, 11% trainees)[10] IBD was found in 14% of their patients (6.8% UC, 7.1% CD). This study showed that physicians believe that although stress and psychosocial factors do not contribute to the etiology of IBD, they are important in the clinical exacerbation of symptoms (more so in CUC than CD). Physicians also believe that these factors are more important than what they had learned from the scientific literature (which in the 1980s tended to discount psychosocial influences). Also, the respondents did not believe that IBD patients had a characteristic personality style, and the psychosocial impact of IBD was considered no different from that of other chronic diseases (such as diabetes mellitus or arthritis). Notably, more than half of the patients with IBD believe that stress or their own personality is a major contributor to the development of their disease, and more than 90% think that it influences their disease activity.[11,12]

# EMOTIONAL DISTRESS AND ALTERED GI FUNCTION AND SYMPTOMS

For centuries, clinical experience[1] and also epidemiological evidence[13] supported the contention that emotional distress can produce changes in bowel function and lead to abdominal discomfort in almost everyone, and particularly in patients with functional gastrointestinal disorders.[14] Many of the stress-related symptoms that patients with IBD experience may relate to stress-induced changes in motility and pain sensation independent of their disease activity.[4,6] Psychological and emotional stresses can affect the GI motor, sensory and secretory function directly or indirectly through the richly innervated nerve plexuses existing between the enteric nervous system and its spinal and autonomic connections to the central nervous system (the 'brain–gut axis'),[15] and mediated by various peptides having neurotransmitter and endocrine-like actions: VIP, TRH, 5HT, CCK, substance P, CGRP and the enkephalins.[16]

Stress effects on intestinal function have been reported in both humans and laboratory animals. For example, anger has been shown to significantly alter colonic[17] and gastric[18] motor activity in patients with IBS and healthy controls. Other preliminary observations show that psychological stressors can also increase colonic or rectosigmoid sensitivity to distension[19] in healthy volunteers. Animal studies have also demonstrated stress-induced alterations in intestinal myoelectric activity[20–23] and sensory function.[24] Furthermore, maternal separation in newborn rats can lead to permanent visceral hyperalgesia, somatic hypoalgesia and enhanced colonic activity in response to psychological stress.[25]

The association between psychological stress and symptom exacerbation is well recognized for individuals with functional gastrointestinal disorders,[14,16] and basic investigational studies are providing the mechanisms for these observations.[26] Furthermore, IBS symptoms may coexist with IBD. In a recent study[6] of 43 UC and 40 CD patients in long-standing (at least 1 year ) remission, 30% of UC and 57% of CD patients reported GI symptoms compatible with irritable bowel syndrome (IBS). Notably, these symptoms were predicted by anxiety (Spielberger State Trait Anxiety Inventory) and depression (the Hospital Anxiety and Depression Scale). Thus symptoms, such as abdominal pain and change in bowel function, may occur in IBD without significant disease activity. This might relate to alterations in motor and sensory function[4] resulting from previous inflammation[27] or psychological distress.[15]

## ANIMAL RESEARCH LINKING STRESS WITH GASTROINTESTINAL INFLAMMATION

Animal studies can provide a link between environmental stress and the development of gastrointestinal inflammation and inflammatory disease. Physical restraint, prolonged swimming or premature weaning can produce acute gastric erosions ('stress ulcers') in rats.[16] Physical restraint or conditioned anxiety were reported to produce chronic gastroduodenitis in 11/19 Rhesus monkeys (and two monkeys also developed chronic colitis).[28] In another study, other major social disruptions (e.g. death of a mate) led to fatal colitis in four Siamang gibbons.[29,30]

The cotton-top tamarin, a New World monkey from Colombia, develops ulcerative colitis and colon carcinoma only in captivity.[31,32] Interestingly, these animals naturally live in an unusual social unit in the jungles, with one breeding female, several non-breeding females, and one to three reproductively active males who care for the offspring. It is proposed that capturing these animals and caging them in male–female pairs, usually at lower temperatures than the jungle habitat, produces enough environmental disruption (social isolation and cold stress) to influence the development of these diseases.[32–34] No other environmental factors, such as infection, diet or radiation, have been found to explain why these diseases occur in captivity. Thus, this species may be the closest colitis model to humans that implicates disruption of brain–gut interactions in the pathogenesis of the inflammation.

More recent studies in animal models have shown that stress can also augment the inflammatory response to 2,4,6-trinitrobenzenesulfonic acid (TNB)-induced colitis and to reactivate the inflammatory process in rats recovered from TNB-induced colitis.[35–38] Animal models can increase our understanding of the association between stress and intestinal inflammation by studying specific determinants of intestinal stress-induced inflammatory response and its possible pathophysiological mediators.[38]

## CLINICAL RESEARCH RELATING PSYCHOSOCIAL STRESS TO INFLAMMATORY BOWEL DISEASE

Persons who experience social disorganization are considered more susceptible to a variety of medical disorders,[39] and major changes in a person's lifestyle have been shown to correlate with the subsequent incidence of illness or injury.[40,41] These observations have led to a variety of epidemiologic investigations linking psychosocial stress in humans to many chronic diseases.

The older clinical and epidemiological studies in IBD that relate life stress to symptom exacerbation generally show a positive association,[42–44] but are flawed because of methodological

limitations:[45–48] 1) the bias of the investigators, 2) retrospective design, 3) small sample size, 4) lack of control groups, 5) naive approach to stress measurement with inappropriate selection of psychological instruments, or analysis of data, 6) referral bias, and 7) inaccurate medical diagnosis. These limitations have led some authors to conclude that no relationship between stress and illness exacerbation in IBD exists, as the positive studies are poorly designed.[45] However, the complex relationship between psychosocial factors and human illness makes even a well-designed negative study insufficient to support this conclusion. For example, most studies evaluating the effect of stressors on illness exacerbation in IBD have not included measures of the effect of these stressors on the individual modulating factors, such as social support and coping style, in the design (Fig. 24.1).[16] So, a non-significant study might only mean that it failed to consider all the relevant psychosocial measures in the analysis.

A few prospective studies have used sophisticated methods such as time lag analysis to determine whether stress precedes symptom exacerbation. North et al.[48] studied the effects of major life events and mood on bowel symptoms and pain in 32 patients with IBD. They found no association between these life events and mood with symptoms 1 or 2 months later, although an association was found between depressive symptoms and symptom severity.

However, this lack of association between psychosocial events and later symptom exacerbation is not surprising. To presume an effect of pre-existing major life events on bowel symptoms a month or two later may be unrealistic, as there is ample time for psychosocial (e.g. social support, coping) adaptation,[16] which can affect the outcome.[49]

In a more rigorous study using a larger sample of 124 IBD patients, Duffy et al.[50] also evaluated monthly major life events with symptoms of pain, bowel dysfunction and bleeding. The authors did find a strong relationship between major life events, particularly health-related events, and symptom exacerbation. At baseline, patients with a history of life events had a greater risk of active disease than did those without (RR = 1.97, 95% CI 1.13–3.43), and there was a twofold increased risk at 6-month follow-up (RR = 2.56, 95% CI 1.34–4.86). Furthermore, a significant but weaker association also existed for life events that predated symptom exacerbation by 1 month (correlation range 0.24–0.37). Using a time series regression of bowel symptoms recorded over a 28-day period, another research group[43] found a significant association between acute daily stress and bowel symptoms (e.g. pain, nausea, diarrhea) even after controlling for major life events. However, the limitation of these studies with regard to IBD is the short period of follow-up evaluation, and also that the symptoms studied (e.g. pain, diarrhea) can be physiologic responses of the gut to acute stress, rather than measures of increased disease activity.

A more recent prospective cohort study addressed some of these limitations. Levenstein et al.[51] evaluated 62 patients with known UC who were enrolled while in clinical remission. They were followed for up to 45 months and exacerbation status (defined as ≥10 days of symptoms associated with intensified therapy by a physician and/or rectal inflammation on endoscopy), as the study endpoint, was monitored for up to 68 months. The investigators found that high scores for long-term perceived stress tripled the risk of UC exacerbation during the next 8 months. Exacerbation was not associated with short-term (past month) perceived stress or depressive symptoms.

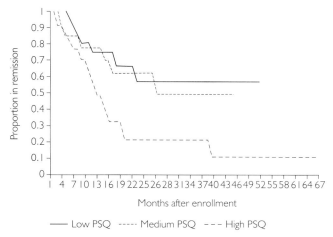

**Fig. 24.2** Kaplan–Meier analysis of cumulative rates of exacerbation in ulcerative colitis patients with high, middle, and low tertile scores on long-term Perceived Stress Questionnaire Scores (PSQ) at enrollment. Risk of exacerbation was higher among patients with high long-term stress levels than among those with low levels ($P = 0.03$ by log-rank test).[51]

The advantages of this study were its prospective design, reasonable clinical endpoints of exacerbation, and attention to the use of a more rigorous perceived stress questionnaire[52] that assesses the individual experience associated with the stressful event (Fig. 24.2).

From these and other studies we can conclude that: 1) epidemiologic and clinical data have historically indicated an association between various psychosocial stressors and illness exacerbation, not unique to IBD; 2) data linking life events and daily stressors with physiological effects (e.g. pain, diarrhea) are generally supported; 3) for IBD, data relating major life events with disease exacerbation are conflicting and not well studied, although better-designed prospective studies suggest a positive association; 4) the major stressors identified in life events research are not unique or condition specific: they can include illness or death in the family, abuse, divorce or separation, interpersonal conflict, or other major loss unique to the individual. Future studies will need to be more rigorous in their design, and must also evaluate psychosocial modulators (e.g. social support and coping) and differentiate acute (e.g. daily 'hassles') from chronic (e.g. life event) stressors, and acute physiological responses (e.g. diarrhea, pain) from more chronic effects associated with inflammatory responses and disease activation.

## MECHANISMS MEDIATING STRESS, NEUROENDOCRINE IMMUNE FUNCTION AND IBD

An understanding of how psychosocial factors could lead to the onset or exacerbation of IBD has been advanced with new knowledge of the relationships between CNS, endocrine and immune function.[53–58]

## PSYCHOSOCIAL STRESS AND NEUROENDOCRINE–IMMUNE REGULATION

Environmental stress can influence disease susceptibility via the central nervous system and its humoral and cellular inflammatory/immune connections. Associations between stressful experiences, such as bereavement, marital disruption or stress-inducing experiments, and in vivo effects on immune function have been recognized for at least two decades and include decreased responsiveness to mitogens and antigens, reduced lymphocyte-mediated cytotoxicity, reduced delayed hypersensitivity, diminished skin graft rejection and graft-versus-host reactivity and suppressed antibody response.[16] Only in the last several years have the mechanisms for these associations been studied and are beginning to be understood.

The central neuroendocrine system serves as an interface between environmental factors (e.g. stress) and the body's physiological response. Several regions of the brain (including the paraventricular nucleus in the hypothalamus, the CRH (corticotropin-releasing hormone) subsystem, amygdala and periaquaductal gray) are involved in the body's homeostatic adaptation to stress. These structures receive input from peripheral visceral and somatic afferents and from cortical structures (e.g. the anterior cingulate and medial prefrontal cortex).[59,60]

The stress responses are enabled via two primary interconnected subsystems, which are the limbs of the body's homeostatic stress adaptation system. Together they coordinate both the peripheral and the behavioral components of the stress response and related neuroendocrine–immune pathways.[53,54] The CRH subsystem has at its rostral end the paraventricular nucleus of the hypothalamus, and activates distally the hypothalamopituitary–adrenal (HPA) axis. The sympathetic subsystem, which has rostrally the locus ceruleus of the brain stem, activates the sympathetic adrenomedullary system. These two systems are reciprocally communicating and are also in close interaction with the immune system, which in turn reciprocally provides feedback, thus creating a neuroendocrine–immune axis (Table 24.1).[15] Lymphocytes and macrophages contain receptors for, and respond to, neurotransmitters, neuropeptides and hormones, and also produce many of these substances.[61] The CNS contains neuronal pathways and receptors for cytokines, such as interleukin-1 (IL-1). Peripheral nerves and the autonomic nervous system also innervate the immune system organs.[62] These feedback systems of the neuroendocrine–immune axis make it possible for stressors, via their neural and endocrine connections, to influence the immune/inflammatory response in a variety of systems, including the colon,[53] and for immune/inflammatory mediators such as cytokines present in the colon to modulate higher neural function and behavior.[57,63]

With regard to the CRH subsystem, immune/inflammatory mediators constitute the afferent limb of the HPA axis and are potent activators of this system.[53,57] As shown in Figure 24.3, the cytokines – interleukins, tumor necrosis factor-α and prostaglandin E$_2$ – and platelet-activating factor stimulate the hypothalamus to secrete CRH.[53] CRH in turn stimulates the pituitary gland to release corticotropin (ACTH), which stimulates the adrenal glands to release glucocorticoids. The corticosteroids suppress inflammation and the production of cytokines, thereby completing the negative feedback circuit. Homeostasis is achieved through dynamic and integrated responses of these systems in response to intrinsic or extrinsic forces (e.g. stress, infection, other illnesses) that could disturb the steady state. Furthermore, as noted, peripheral cytokines also have central effects that may contribute to the behavioral features of chronic inflammatory conditions (see below).

Given these associations, many chronic conditions are being linked to disruption or dysregulation of this stress-response

**Table 24.1 Components of the immune, CNS and neuroendocrine systems[52]**

| System | Anatomic structure | Mediators |
| --- | --- | --- |
| Immune | Lymphocytes<br>Macrophages<br>Thymus/spleen<br>Bone marrow | Interleukins (IL-1, IL-2)<br>(IL-3, IL-6)<br>Cytokines (IC-4, IC-8, IC-10)<br>Transforming growth factor-β<br>Tumor necrosis factor-α<br>Interferon-γ |
| Neural | Central nervous system<br>Peripheral nervous system | Serotonin (5-HT)<br>Acetylcholine (ACh)<br>Norepinephrine (NE)<br>Dopamine<br>γ-Aminobutyric acid (GABA)<br>Opioids<br>Neuropeptides (substance P, VIP) |
| Neuroendocrine | Hypothalamus<br>Pituitary<br>Adrenal<br>Thyroid | Corticotropin-releasing hormone (CRH)<br>Corticotropin (ACTH)<br>Corticosteroids<br>Follicle-stimulating hormone (FSH)<br>Luteinizing hormone (LH)<br>Thyroid-stimulating hormone (TSH)<br>Growth hormone (GH) |

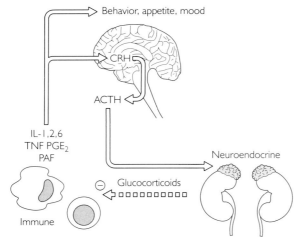

**Fig. 24.3** The immune–central nervous system–endocrine feedback system. Stimulation by immune cytokines and inflammatory mediators facilitates a hypothalamopituitary–adrenal (HPA) response, beginning with release of corticotropin-releasing hormone (CRH). This, in turn, will lead to release of ACTH, which stimulates glucocorticoid release from the adrenal glands. Finally, the glucocorticoids will suppress (hatched line) inflammation and the immune response, thereby completing the negative feedback circuit. Homeostasis is maintained through dynamic and integrated responses of these systems in response to intrinsic or extrinsic forces (e.g. stress, infection, other illnesses) that could disturb the steady state. (With permission from[53].)

system.[53,54] For example, it has been proposed that increased HPA-axis reactivity can mimic hypercortisolemia (e.g. Cushing's syndrome), and also increase susceptibility to infectious agents and tumors while resisting the development of autoimmune or inflammatory disease. Conversely, decreased HPA-axis reactivity would lead to resistance to infections and neoplasms, but an increased susceptibility to certain functional somatic disorders (e.g. fibromyalgia, chronic fatigue syndrome), psychiatric conditions (post-traumatic stress disorder) or autoimmune/inflammatory conditions, such as rheumatoid arthritis, or autoimmune thyroiditis and possibly even inflammatory bowel disease.[53,54,64] Evidence for centrally altered HPA reactivity and susceptibility to inflammatory conditions exists with certain animal models. Lewis rats are genetically susceptible, and Fischer rats resistant to the induction of various inflammatory conditions (e.g. experimental arthritis).[65] The presence or absence of an inflammatory response is related to species-specific differences in the responsiveness of the HPA axis to stress. Lewis rats have a genetic defect in the synthesis and release of CRH. So, when challenged with bacterial cell-wall peptidoglycans, cytokines or other inflammatory stimuli, they mount a poor ACTH response and have a diminished corticosterone output, thus leading to increased inflammation. Conversely, Fischer rats have genetically intact CRH reactivity and are able to resist the development of inflammatory conditions. Moreover, transplantation of hypothalamic tissue from inflammatory resistant rats to Lewis rats provides protection against inflammation,[66] thus supporting a role for central mediation of inflammation.

## EVIDENCES IMPLICATING NEUROENDOCRINE–IMMUNE MECHANISMS IN IBD

With regard to IBD in humans, there are several lines of evidence that implicate a possible relationship between neuroendocrine–immune dysfunction and the pathophysiology or clinical expression of IBD.

### Eosinophilia–myalgia syndrome

This is an inflammatory disease associated with diarrhea due to a chronic colitis (eosinophilic and mononuclear colonic mucosal infiltration).[67] The disorder results from ingestion of impure L-tryptophan, and administering this substance to Lewis rats produces the same immune cell activation effects and gastrointestinal findings as in humans.[67] This is associated with the suppression of hypothalamic CRH mRNA expression,[68] and the L-tryptophan impurity implicated in the disease appears to have neurotransmitter-like properties that suppress CRH release. Thus, decreased CRH reactivity in this situation is associated with development of the condition, presumably related to unopposed activity of gut inflammatory/immune mediators.

## Stress-induced effects on HPA-axis activity and intestinal inflammation

Animal studies of strains with genetically impaired HPA-axis reactivity demonstrate the role for central (HPA axis and CRH) influences on gut inflammation. Sartor et al.[69] used subserosal injections of streptococcal peptidoglycan–polysaccharide (PG–PS) to induce chronic relapsing granulomatous enterocolitis (bowel disease, arthritis and extraintestinal manifestations), which is morphologically similar to human Crohn's disease.[69] Notably, the disease develops in Lewis and Sprague–Dawley rats (which have genetically deficient HPA-axis reactivity), but not in Fischer or Buffalo rats (having increased HPA-axis reactivity). In addition to HPA-axis dysfunction, increased tissue IL-1/IL-1 receptor antagonist ratio and increased activation of the kallikrein–kinin system have been implicated in the pathogenesis of the disease.[70,71]

Furthermore, the relationship of psychosocial stress (e.g. physical restraint and water avoidance) to HPA-axis reactivity and intestinal inflammation has been supported by a recent study using a trinitrobenzene (TNB)-induced colitis in Lewis and Fischer rats.[35] In this study both strains (i.e. Lewis and Fischer) exhibit a similar degree of mucosal inflammation in response to TNB. However, the instillation of superimposed stress, before TNB, was associated with more pronounced and worsening of the colitis in the Lewis rats, because of their greater genetic susceptibility to HPA hyporeactivity, as previously discussed. Furthermore, daily intracerebroventricular administration of CRF inhibits the TNB-induced inflammation in both Lewis and Fischer rats, and intracerebroventricular injection of a CRF antagonist, astressin, resulted in enhancement of the inflammation.

## Stress-induced, immune-mediated mucosal inflammation

As noted, stress can produce an inflammatory response in the intestinal mucosa. The evidence suggests this to be immune mediated. Collins and Qiu et al.[36,72] induced a reactivation of colonic inflammation by restraint stress in Wistar–Kyoto and Sprague–Dawley rats that were previously sensitized by TNB colitis. This stress-induced reactive inflammation did not occur in athymic mice, severe combined immune deficiency (SCID) mice, or in CD4+ depleted Balb/c knockout mice, yet inflammation occurred with the transfer of CD4+ enriched cells from mice with acute colitis to SCID mice placed under the same stress paradigm. This suggests that stress can reactivate previously induced intestinal inflammation in quiescence, and that this event is immune mediated and may involve CD4+ lymphocytes.

Mast cells may also mediate the intestinal inflammatory response to stress. Water avoidance stress in rats induces mucosal inflammation (as evidenced by mucus depletion, enlarged mitochondria, neutrophil/monocytic infiltration, auto-

phagosomes and increased myeloperoxidase activity) and increased mucosal permeability to macromolecules.[73] These alterations occurred in wildtype (+/+) control rats but not in mast cell-deficient (Ws/Ws) rats. Furthermore, in humans, cold water stress can induce jejunal mast cell activation.[74]

## Stress-induced increase in gut mucosal permeability

It is believed that in a biologically susceptible host IBD is initiated with the transmigration of antigenic macromolecules through leaky epithelia. When Wistar–Kyoto rats are physically restrained there is an increase in their intestinal permeability, stimulating $Cl^-$ ion secretion and reducing mucosal barrier function, thereby allowing for transmural migration of macromolecules.[75]

The mechanisms associated with the stress-mediated effects on mucosal permeability are not yet clear. Some studies suggested enhanced cholinergic activity on epithelial function in a genetically susceptible strain that has reduced cholinesterase activity.[43,75,76] Others have demonstrated the involvement of inflammation and mast cell reactivity.[73]

## Alteration of mucosal neuropeptide activity in IBD

The enteric nervous system (ENS) neuropeptides (e.g. VIP, somatostatin) present in the gut lamina propria are not only involved in the regulation of motor function and sensation within the gut, but (by also being present on lymphoid cell populations) can influence mucosal immune and inflammatory function via cytokine activation.[55] In fact, these neuropeptides are reduced in IBD and correlate with the degree of tissue inflammation.[55] There is even evidence that the reduction in ENS neurotransmitter content and release may be immunologically mediated.[63] In addition, peripheral (i.e. mucosal) CRH, which has pro-inflammatory effects, is increased in patients with UC.[77] So, it is possible that stress-induced alteration in neuropeptides, leading to the lack of availability of local neuropeptides (VIP, SMS) and the increased activity of others (e.g. CRH), may contribute to unopposed cytokine production, thereby locally upregulating the inflammatory state.

## Behavioral conditioning of the stress–inflammatory response

Several studies during the past 25 years have provided evidence for possible behavioral conditioning of the immune function. Using a classic (pavlovian) conditioning model linking the taste of saccharin to cyclophosphamide in NZB-NZW mice, Ader and Cohen were able to suppress immune function. Compared to controls, the conditioned animals taking only saccharin showed a significant delay in the development of murine lupus erythematosus as well as increased survival time.[78] With regard to GI inflammation, a more recent study has shown that mucosal mast cells can be conditioned to secrete an immune mediator (protease II) in response to an audiovisual cue,[79] thus providing evidence for mucosal immune (mast cell) system conditioning by environmental stimuli via a CNS–immune system interaction.

These data help explain how stress may exacerbate or 'rekindle' an inflammation response in a host previously conditioned by chemical inflammation. Thus Wistar–Kyoto and Sprague–Dawley rats that recover from experimental colitis induced by TNBS, when subsequently stressed by physical restraint, become conditioned to show an increased tissue inflammatory response.[36]

## Effects of gut inflammation on enteric neural function

Once inflammation is produced, there can be further effects on neural function peripherally or centrally. In animals, intestinal inflammation can alter the function of the enteric smooth muscle,[80,81] the myenteric plexus[82] and interstitial cells of Cajal.[83] These inflammatory induced alterations in intestinal motor[84–87] and sensory[30,36,88] function may sensitize enteric nerve and smooth muscle function, thereby leading to symptoms of abdominal pain or bowel dysfunction.

## Effects of inflammation on CNS function and behavior

Intestinal inflammation via cytokine activation can also affect CNS function, leading to behavioral effects. It is now recognized that many of the behavioral features of chronic inflammatory diseases, called 'sickness behavior' (e.g. fever, fatigue, anorexia, depression), may result from the central effects of peripherally activated inflammatory cytokines.[14,60,89] Proinflammatory cytokines (e.g. IL-1, IL-6, TNF and interferons), released by activated monocytes and macrophages during inflammation, can activate vagal afferent pathways to the brain[89] or induce the synthesis and release of inflammatory cytokines within the brain.[90] These locally and centrally produced cytokines can lead to sickness behavior. For example, recent studies have shown that systemic (at the periphery) or central (lateral ventricle of the brain) injection of cytokines can induce a variety of non-specific behavioral symptoms in experimental animals.[91,92]

Given these observations, perturbations of the neuroenteric circuitry (either genetic, physiologically or behaviorally conditioned) may help explain the variation in the frequency and severity of disease activity or the inflammatory responses to induction of viral or bacterial agents. The host's immune system will contribute to disease pathogenesis and chronicity, either by a failure to clear the antigen(s) and/or because of an inappropriate immune response to the infectious agent(s). Disease activity would be influenced by alterations in circulating and tissue neuropeptides, or in the sensitivity of immune–inflammatory effector cells to these peptides. Furthermore, if subsets of IBD patients have dysregulation of the HPA axis, or other neuroendocrine systems that perpetuate the inflammatory response, then there is potential benefit for the use of psychotropic agents[53] and psychological treatments, not only to improve psychologic comorbidity, but to also alter the activity of the disease.

# THE PSYCHOSOCIAL CONCOMITANTS AND CONSEQUENCES OF IBD

Once IBD develops, there are psychosocial concomitants and consequences unique to the individual that must be understood in order to effect proper care.

## PERSONALITY

A major and somewhat naive focus of research during the psychoanalytically dominated era of psychosomatic medicine (1920–1955) was to understand certain diseases as being linked to specific personality features or conflicts.

## Psychosomatic specificity

The predominant theory during this era was that of 'psychosomatic specificity', which assumed that specific psychologic features were associated with, and necessary for, the development of a particular disease. Beginning with the belief that distinct personality profiles existed, later work was directed at the role of unconscious conflicts as stressors leading to the onset of disease. Alexander and his associates[93] emphasized that psychodynamic conflicts and specific personality features, in addition to a biologic predisposition (factor X) contributed to the development of a disease: '…some specific local somatic factor (factor X) may be responsible for the fact that in some patients anal regression produces ulceration in the bowels'. Therefore, the proper environmental stimulus could activate the psychologic conflict, and the biologically predisposed individual would develop or exacerbate the disease. Seven medical diseases, including ulcerative colitis and peptic ulcer, were thought to be representative of this hypothesis.[93]

To develop ulcerative colitis, the proposed antecedent conflict was the need to carry out certain obligations coupled with unwillingness or inability to do so. When this conflict was activated, such as when needing to leave home to go to school but feeling unprepared, the disease might become clinically expressed. In psychodynamic terms, the patient regresses to the time of the first environmental demand for accomplishment, the period of bowel control development. At this stage of life, the child perceives bowel function and stools as achievements: defecation is both giving up a cherished possession, and an accomplishment. In the person predisposed to develop UC, the conflict and this regression would activate neural (presumed to be parasympathetic) pathways in the colon. The physiologic effect would be to alter bowel motility (producing diarrhea) while also breaking the protective mucosal barrier, making it vulnerable to digestion and bacterial invasion. Interestingly, this hypothesis, proposed almost 50 years ago, is consistent with the previously described reports of cholinergically mediated stress-induced increases in mucosal permeability in rats.[75,76,94]

Further elaboration of the psychodynamic hypothesis occurred when the research shifted from intrapsychic conflicts to problems with interpersonal relationships. Ulcerative colitis patients were described as dependent on parents or parent substitutes, and overly sensitive to personal rejection. Relationship difficulties were manifest either as extreme dependence and unrealistic demands on others, or as reluctance to develop any trusting relationships.[95] Illness exacerbation would occur when a key relationship was lost through separation or bereavement. Thus, it was concluded that the personality structure and intrapsychic conflicts could cause these people to evolve to certain relationships or gravitate toward certain kinds of life situations, disruption of which might be followed by onset or relapse of the disease. Given this construct, it was recommended that the physician establish a predictable and consistent relationship with such patients.[96]

Although there were attempts to validate the specificity of these personality factors for medical diseases,[97,98] the methodology and results were not convincing because of small sample sizes, skewed sampling (using only psychiatric patients), uncontrolled psychologic assessment, and poor validation of disease (patient samples often included those with CD and infectious colitis).[47,99] In retrospect, the theory of psychosomatic specificity is too simplistic, as it proposes that emotional factors are causative, rather than a modulating component of the illness. Furthermore, attention was directed solely at psychodynamic factors. Life stress, the social environment and the patient's coping style were not considered. We now believe that the reported results related more to a generalized effect of psychologic distress on illness, or to the psychosocial effects of chronic illness, rather than being specific for any disease. By the 1960s this theory had become unpopular among patients and physicians because of its stigmatizing features, and in the 1980s it was replaced by the more general systems or biopsychosocial understanding of disease.[2]

## Alexithymia

One personality construct studied by psychiatrists and psychosomaticists over the last 25 years for a variety of medical conditions, including IBD, is that of alexithymia (from the Greek: 'absence of words for emotions').[97] Patients with alexithymia have chronic difficulty in recognizing and verbalizing emotions, are concrete in their thinking, and have a reduced capacity for fantasy, which limits their ability to regulate emotions or use coping strategies effectively, and is associated with decreased quality of life.[100] Clinicians may observe that although patients with alexithymia might express emotions, such as anger or sadness, in relation to their illness, they know little about the psychological basis for these feelings and cannot link them with memories or specific situations.[101] One epidemiological study[102] showed that IBD patients seen in a referral setting exhibited alexithymic features greater than controls but less so than patients with functional gastrointestinal disorders. These findings are not thought to be characteristic of the disorder, but may reflect the long-term effects of chronic illness or result from ascertainment bias relating to the high healthcare-seeking subset of patients evaluated in this study.

It is believed that alexithymia, possibly developing in response to severe illness or other early trauma, may lead patients to 'reroute' the communication of psychological distress through somatic and behavioral, rather than verbal, communication. This can occur through physiologic (sympathetic) arousal, increased vigilance to and reporting of physical sensations (somatization), unhealthy behaviors (e.g. cigarette and alcohol use, disordered eating patterns, non-adherence to medical treatments), or increased healthcare-seeking behaviors.[103] Alexithymia is not specific to IBD, but may reflect behavioral adaptations to chronic illness, and become operative when patients have limited psychologic resources to adjust to their chronic condition. Their tendency to communicate emotional distress through somatic symptoms rather than verbally may be associated with more frequent physician visits and a poorer prognosis. The clinical relevance of this observation is that patients with these behavioral features may not respond well to psychological 'insight' or 'talk therapy'. Behavioral or psychopharmacologic treatments are therefore recommended.[101]

## PSYCHIATRIC DIAGNOSES AND PSYCHOLOGIC DISTURBANCES

Although many clinicians and investigators have noted a close relationship between disease activity and psychological disorders, associations are bidirectional and strongly influenced by the severity and chronicity of the disease. In general, the prevalence of psychological disorders in patients with IBD is understandably higher than in the general population.[12,104,105] In one study of 116 consecutive patients with IBD, 25.9% showed 'probable psychological disorder' on the clinical depression and anxiety scales of the Hospital Anxiety and Depression Scale (HADS).[105] A retrospective epidemiological study[106] found that both depression and anxiety preceded the first diagnosis of UC more often than would be predicted from control data (no such association was found with CD), and patients with either UC or CD are at an increased risk of a subsequent diagnosis of depression or anxiety. This association was strongest during the first year after the initial diagnosis of UC or CD. Overall the frequency of psychiatric diagnoses in past studies of IBD range from 13 to 100%,[46] and no fixed prevalence of specific diagnostic profile can be found. This relates to: 1) differing study samples: for example, psychiatric IBD patients or those studied at medical referral centers will have more psychosocial disturbance than those in the community; 2) use of different (at times inappropriate) assessment methods; 3) inappropriate registration and comparisons between current and lifetime psychiatric diagnosis; 4) failure to control for disease severity; and 5) investigator bias in the interpretation of the data. Although these methodological limitations have led some authors to conclude that psychosocial disturbances do not exist,[45] it is more reasonable to understand the findings as varying elaborations related to differing populations and study designs.

Given these limitations, it is still possible to derive some conclusions:

1. Studies drawn from subjects in non-referral settings indicate that the psychological profiles are similar to normal subjects, although with wide variation.
2. IBD patients have slightly higher frequencies of psychiatric diagnosis and slightly greater psychological distress than normal controls, at a level comparable to patients with other chronic diseases, and significantly fewer psychological difficulties than patients with irritable bowel syndrome.[104–111]
3. The psychiatric diagnoses are non-specific and most often relate to anxiety and depression, particularly in patients with chronic disease.[44,106]
4. Patients with CD have greater psychological disturbances than those with UC.[46,109,112–116]
5. The degree of psychological disturbance appears to correlate with the severity of the disease,[109,112,117–119] and this may explain the greater prevalence of these diagnoses in CD. In a national random study of persons belonging to the Crohn's and Colitis Foundation of America,[109] patients with CD had greater psychological dysfunction (SIP, 8.0 +0.4 SE) and psychological distress (SCL-90) than those with UC (SIP, 6.1 +0.6 SE; SCL-90, 53.7 +0.63 SE). Yet, after controlling for disease severity, these differences were no longer significant.[109] Furthermore, comparisons between IBD members with active (CDAI >182) and inactive disease confirmed that all psychosocial measures were significantly higher in those with more active disease.
6. Psychological disturbances appear to be successfully mediated through the use of problem-based coping strategies such as social support, education, problem solving and positive reappraisal of distressing experiences.[49,109,120]

These findings suggest that psychological disturbances are a component of the illness that modulates its clinical expression, rather than being etiologic or specific to IBD.

# THE PSYCHOLOGICAL IMPACT OF INFLAMMATORY BOWEL DISEASE: HEALTH-RELATED QUALITY OF LIFE (HRQOL)

Laboratory studies, histopathology and endoscopic/radiologic findings do not adequately explain the psychosocial impact of chronic illness such as IBD,[2,7] which also depends on previous experiences, the person's psychological state and their socio-cultural environment. For example, daily functional status related to IBD correlates better with scores of wellbeing and healthcare utilization than the physician's rating of disease activity.[112]

Health-related quality of life (HRQOL) incorporates the patient's perceptions, illness experience and functional status as related to the medical condition.[121] It is influenced by social, cultural, psychological and disease-related factors.[7] Its measurement differs from disease measurement by incorporating psychosocial (e.g. daily function, recreation, sexual function etc.) as well as biological factors, and as shown in one study, both disease severity and psychological distress contribute to poor HRQOL.[105] The validation of these instruments rests with the patient.[7] Recently standardized instruments have been developed to measure various aspects of HRQOL.[122]

## Global measure

The simplest measure of HRQOL employs a 'global' question (e.g. 'How would you rate your general wellbeing'?), and the patient incorporates the multiple domains of HRQOL into a single response (usually rated on a five-point scale: 'excellent, very good, good, fair or poor'). Whereas this measure is a strong predictor of physician visits for patients with IBD[109] it yields no information about the underlying factors leading to the response, and may be contaminated by the person's level of psychological distress.

## Generic measures

Generic measures assess HRQOL independent of the specific features of the disease. They can provide a range of responses for a patient group, and be compared across groups, even with different diseases. There are two types of generic measure.[121,123] Multi-item health profiles incorporate several dimensions of the patient's experience and behavior, such as physical or psychosocial functioning, or perceptions of disease impact. For example, the Sickness Impact Profile (SIP)[124] encompasses 12 discrete areas of daily function (e.g. eating, communication, bodily care, home management etc.) which can be reduced to an overall score, as well as physical and psychosocial summary scores. Figure 24.4 compares the SIP overall scores for patients with CUC and CD[112] with other diseases.[123] Another generic measure is the SF-36,[125] which encompasses eight domains of physical and social function and roles, bodily pain, vitality, general and mental health.

*Utility measures* can determine patient preferences for a type of treatment. The 'time trade-off technique' (TTOT) evaluates the patient's perception of existing health compared to death. A score ranging from 0.0 (equal to death) to 1.0 (full health) is obtained by having the patient choose between living in the present state of health, with all its physical and psychosocial limitations, or choosing a shorter lifespan but in perfect health. For example, two 30-year-old patients with Crohn's disease

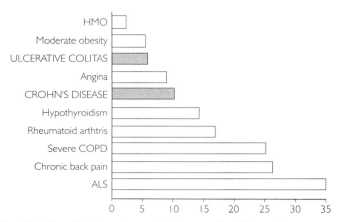

**Fig. 24.4** Overall Sickness Impact Profile scores for different diseases. It can be seen that patients with IBD have functional impairment that is greater than that of a health maintenance organization (HMO) population, but much less than in patients with chronic back pain or amyotrophic lateral sclerosis. (Adapted from Patrick et al.[123].)

might be expected to live until 75 (life expectancy is determined by actuarial tables). The patient who is in fair health may feel well enough to only trade 5 years of life (and live until age 70) in full health. This person would have a utility score of 70/75 = 0.93. In comparison, the other patient who experiences very poor health may be willing to trade off 30 years of life (and live until age 45 in full health, and the utility score would be 45/75 = 0.60. The change in a utility score can also be used to determine patient preferences for a treatment. For example, McLeod et al.[126] have shown an increase in the TTOT from 0.58 +0.34 SD to 0.98 +0.07 SD for CUC patients 1 year after colectomy. Like other single-item measures, the utility score cannot show the domains within which improvement or deterioration occurs.

## Disease (condition)-specific measures

These measures assess the special states and concerns of patients with a particular disease. One for Crohn's disease might have questions about bowel habit, abdominal pain and sexual functioning, whereas one for rheumatoid arthritis might assess hand strength and mobility. These measures are more responsive to clinical changes that occur over time,[127] and the questions are often routinely asked in clinical care, so they are particularly useful for treatment trials. One disease-specific measure for IBD, the Inflammatory Bowel Disease Questionnaire (IBDQ),[128] was shown to be reliable, valid and responsive to changes relating to medical treatment.[129] Table 24.2 lists the features of this and other specific instruments developed for IBD, and this information is found elsewhere.[122]

# HEALTHCARE UTILIZATION

The frequency of IBD seen in GI practice is about 14% (7% UC and 7% CD).[10,130] The determinants of why patients with IBD go to the physician are many and are based on both medical and psychosocial influences. In a national sample of 320 patients with UC and 671 with CD, Drossman et al.[109] found that although the number of hospitalizations and surgeries was related primarily to physical health factors (e.g. weight loss, number of stool per week, physical dysfunction), the number of physician visits was related to both psychosocial and physical health factors. Similarly, physician visits and hospitalization, in

## Table 24.2. Specific health status instruments for IBD[141]

| Name | Scales | Comments |
|---|---|---|
| Inflammatory Bowel Disease Questionnaire (IBDQ)[129]<br>32-item Likert Scale<br>Interview format | Bowel symptoms<br>Systemic symptoms<br>Social function<br>Emotional function | Well standardized<br>Designed for clinical trials<br>Developed on 'sick' patients–<br>GI referrals and inpatients |
| Modified IBDQ[141]<br>36-item Likert Scale<br>Self-administered | Bowel symptoms<br>Systemic symptoms<br>Social function<br>Emotional function<br>Functional impairment | Derived from IBDQ<br>Developed on 'well' patients–<br>Local chapter of NFIC |
| Cleveland Clinic IBD Questionnaire[142]<br>47-item Likert Scale<br>Interview format | Functional/economic<br>Social/recreational<br>Affect/life in general<br>Medical/symptoms | Correlates with SIP<br>Developed on UC/CD<br>Surg/non-surg groups<br>Quality of life index<br>distinguishes groups |
| Rating Form of IBD Patient Concerns (RFIPC)[132]<br>25-item Visual Analog Scale self-administered | Impact of disease<br>Sexual intimacy<br>Complications<br>Body stigma | Correlates with SIP and SCL-90<br>Developed on 'well' patients–<br>CCFA national sample |
| UC/CD Health Status Scales[142a]<br>9 or 10-item Likert Scale<br>Physician/patient scoring | Ulcerative colitis<br>Crohn's disease | Standardized to healthcare use, function, psych. distress in CCFA national sample<br>Designed to discriminate mild/severe illness and predict outcome<br>Better predictor than CDAI |

both GI and primary care practices, are predicted by the patients' emotional state, such as depression, and the severity of the disease.[105,131]

## DISEASE-RELATED CONCERNS WITH IBD

Physicians also need to be sensitive and responsive to their patients' concerns about IBD, which may include the personal meaning of the illness and its possible consequences, fears about pain or incontinence, adjustment to perineal disease or an ostomy, or the prospect of future surgery or cancer. For example, symptoms of diarrhea might lead to major concerns about incontinence, body image, feeling of isolation, feeling dirty, or feeling a burden on others, and these concerns may have behavioral consequences that are greater than the physical symptom itself. Physicians must be sensitive and responsive to these concerns, as their nature and degree can affect adjustment to the illness, and health status. Furthermore, such knowledge can help in educating the patient properly about their condition, and in the planning of treatment.

One measure that helps to obtain and quantify this type of information for research and clinical care is the Rating Form of IBD Concerns (RFIPC), which includes the 25 most frequent concerns of patients with IBD.[132] A random sample of 991 patients belonging to the Crohn's and Colitis Foundation of America were evaluated, and the mean scores (0 to 100 scale) and relative rankings for the UC and CD samples are shown in Table 24.3. The most important concerns related to the uncertain future of the disease, the effects of medication, energy levels, surgery (and having an ostomy bag), being a burden on

others, loss of bowel control, and developing cancer. Greater differences in concerns are also seen between CD (e.g. pain and financial difficulties) and UC (e.g. cancer) patients. The identification of these concerns has been operationalized into a management approach based on their frequency, pattern and severity.[133] IBD concerns are also influenced by a variety of sociocultural and psychosocial factors: they 1) are greater in African-Americans than Caucasians;[134] 2) are greater when levels of knowledge about the disease are lower[135] (so addressing concerns through education and counseling may improve health status); 3) correlate directly with patient self-perceptions of wellbeing and other quality of life measures[132,135–137] (giving it construct validity); 4) do not necessarily correlate with physical symptoms (so it represents a separate domain of health status); and 5) improve after surgery[136,138] (and is therefore responsive to clinical changes).

A recent comparison of the RFIPC in eight different countries (USA, Canada, Italy, France, Italy, Austria, Israel and Portugal)[139] shows that severity scores differ across countries and cultures (from 51 in Portugal to 19 in Sweden), and were generally greater in southern than northern countries. Furthermore, there were some country-related differences on individual items. For example, concerns about pain and suffering were highest in France and Portugal.

## SUMMARY OF PSYCHOSOCIAL CONSEQUENCES AND HRQOL IN IBD

Despite the potential adverse consequences of having IBD, several studies of HRQOL show that most patients maintain

**Table 24.3 IBD concerns:  mean scores and comparison of UC and CD rankings**

| | All (n=991) Mean (SD) | UC (n=320) Mean (rank) | CD (n=671) Mean (rank) | P |
|---|---|---|---|---|
| Uncertain nature of my disease | 58.6 (31.2) | 54.3 (4) | 60.6 (1) | 0.0038 |
| Effects of medication | 56.3 (34.3) | 54.7 (3) | 57.0 (3) | 0.3256 |
| Energy level | 55.4 (33.7) | 48.9 (6) | 58.5 (2) | 0.0000* |
| Having surgery | 52.9 (33.1) | 50.8 (5) | 54.0 (4) | 0.1471 |
| Having an ostomy bag | 52.1 (36.9) | 55.6 (1) | 50.5 (5) | 0.0430 |
| Being a burden on others | 47.8 (33.0) | 42.6 (8) | 50.3 (6) | 0.0005* |
| Loss of bowel control | 46.1 (34.1) | 47.7 (7) | 45.3 (8) | 0.2916 |
| Developing cancer | 45.4 (33.1) | 55.5 (2) | 40.6 (12) | 0.0000* |
| Ability to achieve full potential | 43.8 (33.3) | 38.6 (9) | 46.2 (7) | 0.0008* |
| Producing unpleasant odors | 41.7 (34.6) | 37.4 (12) | 43.9 (9) | 0.0062 |
| Feelings about my body | 40.4 (32.7) | 38.1 (10) | 41.5 (11) | 0.1220 |
| Pain or suffering | 39.5 (28.5) | 34.3 (14) | 42.0 (10) | 0.0001* |
| Feeling out of control | 38.0 (32.6) | 37.7 (11) | 38.2 (13) | 0.8295 |
| Attractiveness | 35.8 (32.0) | 32.1 (16) | 37.6 (14) | 0.0126 |
| Having access to quality medical care | 34.5 (35.2) | 33.2 (15) | 35.1 (15) | 0.4334 |
| Dying early | 33.5 (30.5) | 36.9 (13) | 31.8 (20) | 0.0176 |
| Intimacy | 32.2 (32.6) | 31.2 (17) | 32.6 (17) | 0.5302 |
| Loss of sexual drive | 31.6 (32.9) | 30.5 (18) | 32.1 (19) | 0.4836 |
| Feeling alone | 31.0 (31.5) | 28.3 (19) | 32.3 (18) | 0.0654 |
| Financial difficulties | 30.3 (30.2) | 25.5 (21) | 32.8 (16) | 0.0002* |
| Ability to perform sexually | 27.6 (31.0) | 26.2 (20) | 28.3 (22) | 0.3294 |
| Passing the disease to others | 27.1 (33.3) | 22.5 (23) | 29.4 (21) | 0.0016* |
| Feeling "dirty" or "smelly" | 26.1 (30.3) | 24.6 (22) | 26.8 (23) | 0.2786 |
| Being treated as different | 21.6 (27.2) | 19.7 (24) | 22.5 (24) | 0.1341 |
| Ability to have children | 18.1 (28.9) | 18.7 (25) | 18.0 (25) | 0.7294 |
| Sum score | 38.7 (20.4) | 37.0 | 39.6 | 0.0676 |

* Significant difference (P<0 .002), adjusting for multiple comparisons.
** Scores range from 0 = 'Not at all', to 100 = 'A great deal'.

good physical and social functioning,[109,112,128,140,141] at least comparable to other ambulatory patients with disease (Fig. 24.4). Several specific features are noted:

1. Impairment in HRQOL is greater in the psychologic and social than the physical dimension.[109,112,142]
2. Psychosocial impairment is greater for CD than UC,[109,112,141] probably because CD patients have more severe disease.[109,141]
3. Sexual dysfunction may be no different than in the general population; it is reported in 30% of women with IBD, compared to 83% of those with irritable bowel.[143]
4. There is no increased risk of infertility or pregnancy loss in patients with IBD, but there is a higher rate of preterm births than in healthy subjects.[144]
5. The consequences of surgery on HRQOL will depend on the disease. One study showed that CD patients who had surgery reported a poorer quality of life (i.e. continued medical symptoms and social/recreational effects) than those who had not had surgery.[141] This may be because patients with more severe disease eventually have an operation. However, a more recent prospective study of CD patients reported improvement in HRQOL postoperatively compared to baseline values.[138]

For UC patients, colectomy generally leads to an improvement in HRQOL regardless of surgical method.[126,136] However, in one study[145] some differences based on the restorative procedure were noted: patients with ileal pouch–anal anastomoses had fewer restrictions in sports and sexual activities than those with Kock pouches, whereas those with Kock pouches had fewer restrictions in these activities but more restrictions in travel than those with conventional (Brooke) ileostomies. No differences between surgical groups were seen with regard to social life, recreation, work and family activities.

## ILLNESS BEHAVIOR

Throughout life, society, family, prior experiences with illness, and psychologic status will shape an individual's attitudes, expectations and behavior related to an illness.[146] For example, a patient with Crohn's disease having abdominal pain may not go to the physician if he or she has previously experienced the symptoms without consequence, is worried about losing time from work, grew up in a family where attention to illness was minimized, or believes that complaining is a 'weakness'. Another patient with the same disease activity and symptoms may frequently seek medical assistance if he/she perceives symptoms as potentially dangerous, is seeking disability, is dependent on physicians for health management, or comes from a family where greater attention was paid to illness. This section will review certain factors that affect illness behavior.

### Sociocultural and family attitudes

Social and cultural factors can shape later attitudes and behaviors relating to illness. In Western society women are more likely to see physicians, perhaps because males have traditionally been encouraged to be more stoic. With regard to ethnicity, first- and second-generation Jews and Italians were reported to be more dramatic in their response to pain, whereas the Irish tended to deny their symptoms, and the 'Old American' Protestants remained more stoic.[147] Furthermore, whereas Italians were satisfied with relief of pain, the Jewish patients needed to understand the meaning of the pain and its future consequences to be satisfied.

Early family attitudes toward illness may also affect later behaviors. Patients who develop chronic or severe diseases early in childhood may not be afforded the opportunity to develop self-reliance because of an imposed dependence on family and physicians for their wellbeing. Similarly, when family members experience guilt or feel high levels of responsibility for the child's welfare, they may overindulge or control the patient's behaviors, which impedes the child's ability to function in an autonomous manner. Therefore, it is not surprising that patients who develop illnesses early in life (e.g. asthma, diabetes mellitus, IBD) are observed in later years to rely heavily on family and healthcare staff, and efforts often need to be made to help patients in self-management strategies.

## Psychologic status

A patient's psychologic status, including psychiatric diagnosis (DSM Axis I), personality disturbance (DSM Axis II) or current mood state, will affect the illness experience and response to treatment. Psychiatric diagnoses commonly seen in medical patients include depressive disorder, anxiety disorder, somatization (somatoform) disorder and factitious illness.[148] Even without a psychiatric diagnosis, daily distressing experiences or the experience of illness itself can produce symptoms of anxiety or depression. Psychologic distress lowers pain threshold, and for IBD can influence healthcare seeking.[109]

Major life events, such as the loss of a loved one, may lead to adverse health outcomes. A history of physical or sexual abuse, commonly reported among patients with chronic medical and gastrointestinal illnesses,[149-151] is associated with an increased frequency of pain reports and functional disability, greater psychologic distress, and more physician visits and surgical procedures.[151]

## Social support and coping

The availability of social support networks can serve to 'buffer' the adverse effects of these stresses on one's health status. Patients with strong social support systems report a sense of control over illness, and have lower stress levels than those who do not.[152,153]

Similarly, coping, which involves efforts to appraise or manage the illness,[154] can be adaptive or maladaptive. 'Catastrophizing' is a maladaptive coping style where the individual views his or her health state with pessimism, and with little perceived control.[155] This style among GI patients is associated with poor health outcome.[49] However, more effective coping strategies, such as problem solving or seeking social support, improve health status and daily function.[109,120,156] Behavioral treatment methods may improve coping style in IBD patients.[157]

## EFFECTS ON OUTCOME

The preceding paragraphs indicate that psychosocial factors must be understood in terms of their modulating role on the per-

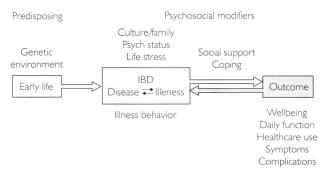

**Fig. 24.5** The relationship of psychosocial factors with health outcome in IBD. Genetic and environmental (possibly including psychosocial) factors early in life determine susceptibility to IBD. Psychosocial modifiers later in life influence the illness experience, subsequent illness behaviors and the clinical outcome. Outcome is understood in terms of health-related quality of life (wellbeing, daily function), healthcare use, symptoms and complications. These factors may, in turn, reciprocally affect the illness and activity of the disease.

sonal experience of IBD, and its clinical outcome. As shown in Figure 24.5, genetic and environmental factors early in life determine susceptibility to IBD. Then, psychosocial modifiers will influence when and how the disease is experienced, the individual's behavior and, ultimately, the clinical outcome. So negative factors such as life stress or concurrent psychiatric diagnosis will lead to more severe illness or, potentially, disease activation. Conversely, health-promoting factors such as strong social support networks or an effective coping style will ameliorate the effects of disease and improve outcome (wellbeing, daily function, healthcare use, symptoms and complications): the patient's health-related quality of life. Note that these outcome factors may in turn reciprocally affect the illness and the activity of the disease.

The varying effects of psychosocial factors among individuals, or at different points in time in the same individual, help explain the variation in the illness condition and clinical outcome. Some patients may have poor health status with little evidence of active disease, whereas others with severe disease function well because of little psychologic morbidity, good social support and effective coping methods.

# INTEGRATING PSYCHOSOCIAL FACTORS IN DIAGNOSIS AND TREATMENT

## ESTABLISH AN EFFECTIVE THERAPEUTIC RELATIONSHIP

An effective therapeutic relationship occurs when the physician actively listens to and appraises the patient's thoughts and concerns empathically, and responds to them non-judgmentally, provides information consistent with the patient's interests and needs, and serves as a knowledgeable adviser to decide with the patient on the plan of care. Additional information on the therapeutic relationship is given elsewhere.[158-160]

## DATA COLLECTION

Data collection involves active listening, and communicating a willingness to address both the biologic and the psychosocial aspects of the illness.[158] This is achieved by encouraging the patient to tell the story in his or her own way, so that the events contributing to the illness unfold naturally.[161,162] The traditional 'medical' and 'social' histories should be elicited together, so that the symptoms are understood in the context of the psychosocial events surrounding the illness. Initially, open-ended questions are used to generate hypotheses and obtain the most accurate data. Facilitating remarks such as: 'Yes?', 'Can you tell me more?', repeating the patient's previous statements, head nodding, or even silence with an expectant look, encourage the patient to say more. More directed (e.g. yes/no) questions should be avoided initially, though they may be used later in the interview to further characterize the symptoms. Multiple-choice or leading questions are to be avoided because the patient's desire to comply may bias the responses.

## EVALUATING THE DATA

After the history and physical examination are completed, the physician should assess the relative influences of the medical and psychosocial dimensions to establish priorities for further evaluation or treatment. When ordering diagnostic studies, safety, cost-effectiveness and clinical utility (i.e. will the results make a difference in treatment?) should be considered. The patient's report must be appraised along with the results of objective studies. Frightened of the implications of a disease flare-up, some patients minimize or ignore their symptoms; others challenge the physician to 'do something!', which may lead to the ordering of unnecessary studies or even surgical intervention.[163]

The physician should also explore the patient's perceptions and fears about the disease, and their treatment expectations. IBD patients commonly express concern about the uncertainty of their disease, medication effects, or the prospect of surgery or cancer.[132] Other fears less often volunteered include: loss of physical attractiveness or sexual function, transmitting the disease to others, premature death, financial hardship, and fear of losing control (bowel or otherwise). The physician can gain the patient's trust by asking supportive and non-threatening questions, such as: 'What concerns or worries do you have about your illness?' 'What do you think is affecting the problem now?' 'What kind of treatment do you think you should receive?' and 'What are your expectations of me in helping you?'

It is also important to corroborate the patient's reports with that of the family. Some patients may hold back on disclosing the degree of functional impairment ('to be strong'), whereas others, at risk of losing family attention, work relief or compensation, may amplify the degree of disability, at least at first. In all cases the physician must realistically apprise the patient of the status of his or her clinical condition and encourage 'well' behavior.

## HELP THE PATIENT LEARN

Helping the patient learn about IBD involves the provision of education and reassurance.[164] Education means: 1) eliciting the patient's understanding, 2) addressing misunderstandings, 3) providing information that is consistent with the patient's knowledge, and 4) checking the patient's understanding of what was discussed. Several excellent resources are available through the Crohn's and Colitis Foundation of America (CCFA), New York. Reassurance involves: 1) identifying the patient's worries and concerns, 2) acknowledging and validating them, 3) respond-

ing to specific concerns, and 4) avoiding 'false' reassurances (e.g. 'Don't worry, everything's fine'), particularly before the medical evaluation is complete. Some patients will benefit from talking with others who share the same experiences.

## HELP THE PATIENT APPRAISE AND ADAPT TO STRESSORS

Many patients recognize that their bowel symptoms follow some psychosocial upset, and this knowledge helps them to manage their illness more effectively. Others may be unwilling to address this association, for they may attribute it to 'mental illness' or a personal 'weakness'. The physician can point out that psychosocial stress may produce symptoms in healthy subjects as well as in patients with various types of illnesses. So the effort is to understand and try to modify all factors affecting the illness condition.

## HELP THE PATIENT TAKE RESPONSIBILITY FOR THE HEALTH CARE

Patients need to actively participate in healthcare decisions. For example, a young woman with UC and recurrent episodes of diarrhea and bleeding over many years that is controlled by steroids and 6-MP or other immunosuppressants, should be apprised of the risks and benefits of continued medication control versus colectomy. The patient can then decide whether and when surgical intervention may be indicated. By taking this level of responsibility, the patient achieves a greater sense of control over the illness, and this is associated with improved health outcome.

## INVOLVE THE FAMILY

The support and encouragement provided by the patient's family are important in any plan of care. With a young child, the parents must be involved in all aspects of diagnosis and care, and for many adult patients communication with the spouse is strongly recommended. However, the patient's autonomy should also be maintained, and it is countertherapeutic to treat the adolescent or adult patient through the family.

Family members may also have concerns. They may feel helpless, guilty or angry, yet expressing such feelings is not usually acceptable. The physician can help ameliorate these feelings by acknowledging them, enlisting the family's participation in the treatment, and recommending family counseling when necessary.

## REINFORCE HEALTH-PROMOTING BEHAVIORS

Particularly in referral practices, maladaptive illness behaviors, which might include failing to take responsibility for one's health care with the expectation of being cared for by others, or denying the psychosocial impact of the illness, may occur, and physicians may unwittingly support these behaviors by attending to physical complaints to the exclusion of other issues, acting on each complaint by ordering unneeded diagnostic studies and treatments, or conversely, ignoring or rejecting the psychosocial aspects of the illness. Instead, the physician should explore the psychosocial factors contributing to these behaviors, encourage the patient to take responsibility and learn to cope with a chronic illness (rather than to expect cure), and limit discussion of symptoms to no more than is needed to satisfy medical concerns.

## OTHER BEHAVIORAL ISSUES

### Antidepressants for pain control

Patients with IBD may experience recurrent chronic abdominal pain that at times is disabling. Assuming the evaluation does not show evidence of an obstruction, abscess or other medically treatable source, the pain may be related to sensitization of neural pathways due to inflammation, injury or emotional distress, and an antidepressant may be considered both for central and peripheral[165] analgesic[166] effects.[159,167] The tricyclic (TCA) antidepressants (e.g. amitriptyline, doxepin, desipramine, nortriptyline) appear effective[168–170] but can produce anticholinergic side effects such as orthostatic hypotension, sedation, fluid retention and cardiac arrhythmias (desiprimine and nortriptyline have fewer of these effects than amitriptyline or doxepin). The selective serotonin reuptake inhibitors (SSRI) (e.g. fluoxetine, sertraline, paroxetine, luvoxamine) have not been as well studied and are more expensive, but are empirically helpful. They have different side effects (agitation, sleep disturbance, vivid dreams, sexual dysfunction, night sweats, diarrhea), which are generally safer and better tolerated than those of the TCA, as they produce little sedation and have no cardiac effects.

Treatment may begin at low doses (one-third to half the full dose) and be maintained for 6–12 months before tapering. The patient should be informed that, independent of effects on mood, the drug acts as a central analgesic by reducing visceral afferent function or facilitating descending pain inhibitory pathways. Patients should also be informed that it can take up to several weeks to work, is not addictive, and side effects, if they occur, ameliorate over 1–2 weeks. A poor clinical response may be due to non-compliance, or a lower than adequate dose.[171]

### Narcotic use

Prescribing narcotics in IBD is a complex issue.[158] Although they are effective, and often indicated for acute painful complications, they are contraindicated when the pain is chronic: narcotics can produce tachyphylaxis and also interfere with the therapeutic relationship, and even produce a narcotic bowel syndrome, with worsening abdominal pain and secondary pseudo-obstruction.[172] A negotiated understanding must be reached to avoid ongoing conflicts where narcotics become the focus of future clinical visits. The physician must understand and address the patient's concerns (e.g. the need for pain relief, the attitude of physicians who may believe the patient is addicted or who has illegitimate complaints), then offer information on how continued narcotic use may impair long-term benefits, and finally engage with the patient on alternative treatment strategies.[148]

### Psychiatric referral

Psychiatric consultation should be considered when: 1) the patient has a psychiatric illness requiring treatment, 2) the patient's daily functioning (e.g. ability to work) or family relationships are seriously impaired, or 3) diagnostic and therapeutic strategies are being considered based on patient complaints without supportive medical data.

## CONCLUSION

An understanding of the role of psychosocial factors in IBD follow clinical experience as molded by prevailing societal views of illness and disease.[1,2] Clinicians have always recognized the importance of psychosocial factors as consequences of IBD, and as predeterminants for symptom exacerbation.[10] However, the influence of psychosocial stress on the onset and activation of these diseases has previously not been accepted, nor supported in the literature. Furthermore, from a reductionistic, biomedical perspective, the possibility of stress 'causing' disease is difficult to conceive. However, over the last decade, improvements in psychosocial assessment and clinical research design methodology, coupled with new data in brain–gut physiology, psychoneuroendocrinology and psychoimmunology, have led clinicians and investigators to make a conceptual shift in their understanding of illness and disease.

From this perspective, and as evidenced by this review, we can make several conclusions:

1. The pathophysiology of IBD is best understood in terms of dysregulation of homeostatic systems (neural, endocrine, immune, inflammatory) in a biologically predisposed host (biopsychosocial model), rather than as conditions caused by specific etiological factor(s).
2. Psychosocial factors contribute to the onset, severity, clinical expression and outcome (HRQOL, therapeutic response) of IBD. The precise role for these factors requires further study.
3. Identifiable psychosocial factors (e.g. psychiatric diagnosis, personality, life stress, coping, social support etc.) correlate with the overall severity of the condition: they are not specific for IBD.
4. The physician must identify those psychosocial factors unique to each individual that contribute to the clinical expression of the disorder.
5. Optimal care requires the establishment of an effective physician–patient relationship.

## REFERENCES

1. Drossman DA. Psychosocial and psychophysiologic mechanisms in GI illness. In: Kirsner JB, ed. The growth of gastroenterologic knowledge in the 20th century. Philadelphia: Lea & Febiger; 1993;419–432.
2. Drossman DA. Presidential address: Gastrointestinal illness and biopsychosocial model. Psychosom Med 1998;60:258–267.
3. Kroenke K, Mangelsdorff AD. Common symptoms in ambulatory care: incidence, evaluation, therapy, and outcome. Am J Med 1989;86:262–266.
4. Bayless TM. Inflammatory bowel disease and irritable bowel syndrome. Med Clin North Am 1990;49:21–28.
5. Isgar B, Harman M, Kaye MD, Whorwell PJ. Symptoms of irritable bowel syndrome in ulcerative colitis in remission. Gut 1983;24:190–192.
6. Simren M, Axelsson J, Gillberg R, Abrahamsson H, Svedlund J, Bjornsson ES. Quality of life in inflammatory bowel disease in remission: The impact of IBS-like symptoms and associated psychological factors. Am J Gastroenterol 2002;97:389–396.
7. Garrett JW, Drossman DA. Health status in inflammatory bowel disease: biological and behavioral considerations. Gastroenterology 1990;99:90–96.
8. Engel GL. The need for a new medical model: A challenge for biomedicine. Science 1977;196:129–136.
9. Drossman DA. Gastrointestinal illness and the biopsychosocial model. J Clin Gastroenterol 1996;22:252–254.
10. Mitchell CM, Drossman DA. Survey of the AGA membership relating to patients with functional gastrointestinal disorders. Gastroenterology 1987;92:1282–1284.
11. Lewis MC. Attributions and inflammatory bowel disease: patients' perceptions of illness causes and the effects of these perceptions on relationships. AARN News Lett 1988;44:16–17.
12. Robertson DAF, Ray J, Diamond I, Edwards JG. Personality profile and affective state of patients with inflammatory bowel disease. Gut 1989;30:623–626.
13. Drossman DA, Sandler RS, McKee DC, Lovitz AJ. Bowel patterns among subjects not seeking health care. Use of a questionnaire to identify a population with bowel dysfunction. Gastroenterology 1982;83:529–534.

14. Drossman DA, Creed FH, Olden KW, Svedlund J, Toner BB, Whitehead WE. Psychosocial aspects of the functional gastrointestinal disorders. In: Drossman DA, Corazziari E, Talley NJ, Thompson WG, Whitehead WE, eds. . The functional gastrointestinal disorders: diagnosis, pathophysiology and treatment. A multinational consensus. Rome II: Degnon and Associates; 2000:157–245.

15. Mayer EA, Naliboff BD, Chang L, Coutinho SV. Stress and the gastrointestinal tract v. stress and irritable bowel syndrome. Am J Physiol Gastrointest Liver Physiol 2001;280:G519–G524.

16. Drossman DA. A biopsychosocial understanding of gastrointestinal illness and disease. In: Feldman M, Scharschmidt B, Sleisenger MH, eds. Sleisenger and Fordtrans's gastrointestinal disease. Philadelphia: WB Saunders; 2002:2371–2380.

17. Welgan P, Meshkinpour H, Beeler M. Effect of anger on colon motor and myoelectric activity in irritable bowel syndrome. Gastroenterology 1988;94:1150–1156.

18. Welgan P, Meshkinpour H, Ma J. Role of anger in antral motor activity in irritable bowel syndrome. Dig Dis Sci 2000;45:248–251.

19. Delvaux MM. Stress and visceral perception. Can J Gastroenterol 1999;13(Suppl A):32A–36A.

20. Muelas MS, Ramirez P, Parrilla P et al. Vagal system involvement in changes in small bowel motility during restraint stress: an experimental study in the dog. Br J Surg 1993;80:479–483.

21. Gue M, Junien JL, Bueno L. Conditioned emotional response in rats enhances colonic motility through the central release of corticotropin-releasing factor. Gastroenterology 1991;100:964–970.

22. Wittmann T, Crenner F, Angel F. Long duration stress: Immediate and late effects on small and large bowel motility in rats. Dig Dis Sci 1990;35:495.

23. Stam R. Neurogastroenterol Motil 2000;12:407.

24. Stam R, Ekkelenkamp K, Frankhuijzen AC, Bruijnzeel AW, Akkermans LM, Wiegant VM. Long-lasting changes in central nervous system responsivity to colonic distension after stress in rats. Gastroenterology 2002;123:1216–1225.

25. Coutinho SV, Plotsky PM, Sablad M et al. Neonatal maternal separation alters stress-induced responses to viscerosomatic nociceptive stimuli in rat. Am J Physiol Gastrointest Liver Physiol 2001;282:G307–G316.

26. Wood JD. Neuropathophysiology of irritable bowel syndrome. J Clin Gastroenterol 2002;35(Suppl):11–22.

27. Collins SM, Assche GV, Hogaboam C. Alterations in enteric nerve and smooth-muscle function in inflammatory bowel diseases. Inflamm Bowel Dis 1997;3:38–48.

28. Porter RW, Brady JV, Conrad D, Mason JW, Galambos R, Rioch D. Some experimental observations on gastrointestinal lesions in behaviorally conditioned monkeys. Psychosom Med 1958;20:379–394.

29. Stout C, Snyder RL. Ulcerative colitis-like lesions in Siamang gibbons. Gastroenterology 1969;57:256–260.

30. Engel GL. Psychological factors in ulcerative colitis in man and gibbon. Gastroenterology 1969;57:362–364.

31. Chalifoux LV, Bronson RT. Colonic adenocarcinoma associated with chronic colitis in cotton top marmosets, *Saguinus oedipus*. Gastroenterology 1981;80:942–947.

32. Wood JD, Peck OC, Tefend KS et al. Colitis and colon cancer in cotton-top tamarins (*Saguinus oedipus oedipus*) living wild in their natural habitat. Dig Dis Sci 1998;33:1443–1453.

33. Drossman DA. Is the cotton-topped tamarin a model for behavioral research? Dig Dis Sci 1985;30:24S–27S.

34. Gozalo A, Montoya E. Mortality causes of the moustached tamarin (*Saguinus mystax*) in captivity. J Med Primatol 1992;21:35–38.

35. Million M, Tache Y, Anton P. Susceptibility of Lewis and Fischer rats to stress-induced worsening of TNB-colitis: protective role of brain CRF. Am J Physiol 1999;276:G1027–G1036.

36. Collins SM, McHugh K, Jacobson K et al. Previous inflammation alters the response of the rat colon to stress. Gastroenterology 1996;111:1509–1515.

37. Gue M, Bonbonne C, Fioramonti J et al. Stress-induced enhancement of colitis in rats: CRF and arginine vasopressin are not involved. Am J Physiol 1997;272:G84–G91.

38. Collins SM. Stress and the gastrointestinal tract IV. Modulation of intestinal inflammation by stress: basic mechanisms and clinical relevance. Am J Physiol Gastrointest Liver Physiol 2001;280:G315–G318.

39. Cassell J. The contribution of the social environment to host resistance. Am J Epidemiol 1976;104:107–123.

40. Holmes TH, Rahe RH. The social readjustment rating scale. J Psychosom Res 1967;11:213–218.

41. Fava GA, Sonino N. Psychosomatic medicine: emerging trends and perspectives. Psychother Psychosom 2000;69:184–197.

42. Hislop IG. Onset setting in inflammatory bowel disease. Med J Aust 1974;1:981–984.

43. Garrett VD, Brantley PJ, Jones GN, McKnight GT. The relation between daily stress and Crohn's disease. J Behav Med 1991;14:87.

44. Robertson DAF, Ray J, Diamond I, Edwards JG. Personality profile and affective state of patients with inflammatory bowel disease. Gut 1989;30:623–626.

45. North CS, Clouse RE, Spitznagel EL, Alpers DH. The relation of ulcerative colitis to psychiatric factors: a review of findings and methods. Am J Psychiatry 1990;147:974–981.

46. Schwarz SP, Blanchard EB. Inflammatory bowel disease: a review of the psychological assessment and treatment literature. Ann Behav Med 1990;12:95–105.

47. Drossman DA. Psychosocial aspects of inflammatory bowel disease. Stress Med 1986;2:119–128.

48. North CS, Alpers DH, Helzer JE, Spitznagel EL, Clouse RE. Do life events or depression exacerbate inflammatory bowel disease? Ann Intern Med 1991;114:381–386.

49. Drossman DA, Li Z, Leserman J, Keefe FJ, Hu YJ, Toomey TC. Effects of coping on health outcome among female patients with gastrointestinal disorders. Psychosom Med 2000;62:309–317.

50. Duffy LC, Zielezny MA, Marshall JR et al. Relevance of major stress events as an indicator of disease activity prevalence in inflammatory bowel disease. Behav Med 1991;17:101–110.

51. Levenstein S, Prantera C, Varvo V et al. Stress and exacerbation in ulcerative colitis: a prospective study of patients enrolled in remission. Am J Gastroenterol 2000;95:1213–1220.

52. Levenstein S, Prantera C, Varvo V et al. Development of the perceived stress questionnaire a new tool for psychosomatic research. J Psychosom Res 1993;37:19–32.

53. Sternberg EM, Chrousos GP, Wilder RL, Gold PW. The stress response and the regulation of inflammatory disease. Ann Intern Med 1992;117:854–866.

54. Chrousos GP. The hypothalamic–pituitary–adrenal axis and immune-mediated inflammation. N Engl J Med 1995;332:1351–1362.

55. Ottoway CA. Role of the neuroendocrine system in cytokine pathways in inflammatory bowel disease. Aliment Pharmacol Ther 1996;10:10–15.

56. Sternberg EM. Emotions and disease: from balance of humors to balance of molecules. Nature Med 1997;3:264–267.

57. Sternberg EM. Perspectives series: cytokines and the brain. J Clin Invest 1997;100:2641–2647.

58. Niess JH, Monnikes H, Dignass A, Klapp BF, Arck P. Effects of stress on immune mediators, neuropeptides and hormones with established relevance for idiopathic inflammatory bowel disease (IBD). Digestion 2002;65:131–140.

59. Bandler R, Keay KA, Floyd N, Price J. Central circuits mediating patterned autonomic activity during active vs. passive emotional coping. Brain Res Bull 2000;53:95–104.

60. Vogt B, Gabriel M. Neurobiology of cingulate cortex and limbic thalamus: A comprehensive handbook. Boston, MA: Birkhaeuser; 1993:313–344.

61. Sternberg EM, Parker CW. Pharmacologic aspects of lymphocyte regulation. In: Marchalonis JJ, ed. The lymphocyte: structure and function. New York: Marcel Dekker; 1988:1–54.

62. Bellinger DL, Lorton D, Romano TD, Olschowka JA, Felten SY, Felten DL. Neuropeptide innervation of lymphoid organs. Ann NY Acad Sci 1990;594:17–33.

63. Collins SM, Hurst SM, Main C et al. Effect of inflammation of enteric nerves: cytokine-induced changes in neurotransmitter content and release. Ann NY Acad Sci 1992;664:415–424.

64. Clauw DJ, Chrousos GP. Chronic pain and fatigue syndromes: Overlapping clinical and neuroendocrine features and potential pathogenic mechanisms. Neuroimmunomodulation 1997;4:134–153.

65. Sternberg EM, Young WS, Bernardini R et al. A central nervous system defect in biosynthesis of corticotropin-releasing hormone is associated with susceptibility to streptococcal cell wall-induced arthritis in Lewis rats. Proc Natl Acad Sci USA 1989;86:4771–4775.

66. Sternberg EM. Neuroendocrine factors in susceptibility to inflammatory disease: focus on the hypothalamic–pituitary–adrenal axis. Horm Res 1995;43:159–161.

67. De Schryver-Kecskemeti K, Bennert KW, Cooper GS, Yang P. Gastrointestinal involvement in L-tryptophan (L-Trp) associated eosinophilia–myalgia syndrome (EMS). Dig Dis Sci 1992;37:697–701.

68. Crofford LJ, Rader JI, Dalakas MC, Hill RHJ, Page SW, Needham LL. L-Tryptophan implicated in human eosinophilia–myalgia syndrome causes fasciitis and perimyositis in the Lewis rat. J Clin Invest 1990;86:1757–1763.

69. Sartor RB, Cromartie WJ, Powell DW, Schwab JH. Granulomatous enterocolitis induced in rats by purified bacterial cell wall fragments. Gastroenterology 1985;89:587–595.

70. McCall RD, Haskill S, Zimmerman EM, Lund PK, Thompson RC, Sartor RB. Tissue interleukin 1 and interleukin-1 receptor antagonist expression in enterocolitis in resistant and susceptible rats. Gastroenterology 1994;106:960–972.

71. Sartor RB, DeLa Cadena RA, Green KD et al. Selective kallikrein–kinin system activation in inbred rats differentially susceptible to granulomatous enterocolitis. Gastroenterology 1996;110:1467–1481.

72. Qiu BS, Vallance BA, Blennerhassett PA, Collins SM. The role of CD4+ lymphocytes in the susceptibility of mice to stress-induced reactivation of experimental colitis. Nature Med 1999;5:1178–1182.

73. Soderholm JD, Yang PC, Ceponis P et al. Chronic stress induces mast cell-dependent bacterial adherence and initiates mucosal inflammation in rat intestine. Gastroenterology 2002;123:1099–1108.

74. Santos J, Saperas E, Nogueiras C et al. Release of mast cell mediators into the jejunum by cold pain stress in humans. Gastroenterology 1998;114:640–648.

75. Kiliaan AJ, Saunders PR, Bijlsma PB et al. Stress stimulates transepithelial macromolecular uptake in rat jejunum. Am J Physiol 1998;275:G1037–G1044.

76. Saunders PR, Hanssen NPM, Perdue MH. Cholinergic nerves mediate stress-induced intestinal transport abnormalities in Wistar–Kyoto rats. Am J Physiol 1997;273:G486–G490.

77. Kawahito Y, Sano H, Mukai S et al. Corticotropin releasing hormone in colonic mucosa in patients with ulcerative colitis. Gut 1995;37:544–551.

78. Ader R, Cohen N. Behaviorally conditioned immunosuppression and murine systemic lupus erythematosus. Science 1982;215:1534–1536.

79. MacQueen G, Marshall J, Perdue M, Siegel S, Bienenstock J. Pavlovian conditioning of rat mucosal mast cells to secrete rat mast cell Protease II. Science 1989;243:83–85.

80. Vallance BA, Galeazzi F, Collins SM, Snider DP. CD4 T cells and major histocompatibility complex class II expression influence worm expulsion and increased intestinal muscle contraction during Trichinella spiralis infection. Infect Immun 1999;67:6090–6097.

81. Collins SM. The immunomodulation of enteric neuromuscular function: implications for motility and inflammatory disorders. Gastroenterology 1996;111:1683–1699.

82. Galeazzi F, Haapala EM, van Rooijen N, Vallance BA, Collins SM. Inflammation-induced impairment of enteric nerve function in nematode-infected mice is macrophage dependent. Am J Physiol Gastrointest Liver Physiol 2000;278:G259–G265.

83. Der T, Bercik P, Donnelly G et al. Interstitial cells of Cajal and inflammation-induced motor dysfunction in the mouse small intestine. Gastroenterology 2000;119:1590–1599.

84. Collins SM, Blennerhassett P, Vermillion DL, Davis K, Langer J, Ernst PB. Impaired acetylcholine release in the inflamed rat intestine is T cell independent. Am J Physiol 1992;263:G198–G201.

85. Kishimoto S, Kobayashi H, Shimizu S et al. Changes of colonic vasoactive intestinal peptide and cholinergic activity in rats with chemical colitis. Dig Dis Sci 1992;37:1729–1737.

86. Miampamba M, Sharkey KA. Distribution of calcitonin gene-related peptide, somatostatin, substance P and vasoactive intestinal polypeptide in experimental colitis in rats. Neurogastroenterol Motil 1998;10:315–329.

87. Mashimo H, Kjellin A, Goyal RK. Gastric stasis in neuronal nitric oxide synthase-deficient knockout mice. Gastroenterology 2000;119:766–773.

88. Fava GA, Pavan L. Large bowel disorders: II. Psychopathology and alexithymia. Psychother Psychosom 1977;27:100–105.

89. Dantzer R. Cytokine-induced sickness behavior: where do we stand? Brain Behav Immun 2001;15:7–24.

90. Berkow R. Medical education: creating physicians or medical technicians? Croatian Med J 2002;43:45–49.

91. Dautzer R. Cytokine-induced sickness behavior: where do we stand? Brain Behav Immun 2001;15:7–24.

92. Sternberg EM. Perspectives series: Cytokines and the brain. J Clin Investig 1997;100:2641–2647.

93. Alexander F. Psychosomatic medicine: its principles and applications. New York: WW Norton; 1950.

94. Saunders PR, Kosecka U, McKay DM, Perdue MH. Acute stressors stimulate ion secretion and increase epithelial permeability in rat intestine. Am J Physiol 1994;267:G794–G799.

95. Weiner H. Psychobiology and human disease. New York: Elsevier Science; 1977.

96. Engel GL. Studies of ulcerative colitis V. Psychological aspects and their implications for treatment. Am J Dig Dis 1958;3:315–337.

97. Sifneos PE. The prevalence of 'alexyithmic' characteristics in psychsomatic patients. Psychother Psychosom 1973;22:255–262.

98. Alexander F, French TM, Pollack G. Psychosomatic specificity: experimental study and results. Chicago: University of Chicago Press; 1968.

99. Aronowitz R, Spiro HM. The rise and fall of the psychosomatic hypothesis in ulcerative colitis. J Clin Gastroenterol 1988;10:298–305.

100. Verissimo R, Mota-Cardoso R, Taylor G. Relationships between alexithymia, emotional control, and quality of life in patients with inflammatory bowel disease. Psychother Psychosom 1998;67:75–80.

101. Taylor GJ, Bagby RM, Parker JD. The alexithymia construct. A potential paradigm for psychosomatic medicine. Psychosomatics 1991;32:153–164.

102. Porcelli P, Taylor GJ, Bagby RM, De Carne M. Alexithymia and functional gastrointestinal disorders. A comparison with inflammatory bowel disease. Psychother Psychosom 1999;68:263–269.

103. Lumley MA, Stettner L, Wehmer F. How are alexithymia and physical illness linked? A review and critique of pathways. J Psychosom Res 1996;41:505–518.

104. Magni G, Bernasconi G, Mauro P et al. Psychiatric diagnoses in ulcerative colitis: A controlled study. Br J Psychiatry 1991;158:413–415.

105. Guthrie E, Jackson J, Shaffer J, Thompson D, Tomenson B, Creed F. Psychological disorder and severity of inflammatory bowel disease predict health-related quality of life in ulcerative colitis and Crohn's disease. Am J Gastroenterol 2002;97:1994–1999.

106. Kurina LM, Goldacre MJ, Yeates D, Gill LE. Depression and anxiety in people with inflammatory bowel disease. J Epidemiol Commun Health 2001;55:716–720.

107. Mendeloff AI, Monk M, Siegel CI, Lilienfeld A. Illness experience and life stresses in patients with irritable colon and with ulcerative colitis. An epidemiologic study of ulcerative colitis and regional enteritis in Baltimore, 1960–1964. N Engl J Med 1970;282:14–17.

108. Clouse RE, Alpers DH. The relationship of psychiatric disorder to gastrointestinal illness. Annu Rev Med 1986;37:283–295.

109. Drossman DA, Leserman J, Mitchell CM, Li Z, Zagami EA, Patrick DL. Health status and health care use in persons with inflammatory bowel disease: A national sample. Dig Dis Sci 1991;36:1746–1755.

110. Walker EA, Katon W, Roy-Byrne PP, Li L, Amos D. Psychiatric illness and irritable bowel syndrome: a comparison with inflammatory bowel disease. Am J Psychiatry 1990; 147:1656–1661.

111. Schwarz SP, Blanchard EB, Berreman CF et al. Psychological aspects of irritable bowel syndrome: comparisons with inflammatory bowel disease and nonpatient controls. Behav Res Ther 1993;31:297–304.

112. Drossman DA, Patrick DL, Mitchell CM, Zagami EA, Appelbaum MI. Health related quality of life in inflammatory bowel disease: functional status and patient worries and concerns. Dig Dis Sci 1989;34:1379–1386.

113. Tarter RE, Switala J, Carra J, Edwards KL, Van Thiel DH. Inflammatory bowel disease: psychiatric status of patients before and after disease onset. Int J Psychiatry Med 1987;17:173.

114. Helzer JE. A controlled study of the association between ulcerative colitis and psychiatric diagnoses. Dig Dis Sci 1982;27:513–518.

115. Helzer JE. A study of the association between Crohn's disease and psychiatric illness. Gastroenterology 1984;86:324–330.

116. Andrews H, Barczak P, Allan RN. Psychiatric illness in patients with inflammatory bowel disease. Gut 1987;28:1600–1604.

117. McKegney FP, Gordon RO, Levine SM. A psychosomatic comparison of patients with ulcerative colitis and Crohn's disease. Psychosom Med 1970;32:153–166.

118. Engel CCJ, Walker EA, Katon WJ. Factors related to dissociation among patients with gastrointestinal complaints. J Psychosom Res 1996;40:643–653.

119. Porcelli P, Zaka S, Centonze S, Sisto G. Psychological distress and levels of disease activity in inflammatory bowel disease. Ital J Gastroenterol 1994;26:111–115.

120. Kinash RG, Fischer DG, Lukie BE, Carr TL. Coping patterns and related characteristics in patients with IBD. Rehab Nurs 1993;18:12–19.

121. Guyatt GH, Feeny DH, Patrick DL. Measuring health-related quality of life. Ann Intern Med 1993;118:622–629.

122. Drossman DA. Inflammatory bowel disease. In: Spilker B, ed. Quality of life and pharmacoeconomics in clinical trials. New York: Raven Press; 1996:925–935.

123. Patrick DL, Deyo RA. Generic and disease-specific measures in assessing health status and quality of life. Med Care 1989;27:S217–S232.

124. Bergner M, Bobbitt RA, Carter WB. The Sickness Impact Profile: development and final revision of a health status measure. Med Care 1981;19:787–805.

125. Ware JE, Sherbourne CD. The MOS 36-item short form Health Survey (SF-36): I. Conceptual framework and item selection. Med Care 1992;30:473–483.

126. McLeod RS, Churchill DN, Lock AM, Vanderburgh S, Cohen Z. Quality of life of patients with ulcerative colitis preoperatively and postoperatively. Gastroenterology 1991;101:1307–1313.

127. Guyatt GH, Walter S, Norman G. Measuring change over time: assessing the usefulness of evaluative instruments. J Chronic Dis 1987;40:171–178.

128. Guyatt G, Mitchell A, Irvine EJ, Singer J, Williams N, Goodacre R et al. A new measure of health status for clinical trials in inflammatory bowel disease. Gastroenterology 1989;96:804–810.

129. Irvine EJ, Feagan B, Rochon J et al. Quality of life: A valid and reliable measure of therapeutic efficacy in the treatment of inflammatory bowel disease. Gastroenterology 1994;106:287–296.

130. Russo MW, Gaynes BN, Drossman DA. A national survey of practice patterns of gastroenterologists with comparison to the past two decades. J Clin Gastroenterol 1999;29:339–343.

131. de Boer AG, Sprangers MA, Bartelsman JF, de Haes HC. Predictors of health care utilization in patients with inflammatory bowel disease: a longitudinal study. Eur J Gastroenterol Hepatol 1998;10:783–789.

132. Drossman DA, Leserman J, Li Z, Mitchell CM, Zagami EA, Patrick DL. The rating form of IBD patient concerns: A new measure of health status. Psychosom Med 1991;53:701–712.

133. Casati J, Toner BB, de Rooy E, Drossman DA, Maunder RG. Concerns of patients with inflammatory bowel disease: A review of emerging themes. Dig Dis Sci 2000;45:26–31.

134. Straus WL, Eisen GM, Sandler RS, Murray SC, Sessions JT. Crohn's disease: does race really matter? Am J Gastroenterol 2000;95:479–483.

135. Moser G, Tillinger W, Sachs G et al. Disease-related worries and concerns: a study on outpatients with inflammatory bowel disease (IBD). Eur J Gastroenterol Hepatol 1995;7:853–858.

136. Provenzale D, Shearin M, Phillips-Bute B et al. Health-related quality of life after ileoanal pull-through: evaluation and assessment of new health status measures. Gastroenterology 1997;113:7–14.

137. de Rooy EC, Toner BB, Maunder RG et al. Concerns of outpatients with inflammatory bowel disease: results from a clinical population. Am J Gastroenterol 2001;96:1816–1821.

138. Yazdanpanah Y, Klein O, Gambiez L et al. Impact of surgery on quality of life in Crohn's disease. Am J Gastroenterol 1997;92:1897–1900.

139. Levenstein S, Li Z, Almer S et al. Cross-cultural variation in disease-related concerns among patients with inflammatory bowel disease. Am J Gastroenterol 2001;96:1822–1830.

140. Drossman DA. Quality of life in IBD: methods and findings. In: Rachmilewitz D, ed. Falk Symposium #72; Inflammatory Bowel Diseases – 1994. Dordrecht: Kluwer Academic Publishers; 1994:105–116.

141. Farmer RG, Easley KA, Farmer JM. Quality of life assessment by patients with inflammatory bowel disease. Cleve Clin J Med 1992;59:35–42.

142. Love JR, Irvine EJ, Fedorak RN. Quality of life in inflammatory bowel disease. J Clin Gastroenterol 1992;14:15–19.

142a. Drossman DA, Li Z, Leserman J, Patrick DL. Ulcerative colitis and Crohn's disease health status scales for research and clinical practice. J Clin Gastroenterol 1992;15:104–112.

143. Guthrie E, Creed FH. Severe sexual dysfunctioning in women with IBS: comparison with IBD and duodenal ulceration. Br Med J 1987;2:577–578.

144. Baird DD, Narendranathan M, Sandler RS. Increased risk of pre-term birth for women with inflammatory bowel disease. Gastroenterology 1990;99:987–994.

145. Kohler LW, Pemberton JH, Zinsmeister AR, Kelly KA. Quality of life after proctocolectomy. A comparison of Brooke ileostomy, Kock pouch, and ileal pouch–anal anastomosis. Gastroenterology 1991;101:679–684.

146. Mechanic D. The concept of illness behavior: culture, situation and personal predisposition. Psychol Med 1986;16:1–7.

147. Zborowski M. Cultural components in responses to pain. J Social Issues 1952;8:16–30.

148. Drossman DA, Chang L. Psychosocial factors in the care of patients with gastrointestinal disorders. In: Yamada T, ed. Textbook of gastroenterology. Philadelphia: Lippincott-Raven; 2003:636–654.

149. Laws A. Does a history of sexual abuse in childhood play a role in women's medical problems? A review. J Women's Health 1993;2:165–172.

150. Drossman DA, Talley NJ, Olden KW, Leserman J, Barreiro MA. Sexual and physical abuse and gastrointestinal illness: review and recommendations. Ann Intern Med 1995;123:782–794.

151. Drossman DA, Li Z, Leserman J, Toomey TC, Hu Y. Health status by gastrointestinal diagnosis and abuse history. Gastroenterology 1996;110:999–1007.

152. Cohen S, Syme SL. Issues in the study and application of social support. In: Cohen S, Syme SL, eds. Social support and health. Orlando: Academic Press; 1985:3–22.

153. Sewitch MJ, Abrahamowicz M, Bitton A et al. Psychological distress, social support, and disease activity in patients with inflammatory bowel disease. Am J Gastroenterol 2001;96:1470–1479.

154. Lazarus RS, Folkman S. Stress, appraisal and coping. New York: Springer Verlag; 1984.

155. Keefe FJ, Williams DA. A comparison of coping strategies in chronic pain patients in different age groups. J Gerontol Psychol Sci 1990;45:161–165.

156. Lazarus RS. Coping theory and research: past, present, and future. Psychosom Med 1993;55:234–247.

157. Schwarz SP, Blanchard EB. Evaluation of a psychological treatment for inflammatory bowel disease. Behav Res Ther 1991;29:167–177.

158. Drossman DA. Psychosocial sound bites: exercises in the patient–doctor relationship. Am J Gastroenterol 1997;92:1418–1423.

159. Drossman DA, Chang L. Psychosocial factors in the care of patients with GI disorders. In: Yamada T, ed. Textbook of gastroenterology. Philadelphia: Lippincott-Raven; 2002:636–654.

160. Drossman DA. Challenges in the physician–patient relationship: Feeling 'drained'. Gastroenterology 2001;121:1037–1038.

161. Morgan WL Jr, Engel GL. The approach to the medical interview. In: Morgan WL Jr, Engel GL, eds. The clinical approach to the patient. Philadelphia: WB Saunders; 1969:26–79.

162. Lipkin M Jr, Kaplan C, Clark W, Novack DH. Teaching medical interviewing: the Lipkin model. In: Lipkin M Jr, Putnam SM, Lazare A, eds. The medical interview: clinical care, education, and research. New York: Springer Verlag; 1995:422–435.

163. DeVaul RA, Faillace LA. Persistent pain and illness insistence – a medical profile of proneness to surgery. Am J Surg 1978;135:828–833.

164. Drossman DA. The physician–patient relationship. In: Corazziari E, ed. Approach to the patient with chronic gastrointestinal disorders. Milan: Messaggi; 1999:133–139.

165. Caset S, Bertrand C, Doherty AM, Diop L. Anti-allodynic effects of tricyclic antidepressants in TNBS-induced chronic colonic hypersensitivity. Gastroenterology 2001;120: A329.

166. Blier P, Abbot FV. Putative mechanisms of action of antidepressant drugs in affective and anxiety disorders and pain. J Psychiatry Neurosci 2001;26:37–43.

167. Clouse RE. Antidepressants for functional gastrointestinal syndromes. Dig Dis Sci 1994;39:2352–2363.

168. Jackson JL, O'Malley PG, Tomkins G, Balden E, Santoro J, Kroenke K. Treatment of functional gastrointestinal disorders with anti-depressants: A meta-analysis. Am J Med 2000;108:65–72.

169. Drossman DA, Creed FH, Fava GA et al. Psychosocial aspects of the functional gastrointestinal disorders. Gastroenterol Int 1995;8:47–90.

170. Drossman DA, Toner BB, Whitehead WE et al. Cognitive–behavioral therapy vs. education and desipramine vs. placebo for moderate to severe functional bowel disorders. Gastroenterology 2003; (in press).

171. Cakkues AL, Popkin MK. Antidepressant treatment of medical–surgical inpatients by nonpsychiatric physicians. Arch Gen Psychiatry 1987;44:157–160.

172. Rogers M, Cerda JJ. Editorial: The narcotic bowel syndrome. J Clin Gastroenterol 1989;11:132–135.

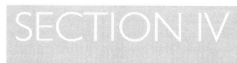

# DIAGNOSIS AND EVALUATION

## CHAPTER 25

# Differential diagnosis of inflammatory bowel disease

David G Forcione and Bruce E Sands

## INTRODUCTION

Crohn's disease (CD) and ulcerative colitis (UC) are the most common of the chronic idiopathic inflammatory bowel diseases (IBD). New insights into the pathogenesis of these diseases, particularly from genetics, offer the best hope for the future of definitive diagnostic testing. At present, however, there is no gold standard test to establish a diagnosis of IBD or to differentiate Crohn's disease and ulcerative colitis with complete certainty. Whereas many disease entities need to be considered in the differential diagnosis of IBD, a definitive diagnosis may nearly always be established through methodical assessment of clinical, laboratory, radiographic, endoscopic and histologic findings. Nevertheless, the protean gastrointestinal and extraintestinal manifestations of IBD may at times make the diagnosis challenging even for the most experienced clinician.

Like most tissues, the gastrointestinal tract is capable of manifesting a response to injury in a limited number of ways. Accordingly, infectious, inflammatory, ischemic and neoplastic processes may imitate IBD by virtue of similar clinical presentations and objective evaluations. Furthermore, few processes have pathognomonic features. It is therefore essential to maintain a broad differential diagnosis while evaluating a patient with suspected IBD. A careful evaluation with focus on history and physical examination must be completed in each case to establish the correct diagnosis, as all too often incomplete evaluations result in erroneous treatment for mistaken diagnoses.

A wide spectrum of entities may be considered in the differential diagnosis of IBD (Tables 25.1 and 25.2). From a diagnostic perspective these may be organized by anatomic localization in the gastrointestinal tract or by etiology and mechanism. Despite the long list of potential entities, some diagnoses commonly imitate IBD in their clinical presentation and endoscopic or radiographic appearances (Table 25.3).

A variety of medications, some in very common use, are capable of causing injury in the gastrointestinal tract, thereby mimicking IBD. A careful review of prescribed and over-the-counter medications is advisable in all cases of suspected IBD. Neoplastic processes, both primary and metastatic, commonly involve the gastrointestinal tract. These may occasionally present in a manner similar to IBD, and should be considered, particularly among elderly patients. Inflammatory conditions, including celiac sprue, microscopic colitis, and eosinophilic gastroenteritis, may resemble IBD in their presentations, and require careful consideration for clinical and histologic clues to distinguish these alternative diagnoses from IBD. Gynecologic disease should be considered in the differential diagnosis of all women suspected to have IBD. Vascular syndromes, ranging from radiation injury to acute thrombosis and vasculitis, may also be mistaken for IBD at times. Infectious causes of enterocolitis remain perhaps the most important consideration in all patients who are evaluated for IBD, with major treatment implications. A spectrum of inherited conditions has been associated with gastrointestinal syndromes akin to IBD. Functional gastrointestinal disease remains a common diagnostic entity in patients with a high prior probability than IBD among most patients presenting with chronic diarrhea and abdominal pain. In summary, the sheer variety of processes that may be mistaken for IBD is startlingly large.

## DRUG-INDUCED ENTEROCOLITIS

### SODIUM PHOSPHATE BOWEL PREPARATION

In addition to reports of significant electrolyte disturbances (hypokalemia, hyperphosphatemia, hypocalcemia), sodium phosphate (NaP)-induced colonic ulceration has also been described.[1] The incidence of apthoid-like colonic ulceration in patients who have undergone bowel preparation with NaP has ranged from 2.6% to 24.5%.[2,3]

The best-described endoscopic abnormalities seen in patients who have undergone bowel preparation with NaP include

**Table 25.1 Differential diagnosis of ileitis**

| Category | | Category | |
|---|---|---|---|
| **Inflammatory** | Acute appendicitis | **Infections** | Salmonella enteriditis |
| | Appendiceal abscess | | Shigella sonnei |
| | Cecal diverticulitis | | Campylobacter jejuni |
| | Graft vs. host disease | | Yersinia enterocolitica |
| | | | Typhlitis |
| **Neoplastic** | Cecal adenocarcinoma | | Mycobacterium tuberculosis |
| | Carcinoid tumor | | Atypical mycobacteria |
| | Lymphoma | | Histoplasma capsulatum |
| | Metastatic cancer | | Cytomegalovirus |
| | | | Cryptospordium parvum |
| **Gynecologic** | Endometriosis | | Entamoeba histolytica |
| | Pelvic inflammatory disease | | |
| | Tubo-ovarian abscess | **Functional** | Irritable bowel syndrome |
| | Tubo-ovarian cysts/neoplasia | | Anorexia nervosa |
| | Ectopic pregnancy | | Sexual abuse |
| **Infiltrative** | Amyloidosis | | |
| | Eosinophilic gastroenteritis | | |
| **Vascular** | Mesenteric ischemia | **Miscellaneous** | Mucocele |
| | Malrotation | | Meckel's diverticulum |
| | Wegener's granulomatosis | | Lipomatosis of ileocecal valve |
| | Necrotizing angiitis | | Appendicea epiploica infarction |
| | Behçet's syndrome | | Adhesions |
| | Cryoglobulinemia | | Ileocolic anastamotic ulcers |
| | Radiation injury | | Blunt trauma |
| | Systemic lupus erythematosus | | Infected urachal cysts |
| | Polyarteritis nodosa | | Foreign body |
| | Henoch–Schönlein purpura | | Non-steroidal |
| | Churg–Strauss syndrome | | anti-inflammatory drugs |

superficial ulcerations, and a pigmented halo with leopardskin markings on a normal background mucosa. NaP-induced ulcers are found predominantly in the left colon. Histologic landmarks of NaP injury include focal basal cryptitis, crypt apoptotic bodies, and normal background mucosa. Chronic inflammatory infiltrates, granulomas and/or distortion of crypt architecture are notably absent and should raise suspicion of underlying IBD. Given some of the overlapping features between NaP-induced colonic injury and those of inflammatory bowel diseases, NaP bowel preparations should be avoided in patients undergoing colonoscopy or flexible sigmoidoscopy for suspected IBD.

## NON-STEROIDAL ANTI-INFLAMMATORY DRUGS

Proximal gastrointestinal tract ulceration is a well-known potential consequence of NSAID use. Small intestinal and colonic injury from NSAIDs has been increasingly described. In addition, NSAIDs have been associated with small bowel strictures and membranous webs. Ileal involvement occurs, with ulcerations resembling those seen in Crohn's disease.[4,5] Colitis, colonic ulcerations and colonic strictures have all been reported in patients taking NSAIDs.[6–8] NSAIDs have also been implicated as a precipitant of IBD flares.[9]

Studies with indium-111 labeled white blood cells have shown that most patients taking NSAIDs have evidence of ileocecal inflammation.[10] However, the vast majority of these patients are asymptomatic and have no recognizable abnormalities on further imaging or endoscopy. Symptomatic presentations may include overt or occult gastrointestinal bleeding, abdominal pain, nausea, vomiting and diarrhea. Given the widespread use of these medications and the overlapping features with IBD, a thorough drug history must be taken when evaluating patients with symptoms suggestive of intestinal inflammation, gastrointestinal bleeding or obstructive lesions.

## GOLD

Enterocolitis is a rare but potentially fatal complication of gold therapy, now uncommonly used in rheumatoid arthritis.[11,12] Typically, patients present with bloody diarrhea, fever, rash and abdominal pain. Colonoscopy reveals a diffusely friable, erythematous and edematous mucosa. Histology demonstrates a mixed inflammatory infiltrate with rare findings of crypt abscesses. Mortality rates as high as 40% were reported in the early literature.[6,13] Systemic glucocorticoids are used in severe cases, but have an unproven efficacy.

## ENTERIC-COATED POTASSIUM SUPPLEMENTS

Small intestinal ulceration, jejunal perforation and stenosis mimicking CD have been reported with enteric-coated potassium supplements.[14,15] The estimated incidence is 3/100 000 patient-

## Table 25.2 Differential diagnosis of colitis

| Inflammatory | Ulcerative colitis | | Infections | | |
| --- | --- | --- | --- | --- | --- |
| | Crohn's disease | | Bacterial | | *Clostridium difficile* |
| | Indeterminate colitis | | | | *Yersinia enterocolitica* |
| | Microscopic colitis | | | | *Escherchia coli* species |
| | (collagenous and lymphocytic) | | | | *Campylobacter jejuni* |
| | Diversion colitis | | | | *Salmonella enteritidis* |
| | Segmental colitis | | | | *Shigella sonnei* |
| | Graft vs. host disease | | | | *Treponema pallidum* |
| | Diverticulitis | | | | *Mycobacterium tuberculosis* |
| | | | | | Atypical mycobacterium |
| Neoplastic | Adenocarcinoma | | | | *Neisseria gonorrhea* |
| | Metastatic cancer | | | | *Chlamydia* species |
| | Mycosis fungoides | | | | *Aeromonas hydrophilia* |
| | Malignant histiocytosis | | | | *Pleisiomonas shigelloides* |
| | Lymphoma | | | | *Actinomyces isreaelli* |
| | Multiple lymphomatosis polyposis | | | | |
| | | | Protozoal | | *Entamoeba histolytica* |
| Vascular | Ischemic colitis | | | | *Isospora belli* |
| | Polyarteritis nodosa | | | | *Cryptosporidium parvum* |
| | Systemic lupus erythematosus | | | | *Endolimax nana* |
| | Rheumatoid arthritis | | | | *Schistosoma mansoni* |
| | Wegener's granulomatosis | | | | |
| | Henoch–Schönlein purpura | | Fungal | | *Basidiobola ranarum* |
| | Cryoglobulinemia | | | | |
| | Dermatomyositis | | Viral | | *Cytomegalovirus* |
| | Behçet's syndrome | | | | *Herpes simplex* |
| | Solitary rectal ulcer syndrome | | | | |
| | Radiation colitis | | Helminthic | | *Strongyloides stercolis* |
| | | | | | *Angiostrongylus costaricensis* |
| Drug-related | Non-steroidal anti-inflammatory drugs | | | | *Anisakiasis* species |
| | Gold | | | | *Trichuris trichuria* |
| | Penicillamine | | | | |
| | Oral contraceptives | | | | |
| | Potassium chloride | | | | |
| | Pancreatic enzyme replacement | | | | |
| | Cathartic colon | | | | |
| | Phosphasoda bowel preparations | | | | |
| | Thermal injury from colostomy irrigation | | | | |
| Genetic syndromes | X-linked agammaglobulinemia | | | | |
| | Common variable immunodeficiency | | | | |
| | Glycogen storage disease type IB | | | | |
| | Chronic granulomatous disease | | | | |
| | Turner's syndrome | | | | |
| | Hermansky–Pudlak syndrome | | | | |
| Miscellaneous | Irritable bowel syndrome | | | | |
| | Factitious diarrhea | | | | |
| | Pneumatosis cystoides intestinalis | | | | |
| | Hidradenitis suppurativa | | | | |
| | Castleman's syndrome | | | | |
| | Linear IgA disease | | | | |

years of slow-release tablet use. Microencapsulated potassium chloride tablets appear to be less injurious.

## CATHARTIC COLON

Chronic use of laxatives may rarely cause inflammatory lesions in the colon ('cathartic colon').[16] In most reports patients also have evidence of melanosis coli, with a distinct endoscopic appearance like 'worn leather'. Most patients have right colon-predominant findings. Histology demonstrates evidence of a mild inflammatory infiltrate with hypertrophy of the muscularis mucosa. Granulomas or architectural changes in the crypts are not seen.

**Table 25.3 Most common 'impostors' in the differential diagnosis of inflammatory bowel disease**

Infectious colitis (including *Clostridium difficile*)
Ischemic colitis
Drug-induced enterocolitis
Solitary rectal ulcer syndrome
Radiation enterocolitis
Diversion colitis
Segmental colitis
Microscopic colitis
Endometriosis
Malignancy
Functional (irritable bowel syndrome)
Diverticular disease

## ORAL CONTRACEPTIVES

The association between oral contraceptive use and transient colitis was first reported by Kilpatrick et al. in 1968.[17] Patients are often young healthy women on oral contraceptive pills containing estrogen and progesterone who abruptly develop abdominal pain and bloody diarrhea. The syndrome has also been described in postmenopausal women on hormone replacement therapy. The enterocolitis of oral contraceptive use is believed to be ischemic. In many cases small and large vessel thrombi have been demonstrated. The duration of hormonal use has ranged from 10 days to 11 years before the event. Rectosigmoid and splenic flexure disease predominates, although the location may vary. Patchy involvement is most common, leading some cases to be misconstrued as presentations of Crohn's disease. Spontaneous resolution upon discontinuation of the medication and with supportive measures is the expected course.[18]

## CANCER CHEMOTHERAPEUTICS

An increasing number of chemotherapeutic agents have been reported in association with the development of an enterocolitis. These include cytosine arabinoside,[19] 5-fluorouracil,[20] cyclophosphamide,[21] methotrexate[22] and flucytosine.[23] Confounding factors in some of these reports include concurrent sepsis and the use of other drugs. Typhlitis, also known as neutropenic ileocolitis, can develop as a result of severe bone marrow suppression due to chemotherapy (see below).

## MISCELLANEOUS DRUGS

A number of other agents have been reported to cause enterocolitis. Ergot and vasopressin are well-known vasoactive medications reported to cause episodes of acute colitis.[24,25] In some cases strictures may develop. Several cases of methyldopa-related colitis have been described.[26] Water-soluble contrast media (Gastrografin, Hypaque, Renografin) have been reported rarely to cause colitis and this may be related to direct mucosal contact with the additive, Tween-80.[27–29] Soapsud enemas have been reported to cause an acute, self-limited colitis, probably from caustic injury to the mucosa.[30] Inadvertent hydrogen peroxide or ethyl alcohol enemas have also been reported to cause a non-specific colitis.[31,32] Ulceration and necrosis in the esophagus, stomach, small intestine, terminal ileum and colon has been described in association with sodium polystyrene sulfonate, an ion exchange resin used to treat hyperkalemia.[33–35]

Nearly all patients described had acute or chronic renal failure. Biopsy may aid in the diagnosis as occasionally resin crystals may be seen. Penicillamine rarely has been reported in association with colitis.[36,37] An ulcerative colitis-like picture with interstitial fibrosis and colonic structuring has been described in patients with cystic fibrosis using high-strength enteric-coated pancreatic enzyme replacement.[38] Colostomy irrigation has been reported to cause colonic thermal injury and stricture.[39]

# NEOPLASTIC PROCESSES

## GASTROINTESTINAL CARCINOID TUMORS

Occurring in only 15/100 000 people, gastrointestinal carcinoid tumors are the most common of the gastrointestinal neuroendocrine tumors.[40,41] Many reports of carcinoid tumors of the gastrointestinal tract mimicking IBD may be found, primarily because of the predilection to involve the distal small intestine and right colon.[42,43] Like lymphoma and primary adenocarcinoma, carcinoid may also complicate underlying ileal Crohn's disease.[44] In one series, 2.3% of patients ultimately diagnosed with ileal carcinoid tumors were initially felt to have Crohn's disease.[45]

In this study, the mean time to a diagnosis of carcinoid tumor was 24 months. The authors describe several clues leading to the diagnosis of carcinoid tumor. These include advanced age at presentation (typically between the ages of 50 and 70), atypical radiologic features (liver lesions should not be found in uncomplicated Crohn's disease, unlike metastatic carcinoid), lack of extraintestinal manifestations (present among 25% of patients with Crohn's disease), and lack of response to standard IBD therapy. A urinary 5-HIAA test is only 75% sensitive for a diagnosis of carcinoid and therefore should not be used in isolation. Nevertheless, in the appropriate clinical scenario an elevated urinary 5-HIAA has a 98% specificity for a diagnosis of carcinoid.[41] Ileal intubation during colonoscopy, although quite helpful in evaluating the presence of involvement with Crohn's disease, often misses a carcinoid tumor as most are located within 60 cm of the ileocecal valve, and in up to 30% of patients multiple tumors can be found. Octreotide or metaiodobenzylguanidine (MIBG) scans may be useful radiologic adjuncts. Biopsy remains the gold standard and should be pursued in all cases.

Clinically, less than 10% of patients suffer from the classic manifestations of carcinoid syndrome – flushing, bronchospasm and diarrhea. Appendiceal carcinoid is most often asymptomatic, as these tend to occur in the distal third of the appendix. Only 10% are found in the base, and this may lead to obstruction causing acute appendicitis. Small intestine carcinoid tumors are the most common ileal tumor and tend to be more symptomatic. Abdominal pain may be related to obstruction in the setting of an intussusception or mass effect, and rarely may be ischemic in origin due to paracrine effects upon the microvasculature of the small bowel.[46] Carcinoid tumors of the colon are most commonly found in the cecum, and unfortunately may present late owing to a prolonged asymptomatic phase.[47] Some patients, however, will have abdominal pain, hematochezia, anorexia or weight loss. In contrast, rectal carcinoid is often discovered during screening digital rectal examination or screening endoscopy as a submucosal mass.

# GASTROINTESTINAL LYMPHOMA

The wide array of non-specific signs and symptoms with which primary gastrointestinal lymphomas may present warrants their consideration in nearly all patients with gastrointestinal disease.[48-51] Furthermore, lymphoma may complicate long-standing intestinal Crohn's disease and ulcerative colitis.[52-54] Multiple lymphomatous polyposis (MLP), a variant of mantle cell lymphoma, can also be seen throughout the gastrointestinal tract, although more commonly in the colon.[55,56] The stomach is the most frequent site of involvement, accounting for 75% of cases, and may present with epigastric pain, anorexia, nausea and vomiting, early satiety, weight loss and gastrointestinal bleeding.[57,58] One variant, mucosa-associated lymphoid tissue tumor (MALToma), is thought to develop in the setting of chronic *Helicobacter pylori* infection. Immunodeficiency related to HIV and transplantation is also a risk factor. Endoscopically, these lesions may be manifest as focal polypoid masses (occasionally with ulceration), enlarged folds and nodular mucosa. The early appearance may resemble a benign gastric ulcer. Diffuse cobblestoning of the proximal small intestinal mucosa is more common among patients of Middle Eastern or Mediterranean descent. Biopsy is diagnostic.

Small intestine lymphoma is much more common among patients of Middle Eastern and Mediterranean descent than in northern Europeans.[59] Abdominal pain (often associated with obstruction due to intussusception), malabsorption (marked by weight loss, diarrhea, nutritional deficiencies) and occult gastrointestinal bleeding are typical patterns of clinical presentation. The terminal ileum is the most common location in the United States, compared to the proximal small bowel in the Middle East. Infiltrating mass lesions, focal ulcerations and nodularity are the most common endoscopic findings if amenable to small bowel enteroscopy or colonoscopy with ileal intubation. Biopsy is diagnostic.

Lymphoma of the colon and rectum may arise de novo, but may also complicate long-standing ulcerative colitis or Crohn's disease. Diarrhea and hematochezia are the most common presentations. Colitis-like changes have been described, making this an important diagnosis to entertain in the differential of new colitis or established colitis that is refractory to treatment.

Mycosis fungoides and Sézary syndrome are extranodal non-Hodgkins lymphomas of T-cell origin that present with cutaneous involvement, predominantly erythroderma. In Sézary syndrome there is also generalized lymphadenopathy, and circulating 'Sézary' cells. None the less, there have been rare case reports of gastrointestinal involvement, including hemorrhage, malabsorption, small bowel perforation and diarrhea.[60-62]

# GASTROINTESTINAL ADENOCARCINOMA

Primary adenocarcinoma, and hamartomatous and adenomatous polyps of the colon, may imitate IBD, particularly in the cecum.[63-68] Variants of colon adenocarcinoma in which there is a diffuse infiltrative submucosal process are also notable imitators of IBD (Fig. 25.1). When malignancy is suspected, multiple biopsies should be taken to avoid sampling error.

# METASTASES

In addition to primary adenocarcinoma of the colon and gastrointestinal carcinoid tumors and lymphomas, metastatic lesions may sometimes present in the gastrointestinal tract as mimics of IBD. Breast cancer and gastric cancer have been reported to present in this way.[69-71] Specifically, linitis plastica of the stomach may metastasize to the colon and present with bloody diarrhea. The findings may be typical of ischemic colitis. Kaposi's sarcoma may also present in the gastrointestinal tract, often with overt or occult gastrointestinal bleeding, and should be considered in the differential diagnosis, particularly in HIV-positive patients.[72-74] Gastrointestinal malignant histiocytosis has also been reported to simulate Crohn's disease.[75]

# INFLAMMATORY CONDITIONS

# GASTROINTESTINAL SARCOIDOSIS

Sarcoidosis, an idiopathic systemic disease characterized by non-caseating granulomas, may manifest in the gastrointestinal tract

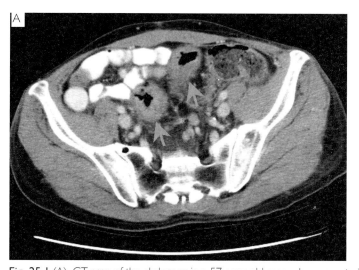

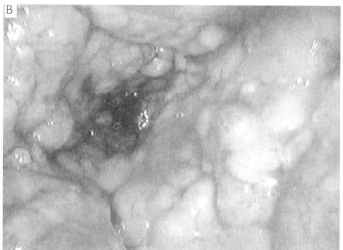

**Fig. 25.1** (A) CT scan of the abdomen in a 57-year-old man who presented with 4 months of lower abdominal pain, bloody diarrhea and weight loss. There is evidence of concentric wall thickening of the sigmoid colon (arrows). (B) Colonoscopy performed on the same patient as in A demonstrated diffuse nodular congestion and erythema from the rectum to 30 cm from the anal verge. Multiple endoscopic biopsies revealed a colon adenocarcinoma with prominent lymphatic invasion and submucosal infiltration.

in less than 1% of cases.[76] However, subclinical involvement is believed to be much more common. The granulomatous nature of this disease makes it a particularly important consideration in the differential diagnosis of Crohn's disease. Interestingly, a number of case reports describe patients with both IBD (UC and Crohn's disease) and sarcoidosis, suggesting the possibility of similar pathogenetic mechanisms.[77]

The stomach is the most frequently involved site and may manifest with frank bleeding, abdominal pain or weight loss. On endoscopy, a variety of non-specific findings may be evident, including nodularity, thickened folds, ulceration and deformities of the antrum and pylorus.[78] Esophageal sarcoidosis,[79] with focal ulcerations and nodularity, may be particularly difficult to distinguish from esophageal Crohn's disease. Small bowel sarcoidosis is rare and may manifest with weight loss, abdominal pain, fever and gastrointestinal bleeding. Protein-losing enteropathy, malabsorption and obstruction are uncommonly seen. Colonic sarcoidosis may manifest with bleeding and abdominal pain.[80] Most patients with sarcoidosis will have significant pulmonary and multisystem involvement, with granulomatous inflammation, distinguishing the diagnosis from IBD

## CELIAC SPRUE

Celiac sprue ('gluten-sensitive enteropathy') is a malabsorptive disorder characterized by small bowel inflammation due to an immune response against gluten-derived gliadin peptides.[81] It has been estimated to affect as many as 1 in every 120–300 persons in North America. As in IBD, many individuals are diagnosed as children or young adults. Only 20% of celiac sprue cases occur in patients who are over 60 years of age.

Celiac sprue is associated with a wide array of gastrointestinal and systemic manifestations that may resemble those of IBD. Iron deficiency anemia is the most common clinical presentation in adults. Abdominal pain, malaise, diarrhea, bloating and weight loss are also common. Less common nutritional deficiencies include those of vitamin D, vitamin K and folate. Steatorrhea and vitamin $B_{12}$ deficiency are seen only in patients with extensive small bowel disease.

Fortunately, the diagnosis of celiac sprue has been facilitated by sensitive and specific serologic and histologic hallmarks. Antibodies directed against endomysium, tissue transglutaminase and gliadin have sensitivity and specificity as high as 85–100%. Imaging studies may show lymphadenopathy, small bowel thickening and, less commonly, hyposplenism or ascites. Involvement of the terminal ileum is quite unusual. Endoscopic small bowel biopsy classically demonstrates villous atrophy and hyperplastic crypts, with an increased number of intraepithelial lymphocytes and plasma cells. Granulomas are not seen.

## EOSINOPHILIC GASTROENTERITIS

Eosinophilic infiltration in the gastrointestinal tract, although rare, may produce a wide array of symptoms, making it a part of many gastrointestinal differential diagnoses, including IBD. Eosinophilic gastroenteritis may be focal or diffuse, with a predilection for gastric antrum and for the proximal small intestine. Involved layers may range from the mucosa to the subserosa.[82,83]

Concurrent upper and lower gastrointestinal tract symptoms are common, and include nausea, vomiting, abdominal pain and diarrhea. Malabsorption with weight loss and nutritional

deficiencies may develop in small bowel involvement. Subserosal disease can also manifest with an eosinophilic ascites, which may be quite specific in the appropriate clinical scenario. Small and large bowel obstructions have been described, as have episodes of hematochezia due to focal rectal involvement. A mild to moderate peripheral blood eosinophilia may be present, but is not universal, being absent in up to 20% of cases.[84] A number of case reports have described focal ileocecal and colonic involvement misdiagnosed as Crohn's disease.[85–87] Naylor et al.[88] reviewed the case reports of 22 patients with eosinophilic colitis, with four of the patients initially misdiagnosed as having IBD. The mean age at diagnosis was 41, and there was no race or gender predilection. Approximately a third of patients had a history of an 'allergic' disorder. In this series the right colon was most commonly involved, with common endoscopic features of erythema, granularity, nodularity, and occasionally mucosal ulceration. Abdominal pain (68%), diarrhea (45%), and nausea, vomiting or weight loss (55%) were the predominant symptoms. Occasionally, constipation (13%) and hematochezia (22%) were also described. The finding of perianal disease in 4% adds to the complexity of the differential diagnosis. Laparotomy was required for diagnosis in slightly over half the cases.

None the less, the findings of significant peripheral eosinophilia, tissue eosinophilia (>20 eosinophils per high-power field), and the absence of chronic crypt changes increase the likelihood of eosinophilic gastroenteritis, after careful exclusion of parasitic infestation (particularly *Eustoma rotundatum*, *Trichuris trichura* and *Oxypuris* species). Although some patients with Crohn's disease may have a tissue eosinophilia, it is uniformly less than that seen in eosinophilic gastroenteritis. Furthermore, in eosinophilic gastroenteritis the eosinophilic infiltrate predominates in the mucosa, in contrast to the usually milder and submucosal eosinophilic infiltrate sometimes seen in Crohn's disease. Radiologically, IBD and eosinophilic gastroenteritis share many features in regard to location and characteristics (wall thickening). An ileocecal valve which appears open in a fixed position with a patulous terminal ileum is more typical of eosinophilic ileocolitis.[86]

## MESENTERIC PANNICULITIS

A number of names have been used to describe mesenteric panniculitis, including mesenteric Weber–Christian disease, mesenteric lipogranuloma, sclerosing mesenteritis and mesenteric lipodystrophy.[89–91] The nature of the mesenteric inflammatory process may mimic Crohn's disease.[92]

Most patients are diagnosed in their 60s, and there are no gender or ethnic predilections. Abdominal pain, fever of unknown origin, diarrhea, constipation and bowel obstruction have been reported as prominent symptoms. Patients may have a palpable mass on abdominal examination, and may give a history of abdominal trauma. Most lesions are focal masses in the small bowel mesentery, and less commonly a diffuse mesenteric thickening. Surgical biopsy reveals fibrosis, chronic inflammatory infiltrates and fat necrosis.

## DIVERTICULAR DISEASE

Small bowel diverticula are uncommon, and largely discovered incidentally. Most (79%) are duodenal, and these may come to attention during endoscopic retrograde cholangiopancreatography (ERCP).[93,94] Most complications arising from small bowel diverticula, however, are found in the 18% of patients with jejunoileal involvement. Manifestations may include overt bleeding, diverticulitis, small bowel obstruction and, rarely, fistula.

Colonic diverticulosis is one of the most common of gastrointestinal disorders. Over 65% of individuals aged 85 and over have evidence of colonic diverticulosis. Nearly 70% of patients with colonic diverticulosis are asymptomatic. However, hematochezia, which occurs in as many as 15%, and diverticulitis, which occurs in another 15%, are associated with significant morbidity. In most patients these are acute presentations, developing over 1–3 days. Diverticular bleeding is nearly always painless and ceases spontaneously in over 80% of patients. Colonoscopy is indicated largely to exclude alternative causes, including neoplasia, vascular lesions and, rarely, colitis.

Diverticulitis, which represents a micro- or macroperforation of the bowel wall, occurs in the sigmoid colon in the vast majority of cases. Left lower quadrant pain developing over 2–3 days, fever and leukocytosis are cardinal manifestations. Computed tomography (CT) illustrates segmental colonic thickening with stranding in the surrounding fat, as well as uninvolved diverticula in most cases. Extensive bowel involvement should raise the suspicion of an alternative diagnosis.[95]

Cecal diverticulitis is notably uncommon, occurring in 1.5% of cases.[96] However, this is an important part of the differential diagnosis of IBD, as well as appendicitis and cecal carcinoma. Epidemiologic studies have found that individuals of Asian descent are more prone to this presentation. Unfortunately, in most series a preoperative diagnosis is made in fewer than 25% of cases.

'Complicated' diverticulitis occurs in 25% of patients, and may include fistula (colocolonic, colovesicular, colovaginal or colocutaneous), obstruction, or frank perforation with abscess formation. Fistulous complications may present with pyuria, pneumaturia or fecaluria. Prolonged pain, fever or peritonitis warrant evaluation for abscess.

## SEGMENTAL COLITIS

Segmental colitis, an inflammatory process involving the colonic mucosa adjacent to diverticula, is an evolving clinical entity first described by Cawthorn et al. in 1983.[97] Since then, a number of small case series have reviewed the pertinent clinicopathologic findings.[98–101] In the largest series to date, Imperiali et al.[102] reported on 14 cases discovered during 5457 consecutive colonoscopies. Three other patients initially diagnosed with segmental colitis were ultimately given a diagnosis of Crohn's disease. In this series the mean age was 67. Hematochezia was the presenting symptom in 86%, with half reporting abdominal pain or diarrhea. Thirty-five per cent of patients had had similar episodes in the past. Acute-phase reactants were remarkably normal in 86%. Defining endoscopic features included edema, erythema, friability, erosions and frank ulcerations in the presence of usually extensive sigmoid diverticulosis. Rectal sparing was noted in all cases. Non-specific inflammation was noted on histology. On a regimen of oral and topical 5-aminosalicylates, clinical and endoscopic remission was noted in 86% of patients at 12 months.

The true nature and prevalence of this disease remains to be seen. Some have argued that the syndrome may represent one variant in the spectrum of Crohn's disease. Others postulate an ischemic or iatrogenic etiology. Regardless, the high prevalence of diverticular disease in Western society should prompt greater consideration of this clinical entity.

## DIVERSION COLITIS

Diversion colitis has been a well-described entity since 1981.[103] It has come to be defined by an inflammatory process in the colorectal remnant of patients without pre-existing IBD who have undergone a surgical ostomy for benign or malignant colorectal disease.[104] The resulting segmental fecal diversion results in clinical, endoscopic and histologic evidence of inflammation in over 90% of patients.

Disruption of the fecal stream appears to cause colitis from a deficiency in short-chain fatty acids, particularly butyrate and propionate, derived from commensal flora. In vitro experiments have demonstrated the role of these compounds in maintaining colonic epithelial integrity. Furthermore, instillation of short-chain fatty acids results in a dramatic clinical, endoscopic and histologic response.

Clinically, most patients have mild symptoms, including rectal bleeding, mucous discharge and tenesmus. In one series, only 4% had severe symptoms.[105] On biopsy, hyperplastic lymphoglandular expansion in the submucosa with cryptitis is observed. Granulomas are unusual. Given the clear overlap of clinicopathologic findings with IBD, it is critical to ensure that there is no pre-existing IBD, the surgical specimen is free of findings consistent with IBD, and the intestine proximal to the stoma remains free of involvement.

Although enemas containing short-chain fatty acids or 5-aminosalicylates are usually quite effective in controlling symptoms,[106] early restoration of intestinal continuity remains curative.

## BYPASS ENTERITIS

First described by Passaro and colleagues in 1975,[107] bypass enteritis has been found frequently as a complication of jejunoileal bypass surgery for morbid obesity. The syndrome has been reported in 18–54% of patients after jejunoileal bypass, manifesting from 18 months to 7 years from surgery.[108] Patients may develop abdominal bloating, hematochezia, diarrhea, nausea and vomiting. Some may manifest with severe electrolyte imbalances, specifically with carpopedal spasm from hypocalcemia. Extraintestinal manifestations are also common, including anemia, arthritis, fever, weight loss and dermatitis.

The mechanism of disease is poorly understood, although most authorities regard bacterial overgrowth in the bypassed ileal segment,[109] with consequent release of endotoxins, as the most likely inciting factor. On endoscopic evaluation one may see large ulcerations with edema. Evidence of acute and chronic inflammation with elongation of crypts and loss of villi is visible on microscopy. Although broad-spectrum antibiotics may be efficacious, restitution of alimentary continuity is the treatment of choice.

## GRAFT-VERSUS-HOST DISEASE

Bone marrow transplantation has been an evolving and increasingly successful treatment for hematologic and solid organ malignancies. Graft-versus-host disease (GVHD) is the major complication seen after allogeneic bone marrow transplantation. GVHD is an immune disease characterized by graft effector cells (T cells) and the cytokine milieu they create (interleukin-1, interleukin-2, tumor necrosis factor-$\alpha$) causing end organ damage. A small amount of GVHD is desirable as it may induce a graft-versus-tumor effect and increase the chance of survival.

However, the line between a helpful response and one that results in significant host organ injury is a fine one. Acute and chronic forms of GVHD exist, with symptoms before 100 days after transplantation being indicative of the acute form. The skin, liver and gastrointestinal tract are the main organs of involvement.

Gastrointestinal GVHD[110] may be associated with a significant amount of morbidity. Symptoms may include abdominal pain, ileus, gastrointestinal bleeding, profuse watery diarrhea, anorexia, nausea and vomiting. In the chronic setting, oral mucositis, malabsorption with diarrhea, and esophageal stricturing have been described. Radiographic identification of gastrointestinal GVHD is variable, including diffuse small bowel thickening, ileitis, colon thickening, segmental colitis and ileus. Endoscopic appearances similarly range from normal-appearing mucosa to mucosal sloughing and deep ulceration. Proximal gastrointestinal involvement is increasingly being reported. Apoptotic cells are the histologic hallmark of GVHD, with a notable absence of distorted crypts, granulomas and crypt abscesses.

## MICROSCOPIC COLITIS

Microscopic colitis may be divided into two histologic types: lymphocytic and collagenous.[111] In contrast to the major forms of IBD, these entities are associated with minimal or absent endoscopic evidence of inflammation. For a complete overview of these conditions, see Chapter 48.

## NON-GRANULOMATOUS ULCERATIVE JEJUNOILEITIS

Non-granulomatous ulcerative jejunoileitis (NGUJI) is a rare gastrointestinal disorder characterized by progressive small bowel ulceration, predominantly in the duodenum and jejunum.[112] Most individuals are middle-aged and present with chronic diarrhea, abdominal pain, fever or malabsorption. On histology there is evidence of villous atrophy and a chronic inflammatory infiltrate, without granulomas.

## IDIOPATHIC GRANULOMATOUS GASTRITIS

Granulomatous gastritis has been reported to account for 0.35% of all gastric biopsy or resection specimens.[113,114] Crohn's disease and sarcoidosis account for 75% of these cases. A number of other conditions have been associated with granulomatous gastritis, including infections (*Tropheryma whippellii*, *Helicobacter pylori*, *Mycobacterium tuberculosis*, *Treponema pallidum*, *Taenia saginata*), malignancy (adenocarcinoma, lymphoma, histiocytosis), and inflammatory (Wegener's granulomatosis, chronic granulomatous disease, foreign body, gastric perforation). Idiopathic granulomatous gastritis appears to be quite rare.

## GYNECOLOGIC CONDITIONS

### ENDOMETRIOSIS

Endometriosis is a common disorder of premenopausal women and is characterized by the presence of ectopic endometrial tissue outside the uterus. In the UK it is reportedly found in up to 25% of patients who undergo laparoscopy for persistent pelvic pain.[115]

The gastrointestinal tract is a common site of implantation. In some series, up to 50% of patients with extensive pelvic endometriosis may have gastrointestinal involvement.[116] The rectosigmoid, appendix and terminal ileum are most often affected. Most lesions are serosal, and are discovered when hemorrhage ensues or adhesions develop. Rarely, muscular involvement may manifest as fibrosis and lead to abdominal pain and obstruction. There are a few reports of ileocecal endometriosis manifesting as ulcerative mucosal lesions.[117-119] A retrospective series of 7500 patients with endometriosis from the Mayo Clinic revealed that the small intestine was involved in 0.5%.[120] Terminal ileum was the most common site of involvement. Ileal endometriosis and Crohn's disease may also occur simultaneously.[121]

The diagnosis of gastrointestinal endometriosis is most often made at laparotomy. Imaging is suggestive if implants are defined in the pelvis as well, but is otherwise neither specific nor sensitive. Although a clinical pattern of worsening symptoms in the perimenstrual time frame seems physiologically sensible, this cannot be used as a distinguishing characteristic as this finding was only evident in 10% of patients in the Mayo Clinic series. None the less, given the clinical and radiologic similarities, endometriosis should be entertained in the differential diagnosis of female patients suspected of having IBD.

## VASCULAR DISORDERS

### RADIATION EXPOSURE

External beam radiation may cause multiple potential gastrointestinal complications leading to significant morbidity.[122] Any part of the gastrointestinal tract may be involved depending upon radiation dose, exposure field, fractionation and type of radiation. An obliterative vasculopathy is demonstrated on histology in the chronic phase.

In general, radiation doses over 40 Gy – a common dose for the treatment of thoracic and intra-abdominal malignancies – may be associated with gastrointestinal involvement.[123] Although most cases of acute radiation injury are difficult to confuse with IBD, the varied nature and delayed onset of manifestations (often decades later) raises a wide range of putative alternative diagnoses, including IBD. Furthermore, it is known that adjunctive chemotherapy or underlying enterocolitis predispose patients to more significant injury at a lower radiation dose.[124] Other risk factors are lean body habitus, diabetes mellitus and hypertension.[125] Thus, a history of radiation exposure should be sought in all patients who are being evaluated for IBD.

In the esophagus, acute radiation injury may present with severe esophagitis, and rarely fistula formation. Over time, strictures and occasionally squamous cell cancer may evolve.[126] Acute gastric involvement may be in the form of a hemorrhagic gastropathy, which may lead to fibrosis and outlet obstruction. Small bowel manifestations may include vomiting, diarrhea, weight loss and fistula formation. Recurrent small bowel obstructions can develop as a result of a fixed stenosis.[127]

Acute and chronic colorectal disease mimics ulcerative colitis, with predominant symptoms of hematochezia, tenesmus and diarrhea. Proctitis is a particularly troublesome symptom in those receiving radiation for prostate cancer. Colonic strictures and ischemic ulceration may develop. The visualization of numerous telengiectasias should raise suspicion for this entity.

## MESENTERIC ISCHEMIA

Ischemic injury to the gastrointestinal tract is a common and potentially life-threatening clinical entity. In general, patients are acutely ill and have a clear long-standing history of or risk factors for atherosclerosis. The differential diagnosis of chronic IBD may enter the picture in rare patients with atypical presentations or chronic gastrointestinal manifestations.

Ischemic small bowel disease is potentially devastating.[128,129] Acute presentations are associated with embolic or thrombotic occlusion of the superior mesenteric artery in 65% of cases. Mesenteric venous thrombosis comprises only 5% of cases, and non-occlusive disease another 30%. Acute abdominal pain out of proportion to physical findings in the patients at risk (with atherosclerosis, hypercoaguable conditions, cocaine use or an abdominal bruit) should alert the clinician to this disorder. Chronic mesenteric ischemia is usually associated with multivessel (celiac artery, superior mesenteric artery, inferior mesenteric artery) atherosclerosis. The clinical manifestations of chronic postprandial pain, early satiety, weight loss and food aversion may be mistaken for those of proximal Crohn's disease. However, the near-universal prevalence of severe vascular disease, elderly age and abdominal bruit on examination should suggest the correct diagnosis.

Ischemic colitis is the most common form of gastrointestinal ischemia, accounting for more than half of cases.[130,131] Non-occlusive vascular disease is the most common etiology. The spectrum of clinical manifestations is broad, ranging from the most common, a reversible colopathy, to the less common, including 20% of patients who may develop chronic ischemic colitis, ischemic strictures and, rarely, gangrene. In contrast to IBD, ischemic colitis is a disease of the elderly, with more than 90% of patients being over 70. In younger patients, vasculitic syndromes, drug-induced ischemia (cocaine, estrogens, danazol and psychotropic medications), sickle cell disease, thrombophilic syndromes and long-distance running should be entertained as causes. The most common predisposing factors in usual ischemic colitis include an acute hypotensive episode (drug related, myocardial ischemia, congestive heart failure, cardiac arrhythmias), or vascular surgery such as bypass grafting. Distal colonic obstructing lesions, including colorectal cancer, may also induce acute ischemic colitis.

The classic presentation of ischemic colitis is that of bloody diarrhea associated with crampy lower abdominal pain and the urge to defecate. In most patients there is no significant change in the hematocrit. CT scans outline the most commonly affected areas ('watershed' areas with limited collateral flow from the inferior mesenteric artery), including the splenic flexure, rectosigmoid and hepatic flexure (Fig. 25.2A). The rectum is generally spared. Bowel wall thickening, a non-specific finding, may be noted. At colonoscopy there are typically patchy submucosal hemorrhages, ulcerated mucosa and increased pallor (Fig. 25.2B). Frank gangrene is a rare but ominous finding. Histology may reveal submucosal edema and hemorrhage, fibrinopurulent exudates and glandular dropout.

In 80% of patients colopathy is transient, reversed by restoration of intravascular blood volume and blood pressure, often within 48 hours. However, recurrent episodes or a single severe episode may lead to a chronic colitis marked by recurrent bloody diarrhea, fevers, protein-losing enteropathy, colonic strictures and, rarely, perforation.

## GASTROINTESTINAL ANGIOEDEMA

Gastrointestinal angioedema is a rare clinical entity that may develop in the setting of hereditary angioneurotic edema (deficiency in C1 inhibitor), acquired C1 esterase deficiency due to autoimmune disease, neoplasia or lymphoproliferative disease.[132] Medications may rarely cause this entity, with angiotensin-

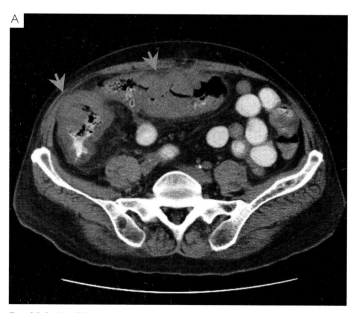

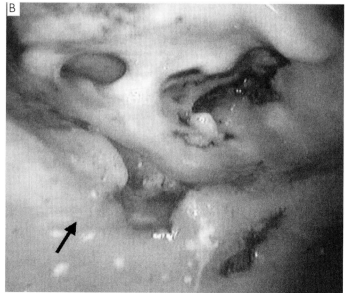

**Fig. 25.2** (A) CT scan of the abdomen in a 67-year-old man who presented with diffuse abdominal pain and bloody diarrhea 10 days after a coronary artery bypass graft procedure. There is evidence of significant concentric wall thickening of the ascending and transverse colon. (B) Colonoscopy demonstrated severe patchy ulceration beginning in the mid-distal transverse colon, with areas of exudates. Biopsies from the periphery of the ulcers (arrow) revealed submucosal hemorrhage and gland dropout, consistent with ischemic colitis.

converting enzyme inhibitors the most commonly reported drug class.[133–135] Typically, patients develop abdominal pain within a few days of initiating therapy, although there have been reports of patients developing this syndrome as long as 9 weeks from the start of therapy. Markers of acute inflammation are noted, including fever, rigors, peritoneal signs and leukocytosis. Imaging demonstrates diffuse small bowel edema and ascites. Removal of the offending drug and supportive therapy are curative in most instances.

## GASTROINTESTINAL VASCULITIS

The gastrointestinal complications of systemic vasculitis usually present with diarrhea, abdominal pain or gastrointestinal bleeding, and often may be clinically indistinguishable from ulcerative colitis or Crohn's disease. Based upon a number of series, approximately 25% of patients with systemic vasculitis will have clinically evident gastrointestinal involvement.[136] In nearly all patients, renal and cutaneous manifestations have predominated for months to years before gastrointestinal disease.

*Polyarteritis nodosa* is a necrotizing vasculitis involving the small and medium-sized blood vessels.[137–139] Up to 50% of patients will have abdominal angina, bowel perforation, diarrhea or gastrointestinal bleeding. *Churg–Strauss syndrome* is also a systemic vasculitis that predominantly affects small and medium-sized blood vessels. Patients typically also have evidence of asthma, peripheral eosinophilia and allergic rhinitis. Patients with diarrheal syndromes have been identified, with evidence of proctocolitis on colonoscopy and eosinophilic infiltrates on biopsy in addition to vasculitis.[140,141]

*Behçet's syndrome* is a rare, chronic relapsing vasculitis most classically associated with recurrent oral and genital ulcerations, although all organs may be affected.[142] Behçet's is most common in the Middle East, Mediterranean and Far East. Mean age of onset is 25–35 years. Although no consistent immune alterations have been discovered, an autoimmune etiology is postulated. The gastrointestinal tract is one of the more commonly affected sites.[143] Typical lesions include aphthous ulcerations, esophagitis, fistula, strictures and varices. Gastric and duodenal involvement may manifest as erosions and ulcers. The most frequent extraoral sites of gastrointestinal involvement are the ileocecal region and the colon. Anorectal involvement is quite rare. The clinical presentation is similar to that of Crohn's disease, including many shared extraintestinal manifestations. Patchy ulcerations may be aphthoid or, less commonly, longitudinal in appearance. Histologic hallmarks are crypt abscesses, submucosal fibrosis, vasculitis, and the notable rarity of granulomas. Treatment strategies have included glucocorticoids, colchicine, 5-aminosalicylates, thalidomide, azathioprine and infliximab.[144] Surgery is ultimately required in 10% of cases.

*Wegener's granulomatosis* is a small vessel systemic vasculitis primarily affecting the kidney, lungs and upper respiratory tract. Most patients have evidence of circulating antibodies to proteinase 3, a protease contained in the azurophil granules found in the cytoplasm of neutrophils (also known as c-ANCA, cytoplasmic—antineutrophil cytoplasmic antibodies). These antibodies and antigenic targets are distinct from the perinuclear ANCA associated with UC. Gastrointestinal involvement has been reported rarely.[145–150] In six clinical series describing 326 patients with Wegener's disease, none of the patients had documented symptomatic or histologic involvement of the gastrointestinal tract.[151] In contrast, in autopsy series of 39 patients, 33% showed evidence of vasculitic involvement by histology in the small and large bowel.[152] Furthermore, there have been case reports of Wegener's disease in association with esophageal ulceration, granulomatous gastritis due to Wegener's,[153] small bowel perforation, intestinal infarction, colitis and overt gastrointestinal bleeding. Although the granulomatous histologic pattern may make it difficult to distinguish this entity from Crohn's disease, most patients with Wegener's disease will have circulating c-ANCA and evidence of renal, upper airway or pulmonary involvement. *Microscopic polyangiitis* may have a similar gastrointestinal presentation, including abdominal pain, diarrhea and gastrointestinal bleeding. Up to 80% of these patients, however, will have evidence of circulating p-ANCA, with myeloperoxidase as the primary neutrophil antigen.

*Henoch–Schönlein purpura* is a small vessel systemic vasculitis that typically presents in children with gross hematuria, palpable purpura and arthritis, although individuals of any age may develop it.[154,155] In nearly 90% of cases an upper respiratory tract infection precedes the development of vasculitis. Gastrointestinal involvement is seen in nearly 50% of patients, including gastrointestinal bleeding, abdominal pain and diarrhea. Acute abdominal pain, often described as a crampy, diffuse pain associated with nausea, vomiting and bloody diarrhea after a meal, may be the most common presenting symptom in Henoch–Schönlein purpura, occurring in 65% of cases. Rarely, patients may go on to develop intussusception (usually ileocolic), perforation, bowel necrosis or ileal stricture.[156,157] Diagnosis is based on the clinical spectrum and the detection of IgA-containing immune complex depositions on renal or cutaneous biopsies.

Although *systemic lupus erythematosus* (SLE) may involve the gastrointestinal tract in as many as half of patients, only approximately 2% will have symptoms. Patients may manifest with nausea, vomiting, serositis, and overt or occult gastrointestinal bleeding.[158–160] Mesenteric vasculitis may be most worrisome, as it may lead to transmural necrosis. Most such patients will have had intermittent symptoms for up to 4 weeks prior to diagnosis, including abdominal pain, anorexia and gastrointestinal bleeding. *Rheumatoid arthritis* (RA) is rarely associated with gastrointestinal involvement.[161] However, some investigators have described asymptomatic rectal vasculitis in 25% of patients with RA.[162] Up to 90% of patients with *systemic sclerosis* (scleroderma) have gastrointestinal involvement.[163,164] Deposition of submucosal collagen, expansion of fibroblast populations and vasculopathy may lead to abnormal gastrointestinal motility, resulting in severe dysphagia, reflux esophagitis, malabsorption, diarrhea due to bacterial overgrowth, or constipation. *Buerger's disease* (thrombangitis obliterans),[165] *Takayasu's arteritis*[165] and *dermatomyositis*[166,167] have rarely been reported in association with gastrointestinal ischemia and perforation. *Essential cryoglobulinemia* may present with gastrointestinal bleeding and chronic diarrhea.[168]

## GASTROINTESTINAL INFECTIONS

Because of the variable manifestations and time courses with which gastrointestinal infections may present, they represent one of the most common and important disease groups in the differential diagnosis of IBD. Infection must be considered and evaluated for in each patient presenting with signs and symptoms suggesting IBD, despite the fact that the frequency of isolating an organism from a stool culture is far less than 40%.[169] Bacterial, viral, fungal, protozoal and helminthic infections have all been reported to masquerade as IBD. One must assess a patient carefully for susceptibility to these potential pathogens based upon travel history, recent antibiotic exposures, occupational exposures and sick contacts, comorbid medical conditions and immunocompetence.

## BACTERIAL PATHOGENS

There are many bacterial infections that may simulate IBD, chief among them being the common enteric pathogens, including *Salmonella enteritidis*, *Shigella sonnei*, *Camplyobacter jejuni*, *Escherichia coli* and *Yersinia enterocolitica*. Antibiotic-associated colitis, most commonly due to *Clostridium difficile*, must also be considered, particularly among patients who have had recent antibiotic exposure, or who have been recently hospitalized or in a healthcare facility.

In the US salmonellosis is one of the most common foodborne diseases.[170] Ingestion of contaminated poultry, eggs or milk products is the most common mode of transmission. Young age and immunodeficiency states appear to be risk factors for acquiring infection. Despite a colonic predilection of infection, ileocolitis and isolated ileitis have been described.[171–73] Most cases are self-limited, lasting 3–70 days; however, <1% will maintain a chronic, asymptomatic carriage state.

*Shigella* infection is the next most common foodborne illness in the US. The agent may also be spread by person-to-person contact. *Shigella* is the cause of classic dysentery.[174] Over half of patients will have fever, abdominal pain, and frequent (10–20 movements/day) bloody diarrhea as major manifestations. Although *Shigella* infections are largely self-limited, some patients develop severe proctocolitis resembling ulcerative colitis, bowel obstruction, colonic perforation and toxic megacolon.

*Yersinia enterocolitica*, another foodborne pathogen, is particularly important to consider because of its propensity to cause a protracted symptom course with fever (often high), right lower quadrant abdominal pain and, at times, extraintestinal manifestations, including a reactive arthropathy, oral ulcers, Reiter's syndrome (particularly in patients with HLA-B27) and erythema nodosum.[175] This organism tends to invade Peyer's patches and mesenteric lymph nodes, often resulting in clinical signs, symptoms and imaging consistent with appendicitis or Crohn's ileitis.[176–179] Extensive ileocolic ulceration is often found at endoscopy in infected patients.

*Campylobacter jejuni* may account for the most cases of acute bacterial enterocolitis in the US. Up to a third of patients may present with a flu-like syndrome marked by malaise, fevers, and generalized body aches lasting several days before the gastrointestinal symptoms predominate.[180] Diarrhea, often bloody and frequent, lasts up to 10 days. As this organism may involve primarily the distal small bowel and ileum, it may mimic acute appendicitis and Crohn's ileitis. Toxic megacolon and acute colitis may also occur, and may resemble ulcerative colitis. A number of different strains of *Escherichia coli* may produce acute diarrheal syndromes. Most notable as IBD imposters are the so-called enterohemorrhagic *E. coli* (EHEC) and the enteroinvasive *E. coli* (EIEC).[181] EHEC may produce a rapidly progressive clinical course marked by bloody diarrhea, renal failure and microangiopathic anemia.[182]

Infection with *Clostridium difficile* may produce a wide spectrum of clinical manifestations, ranging from an asymptomatic carriage state to symptomatic colitis, and rarely to toxic megacolon.[183] A history of recent (days to 8 weeks) antibiotic exposure is usual. Nearly all antibiotics have been implicated. Recent hospitalization or healthcare facility contact are expected exposures, although community-acquired infection has also been reported. Most patients suffer from watery diarrhea. Progression to colitis, pseudomembranous colitis or fulminant colitis with toxic megacolon (2–3% of patients) is clearly associated with significant morbidity and mortality.[184] Infection with *Clostridium difficile* may be a cause of relapse in patients with an established diagnosis of IBD.[185] One clue to the diagnosis of *Clostridium difficile* infection is the often profound leukocytosis associated with this infection. CT scans may show diffuse colonic thickening and thumbprinting (Fig. 25.3A). Endoscopic findings range from patchy colitis to large exudative plaques consistent with pseudomembranes (Fig. 25.3B). Rapid and early identification of the cytotoxin in the stool remains the best diagnostic measure.

A number of less common bacterial pathogens must also be considered in the evaluation. Sexually transmitted organisms, including *Chlamydia trachomatis* and *Neisseria gonorrhoeae*, may result in a severe proctitis in individuals exposed to anal intercourse.[186] *Plesiomonas shigelloides* and *Aeromonas hydrophilia* are Gram-negative organisms commonly found in fresh water.[187,188] A spectrum of infection has been demonstrated for both organisms, ranging from asymptomatic carriage to dysentery and, rarely, protracted diarrheal syndromes resembling IBD.[189–192] The microbiology laboratory should be directed to investigate for these agents in suspect cases, particular in recent travelers or those who may have ingested raw seafood.

*Actinomyces israelii* is a Gram-positive commensal organism in the gastrointestinal tract.[193,194] It may rarely produce actinomycosis, a chronic granulomatous disease most often occurring in middle-aged men. Trauma, recent abdominal surgery and the use of intrauterine contraceptive devices are risk factors. Although cervicofacial involvement is most common, intraabdominal disease predominates in 20% of patients, with the ileocecal area and appendiceal regions being targeted. A chronic presentation of weight loss, anorexia, abdominal pain and diarrhea may be mistaken for gastrointestinal tuberculosis, neoplasia or Crohn's disease.[195,196] Imaging often reveals a destructive ileocecal mass. Culture and biopsy with identification of so-called 'sulfur granules' may be diagnostic, although exploratory laparotomy for presumed neoplasia is the most common means of diagnosis.

Spirochetes may rarely affect the GI tract in a manner to arouse suspicion for IBD. *Treponema pallidum*, the agent of syphilis, has been reported in association with a granulomatous gastropathy in the tertiary form of the illness.[197–199] *Treponema pallidum* may also cause proctitis. Often, patients may have concurrent perianal condyloma latum, and painful inguinal lymphadenopathy.[200] Biopsy may reveal the organism on dark-field microscopy. A positive serum rapid plasma reagin (RPR) is also found.

Recognition of enterocolitis due to *Mycobacterium tuberculosis* has increased since the emergence of HIV/AIDS, the broader use of immunosuppressants, and the influx of immigrants from highly endemic areas of Africa and Southeast Asia.[201] The ileocecal region has a predilection for involvement because of

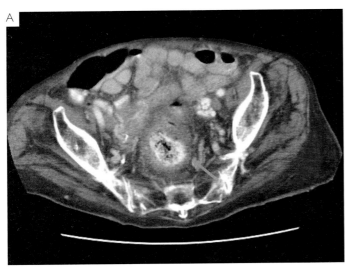
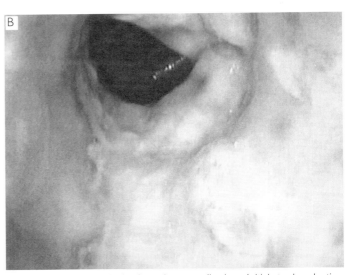

**Fig. 25.3** (A) CT scan of the abdomen in an 84-year-old woman who presented with lower abdominal pain and watery diarrhea. Initial stool evaluation for microbial pathogens and *Clostridium difficile* toxin was negative. The image demonstrates focal, concentric thickening of the rectosigmoid colon (arrow). (B) Colonoscopy revealed diffuse pseudomembrane formation from the rectum to mid-sigmoid colon. Colon biopsies demonstrated pseudomembranes with an acute polymorphonuclear infiltrate in the submucosa. Repeat stool analysis for *Clostridium difficile* toxin was positive.

the abundance of lymphoid tissue. Patients may have protracted symptoms marked by weight loss, anorexia, fevers, night sweats, abdominal pain and diarrhea.[202] Ascites may be seen, setting it apart from IBD.

The true diagnosis will often be evident from an abnormal chest X-ray or positive PPD skin test. Abdominal CT may reveal concentric ileocecal thickening, regional lymphadenopathy, ascites, and often evidence of pulmonary involvement. Stricture and fistula may also develop, and may further confound the diagnosis with Crohn's disease. One study evaluating 200 patients with known ileocecal tuberculosis in India concluded that an isolated, short-segment terminal ileal stricture was specific for mycobacterial disease.[203] Endoscopic evaluation demonstrates ileocecal deformities, often with extensive ulceration. A gaping ileocecal valve is an often-cited finding. Biopsy should reveal large caseating granulomas, with evidence of organisms on Ziehl–Nielsen staining. Genetic probes have also been used to confirm the diagnosis. In addition to causing gastrointestinal symptoms that mimic IBD, systemic infection with *Mycobacterium tuberculosis* may complicate immunosuppressive therapy in patients with IBD. A high degree of suspicion and a careful evaluation for latent tuberculous infection should be sought in patients with IBD beginning immunosuppressive therapy, as glucocorticoid administration and anti-TNF therapy may result in devastating outcomes.[204] Multidrug regimens are used initially until sensitivities are noted.

Non-tuberculous mycobacteria (particularly *Mycobacterium avium intracellulare*) have rarely been reported to cause an ileocolitis in immunocompromised hosts. Most of these patients will have systemic manifestations of disseminated infection, including hepatosplenomegaly, cytopenias due to bone marrow involvement, and fevers from bacteremia.

*Whipple's disease* is very rare, with an average of 30 cases being reported annually.[205,206] Most patients are white males of European ancestry, with a mean age at diagnosis of 49. Most patients have either been farmers or have had occupational exposure to soil or animals. Despite the identification of *Tropheryma whippellii* in 1992, the pathogenetic mechanisms remain poorly defined. Most investigators favor an important role for a subtle

host immune deficiency, which permits massive accumulation of *Tropheryma whippellii* throughout the body. The manifestations of Whipple's disease are protean and require a high degree of clinical suspicion to be diagnosed. Although almost every organ system has been implicated as a target for *Tropheryma whippellii*, migratory polyarthralgias, abdominal pain, diarrhea, lymphadenopathy, fevers, weight loss and nutritional deficiencies dominate the clinical presentation. Central nervous system (dementia) and cardiac (pericarditis) manifestations are less common. The wide spectrum of symptoms and signs unfortunately results in a diagnostic delay of 6 years on average and raises a broad differential diagnosis, with IBD often invoked.

The diagnosis of Whipple's disease requires demonstration of *Tropheryma whippellii* in tissue. Currently, upper gastrointestinal endoscopy with small bowel biopsy is the gold standard for diagnosis. Demonstration of abundant PAS-positive organisms in the submucosa in the setting of villous atrophy is diagnostic. Granulomas are a reported, but uncommon, histologic observation. More recently, PCR techniques have been used to make the diagnosis, with a very high sensitivity and specificity. Granulomas or chronic archictectural changes in the crypts are not seen.

## VIRAL PATHOGENS

Cytomegalovirus (CMV) and herpes simplex (HSV) may be associated with severe infections in immunocompromised hosts and may simulate IBD. Furthermore, CMV may also complicate IBD at a higher frequency, probably because of the common presence of drug-induced immunosuppression.

Both viruses may result in a diffuse colitis, proctitis, perforation, obstruction and gastrointestinal bleeding.[207–212] Fever, bloody diarrhea, weight loss and abdominal pain are common. About half of patients with HSV-2 proctitis will also experience neurologic symptoms, including sacral parasthesias and difficulties with micturition. One may also see the common vesicular eruption associated with HSV, both cutaneous and mucosal.

Proximal gastrointestinal symptoms, including odynophagia, dysphagia, nausea and epigastric pain, may be seen and may

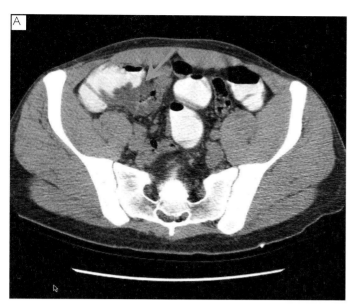
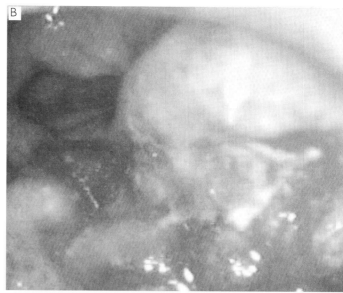

**Fig. 25.4** (A) CT scan of the abdomen in a 26-year-old man who presented with right lower quadrant abdominal pain and bloody diarrhea. Four weeks prior to presentation he had been traveling in South America. Images demonstrate a mass in the ileocecal region (arrow). (Courtesy of Dr Robert Schapiro.) (B) Colonoscopy demonstrated hemorrhagic ulceration in the terminal ileum (image). Ileal biopsies demonstrated trophozoites consistent with *Entamoeba histolytica* infection. (Courtesy of Dr Robert Schapiro.)

dominate the presentation. Both viruses may involve the entire gastrointestinal tract, often making panendoscopy necessary to establish the diagnosis. At endoscopy, one typically finds discrete ulcers with edematous and friable mucosa. Histology is critical in identifying viral inclusions in the setting of inflammation. Virus-specific immunostains are often used to confirm the diagnosis. One may also attempt culture of the virus. In addition to causing gastrointestinal symptoms that mimic IBD, systemic infection with HSV or CMV may complicate immunosuppressive therapy of patients with IBD.[213] Specific antiviral therapy and reconstitution of the immune system are the mainstays of therapy.

## FUNGAL PATHOGENS

Fungal disease of the gastrointestinal tract is unusual. *Histoplasma capsulatum* is the most common endemic mycosis in the US, with particular foci in the Ohio River valley. Gastrointestinal involvement is especially common in the immunocompromised host and may present with ulcerative disease or focal masses, predominantly of the ileum and colon.[214–216] In up to 33% of patients with gastrointestinal involvement one may find isolated terminal ileum involvement.[217] Symptoms include anorexia, weight loss, abdominal pain and diarrhea. Perforation and frank bleeding are rare. Proximal involvement with esophageal, gastric and jejunal ulceration has also been reported. Biopsy reveals parasitized submucosal macrophages, and at times granulomas. Detection of histoplasma urinary antigen may aid in the diagnosis. In addition to causing gastrointestinal symptoms that mimic IBD, systemic infection with *Histoplasma capsulatum* may complicate immunosuppressive therapy of patients with IBD. An uncommon fungus, *Basidiobola ranarum*, has also rarely been reported to mimic IBD.[218,219]

## PROTOZOAL PATHOGENS

Of the human protozoal infections, *Entamoeba histolytica* is most notorious for imitating IBD.[220,221] The highest rates of infection are in Central and South America, Africa and India. Patients may be asymptomatic, or may report fevers, weight loss and bloody diarrhea. Colitis with aphthoid ulcerations, focal masses ('ameboma'), perforation and toxic megacolon have all been described (Fig. 25.4). There are also rare reports of perianal amebiasis and colonic involvement complicated by fistula. Isolated ileal involvement is unusual. Extraintestinal manifestations are generally not seen. Diagnosis can be made by biopsy, stool evaluation, or by serology (indirect fluorescent antibody). Although the cecum is the most common site of involvement, rectal ulceration is common enough to permit diagnosis by sigmoidoscopy in most cases.

Less common organisms that may cause protracted diarrheal syndromes include *Isospora belli*, *Cyclospora*, *Cryptosporidium parvum*, *Giardia lamblia* and *Endolimax nana*.[222–224] Although there is a greater predilection for these organisms to infect immunocompromised hosts, they are often seen in otherwise healthy individuals as they are generally waterborne. In suspected cases stool analysis should be done for these specific organisms.

## HELMINTHS

Several helminths are associated with acute and chronic diarrheal syndromes that may resemble IBD. Peripheral eosinophilia (at times up to 50%) is common to each of these, and may help distinguish these syndromes from IBD. Stool analysis for ova, and a detailed travel and dietary history are important in evaluating for these pathogens.

Intestinal capillariasis, caused by *Capillaria philippinensis*, is seen largely in the Philippines and Thailand. Clinically, it is associated with fever, abdominal pain, diarrhea, and at times malabsorption and weight loss.[225] Trichostrongyliasis (*Trichostrongylus* species) occurs with the ingestion of unwashed vegetables contaminated with animal manure. Anemia, abdominal pain, diarrhea and malabsorption may be seen.[226] Anisakiasis is caused by *Anisakis simplex* or *Anisakis physeteris*. It has been most widely seen in Japan, perhaps owing to the frequent ingestion of raw fish. Manifestations include abdominal pain and diarrhea. Focal ileocecal involvement has been described, and because of an associated tissue eosinophilia the infestation may mimic eosinophilic gastroenteritis.[227–230] Rarely, the worm may be seen emanating from an ulcer base. *Angiostrongylus costaricensis* may cause a granulomatous inflammation in the distal ileum, appendix and right colon.[231]

Finally, gastrointestinal infection with *Strongyloides stercolis*, *Schistosoma mansoni* and *Trichuris trichuria* may also simulate IBD, and in particular these helminths have been associated with intestinal granuloma formation.[232–234]

## GENETIC SYNDROMES

**Turner's syndrome** is caused by absence of an X chromosome, leading to a 45 XO karyotype in 1 in 5000 live female births. In addition to typical features of short stature, a webbed neck and bicuspid aortic valve, there is an increased risk of both UC and Crohn's disease compared to an age-matched population.[235–237]

**Glycogen storage disease type 1b** is associated with deficiency of a glucose-6-phosphatase transport protein. In addition to growth retardation, hepatomegaly and recurrent attacks of hypoglycemia, these children develop a granulomatous colitis which, interestingly, often responds to granulocyte colony-stimulating factor.[238,239]

**Hermansky–Pudlak syndrome**, an autosomal recessive disease associated with pulmonary fibrosis, bleeding diathesis due to abnormal platelet aggregation, and oculocutaneous albinism, has also been associated with a granulomatous colitis (approximately 20%).[240]

**Chronic granulomatous disease** (CGD) is associated with impaired phagocyte killing due to a diminished ability to generate oxidative radicals. In addition to recurrent bacterial infections, these patients have a propensity for visceral granuloma formation, including the gastrointestinal tract, rarely leading to obstruction.[241–243] **Chediak–Higashi syndrome** is associated with recurrent pyogenic infections, a variety of neurologic abnormalities, including nystagmus and neuropathy, and partial oculocutaneous albinism. There have also been rare case reports of patients developing ileal and right colon lesions resembling Crohn's disease, which at biopsy demonstrate a non-specific lymphocytic infiltration.[244]

Patients with **X-linked agammaglobulinemia** and **common variable immunodeficiency** also carry a higher risk of gastrointestinal disease similar to IBD.[245–247]

## MISCELLANEOUS CONDITIONS

**Irritable bowel syndrome (IBS)** is an extremely common diagnostic category, making up the majority of outpatient visits in many community-based gastrointestinal practices.[248] Given the commonly cited symptom complex of abdominal pain, diarrhea or constipation, bloating, and the lack of a specific test to identify this syndrome, IBS remains a diagnosis of exclusion. IBD should be considered in all cases. Clues favoring a diagnosis of IBS include lack of fever, weight loss, extraintestinal manifestations, nighttime symptoms, or overt or occult gastrointestinal bleeding. Laboratory studies should be normal. None the less, these patients should be followed over time to look for evolving signs of a true inflammatory process.

**Factitious diarrhea** should be considered in all patients referred for evaluation of chronic diarrhea. In some series as many as 15% of patients with chronic diarrhea will ultimately be found to be abusing laxatives.[249] Patients tend to be female, have a high socioeconomic status, and are often employed in the healthcare industry. Clues to this diagnosis include the presence of a low stool osmolarity suggesting the addition of water to augment the stool volume, and the detection of laxatives by thin-layer chromatography.

**Hidradenitis suppurativa** is a chronic and recurrent suppurative disorder in which the hair follicles become occluded, with resultant secondary inflammation of the aprocrine sweat glands, most commonly in the axillary, inguinal and perianal areas. There have been several case reports describing a higher prevalence of Crohn's disease among patients with hidradenitis suppurativa. Some patients with hidradenitis suppurativa have evidence of granuloma on skin biopsy, and later develop evidence of Crohn's disease. Occasionally, the draining sinuses of hidradenitis suppurativa may be confused for perianal fistulae arising in Crohn's disease.[250,251]

**Marathon running** has been associated with occult and overt gastrointestinal bleeding which, in extreme cases, manifests as an acute, self-limited colitis.[252,253] Ischemia, because of the diversion of splanchnic blood flow, is the postulated mechanism.[254]

**Pneumatosis cystoides intestinalis** is an unusual condition in which there are small and large gas-filled submucosal cysts throughout the colon. These may manifest by occult gastrointestinal blood loss.[255,256] The presence of submucosal cysts, however, is pathognomonic.

**Solitary rectal ulcer syndrome** is commonly misdiagnosed. It is characterized by varied lesions located along the anterior wall of the rectum, most often within 10 cm of the anal verge.[257] Lesions may be unifocal or multiple, and may be ulcerated, erythematous or polypoid. Clinically, patients may present with rectal bleeding, straining and pelvic fullness. The histologic hallmarks of solitary rectal ulcer syndrome include a collagenous and muscular infiltration of the lamina propria and a thickened mucosal layer with crypt architectural distortion, distinguishing this entity from chronic IBD.[258]

**Cystica profunda**, a similar entity, is characterized by submucosal mucus-filled cysts, and is most commonly found in the rectum. An enterocolitic form has also been described, with skip lesions in the colon and terminal ileum.[259]

There are few reports in the literature describing the entity of **foreign-body ileitis** mimicking IBD. The first description was that of Iannuccilli in 1973, in which he reported a 17-year-old boy as having 'regional enteritis with foreign body.'[260] He had accidentally swallowed a penny that lodged in the terminal ileum and ultimately eroded through, causing peritonitis. The small bowel series revealed severe ileocolitis, indistinct from Crohn's disease. Other case reports describe toothpick, bottle cap and fruit pit ileitis.[261–263]

This diagnosis should be entertained particularly in those patients with acute onset of symptoms, and in those with a propensity for unusual ingestions (mentally ill patients). A flat film of the abdomen may clinch the diagnosis early in the evaluation and avoid a large and expensive search for other diseases.

The urachus is a fibrous cord that emanates from the anterior bladder wall cranially towards the umbilicus. Rarely, these tracts may become infected and present as an acute or chronic abdominal pain syndrome, often with fevers. A misdiagnosis of Crohn's disease has been reported in the setting of an **infected urachal cyst** based upon similar presenting features.[264]

**Lipomatosis of the ileocecal valve**, also known as lipohyperplasia, is characterized by an intense fatty infiltration of the ileocecal valve.[265–267] Unlike a lipoma, there is no evident encapsulation. Associated factors include age over 40, female gender and obesity. In as many as 50% of patients an 'ileocecal valve syndrome' may evolve, characterized by abdominal pain, nausea, vomiting, diarrhea and, rarely, overt gastrointestinal bleeding. Some of these symptoms presumably occur in the setting of intermittent intussusception with partial obstruction. Crohn's disease has been initially considered in rare patients presenting with these manifestations.[268]

**Typhlitis**, also known as 'neutropenic enterocolitis' and 'ileocecal syndrome', is a potentially life-threatening complication in the immunocompromised host. The predilection for ileocecal involvement has been suggested to be related to the relative distensibility and diminished vascular supply of the cecum.[269]

Patients may present with fever, abdominal pain, nausea, vomiting, diarrhea and, in up to 35% of cases, overt gastrointestinal bleeding. Most patients will be profoundly neutropenic (<500/mL), although a small minority may have relatively normal absolute neutrophil counts. Peritoneal signs may occur late in the presentation and are predictive of a more severe course. CT of the abdomen can help distinguish between appendicitis and typhlitis. In the latter, ileocecal thickening, often with intramural air, is seen. Stool studies must be done to exclude specific infectious etiologies.

Appendiceal **mucoceles** are rare lesions in which the appendix becomes distended with mucus.[270] Because of their location and the non-specific symptoms with which they may present (such as right lower quadrant abdominal pain, obstruction, intussusception and, rarely, bleeding), they are considered in the differential diagnosis of IBD.[271]

**Melkersson–Rosenthal syndrome** is an unusual condition characterized by recurrent orofacial swelling (usually lips, known as Miescher's cheilitis granulomatosa), intermittent facial nerve palsy and a fissured tongue (lingua plicata).[272] Non-caseating granulomas, as in Crohn's disease and sarcoidosis, are typical. There have now been several reports in which extrafacial manifestations of Melkersson–Rosenthal syndrome have been described, involving the chest, dorsum of the hands and feet, buttocks, vulva and perianal soft tissue. Although the distinction between Melkersson–Rosenthal syndrome and Crohn's disease may not always be evident, the lack of luminal involvement should raise suspicion of the former. The **systemic amyloid** syndromes include AL amyloidosis (related to an underlying plasma cell dyscrasia), AA amyloidosis (related to an underlying chronic inflammatory disease), familial amyloidosis, dialysis-related amyloidosis and senile amyloidosis. Autopsy series have demonstrated gastrointestinal involvement in 70–100% of patients with systemic amyloidosis, although only approximately 50% had referable symptoms during life.[273] The entire gastrointestinal tract may be involved, and non-specific symptoms may include nausea, vomiting, anorexia, weight loss, diarrhea or constipation. There is a recognized association of IBD with systemic amyloidosis (usually AA variant), affecting 0.9% of patients with Crohn's disease and 0.07% with ulcerative colitis. In some autopsy series, however, as many as 29.4% of patients with Crohn's disease were noted to have amyloid deposits, mostly with renal involvement.[274]

Small intestine amyloid deposits may result in bleeding or pain from ischemia, infarction or perforation, malabsorption from dysmotility and bacterial overgrowth, and pseudo-obstruction. There have been rare reports of ischemic colonic ulceration and frank colitis. Endoscopic observations are non-specific. Biopsies are diagnostic if they demonstrate characteristic amyloid deposits on Congo red staining under polarized light microscopy. Fat pad biopsies may also provide evidence of amyloid deposition if necessary.

**Appendicitis** should be a part of the differential diagnosis for all patients with abdominal pain, whether acute or chronic. Each year in the United States there are 250 000 cases diagnosed, with the majority being in their teens.[275]

In addition to cecal diverticulitis, Meckel's diverticulitis, infectious ileitis and gynecologic disease, Crohn's ileitis should be considered in the differential diagnosis, particularly in those cases where there is radiologic evidence of more extensive bowel disease, chronic diarrhea, constitutional symptoms or family history. In one series, patients with Crohn's disease were more often afebrile and had symptoms of chronic diarrhea.[276] Furthermore, laboratory testing more often revealed normal leukocyte counts, anemia and hypoalbuminemia, suggestive of chronic inflammation. The finding of 'creeping fat' at laparotomy, in which thickened mesenteric fat wraps around ileal loops, is highly suggestive of Crohn's disease.

Subacute cases of appendicitis and complicated cases of appendicitis in which there may be periappendiceal abscesses may be particularly difficult to distinguish from Crohn's disease. Chronic appendicitis, in which there is a recurring symptom complex of right lower quadrant pain and fever in the setting of intermittent appendiceal obstruction, is another challenging diagnostic dilemma.[277] Distinction from Crohn's disease is often not possible without clear extra-appendiceal disease or other characteristic findings by history or examination.[278] Most patients are correctly diagnosed at the time of laparotomy.

For unclear reasons, acute appendicitis and Crohn's disease rarely coexist. In fact, in Crohn's initial description, he stated '...the appendix is always free from guilt and changes'.[279] Granulomatous inflammation of the appendix, however, is seen in up to 50% of patients with colonic Crohn's disease.[280–282] Although the preoperative diagnosis of Crohn's disease is not often feasible in patients presenting with signs and symptoms of appendicitis, failure to do so may have important consequences, including fistula formation in 33%.

**Meckel's diverticulum**, a true congenital diverticulum, is found in the ileum of 3% of the normal population. Case reports describe peridiverticular ileal ulceration, presumably due to gastric acid-induced injury. In addition, there are reports of ileal stricture and extensive terminal ileal and ileocecal valve involvement in patients with Meckel's diverticulum bearing ectopic gastric mucosa, making for a difficult distinction from Crohn's disease.[283] Granulomas were not observed in these cases.

**Linear IgA dermatosis** and **Castleman's syndrome** also carry a higher risk of gastrointestinal disease similar to IBD.[284,285]

# DISTINGUISHING CROHN'S DISEASE AND ULCERATIVE COLITIS

In each suspected case of IBD, distinguishing Crohn's disease from ulcerative colitis remains important and at times difficult. This distinction has a significant impact on the choice of medical and surgical therapies, and on the prognosis. In most cases the correct diagnosis can be made after careful evaluation of clinical, endoscopic, radiologic and histologic findings (Table 25.4 A and B).

From an epidemiologic perspective UC and CD have many similarities. In both conditions men and women are nearly equally affected. In both conditions there is usually a predominance of presentation in the second and third decades of life, with a second peak in the 60s and 70s reported by some. In general, both follow a chronic relapsing and remitting course. Familial occurrences are more frequent in Crohn's disease (20–40%) than in ulcerative colitis (10–15%).[286] Patients with UC are more likely to be former or non-smokers, as opposed to the higher prevalence of active smokers in CD.

Clinical presentations, although overlapping in many instances, are helpful in guiding the clinician towards a diagnosis. In UC, the most typical presentations include recurrent episodes of bloody diarrhea. Tenesmus is a common feature of UC of varying anatomic extents, reflecting the nearly universal involvement of the rectum in the inflammatory process. Patients with Crohn's disease tend to have more varied presentations. Although bloody diarrhea may be seen, non-bloody diarrhea is more commonly observed. Abdominal pain, fevers, weight loss, nausea, vomiting and anorexia may be evident. Up to 25% of patients with either condition will have one or more extraintestinal manifestations, including arthritic, dermatologic, hepatobiliary and ocular conditions.[287] Although such manifestations have low specificity, primary sclerosing cholangitis and pyoderma gangrenosum are more commonly found in patients with UC, whereas erythema nodosum, clubbing and aphthous stomatitis are more prevalent among those with CD. The physical examination should focus on findings associated with these extraintestinal manifestations. In addition, the presence of fistula, perianal disease and a focal abdominal mass (particularly in the right lower quadrant) strongly implicates Crohn's disease.

Laboratory studies do not reliably distinguish between UC and CD. Anemia and elevated markers of inflammation (C-reactive protein (C-RP) and erythrocyte sedimentation rate (ESR)) are common in both diseases. However, elevated ESR and C-RP are more often seen in CD, perhaps reflecting the transmural nature of the inflammation. Such findings may also raise the possibility of one or more pyogenic complications of CD. Findings of hypocalcemia and cobalamin (vitamin $B_{12}$) deficiency should prompt consideration of Crohn's disease, reflecting small intestinal malabsorption. More recently, serologic markers have been added to the diagnostic armamentarium as non-invasive ways of distinguishing CD and UC. Antibodies directed against *Saccharamyces cerevisiae* (ASCA)

**Table 25.4A Differentiating ulcerative colitis from Crohn's disease: clinical and serologic features**

|  | Ulcerative colitis | Crohn's disease |
|---|---|---|
| Clinical features |  |  |
| Abdominal pain | Occasionally | Frequently |
| Bloody diarrhea | Frequently | Occasionally |
| Perianal disease | Rarely | Frequently |
| Constitutional symptoms (fevers, weight loss, night sweats) | Occasionally | Freqeuntly |
| Palpable abdominal mass | Rarely | Common |
| Perianal fistulae | Rarely | Frequently |
| Rectovaginal fistulae | Occasionally | Commonly |
| Intra-abdominal abscess | Rarely | Commonly |
| Bowel obstruction | Rarely | Frequently |
| Antibiotic response | Rarely | Frequently |
| Disease distribution | Continuous colonic involvement from rectum | Segmental involvement from mouth to anus |
| Effect of smoking | Often improved | Often worsened |
| Postoperative recurrence | Pouchitis in ileal puch | Frequently |
| Serologic features |  |  |
| ASCA | 15% | 65% |
| pANCA | 70% | 20% |

ASCA, anti-Saccharomyces cerevisiae antibodies; pANCA, perinuclear antineutrophil antibodies.

**Table 25.4B Differentiating ulcerative colitis and Crohn's disease: radiologic, endoscopic, and histologic features**

|  | Ulcerative colitis | Crohn's disease |
|---|---|---|
| Radiologic features |  |  |
| Proximal small bowel thickening | Not seen | Commonly |
| Terminal ileal thickening | Rarely | Frequently |
| Rectal sparing | Rarely | Frequently |
| Fistulae | Rarely | Commonly |
| Strictures | Rarely | Commonly |
| Pancolitis | Commonly | Occasionally |
| Intra-abdominal abscesses | Rarely | Commonly |
| Mesenteric inflammation | Occasionally | Frequently |
| Endoscopic features |  |  |
| Mucosal involvement | Continuous | Segmental |
| Mucosal bridging | Commonly | Rarely |
| Cobblestoning | Rarely | Frequently |
| Rectal involvement | Frequently | Rarely |
| Strictures | Rarely | Commonly |
| Fistulae | Rarely | Commonly |
| Pseudopolyps | Commonly | Commonly |
| Serpiginous or linear ulcers | Rarerly | Frequently |
| Terminal ileal involvement | Rarely (backwash ileitis) | Frequently |
| Histologic features |  |  |
| Crypt abscesses | Frequently | Occasionally |
| Mucin depletion | Commonly | Commonly |
| Non-caseating granulomas | Rarely (pouchitis) | Commonly (30% biopsy specimens, 50% surgical specimens) |

and perinuclear antineutrophil cytoplasmic antibodies (p-ANCA) have been investigated. In general, ASCA are more commonly found in patients with Crohn's disease, whereas p-ANCA are more common in patients with UC. The clinical role of these antibodies is still under investigation (see Chapter 29).

Radiography remains an essential part of the evaluation. Approximately two-thirds of patients with Crohn's disease will have small bowel or ileocolonic disease. Thus, radiologic assessment of the small intestine is routine in evaluating and staging disease. Identification of fistulae on barium studies and intra-abdominal abscesses on CT is more suggestive of Crohn's disease. Despite being far more common in Crohn's disease, strictures may be found in either disease and should always prompt evaluation for underlying malignancy.

Endoscopy is a key component of the evaluation of suspected IBD. Rectal involvement is nearly uniform in UC. Typically, in UC there is evidence of mucosal friability, granularity and superficial ulceration. So-called backwash ileitis may be seen in pancolitis. In contrast, ileocecal involvement is most characteristic of CD. The pattern seen in CD is often a discontinuous or patchy distribution, and late in the disease deep serpiginous ulcers and cobblestoning may be seen. Although noted in less than half of cases, the presence of granulomas on biopsy is relatively specific for Crohn's disease, and should not be seen in UC. Surgical specimens may corroborate a diagnosis of Crohn's disease by demonstrating the transmural, yet focal, nature of Crohn's disease.

In approximately 10% of cases of colitis it is not possible to distinguish between Crohn's and UC.[288] Such patients are deemed to have indeterminate colitis. Most of these patients will ultimately become more clinically congruent with Crohn's disease or ulcerative colitis. However, this diagnosis carries a higher rate of pouch failure and intra-abdominal infection following ileal pouch–anal anastamosis.[289] Genetic analysis may eventually assist in diagnosis and prognosis, and may indeed finally establish whether patients with indeterminate colitis have CD, UC, or an altogether distinct variety of IBD.

## CONCLUSIONS

The protean manifestations of Crohn's disease and ulcerative colitis render them challenging diagnostic entities. Furthermore, many of the same features that are commonly seen with IBD may also be manifestations of a wide spectrum of alternative diagnoses. Among these are common entities with atypical presentations, and more rare syndromes that may have a primarily gastrointestinal presentation.

In most cases a correct diagnosis can be made after consideration of the history and physical examination, laboratory data, stool examination, abdominal imaging and endoscopic visualization with biopsy. Clinicopathologic correlation is an essential component of the diagnostic evaluation, and will enable appropriate therapeutic interventions to be made.

## REFERENCES

1. Watts DA, Lessells AM, Penman ID, Ghosh S. Endoscopic and histologic features of sodium phosphate bowel preparation-induced colonic ulceration: case report and review. Gastrointest Endosc 2002;55:584–587.

2. Preiksaitis HG, Zwas FR. Colonic mucosal abnormalities associated with oral sodium phosphate solution. Hum Pathol 1998;29:972–978.

3. Cirillo NW, el-Serag HB, Eisen RN, Driman DK. Colorectal inflammation and increased cell proliferation associated with oral sodium phosphate bowel preparation solution. Gastrointest Endosc 1996;43:463–466.

4. Aabakken L, Osnes M. Non-steroidal anti-inflammatory drug-induced disease in the distal ileum and large bowel. Scand J Gastroenterol 1989;163:48–55.

5. Kirsch M. Drug-induced ileal disease: a new entity in the differential diagnosis of Crohn's disease. South Med J 1994;87:546–548.

6. Fortson WC, Tedesco FJ. Drug-induced colitis: a review. Am J Gastroenterol 1984;79:878–883.

7. Hebuterne X, Dreyfus G, Fratini G, Rampal P. Nonsteroidal antiinflammatory drug-induced colitis and misoprostol. Dig Dis Sci 1996;41:520–521.

8. Robinson MH, Wheatley T, Leach IH. Nonsteroidal antiinflammatory drug-induced colonic stricture. An unusual cause of large bowel obstruction and perforation. Dig Dis Sci 1995;40:315–319.

9. Miner PB Jr. Factors influencing the relapse of patients with inflammatory bowel disease. Am J Gastroenterol 1997;92:1S–4S.

10. Bjarnason I, Zanelli G, Smith T et al. Nonsteroidal antiinflammatory drug-induced intestinal inflammation in humans. Gastroenterology 1987;93:480–489.

11. Langer HE, Hartmann G, Heinemann G, Richter K. Gold colitis induced by auranofin treatment of rheumatoid arthritis: case report and review of the literature. Ann Rheum Dis 1987;46:787–792.

12. White RF, Major GA. Gold colitis. Med J Aust 1983;1:174–175.

13. Sckolnick BR, Katz LA, Kozower M. Life-threatening enterocolitis after gold salt therapy. J Clin Gastroenterol 1979;1:145–148.

14. Hillemand P, Bensaude A, Delavierre P, Debbasch L. Ulcerous stenosis of the small intestine after absorption of potassium. Bull Mem Soc Med Hop Paris 1968;119:241–245.

15. Teniere P, Le Douarec P, Koytcha F, Testart J. Ulcerous stenosis of the small intestine caused by absorption of potassium chloride tablets. J Chir (Paris) 1973;106:271–280.

16. Urso FP, Urso MJ, Lee CH. The cathartic colon: pathological findings and radiological/pathological correlation. Radiology 1975;116:557–559.

17. Kilpatrick ZM, Silverman JF, Betancourt E, Farman J, Lawson JP. Vascular occlusion of the colon and oral contraceptives. Possible relation. N Engl J Med 1968;278:438–440.

18. Deana AD, Calderan A, Pavanetto M et al. Reversible ischemic colitis in young women. Association with oral contraceptive use. Int J Peptide Protein Res 1995;46:535–546.

19. Slavin RE, Dias MA, Saral R. Cytosine arabinoside induced gastrointestinal toxic alterations in sequential chemotherapeutic protocols: a clinical–pathologic study of 33 patients. Cancer 1978;42:1747–1759.

20. Zilling TL, Ahren B. Ischaemic pancolitis: a serious complication of chemotherapy in a previously irradiated patient. Case report. Acta Chir Scand 1989;155:77–78.

21. Mehrotra T. Haemorrhagic colitis after cyclophosphamide. Lancet 1966;2:345.

22. Atherton LD, Leib ES, Kaye MD. Toxic megacolon associated with methotrexate therapy. Gastroenterology 1984;86:1583–1588.

23. Bennet JE. Flucytosine. Ann Intern Med 1977;86:319–321.

24. Weinberg EJ, Boudreau RJ, Kuni CC, Engeler CE, Stillman AE. Ischemic bowel disease attributable to ergot. Clin Nucl Med 1994;19:924–925.

25. de Peyer R, Muller AF, Lambert M. Reversible ischemic colitis after intravenous vasopressin therapy. JAMA 1982;247:666–667.

26. Graham CF, Gallagher K, Jones JK. Acute colitis with methyldopa. N Engl J Med 1981;304:1044–1045.

27. Burry VF, Fellows RA, Beatty EC, Leonidas JC. Possible adverse effect of methylglucamine diatrizoate compounds on the bowel of newborn infants with meconium ileus. Radiology 1976;121:693–696.

28. Jones B, Seltzer SE. Cecal perforation associated with Gastrografin enema. Am J Roentgenol 1978;130:997–998.

29. Creteur V, Douglas D, Galante M, Margulis AR. Inflammatory colonic changes produced by contrast material. Radiology 1983;147:77–78.

30. Pike BF, Phillippi PJ, Lawson EH Jr. Soap colitis. N Engl J Med 1971;285:217–218.

31. Meyer CT, Brand M, DeLuca VA, Spiro HM. Hydrogen peroxide colitis: a report of three patients. J Clin Gastroenterol 1981;3:31–35.

32. Herrerias JM, Muniain MA, Sanchez S, Garrido M. Alcohol-induced colitis. Endoscopy 1983;15:121–122.

33. Cheng ES, Stringer KM, Pegg SP. Colonic necrosis and perforation following oral sodium polystyrene sulfonate (Resonium A/Kayexalate) in a burn patient. Burns 2002;28:189–90.

34. Rogers FB, Li SC. Acute colonic necrosis associated with sodium polystyrene sulfonate (Kayexalate) enemas in a critically ill patient: case report and review of the literature. J Trauma. 2001;51:395–7.

35. Dardik A, Moesinger RC, Efron G, et al. Acute abdomen with colonic necrosis induced by Kayexalate-sorbitol. South Med J. 2000;93:511–13.

36. Hickling P, Fuller J. Penicillamine causing acute colitis. Br Med J 1979;2:367.

37. Houghton AD, Nadel S, Stringer MD. Penicillamine-associated total colitis. Hepatogastroenterology 1989;36:198.

38. Ablin DS, Ziegler M. Ulcerative type of colitis associated with the use of high strength pancreatic enzyme supplements in cystic fibrosis. Pediatr Radiol 1995;25:113–115.

39. Ott DJ, Gelfand DW, Jackson FR. Thermal injury of the colon due to colostomy irrigation. Gastrointest Radiol 1981;6:231–233.
40. Godwin JD II. Carcinoid tumors. An analysis of 2,837 cases. Cancer 1975;36:560–569.
41. Mayer RJ, Kulke MH. Carcinoid tumors. N Engl J Med 1999;340:858–868.
42. Mir-Madjlessi SH, Winkelman EI, Davis GA. Carcinoid tumors of the terminal ileum simulating Crohn's disease. Cleveland Clin J Med 1988;55:257–262.
43. Verma VK. Multiple carcinoid tumour mimicking Crohn's disease: a case report. J Ir Med Assoc 1972;65:412–413.
44. Greenstein AJ, Balasubramanian S, Harpaz N, Rizwan M, Sachar DB. Carcinoid tumor and inflammatory bowel disease: a study of eleven cases and review of the literature. Am J Gastroenterol 1997;92:682–685.
45. Hsu EY, Feldman JM, Lichtenstein GR. Ileal carcinoid tumors simulating Crohn's disease: incidence among 176 consecutive cases of ileal carcinoid. Am J Gastroenterol 1997;92:2062–2065.
46. Argenta LC, Strodel WE, Wheeler RH et al. Mesenteric angiopathy, intestinal gangrene, and midgut carcinoids. Surgery 1981;90:720–728.
47. Welch JP, Macaulay WP, Rosenberg JM. Carcinoid tumors of the colon. A study of 72 patients. J Surg Oncology 1985;28:217–221.
48. Weir AB, Poon MC, Groarke JF, Wilkerson JA. Lymphoma simulating Crohn's colitis. Dig Dis Sci 1980;25:69–72.
49. Friedman HB, Silver GM, Brown CH. Lymphoma of the colon simulating ulcerative colitis. Report of four cases. Am J Dig Dis 1968;13:910–917.
50. Haber DA, Mayer RJ. Primary gastrointestinal lymphoma. Semin Oncol 1988;15:154–169.
51. Crump M, Gospodarowicz M, Shepherd FA. Lymphoma of the gastrointestinal tract. Semin Oncol 1999;26:324–337.
52. Perosio PM, Brooks JJ, Saul SH, Haller DG. Primary intestinal lymphoma in Crohn's disease: minute tumor with a fatal outcome. Am J Gastroenterol 1992;87:894–898.
53. Brown I, Schofield JB, MacLennan KA, Tagart RE. Primary non-Hodgkin's lymphoma in ileal Crohn's disease. Eur J Surg Oncol 1992;18:627–631.
54. Wagonfeld JB, Platz CE, Fishman FL, Sibley RK, Kirsner JB. Multicentric colonic lymphoma complicating ulcerative colitis. Am J Dig Dis 1977;22:502–508.
55. Srivastava A, Mehrotra P, Aggarwal R, Pandey R, Khanna S, Naik SR. Multiple lymphomatous polyposis presenting as inflammatory bowel disease. Indian J Gastroenterol 1998;17:151–152.
56. Delmer A, Lavergne A, Molina T et al. Multiple lymphomatous polyposis of the gastrointestinal tract: prospective clinicopathologic study of 31 cases. Groupe D'etude des Lymphomes Digestifs. Gastroenterology 1997;112:7–16.
57. Freeman C, Berg JW, Cutler SJ. Occurrence and prognosis of extranodal lymphomas. Cancer 1972;29:252–260.
58. Cogliatti SB, Schmid U, Schumacher U et al. Primary B-cell gastric lymphoma: a clinicopathological study of 145 patients. Gastroenterology 1991;101:1159–1170.
59. Salem P, el-Hashimi L, Anaissie E et al. Primary small intestinal lymphoma in adults. A comparative study of IPSID versus non-IPSID in the Middle East. Cancer 1987;59:1670–1676.
60. Delmer A, Lavergne A, Molina T et al. Mycosis fungoides with gastrointestinal involvement. Gastroenterology 1997;112:7–16.
61. Olinger E, Variakojis D, Gordon L, Slater DN. Gastrointestinal complications of mycosis fungoides. Gastrointest Endosc 1988;34:478–481.
62. Cohen MI, Widerlite LW, Schechter GP et al. Gastrointestinal involvement in the Sezary syndrome. Gastroenterology 1977;73:145–149.
63. Andreson JL, Banks PA. Tumor of the ileocecal region: differentiation from Crohn's disease. Am J Gastroenterol 1982;77:910–912.
64. Tandon R, Buhac I, Rodgers JB Jr. Obstruction of the ileocecal valve by an adenomatous polyp mimicking regional enteritis. Am J Dig Dis 1972;17:929–933.
65. Taves DH, Probyn L. Cecal carcinoma: initially diagnosed as Crohn's disease on small bowel follow-through. Can J Gastroenterol 2001;15:337–340.
66. Tanaka M, Miyakawa S, Perez C. Carcinoma of the hepatic flexure with proximal lymphatic invasion mimicking Crohn's disease. Br J Dermatol 1998;138:522–525.
67. Caceres J, Valls J, Milman PJ. Primary ileal adenocarcinoma simulating Crohn's disease. Gastrointest Radiol 1984;9:365–367.
68. Smith CE, Filipe MI, Owen WJ. Neuromuscular and vascular hamartoma of small bowel presenting as inflammatory bowel disease. Gut 1986;27:964–969.
69. Katon RM, Brendler SJ, Ireland K. Gastric linitis plastica with metastases to the colon: a mimic of Crohn's disease. J Clin Gastroenterol 1989;11:555–560.
70. Koos L, Field RE. Metastatic carcinoma of breast simulating Crohn's disease. Int Surg 1980;65:359–362.
71. Lammer J, Dirschmid K, Hugel H. Carcinomatous metastases to the colon simulating Crohn's disease. Gastrointest Radiol 1981;6:89–91.
72. Weber JN, Carmichael DJ, Boylston A, Munro A, Whitear WP, Pinching AJ. Kaposi's sarcoma of the bowel presenting as apparent ulcerative colitis. Gut 1985;26:295–300.
73. Biggs BA, Crowe SM, Lucas CR, Ralston M, Thompson IL, Hardy KJ. AIDS related Kaposi's sarcoma presenting as ulcerative colitis and complicated by toxic megacolon. Gut 1987;28:1302–1306.
74. Roth JA, Schell S, Panzarino S, Coronato A. Visceral Kaposi's sarcoma presenting as colitis. Am J Surg Pathol 1978;2:209–214.
75. Sakanoue Y, Kusunoki M, Shoji Y et al. Malignant histiocytosis of the intestine simulating Crohn's disease. Report of a case. Dis Colon Rectum 1992;35:266–269.
76. Sprague R, Harper P, McClain S, Trainer T, Beeken W. Disseminated gastrointestinal sarcoidosis. Case report and review of the literature. Gastroenterology 1984;87:421–425.
77. Fries W, Grassi SA, Leone L et al. Association between inflammatory bowel disease and sarcoidosis. Report of two cases and review of the literature. Scand J Gastroenterol 1995;30:1221–1223.
78. Levine MS, Ekberg O, Rubesin SE, Gatenby RA. Gastrointestinal sarcoidosis: radiographic findings. Am J Roentgenol 1989;153:293–295.
79. Lukens FJ, Machicao VI, Woodward TA, DeVault KR. Esophageal sarcoidosis: an unusual diagnosis. J Clin Gastroenterol 2002;34:54–56.
80. Hilzenrat N, Spanier A, Lamoureux E, Bloom C, Sherker A, Oren R. Colonic obstruction secondary to sarcoidosis: nonsurgical diagnosis and management. Gastroenterology 1995;108:1556–1559.
81. Farrell RJ, Kelly CP. Celiac sprue. N Engl J Med 2002;346:180–188.
82. Klein NC, Hargrove RL, Sleisenger MH, Jeffries GH. Eosinophilic gastroenteritis. Medicine 1970;49:299–319.
83. Redondo-Cerezo E, Cabello MJ, Gonzalez Y, Gomez M, Garcia-Montero M, de Teresa J. Eosinophilic gastroenteritis: our recent experience: one-year experience of atypical onset of an uncommon disease. Scand J Gastroenterol 2001;36:1358–1360.
84. Talley NJ, Shorter RG, Phillips SF. Eosinophilic gastroenteritis: a clinicopathological study of patients with disease of the mucosa, muscle layer, and subserosal tissues. Mayo Clin Proc 1990;65:187–191.
85. Tedesco FJ, Huckaby CB, Hamby-Allen M, Ewing GC. Eosinophilic ileocolitis: expanding spectrum of eosinophilic gastroenteritis. Dig Dis Sci 1981;26:943–948.
86. Schulze K, Mitros FA. Eosinophilic gastroenteritis involving the ileocecal area. Dis Colon Rectum 1979;22:47–50.
87. Haberkern CM, Christie DL, Haas JE. Eosinophilic gastroenteritis presenting as ileocolitis. Gastroenterology 1978;74:896–899.
88. Naylor AR, Pollet JE. Eosinophilic colitis. Dis Colon Rectum 1985;28:615–618.
89. Durst AL, Freund H, Rosenmann E, Birnbaum D. Mesenteric panniculitis: review of the literature and presentation of cases. Surgery 1977;81:203–211.
90. Nyamekye I, Reed MW, Polacarz S, Wilkinson JM. Advanced gastrointestinal malignancy or benign inflammatory disease? An unusual presentation of sclerosing mesenteritis. Report of a case. Dis Colon Rectum 1994;37:1155–1157.
91. Parra-Davila E, McKenney MG, Sleeman D et al. Mesenteric panniculitis: case report and literature review. Am Surg 1998;64:768–771.
92. Rosa I, Benamouzig R, Guettier C et al. Mesenteric panniculitis simulating Crohn disease. Gastroenterol Clin Biol 1996;20:905–908.
93. Akhrass R, Yaffe MB, Fischer C, Ponsky J, Shuck JM, Hay WW Jr. Small-bowel diverticulosis: perceptions and reality. J Am Coll Surg 1997;184:383–388.
94. Leivonen MK, Halttunen JA, Kivilaakso EO. Duodenal diverticulum at endoscopic retrograde cholangiopancreatography, analysis of 123 patients. Hepato-Gastroenterology 1996;43:961–966.
95. Goldstein NS, Leon-Armin C, Mani A. Crohn's colitis-like changes in sigmoid diverticulosis specimens is usually an idiosyncratic inflammatory response to the diverticulosis rather than Crohn's colitis. Am J Surg Pathol 2000;24:668–675.
96. Randle PM, Matz LR. Caecal diverticulitis. Aust NZ J Surg 1989;59:391–394.
97. Cawthorne S, Gibbs N, Marks C. Segmental colitis: A new complication of diverticular colitis. Gut 1983;24.
98. Jani N, Finkelstein S, Blumberg D, Regueiro M. Segmental colitis associated with diverticulosis. Dig Dis Sci 2002;47:1175–1181.
99. Van Rosendaal GM, Andersen MA. Segmental colitis complicating diverticular disease. Can J Gastroenterol 1996;10:361–364.
100. Peppercorn MA. Drug-responsive chronic segmental colitis associated with diverticula: a clinical syndrome in the elderly. Am J Gastroenterol 1992;87:609–612.
101. Polit SA. Chronic segmental colitis in association with diverticulosis: a clinical syndrome in the elderly? J Am Geriatr Soc 1993;41:1155–1156.
102. Imperiali G, Meucci G, Alvisi C et al. Segmental colitis associated with diverticula: a prospective study. Gruppo di Studio per le Malattie Infiammatorie Intestinali (GSMII). Am J Gastroenterol 2000;95:1014–1016.
103. Glick ME, Goldman H, Glotzer DJ. Proctitis and colitis following diversion of the fecal stream. Gastroenterology 1981;80:438–441.
104. Haque S, West AB. Diversion colitis – 20 years a-growing. J Clin Gastroenterol 1992;15:281–283.
105. Abramson D, Kim DS, Hashmi HF, Whelan RL. Diversion colitis. A prospective study. Surg Endosc 1994;8:19–24.
106. Harig JM, Soergel KH, Komorowski RA, Wood CM. Treatment of diversion colitis with short-chain-fatty acid irrigation. N Engl J Med 1989;320:23–28.
107. Passaro E Jr. Bypass enteritis. A new complication of jejunoileal bypass for obesity. Am J Surg 1975;129:62–66.
108. Brolin RE, Mendelow H, Ravitch MM. The manifestations of bypass enteritis following jejunoileal bypass. Surg Gynecol Obstet 1980;151:209–214.
109. Ament ME, Finegold SM, Corrodi P, Passaro E. Bacterial flora of the small bowel before and after bypass procedure for morbid obesity. JAMA 1976;236:269–272.
110. Salzman D, Lazenby AJ, Wilcox CM, Iqbal N. Diagnosis of gastrointestinal graft-versus-host disease. Am J Gastroenterol 2000;95:3034–3038.
111. Smyrk TC, Tremaine WJ, Sandborn WJ, Pardi DS. Microscopic colitis: a review. Am J Gastroenterol 2002;97:794–802.

112. Ruan EA, Komorowski RA, Hogan WJ, Soergel KH. Nongranulomatous chronic idiopathic enterocolitis: clinicopathologic profile and response to corticosteroids. Gastroenterology 1996;111:629–637.

113. Uygur-Bayramicli O, Yavuzer D, Dolapcioglu C, Sensu S, Tuncer K. Granulomatous gastritis due to taeniasis. J Clin Gastroenterol 1998;27:351–352.

114. Shapiro JL, Goldblum JR, Petras RE. A clinicopathologic study of 42 patients with granulomatous gastritis. Is there really an 'idiopathic' granulomatous gastritis? Am J Surg Pathol 1996;20:462–470.

115. Boulton R, Chawla MH, Poole S, Hodgson HJ, Barrison IG. Ileal endometriosis masquerading as Crohn's ileitis. J Clin Gastroenterol 1997;25:338–342.

116. Yantiss RK, Clement PB, Young RH. Endometriosis of the intestinal tract: a study of 44 cases of a disease that may cause diverse challenges in clinical and pathologic evaluation. Am J Surg Pathol 2001;25:445–454.

117. Cappell MS, Friedman D, Mikhail N. Endometriosis of the terminal ileum simulating the clinical, roentgenographic, and surgical findings in Crohn's disease. Am J Gastroenterol 1991;86:1057–1062.

118. Langlois NE, Park KG, Keenan RA. Mucosal changes in the large bowel with endometriosis: a possible cause of misdiagnosis of colitis? Hum Pathol 1994;25:1030–1034.

119. Minocha A, Davis MS, Wright RA. Small bowel endometriosis masquerading as regional enteritis. Dig Dis Sci 1994;39:1126–1133.

120. Martimbeau PW, Pratt JH, Gaffey TA. Small-bowel obstruction secondary to endometriosis. Mayo Clin Proc 1975;50:239–243.

121. Cameron IC, Rogers S, Collins MC, Reed MW. Intestinal endometriosis: presentation, investigation, and surgical management. Int J Colorectal Dis 1995;10:83–86.

122. Hauer-Jensen M. Late radiation injury of the small intestine. Clinical, pathophysiologic and radiobiologic aspects. A review. Acta Oncol 1990;29:401–415.

123. Yeoh E, Horowitz M. Radiation enteritis. Br J Hosp Med 1988;39:498–504.

124. Ooi CJ, Zietman AL, Menon V et al. Morbidities of adjuvant chemotherapy and radiotherapy for resectable rectal cancer: an overview. Int J Radiat Oncol Biol Phys 2000;46:995–998.

125. Rodier JF. Radiation enteropathy – incidence, aetiology, risk factors, pathology and symptoms. Tumori 1995;81:122–125.

126. Vanagunas A, Jacob P, Olinger E. Radiation-induced esophageal injury: a spectrum from esophagitis to cancer. Am J Gastroenterol 1990;85:808–812.

127. Galland RB, Spencer J. Natural history and surgical management of radiation enteritis. Br J Surg 1987;74:742–747.

128. Cappell MS. Intestinal (mesenteric) vasculopathy. I. Acute superior mesenteric arteriopathy and venopathy. Gastroenterol Clin North Am 1998;27:783–825.

129. Hassan HA, Raufman JP. Mesenteric venous thrombosis. South Med J 1999;92:558–562.

130. Cappell MS. Intestinal (mesenteric) vasculopathy. II. Ischemic colitis and chronic mesenteric ischemia. Gastroenterol Clin North Am 1998;27:827–860.

131. Greenwald DA, Brandt LJ. Colonic ischemia. J Clin Gastroenterol 1998;27:122–128.

132. Burak KW, May GR. C1 inhibitor deficiency and angioedema of the small intestine masquerading as Crohn's disease. Can J Gastroenterol 2000;14:349–451.

133. Abdelmalek MF, Douglas DD. Lisinopril-induced isolated visceral angioedema: review of ACE-inhibitor-induced small bowel angioedema. Dig Dis Sci 1997;42:847–850.

134. Smoger SH, Sayed MA. Simultaneous mucosal and small bowel angioedema due to captopril. South Med J 1998;91:1060–1063.

135. Chase MP, Fiarman GS, Scholz FJ, MacDermott RP. Angioedema of the small bowel due to an angiotensin-converting enzyme inhibitor. J Clin Gastroenterol 2000;31:254–257.

136. Camilleri M, Pusey CD, Chadwick VS, Rees AJ. Gastrointestinal manifestations of systemic vasculitis. Q J Med 1983;52:141–149.

137. Williams DH, Kratka CD, Bonafede JP, Katon RM. Polyarteritis nodosa of the gastrointestinal tract with endoscopically documented duodenal and jejunal ulceration. Gastrointest Endosc 1992;38:501–503.

138. Perez RA, Silver D, Banerjee B. Polyarteritis nodosa presenting as massive upper gastrointestinal hemorrhage. Surg Endosc 2000;14:87.

139. Roikjaer O. Perforation and necrosis of the colon complicating polyarteritis nodosa. Case report. Acta Chir Scand 1987;153:385–386.

140. Fraioli P, Barberis M, Rizzato G. Gastrointestinal presentation of Churg–Strauss syndrome. Sarcoidosis 1994;11:42–45.

141. Shimamoto C, Hirata I, Ohshiba S, Fujiwara S, Nishio M. Churg–Strauss syndrome (allergic granulomatous angiitis) with peculiar multiple colonic ulcers. Am J Gastroenterol 1990;85:316–319.

142. Bang D. Clinical spectrum of Behçet's disease. J Dermatol 2001;28:610–613.

143. Bayraktar Y, Ozaslan E, Van Thiel DH. Gastrointestinal manifestations of Behçet's disease. J Clin Gastroenterol 2000;30:144–154.

144. Hidalgo V, Fernandez-Melon J, Schlincker A, Martin-Mola E, Travis SP. Treatment of intestinal Behçet's syndrome with chimeric tumour necrosis factor alpha antibody. Lancet 2001;358:1644.

145. Steele C, Bohra S, Broe P, Murray FE. Acute upper gastrointestinal haemorrhage and colitis: an unusual presentation of Wegener's granulomatosis. Eur J Gastroenterol Hepatol 2001;13:993–995.

146. Fallows GA, Hamilton SF, Taylor DS, Reddy SB. Esophageal involvement in Wegener's granulomatosis: a case report and review of the literature. Can J Gastroenterol 2000;14:449–451.

147. Pinkney JH, Clarke G, Fairclough PD. Gastrointestinal involvement in Wegener's granulomatosis. Gastrointest Endosc 1991;37:411–412.

148. Tupler RH, McCuskey WH. Wegener granulomatosis of the colon: CT and histologic correlation. J Comput Assist Tomogr 1991;15:314–316.

149. Srinivasan U, Coughlan RJ. Small intestinal perforation complicating Wegener's granulomatosis. Rheumatology (Oxford) 1999;38:289–290.

150. Wilson RH, Kerr PP, McLoughlin J, Gormley M. Symptomatic colitis as the initial presentation of Wegener's granulomatosis. Br J Clin Pract 1993;47:315–318.

151. Temmesfeld-Wollbrueck B, Heinrichs C, Szalay A, Seeger W. Granulomatous gastritis in Wegener's disease: differentiation from Crohn's disease supported by a positive test for antineutrophil antibodies. Gut 1997;40:550–553.

152. Fauci AS, Wolff SM. Wegener's granulomatosis: studies in eighteen patients and a review of the literature. Arthritis Rheum 1973;16:657–664.

153. Sokol RJ, Farrell MK, McAdams AJ. An unusual presentation of Wegener's granulomatosis mimicking inflammatory bowel disease. Gastroenterology 1984;87:426–432.

154. Saulsbury FT. Henoch–Schonlein purpura in children. Report of 100 patients and review of the literature. Medicine (Baltimore) 1999;78:395–409.

155. Patrignelli R, Sheikh SH, Shaw-Stiffel TA. Henoch–Schonlein purpura. A multisystem disease also seen in adults. Postgrad Med 1995;97:123–124, 127, 131–134.

156. Klein GL, Stafford S III. Unusual gastrointestinal manifestations of Henoch–Schonlein purpura [Letter]. Am J Dis Child 1975;129:1238–1239.

157. Scherbaum WA, Kaufmann R, Vogel U, Adler G. Henoch–Schonlein purpura with ileitis terminalis. Clin Investig 1993;71:564–567.

158. Hallegua DS, Wallace DJ. Gastrointestinal manifestations of systemic lupus erythematosus. Curr Opin Rheumatol 2000;12:379–385.

159. Edmunds SE, Ganju V, Beveridge BR, French MA, Quinlan MF. Protein-losing enteropathy in systemic lupus erythematosus. Aust NZ J Med 1988;18:868–871.

160. Hoffman BI, Katz WA. The gastrointestinal manifestations of systemic lupus erythematosus: a review of the literature. Semin Arthritis Rheum 1980;9:237–247.

161. Hurd ER. Extraarticular manifestations of rheumatoid arthritis. Semin Arthritis Rheum 1979;8:151–176.

162. Schneider RE, Dobbins WO III. Suction biopsy of the rectal mucosa for diagnosis of arteritis in rheumatoid arthritis and related diseases. Ann Intern Med 1968;68:561–568.

163. Rose S, Young MA, Reynolds JC. Gastrointestinal manifestations of scleroderma. Gastroenterol Clin North Am 1998;27:563–594.

164. Sjogren RW. Gastrointestinal features of scleroderma. Curr Opin Rheumatol 1996;8:569–575.

165. Burke AP, Sobin LH, Virmani R. Localized vasculitis of the gastrointestinal tract. Am J Surg Pathol 1995;19:338–349.

166. Eshraghi N, Farahmand M, Maerz LL, Campbell SM, Deveney CW, Sheppard BC. Adult-onset dermatomyositis with severe gastrointestinal manifestations: case report and review of the literature. Surgery 1998;123:356–358.

167. Leibowitz G, Eliakim R, Amir G, Rachmilewitz D. Dermatomyositis associated with Crohn's disease. J Clin Gastroenterol 1994;18:48–52.

168. Baxter R, Nino-Murcia M, Bloom RJ, Kosek J. Gastrointestinal manifestations of essential mixed cryoglobulinemia. Gastrointest Radiol 1988;13:160–162.

169. Rickert RR. The important 'impostors' in the differential diagnosis of inflammatory bowel disease. J Clin Gastroenterol 1984;6:153–163.

170. Mishu B, Koehler J, Lee LA et al. Outbreaks of *Salmonella enteritidis* infections in the United States, 1985–1991. J Infect Dis 1994;169:547–552.

171. Wagner JE, Owens DR, Balthazar EJ. *Salmonella*- and *Shigella*-induced ileitis: CT findings in four patients. Infect Immun 1981;31:1232–1238.

172. Vender RJ, Marignani P. *Salmonella* colitis presenting as a segmental colitis resembling Crohn's disease. Dig Dis Sci 1983;28:848–851.

173. Wong SY, Ng FH, Kwok KH, Chow KC. Skip colonic ulceration in typhoid ileo-colitis. J Gastroenterol 1999;34:700–701.

174. Stoll BJ, Glass RI, Huq MI, Khan MU, Banu H, Holt J. Epidemiologic and clinical features of patients infected with *Shigella* who attended a diarrheal disease hospital in Bangladesh. J Infect Dis 1982;146:177–183.

175. Cover TL, Aber RC. *Yersinia enterocolitica*. N Engl J Med 1989;321:16–24.

176. Tuohy AM, O'Gorman M, Byington C, Reid B, Jackson WD. *Yersinia* enterocolitis mimicking Crohn's disease in a toddler. Pediatrics 1999;104:e36.

177. Macfarlane PI, Miller V. *Yersinia enterocolitica* mimicking Crohn's disease. J Pediatr Gastroenterol Nutr 1986;5:671.

178. Sandler M, Girdwood AH, Kottler RE, Marks IN. Terminal ileitis due to *Yersinia enterocolitica*. A case report and review of the literature. S Africa Med J 1982;62:573–576.

179. Vantrappen G, Geboes K, Ponette E. *Yersinia* enteritis. Med Clin North Am 1982;66:639–653.

180. Pitkanen T, Ponka A, Pettersson T, Kosunen TU, Mattila J. *Campylobacter* enteritis in 188 hospitalized patients. Arch Intern Med 1983;143:215–219.

181. Ilnyckyj A, Greenberg H, Bernstein CN. *Escherichia coli* O157:H7 infection mimicking Crohn's disease. Gastroenterology 1997;112:995–999.

182. Nataro JP, Kaper JB, Tacket CO. Diarrheagenic *Escherichia coli*. Clin Microbiol Rev 1998;11:403.

183. Farrell RJ, Kelly CP, Kyne L. *Clostridium difficile*. Gastroenterol Clin North Am 2001;30:753–777.

184. Rubin MS, Bodenstein LE, Kent KC. Severe *Clostridium* difficile colitis. Dis Colon Rectum 1995;38:350–354.

185. Meyers S, Mayer L, Bottone E, Desmond E, Janowitz HD. Occurrence of *Clostridium difficile* toxin during the course of inflammatory bowel disease. Gastroenterology 1981;80:697–670.

186. Barlow D, Moran JS. Treating uncomplicated *Neisseria gonorrhoeae* infections: is the anatomic site of infection important? Genitourinary Med 1996;72:422–426.

187. Brenden RA, Miller MA, Janda JM. Clinical disease spectrum and pathogenic factors associated with *Plesiomonas shigelloides* infections in humans. Sexually Transmitted Dis 1995;22:39–47.

188. Hanson PG, Standridge J, Jarrett F, Maki DG. Freshwater wound infection due to *Aeromonas hydrophila*. JAMA 1977;238:1053–1054.

189. Holmberg SD, Farmer JJ III. *Aeromonas hydrophila* and *Plesiomonas shigelloides* as causes of intestinal infections. Rev Infect Dis 1984;6:633–639.

190. Doman DB, Golding MI, Goldberg HJ, Doyle RB. *Aeromonas hydrophila* colitis presenting as medically refractory inflammatory bowel disease. Am J Gastroenterol 1989;84:83–85.

191. Wedzina W, Yarze JC. *Aeromonas* as a cause of segmental colitis. Am J Gastroenterol 1997;92:2104–2106.

192. Willoughby JM, Rahman AF, Gregory MM. Chronic colitis after *Aeromonas* infection. Gut 1989;30:686–690.

193. Weese WC, Smith IM, Weese-Mayer DE. A study of 57 cases of actinomycosis over a 36-year period. A diagnostic 'failure' with good prognosis after treatment. Arch Intern Med 1975;135:1562–1568.

194. Burden SJ, Burden P. Actinomycosis. Nature 1989;341:716–720.

195. Spencer TE, Brewer JM, Brewer NS. Primary anorectal actinomycosis. Arch Biochem Biophys 1971;142:122–131.

196. Gonor S, Allard M, Boileau GR. Appendicovesical fistula caused by ileocecal actinomycosis. Can J Surg 1982;25:23–24.

197. Ikebe M, Oiwa T, Mori M, Kuwano H, Sugimachi K, Yao T. Gastric syphilis: case report and review of the literature. Radiat Med 1994;12:171–175.

198. Fyfe B, Poppiti RJ Jr, Lubin J, Robinson MJ. Gastric syphilis. Primary diagnosis by gastric biopsy: report of four cases. Arch Pathol Lab Med 1993;117:820–823.

199. Reisman TN, Leverett FL, Hudson JR, Kalser MH. Syphilitic gastropathy. Am J Dig Dis 1975;20:588–593.

200. Kleiner RC, Najarian L, Levenson J, Kaplan HJ. AIDS complicated by syphilis can mimic uveitis and Crohn's disease. Case report. Arch Ophthalmol 1987;105:1486–1487.

201. Marshall JB. Tuberculosis of the gastrointestinal tract and peritoneum. Am J Gastroenterol 1993;88:989–999.

202. Panton ON, Sharp R, English RA, Atkinson KG. Gastrointestinal tuberculosis. The great mimic still at large. Dis Colon Rectum 1985;28:446–450.

203. Shah P, Ramakantan R. Differentiating tuberculosis from Crohn's disease of the small bowel. Dis Colon Rectum 1989;32:905.

204. Keane J, Gershon S, Wise RP et al. Tuberculosis associated with infliximab, a tumor necrosis factor alpha-neutralizing agent. N Engl J Med 2001;345:1098–1104.

205. Ratnaike RN. Whipple's disease. Postgrad Med J 2000;76:760–766.

206. Ramaiah C, Boynton RF. Whipple's disease. Gastroenterol Clin North Am 1998;27:683–695, vii.

207. Diepersloot RJ, Kroes AC, Visser W, Jiwa NM, Rothbarth PH. Acute ulcerative proctocolitis associated with primary cytomegalovirus infection. Arch Intern Med 1990;150:1749–1751.

208. Wajsman R, Cappell MS, Biempica L, Cho KC. Terminal ileitis associated with cytomegalovirus and the acquired immune deficiency syndrome. Am J Gastroenterol 1989;84:790–793.

209. Caroline DF, Hilpert PL, Russin VL. CMV colitis mimicking Crohn's disease in a patient with acquired immune deficiency syndrome (AIDS). Can Assoc Radiol J 1987;38:227–228.

210. Colemont LJ, Pen JH, Pelckmans PA, Degryse HR, Pattyn SR, Van Maercke YM. Herpes simplex virus type 1 colitis: an unusual cause of diarrhea. Am J Gastroenterol 1990;85:1182–1185.

211. Goodell SE, Quinn TC, Mkrtichian E, Schuffler MD, Holmes KK, Corey L. Herpes simplex virus proctitis in homosexual men. Clinical, sigmoidoscopic, and histopathological features. N Engl J Med 1983;308:868–871.

212. Sperling HV, Reed WG. Herpetic gastritis. Am J Dig Dis 1977;22:1033–1034.

213. Papadakis KA, Tung JK, Binder SW et al. Outcome of cytomegalovirus infections in patients with inflammatory bowel disease. Am J Gastroenterol 2001;96:2137–2142.

214. Morrison YY, Rathbun RC, Huycke MM. Disseminated histoplasmosis mimicking Crohn's disease in a patient with the acquired immunodeficiency syndrome. Am J Gastroenterol 1994;89:1255–1257.

215. Gonzalez Keelan CG, Imbert M. Colonic histoplasmosis simulating Crohn's disease in a patient with AIDS: case report and review of the literature. Bol Asoc Med P R 1988;80:248–250.

216. Cappell MS, Mandell W, Grimes MM, Neu HC. Gastrointestinal histoplasmosis. Dig Dis Sci 1988;33:353–360.

217. Alberti-Flor JJ, Granda A. Ileocecal histoplasmosis mimicking Crohn's disease in a patient with Job's syndrome. Digestion 1986;33:176–180.

218. Khan ZU, Prakash B, Kapoor MM, Madda JP, Chandy R. Basidiobolomycosis of the rectum masquerading as Crohn's disease: case report and review. Clin Infect Dis 1998;26:521–523.

219. Pasha TM, Leighton JA, Smilack JD, Heppell J, Colby TV, Kaufman L. Basidiobolomycosis: an unusual fungal infection mimicking inflammatory bowel disease. Gastroenterology 1997;112:250–254.

220. Patel AS, DeRidder PH. Amebic colitis masquerading as acute inflammatory bowel disease: the role of serology in its diagnosis. J Clin Gastroenterol 1989;11:407–410.

221. Tucker PC, Webster PD, Kilpatrick ZM. Amebic colitis mistaken for inflammatory bowel disease. Arch Intern Med 1975;135:681–685.

222. Manthey MW, Ross AB, Soergel KH. Cryptosporidiosis and inflammatory bowel disease. Experience from the Milwaukee outbreak. Dig Dis Sci 1997;42:1580–1586.

223. Alfandari S, Ajana F, Senneville E, Beuscart C, Chidiac C, Mouton Y. Haemorrhagic ulcerative colitis due to Isospora belli in AIDS. Int J STD AIDS 1995;6:216.

224. Gunasekaran TS, Hassall E. Giardiasis mimicking inflammatory bowel disease. J Pediatr 1992;120:424–426.

225. Cross JH. Intestinal capillariasis. Clin Microbiol Rev 1992;5:120–129.

226. Markell EK. Intestinal nematode infections. Pediatr Clin North Am 1985;32:971–986.

227. Bouree P, Paugam A, Petithory JC. Anisakidosis: report of 25 cases and review of the literature. Comp Immunol Microbiol Infect Dis 1995;18:75–84.

228. Ishiguro A, Uno Y, Ishiguro Y, Sakuraba H, Munakata A. Anisakiasis of the ileocecal valve. Gastrointest Endosc 2001;53:677–679.

229. Kanisawa Y, Kawanishi N, Hisai H, Araya H. Colonic anisakiasis: an unusual cause of intussusception. Endoscopy 2000;32:S55.

230. Eskesen A, Strand EA, Andersen SN, Rosseland A, Hellum KB, Strand OA. Anisakiasis presenting as an obstructive duodenal tumor. A Scandinavian case. Scand J Infect Dis 2001;33:75–76.

231. Liacouras CA, Bell LM, Aljabi MC, Piccoli DA. *Angiostrongylus costaricensis* enterocolitis mimics Crohn's disease. J Pediatr Gastroenterol Nutr 1993;16:203–207.

232. Hung HC, Jan SE, Cheng KS, Chu KC, Chien TC. Gastrointestinal bleeding due to whipworm (*Trichuris trichiura*) infestation: a case report. Zhonghua Yi Xue Za Zhi (Taipei) 1995;55:408–411.

233. Strickland GT. Gastrointestinal manifestations of schistosomiasis. Gut 1994;35:1334–1337.

234. Weight SC, Barrie WW. Colonic *Strongyloides stercoralis* infection masquerading as ulcerative colitis. J R Coll Surg Edin 1997;42:202–203.

235. Knudtzon J, Svane S. Turner's syndrome associated with chronic inflammatory bowel disease. A case report and review of the literature. Acta Med Scand 1988;223:375–378.

236. Price WH. A high incidence of chronic inflammatory bowel disease in patients with Turner's syndrome. J Med Genet 1979;16:263–266.

237. Weinrieb IJ, Fineman RM, Spiro HM. Turner syndrome and inflammatory bowel disease. N Engl J Med 1976;294:1221–1222.

238. Yamaguchi T, Ihara K, Matsumoto T et al. Inflammatory bowel disease-like colitis in glycogen storage disease type 1b. Inflamm Bowel Dis 2001;7:128–132.

239. Franceschini R, Gianetta E, Pastorino A et al. Crohn's-like colitis in glycogen storage disease Ib: a case report. Hepatogastroenterology 1996;43:1461–1464.

240. Gahl WA, Brantly M, Kaiser-Kupfer MI et al. Genetic defects and clinical characteristics of patients with a form of oculocutaneous albinism (Hermansky–Pudlak syndrome). N Engl J Med 1998;338:1258–1264.

241. Werlin SL, Chusid MJ, Caya J, Oechler HW. Colitis in chronic granulomatous disease. Gastroenterology 1982;82:328–331.

242. Sloan JM, Cameron CH, Maxwell RJ, McCluskey DR, Collins JS. Colitis complicating chronic granulomatous disease. A clinicopathological case report. Gut 1996;38:619–622.

243. Lindahl JA, Williams FH, Newman SL. Small bowel obstruction in chronic granulomatous disease. J Pediatr Gastroenterol Nutr 1984;3:637–640.

244. Ishii E, Matui T, Iida M, Inamitu T, Ueda K. Chediak–Higashi syndrome with intestinal complication. Report of a case. J Clin Gastroenterol 1987;9:556–558.

245. Washington K, Stenzel TT, Buckley RH, Gottfried MR. Gastrointestinal pathology in patients with common variable immunodeficiency and X-linked agammaglobulinemia. Am J Surg Pathol 1996;20:1240–1252.

246. Kutukculer N, Yagci RV, Aydogdu S, Aksu G, Genc B. Chronic inflammatory bowel disease in a patient with common variable immunodeficiency. Turk J Pediatr 2001;43:88–90.

247. Lederman HM, Winkelstein JA. X-linked agammaglobulinemia: an analysis of 96 patients. Medicine (Baltimore) 1985;64:145–156.

248. Olden KW. Diagnosis of irritable bowel syndrome. Gastroenterology 2002;122:1701–1714.

249. Bytzer P, Stokholm M, Andersen I, Klitgaard NA, Schaffalitzky de Muckadell OB. Prevalence of surreptitious laxative abuse in patients with diarrhoea of uncertain origin: a cost benefit analysis of a screening procedure. Gut 1989;30:1379–1384.

250. Tsianos EV, Dalekos GN, Tzermias C, Merkouropoulos M, Hatzis J. Hidradenitis suppurativa in Crohn's disease. A further support to this association. Pediatr Clin North Am 1985;32:971–986.

251. Gower-Rousseau C, Maunoury V, Colombel JF et al. Hidradenitis suppurativa and Crohn's disease in two families: a significant association? Am J Gastroenterol 1992;87:928.

252. Fisher RL, McMahon LF Jr, Ryan MJ, Larson D, Brand M. Gastrointestinal bleeding in competitive runners. Dig Dis Sci 1986;31:1226–1228.

253. Halvorsen FA, Lyng J, Glomsaker T, Ritland S. Gastrointestinal disturbances in marathon runners. Br J Sports Med 1990;24:266–268.

254. Oktedalen O, Lunde OC, Opstad PK, Aabakken L, Kvernebo K. Changes in the gastrointestinal mucosa after long-distance running. Scand J Gastroenterol 1992;27:270–274.

255. Pieterse AS, Leong AS, Rowland R. The mucosal changes and pathogenesis of pneumatosis cystoides intestinalis. Hum Pathol 1985;16:683–688.

256. Galandiuk S, Fazio VW. Pneumatosis cystoides intestinalis. A review of the literature. Dis Colon Rectum 1986;29:358–363.

257. Ford MJ, Anderson JR, Gilmour HM, Holt S, Sircus W, Heading RC. Clinical spectrum of 'solitary ulcer' of the rectum. Gastroenterology 1983;84:1533–1540.

258. Levine DS, Surawicz CM, Ajer TN, Dean PJ, Rubin CE. Diffuse excess mucosal collagen in rectal biopsies facilitates differential diagnosis of solitary rectal ulcer syndrome from other inflammatory bowel diseases. Dig Dis Sci 1988;33:1345–1352.

259. Walker JP, Wiener I, Rowe EB. Colitis cystica profunda: diagnosis and management. South Med J 1986;79:1167–1170.

260. Iannuccilli EA, Migliaccio AJ. Regional enteritis with foreign body. JAMA 1973;223:1288.

261. O'Gorman MA, Boyer RS, Jackson WD. Toothpick foreign body perforation and migration mimicking Crohn's disease in a child. J Pediatr Gastroenterol Nutr 1996;23:628–630.

262. Catucci V, Albrizio M, Sebastiani R, Martinelli G, Florio C. Ileal stenosis caused by chronic granulomatous inflammation secondary to a foreign body simulating Crohn disease. Minerva Chir 1990;45:419–424.

263. Segal I, Nouri MA, Hamilton DG et al. Foreign-body ileitis. A case report. S Africa Med J 1980;58:421–422.

264. Goldman IL, Caldamone AA, Gauderer M, Hampel N, Wesselhoeft CW, Elder JS. Infected urachal cysts: a review of 10 cases. J Urol 1988;140:375–378.

265. Tatsuguchi A, Fukuda Y, Moriyama T, Yamanaka N. Lipomatosis of the small intestine and colon associated with intussusception in the ileocecal region. Gastrointest Endosc 1999;49:118–121.

266. Tani T, Abe H, Tsukada H, Kodama M. Lipomatosis of the ileum with volvulus: report of a case. Surg Today 1998;28:640–642.

267. Mylonakis BJ, Karkanias GG, Katergiannakis VA, Manouras AJ, Apostolidis NS. Lipomatosis of the ileocecal valve leading to episodes of partial small bowel obstruction. Mt Sinai J Med 1995;62:302–304.

268. Bhupalan AJ, Forbes A, Lloyd-Davies E, Wignall B, Murray-Lyon IM. Lipomatosis of the ileocaecal valve simulating Crohn's disease. Postgrad Med J 1992;68:455–456.

269. Dworkin B, Winawer SJ, Lightdale CJ. Typhlitis. Report of a case with long-term survival and a review of the recent literature. Dig Dis Sci 1981;26:1032–1037.

270. Isaacs KL, Warshauer DM. Mucocele of the appendix: computed tomographic, endoscopic, and pathologic correlation. Am J Gastroenterol 1992;87:787–789.

271. Mourad FH, Hussein M, Bahlawan M, Haddad M, Tawil A. Intestinal obstruction secondary to appendiceal mucocele. Dig Dis Sci 1999;44:1594–1599.

272. Ilnyckyj A, Aldor TA, Warrington R, Bernstein CN. Crohn's disease and the Melkersson–Rosenthal syndrome. Can J Gastroenterol 1999;13:152–154.

273. Friedman S, Janowitz HD. Systemic amyloidosis and the gastrointestinal tract. Gastroenterol Clin North Am 1998;27:595–614, vi.

274. Greenstein AJ, Sachar DB, Panday AK et al. Amyloidosis and inflammatory bowel disease. A 50-year experience with 25 patients. Medicine 1992;71:261–270.

275. Addiss DG, Shaffer N, Fowler BS, Tauxe RV. The epidemiology of appendicitis and appendectomy in the United States. Am J Epidemiol 1990;132:910–925.

276. Oren R, Rachmilewitz D. Preoperative clues to Crohn's disease in suspected, acute appendicitis. Report of 12 cases and review of the literature. J Clin Gastroenterol 1992;15:306–310.

277. Savrin RA, Clausen K, Martin EW Jr., Cooperman M. Chronic and recurrent appendicitis. Am J Surg 1979;137:355–357.

278. Huang JC, Appelman HD. Another look at chronic appendicitis resembling Crohn's disease. Mod Pathol 1996;9:975–981.

279. Crohn B, Ginzburg L, Oppenheimer G. Regional ileitis. J Clin Gastroenterol 1932;21:249–253.

280. Agha FP, Ghahremani GG, Panella JS, Kaufman MW. Appendicitis as the initial manifestation of Crohn's disease: radiologic features and prognosis. Am J Roentgenol 1987;149:515–518.

281. Higgins MJ, Walsh M, Kennedy SM, Hyland JM, McDermott E, O'Higgins NJ. Granulomatous appendicitis revisited: report of a case. Dig Surg 2001;18:245–248.

282. Yang SS, Gibson P, McCaughey RS, Arcari FA, Bernstein J. Primary Crohn's disease of the appendix: report of 14 cases and review of the literature. Ann Surg 1979;189:334–339.

283. Andreyev HJ, Owen RA, Thomas PA, Wright PL, Forbes A. Acid secretion from a Meckel's diverticulum: the unsuspected mimic of Crohn's disease? Am J Gastroenterol 1994;89:1552–1554.

284. Chi HI, Arai M. Linear IgA bullous dermatosis associated with ulcerative colitis. J Dermatol 1999;26:150–153.

285. Rodefeld MD, Sterkel R, Keating JP, Kane RE, deMello DE, Langer JC. Mesenteric Castleman's disease masquerading as inflammatory bowel disease. J Pediatr Gastroenterol Nutr 1998;27:589–592.

286. Tysk C, Lindberg E, Jarnerot G, Floderus-Myrhed B. Ulcerative colitis and Crohn's disease in an unselected population of monozygotic and dizygotic twins. A study of heritability and the influence of smoking. Gut 1988;29:990–996.

287. Rankin GB. Extraintestinal and systemic manifestations of inflammatory bowel disease. Med Clin North Am 1990;74:39–50.

288. Geboes K. Crohn's disease, ulcerative colitis or indeterminate colitis – how important is it to differentiate? Acta Gastroenterol Belg 2001;64:197–200.

289. Yu CS, Pemberton JH, Larson D. Ileal pouch–anal anastomosis in patients with indeterminate colitis: long-term results. Med Clin North Am 1990;74:39–50.

## CHAPTER 26

# Endoscopy in inflammatory bowel disease

Richard J Farrell and Mark A Peppercorn

## INTRODUCTION

The development of fiberoptic and video endoscopy has improved the accurate diagnosis of chronic ulcerative colitis (UC) and Crohn's disease (CD), allowed ready assessment of disease activity and defined the consequences of the inflammatory process, including strictures, mass lesions, bleeding and the development of dysplasia or malignancy.[1] To this end, direct mucosal visualization of the colon, particularly in conjunction with biopsy, has both complemented and supplanted barium X-ray studies. Endoscopy also plays a key role in the management of inflammatory bowel disease (IBD), particularly in the evaluation of patients with disease refractory to conventional medical therapy and in defining the severity and location of disease in order to choose appropriate treatment options. Moreover, flexible sigmoidoscopy, ileocolonoscopy and endoscopic retrograde cholangiopancreatography (ERCP) play an important role in managing the complications of inflammatory bowel disease, such as gastrointestinal bleeding, strictures and primary sclerosing cholangitis. This chapter will review the role of endoscopy in diagnosis and the management of complications in patients with inflammatory bowel disease.

## INDICATIONS FOR ENDOSCOPY

Endoscopy plays a key role in the diagnosis and management of inflammatory bowel disease and adds crucial mucosal and histological information to the constellation of history, physical examination, radiographic findings and laboratory values. Table 26.1 lists current indications for ileocolonoscopy in inflammatory bowel disease. Differentiation between Crohn's disease and ulcerative colitis has important ramifications for medical therapy, surgical options and prognosis. This distinction can be made accurately in at least 85% of patients, and accuracy increases to 95% with re-examination and the passage of time.

In the acutely ill patient colonoscopy can identify deep ulcerations consistent with severe colitis, and thereby adds to the clinical determination of the need for more aggressive medical therapy or surgery. Although it is not done routinely, colonoscopy can be performed safely in acutely ill patients and may prove to play an important role in the evaluation of patients with acute or severe inflammatory bowel disease. Carbonnel et al.[2] performed colonoscopy without complication, except for one colonic dilatation, in 85 consecutive patients with acute flares of ulcerative colitis, 46 of whom had severe endoscopic colitis characterized by extensive deep colonic ulcerations, and the remaining 39 patients having moderate endoscopic colitis. Forty-three of the 46 patients (94%) with severe endoscopic colitis were operated upon; 38 of them failed to improve with high-dose corticosteroids and five had a toxic megacolon. Extensive ulcerations reaching at least the circular muscle layer were found on pathological examination of colectomy specimens in 42 of the 43 patients. Conversely, 30 of 39 patients with moderate endoscopic colitis went into clinical remission with medical treatment, and only nine needed further surgery because of medical treatment failure. Six of these nine patients underwent another colonoscopy prior to colectomy, and all six showed features of severe endoscopic colitis with deep ulcerations. In the emergency setting, uncontrollable bleeding, toxic megacolon and bowel perforation remain the most common indications for surgery, and endoscopy plays a limited role in evaluating these situations. Decisions regarding elective surgery are based on clinical as well as endoscopic parameters that include response to steroids, other immunosuppressants including biological therapies, the need for their prolonged use, and the overall condition of the patient.

When colonoscopy is indicated, complete inspection of the colon and terminal ileum is the goal except in predetermined cases, i.e. patients with severe inflammation in whom partial examination may provide the necessary information with less risk of perforation. Poor bowel preparation is the commonest reason for incomplete colonoscopy in ulcerative colitis, whereas in Crohn's disease termination of the examination is usually

## Table 26.1 Indications for ileocolonoscopy in inflammatory bowel disease

Diagnosis of ileocolitis
Differentiating between ulcerative colitis and Crohn's colitis
Assessment of disease extent
Assessment of disease activity
Assessment of disease recurrence
Assessment of efficacy of medical therapy
Assessment of disease complications and radiographic abnormalities
Screening/surveillance for dysplasia and cancer
Evaluation of unexplained diarrhea
Therapeutic endoscopy for disease complications
Perioperative endoscopy

related to the presence of strictures or severe inflammation with large, deep ulcerations, which carry an increased risk of perforation. Complete inspection of the colon is particularly important when the goal is surveillance for dysplasia or cancer. Earlier studies reported that complete examinations are achieved in 95% of patients with ulcerative colitis and 75% of patients with Crohn's disease.[3,4] Although not formally evaluated in Crohn's disease, the advent of variable-stiffness colonoscopes that combine pediatric shaft characteristics with the ability to stiffen when needed has recently been shown in randomized trials to significantly reduce intubation time and patient discomfort, as well as the ability to visualize beyond obstructive bowel lesions.[5]

# ENDOSCOPY FOR DIAGNOSIS OF INFLAMMATORY BOWEL DISEASE

## ULCERATIVE COLITIS

None of the endoscopic features of inflammatory bowel disease is completely specific, and the diagnosis should be based on a combination of clinical, endoscopic and histological findings. Table 26.2 outlines the typical endoscopic features of ulcerative colitis and Crohn's disease as seen at various stages in the disease course. In active ulcerative colitis the most typical appearance is that of diffusely erythematous, friable and granular mucosa,

## Table 26.2 Diagnostic colonoscopic features of ulcerative colitis and Crohn's disease

| | Ulcerative colitis | Crohn's disease |
|---|---|---|
| **Early findings** | Edema | Aphthous ulceration |
| | Confluent erythema | Discontinuous erythema |
| | Rectal involvement | Rectal sparing |
| | | Perianal disease |
| **Intermediate changes** | Granularity | Linear ulcers |
| | Contact bleeding | Cobblestoning |
| | | Skip lesions |
| **Late changes** | Discrete ulcers | Contact bleeding |
| | Pus/exudate | Confluent ulcers |
| | Loss of haustral folds | Strictures |
| | | Mucosal bridging |

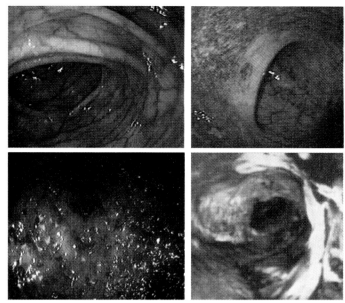

Fig. 26.1 Endoscopic spectrum of severity in ulcerative colitis. In the normal colon the mucosa is shiny, pale pink, and retains a delicate reticulated vascular pattern (upper left). In mild ulcerative colitis the mucosa becomes duller and erythematous, often with a 'granular' texture, and the vascular pattern is blurred (upper right). In moderate ulcerative colitis gross pitting of the mucosa is seen and the lining may crumble away and bleed at the lightest touch (friability) (lower left). In severe ulcerative colitis macroulceration, occasionally deep, with mucopurulent exudate and spontaneous hemorrhage is seen (lower right). (Reproduced with permission from American Gastroenterology Association, Gastroenterology Teaching Project 002, Inflammatory Bowel Disease, 3rd Edition.)

with loss of the normal vascular pattern.[3,6] Figure 26.1 illustrates the endoscopic spectrum of disease severity in ulcerative colitis. The lesions begin at the anorectal junction and spread arborally in a homogeneous fashion. The upper limit of the diseased mucosa may be anywhere from the rectum to the ileocecal valve. Although a normal rectum at endoscopy is a strong argument against ulcerative colitis unless the patient has recently been given topical treatments,[7,8] the rectum should be always be biopsied as a histologically normal rectum theoretically excludes ulcerative colitis.[9] Contrary to traditional teaching, endoscopic and histological patchiness of inflammation and rectal sparing are common during the course of disease in treated ulcerative colitis, and seem to be unrelated to specific therapy.[10] A study by Bernstein et al.[11] prospectively evaluated the prevalence of patchiness, including rectal sparing, in treated patients with ulcerative colitis. Patchiness was defined endoscopically as frank rectal sparing with a normal endoscopic appearance, and histologically by absence of inflammation in the lamina propria and crypts. Discrete endoscopic areas of patchiness and inflammation that were larger proximally than distally were also considered to represent patchy mucosal inflammation. None of the 39 patients evaluated had features that would suggest a diagnosis of Crohn's disease, such as perianal disease, small bowel involvement, large skip lesions or granulomas. On endoscopic criteria, 17 patients (44%) had endoscopic evidence of patchiness, including five (13%) with rectal sparing. Thirteen (33%) had histologic evidence of patchiness, including six (15%) with rectal sparing. Both endoscopic and histologic patchiness were seen in nine patients (23%). The patchy and non-patchy groups did not differ in regard to the use of rectal therapy. The authors

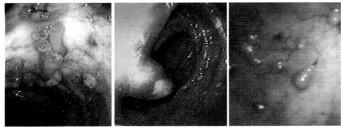

**Fig. 26.2** Pseudopolyps in ulcerative colitis and Crohn's disease. Chronic inflammation often leads to diffuse mucosal atrophy, leaving behind hypertrophic islands of swollen edematous tissue and granulation tissue that assume a polypoid shape. These inflammatory polyps, known as pseudopolyps, have no malignant potential and occur in both ulcerative colitis and Crohn's disease. The endoscopic appearance of pseudopolyps may vary from tiny diffuse bumps (left), to large fleshy protuberances with white tips (middle) to scattered pearly 'teardrop' shapes (right). (Reproduced with permission from American Gastroenterology Association, Gastroenterology Teaching Project 002, Inflammatory Bowel Disease, 3rd Edition.)

concluded that in patients with treated ulcerative colitis, the finding of rectal sparing or patchiness should not necessarily indicate a change in the diagnosis to Crohn's disease.

Although deep ulcerations may occur in ulcerative colitis, especially in severe colitis,[2] they are confined to areas of mucosal inflammation. Aphthoid ulcers are never seen in ulcerative colitis. Chronic inflammation often leads to diffuse mucosal atrophy, leaving behind hypertrophic islands of swollen, edematous tissue and granulation tissue that assume a polypoid shape. Inflammatory polyps, known as pseudopolyps, have no malignant potential and occur in both ulcerative colitis and Crohn's disease. As illustrated in Figure 26.2, the endoscopic appearance of pseudopolyps may vary from tiny diffuse bumps, to fleshy protuberences with white tips, to scattered pearly 'teardrop' shapes. Narrowing of the lumen and loss of the haustral folds are seen in long-standing ulcerative colitis, defining the microcolonic appearance. The terminal ileum is usually normal in ulcerative colitis. Nevertheless, patients with extensive ulcerative colitis occasionally have patchy mild inflammation in the terminal ileum, known as 'backwash ileitis'.[12] Furthermore, in so-called 'left-sided' ulcerative colitis distal involvement may be accompanied by more proximal areas of inflammation, particularly in the periappendiceal area of the cecum characterized by reddish mucosa with mucinous exudate.[13] A recent study compared the clinical activity, histologic grade of inflammation and subsequent clinical course in 23 patients with active distal ulcerative colitis with patchy involvement at the appendiceal orifice with that of 17 patients with left-sided ulcerative colitis and no involvement at the appendiceal orifice.[14] Whereas patients with distal ulcerative colitis and involvement at the appendiceal orifice had more histologically active disease, their endoscopic remission rate at 12 months was higher (84% versus 40%, $P<0.05$), suggesting that appendiceal involvement may be indicative of disease which responds reasonably well to pharmacotherapy.

Sigmoidoscopy establishes the diagnosis of ulcerative colitis in more than 95% of cases.[15–17] In a patient with signs and symptoms of colitis (diarrhea, rectal bleeding, tenesmus), a flexible sigmoidoscopy with biopsy and stool studies for ova and parasites plus bacterial culture may be all that is required. This is particularly true if the inflammatory process is distal and the sigmoidoscope can be passed above the inflamed segment. To this end, as well as that of patient and endoscopist comfort, the flexible sigmoido-

scope has virtually replaced the rigid sigmoidoscope or proctoscope. In patients with diffuse inflammation and suspected ulcerative proctitis or proctocolitis, at least two biopsies should be taken above the endoscopic demarcation line to ensure the absence of more proximal disease, which requires systemic as opposed to topical therapy. Although some authors prefer the use of a cupped bronchoscopic biopsy forceps through a rigid sigmoidoscope, small tissue samples obtained through a flexible instrument are equally interpretable and may be associated with a lower incidence of post-biopsy bleeding. To minimize the risk of perforation, the extent of scope passage and the amount of air insufflation should be limited in the extremely ill patient.

## CROHN'S DISEASE

In Crohn's disease the endoscopic lesions are patchy, asymmetrical and heterogeneous.[3,18] Figure 26.3 illustrates the endoscopic appearance of mild and severe active Crohn's disease. Ulcers, whether aphthoid, superficial or deep, are frequently surrounded by normal mucosa. Typically, segments of normal mucosa are interspersed between abnormal areas, a finding that should be confirmed by biopsies. The rectum is spared in approximately 50% of cases. The presence of small ulcerations on the ileocecal valve or in the terminal ileum is virtually pathognomonic of Crohn's disease. While ileocolic fistulous tracts are more frequently identified by barium contrast studies, occasionally coloscopy may reveal the site of entry of a fistulous tract into the colon as descrete nodular excrescences in an area of relatively less involved mucosa (Fig. 26.4) In the setting of Crohn's disease there has been some debate about the best biopsy site to delineate granulomas for definitive diagnosis.[19,20] Incidences of gran-

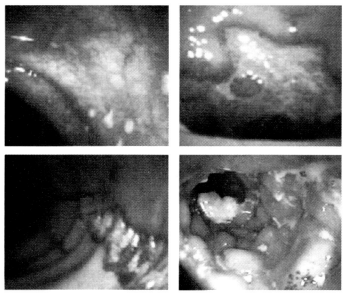

**Fig. 26.3** Endoscopic appearnces of mild and severe active luminal Crohn's disease. The most characteristic early endoscopic lesions of Crohn's disease are discrete 'punched-out' aphthous ulcers with erythematous borders and relatively normal intervening mucosa (upper left). Irregular 'punched out' stellate ulcers (upper right) and long longitudinal ulcers (lower left) are frequently seen in active Crohn's disease. Deep macroulcerations, exudate and nodularity with pseudopolyps all contribute to the luminal narrowing seen in advanced Crohn's disease (lower right). (Reproduced with permission from American Gastroenterology Association, Gastroenterology Teaching Project 002, Inflammatory Bowel Disease, 3rd Edition.)

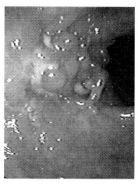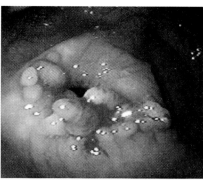

**Fig. 26.4** Endoscopic features of ileosigmoid fistulae in Crohn's disease. Fistulae into the signoid colon often arise from adjacent active ileal disease and may appear on endoscopy as subtle, discrete lesions against a background of relatively less involved mucosa. The site of entry of the fistula into the sigmoid may be marked by a subtle cluster of pearly excrescences to the left of the lumen (left), or the fistulous opening may be more identifiable surrounded by nodular mucosal excresences (right). (Reproduced with permission from American Gastroenterology Association, Gastroenterology Teaching Project 002, Inflammatory Bowel Disease, 3rd Edition.)

ulomata between 16% and 36% have been reported. Whereas some authors recommend three or four biopsies of endoscopically normal rectal mucosa,[19,21] a study by Potzi et al.[20] demonstrated that ulcer biopsies were more likely to demonstrate granulomas (29 of 85) than aphthoid lesions (7 of 32) or cobblestone areas (0 of 21). In this study, histology was consistent with, but not diagnostic of, Crohn's disease in 55% of cases, and non-diagnostic in another 21%.

Whereas barium contrast studies may be complementary to sigmoidoscopy in both diseases, the European Cooperative Crohn's Disease Study noted that only 36% of patients with Crohn's colitis (25% of total) had rectal involvement, and that 39% had isolated involvement above the sigmoid colon.[22] Many of these patients had aphthoid ulcers that would have been missed with barium contrast X-rays. Consequently, ileocolonoscopy plays a more important role in the diagnosis of Crohn's disease than in chronic ulcerative colitis, and ileoscopy should be part of standard colonoscopy in any patient with suspected Crohn's disease.[23]

However, there have been conflicting results when ileoscopy has been compared to small bowel barium studies. During an 18-month period Marshall et al.[24] retrospectively compared the diagnostic accuracy of ileoscopy and small bowel meal with pneumocolon in 48 consecutive patients who had both ileocolonoscopy and small bowel meal with pneumocolon. All ileocolonoscopy reports, radiographs and ileal biopsies were reviewed blindly by paired gastroenterologists, radiologists and pathologists, respectively, and a gold standard diagnosis was determined for each patient by consensus. Fourteen patients (29%) had Crohn's disease, five (10.4%) had lymphoid nodular hyperplasia and 29 (60%) were normal. The sensitivity for a diagnosis of Crohn's ileitis was 93% for ileocolonoscopy and 100% for small-bowel X-ray, and their specificities were 100% and 97%, respectively. The gold standard diagnosis confirmed ileocolonoscopic findings in 45 patients (94%) and radiographic findings in 42 (88%). Agreement between ileocolonoscopy and small bowel meal occurred in 39 cases (81%). By combining histology with ileocolonoscopy, the sensitivity and specificity increased to 100% for all diagnoses. The authors concluded that ileocolonoscopy and small bowel meal with pneumocolon are complementary techniques for imaging the terminal

ileum. In contrast, a recent retrospective study comparing the diagnostic accuracy of small bowel barium examination with that of ileoscopy in 55 patients with Crohn's disease concluded that ileoscopy was superior to barium examination in the evaluation of Crohn's disease of the terminal ileum.[25] Using ileoscopy findings as the gold standard, the sensitivity and specificity of routine radiology reports for detecting inflammatory changes of the terminal ileum by small bowel barium study were 66% and 82%, respectively. Sensitivity and specificity increased to 68% and 91% with double reading by experienced radiologists. The sensitivity and specificity of barium studies were influenced by the quality of the examination, with a sensitivity of 91% and specificity of 100% when the quality was good. The conflicting data comparing ileoscopy and small bowel X-ray may reflect the retrospective nature of the studies, operator dependence, and the variable quality and technique of barium examinations. In a prospective study by Coremans et al.[26] 110 patients with a radiologic diagnosis of Crohn's terminal ileitis were subsequently evaluated with ileocolonoscopy. Twenty-eight (25%) were found to have other causes for their radiographic abnormalities, including nodular lymphoid hyperplasia. The authors concluded that ileocolonoscopy plus biopsy was a valuable tool to confirm the presence and diagnosis of Crohn's ileitis, and can provide useful information about the nature and extent of the inflammation as well as alternative diagnoses for radiological abnormalities of the ileum.

Although the data comparing the diagnostic benefits of initial flexible sigmoidoscopy against initial colonoscopy in adults with suspected inflammatory bowel disease are limited, there are a number of studies in the pediatric and adolescent population.[27,28] A recent nationwide survey assessed practice behavior, procedure charges and costs for either flexible sigmoidoscopy or colonoscopy in pediatric patients presenting with colitis, suggestive of inflammatory bowel disease.[28] The vast majority of survey respondents would proceed with colonoscopy if colitis suggestive of Crohn's disease was noted in the rectosigmoid area (81%), or if ulcerative colitis extended proximal to the rectosigmoid area (70%). If colonoscopy were to follow if flexible sigmoidoscopy suggested either ulcerative colitis or Crohn's disease (67%), then colonoscopy would result in a savings of 23%. If the evaluation was predetermined to be limited to flexible sigmoidoscopy (16%), then flexible sigmoidoscopy was the cost-effective strategy, with savings of 29%. If colonoscopy were to follow flexible sigmoidoscopy for Crohn's colitis only (13%), there was no clear cost advantage. The authors concluded that the most cost-effective strategy depends on the physician's need to know the disease location. When knowledge of disease distribution is not essential for patient care, flexible sigmoidoscopy can lead to substantial cost savings. However, as most physicians want to establish the extent of disease at index endoscopy in both suspected ulcerative colitis and Crohn's disease, initial colonoscopy is the more cost-effective strategy.

# ENDOSCOPIC DIFFERENTIATION OF ULCERATIVE COLITIS AND CROHN'S COLITIS

Ileocolonoscopy plus biopsy not only makes a definitive diagnosis in the vast majority of cases of inflammatory bowel disease, but also helps differentiate between ulcerative colitis and Crohn's

**Table 26.3 Differentiating colonoscopic features of ulcerative colitis and Crohn's colitis**

**Table 26.3 Differentiating colonoscopic features of ulcerative colitis and Crohn's colitis**

|  | Ulcerative colitis | Crohn's disease |
|---|---|---|
| **Nature of mucosal lesions** | | |
| Erythema | +++ | ++ |
| Blurred vascular pattern | +++ | + |
| Granularity, friability | +++ | + |
| Cobblestoning | – | ++ |
| Pseudopolyps | +++ | ++ |
| Aphthoid ulcers | – | +++ |
| Superficial ulcers | + | +++ |
| Serpiginous deep ulcers | – | +++ |
| Strictures | ++ | +++ |
| Mucosal bridges | ++ | ++ |
| **Distribution of lesions** | | |
| Rectal involvement | ++++ | ++ |
| Continuous and symmetrical involvement | ++++ | + |
| Patchiness | * | +++ |
| Skip areas | – | +++ |
| Ileal ulcerations (including ileocecal valve) | – | +++ |

Key: – almost never; + rare; ++ possible; +++ frequent; ++++ almost constant

*With the exception of periappendicular or cecal inflammation and occasionally patients receiving oral anti-inflammatory therapy as well as topical treatment with suppositories or enemas. (Adapted from Bouhnik Y et al. Inflammatory bowel diseases. In: Classen M, Tytgat GNJ, Lightdale CJ, eds. Gastroenterological endoscopy. Stuttgart: Thieme; 2002:575–597.)

disease. A recent Belgian study has confirmed that routine ileoscopy with biopsy is useful in patients with symptoms of inflammatory bowel disease, the main indications being diagnosis of isolated ileal disease in the presence of a normal colon, and differential diagnosis in patients with extensive colitis and predominantly left-sided colitis.[29] However, in approximately 10% of cases Crohn's colitis and ulcerative colitis may look strikingly similar. Table 26.3 outlines the differentiating endoscopic features of ulcerative colitis and Crohn's colitis. Pera et al.[30] prospectively assessed 357 patients who had 606 colonoscopies performed over 22 months and in whom the endoscopic appearances were those of ulcerative colitis, Crohn's colitis or indeterminate colitis. After a mean follow-up of 22 months, a final, definite, endoscopy-independent diagnosis was reached by means of autopsy, surgery, or histology on biopsy in 71% of patients. The accuracy of colonoscopy was 89% and 7% of patients were diagnosed as having indeterminate colitis. Diagnostic errors occurred in 4% of cases and were more frequent in patients with severe inflammatory activity (9%). The most useful endoscopic features in differentiating ulcerative colitis from Crohn's colitis were discontinuous involvement, anal lesions, and cobblestoning of mucosa for Crohn's disease, and erosions or microulcers and granularity for ulcerative colitis. A large population-based cohort of Norwegian patients with a new diagnosis of inflammatory bowel disease (527 cases of ulcerative colitis, 228 cases of Crohn's disease, 36 cases of indeterminate colitis, and 55 cases of possible inflammatory bowel disease) were offered a clinical follow-up in which the initial diagnosis was assessed.[31] After 1–2 years 98% (814/830) were available for follow up, which included a colonoscopy in 77% (637/830). Approximately 17% of the patients presenting with

colitis were reclassified. Twenty-seven patients were reclassified as not having inflammatory bowel disease (3%), and 65 patients were characterized as possible inflammatory bowel disease (8%). Of the patients initially classified as ulcerative colitis, 88% had their diagnosis confirmed, compared to 91% with an initial diagnosis of Crohn's disease. In patients with indeterminate colitis, 33% were classified as definite ulcerative colitis and 17% as Crohn's disease. Although overall the initial incidence was only marginally altered, the study illustrates the importance of endoscopic re-evaluation of the initial diagnosis, as at least one in six patients, including those with a diagnosis of ulcerative colitis and Crohn's disease, were reclassified at follow-up. This uncertainty is especially distressing when surgery is contemplated, as the preoperative diagnosis will in most cases dictate the type of surgery performed. In addition, overlapping features may prevail in young adult patients presenting with acute and very severe extensive colitis.[30,32] In this clinical setting, the usefulness of combined measurements of the serological markers pANCA and anti-*Saccharomyces cerevisiae* antibody (ASCA) needs to be evaluated.[33,34] This situation has been further complicated by the observation that perinuclear antineutrophil cytoplasmic antibodies (pANCA) are a marker for a subset of patients with Crohn's disease whose disease is confined to the left colon and who have endoscopic and/or histological features typical of ulcerative colitis.[35] This is dealt with in more detail in Chapter 29.

# ENDOSCOPIC DIFFERENTIATION OF INFLAMMATORY BOWEL DISEASE FROM OTHER CAUSES OF COLITIS

The symptoms of inflammatory bowel disease are not specific for these diseases and endoscopy plays an important role in distinguishing inflammatory bowel disease from other diseases with similar symptoms. The classic endoscopic features of ulcerative colitis, as well as the typical anorectal features of Crohn's disease, can sometimes be mimicked by several infectious colitides, as well as non-infectious diseases including ischemic colitis, radiation colitis and colitis secondary to NSAID use. Table 26.4 lists the infections that mimic inflammatory bowel disease, the typical clinical and/or endoscopic features, and the corresponding diagnostic tests. Table 26.5 lists non-infectious diseases that mimic inflammatory bowel disease. The differential diagnosis of inflammatory bowel disease is covered extensively in Chapter 25.

Infectious diarrhea with rectal bleeding is common and approximately one-third of patients with mucoid bloody diarrhea and suspected inflammatory bowel disease will have an infectious cause for their diarrhea.[36] Differential diagnosis between inflammatory bowel disease and acute self-limited colitis (ASLC), which is usually infectious in etiology, is particularly important in the case of a severe first attack for which corticosteroid therapy or surgery is contemplated. Distinguishing inflammatory bowel disease from infectious causes requires a careful history, stool studies, and endoscopy with biopsies. However, stool cultures require 48–72 hours, and grow pathogens in only 40–60% of ASLC cases, and patients with inflammatory bowel disease can occasionally have concurrent bacterial infection. The endoscopic features of ASLC overlap considerably with those of idiopathic inflammatory bowel disease.[37] Endoscopic features more common in infections of the

## Table 26.4. Infectious colitis pathogens mimicking inflammatory bowel disease

| Infectious agent | Clinical and/or endoscopic features | Diagnostic test | | Mimics |
|---|---|---|---|---|
| | | UC | CD | |
| **Bacterial pathogens** | | | | |
| Salmonellosis | Mean duration 3 weeks; friabile mucosa with petechiae, may be segmental | + | + | Stool culture |
| Shigellosis | Anal intercourse; patchy, intense magenta-colored erythema, rectal sparing rare | + | − | Stool culture |
| *Campylobacter* | Abdominal pain worse than endoscopic findings; acute like CD/chronic like UC | + | + | Stool culture |
| *E. coli* O157:H7 | Range from non-bloody diarrhea to fulminant colitis; RLQ pain/mass, R>L | + | + + | Stool culture or biopsy |
| Yersinia | Mean duration 2 weeks but 14% prolonged; patchy, R>L, ileal aphthoid ulcers | + | + + | Stool culture or serology |
| *C. difficile* | Prior antibiotics; pseudomembranes, L>R but rectal sparing in 30% cases | + | + | Stool toxins |
| *Klebsiella oxytoca* | Hemorrhagic colitis in association with penicillin, synergistins and quinolones | + | − | Withdraw antibiotics |
| Tuberculosis | No rectal/perianal lesions, transverse/circumferential ulcers, cecal narrowing | − | + + | Ziehl–Nielsen stain of biopsy |
| Gonorrhea | Anal intercourse; proctitis, perianal and low rectal friability and ulcers | + | − | Culture (rectal swab) |
| Chlamydia | Anal intercourse; lymphogranuloma venereum; perianal stricture, abscess, fistula | + | − | Serology, Frei test |
| Syphilis | Anal intercourse; proctitis; perianal vesicles and low rectal ulcers | + | + | Serology, Silver stain of rectal biopsy |
| **Parasitic pathogens** | | | | |
| Schistosomiasis | Travel; extensive colitis, segmental lesions including large proliferative polyps | + | − | Stool exam, rectal biopsy |
| Amebiasis | Travel, immigrants, homosexual, institutionalized; acute like UC/chronic like CD | + | + | Fresh stool for trophozoites, serology or rectal biopsy |
| **Viral pathogens** | | | | |
| Herpes simplex | Anal intercourse; painful proctitis; perianal vesicles, deep ulcers in lower rectum | + | + | Biopsy |
| Cytomegalovirus | Immunocompromised; fulminant R>L colitis, discrete punched-out shallow ulcers | + | + | Biopsy ulcer edge for viral inclusion bodies, serology |
| **Fungal pathogens** | | | | |
| Candida | Immunocompromised, neutropenic and AIDS patients; esophageal > colon | − | + | Biopsy evidence of invasion |
| Aspergillus | Immunocompromised, neutropenic and AIDS patients; bleeding ulcers | − | + | Biopsy evidence of invasion |
| Histoplasmosis | Immunocompromised, midwestern USA; pulmonary > GI symptoms, R>L | − | + | Special stain, culture |

UC, ulcerative colitis; CD, Crohn's disease, RLQ, right lower quadrant; >, greater than; R, right-sided; L, left-sided; GI, gastrointestinal

colon include a yellowish exudate partially or completely covering the mucosal surface, patchy petechial hemorrhage, focal edema, and erythema. Rectal sparing and a patchy and uneven distribution of lesions in the more proximal colon are not found in ulcerative colitis, and should alert the endoscopist to the possibility of an infectious origin.[12,38] Mucosal edema, responsible for the granular appearance so characteristic of inflammatory bowel disease, may also be present in specific infections of the colon. In the evolution of any colonic infection the mucosal response can vary from diffuse involvement to residual patches of inflammation, resulting in the panorama of endo-scopic findings related to the inoculating dose of infection, the aggressiveness of the particular organism in the individual patient, the host's response to inflammation, the duration of infection, and whether the patient is receiving concurrent immunosuppressant or antomicrobial therapy.[12]

Histological examination of rectal and colonic biopsies can be helpful in distinguishing idiopathic inflammatory bowel disease from infectious diseases. However, although biopsies are helpful in the setting of acute or chronic colitis,[3,39] the bowel has a limited repertoire of histologic responses to a variety of immunologic, infectious and vascular insults. Biopsy is therefore

**Table 26.5 Non-infectious diseases mimicking inflammatory bowel disease**

Ischemic colitis
Diverticular disease
Radiation colitis
Solitary rectal ulcer/mucosal prolapse
Drug-induced colitis
NSAIDs
Chemotherapy
Gold salts
Methotrexate
Isotretinoin
Pancreas enzyme supplements
Colonoscopy-related colitis
Oral sodium phosphate preparation
Hydrogen peroxide disinfectant
Glutaraldehyde disinfectant
Miscellaneous
Diversion colitis
Acute graft-versus-host disease
Kaposi's sarcoma of the bowel
Portal colopathy
Cap polyposis

most helpful in defining unexpected pathologies, such as granulomas, pseudomembranes, viral inclusion bodies or amebic trophozoites, rather than excluding the diagnosis of ulcerative proctitis or proctosigmoiditis.[39,40] Surawicz and Belic described seven histological features that have a predictive probability of 87–100% for ulcerative colitis and Crohn's disease.[41] These were distorted crypt architecture, increased numbers of both round cells and neutrophils in the lamina propria, a villous surface, epithelioid granuloma, crypt atrophy, basal lymphoid aggregates, and basally located isolated giant cells. Although one or more of these features was present in 79% of all idiopathic inflammatory bowel disease cases, the study examined diseases of less than 1 month's duration. Hence, the discriminative value of these features may be less for chronic infections. Some causes of colitis unfortunately cannot always be distinguished from inflammatory bowel disease by their appearance on endoscopy. Even with biopsies, it is sometimes impossible to distinguish between inflammatory bowel disease and these other conditions.

Occasionally the history or specific features of examination may suggest that an infectious pathogen is likely. Although a prolonged history of ileocolitis is against a diagnosis of salmonellosis or shigellosis, a small minorty of patients can develop colitis with an average duration of 3 weeks. Similarly, whereas most patients with Yersinia enterocolitica infection have a self-limited course that resolves within 2 weeks, one long-term study reported that 14% of patients were readmitted for abdominal pain or diarrhea.[42] The search for an infectious agent should especially be undertaken in homosexual males or people who engage in anal intercourse, as they are susceptible to infectious proctitis (Neisseria gonorrhoeae, herpes simplex, syphilis, Chlamydia) and colitis (shigellosis, amebiasis). The combination of painful perianal vesicles, mucosal friability and ulceration in the distal 10 cm of the rectum is highly suggestive of herpetic proctitis, although similar findings can be seen with other forms of sexually transmitted proctitis, such as lymphogranuloma venereum, gonorrhea and syphilis.[43,44] Although Mycobacterium tuberculosis, Yersinia enterocolitica and

cytomegalovirus infection can present with patchy, right-sided distribution, including involvement of the terminal ileum resembling Crohn's disease, fistulae, abscesses, stenoses and skip lesions are rare. By contrast, Chlamydia trachomatis, the etiological agent for lymphogranuloma venereum, may be complicated by strictures, abscesses and fistulae similar to perianal Crohn's disease.

# ENDOSCOPIC ASSESSMENT OF DISEASE EXTENT

Definition of disease extent allows categorization of subsequent carcinoma risk in chronic ulcerative colitis and defines the likelihood of therapy per rectum controlling colitic symptoms. Definition of disease extent by colonoscopy may also define the likelihood of surgical success in a patient being considered for large bowel resection for Crohn's disease. Whereas most authors feel that colonoscopy in acute or severe disease risks perforation or precipitation of toxic megacolon, its use in chronic inflammatory bowel disease has become increasingly accepted.[3] It is significantly more sensitive in defining disease extent than barium contrast studies, and even more sensitive when used in conjunction with mucosal biopsy.[45,46] For instance, Floren et al.[47] prospectively colonoscoped patients with chronic ulcerative colitis, defining pancolitis endoscopically in 40 patients but histologically in 70. In 34 of 107 examinations (31%) the disease extent was underestimated by gross visualization alone. Delpre et al.,[48] in turn, demonstrated electron microscopic changes in parts of the colon that were both endoscopically and histologically normal in 15 ulcerative colitis patients. These authors suggested that mucosal involvement is universal in many patients, even without histologic changes on light microscopy. Such reasoning may explain the clinical fact that 5–15% of patients with left-sided colitis develop more proximal disease. Moreover, there is increasing evidence that disease extent in ulcerative colitis is not static but changes with time in approximately half of the patients. This has important implications for initiating cancer surveillance programs. Niv et al.[49] reported on 31 patients with ulcerative colitis, of whom 77% had either regression or extension of disease over a 17-month period. These authors felt that change in disease extent in chronic ulcerative colitis was part of the natural history and not the exception. In the largest study to date, an inception cohort of 1161 patients with ulcerative colitis was examined by actuarial analysis and by multivariate regression analysis of a subgroup of 467 patients diagnosed in 1979–87 for changes in disease extent.[50] The probability for further progression of proctosigmoiditis, evaluated by sigmoidoscopy and radiology, was 53% after 25 years. The probability for regression was 76.8% for left-sided colitis and 75.7% for extensive colitis after 25 years. Age influenced the regression probability in extensive disease.

# ENDOSCOPIC ASSESSMENT OF DISEASE SEVERITY

## ULCERATIVE COLITIS

Quantifying disease severity in ulcerative colitis is less complicated than in Crohn's disease, and several scores have been used in therapeutic trials in ulcerative colitis. Although these scores

**Table 26.6 Endoscopic grading of ulcerative colitis**

| | |
|---|---|
| Grade 0 | Pale clonic mucosa with well-demarcated areas |
| | Fine submucosal nodularity with nodules identifiable beneath the normal-colored mucosa (in healed or resolved colitis) |
| | Tertiary arborization (neovascularization of the terminal arterioles) |
| Grade 1 | Edematous, erythematous, smooth, and glistening mucosa with masking of the normal pattern |
| Grade 2 | Edematous, erythematous mucosa with a fine granular surface |
| | Sporadic areas of spontaneous mucosal hemorrhage (petechiae) |
| | Friability to gentle endoscopic pressure |
| Grade 3 | Edematous, erythematous, granular, and friable mucosa with spontaneous hemorrhage and mucopus in the lumen |
| | Occasional mucosal ulceration |

(Adapted from Baron JH, Connell AM, Lennard-Jones JE. Variation between observers in describing mucosal appearance in proctocolitis. Br Med J 1964;1:89.)

are less frequently used in clinical practice, one of the more widely used is presented in Table 26.6.[51] Although the use of colonoscopy to define the severity of ulcerative colitis is limited in the acutely ill patient, rigid or flexible sigmoidoscopy in conjunction with biopsy remains a fairly accurate way to determine activity of ulcerative proctitis or colitis in more chronic disease.[39] Powell-Tuck et al.[52] cross-tabulated 222 observations of each of 10 symptoms and signs with the sigmoidoscopic appearances in patients with ulcerative colitis. They observed that the subdivision of hemorrhagic mucosae into those that bleed spontaneously and those that bleed only on light touching or scraping was meaningful clinically, and developed an activity index that comprised four variables in addition to the sigmoidoscopic appearance. Subsequently, Seo et al.[53] evaluated the sigmoidoscopic severity and colitis activity index in 37 patients with distal ulcerative colitis, 23 with left-sided ulcerative colitis, and 36 with extensive ulcerative colitis, in which the severity was divided into three categories: grade 1 = mildly active, grade 2 = moderately active, and grade 3 = severely active. The authors found that the colitis activity index correlated well with sigmoidoscopic activity, so that high activity index values with a low sigmoidoscopic severity are thus considered to reflect extensive involvement, whereas a high sigmoidoscopic severity with low activity index values is thought to indicate the involvement of the distal colon. In clinical practice, endoscopic visualization allows the formulation of a treatment plan and provides a means to monitor either local or systemic therapies. Sigmoidoscopic changes often lag behind clinical response, however, and histologic abnormalities may persist 6 months or longer despite an endoscopically normal rectum.[54,55]

## CROHN'S DISEASE

Although the role of colonoscopy in defining disease extent in chronic ulcerative colitis and Crohn's disease is clear, there are conflicting data about its role in documenting the severity of inflammatory bowel disease. There have been several attempts to define an endoscopic index that correlates with the severity of Crohn's disease. Gomes et al.[56] prospectively studied 22 patients and concluded that there was poor correlation between endoscopy and histology and clinical disease indices. Subsequently, the GETAID group developed a quantitative Crohn's disease endoscopic index of severity (CDEIS).[57] To calculate the CDEIS, the bowel was divided into five segments

(rectum, sigmoid and left colon, transverse colon, right colon and ileum) and a numerical score based on surface involvement by disease or ulceration, and the presence or absence of deep or superficial ulcerations was assigned. The method of calculating the index is demonstrated in Table 26.7. Using this index, no correlation was found between the clinical Crohn's disease activity index (CDAI) and endoscopically demonstrated disease. Likewise, no correlation was observed between any laboratory values and endoscopic parameters of activity. The GETAID also evaluated interobserver variation in colonic Crohn's disease and found that whereas pseudopolyps, superficial and deep ulcerations, and stenosis were reproducibly recognized, reproducibility was somewhat less for aphthoid ulcers, and quite low for erythema and mucosal edema.[58]

# ENDOSCOPIC ASSESSMENT OF RESPONSE TO MEDICAL THERAPY

## ULCERATIVE COLITIS

Drug-induced clinical remission is associated with endoscopic and histological remission in approximately 70% and 50% of patients with active ulcerative colitis.[7,59-62] However, there are limited data on whether endoscopic remission delayed the subsequent relapse. A study by Courtney et al.[63] reported a 1-year relapse rate for ulcerative colitis patients in endoscopic remission of 4% (one of 26 patients), compared to a 30% relapse rate (17 of 56) in those with mucosal erythema and edema. Although this study found no correlation between the histological grade and subsequent relapse rate, Riley et al.[64] found that histological activity, particularly features of acute inflammation such as crypt abscesses, epithelial mucus depletion and neutrophil infiltrate rather than lymphocyte infiltrate, were predictive of relapse. Similarly, Bitton et al.[65] prospectively followed 74 patients with inactive ulcerative colitis for 1 year to assess whether clinical, biological and histologic parameters could predict time to clinical relapse. They found that although there were no specific endoscopic features of quiescent disease that helped predict relapse, younger age, multiple previous relapses (for women), and basal plasmacytosis on rectal biopsy specimens were independent predictors of earlier relapse. Hence, repeated sigmoidoscopies and biopsies are usually

**Table 26.7 Format for calculating the Crohn's disease endoscopic index of severity (CDEIS)**

| | Rectum | Sigmoid and Left colon | Transverse colon | Right colon | Ileum | Score | Totals |
|---|---|---|---|---|---|---|---|
| **Deep ulceration**<br>Score 12 if present in the segment<br>Score 0 if absent in the segment | 0 | 0 | 12 | 0 | – | = 12 | Total 1 |
| **Superficial ulceration**<br>Score 12 if present in the segment<br>Score 0 if absent in the segment | 0 | 0 | 6 | 6 | – | = 12 | Total 2 |
| **Surface involved by the disease (cm)*** | 0.0 | 2.0 | 8.0 | 6.0 | – | = 16.0 | Total 3 |
| **Ulcerated surface (cm)*** | 0.0 | 0.0 | 6.0 | 1.5 | – | = 7.5 | Total 4 |
| | | Total 1 + Total 2 + Total 3 + Total 4 | | | | = 47.5 | Total A |
| | | No. of segments (n) totally or partially explored (1–5) | | | | = 4 | n |
| | | Total A divided by n | | | | = 11.9 | Total B |
| | | Score 3 if ulcerated stenosis at any site, 0 if not | | | | = 0 | Total C |
| | | Score 3 if nonulcerated stenosis at any site, 0 if not | | | | = 0 | Total D |
| | | **TOTAL B + TOTAL C + TOTAL D** | | | | = **14.9** | CDEIS SCORE |

(Adapted from Mary J, Modigliani R. Development and validation of an endoscopic index of the severity for Crohn's disease: a prospective, multicenter study. Groupe d'Etudes Therapeutiques des Affections Inflammatoires Digestives (GETAID). Gut 1989;30:983–9.)

The findings at this example colonoscopy were as follows: a) normal rectum; b) presence of non-ulcerative lesions involving 20% of the sigmoid and left colon area; c) 80% of the transverse colon was diseased, including superficial and deep ulcerations; the ulcerations represented 60% of the segmental surface; d) the right colon was incompletely explored, due to a non-ulcerated stenosis, and 60% of the explored right colon was diseased, 15% being accounted for by superficial ulcerations; the ileum was not reached. No ulcerated stenoses were seen at any site.

recommended in ulcerative colitis, and to continue drug therapy until endoscopic and histological remission is achieved.

## CROHN'S DISEASE

Few early medical trials used endoscopic improvement as an endpoint for clinical success. This largely reflected the inability of anti-inflammatory agents and corticosteroids to effectively induce mucosal healing in Crohn's disease. In the European Cooperative Crohn's Disease Study, colonoscopy was performed in 130 of 221 patients from four study centers, but only 52 had repeat procedures at the end of the study period.[22] Although aphthoid lesions and cobblestoning tended to decrease in patients treated respectively with sulfasalazine and combined prednisone and sulfasalazine, no consistent findings were noted and no drug was associated with statistically significant endoscopic improvement. Korelitz and Sommers used sigmoidoscopy and biopsy in a number of patients treated for distal Crohn's disease and found that crypt abscesses, acute inflammation, granulomas and lymphangiectasia improved.[66] Microgranulomas and chronic inflammation were usually unchanged, and fibrosis and edema were actually more common after therapy. In a prospective trial, the GETAID group assessed the value of colonoscopic monitoring of treatment in Crohn's disease.[67,68] Clinical remission was achieved in 136 of 147 patients (92%) with an acute flare of colonic or ileocolonic Crohn's disease (CDAI > 200) who received 1 mg/kg/day of prednisolone orally for at least 3 and at most 7 weeks' duration until clinical remission (CDAI < 150 and a reduction in CDAI of at least 100 points compared to baseline) was achieved. There was clear overall endoscopic improvement, as the mean CDEIS dropped from an initial value of $13.7 \pm 6.4$ to $6.9 \pm 5.5$ ($P < 0.01$), but only 40 of these patients (27%) were in endoscopic remission, whereas the remaining 96 (65%) still had active endoscopic lesions. These 96 patients were randomly assigned to either immediate prednisolone tapering or prolonga-

tion of prednisolone (1 mg/kg/day) for a further 5 weeks. The extra course of prednisolone significantly improved the CDEIS, and 30% of patients achieved endoscopic remission. Nevertheless, the two groups had an identical subsequent course, in terms of both weaning from prednisolone (82% and 80%, respectively) and the cumulative clinical relapse rate 18 months after weaning (69% and 70%, respectively). The outcome for patients with endoscopic remission after the initial phase of treatment was similar. These results suggest that persistent endoscopic lesions in patients with Crohn's disease who achieve corticosteroid-induced clinical remission are not predictive of early relapse. Hence, it appears that endoscopic monitoring of Crohn's disease patients receiving corticosteroids is not worthwhile.[69] However, this conclusion should be qualified by the observation that induction of remission therapy with corticosteroids in this study was not followed by an effective maintenance of remission therapy. Endoscopic monitoring of induction therapy with corticosteroids as a bridge to maintenance therapy with azathioprine, 6-mercaptopurine or methotrexate might be a useful strategy (see below). Preliminary studies have suggested that endoscopic monitoring may have a role in Crohn's disease patients treated with biological agents or long-term immunomodulator therapies. D'Haens et al.[70] performed ileocolonoscopy in 20 consecutive patients with Crohn's colitis or ileocolitis in clinical remission who had been taking azathioprine for a mean of 2 years. Complete healing was observed in 14 of the 20 (70%), and in the ileum in seven of 13 (54%). Histological examination showed disappearance of the inflammatory infiltrate, with a certain degree of architectural distortion remaining. Of 14 patients treated with 25 mg of intramuscular methotrexate for 12 weeks, five had complete colonoscopic healing.[71] This included areas of deep ulceration and pseudopolyposis that occasionally healed into non-obstructing stenoses. Additional patients had significant healing of the colon but were left with ongoing rectal disease, something that has also been noted in patients treated with 6-mercaptopurine. Clinical improvement after infliximab therapy was also accompanied by significant healing of endoscopic lesions, with a good correlation between the changes in CDEIS and CDAI.[72] At the histological level, disappearance of the inflammatory infiltrate was observed in infliximab-treated patients. Recent data suggest that lack of endoscopic remission in Crohn's disease is predictive of subsequent relapse. A subgroup analysis of 19 patients who completed the 54-week ACCENT-1 study demonstrated that if significant mucosal healing can be achieved with infliximab therapy for Crohn's disease, the time to relapse is significantly prolonged.[73] Nine patients who had complete disappearance of ulcers remained relapse free for a median of 20 weeks (range 14–78), six patients who had significant but incomplete endoscopic healing had no relapse for a median of 19 weeks (range 17–50), and four patients who had no healing at all developed clinical relapse after a median of 4 weeks (range 0–8). The authors concluded that endoscopic appearance is a better predictor of the further clinical course than CDAI, and that endoscopic healing should probably become a standard treatment goal in Crohn's disease.

# ENDOSCOPIC ASSESSMENT OF DISEASE RECURRENCE

## ULCERATIVE COLITIS

After total colectomy with ileorectal anastomosis the rectum is at risk for carcinoma, and requires the same endoscopic surveillance as an intact colon. Endoscopy is also useful in establishing the diagnosis of pouchitis or inflammation of the Koch or J, S or W pouch post proctocolectomy.[74] Described in detail in Chapter 46, the cumulative risks for a first episode of pouchitis have been reported to be respectively 15%, 36% and 46% at 1, 5 and 10 years after ileoanal anastomosis.[39] Pouchitis presents endoscopically similarly to active ulcerative colitis, with a diffusely erythematous mucosa. Granularity, loss of vascular markings and friability are common. Although small superficial ulcerations are typical, occasionally deep and sometimes irregular ulcers may be seen. The mucosa of the terminal ileum above the ileal reservoir is normal and there is a gradation of inflammation within the ileal reservoir; this is more severe in the distal than in proximal zones.[75] Endoscopy findings often correlate with both acute and chronic histological changes,[75] which include infiltration of polymorphonuclear leukocytes or chronic inflammatory cells in the lamina propria, crypt abscesses, goblet cell dystrophia, and villous atrophy.[76] The diagnosis of pouchitis relies on clinical, endoscopic and histological criteria,[77] and in some cases may be difficult to differentiate from misdiagnosed Crohn's disease.[78] Minor endoscopic abnormalities may be present in asymptomatic patients, whereas patients with increased stool frequency, urgency and abdominal pain may have no endoscopic abnormalities. A recent study assessed the etiology of bowel symptoms using the Pouchitis Disease Activity Index (PDAI) in 61 consecutive symptomatic patients with ulcerative colitis after ileal pouch–anal anastomosis.[79] Pouchitis was defined as a PDAI score of 7 or more, cuffitis was defined as endoscopic and histological inflammation of the rectal cuff and no inflammation of the pouch, and irritable pouch syndrome was defined as symptoms with a PDAI of 3 or less. All four patients with cuffitis responded to topical hydrocortisone or mesalamine, whereas 12 patients with irritable pouch syndrome

(46%) responded to antidiarrheal, anticholinergic and/or antidepressant therapies. The authors concluded that there is an overlap of symptoms among patients with pouchitis, cuffitis and irritable pouch syndrome, and that endoscopic evaluation can differentiate among these groups.

## CROHN'S DISEASE

Colonoscopy can also be used to assess the development of diversion colitis or recurrent disease in patients who have undergone previous bowel resection for Crohn's disease. Clinical relapse post resection of all diseased tissue has been reported in 33% and 44% of Crohn's patients at 5 and 10 years, respectively.[80] Rutgeerts et al.[81] studied 114 patients who underwent 'curative' ileocolonic resection with colonoscopy. Although 40% were asymptomatic, endoscopy revealed ileal recurrence in about 70% of patients within 1 year after surgery, disease recurrence that was usually missed radiographically. Eighty-eight per cent of these recurrences were at the anastomosis or in the neoterminal ileum. In a subsequent prospective study, 50 patients who had undergone an ileocecal or ileocolonic resection were colonoscoped at a median time of 6 weeks post surgery.[82] Only eight of the 50 patients were endoscopically free of recurrent disease. Most of these recurrences also occurred proximal to or at the level of the anastomosis. The GETAID group reported a 60% endoscopic recurrence rate 3 months postoperatively.[83] Most significantly, the course of the disease was well predicted by the severity of the early ileal postoperative lesions, suggesting that it may be possible to define a subgroup of patients in the early postoperative period who are at high risk of clinical recurrence and are especially suited for prophylactic therapy. Rutgeerts et al. developed a postoperative ileal endoscopic score for this purpose (Table 26.8).[84]

Diversion colitis has been described primarily in the rectal stump and distal colon.[85] Korelitz et al.[86] described 16 patients with Crohn's disease who developed inflammatory mucosal changes in the bypassed segment 3–36 months after diversion. Whereas a subset of these patients was felt to have rectal Crohn's disease, four had mucosal normalization after reanastomosis. Although endoscopic evidence of diversion colitis may be considered unimportant in the absence of symptoms, it is possible that treatment at a preclinical stage, as in recurrent Crohn's disease, may delay or ameliorate the subsequent development of symptoms.

Direct mucosal visualization can also define recurrent disease through a conventional ileostomy or colostomy stoma. It is particularly useful in the evaluation of patients with chronic peristomal ulcers in whom the diagnosis of recurrent or de novo

| Score | Description of lesions |
|---|---|
| 0 | No lesions |
| 1 | Fewer than five aphthous lesions |
| 2 | Five or more aphthous lesions with normal mucosa between the lesions, or skip areas of larger lesions, or lesions confined to the ileocolonic anastomosis (i.e. > 1 cm in length) |
| 3 | Diffuse aphthous ileitis, with diffusely inflamed mucosa |
| 4 | Diffuse inflammation, already with larger ulcers, nodules, and/or narrowing |

Table 26.8 Rutgeert's score for assessing postoperative ileal endoscopic lesions in Crohn's disease

disease is entertained.[87] It may also reveal ileal or colonic varices in patients with cirrhosis secondary to primary sclerosing cholangitis, although periostomal hypervascularity and stomal nodularity are more typically evident.[88]

# ENDOSCOPIC ASSESSMENT OF COMPLICATIONS

Although the recognition of dysplasia as a precursor to cancer in ulcerative colitis and Crohn's colitis supports the rationale for performing colonoscopic surveillance, there remains significant debate regarding the utility (benefits, reliability and cost) of surveillance programs.[89,90] Randomized controlled clinical trials have yet to be performed assessing the efficacy of surveillance, and the appropriate endpoints for recommending colectomy remain undefined.[91] Despite published guidelines and a general consensus that patients with extensive ulcerative colitis for 7–8 years and those with left-sided disease for 15 years should be enrolled in surveillance programs, tremendous inconsistencies exist in clinical practice. The numerous and often conflicting recommendations regarding colonoscopic surveillance for dysplasia and early carcinoma are covered extensively in Chapter 43. These chapters overlap, however, in that endoscopy is often used in the evaluation of local strictures, mass lesions, and acute or chronic bleeding.

In the setting of long-standing ulcerative colitis or Crohn's colitis, mass lesions or strictures are ominous and must be considered malignant until proved otherwise.[3] Direct visualization and multiple biopsies are required. Although some mass lesions are pseudopolyps without premalignant potential, a true dysplasia-associated lesion or mass (DALM) (Fig. 26.5) that does not resemble an adenoma – i.e. a mass lesion, stricture or broad-based tumor – was associated with a 38% incidence of carcinoma (5/13) in one study, a finding independent of dysplasia in the remainder of the colon.[92] Although a true DALM is an indication for colectomy, two recent studies have demonstrated that an adenoma-like DALM can be treated safely by endoscopic

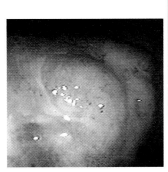
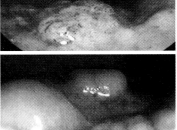

**Fig. 26.5** Dysplasia-associated lesions or mass (DALM). Although some mass lesions are pseudopolyps without premalignant potential, a true dysplasia-associated lesion or mass (DALM) that does not resemble an adenoma, i.e. a mass lesion, stricture or broad-based tumor, is associated with a very high incidence of synchronous or subsequent carcinoma. The finding of any degree of dysplasia in the broad-based, nodular mucosal elevations in these three patients with long-standing ulcerative colitis mandates immediate colectomy. (Reproduced with permission from American Gastroenterology Association, Gastroenterology Teaching Project 002, Inflammatory Bowel Disease, 3rd Edition.)

resection. The studies showed that an adenoma-like DALM in patients with chronic colitis, regardless of its location (either within or outside areas of documented colitis), may be resected at polypectomy just as in non-colitic colons, and followed by annual surveillance colonoscopy, provided there is no dysplasia in the adjacent flat mucosa or other surveillance biopsies.[93,94] In Crohn's disease, the majority of mass lesions tend to be local edema in conjunction with pseudopolyps. In general, only exceptionally large or friable pseudopolyps, or those associated with mucosal discoloration, warrant biopsy.

The use of endoscopy to define the site of acute bleeding in ulcerative colitis is often confined to rigid or flexible sigmoidoscopy, which is used to confirm a disease flare. In Crohn's disease, colonoscopy is often used to define active disease sites associated with a chronic, low-grade bleeding pattern. Occasionally, colonoscopy may help in acutely and massively bleeding patients to attempt endoscopic control of the site or to localize it for the surgeon.[94a]

# ENDOSCOPIC THERAPY IN INFLAMMATORY BOWEL DISEASE

## STRICTURE

The past 15 years have seen an expanding application for therapeutic endoscopy in inflammatory bowel disease, particularly in patients with fibrotic strictures secondary to Crohn's disease. Although most inflammatory strictures will respond to conservative therapy, including corticosteroids, obstruction secondary to fibrotic strictures is the precipitating event for surgical intervention in one-third of patients with ileocolonic disease and half of patients with disease limited to the small bowel, and has a high risk of recurrence following surgical resection. A subset of these patients may benefit from endoscopic therapy, particularly those who have undergone extensive bowel resection. Following the experience with polyvinyl dilators and hydrostatic or pneumatic balloon dilation for ischemic or anastomotic strictures, there have been an increasing number of reports of successful dilation of benign strictures in Crohn's disease. Brower was the first to report successful dilation of an obstructed ileum with a 15 mm balloon, which left the patient asymptomatic for 6 months post procedure.[95] Kirtley et al.[96] subsequently described a single patient with a terminal ileal stricture whose obstructive symptoms were dramatically improved following colonoscopic dilation with a 12 mm balloon, and Linares et al.[97] studied 44 patients with anorectal Crohn's strictures over a 10-year period. Strictures were located in the rectum in 22, the anal canal in 15 and the anorectum in 11, with four patients having strictures at two sites. Thirty-three patients had relief of distal obstructive symptoms with a single dilation using a variety of dilating modalities. Eight patients required two dilations and 10 required more than two treatments. Proctocolectomy was eventually required in 19 of the 44 patients, and three additional patients had various types of diverting ileostomies.

The majority of more recent series report successful dilation with through-the-scope (TTS) pneumatic balloons being passed through the colonoscope's instrument channel, especially in Crohn's disease patients with strictures at the ileocolonic anastomosis (Fig. 26.6). The procedure is performed under direct vision, with dilation of the TTS balloon to a diameter of 18 mm being possible in the majority of cases without compli-

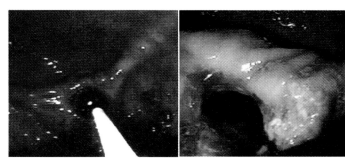

**Fig. 26.6** Balloon dilation of Crohn's disease strictures. Successful dilation of Crohn's disease strictures can be achieved using through-the-scope (TTS) pneumatic balloons passed through the colonsocope's instrument channel. The procedure is performed under direct vision, with dilation of the TTS balloon to a diameter of 18 mm possible in the majority of cases without complications. Duration of insufflation of the TTS balloon in the series varies from multiple 15–60 second inflation periods up to 4 minutes, although longer inflation periods tend to be associated with more pain. One large series reported a success rate of completetly relieving obstructive symptoms in 34 of 55 patients (62%) at mean follow-up of 34 months, with 19 of 55 patients (38%) requiring reoperation for persistant obstructive symptoms. Six of 55 (11%) patients suffered a perforation, two of whom needed surgical intervention. Ileocolonic anastomoses were more successfully dilated, whereas ileosigmoid and ileorectal anastomoses were associated with more complications. (Reproduced with permission from American Gastroenterology Association, Gastroenterology Teaching Project 002, Inflammatory Bowel Disease, 3rd Edition.)

cations.[98] Duration of insufflation of the TTS balloon in the series varies from multiple 15–60-second inflation periods up to 4 minutes,[98,99] although longer periods tend to be associated with more pain. Although immediate symptom relief is usual when the dilation is technically successful, long-term symptomatic improvement is observed in 45–65% of cases.[98,99] Pain during balloon dilation is variable but rarely necessitates additional analgesia. Whereas most series demonstrate that endoscopic dilation of colonic or ileocolonic strictures can be undertaken safely, even in cases of active Crohn's disease, Bloomberg et al.[99] reported moderate bleeding in two patients (7.4%) who were treated with large 25 mm balloons, and perforations in two of 27 patients, both of which required surgical intervention. Although only one of the perforations was felt to be directly related to dilatation (3.7%), the bleeding resolved in both cases without further intervention, but blood transfusions were required. In the largest published series to date, Gevers et al.[100] prospectively followed 55 patients with 59 ileocolonic Crohn's strictures who underwent 78 hydrostatic balloon dilations with Gruentzig balloon catheters. Twenty-eight were ileocolonic anastomotic strictures, seven ileosigmoid or ileorectal anastomotic strictures, 12 strictures of the neo-terminal ileum, three of the terminal ileum, and four of the ileocecal valve. The mean length of stenosis was 4 cm (range 0.5–20 cm). A long-term success rate of complete relief of obstructive symptoms was achieved in 34 of 55 patients (62%); mean follow-up was 34 months. Nineteen of 55 (38%) required reoperation for ongoing or recurrent obstructive symptoms. Six of 55 (11%) suffered a perforation, two of whom needed surgical intervention, whereas the other four were treated with intravenous fluids and antibiotics. Ileocolonic anastomoses were more often successfully dilated, whereas ileosigmoid and ileorectal anastomoses gave more complications.

In another Belgian study, 13 patients with symptomatic strictures were treated with balloon dilation combined with local corticosteroid (betamethasone) injection. Almost all of the patients experienced immediate relief of their symptoms, and none required surgery at 47 months of follow-up.[101] After 52 treatment sessions in the 13 patients, no perforation or any other complication occurred that was directly related to the treatment. In a recent controlled study published in abstract form, Raedler et al.[102] randomly assigned 30 patients with ileocecal ($n=22$) or rectosigmoid ($n=8$) Crohn's disease strictures who were treated with endoscopic dilation to receive either a combination of budesonide and azathioprine or placebo immediately after the therapeutic endoscopy. The budesonide–azathioprine group had a significantly lower symptomatic recurrence rate at 1 year than the placebo group – 20% versus 55%, $P=0.02$. Although the risk of major bleeding and perforation is minimized if one avoids overaggressive or repeated dilation, the best results after TTS balloon dilation are in short strictures with a length of less than 8 cm.[98] Whereas patients with a short anastomotic stricture may be amenable to endoscopic dilation, patients with multiple short stenoses may be better served by surgical stricturoplasty.

## TOXIC MEGACOLON

Toxic megacolon, reported to occur in 2.5% of patients with ulcerative colitis and a smaller percentage of patients with Crohn's colitis, has historically been felt to be an absolute contraindication to endoscopy.[103] Because of successful reports of colonoscopic decompression in Ogilvie's syndrome, several authors have attempted similar treatment in IBD patients with megacolon. Riedler et al.[104] undertook colonoscopic decompression as a preoperative procedure and felt that subsequent colectomy was facilitated. Banez et al.[105] described its use in three patients with ulcerative colitis and a single patient with Crohn's disease, and Hoashi et al.[106] described successful colonoscopic decompression of toxic megacolon in a patient with ulcerative colitis. All had successful colonoscopic placement of a long tube and steroid 'colonoclysis'. The authors stress that their results should not be interpreted as definitive therapy for inflammatory bowel disease-related megacolon, and previous series suggest that approximately half the patients with toxic megacolon will require surgery, three-quarters of these as an emergency.[103] While acknowledging the very significant risk of initiating free perforation, colonoscopic decompression could be considered in the extremely high-risk surgery patient.

## BLEEDING

Acute lower gastrointestinal bleeding is more frequently associated with active ulcerative colitis but is a rare complication of Crohn's disease. Although massive bleeding occasionally occurs in ulcerative colitis and is an indication for coloectomy, most bleeding in ulcerative colitis is secondary to diffuse mucosal friability.[94a] In contrast, most patients with Crohn's disease often have chronic, low-grade bleeding. Major lower gastrointestinal bleeding in Crohn's disease is occasionally the result of deep ulceration into a large vessel, often in the setting of recurrent ileal disease in patients with colectomy or ileostomy.[107] Although data are available that demonstrate that coagulative and injection modalities can stop acute bleeding and prevent recurrent hemorrhage in the upper gastrointestinal tract, there are limited data describing similar modalities for an actively bleeding Crohn's ulceration. Belaiche et al.[108] recently retrospectively reviewed 34 cases of acute lower gastrointestinal bleeding in Crohn's disease. The bleeding occurred during a flare-up of the disease in 35% of cases, and was a presenting feature of the diagnosis in 24% of cases. The bleeding was more frequent in colonic disease (85%) than in isolated small bowel disease (15%). The origin of the bleeding was identified by ileocolonoscopy in 60% of cases, and the bleeding lesion was an ulcer in 95% of cases, most frequently in the left colon. Treatment was medical in the vast majority of cases (almost 80%), assisted by endoscopy in seven patients (21%). Given the potential efficacy of medical or endoscopic therapy, as well as the absence of mortality or significant morbidity, the authors recommended that a conservative approach should be the first-line therapy in the majority of patients. Although therapeutic endoscopy currently has a limited role in active lower gastrointestinal bleeding in the setting of inflammatory bowel disease, there may soon be a time in which a directed anti-inflammatory or biological therapy might be sprayed or injected directly into a chronically inflamed bowel segment.

# UPPER GASTROINTESTINAL AND BILIARY TRACT DISEASE

With the exception of the hepatobiliary manifestations, upper gastrointestinal tract lesions in IBD are limited to Crohn's disease. The exception is a colectomized patient with ulcerative colitis reported by Zimmerman et al.[109] who presented with dysphagia and odynophagia and was found to have multiple aphthoid ulcers of the mouth, pharynx and esophagus. No viral studies were performed. When the esophagus, stomach or duodenum are involved in Crohn's disease, the condition usually occurs in association with disease elsewhere.[110,111] The prevalence of upper gastrointestinal Crohn's disease is difficult to determine, as series are not population based. Jouin et al.[112] carried out endoscopic examinations in 129 patients from a cohort of 195 patients with Crohn's disease. Upper gastrointestinal tract lesions were observed in 28%, with granulomas detected in 19%. Higher prevalences of up to 60% have been reported, especially in children.[113]

## ESOPHAGUS

Esophageal involvement has been infrequently reported in Crohn's disease and may be underdiagnosed.[114,115] Patients with Crohn's disease complaining of esophageal symptoms should undergo upper endoscopy with biopsies. Although there are no specific endoscopic appearances, the diagnosis of esophageal Crohn's disease should be entertained if aphthous or deep ulcers or strictures are present. Strictures, fistulae and mucosal bridging in the esophagus have occasionally been described. Of the 52 cases reported between 1980 and 1986, 80% presented with dysphagia and two had an associated esophagobronchial fistula.[116] Esophageal involvement presents most commonly as aphthoid ulceration (40%), deep and discrete ulcers (21%), strictures (19%), and cobblestoning (6%). In a prospective study correlating the clinical, radiologic, endoscopic and histologic features of the upper gastrointestinal tract in 31 adolescents and children with small bowel or colonic Crohn's disease, Mashako et al.[113] found upper gastrointestinal tract symptoms in only five patients (16%). Endoscopy revealed macroscopic lesions in

13 children (42%) and these were confirmed histologically in 39% (granulomas 39%, non-specific inflammation 48%). Aphthoid ulcerations were most common, but polypoid and inflammatory gastroduodenitis were also seen. Eight patients had esophageal, six gastric and eight duodenal lesions, and most had multiple sites of involvement. These figures are considerably higher than the 1.5–5% incidence of upper gastrointestinal involvement in Crohn's disease reported by other authors.[112]

## STOMACH

Gastric Crohn's disease can cause cobblestoning and thickened folds, aphthoid ulcers, and tubular stenosis of the antrum and pyloric channel.[117,118] More commonly, gastric Crohn's disease is endoscopically visualized as antral or fundal erythema, edema or erosions. In a study of 225 patients with distal small bowel or colonic Crohn's disease, Schmitz-Moorman et al.[119] found erosive or erythematous gastric changes in 49%, and approximately one-third of these had granulomas found on biopsy. Mashako et al.[113] and Danzi et al.[120] reported 19% and 18% incidences of gastric lesions, respectively, in patients with Crohn's disease who were systemically evaluated with endoscopy despite the absence of upper gastrointestinal tract symptoms. More recent studies suggest that systematic upper endoscopy with gastric mucosal biopsy, even in the absence of endoscopic lesions, may be valuable in cases of indeterminate colitis. Completely normal-appearing mucosa may reveal granulomas. A particular form of gastritis characterized by a focal infiltration of CD3+ lymphocytes, histiocytes and granulocytes has been described in Crohn's disease.[121] In another series, focal gastritis had a specificity of 84% and a positive predictive value of 71% for Crohn's disease compared to ulcerative colitis and non-inflammatory bowel disease patients with dyspepsia.[122]

Antral stenosis occasionally requires bypass or, less frequently, resection. Although balloon dilation is widely used in non-malignant pyloric stenosis, limited data are available on either the short-term or long-term results of endoscopic balloon dilation for obstructive gastroduodenal Crohn's disease. Matsui et al.[123] reported on five patients with Crohn's disease who had obstructive gastroduodenal lesions that were treated using endoscopic balloon dilation. Although all initial dilations successfully provided symptomatic relief, three of the five patients (60%) developed recurrent obstructive symptoms during a mean follow-up period of 4.2 years. Owing to symptomatic recurrence, three patients required successive or regularly scheduled repeat balloon dilations, which were successful without any complications, and all of the patients were able to avoid surgical intervention. The authors concluded that patients who have undergone balloon dilation for obstructive gastroduodenal Crohn's disease have a high rate of recurrence of symptomatic gastric obstruction. However, repeat dilations are successful in continuing to prevent the need for surgery.

## DUODENUM

The duodenum has been identified as the most frequent location of upper gastrointestinal tract involvement in Crohn's disease in many studies.[110,117,118] As with esophageal and gastric lesions, reported incidences vary widely depending on the clinical criteria (symptomatic or not) and the investigational modality used. In a review of 89 patients with duodenal Crohn's disease diagnosed between 1952 and 1986, 93% had abnormal radiographs with mucosal thickening, edema, ulceration and nodularity.[124] Claiming an incidence of duodenal Crohn's disease of 1–2%, the authors noted gastric involvement in 60% of their patients with duodenal lesions. They reported various degrees of diminished duodenal distensibility or stenosis; aphthoid, linear, stellate or serpiginous ulceration; and friability in their patients who underwent upper endoscopy. More than 60% presented with upper abdominal pain, weight loss, or nausea and vomiting, and approximately one-fifth had significant bleeding. Thirty-seven per cent of patients had clinically significant duodenal lesions that required surgical intervention.

Gastroduodenal Crohn's disease may be associated with serious complications. In a series of 54 patients, Yamamoto et al.[111] reported that the commonest complications were stricture in 41 (76%), followed by ulceration in four and duodenocutaneous fistula in two. Thirty-three patients (61%) eventually required surgery. Similar severe inflammatory lesions of the duodenal sweep (C-loop) have been purported to be associated with pancreatitis and biliary ductal dilation, perhaps related to involvement of the papillary area of the sphincter of Oddi.[125] Duodenal lesions occasionally fistulize into the small bowel or colon. More frequently, however, it is Crohn's lesions of the distal small bowel that fistulize into the stomach or duodenum, and no intrinsic gastroduodenal Crohn's disease is noted.[126] In contrast, if patients with Crohn's disease are systematically studied despite the absence of symptoms, duodenal lesions are found more frequently. Duodenal involvement occurs most commonly in the first and second portions of the duodenum and consists of spotty inflammation, edema or erosive disease. Lesions have been noted in 26–53% of patients in reported series, with biopsies being confirmatory in a smaller number.[110,113,118]

The preceding data suggest the importance of multiple biopsies in Crohn's disease patients with upper gastrointestinal tract symptoms, perhaps after an initial trial of $H_2$-blocking agents or proton pump inhibitors. Aphthoid ulcers, areas of mucosal edema or erythema and cobblestone areas seem to have the greatest histological yield,[118] although as in the rectum, even biopsies of endoscopically normal areas may reveal granulomas. However, there is no indication to endoscope and biopsy asymptomatic Crohn's disease patients unless it is felt that the information obtained will change the subsequent management.

## HEPATICOBILIARY TREE AND PANCREAS

Although a variety of hepatobiliary tract lesions have been descibed in association with inflammatory bowel disease, primary sclerosing cholangitis presents a particular challenge to therapeutic endoscopy. Consisting of multiple intra- and extrahepatic strictures and ectasias of the biliary tree, and presenting with cholestasis or recurrent cholangitis, primary sclerosing cholangitis is covered in detail in Chapter 44. Primary sclerosing cholangitis occurs in approximately 3–5% of patients with ulcerative colitis and in a smaller number of patients with Crohn's disease.[127] Endoscopic retrograde cholangiopancreatography (ERCP) plays an important role in displaying the characteristic features, including diminished arborization, ectasia and stenosis. Recent studies suggest that magnetic resonance cholangiography (MRC) has replaced ERCP for diagnosis.[128,129] Ferrara et al.[130] recently evaluated the clinical usefulness of MRC in the diagnosis of 21 children with clinical and laboratory suspicion of primary sclerosing cholangitis. In 13 cases (62%) MRC showed abnormalities of the biliary tree that were considered positive for primary sclerosing cholangitis, whereas in eight cases there were no signs of primary sclerosing cho-

langitis. Both MRC and ERCP correctly identified changes in 13 cases and excluded abnormalities in five. MRC had a sensitivity of 81%, a specificity of 100%, a negative predictive value of 62%, positive predictive value of 100% and an accuracy of 85%. The authors proposed that MRC should be the preliminary imaging modality of choice for the diagnosis of primary sclerosing cholangitis in children.

Nevertheless, ERCP will remain useful for biopsies or cytological examination, to exclude cholangiocarcinoma, and for stenting.[131,132] Endoscopy is indicated not only to assess and diagnose this condition by demonstrating the classic appearance of strictures, pseudodiverticula and local areas of ductal dilation, but also to rule out primary and secondary cholangiocarcinoma. The latter may require direct transpapillary brushing or biopsy of a dominant stricture. Endoscopic therapy includes biliary sphincterotomy, balloon extraction of pigment debris, and hydrostatic and pneumatic balloon dilation of strictures using balloons ranging from 4 to 10 mm.[131] Nasobiliary drains have also been placed to allow duct lavage with saline, ursodeoxycholic acid or corticosteroids. In a prospective trial, patients with primary sclerosing cholangitis were treated with biliary sphincterotomy and balloon dilation with or without plastic stent placement. These patients had significantly improved levels of bilirubin and fewer episodes of cholangitis during the 1-year follow-up period.[133] The authors concluded that endoscopic therapy was an effective temporizing therapy in sclerosing cholangitis, although they have since abandoned stent placement because of stent-related cholangitis.

Pancreatitis is a rare extraintestinal manifestation of inflammatory bowel disease. Chronic pancreatitis associated with ulcerative colitis differs from that observed in Crohn's disease by the presence of more frequent bile duct involvement, weight loss and pancreatic duct stenosis, possibly giving a pseudotumor pattern.[134] Diagnostic ERCP has also been claimed to show changes consistent with chronic pancreatitis in 15–20% of patients with primary sclerosing cholangitis.[135] Because it occurs most commonly in patients with the sicca syndrome, a number of these patients have been diagnosed with chronic pancreatic insufficiency. ERCP has been used therapeutically, particularly in patients with recurrent cholangitis or progressive cholestasis and one or more endoscopically amenable stenoses.

# ENTEROSCOPY

The development of new semilong push enteroscopes has improved the diagnostic and therapeutic approach to intestinal diseases, owing to the biopsy and therapeutic capabilities they offer. In Crohn's disease, push enteroscopy is useful in atypical clinical presentations of the disease and for the treatment by dilation of jejunal and ileal strictures.[136] The diagnostic yield of push-type enteroscopy has been evaluated in eight patients with clinical symptoms suggestive of Crohn's disease, but without specific abnormalities on lower and upper endoscopy and small bowel barium contrast studies.[137] Four patients (50%) were found to have macroscopic and/or microscopic lesions of Crohn's disease in the small intestine. In another series, Crohn's disease represented two of 26 diagnoses (8%) in 131 patients referred for unexplanied occult anemia, and 10 of 34 diagnoses (29%) in 110 patients referred for investigations after upper and lower endoscopies and a small bowel barium follow-through in which the findings were considered normal or abnormal but without a definite diagnosis.[138]

# INTRAOPERATIVE ENDOSCOPY

Although the indications for intraoperative endoscopy have diminished over recent years during the development of push enteroscopy, intraoperative evaluation of the small bowel can be accomplished safely by inserting the endoscope in a retrograde fashion from the distal opening of the small intestine up to the ligament of Treitz.[139] Although intraoperative endoscopy revealed lesions missed preoperatively in seven of 20 patients (65%), the additional endoscopic information modified the surgical treatment in only two (10%).[140] A study by Smedh et al.[141] compared the extent of mucosal inflammation evaluated by intraoperative endoscopy with changes in the external bowel wall observed at laparotomy, including creeping fat, mural thickening and serositis. Mucosal inflammation was generally more extensive than serositis ($P<0.01$), but less than mural thickening ($P<0.001$). The extent of creeping fat was similar to the extent of mucosal lesions. The endoscopic findings modified surgical decisions in 20 of the 33 patients (61%). In a prospective study of 21 patients undergoing ileocolectomy, intraoperative endoscopy revealed mild lesions distributed at random along the small intestine 30 cm beyond the resection margin in 10 cases (47%).[142] At colonoscopy performed 12 weeks later, lesions were found in 11 of the 21 patients (52%) between the section margins, and were estimated to be 25 cm over the anastomosis. However, small bowel endoscopic lesions left in place after 'curative' surgery had no influence on early endoscopic anastomotic recurrences in Crohn's disease. A recent study by Esaki et al.[143] corroborated the poor correlation between small intestinal lesions demonstrated at intraoperative endoscopy and risk of postoperative recurrence. In the study, 27 patients with Crohn's disease requiring surgery were examined by both preoperative radiography and intraoperative endoscopy. Intestinal lesions were identified in 23 patients by intraoperative endoscopy, and in 19 by radiography. Longitudinal ulcers were equivalently detected by intraoperative endoscopy (63%) and radiography (56%), whereas small ulcers and inflammatory polyps were less frequently detected by radiography than by intraoperative endoscopy (37% vs. 74% and 19% vs. 33%, respectively). Neither the presence nor the distribution of intraoperative endoscopy findings was related to postoperative recurrence.

# ENDOSCOPIC ULTRASOUND

Anorectal pathology is common in Crohn's disease. Transrectal enodscopic ultrasound (EUS) may provide information about the rectal wall and pararectal tissues. Mucosal inflammation is endosonographically characterized by the preservation of the five-layered wall structure, with superficial thickening of the rectal wall. In ulcerative colitis wall changes mainly involve the first three layers, corresponding to inflammation of the mucosa and submucosa. By contrast, transmural inflammation characterized by focal interruption or loss of the five-layered wall structure may be a distinctive finding in patients with Crohn's disease.[144] In a recent blinded prospective study in 20 normal subjects, 26 patients with ulcerative colitis, 39 patients with Crohn's disease and four with infectious colitis, Gast and Belaiche concluded that rectal EUS could help differentiate acute Crohn's disease and ulcerative colitis, and predict remission in Crohn's disease.[145] During a 14-month period they studied several parameters on rectal EUS, including total wall thickness, mucosal appearance, submucosal thickness, number of enlarged vessels in the submucosa, and number of pathological lymph nodes around the rectum and sigmoid colon. Normal subjects showed some features that were significantly different from those in Crohn's disease or ulcerative colitis patients. A greater number of pathological lymph nodes was characteristic for acute ulcerative colitis, whereas the number of enlarged vessels was increased in acute Crohn's disease. Although quiescent Crohn's disease showed a lower amount of wall thickening than acute Crohn's disease, they found no significant alterations of the five parameters in quiescent ulcerative colitis compared to acute ulcerative colitis.

Transrectal ultrasound can also demonstrate some perianal Crohn's lesions missed by routine proctoscopy, such as pararectal and perianal abscesses and fistulae,[146,147] although magnetic resonance examination provides similar information with less discomfort to the patient. Schratter-Sehn et al.[148] compared endoscopic ultrasound (EUS) with computed tomography (CT) in the differential diagnosis of perianorectal complications in 25 patients with Crohn's disease. They found that EUS was superior to CT in diagnosing fistulae (14 versus 4 correct diagnoses) and inflammatory infiltration of the lower pelvic muscles (11 versus 2 correct diagnoses). Both methods were equivalent in diagnosing perianorectal abscesses, but CT was superior in the detection of inflammatory changes in the pararectal fasciae and fatty tissue that could not be detected by EUS. Although the authors concluded that EUS should be used as the primary method for diagnosing perianorectal changes in patients with Crohn's disease, especially in the case of fistulae and abscesses, having the added advantage of lack of radiation for the patient, magnetic resonance imaging (MRI) has largely superseded CT as the cross-sectional imaging modality of choice for assessing perianal disease. Schwartz et al.[149] prospectively enrolled 34 patients with suspected Crohn's disease perianal fistulae in a blinded study comparing EUS, MRI and examination under anesthesia (EUA). Three patients did not undergo MRI, and one patient did not undergo EUS or EUA. Thirty-two patients had 39 fistulae (20 trans-sphincteric, five extrasphincteric, six recto-vaginal, eight others) and 13 abscesses. The accuracy of all three modalities when assessed individually was 85% or greater: EUS 29 of 32 (91%), MRI 26 of 30 (87%), and EUA 29 of 32 (91%). The authors concluded that whereas EUS, MRI and EUA are all accurate tests for determining fistula anatomy, the optimal approach may be to combine any two of the three methods, as accuracy was 100% when this was done.

Higaki et al.[150] recently demonstrated that catheter probe-assisted endoluminal ultrasonography may predict the occurrence of relapse of ulcerative colitis. In a 1-year prospective study of 23 ulcerative colitis patients who had not suffered a relapse for 1 month, the thickness of the first to the third layers of the rectal wall, as evaluated by EUS at the beginning of the study, was found to be significantly greater in the group who had relapses within a year than in the non-relapse group (mean thickness 2.73 mm vs. 1.79 mm, $P = 0.0001$).

# EMERGING ENDOSCOPIC TECHNOLOGY

A recent innovation in colonoscopy has been the use of chromoscopy. This technique allows better visualization of mucosal lesions by applying dyes to the mucosal surface.[151] Dye-spraying techniques, and fluoresecence combined with magnifying endoscopes, have been used to detect early lesions in Crohn's disease. Using indigo carmine, Okada et al.[152] were able to detect aphthoid ulcers, erythema and small ulcers in 90% of Crohn's disease patients and 0% of healthy volunteers. Incorporating methylene blue into the colonic lavage solution, Makiyama et al.[153] described a worm-eaten appearance, and biopsies of these areas had a high incidence of granulomas in Crohn's disease. Using magnifying colonoscopy in combination with electron microscopy and immunohistochemistry, Fujimura et al.[154] observed a red halo appearance surrounding lymphoid follicles, which seemed to precede visible aphthoid ulcers in the colon of Crohn's disease patients. Maunoury et al.[155] established a method of combining endoscopy and fluorescence angiography to study submucosal microcirculation in the neoterminal ileum after ileocolonic resection for Crohn's disease. Endoscopic lesions were associated with large fluorescent spots corresponding to aphthoid lesions, or fluorescent rims surrounding a dark zone corresponding to stellar deep ulcers. Small spots producing bright fluorescence were distributed singly in mucosal areas that appeared normal at routine endoscopy. These fluorescent spots may indicate increased mucosal blood flow or enhanced transcapillary diffusion of fluorescein, associated with inflammation or genuine microvascular injury. A recent pilot study of 20 patients, including those with inflammatory bowel disease, reported that the use of light-induced fluorescence endoscopy (LIFE) combined with conventional white-light colonoscopy can improve the detection of colonic dysplasia.[156] Of the 22 dysplastic lesions found by conventional colonoscopy 20 were detected by LIFE (sensitivity 91%). However, whereas the specificity of conventional white-light colonoscopy was 80%, the specificity of LIFE was 90% (two false positive results).

In 1984, Makiyama et al.[157] first reported the endoscopic appearances of the rectal mucosa of patients with Crohn's disease as visualized with a magnifying colonoscope.[157] More recently, magnifying colonoscopy was carried out in 41 patients with ulcerative colitis, and the findings in the rectum were graded according to the network pattern and cryptal openings.[158] Magnifying colonoscopy did not detect network pattern in 37% and cryptal opening in 24% of the patients. When each finding was considered separately, there was no correlation with clinical, endoscopic or histological grades of activity. However, when the two features were coupled, patients with visible network pattern and cryptal opening had a lower clinical activity index and lower grade of histologic inflammation than those in whom neither finding could be visualized.

Jaramillo et al.[159] investigated 85 patients with extensive ulcerative colitis with a disease duration of at least 10 years who were taking part in a cancer surveillance program. Using high-resolution video endoscopy and chromoscopy they discovered 104 polyps in 38 patients, 77 of which (74%) were flat.

## CONCLUSION

The major indications for endoscopy in inflammatory bowel disease have been in establishing the diagnosis, differentiating ulcerative colitis from Crohn's disease, defining complications, and defining the extent, activity and severity of disease. More recently, endoscopy has also been used therapeutically. Despite initially being limited to anecdotal reports describing its use for inflammatory strictures and bleeding and small series defining its application in sclerosing cholangitis, there are now numerous reports and published trials highlighting the important role of therapeutic endoscopy in managing the complications of inflammatory bowel disease. Therapeutic endoscopy may ultimately play a role in delivering anti-inflammatory or biological agents, as well as anti-inflammatory gene therapy, directly to local areas of inflamed bowel, and emerging endoscopy technology may significantly improve our ability to detect dysplastic lesions.

## REFERENCES

1. Kozarek R. Endoscopy in inflammatory bowel disease. In: MacDermott RP Stenson WF, eds. Inflammatory bowel disease. New York: Elsevier; 1992:439–451.
2. Carbonnel F, Lavergne A, Lemann M et al. Colonoscopy of acute colitis. A safe and reliable tool for assessment of severity. Dig Dis Sci 1994;39:1550–1557.
3. Waye JD. Endoscopy in inflammatory bowel disease: indications and differential diagnosis. Med Clin North Am 1990;74:51–65.
4. Granqvist S, Gabrielsson N, Sundelin P, Thorgeirsson T. Precancerous lesions in the mucosa in ulcerative colitis. A radiographic, endoscopic, and histopathologic study. Scand J Gastroenterol 1980;15:289–296.
5. Brooker JC, Saunders BP, Shah SG, Williams CB. A new variable stiffness colonoscope makes colonoscopy easier: a randomised controlled trial. Gut 2000;46:801–805.
6. Hunt RH WJ. Colonoscopy, techniques, clinical practice and colour atlas, vol. 348. London: Chapman & Hall;1981.
7. Geboes K, Desreumaux P, Jouret A, Ectors N, Rutgeerts P, Colombel JF. Histopathologic diagnosis of the activity of chronic inflammatory bowel disease. Evaluation of the effect of drug treatment. Use of histological scores. Gastroenterol Clin Biol 1999;23:1062–1073.
8. Odze R, Antonioli D, Peppercorn M, Goldman H. Effect of topical 5-aminosalicylic acid (5-ASA) therapy on rectal mucosal biopsy morphology in chronic ulcerative colitis. Am J Surg Pathol 1993;17:869–875.
9. Spiliadis CA, Lennard-Jones JE. Ulcerative colitis with relative sparing of the rectum. Clinical features, histology, and prognosis. Dis Colon Rectum 1987;30:334–336.
10. Kim B, Barnett JL, Kleer CG, Appelman HD. Endoscopic and histological patchiness in treated ulcerative colitis. Am J Gastroenterol 1999;94:3258–3262.
11. Bernstein CN, Shanahan F, Anton PA, Weinstein WM. Patchiness of mucosal inflammation in treated ulcerative colitis: a prospective study. Gastrointest Endosc 1995;42:232–237.
12. Chutkan RK, Waye JD. Endoscopy in inflammatory bowel disease. In: Kirsner JB, ed. Inflammatory bowel disease. Baltimore: Williams & Wilkins;2000:453–477.
13. D'Haens G, Geboes K, Peeters M, Baert F, Ectors N, Rutgeerts P. Patchy cecal inflammation associated with distal ulcerative colitis: a prospective endoscopic study. Am J Gastroenterol 1997;92:1275–1279.
14. Matsumoto T, Nakamura S, Shimizu M, Iida M. Significance of appendiceal involvement in patients with ulcerative colitis. Gastrointest Endosc 2002;55:180–185.
15. Freeny PC. Crohn's disease and ulcerative colitis. Evaluation with double-contrast barium examination and endoscopy. Postgrad Med 1986;80:139–146, 149, 152–156.
16. Oshitani N, Kitano A, Nakamura S et al. Clinical and prognostic features of rectal sparing in ulcerative colitis. Digestion 1989;42:39–43.
17. Newman SL. Ileoscopy, colonoscopy, and backwash ileitis in children with inflammatory bowel disease: quid pro quo? J Pediatr Gastroenterol Nutr 1987;6:325–327.
18. Allison JG, Brown FM. Majeski JA. Pillars in the colon. Crohn's colitis with unusual endoscopic and morphologic appearances: report of a case. Dis Colon Rectum 1987;30:712–714.
19. Korelitz BI, Sommers SC. Rectal biopsy in patients with Crohn's disease. Normal mucosa on sigmoidoscopic examination. Jama 1977;237:2742–2744.
20. Potzi R, Walgram M, Lochs H, Holzner H, Gangl A. Diagnostic significance of endoscopic biopsy in Crohn's disease. Endoscopy 1989;21:60–62.
21. Surawicz CM, Meisel JL, Ylvisaker T, Saunders DR, Rubin CE. Rectal biopsy in the diagnosis of Crohn's disease: value of multiple biopsies and serial sectioning. Gastroenterology 1981;80:66–71.
22. Lorenz-Meyer H, Malchow H, Miller B, Stock H, Brandes JW. European Cooperative Crohn's Disease Study (ECCDS): colonoscopy. Digestion 1985;31:109–119.
23. Lewis BS. Ileoscopy should be part of standard colonoscopy: a comparison of radiographic and endoscopic evaluation of the ileum. J Clin Gastroenterol 2000;31:103–104.
24. Marshall JK, Hewak J, Farrow R et al. Terminal ileal imaging with ileoscopy versus small-bowel meal with pneumocolon. J Clin Gastroenterol 1998;27:217–222.
25. Tribl B, Turetschek K, Mostbeck G et al. Conflicting results of ileoscopy and small bowel double-contrast barium examination in patients with Crohn's disease. Endoscopy 1998;30:339–344.

26. Coremans G, Rutgeerts P, Geboes K, Van den Oord J, Ponette E, Vantrappen G. The value of ileoscopy with biopsy in the diagnosis of intestinal Crohn's disease. Gastrointest Endosc 1984;30:167–172.

27. Holmquist L, Rudic N, Ahren C, Fallstrom SP. The diagnostic value of colonoscopy compared with rectosigmoidoscopy in children and adolescents with symptoms of chronic inflammatory bowel disease of the colon. Scand J Gastroenterol 1988;23:577–584.

28. Deutsch DE, Olson AD. Colonoscopy or sigmoidoscopy as the initial evaluation of pediatric patients with colitis: a survey of physician behavior and a cost analysis. J Pediatr Gastroenterol Nutr 1997;25:26–31.

29. Geboes K, Ectors N, D'Haens G, Rutgeerts P. Is ileoscopy with biopsy worthwhile in patients presenting with symptoms of inflammatory bowel disease? Am J Gastroenterol 1998;93:201–206.

30. Pera A, Bellando P, Caldera D et al. Colonoscopy in inflammatory bowel disease. Diagnostic accuracy and proposal of an endoscopic score. Gastroenterology 1987;92:181–185.

31. Moum B, Ekbom A, Vatn MH et al. Inflammatory bowel disease: re-evaluation of the diagnosis in a prospective population based study in south eastern Norway. Gut 1997;40:328–332.

32. Price AB. Overlap in the spectrum of non-specific inflammatory bowel disease – 'colitis indeterminate'. J Clin Pathol 1978;31:567–577.

33. Quinton JF, Sendid B, Reumaux D et al. Anti-*Saccharomyces cerevisiae* mannan antibodies combined with antineutrophil cytoplasmic autoantibodies in inflammatory bowel disease: prevalence and diagnostic role. Gut 1998;42:788–791.

34. Ruemmele FM, Targan SR, Levy G, Dubinsky M, Braun J, Seidman EG. Diagnostic accuracy of serological assays in pediatric inflammatory bowel disease. Gastroenterology 1998;115:822–829.

35. Vasiliauskas EA, Plevy SE, Landers CJ et al. Perinuclear antineutrophil cytoplasmic antibodies in patients with Crohn's disease define a clinical subgroup. Gastroenterology 1996;110:1810–1819.

36. Tedesco FJ, Hardin RD, Harper RN, Edwards BH. Infectious colitis endoscopically simulating inflammatory bowel disease: a prospective evaluation. Gastrointest Endosc 1983;29:195–197.

37. Rutgeerts P, Geboes K, Ponette E, Coremans G, Vantrappen G. Acute infective colitis caused by endemic pathogens in western Europe: endoscopic features. Endoscopy 1982;14:212–219.

38. Farrell RJ, LaMont JT. Role of microbial factors in inflammatory bowel disease. In: Regueiro MD, ed. Gastroenterol Clin North Am Philadelphia: WB Saunders;2002 (in press).

39. Fochios SE, Korelitz BI. The role of sigmoidoscopy and rectal biopsy in diagnosis and management of inflammatory bowel disease: personal experience. Am J Gastroenterol 1988;83:114–119.

40. Van Ness MM, Cattau EL Jr. Fulminant colitis complicating antibiotic-associated pseudomembranous colitis: case report and review of the clinical manifestations and treatment. Am J Gastroenterol 1987;82:374–377.

41. Surawicz CM, Belic L. Rectal biopsy helps to distinguish acute self-limited colitis from idiopathic inflammatory bowel disease. Gastroenterology 1984;86:104–113.

42. Matsumoto T, Iida M, Matsui T et al. Endoscopic findings in *Yersinia enterocolitica* enterocolitis. Gastrointest Endosc 1990;36:583–587.

43. Quinn TC, Lukehart SA, Goodell S, Mkrtichian E, Schuffler MD, Holmes KK. Rectal mass caused by *Treponema pallidum*: confirmation by immunofluorescent staining. Gastroenterology 1982;82:135–139.

44. Lebedeff DA, Hochman EB. Rectal gonorrhea in men: diagnosis and treatment. Ann Intern Med 1980;92:463–466.

45. ASGE, AGA, and ACG Consensus Committee. The role of colonoscopy in the management of patients with inflammatory bowel disease. Guidelines for clinical application. Gastrointest Endosc 1988;34:10S–11S.

46. Gabrielsson N, Granqvist S, Sundelin P, Thorgeirsson T. Extent of inflammatory lesions in ulcerative colitis assessed by radiology, colonoscopy, and endoscopic biopsies. Gastrointest Radiol 1979;4:395–400.

47. Floren CH, Benoni C, Willen R. Histologic and colonoscopic assessment of disease extension in ulcerative colitis. Scand J Gastroenterol 1987;22:459–462.

48. Delpre G, Avidor I, Steinherz R, Kadish U, Ben-Bassat M. Ultrastructural abnormalities in endoscopically and histologically normal and involved colon in ulcerative colitis. Am J Gastroenterol 1989;84:1038–1046.

49. Niv Y, Bat L, Ron E, Theodor E. Change in the extent of colonic involvement in ulcerative colitis: a colonoscopic study. Am J Gastroenterol 1987;82:1046–1051.

50. Langholz E, Munkholm P, Davidsen M, Nielsen OH, Binder V. Changes in extent of ulcerative colitis: a study on the course and prognostic factors. Scand J Gastroenterol 1996;31:260–266.

51. Baron JH, Connell AM, Lennard-Jones JE. Variation between observers in describing mucosal appearances in proctocolitis. Br Med J 1964;1:89–92.

52. Powell-Tuck J, Day DW, Buckell NA, Wadsworth J, Lennard-Jones JE. Correlations between defined sigmoidoscopic appearances and other measures of disease activity in ulcerative colitis. Dig Dis Sci 1982;27:533–537.

53. Seo M, Okada M, Maeda K, Oh K. Correlation between endoscopic severity and the clinical activity index in ulcerative colitis. Am J Gastroenterol 1998;93:2124–2129.

54. Dick AP, Holt LP, Dalton ER. Persistence of mucosal abnormality in ulcerative colitis. Gut 1966;7:355–360.

55. Korelitz BI, Sommers SC. Responses to drug therapy in ulcerative colitis. Evaluation by rectal biopsy and histopathological changes. Am J Gastroenterol 1975;64:365–370.

56. Gomes P, du Boulay C, Smith CL, Holdstock G. Relationship between disease activity indices and colonoscopic findings in patients with colonic inflammatory bowel disease. Gut 1986;27:92–95.

57. Mary JY, Modigliani R. Development and validation of an endoscopic index of the severity for Crohn's disease: a prospective multicentre study. Groupe d'Etudes Therapeutiques des Affections Inflammatoires du Tube Digestif (GETAID). Gut 1989;30:983–989.

58. Modigliani R MJ. Reproducibility of colonoscopic findings in Crohn's disease: a prospective multicenter study of interobserver variation. Groupe d'Etudes Therapeutiques des Affections Inflammatoires du Tube Digestif (GETAID). Dig Dis Sci 1987;32:1370–1379.

59. Campieri M, Gionchetti P, Belluzzi A et al. Topical treatment with 5-aminosalicylic in distal ulcerative colitis by using a new suppository preparation. A double-blind placebo controlled trial. Int J Colorectal Dis 1990;5:79–81.

60. Bansky G, Buhler H, Stamm B, Hacki WH, Buchmann P, Muller J. Treatment of distal ulcerative colitis with beclomethasone enemas: high therapeutic efficacy without endocrine side effects. A prospective, randomized, double-blind trial. Dis Colon Rectum 1987;30:288–292.

61. Halpern Z, Sold O, Baratz M, Konikoff F, Halak A, Gilat T. A controlled trial of beclomethasone versus betamethasone enemas in distal ulcerative colitis. J Clin Gastroenterol 1991;13:38–41.

62. Campieri M, Paoluzi P, D'Albasio G, Brunetti G, Pera A, Barbara L. Better quality of therapy with 5-ASA colonic foam in active ulcerative colitis. A multicenter comparative trial with 5-ASA enema. Dig Dis Sci 1993;38:1843–1850.

63. Courtney MG, Nunes DP, Bergin CB. Colonoscopic but not histological appearance determines likelihood of relapse of ulcerative colitis. Am J Gastroenterol 1991;86:243A.

64. Riley SA, Mani V, Goodman MJ. Why do patients with ulcerative colitis relapse? Gut 1991;32:832.

65. Bitton A, Peppercorn MA, Antonioli DA et al. Clinical, biological, and histologic parameters as predictors of relapse in ulcerative colitis. Gastroenterology 2001;120:13–20.

66. Korelitz BI, Sommers SC. Response to drug therapy in Crohn's disease: evaluation by rectal biopsy and mucosal cell counts. J Clin Gastroenterol 1984;6:123–127.

67. Modigliani R, Mary JY, Simon JF et al. Clinical, biological, and endoscopic picture of attacks of Crohn's disease. Evolution on prednisolone. Groupe d'Etude Therapeutique des Affections Inflammatoires Digestives. Gastroenterology 1990;98:811–818.

68. Landi B, Anh TN, Cortot A et al. Endoscopic monitoring of Crohn's disease treatment: a prospective, randomized clinical trial. The Groupe d'Etudes Therapeutiques des Affections Inflammatoires Digestives. Gastroenterology 1992;102:1647–1653.

69. Modigliani R. Endoscopic management of inflammatory bowel disease. Am J Gastroenterol 1994;89:S53–65.

70. D'Haens G, Geboes K, Rutgeerts P. Endoscopic and histologic healing of Crohn's (ileo-) colitis with azathioprine. Gastrointest Endosc 1999;50:667–671.

71. Kozarek RA, Patterson DJ, Gelfand MD, Botoman VA, Ball TJ, Wilske KR. Methotrexate induces clinical and histologic remission in patients with refractory inflammatory bowel disease. Ann Intern Med 1989;110:353–356.

72. D'Haens G, Van Deventer S, Van Hogezand R et al. Endoscopic and histological healing with infliximab anti-tumor necrosis factor antibodies in Crohn's disease: A European multicenter trial. Gastroenterology 1999;116:1029–1034.

73. D'Haens G, Noman M, Baert F et al. Endoscopic healing after infliximab treatment for Crohn's disease provides a longer time to relapse. Gastroenterology 2002;122:100A.

74. Stocchi L, Pemberton JH. Pouch and pouchitis. Gastroenterol Clin North Am 2001;30:223–241.

75. Setti Carraro PG, Talbot IC, Nicholls JR. Patterns of distribution of endoscopic and histological changes in the ileal reservoir after restorative proctocolectomy for ulcerative colitis. A long-term follow-up study. Int J Colorectal Dis 1998;13:103–107.

76. Lieskovsky G, Skinner DG, Boyd SD. Complications of the Kock pouch. Urol Clin North Am 1988;15:195–205.

77. Di Febo G, Miglioli M, Lauri A et al. Endoscopic assessment of acute inflammation of the ileal reservoir after restorative ileo-anal anastomosis. Gastrointest Endosc 1990;36:6–9.

78. Goldstein NS, Sanford WW, Bodzin JH. Crohn's-like complications in patients with ulcerative colitis after total proctocolectomy and ileal pouch–anal anastomosis. Am J Surg Pathol 1997;21:1343–1353.

79. Shen B, Achkar JP, Lashner BA et al. Irritable pouch syndrome: a new category of diagnosis for symptomatic patients with ileal pouch–anal anastomosis. Am J Gastroenterol 2002;97:972–977.

80. Bernell O, Lapidus A, Hellers G. Risk factors for surgery and postoperative recurrence in Crohn's disease. Ann Surg 2000;231:38–45.

81. Rutgeerts P, Geboes K, Vantrappen G, Kerremans R, Coenegrachts JL, Coremans G. Natural history of recurrent Crohn's disease at the ileocolonic anastomosis after curative surgery. Gut 1984;25:665–672.

82. Tytgat GN, Mulder CJ, Brummelkamp WH. Endoscopic lesions in Crohn's disease early after ileocecal resection. Endoscopy 1988;20:260–262.

83. Florent C, Cortot A, Quandale P et al. Placebo-controlled clinical trial of mesalazine in the prevention of early endoscopic recurrences after resection for Crohn's disease. Groupe d'Etudes Therapeutiques des Affections Inflammatoires Digestives (GETAID). Eur J Gastroenterol Hepatol 1996;8:229–233.

84. Rutgeerts P, Geboes K, Vantrappen G, Beyls J, Kerremans R, Hiele M. Predictability of the postoperative course of Crohn's disease. Gastroenterology 1990;99:956–963.

85. Glotzer DJ, Glick ME, Goldman H. Proctitis and colitis following diversion of the fecal stream. Gastroenterology 1981;80:438–441.

86. Korelitz BI, Cheskin LJ, Sohn N, Sommers SC. The fate of the rectal segment after diversion of the fecal stream in Crohn's disease: its implications for surgical management. J Clin Gastroenterol 1985;7:37–43.

87. Wolfsen HC, Brubacher LL, Ng CS, Kayne AL, Kozarek RA. Refractory parastomal ulcers: a multidisciplinary approach. J Clin Gastroenterol 1990;12:651–655.

88. Wolfsen HC, Kozarek RA, Bredfeldt JE, Fenster LF, Brubacher LL. The role of endoscopic injection sclerotherapy in the management of bleeding peristomal varices. Gastrointest Endosc 1990;36:472–474.

89. Bernstein CN, Shanahan F, Weinstein WM. Are we telling patients the truth about surveillance colonoscopy in ulcerative colitis? Lancet 1994;343:71–74.

90. Provenzale D, Onken J. Surveillance issues in inflammatory bowel disease: ulcerative colitis. J Clin Gastroenterol 2001;32:99–105.

91. Zack MM, Ekbom A, Persson PG, Adami HO. Evaluation of surveillance programmes for colorectal cancer in ulcerative colitis patients by case–control studies: methodological considerations. J Med Screen 1997;4:137–141.

92. Rosenstock E, Farmer RG, Petras R, Sivak MV Jr, Rankin GB, Sullivan BH. Surveillance for colonic carcinoma in ulcerative colitis. Gastroenterology 1985;89:1342–1346.

93. Engelsgjerd M, Farraye FA, Odze RD. Polypectomy may be adequate treatment for adenoma-like dysplastic lesions in chronic ulcerative colitis. Gastroenterology 1999;117:1288–1294; discussion 1488–1491.

94. Rubin PH, Friedman S, Harpaz N et al. Colonoscopic polypectomy in chronic colitis: conservative management after endoscopic resection of dysplastic polyps. Gastroenterology 1999;117:1295–1300.

94a. Pardi DS, Loftus EV Jr, Tremaine WJ et al. Acute major gastrointestinal hemorrhage in inflammatory bowel disease. Gastrointest Endosc 1999;49:153–157.

95. Brower RA. Hydrostatic balloon dilation of a terminal ileal stricture secondary to Crohn's disease. Gastrointest Endosc 1986;32:38–40.

96. Kirtley DW, Willis M, Thomas E. Balloon dilation of recurrent terminal ileal Crohn's stricture. Gastrointest Endosc 1987;33:399–400.

97. Linares L, Moreira LF, Andrews H, Allan RN, Alexander-Williams J, Keighley MR. Natural history and treatment of anorectal strictures complicating Crohn's disease. Br J Surg 1988;75:653–655.

98. Breysem Y, Janssens JF, Coremans G, Vantrappen G, Hendrickx G, Rutgeerts P. Endoscopic balloon dilation of colonic and ileo-colonic Crohn's strictures: long-term results. Gastrointest Endosc 1992;38:142–147.

99. Blomberg B, Rolny P, Jarnerot G. Endoscopic treatment of anastomotic strictures in Crohn's disease. Endoscopy 1991;23:195–198.

100. Gevers AM, Couckuyt H, Coremans G, Hiele M, Rutgeerts P. Efficacy and safety of hydrostatic balloon dilation of ileocolonic Crohn's strictures. A prospective long-term analysis. Acta Gastroenterol Belg 1994;57:320–322.

101. Ramboer C, Verhamme M, Dhondt E, Huys S, Van Eygen K, Vermeire L. Endoscopic treatment of stenosis in recurrent Crohn's disease with balloon dilation combined with local corticosteroid injection. Gastrointest Endosc 1995;42:252–255.

102. Raedler A PI, Schreiber S. Traetment with azathioprine and budesonide prevents recurrence of ileocolonic stenosis after endoscopic dilation in Crohn's disease. Gastroenterology 1997;112:1067A.

103. Sheth SG, LaMont JT. Toxic megacolon. Lancet 1998;351:509–513.

104. Riedler L, Wohlgenannt D, Stoss F, Thaler W, Schmid KW. Endoscopic decompression in 'toxic megacolon'. Surg Endosc 1989;3:51–53.

105. Banez AV, Yamanishi F, Crans CA. Endoscopic colonic decompression of toxic megacolon, placement of colonic tube, and steroid colonclysis. Am J Gastroenterol 1987;82:692–694.

106. Hoashi T, Tsuda S, Yao T et al. [A case of ulcerative colitis with toxic megacolon, successfully treated with colonoscopic decompression]. Nippon Shokakibyo Gakkai Zasshi 1991;88:91–95.

107. Bayless TM, Harris ML, O'Brien J. Crohn's disease of the colon. In: Bayless TM, ed. Current therapy in gastrointestinal and liver disease. St. Louis: Mosby;1990:345–350.

108. Belaiche J, Louis E, D'Haens G et al. Acute lower gastrointestinal bleeding in Crohn's disease: characteristics of a unique series of 34 patients. Belgian IBD Research Group. Am J Gastroenterol 1999;94:2177–2181.

109. Zimmerman HM, Rosenblum G, Bank S. Apthous ulcers of the esophagus in a patient with ulcerative colitis. Gastrointest Endosc 1984;30:298–299.

110. Reynolds HL Jr, Stellato TA. Crohn's disease of the foregut. Surg Clin North Am 2001;81:117–135, viii.

111. Yamamoto T, Allan RN, Keighley MR. An audit of gastroduodenal Crohn disease: clinicopathologic features and management. Scand J Gastroenterol 1999;34:1019–1024.

112. Jouin H, Baumann R, Abbas A, Duclos B, Weill-Bousson M, Weill JP. [Esophagogastroduodenal localizations of Crohn's disease are frequent]. Gastroenterol Clin Biol 1986;10:549–553.

113. Mashako MN, Cezard JP, Navarro J et al. Crohn's disease lesions in the upper gastrointestinal tract: correlation between clinical, radiological, endoscopic, and histological features in adolescents and children. J Pediatr Gastroenterol Nutr 1989;8:442–446.

114. Decker GA, Loftus EV Jr, Pasha TM, Tremaine WJ, Sandborn WJ. Crohn's disease of the esophagus: clinical features and outcomes. Inflamm Bowel Dis 2001;7:113–119.

115. Fefferman DS, Shah SA, Alsahlil M, Gelrud A, Falchuk KR, Farrell RJ. Successful treatment of refractory esophageal Crohn's disease with infliximab. Dig Dis Sci 2001;46:1733–1735.

116. Kuboi H, Yashiro K, Shindou H, Sasaki H, Hayashi N, Nagasako K. Crohn's disease in the esophagus – report of a case. Endoscopy 1988;20:118–121.

117. Rutgeerts P, Onette E, Vantrappen G, Geboes K, Broeckaert L, Talloen L. Crohn's disease of the stomach and duodenum: A clinical study with emphasis on the value of endoscopy and endoscopic biopsies. Endoscopy 1980;12:288–294.

118. van Hogezand RA, Witte AM, Veenendaal RA, Wagtmans MJ, Lamers CB. Proximal Crohn's disease: review of the clinicopathologic features and therapy. Inflamm Bowel Dis 2001;7:328–337.

119. Schmitz-Moormann P, Malchow H, Pittner PM. Endoscopic and bioptic study of the upper gastrointestinal tract in Crohn's disease patients. Pathol Res Pract 1985;179:377–387.

120. Danzi JT, Farmer RG, Sullivan BH Jr, Rankin GB. Endoscopic features of gastroduodenal Crohn's disease. Gastroenterology 1976;70:9–13.

121. Oberhuber G, Puspok A, Oesterreicher C et al. Focally enhanced gastritis: a frequent type of gastritis in patients with Crohn's disease. Gastroenterology 1997;112:698–706.

122. Parente F, Cucino C, Bollani S et al. Focal gastric inflammatory infiltrates in inflammatory bowel diseases: prevalence, immunohistochemical characteristics, and diagnostic role. Am J Gastroenterol 2000;95:705–711.

123. Matsui T, Hatakeyama S, Ikeda K, Yao T, Takenaka K, Sakurai T. Long-term outcome of endoscopic balloon dilation in obstructive gastroduodenal Crohn's disease. Endoscopy 1997;29:640–645.

124. Nugent FW, Roy MA. Duodenal Crohn's disease: an analysis of 89 cases. Am J Gastroenterol 1989;84:249–254.

125. Spiess SE, Braun M, Vogelzang RL, Craig RM. Crohn's disease of the duodenum complicated by pancreatitis and common bile duct obstruction. Am J Gastroenterol 1992;87:1033–1036.

126. Jacobson IM, Schapiro RH, Warshaw AL. Gastric and duodenal fistulas in Crohn's disease. Gastroenterology 1985;89:1347–1352.

127. Bernstein CN, Blanchard JF, Rawsthorne P, Yu N. The prevalence of extraintestinal diseases in inflammatory bowel disease: a population-based study. Am J Gastroenterol 2001;96:1116–1122.

128. Ernst O, Asselah T, Sergent G et al. MR cholangiography in primary sclerosing cholangitis. Am J Roentgenol 1998;171:1027–1030.

129. Oshitani N, Iimuro M, Kawashima D et al. Three cases of primary sclerosing cholangitis associated with ulcerative colitis; diagnostic usefulness of magnetic resonance cholangiopancreatography. Hepatogastroenterology 2002;49:317–321.

130. Ferrara C, Valeri G, Salvolini L, Giovagnoni A. Magnetic resonance cholangiopancreatography in primary sclerosing cholangitis in children. Pediatr Radiol 2002;32:413–417.

131. Ponsioen CY, Lam K, van Milligen de Wit AW, Huibregtse K, Tytgat GN. Four years experience with short term stenting in primary sclerosing cholangitis. Am J Gastroenterol 1999;94:2403–2407.

132. Ponsioen CY, Vrouenraets SM, van Milligen de Wit AW et al. Value of brush cytology for dominant strictures in primary sclerosing cholangitis. Endoscopy 1999;31:305–309.

133. Johnson GK, Geenen JE, Venu RP, Hogan WJ. Endoscopic treatment of biliary duct strictures in sclerosing cholangitis: follow-up assessment of a new therapeutic approach. Gastrointest Endosc 1987;33:9–12.

134. Barthet M, Hastier P, Bernard JP et al. Chronic pancreatitis and inflammatory bowel disease: true or coincidental association? Am J Gastroenterol 1999;94:2141–2148.

135. Epstein O, Chapman RW, Lake-Bakaar G, Foo AY, Rosalki SB, Sherlock S. The pancreas in primary biliary cirrhosis and primary sclerosing cholangitis. Gastroenterology 1982;83:1177–1182.

136. Gay GJ, Delmotte JS. Enteroscopy in small intestinal inflammatory diseases. Gastrointest Endosc Clin North Am 1999;9:115–123.

137. Perez-Cuadrado E, Macenlle R, Iglesias J, Fabra R, Lamas D. Usefulness of oral video push enteroscopy in Crohn's disease. Endoscopy 1997;29:745–747.

138. Bouhnik Y, Bitoun A, Coffin B, Moussaoui R, Oudghiri A, Rambaud JC. Two way push videoenteroscopy in investigation of small bowel disease. Gut 1998;43:280–284.

139. Delmotte JS, Gay GJ, Houcke PH, Mesnard Y. Intraoperative endoscopy. Gastrointest Endosc Clin North Am 1999;9:61–69.

140. Lescut D, Vanco D, Bonniere P et al. Perioperative endoscopy of the whole small bowel in Crohn's disease. Gut 1993;34:647–649.

141. Smedh K, Olaison G, Nystrom PO, Sjodahl R. Intraoperative enteroscopy in Crohn's disease. Br J Surg 1993;80:897–900.

142. Klein O, Colombel JF, Lescut D et al. Remaining small bowel endoscopic lesions at surgery have no influence on early anastomotic recurrences in Crohn's disease. Am J Gastroenterol 1995;90:1949–1952.

143. Esaki M, Matsumoto T, Hizawa K et al. Intraoperative enteroscopy detects more lesions but is not predictive of postoperative recurrence in Crohn's disease. Surg Endosc 2001;15:455–459.

144. Shimizu S, Tada M, Kawai K. Value of endoscopic ultrasonography in the assessment of inflammatory bowel diseases. Endoscopy 1992;24 (Suppl 1):354–358.

145. Gast P, Belaiche J. Rectal endosonography in inflammatory bowel disease: differential diagnosis and prediction of remission. Endoscopy 1999;31:158–166.

146. Van Outryve MJ, Pelckmans PA, Michielsen PP, Van Maercke YM. Value of transrectal ultrasonography in Crohn's disease. Gastroenterology 1991;101:1171–1177.

147. Tio TL, Kallimanis GE. Endoscopic ultrasonography of perianorectal fistulas and abscesses. Endoscopy 1994;26:813–815.

148. Schratter-Sehn AU, Lochs H, Vogelsang H, Schurawitzki H, Herold C, Schratter M. Endoscopic ultrasonography versus computed tomography in the differential diagnosis of perianorectal complications in Crohn's disease. Endoscopy 1993;25:582–586.

149. Schwartz DA, Wiersema MJ, Dudiak KM et al. A comparison of endoscopic ultrasound, magnetic resonance imaging, and exam under anesthesia for evaluation of Crohn's perianal fistulas. Gastroenterology 2001;121:1064–1072.

150. Higaki S, Nohara H, Saitoh Y et al. Increased rectal wall thickness may predict relapse in ulcerative colitis: a pilot follow-up study by ultrasonographic colonoscopy. Endoscopy 2002;34:212–219.

151. Kim CY, Fleischer DE. Colonic chromoscopy. A new perspective on polyps and flat adenomas. Gastrointest Endosc Clin N Am 1997;7:423–437.

152. Okada M, Maeda K, Yao T, Iwashita A, Nomiyama Y, Kitahara K. Minute lesions of the rectum and sigmoid colon in patients with Crohn's disease. Gastrointest Endosc 1991;37:319–324.

153. Makiyama K, Tanaka T, Senju M, Itsuno M, Murata I, Hara K. Clinical course and magnifying endoscopic findings of fine lesions of the large intestinal mucosa in Crohn's disease. Gastroenterol Jpn 1989;24:120–126.

154. Fujimura Y, Kamoi R, Iida M. Pathogenesis of aphthoid ulcers in Crohn's disease: correlative findings by magnifying colonoscopy, electron microscopy, and immunohistochemistry. Gut 1996;38:724–732.

155. Maunoury V, Mordon S, Klein O, Colombel JF. Fluorescence endoscopic imaging study of anastomotic recurrence of Crohn's disease. Gastrointest Endosc 1996;43:603–604.

156. Brand S, Stepp H, Ochsenkuhn T et al. Detection of colonic dysplasia by light-induced fluorescence endoscopy: a pilot study. Int J Colorectal Dis 1999;14:63–68.

157. Makiyama K, Bennett MK, Jewell DP. Endoscopic appearances of the rectal mucosa of patients with Crohn's disease visualised with a magnifying colonoscope. Gut 1984;25:337–340.

158. Matsumoto T, Kuroki F, Mizuno M, Nakamura S, Iida M. Application of magnifying chromoscopy for the assessment of severity in patients with mild to moderate ulcerative colitis. Gastrointest Endosc 1997;46:400–405.

159. Jaramillo E, Watanabe M, Befrits R, Ponce de Leon E, Rubio C, Slezak P. Small, flat colorectal neoplasias in long-standing ulcerative colitis detected by high-resolution electronic video endoscopy. Gastrointest Endosc 1996;44:15–22.

## CHAPTER 27

# Pathology of idiopathic inflammatory bowel disease

Robert H Riddell

## INTRODUCTION

This chapter reviews the pathology of ulcerative colitis (UC) and Crohn's disease (CD) and discusses features useful in distinguishing them from each other and from other forms of inflammatory bowel disease. The emphasis throughout is to indicate which features are reliable or relatively definitive indicators of the underlying disease. The literature on the subject is supplemented by personal experience. The complications of hemorrhage, toxic dilatation and perforation developing as a consequence of severe or fulminant colitis, and less severe complications such as inflammatory polyps and benign fibromuscular strictures, are also considered. The role of upper endoscopy in the differential diagnosis of IBD is evolving with the recognition of apparent changes in patients with ulcerative colitis. The pathology of the appendix in IBD, as well as its potential role in the genesis of these diseases, is also included. The important topics of dysplasia and cancer (see Chapter 26) in UC, as well as extraintestinal manifestations of UC (see Chapter 26), are discussed elsewhere.

## BIOPSY DIAGNOSIS OF INFLAMMATORY BOWEL DISEASE

### ROLE OF THE ENDOSCOPIST

The role of the endoscopist is to provide the pathologist with the most representative biopsy tissues for the most accurate diagnosis. The endoscopist must:

1. Be aware of the diagnostic histologic criteria in IBD and in the diseases considered in the differential diagnosis;
2. Provide biopsy samples taken specifically to identify these changes;
3. Indicate to the pathologist the reason for taking the biopsies and which question(s) specifically need to be answered.

There is everything to be gained by the pathologist's arriving at a specific independent diagnosis by looking at slides 'blindly' initially; however, it makes no sense to put a report in the patient's chart without knowing the clinical issues and having some notion of the endoscopic appearances. These can have huge implications for subsequent management, prognosis, cancer risk, ileoanal. For example, when endoscopic features highly suggestive of CD are present, biopsies should document the distribution of disease and any focal tendency, including aphthoid ulcers. A series of biopsies should therefore be obtained, beginning in the terminal ileum at full colonoscopy, or as proximal as possible at flexible sigmoidoscopy, demonstrating inflammation and particularly the presence of ulceration against the background of a relatively normal mucosa from all parts of the bowel viewed. If the endoscope cannot be introduced into the terminal ileum, it may be possible to advance the endoscopic forceps into the terminal ileum and take random biopsy specimens. Also, if endoscopy demonstrates disease limited to one or more segments of the large bowel, then that area should be biopsied, together with the apparently normal mucosa above and/or below.

The rationale for these suggestions can be readily appreciated. Consider a patient with what appears to be proctitis. At flexible sigmoidoscopy the temptation is to take one or two biopsies of the diseased rectum only. If the patient proves to have ulcerative proctitis, the immediate concern is whether they actually have more proximal quiescent disease. Demonstration that the proximal left colon is normal confirms the diagnosis of ulcerative proctitis. However, demonstration of quiescent disease as far as the splenic flexure immediately raises the question of how far proximally the disease actually extends and, if the patient has had similar symptoms previously, of an increased risk of colorectal cancer. In a patient with what appears to be a lesion in the sigmoid with a differential diagnosis that includes CD and ischemia, biopsies of the terminal ileum or remaining colon may provide evidence of inflammatory bowel disease elsewhere, and with documented rectal sparing may firmly exclude an underlying ulcerative colitis.

Throughout, areas of ulceration should be targeted for biopsy, but the art also is to demonstrate whether ulceration is occurring on a background mucosa that is largely uninflamed, a feature that is typical of CD but not seen in UC unless the disease is fulminating. Biopsies of ulcers should therefore be taken from their periphery to include part of the adjacent mucosa if possible. If this is not readily achieved, then sample both normal and abnormal areas with two biopsies from the same site a few millimeters apart, one biopsy from the edge of the ulcer, the other from the relatively normal mucosa. Biopsies from terminal ileum and throughout the large bowel provide the best return in terms of diagnostic accuracy.[1,2]

## ROLE OF THE PATHOLOGIST

To document the correct histologic diagnosis of UC versus CD, fundamental requirements also apply to the pathologist, who needs to understand the following.

- Although the diagnostic features of chronic IBD and its major subtypes UC and CD are not absolutely definitive, certain morphologic combinations are highly suggestive of each of these diseases.
- Other morphologic combinations are so unlike the diseases under consideration in their differential diagnosis as to be readily excluded – a negative but clinically useful piece of information.
- The diagnosis of 'non-specific acute and chronic inflammation' for all biopsies having acute and chronic inflammation is purely descriptive and therefore not a diagnosis, but must be interpreted diagnostically within the clinical context and the information provided by the endoscopist. Nevertheless, combinations of histologic changes are frequently highly characteristic of one or other major forms of disease.

The pathologist has a challenging role. Initially the objective is to examine the series of biopsies and attempt to visualize what the endoscopist has seen in the clinical context and the questions to be answered. It may be advisable to examine a series of biopsy specimens initially without clinical data to reduce expectation bias (for example, if the clinical diagnosis states 'probable CD' the tendency is to look for features to support that diagnosis, rather than to reach that conclusion independently). A common problem is the temptation to report biopsy results descriptively without diagnostic interpretation. Thus, unless granulomas are found, a diagnosis of CD is not considered seriously.

## DIAGNOSIS OF IBD VERSUS NON-IBD

The two criteria used previously for the diagnosis of IBD remain, namely, the combination of architectural distortion indicating prior crypt destruction and a deep plasmacytic infiltrate reaching the muscularis mucosae, usually accompanied by a diffuse increase in lymphocytes. This combination is virtually limited to UC and CD.[3–5] A recent study used multiple logistic regression analysis of 70 histologic features to distinguish IBD from non-IBD and UC from CD. For IBD, the statistically significant histologic features were crypt architectural abnormalities, basal plasmacytosis with severe chronic inflammation, and distal Paneth cell metaplasia. The features of CD were segmental crypt architectural abnormalities and mucin depletion, mucin preservation at the active sites, and focal chronic inflammation without crypt atrophy. For IBD and non-IBD, both sensitivities

### Table 27.1 Criteria for the biopsy diagnosis of Crohn's disease

Large bowel or terminal ileal biopsy granulomas
Aphthoid ulcers
Markedly focal cryptitis
Markedly focal chronic inflammation
Ileal biopsy
Pyloric metaplasia
Acute terminal ileitis, especially without contiguous colonic disease
Jejunalization of villi
Multiple large bowel biopsies
Proximal or focal distribution of ulceration
Evidence of prior proximal or focal distribution of ulceration
Proximal architectural distortion with distal architectural preservation
Random foci of architectural distortion

*Note:* A false impression of focal disease can be obtained from biopsies of inflammatory polyps, granulation tissue at anastomotic lines, and the excess inflammation occurring normally at the ileocecal valve.
*Source:* Modified from Tanaka M, Riddell RH. The pathological diagnosis and differential diagnosis of Crohn's disease. Hepatogastroenterology 1990;37:18.

and specificities exceeded 97%. Probable CD and UC both had specificities of >97%, and sensitivities of 94% and 89%, respectively.[6] This study was for active disease and clearly requires multiple colonoscopic biopsies. Other features useful in distinguishing CD from other diseases are shown in Table 27.1. Diagnostic features are discussed in the following paragraphs. However, it needs to be remembered that all aspects of the pathology are dynamic and that remodeling occurs continuously in all parts of the process, and can therefore change with time as healing and exacerbations occur. Whereas the diagnosis of IBD itself is based on what is almost an 'all or none' series of changes and can be made on a single biopsy if the criteria are present, the distinction of different subtypes of IBD is often more difficult and depends on the distribution of the disease throughout the large bowel as well as specific morphological features, and therefore is much more dependent on a series of biopsies from terminal ileum to rectum.[4,5]

In UC, architectural changes always follow the pattern of active disease and are more pronounced distally. The architectural damage and the severity of the inflammatory infiltrate are highly variable. Such findings in a haphazard pattern document the focal nature of CD and establish the diagnosis. The information obtained in this manner is proportional to the number of biopsies taken, and the 'one every 10 cm' rule works well but also is open to two distinct patterns of misinterpretation. The first is that inflammatory polyps must always be excluded from this assessment, for knobs of granulation tissue can exist in otherwise quiescent ulcerative colitis and lead to a false impression of focally active disease. The second is that some patients with ulcerative colitis by all other parameters have a focus of inflammation in the vicinity of the ileocecal valve.[7,8] The significance of this finding is not clear: apparently it does not indicate either Crohn's disease or total involvement with ulcerative colitis.

Acute inflammation of the terminal ileum only occurs in UC in continuity with active disease of the involved right colon. Isolated terminal ileal disease therefore precludes a diagnosis of UC or indicates that a second disease is present. Pyloric metaplasia indicates prior deep ulceration in CD and is not seen in

UC. Adaptive changes such as jejunalization of villi may be present particularly in CD, but this is unreliable if terminal ileal resection has been performed.

Ulceration in CD is focal and on a background of little or no excess chronic inflammation; ulceration in ulcerative colitis is on a background of an inflamed mucosa. Acute inflammation tends to be crypt sparing in CD, so that neutrophils remain in the lamina propria in CD, but involve crypts, usually diffusely, in UC. Granulomatous inflammation is indicative of CD but unacceptable in UC unless immediately adjacent to a ruptured crypt, or to some other obvious cause. However, patients with CD also have increased numbers of macrophages; conversely, a villous or irregular surface supports a diagnosis of UC.[3]

# ULCERATIVE COLITIS

Ulcerative colitis is an acute and chronic inflammatory disease of unknown etiology but probably reflects a failure to down-regulate what should be a normal immune response. It affects primarily the mucosa of the large bowel with symptoms of rectal bleeding, diarrhea and tenesmus, and is characterized by exacerbations and remissions of bloody diarrhea. Histologically, exacerbations are characterized by a predominantly acute inflammatory process associated with destruction of mucosal elements, primarily epithelial cells. Loss of crypts (atrophy) and/or distortion of crypt architecture are present at all stages of the disease. The rectum is invariably involved. The disease extends proximally in a symmetric manner and, in some patients, involves the entire large bowel and occasionally the terminal ileum, sometimes at the onset. Patients in this group are at increased risk of colorectal carcinoma. The pathologic appearance reflects all stages and complications of the disease, as well as responses to therapy.

Most patients with acute ulcerative colitis develop mild to moderately active disease; occasionally the disease is severely active at onset and may require urgent colectomy.[9] A late indication for surgery is suspicion of colorectal carcinoma. Because colonic resection today is limited to a small proportion of patients who are unresponsive to medical therapy, macroscopic examination of the colon is most frequently a function of the endoscopist, and the material submitted to the pathologist is limited to mucosal biopsies.

## DISTRIBUTION OF THE DISEASE

The distribution of the disease is a useful diagnostic feature for both the endoscopist and the pathologist, especially when the pathologist is provided with multiple, separately identified biopsies. The disease invariably involves the rectum, either macroscopically or with architectural distortion, but if the latter is absent from the rectum it is rarely found proximally. The exception is that in those with diverticular disease a rare patient may have an associated colitis that goes on to apparent typical ulcerative proctosigmoiditis that extends distally over some months from the area of diverticular inflammation.[10] However, there may be apparent changes in the distribution of UC, depending on the activity of the disease. Traditional descriptions of the distribution of ulcerative colitis were made on resected specimens and are not necessarily representative of the ulcerative colitis population in general. In major centers this has been particularly

apparent in patients with quiescent disease undergoing surveillance for dysplasia, when full series of colonoscopic biopsies sometimes are unremarkable, with little or no evidence of prior disease. A similar lack of architectural distortion can be found in patients diagnosed and treated early in the disease, when there has been no time for architectural abnormalities to occur.[11,12] A further potential trap is the finding of a skip lesion with a focus of inflammation around the ileocecal valve, sometimes called the cecal patch.[7,8] Histologically, even in normal patients this is very similar to microscopic colitis with transmucosal plasma cells, but in patients with distal colitis only must not be misinterpreted as the skip lesion of Crohn's disease.

The importance of fully documenting the nature and distribution of the underlying disease cannot be overemphasized. In some patients the disease appears to involve much or all of the colon. In others an endoscopically and histologically indistinguishable disease remains limited to the rectum.[13] A small group of patients develop an apparently intractable proctosigmoiditis, but the histologic picture is identical to that of UC, although more severe histologically.[14] In patients with limited colonic involvement the transition from diseased to normal mucosa usually is gradual but occasionally abrupt. Proximal spread occurs in continuity without intervening areas of uninvolved mucosa, contrasting with the discontinuous pattern of involvement in Crohn's colitis. Variation in macroscopic activity and severity may falsely suggest the presence of skip areas. However, unless fulminant disease is present, biopsies from such skip areas are invariably abnormal, showing chronic inflammation with deep plasma cells reaching the muscularis mucosae (this is normal around the ileocecal valve), architectural abnormalities, or both. Likewise, apparently uninvolved rectal mucosa is occasionally observed endoscopically in the presence of active disease proximally, yet is abnormal when examined histologically.[12] This observation emphasizes the importance of always obtaining a biopsy from seemingly uninvolved mucosa, whether proximal or distal.

## HISTOLOGIC FINDINGS

In UC the spectrum of changes correlates reasonably well with the clinical course of the disease and the endoscopic appearance. Endoscopic examination demonstrates mucosal hyperemia, granularity, friability, ulceration and bleeding, depending on the severity of the disease. Although there is an overall correlation between histology and symptoms, particularly between the presence of neutrophils (active disease) and symptoms, this is not absolute.

Histologically, UC is characterized by two major features (Fig. 27.1) indicative of prior mucosal destruction and chronicity.[15] Paradoxically, CD may manifest similar features, but they are typically focal in distribution.[5,16] Most of the histopathologic findings in UC are limited to the mucosa and superficial submucosa, with the deeper layers being unaffected except in fulminant disease. Features of UC are as follows:

- Alterations of crypt architecture include distortion of crypts, which may be bifid, irregular, reduced in number, with a gap between the crypt bases and the muscularis mucosae. They may also contain Paneth cells distal to the hepatic flexure (proximal to this they are normal) and are usually indicative of prior crypt destruction and subsequent regeneration. These features are most pronounced distally.

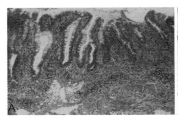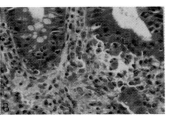

**Fig. 27.1** (A) Active ulcerative colitis. The normal mucosal architecture is distorted with a reduced number of irregular crypts, which also fail to reach the muscularis mucosae. Small basal lymphoid aggregates also are present immediately above the muscularis mucosae. Increased numbers of inflammatory cells are present in the lamina propria. Note the uniformity of the inflammatory infiltrate. (B) Detail of active ulcerative colitis showing neutrophils in the lamina propria, which attack the adjacent crypts.

- Basal plasma cells and multiple basal lymphoid indicate chronicity. Basal plasma cells also may be seen in other chronic colitides, including CD and microscopic and collagenous colitis, but rarely in acute infectious colitis. They can be normal around the ileocecal valve.
- Minor features include hyperplasia of argentaffin cells, mucosal vascular congestion with edema, and focal hemorrhage.
- Features of disease activity include neutrophils with crypt abscesses, depletion of goblet cell mucin and erosions (Fig. 27.1). Shallow superficial mucosal ulcers (erosions) are frequently seen in active disease. Deeper ulcers penetrating the muscularis mucosae into the superficial submucosa are noted principally in severe cases.

## ACTIVE ULCERATIVE COLITIS

### Macroscopic appearance

In active UC, endoscopically the mucosa is typically red, friable and granular, with contact bleeding. In long-standing disease features include erythema, loss of vascular pattern and friability.[17] In milder cases, friability may be evident only when pressure of the endoscope against the colonic wall induces petechiae with oozing of blood. Redness probably is caused by a combination of mucin depletion and capillary dilatation, perhaps also including hemorrhage into the lamina propria. The granular appearance of the mucosa may be due to enhancement of the innominate lines[18,19] as a result of increased cell numbers and edema in the lamina propria. Surface ulceration usually is relatively superficial (erosions) and may be obscured by an overlying mucopurulent exudate. The finding of ulcers indicates severe UC or some other form of IBD. With rare exceptions epithelial destruction in UC occurs against the background of an inflamed mucosa, in contrast to CD, in which sudden transitions from ulcers to normal mucosa are typical. In contrast to CD, a cobblestone-like appearance rarely is seen in UC, produced when inflamed residual mucosa is spared from surrounding anastomosing erosions.

### Histologic features

The mucosal changes in active colitis include:

- Usually some degree of architectural distortion (i.e. not test tube-like crypts).
- A chronic component more diffusely involving the lamina propria, usually with a deep plasmacytosis (remember, this can be normal around the ileocecal valve).

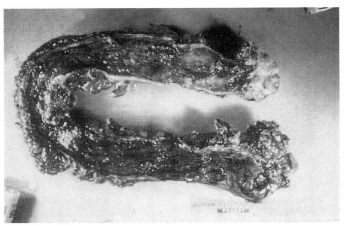

**Fig. 27.2** Haustra-less bowel with marked shortening typical of chronic ulcerative colitis.

- An acute component associated with crypt abscesses – neutrophils invading the crypt epithelium form crypt abscesses that are a characteristic and reliable indicator of activity (Fig. 27.2).
- Neutrophilic infiltration ranges from small accumulations within crypt epithelium (cryptitis) to invasion of crypt lumina (crypt abscess) and ultimately, if crypt ulceration occurs, progression to large intramucosal abscesses that can completely destroy the crypt epithelium and extend into the lamina propria and submucosa. Neutrophilic infiltrate with crypt abscesses is an important characteristic of UC, although not pathognomonic. Crypt abscesses also are a feature of acute colitis of other causes and reflect the activity of the acute inflammatory process rather than the underlying etiology.
- It is unusual in ulcerative colitis for a neutrophilic infiltrate to occur without epithelial invasion, and should lead to consideration of superimposed infection or the possibility that the underlying disease is Crohn's disease.
- Most crypts in a diseased segment show a similar degree of involvement.
- The mid and deeper parts of the crypts usually are the most affected, in contrast to acute infectious colitis, where the acute inflammation affects primarily the luminal epithelium and the superficial portion of the crypts.
- The presence of chronic disease in which isolated crypt abscesses are intermixed with completely uninvolved crypts is more typical of CD.
- Depletion of goblet cell mucin is a characteristic and consistent finding in active UC and, except where dysplasia is present, is another reliable indicator of activity. However, it is not specific and is found in CD and acute infectious colitis. Mucin depletion in UC tends to affect all crypts and is pronounced when there is an intense inflammatory infiltrate. Restoration of normal mucin content, usually beginning in the most superficial portion of the crypts, occurs with resolution and returns to normal levels when disease is quiescent.
- An increased rate of epithelial cell proliferation is reflected in the increased numbers of mitotic figures, from the usual of one per three crypts to one or more per crypt. Epithelial regeneration also may be seen in active disease. When the acute attack is resolving, epithelial regeneration becomes a prominent histologic feature characterized by a decrease in

the number of nuclei (cells) per unit area of crypt or luminal epithelium, and accompanied by atypical nuclei that may be mistaken for dysplasia.[20]

## Grading activity in UC

In clinical practice there is little to be gained from quantitatively grading activity in UC, but it may be useful in clinical trials. When necessary, a six-grade classification system for inflammation has been developed which could also be fine tuned within each grade and appears to have good reproducibility. The grades are:

0, structural (architectural) change only with no excess of inflammatory cells
1, increased chronic inflammation in the lamina propria
2, lamina propria neutrophils
3, neutrophils in epithelium
4, crypt destruction
5, erosions or ulcers.

Initially, κ values between the observers were too low to be useful. Following the development of a semiquantitative pictorial scale for each criterion, κ values improved to 0.62, 0.70 and 0.59. For activity defined by neutrophils between epithelial cells, κ values were 0.903, 1.000 and 0.907. Complete agreement was reached in 64% of samples of endoscopically normal and in 66% of endoscopically inflamed tissue. Neutrophils in epithelium correlated with the presence of crypt destruction and ulceration. This system had modest agreement with the endoscopic grading system, which it complemented, but clearly needs baseline illustrations as landmarks.[21]

# QUIESCENT ULCERATIVE COLITIS

## Macroscopic appearance

The mucosa may appear relatively normal or may be smooth and atrophic. Inflammatory polyps often are present and may be numerous. Small nodules, villous foci or flat plaque-like areas suggest dysplasia and the concomitant risk of underlying invasive carcinoma or a small carcinoma. Shortening and reduction in the diameter of the bowel and bowel thickening are attributed to fibromuscular proliferation, reduplication of the muscularis mucosae, and submucosal fibrosis (Fig. 27.2). These changes are most likely the result of previous severe inflammation and ulceration extending into the submucosa. Radiologic manifestations of these muscular changes include loss of haustra, reduction in transverse diameter, and increased sacrorectal distance. A total lack of haustra ultimately may produce a tube-like appearance. These radiologic findings occasionally revert to normal if the disease remains quiescent for a long period.[22]

## Histologic features

Quiescent disease is variable in its histologic appearances but usually retains the three components, namely: architectural change, chronic inflammation and a neutrophilic infiltrate.

The degree of architectural change varies from minor abnormalities to severe mucosal atrophy, and is related to the severity of the previously active disease. The normal parallel arrangement of closely packed crypts is lost; crypts are reduced in number, more widely separated, and often branched (Fig. 27.3). Shortening of crypts leaves a prominent gap between

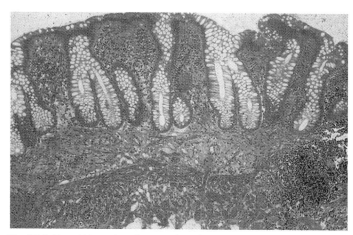

**Fig. 27.3** Rectal biopsy in quiescent ulcerative colitis shows a marked reduction in the number of crypts, whch are distorted and fall well short of the muscularis mucosae. These changes are indicative of chronic inflammatory diseases which have caused full-thickness mucosal ulceration. Similar biopsies can be found in patients with Crohn's disease, with ischemia, or following irradiation.

the crypt bases and the muscularis mucosae. Shortening and branching of crypts are useful in the differential diagnosis frequently seen in UC, less common in CD, and rare in other diseases. Some patients show only minimal loss of parallelism, slightly increased separation and occasional branching of crypts. Complete regeneration of the mucosa, including the crypt architecture, occurs in approximately 30% of patients with ulcerative colitis on maintenance therapy.[11] However, it is unclear whether these patients ever had an unequivocally abnormal architecture. In the quiescent state the goblet cell population is restored to normal and the inflammatory infiltrate is diminished. Neutrophils are usually absent and their re-emergence indicates an increased risk of recurrence, especially during the following 12 months. The risk increases to 75% if crypt abscesses are present.[23] Paneth cells, almost never found in the normal colon except in the vicinity of the ileocecal valve, may appear in any region of the colon or rectum. They are usually located at the base of crypts and are occasionally numerous. Argentaffin cells may also be increased.

## Specificity of atrophic or regenerative changes

These changes are indicative of previous complete mucosal ulceration or crypt destruction. Although idiopathic UC is the most frequent cause, identical changes also can be seen in other diseases, especially CD, chronic ischemia, irradiation damage, or the solitary rectal ulcer syndrome and rarely pseudomembranous colitis or severe shigellosis.[24,25] In resections there is invariably regenerative hyperplasia or duplication of the muscularis mucosae.

There may be hypertrophy of the muscularis mucosae accompanied by separation of fibers. It is generally most prominent in the rectum, where the muscularis mucosae is normally thickest (Fig.27.3). Repeated episodes of activity may produce a multilayered muscularis mucosae, which may be a factor in the benign strictures observed in UC.[26] Similar thickening of the muscularis mucosae is present in chronic colitides of other etiologies and thus represents a non-specific feature of chronic inflammation of the colon.

# LESS COMMON FINDINGS ON BIOPSY

Although the patterns described above are classic, exceptions occur. Further, these exceptions have clinical and therapeutic significance, as discussed in the following paragraphs.

## Lack of atrophic or regenerative changes

The finding of an atrophic mucosa with typical regenerative features in patients with long-standing UC is always reassuring because it tends to confirm the correctness of that diagnosis. Further, in patients who are being investigated for bloody diarrhea, the presence of these features with the addition of acute inflammatory changes involving the crypts is strong supportive evidence of UC.[15,27] Nevertheless, such changes are not always present in patients with known UC. For example:

- Patients with active disease treated very promptly may not develop the crypt destruction or erosions that result in architectural distortion. Resolution of the inflammation therefore may result in a return to normal mucosa. In a first attack in particular there may have been insufficient time for architectural distortion to have taken place.[11]
- In patients with known extensive or total disease previously and either radiologic or endoscopic evidence of activity, only distal biopsies may show typical changes. This finding implies that the extent of disease needs to be assessed relatively early after a flare so that patients at subsequent cancer risk are identified.
- In patients with quiescent disease for long periods – often a decade or more – biopsies from all parts of the large bowel may fail to show regenerative changes. This finding has been documented in rectal biopsies.[23]
- In patients developing carcinoma in UC, not only may there be no regenerative changes, but crypts may be packed tightly together. Apparently the architectural changes so typical of UC either never develop in some patients or reflect the ability of the mucosa over time to revert to a more normal pattern. A further possibility is that there is a trophic growth factor at work, possibly gastrin-like, that results in hypertrophy and hyperplasia of crypts and possibly facilitates the development of dysplasia or carcinoma. Persistent Paneth cell metaplasia may be the only marker of previous disease, but even this may be absent.
- In the pediatric population the initial presentation is frequently atypical, and the first series of colonoscopic biopsies are sometimes difficult to distinguish from infectious colitis. Rectal sparing may also be part of this picture.[28,29]
- In some patients diverticular-associated inflammation can extend distally, subsequently producing a picture indistinguishable from that of ulcerative colitis.[10] Such patients may therefore initially have entirely normal rectal biopsies.

The importance of recognizing apparently normal rectal biopsies is to be aware that lack of architectural changes can never completely exclude underlying IBD. That is, because involved bowel may be architecturally normal, quiescent colitis in biopsies may fail to show architectural changes. Conversely, pathologists must not overinterpret this lack of microscopic involvement to suggest that the patient never had UC. Nevertheless, patients undergoing periodic surveillance colonoscopy who change their clinician clearly need some evidence of their former colitis, especially prior biopsy documentation, provided to their new gastroenterologist.

## Follicular proctitis

Typically, in active ulcerative colitis a chronic inflammatory infiltrate, composed mostly of lymphocytes and plasma cells, accompanied by variable numbers of eosinophils and mast cells, extends diffusely throughout the lamina propria. Indeed, the presence of basal lymphoid or plasma cell aggregates (Fig. 27.1) is very useful in distinguishing IBD from acute infectious colitis, in which it is not seen. In the normal colonic mucosa occasional lymphoid follicles are present adjacent to or straddling the muscularis mucosae. In some diseases the follicles may become large and numerous in the rectum and, less commonly, throughout the colon. They are invariably situated above the muscularis mucosae, a pattern designated as follicular proctitis or colitis and often accompanied by regenerative epithelium. This finding is usually a variant of active UC and resolves with therapy. However, it also is found in diversion disease, and at most centers diversion disease is by far the most common cause of follicular proctitis. However, it can also be seen in UC, CD, infectious colitis from *Chlamydia* or lymphogranuloma venereum, and in some instances is idiopathic.[30] Despite a clinical similarity to ulcerative proctitis or colitis, patients with lymphoid follicular proctitis unresponsive to UC therapy have biopsies not typical of UC (no architectural distortion or neutrophilic infiltrate).[31]

## Eosinophils dominating biopsies

The intensity of inflammation in UC varies, particularly during the resolving phase of the disease, and may result in a patchy distribution but not the clearly focal distribution of CD.[12,32] Eosinophils may be so numerous in treated ulcerative colitis that they completely dominate the lamina propria inflammation, particularly when the disease is quiescent, and may lead to the descriptive diagnosis of eosinophilic colitis. Eosinophilic colitis in patients not having IBD is a relatively poorly described entity[9,33] and is far less common than ulcerative colitis. Because many eosinophils are found throughout the gastrointestinal tract in inflammatory bowel disease of both major types, a correlation with therapy has been suggested.[9] Allergic proctitis, most common in children, usually is the result of allergy to cow's milk, soy protein or both, and in this situation the architectural changes of UC are absent.[34] Clinically, this condition is often accompanied by a peripheral eosinophilia and is steroid responsive.[9,35] A pericrypt eosinophilic infiltrate may be seen in patients with connective tissue disorders[36] and in those with allergic reactions to non-steroidal anti-inflammatory drugs (NSAIDs).[37] An eosinophilic cryptitis also has been noted in acute radiation colitis and in several other conditions, such as food allergy, parasitic infection with *Strongyloides*, *Ascaris* or *Enterobius*, UC, CD, reactive arthropathies, and in some instances as an idiopathic condition. Eosinophils are common in all biopsies of patients with IBD, including duodenal and terminal ileal biopsies. It is a moot point as to whether this might reflect a low-grade reaction to sulfas used for therapy, but as it can be seen in patients not undergoing therapy,[1] as well as experimentally,[38] it seems to be an intrinsic part of the disease.

## Granulomas

A recurring question is whether the presence of granulomas is consistent with ulcerative colitis. One rule of thumb is that well-formed sarcoid-like granulomas are not part of the spectrum of ulcerative colitis, and if they are present an alternative explanation must be found. However, crypt abscesses may rupture, causing extravasation of mucin into the lamina propria, and this rupture can elicit foreign body giant cells and a few histiocytes.[32,39] Sarcoid-like granulomas are very rare, although a mucin stain, such as alcian blue at pH 2.5, PAS, or a combination of the two, is worth performing if there is a suspicion that a 'granuloma' may have developed after extravasation of mucin. The finding of granulomas therefore requires the exclusion of other diseases known to result in granuloma formation. Granulomas immediately adjacent to foci of acute inflammation, usually ulcers, may represent a response to foreign material. Occasional giant cells can be found in all subtypes of IBD and are therefore unhelpful except for prompting a search for well-formed granulomas.[39]

## CECAL PATCH

It has long been recognized that patients with distal UC may have a focus of acute inflammation in the ileocecal region.[40] This is of interest given the frequent involvement of the appendix as a skip lesion in fulminant disease and the potential protective effect of appendectomy for UC (see Chapter 17). It is important to recognize that this does not imply total involvement of the large bowel, an increased cancer risk, or a skip lesion of CD.[7,8] However, in one series a discontinuous cecal/periappendiceal lesion was found in about 20% of patients, and in 80% of these had similar activity to the distal disease; the patients also tended to be younger and have a longer history than those without the lesion.[41]

## CHANGES FOLLOWING THERAPY, PATCHINESS AND RELATIVE RECTAL SPARING

Neutrophils disappear as the acute inflammation subsides, but may persist in and around the crypts in the early stages of resolution. As the epithelium matures, the goblet cell population is restored and mitotic figures decrease. The final feature of resolution is the gradual decline in the diffuse infiltrate of lymphocytes and plasma cells. Uneven resolution of chronic inflammation may produce a patchy infiltrate that could be misinterpreted as CD. However, in ulcerative colitis marked focal change is unusual, and erosions with virtually normal adjacent mucosa are only seen in UC when fulminant disease is present or a nodule of granulation is biopsied and, as such, is a good marker of Crohn's disease. Complete histologic resolution may take several months after the symptoms have subsided and the endoscopic appearance has returned to normal. In some patients low-grade activity persists endoscopically and histologically. However, healing may be distinctly patchy, not only with rectal healing occurring initially with therapy, resulting in relative rectal sparing, but with some degree of patchiness in the remainder of the large bowel.[11,42-44] The difficulty is in knowing how much focality is permissible before a diagnosis of Crohn's disease should be seriously entertained. My personal opinion is that one needs an erosion or marked focal chronic active inflammation in one part of the biopsy with adjacent virtually normal mucosa in the same biopsy to consider CD seriously. Similar changes are only seen in UC if fulminant disease is present (see subsequent discussion).

## FULMINANT COLITIS

Some patients with UC experience a particularly severe or fulminant episode that is unresponsive to intensive medical therapy and accompanied by massive uncontrollable hemorrhage or toxic

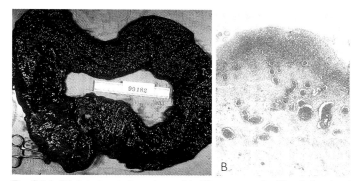

**Fig. 27.4** (A) Fulminant ulcerative colitis. The mucosa is diffusely involved down to the anorectal junction (bottom right). (B) Histology of fulminant colitis, here showing complete denudation of the mucosa and submucosa and myocytolysis of the muscularis propria. The amount of inflammation can vary from minimal, as seen here, to pronounced.

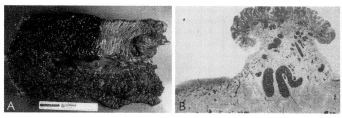

**Fig. 27.5** (A) Fulminant ulcerative colitis with mucosal islands. The deep ulcers extend down to the muscularis propria, leaving islands of residual mucosa with a polypoid configuration – 'true' pseudopolyps. (B) Pseudopolyp, created by deep ulceration into the submucosa, the 'polyp' being formed by an island of residual mucosa.

dilatation requiring urgent colectomy. These fulminant attacks tend to occur early in the course of the disease but occasionally develop in patients with long-standing colitis. Ulcerative colitis confined to the mucosa rarely, if ever, causes illness sufficiently severe to require colectomy.[45] Severe UC always includes rectosigmoid involvement with variable degrees of proximal extension in continuity. The resected bowel from such cases has become the source of most of the macroscopic descriptions of UC. Examination of resected specimens demonstrates only minimal external changes, as might be expected in a disease that predominantly involves the mucosa. In contrast to the minimal change on the serosal surface, the mucosal changes are dramatic (Fig. 27.4). The most severely involved mucosa is dark red or purple, hemorrhagic and friable, with extensive ulceration; it is covered with a mixture of blood, mucus, pus, necrotic debris and liquid stool. Extensive, deep ulcerations, exposing the underlying submucosa or circular internal portion of the muscularis propria, are common. Confluence of ulcers produces longitudinal furrows with residual isolated polypoid islands of mucosa (Fig. 27.5). This perhaps is the only occasion when the term 'pseudopolyp' is appropriate. Because of the ambiguity of the term 'polyp' the designation 'mucosal islands' is preferred. Deep fissuring, more characteristic of CD, is rarely seen except in toxic dilatation. A confusing but rare change endoscopically is apparent rectal sparing with an irregular and patchy transition to active disease, suggesting CD. Histologic examination demonstrates the characteristic findings of ulcerative colitis architecturally, but variable inflammation (Fig. 27.4A).

Histologically, the inflammatory infiltrate is frequently restricted to the mucosa and submucosa. Extension of disease that exposes the muscularis propria tends to be focal and inter-mixed with residual areas of mucosa. Occasionally, patients with severe active UC, without toxic dilatation, are unresponsive to medical therapy such as cyclosporin, and may be complicated by colonic perforation. Focal cleft-like extension of the mucosal ulcers into and through the muscularis propria creates potential sites of perforation. The penetration of the muscularis propria is usually less extensive than in toxic megacolon, and the mus-cular inflammation and destruction are confined to the imme-diate vicinity of the deep ulcers. Unlike in patients with toxic megacolon, the inflammatory infiltrate tends to be more promi-nent in relation to the degree of vascular dilatation. V-shaped ulcers in fulminant UC may penetrate into, although rarely through, the muscularis propria and may be interpreted as the transmural inflammation of CD. These ulcers can be found in the very active or fulminant phase of any of the inflammatory diseases, and therefore are not specific. They may be accompa-nied by a chronic inflammatory infiltrate which, if it extends through the muscularis propria, generally can be incorporated into the term 'transmural inflammation', even though the hyper-plastic lymphoid aggregates so characteristic of CD are absent (see subsequent discussion of Crohn's disease).

Changes in the remainder of the submucosa usually are limited to vascular dilatation and edema. Fibrosis, lymphocytic aggregates and other features of CD are absent. Occasional foreign body granulomas may be found adjacent to deep ulcers that extend into the submucosa, one of the few occasions when granulomas may be seen in UC. These granulomas should not be confused with the sarcoid-like granulomas seen in CD, which are independent of overlying ulcers. The foreign body granulo-mas in UC are usually associated with foreign material, identifiable by the use of polarized light. Occasionally a diffuse submucosal periarteritis-like vasculitis is present.[46,47] More fre-quently, involvement of vessels occurs in the base of an ulcer, with ischemic necrosis of its wall.

## TOXIC DILATATION AND PERFORATION

Toxic dilatation is a complication of fulminant colitis that may result in perforation. Toxic megacolon occurs in 2–4% of all patients with UC[48,49] and in up to 13% of hospital patients.[49,50] It may develop at any time but is most common early in the course of the disease, and may be the presenting manifestation. Overall, the mortality rate approximates 15%; the presence of perforation is the single most important determinant of prognosis, with a mortality rate of about 50%.[50,51] This may be true for overt perforation with spillage of gut contents into the peritoneal cavity. However, the overall mortality rate of UC is slightly higher than that of the general population (see Chapter 8). Although no definite explanation is yet available for the state of toxic megacolon, of the particular factors studied the extent and depth of ulceration have the strongest correla-tion with the area of dilatation.[45,51] Hypokalemia and drugs, such as narcotics and anticholinergics, which decrease motility, are aggravating factors but not primary etiologic agents.[51]

Dilatation is most often greatest in the transverse colon or flexures, but involves other parts of the colon (Fig. 27.6) and occasionally almost the entire colon; it involves all layers, includ-ing the muscularis propria and serosa. The serosa is congested, dull, opaque, and often covered by a fibrinous or fibrinopurulent exudate. The thin friable wall, which has been compared to wet

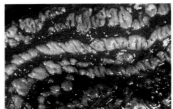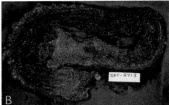

**Fig. 27.6** Examples of indeterminate colitis. (A) Longitudinal ulcers mim-icking the cobblestone phase of Crohn's disease (biopsies may show an identical focal ulceration on a background of relatively normal mucosa in both Crohn's disease and fulminant colitis of any etiology). (B) Fulminant ulcerative colitis. There is relative rectal sparing distally (bottom). Note also the transition at either end (the ileocecal valve is in the outer); ulceration is focal proximally and more uniform distally, but either form may be present at either end. If focal ulceration is present distally, this can enhance the impression of Crohn's disease.

tissue paper, is easily ruptured, and perforation may occur spon-taneously or with the most gentle surgical handling. Mucosal ulceration is severe, with frequent cleft-like extensions into the muscularis propria accompanied by extensive destruction of muscle fibers. Vascular engorgement may be more prominent than the inflammatory cell infiltrate.

In patients who successfully negotiate an episode of toxic dilatation and then recover temporarily, in whom colectomy is performed subsequently, specimens may demonstrate a regene-rated mucosa extending into the muscularis propria, presumably representing re-epithelialization of previously deep ulcerations. The intense inflammation and destruction of muscle fibers undoubtedly interrupt normal neuromuscular networks con-trolling the tone of the colon, accounting for the dilatation. Increasingly, patients with severe disease are being treated with cyclosporin or tacrolimus, obviating surgery in the short term, and for approximately half of these patients in the long term as well.[52-54] Patients successfully treated conservatively for several weeks may regenerate the mucosa deep in the muscularis propria or develop colitis cystica profunda. However, permanent recovery from fulminant colitis is rarely complete, and these patients ultimately require colectomy.

## BENIGN STRICTURES

Strictures always are a concern in UC because of the possibility of underlying neoplasia. Benign strictures are local sequelae of ulcerative colitis and are usually of little consequence to the patient and not an indication for colectomy. However, colectomy is sometimes considered if there is doubt as to their underlying pathologic significance, or if they prevent the colonoscopist from reaching the proximal colon in cancer surveillance programs. They usually are smooth, may be multiple, are sometimes reversible, and are rarely sufficiently narrow to cause obstruc-tion. Benign strictures have been attributed to hypertrophy of the muscularis mucosae.[26] Hypertrophy of the muscularis mucosae, sometimes with duplication (a second layer) and with intervening fibrosis, is an indicator of previous ulceration. Strictures that are not reversible frequently are malignant but may be the result of fibrosis of the submucosa or muscularis propria. Benign strictures are most commonly seen in patients with long-standing disease, although occasionally they are observed early.[26,55,56]

## BACKWASH ILEITIS

Total colonic involvement is accompanied by extension of mucosal inflammation into the distal terminal ileum in 10–20% of patients. It is usually associated with a dilated patulous ileocecal valve. Whether this lesion represents a reaction to the reflux of colonic content into the terminal ileum[57] or primary ileal involvement has not been established. Morphologically the ileitis clearly resembles the colonic disease,[58] implicating the intestinal contents in its origin. 'Backwash ileitis' has no prognostic significance and resolves following colectomy. Despite the ileitis and rare instances of ileal perforation in UC[59] the affected ileum can be utilized for ileostomy or the formation of a pouch in patients requiring surgery. The differential diagnosis is with terminal ileal Crohn's disease. Backwash ileitis must be in continuity with colonic ulcerative colitis, whereas Crohn's disease ileitis should have typical endoscopic features in the large as well as the small bowel (or there would not be a problem). Possibly because backwash ileitis invariably indicates active total ulcerative colitis, it appears to be an additional risk factor for colorectal carcinoma in UC[60] and may also predict pouchitis in patients undergoing ileoanal pouch anastomosis.[61]

## INFLAMMATORY POLYPS

Polypoid mucosal tags are a relatively common sequela of all forms of inflammatory bowel disease, including UC. The term 'pseudopolyp' is commonly used for mucosal projections to avoid confusion with adenomas. These mucosal tags, unlike the 'mucosal islands' in acute disease, fit the definition of polyp and so the term 'inflammatory polyp' is preferred.[9,62] In active disease they consist of isolated congested mucosal remnants, resulting from undermining ulcers or from nodules of granulation tissue. Although they may result from undermining ulcers with re-epithelialization of the undermined surface, they may also result from epithelialization of nodules of granulation tissue.

Inflammatory polyps are distributed in a diffuse or irregular fashion throughout the colon but are relatively uncommon in the rectum, especially close to the anal verge.[56] They are not exclusive to UC and may follow ulceration in inflammatory bowel disease of other causes. True adenomatous polyps may occur as a coincidental finding in patients with UC, although their incidence is low.

Inflammatory polyps assume many shapes and occasionally form mucosal bridges; they may be bifid or trifid. Most inflammatory polyps are less than 1.5 cm long, although they vary considerably in size and occasionally may reach several centimeters in length or diameter. They persist in the quiescent stage after re-epithelialization and often remain as indicators of the preceding severe ulceration. When especially numerous they can form a forest of polyps, for which the term 'colitis polyposa' has been used; however, localization to one region of the large bowel usually indicates underlying CD.

The histologic appearance of inflammatory polyps varies, depending on whether the mucosa originated from a mucosal island, in which case their mucosa may be virtually normal, or from regenerated mucosa, with the typical features of regeneration. Polyps resulting from proliferation of granulation tissue may resemble juvenile polyps histologically. Although there has been controversy concerning the precancerous potential of inflammatory polyps[58,59] current opinion considers them benign.[25,56,63]

Nevertheless, there is no reason why they could not become dysplastic. Some inflammatory polyps become so large as to create suspicion of carcinoma or even cause obstruction.[63,64] Indeed, prevention from carrying out surveillance colonoscopy in patients in the high-risk group for carcinoma is one of the more uncommon reasons for prophylactic colectomy. Most commonly, large inflammatory polyps occur in patients with severe total colonic involvement. This is the probable basis for the reported positive association of inflammatory polyps with toxic megacolon and the arthropathy of UC,[25] as both tend to occur with severe total colitis. Patients with mild disease rarely develop inflammatory polyposis.

## ANAL LESIONS

Anal lesions occur in a minority of patients with UC and are secondary to the diarrhea. They include anal fissure, rectal prolapse, hemorrhoids, perianal excoriations and perirectal abscesses. In UC the anal complications are considerably less frequent and less severe than in CD. Rectovaginal fistulas are rare in UC and should always raise the suspicion of CD.

## THE APPENDIX IN IBD

The appendix is frequently involved in IBD, although most frequently it is a mucosal appendicitis in patients with severe disease but which appears never to be symptomatic. Appendiceal involvement in patients undergoing proctocolectomy for ulcerative colitis or Crohn's disease is common, occurring in at least half of all resections for IBD, and is well above control levels if right hemicolectomy for carcinoma is used. Clinically these patients behave as those without this feature.[65–67] Appendiceal inflammation, like the cecal patch, may not be in continuity with more distal disease.

In both ulcerative and indeterminate colitis the appendix is usually involved in continuity with large bowel disease, but sometimes as a skip lesion that has no implications for Crohn's disease. Quite frequently this is in continuity with disease around the ileocecal valve. In resections for ulcerative colitis the appendix is frequently inflamed even in patients with disease otherwise limited to the left colon,[68,69] although in other studies involvement is present in continuity.[70] Interestingly, even though quite severe, the submucosa is invariably either not involved or only involved superficially, and symptoms of appendicitis are either non-existent or buried in the more severe symptoms of the colitis.[71]

In patients with Crohn's disease there may be the typical transmural lymphoid hyperplasia and occasional granulomas as part of granulomatous appendicitis. However, virtually identical changes can be seen as part of otherwise unremarkable resolving appendicitis with prior transmural inflammation and Crohn's-like lymphoid hyperplasia following abscess formation, in a manner similar to that seen following diverticulitis, which can also mimic Crohn's disease. However, patients with granulomatous appendicitis may have evidence of other infections, especially *Yersinia*, which may have necrotizing granulomas. However, by PCR 25% of granulomatous appendicitis with no other evidence of IBD has evidence of *Yersinia*, either *Y. enterocolitica* or *Y. pseudotuberculosis*, or both.[72]

## PRECLINICAL ULCERATIVE COLITIS

Knowledge of the pathophysiology of an initial episode of UC is limited, even though the architectural distortion and the basal lymphoid or plasma cell aggregates in UC are present during the initial episode.[73] UC treated promptly with complete clinical and endoscopic resolution may not develop these features.[11] Because the inflammatory features of UC take time to develop, the preclinical phase may be longer than that of an acute infectious colitis, i.e. weeks or months. Two pieces of data provide an insight into this phase of ulceration. In one study published in abstract only, patients in relapse manifested an increased number of mononuclear cells in the lamina propria.[74] The second study indicated that patients with neutrophils accumulating as crypt abscesses were more likely to undergo relapse.[23] The sequence of events may be an increase in chronic inflammatory cells, and the elaboration of an appropriate cytokine initiates the recruitment of neutrophils into the lamina propria, culminating in a clinical attack. Another more likely mechanism is represented by a group of colitides in which disease seems to date from an episode of acute infection acting as the 'trigger' for the development of ulcerative colitis. Exactly when these patients relinquish the label of postinfectious diarrhea and are then considered to have IBD (UC or CD) usually coincides with a subsequent exacerbation unaccompanied by a detectable pathogen.

## CROHN'S DISEASE

Crohn's disease is characterized in its active phase by aphthoid ulceration, often with adjacent cobblestoning, by a chronic inflammatory process that varies from mucosal to transmural disease, the latter being composed of lymphoid hyperplasia in aggregates and sometimes granulomas, by fissures, abscesses and fistulous tracts. In the resolving phase fibrosis may result in strictures. CD is characteristically a focal or multifocal disease radiologically, endoscopically and pathologically, and has a remarkable capacity to recur following intestinal resection. As with UC there may be a variety of accompanying extraintestinal diseases, but unlike UC CD per se, as manifested by granulomatous disease, may sometimes affect other organs.[9] Although the most severe areas may display transmural inflammation, areas of cobblestoning tend to be mucosal and submucosal in extent.

Crohn's disease can affect any part of the gastrointestinal tract. Ileocolic, small intestinal and upper gastrointestinal Crohn's disease occurs in approximately 30–55%, 25–35% and 5–10% of patients, respectively, and disease limited to the colon accounts for 15–25%.[75–80] Anal or anorectal disease includes fissures, fistulae and ulcers. Disease often extends to the perianal skin, resulting in the openings of fissures or fistulae and resulting nodules of granulation tissue and skin tags that can become enormous ('elephant ears').

The diagnosis of CD rests upon the demonstration of a constellation of appropriate clinical, gross (radiologic, endoscopic or resections) and microscopic features, any of which may strongly suggest the diagnosis. In the pathologic differential diagnosis from other forms of inflammatory bowel disease the gross appearances, however viewed, may be worth any number of histologic sections in demonstrating focality, cobblestoning or aphthoid ulcers, all of which can be difficult to establish when reviewing a series of slides. Because resections are carried out only for complications of the disease, the range of changes encountered grossly by the pathologist is relatively limited. Indications for surgery include strictures causing obstructive symptoms (which can sometimes be managed by strictureplasty or dilatation) or fistulae, active disease that has been unresponsive to treatment, sometimes with bleeding, fulminant colitis, and rarely carcinoma can also occur, although carcinomas are sometimes unexpected 'incidental' findings (see Chapters 38 and 39).

## EARLY LESIONS OF CROHN'S DISEASE

The prototype lesion of Crohn's disease is the aphthoid ulcer, a focus of mucosal erosion or ulceration ideally located in the M-cell region over lymphoid nodules in the small bowel.[81] However, erosions may occur anywhere.[82] Histologically they may be entirely non-specific and may also stimulate an underlying histiocytic, lymphocytic or plasmacytic reaction. Characteristically they occur in a mucosa that is relatively uninflamed, and it is the combination of erosions on a background of relatively uninflamed mucosa that is the hallmark of CD, and very useful in the distinction from ulcerative colitis. Further, an excess of chronic inflammatory cells of any or all of these types can be an incidental histological finding. Incidental microscopic inflammation in endoscopically normal mucosa, such as Helicobacter-negative gastritis, an enteritis, colitis, an intraepithelial lymphocytosis or incidental granulomas, are all part of what may be early disease. However, it is the focal chronic active lesion on a background of relatively normal mucosa that is the characteristic histological lesion, and this may be visible endoscopically but may also be an incidental biopsy finding.[83,84] The typical thickened bowel with transmural inflammation is very much an old-established lesion, and even in resections transmural disease may only be found at the site of bowel thickening or strictures. Whereas acute lesions are much more likely to be superficial, erosions and ulcers are invariably found within strictures and proximal to strictures, and both may resolve when the stricture is dealt with.

When spraying with indigo carmine, minute lesions such as aphthoid lesions, small lesions, areas of erythema and small ulcers were found in 90% of patients with CD and in 0% of healthy volunteers.[82] Histologically, granulomas can be found in 15–20% of patients with CD,[82,85] although in large centers these tend to be uncommon, possibly reflecting referral bias. In the large intestine the lymphoepithelial complex, of which the M cell is a part in the small intestine, clearly has a counterpart that similarly is predisposed to the development of aphthoid ulcers.[86] This relationship offers at least a partial explanation for the frequent association of aphthoid ulcers with underlying lymphoid tissue.

Whether aphthoid ulcers really are the earliest lesions in CD has been questioned. Some suggest that the initial early lesion may be damage and rupture of small mucosal capillaries, presumably preceding infiltration of the lamina propria by inflammatory cells; loss of the overlying epithelium follows this vascular damage.[87] However, the same group did not consider this finding a useful feature in the distinction of IBD from acute infection. Also, the presence of capillary thrombi was not related to the severity of inflammation.[88] Because bacterial toxins, such as those produced in pseudomembranous colitis, affect endothelium, the possibility of a partially shared final common pathway with infectious colitis in at least some patients with CD seems reasonable.

Aphthoid ulcers develop relatively quickly and seem to be related to mucosal contact with the intestinal content. One uncontrolled endoscopic study examined 50 consecutive patients 6 weeks to 6 months after surgical resection of the terminal ileum and found that 70% had lesions in the neoterminal ileum. All were in the form of aphthoid ulcers, some large or multiple. Half of the anastomotic junctions were also ulcerated, and one-third of these had large ulcers involving much of the circumference of the bowel.[89] A similar study found a 72% recurrence rate in those undergoing endoscopy within 1 year of ileocolonic resection.[90] Not surprisingly, patients without recurrence were asymptomatic, and 27% of those with mucosal or submucosal disease had symptoms, compared to 87% of those with transmural disease, who did not.[91] The relationship of aphthoid ulcer formation to the fecal stream is further indicated by the disappearance of these ulcers following diversion of the fecal stream, and their reappearance at the anastomosis when the continuity of the fecal stream is re-established.[92] Infusion of intestinal contents into an excluded loop of ileum in one patient (clearly an uncontrolled study) rapidly resulted in recurrent disease.[38]

## DEVELOPMENT AND RESOLUTION OF COBBLESTONE MUCOSA AND LINEAR ULCERATION

Although the long-term natural history of CD is well known, its evolution over a brief timespan is less defined. The fact that foci of localized mucosal architectural distortion may be found in resected specimens strongly suggests that aphthoid ulcers can completely heal locally. Indeed, focal architectural distortion in biopsies is one of the diagnostic criteria on which a diagnosis of Crohn's disease can be made.[5]

In some patients this is accompanied by duplication of the muscularis mucosae and submucosal fibrosis with or without local chronic inflammation. This pattern suggests that CD undergoes cycles of formation and healing of aphthoid ulcers, which may completely resolve. This delicate pathophysiologic homeostatic mechanism sometimes decompensates, resulting in severe clinical disease, the first stage of which is the extension of pinpoint aphthoid ulcers to form the longitudinal and transverse ulcers that constitute the islands of cobblestoning so characteristic of the disease. In examining resected specimens one can invariably find in the least affected areas small, well-circumscribed aphthoid ulcers. However, progressing into more severely affected mucosa, aphthoid ulcers often enlarge and develop a more stellate appearance (Fig. 27.7). These stellate ulcers tend to fuse primarily in a longitudinal direction, and also transversely, to form cobblestoned islands of mucosa that often are histologically normal, surrounded on all sides by fused aphthoid ulcers. The mucosa is slightly edematous, but the underlying submucosa is very edematous with severe lymphangiectasia. It is the submucosal disease that results in the cobblestone appearance. The mucosa is frequently normal, although a spectrum of changes from architecturally normal to atrophic mucosa can be found in which the inflammatory component varies from normal to an excess of either acute or chronic inflammatory cells, often both. Mast cells are present in large

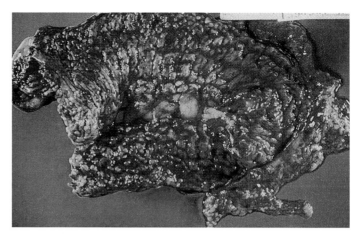

**Fig. 27.7** Crohn's disease. Total colectomy; the ileocecal valve is top left and the sigmoid colon is lower left. The the right colon, numerous aphthoid ulcers are visible, some of which have enlarged and fused with formation of transverse and longitudinal ulcers, giving a typical 'cobblestone' appearance.

numbers in this phase of the disease, both in the submucosa and in the muscle.[93]

Mucosal ulceration ultimately resolves by the development of typical regenerative changes similar to those described for UC. In the small intestine, metaplasia to pyloric-type glands is a frequent but non-specific finding; architectural and active regenerative changes also can be found. These metaplastic glands are strongly immunoreactive to epidermal growth factor and form as buds from the regenerating epithelium.[94] Trefoil peptide gene expression in these pyloric-like glands is presumably a protective cellular response also involving heat-shock proteins (e.g. pS2 mRNA) and various growth factors.

Ultrastructural immunolocalization showed the pS2 to be co-packaged in the mucus cell granules. pS2 peptide was demonstrated in local neuroendocrine cells and was also co-packaged with the neuroendocrine granules. The co-packaging of the same secretory protein in both mucus and neuroendocrine granules, which have different functions, is unusual and may indicate an important role for pS2 in the secretory process itself, or as a ligand delivered to its receptor via multiple routes.[95] The crypts associated with the metaplastic lineage also showed pronounced neuroendocrine cell hyperplasia. In addition, patients who have undergone ileal resection frequently show adaptive changes in the neoterminal ileum, which develops the invaginations and absorptive cells resembling those seen in jejunal rather than ileal villi.[24] Edema can either be reabsorbed or may undergo gradual fibrosis. The latter would explain some of the tight strictures (Fig. 27.8) that seem to involve the submucosa rather than the full thickness of the bowel wall.

## TRANSMURAL INFLAMMATION, FIBROSIS AND STRICTURES

Transmural inflammation, fibrosis and strictures occur much less frequently in CD than the mucosal and submucosal lesions described in the previous section, but may be found focally in resected specimens. The notion that CD is by definition a transmural disease is an acceptable generalization and appropriate when dealing with resected specimens. However, it has become increasingly apparent that much of clinical disease being treated today is chiefly mucosal, and that in some patients intestinal

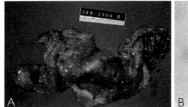
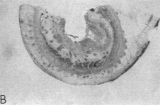

Fig. 27.8 (A) Typical terminal ileal stricture from Crohn's disease, causing obstructive symptoms. Note that ulcerations are present not only within the stricture but also within the diseased mucosa proximally. (B) Whole mount of ileal stricture showing mucosal ulceration and the typical transmural inflammatory infiltrate in the form of a rosary bead-like appearance on both sides of the muscularis propria.

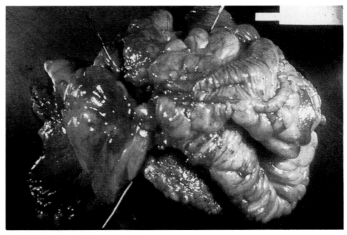

Fig. 27.9 Inflammatory mass in Crohn's disease caused by matted loops of small bowel with abscess formation and numerous fistulae, some of which are demarcated by probes.

resections may show only disease limited to the mucosa or submucosa. Transmural inflammation is uncommon in resections carried out during the acute or active phase of Crohn's disease, when fulminant disease is present in resections for uncontrollable bleeding. It is also relatively uncommon when rectal stumps are excised for persistent anorectal disease. Even in resections for otherwise unremarkable Crohn's disease a considerable search is required to identify transmural disease; occasionally it is not found. Some observers have called this superficial CD.[96,97] In the absence of non-caseating granulomas or transmural disease, the presence of numerous submucosal lymphoid aggregates in the submucosa is probably the minimal change on which a diagnosis of Crohn's disease can established confidently (superficial Crohn's disease).

Transmural disease invariably takes the form of lymphoid aggregates and fibrosis of the bowel wall, which may result in strictures. Lymphoid aggregates, whether submucosal or transmural, tend to develop rather quickly after the formation of aphthoid ulcers.[98] They are most dense in an expanded submucosa, with a second row immediately external to the muscularis propria, forming a double 'rosary-bead' effect. When both are well developed the diagnosis of CD can made with ease, even in the absence of granulomas. Occasional lymphoid aggregates may also occur within the muscularis propria, particularly along the myenteric plexus. However, although virtually diagnostic of CD, transmural lymphoid aggregates do have 100% specificity, and other local inflammatory lesions, such as chronic *Chlamydia* infection (lymphogranuloma venereum) and peridiverticulitis, also cause numerous lymphoid aggregates, although not in the exquisite rosary-bead arrays so typical of Crohn's disease. Nevertheless, both diseases are focal and tend to involve the rectum and sigmoid colon, respectively.

Granulomas may accompany the lymphoid aggregates and, when present, are often situated adjacent to dilated lymphatics and to nerves, sometimes forming a row within the myenteric plexus. Ulceration within tight strictures is the rule, regardless of the underlying disease, and therefore is unhelpful diagnostically. Focal ulcers outside the strictured segment bowel (Fig. 27.8) and immediately proximal to narrowed segment of bowel (prestenotic ulceration) are useful indicators of CD. Neuronal hyperplasia also is a characteristic finding in resections for CD.[99]

## DEVELOPMENT OF FISSURES AND FISTULAE

Fissures and fistulae are characteristic of Crohn's disease. Fissures are always observed to arise from the bases of

aphthoid ulcers, invariably one of the lateral edges; and fistula tracts represent extensions of these lesions. Because free perforation in the absence of toxic dilatation is rare in Crohn's disease, it seems unlikely that these develop very quickly. Instead, there is sufficient time for a serositis to develop on the external surface of the bowel, producing adhesions to adjacent loops of bowel into which fissures may pass. Occasionally, large inflammatory masses are encountered that are the result of adherent loops of bowel encompassing fistulae and abscesses (Fig. 27.9).

Fissures are invariably lined by neutrophils with a surrounding infiltrate of histiocytes and other mononuclear cells. Yet, with time, it is not uncommon to observe attempts to re-epithelialize these tracts, at least in part. This has important clinical connotations, presuming that the driving force causing tracts is removed, whether by diversion of intestinal contents, parenteral nutrition, antibiotics or combinations of these, the fissures might undergo some degree of healing.

The few studies examining the chronology of different lesions in CD suggest that large ulcers, sinuses and strictures are the final features, appearing after aphthoid ulcers and transmural inflammation and requiring the longest time to develop.[98] Fissures and fistulae are considered to develop chiefly proximal to sites of obstruction, supporting the conclusion that they are a late feature of the disease.[100,101] However, they are frequently found distal to strictures, and in some patients are present both proximal and distal to strictures, although in one study almost half were completely unrelated to strictures.[102] These studies suggest that if a relationship exists between the formation of fissures, fistulae and strictures, the latter may be a secondary reaction. In attempting to predict which patients might have abscesses or fistulae, one study found that features such as the extent of disease, the number of stenoses and the caliber of the stenotic bowel bore no relationship. In ileal CD, the thickness of the bowel wall in stenoses was significantly different: 12.0 ' 3.4 mm versus 7.6 ' 3.1 mm in those with stenosis but no extramural complications. In colonic CD the length of stenosis was significantly greater in patients with complications, but there was no correlation with duration of symptoms, age at surgery or sex.[103]

## CORRELATIONS OF EXTERNAL FAT-WRAPPING WITH MUCOSAL DISEASE: SURGICAL IMPLICATIONS

Fat-wrapping has traditionally been relied upon by surgeons to estimate the extent of underlying disease. Until recently this approach had never been questioned, often because surgeons palpated the bowel to detect areas of thickening or rigidity, and also examined freshly resected opened bowel to ensure that anastomoses were not being established through areas of gross disease. The assumption was that the inflammation would recur more quickly in this circumstance instead of with anastomoses made through normal-appearing mucosa. Surgical therapy was based on the assumption that CD was widely distributed and that resection for cure therefore was unrealistic. Microscopic disease appears to play no role in predicting early recurrence.[104,105] Several studies have clarified these issues by examining the extent of disease at operation. Retrograde panendoscopy of the entire small bowel at laparotomy for surgical resection demonstrated disease scattered throughout the small bowel in two-thirds (13 of 20) of patients. In half of these cases the lesion was not detected by palpation or other investigations prior to the endoscopy.[106] A second study evaluated a consecutive unselected series of 27 resections for CD in 25 patients and found that fat-wrapping correlated closely with transmural inflammation, and also with intestinal fibrosis, muscularization and stricture formation. Macroscopic ulceration extended beyond the fat-wrapping in 11 instances and to surgical resection margins in six cases. In a pathologic study of 225 small intestine resections, fat-wrapping was seen only in CD.[107]

In a third study, radiologically diagnosed disease was not identified by the surgeon at laparotomy and resection was deferred. Ultimately, the disease was shown to be superficial (limited to the mucosa and submucosa), confirming the lack of sensitivity of surgical palpation in determining the extent of disease.[108] A further study utilizing intraoperative endoscopy found a similar relationship between mucosal inflammation and fat-wrapping or serositis, but also noted a possible exception. In 23 patients undergoing resection for fistula or abscess, eight had serositis and/or fat-wrapping in bowel segments without mucosal inflammation. Endoscopic findings influenced surgical decisions in 20 of the 33 operations, limiting planned resection in 14, identifying strictures for repair in one, deciding against resection in two cases and for extended resection in three. Intraoperative enteroscopy can provide information for more precise surgery, thereby limiting the extent of resection.[109]

## HISTOLOGICAL FINDINGS

### Granulomas

There are pronounced variations between series concerning the presence of granulomas in biopsies or resected specimens. Even if granulomas are present, the chances of finding them in biopsies depend on their frequency and size, the number of slides examined, and the number of sections on each slide. The diligence of the examiner and the criteria employed are important.[7] Personal preference is for a localized well-formed aggregate of epithelioid histiocytes; the presence of giant cells or a surrounding cuff of lymphocytes is not required. Single giant cells and indefinite aggregates of histiocytes are excluded, but prompt a search in adjacent sections or further slides from the same block for better-formed granulomas. Central necrosis can occasionally be seen in granulomas in Crohn's disease, but true caseation should raise the question of an alternative diagnosis, particularly tuberculosis. Granulomas less than four cells in diameter are of questionable significance. In practice, this is rarely a problem with the availability of multiple sections. If there is any doubt, this is stated in the report, usually that a poorly formed granuloma may be present. Depending on the clinical circumstances, if multiple levels throughout the block are unrevealing, a repeat biopsy may be requested or a simple inquiry may be made as to whether there is any other clinical evidence to suggest CD. Some observers have found that biopsies from the edges of aphthoid ulcers have a high yield of granulomas. Overall, granulomas are found in CD at some time in about two-thirds of patients, and careful examination of rectal biopsies may increase the yield.

The differential diagnosis of granulomas depends to a large extent on which part of the gastrointestinal tract is biopsied. Infections causing granulomas include tuberculosis, fungi, *Yersinia* or *Chlamydia* infection, rarely syphilis, and foreign material and mucus. Sarcoid is similarly uncommon. In the stomach, food, idiopathic granulomatous gastritis and reactions to tumors are all rare causes of granulomas. Chronic active *Helicobacter pylori*-negative gastritis is the hallmark of gastric CD.[83,84] In a patient with known Crohn's disease granulomas can be found in any part of the gastrointestinal tract, including minor salivary glands, and are infrequent in the esophagus. The incidental finding of a granuloma in an otherwise normal biopsy in a patient with Crohn's disease poses a problem of interpretation. It may represent a completely different pathologic process, especially if the patient comes from an area where other granulomatous diseases are a consideration. Only long-term follow-up will provide the answer as to whether this represents early involvement by CD. There have been suggestions that granulomatous CD may be less aggressive than its non-granulomatous counterpart in other diseases, such as leprosy and primary biliary cirrhosis.

### Aphthoid ulcers

These produce a characteristic biopsy appearance with an ulcer on one edge of the biopsy, invariably with adjacent crypts that are uninvolved by an acute inflammatory process, nor are they mucin depleted[24,110] (Fig. 27.10). In the large bowel this is in direct contrast to ulcerative colitis, in which ulceration or erosion invariably occurs on a background of significant inflammation, with diffuse mucin depletion and a neutrophil infiltrate involving the crypts. In the upper gastrointestinal tract localized ulcer disease, particularly that associated with aspirin or NSAIDs, can produce virtually identical biopsy findings. The endoscopic finding of cobblestoning disease in the distal duodenum or combined gastroduodenal disease increases the index of suspicion of CD. Because upper gastrointestinal disease invariably occurs in patients with documented disease elsewhere in the gastrointestinal tract, a primary diagnosis of CD in the upper part of the gastrointestinal tract is extremely unlikely. Oral sodium phosphate bowel preparation solution can cause aphthoid ulcers focally, or throughout the large bowel endoscopically. Biopsy of these lesions can show focal active colitis or erosion, mimicking biopsies from aphthoid ulcers of CD.[83]

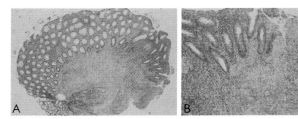

**Fig. 27.10** (A) Sigmoid biopsy in Crohn's disease. Crypts on the left are relatively preserved with normal architecture and mucus production; on the right, both are abnormal. Multiple basal lymphoid aggregates confirm chronic disease. (B) Detail from right edge of A shows the edge of an ulcer (right). The combination of an ulcer on one part of the biopsy with realtively preserved mucosa in another part is characteristic of a biopsy from an aphthoid ulcer.

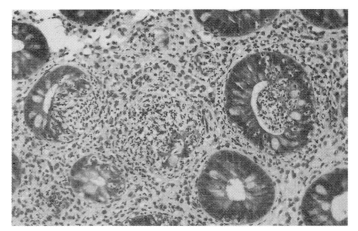

**Fig. 27.11** Focal mucosal disease in which there is a focus of heavy inflammation with an obvious crypt abscess. This pattern is typical of the focal pattern of inflammation that characterizes Crohn's disease and is almost never seen in ulcerative colitis.

## Focal mucosal disease

This consists of a marked variability in the quantity of inflammation in different parts of the same biopsy (Fig. 27.11) or between biopsies. In the upper gastrointestinal tract similar changes also can be seen in a variety of inflammatory conditions, including peptic ulcer; therefore, it is most useful when present in the more distal duodenum, where peptic ulcer- and drug-induced disease is less frequent. In the large bowel, similar changes can be seen in active or resolving infections and in ulcerative proctitis or colitis near the transition with normal mucosa. As a finding in a single biopsy, this change is relatively unhelpful other than to identify that part of the bowel as having inflammatory disease, although pronounced focality does not occur in UC. Indeed, focal disease, whether manifest by acute or chronic inflammation or architectural changes focally within the large bowel, is a very good marker of Crohn's disease; conversely, diffuse disease most marked distally (with occasional exceptions indicated previously) but including a cecal patch, is a very good indicator of ulcerative colitis.[4,5,16,111]

## Terminal ileal biopsy

The presence of an acute terminal ileitis in an appropriate clinical setting strongly favors Crohn's disease (Fig. 27.12). Occasionally granulomas are found, but these are uncommon (Fig. 27.13A). Adaptive changes are limited to biopsies of neoterminal ileum

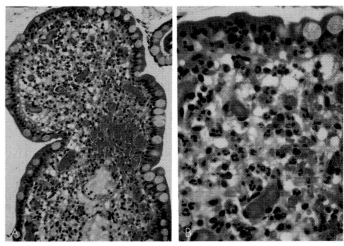

**Fig. 27.12** Acute terminal ileitis. (A) Terminal ileal biopsy with a bulbous and inflamed villus. (B) Detail shows numerous neutrophils in the lamina propria. These features are those of an acute terminal ileitis; in Western society, however, involvement by Crohn's disease is by far the most common cause of changes such as these in a patient coming to colonoscopy.

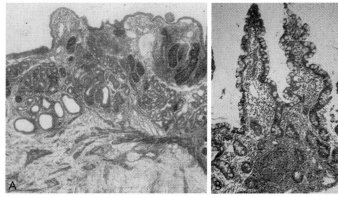

**Fig. 27.13** Other features that may be found in terminal ileal biopsies. (A) Focus of pyloric metaplasia that is indicative of prior ulceration at this site, albeit of any cause. (B) Focus of chronic inflammation in the deep lamina propria with a well-formed granuloma.

following prior ileocecal resection, and consist of relative 'jejunalization' of terminal ileal villi. If extensive small bowel resection has been carried out, some may argue that this merely indicates normal mid-ileal villi. However, it has been noted in patients with extensive small bowel disease and limited resections, and is therefore a significant finding. The role of ileoscopy in patients with terminal ileal Crohn's disease is self-evident, but when colitis is present it can increase diagnostic accuracy. In one study of 257 patients with persistent diarrhea, ileal disease without colonic involvement was present in 44 of 123 patients. Microscopic lesions of the ileum were present in 125 (49%). Two of these had a normal endoscopy. Thirteen patients had a diffuse colitis and 11 had a predominantly left-sided colitis, both originally suggestive of ulcerative colitis. Crohn's disease was diagnosed in 88 patients and infectious disease in 17. Ileal biopsies were assessed as being essential for the diagnosis in 15 patients and contributory in 53. Granulomas, solitary giant cells, pseudopyloric gland metaplasia, eosinophils and a disturbed villous architecture were the most important lesions observed in Crohn's disease.[1]

*Pyloric metaplasia*

Although of no value in the upper gastrointestinal tract, pyloric metaplasia may be found particularly in biopsies from the terminal ileum (Fig. 27.13B). Although merely an indicator of pre-existing chronic inflammatory disease, in North America this differentiates CD from UC. In other parts of the world this is a less definitive finding.

## DISPROPORTIONATE SUBMUCOSAL INFLAMMATION

This situation applies only to large bowel biopsies and consists of a heavy submucosal infiltrate with a relatively normal overlying mucosa.[112] The clinical correlation of this observation is a biopsy taken from an apparently inflamed mucosa. If only normal-appearing mucosa is obtained, the possibility of disproportionate submucosal disease indicative of CD always should be considered. This does not include either a large solitary lymphoid nodule, which may be normal but always either straddles or is located immediately below the muscularis mucosae, or a multiple small lymphoid aggregates on either side of the muscularis mucosae.

## DIFFERENTIAL DIAGNOSIS OF UNUSUAL DISEASE

Occasionally CD occurs with unusual clinical or pathologic features, such as single or multiple large but otherwise non-specific serpiginous or longitudinal ulcers of the large or small bowel. Even in the presence of granulomas the diagnosis may be difficult because of their unusual appearance. In the absence of granulomas the differential diagnosis includes non-specific ulceration, including ischemia; infections; resolving (non-granulomatous) tuberculosis; drug-induced disease (e.g. by potassium chloride or digoxin); ulcerative jejunoileitis; ulcers in celiac sprue; or lymphoma. In the absence of a likely cause or other evidence of CD such ulcers are usually classified as idiopathic. Those associated with other diseases depend on the demonstration of that condition or documented ingestion of the damaging drug. The distinction from other types of IBD, primarily UC, as well as acute infectious colitis and microscopic colitis, needs to be appreciated. Finally some diseases mimic CD even to the point of histologic overlap, including the following:

- Oral sodium phosphate bowel preparation[113]
- Behçet's disease[114,115]
- Enterocolitis associated with seronegative spondyloarthropathies[116,117]
- In children, glycogen storage disease type IIb[116–118]
- Possibly Hermansky–Pudlak syndrome[119]
- Possibly chronic granulomatous disease[120,121]
- Lymphogranuloma venereum[122]
- Diversion proctitis and colitis (see subsequent discussion).

## INDETERMINATE COLITIS

The term 'indeterminate colitis' was proposed originally for those instances of fulminant colitis with maximal overlap of the pathologic features of both UC and CD.[123,124] However, the term has become used in a second sense for patients who appear to have inflammatory bowel disease but who do not readily fall into either of the major forms. A firm diagnosis of either UC or CD often depends on a review of all previous material, or may await the evidence from resection or subsequent follow-up. In resected specimens this essentially depends on the number of features that are not acceptable for fulminant disease of undetermined etiology, features that are unlike those of ulcerative colitis, and which raise the likelihood of CD. Clearly, there are degrees of certainty with which a diagnosis of CD can be made, e.g. definite, probable, possible, no evidence. The first and last of these do not pose diagnostic problems; however, the others (possible and probable) can be managed in two ways. Either or both can be submerged into 'indeterminate colitis'; alternatively, a diagnosis of 'inflammatory bowel disease, possibly/probably Crohn's disease', also can be rendered.

The real questions are in determining the criteria used for either of these diagnoses, how sensitive these criteria are for the development of subsequent CD, and most important, any implications for the patient's management. The latter is a key issue for patients in whom any form of surgery is being considered, as the type of surgery considered or offered may depend entirely on the likelihood of CD being the underlying disease. The simplest example is a fulminant colectomy specimen in which a solitary granuloma is present, for which no apparent cause is found in 20 sections of bowel. Assuming that this is not a reaction to mucin, other demonstrable foreign material or another definable cause, is this sufficient basis for a diagnosis of Crohn's disease? Most pathologists would be hesitant, even if the granuloma is present in the serosa and away from all areas of inflammation. Similarly, most also would hesitate to make an unequivocal diagnosis of UC. This problem can be resolved either as 'indeterminate colitis' or inflammatory bowel disease, possibly/probably (depending on the degree of certainty) CD. The term 'fulminant colitis of undetermined etiology' may be preferable because 'indeterminate colitis' implies that the underlying disease is either UC or CD. In practice, virtually every diffuse inflammatory disease of the bowel, including those caused by infections and medications, has been complicated by fulminant disease. Because about half of all instances of classic acute infectious colitis based upon all criteria, including histologic assessment, have an unidentified cause, it is possible for infections in which no pathogen is found to develop fulminant complications.

The major questions therefore become:

1. What features are acceptable as part of fulminant colitis, regardless of the etiology?
2. Are any of these features predictive of an increased likelihood of pouchitis in patients undergoing ileoanal pouch formation?
3. What features are acceptable as part of fulminant colitis, regardless of the etiology? These features include the following:[110]
   - A macroscopic appearance that may include rectal sparing with a transition to focal ulcers which may be aphthoid. A similar area of transition to relatively normal mucosa may also be present proximally.
   - Ulcers, which macroscopically may be 'tramtrack' or 'bear-claw', and cobblestoning may be present.
   - Fissuring ulcers that may penetrate any distance into or through the submucosa, muscularis propria and serosa, with or without perforation, in a tissue reaction that is necessarily transmural but which consists of an admixture

of inflammatory cells, including neutrophils, macrophages, plasma cells and lymphocytes.

- Intervening mucosa between ulcers may vary from normal to inflamed, with architectural distortion. If the distribution of the architectural distortion is similar to that expected in UC, this is presumptive evidence that UC is the underlying disease, although not necessarily the cause of the fulminant disease.
- Vasodilatation, congestion and hemorrhage that may 'dissolve' the muscularis propria and ultimately result in perforation.

Features that tend to lead to a diagnosis of indeterminate colitis include typical features of IBD so that this is not in doubt (e.g. architectural abnormalities and a plasmacytosis down to the muscularis mucosae – i.e. clearly IBD, but also with:

- Rectal sparing with proximal disease that looks like UC;
- Diffuse Crohn's disease – ultimately these patients develop terminal ileal disease or typical Crohn's disease strictures of the large bowel, and may even cause consideration of whether both UC and CD are present together;
- Some degree of focality or apparent discontinuous disease endoscopically other than a cecal patch.

Morphologically this includes:

- Fulminant disease with transmural inflammation but not in the form of typical lymphoid hyperplasia;
- Minimal lymphoid aggregates in the subserosa in fulminant disease;
- Mucosal granulomas that are usually clearly mucin (i.e. adjacent destroyed crypts) or poorly formed so that they are not clearly sarcoid-like.
- Some form of upper intestinal disease (see subsequent discussion).

In patients with only a short history of colitis that quickly becomes fulminant but unresponsive to therapy in whom there is little architectural distortion, it may be better to use the term 'colitis of uncertain etiology'. Some of these may well be fulminant infections in which an organism such as non-verotoxin toxigenic *Escherichia coli* would elude culture.

The corollary is which features suggest that the underlying disease may be CD? These include:

- Submucosal or subserosal lymphoid aggregates, particularly away from areas of ulceration;
- Well-formed non-caseating granulomas that are not a reaction to mucin or ruptured crypts, or a foreign body reaction;
- Skip areas grossly (helpful but not pathognomonic);

In the absence of these features, usually it is impossible to suggest CD. Nevertheless, in most patients with apparent UC who have undergone resection and subsequently developed evidence of CD one or more of these features often can be found in the previously resected specimen.

## UPPER INTESTINAL TRACT FINDINGS IN IBD

The presence of upper GI lesions has been used to distinguish CD from UC (and potentially indeterminate colitis), in view of involvement by CD that can be seen endoscopically while his-

tologically resulting in typical focal, chronic active *Helicobacter*-negative inflammation in both stomach and duodenum.[83,84] Some patients do have granulomas but they are relatively uncommon. Many patients also have a mild superficial diffuse *Helicobacter*-negative pangastritis that probably represents an upregulated gastric immune system, but this is not well documented. The use of upper endoscopy as a differential diagnostic tool, especially in patients undergoing consideration for ileoanal pouch anastomosis when the nature of the underlying disease was uncertain, was one avenue of investigation. However, a series of papers, primarily in the pediatric literature, have suggested that upper intestinal tract lesions can also occur in patients with what seems to be unequivocal ulcerative colitis. A diffuse duodenitis is the most common lesion (in itself unlike CD, which usually has a distinctly focal appearance on biopsy).[125-130] Although one is intrinsically skeptical about this association it does seem to be genuine, and the histology illustrated looks like very typical large bowel ulcerative colitis – often including resections.

## OTHER DIFFERENTIAL DIAGNOSES

### FOCAL ACTIVE COLITIS

There are really two distinct morphological entities represented here, one being focal active colitis (simply neutrophils in the lamina propria, often around or within crypt epithelium). This is associated with acute infectious colitis or oral sodium phosphate (Fleet's) preparation, and may also have endoscopic aphthoid-like ulcers.[113,131] Also included is focal chronic active colitis which, having a chronic component (an excess of plasma cells), is clearly a much longer-lived entity and is also sometimes associated with architectural abnormalities, immediately suggesting IBD as a cause. Being a descriptive diagnosis, the issue is the causes of such lesions. These include Crohn's colitis, and UC undergoing therapy.[111,132]

### ISCHEMIA

It may be difficult to differentiate histologically between acute UC and low-grade ischemic colitis in the elderly patient. The subsequent clinical course provides better differentiation than does evolution of the histologic changes. Although the deposition of hemosiderin may indicate ischemic colitis, it is in fact a non-specific finding.[133] Attention has been drawn to two issues. The first is the continuing association of ischemia with drugs, particularly those potentially able to cause vasoconstriction, such as amphetamines[134,135] and crack cocaine.[136] The second is that intimal proliferation of mesenteric veins, possibly caused by a primary phlebitis, may be a primary cause of ischemia.[137,138] From a histologic viewpoint, by far the most useful features of chronic ischemia are fibrosis of the lamina propria, which is rare other than in ischemia, and dilatation of superficial lamina propria capillaries, presumably as a compensatory feature.[24] An ischemic colitis apparently resulting from oral phosphosoda bowel preparation has also been reported.[139]

### INFECTION (ACUTE SELF-LIMITED COLITIS)

Some forms of infective colitis resemble UC clinically. For example, bacillary dysentery and gonococcal proctitis produce mucosal inflammation with a macroscopic distribution similar to that of UC or proctitis. However, the clinical picture and

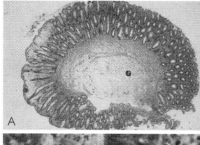
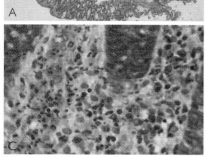
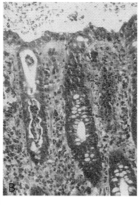

**Fig. 27.14** (A) Acute self-limited colitis. There is no architectural distortion, although crypts are pushed apart slightly by either edema (left) or the inflammatory infiltrate. There are no basal lymphoid infiltrates indicative of longstanding inflammatory bowel disease. (B) Detail showing a superficial crypt abscess: although neutrophils in the lamina propria are plentiful, they show little tendency to infiltrate crypts. (C) Higher power; numerous neutrophils in the lamina propria.

microbiologic studies of the stool or mucus usually establish the correct diagnosis. Standard microbiologic methods may be inadequate and special methods are necessary to isolate organisms such as *Campylobacter* or *Yersinia*. Furthermore, a predisposition for *Salmonella* infection has been reported in patients with UC and CD.[140] In some patients exacerbations of UC occur with stools that contain *Campylobacter*[141] or *Clostridium difficile* toxin.[142] It is not clear whether the apparent predisposition to infection with these organisms is peculiar to ulcerative colitis, a consequence of antibiotics or steroid therapy, or represents a carrier state.

The characteristic histologic features of acute infective colitis differ from those of UC.[15,27] In infective colitis the architecture is preserved. Neutrophils typically tend to be superficial, and acute inflammation primarily in the lamina propria (Fig. 27.14), in contrast to UC, in which the acute inflammation and crypt abscesses are usually prominently basal.[142] In infective colitis, mucin depletion and accompanying chronic inflammatory cell infiltration are often less than in UC. Basal lymphoid or plasma cell aggregates are conspicuously absent. Recovery from infective colitis is usually followed by restoration of histologically normal mucosa. The diffuse mucosal atrophy and crypt distortion indicative of previously active disease, typical of quiescent UC, are absent, unless infection is superimposed on an underlying UC. Gram stains rarely demonstrate the infecting organisms and are usually of little value in the differential diagnosis.

## DIVERSION COLITIS

Diversion colitis appears within approximately 3 months following any diversion procedure, and the tissue reaction resolves when bowel continuity is re-established.[143] The pathologic features are well known; lymphoid follicular hyperplasia is a major pathologic feature. In arriving at an appropriate diagnosis, this is not an issue in patients without a prior history of IBD: problems arise in patients with IBD. Lymphoid follicular hyperplasia is

found in almost all cases of IBD and may be pronounced. Other changes diagnostic of UC are present, including surface epithelial degeneration and ulceration, mucosal inflammation with crypt abscesses, and crypt branching.[144,145] Of much greater concern is that in some proctectomy specimens the lymphoid hyperplasia is so severe that the appearance may be indistinguishable from that of the transmural lymphoid aggregates seen in CD, including granulomas, most likely a reaction to extruded mucin or foreign (suture) material. Review of 15 colectomy specimens demonstrated unequivocal UC, and none of the patients subsequently showed any clinical, radiologic or pathologic evidence to support a diagnosis of CD. In this study four patients also had changes suggestive of pseudomembranous colitis.[146,147] Also, granulomas are usually found in patients with Crohn's disease or indeterminate colitis, but not ulcerative colitis in the prior colectomy specimens, but did not seem to be associated with an increased risk of Crohn's-like disease clinically.[148] In one study of children with Hirschsprung's disease undergoing colectomy the presence of lymphoid follicles, and often collections of eosinophils, was likened to an iatrogenic appendix, in which both were also seen frequently.[149] Given the involvement of the appendix in IBD, and the IBD-like features in these diverted bowels, the similarities are not without interest. Some patients undergoing resections have had a granulomatous vasculitis, but its significance is uncertain.[150,151] Although initial hopes were high that this was a deficiency disease curable by rectal administration of short-chain fatty acids, subsequent reports have been less enthusiastic.[152] The possibility that microcarcinoids might develop as a long-term complication of this disorder, perhaps akin to the ECL hyperplasia seen in atrophic gastritis, seems to be unlikely.[153]

## POUCHITIS

The situation with inflammation in Kock or ileoanal J or S pouches is similar; the major questions are the cause of the entity, its pathologic features, and how many of these changes are due to recurrent, previously unrecognized CD. Like diversion colitis, pouchitis occurs in IBD patients and is uncommon in those with familial polyposis undergoing the same operation (see Chapter 44).[154] The process is most pronounced at the point of contact of the fecal stream with the pouch (usually posteriorly),[155] and appears to be related to the numbers of anaerobes present.[156,157] Possible mechanisms include lack of nutrient short-chain fatty acids[158] and damage by oxygen-derived free radicals, which may cause transient mucosal ischemia, preventable or alleviated by allopurinol.[159] Patients who have had indeterminate colitis may be particularly predisposed. There is modest correlation between symptoms, endoscopic appearance and the histologic picture. Patients with a history of clinical pouchitis have more acute inflammation than those without symptoms, and this is reversed with metronidazole.[156,160] A significant correlation exists between acute and chronic inflammation and the number of anaerobes present, and bacterial overgrowth in the pouch is probably an important pathogenic factor.[156]

Inflammatory changes in pouchitis are related in part to the length of time the pouch has been functioning. In one study, after 3 months of pouch function the scores for acute and chronic inflammation, the degree of sulfomucin (indicating change to a large bowel mucin phenotype) and crypt cell proliferation were significantly higher[155,161,162] and the index of villous atrophy was significantly lower (indicating a greater degree of villous atrophy) than at pouch formation or at ileostomy closure.

The changes seen at 6 and 12 months were not significantly different from those at 3 months. There was no significant correlation between the efficiency of pouch evacuation and any of the mucosal changes. Again, exposure to the fecal stream appeared to be necessary for changes to take place in the pouch mucosa, although the amount of stasis, as measured by radioisotopic evacuation studies, seemed to be irrelevant.[155] Although inflammation may be severe, the number of intraepithelial lymphocytes is often reduced. Fistulae may develop as the result of anastomotic leakage. As in diversion colitis some patients also develop granulomas, perhaps as a reaction to extruded mucin or foreign material but suggestive of CD. The degenerative axonal changes originally described in CD also can be present in pouches.[163] Overall, however, the diagnostic role of biopsy in pouchitis is limited.

Inevitably, particularly when pouches are fashioned at the same time as colectomy, a small number – probably in the range of 3–5% – are created in patients who have or develop CD. The pouch requires removal in approximately 50% of cases. Interestingly, in one-third of patients the pouch appears to function relatively normally.[164] In patients with long-standing disease biopsies may be carried out to ensure that dysplasia is not present.[165,166] Because a cuff of rectal mucosa inevitably remains to preserve anal function, this is susceptible both to recurrent proctitis (cuffitis) as well as dysplasia.[167]

A common problem can be defining whether a specific biopsy from the pouch outlet really represents inflamed flat pouch mucosa or is actually from the cuff, as a surface villous appearance is not uncommon in active UC. Despite the fact that Paneth cell metaplasia occurs in UC, the Paneth cell numbers rarely match those seen in the small bowel, so the distinction is usually readily apparent on these grounds. It is important because small bowel nuclei are larger than those from the large bowel, so one is likely to acquire increased numbers of biopsies indefinite for dysplasia in biopsies actually originating from the distal inflamed pouch.

# MICROSCOPIC, LYMPHOCYTIC AND COLLAGENOUS COLITIS

These diseases do not enter into the differential diagnosis of idiopathic inflammatory bowel disease; however, they require consideration in the differential diagnosis of patients with diarrhea. Clinically, they are the most likely diagnoses in middle-aged to elderly women presenting with watery diarrhea. The endoscopic appearances are those of a virtually normal mucosa, although mild reddening, friability or pinpoint mucosal hemorrhages may be present (see also Chapter 28).

The major problem is that none of these descriptive colitides are well-defined clinicopathologic entities. Microscopic colitis can include any excess of inflammation associated with normal endoscopy; the addition of a collagen band to this establishes a diagnosis of collagenous colitis. Some resolve dramatically; others persist or recur.

## MICROSCOPIC COLITIS

Microscopic colitis is a non-specific descriptive term applied to patients presenting with watery diarrhea in the absence of radiologic or endoscopic abnormalities but with an excess of chronic

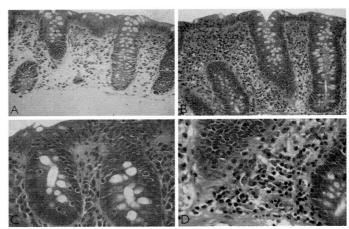

**Fig. 27.15** Microscopic colitis. (A) Normal inflammatory infiltrate in the large bowel compared to that seen in microscopic colitis. (B) Note not only the obvious increase in inflammation of the latter but its extension to the muscularis mucosae (transmucosal inflammation). (C) Surface epithelium and superficial crypts showing the increased inflammatory infiltrate but also an intraepithelial lymphocytosis, a component that some have selected as a defining characteristic of lymphocytic colitis. (D) The muscularis mucosae is shown along the bottom of the micrograph with numerous plasma cells immediately above it. Plasma cells as abundant as these, deep in the mucosa, are confied to ulcerative colitis, Crohn's disease, and microscopic and collagenous colitis.

inflammatory cells on biopsy.[168] It is also not unreasonable to include other histologic abnormalities that do not readily fit other recognizable patterns of inflammation (such as collagenous colitis, lymphocytic colitis, melanosis coli, infections and amyloid, although the latter is usually not associated with colitis) to represent the concept of diarrhea with a normal endoscopic appearance. Actually, abnormalities can be found in 15–20% of patients with diarrhea if biopsies are taken.[163,169] Histologic findings are dependent on the underlying disease. It is currently unclear whether microscopic colitis is a relatively specific entity[170] or merely the rediscovery of the fact that biopsies of endoscopically apparently normal mucosa may show a variety of changes, including inflammation. The underlying physiologic defect appears to be a failure to absorb sodium chloride and water. Symptoms appear to be related quantitatively to the inflammatory infiltrate.[171]

There are no agreed histologic criteria for microscopic/lymphocytic colitis. However, the following are useful[24] (Fig.27.15):

- Normal crypt architecture – an occasional bifid crypt is allowable and sometimes crypts do not extend to the muscularis mucosae.
- Usually some degree of mucin depletion.
- Surface epithelium may be attenuated and cuboidal to columnar, and may be infiltrated lymphocytes, neutrophils, or eosinophils or any combination. Most initial biopsies do have an intraepithelial lymphocytosis, to which in the absence of a thickened subepithelial collagen band the name 'lymphocytic colitis' is frequently applied (see below). Sometimes the lymphocytosis may involve primarily crypt epithelium.[172]
- Diffuse increase in plasma cells that usually extends to the muscularis mucosae, especially if it has not been treated.

- A subepithelial collagen band not exceeding 7 m (>10 m indicates collagenous colitis).
- Colitis that is diffuse throughout the large bowel but which may spare the rectum.
- Rarely basal giant cells may be present.[173]
- An increase in apoptotic bodies may be apparent.

In contrast to UC, microscopic colitis is associated with a more pronounced infiltration with eosinophils and an increase in intraepithelial lymphocytes.[174] When inflammation is pronounced, plasma cells reach the muscularis propria, thereby mimicking idiopathic inflammatory bowel disease; this seems to be one of the most reliable features of this disease. Focality, particularly within a biopsy, immediately raises the question of CD, and an increase in the number of basal lymphocytes or lymphoid aggregates suggests idiopathic inflammatory bowel disease.

## LYMPHOCYTIC COLITIS

It has been suggested that this term replace microscopic colitis in view of the identical morphologic features, but with emphasis on intraepithelial lymphocytes, primarily in the luminal epithelium.[175,176] That is, the term can be used as a synonym for any biopsy demonstrating an excess of intraepithelial lymphocytes, and could include biopsies in patients with known Crohn's disease (in whom it is common), Brainerd diarrhea, and even proximal colonic biopsies in patients with celiac disease. Ideally there is an excess of plasma cells in the lamina propria. Although a proportion of patients with microscopic colitis have an excess of intraepithelial lymphocytes, this is only one of many features in these patients. Furthermore, this criterion is neither sensitive nor specific; and similar changes can be seen in patients with collagenous colitis elsewhere in the bowel.[175] In some patients it is closely related to the amount of lamina propria inflammation.[177] The author and other pathologists have noted similar changes in patients with idiopathic inflammatory bowel disease, particularly CD, in large bowel biopsies from patients with celiac sprue, and occasionally in infections. It is therefore not a specific diagnosis. Given this potential lack of specificity, it is still possible to define a subgroup of microscopic colitis characterized by a diffuse increase in lymphocytes, although its clinical significance is not evident.[178]

## COLLAGENOUS COLITIS

This clinicopathologic syndrome is characterized by chronic watery diarrhea, by a virtually normal endoscopic appearance, and histologically by inflammation virtually identical to that seen in microscopic colitis, but with a significant increase in the thickness of the subepithelial collagen table immediately beneath the surface epithelium (Fig. 27.16). However, the intraepithelial lymphocytosis may be less marked or absent and other intraepithelial inflammatory cells, especially neutrophils and eosinophils, may be present. It is the only member of this group of related disorders in which there is a reasonably objective morphologic criterion on which at least part of the diagnosis can be based. It is a true colitis, and a prominent collagen band alone does not indicate collagenous colitis. A thickened collagen table without inflammation has been noted in hyperplastic polyps, and in patients with diverticular disease, megacolon,[179] colonic carcinoma,[180] Crohn's disease,[181,182] and possibly pseudomembranous colitis.[183,184] This disease is not as uncommon as was originally thought and is increasing in incidence.[163,181,183,185,186]

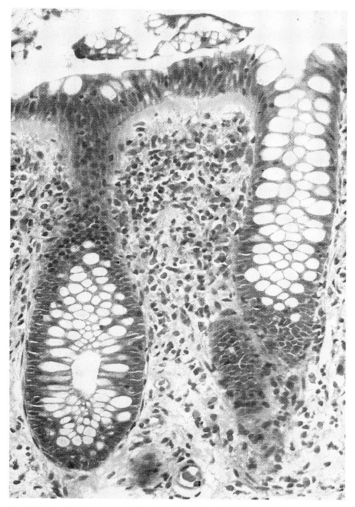

**Fig. 27.16** Collagenous colitis. This has all of the features of microscopic colitis as shown in Figure 27.15 but with a subtle subepithelial collagen band immediately beneath the luminal epithelium. In the presence of a colitis, all patients with a collagen band this thick (about 15 μm) will have symptoms. However, unless specifially looked for, it is easily missed and is here emphasized with a trichrome stain.

It affects mainly middle-aged to elderly women, with less than 20% of cases occurring in men. Apart from the typical non-bloody chronic watery diarrhea, often present for months or years, symptoms include colicky abdominal pain, nausea, vomiting and flatulence. One patient had lifelong intractable idiopathic constipation.[187] The histologic features of collagenous colitis resemble those of microscopic colitis, except for the thickened collagen band. The normal subepithelial basement membrane has a minimum thickness of 0.4 μm,[179,188-190] although the normal upper limit varies from 3 to 7 μm. Diarrhea does not seem to result until this thickness exceeds 7–10 μm; at 15 μm thickness all patients have diarrhea,[179] and it may affect up to one-third of the mucosa superficially (about 100 μm). Because it is so tedious to actually measure the collagen band, when it is prominent a useful indicator is that lymphocyte or plasma cell nuclei are about 5 μm in diameter. If two nuclei would fit into the collagen band in a well oriented part of the biopsy it is probably pathologically thickened.

The thickened collagen band is frequently visible on scanning the slide. However, sometimes it is very subtle, so that its detection is dependent on a deliberate search of the subepithelial region of the biopsy. A further indication of the possible presence of the disease is that the surface epithelium is very fragile and strips easily, so that it may be artefactually absent. When this artefact occurs, the 'exposed' lamina propria should always be examined for evidence of a thickened collagen band. The subepithelial collagen plate is obviously thickened and frequently includes numerous small blood-filled capillaries, often accompanied by neutrophils or nuclear dust within and beneath it. Small vascular channels are often prominent within the collagen band, and their walls are hyalinized early in the disease. If the diagnosis is in question, an area of the biopsy where crypts have been cut longitudinally should be examined.

In some patients, biopsies taken prior to the formation of a thickened collagen table show a mild to moderate colitis, accompanied by a gradual thickening of the collagen table over several years.[183,191,192] Although these reports also support this condition initially as an inflammatory disease with subsequent formation of a thickened collagen layer, the collagen band can be very focal.[177,193] The distribution of the disease is usually diffuse throughout the colon, but there is considerable variation between specimens, with disease being more severe in some areas than others, yet some parts of the bowel are spared.[177,181,193–195] We have examined rectal biopsies without a thickened collagen band in about 25% of patients. Other sites are involved 70–80% of the time but may be focally involved. Rectal biopsies also may show no increase in inflammation, but the rectosigmoid and the remaining colon are invariably inflamed. Flexible sigmoidoscopy with biopsies from several separate sites (e.g. descending colon, sigmoid colon, rectum) will allow the thickened collagen band to be detected in about 80% of patients with an excess of chronic inflammation in virtually all instances.[177] Although full colonoscopy with multiple biopsies may be required to detect the focal thickening of the basement membrane, if multiple biopsies from the descending colon, sigmoid colon and rectum are not inflamed, collagenous colitis is extremely unlikely to be found on full colonoscopy.[177]

A major problem is a false-positive diagnosis when the mucosa is cut tangentially, causing an artificial thickening of the collagen. Another potential problem is that nuclei of luminal epithelial cells may be located in the middle of the cell, causing the eosinophilic basal third of the cells to be misinterpreted as a collagen band. This problem is avoided if the diagnosis is always confirmed with collagen stains or is examined carefully. Other diseases causing mucosal fibrosis, such as ischemia or solitary rectal ulcer syndrome, usually involve the full thickness of the mucosa.

Several diseases are associated with collagenous colitis – those involving the large or small bowel and those affecting other organs. An enteritis seems to occur more frequently in association with collagenous colitis than would be expected by chance; in some patients this is celiac sprue, but in others it is an enteritis best described as partial villous atrophy.[196,197] In one patient the terminal ileum was involved.[198] We also have seen patients with both collagenous colitis and celiac disease who differ by being male and having maximal involvement in the rectum.[196] Jejunal biopsies in 10 patients with collagenous colitis demonstrated celiac disease in several.[199] Not surprisingly, the colitis does not respond to gluten withdrawal, although symptoms may diminish. The association was sometimes discovered because of failure of the disease to respond fully to therapy, prompting

**Table 27.2 Some causes of microscopic/lymphocytic/non-specific colitis**

Infection (culture negative)
Idiopathic inflammatory bowel disease (usually non-lymphocytic)
Crohn's disease
Proximal biopsies in ulcerative colitis
Distal biopsies in healed ulcerative colitis
(?) Collagenous colitis (sampling problems)
Oral sodium phosphate bowel preparation
Drugs/medications, especially NSAIDs
Bile salts
Chronic ischemia
Diverticulitis
Reactive arthropathies
Idiopathic colitis (exclude: specific infections, pseudomelanosis, solitary rectal ulcer syndrome)
? Following enteric infections used for vaccination
? Irritable bowel syndrome

investigation of the colon. There also have been numerous patients with IBD and a severely thickened collagen band.[200] Collagenous colitis is also associated with a variety of extra-intestinal diseases – severe arthritis and thyroid disease in particular[181,183] – raising the question of a broader immunologic spectrum of diseases. Many patients have a long-standing history of chronic ingestion of enteric-coated aspirin or other NSAID, and symptoms often have stopped dramatically upon withdrawal of the medication. In one patient a 'toxin' was reported in the stool.[201] Different causes of microscopic/lymphocytic colitis are shown in Table 27.2.

## VARIANTS OF MICROSCOPIC COLITIS

Occasionally in clinical situations consistent with microscopic colitis, biopsies demonstrate an obvious histologic abnormality that does not fit readily into any of the recognized diagnostic patterns. For instance, in the absence of any pathogen, patients with a chiefly neutrophilic infiltration affecting the right side of the colon, maximal in the region of the ileocecal valve, diminishing distally and disappearing in the transverse colon, may represent a variant of microscopic colitis. In some forms of microscopic colitis the distribution of the findings suggests the underlying etiology. Right-sided colonic disease may occasionally be associated with bile salt colitis or the ileocolitis noted in patients with seronegative reactive arthropathies (see subsequent discussion). However, infections and CD remain the most likely background entities. An intraepithelial lymphocytosis, usually less than that seen in the colon, can be seen in the terminal ileum. Some patients have what appears to be a picture resembling some of the variants associated with infection (an infectious colitis-type picture), except that it is chronic. Given that known infections such as amebic colitis and pseudomembranous colitis can be chronic, and that entities such as Brainerd diarrhea has some of the appearances of an infection without a demonstrable pathogen, it is also possible that some of these represent chronic infections of unknown etiology.

- **Brainerd-type diarrhea** Named after the town in which it was described, these long-standing diarrheas that take months or even years to resolve have all of the hallmarks of infection without an agent being identified. Other outbreaks have included cruise ships. Morphologically, some biopsies appear to resemble low-grade infection, or simply an intraepithelial lymphocytosis.[202] It is always disconcerting to attribute diarrhea simply to an intraepithelial lymphocytosis in the absence of other abnormalities, but the occasional patient whose biopsies have come my way did resolve over the ensuing year.

- **Microscopic enteritis/colitis associated with autism** A new syndrome has been reported in children with autism who exhibited developmental regression and gastrointestinal symptoms (autistic enterocolitis). In some children this has been soon after MMR (measles, mumps, rubella) vaccination. The question is whether there is a connection between these, with the cytokines produced during the inflammatory process affecting development of the brain and resulting in variants of autism. The inflammation in the gut is subtle, with a mild intraepithelial lymphocytosis throughout the intestines, a low-grade microscopic colitis, and apparent lymphoid hyperplasia with polyp formation in some children, and possibly aphthoid ulcers.[203,204] Attempts to recover the virus have been variable, with some failing to find any virus.[205] Needless to say, this is highly contentious, having a direct impact on the possible use or not of MMR vaccination in infants.

- **Microscopic colitis associated with irritable bowel syndrome** Although classically biopsies have been used to exclude underlying pathology, on both theoretical and experimental data,[206] and when inflammatory cells are counted, there is often a minor increase in cells that are readily overlooked, such as mast cells.[207] In some instances inflammation has been in the form of inflammation in the myenteric plexus[208,209] or mucosa. In one study histologic and immunohistochemical examination of colonoscopic biopsy specimens from 77 patients with symptoms satisfying the Rome criteria and 28 asymptomatic control patients indicated three different groups:[209]

    1. The first (38 of 77) had normal conventional histology; however, immunohistochemistry showed increased intraepithelial lymphocytes, lamina propria CD3+ T cells and CD25+ cells compared with asymptomatic controls.
    2. The second group (31 of 77) had non-specific microscopic inflammation, and immunohistochemistry showed similar increases in lymphocyte populations (not significant compared with the uninflamed group) as well as increased numbers of neutrophils and mast cells compared to controls and the uninflamed group.
    3. The third group (8 of 77) fulfilled the criteria for classic lymphocytic colitis.

- **Apoptotic colopathy** In some patients with apparently normal biopsies there are numerous apoptotic bodies (nuclear fragments) either beneath the surface epithelium, which may be at least in part physiological and is found especially around the ileocecal valve, or in the crypts. Although there are well-recognized associations, such as graft-versus-host disease,[210] common variable immunodeficiency disease,[211] HIV-associated colitis[212] and even oral sodium phosphate enemas (Fleet's),[113] it has also become apparent that medications in particular, including NSAIDs[213] and ticlopidine,[214] can result in an apparent excess of apoptotic bodies. It is also quite common in ulcerative colitis, when it is probably the way that initial loss of crypt epithelium occurs.[215] The concept of apoptotic bodies

as an indication of drug-associated disease is novel, other than for cytotoxic drugs. In one study under normal conditions apoptotic bodies seldom were seen and the mean apoptotic count was less than 1.0. In untreated inflammatory bowel disease the mean apoptotic count was marginally increased (2.3), but during a partial response to drug treatment the apoptotic count rose to 13.1. In colonic lesions directly attributable to drugs the apoptotic count always was increased, reaching its highest level (106) with 5-fluorouracil.[113,213] There as been a suggestion that the apoptosis may represent chicken rather than egg, but this still awaits full publication.[216]

Whether such changes will be useful practically remains to be determined.

# DRUG-INDUCED PROCTITIS AND COLITIS

A medication history is indispensable in the investigation of patients with diarrhea. Ingestion of laxatives remains a relatively common cause of diarrhea, and one of the best reasons for advocating routine biopsies in patients with diarrhea undergoing colonoscopy is that evidence of anthraquinone ingestion, as manifested by pseudomelanosis coli, remains relatively common, may be denied by the patient, and may not be obvious endoscopically. Further, small amounts of anthraquinone can be overlooked unless a deliberate search is made of all large bowel biopsies from patients with diarrhea without obvious cause. Enemas and laxatives can cause mucin depletion, superficial epithelial damage, and even a superficial neutrophilic infiltrate.[113] A variety of drugs given either topically or systemically can cause colitis or proctitis, including penicillamine, sulfasalazine, methyldopa[217] and gold.

## NSAIDS

These appear to be responsible for considerable gastrointestinal morbidity and mortality. In many patients NSAIDs result in pooling of labeled neutrophils to the terminal ileum, presumably causing acute inflammation in this location. They may also induce severe small bowel ulcerations, which can perforate or bleed or cause protein loss, steatorrhea or, rarely, induce the formation of multiple diaphragms in the small intestine[218] and large intestine, as well as a colitis.[219,220] NSAIDs can cause a similar spectrum of diseases in the large bowel. The fenemates (mefenamic acid in particular) are associated with bloody diarrhea and an endoscopic appearance that mimics UC, although histologically only a mild colitis has been reported.[221,222] NSAIDs are also implicated in collagenous colitis.[223] One study reported an increased number of inflammatory cells, primarily lymphocytes, in the lamina propria, suggestive of microscopic colitis.[103] There also are case reports of eosinophilic colitis caused by naproxen,[217] and of pseudomembranous colitis resulting from diclofenac,[224,225] and increasingly 'non-specific' ulcers of the right colon in particular, but occasionally in the transverse and sigmoid colons[226,227] (Fig. 27.17). The changes in diffuse colitis, whether lymphocytic[228] or plasmacytic, as seen in collagenous colitis, closely resemble CD. NSAIDs also can cause exacerbations of established inflammatory bowel disease[229,230] and induce

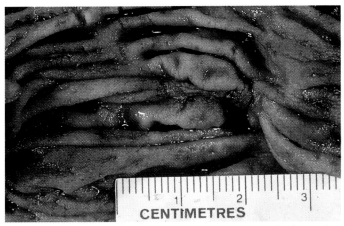

**Fig. 27.17** Ulcer in the right colon just above the ileocecal valve in a patient taking NSAIDs.

perforation, bleeding and fistula formation in other pre-existing diseases, such as diverticulitis.[218]

## ISCHEMIA

Recently it has become apparent that vasoconstriction from recreational drugs, particularly crack cocaine, can result in ischemic ulcers of the large bowel, often the rectum. The presence of 'non-specific' ulcers with lamina propria fibrosis or hyalinization suggests ischemia. In young patients in particular, in whom it is unexpected, this should lead to consideration of substance abuse.[136,231–233] Ergot taken for migraine can also induce ischemic lesions, and because of the lamina propria fibrosis this can also resemble solitary rectal ulcer syndrome.[234–236] In women, oral contraceptive use still has to be borne in mind.[237]

## COLITIS ASSOCIATED WITH IMMUNE DEFICIENCY

Immune deficiency can be hereditary, iatrogenic, a result of chemotherapy or immune suppression and graft-versus-host disease (GVH) following transplantation, or acquired either as a result of toxins or viruses such as the human immuno-deficiency virus (HIV) causing AIDS. All of these can affect the gut in different ways. The spectrum of disease is broad and includes the following areas.[24]

Immunodeficiency diseases can result in or be associated with:

1. Decreased plasma cells, lymphoid hyperplasia, secondary infection (e.g. giardiasis), secondary neoplasia (e.g. carcinoma and lymphoma of the intestinal tract, thymoma);
2. Decreased plasma cells (Bruton's) or plasma cells and lymphocytes (severe combined immunodeficiency syndrome);
3. Chronic granulomatous disease – brownish yellow histiocytes, poorly formed granulomas, CD-like colitis.

The enterocolitis associated with these immune deficiency states can be caused by or related to the following:

- Overgrowth of aerobic Gram-negative bacteria;
- Fungi, including Candida, Aspergillus, Torulopsis;
- Viruses such as cytomegalovirus (CMV);
- Pseudomembranous colitis (C. difficile);

- Neutropenic enterocolitis ('typhlitis');
- Parasitic infection such as Giardia, Cryptosporidium, disseminated Strongyloides infection;
- AIDS: numerous organisms, including Candida, CMV and herpesvirus, Cryptosporidium, Microsporidium including Isospora, Mycobacterium avium-intracellulare, Toxoplasma[238] Pneumocystis; AIDS enteropathy and colitis; Kaposi's sarcoma, lymphoma, anal condylomata and squamous carcinoma.

In patients with AIDS, some of the newer infections include Toxoplasma colitis occurring with disseminated toxoplasmosis,[238] histoplasma and HIV colitis.

Histoplasma infection has been described in an HIV-positive male who presented with acute diarrhea. The diagnosis was made by flexible sigmoidoscopy with biopsy, which revealed organisms morphologically consistent with Histoplasma capsulatum, confirmed by culture. At colonoscopy, skip areas with plaques, ulcers and a pseudopolyp were observed. The colitis resolved endoscopically after a 6-week course of intravenous amphotericin B, and the patient has had no recurrence of symptoms while on maintenance therapy with amphotericin B. However, the organisms continue to be noted on biopsies of normal-appearing areas in the rectum and sigmoid.[239]

HIV colitis is increasingly recognized in both the small and the large bowel and is characterized by an increase in chronic and sometimes acute inflammatory cells in the absence of an identifiable pathogen. Chronic diarrhea for longer than 6 months is common; other symptoms include rectal bleeding and abdominal pain. The mucosal pattern on colonoscopy may show a diffuse proctocolitis, consisting of contact bleeding, superficial ulcerations, exudates, or loss of vascular pattern. The inflammatory cell infiltrate with preserved crypt architecture may persist for years. HIV nucleic acid can be identified by in situ hybridization in colonic biopsies and HIV DNA confirmed by Southern blot analysis, although AIDS-positive control subjects without colitis can yield similar results.

## CYTOMEGALOVIRUS

Cytomegalovirus (CMV) may complicate almost any form of severe colitis, but is particularly seen in patients with AIDS and those receiving allografts of virtually any organ. It has been described following renal transplantation and following heart transplantation. In many instances it follows an episode of rejection treated by raising the dose of steroids.[240] It can also complicate drug-associated colitis (6200)and is associated with neutropenic enterocolitis (6202). In most instances it takes the form of multiple lesions varying from superficial erosions with a pseudomembranous appearance to large deep irregular serpiginous punched-out ulcers that may perforate. CMV inclusions are particularly found in the endothelium but are observed in virtually all mesenchymal, epithelial and neural tissue.

Among 44 male homosexuals who had CMV on colonic biopsy, CMV colitis was the index diagnosis for AIDS in 11 (25%). CMV colitis therefore can present early in AIDS, with such non-specific signs as fever, intermittent diarrhea, weight loss and hematochezia. Colonoscopy can appear normal and several biopsies may be required for accurate diagnosis. Colonoscopic biopsies positive for CMV were found only in the cecum in seven (39%) of 18 patients. The median time to the development of CMV colitis after the diagnosis of AIDS was 16 months in those patients who had received zidovudine and 3 months in those who had not.[241]

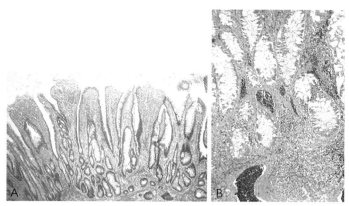

**Fig. 27.18** (A) Solitary rectal ulcer syndrome. The lamina propria obliterated by fibromuscular tissue derived form the hyperplastic muscularis mucosae. Note the early superficial ulceration. (B) Fibromuscular tissue in the lamina propria.

There has been a resurgence of interest in whether superimposed infection in patients with colitis is associated with more severe disease,[242–244] as well as in immunocompetent individuals,[242,245,246] and this is important because ganciclovir appears to have a role in the treatment of these patients.[247]

## SOLITARY RECTAL ULCER SYNDROME

The clinicopathologic spectrum of this disease is well described[248–251] and has a characteristic histologic appearance (Fig. 27.18). Nevertheless, it may escape diagnosis if the pathologist or clinician is not familiar with the typical appearances or if the biopsy is taken from an area of mucosa that is minimally involved, and still causes problems in diagnosis.[207,252] Solitary rectal ulcer syndrome is considered only in the differential diagnosis of idiopathic IBD limited to the rectum and distal sigmoid colon, and not in the differential diagnosis of more extensive disease.

## REFERENCES

1. Geboes K, Ectors N, D'Haens G, Rutgeerts P. Is ileoscopy with biopsy worthwhile in patients presenting with symptoms of inflammatory bowel disease? Am J Gastroenterol 1998;93:201–226.
2. Yusoff IF, Ormonde DG, Hoffman NE. Routine colonic mucosal biopsy and ileoscopy increases diagnostic yield in patients undergoing colonoscopy for diarrhea. J Gastroenterol Hepatol 2002;17:276–280.
3. Seldenrijk CA, Morson BC, Meuwissen SG, Schipper NW, Lindeman J, Meijer CJ. Histopathological evaluation of colonic mucosal biopsy specimens in chronic inflammatory bowel disease: diagnostic implications. Gut. 1991;32:1514–1520.
4. Tanaka M, Masuda T, Yao T et al. Observer variation of diagnoses based on simple biopsy criteria differentiating among Crohn's disease, ulcerative colitis, and other forms of colitis. J Gastroenterol Hepatol. 2001;16:1368–1372.
5. Tanaka M, Saito H, Fukuda S, Sasaki Y, Munakata A, Kudo H. Simple mucosal biopsy criteria differentiating among Crohn disease, ulcerative colitis, and other forms of colitis: measurement of validity. Scand J Gastroenterol 2000;35:281–226.
6. Allison MC, Hamilton-Dhillon AP, Pouncer RE. The value of rectal biopsy in distinguishing self-limited colitis from early inflammatory bowel disease. Q J Med 1987;65:985–995.
7. Ang ST, Bernstein CN, Robert ME, Weinstein WF. Cecal inflammation occurs in health and may result in false diagnoses of pancolitis: a prospective study (Abstract). Gastroenterology 1993;104:A1028.
8. D'Haens G, Geboes K, Peeters M, Baert F, Ectors N, Rutgeerts P. Patchy cecal inflammation associated with distal ulcerative colitis: A prospective endoscopic study. Am J Gastroenterol 1997;92:1275–1279.
9. Lewin KJ, Riddell RH, Weinstein WM. Gastrointestinal pathology and its clinical implications. New York: Igaku-Shoin; 1992.
10. Makapugay LM, Dean PJ. Diverticular disease-associated chronic colitis. Am J Surg Pathol 1996;20:94–102.
11. Odze R, Antonioli D, Peppercorn M, Goldman H. Effects of topical 5-aminosalicylic acid (5-ASA) therapy on rectal mucosal biopsy morphology in chronic ulcerative colitis. Am J Surg Pathol 1993;17:869–875.
12. Bernstein CN, Shanahan F, Weinstein WM. Histological patchiness and sparing of the rectum in ulcerative colitis: Refuting the dogma. J Clin Pathol 1997;50:354–355.
13. Farmer RG. Longterm prognosis for patients with ulcerative proctosigmoiditis (ulcerative colitis confined to the rectum and sigmoid colon). J Clin Gastroenterol 1979;1:47–50.
14. Jenkins D, Goodall A, Scott BB. Ulcerative colitis: one disease or two? (Quantitative histological differences between distal and extensive disease). Gut. 1990;31:426–430.
15. Schumacher G, Sandstedt B, Mollby R, Kollberg B. Clinical and histologic features differentiating non-relapsing colitis from first attacks of inflammatory bowel disease. Scand J Gastroenterol 1991;26:151–161.
16. Tanaka M, Riddell RH, Saito H, Soma Y, Hidaka H, Kudo H. Morphologic criteria applicable to biopsy specimens for effective distinction of inflammatory bowel disease from other forms of colitis and of Crohn's disease from ulcerative colitis. Scand J Gastroenterol 1999;34:55–67.
17. Baron JH, Connell AM, Lennard-Jones JE. Variation between observers in describing mucosal appearances in proctocolitis. Br Med J 1964;1:89–92.
18. Matsuura K, Wakata H, Takeda N et al. Innominate lines of the colon. Radiology 1977;123:581–584.
19. Cole FM. Innominate grooves of the colon: morphological characteristics and etiological mechanisms. Radiology 1978;128:41–43.
20. Riddell RH, Goldman H, Ransohoff DF et al. Dysplasia in inflammatory bowel disease: standardized classification with provisional clinical applications. Hum Pathol 1983;14:931–968.
21. Geboes K, Riddell R, Ost A, Jensfelt B, Persson T, Lofberg R. A reproducible grading scale for histological assessment of inflammation in ulcerative colitis. Gut 2000;47:404–449.
22. Kirsner JB, Palmer WL, Klotz AP. Reversibility in ulcerative colitis: clinical and radiological observations. Radiology 1951;57:1–14.
23. Riley SA, Mani V, Goodman MJ, Dutt S, Herd ME. Microscopic activity in ulcerative colitis: what does it mean? Gut 1991;32:174–178.
24. Heatley RV, James PD. Eosinophils in the rectal mucosa. A simple method of predicting the outcome of ulcerative proctocolitis? Gut 1979;20:787–791.
25. Jalan KN, Walker RJ, Sircus W, McManus JPA, Prescott RJ, Card WI. Pseudopolyposis in ulcerative colitis. Lancet 1969;2:555–559.
26. Goulston SJM, McGovern VJ. The nature of benign strictures in ulcerative colitis. N Engl J Med 1969;281:3290–3295.
27. Wheeler MH, Curley IR, Williams ED. The association of neurofibromatosis, pheochromcytoma, and somatostatin-rich duodenal carcinoid tumor. Surgery 1986;100:1163–1169.
28. Markowitz J, Kahn E, Grancher K, Hyams J, Treem W, Daum F. Atypical rectosigmoid histology in children with newly diagnosed ulcerative colitis. Am J Gastroenterol 1993;88:2034–2207.
29. Washington K, Greenson JK, Montgomery E et al. Histopathology of ulcerative colitis in initial rectal biopsy in children. Am J Surg Pathol 2002;26:1441–1449.
30. de la Monte SM, Hutchins GM. Follicular proctocolitis and neuromatous hyperplasia with lymphogranuloma venereum. Hum Pathol 1985;16:1025–1032.
31. Flejou JF, Potet F, Bogomoletz VV et al. Lymphoid follicular proctitis. A condition different from ulcerative proctitis? Dig Dis Sci. 1988;33:314–320.
32. Haggitt RC. The differential diagnosis of inflammatory bowel disease. In: Norris HT, ed. Pathology of the colon, small intestine and anus. New York: Churchill Livingstone; 1983:21–60.
33. Naylor AR, Pollet JE. Eosinophilic colitis. Dis Colon Rectum 1985;28:615–618.
34. Odze RD, Bines J, Leichtner AM, Goldman H, Antonioli DA. Allergic proctocolitis in infants: a prospective clinicopathologic biopsy study. Hum Pathol 1993;24:668–674.
35. Falade AG, Darbyshire PJ, Raafat F, Booth IW. Hypereosinophilic syndrome in childhood appearing as inflammatory bowel disease. J Pediatr Gastroenterol Nutr 1991;12:276–279.
36. Clouse RE, Alpers DH, Hockenbery DM, De Schryver-Kecskemeti K. Pericrypt eosinophilic enterocolitis and chronic diarrhea. Gastroenterology 1992;103:168–176.
37. Anttila VJ, Valtonen M. Carbamazepine-induced eosinophilic colitis. Epilepsia 1992;33:119–121.
38. D'Haens GR, Geboes K, Peeters M, Baert F, Pennickx F, Rutgeerts P. Early lesions of recurrent Crohn's disease caused by infusion of intestinal contents in excluded ileum. Gastroenterology 1998;114:262–267.
39. Mahadeva U, Martin JP, Patel NK, Price AB. Granulomatous ulcerative colitis: a reappraisal of the mucosal granuloma in the distinction of Crohn's disease from ulcerative colitis. Histopathology 2002;41:50–55.
40. Matsumoto T, Nakamura S, Shimizu M, Iida M. Significance of appendiceal involvement in patients with ulcerative colitis. Gastrointest Endosc 2002;55:180–185.
41. Yamagishi N, Iizuka B, Nakamura T, Suzuki S, Hayashi N. Clinical and colonoscopic investigation of skipped periappendiceal lesions in ulcerative colitis. Scand J Gastroenterol 2002;37:177–182.

42. Bernstein CN, Shanahan F, Anton PA, Weinstein WM. Patchiness of mucosal inflammation in treated ulcerative colitis: A prospective study. Gastrointest Endosc 1995;42:232–237.

43. Kim B, Barnett JL, Kleer CG, Appelman HD. Endoscopic and histological patchiness in treated ulcerative colitis. Am J Gastroenterol 1999;94:3258–3362.

44. Kleer CG, Appelman HD. Ulcerative colitis: patterns of involvement in colorectal biopsies and changes with time. Am J Surg Pathol 1998;22:983–999.

45. Buckwell NA. Depth of ulceration in acute colitis. Gastroenterology 1980;79:19.

46. Edwards FC, Truelove SC. The course and prognosis of ulcerative colitis. Gut 1964;5:1–22.

47. Warren S, Sommers SC. Pathogenesis of ulcerative colitis. Am J Pathol 1949;25:657–679.

48. Lumb G, Protheroe RHB. Biopsy of the rectum in ulcerative colitis. Lancet 1955;2:1208–1215.

49. Jalan KN, Sircus W, Card WI et al. An experience in ulcerative colitis. I. Toxic dilatation in 55 cases. Gastroenterology 1969;57:68–82.

50. Greenstein AJ, Sachar DB, Gibas A et al. Outcome of toxic dilatation in ulcerative and Crohn's colitis. J Clin Gastroenterol 1985;7:137–143.

51. Norland CC, Kirsner JB. Toxic dilatation of colon (toxic megacolon): etiology, treatment and prognosis in 42 patients. Medicine 1969;48:229–250.

52. Lichtiger S, Present DH, Kornbluth A et al. Cyclosporine in severe ulcerative colitis refractory to steroid therapy [see comments]. N Engl J Med 1994;330:1841–1845.

53. Carbonnel F, Boruchowicz A, Duclos B et al. Intravenous cyclosporine in attacks of ulcerative colitis – short-term and long-term responses. Dig Dis Sci 1996;41:2471–2476.

54. Aiko S, Conner EM, Fuseler JA, Grisham MB. Effects of cyclosporine or FK506 in chronic colitis. J Pharmacol Exp Ther 1997;280:1075–1084.

55. Gumaste V, Sachar DB, Greenstein AJ. Benign and malignant colorectal strictures in ulcerative colitis. Gut 1992;33:938–941.

56. DeDombal FT, Watts JMcK, Watkinson G, Goligher JC. Local complications of ulcerative colitis: stricture, pseudopolyposis, and carcinoma of colon and rectum. Br Med J 1966;1:1442–1447.

57. Fries J. Experiences with allergy to soybean in the United States. J Asthma Res 1966;3:209–211.

58. Saltzstein SI, Rosenberg BF. Ulcerative colitis of the ileum and regional enteritis of the colon, a comparative histologic study. Am J Clin Pathol 1963;40:610–623.

59. Markowitz AM. The less common perforations of the small bowel. Ann Surg 1960;152:240–257.

60. Heuschen UA, Hinz U, Allemeyer EH et al. Backwash ileitis is strongly associated with colorectal carcinoma in ulcerative colitis. Gastroenterology 2001;120:841–887.

61. Schmidt CM, Lazenby AJ, Hendrickson RJ, Sitzmann JV. Preoperative terminal ileal and colonic resection histopathology predicts risk of pouchitis in patients after ileoanal pull-through procedure. Ann Surg 1998;227:654–662.

62. Morson BC, Dawson IMP. Gastrointestinal pathology, 2nd edn. Oxford: Blackwell; 1979:732.

63. Hinrichs RH, Goldman H. Localized giant pseudopolyposis of the colon. JAMA 1968;205:108–109.

64. Kelly JK, Langerin JM, Price LM, Hershfield NB, Share S, Bluestein P. Giant and symptomatic inflammatory polyps of the colon in idiopathic inflammatory bowel disease. Am J Surg Pathol 1986;10:420–428.

65. Mery CM, Carmona-Sanchez R, Suazo-Barahona J, Ponce-de Leon S, Robles-Diaz G. Appendectomy and the development of ulcerative colitis. Am J Gastroenterol 2000;95:1850–1851.

66. Perry WB, Opelka FG, Smith D et al. Discontinuous appendiceal involvement in ulcerative colitis: pathology and clinical correlation. J Gastrointest Surg 1999;3:141–144.

67. Davison AM, Dixon MF. The appendix as a 'skip lesion' in ulcerative colitis [see comments]. Histopathology 1990;16:93–95.

68. Groisman GM, George J, Harpaz N. Ulcerative appendicitis in universal and nonuniversal ulcerative colitis. Mod Pathol 1994;7:322–325.

69. Kroft SH, Stryker SJ, Rao MS. Appendiceal involvement as a skip lesion in ulcerative colitis. Mod Pathol 1994;7:912–914.

70. Goldblum JR, Appelman HD. Appendiceal involvement in ulcerative colitis. Mod Pathol 1992;5:607–610.

71. Jahadi MR, Faus ML, Shaw ML. The pathology of the appendix in ulcerative colitis. Dis Colon Rectum 1976;19:345–349.

72. Lamps LW, Madhusudhan KT, Greenson JK et al. The role of Yersinia enterocolitica and Yersinia pseudotuberculosis in granulomatous appendicitis: a histologic and molecular study. Am J Surg Pathol 2001;25:508–515.

73. Saebo A, Lassen J. A survey of acute and chronic disease associated with Yersinia enterocolitica infection. A Norwegian 10-year follow-up study on 458 hospitalized patients. Scand J Infect Dis 1991;23:517–527.

74. Pontes EL, Piris J, Jewell DP, Truelove SC. Local immune responses preceding clinical relapse in ulcerative colitis: changes in Ig-containing cells, T-lymphocytes and eosinophils (Abstract). Gut 1982;23:895–899.

75. Lockhart-Mummery HE, Morson BC. Crohn's disease of the large intestine. Gut 1964;5:493–509.

76. Price AB, Morson BC. Inflammatory bowel disease: The surgical pathology of Crohn's disease and ulcerative colitis. Hum Pathol 1975;6:7–29.

77. Farmer RG, Hawk WA, Turnbull RB. Clinical patterns in Crohn's disease: A statistical study of 615 cases. Gastroenterology 1975;68:627–635.

78. Truelove SC, Pea AS. Course and prognosis of Crohn's disease. Gut 1976;17:192–201.

79. Higgens CS, Allan RN. Crohn's disease of the distal ileum. Gut 1980;21:933–940.

80. Okada M, Yao T, Fuchigami T, Iida M, Date H. Anatomical involvement and clinical features in 91 Japanese patients with Crohn's disease. J Clin Gastroenterol 1987;9:165–171.

81. Owen RL. And now pathophysiology of M cells – good news and bad news from Peyer's patches. Gastroenterology 1983;85:468–470.

82. Okada M, Maeda K, Yao T, Iwashita A, Nomiyama Y, Kitahara K. Minute lesions of the rectum and sigmoid colon in patients with Crohn's disease. Gastrointest Endosc 1991;37:319–324.

83. Oberhuber G, Püspök A, Oesterreicher C et al. Focally enhanced gastritis: A frequent type of gastritis in patients with Crohn's disease. Gastroenterology 1997;112:698–706.

84. Wright C, Riddell RH. Histology of the stomach and duodenum in Crohn's disease. Am J Surg Pathol 1998, 22:383–390.

85. Surawicz CM, Meisel JL, Ylvisaker T, Saunders DR, Rubin CE. Rectal biopsy in the diagnosis of Crohn's disease: value of multiple biopsies and serial sectioning. Gastroenterology 1981;81:66–71.

86. O'Leary AD, Sweeney EC. Lymphoglandular complexes of the colon: structure and distribution. Histopathology 1986;10:267–283.

87. Sankey EA, Dhillon AP, Anthony A et al. Early mucosal changes in Crohn's disease. Gut 1993;34:375–381.

88. Dhillon AP, Anthony A, Sim R et al. Mucosal capillary thrombi in rectal biopsies. Histopathology 1992;21:127–133.

89. Tytgat GNJ, Muider CJJ, Brummelkamp WH. Endoscopic lesions in Crohn's disease early after ileocecal resection. Endoscopy 1988;20:260–262.

90. Rutgeerts P, Geboes K, Vantrappen G, Kerremans R, Coenegrachts JL, Coremans G. Natural history of recurrent Crohn's disease at the ileocolonic anastomosis after curative surgery. Gut 1984;25:665–672.

91. Ekberg O, Fork F-T, Hildell J. Predictive value of small bowel radiography for recurrent Crohn's disease. Am J Radiol 1980;135:1051–1055.

92. Rutgeerts P, Goboes K, Peeters M et al. Effect of faecal stream diversion on recurrence of Crohn's disease in the neoterminal ileum [see comments]. Lancet 1991;338:771–774.

93. Dvorak AM, Monahan RA, Osage JE, Dickersin GR. Crohn's disease. Transmission electron microscopic studies. II. Immunologic inflammatory response. Alterations of mast cells, basophils, eosinophils and the microvasculature. Hum Pathol 1980;11:606–619.

94. Wright NA, Pike C, Elia G. Induction of a novel epidermal growth factor-secretory cell lineage by mucosal ulceration in human gastrointestinal stem cells. Nature 1990;343:82–86.

95. Poulsom R, Chinery R, Sarraf C et al. Trefoil peptide expression in intestinal adaptation and renewal. Scand J Gastroenterol 1992;192:17–28.

96. McQuillan AC, Appelman HD. Superficial Crohn's disease – a study of 10 patients. Surg Pathol 1989;2:231–239.

97. Cook MG, Dixon MF. An analysis of the reliability of detection and diagnostic value of various pathological features in Crohn's disease and ulcerative colitis. Gut 1973;14:255–262.

98. Kelly JK, Sutherland LR. The chronological sequence in the pathology of Crohn's disease. J Clin Gastroenterol 1988;10:28–33.

99. Dvorak AM, Osage JE, Monahan RA, Dickersin GR. Crohn's disease. Transmission electron microscopic studies. III. Target tissues. Proliferation of and injury to smooth muscle and the autonomic nervous system. Hum Pathol 1980;11:620–634.

100. Kelly JK, Preshaw RM. Origin of fistulas in Crohn's disease. J Clin Gastroenterol 1989;11:193–196.

101. Kelly JK, Siu TO. The strictures, sinuses, and fissures of Crohn's disease. J Clin Gastroenterol 1986;8:594–598.

102. Kahn E, Markowitz J, Blomquist K, Daum F. The morphologic relationship of sinus and fistula formation to intestinal stenoses in children with Crohn's disease. Am J Gastroenterol 1993;88:1395–1398.

103. Tonelli F, Ficari F. Pathological features of Crohn's disease determining perforation. J Clin Gastroenterol 1991;13:226–230.

104. Kotanagi H, Kramer K, Fazio VW, Petras RE. Do microscopic abnormalities at resection margins correlate with increased anastomotic recurrence in Crohn's disease? Retrospective analysis of 100 cases. Dis Colon Rectum 1991;34:909–916.

105. Fazio VW, Marchetti F, Church JM et al. Effect of resection margins on the recurrence of Crohn's disease in the small bowel – a randomized controlled trial. Ann Surg 1996;224:563–571.

106. Lescut D, Vanco D, Bonniere P et al. Perioperative endoscopy of the whole small bowel in Crohn's disease [see comments]. Gut 1993;34:647–649.

107. Sheehan AL, Warren BF, Gear MW, Shepherd NA. Fat-wrapping in Crohn's disease: pathological basis and relevance to surgical practice. Br J Surg 1992;79:955–958.

108. Butterworth RJ, Williams GT, Hughes LE. Can Crohn's disease be diagnosed at laparotomy? Gut 1992;33:140–142.

109. Smedh K, Olaison G, Nystrom PO, Sjodahl R. Intraoperative enteroscopy in Crohn's disease. Br J Surg 1993;80:897–900.

110. Tanaka M, Riddell RH. The pathological diagnosis and differential diagnosis of Crohn's disease. Hepatogastroenterology 1990;37:18–31.

111. Volk EE, Shapiro BD, Easley KA, Goldblum JR. The clinical significance of a biopsy-based diagnosis of focal active colitis: a clinicopathologic study of 31 cases. Mod Pathol 1998;11:789–794.

112. Dyer NH, Stansfeld AG, Dawson AM. The value of rectal biopsy in the diagnosis of Crohn's disease. Scand J Gastroenterol 1970;5:494–497.

113. Driman DK, Preiksaitis HG. Colorectal inflammation and increased cell proliferation associated with oral sodium phosphate bowel preparation solution. Hum Pathol 1998;29:972–978.

114. Kasahara Y, Tanaka S, Nishino M, Umemura H, Shiraha S, Kuyama T. Intestinal involvement in Behcet's disease: review of 136 surgical cases in the Japanese literature. Dis Colon Rectum 1981;24:103–106.

115. Jung HC, Rhee PL, Song IS, Choi KW, Kim CY. Temporal changes in the clinical type or diagnosis of Behcet's colitis in patients with aphthoid or punched-out colonic ulcerations. J Korean Med Sci 1991;6:313–318.

116. Couper R, Kapelushnik J, Griffiths AM. Neutrophil dysfunction in glycogen storage disease Ib: association with Crohn's-like colitis. Gastroenterology 1991;100:549–554.

117. Roe TF, Coates TD, Thomas DW, Miller JH, Gilsanz V. Brief report: treatment of chronic inflammatory bowel disease in glycogen storage disease type Ib with colony-stimulating factors. N Engl J Med. 1992;326:1666–1669.

118. Yamaguchi T, Ihara K, Matsumoto T et al. Inflammatory bowel disease-like colitis in glycogen storage disease type Ib. Inflamm Bowel Dis 2001;7:128–132.

119. Schinella RA, Greco MA, Garay SM, Lackner H, Wolman SR, Fazzini EP. Hermansky–Pudlak syndrome: a clinicopathologic study. Hum Pathol 1985;16:366–376.

120. Werlin SL, Chusid MJ, Caya J, Oechler HW. Colitis in chronic granulomatous disease. Gastroenterology 1982;82:328–331.

121. Isaacs D, Wright VM, Shaw DG, Raafat F, Walker-Smith JA. Chronic granulomatous disease mimicking Crohn's disease. J Pediatr Gastroenterol Nutr 1985;4:498–501.

122. Warren BF, Shepherd NA. The role of pathology in pelvic ileal reservoir surgery. Int J Colorectal Dis 1992;7:68–75.

123. Lee KS, Medline A, Shockey S. Indeterminate colitis in the spectrum of inflammatory bowel disease. Arch Pathol Lab Med 1979;103:173–176.

124. Price AB. Overlap in the spectrum of non-specific inflammatory bowel disease: colitis indeterminate. J Clin Pathol 1978;31:567–577.

125. Valdez R, Appelman HD, Bronner MP, Greenson JK. Diffuse duodenitis associated with ulcerative colitis. Am J Surg Pathol 2000;24:1407–1413.

126. Mitomi H, Atari E, Uesugi H et al. Distinctive diffuse duodenitis associated with ulcerative colitis. Dig Dis Sci 1997;42:684–693.

127. Sasaki M, Okada K, Koyama S et al. Ulcerative colitis complicated by gastroduodenal lesions. J Gastroenterol 1996;31:585–589.

128. Kaufman SS, Vanderhoof JA, Young R, Perry D, Raynor SC, Mack DR. Gastroenteric inflammation in children with ulcerative colitis. Am J Gastroenterol 1997;92:1209–1212.

129. Terashima S, Hoshino Y, Kanzaki N, Kogure M, Gotoh M. Ulcerative duodenitis accompanying ulcerative colitis. J Clin Gastroenterol 2001;32:172–175.

130. Tobin JM, Sinha B, Ramani P, Saleh AR, Murphy MS. Upper gastrointestinal mucosal disease in pediatric Crohn disease and ulcerative colitis: a blinded, controlled study. J Pediatr Gastroenterol Nutr 2001;32:443–448.

131. Wong NA, Penman ID, Campbell S, Lessells AM. Microscopic focal cryptitis associated with sodium phosphate bowel preparation. Histopathology 2000;36:476–478.

132. Greenson JK, Stern RA, Carpenter SL, Barnett JL. The clinical significance of focal active colitis. Hum Pathol 1997;28:729–733.

133. Mitros F, Johlin F. Relative nonspecificity of hemosiderin deposition in colon as a marker for ischemia. Lab Invest 1986;54:44A.

134. Johnson TD, Berenson MM. Methamphetamine-induced ischemic colitis. J Clin Gastroenterol 1991;13:687–689.

135. Bravo AJ, Lowman RM. Benign ulcer of the sigmoid colon. An unusual lesion that can simulate carcinoma. Radiology 1968;90:113–115.

136. Yang RD, Han MW, McCarthy JH. Ischemic colitis in a crack abuser. Dig Dis Sci 1991;36:238–240.

137. Miyazaki K, Funakoshi A, Nishihara S, Wasada T, Koga A, Ibayashi H. Aberrant insulinoma in the duodenum. Gastroenterology 1986;90:1280–1285.

138. Flaherty MJ, Lie JT, Haggitt RC. Mesenteric inflammatory veno-occlusive disease. A seldom recognized cause of intestinal ischemia. Am J Surg Pathol 1994;18:779–784.

139. Ullah N, Yeh R, Ehrinpreis M. Fatal hyperphosphatemia from a phosphosoda bowel preparation. J Clin Gastroenterol 2002;34:457–458.

140. Lindeman RJ, Weinstein L, Levitan R, Patterson JF. Ulcerative colitis and intestinal salmonellosis. Am J Med Sci 1967;254:855–861.

141. Newman A, Lambert JR. *Campylobacter jejuni* causing flare-up of inflammatory bowel disease. Lancet 1980;2:919.

142. Bolton RP, Sheriff RJ, Read AD. *Clostridium difficile* associated diarrhoea: a role in inflammatory bowel disease. Lancet 1980;1:383–384.

143. Glotzer DJ, Glick ME, Goldman H. Proctitis and colitis following diversion of the fecal stream. Gastroenterology 1981;80:438–441.

144. Yeong ML, Bethwaite PB, Prasad J, Isbister WH. Lymphoid follicular hyperplasia – a distinctive feature of diversion colitis. Histopathology 1991;19:55–61.

145. Geraghty JM, Talbot IC. Diversion colitis: histological features in the colon and rectum after defunctioning colostomy. Gut 1991;32:1020–1023.

146. Warren BF, Shepherd NA, Bartolo DC, Bradfield JW. Pathology of the defunctioned rectum in ulcerative colitis. Gut 1993;34:514–516.

147. Warren BF, Shepherd NA. Diversion proctocolitis. Histopathology 1992;21:91–93.

148. Asplund S, Gramlich T, Fazio V, Petras R. Histologic changes in defunctioned rectums in patients with inflammatory bowel disease: a clinicopathologic study of 82 patients with long-term follow-up. Dis Colon Rectum 2002;45:1206–1213.

149. Vujanic GM, Dojcinov SD. Diversion colitis in children: an iatrogenic appendix vermiformis? Histopathology 2000;36:41–46.

150. Feakins RM. Diversion proctocolitis with granulomatous vasculitis in a patient without inflammatory bowel disease. Histopathology 2000;36:88–89.

151. Rice AJ, Abbott CR, Mapstone NM. Granulomatous vasculitis in diversion procto-colitis. Histopathology 1999;34:276–277.

152. Guillemot F, Colombel JF, Neut C et al. Treatment of diversion colitis by short-chain fatty acids. Prospective and double-blind study [see comments]. Dis Colon Rectum 1991;34:861–864.

153. Griffiths AP, Dixon MF. Microcarcinoids and diversion colitis in a colon defunctioned for 18 years. Report of a case. Dis Colon Rectum 1992;35:685–688.

154. Shepherd NA, Healey CJ, Warren BF, Richman PI, Thomson WH, Wilkinson SP. Distribution of mucosal pathology and an assessment of colonic phenotypic change in the pelvic ileal reservoir. Gut 1993;34:101–105.

155. de Silva HJ, Jones M, Prince C, Kettlewell M, Mortensen NJ, Jewell DP. Lymphocyte and macrophage subpopulations in pelvic ileal pouches [see comments]. Gut 1991;32:1160–1165.

156. Santavirta J, Mattila J, Kokki M, Matikainen M. Mucosal morphology and faecal bacteriology after ileoanal anastomosis. Int J Colorectal Dis 1991;6:38–41.

157. Onderdonk AB, Dvorak AM, Cisneros RL et al. Microbiologic assessment of tissue biopsy samples from ileal pouch patients. J Clin Microbiol 1992;30:312–317.

158. Clausen MR, Tvede M, Mortensen PB. Short-chain fatty acids in pouch contents from patients with and without pouchitis after ileal pouch–anal anastomosis. Gastroenterology 1992;103:1144–1153.

159. Levin KE, Pemberton JH, Phillips SF, Zinsmeister AR, Pezim ME. Role of oxygen free radicals in the etiology of pouchitis. Dis Colon Rectum 1992;35:452–456.

160. Kmiot WA, Hesslewood SR, Smith N, Thompson H, Harding LK, Keighley MR. Evaluation of the inflammatory infiltrate in pouchitis with 111In-labeled granulocytes [see comments]. Gastroenterology 1993;104:981–988.

161. de Silva HJ, Millard PR, Kettlewell M, Mortensen NJ, Prince C, Jewell DP. Mucosal characteristics of pelvic ileal pouches. Gut 1991;32:61–65.

162. Bahia SS, McMahon RF, Hobbiss J, Taylor TV, Stoddart RW. Pelvic ileo-anal reservoirs: a lectin histochemical study. Histochem J 1993;25:392–400.

163. Prior A, Lessels AM, Whorwell PJ. Is biopsy necessary if colonoscopy is normal? Dig Dis Sci 1987;32:673–676.

164. Deutsch AA, McLeod RS, Cullen J, Cohen Z. Results of the pelvic-pouch procedure in patients with Crohn's disease. Dis Colon Rectum 1991;34:475–477.

165. Thompson-Fawcett MW, Marcus V, Redston M, Cohen Z, McLeod RS. Risk of dysplasia in long-term ileal pouches and pouches with chronic pouchitis. Gastroenterology 2001;121:275–281.

166. Veress B, Reinholt FP, Lindquist K, Lofberg R, Liljeqvist L. Long-term histomorphological surveillance of the pelvic ileal pouch: dysplasia develops in a subgroup of patients. Gastroenterology 1995;109:1090–1097.

167. Thompson-Fawcett MW, Mortensen NJ, Warren BF. 'Cuffitis' and inflammatory changes in the columnar cuff, anal transitional zone, and ileal reservoir after stapled pouch–anal anastomosis. Dis Colon Rectum 1999;42:348–355.

168. Bo-Linn GW, Vendrell DD, Lee E, Fordtran JS. An evaluation of the significance of microscopic colitis in patients with chronic diarrhea. J Clin Invest 1985;75:1559–1569.

169. Sanderson IR, Boyle S, Williams CB, Walker-Smith JA. Histological abnormalities in biopsies from macroscopically normal colonoscopies. Arch Dis Child 1986;61:274–277.

170. Kinghan JGC, Levison DA, Ball JA, Dawson AM. Microscopic colitis – a cause of chronic watery diarrhea. Br Med J 1982;285:1601–1604.

171. Lee E, Schiller LR, Vendrell D, Santa Ana CA, Fordtran JS. Subepithelial collagen table thickness in colon specimens from patients with microscopic colitis and collagenous colitis. Gastroenterology 1992;103:1790–1796.

172. Rubio CA, Lindholm J. Cryptal lymphocytic coloproctitis: a new phenotype of lymphocytic colitis? J Clin Pathol 2002;55:138–140.

173. Libbrecht L, Croes R, Ectors N, Staels F, Geboes K. Microscopic colitis with giant cells. Histopathology 2002;40:335–338.

174. Fasoli R, Talbot I, Reid M, Prince C, Jewell DP. Microscopic colitis: can it be qualitatively and quantitatively characterized? Ital J Gastroenterol 1992;24:393–396.

175. Lazenby AJ, Yardley JH, Giardiello FM, Jessurun J, Bayless TM. Lymphocytic ('microscopic') colitis: A comparative histologic study with particular reference to collagenous colitis. Hum Pathol 1989;20:18–28.

176. Giardiello FM, Lazenby AJ, Bayless TM et al. Lymphocytic (microscopic) colitis. Clinicopathologic study of 18 patients and comparison to collagenous colitis. Dig Dis Sci 1989;34:1730–1738.

177. Tanaka M, Mazzoleni G, Riddell RH. Distribution of collagenous colitis: utility of flexible sigmoidoscopy. Gut 1992;33:65–70.

178. Mills LR, Schuman BM, Thompson WO. Lymphocytic colitis. A definable clinical and histological diagnosis. Dig Dis Sci 1993;38:1147–1151.

179. Gledhill A, Cole FM. Significance of basement membrane thickening in the human colon. Gut 1984;25:1085–1088.

180. Gardiner GW, Goldberg R, Currie D, Murray D. Colonic carcinoma associated with an abnormal collagen table. Cancer 1984;54:2973–2977.

181. Jessurum J, Yardley JG, Giardiello FM, Hamilton SR, Bayless TM. Chronic colitis with thickening of the subepithelial collagen layer (collagenous colitis). Histopathologic findings in 15 patients. Hum Pathol 1987;18:839–848.

182. Chandratre S, Bramble MG, Cooke WM, Jones RA. Simultaneous occurrence of collagenous colitis and Crohn's disease. Digestion 1987;36:55–60.

183. Fausa O, Foerster A, Hovig T. Collagenous colitis. A clinical, histological, and ultrastructural study. Scand J Gastroenterol 1985;107:8–23.

184. Danzi JT, McDonald TJ, King J. Collagenous colitis. Am J Gastroenterol 1988;83:83–85.

185. Lindstrom CG. 'Collagenous colitis' with watery diarrhoea – a new entity? Pathol Eur 1976;11:87–89.

186. Kingham JGC, Levison DA, Morson BC, Dawson AM. Collagenous colitis. Gut 1986;27:570–577.

187. Leigh C, Alahmady A, Mitros FA, Metcalf A, Al-Jurf A. Collagenous colitis associated with chronic constipation. Am J Surg Pathol 1993;17:81–84.

188. Bogomoletz WV, Adnet JJ, Birembaut P, Feydy P, Dupon P. Collagenous colitis: an unrecognized entity. Gut 1980;21:164–168.

189. van den Oord JJ, Geboes K, Desmet VJ. Collagenous colitis: an abnormal collagen table? Two new cases and review of the literature. Am J Gastroenterol 1982;77:377–381.

190. Flejou JF, Grimand JA, Molas G, Baviera G, Potet F. Collagenous colitis. Ultrastructural study and collagen immunotyping in four cases. Arch Pathol Lab Med 1984;108:977–982.

191. Teglbjaerg PS, Tahysen EH, Jensen HH. Development of collagenous colitis in sequential biopsy specimens. Gastroenterology 1984;87:703–709.

192. Giardiello FM, Bayless TM, Kessurun J, Hamilton SR, Yardley JH. Collagenous colitis: physiologic and histopathologic studies in seven patients. Ann Intern Med 1987;106:46–49.

193. Carpenter HA, Tremaine WJ, Batts KP, Czaja AJ. Subepithelial collagen table thickness in colon specimens from patients with microscopic colitis and collagenous colitis. Gastroenterology 1992;103:1790–1796.

194. Carpenter HA, Tremaine WJ, Batts KP, Czaja AJ. Sequential histologic evaluations in collagenous colitis. Correlations with disease behavior and sampling strategy. Dig Dis Sci 1992;37:1903–1909.

195. Rams H, Rogers AI, Ghandur-Mnaymneh L. Collagenous colitis. Ann Intern Med 1987;106:108–113.

196. Riddell RH, Croitoru K, Irvine EJ. Association of collagenous colitis and celiac sprue. A further cause of failure to respond to gluten withdrawal. Gastroenterology 1990;98:A198.

197. Eckstein RP, Dowsett JF, Riley JW. Collagenous colitis: a case of collagenous colitis with involvement of the small intestine. Am J Gastroenterol 1988;83:767–771.

198. Lewis FW, Warren GH, Goff JS. Collagenous colitis with involvement of terminal ileum. Dig Dis Sci 1991;36:1161–1163.

199. Armes J, Gee DC, Macrae FA, Schroeder W, Bhathal PS. Collagenous colitis: jejunal and colorectal pathology. J Clin Pathol 1992;45:784–787.

200. Giardiello FM, Jackson FW, Lazenby AJ. Metachronous occurrence of collagenous colitis and ulcerative colitis. Gut 1991;32:447–449.

201. Griesser GH, Schumacher U, Eifeldt R, Horny H-P. Adenosquamous carcinoma of the ileum. Report of a case and review of the literature. Virchows Arch [Pathol Anat]. 1985;406:483–487.

202. Bryant DA, Mintz ED, Puhr ND, Griffin PM, Petras RE. An outbreak of Brainerd diarrhea associated with colonic epithelial lymphocytosis resembling lymphocytic colitis. Am J Surg Pathol 1996;20:1102–1109.

203. Torrente F, Ashwood P, Day R et al. Small intestinal enteropathy with epithelial IgG and complement deposition in children with regressive autism. Mol Psychiatry 2002;7:375–382, 334.

204. Wakefield AJ, Murch SH, Anthony A et al. Ileal–lymphoid–nodular hyperplasia, non-specific colitis, and pervasive developmental disorder in children. Lancet 1998;351:637–641.

205. Thjodleifsson B, Davidsdottir K, Agnarsson U, Sigthorsson G, Kjeld M, Bjarnason I. Effect of Pentavac and measles-mumps-rubella (MMR) vaccination on the intestine. Gut 2002;51:816–817.

206. Collins SM. A case for an immunological basis for irritable bowel syndrome. Gastroenterology 2002;122:2078–2080.

207. O'Sullivan M, Clayton N, Breslin NP et al. Increased mast cells in the irritable bowel syndrome. Neurogastroenterol Motil 2000;12:449–457.

208. Tornblom H, Lindberg G, Nyberg B, Veress B. Full-thickness biopsy of the jejunum reveals inflammation and enteric neuropathy in irritable bowel syndrome. Gastroenterology 2002;123:1972–1979.

209. Chadwick VS, Chen W, Shu D et al. Activation of the mucosal immune system in irritable bowel syndrome. Gastroenterology 2002;122:1778–1783.

210. Washington K, Bentley RC, Green A, Olson J, Treem WR, Krigman HR. Gastric graft-versus-host disease: a blinded histologic study. Am J Surg Pathol 1997;21:1037–1046.

211. Washington K, Stenzel TT, Buckley RH, Gottfried MR. Gastrointestinal pathology in patients with common variable immunodeficiency and X-linked agammaglobulinemia. Am J Surg Pathol 1996;20:1240–1252.

212. Orenstein JM, Dieterich DT. The histopathology of 103 consecutive colonoscopy biopsies from 82 symptomatic patients with acquired immunodeficiency syndrome: original and look-back diagnoses. Arch Pathol Lab Med 2001;125:1042–1046.

213. Lee FD. Importance of apoptosis in the histopathology of drug related lesions in the large intestine. J Clin Pathol 1993;46:118–122.

214. Berrebi D, Sautet A, Flejou JF, Dauge MC, Peuchmaur M, Potet F. Ticlopidine induced colitis: a histopathological study including apoptosis. J Clin Pathol 1998;51:280–283.

215. Iwamoto M, Koji T, Makiyama K, Kobayashi N, Nakane PK. Apoptosis of crypt epithelial cells in ulcerative colitis. J Pathol 1996;180:152–159.

216. McKenna BJ, Eldeiry D, Odze RD, Brian TP, Appelman HD. Apoptotic colopathy: a new variant of microscopic diarrheal disease? Lab Invest 2001;81:91A [Abstract].

217. Bridges AJ, Marshall JB, Diaz-Arias AA. Acute eosinophilic colitis and hypersensitivity reaction associated with naproxen therapy. Am J Med 1990;89:526–527.

218. Bjarnason I, Hayllar J, Mac Pherson AJ, Russell AS. Side effects of nonsteroidal anti-inflammatory drugs on the small and large intestine in humans [see comments]. Gastroenterology 1993;104:1832–1847.

219. Byrne MF, McGuinness J, Smyth CM et al. Nonsteroidal anti-inflammatory drug-induced diaphragms and ulceration in the colon. Eur J Gastroenterol Hepatol 2002;14:1265–1269.

220. Katsinelos P, Christodoulou K, Pilpilidis I et al. Colopathy associated with the systemic use of nonsteroidal antiinflammatory medications. An underestimated entity. Hepatogastroenterology 2002;49:345–348.

221. Hall RI, Petty AH, Cobden I, Lendrum R. Enteritis and colitis associated with mefenamic acid. Br Med J [Clin Res Ed] 1983;287:1182.

222. Tanner AR, Raghunath AS. Colonic inflammation and non-steroidal anti-inflammatory drug administration. An assessment of the frequency of the problem. Digestion 1988;41:116–120.

223. Bunney RG. Non-steroidal anti-inflammatory drugs and the bowel. Lancet 1989;2:1047.

224. Gentric A, Pennec YL. Diclofenac-induced pseudomembranous colitis [letter]. Lancet 1992;340:126–127.

225. Ravi S, Keat AC, Keat ECB. Colitis caused by non-steroidal anti-inflammatory drugs. Postgrad Med J 1986;62:773–776.

226. Debenham GP. Ulcer of the cecum during oxyphenbutazone (tandearil) therapy. Can Med Assoc J 1966;94:1182–1184.

227. Schonberger B, Nickl S, Schweiger F. Colonic ulcerations associated with diclofenac treatment. Can J Gastroenterol 1992;6:15.

228. de Silva HJ, Gatter KC, Millard PR, Kettlewell M, Mortensen NJ, Jewell DP. Crypt cell proliferation and HLA-DR expression in pelvic ileal pouches. J Clin Pathol 1990;43:824–828.

229. Kaufman HJ, Taubin HL. NSAID activate quiescent inflammatory bowel disease. Ann Intern Med 1987;107:513.

230. Rampton DS, McNeil NI, Sarner M. Analgesic ingestion and other factors preceding relapse in ulcerative colitis. Gut 1983;24:187–189.

231. Yang RD, Han MW, McCarthy JH. Ischemic colitis in a crack abuser. Dig Dis Sci 1991;36:238–240.

232. Boutros HH, Pautler S, Chakrabarti S. Cocaine-induced ischemic colitis with small-vessel thrombosis of colon and gallbladder. J Clin Gastroenterol 1997;24:49–53.

233. Niazi M, Kondru A, Levy J, Bloom AA. Spectrum of ischemic colitis in cocaine users. Dig Dis Sci 1997;42:1537–1541.

234. Greene FL, Ariyan S, Stansel HC Jr. Mesenteric and peripheral vascular ischemia secondary to ergotism. Surgery 1977;81:176–179.

235. Stillman AE, Weinberg M, Mast WC, Palpant S. Ischemic bowel disease attributable to ergot. Gastroenterology 1977;72:1336–1337.

236. Eckardt VF, Kanzler G, Remmele W. Anorectal ergotism: another cause of solitary rectal ulcer syndrome. Gastroenterology 1986;91:1123–1127.

237. Frossard JL, Spahr L, Queneau PE, Armenian B, Brundler MA, Hadengue A. Ischemic colitis during pregnancy and contraceptive medication. Digestion 2001;64:125–127.

238. Pauwels A, Meyohas MC, Eliaszewicz M, Legendre C, Mougeot G, Frottier J. Toxoplasma colitis in the acquired immunodeficiency syndrome [see comments]. Am J Gastroenterol 1992;87:518–519.

239. Clarkston WK, Bonacini M, Peterson I. Colitis due to Histoplasma capsulatum in the acquired immune deficiency syndrome. Am J Gastroenterol 1991;86:913–916.

240. Escudero-Fabre A, Cummings O, Kirklin JK, Bourge RC, Aldrete JS. Cytomegalovirus colitis presenting as hematochezia and requiring resection. Arch Surg 1992;127:102–104.

241. Dieterich DT, Rahmin M. Cytomegalovirus colitis in AIDS: presentation in 44 patients and a review of the literature. J AIDS 1991;4:S29–S35.

242. Crowley B, Dempsey J, Olujohungbe A, Khan A, Mutton K, Hart CA. Unusual manifestations of primary cytomegalovirus infection in patients without HIV infection and without organ transplants. J Med Virol 2002;68:237–240.

243. Bloomfeld RS. Are we missing CMV infections in patients hospitalized with severe colitis? Inflamm Bowel Dis 2001;7:348–349.

244. Caserta L, Riegler G. Cytomegalovirus and herpes simplex virus antibodies in patients with idiopathic ulcerative colitis. Am J Gastroenterol 2001;96:3036–3037.

245. Sakamoto I, Shirai T, Kamide T et al. Cytomegalovirus enterocolitis in an immunocompetent individual. J Clin Gastroenterol 2002;34:243–246.

246. Karakozis S, Gongora E, Caceres M, Brun E, Cook JW. Life-threatening cytomegalovirus colitis in the immunocompetent patient: report of a case and review of the literature. Dis Colon Rectum 2001;44:1716–1720.

247. Dieterich DT, Kotler DP, Busch DF et al. Ganciclovir treatment of cytomegalovirus colitis in AIDS: a randomized, double-blind, placebo-controlled multicenter study. J Infect Dis 1993;167:278–282.

248. Vora IM, Sharma J, Joshi AS. Solitary rectal ulcer syndrome and colitis cystica profunda – a clinicopathological review. Indian J Pathol Microbiol 1992;35:94–102.

249. Vaizey CJ, Roy AJ, Kamm MA. Prospective evaluation of the treatment of solitary rectal ulcer syndrome with biofeedback. Gut 1997;41:817–820.

250. Kang YS, Kamm MA, Engel AF, Talbot IC. Pathology of the rectal wall in solitary rectal ulcer syndrome and complete rectal prolapse. Gut 1996;38:587–590.

251. Rutter KR, Riddell RH. The solitary ulcer syndrome of the rectum. Clin Gastroenterol 1975;4:505–530.

252. Ertem D, Acar Y, Karaa EK, Pehlivanoglu E. A rare and often unrecognized cause of hematochezia and tenesmus in childhood: solitary rectal ulcer syndrome. Pediatrics 2002;110:79.

## CHAPTER 28

# Imaging of the idiopathic inflammatory bowel diseases

Karen M Horton, Bronwyn Jones and Elliot K Fishman

## INTRODUCTION

Despite the widespread use of fiberoptic endoscopy, radiologic imaging continues to play a significant role in the diagnosis, evaluation and management of patients with inflammatory bowel disease. In the past, barium studies were the primary method available for examining the small bowel and colon. However, today's radiologist can employ a variety of state-of-the-art imaging modalities to evaluate the gastrointestinal tract, as well as the extraintestinal manifestations of many gastrointestinal diseases. This chapter will discuss the variety of radiologic imaging techniques currently utilized in the evaluation of patients with Crohn's disease and ulcerative colitis. Important radiologic features will be reviewed and illustrated.

## CURRENT IMAGING MODALITIES

### CONTRAST STUDIES

Contrast studies are the cornerstone in radiologic diagnosis of inflammatory bowel disease and are sensitive in demonstrating the mucosal extent of disease. The most common contrast examinations performed today include small bowel series, enteroclysis, barium enema, and the upper gastrointestinal series.

### The small bowel series versus the enteroclysis

Two methods are available for radiographic examination of the small intestine: small bowel series and enteroclysis. Over the last several years there has been considerable debate in the radiologic literature as to which of these procedures is superior. The traditional small bowel series is faster, safer, and involves considerably less radiation than enteroclysis.[1] Enteroclysis is more sensitive for focal lesions such as adhesions and Meckel's diverticulum,[2] but has a higher complication rate and is technically more demanding. Overall, the accuracy of the two techniques

for Crohn's disease is probably similar, as long as both are performed with careful attention to detail.[2,3] However, enteroclysis is more sensitive in patients with low-grade or early small bowel obstruction.

In the standard small bowel series, the patient drinks two to four 12-ounce cups of a relatively thin barium suspension. At regular intervals (20–30 minutes on average) an overhead abdominal radiograph is taken in order to follow the progression of the barium through the small intestine. When the barium reaches the right colon (typically 30–90 minutes), the patient is taken into the fluoroscopy suite. Under fluoroscopic control, the radiologist vigorously compresses the small bowel while moving the patient into various positions in order to unwind superimposed loops. A series of compression spot radiographs is obtained, with special attention paid to the terminal ileum.

In cases where the terminal ileum is not well visualized, air can be administered through a rectal tube until it reaches the ileocecal region. This technique is a valuable adjunct to the routine small bowel series. Alternatively, a special radiograph called the prone-angled compression view can be obtained to allow better visualization of the pelvic small bowel loops which often are overlapped on routine AP radiographs.[4]

During enteroclysis, a tube is passed through the nose and advanced through the esophagus and stomach, into the jejunum, just past the ligament of Treitz. A small balloon is then inflated to keep the tube in place and to prevent regurgitation of contrast. In some centers the patient is given a mild sedative, such as Valium.[5] Under fluoroscopic guidance, 200–250 mL of specially formulated barium is infused through the tube at a rate of 50–100 mL/min. Next, the radiologist infuses 750–1000 mL of a methylcellulose solution. This combination of barium and methylcellulose results in distension and coating of the small bowel loops (Fig. 28.1). The appearance is similar to that of a double-contrast enema. Thus, this technique is sometimes referred to as a small bowel enema. Some advocate single-contrast enteroclysis, and would therefore not use methylcellulose.

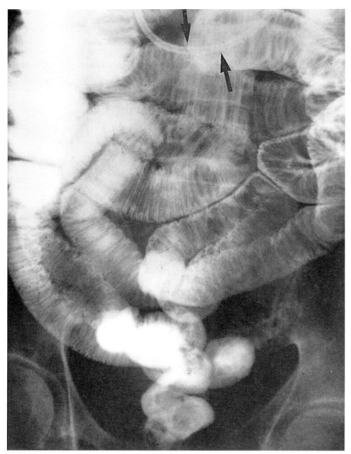

**Fig. 28.1** The appearance of normal small bowel on enteroclysis. The combination of barium and methylcellulose administered rapidly results in distension and coating of small bowel loops, appearing similar to an air contrast enema. Therefore, enteroclysis is sometimes referred to as a small bowel enema. The enteroclysis tube is present in the duodenum (arrows).

## The barium enema

The double-contrast barium enema is a safe and effective imaging tool for the evaluation of patients with inflammatory bowel disease. Its ability to demonstrate the diameter and extent of colonic strictures and the presence of fistulae is an advantage over colonoscopy in selected clinical settings. In addition, a barium enema is usually able to effectively image areas of colon that cannot be reached in cases of incomplete colonoscopy,[6] which occurs in almost 10% of colonoscopic examinations.[7] Therefore, barium enema and colonoscopy with biopsy should be considered complementary studies.

The double-contrast barium enema is performed by carefully administering a viscous high-density barium sulfate suspension through a rectal tube. Next, under fluoroscopic guidance and with various patient positioning, air is gently introduced through the tube until the entire colon is distended with air and coated with barium. This examination requires careful attention to technique so that optimal coating of the colon is achieved. Excess barium or air will result in inadequate visualization of the colon.

Spot films are often taken by the radiologist during filling of the colon. Next, a series of overhead films is taken by the technologist after the patient has been positioned appropriately to demonstrate the entire colon. Finally, a postevacuation film com-pletes the study. Often, the terminal ileum will be demonstrated best or only on the postevacuation film, after the colon has actively contracted.

Single-contrast examination of the colon is also helpful in cases of suspected obstruction or fistula, but cannot demonstrate subtle mucosal involvement or shallow ulceration. During this examination, the radiologist administers a thinner barium suspension or, in some cases, a water-soluble solution through a rectal tube. Under fluoroscopic guidance the radiologist palpates/compresses the colon and takes spot films. The technologist will then take a standard series of overhead films after careful positioning of the patient. Finally, a radiograph is taken after the patient has evacuated the barium. Again, careful attention to technique is essential to obtain high-quality radiographs.

## Upper gastrointestinal series

The upper gastrointestinal series allows evaluation of the esophagus, stomach and duodenal C-loop. The examination can be performed by either single- or double-contrast techniques.

The single-contrast examination involves the patient drinking a thin suspension of barium or a water-soluble contrast solution. Fluoroscopic spot radiographs of the esophagus, stomach and duodenum are taken by the radiologist. Subtle mucosal involvement is not reliably detected using single-contrast techniques.

During the double-contrast examination the patient ingests 4–6 g of effervescent gas crystals followed by a thick barium suspension. This results in air distension of the upper gastrointestinal tract, which is coated with barium. The radiologist then positions the patient appropriately and obtains a series of spot radiographs. Esophageal peristalsis is also assessed in the prone, right anterior oblique position using a thin barium suspension.

## Computed tomography (CT)

CT has become a valuable diagnostic tool in the evaluation of patients with inflammatory bowel disease and is considered complementary to traditional contrast examinations. Although barium contrast studies are superior in demonstrating mucosal extent of disease, CT can accurately image the bowel wall as well as extraluminal extension of disease.[8] Therefore, CT can significantly affect patient management.[9] In addition, it is important to recognize the CT features of inflammatory bowel disease, as CT may be the first imaging study performed in a patient presenting with non-specific abdominal pain.

Accurate CT imaging of the small bowel and colon requires careful attention to technique. The following is the authors' protocol.

Traditionally, the patient routinely drinks approximately 750–1000 mL of a 3% oral iodinated contrast solution 60–90 minutes before the scan and an additional 250 mL of oral contrast immediately before the study. This allows adequate contrast opacification of the stomach and small bowel. These iodinated agents will appear white on a CT scan owing to the density of the iodine. If colonic pathology is suspected, it is important to opacify the entire colon adequately. In these cases, oral contrast is administered the night before the study as well as prior to the scan, to ensure that contrast opacifies the colon as well as the small bowel. Alternatively, in urgent cases, or in patients in whom limited rectosigmoid disease is suspected, a 3–4% iodinated contrast solution can be administered gently through a rectal tube. The use of air and/or water to distend the colon has also been reported.[10]

Recently, there has been interest in using alternative oral contrast agents for CT. Although traditional iodinated or dilute barium agents opacify the intestines well, they appear white on CT and may therefore obscure subtle changes in the small bowel wall or subtle differences in enhancement.[11–13] Water may be a superior oral contrast agent for CT, especially when rapid imaging is performed after IV contrast administration. Water is safe, well tolerated, and allows excellent visualization of the enhancing bowel wall. The use of water as a CT contrast agent has been well described in the literature and is especially helpful for the stomach and upper gastrointestinal tract.[14,15] Opacification of the distal ileum may be suboptimal with water, but even if the distal loops are not maximally distended, pathology can still be appreciated because of the changes in enhancement and wall thickness.

In patients with Crohn's disease, subtle areas of increased enhancement can be easily identified. Also, wall thickening is well visualized. Unlike the high-density oral contrast agents, water will not interfere with 3D imaging. The use of the high-density oral contrast agents requires extensive editing if 3D imaging is performed.

The administration of intravenous contrast is essential for complete evaluation of patients with inflammatory bowel disease, especially if extracolonic extension of disease is suspected. We routinely administer 100–120 mL of Omnipaque 350 (Amersham Health, Princeton, NJ) at a rate of 2–3 mL/s injected through a peripheral vein.

On standard non-spiral CT scanners the abdomen should be routinely imaged from the level of the diaphragm through the perineum.[16] Consecutive slices with 5 mm collimation are obtained contiguously at 5 mm intervals. Additional scans are then performed through specific areas of concern.

The introduction of spiral CT technology in the 1990s allowed faster, subsecond scanning, which could be combined with rapid contrast infusion and narrow collimation (2–5 mm). The entire upper abdomen could be imaged in a single 30-second breath hold. This essentially eliminated misregistration artifacts due to patient movement or respiration. Using spiral CT, 5 mm collimation can be performed with a table speed of 8 mm/s, with reconstruction every 5 mm. Our standard single detector spiral CT protocol is to begin scanning 45–50 seconds after initiation of contrast injection. This corresponds to the portal venous phase of enhancement.

Today, multidetector-row CT (MDCT) represents the latest technical advancement in CT scanning and has completed the evolution from a slice-based technique to a volume-based one.[17] Eight- and 32-detector-row scanners are now widely available and allow four-16 slices to be obtained in less than 500 ms with thinner collimation (0.5–1.0 mm). The 32-detector-row scanners which are now being introduced offer at least a threefold increase in speed and a doubling of resolution compared with current systems. The speed, thinner collimation and increased resolution availability of MDCT, along with advancements in 3D CT imaging systems, has greatly expanded the role of CT in evaluation of patients with suspected bowel pathology, including Crohn's disease. With MDCT scanning is faster, which allows more accurate timing of the bolus during the arterial and venous phases. This results in better CT angiography images of the mesenteric arteries and veins. In patients with active Crohn's disease, enlargement of the vessels supplying the disease loops can often be visualized. In addition, this faster scanning allows better visualization of the enhancing bowel wall. Little has been published about this technique, but the ability to measure the enhancement of the bowel over time could be helpful in the diagnosis of certain diseases such as ischemia or Crohn's.

## 3D Imaging

Three-dimensional reconstruction of CT data has been possible for almost 20 years. However, early systems were crude and offered only simplistic renderings of the surface of structures (shaded surface) such as the bone. They offered few applications for imaging of the gastrointestinal tract. Fortunately, major advancements in both CT scanner technology and computer hardware/software have now made powerful and affordable 3D imaging systems widely available. Current systems offer real-time volume-rendering software which is easy to use and simple to incorporate into existing practice, and allows comprehensive visualization of the gastrointestinal tract. We currently use the Siemens 3D-Virtuoso (Siemens Medical Solutions, Iselin, NJ). This volume-rendering software allows real-time manipulation of the 3D dataset. The data can be viewed from any angle, and settings (brightness, opacity, window width and window level) can be manipulated to allow optimal visualization of the pathology. Because the CT findings in Crohn's disease can be complicated owing to extraintestinal manifestations such as fistulae, abscess, bone or muscle involvement, as well as bowel disease, 3D imaging is often helpful for a comprehensive understanding of the disease process.

There is not much written in the literature about the value of 3D imaging in patients with Crohn's disease. However, in 1997, Raptopoulos et al. studied 22 patients with Crohn's disease to determine the usefulness of multiplanar reconstructions in revealing complications.[18] In this study, the use of multiplanar reconstructions significantly improved the observer's confidence in their interpretation of the findings and in their understanding of the disease. The use of multiplanar reconstructions also improved their ability to detect the extent of the bowel involvement. Also in that study, the authors compared the CT findings with barium studies and found that the CT and barium studies were comparable in 9/14 patients.[18] In 4/14 patients the CT was thought to be superior to the barium studies.[18] The CT study was thought to be inferior to the barium study in one patient. Since 1997 the quality of multiplanar reconstructions has significantly improved owing to the improvements in scanner technology and the ability to obtain thinner collimation (Fig. 28.2). It has been our experience that 3D imaging with its flexibility and speed adds definite value when evaluating patients with Crohn's disease. Complex disease can be better understood. In addition, 3D imaging is well received by clinicians, who find it easier to visualize the disease process in the coronal or sagittal plane, in contrast to axial imaging. In many cases a single or a few coronal 3D images will display the pathology, compared with many axial images.

## MAGNETIC RESONANCE IMAGING (MRI)

Multiplanar capability, high contrast resolution and the lack of ionizing radiation make MRI an ideal abdominal imaging modality. However, its application in gastrointestinal tract imaging has been limited. In the past, image acquisition times

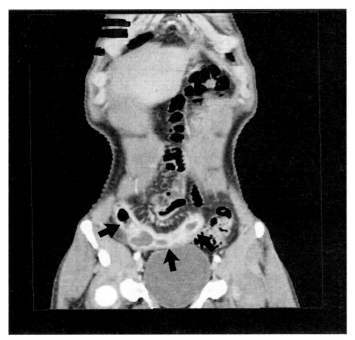

**Fig. 28.2** Coronal multiplanar reconstruction in a patient with Crohn's disease demonstrates a thickened loop of small bowel in the right lower quadrant (arrows). Water has been used as oral contrast. The thickened bowel wall has a layered appearance due to mucosal hyperemia.

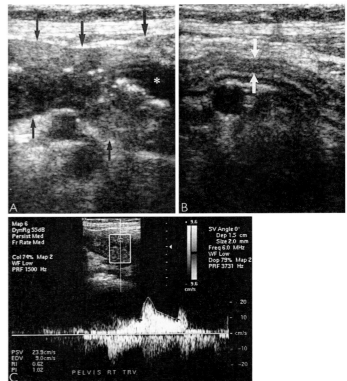

**Fig. 28.3** Crohn's disease. (A) Ultrasound examination reveals marked circumferential thickening of a small bowel loop in the mid abdomen in this patient with Crohn's disease. (*,lumen; arrows, thickened bowel wall). (B) Ultrasound of a normal collapsed small bowel loop for comparison (arrows). The normal bowel wall on sonography is less than 3 mm thick. (C) Doppler examination of the thickened small bowel demonstrates increased blood flow compatible with active inflammation and hyperemia. (Images courtesy of Dr Sheila Sheth, Baltimore, MD.)

were prohibitively long, image quality was significantly degraded by movement and bowel peristalsis, and there was no adequate oral contrast agent available.

Currently, recent technical advancements have reduced imaging times significantly, thereby reducing artifacts caused by motion. In addition, there is active ongoing research in a variety of possible MRI intraluminal contrast agents, including water, barium,[19] perflubron (perfluorooctylbromide)[20] and per-rectal vegetable oil.[21]

Because of these recent advancements there is now increasing interest in the application of MRI for imaging inflammatory bowel disease, including Crohn's disease and ulcerative colitis.

Several studies of MRI in Crohn's disease suggest that it may be useful in evaluating the severity of disease and may provide information complementary to the clinical evaluation.[22] Bowel wall thickening can be detected and is considered a reliable sign of disease, as is marked enhancement.[23] One recent study was published comparing MRI and CT for imaging bowel disease in patients with Crohn's disease. Overall, MRI was more sensitive (80–85%) than single-phase CT (60–65%) for visualizing bowel thickening.[24] However, MRI and CT performed equally well in patients with moderate to marked thickening. MRI identified more patients with minimal wall thickening than CT, although this could not always be correlated on endoscopy or small bowel series.[24]

Although direct MR imaging of the bowel is currently limited, MRI is an effective modality for the evaluation of complications of Crohn's disease, including sinus tracts, fistulae and abscesses,[25,26] and has been found to be especially useful in the evaluation of perianal and perirectal disease.[25] MRI is the imaging modality of choice for perianal fistulae and abscesses, and for pregnant patients.

However, further advancements will be necessary before MRI becomes a practical GI tract imaging modality for inflammatory bowel disease.

## ULTRASONOGRAPHY

Ultrasonography is a safe, non-invasive imaging modality that is gaining wider acceptance as a technique for imaging the gastrointestinal tract, especially in children. In Europe ultrasound is extensively used as a screening technique for disease of the gastrointestinal tract. Right lower quadrant sonography, using modern 3.5 or 5.0 MHz transducers, allows accurate visualization of the distal small bowel. Wall thickening and echotexture can therefore be evaluated. In addition, ultrasound of the colon can also be performed after water enema in patients with Crohn's disease or ulcerative colitis in order to evaluate wall thickening. The application of color Doppler imaging and power Doppler may allow differentiation of active bowel thickening (increased blood flow) from chronic wall thickening/fibrosis (no increased flow).[27] Similarly, Doppler ultrasound can also demonstrate hemodynamic changes in patients with active inflammatory bowel disease which are not present in those with quiescent disease[28] (Fig. 28.3).

A recent study by Solvig et al. compared ultrasound and enteroclysis findings in patients with Crohn's disease. In 18/20 patients the ultrasound and enteroclysis findings correlated, and also the ultrasound examination was normal in 37 of 39 patients with a normal enteroclysis.[29] Another study by Hata[30] concluded that ultrasound has a sensitivity of 86% for Crohn's disease and 89% for ulcerative colitis.

The role of ultrasound in the gastrointestinal tract is still evolving. Although recent work is promising, ultrasound continues to be very operator dependent and is adversely affected by such factors as obesity and intraluminal gas. This will probably limit its widespread application for imaging the bowel in the USA.

## NUCLEAR MEDICINE

With the availability of radionuclide-labeled white blood cells, nuclear scintigraphy is quickly emerging as a promising technique for visualizing actively inflamed bowel. In the past, the major radionuclide used in evaluating patients with active inflammatory bowel disease was gallium-67.[31–33] Although this agent was considered sensitive and specific for the diagnosis of active bowel disease, gallium is normally excreted by the bowel, making interpretation of studies very difficult, even after adequate bowel preparation.

Today, new radionuclides are available, including indium- and technetium-labeled white blood cells. In these studies, blood is removed from the patient and the white blood cells are separated and labeled, then reinjected. The radionuclide accumulates at sites of acute inflammation or infection. On imaging, typically performed at 6, 12 and 24 hours, any bowel activity is abnormal and signifies active inflammation/infection (Fig. 28.4). Focal intra-abdominal activity is suggestive of abscess.

Several studies have demonstrated good correlation between the results of indium-labeled white cell studies and colonoscopy, barium enema and clinical symptoms in patients with active inflammatory bowel disease.[34–37] Technetium-99m-hexamethyl-propylamine-oxime (HMPAO) is another white blood cell labeling agent which is less expensive and results in decreased patient radiation dose and better image quality. This agent has also been shown to be helpful in assessment of the existence, extent and intensity of active inflammation in inflammatory bowel disease patients,[38] and is likely to replace indium in the future. In a study of 115 patients with Crohn's disease and 21 with ulcerative colitis, sensitivities for active disease were 98% and 98% at 1 and 3 hours, respectively.[38] Specificity was 100% and 83% at 1 and 3 hours, respectively. Both indium- and technetium-labeled white blood cells have been shown to be useful in screening patients for active inflammatory bowel disease.[39,40]

As new, more selective radionuclides become available, the role of nuclear scintigraphy in the evaluation of patients with inflammatory bowel disease will probably expand. At present, the strength of these radionuclides lies in the ability to screen patients for disease and to differentiate active from inactive disease. However, because of the limited spatial resolution and the current difficulty in differentiating between inflammatory and infectious bowel diseases, the use of scintigraphy is limited to problem cases where other imaging modalities are equivocal.

## RADIOGRAPHIC FINDINGS IN CROHN'S DISEASE

### CONTRAST STUDIES

#### Site of involvement

Crohn's disease can affect any portion of the gastrointestinal tract.

The terminal ileum is the most common site of involvement and in up to 30% of patients is the only site. However, ileal disease often occurs in combination with right colon involvement.[43] The combination of small bowel and colon involvement occurs in 50% of patients.[44,45]

Disease limited to the colon occurs in only 19% of patients. The rectum is involved in approximately 50% of patients and spared in the remaining 50%, but isolated anal and perianal involvement is rare and only found in 2%. Anorectal disease can include erosions, ulcers, hemorrhoids, perineal abscess, fissures and fistulae.[46,47]

With double-contrast techniques up to 13% of patients with Crohn's disease will show early signs of involvement of the upper gastrointestinal tract.[48] These patients typically will also have concomitant disease in the small bowel or colon.[48] Duodenal involvement is commoner in young patients than in older ones.

### SMALL BOWEL AND COLON

#### Mucosal granularity

The earliest radiographic finding on contrast studies in Crohn's disease is a diffuse granular appearance to the normally smooth mucosa of an involved bowel segment.[50] This pattern is most commonly seen in the small bowel, but rarely can be detected in the esophagus as well.

This distinctive radiographic appearance is produced by a network of radiolucent foci which measure 0.5–1 mm in diameter, and represents edema and lymphocytic infiltration of the villi.[51] Electron microscopic studies of early Crohn's disease show that the villi are not only edematous but also clubbed and branching, thereby also contributing to the granularity.

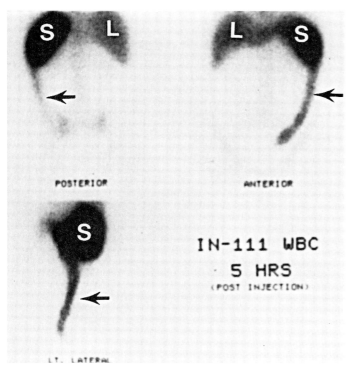

**Fig. 28.4** Ulcerative colitis. In[111]-labeled white blood cell scan obtained 5 hours post injection demonstrates marked accumulation of the tracer in the left colon (arrow), compatible with active inflammation. The liver (L), spleen (S) and bones are also visualized, as they are normal sites of white blood cell accumulation. (Images courtesy of Dr Cahid Civelek, Baltimore, MD.)

## Fold and wall thickening

Thickening of the bowel wall is a common radiographic finding in Crohn's disease involving both the small bowel and colon.

On contrast studies, the normal small bowel fold and wall thickness should be <3 mm. In Crohn's disease – a transmural disease – as the edema and inflammation involve deeper portions of the wall, thickening of the small bowel folds occurs which can be detected on contrast studies. The fold thickening is often eccentric, discontinuous and irregular ('skip areas'), reflecting the underlying pathology. Small bowel wall thickening can also be seen as parallel separation of adjacent loops (Fig. 28.5).

Colonic wall thickening also occurs in patients with Crohn's disease and, as in the small bowel, typically appears patchy, discontinuous and asymmetric, reflecting the underlying pathology. The asymmetry of the disease involvement can result in the formation of pseudodiverticula. This discontinuous appearance ('skip areas') is an important feature that distinguishes Crohn's disease from ulcerative colitis, which usually appears confluent, continuous and circumferential.

## Strictures

Rigid wall thickening and fibrosis can also occur in the small bowel and colon in Crohn's patients and presents as segmental areas of luminal narrowing. The deformity may affect only a portion of the bowel wall or may be circumferential, resulting in the formation of a stricture. On contrast examination these strictures typically appear as segmental narrowing, without normal mucosal pattern and with smooth tapered ends. The stricturing can be marked, especially in the terminal ileum. This is sometimes referred to as the 'string sign'. Marked stricturing in the small bowel or colon may result in obstruction.

## Lymphoid hyperplasia

Extensive 'lymphoid hyperplasia' may be an early sign of Crohn's disease in the small bowel and colon. True lymphoid hyperplasia shows small regular 2–3 mm filling defects in a carpet-like pattern (Fig. 28.6). Variability in size or lymphoid follicles larger than 3 mm should suggest inflammation of the lymphoid follicle, and is suggestive of Crohn's disease. The aphthoid ulcer is actually an ulcerated lymphoid follicle. Sometimes there is marked enlargement of these lymphoid follicles in patients with Crohn's disease, mimicking lymphoma.

## Ulceration

Aphthoid or discrete ulcers are among the earliest mucosal lesions to be demonstrated on contrast studies. They often occur on a background of normal mucosa or, less commonly, at the margin of a severely diseased segment.[52] These lesions often appear on double-contrast studies as round or oval well-defined barium collections measuring a few millimeters in size. The

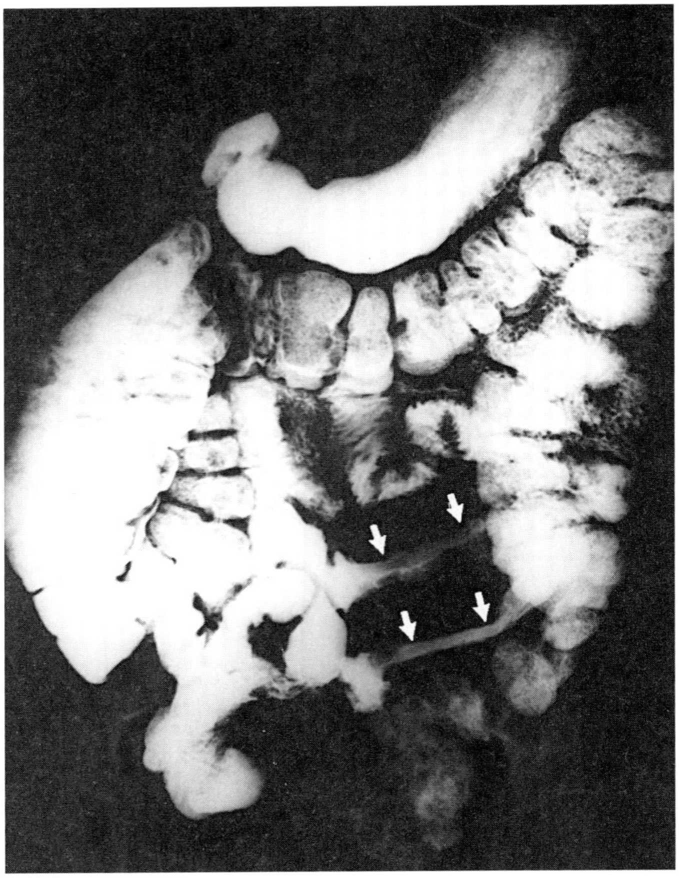

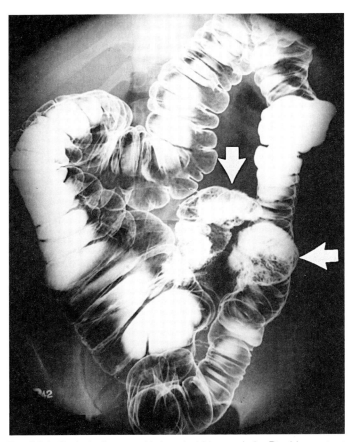

**Fig. 28.5** Crohn's disease with bowel wall thickening. Small bowel series reveals luminal narrowing and fold destruction of two adjacent small bowel loops in the left lower abdomen (arrows). There is wide separation between these two loops and adjacent small bowel, indicating significant wall thickening.

**Fig. 28.6** Crohn's disease with lymphoid hyperplasia. Double-contrast barium enema in a patient with Crohn's disease reveals many small (2–3 mm) filling defects in the terminal ileum (arrows) compatible with lymphoid hyperplasia.

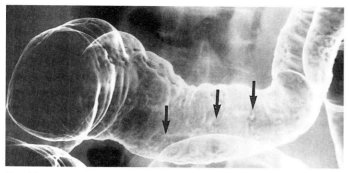

Fig. 28.7 Crohn's disease with aphthous ulcers. Double-contrast barium enema reveals many discrete aphthoid ulcers (arrows) within the transverse colon. The remainder of the colon appears normal, reflecting the segmental nature of the disease.

borders of the ulcers are typically well defined, often with a surrounding halo of edema (Fig. 28.7).

Aphthoid ulcers are seen on double-contrast barium enemas in up to 70% of patients with Crohn's disease.[52,53] These lesions typically are not shown with single-contrast studies except for exquisite compression studies, as typically they are shallow and do not give a profile abnormality. Ulcers more than 3 mm deep are more commonly seen in Crohn's disease than in ulcerative colitis. Other descriptive terms have been used, such as the 'rose thorn' and 'collar button' ulcers. Originally it was thought that the rose thorn signified Crohn's and the collar button was specific for ulcerative colitis. It was then realized that these ulcers reflect depth: the rose thorn ulcer is deeper and is typically seen in Crohn's disease, whereas the collar button ulcer is more shallow and thus seen in ulcerative colitis.

Aphthous ulcers can be detected in inflammatory colitides (i.e. Shigellosis, amebic colitis) and therefore are not pathognomonic of Crohn's disease.[54]

## Cobblestoning

Cobblestoning is another radiographic feature that is very characteristic of Crohn's disease, and often considered pathognomonic (Fig. 28.8). Cobblestoning consists of a combination of submucosal edema and deep transverse and longitudinal fissuring which collects barium. This combination gives an appearance similar to that of a cobbled street.

## Fistulae

Fistulae are a frequent complication of Crohn's disease. They may be grouped into three general categories: enterocutaneous, enteroenteric, and those involving the bowel and adjacent organs, such as the bladder (enterovesical) or psoas muscles.

Enterocutaneous fistulae can be diagnosed using radiographic contrast studies and appear as extraluminal contrast collections. If an enterocutaneous fistula is suspected, water-soluble contrast should be used, as barium may remain, coating the fistulous tract, indefinitely. The fistula can be visualized leading from the diseased contrast-filled bowel loop to the skin surface. Cross-table lateral views may be necessary to visualize fistulae. In other cases, water-soluble contrast can be injected directly into the skin opening (this radiographic examination is sometimes referred to as a fistulogram or a sinogram). If the contrast fills a bowel loop, the presence of an enterocutaneous fistula is confirmed.

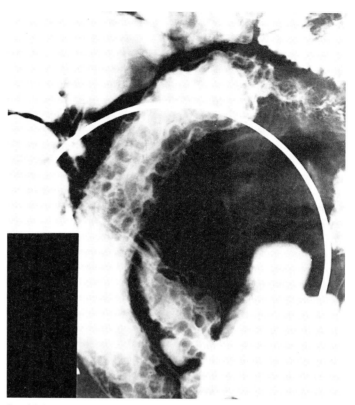

Fig. 28.8 Crohn's disease with cobblestoning. Compression spot views of two distal small bowel loops reveals a classic example of cobblestoning. This appearance is created by a combination of deep transverse and longitudinal ulcerations surrounding islands of inflamed but non-ulcerated mucosa (pseudopolyps).

Enteroenteric fistulae can also be diagnosed with contrast studies and require careful attention to detail. Small bowel to small bowel fistulae are especially difficult to diagnose and demand vigorous compression and high-quality radiographs. Fistulae appear as linear contrast collections between bowel loops. When multiple, they can form a 'starburst' pattern (Fig. 28.9).

Enterocolic fistulae are diagnosed when contrast appears in the colon prematurely during a small bowel series. For example, if contrast appears in the left colon before the right colon fills, there must be an enterocolic communication. Anovaginal, rectovaginal, rectourethral, gastrocolic and duodenal colic fistulae have been reported.[55–58] If a perianal or a colorectal fistula is suspected, a single-contrast water-soluble enema is usually performed to demonstrate it. Linear extraluminal collections of contrast may be seen in the pericolic tissues, sometimes opacifying adjacent structures (i.e. the vagina).

Enterovesical fistulae are difficult to demonstrate by conventional radiographic methods, but can be identified during a small bowel examination when contrast or air is identified within the bladder. However, CT is more sensitive.[59]

## Polyps

Inflammatory polyps, postinflammatory polyps and pseudopolyps can all occur in Crohn's disease, although they are more common in ulcerative colitis. The colon is the most common location for polyp formation.

Inflammatory polyps can occur in the setting of any active inflammatory disease. On contrast examination inflammatory

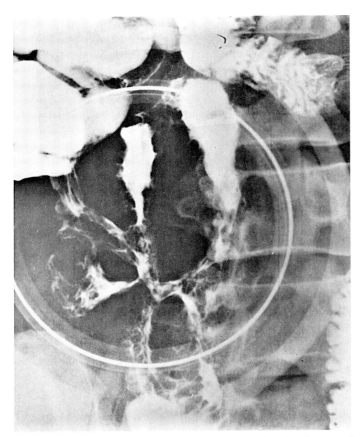

**Fig. 28.9** Crohn's disease with fistulae. Spot compression view from small bowel series demonstrates multiple interconnecting fistulae in the distal small bowel. This appearance is likened to a spiderweb or starburst pattern.

polyps appear as polypoid fillings defects which cannot be differentiated from adenomatous polyps. Endoscopy and biopsy are necessary for diagnosis.

Postinflammatory polyps can occur in Crohn's disease or ulcerative colitis and merely reflect previous extensive ulceration with sparing of some of the mucosa. Postinflammatory polyps form when extensive ulcerations heal, leaving a round or finger-like projection of submucosa covered by mucosa on all sides.[60] On barium enema they appear as multiple filiform filling defects. Also, bridging postinflammatory polyps may be formed by ulceration undermining a patch of non-ulcerated mucosa.

Pseudopolyp is a term given to an area of inflamed mucosa surrounded by extensive ulceration. Owing to the surrounding ulceration, this area may give the appearance of a filling defect or polyp. In Crohn's disease pseudopolyps may occur in the small bowel or colon and, when multiple, may produce an appearance similar to true cobblestoning[60] (Fig. 28.8). Although pseudopolyps are benign, they may bleed and occasionally become so large that they obstruct the colon.[61]

## Extraluminal disease

CT is currently the imaging modality of choice to evaluate the extraluminal extent of disease in patients with Crohn's disease. However, extraluminal inflammatory masses can be suggested on small bowel series or barium enema when extrinsic compression of bowel is present. Similarly, the separation/displacement of small bowel loops may indicate the presence of adenopathy, mesenteric inflammation, mesenteric fatty replacement (creeping fat) or an interloop abscess. In addition, complications of Crohn's disease, such as perforation or intussusception, can be demonstrated on contrast studies, although CT examination is more sensitive (see CT – complications).

# UPPER GASTROINTESTINAL TRACT

## ESOPHAGUS

Crohn's disease of the esophagus is not common and occurs only rarely as an isolated finding. Crohn's disease elsewhere in the gastrointestinal tract is usually evident.

As in the small bowel and colon, aphthoid ulcers are the earliest radiographic findings in Crohn's disease of the esophagus, appearing radiographically as punctate, linear or ring-like collections of barium with a radiolucent halo.[62] These ulcers can be subtle and will only be recognized with optimal double-contrast technique.

As the disease progresses, the ulcers may enlarge and deepen (Fig. 28.10). A diffuse esophagitis may occur and results in fold thickening or a diffusely cobblestoned mucosa.[63] Rarely intramural or extraesophageal fistulae can occur. Progressive fibrosis can lead to esophageal stricturing.[64]

Filiform polyps have also been reported in the esophagus.[65] On occasion these have been very large, producing severe dysphagia.

## STOMACH

When Crohn's disease occurs in the stomach, it typically involves the antrum or the body and antrum.[66] If the stomach is involved, the duodenum is also usually affected.[62]

Radiographic features of gastric Crohn's disease include aphthous ulcers that tend to be localized to the antrum or body and antrum, fold thickening, larger ulcers or, occasionally, cobblestoning of the mucosa. Scarring and fibrosis may result in antral narrowing, which is often referred to as a 'ram's horn'[67] appearance (Fig. 28.11). Fistulae involving the stomach are very rare but do occur.[62] Occasionally, a focal area of Crohn's may simulate a mass lesion.

## DUODENUM

The radiographic findings in Crohn's disease involving the duodenum are similar to those found elsewhere and include aphthous ulcers, larger ulcers and fold thickening. The appearance may mimic peptic ulcer disease. As the disease progresses there may be effacement of the mucosa, or stenosis due to fibrosis and scarring. If the scarring is asymmetric pseudodiverticula may be visualized.[68]

# CT FINDINGS

## PRIMARY DISEASE

The most characteristic finding on CT in Crohn's disease is wall thickening involving the distal small bowel and/or colon (Fig. 28.2). Wall thickening can be diffuse or eccentric with skip areas. In advanced cases of Crohn's disease the wall often measures more than 1 cm in thickness[69] (Fig. 28.12). In a study by Philpotts et al. the mean colon wall thickness in Crohn's colitis was 13 mm and the appearance was homogeneous. This was

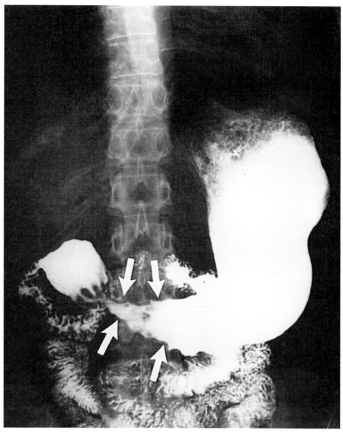

Fig. 28.11 Crohn's disease affecting the stomach. Upper GI series reveals narrowing and rigidity of the gastric antrum (arrows). This appearance is often referred to as a 'ram's horn' antrum, which can been seen in Crohn's disease as well as in other inflammatory conditions.

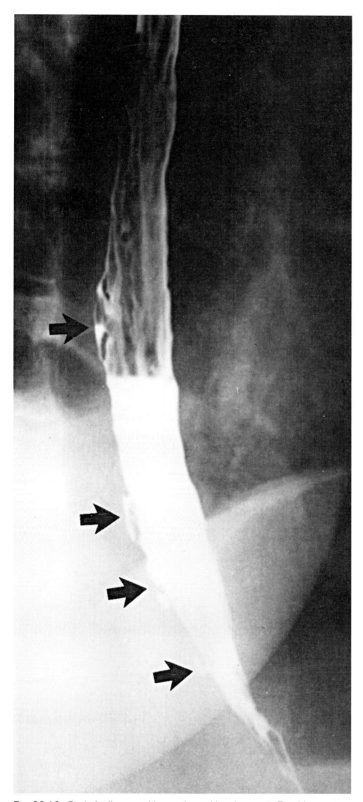

Fig. 28.10 Crohn's disease with esophageal involvement. Double-contrast esophagogram demonstrates several discrete ulcers in the mid and distal esophagus. Esophageal involvement in Crohn's disease is not common.

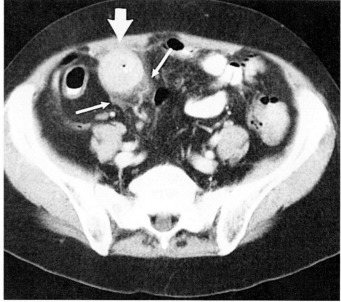

Fig. 28.12 Crohn's disease with wall thickening. CT scan with intravenous and oral contrast medium demonstrates marked thickening of the wall of the terminal ileum (large arrow). The wall measures 15 mm in thickness. In addition, increased density and stranding are identified in the adjacent mesenteric fat (little arrows), compatible with active inflammation.

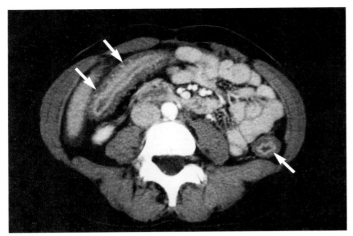

Fig. 28.13 Contrast-enhanced MDCT in a patient with Crohn's colitis. Water was used as rectal contrast. Moderate colonic thickening (arrows) is present. Also, the use of water allows visualization of the bowel wall layers, which appear distinct owing to inflammation and mucosal hyperemia.

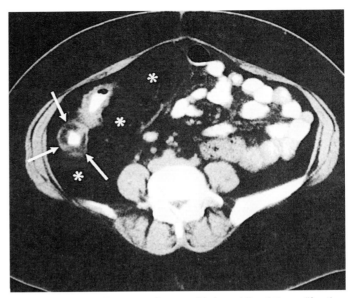

Fig. 28.14 Crohn's disease – submucosal halo and fibrofatty proliferation. CT scan with oral contrast medium demonstrates low-attenuation submucosal fat in the ascending colon (arrows) and fibrofatty proliferation of adjacent mesenteric fat (asterisks).

significantly greater than in ulcerative colitis, where the mean wall thickness was 7.8 mm and the appearance heterogeneous.[70] Although wall thickening in Crohn's disease is commonly the result of submucosal inflammation, edema, fibrosis or fat, hypertrophy of the muscularis propria also occurs. The use of water as an oral contrast agent allows excellent visualization of the enhancing bowel wall. In some cases the wall may enhance homogeneously, whereas in others distinct layers may be visualized, creating a halo or layered appearance to the wall (Figs 28.3. 28.13). Gore et al. suggested that preservation of the bowel layers may indicate reversible disease, in contrast to a homogeneous thickened wall, which may indicated fibrotic disease.[71]

In patients with active disease and hyperemia, 3D imaging may be useful to detect alterations in the mesenteric vasculature. Dilated or beaded mesenteric artery branches may be visualized as they supply the diseased and hyperemic segments.

In cases of significant persistent segmental wall thickening, the possibility of stricture should be considered. In some patients, a layer (halo) of low density representing submucosal edema[72] or fat deposition[73] can be identified within the bowel wall (Fig. 28.14). Although more commonly seen in patients with ulcerative colitis, this submucosal halo can also be present in Crohn's disease. In addition to the bowel wall thickening, inflammatory stranding in the adjacent mesenteric or pericolonic fat can be present and usually signifies active inflammation (Fig. 28.12).

It is important that CT scanning extend to the perineum, as perirectal/perianal abnormalities are demonstrated on CT in up to 37% of Crohn's patients.[16] Findings include inflammation of perirectal fat, bowel wall thickening, fistulae or sinus tracts, and abscesses[16] (Fig. 28.15).

## MESENTERIC DISEASE

Another characteristic CT finding in patients with Crohn's disease is fibrofatty proliferation ('creeping fat'), which appears as an increased quantity of mesenteric fat that can be extensive (Fig. 28.14). Fibrofatty proliferation can displace bowel and sometimes simulates a mass or abscess on plain abdominal radiographs or barium studies. Small mesenteric lymph nodes and mesenteric inflammation can also result in separation of bowel loops.

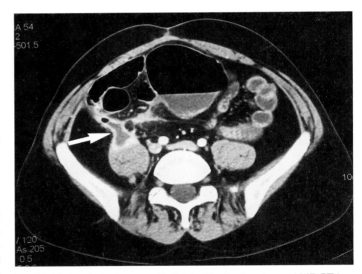

Fig. 28.15 Crohn's disease with fistula. Contrast-enhanced MDCT in a patient with Crohn's disease demonstrates a fistula (arrow) between the distal small bowel and the right psoas muscle.

Intra-abdominal abscess often appears as a soft tissue density or low-density mass which often contains air and/or extravasated oral contrast. An abscess can be confined to the bowel wall, can extend into the mesentery, or can involve adjacent structures such as the bladder, psoas muscle or pelvic sidewall (Fig. 28.16). Percutaneous drainage of intra-abdominal abscesses can be safely performed by the radiologist under CT guidance.[74]

## COMPLICATIONS

Because CT can accurately demonstrate the bowel wall as well as extraluminal extension of disease, a variety of complications of Crohn's disease can be effectively diagnosed with CT.[75] In fact, CT was shown to affect patient management in 28% of

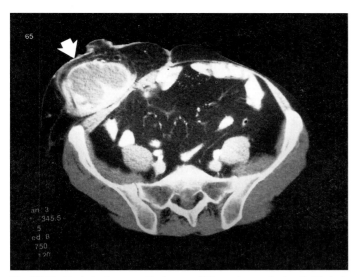

Fig. 28.16 Crohn's disease with abscess. CT scan in a patient with Crohn's disease and abdominal pain reveals a large abscess (arrow) in the right anterior abdominal wall at the site of the patient's ileostomy. CT or ultrasound could be used for guidance during drainage if necessary.

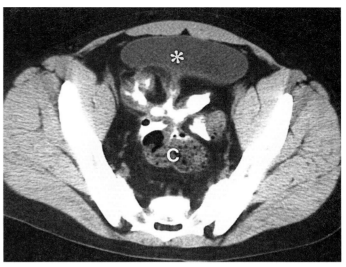

Fig. 28.17 Crohn's disease with fistula. CT scan with oral contrast material in a patient with Crohn's disease demonstrates multiple fistulae in the pelvis involving several contrast-filled small bowel loops and colon (C), and possibly bladder (asterisk).

cases with symptomatic Crohn's disease.[9] In this study, in 22 of 80 patients CT revealed previously unexpected findings that subsequently led to a change in medical or surgical management. These findings included fistulae, abscess, avascular necrosis of the femoral head, osteomyelitis and venous thrombosis.

Complications commonly imaged with CT include:

(1) **Obstruction** CT is valuable in patients with suspected small bowel obstruction, and can frequently determine the cause of obstruction and whether there is evidence of strangulation.[76] In patients with Crohn's disease, small bowel obstruction can result from stricture, inflammatory masses or adhesions following surgical resections. CT is also helpful in distinguishing obstruction from ileus.

(2) **Fistulae** In addition to enterovesical fistulae, enterocutaneous, perianal and rectovaginal fistulae can all be reliably detected with CT. They appear as extraluminal linear contrast collections with surrounding inflammation (Fig. 28.17). If a rectovaginal or perianal fistula is suspected, contrast can be administered via the rectum for better visualization.

(3) **Genitourinary complications** CT is a sensitive method for evaluating the bladder and can reliably detect bladder involvement in Crohn's disease.[77] Bladder involvement may consist of focal bladder wall thickening with or without an adjacent extravesical soft tissue inflammatory mass.[59] Enterovesical fistulae can also be imaged and appear as intravesical air, usually with associated bladder wall thickening and/or extravesical inflammatory mass[59] (Fig. 28.18). If an enterovesical fistula is suspected, intravenous contrast should not be administered. Then, if contrast is detected in the bladder, it must be oral contrast that entered the bladder though a enterovesical fistula.

Ureteral obstruction, commonly of the right ureter, can also result from mesenteric inflammation or abscess. This can easily be detected on CT performed with intravenous contrast.

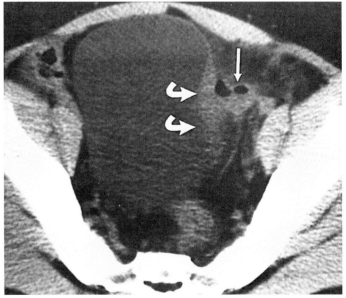

Fig. 28.18 Crohn's disease with enterovesical fistula. CT scan in a patient with long-standing Crohn's disease demonstrates moderate thickening of the left lateral bladder wall (curved arrows), adjacent to an inflamed small bowel loop (straight arrow). Air was present in the bladder on different slices (not shown). These findings confirm the presence of an enterovesical fistula.

(4) **Cancer** Over the years, numerous studies have attempted to determine the relationship between Crohn's disease and the development of malignancies. A recent extensive review of the literature supports the concept that there is an increased risk of small bowel adenocarcinoma, colorectal cancer, and possibly cholangiocarcinomas in patients with Crohn's disease.[78] Although screening for dysplasia and cancer in patients with Crohn's disease is controversial at present, it is clear that CT should play an important role in cancer detection and staging.

# RADIOGRAPHIC FINDINGS IN ULCERATIVE COLITIS

## CONTRAST STUDIES

### Site of involvement

Classically, ulcerative colitis involves the rectosigmoid colon and extends proximally, involving the colon continuously. Although the rectum appears radiographically normal in up to 20% of patients, rectosigmoid involvement is present in 95% at proctosigmoidoscopy.[51] Isolated disease in the right colon does not occur.

The involved portions of the colon are symmetrically, concentrically diseased, which is distinct from the segmental, eccentric and asymmetric pattern of involvement in Crohn's disease.

Terminal ileal disease is demonstrated in 10–25% of patents with ulcerative colitis[51] and is often referred to as 'backwash ileitis'. Typically only a segment of ileum – usually the distal 5–25 cm – is involved and appears patulous and inflamed. Extensive ulceration or stricturing of the terminal ileum, as seen in Crohn's disease, does not occur. This backwash ileitis only occurs in the presence of pancolitis and is thought to be related to reflux of colonic contents into the small bowel.

## COLON

### Mucosal granularity

The earliest radiographically detectable evidence of disease in ulcerative colitis is a granularity of the colon surface which is associated with edema and hyperemia[79] (Fig. 28.19). The granular pattern is thought to result from abnormalities in the quality and quantity of mucus produced by the affected mucosa.[80] The granularity usually diffusely involves the affected portion of colon. This will be demonstrated on double-contrast enema but will not be appreciated on single-contrast studies that underestimate the extent of early disease.

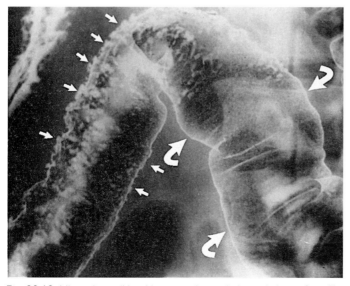

Fig. 28.19 Ulcerative colitis with mucosal granularity and ulcers. Spot film from an air contrast barium enema demonstrates a fine granular appearance to the mucosa in the right portion of the transverse colon (curved arrows). The mid and left transverse colon demonstrates numerous ulcerations (small arrows).

### Ulceration

Early ulcers in ulcerative colitis appear as fine speckled barium collections superimposed on a granular-appearing mucosa. These fine ulcerations, also called mucosal stippling, may also produce a shaggy, spiculated contour to the bowel wall. This is sometimes best appreciated on the postevacuation radiograph.

Although more characteristic of Crohn's disease or infectious colitis, discrete isolated ulcers can occur in patients with ulcerative colitis.[81] These small ulcers appear as small round contrast collections surrounded by lucent halos of edema. They are generally diffusely and symmetrically distributed over the involved region. This is in contrast to the ulcerations in Crohn's disease, which are typically asymmetric and patchy in distribution. As the disease progresses, ulcerations can penetrate deeper into the wall of the colon and produces a variety of sizes and shapes. When the ulceration undermines the submucosal layer, a collar button ulcer can be seen.[80] However, the collar button ulcer is not unique to ulcerative colitis.

### Folds

Early in ulcerative colitis, haustral folds appear thickened and nodular due to inflammation and edema. However, as the disease progresses the haustral fold become blunted, or may be completely lost due to relaxation of the taeniae coli muscle.[82] Such an appearance is sometimes referred to as a 'lead pipe' colon. The haustra may reappear after the colon has healed and the taeniae have regained tonus.[82,83]

### Colonic shortening

Colonic shortening, as demonstrated by barium enema, is characteristic of ulcerative colitis. The exact cause of the shortening has not been ascertained. However, Gore[83] believes that it may be produced by thinning and relaxation of the muscularis mucosae in conjunction with luminal narrowing and loss of haustra.

### Polyps

Postinflammatory polyps can occur in patients with ulcerative colitis, and appear as multiple thin filiform filling defects on barium enema. In most cases when postinflammatory polyps are present, there is no evidence of active colitis. Postinflammatory polyps are benign and are not associated with malignant transformation.

Pseudopolyps, areas of inflamed mucosa surrounded by extensive ulceration, also occur in patients with severe ulcerative colitis.

### Stricture

Colonic strictures are not uncommon in patients with ulcerative colitis, and are usually associated with long-standing total colonic disease. The rectum and sigmoid are most commonly involved.[84] Most of the narrowings seen in ulcerative colitis are benign and in most cases are due to smooth muscle hypertrophy and are therefore potentially reversible.[84]

On barium enema, a stricture appears as a symmetric segment of narrowing with tapered margins. However, because carcinoma in ulcerative colitis tends to be plaque-like and flat rather than polypoid in appearance, narrowings detected on barium enema in patients with ulcerative colitis are referred for colonoscopy and biopsy to confirm or deny the possibility of cancer.

## Dysplasia

Mucosal dysplasia is a premalignant histologic condition that occurs in the colon of patients with ulcerative colitis. It is usually diagnosed on surveillance biopsy, as it frequently is not recognized grossly at colonoscopy.[85]

Mucosal dysplasia has been detected using double-contrast barium enema, although not consistently.[86–88] According to Frank et al.,[87] dysplasia may appear as an irregular area of nodularity with sharply angled edges. Other authors have described fine granularity, minute spiculations or a reticular mucosal pattern. If the double-contrast barium enema detects possible dysplasia, that area can be targeted for colonoscopy and biopsy. However, barium enema is not considered a sensitive method for dysplasia detection, and regular colonoscopy and biopsy is the recommended surveillance regimen.

## Colon cancer

The association of chronic ulcerative colitis with the development of colorectal cancer is well known. The carcinoma which develops is often flat and infiltrating and can be difficult to detect on barium enema[89,90] (Fig. 28.20). Some carcinomas may infiltrate the submucosa and muscular wall without demonstrating a significant mucosal or intraluminal component. This type of lesion can produce very subtle contour abnormalities or luminal narrowing. Therefore, at barium enema any non-distensible segment of colon should be referred for endoscopy and biopsy.

## Toxic dilatation

Toxic dilatation of the colon is a serious, life-threatening complication of inflammatory bowel disease. It is most commonly recognized as a complication of ulcerative colitis, although it may occur in Crohn's disease or infectious colitis. Toxic dilatation is the result of acute transmural inflammation and is usually associated with fever, elevated sedimentation rate and leukocytosis.

Radiographically, the most prominent radiographic feature of toxic megacolon is dilatation of the colon, most commonly observed in the transverse colon, the most anterior portion of the colon in the supine position. The average width of the transverse colon in toxic megacolon is >9 cm, compared with the normal transverse colon which measures <6 cm.[91] In addition to the dilation, the haustral folds are typically edematous, giving the bowel wall a nodular contour.

The diagnosis of toxic megacolon is usually made on plain films of the abdomen (Fig. 28.21). By repositioning the patient and redistributing the air column, different portions of the colon can be evaluated. Because the colon is acutely inflamed and at risk for perforation, a contrast enema is contraindicated. Plain films at 12 hour intervals (or more frequently, depending on the patient's clinical condition) should be taken to monitor the size of the bowel lumen and to check for pneumoperitoneum. Bowel perforation may be silent as the patient is typically receiving high-dose steroids to reduce the inflammation.

## Ileal pouch–anal anastomosis

The ileal pouch is a well-accepted surgical option for patients who require a total colectomy for chronic ulcerative colitis or familial adenomatous polyposis. The surgery consists of the construction of an ileal reservoir that is anastomosed to the anus

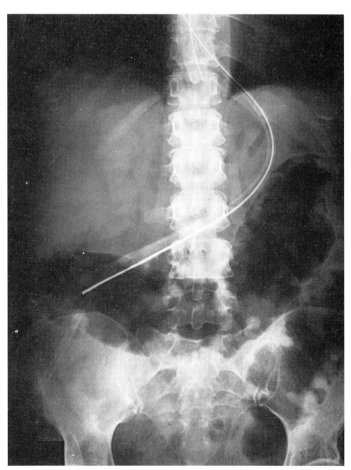

**Fig. 28.21** Ulcerative colitis with toxic megacolon. Abdominal radiograph reveals moderate air distension of the transverse and descending colon, with numerous polypoid masses that represent inflammatory polyps and edematous mucosa. Contrast studies are contraindicated in cases of toxic megacolon because the intense active inflammation of the colon increases the potential for perforation.

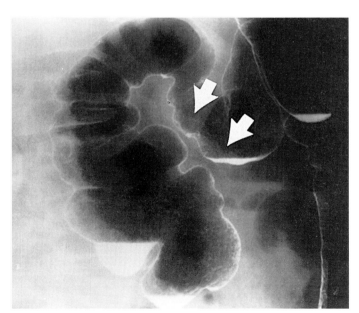

**Fig. 28.20** Ulcerative colitis and cancer. Coned view of the cecum and hepatic flexure during double-contrast barium demonstrates a subtle mass in the transverse colon. This was found to be an adenocarcinoma at surgery.

after total colectomy. This avoids the creation of a permanent external stoma and usually leads to good functional results. The procedure is associated with a variety of complications that can be effectively imaged using contrast radiography.

Radiographic examination of the ileoanal pouch is routinely performed to exclude leakage and to evaluate pouch size and function. At the authors' institution, the reservoir examination is performed in a retrograde fashion through a 12 Fr red rubber catheter using thin barium or water-soluble contrast. Antero-posterior, oblique and lateral spot radiographs of the distended pouch are obtained. Postevacuation anteroposterior and lateral radiographs are also taken. If functional measurements are desired, a simple radiographic evaluation of ileoanal pouch volume can be performed.[92] With this technique, barium is instilled into the pouch via the rectum while the patient is in the standing position. The total volume infused, volume until reflux into the small bowel and volume voided can be measured. This test gives useful information about pouch function and capacity.

Complications which can be diagnosed with pouch contrast radiography include small bowel obstruction, pouch fistula, anastomotic leak, pouchitis and stricture.[93] Continent ileostomy (also called a Kock pouch) is an alternative to the ileal pouch procedure.[94] An ileal reservoir is created and then an intussusception created at the stoma itself, resulting in a one-way valve effect (nipple valve). The patient can intubate the pouch at regular intervals to empty the reservoir of fluid. Slippage of the nipple valve is common, and can be diagnosed radiographically with a contrast study of the continent ileostomy.

# CT

## PRIMARY DISEASE

Ulcerative colitis is typically left-sided or diffuse, and rarely if ever involves the right colon exclusively. On CT scan the most frequent finding is colonic wall thickening, which is present in up to 75% of patients and has a mean thickness of 7.8 mm.[69,70] This is significantly less thick than in Crohn's disease. The bowel wall thickening in ulcerative colitis is diffuse and symmetric, whereas Crohn's disease classically appears irregular and asymmetric, owing to the transmural nature of the disease (Figs 28.22, 28.23). It can also appear smooth and featureless. Ulcers, as documented on endoscopy or barium studies, are not typically visualized on CT because of the spatial resolution. The full extent of colonic involvement may be better appreciated if 3D imaging is available (Fig. 28.24).

The attenuation of the thickened bowel wall in ulcerative colitis is typically more heterogeneous than in Crohn's disease.[70] The halo sign, a low-attenuation ring in the bowel wall due to deposition of submucosal fat,[73] or edema[72] may be present. Submucosal fat deposition is seen more commonly in ulcerative colitis than in Crohn's, and can be especially dramatic in the rectum (Fig. 28.25). It has not been observed in the acute colitides such as pseudomembranous colitis, ischemic colitis or infectious colitis.[70] However, submucosal edema has been seen in patients with graft-versus-host disease and viral enteritis.[95]

Other features which can help distinguish ulcerative colitis from Crohn's are the lack of small bowel involvement, abscess or mesenteric fibrofatty proliferation, which are all characteristic findings in Crohn's disease. In addition, rectal and perirectal

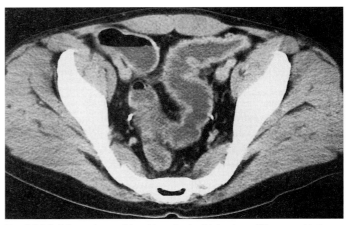

Fig. 28.22 Ulcerative colitis with colonic thickening. CT scan with intravenous contrast demonstrates diffuse symmetric thickening of the rectosigmoid colon in this patient with ulcerative colitis.

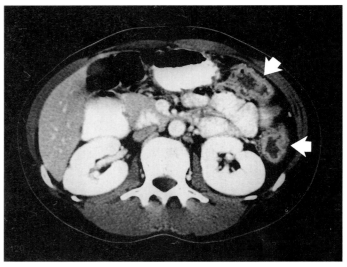

Fig. 28.23 Ulcerative colitis with colonic thickening. Contrast-enhanced CT scan in a patient with ulcerative colitis demonstrates diffuse irregular thickening of the descending colon (arrows). The ascending colon is not involved.

abnormalities are often prominent features of ulcerative colitis. Marked rectal wall thickening can be seen which results in luminal narrowing. Also, prominent perirectal fibrofatty proliferation and widening of the presacral space has been reported in ulcerative colitis (Fig. 28.25), as well as in Crohn's, pseudomembranous colitis, radiation colitis, pelvic lipomatosis etc.[96]

# COMPLICATIONS

## TOXIC MEGACOLON

Toxic megacolon is a severe, life-threatening fulminant transmural colitis most commonly associated with ulcerative colitis. The patient typically presents with profuse bloody diarrhea, abdominal pain, fever and leukocytosis. On CT there is distension of the colon, most commonly involving the transverse colon which contains large amounts of fluid and air. The haustra appear edematous and distorted, or may be absent. The presence of pneumatosis signifies ischemia and necrosis. The major complication of toxic megacolon is perforation, with resulting sepsis,

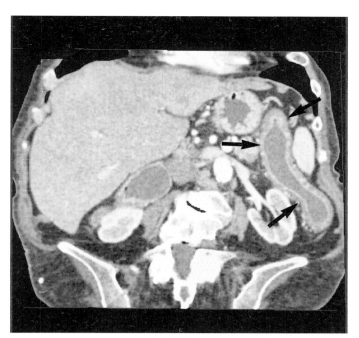

**Fig. 28.24** Coronal 3D CT in a patient with ulcerative colitis shows diffuse thickening of the descending colon (arrow). Water was used as oral contrast and allows good visualization of the inflamed colonic wall.

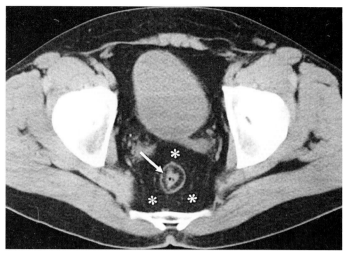

**Fig. 28.25** Ulcerative colitis with submucosal halo and perirectal fibrofatty proliferation. CT scan in a patient with long-standing ulcerative colitis demonstrates a submucosal halo of fat within the rectal wall (arrow) as well as perirectal fibrofatty proliferation (asterisks).

shock, and possibly death. Perforation can be detected as extraluminal air on plain films and CT.

## MALIGNANCY

The association of ulcerative colitis with colorectal cancer is well established. CT is particularly valuable for characterization of primary colonic malignancies and remains the study of choice for the staging of colonic malignancies, as it can reliably demonstrate regional extension of tumor and well as adenopathy and distant metastases.

On CT, adenocarcinoma of the colon usually appears as a soft tissue attenuation mass with irregular borders. Larger masses may have a low-density necrotic center, or occasionally may contain gas, resembling an abscess. Rectal cancers may appear as asymmetric wall thickening which narrows the lumen.

CT is able to detect extension of tumor into the pericolonic fat, invasion of adjacent organs such as bladder or pelvic muscles, and adenopathy. It is the study of choice for the detection of liver metastases, which will appear as multiple hypodense lesions within the liver after the injection of intravenous contrast.

## EXTRAINTESTINAL COMPLICATIONS OF INFLAMMATORY BOWEL DISEASE

Patients with inflammatory bowel disease experience a variety of extraintestinal complications, which can result in considerable morbidity and in some cases mortality. Many of these conditions are encountered by radiologists. For instance, musculoskeletal complications such as sacroiliitis, arthritis, osteoporosis and osteomyelitis can be effectively imaged with plain radiographs, bone scintigraphy and MRI. Hepatobiliary conditions, including fatty infiltration, sclerosing cholangitis, cholangiocarcinoma and cholelithiasis, can be evaluated with CT, MRI, US and/or cholangiography. Radiologists must be famil-

iar with these and the many other associated multisystem complications.

## CONCLUSION

Although contrast studies remain the principal tools for the diagnosis and evaluation of suspected inflammatory bowel disease, other imaging modalities are now playing a larger role. CT, in particular, is useful for evaluation of the extraluminal extent of disease, and for complications. In addition, because CT plays an important role in the evaluation of patients with abdominal pain, it may be the initial imaging study performed in those with inflammatory bowel disease.

In summary, the diagnosis and management of inflammatory bowel disease is complex and requires the cooperation of many medical specialties. Radiologists continue to play a vital role in the evaluation of Crohn's disease and ulcerative colitis, as radiographic studies are considered complementary to endoscopy.

## REFERENCES

1. Theoni R, Gould R. Enteroclysis and small bowel series: comparison of radiation dose and examination time. Radiology 1991;178:659–662.
2. Ott DJ, Chen YM, Gelfand DW, Van Swearingen F, Munitz HA. Detailed per-oral small bowel examination vs. enteroclysis. Part II: Radiographic accuracy. Radiology 1985;155:31–34.
3. Carlson HC. Perspective: the small bowel examination in the diagnosis of Crohn's disease. AJR 1986;147:63–65.
4. Yue NC, Jones B. Crohn disease: prone-angled compression view in radiographic evaluation. Radiology 1993;187:577–580.
5. Maglinte D, Lappas J, Chernish S et al. Improved tolerance of enteroclysis by use of sedation. AJR 1988;151:951–952.
6. Hagenthau P, Wagner H, Stinner B, Klose K. The value of double contrast colon imaging in inadequate colonoscopic diagnosis. (German). Radiologe 1995;35:356–360.
7. Cirocco W, Rusin L. Factors that predict incomplete colonoscopy. Dis Colon Rectum 1995;38:964–968.
8. Orel SG, Rubesin SE, Jones B et al. Computed tomography vs. barium studies in the acutely symptomatic patient with Crohn disease. J Comput Assist Tomogr 1987;11:1009–1016.
9. Fishman E, Wolf E, Jones B, Bayless T, Siegelman S. CT evaluation of Crohn's disease: effect on patient management. AJR 1987;148:537–540.
10. Amin Z, Boulos P, WB L. Technical report: spiral CT pneumocolon for suspected colonic neoplasms. Clinical Radiology 1996;51:56–61.

11. Horton KM, Eng J, Fishman EK. Normal enhancement of the small bowel: Evaluation with spiral CT. J Comput Assist Tomogr 2000;24:67–71.

12. Horton KM, Fishman EK. Multidetector CT in the evaluation of mesenteric ischemia: Can it be done? RadioGraphics 2001;21:1463–1473.

13. Horton KM, Fishman EK. Helical CT of the stomach: evaluation with water as an oral contrast agent. AJR 1998;171:1373–1376.

14. Rossi M, Broglia L, Maccioni F et al. Hydro-CT in patients with gastric cancer: preoperative radiologic staging. Eur Radiol 1997;7:659–664.

15. Winter TC, Ager JD, Nghiem HV, Hill RS. Upper gastrointestinal tract and abdomen: water as an orally administered contrast agent for helical CT. Radiology 1996;201:365–370.

16. Yousem DM, Fishman EK, Jones B. Crohn disease: perirectal and perianal findings at CT. Radiology 1988;167:331–334.

17. Horton KM, Sheth S, Corl F, Fishman EK. Multidetector row CT: principles and clinical applications. Crit Rev Comput Tomogr 2002;43:143–181.

18. Raptopoulos V, Schwartz RK, McNicholas MM et al. Multiplanar helical CT enterography in patients with Crohn's disease. AJR 1997;169:1545–1550.

19. Burton SS, Liebig T, Frazier SD, Ros PR. High density oral barium sulfate in abdominal MRI: efficacy and tolerance in a clinical setting. Magn Reson Imaging 1997;15:1033–1036.

20. Anderson CM, Brown JJ, Balfe DM et al. MRI imaging of Crohn disease: use of perflubron as a gastrointestinal contrast agent. J Magn Reson Imaging 1994;4:491–496.

21. Pokiesser P, Schober E, Hittmair K et al. Vegetable oil as an MR contrast agent for rectal applications. Magn Reson Imaging 1995;13:979–984.

22. Kettriz U, Isaacs K, Warshauer DM, Semelka RC. Crohn's disease. Pilot study comparing MRI of the abdomen with clinical evaluation. J Clin Gastroenterol 1995;21:249–253.

23. Rollandi GA, Martinolli C, Conzi R et al. Magnetic resonance imaging of the small intestine and colon in Crohn's disease. Radiol Med 1996;91:81–85.

24. Low RN, Francis IR, Politoske D, Bennett M. Crohn's disease evaluation: comparison of contrast-enhanced MR imaging and single-phase helical CT scanning. J Magn Reson Imaging 2000;11:127–135.

25. O'Donovan AN, Somers S, Farrow R, Mernagh JR, Sridhar S. MR imaging of anorectal Crohn disease: a pictorial essay. Radiographics 1997;17:101–107.

26. Koelbel G, Schmiedl U, Majer MC et al. Diagnosis of fistulae and sinus tracts in patients with Crohn disease: value of MR imaging. Am J Roentgenol 1989;152:999–1003.

27. Sarrazin J, Wilson SR. Manifestations of Crohn disease at US [Review]. Radiographics 1996;16:499–520; discussion 520–521.

28. Maconi G, Imbesi V, Bianchi Porro G. Doppler ultrasound measurement of intestinal blood flow in inflamamtory bowel disease. Scand J Gastroenterol 1996;31:590–593.

29. Solvig J, Ekberg O, Lindgren S, Floren CH, Nilsson P. Ultrasound examination of the small bowel: comparison with enteroclysis in patients with Crohn disease. Abdom Imaging 1995;20:323–326.

30. Hata J, Haruma K, Suenaga K et al. Ultrasonographic assessment of inflammatory bowel disease. Am J Gastroenterol 1992;87:443–447.

31. Holdstock G, Ligorria JE, Kramitt EL. Gallium 67 scanning in patients with Crohn's disease : an aid to the diagnosis of abdominal abscess. Br J Surg 1982;69:277–278.

32. Jones B, Abbruzzese AA, Hill TC et al. Gallium 67 citrate scintigraphy in ulcerative colitis. Gastrointest Radiol 1980;5:267–272.

33. Rheingold OJ, Tedesco FJ, Block FE et al. Gallium 67 citrate scintiscanning in active inflammatory bowel disease. Dig Dis Sci 1979;24:363–368.

34. Saverymuttu SH, Peters AM, Hodgson JH et al. Indium-111 autologous leukocyte scanning; comparison with radiology for imaging of the colon in inflammatory bowel disease. Br Med J 1982;285:255–257.

35. Saverymuttu SH, Peters AM, Hodgson JH et al. Indium-111 leukocyte scanning in small bowel Crohn's disease. Gastrointest Radiol 1983;8:157–161.

36. Sehal AW, Munro JM, Ensell J et al. Indium-111 tagged leukocytes in the diagnosis of inflammtory bowel disease. Lancet 1981;1:230–233.

37. Stein DT, Gray GM, Gregory PB. Indium-111 leukocyte scanning in ulcerative colitis and Crohn's colitis, a comparison study. Gut 1981;22:876.

38. Arndt JW, Grootscholten MI, van Hogezand RA et al. Inflammatory bowel disease activity assessment using technetium-99m-HMPAO leukocytes. Dig Dis Sci 1997;42:387–393.

39. Giaffer MH, Tindale WB, Holdworth D. Value of technetium-99m HMPAO-labeled leukocyte scintigraphy as an initial screening test in patients suspected of having inflammatory bowel disease. Eur J Gastrenterol Hepatol 1996;8:1195–1200.

40. Weldon MJ, Masoomi AM, Britten AJ et al. Quantification of inflammatory bowel disease activity using technetium-99m HMPAO labeled leucocyte single photon emission computerized tomography (SPECT). Gut 1995;36:243–250.

41. Caroline D, Friedman A. The radiology of inflammatory bowel disease. Med Clin North Am 1994;78:1353–1385.

42. Farmer RG, Whelan G, Fazio VW. Long term follow-up of patients with Crohn's disease. Relationship between clinical pattern and prognosis. Gastroenterology 1985;88:1818–1825.

43. Mekhijan HS, Switz DM, Melnyk CS, Rankin GB, Brooks RK. Clinical features and natural history of Crohn's disease. Gastroenterology 1979;77:898.

44. Ogorek C, Fisher R. Differentiation between Crohn's disease and ulcerative colitis. Med Clin North Am 1994;78:1249–1258.

45. Gore R, Laufer I. Ulcerative colitis and granulomatous colitis: idiopathic inflammatory bowel disease. In: Gore RM, Laufer I, eds. Textbook of gastrointestinal radiology. Philadelphia: WB Saunders; 1994:1098–1141.

46. Wagtmans M, vanHogezand R, Griffioen G, Verspaget H, Lamers C. Crohns disease of the upper gastrointestinal tract. Neth J Med 1997;50:S2–7.

47. Glick SN, Teplick SK. Crohn disease of the small intestine: diffuse mucosal granularity. Radiology 1985;154:313–317.

48. Eisenberg RL. Gastrointestinal radiology: a pattern approach. Philadelphia: Lippincott-Raven; 1996.

49. Elvin FM, Oddson TA, Rice RP, Garbutt JT, Bradenham BP. Double contrast barium enema in Crohn's disease and ulcerative colitis. Am J Roentgenol 1978;131:207–213.

50. Laufer I, Hamilton J. The radiologic differentiation between ulcerative and granulomatous colitis by double contrast radiology. Am J Gastroenterol 1976;66:259–269.

51. Kelvin FM, Gedgaudas RK. Radiologic diagnosis of Crohn disease (with emphasis on its early manifestations) [Review]. Crit Rev Diagn Imaging 1981;16:43–91.

52. Scott N, Nair A, Hughes L. Anovaginal and rectovaginal fistula in a patient with Crohn's disease. Br J Surg 1992;79:1379–1380.

53. Pichney L, Fantry G, Graham S. Gastrocolic and duodenocolic fistulas in Crohn's disease. J Clin Gastroenterol 1992;15:205–211.

54. Santoro G, Bucci L, Frizelle FA. Management of rectourethral fistulas in Crohn's disease. Int J Colorectal Dis 1995;10:183–188.

55. Annibali R, Pietri P. Fistulous complications of Crohn's disease. Int Surg 1992;77:19–27.

56. Goldman SM, Fishman EK, Gatewood OM, Jones B, Siegelman SS. CT in the diagnosis of enterovesical fistulae. Am J Roentgenol 1985;144:1229–1233.

57. Buck JL, Dachman AH, Sobin LH. Polypoid and pseudopolypoid manifestations of inflammatory bowel disease [Review]. Radiographics 1991;11:293–304.

58. Jones B, Abbruzzese AA. Obstructing giant pseudopolyps in granulomatous colitis. Gastrointest Radiol 1978;3:437–438.

59. Levine M. Crohn's disease of the upper gastrointestinal tract. In: Feczko P, Halpert R, eds. The Radiologic Clinics of North America: radiology of inflammatory bowel disease, vol. 25. Philadelphia: WB Saunders; 1989:79–91.

60. Ghahremani G, Gore R, Breuer R et al. Esophageal manifestations of Crohn's disease. Gastrointest Radiol 1982;7:199–203.

61. Davidson JT, Sawyers JL. Crohn's disease of the esophagus. Am Surg 1983;49:168–172.

62. Cockey BM, Jones B, Bayless TM, Shauer A. Filiform polyps of the esophagus with inflammatory bowel disease. 1985;144:1207–1208.

63. Marshak R, Maklansky D, Kurzban J et al. Crohn's disease of the stomach and duodenum. Am J Gastroenterol 1982;77:340–343.

64. Farman J, Faegenburg D, Dallemand S, Chen CK. Crohn's disease of the stomach: the 'ram's horn' sign. Am J Roentgenol Radium Ther Nucl Med 1975;123:242–251.

65. Thompson W, Cockrill H, Rice R. Regional enteritis of the duodenum. 1975;123:252–261.

66. Gore RM, Marn CS, Kirby DF, Vogelzang RL, Neiman HL. CT findings in ulcerative, granulomatous, and indeterminate colitis. AJR Am J Roentgenol 1984;143:279–284.

67. Philpotts LE, Heiken JP, Westcott MA, Gore RM. Colitis: use of CT findings in differential diagnosis. Radiology 1994;190:445–449.

68. Gore RM, Balthazar EJ, Ghahremani GG, Miller FH. CT features of ulcerative colitis and Crohn's disease [Review]. Am J Roentgenol 1996;167:3–15.

69. Frager DH, Goldman M, Beneventano TC. Computed tomography in Crohn disease. J Comput Assist Tomogr 1983;7:819–824.

70. Jones B, Fishman EK, Hamilton SR et al. Submucosal accumulation of fat in inflammatory bowel disease: CT/pathologic correlation. J Comput Assist Tomogr 1986;10:759–763.

71. Gazelle CS, Mueller PR. Abdominal abscess: imaging and intervention. Radiol Clin North Am 1994;32:913–932.

72. Kerber G, Greenberg M, Rubin J. Computed tomography evaluation of local and extraintestinal complications of Crohn's disease. Gastrointest Radiol 1984;9:143–148.

73. Taourel P, Fabre J, Pradel J et al. Value of CT in the diagnosis and management of patients with suspected acute small bowel obstruction. AJR 1995;165:1187–1192.

74. Merine D, Fishman EK, Kuhlman JE et al. Bladder involvement in Crohn disease: role of CT in detection and evaluation. J Comput Assist Tomogr 1989;13:90–93.

75. Berstein D, Rogers A. Malignancy in Crohn's disease. Am J Gastroenterol 1996;91:434–440.

76. Laufer I, Mullens JE, Hamilton J. Correlation of endoscopy and double-contrast radiography in the early stages of ulcerative and granulomatous colitis. Radiology 1976;118:1–6.

77. Lichtenstein J. Radiologic–pathologic correlation of inflammatory bowel disease. Radiol Clin North Am 1987;25:3–24.

78. Williams HJ Jr, Stephens DH, Carlson HC. Double-contrast radiography: colonic inflammatory disease. Am J Roentgenol 1981;137:315–322.

79. Bartram C. Radiology in inflammatory bowel disease. New York: Marcel Dekker; 1983:31–62.

80. Gore RM. Colonic contour changes in chronic ulcerative colitis: reappraisal of some old concepts [Review]. Am J Roentgenol 1992;158:59–61.

81. Caroline D, Evers K. Colitis: radiographic features and differentiation of idiopathic inflammatory bowel disease. In: Feczko P, Halpert R, eds. The Radiologic Clinics of North America: radiology of inflammatory bowel disease, vol. 25. Philadelphia: WB Saunders; 1987:47–65.

82. Granqvist S, Gabrielsson N, Sundelin P, Thorgeirsson T. Precancerous lesions in the mucosa in ulcerative colitis. Scand J Gastroenterol 1980;15:289–296.

83. Frank P, Riddell R, Feczko P, Levin B. Radiological detection of colonic dsyplasia (precarcinoma) in chronic ulcerative colitis. Gastrointest Radiol 1978;3:209–219.

84. Matsumoto T, Iida M, Kuroki F et al. Dysplasia in ulcerative colitis: is radiography adequate for diagnosis? [see comments]. Radiology 1996;199:85–90.

85. Kelvin FM, Woodward BH, McLeod ME, Fetter BF, Jones RS. Prospective diagnosis of dysplasia (precancer) in chronic ulcerative colitis. Am J Roentgenol 1982;138:347–349.

86. Feczko P. Malignancy complicating inflammatory bowel disease. In: Feczko P, Halpert R, eds. The Radiologic Clinics of North America, vol. 25. Philadelphia: WB Saunders; 1989:157–172.

87. Butt J, Morson B. Dysplasia and carcinoma in inflammatory bowel disease. Gastroenterology 1981;80:865–868.

88. Norland C, Kirsner J. Toxic dilatation of the colon (toxic megacolon): etiology, treatment and prognosis in 42 patients. Medicine 1969;48:229–250.

89. Schmidt CM, Horton KM, Sitzmann JV, Jones B, Bayless T. Simple radiographic evaluation of ileoanal pouch volume. Dis Colon Rectum 1996;39:66–73.

90. Alfisher MM, Scholz FJ, Roberts PL, Counihan T. Radiology of ileal pouch–anal anastomosis: normal findings, examination pitfalls, and complications. Radiographics 1997;17:81–98; discussion 98–99.

91. Hastings G, Weber R. Inflammatory bowel disease: Part II. Medical and surgical management. Am Fam Phys 1993;47:811–818.

92. Jones B, Kramer SS, Saral R et al. Gastrointestinal inflammation after bone marrow transplantation: graft-versus-host disease or opportunistic infection? Am J Roentgenol 1988;150:277–281.

93. Krestin G, Beyer D, Steinbrich W. Computed tomography in the differential diagnosis of the enlarged retrorectal space. Gastrointest Radiol 1986;11:364–369.

## CHAPTER 29

# Serology and laboratory markers of disease activity

Stephan R Targan and Loren C Karp

## INTRODUCTION

The role of laboratory evaluations of disease activity in inflammatory bowel diseases, ideally, is to identify specific forms of the disease, indicate degree of disease activity, suggest disease course, and predict response to therapeutic interventions in a clinically non-invasive manner. Numerous laboratory markers have been advanced over the last half-century, including fecal indicators and those that are serologically expressed. To date, no single method has been developed with the requisite specificity and sensitivity to be of absolute clinical utility. In research trials, and to some extent in clinical practice, disease activity is measured radiologically, endoscopically, histologically, and through the use of indices such as Truelove and Witts' Ulcerative Colitis Activity Index[1] and the Crohn's Disease Activity Index (CDAI).[2] Rarely are the activity indices applied with any regularity in clinical practice. What remains are several disease markers and inflammatory parameters which, used together, can approach the objectives listed above. New technologies, however, currently being evaluated for utility, such as wireless video capsule endoscopy, will further refine our ability to diagnose and assess degree of activity in inflammatory bowel disease and will probably stimulate dramatic changes in the way we use laboratory markers to determine treatment approaches. This chapter reviews the history of the various disease indicators employed in the treatment of patients with inflammatory bowel diseases, offers insights into the most efficacious use of those currently available, describes the proposed use of new markers, and suggests directions for future research and the application of technology in patient management. Common laboratory tests will be considered, as will be those that appear to be relevant specifically for inflammatory bowel diseases.

The literature on serologically defined immunologic markers for the inflammatory bowel diseases dates back to 1959, when Broberger and Perlmann reported that precipitating and hemagglutinating immunoglobulin (Ig)-G antibodies were detectable in serum of the majority of patients with ulcerative colitis.[3]

Broberger and Perlmann's hypothesis was that these antibodies were produced at the site of the ulcerative lesions, and that ulcerative colitis may be an indirect response to commensal antigens. In the ensuing years a multitude of other potential immune markers were advanced, including carcinoembryonic antigen activity,[4,5] $\beta_2$-microglobulin,[6] angiotensin-converting enzyme,[7,8] $\alpha_1$-antitrypsin,[9-12] somatomedin-C,[13] interleukin (IL)-2 and IL-2 receptor,[14-17] none of which emerged as useful in clinical practice.

## MARKER ANTIBODIES

Nearly a quarter of a century ago, Das and colleagues reported the presence of colonic tissue-bound antibodies in patients with ulcerative colitis and that this antibody recognized a 40 kDa colonic protein.[18] Lack of reproducible results has stimulated much controversy around this finding. More recently, using more advanced technology, the same group demonstrated the presence of antibodies to tropomyosin in the serum and mucosa of patients with ulcerative colitis.[19,20] The reactivity to tropomyosin, however, potentially can be explained by the possibility that some motif within the molecule is cross-reacting with an environmental bacterial protein. Thus, this reactivity to tropomyosin may only represent a tiny fragment of the reactive potential to components of the microflora.

In the late 1980s and early 1990s Main et al. and Barnes et al. began to investigate the potential utility of antibodies to *Saccharomyces cerevisiae* (ASCA) for Crohn's disease,[21-24] and Saxon et al. and Rump et al. identified antinuclear cytoplasmic antibodies (ANCA) in the serum of patients with ulcerative colitis.[25-27] In addition to ANCA and ASCA, other immune markers have been advanced, including pancreatic autoantibody[28-30] and anti-endothelial cell antibody,[8,19,31] which vary in the degree to which they have been shown to reflect underlying immune responses or interactions with factors in the intestinal environment.

Spurred by progress in studies of animal models in recent years, greater attention has been paid to the role of bacterial antigens in human inflammatory bowel disease. Other evidence of this role is provided in clinical experience in which some patients with Crohn's disease experience improvement in their symptoms from treatment with antibiotics,[32,33] and post-operative ulcerative colitis patients with inflammation of the ileal pouch can be treated successfully with antibiotics.[34] Investigation of the role of bacterial antigens and the antibodies that reflect them has been and continues to be pursued in parallel.

Many serum markers have been proposed for use in the diagnosis of inflammatory bowel disease. In addition to ANCA and ASCA, which are becoming increasingly well characterized, two additional markers have been identified which react to products of bacteria, i.e. the *Escherichia coli*-related outer membrane porin C (omp-C)[35] and I2,[36,37] which is related to *Pseudomonas fluorescens*. These markers have been shown to be associated with Crohn's disease and a subset of patients with ulcerative colitis. Although current technology may limit the sensitivity of these markers at present, they have great potential to be useful, as is described below. It is likely that over the next several years the utility of such markers will remain controversial. Recent studies suggest that the novel technique of wireless video capsule endoscopy may be a more sensitive tool for diagnosis and determination of the extent of involvement than the conventional endoscopic techniques.[38,39]

Much attention also has been paid to the specificity of such serologic evaluations in diagnosing Crohn's disease and/or ulcerative colitis. Ongoing research will continue to elucidate more phenotypic overlaps within classically defined disease populations, as in the case of ulcerative colitis-like Crohn's disease.[40,41] For example, those patients thought to have ulcerative colitis yet who express markers considered standard for Crohn's disease may well have a different form of disease with its own unique immunogenetic mechanisms. Overlapping serological markers and disease manifestations probably account for what at present appears to be weak specificity values for these tests. This potential is suggested in an abstract, in which serum ASCA was shown to correlate with the ultimate development of Crohn's disease in patients who underwent ileal pouch–anal anastomosis (IPAA).[42]

Immune responsiveness to several specific microbial antigens in patients with Crohn's disease and ulcerative colitis has recently been described by Targan and colleagues.[36,37,40,43–45] In addition, monoclonal antibodies were developed with similar reactivity to polyclonal antibodies seen in ulcerative colitis patients expressing serum pANCA,[46–49] and these monoclonal antibodies cross-react with specific bacterial antigens.[43] The study demonstrates that a subset of patients with Crohn's disease develops an IgA response to Omp-C.[35] The author's group also recently reported that reactivity to the bacterial sequence of I2 as measured by IgA is far more frequent in Crohn's disease than ulcerative colitis or control inflammatory conditions.[35,37,45] The significance of these antibodies for diagnosis, disease stratification and treatment is discussed in the following sections.

# ANTINEUTROPHIL CYTOPLASMIC ANTIBODIES (ANCA) AND ANTI-SACCHAROMYCES CEREVISIAE ANTIBODIES (ASCA)

It is no longer a question as to whether inflammatory bowel disease represents heterogeneous groups of diseases, manifesting ultimately as mucosal inflammation.[50,51] Clinical, subclinical and genetic evidence, well covered in other chapters, supports this hypothesis. By far the most extensively studied serum markers for inflammatory bowel diseases are ANCA and ASCA, which have been used to classify these diseases into more homogeneous subgroups. These antibodies also provide clues to pathogenesis, and can therefore be predictive of response to new biologic therapeutic modalities. Panels of marker antibodies, or marker antibody *profiles*, have been demonstrated to represent underlying and distinct inflammatory mechanisms.[40,41] Despite initially being thought to be simply tools to aid in differentiating Crohn's disease and ulcerative colitis and to further clarify cases of 'indeterminate colitis', these markers appear to reflect distinct cytokine profiles and varying underlying inflammatory mechanisms.[40,41,51,52]

## Antineutrophil cytoplasmic antibodies (ANCA)

Over the last decade, disease-specific markers analogous to those used in rheumatological disorders have begun to be applied to inflammatory bowel diseases. Early reports in inflammatory bowel disease included an association between a subtype of ANCA and patients with ulcerative colitis. This subtype, pANCA, differs from the ANCA associated with Wegener's granulomatosis and other vasculitides in that it reacts to different antigens. These antibodies are further distinguished from other ANCA by sensitivity of their antigen to DNase I treatment, and localization to the inner nuclear membrane.[53,54] The pANCA associated with inflammatory bowel disease is produced by mucosal B cells and represents a response to different cross-reactive antigens.[55] A recent study employed high-titer pANCA sera to isolate a 50 kDa nuclear envelope protein, which was able to discriminate patients with ulcerative colitis, primary sclerosoing cholangitis and autoimmune hepatitis.[56,57] Other antigenic candidates include nuclear high-mobility group proteins (HMG-1 and -2)[58,59] and members of the histone $H_1$ family.[55,60,61] Much of the controversy regarding the utility of pANCA is a result of differing detection technologies. Controlled, comparative studies have shown that the most sensitive and specific method for detection of ANCA in serum is by fixed neutrophil enzyme-linked immunosorbent assay (ELISA) in combination with immunofluorescent microscopy and confirmation of loss of the perinuclear pattern following DNAse digestion of neutrophils (Table 29.1).[62]

## Anti-Saccharomyces cerevisiae antibodies (ASCA)

ASCA is a serum marker for Crohn's disease which was first reported in the late 1980s.[21] The antigenic stimulus for ASCA is unknown. Sendid et al. reported that the epitopes responsible for the antigenic reactivity in ASCA were yeast cell wall phosphopeptidomannans.[63] Mannans are an important antigenic constituent of mycobacteria and other microorganisms, and are thought to be the major antigenic component of yeast cell walls.[22] Taylor et al.[64] described the association of ASCA with the TNF microsatellite haplotype a11b4c1d3e3 in patients with inflammatory bowel disease, suggesting that a gene related to ASCA expression resides on chromosome 6 within the MHC in the vicinity of this haplotype. A mutation located on the haplotype may be contributing to ASCA expression. Together, these findings suggest that ASCA, like pANCA, reflect specific mucosal immune mechanisms.

**Table 29.1 Sensitivity of ANCA for ulcerative colitis and of ASCA and antipancreatic antibody (PAB) for Crohn's disease among laboratories**

| Variable | Sensitivity (%) | Specificity (%) | Positive predictive value (%) |
|---|---|---|---|
| Ulcerative colitis | Value | Value | Value (95% CI) |
| Prometheus ANCA | 63 | 75 | 72 (60%, 82%) |
| Oxford ANCA | 39 | 78 | 65 (50%, 78%) |
| Wuerzburg ANCA | 31 | 86 | 70 (53%, 84%) |
| Mayo ANCA | 48 | 81 | 73 (53%, 84%) |
| Smith Kline Beecham ANCA | 0 | 100 | 0 |
| Crohn's disease | | | |
| Prometheus ASCA | 44 | 87 | 76 (61%, 87%) |
| Lille ASCA | 39 | 87 | 74 (61%, 86%) |
| Wuerzburg PAB | 15 | 100 | 100 (74%, 100%) |

Reproduced with permission from[62].

## ANCA AND ASCA IN DIAGNOSIS

Ongoing study has contributed evidence in support of using the combined results of these two assays as a screen for inflammatory bowel disease, and as a means for differentiating among the various forms of the disease. The combined approach, in which positive results are followed by secondary, more specific assays, has been demonstrated to be 80% sensitive in a pediatric population and >90% specific when positive screening was followed by the confirmatory tests.[65] For the purposes of comparison, the sensitivity of rheumatoid factor (15–20% sensitive) or antinuclear antibody (ANA) (24–66% sensitive) for juvenile rheumatoid arthritis is far less than that of combined ANCA and ASCA screening for inflammatory bowel disease. pANCA and ASCA can be used as a first-line screen for patients who present with symptoms that could be due to inflammatory bowel disease, and therefore define those patients who would benefit by further evaluation in this vein. Furthermore, mounting evidence suggests that these tests can be employed to predict the natural history of Crohn's disease and assist in differentiating Crohn's disease from ulcerative colitis.

pANCA are detected in the sera of 60–70% of patients with ulcerative colitis. Serum pANCA are also expressed in 15% of patients diagnosed with Crohn's disease.[25,65–67] Serum pANCA in Crohn's disease represent a disease subtype with distinct clinical and subclinical characteristics.[40] Patients with Crohn's disease who express pANCA have an ulcerative colitis-like left-sided disease with associated ulcerative colitis-like endoscopic and histopathologic presentation. ASCA have been detected in the serum of 50–60% of patients with Crohn's disease.[40,65,68] IgG and/or IgA ASCA expression distinguishes different subgroups of patients with Crohn's disease. Levels of ASCA are independently associated with earlier age of onset of disease and a tendency towards developing classic fibrostenosing and internal penetrating small bowel complications. Two large studies, using well-characterized cohorts of patients with inflammatory bowel disease, showed that pANCA expression in the absence of ASCA expression has a positive predictive value of 88–92.5% for ulcerative colitis.[67,69] For Crohn's disease, expression of serum ASCA in the absence of pANCA has a positive predictive value of 95–96%. In a pediatric cohort, Ruemmele et al. showed that IgA +/– IgG ASCA were 95–100% specific for Crohn's disease, and that pANCA were 92% specific for ulcerative colitis.[65] Also in children, Dubinsky et al. showed that a sequential diagnostic strategy using these markers was 84% accurate for differentiating patients with inflammatory bowel disease from those without (Table 29.2).[70]

Joossens et al. performed a study of patients whose disease had been categorized as indeterminate.[71] Based on these serum markers, a differential diagnosis of Crohn's disease was achieved by detecting the presence of ASCA and the lack of pANCA in 80% of patients. The presence of pANCA and the absence of ASCA diagnosed ulcerative colitis in 63.6% of patients in this population with indeterminate colitis. We have shown that serum pANCA and ASCA levels do not vary over time, nor do they vary with disease activity.[35] It is important, therefore, to note that these patients were followed for a mean of 5 years prior to the development of clinical characteristics consistent with either Crohn's disease or ulcerative colitis. An interesting finding of this study was that 48.5% of patients had no seroreactivity to pANCA or ASCA, suggesting another potential subgroup(s) of patients with IBD.

## ANCA AND ASCA FOR DISEASE STRATIFICATION AND THERAPEUTIC MANAGEMENT

Autoantibodies also have been used to predict disease course. For example, in rheumatoid arthritis a high titer of rheumatoid factor in conjunction with expression of the homozygote HLA-DRB1*0401/0404 MHC class II allele is associated with very aggressive, nodular, erosive joint disease.[72] Similarly, the combination of ASCA and ANCA evaluations predicts certain manifestations of Crohn's disease.[40] The serum expression of both IgG and IgA, particularly at higher levels, is associated with small bowel involvement rather than colonic disease.[40] As described above, high levels of pANCA in patients with Crohn's disease are associated with an ulcerative colitis-like phenotype. Homogeneous autoantibody expression and the magnitude thereof further stratifies subgroups of Crohn's disease. Higher levels of both IgG and IgA ASCA and the absence of pANCA correlate with fibrostenotic and perforating disease. In contrast, higher levels of pANCA and the absence ASCA are associated with patients who do not have fibrostenotic or fistulizing disease. Among patients with small bowel disease, an increased frequency and number of surgeries has been demonstrated in those with high levels of IgG and IgA ASCA and no pANCA, compared to patients with high levels of pANCA and no ASCA. A

**Table 29.2 Overall accuracy of hypothetical sequential diagnostic testing strategy for suspected IBD in 128 pediatric patients**

| Modified | Traditional * | Invasive work-up recommended | n | Diagnostic accuracy | |
|----------|---------------|------------------------------|---|---------------------|--|
| IBD | | | | | |
| + | + | + | 37 | correct | |
| + | – | – | 7 | incorrect | 37/54 (69%) |
| – | not done | – | 10 | incorrect | |
| | | | 54 | | |
| Non-IBD | | | | | |
| + | + | + | 4 | incorrect | |
| + | – | – | 17 | correct | 70/74 (95%) |
| – | not done | – | 53 | correct | |
| | | | 74 | | |
| | Total correct 107/128 (84%) | | | | |

\* Only positive modified assays were sequenced to the traditional assay for confirmation.
Reproduced with permission from [70].

recent prospective study in children showed preliminary results that corroborate these findings.[73]

Recent studies have shown that patients with Crohn's disease who expressed pANCA are less likely to respond to infliximab (anti-TNF-$\alpha$) than are those who expressed serum ASCA or who were unreactive.[64,74] This finding suggests a disease process in this group of Crohn's patients that is not influenced as strongly by overproduction of TNF. An additional environmental factor that may be relevant in this subgroup of patients is smoking. Parsi et al. showed recently that smoking behavior in patients with Crohn's disease is associated with poor response to infliximab.[75] In this study, 73% of non-smokers responded well to infliximab, compared to 22% of smokers. A response greater than 2 months in duration was achieved by 59% of non-smokers, compared to 6% of smokers. Vermiere et al.[76] did not corroborate this finding in a similar study. As mentioned above, in ulcerative colitis pANCA expression is associated with treatment-resistant left-sided disease and the need for surgery early in the disease course.[77] The implication of these findings is that there is a strong likelihood that this group of patients will require treatment with more aggressive, immunomodulating agents.

The association between pANCA and more severe disease and early surgery makes this serum marker a potentially important prognostic tool. The most commonly performed surgical procedure for ulcerative colitis is IPAA (ileal pouch–anal anastomosis). Fleshner et al. demonstrated that 56% of patients with a high level of pANCA (>100 EU/mL) prior to surgery are strongly associated with the development of antibiotic-dependent or -resistant pouchitis after IPAA, compared to 20% of patients with low pANCA or no pANCA expression.[78] Pouchitis is a response to resident microflora and pANCA represent a response to certain bacterial antigens; therefore, patients expressing high levels of pANCA may be particularly susceptible to luminal bacteria, resulting in pouchitis. Awareness of a particular patient's susceptibility to pouchitis may be an indication for more aggressive medical therapy before recommendation of IPAA. When surgery is necessary, high levels of pANCA may suggest preoperative prophylaxis with probiotics, or the use of probiotics early in pouchitis treatment.[79]

## ANCA AND ASCA IN COMBINATION WITH AUTO- OR OTHER BACTERIAL AGENTS

What is emerging is a panel of serological markers by which to classify subgroups of inflammatory bowel disease. Antipancreatic antibodies can be used as an element of such a panel. Antipancreatic antibodies are highly specific for Crohn's disease, but their incidence is only 15–31%.[29,62] Unlike pANCA, antipancreatic antibody expression is not found in family members of patients with ulcerative colitis. Seibold et al. found no association among control populations.[30] Antipancreatic antibody expression does not appear to be affected by disease severity.[30] As part of a panel, antipancreatic antibodies can enhance the diagnostic sensitivity of these combined tests for ulcerative colitis and Crohn's disease.[62]

Further refinements to the panel have emerged recently in the form of immune responses to certain bacterial antigens. In a study designed to define the immunoglobulin immune response to Saccharomyces cerevisiae, Omp-C, I2 and pANCA, we demonstrated heterogeneity in immune responses as well as the magnitude of that response within patients with Crohn's disease.[35] The results of this study demonstrate a variety of patterns of immune responses to microbial and autoantigens that differ widely among groups of patients. Based on these findings, it becomes feasible to suggest that certain antibiotics might be most effective in those patients who have the greatest number and intensity of responses to bacterial antigens. Similarly, the most intense responses to the broadest number of these antigens may define those patients who can best be treated by manipulation of the bacterial content of the gut by antibiotics or probiotics. Figure 29.1 shows the relationships between marker antibodies in a cohort by presence versus absence. Panel A shows the percentage of the Crohn's disease cohort that is positive for each marker. Panels B, C and D depict the intersections of those groups. In each panel, the percentage of the entire cohort defined by the Venn diagram is shown. Broad usage of these antibody patterns for clinical stratification will require clinical studies to define the phenotypes associated with the patterns. In one preliminary such study, patients with the I2/Omp-C antibody profiles were demonstrated to be more likely to achieve

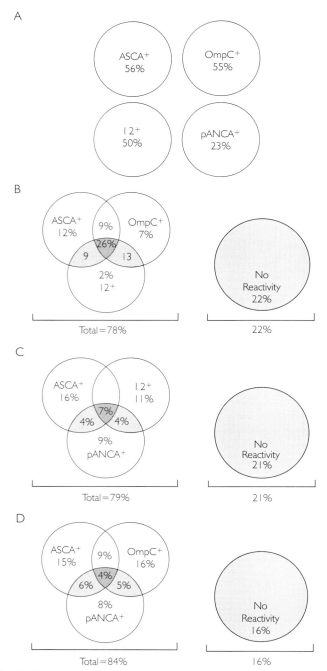

**Fig. 29.1** Relationships between marker antibodies in Crohn's disease. (Reproduced with permission from [35].)

remission from treatment with antibiotics than patients without these responses or with a different antibody profile.[80] These findings will need to be confirmed in larger studies.

## STANDARD LABORATORY PARAMETERS

Standard laboratory parameters in association with other more sophisticated measures of immune activation or increased inflammation are used to measure disease activity in both ulcerative colitis and Crohn's disease. None of these is predictive of active inflammation in all patients with either disease. As suggested by research in a multitude of animal models, it is likely that there is vast heterogeneity in inflammatory repertoires (cytokine profiles and cytokine gene regulation) in the mucosa of patients, with Crohn's disease and ulcerative colitis being the extreme ends of a spectrum. Stratification of subgroups of patients based on such inflammatory repertoires will help correlate specific repertoires with specific disease types – as yet, no single measure proves adequate.

Experience with these markers used as a panel more closely approaches the needs of physicians and patients for disease diagnosis, assessment and treatment planning.[69,74] Ideally, such a laboratory marker panel would be performed at the time a patient presents with active disease in an attempt to generate an 'inflammatory profile'. At the time of presentation the patient is on no medications that could alter results and make them very difficult to interpret, as is the case in the example of prednisone, which elevates the white blood cell count. These tests complement the initial evaluation, which includes colonoscopy with ileal intubation, upper endoscopy with jejunal intubation and, more recently, wireless video capsule endoscopy.[38] Although no specific test correlates in every, or even most, cases of inflammatory bowel disease, any one or more of these indicators may be useful in a particular patient, followed over time as a monitor of disease activity.

## PERIPHERAL BLOOD

### White blood cell count

The absolute white cell count can be elevated in both ulcerative colitis and Crohn's disease. This is generally reflective of neutrophilia. In many patients the absolute count is not elevated, yet there is a 'shift to the left with earlier elements being predominant'. Patients with Crohn's disease can present with an extremely high fever, in which case a shift to the left may be indicative of a complication of the disease and not simply active disease. In severe ulcerative colitis we have found that the percentage of neutrophils correlated with disease severity as well as aiding in the prediction of response to agents such as cyclosporin. The higher the number of band neutrophils, the more severe the colitis and the less likely the patient is to respond to cyclosporin.[81] Band neutrophils alone are not indicative of inflammation in all patients with Crohn's disease.

### Platelets

Platelet count can be seen to represent disease activity, as it has been shown that high levels of these cells are found more commonly in patients with active disease. In a large percentage of Crohn's disease patients, platelets are elevated above normal. It is not only important as a measure of disease activity, but can help differentiate between Crohn's disease and ulcerative colitis inflammation. Most patients with an indeterminate inflammatory bowel disease that cannot be readily categorized and who present with elevated platelets are eventually diagnosed with Crohn's disease and not ulcerative colitis (personal observation). Elevated platelets are also seen in patients with severe ulcerative colitis accompanied by profound iron deficiency. Therefore, platelet count alone is insufficient to determine disease activity. With treatment, platelet counts return to normal ranges. In Crohn's disease, platelet count mirrors the CDAI.[82,83] Elevated platelets are a manifestation of acute blood loss, which can confound the use of platelet counts as a measure of disease activity.

## Albumin

Serum levels of albumin decrease in the setting of active inflammatory bowel diseases; however, albumin levels are influenced by protein loss and malnutrition.[84] In severe ulcerative colitis, very low albumin has been suggested to predict outcome and the requirement for surgery.[85]

## Erythrocyte sedimentation rate (ESR)

ESR is a classic measure of inflammation, although it is not specific to any one part of the body. In IBD, the ESR can identify the acute phase response in very general and flawed terms. ESRs do not adjust in direct correlation to disease improvement. In Crohn's disease, ESR seems to correlate differently depending upon disease location, making it an unreliable indicator. There are patients with active disease whose only indication is elevated ESR, and this is consistent with Crohn's disease and ulcerative colitis.

## C-reactive protein (CRP) and orosomucoid

CRP and orosomucoid are acute-phase proteins that correlate with disease activity in IBD. The protein in orosomucoid has been the most commonly employed standard laboratory test for the measurement of activity, particularly in Crohn's disease. This particular protein may represent increased IL-6 levels generated by mucosal inflammation (see below). CRP has been used in many clinical trials to determine the decrease in inflammatory response, but may be reflective of a subtype of disease. The level of CRP may not be indicative of the level of inflammation as is bandemia in ulcerative colitis, but it is consistent with a particular level of inflammation. Despite being an important marker, it is not useful on its own.[86–88]

## FECAL/PERMEABILITY MARKERS

There has been a very recent interest in the use of fecal markers for the prediction of disease activity. These have been used to determine whether there is active inflammatory disease and to differentiate this from conditions that may mimic inflammatory bowel disease, such as irritable bowel syndrome. More recent studies have shown a high degree of positivity in patients with known Crohn's disease and ulcerative colitis, but the sensitivity of these tests to pick up minimally active Crohn's disease compared to what might be seen with wireless video capsule endoscopy is not known. These tests may be a good indicator of disease activity in patients with known Crohn's disease, but we do not yet know whether and how these markers change in settings of treatment and remission.[89]

Recently, interest has refocused on various protein fecal markers of disease activity. Inflammation renders the mucosa of patients with IBD far more permeable than healthy mucosa, and this results in loss of protein to the lumen.[90] Studies have demonstrated that clearance of $\alpha_1$-antitrypsin can be used as a measure of disease activity.[91,92]

Numerous studies have indicated that fecal calprotectin offers an accurate view of disease activity.[93–98] Bunn et al., in a study of 22 pediatric cases, demonstrated that calprotectin correlated closely with macroscopic and histologic inflammation.[99,100] In a recently published study, Tibble et al. found that the combination of fecal calprotectin, Rome I criteria and intestinal permeability was 50% sensitive and 92% specific in differentiating between patients with irritable bowel syndrome and those with inflammatory bowel disease.[89] Significantly, fecal calprotectin has been shown to be a very specific predictor of clinical relapse.[94] Fecal calprotectin, therefore, is a promising non-invasive indicator of disease activity in both Crohn's disease and ulcerative colitis. Another factor, lactoferrin, detected in whole gut lavage fluid, has been shown to correlate well with other measures of disease activity for ulcerative colitis and Crohn's disease.[101]

## CYTOKINE MARKERS

Other cytokine markers are also under investigation for their utility in diagnosis and management of Crohn's disease and ulcerative colitis. IL-6 has been shown to correlate with platelet counts in patients with ulcerative colitis.[102] Louis et al. tested serum samples from 36 patients with Crohn's disease for expression several factors, including tumor necrosis factor-α, soluble TNF receptors and IL-6, to determine whether any were predictive of relapse. IL-6 had the greatest ability to predict relapse in parallel to clinical characteristics and other laboratory parameters. In a later study, the same group showed that both IL-6 and IL-2r are associated with frequently relapsing Crohn's disease.[103] Reinisch et al. also found an association with Crohn's disease and IL-6, suggesting that IL-6 expression correlates not only with inflammatory activity, but also reflected the clinical course of disease during treatment with steroids, as well as predicted clinical relapse.[104] Very recently, Brown et al. reported that expression of IL-6 in the serum and mucosa of pediatric patients is predictive or confirmatory of inflammatory bowel disease.[105]

Tumor necrosis factor-α (TNF-α) production is elevated in the inflamed mucosa of patients with inflammatory bowel disease, and particularly Crohn's disease,[106] and it corresponds that antibodies to TNF-α have been used successfully to treat certain patients with this disease.[107–110] Furthermore, increased levels of TNF-α are also found in uninvolved areas of mucosa in these patients.[111,112] However, conflicting data make it hard to appreciate the potential use for this cytokine and its receptors in the clinical setting. Maeda et al. showed that increased levels of serum TNF-α are associated with both ulcerative colitis and Crohn's disease.[113] Although several studies have also shown that elevated serum TNF-α correlates with both laboratory and clinical indices of disease activity,[113–116] other groups have not found a significant correlation.[117,118] Similarly conflicting reports have resulted from studies measuring TNF-α in stool samples from patients with inflammatory bowel diseases.[119–121] Increased levels of circulating receptors to TNF, TNF-RI and TNF-RII, have been reported to correlate with both Crohn's disease and ulcerative colitis,[116,122] but this result could not be confirmed by another group.[123] One recent study has reported that high levels of serum TNF-α are associated with poor response to infliximab (anti-TNF-α) in patients with fistulizing Crohn's disease,[124] suggesting that this measurement could be a way of identifying patients likely to respond to this treatment. Further studies regarding the utility of TNF-related proteins are needed to

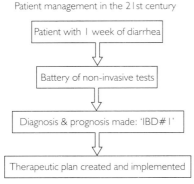

Patient management in the 21st century

Patient with 1 week of diarrhea

↓

Battery of non-invasive tests

↓

Diagnosis & prognosis made: 'IBD#1'

↓

Therapeutic plan created and implemented

**Fig. 29.2** The goal of laboratory and serological markers in inflammatory bowel disease. Tests performed early in evaluation suggest specific types of inflammation and indicate the most efficacious treatment regimen.

determine whether this measurement would enhance a panel of markers for use in inflammatory bowel diseases.

Interleukin-1 (IL-1) and its receptor, IL-1 receptor agonist (IL-1ra), like TNF-α, play major roles in the immune response leading to inflammation. It has been reported that the IL-1/IL-1ra ratio has an inverse relationship to increased levels of disease activity.[125] In a pediatric study, Hyams et al. have shown that circulating IL-1ra is increases in corresponding increments to disease activity as measured by activity indices.[126] Guimbaud et al. found that IL-1β correlated well with disease activity in ulcerative colitis.[102] Overall, these markers have been studied in heterogeneous populations of patients. As homogeneous subpopulations and disease phenotypes are further defined, careful studies may demonstrate a use for one or all of these markers within a specific group of patients.

## CONCLUSIONS

The current goal of research on serological and laboratory parameters for inflammatory bowel diseases is to identify markers which, in combination, can predict patient response to specific therapeutic modalities. Such a panel of markers would prevent the long-term use of ineffectual therapies in patients unlikely to respond and avoid side effects, such as those associated with corticosteroids and infliximab. Predictions made upon these parameters may be further refined with the addition of genotyping, as is being done with TMPT for the use of 6-mercaptopurine. Genotypes, in combination with serum markers, reflect underlying inflammatory patterns, which in turn provide specific targets for therapeutic development and intervention. In a current example, Crohn's patients with high-level pANCA have been shown to respond poorly to treatment with infliximab,[64,76] and ulcerative colitis patients with elevated band neutrophil counts have been shown to develop more severe disease and respond poorly to cyclosporin.[81] The insight afforded by these two simple test results can save patients from ineffective trials of medications and allow them to avoid the potential serious side effects associated with these treatments.

Early in the 21st century, as depicted in Figure 29.2, it is conceivable that our approach to patients who present with symptoms suggestive of inflammatory bowel disease would be based on the immediate performance of a panel of genetic, serologic

and standard laboratory tests performed in conjunction with the use of esophagogastroduodenoscopy, colonoscopy with ileal intubation, and wireless video capsule endoscopy. Such early evaluations would indicate a particular inflammatory bowel disease phenotype, and the likely course of disease on an individual patient basis. In many instances, the same information will identify which treatment modalities would be most efficacious. Those patients likely to encounter severe courses would undergo early intervention with immunomodulatory regimens.

Although the scholarship on peripheral blood and fecal markers for measuring disease activity is quite dynamic at present, they too should be employed at the time of patient presentation. Clinical studies are required to evaluate whether the combination of activity markers with diagnostic markers will allow for further subclassification of patient groups, and correlate these with specific cytokine patterns and types of mucosal inflammation.

## REFERENCES

1.  Truelove SC. The treatment of ulcerative colitis. Schweiz Med Wochenschr 1981;111:1342–1346.
2.  Best WR, Becktel JM, Singleton JW, Kern F Jr. Development of a Crohn's disease activity index. National Cooperative Crohn's Disease Study. Gastroenterology 1976;70:439–444.
3.  Broberger O, Perlmann P. Autoantibodies in human ulcerative colitis. J Exp Med 1959;110:657–674.
4.  Khoo SK, Hunt PS, Mackay IR. Studies of carcinoembryonic antigen activity of whole and extracted serum in ulcerative colitis. Gut 1973;14:545–548.
5.  Turner MD, Kleinman MS, Thayer W. Serum carcinoembryonic antigen (CEA) in patients with chronic inflammatory bowel disease. Digestion 1973;9:116–123.
6.  Descos L, Andre C, Beorghia S, Vincent C, Revillard JP. Serum levels of beta-2-microglobulin - a new marker of activity in Crohn's disease. N Engl J Med 1979;301:440–441.
7.  Silverstein E, Fierst SM, Simon MR, Weinstock JV, Friedland J. Angiotensin-converting enzyme in Crohn's disease and ulcerative colitis. Am J Clin Pathol 1981;75:175–178.
8.  Sommer H, Schweisfurth H, Schulz M. Serum angiotensin-I-converting enzyme and carboxypeptidase N in Crohn's disease and ulcerative colitis. Enzyme 1986;35:181–188.
9.  Karbach U, Ewe K, Dehos H. Antiinflammatory treatment and intestinal alpha 1-antitrypsin clearance in active Crohn's disease. Dig Dis Sci 1985;30:229–235.
10. Karbach U, Ewe K, Bodenstein H. Alpha 1-antitrypsin, a reliable endogenous marker for intestinal protein loss and its application in patients with Crohn's disease. Gut 1983;24:718–723.
11. Fischbach W, Becker W, Mossner J, Koch W, Reiners C. Faecal alpha-1-antitrypsin and excretion of 111 indium granulocytes in assessment of disease activity in chronic inflammatory bowel diseases. Gut 1987;28:386–393.
12. Fischbach W, Becker W. Clinical relevance of activity parameters in Crohn's disease estimated by the faecal excretion of 111In-labeled granulocytes. Digestion 1991;50:149–152.
13. Kirschner BS, Sutton MM. Somatomedin-C levels in growth-impaired children and adolescents with chronic inflammatory bowel disease. Gastroenterology 1986;91:830–836.
14. Brynskov J, Tvede N. Plasma interleukin-2 and a soluble/shed interleukin-2 receptor in serum of patients with Crohn's disease. Effect of cyclosporin. Gut 1990;31:795–799.
15. Crabtree JE, Juby LD, Heatley RV, Lobo AJ, Bullimore DW, Axon AT. Soluble interleukin-2 receptor in Crohn's disease: relation of serum concentrations to disease activity. Gut 1990;31:1033–1036.
16. Duclos B, Reimund JM, Lang JM, Coumaros G, Lehr L, Chamouard P. Elevated levels of soluble interleukin-2 receptors in Crohn's disease. Gastroenterol Clin Biol 1990;14:104–105.
17. Mueller C, Knoflach P, Zielinski CC. T-cell activation in Crohn's disease. Increased levels of soluble interleukin-2 receptor in serum and in supernatants of stimulated peripheral blood mononuclear cells. Gastroenterology 1990;98:639–646.
18. Das KM, Dubin R, Nagai T. Isolation and characterization of colonic tissue-bound antibodies from patients with idiopathic ulcerative colitis. Proc Natl Acad Sci USA 1978;75:4528–4532.
19. Kesari KV, Yoshizaki N, Geng X, Lin JJ, Das KM. Externalization of tropomyosin isoform 5 in colon epithelial cells. Clin Exp Immunol 1999;118:219–227.
20. Onuma EK, Amenta PS, Ramaswamy K, Lin JJ, Das KM. Autoimmunity in ulcerative colitis (UC): a predominant colonic mucosal B cell response against human tropomyosin isoform 5. Clin Exp Immunol 2000;121:466–471.

21. Main J, McKenzie H, Yeaman GR, Kerr MA, Robson D, Pennington CR, Parratt D. Antibody to *Saccharomyces cerevisiae* (bakers' yeast) in Crohn's disease. Br Med J 1988;297:1105–1106.

22. McKenzie H, Main J, Pennington CR, Parratt D. Antibody to selected strains of *Saccharomyces cerevisiae* (baker's and brewer's yeast) and *Candida albicans* in Crohn's disease. Gut 1990;31:536–538.

23. McKenzie H, Parratt D, Main J, Pennington CR. Antigenic heterogeneity of strains of *Saccharomyces cerevisiae* and *Candida albicans* recognised by serum antibodies from patients with Crohn's disease. FEMS Microbiol Immunol 1992;4:219–224.

24. Barnes RM, Allan S, Taylor-Robinson CH, Finn R, Johnson PM. Serum antibodies reactive with *Saccharomyces cerevisiae* in inflammatory bowel disease: is IgA antibody a marker for Crohn's disease? Int Arch Allergy Appl Immunol 1990;92:9–15.

25. Saxon A, Shanahan F, Landers C, Ganz T, Targan S. A distinct subset of antineutrophil cytoplasmic antibodies is associated with inflammatory bowel disease. J Allergy Clin Immunol 1990;86:202–210.

26. Rump JA, Worner I, Roth M, Scholmerich J, Hansch M, Peter HH. p-ANCA of undefined specificity in ulcerative colitis: correlation to disease activity and therapy. Adv Exp Med Biol 1993;336:507–513.

27. Rump JA, Scholmerich J, Gross V et al. A new type of perinuclear anti-neutrophil cytoplasmic antibody (p-ANCA) in active ulcerative colitis but not in Crohn's disease. Immunobiology 1990;181:406–413.

28. Stocker W, Otte M, Ulrich S et al. Autoimmunity to pancreatic juice in Crohn's disease. Results of an autoantibody screening in patients with chronic inflammatory bowel disease. Scand J Gastroenterol 1987;Suppl 139:41–52.

29. Seibold F, Weber P, Jenss H, Wiedmann KH. Antibodies to a trypsin sensitive pancreatic antigen in chronic inflammatory bowel disease: specific markers for a subgroup of patients with Crohn's disease. Gut 1991;32:1192–1197.

30. Seibold F, Mork H, Tanza S et al. Pancreatic autoantibodies in Crohn's disease: a family study. Gut 1997;40:481–484.

31. Berberian LS, Valles-Ayoub Y, Gordon LK, Targan SR, Braun J. Expression of a novel autoantibody defined by the VH3-15 gene in inflammatory bowel disease and *Campylobacter jejuni* enterocolitis. J Immunol 1994;153:3756–3763.

32. Prantera C, Zannoni F, Scribano ML et al. An antibiotic regimen for the treatment of active Crohn's disease: a randomized, controlled clinical trial of metronidazole plus ciprofloxacin. Am J Gastroenterol 1996;91:328–332.

33. Prantera C, Kohn A, Zannoni F, Spimpolo N, Bonfa M. Metronidazole plus ciprofloxacin in the treatment of active, refractory Crohn's disease: results of an open study. J Clin Gastroenterol 1994;19:79–80.

34. Madden MV, McIntyre AS, Nicholls RJ. Double-blind crossover trial of metronidazole versus placebo in chronic unremitting pouchitis. Dig Dis Sci 1994;39:1193–1196.

35. Landers CJ, Cohavy O, Misra R et al. Selected loss of tolerance evidenced by Crohn's disease-associated immune responses to auto- and microbial antigens. Gastroenterology 2002;123:689–699.

36. Dalwadi H, Wei B, Kronenberg M, Sutton CL, Braun J. The Crohn's disease-associated bacterial protein I2 is a novel enteric t cell superantigen. Immunity 2001;15:149–158.

37. Sutton CL, Kim J, Yamane A et al. Identification of a novel bacterial sequence associated with Crohn's disease. Gastroenterology 2000;119:23–31.

38. Mow WS, Lo SK, Abreu MT, Targan SR, Papadakis KA, Vasiliauskas EA. Video capsule enteroscopy can be useful in the diagnosis and management of inflammatory bowel disease. Gastroenterology 2002;122:A218.

39. Costamagna G, Shah SK, Riccioni ME et al. A prospective trial comparing small bowel radiographs and video capsule endoscopy for suspected small bowel disease. Gastroenterology 2002;123:999–1005.

40. Vasiliauskas EA, Plevy SE, Landers CJ et al. Perinuclear antineutrophil cytoplasmic antibodies in patients with Crohn's disease define a clinical subgroup. Gastroenterology 1996;110:1810–1819.

41. Vasiliauskas EA, Kam LY, Karp LC, Gaiennie J, Yang H, Targan SR. Marker antibody expression stratifies Crohn's disease into immunologically homogeneous subgroups with distinct clinical characteristics. Gut 2000;47:487–496.

42. Valentine JF, Lauwers GY, Rout WR. Are ASCA-positive ulcerative colitis patients at higher risk for pouchitis and pouch fistulae. Gastroenterology . 2000;118:A106.

43. Cohavy O, Bruckner D, Gordon LK et al. Colonic bacteria express an ulcerative colitis pANCA-related protein epitope. Infect Immun 2000;68:1542–1548.

44. Cohavy O, Harth G, Horwitz M et al. Identification of a novel mycobacterial histone H1 homologue (HupB) as an antigenic target of pANCA monoclonal antibody and serum immunoglobulin A from patients with Crohn's disease. Infect Immun 1999;67:6510–6517.

45. Sutton CL, Yang H, Li Z, Rotter JI, Targan SR, Braun J. Familial expression of anti-Saccharomyces cerevisiae mannan antibodies in affected and unaffected relatives of patients with Crohn's disease. Gut 2000;46:58–63.

46. Eggena M, Targan SR, Iwanczyk L, Vidrich A, Gordon LK, Braun J. Phage display cloning and characterization of an immunogenetic marker (perinuclear anti-neutrophil cytoplasmic antibody) in ulcerative colitis. J Immunol 1996;156:4005–4011.

47. Gordon LK, Eggena M, Holland GN, Weisz JM, Braun J. pANCA antibodies in patients with anterior uveitis: identification of a marker antibody usually associated with ulcerative colitis. J Clin Immunol 1998;18:264–271.

48. Gordon LK, Eggena M, Targan SR, Braun J. Mast cell and neuroendocrine cytoplasmic autoantigen(s) detected by monoclonal pANCA antibodies. Clin Immunol 2000;94:42–50.

49. Gordon LK, Eggena M, Targan SR, Braun J. Definition of ocular antigens in ciliary body and retinal ganglion cells by the marker antibody pANCA. Invest Ophthalmol Vis Sci 1999;40:1250–1255.

50. Papadakis KA, Targan SR. Current theories on the causes of inflammatory bowel disease. Gastroenterol Clin North Am 1999;28:283–296.

51. Targan SR, Murphy LK. Clarifying the causes of Crohn's. Nature Med 1995;1:1241–1243.

52. Plevy SE, Targan SR, Yang H, Fernandez D, Rotter JI, Toyoda H. Tumor necrosis factor microsatellites define a Crohn's disease-associated haplotype on chromosome 6. Gastroenterology 1996;110:1053–1060.

53. Vidrich A, Lee J, James E, Cobb L, Targan S. Segregation of pANCA antigenic recognition by DNase treatment of neutrophils: ulcerative colitis, type 1 autoimmune hepatitis, and primary sclerosing cholangitis. J Clin Immunol 1995;15:293–299.

54. Billing P, Tahir S, Calfin B et al. Nuclear localization of the antigen detected by ulcerative colitis-associated perinuclear antineutrophil cytoplasmic antibodies. Am J Pathol 1995;147:979–987.

55. Targan SR, Landers CJ, Cobb L, MacDermott RP, Vidrich A. Perinuclear anti-neutrophil cytoplasmic antibodies are spontaneously produced by mucosal B cells of ulcerative colitis patients. J Immunol 1995;155:3262–3267.

56. Terjung B, Worman HJ, Herzog V, Sauerbruch T, Spengler U. Differentiation of antineutrophil nuclear antibodies in inflammatory bowel and autoimmune liver diseases from antineutrophil cytoplasmic antibodies (p-ANCA) using immunofluorescence microscopy. Clin Exp Immunol 2001;126:37–46.

57. Terjung B, Spengler U, Sauerbruch T, Worman HJ. 'Atypical p-ANCA' in IBD and hepatobiliary disorders react with a 50-kilodalton nuclear envelope protein of neutrophils and myeloid cell lines. Gastroenterology 2000;119:310–322.

58. Sobajima J, Ozaki S, Uesugi H et al. Prevalence and characterization of perinuclear anti-neutrophil cytoplasmic antibodies (P-ANCA) directed against HMG1 and HMG2 in ulcerative colitis (UC). Clin Exp Immunol 1998;111:402–407.

59. Sobajima J, Ozaki S, Osakada F et al. Novel autoantigens of perinuclear anti-neutrophil cytoplasmic antibodies (P-ANCA) in ulcerative colitis: non-histone chromosomal proteins, HMG1 and HMG2. Clin Exp Immunol 1997;107:135–140.

60. Eggena M, Cohavy O, Parseghian MH et al. Identification of histone H1 as a cognate antigen of the ulcerative colitis-associated marker antibody pANCA. J Autoimmun 2000;14:83–97.

61. Reumaux D, Meziere C, Colombel JF, Duthilleul P, Mueller S. Distinct production of autoantibodies to nuclear components in ulcerative colitis and in Crohn's disease. Clin Immunol Immunopathol 1995;77:349–357.

62. Sandborn WJ, Loftus EV Jr, Colombel JF et al. Evaluation of serologic disease markers in a population-based cohort of patients with ulcerative colitis and Crohn's disease. Inflamm Bowel Dis 2001;7:192–201.

63. Sendid B, Colombel JF, Jacquinot PM et al. Specific antibody response to oligomannosidic epitopes in Crohn's disease. Clin Diagn Lab Immunol 1996;3:219–226.

64. Taylor KD, Plevy SE, Yang H et al. ANCA pattern and LTA haplotype relationship to clinical responses to anti-TNF antibody treatment in Crohn's disease. Gastroenterology 2001;120:1347–1355.

65. Ruemmele FM, Targan SR, Levy G, Dubinsky M, Braun J, Seidman EG. Diagnostic accuracy of serological assays in pediatric inflammatory bowel disease. Gastroenterology 1998;115:822–829.

66. Targan SR. The utility of ANCA and ASCA in inflammatory bowel disease. Inflamm Bowel Dis 1999;5:61–63; discussion 66–67.

67. Quinton JF, Sendid B, Reumaux D et al. Anti-*Saccharomyces cerevisiae* mannan antibodies combined with antineutrophil cytoplasmic autoantibodies in inflammatory bowel disease: prevalence and diagnostic role. Gut 1998;42:788–791.

68. Sendid B, Quinton JF, Charrier G et al. Anti-*Saccharomyces cerevisiae* mannan antibodies in familial Crohn's disease. Am J Gastroenterol 1998;93:1306–1310.

69. Peeters M, Joossens S, Vermeire S, Vlietinck R, Bossuyt X, Rutgeerts P. Diagnostic value of anti-*Saccharomyces cerevisiae* and antineutrophil cytoplasmic autoantibodies in inflammatory bowel disease. Am J Gastroenterol 2001;96:730–734.

70. Dubinsky MC, Ofman JJ, Urman M, Targan SR, Seidman EG. Clinical utility of serodiagnostic testing in suspected pediatric inflammatory bowel disease. Am J Gastroenterol 2001;96:758–765.

71. Joossens S, Reinisch W, Vermeire S et al. The value of serologic markers in indeterminate colitis: a prospective follow-up study. Gastroenterology 2002;122:1242–1247.

72. Weyand CM, McCarthy TG, Goronzy JJ. Correlation between disease phenotype and genetic heterogeneity in rheumatoid arthritis. J Clin Invest 1995;95:2120–2126.

73. Desir B, Amre DK, Seidman EG. Clinical signficance of ASCA and pANCA levels in IBD and their correlation with disease course and activity. Gastroenterology 2002;122:A177.

74. Esters N, Vermeire S, Joossens S et al. Serological markers for prediction of response to anti-tumor necrosis factor treatment in Crohn's disease. Am J Gastroenterol 2002;97:1458–1462.

75. Parsi MA, Achkar JP, Richardson S et al. Predictors of response to infliximab in patients with Crohn's disease. Gastroenterology 2002;123:707–713.

76. Vermeire S, Louis E, Carbonez A et al. Demographic and clinical parameters influencing the short-term outcome of anti-tumor necrosis factor (infliximab) treatment in Crohn's disease. Am J Gastroenterol 2002;97:2357–2363.

77. Sandborn WJ, Landers CJ, Tremaine WJ, Targan SR. Association of antineutrophil cytoplasmic antibodies with resistance to treatment of left-sided ulcerative colitis: results of a pilot study. Mayo Clin Proc 1996;71:431–436.

78.  Fleshner PR, Vasiliauskas EA, Kam LY et al. High level perinuclear antineutrophil cytoplasmic antibody (pANCA) in ulcerative colitis patients before colectomy predicts the development of chronic pouchitis after ileal pouch-anal anastomosis. Gut 2001;49:671–677.

79.  Abreu MT. Controversies in IBD. Serologic tests are helpful in managing inflammatory bowel disease. Inflamm Bowel Dis 2002;8:224–226; discussion 223, 230–221.

80.  Targan S, Landers CJ, Steinhart H, Seidman EG, Greenberg GR. Crohn's disease: preliminary evidence for the association of high level serum antibodies to bacteria associated antigens with antibiotic induced clinical remission. Gastroenterology 2002;122:A177.

81.  Rowe FA, Walker JH, Karp LC, Vasiliauskas EA, Plevy SE, Targan SR. Factors predictive of response to cyclosporin treatment for severe, steroid-resistant ulcerative colitis. Am J Gastroenterol 2000;95:2000–2008.

82.  Talstad I, Rootwelt K, Gjone E. Thrombocytosis in ulcerative colitis and Crohn's disease. Scand J Gastroenterol 1973;8:135–138.

83.  Philips MS. Platelet count in patients with Crohn's disease. Br Med J (Clin Res Ed) 1983;286:1895–1896.

84.  Bendixen G, Goltermann N, Jarnum S, Jensen KB, Weeke B, Westergaard H. Immunoglobulin and albumin turnover in ulcerative colitis. Scand J Gastroenterol 1970;5:433–441.

85.  Chakravarty BJ. Predictors and the rate of medical treatment failure in ulcerative colitis. Am J Gastroenterol 1993;88:852–855.

86.  Andre C, Descos L, Landais P, Fermanian J. Assessment of appropriate laboratory measurements to supplement the Crohn's disease activity index. Gut 1981;22:571–574.

87.  Fagan EA, Dyck RF, Maton PN et al. Serum levels of C-reactive protein in Crohn's disease and ulcerative colitis. Eur J Clin Invest 1982;12:351–359.

88.  Jensen KB, Jarnum S, Koudahl G, Kristensen M. Serum orosomucoid in ulcerative colitis: its relation to clinical activity, protein loss, and turnover of albumin and IgG. Scand J Gastroenterol 1976;11:177–183.

89.  Tibble JA, Sigthorsson G, Foster R, Forgacs I, Bjarnason I. Use of surrogate markers of inflammation and Rome criteria to distinguish organic from nonorganic intestinal disease. Gastroenterology 2002;123:450–460.

90.  Jeejeebhoy KN. Muscle function and nutrition. Gut 1986;27 Suppl 1:25–39.

91.  Grill BB, Hillemeier AC, Gryboski JD. Fecal alpha 1-antitrypsin clearance in patients with inflammatory bowel disease. J Pediatr Gastroenterol Nutr 1984;3:56–61.

92.  Florent C, L'Hirondel C, Desmazures C, Giraudeaux V, Bernier JJ. [Evaluation of ulcerative colitis and Crohn's disease activity by measurement of alpha-1-antitrypsin intestinal clearance (author's transl)]. Gastroenterol Clin Biol 1981;5:193–197.

93.  Roseth AG, Aadland E, Jahnsen J, Raknerud N. Assessment of disease activity in ulcerative colitis by faecal calprotectin, a novel granulocyte marker protein. Digestion 1997;58:176–180.

94.  Tibble J, Teahon K, Thjodleifsson B et al. A simple method for assessing intestinal inflammation in Crohn's disease. Gut 2000;47:506–513.

95.  Roseth AG, Schmidt PN, Fagerhol MK. Correlation between faecal excretion of indium-111-labelled granulocytes and calprotectin, a granulocyte marker protein, in patients with inflammatory bowel disease. Scand J Gastroenterol 1999;34:50–54.

96.  Roseth AG, Kristinsson J, Fagerhol MK et al. Faecal calprotectin: a novel test for the diagnosis of colorectal cancer? Scand J Gastroenterol 1993;28:1073–1076.

97.  Roseth AG, Fagerhol MK, Aadland E, Schjonsby H. Assessment of the neutrophil dominating protein calprotectin in feces. A methodologic study. Scand J Gastroenterol 1992;27:793–798.

98.  Tibble J, Bjarnason I. Non-invasive investigation of inflammatory bowel disease. World J Gastroenterol 2001;7:460–465.

99.  Bunn SK, Bisset WM, Main MJ, Gray ES, Olson S, Golden BE. Fecal calprotectin: validation as a noninvasive measure of bowel inflammation in childhood inflammatory bowel disease. J Pediatr Gastroenterol Nutr 2001;33:14–22.

100.  Bunn SK, Bisset WM, Main MJ, Golden BE. Fecal calprotectin as a measure of disease activity in childhood inflammatory bowel disease. J Pediatr Gastroenterol Nutr 2000;32:171–177.

101.  Kayazawa M, Saitoh O, Kojima K et al. Lactoferrin in whole gut lavage fluid as a marker for disease activity in inflammatory bowel disease: comparison with other neutrophil-derived proteins. Am J Gastroenterol 2002;97:360–369.

102.  Guimbaud R, Bertrand V, Chauvelot-Moachon L et al. Network of inflammatory cytokines and correlation with disease activity in ulcerative colitis. Am J Gastroenterol 1998;93:2397–2404.

103.  Van Kemseke C, Belaiche J, Louis E. Frequently relapsing Crohn's disease is characterized by persistent elevation in interleukin-6 and soluble interleukin-2 receptor serum levels during remission. Int J Colorectal Dis 2000;15:206–210.

104.  Reinisch W, Gasche C, Tillinger W et al. Clinical relevance of serum interleukin-6 in Crohn's disease: single point measurements, therapy monitoring, and prediction of clinical relapse. Am J Gastroenterol 1999;94:2156–2164.

105.  Brown KA, Back SJ, Ruchelli ED et al. Lamina propria and circulating interleukin-6 in newly diagnosed pediatric inflammatory bowel disease patients. Am J Gastroenterol 2002;97:2603–2608.

106.  Breese EJ, Michie CA, Nicholls SW et al. Tumor necrosis factor alpha-producing cells in the intestinal mucosa of children with inflammatory bowel disease. Gastroenterology 1994;106:1455–1466.

107.  Targan SR, Hanauer SB, van Deventer SJ et al. A short-term study of chimeric monoclonal antibody cA2 to tumor necrosis factor alpha for Crohn's disease. Crohn's Disease cA2 Study Group. N Engl J Med 1997;337:1029–1035.

108.  D'Haens G, Van Deventer S, Van Hogezand R et al. Endoscopic and histological healing with infliximab anti-tumor necrosis factor antibodies in Crohn's disease: A European multicenter trial. Gastroenterology 1999;116:1029–1034.

109.  Rutgeerts P, D'Haens G, Targan S et al. Efficacy and safety of retreatment with anti-tumor necrosis factor antibody (infliximab) to maintain remission in Crohn's disease. Gastroenterology 1999;117:761–769.

110.  Present DH. Review article: the efficacy of infliximab in Crohn's disease - healing of fistulae. Aliment Pharmacol Ther 1999;13 Suppl 4:23–28; discussion 38.

111.  Reimund JM, Wittersheim C, Dumont S et al. Increased production of tumour necrosis factor-alpha interleukin-1 beta, and interleukin-6 by morphologically normal intestinal biopsies from patients with Crohn's disease. Gut 1996;39:684–689.

112.  Reinecker HC, Steffen M, Witthoeft T et al. Enhanced secretion of tumour necrosis factor-alpha, IL-6, and IL-1 beta by isolated lamina propria mononuclear cells from patients with ulcerative colitis and Crohn's disease. Clin Exp Immunol 1993;94:174–181.

113.  Maeda M, Watanabe N, Neda H et al. Serum tumor necrosis factor activity in inflammatory bowel disease. Immunopharmacol Immunotoxicol 1992;14:451–461.

114.  Murch SH, Lamkin VA, Savage MO, Walker-Smith JA, MacDonald TT. Serum concentrations of tumour necrosis factor alpha in childhood chronic inflammatory bowel disease. Gut 1991;32:913–917.

115.  Sategna Guidetti C, Pulitano R. Pulmonary tuberculoma associated with Crohn's disease. J Clin Gastroenterol 1991;13:593–594.

116.  Gardiner KR, Halliday MI, Barclay GR et al. Significance of systemic endotoxaemia in inflammatory bowel disease. Gut 1995;36:897–901.

117.  Hyams JS, Treem WR, Eddy E, Wyzga N, Moore RE. Tumor necrosis factor-alpha is not elevated in children with inflammatory bowel disease. J Pediatr Gastroenterol Nutr 1991;12:233–236.

118.  Nielsen OH, Brynskov J, Bendtzen K. Circulating and mucosal concentrations of tumour necrosis factor and inhibitor(s) in chronic inflammatory bowel disease. Dan Med Bull 1993;40:247–249.

119.  Nicholls S, Stephens S, Braegger CP, Walker-Smith JA, MacDonald TT. Cytokines in stools of children with inflammatory bowel disease or infective diarrhoea. J Clin Pathol 1993;46:757–760.

120.  Braegger CP, Nicholls S, Murch SH, Stephens S, MacDonald TT. Tumour necrosis factor alpha in stool as a marker of intestinal inflammation. Lancet 1992;339:89–91.

121.  Saiki T, Mitsuyama K, Toyonaga A, Ishida H, Tanikawa K. Detection of pro- and anti-inflammatory cytokines in stools of patients with inflammatory bowel disease. Scand J Gastroenterol 1998;33:616–622.

122.  Stronkhorst A., Jansen J, Tytgat G et al. Soluble IL-2 and TNF receptors p55 and p75 in Crohn's disease. Gastroenterology 1994;106: A779.

123.  van Dullemen HM, van Deventer SJ, Hommes DW et al. Treatment of Crohn's disease with anti-tumor necrosis factor chimeric monoclonal antibody (cA2). Gastroenterology 1995;109:129–135.

124.  Martinez-Borra J, Lopez-Larrea C, Gonzalez S et al. High serum tumor necrosis factor-alpha levels are associated with lack of response to infliximab in fistulizing Crohn's disease. Am J Gastroenterol 2002;97:2350–2356.

125.  Casini-Raggi V, Kam L, Chong YJ, Fiocchi C, Pizarro TT, Cominelli F. Mucosal imbalance of IL-1 and IL-1 receptor antagonist in inflammatory bowel disease. A novel mechanism of chronic intestinal inflammation. J Immunol 1995;154:2434–2440.

126.  Hyams JS, Fitzgerald JE, Wyzga N, Treem WR, Justinich CJ, Kreutzer DL. Characterization of circulating interleukin-1 receptor antagonist expression in children with inflammatory bowel disease. Dig Dis Sci 1994;39:1893–1899.

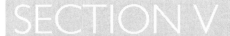

# MEDICAL THERAPY

## CHAPTER 30

# Clinical trial design with an emphasis on indices to measure disease activity

Lloyd R Sutherland and Li Feng Xiao

## INTRODUCTION

The recent passing of Sidney Truelove leads to reflection on the role that well-designed clinical trials have played in the remarkable improvement in the prognosis for patients diagnosed with inflammatory bowel disease. For those of us who trained in the 1970s it is humbling to recall that only 20 years prior to that, ulcerative colitis was associated with a mortality rate of up to 30% per episode. Today a death related to ulcerative colitis is a rarity, requiring a serious review within the appropriate Division or Department.

The history of the therapy of ulcerative colitis is, in part, a journey through the curriculum vitae of Truelove. He designed trials that led to the introduction of corticosteroid therapy for the induction of remission of ulcerative colitis, and provided supportive evidence that the aminosalicylate sulfasalazine was effective in maintenance of remission. He designed one of the few trials of azathioprine for both the induction and maintenance of remission in ulcerative colitis. He encouraged a generation of British gastroenterologists to become involved in clinical trials. His last and perhaps most significant achievement was the elegant demonstration that 5-aminosalicylate was the active moiety of sulfasalazine. Perhaps equally important was his role in the founding of the International Organization for the Study of Inflammatory Bowel Disease (IOIBD), which has provided a means of raising the overall quality of trials in inflammatory bowel disease.

The therapeutic response consists of a variety of components, as shown in Figure 30.1. Although the importance of each factor may vary from disease to disease, all would appear to have a role in the response. They include the natural history of the disease, the placebo effect, the Hawthorne effect (see below), and finally the actual effect due to the medication itself. For most chronic diseases episodes of activity tend to be followed by episodes of inactivity which, unfortunately, are not predictable. The placebo effect used to be dismissed as simply a psychosomatic factor, but a significant body of medical literature has arisen regarding interactions between the mind–gut–immunologic system which provides support for the effect. The Hawthorne effect summarizes the various components within the trial itself that support a positive result. In studies patients are carefully supervised with frequent visits to the supportive environment. Compliance is encouraged by the study nurse. Finally, within the therapeutic response is the effect of the intervention itself. The entire clinical trial can be seen as a complex exercise that isolates the true therapeutic effect of the agent itself.

This chapter will deal briefly with the methodology that has evolved over the decades in the assessment of potential therapies for the assessment of inflammatory bowel disease. Although the standards for clinical trials have risen in the past decades, the essential principles remain unchanged. Everything focuses on providing the most bias-free assessment possible of the new intervention. After a short overview of the basic design methodology for randomized controlled trials, a detailed review of the indices available to those who design clinical trials is presented.

## METHODOLOGY FOR THE CLINICIAN

Acquiring the habit of spending more than 30 seconds perusing the Methods section of any published report of a clinical trial provides the framework to answer the question asked by every clinician: 'will this study change the way I practice medicine?'

The methodologist bases his or her design on the three pillars of any clinical trial: randomization, a control for comparative purposes, and evaluation by individuals, indifferent or masked, to the particular intervention offered. Evaluating the quality of the methodology implementing these principles will determine whether or not the intervention should be incorporated into practice.

Although randomization has a role to play in the theoretical underpinnings of statistics, it is much more important as

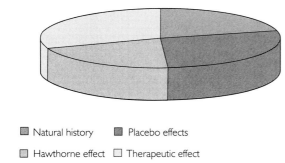

■ Natural history    ■ Placebo effects

■ Hawthorne effect    □ Therapeutic effect

**Fig. 30.1** Components of the therapeutic response

supporting the crucial bias-free assignment of patients to any of the treatment groups. Other forms of 'pseudorandomization' would include randomization by date of birth, clinic day, or any other strategy by which the recruiting clinician has a better than 50% chance of knowing what the next treatment assignment is.

The important role played by the control can be summarized in the statement: 'those who have enthusiasm have no controls and those with controls have no enthusiasm'. The control should mimic the compound being evaluated as closely as possible. If a placebo is to be used it should be of the same color and shape as the new medication and, if possible, even taste like the drug being evaluated. If both study arms contain active drugs then each patient randomized should receive the active medication along with the placebo of the other medication being evaluated ('double-dummy' technique).

Blinding refers to the concept that as few people as possible should have access to the treatment allocation plans. In a single-blind study either the subject or the person doing the evaluation is masked/blinded to the treatment allocation. In a double-blind study both subject and investigator are masked to the treatment assignment.

A variety of instruments are available to assess the overall quality of a randomized controlled trial; however, recent attention has focused on the concealment of allocation as a single item summarizing the quality of the trial. Concealment of allocation refers to the steps taken to prevent anyone from having a better chance of predicting the allocation than chance alone. This would include identical packaging and appearance, restricted access to the allocation code, and a central office for intervention assignment. Concealment of allocation is always possible, whereas double blinding may not be.

## THE STUDY POPULATION

In an ideal world every patient with a particular disease would participate in trials as soon as new therapies were introduced. In the real world the evaluation focuses on a sample drawn from the pool of available patients. Because many of the available patients are drawn from university or tertiary-level hospitals the relevance to patients with moderate disease may be questionable.

A significant amount of time and energy is invested in the attempt to make the study sample as generalizable and representative of the entire population with the disease as possible. Noting the dates of initiation and closure of a trial will assist clinicians in determining the generalizability of the study. For example, of two trials, one took a year to recruit 200 patients and the other

recruited 40 patients over 3 years. It is likely that the trial that recruited 200 patients will be of more assistance (i.e. generalizable) to the patients of the community gastroenterologist.

## AVOIDING RECRUITMENT (SELECTION) BIAS

Recruitment or selection bias occurs primarily in the selection of patients for either inclusion in or exclusion from a trial. It may help to consider the clinician as the gatekeeper for the trial. The knowledge as to what the patient might receive if they enrolled in the trial may be a powerful stimulus to inform or not inform a patient about a trial. Suppose that a gastroenterologist is involved in recruiting patients in a trial of a new agent for irritable bowel syndrome. Patients are 'randomized' alphabetically: those with last names beginning with A–M will receive drug A, and those with last names beginning with N–Z will receive drug B. It is assumed that the letters of the alphabet will be randomly distributed among the population at large. Although the gastroenterologist professes an open mind on the topic, his bias is that IBS is a disease of women, with a strong functional overlay for which there is no effective therapy. In recruiting patients for his center he does not inform any male patients and only enrolls those who have responded to antispasmodics in the past. Because he did not inform all of the patients in his clinic about the trial, many who might have been enrolled never had a chance to participate. This recruitment bias could compromise the generalizability of the study. In the past a certain amount of selection bias was tolerated. Two important groups that were often excluded were women of childbearing age and children.

## SAMPLE SIZE AND POWER

An important part of the Methods section deals with the issues of sample size and statistical power. The focus of any randomized controlled trial is the primary outcome variable. The sample size reflects a number of patients required to detect a significant difference or to detect components between the two compounds being assessed. If a sample size calculation is not reported then one should be very careful in interpreting the results of the study.

Careful attention should be given to whether an intention to treat analysis was performed or a 'per patient' analysis is reported. The intention to treat analysis includes every patient randomized to take medication. This generally gives the most conservative assessment of the medication. The per patient protocol includes only those who completed the trial and often provides the most optimistic evaluation of the effectiveness of the medication.

## SUMMARY

Clinical trials in inflammatory bowel disease will continue to face a variety of challenges. First, most trials in inflammatory bowel disease are less than 12 months in duration and the relevance of such trials to patients with a lifelong disease may be questionable. Second, there are no mutually agreed-upon indices that might lead to a consensus among clinicians, members of the research community and the public. Third, the actual phenotypes and genotypes of Crohn's disease and ulcerative colitis are still unknown. Fourth, certain subgroups of patients with bowel disease are excluded from trials. These include children, women of childbearing age, and patients with disease in unusual locations.

# WHY ASSESS DISEASE ACTIVITY?

The development of instruments to assess disease activity in patients with IBD was an important milestone on the road to evidence-based medicine. The need to identify safe and efficacious medications led to the creation of a variety of scales (or indices) to assess disease activity in IBD. Disease activity indices are most useful in clinical trials, but they may offer opportunities in medical practice for following patients, particularly the indices that do not require diary data. They have also been used as instruments for assessing disease activity for surveys. The introduction of the first disease activity scale for IBD was in the context of a clinical trial. In 1955, Truelove and Witts conducted a placebo-controlled trial of steroid therapy in patients with ulcerative colitis. The need to classify disease severity led to the birth of the first disease activity index, the 'Truelove and Witts Index'. Since then, many indices have been developed and used to evaluate IBD therapeutic programs or strategies in clinical trials. Indices make it possible to make comparisons between patients groups or to examine the impact of any intervention (pre and post intervention).

# CLINICAL DISEASE ACTIVITY INDICES

To date, a number of disease-specific scales for measuring clinical disease activity have been created for Crohn's disease and ulcerative colitis. Although some of them have been evaluated extensively in terms of validity, reliability, responsiveness and feasibility, many would benefit from further evaluation and refinement. The instruments used to measure disease activity for IBD were introduced separately for Crohn's disease and ulcerative colitis, with respect to the indices themselves, their evaluation status and their practical values. A summary table is provided at the end of the section of clinical disease activity indices separately for Crohn's disease and for ulcerative colitis.

## CLINICAL DISEASE ACTIVITY INDICES FOR CROHN'S DISEASE

### Crohn's Disease Activity Index

One of the most commonly used indices is the Crohn's Disease Activity Index (CDAI). This was developed in the early 1970s by the National Cooperative Crohn's Disease Study (NCCDS).[1–3] Today it is one of the most popular instruments in clinical research into Crohn's disease. The CDAI score is determined by eight items, including the number of liquid stools, the extent of abdominal pain, general wellbeing, the occurrence of extraintestinal symptoms, the need for antidiarrheal drugs, the presence of abdominal masses, hematocrit and body weight (Table 30.1). Each of the eight items has a numerical score rating and a preassigned weight (or multiplier). The sum of the eight weighted item scores quantifies the overall disease severity of the patient, with a high score indicating severe disease.

To apply the CDAI to a subject, the patient needs to complete a three-item diary (for the first three items in Table 30.1) over a 7-day period. The values for the remaining five items can be recorded during each patient visit from the history and physical examination, as well as the relevant laboratory record. The overall CDAI scores range from 0 to approximately 600,[4] with 150 being defined as a cut-off value for clinical remission. Compared with the physician's global assessment category (i.e. 'very well' to 'very poor'),[2] 90% of the patients who had a CDAI score below 150 were rated by physicians as 'very well'. Thirty-one per cent and 6% of the patients who had a CDAI score of less than 150 were separately rated as 'fair to good' and 'poor'. No patient with a CDAI score below 150 was rated as 'very poor'. On the other hand, a CDAI score greater than 450 was considered as extremely severe disease.[2,4]

The CDAI is a valid instrument for assessing disease activity, although it does not cover all patient subgroups (e.g. children) or all domains of the disease spectrum (e.g. psychosocial). It has been used as the gold standard for developing and testing other instruments for over a quarter of a century. The CDAI also demonstrates acceptable reliability despite its interrater variability. In one study involving only a few subjects, the calculated CDAI score varied between the observers. Whether the variation was related more to the ability of the subjects to follow instructions, the use of calculators, or to significant deficiencies in the instrument is not clear. The interobserver variability, however, reduces when the observers are educated about the items of the index.[5]

One of the potential benefits or drawbacks of the CDAI is its subjectivity. A substantial proportion of the CDAI score is derived from two subjective items (i.e. the severity of abdominal pain and general wellbeing). Although the two items represent very important aspects of the disease, they depend heavily on the patients' perception of their disease. On the other hand, these items become in a sense a mini quality of life index.

Another major problem with the index is that it is cumbersome and time-consuming to complete, taking 7 days and relying on information from the laboratory and physical examinations. As a result, the CDAI has almost exclusively been used in clinical trials.

### Harvey–Bradshaw Index

Since the creation of the CDAI, other indices that attempt to simplify it have been developed. The Harvey–Bradshaw index (HBI), also known as the Simple Index (Table 30.2), only requires the patient to recall activity data for the previous 24-hours. There are five clinical items in the HBI: general wellbeing, abdominal pain, number of daily liquid stools, abdominal mass and number of complications. The HBI does not collect drug use or laboratory data, and a weight is not required in calculating the scores. The correlation of the HBI with the CDAI has been proved by several studies to be good.[6–8] Compared with the CDAI, the HBI clearly possesses the property of easy application, but its validity and reliability have been questioned.[9,10]

### The OMGE index and the Cape Town Index

Other clinical indices include the Organisation Mondiale de Gatroenterologie (OMGE) index[11] and the Cape Town Index (CTI, also called the South African Index).[9] The OMGE index changed the way the HBI quantifies the frequency of daily liquid stools. The HBI uses the absolute number of daily liquid stools (which may provide an inappropriate weight to the overall HBI score for certain patients). For example, patients who have undergone intestinal resection with subsequent increased numbers of liquid stools would have a falsely high score by the HBI criteria. This stool frequency, however, may not truly reflect

## Table 30.1 Crohn's Disease Activity Index

| Items | | Scores | | Weight | Weighted scores |
|---|---|---|---|---|---|
| 1. | Number of liquid or soft stools | X1= | number of liquid/soft stools for 7 days | 2 | X1x2 |
| 2. | Abdominal pain | X2= | sum of 7 daily ratings (0=none, 1=mild, 2=moderate, 3=severe) | 5 | X2x5 |
| 3. | General wellbeing | X3= | sum of 7 daily ratings (0=well, 1=slightly under par, 2=poor, 3=very poor, 4=terrible) | 7 | X3x7 |
| 4. | Number of complications | X4= | number of listed complications (arthritis or arthralgia, iritis or uveitis, erythema nodosum or pyoderma, gangrenosum or aphthous stomatitis, anal fissure or fistula or abscess, other fistula, fever over 37.8ºC) | 20 | X4x20 |
| 5. | Use of diphenoxylate or loperamide for diarrhea | X5= | rating (0=no, 1=yes) | 30 | X5x30 |
| 6. | Abdominal mass | X6= | rating (0=no, 2=questionable, 5=definite) | 10 | X6x10 |
| 7. | Hematocrit | X7= | rating (47-Hct (male), 42-Hct (female)) | 6 | X7x6 |
| 8. | Percentage below standard weight | X8= | body weight (1-weight/standard weight) x100 (add or subtract according to sign) | 1 | X8x1 |

**Total score = sum of the weighted scores**

Adapted from Best WR, Becktel JM, Singleton JW. Rederived values of the eight coefficients of the Crohn's Disease Activity Index (CDAI). Gastroenterology 1979;77:843–846.

## Table 30.2 Harvey–Bradshaw Index (Simple Index)

| Items | | Scores |
|---|---|---|
| 1. | General wellbeing | 0=very well, 1=slightly under par, 2=poor, 3=very poor, 4=terrible |
| 2. | Abdominal pain | 0=none, 1=mild, 2=moderate, 3=severe |
| 3. | Number of liquid stools daily | Number of liquid stools/day |
| 4. | Abdominal mass | 0=none, 1=dubious, 2=definite, 3= definite and tender |
| 5. | Complications | Arthralgia, uveitis, erythema nodosum, aphthous ulcer, pyoderma gangrenosum, stomatitis, anal fissure, new fistula, abscess (score 1 per item) |

**Total score = sum of the item scores**

Adapted from Harvey RF, Bradshaw JM. A simple index of Crohn's disease activity. Lancet 1980;1:514.

active inflammation. To overcome this, the OMGE index scores the stool frequency on a Likert scale of 0–5 (0 = normal bowel habit and 5 = more than 10 motions per day).

## Cape Town Index

Another derivative of the CDAI, the Cape Town Index (Table 30.3), proposed to further modify the item ratings. Unlike the HBI and the OMGE index (for which the daily bowel frequency and/or complications are scored based on the actual number of events), all the items of the CTI have a predefined value. The CTI contains eight items (or 11 item levels) that cover patient subjective symptoms, physician clinical findings and laboratory data. With each item having a score of 0–3, the CTI has an overall score of 0–33. Because of the overlap in the items used, it is not surprising that the CDAI, the HBI, the OMGE index and the CTI are intercorrelated.

## Table 30.3 Cape Town Index (South African Index)

| Items | Scores 0 | 1 | 2 | 3 |
|---|---|---|---|---|
| 1. Diarrhea (episodes/day) | None | =4 | 5 | =6 |
| 2. Abdominal pain | None | Mild | Moderate | Severe |
| 3. Wellbeing | Normal | Below par | Unwell | Terrible |
| 4. Complications | | | | |
|    Local | None | Skin tag | Sinus | Fistula |
|    Systemic | None | Stomatitis | Arthralgia | A/I/ER** |
|    Fever | Normal (37°C) | =38°C | =39°C | >39°C |
| 5. Weight vs. previous weight | No change | No change | <95% | <90% |
| 6. Abdominal examination | | | | |
|    Mass | None | None | Indefinite | Definite |
|    Tenderness | None | Mild | Moderate | Severe |
| 7. Hemoglobin (g/L) | >120 | =120 | =110 | =100 |
| 8. ESR* (mm/first hour) | =15 | >15 | >25 | >40 |

**Total score = sum of the item scores**

\* ESR = erythrocyte sedimentation rate; \*\* A/I/ER = arthritis/iritis/erythema nodosum.
Adapted from Wright JP, Marks IN, Parfitt A. A simple clinical index of Crohn's disease activity – the Cape Town index. S Africa Med J 1985;68:502–503.

## Table 30.4 Van Hees Index (Dutch Index)

| Items | Scores |
|---|---|
| X1. Serum albumin | Grams per liter |
| X2. Erythrocyte sedimentation rate | Millimeters in the first hour |
| X3. Quetelet index | Weight (kg)×10/height (cm)² |
| X4. Abdominal mass | 1=none, 2=dubious, 3=diameter<6 cm, 4=diameter 6–12 cm, 5=diameter>2 cm |
| X5. Sex | 1=male, 2=female |
| X6. Temperature | Daily average (°C) in 1 week |
| X7. Stool consistency | 1=well-formed, 2=soft, 3=watery |
| X8. Intestinal resection | 1=no, 2=yes |
| X9. Extraintestinal lesions | Number of extraintestinal lesions |

Total score = $-209 - 5.48X_1 + 0.29 X_2 - 0.22 X_3 + 7.83 X_4 - 12.3 X_5 + 16.4 X_6 + 8.46 X_7 - 9.17 X_8 + 10.7 X_9$

Adapted from van Hees PA, van Elteren PH, van Lier HJ, van Tongeren JH. An index of inflammatory activity in patients with Crohn's disease. Gut 1980;21:279–286.

## Present–Korelitz Index

The Present–Korelitz Index[12] is an instrument with specific treatment goals for individual patients (also known as 'Therapeutic Goals' score). The goals are classified into three categories: reduction of steroid dosage, healing of fistulae, and amelioration of other specific clinical symptoms and signs. The degree of improvement (or worsening) in each goal item is recorded on a scale of +3 for excellent improvement to –3 for severe worsening, with 0 representing no change. Although the index incorporates items that distinguish it from other disease activity indices (e.g. the item measuring the effect of reduction of steroid dosage on the disease process) and is easy to score, it has not been widely used or validated.

## Van Hees Index

The CDAI and its derivatives all emphasize subjective components (e.g. general wellbeing and abdominal pain) because these components represent important aspects of the disease. However, other attempts have been made to create 'objective' instruments to measure Crohn's disease activity. The Van Hees Index (VHI, also known as the Dutch Index)[13] has nine items that cover clinical and laboratory aspects (Table 30.4). To calculate the overall VHI score, the nine item scores are directly entered into a multiple regression equation (Table 30.4), with 100, 150 and 210 representing quiescent, mild and severe disease conditions, respectively. The VHI has been prospectively validated, but correlates poorly with the CDAI, the HBI, the

OMGE index and the CTI. This poor correlation may be the result of the extensive incorporation of laboratory-based items by the VHI.[5] It also suggests that the VHI does not measure the same features of Crohn's disease as do other indices.

## Perianal disease activity indices

Investigators have created scales that measure disease activity in patients with specific symptoms or signs, largely because of the inadequacy of other generic indices. For example, the 'Perianal Disease Activity Index' (Table 30.5) was developed to measure the severity of perianal Crohn's disease.[14] The PDAI incorporates five items (i.e. discharge, pain, restriction of sexual activity, type of perianal disease, and degree of induration) that are graded on a 5-point Likert scale (range 0–4), with higher scores indicating severe symptoms. A cut-off value for defining remission is still to be determined.

As another example, a fistula drainage assessment scale has recently been used to categorize perianal fistulae as being open, actively draining or closed. It has been used in several clinical trials.[15] Further studies are, however, needed to determine its repeatability compared with that of the PDAI.

## Disease activity indices for survey and pediatric research

A derivative of the CDAI suitable for population surveys (Table 30.6) was proposed by Sandler et al.[16] in the late 1980s. This index uses only three items (i.e. bowel frequency, abdominal pain and general wellbeing) derived from the original CDAI. The selection of the items was based on multivariate regression analyses using physician's global assessment as the dependent variable. The overall score of this index is determined by the following formula:

$$(3 \times \text{number of stools}) + (10 \times \text{abdominal pain}) + (8 \times \text{general wellbeing})$$

This index correlates well with the CDAI ($r=0.87$, $P<0.0001$) but can easily be perceived as being weak in content

### Table 30.5 Perianal Crohn's Disease Activity Index

| Items | Scores 0 | 1 | 2 | 3 | 4 |
|---|---|---|---|---|---|
| 1. Discharge | No Discharge | Minimal \mucous discharge | Moderate mucous or purulent discharge | Substantial discharge | Gross fecal soiling |
| 2. Pain/restriction of activities | No activity restriction | Mild discomfort, no restriction | Moderate discomfort, some limitation of activities | Marked discomfort, marked limitation | Severe pain, severe limitation |
| 3. Restriction of sexual activity | No restriction sexual activity | Slight restriction sexual activity | Moderate limitation sexual activity | Marked limitation sexual activity | Unable to engage in sexual activity |
| 4. Type of perianal disease | No perianal disease/skin tags | Anal fissure or mucosal tear | <3 perianal fistulae | =3 Perianal fistulae | Anal sphincter ulceration or fistulae with significant undermining of skin |
| 5. Degree of induration | No induration | Minimal induration | Moderate induration | Substantial induration | Gross fluctuance/abscess |

Adapted from Irvine EJ. Usual therapy improves Perianal Crohn's disease as measured by a new disease activity index. McMaster IBD Study Group. J Clin Gastroenterol 1995;20:27–32.

### Table 30.6 Crohn's Disease Activity Index for Survey Research

| Items | | Scores | | Weight | Weighted scores |
|---|---|---|---|---|---|
| 1. | Number of liquid or soft stools | X1 = | number of liquid/soft stools for 7 days | 3 | X1x2 |
| 2. | Abdominal pain | X2 = | sum of 7 daily ratings (0=none, 1=mild, 2=moderate, 3=severe) | 10 | X2x5 |
| 3. | General wellbeing | X3 = | sum of 7 daily ratings (0=well, 1=slightly under par, 2=poor, 3=very poor, 4=terrible) | 8 | X3x7 |

Total score = sum of the weighted scores

Adapted from Sandler RS, Jordan MC, Kupper LL. Development of a Crohn's index for survey research. J Clin Epidemiol 1988;41:451–8.

validity, owing to its inclusion of variables in only one dimension (i.e. patients' self-assessment of their symptoms).

## Pediatric indices

Several clinical disease activity indices have been proposed for children with Crohn's disease. The earlier indices have been criticized for not incorporating growth data[17] or for lacking sigmoidoscopic and radiologic assessment.[18] As a result, they have not been widely used in clinical research. The Pediatric Crohn's Disease Activity Index (PCDAI) (Table 30.7) was proposed by a multicenter study group in the early 1990s. It includes 11 items covering five domains (i.e. patient history, physical examination, laboratory assessment, weight, and height change data). All the items are assigned a score, with higher score indicating a worse condition. The total score ranges from 0 to a maximum of 100. The PCDAI correlates well with the physician global assessment of disease activity ($r=0.77$; $P=0.04$) and

with the modified Harvey–Bradshaw index (i.e. the OMGE index) ($r=0.86$; $P=0.001$).[19]

The clinical disease activity indices for Crohn's disease described above are summarized in Table 30.8.

## CLINICAL DISEASE ACTIVITY INDICES FOR ULCERATIVE COLITIS

Compared to Crohn's disease, there is little agreement as to which activity profile is preferable for the clinical assessment of ulcerative colitis. Since the development of the qualitative measure of disease activity by Truelove and Witts[20] a number of other disease activity indices have been proposed. These indices are all numerical (or quantitative) in nature, because of the need for statistical evaluation in clinical research. Among these, the most frequently used probably includes the Powell-Tuck Index,[21] the Mayo Score,[22] the Disease Activity Index (Sutherland Index),[23] the Clinical Activity Index[24] and the Lichtiger Index.[25]

### Table 30.7 Pediatric Crohn's Disease Activity Index

| Items | Scores 0 | 2.5 | 5 | 10 |
|---|---|---|---|---|
| 1. Abdominal pain | None | – | Mild: brief, does not interfere with activities | Mod/severe-daily, longer lasting, affects activities, nocturnal |
| 2. Stool frequency (per day) | 0–1 liquid tools, no blood | – | Up to 2 semi-formed with small blood, or 2–5 liquid | Gross bleeding, or ≥6 liquid, or nocturnal diarrhea |
| 3. General wellbeing (for past week) | No limitation of activities, well | – | Occasional difficulty in maintaining age-appropriate activities, below par | Frequent limitation of activity, very poor |
| 4. HCT (%) | | | | |
| <10 yrs | >33 | 28–32 | <28 | – |
| 11–14 yrs (M) | ≥ 35 | 30–34 | <30 | – |
| 11–19 yrs (F) | ≥ 34 | 29–33 | <29 | – |
| 15–19 yrs (M) | ≥ 37 | 32–36 | <32 | – |
| 5. ESR (mm/hr) | <20 | 20–50 | >50 | – |
| 6. Albumin (g/dL) | ≥ 3.5 | – | 3.1–3.4 | =3.0 |
| 7. Weight | Weight gain or voluntary weight stable/loss | – | Involuntary weight stable, weight loss 1–9% | Weight loss ≥10% |
| 8. Height | | | | |
| at diagnosis | <1 channel | – | ≥ 1, <2 channel decrease | >2 channel decrease decrease |
| or, at follow-up | Height velocity ≥ –1SD | – | Height velocity <–1SD, >–2SD | Height velocity =–2SD |
| 9. Abdomen | No tenderness, no mass | – | Tenderness, or mass without tenderness | Tenderness, involuntary guarding, definite mass |
| 10. Perirectal disease | None, asymptomatic tags | – | 1–2 indolent fistula, scant drainage, no tenderness | Active fistula, drainage, tenderness, or abscess |
| 11. Extraintestinal manifestations* | None | – | One | ≥ Two |

Total score = sum of the item scores

* Fever ≥38.5°C for 3 days over past week, definite arthritis, uveitis, E. nodosum, or P. gangrenous
Adapted from Hyams JS, Ferry GD, Mandel FS et al. Development and validation of a pediatric Crohn's disease activity index. J Pediatr Gastroenterol Nutr 1991;12:439–447.

## Table 30.8 Summary of clinical disease activity indices for Crohn's disease

| First author | Instruments | Current utility | Scores and definitions | Strengths and limitations |
|---|---|---|---|---|
| Best[3] | Crohn's Disease Activity Index | Adult; clinical research; primary endpoint | Score range: 0 to about 600; clinical remission: =150 | Rigorously validated; most frequently used; 'gold standard' for validating other indices; cumbersome (take 7 days to complete) |
| Harvey[6] | Harvey–Bradshaw Index (Simple Index) | Adult; clinical research; primary endpoint | Score range: depend on daily number of liquid stools; no score defined for clinical remission | Validated; a derivative of CDAI; easy to complete; total score heavily depend on number of liquid stools; not as strong as CDAI in validity |
| Myren[11] | The OMGE index | Adult; clinical research; primary endpoint | Score range: depend on number of local/systemic complications; no score defined for clinical remission | Validated; a derivative of CDAI (modified version of HBI); easy to complete; not as strong as CDAI in validity |
| Wright[9] | Cape Town Index (South African Index) | Adult; clinical research; primary endpoint | Score range: 0 to 33; no score defined for clinical remission | Validated; a derivative of CDAI; easy to complete; all items balanced compared with HBI and OMGE; not as strong as CDAI in validity |
| Present[12] | Present/Korelitz Index | Adult; clinical research; primary endpoint | Score range: −12 to +12 for each treatment period; no score defined for clinical remission | Specific treatment goals individually established; not rigorously developed or progressively validated |
| van Hees[13] | Van Hees Index (Dutch Index) | Adult; clinical research; primary endpoint | Score range: depend on actual ratings of several items; 100, 150 and 210 represent quiescent, mild and severe condition | Validated; objective measure of disease activity; correlate poorly with the CDAI and its derivatives |
| Irvine[14] | Perianal Disease Activity Index | Adult; clinical research; secondary endpoint | Graded on a 5-point scale; cut-off value for defining remission to be determined | Validated; especially useful for perianal Crohn's disease; may need further validation |
| Present[15] | Fistula Drainage Assessment | Adult; clinical research; primary endpoint | Qualitative activity measure; remission defined as closure of all fistulas draining for at least 4 weeks | Validated; especially useful for assessing fistula closure; need further reliability testing |
| Sandler[16] | Crohn's Disease Activity Index for Survey Research | Adult; survey research; primary endpoint | Score range: depend on liquid stool frequency (determined by formula); used for survey purpose | Useful for survey research; correlate well with CDAI; lack of face validity |
| Hyams[19] | Pediatric Crohn's Disease Activity Index | Children; clinical research; primary endpoint | Score range: 0 to 100; no score defined for clinical remission | Useful for clinical research for children; correlate well with OMGE and physician general assessment; need further evaluation |

## Truelove and Witts Index

The earliest attempt to use clinical criteria to assess disease activity for ulcerative colitis was made by Truelove and Witts[20] in their study of corticosteroid therapy in patients with ulcerative colitis. To date, the Truelove and Witts Index (Table 30.9) remains one of the most popular in clinical research for ulcerative colitis. It includes six items that cover clinical parameters and laboratory measurements. The index assesses disease activity qualitatively. Instead of using numerical scoring to rate the severity of disease, the items of the Truelove and Witts Index are rated on the scales of 'mild' and 'severe', with 'moderate' being classified between 'mild' and 'severe'. A potential problem with this index is its inability to classify patients who meet some, but not all of the criteria.

## Powell-Tuck Index

The Powell-Tuck Index (PTI; Table 30.10) was first established in the late 1970s and has been used in clinical trials.[26] It has also

## Table 30.9 Truelove and Witts Index

| Items | Scores* Severe | Scores* Mild |
|---|---|---|
| 1. Bowel frequency | =6 daily | =4 daily |
| 2. Blood in stool | ++ | ± |
| 3. Temperature | >37.5°C on 2 of 4 days | Normal |
| 4. Pulse rate (beats/min) | >90 | Normal |
| 5. Hemoglobin (allow for transfusion) | =75% | Normal or near normal |
| 6. Erythrocyte sedimentation rate (mm/h) | <30 | =30 |

* Moderate disease is intermediate between severe and mild classifications
Adapted from Truelove SC, Witts LJ. Cortisone in ulcerative colitis: final report on a therapeutic trial. Br Med J 1955;2:1041–1048.

**Table 30.10 Powell-Tuck Index**

| | Scores | | | |
|---|---|---|---|---|
| Items | 0 | 1 | 2 | 3 |
| 1. Wellbeing | No impairment | Impaired, but able to continue activities | Activities reduced | Unable to work |
| 2. Abdominal pain | No abdominal pain | With bowel actions | More continuous | – |
| 3. Bowel frequency | <3/24 h | 3–6/24 h | >6/24 h | – |
| 4. Stool consistency | Normal or variably normal | Semiformed | Liquid | – |
| 5. Bleeding | No sign of bleeding | Trace | More than a trace | – |
| 6. Anorexia | Absent | Present | – | – |
| 7. Nausea and vomiting | Absent | Present | – | – |
| 8. Abdominal tenderness | None | Mild | Marked | Rebound |
| 9. Eye, joint, mouth or skin complications | None | Mild on 1 site | Severe or mild on =2 sites | – |
| 10. Temperature | <37.1°C | 37.1–38°C | >38°C | – |

Total score = sum of the item scores

Adapted from Powell-Tuck J, Day DW, Buckell NA, Wadsworth J, Lennard-Jones JE. Correlations between defined sigmoidoscopic appearances and other measures of disease activity in ulcerative colitis. Dig Dis Sci 1982;27:533–537.

been recognized as an established index by the other investigators[27] in developing their own disease activity indices for ulcerative colitis. The PTI includes 10 items that cover general health, physical signs, intestinal and extraintestinal symptoms, body temperature, and macroscopic appearance at sigmoidoscopy. The PTI score ranges from 0 to a maximum of 22. The scoring system of the PTI depends heavily on the patient's general health status, symptoms and signs, and gives little weight to the sigmoidoscopic ratings.

## Disease Activity Index and Mayo Score

Both the Disease Activity Index (DAI, also known as the Sutherland Index) and the Mayo Score (Table 30.11) were proposed in the mid-1980s and have been used in a number of studies[22,23,28,29] since then. The two indices were based on the Truelove and Witts' criteria[30] for classifying the clinical activity and Baron et al.'s[31] criteria for grading the mucosal appearance. The difference between the two indices is that the former is scored on a 1-day basis whereas the latter is scored on a 3-day basis. Both indices ranges in score from 0 to 12, with a score of 2 (with no individual subscore >1) indicating clinical remission, 3–5 indicating mildly active disease, 6–10 indicating moderately active disease, and 11–12 indicating severe disease.

## Clinical Activity Index

The Clinical Activity Index (CAI, Table 30.12) was proposed in 1989 by Rachmilewitz[24] in an international study of drug therapy in active ulcerative colitis. Along with the CAI, a colonoscopic index was also proposed (see endoscopic disease activity section). The clinical disease activity section of the CAI includes seven items covering clinical and laboratory data and has a score ranging from 0 to a maximum of 29. The CAI items used an irregular ordinal score scheme to address the weight of each item. For example, the score for 'blood in stools' is rated as

0 for 'no blood', 2 for 'little blood', and 4 for 'a lot of blood', with no intermediate score (e.g. 1 and 3) being assigned. The body temperature has only two ratings: 0 for 37–38°C and 3 for >38°.

## Lichtiger Index

The Lichtiger Index[25] (Table 30.13) was proposed in a drug treatment trial in severe ulcerative colitis patients in the early 1990s. It consists of eight easily collected items that cover both subjective (degree of pain, degree of cramping, assessment of general wellbeing, and the presence of abdominal tenderness) and objective (number of stools, number of nocturnal bowel movements, frequency of visible blood in stool, frequency of incontinence and the need of antidiarrheal drugs) features. The index does not require laboratory data. With the item scores ranging from 0 to 5, the maximum score is 21. Used in a trial of severe ulcerative colitis patients, a score of less than 10 on 2 consecutive days was considered to indicate a clinical response. The Lichtiger Index has been used in several clinical trials[25,32,33] and was reported to have good validity and interrater reliability.

## Other disease activity indices for ulcerative colitis

Other indices have been described recently. For example, Rutegard et al.[34] proposed a compound index for the assessment of disease activity in ulcerative colitis. The index combines three different scores that evaluate clinical, endoscopic and histological findings. Each score contributes a maximum of three points to the index, with the overall score ranging from 0 to a maximum of 9. The clinical score, however, did not correlate well with the endoscopic scores.[34]

Walmsley et al.[27] proposed a simple clinical colitis activity index in 1998. The index uses a small number of clinical criteria and does not require physical examination, sigmoidoscopic evaluation or laboratory data. It can be easily calculated by a

## Table 30.11 Disease Activity Index (Sutherland Index, Mayo Score)

| | Scores | | | |
|---|---|---|---|---|
| Items | 0 | 1 | 2 | 3 |
| 1. Stool frequency | Normal | 1–2 stools/day > normal | 3–4 stools/day > normal | >5 stools/day > normal |
| 2. Rectal bleeding | None | Streaks of blood | Obvious blood | Mostly blood |
| 3. Mucosal appearance | Normal | Mild friability | Moderate friability | Exudation, spontaneous bleeding |
| 4. Physician's rating of disease activity | Normal | Mild | Moderate | Severe |

Total score = sum of the item scores

Adapted from Sutherland LR, Martin F, Greer S et al. 5-Aminosalicylic acid enema in the treatment of distal ulcerative colitis, proctosigmoiditis, and proctitis. Gastroenterology 1987;92:1894–1898 and Schroeder KW, Tremaine WJ, Ilstrup DM. Coated oral 5-aminosalicylic acid therapy for mildly to moderately active ulcerative colitis. A randomized study. N Engl J Med 1987;317:1625–1629.

## Table 30.12 Clinical Activity Index (clinical section)

| | Scores | | | | |
|---|---|---|---|---|---|
| Items | 0 | 1 | 2 | 3 | 4 |
| 1. Number of stools weekly | <18 | 18–35 | 36–60 | >60 | – |
| 2. Blood in stools (weekly average) | None | – | Little | – | A lot |
| 3. Investigator's global assessment of symptomatic state | Good | Average | Poor | Very poor | – |
| 4. Abdominal pain/cramps | None | Mild | Moderate | Severe | – |
| 5. Temperature due to colitis (°C) | 37–38 | – | – | >38 | – |
| 6. Extraintestinal manifestations (each rated 3 points) | – | – | – | Iritis, Erythema nodosum, Arthritis | – |
| 7. Laboratory findings | – | ESR>50 in 1st hr | ESR>100 In 1st hr | – | Hemoglobin <100 g/l |

Total score = sum of the item scores

* ESR = erythrocyte sedimentation rate.
Adapted from Rachmilewitz D. Coated mesalazine (5-aminosalicylic acid) versus sulphasalazine in the treatment of active ulcerative colitis: a randomised trial. Br Med J 1989;298:82–86.

family physician in a routine office practice. The index reportedly correlated well ($r=0.959$) with the Powell-Tuck Index, but further evaluation is needed.

The clinical disease activity indices for ulcerative colitis described above are summarized in Table 30.14.

## HEALTH-RELATED QUALITY OF LIFE

The disease activity indices generally reflect a medical perception of the disease activity and do not consider patients' views of the impact of IBD on their everyday life. This deficiency led to the development of instruments that measure health-related quality of life (HRQOL). The HRQOL instruments provide measures of health perception in the physical, psychological and social dimensions. As a secondary outcome measure, the HRQOL instruments have been increasingly used in the field of clinical trials for IBD.

## Inflammatory Bowel Disease Questionnaire

The Inflammatory Bowel Disease Questionnaire (IBDQ)[10,35–37] is a disease-specific HRQOL instrument developed as an evaluative instrument for assessment of treatment efficacy in clinical trials.[35] To date, the IBDQ, as a secondary outcome measure, has gained wide acceptance and has been used extensively in clinical trials for Crohn's disease.[38–41] It consists of 32 items

## Table 30.13 Lichtiger Index

| | Scores | | | | | |
|---|---|---|---|---|---|---|
| Items | 0 | 1 | 2 | 3 | 4 | 5 |
| 1. Diarrhea (number of stools daily) | 0–2 | 3 or 4 | 5 or 6 | 7–9 | 10 | – |
| 2. Nocturnal diarrhea | No | Yes | – | – | – | – |
| 3. Visible blood in stool (% of movements) | 0 | <50 | ≥ 50 | 100 | – | – |
| 4. Fecal incontinence | No | Yes | – | – | – | – |
| 5. Abdominal pain or cramping | None | Mild | Moderate | Severe | – | – |
| 6. General wellbeing | Perfect | Very good | Good | Average | Poor | Terrible |
| 7. Abdominal tenderness | No | Mild and localized | Mild to moderate and diffuse | Severe or rebound | – | – |
| 8. Need for antidiarrheal drugs | No | Yes | – | – | – | – |
| Total score = sum of the item scores | | | | | | |

Adapted from Lichtiger S, Present DH, Kornbluth A et al. Cyclosporine in severe ulcerative colitis refractory to steroid therapy. N Engl J Med 1994;330:1841–1845.

## Table 30.14 Summary of clinical disease activity indices for ulcerative colitis

| First author | Instruments | Current utility | Scores and definitions | Strengths and limitations |
|---|---|---|---|---|
| Truelove[20] | Truelove and Witts Index | Adult, clinical research; primary endpoint | Qualitative activity measure; disease activity defined as 'mild', 'moderate', and 'severe' | Most frequently used and referred; inability to classify patients who meet some, but not all of the criteria |
| Powell-Tuck[21] | Powell-Tuck Index | Adult, clinical research; primary endpoint | Score range: 0 to 22; no score defined for clinical remission | Frequently used and referred; heavily depend on general health status, symptoms and signs; need progressive validation |
| Sutherland[23] | Disease Activity Index | Adult, clinical research; primary endpoint | Score range: 0 to 12; <=2 (with no individual subscore>1) defined as clinical remission (1-day basis) | Frequently used and referred; endoscopic assessment included; need progressive validation |
| Schroeder[22] | Mayo Score | Adult, clinical research; primary endpoint | Score range: 0 to 12; <=2 (with no individual subscore>1) defined as clinical remission (3-day basis) | Frequently used and referred; endoscopic assessment included; need progressive validation |
| Rachmilewitz[24] | Clinical Activity Index | Adult, clinical research; primary endpoint | Score range: 0 to 29; no score defined for clinical remission | Frequently used and referred; comes with a endoscopic section; need progressive validation |
| Lichtiger[25] | Lichtiger Index | Adult, clinical research; primary endpoint | Score range: 0 to 21; <10 on 2 consecutive days indicating clinical response | Reported having good validity and interrater reliability; less frequently used or referred |

covering four domains, including bowel function, systemic symptoms, emotional status and social function.[35,42] With each item being scored from 1 to 7, the overall IBDQ score ranges from a minimum of 32 to a maximum of 224 (a higher score indicating better quality of life). For patients with inflammatory Crohn's disease in remission, the overall scores usually range from 170 to 190.[10] The validity, reliability and responsiveness of the IBDQ have been demonstrated to be adequate.[10] The IBDQ correlates well with the CDAI ($r=-0.67$; $P<0.001$)[10] but poorly with physician global assessment ($r=0.35$; $P=0.001$).[43] However, before the IBDQ can be applied to specific IBD subgroups (such as primarily fistulizing Crohn's disease) further validation is needed. The IBDQ was initially an interviewer-administered instrument, although a self-administered version has also been developed and validated.[37] Owing to the rising costs of clinical trials, the self-administered IBDQ may be more desirable in the future. To assure patients with Crohn's disease that they have an improved HRQOL after medical treatment, Sandborn et al.[4] recommended that the IBDQ be routinely used in all prospective randomized controlled trials. Further work may be required before the IBDQ can be used as a primary outcome measure.

## Rating Form of IBD Patient Concerns

Another disease-specific HRQOL instrument for IBD is the Rating Form of IBD Patient Concerns (RFIPC). This was developed by Drossman et al.[44] to measure HRQOL in IBD patients and to compare it with the measures of disease activity. The RFIPC consists of 25 items (or concerns) that address disease, body-, interpersonal- and sexually related concerns. The RFIPC are graded on 10-cm visual analog scales, with 0 cm indicating 'not at all' and 10 cm indicating 'a great deal'. A typical question might be 'Because of your condition, how concerned are you with…?' The RFIPC questionnaire takes 10–15 minutes to complete and the overall score is determined by the mean of the 25 item scores. The RFIPC has been evaluated in a number of studies in different countries,[44–46] but few randomized controlled trails have actually used this instrument as an outcome measure.

# MEASURING ENDOSCOPIC DISEASE ACTIVITY

An objective assessment of disease activity has proved to be one of the great challenges encountered by clinical researchers in IBD. Investigators have attempted to evaluate the potential role of endoscopic assessment of disease activity in providing objective data for disease activity assessment. A number of endoscopic disease activity indices have been proposed and developed, but only a few have been validated.

## Crohn's Disease Endoscopic Index of Severity

The Crohn's Disease Endoscopic Index of Severity (CDEIS) (Table 30.15) was proposed by a French multicenter IBD study group (Groupe D'Etudes Thérapeutiques des Affections Inflammatiores du Tube Digestif, GETAID) and has been progressively developed and validated.[47–50] The index looks at the presence or absence of lesions, their severity and their extent to grade the severity of the disease on a six-item scale.[50] To determine the CDEIS score, a numerical score needs to be calculated for each of the six items, with each having a preassigned weight. The sum of the six weighted item scores constitutes the overall CDEIS score, with a higher score indicating worse disease. A cut-off value that defines clinical remission is still to be determined. The endoscopic remission was, however, defined as the absence of lesions, or the presence of scarring as an indication of lesion healing, or the improvement of lesions by at least two items with

## Table 30.15 Crohn's Disease Endoscopic Index of Severity

| Items | Score | Weight | Weighted scores |
|---|---|---|---|
| 1. Number of rectocolonic segments | $X_1$ = number of deep ulcerations seen divided by number of segments examined (rectum, sigmoid and left colon, transverse colon, right colon, and ileum) | 12 | $X_1 \times 12$ |
| 2. Number of rectocolonic segments | $X_2$ = number of superficial ulcerations seen divided by number of segments examined (rectum, sigmoid and left colon, transverse colon, right colon, and ileum) | 6 | $X_2 \times 6$ |
| 3. Segmental surfaces involved by disease | $X_3$ = sum of each of the individual segmental surfaces involved by disease divided by number of segments examined. The degree of disease involvement in each segment is determined by examining each segment for 9 lesions* and estimating the number of cm of involvement (1 or more lesions present) in a representative 10 cm portion from each segment. | 1 | $X_3 \times 1$ |
| 4. Segmental surfaces involved by ulceration | $X_4$ = sum of each of the individual segmental surfaces involved by ulceration divided by number of segments examined. The degree of ulceration in each segment is determined by examining each segment for ulceration** and estimating the number of cm of intestine involved by ulceration in a representative 10 cm portion from each segment. | 1 | $X_4 \times 1$ |
| 5. Presence of a non-ulcerated stenosis | $X_5$ = presence of an ulcerated stenosis in any of the segments examined<br>0 = absence and 1 = presence | 3 | $X_5 \times 3$ |
| 6. Presence of an ulcerated stenosis | $X_6$ = presence of an ulcerated stenosis in any of the segments examined<br>0 = absence and 1 = presence | 3 | $X_5 \times 3$ |

Total score = sum of the weighted scores

* 9 lesions = pseudopolyps, healed ulcerations, frank erythema, frank mucosal swelling, aphthoid ulcers, superficial ulcers, deep ulcers, non-ulcerated stenosis and ulcerated stenosis.
** Ulceration = aphthoid ulcers, superficial ulcers, deep ulcers, ulcerated stenosis
Adapted from Mary JY, Modigliani R. Development and validation of an endoscopic index of the severity for Crohn's disease: a prospective multicentre study. Groupe d'Etudes Therapeutiques des Affections Inflammatoires du Tube Digestif (GETAID). Gut 1989;30:983–989.

no residual deep ulceration. The CDEIS has been used in several clinical trials as a secondary outcome measure.[47,51]

## Rutgeerts Score

Another validated endoscopic activity index for Crohn's disease is the Endoscopic Scoring System for Postoperative Recurrence (also known as Rutgeerts Score; Table 30.16). The Rutgeerts Score has been used as a tool to assess patients with ileal or ileocolonic Crohn's disease who undergo surgical resection. The index looks at the presence or absence of lesions and the severity of lesions in the neoterminal ileum to determine the patient's postoperative prognosis. The index consists of five items that are graded on scale of 0–4 , with a score of 3–4 being defined as having a greater likelihood of clinical relapse.[52] The Rutgeerts Score has been used in a number of clinical trials[53–59] for such a purpose. There are still other instruments that perform endoscopic assessment for Crohn's disease.[7,60] These, however, have not been validated in randomized controlled clinical trials.

## Baron's Criteria

For ulcerative colitis a number of indices for assessing endoscopic disease activity have been proposed. One of the earliest was created by Baron et al.[31] after examining mucosal appearance in patients during sigmoidoscopy (Table 30.17). Baron's Criteria macroscopically grade the severity of the inflammatory changes using a four-item scale with the score ranging from 0 to 3. Despite grading the severity of the lesions, the criteria do not claim any relation to the disease severity. Today the Baron's

Criteria are the most frequently used/referred-to endoscopic disease activity instrument for ulcerative colitis. Based on these criteria, several other indices have also been developed. For example, the Disease Activity Index and the Mayo Score (see Table 30.11) both derived their endoscopic assessment items from Baron's criteria.

## OTHER ENDOSCOPIC DISEASE ACTIVITY INDICES FOR ULCERATIVE COLITIS

As indicated earlier, Rachmilewitz et al.[24] also proposed a four-item endoscopic disease activity index (Table 30.18) together with the clinical section of the Clinical Disease Indices (Table 30.12). There are still many other endoscopic disease activity indices proposed by different investigators. Most referred to previous published criteria for their self-development. However, although all have been used in clinical trials, few have been progressively validated.

## HISTOLOGICAL DISEASE ACTIVITY

Until recently histological assessment of Crohn's disease activity was not frequently used in the assessment of new drug treatments. One major reason is that the current microscopic grading of lesions (or improvement) does not correlate well with other disease activity indices. As a result, the utility of such instruments for evaluating the severity of Crohn's disease

### Table 30.16 Endoscopic Scoring System for Postoperative Recurrence (Rutgeerts Score)

| Items | Scores |
|---|---|
| 1. No lesions in the distal ileum | 0 |
| 2. =5 Aphthous lesions | 1 |
| 3. >5 Aphthous lesions with normal mucosa between the lesions, or skip areas of larger lesions or lesions confined to ileocolonic anastomosis (i.e. <1 cm in length) | 2 |
| 4. Diffuse aphthous ileitis with diffusely inflamed mucosa | 3 |
| 5. Diffuse inflammation with already larger ulcers, nodules, and/or narrowing | 4 |

Adapted from Rutgeerts P, Geboes K, Vantrappen G, Beyls J, Kerremans R, Hiele M. Predictability of the postoperative course of Crohn's disease. Gastroenterology 1990;99:956–963.

### Table 30.17 Baron's Criteria for Assessing Endoscopic Disease Activity

| Items | Scores |
|---|---|
| 1. Normal: mat mucosa, ramifying vascular pattern clearly visible throughout, no spontaneous bleeding, no bleeding to light touch | 0 |
| 2. Abnormal but not hemorrhagic: appearances between '0' and '2' | 1 |
| 3. Moderately hemorrhagic: bleeding to light touch, but no spontaneous bleeding seen ahead of instrument on initial inspection | 2 |
| 4. Severely hemorrhagic: spontaneous bleeding seen ahead of instrument at initial inspection, and bleeds to light touch | 3 |

Adapted from Baron JH, Connell AM, Lennard-Jones JE. Variation between observers in describing mucosal appearances in proctocolitis. Br Med J 1964;1:89–92.

### Table 30.18 Clinical Activity Index (endoscopic section)

| Items | Scores 0 | 1 | 2 | 4 |
|---|---|---|---|---|
| 1. Granulation scattering reflected light | No | – | Yes | – |
| 2. Vascular pattern | Normal | Faded/ disturbed | Completely absent | – |
| 3. Vulnerability of mucosal | None | – | Slightly increased (contact bleeding) | Greatly increased (spontaneous bleeding) |
| 4. Mucosal damage (mucus, fibrin, exudates, erosions, ulcer) | None | – | Slight | Pronounced |

Total score = sum of the item scores

Adapted from Rachmilewitz D. Coated mesalazine (5-aminosalicylic acid) versus sulphasalazine in the treatment of active ulcerative colitis: a randomised trial. Br Med J 1989;298:82–86.

### Table 30.19 Scoring system for histological abnormalities in Crohn's disease mucosal biopsy specimens

| Items | Scores 0 | 1 | 2 | 3 |
|---|---|---|---|---|
| 1. Epithelial damage | Normal | Focal pathology | Extensive pathology | – |
| 2. Architectural changes | Normal | Moderately disturbed (<50%) | Severely disturbed (>50%) | |
| 3. Infiltration of mononuclear cells in the lamina propria | Normal | Moderate increase | Severe increase | |
| 4. Polymorphonuclear cells in the lamina propria | Normal | Moderate increase | Severe increase | |
| 5. Polymorphonuclear cells in epithelium | – | In surface epithelium | Cryptitis | Crypt abscess |
| 6. Presence of erosion and/or ulcers | No | Yes | | |
| 7. Presence of granuloma | No | Yes | | |
| 8. No. of biopsy specimens | None (0 of 6) | =33% (1 or 2 of 6) | 33–66% (3 or 4 of 6) | >66% (5 or 6 of 6) |

Total score = sum of the item scores

Adapted from D'Haens GR, Geboes K, Peeters M, Baert F, Penninckx F, Rutgeerts P. Early lesions of recurrent Crohn's disease caused by infusion of intestinal contents in excluded ileum. Gastroenterology 1998;114:262–267.

is limited. Although certain histological disease indices, e.g. the scoring system for histological abnormalities in Crohn's disease mucosal biopsy specimens[61] (Table 30.19), were proposed by some investigators, with their current validation status they are not recommended to be used as an outcome measure in drug trials.[4] Further studies are needed to prospectively validate the existing indices and to develop new indices.

For ulcerative colitis, a number of histological disease activity indices have been proposed and used in clinical trials. The earliest microscopic disease activity criteria were created by Truelove and Richards[62] in the mid 1950s in a biopsy study of ulcerative colitis. The criteria assess features such as the nature and distribution of the inflammatory cell infiltrate, as well as the degree of the glandular destruction and ulceration. The criteria are still the most frequently referred-to instrument in today's clinical research. A modified version of the criteria is presented in Table 30.20. Although different histological disease activity indices have been used as secondary outcome measure in clinical trials for ulcerative colitis,[63–66] their validation status and their correlation with the clinical disease indices are, however, largely unknown.

## Table 30.20 Histological Disease Activity Index

| | Scores | | | |
|---|---|---|---|---|
| **Items** | **0** | **1** | **2** | **3** |
| Active inflammation | Normal: Neutrophils not present in crypt or surface epithelium and no exudates, erosion, or ulceration | Low grade: Neutrophils present transmigrating through the crypt epithelium or within crypt lumina in <20% of crypts | Moderate: Neutrophilic infiltration in >20% of crypts or presence of erosions (loss of superficial mucosa accompanied by fibroinflammatory exudate) | High grade: Presence of ulcers (loss of the entire thickness of mucosa and recognized as fragments of inflamed gradation tissue) |
| Chronic inflammation | No increase: Number of chronic inflammatory cells within normal limits and present primarily in the superficial lamina propria | Moderate: Mononuclear cells present in moderate numbers and aggregated between crypts at the base of the lamina propria | Severe: Marked increase in chronic inflammation shown by sheets of chronic cells | – |
| Crypt distortion | None: Crypts had normal outlines with only artifactual irregularities | Mild: Scattered or rare crypts showing irregular (bent, forked) outline | Moderate: Approximately 25–50% of crypts with an irregular outline | Severe: More than 50% of crypts with an irregular outline |

Total score = sum of the item scores

Adapted from Hanauer SB, Robinson M, Pruitt R et al. Budesonide enema for the treatment of active, distal ulcerative colitis and proctitis: a dose-ranging study. US Budesonide enema study group. Gastroenterology 1998;115:525–532.

# REFERENCES

1. Winship DH, Summers RW, Singleton JW et al. National Cooperative Crohn's Disease Study: study design and conduct of the study. Gastroenterology 1979;77:829–842.
2. Best WR, Becktel JM, Singleton JW, Kern F Jr. Development of a Crohn's disease activity index. National Cooperative Crohn's Disease Study. Gastroenterology 1976;70:439–444.
3. Best WR, Becktel JM, Singleton JW. Rederived values of the eight coefficients of the Crohn's Disease Activity Index (CDAI). Gastroenterology 1979;77:843–846.
4. Sandborn WJ, Feagan BG, Hanauer SB et al. A review of activity indices and efficacy endpoints for clinical trials of medical therapy in adults with Crohn's disease. Gastroenterology 2002;122:512–530.
5. de Dombal FT, Softley A. IOIBD report no 1: Observer variation in calculating indices of severity and activity in Crohn's disease. International Organisation for the Study of Inflammatory Bowel Disease. Gut 1987;28:474–481.
6. Harvey RF, Bradshaw JM. A simple index of Crohn's-disease activity. Lancet 1980;1:514.
7. Gomes P, du Boulay C, Smith CL, Holdstock G. Relationship between disease activity indices and colonoscopic findings in patients with colonic inflammatory bowel disease. Gut 1986;27:92–95.
8. Wright JP, Young GO, Tigler-Wybrandi N. Predictors of acute relapse of Crohn's disease. A laboratory and clinical study. Dig Dis Sci 1987;32:164–170.
9. Wright JP, Marks IN, Parfitt A. A simple clinical index of Crohn's disease activity – the Cape Town index. S Africa Med J 1985;68:502–503.
10. Irvine EJ, Feagan B, Rochon J et al. Quality of life: a valid and reliable measure of therapeutic efficacy in the treatment of inflammatory bowel disease. Canadian Crohn's Relapse Prevention Trial Study Group. Gastroenterology 1994;106:287–296.
11. Myren J, Bouchier IA, Watkinson G, Softley A, Clamp SE, de Dombal FT. The OMGE multinational inflammatory bowel disease survey 1976–1986. A further report on 3175 cases. Scand J Gastroenterol 1988;144:11–19.
12. Present DH, Korelitz BI, Wisch N, Glass JL, Sachar DB, Pasternack BS. Treatment of Crohn's disease with 6-mercaptopurine. A long-term, randomized, double-blind study. N Engl J Med 1980;302:981–987.
13. van Hees PA, van Elteren PH, van Lier HJ, van Tongeren JH. An index of inflammatory activity in patients with Crohn's disease. Gut 1980;21:279–286.
14. Irvine EJ. Usual therapy improves perianal Crohn's disease as measured by a new disease activity index. McMaster IBD Study Group. J Clin Gastroenterol 1995;20:27–32.
15. Present DH, Rutgeerts P, Targan S et al. Infliximab for the treatment of fistulas in patients with Crohn's disease. N Engl J Med 1999;340:1398–1405.
16. Sandler RS, Jordan MC, Kupper LL. Development of a Crohn's index for survey research. J Clin Epidemiol 1988;41:451–458.
17. Whittington PF, Barnes HV, Bayless TM. Medical management of Crohn's disease in adolescence. Gastroenterology 1977;72:1338–1344.
18. Lloyd-Still JD, Green OC. A clinical scoring system for chronic inflammatory bowel disease in children. Dig Dis Sci 1979;24:620–624.
19. Hyams JS, Ferry GD, Mandel FS et al. Development and validation of a pediatric Crohn's disease activity index. J Pediatr Gastroenterol Nutr 1991;12:439–447.
20. Truelove SC, Witts LJ. Cortisone in ulcerative colitis: final report on a therapeutic trial. Br Med J 1955;2:1041–1048.
21. Powell-Tuck J, Day DW, Buckell NA, Wadsworth J, Lennard-Jones JE. Correlations between defined sigmoidoscopic appearances and other measures of disease activity in ulcerative colitis. Dig Dis Sci 1982;27:533–537.
22. Schroeder KW, Tremaine WJ, Ilstrup DM. Coated oral 5-aminosalicylic acid therapy for mildly to moderately active ulcerative colitis. A randomized study. N Engl J Med 1987;317:1625–1629.
23. Sutherland LR, Martin F, Greer S et al. 5-Aminosalicylic acid enema in the treatment of distal ulcerative colitis, proctosigmoiditis, and proctitis. Gastroenterology 1987;92:1894–1898.
24. Rachmilewitz D. Coated mesalazine (5-aminosalicylic acid) versus sulphasalazine in the treatment of active ulcerative colitis: a randomised trial. Br Med J 1989;298:82–86.
25. Lichtiger S, Present DH, Kornbluth A et al. Cyclosporine in severe ulcerative colitis refractory to steroid therapy. N Engl J Med 1994;330:1841–1845.
26. Powell-Tuck J, Bown RL, Lennard-Jones JE. A comparison of oral prednisolone given as single or multiple daily doses for active proctocolitis. Scand J Gastroenterol 1978;13:833–837.
27. Walmsley RS, Ayres RC, Pounder RE, Allan RN. A simple clinical colitis activity index. Gut 1998;43:29–32.
28. Biddle WL, Greenberger NJ, Swan JT, McPhee MS, Miner PB Jr. 5-Aminosalicylic acid enemas: effective agent in maintaining remission in left-sided ulcerative colitis. Gastroenterology 1988;94:1075–1079.
29. Sninsky CA, Cort DH, Shanahan F et al. Oral mesalamine (Asacol) for mildly to moderately active ulcerative colitis. A multicenter study. Ann Intern Med 1991;115:350–355.
30. Truelove SC. Treatment of ulcerative colitis with local hydrocortisone hemisuccinate sodium: a report on a controlled therapeutic trial. Br Med J 1958;2:1072–1077.
31. Baron JH, Connell AM, Lennard-Jones JE. Variation between observers in describing mucosal appearances in proctocolitis. Br Med J 1964;1:89–92.
32. Lichtiger S. Cyclosporine therapy in inflammatory bowel disease: open-label experience. Mt Sinai J Med 1990;57:315–319.
33. Lichtiger S, Present DH. Preliminary report: cyclosporin in treatment of severe active ulcerative colitis. Lancet 1990;336:16–19.
34. Rutegard I, Ahsgren L, Stenling R, Nilsson T. A simple index for assessment of disease activity in patients with ulcerative colitis. Hepatogastroenterology 1990;37:110–112.
35. Guyatt G, Mitchell A, Irvine EJ et al. A new measure of health status for clinical trials in inflammatory bowel disease. Gastroenterology 1989;96:804–810.
36. Mitchell A, Guyatt G, Singer J et al. Quality of life in patients with inflammatory bowel disease. J Clin Gastroenterol 1988;10:306–310.
37. Love JR, Irvine EJ, Fedorak RN. Quality of life in inflammatory bowel disease. Clin Gastroenterol 1992;14:15–19.
38. Feagan BG, Fedorak RN, Irvine EJ et al. A comparison of methotrexate with placebo for the maintenance of remission in Crohn's disease. North American Crohn's Study Group Investigators. N Engl J Med 2000;342:1627–1632.
39. Feagan BG, Rochon J, Fedorak RN et al. Methotrexate for the treatment of Crohn's disease. The North American Crohn's Study Group Investigators. N Engl J Med 1995;332:292–297.

40. Greenberg GR, Feagan BG, Martin F et al. Oral budesonide for active Crohn's disease. Canadian Inflammatory Bowel Disease Study Group. N Engl J Med 1994;331:836–841.

41. Greenberg GR, Feagan BG, Martin F et al. Oral budesonide as maintenance treatment for Crohn's disease: a placebo-controlled, dose-ranging study. Canadian Inflammatory Bowel Disease Study Group. Gastroenterology 1996;110:45–51.

42. Guyatt GH, Deyo RA, Charlson M, Levine MN, Mitchell A. Responsiveness and validity in health status measurement: a clarification. J Clin Epidemiol 1989;42:403–408.

43. Irvine EJ. Quality of life measurement in inflammatory bowel disease. Scand J Gastroenterol 1993;199:36–39.

44. Drossman DA, Patrick DL, Mitchell CM, Zagami EA, Appelbaum MI. Health-related quality of life in inflammatory bowel disease. Functional status and patient worries and concerns. Dig Dis Sci 1989;34:1379–1386.

45. Drossman DA, Leserman J, Li ZM, Mitchell CM, Zagami EA, Patrick DL. The rating form of IBD patient concerns: a new measure of health status. Psychosom Med 1991;53:701–712.

46. Hjortswang H, Strom M, Almeida RT, Almer S. Evaluation of the RFIPC, a disease-specific health-related quality of life questionnaire, in Swedish patients with ulcerative colitis. Scand J Gastroenterol 1997;32:1235–1240.

47. Landi B, Anh TN, Cortot A et al. Endoscopic monitoring of Crohn's disease treatment: a prospective, randomized clinical trial. The Groupe d'Etudes Thérapeutiques des Affections Inflammatoires Digestives. Gastroenterology 1992;102:1647–1653.

48. Modigliani R, Mary JY, Simon JF et al. Clinical, biological, and endoscopic picture of attacks of Crohn's disease. Evolution on prednisolone. Groupe d'Etudes Thérapeutiques des Affections Inflammatoires Digestives. Gastroenterology 1990;98:811–818.

49. Mary JY, Modigliani R. Development and validation of an endoscopic index of the severity for Crohn's disease: a prospective multicentre study. Groupe d'Etudes Thérapeutiques des Affections Inflammatoires du Tube Digestif (GETAID). Gut 1989;30:983–989.

50. Reproducibility of colonoscopic findings in Crohn's disease: a prospective multicenter study of interobserver variation. Groupe d'Etudes Thérapeutiques des Affections Inflammatoires du Tube Digestif (GETAID). Dig Dis Sci 1987;32:1370–1379.

51. D'Haens G, Van Deventer S, Van Hogezand R et al. Endoscopic and histological healing with infliximab anti-tumor necrosis factor antibodies in Crohn's disease: A European multicenter trial. Gastroenterology 1999;116:1029–1034.

52. Rutgeerts P, Geboes K, Vantrappen G, Beyls J, Kerremans R, Hiele M. Predictability of the postoperative course of Crohn's disease. Gastroenterology 1990;99:956–963.

53. Hellers G, Cortot A, Jewell D et al. Oral budesonide for prevention of postsurgical recurrence in Crohn's disease. The IOIBD Budesonide Study Group. Gastroenterology 1999;116:294–300.

54. Ewe K, Bottger T, Buhr HJ, Ecker KW, Otto HF. Low-dose budesonide treatment for prevention of postoperative recurrence of Crohn's disease: a multicentre randomized placebo-controlled trial. German Budesonide Study Group. Eur J Gastroenterol Hepatol 1999;11:277–282.

55. Caprilli R, Andreoli A, Capurso L et al. Oral mesalazine (5-aminosalicylic acid; Asacol) for the prevention of post-operative recurrence of Crohn's disease. Gruppo Italiano per lo Studio del Colon e del Retto (GISC). Aliment Pharmacol Ther 1994;8:35–43.

56. Brignola C, Cottone M, Pera A et al. Mesalamine in the prevention of endoscopic recurrence after intestinal resection for Crohn's disease. Italian Cooperative Study Group. Gastroenterology 1995;108:345–349.

57. Florent C, Cortot A, Quandale P et al. Placebo-controlled clinical trial of mesalazine in the prevention of early endoscopic recurrences after resection for Crohn's disease. Groupe d'Etudes Thérapeutiques des Affections Inflammatoires Digestives (GETAID). Eur J Gastroenterol Hepatol 1996;8:229–233.

58. Lochs H, Mayer M, Fleig WE et al. Prophylaxis of postoperative relapse in Crohn's disease with mesalamine: European Cooperative Crohn's Disease Study VI. Gastroenterology 2000;118:264–273.

59. Rutgeerts P, Hiele M, Geboes K et al. Controlled trial of metronidazole treatment for prevention of Crohn's recurrence after ileal resection. Gastroenterology 1995;108:1617–1621.

60. Olaison G, Sjodahl R, Tagesson C. Glucocorticoid treatment in ileal Crohn's disease: relief of symptoms but not of endoscopically viewed inflammation. Gut 1990;31:325–328.

61. D'Haens GR, Geboes K, Peeters M, Baert F, Penninckx F, Rutgeerts P. Early lesions of recurrent Crohn's disease caused by infusion of intestinal contents in excluded ileum. Gastroenterology 1998;114:262–267.

62. Truelove SC, Richards WCD. Biopsy studies in ulcerative colitis. Br Med J 1956;1:1315–1318.

63. Lofberg R, Ostergaard Thomsen O, Langholz E et al. Budesonide versus prednisolone retention enemas in active distal ulcerative colitis. Aliment Pharmacol Ther 1994;8:623–629.

64. Hanauer SB, Robinson M, Pruitt R et al. Budesonide enema for the treatment of active, distal ulcerative colitis and proctitis: a dose-ranging study. US Budesonide enema study group. Gastroenterology 1998;115:525–532.

65. Mulder CJ, Endert E, van der Heide H et al. Comparison of beclomethasone dipropionate (2 and 3 mg) and prednisolone sodium phosphate enemas (30 mg) in the treatment of ulcerative proctitis. An adrenocortical approach. Neth J Med 1989;35:18–24.

66. Sandborn WJ, Tremaine WJ, Schroeder KW et al. A placebo-controlled trial of cyclosporine enemas for mildly to moderately active left-sided ulcerative colitis. Gastroenterology 1994;106:1429–1435.

## CHAPTER 31

# Quality of life and pharmacoeconomics

Brian G Feagan

## INTRODUCTION

Patients with IBD experience important disability from disease-related symptoms and complications. Apart from the common physical complaints of diarrhea, abdominal pain and fatigue, many individuals face impairment of activities of daily living. Patients with IBD must also adjust their life expectations, as education, employment, sexuality, family life and social interactions are frequently affected. Adolescents in particular must cope not only with the physical manifestations of IBD but also with the effects of a chronic illness on social relationships and maturation. Although traditional measures of disease severity, such as the Crohn's Disease Activity Index (CDAI),[1] quantify physical symptoms, they do not adequately evaluate many aspects of life that are important to patients. Measurement of health-related quality of life (HRQL) provides an opportunity to better to assess these issues.

HRQL measurement is also integral to the performance of pharmacoeconomic analysis in these diseases. Crohn's disease and ulcerative colitis generate high costs for society. Although highly effective new treatments[2,3] are now available for use in IBD these new agents are more costly and society must make intelligent choices about resource allocation. Pharmacoeconomic analyses provide valuable information to decision-makers who must choose which new treatments are funded.

This chapter provides an overview of HRQL assessment and discusses the use of these measures in pharmacoeconomic analyses.

## MEASUREMENT OF HEALTH-RELATED QUALITY OF LIFE

HRQL measurement is a rapidly evolving field that has gained widespread acceptance for the study of chronic diseases.[4] The World Health Organization defines health as a state of complete physical, mental and social wellbeing, in contrast to the absence of disease.[5] Accordingly, valid HRQL measures incorporate psychological, functional and social assessments in addition to the assessment of physical symptoms. For this reason HRQL measures provide additional information to patients and caregivers beyond that offered by traditional disease activity indices.[6]

HRQL assessment is integral to the study of IBD for two main reasons. First, although hospitalization, surgery and disease-related complications are important outcomes that can be used to evaluate patients' prognosis and response to new treatments, these events occur infrequently. Thus, a need exists to assess other patient-related outcomes. Second, the burden of physical symptoms and social and psychological morbidity attributable to IBD is, for the most part, lifelong. Thus measures of outcome that have the capacity to be performed repetitively and non-intrusively are highly valuable.

## A HISTORICAL OVERVIEW

Evaluation of HRQL in IBD is a relatively young discipline. An initial study from Oxford[7] in 1963 suggested that approximately one-third of patients with ulcerative colitis showed some degree of social or physical dysfunction. Although a handful of similar studies appeared in the literature throughout the 1970s and 1980s[8-12] these early investigations were performed without the benefit of valid HRQL assessments and used suboptimal sampling techniques. Thus it is not surprising that inconsistent and contradictory results were obtained. Nevertheless, an overview of the data available from this era suggests that whereas the majority of patients with IBD enjoy relatively good HRQL, a minority show some impairment of functional status. For example, Binder and colleagues[12] reported that approximately 20% of patients with Crohn's disease were unable to work at full capacity 20 years from the time of diagnosis. Other investigators, using primarily interview techniques or generic health status questionnaires, confirmed that relevant social and psychological impairment is relatively common in this group of patients.

In the late 1980s the development of disease-specific HRQL questionnaires led to important advances in the field. Guyatt and colleagues, working in Canada, developed the Inflammatory Bowel Disease Questionnaire (IBDQ),[13,14] a disease-specific HRQL measure that has since become a reference standard for use in both randomized controlled trials and epidemiological studies. At approximately the same time, Drossman and colleagues[15] in the United States developed the Rating Form of IBD Patient Concerns (RFIPC). In contrast to the IBDQ, the RFIPC identifies specific concerns of patients regarding the effects of the disease on their health status. This instrument has been used primarily as an epidemiological tool to identify the relative importance of various patient concerns and to determine the best strategies to educate patients regarding specific disease-related problems.

The development of these questionnaires allowed investigators to obtain important new information in many different areas. Accordingly, the number of publications reporting on HRQL in IBD increased rapidly during the 1990s and into the new millennium.

## MEASUREMENT OF HRQL

As noted previously, evaluation of HRQL requires the development of valid measurement tools. Typically these are questionnaires that vary widely in complexity and ease of administration. It is important to recognize that HRQL instruments must be developed and assessed according to the same standards used to appraise other evaluative procedures, such as disease activity indices and diagnostic tests.[16] Before HRQL questionnaires can be used in research they should undergo a rigorous development process. Most importantly, an instrument's operating properties should be comprehensively evaluated.

## OPERATING PROPERTIES OF HRQL MEASURES

The key operating properties are validity, reliability and responsiveness.[17] Validity refers to the concept that an instrument accurately measures the phenomenon of interest. Several different methods are available to assess validity. If a gold standard is available the technique of criterion validity/correlation of the results obtained with the new instrument to the reference standard can be utilized. Unfortunately, because HRQL assessments are by nature subjective, this technique has limited applicability. Alternatively, construct validity can be utilized. In this approach a priori predictions are made regarding the relationship between the new HRQL instruments and existing measures of disease severity, response to treatment or health status. For example, given that the CDAI score is a well-validated measure of disease severity in Crohn's disease, a moderate degree of correlation should be expected between this index and a new HRQL instrument.[17] If such a relationship is not demonstrated the validity of the new measure is suspect. Reliability assesses the consistency of results obtained when the instrument is administered to the same group of individuals, with the same health status, on two separate occasions. Reliable measures show little variability in stable patients. Reliability is usually expressed as an

intraclass correlation coefficient;[18] more reliable instruments show higher intraclass correlation coefficients. Responsiveness assesses the ability of a measurement to detect change in patients who have experienced a clinically meaningful alteration in health status. The most commonly utilized approach is to compare the ratio of the change in mean score differences between patients who have changed (signal) to the standard deviation of the difference in scores in patients who are stable (noise).[19] This property is often referred to as the 'standardized effect size' or the 'reliability ratio'. Evaluative instruments, for example outcome measures used in randomized controlled trials, must have high signal-to-noise ratios if they are to detect small but clinically relevant treatment effects.

## A TAXONOMY OF HRQL INSTRUMENTS

HRQL measures are either generic or disease specific (Fig. 31.1). Generic instruments assess all aspects of HRQL and thus incorporate broad physical, social and mental health evaluations. Because of their comprehensive nature these questionnaires are most appropriate for evaluating differences betweeen different diseases. Although this information is of little relevance to clinical care, it may be highly valuable to decision-makers who must prioritize budget allocations. An important disadvantage of generic HRQL instruments is that they are less sensitive to clinically relevant changes in health status than the disease-specific measures.[20] In contrast, disease-specific measures are highly sensitive to changes in health status but are limited in their scope, as they only assess a single disorder.[21]

### GENERIC INSTRUMENTS

Two major subcategories of generic HRQL assessment can be identified, psychometric questionnaires and utilities.

### Psychometric questionnaires

A large number of generic instruments are currently available that vary tremendously in complexity and comprehension. These include the Sickness Impact Profile (SIP),[22] the McMaster Health Status Questionnaire,[23] the Nottingham Health Profile[24] and the Short Form-36 (SF-36).[25] The latter has gained widespread

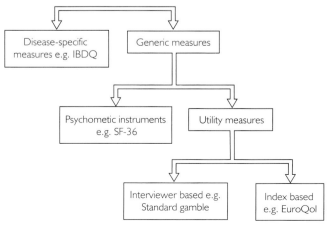

Fig. 31.1 A taxonomy of HRQL instruments.

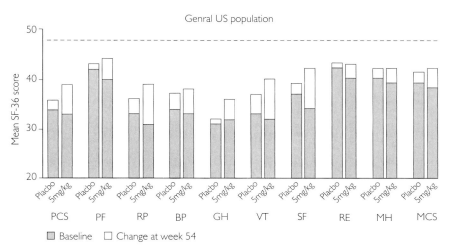

Genral US population

**Fig. 31.2** SF-36 data from the ACCENT I trial The black component of the bars show the baseline values. The shaded areas show the improvement in scores following treatment with either infliximab or placebo. The dotted line shows corresponding scores derived from the general US population. (Reprinted with permission from Elsevier (The Lancet 2002;359:1541–1549).

acceptance because it is straightforward to administer, the operating properties are well characterized, and age-specific population normative data are available for most countries.[26,27] This self-administered tool consists of 36 questions which aggregate into eight domains of health: physical functioning (PF), role physical (RP), bodily pain (BP), general health perceptions (GH), vitality (VT), social functioning (SF), role emotional (RE) and general mental health (MH) (Fig. 31.2). These eight domains are further summarized into two component summary measures: a physical component summary (PCS) and a mental component summary (MCS). Each of the SF-36 scale ranges from 0 to 100; higher scores indicate better function. The SF-36 has been extensively validated in a wide variety of disease states. For patients with IBD both constructional and criterion approaches have shown the SF-36 to be valid for use in clinical studies.[28,29] Although formal responsiveness testing has not been reported, experience with the use of the SF-36 in a recent randomized controlled trial of infliximab therapy for Crohn's disease[30] indicates that it is capable of detecting clinical improvement with treatment. However the SF-36 is unsuitable for use in economic evaluations,[31] and therefore other generic instruments, notably utility measures,[32] must be used for this purpose.

## Utility measures

Three widely accepted techniques exist for utility estimation: the Standard Gamble, the Time Trade-off and the Visual Analog Scale (VAS). Each of these generates a score that ranges from 1.0 (perfect health) to 0.0 (death). Conceptually, utility assessment is an attractive HRQL measurement strategy, as a single score is generated based on patients' preference for different health states.

### Estimating utility

The Standard Gamble is the gold standard procedure for utility estimation.[33–35] In this method patients are asked to consider their current health status and then choose between two possible alternatives: A, to remain in their current health state, or B, to opt for a hypothetical gamble. The gamble has two possible outcomes: (1) a probability (P) of returning to perfect health, or (2) a complementary probability (1 – P) of immediate death. To illustrate this concept consider the following situation based on a patient with Crohn's disease.

If patients with chronically active disease who required corticosteroid therapy to control symptoms were offered a 99%

chance of returning to perfect health, with an associated 1% risk of immediate death, most would accept the gamble. Conversely, most patients would not be enthusiastic about gambling if the complementary probability – a 99% chance of sudden death versus a 1% risk of returning to perfect health – was offered. As the probability P is varied the patient's risk tolerance defines a probability at which it is difficult to decide whether or not to gamble. At this point of equipoise the utility score can be identified. Therefore, patients with more severely impaired quality of life will generate lower utility scores.

The second most commonly used method for calculating utility, the Time Trade-off Technique,[36,37] is based on a variant of the previously described procedure. In this method, the patient identifies the number of years of life in their current health state that they would be willing to trade in exchange for perfect health. The number of years is varied until the respondent is ambivalent about the trade. The utility score is calculated by expressing the number of years traded as a proportion of the patient's calculated life expectancy (estimated from an actuarial table). For example, if a 35-year-old patient with chronically active Crohn's disease is willing to trade 10 of their estimated 43 years of remaining life expectancy, the utility score is estimated to be 35 – 10/43 = 0.58. Finally, using the VAS[38] method the patient identifies a point on a 100-mm visual analog scale, where 0 signifies death and 1.0 indicates perfect health, that best expresses their the current health status. Although the VAS method is easily administered it is sensitive to bias[33] and is therefore the least acceptable method of utility elicitation.

A 1997 publication evaluated 180 patients with Crohn's disease using the three accepted measures of utility estimation (Standard Gamble, Time Trade-off, VAS).[33] Patients were stratified into one of four health states (remission, acute disease exacerbation, corticosteroid-dependent disease, corticosteroid-resistant disease). Utility scores were shown to be both valid and reliable measures of HRQL. Validity was demonstrated by the observation that all three measures of utility ordered hypothetical health states according to a priori predictions (patients with more severe disease scored poorer than those with disease in remission (Fig. 31.3), and all measures had a significant degree of correlation with the other two other accepted measures of disease severity: the IBDQ, which assesses HRQL, and the CDAI, which assesses disease activity. Reliability was demonstrated in stable patients with mild, moderate and severe Crohn's disease. Utility scores were remarkably similar in stable patients at clinic visits 8

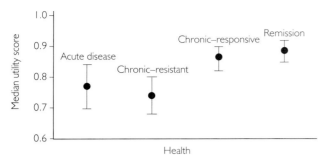

**Fig. 31.3** The Standard Gamble scores derived from a convenience sample of 180 patients with Crohn's disease. (Gregor JC, McDonald JWD, Klar N et al. An evaluation of the utility measurement in Crohn's Disease. Inflamm Bowel Dis 1997;3:265–276.) Higher scores mean better HRQL.

| **Table 31.1  The figure is a representative question from the IBDQ questionnaire** |
| --- |

**How often during the last two weeks have you been unable to attend school or work because of your bowel problem?**

1 = All of the time
2 = Most of the time
3 = A good bit of the time
4 = Some of the time
5 = A little of the time
6 = Hardly any of the time
7 = None of the time

weeks apart. However, these scores were less responsive to changes in disease severity than the CDAI, which indicates that utility assessment is less useful than other instruments detecting small, but clinically important, differences in HRQL.

Elicitation of utility estimates is time-consuming and expensive, as patients must be interviewed by highly trained research associates. Furthermore, variability in interview technique occurs even when standardized 'scripts' are used by inexperienced personnel. In an attempt to address these limitations several 'index-based' utility questionnaires have been developed.[39,40] These generate a score that has been previously correlated with direct utility estimates derived using the Standard Gamble procedure. Although these measures were developed by eliciting scores in a large number of people with various disorders,[41,42] it is necessary to ensure that they are valid for a specific disease. Recently Konig et al.[43] assessed the operating properties of one such measure, the Euro Qol EQ-5D, in 152 patients with IBD. Statistically significant correlations were shown between this measure and VAS-derived utility estimates, CDAI scores and SF-36 scores. The EQ-5D was both reliable, with an intraclass correlation coefficient of 0.77 in stable patients, and responsive to change, as shown by a standardized effect size of 0.79. These data are very promising and suggest that the EQ-5D may be a useful tool for collecting economic information during the conduct of controlled clinical trials. The primary advantage of this approach is that index-based utilities can be obtained with a minimum of respondent burden and do not require the assistance of a skilled interviewer.

Although the abstract nature of utility estimation is a frequent target of derision by clinicians, these critics should recognize that usual medical decision-making requires doctors and patients to make choices under conditions of uncertainty. These choices are associated with measurable risks and have important implications for patient outcomes. For this reason, the Standard Gamble is generally considered to be the most valid technique for utility elicitation, as it incorporates an element of uncertainty into the decision-making process that is not present in either the Time Trade-off or the VAS procedures.

## DISEASE-SPECIFIC INSTRUMENTS

Two well-characterized disease-specific HRQL measures have been developed for use in adults with IBD, the Inflammatory Bowel Disease Questionnaire[13,14] and the Rating Form of Patient Concerns.[44] A disease-specific measure for use in children has also recently been described.[45]

## The Inflammatory Bowel Disease Questionnaire

Measurement of HRQL in Crohn's disease has been greatly advanced through the development of the Inflammatory Bowel Disease Questionnaire (IBDQ). This instrument was created using a methodological paradigm developed by Kirshner and Guyatt.[46] According to this procedure, items of potential importance were identified from a convenience sample of patients with IBD and knowledgeable healthcare providers.[14] The perceived importance of these items was then ranked by 97 patients using a Likert scale. Items which predicted patients' global assessment of HRQL were then selected for incorporation into a multidimensional questionnaire. The operating properties of the prototype questionnaire were subsequently assessed in an independent sample of patients.

Based on this process, a 32-item IBDQ questionnaire was developed that generates a score from 0 to 224 points. (A representative question from this instrument is shown in Table 31.1.) Higher scores are associated with better quality of life. The questionnaire assesses four dimensional subscores: bowel function (e.g. loose stool, abdominal pain), systemic function (e.g. energy level, altered sleep pattern), social function (e.g. ability to attend social events, work attendance) and emotional function (e.g. depression, irritability). Subsequently, validation studies were performed in several patient populations, most notably from data derived from participants in the Canadian Crohn's Relapse Prevention Trial.[17,47] In this large ($n$=305) study the IBDQ showed a high degree of correlation with the CDAI ($r$ = –0.67, $P$ = 0.0001), indicating that it is a valid measure in this population of patients (Fig. 31.4). For patients whose health status was unchanged between visits the intraclass correlation coefficient was estimated to be 0.70, compared to 0.66 for the CDAI. This finding demonstrates that the IBDQ is a reliable instrument. Finally, responsiveness was assessed by calculating the ratio of the mean scores from the baseline value to the time of disease exacerbation in patients who experienced a relapse to the standard deviation of the scores in unchanged patients. Although the responsiveness ratio, 0.81, was inferior to the value calculated for the clinical indices (CDAI,[1] Harvey–Bradshaw[48]), it is consistent with values typically observed for other HRQL measures.

Although it was originally developed as a nurse-administered instrument, Irvine and colleagues have shown that the IBDQ can be self-administered without adversely affecting key operating properties. In a study of 67 patients with Crohn's disease no clinically important differences were observed in the mean IBDQ scores derived using the two different methods of

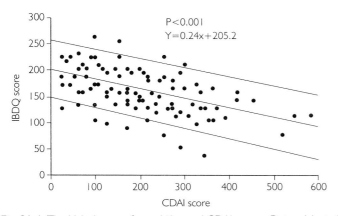

$P<0.001$
$Y=0.24x+205.2$

**Fig. 31.4** The high degree of correlation and CDAI scores. Data originated from a randomized trial of cyclosporine therapy for Crohn's disease. (Reprinted from Gastroenterology, 106, Irvine et al. Quality of life: a valid and reliable measure of therapeutic efficacy in the treatment of inflammatory bowel disease. 287–296, 1994, with permission from the American Gastroenterology Association.)

administration.[49] This was an important observation, as self-administration facilitates the performance of repeated measurements at low cost. Furthermore, mailing questionnaires[50] or the potential use of electronic administration[51] allows performance of large-scale epidemiological studies without the need for the patient to visit the investigational center on repeated occasions.

The IBDQ is now widely used as an outcome measure in randomized controlled trials. As a result, valuable new information regarding the clinical interpretation of IBDQ scores in patients with Crohn's disease has become available. A consistent observation from these studies is that patients in clinical remission generally have scores of 170 or more, whereas those with moderately severe disease activity have scores of 120 or less.[2,30,52,53]

In patients with Crohn's disease the minimum clinically important difference in IBDQ score is estimated to be 16 or more.[52,54] Unfortunately, similar relational data from large-scale studies in patients with ulcerative colitis are lacking.

## The Short Inflammatory Bowel Disease Questionnaire

Following the development of the IBDQ, an abbreviated version, the Short Inflammatory Bowel Disease Questionnaire (SIBDQ), was generated using the previously described CCRPT data. Irvine and colleagues[55] reduced the original 32 IBDQ items to 10 by selecting items that were most responsible for variability. As in the original questionnaire, these items were evaluated on a seven-point Likert scale, yielding a potential range in scores from 10 (poor HRQL) to 70 (optimum HRQL). Subsequently the operating properties of the SIBDQ were evaluated in a group of 150 patients with Crohn's disease and 45 patients with ulcerative colitis. In this study the SIBDQ explained respectively 92% and 90% of the variance in patients' IBDQ scores. The intraclass correlation coefficient in patients with stable Crohn's disease activity was 0.65, indicating that the modified instrument was suitably reliable. In patients who experienced a relapse of disease the average SIBDQ score increased by 9.3 points ($P=0.001$), which suggested that the instrument was responsive to a clinically meaningful change in health status. A second study performed by the same investigators in 109 patients with ulcerative

colitis and Crohn's disease confirmed their initial findings regarding the reliability of the instrument.[56]

Two additional evaluations of the SIBDQ in patients with ulcerative colitis have recently been reported. Han et al.[57] studied 122 outpatients with a diverse range of disease severities. Using the same methodology employed by the original developers of the SIBDQ, these investigators created a unique 'ulcerative colitis-specific' measure based on the SIBDQ. Although only three items were shared between the original SIBDQ and the newly derived instrument, the correlation between the two measures was high. Based on analysis of their data, Han et al. concluded that the original SIBDQ was also appropriate for use in UC and that their modification did not provide any additional value. In a second study, Jowett and colleagues[58] assessed the operating properties of the SIBDQ in 61 patients with UC. A high degree of correlation between the SIBDQ and clinical measures of disease severity was demonstrated ($r = 0.83$). Patients who experienced a minor flare of colitis showed, on average, a reduction of 11.8 points in the total SIBDQ score. The authors concluded that the SIBDQ could be reliably used to evaluate HRQL in ulcerative colitis.

In summary, the SIBDQ appears to be a useful modification of the original instrument that can be used to evaluate patients with both ulcerative colitis and Crohn's disease. However, additional data are required before it can be accepted as a convenient replacement for the IBDQ. Extensive large-scale experience with the SIBDQ in clinical investigation is lacking. A specific concern is the possibility of loss of responsiveness and reliability[59] that is frequently encountered when HRQL instruments undergo extensive item reduction. Nevertheless, this quality of life measure has great promise as an easily administered tool for epidemiological research and, possibly, as a guide to clinical practice.

## The Rating Form of IBD Patient Concerns (RFIPC)

In 1989 Drossman and colleagues[44] described a self-administered questionnaire that evaluated patients' disease-related concerns and worries. The intention was to identify specific concerns so that appropriate educational, psychological, compliance-enhancing or drug therapies could be implemented in patients at risk. The authors interviewed patients and recorded the findings by videotape. A list of 21 potential items was generated and assessed in 150 patients with IBD. Patients with ulcerative colitis were more concerned about the development of cancer or losing control of bowel function, whereas those with Crohn's disease identified pain and fertility as primary concerns (Table 31.2). The items in the RFIPC were grouped into four categories (body related, sex-related, disease related, inter-/intrapersonal). The developers subsequently modified the RFIPC by adding four additional items and scoring the items on a 10 cm visual analog scale. In a revalidation study[15] they administered the modified instrument to 150 patients with IBD. The primary concerns identified by patients who participated in this study were body image, lack of physical energy, requirement for surgery and the need for an ostomy. The modified questionnaire was subsequently administered to both mixed populations with IBD[60] and patients with ulcerative colitis.[61] For the most part the findings in these studies have been similar to the original reports. For example, Blondel-Kuchaski and colleagues[62] preferred a longitudinal evaluation of the instrument in 231 French patients with Crohn's disease. The most important areas of concern were

**Table 31.2 Patient concerns in inflammatory bowel disease: Numerical ranking and comparison of UC and CD outpatients. The data were obtained from a mixed population of patients with Crohn's disease and ulcerative colitis.**

| | ALL (N=150) Mean (S.D.) | UC (N=60) Mean (Rank) | CD (N=77) Mean (Rank) | P< |
|---|---|---|---|---|
| Sumscore | 39.0 (21.1) | 37.5 | 38 | |
| 1. Having ostomy bag | 63.3 (35.2) | 61.2 (1) | 62.1 (1) | |
| 2. Your energy level | 59.1 (31.5) | 57.6 (3) | 61.2 (2) | |
| 3. Having surgery | 55.8 (33.1) | 55.7 (5) | 55.7 (3) | |
| 4. Feelings about body | 55.1 (33.4) | 55.5 (6) | 50.8 (4) | |
| 5. Loss Bowel control | 49.9 (36.1) | 58.5 (2) | 44.9 (6) | .04 |
| 6. Developing cancer | 46.4 (33.6) | 55.9 (4) | 39.1 (9) | .005 |
| 7. Burden on others | 45.4 (36.1) | 45.0 (7) | 42.5 (7) | |
| 8. Pain | 43.2 (29.2) | 36.3 (12) | 46.6 (5) | .05 |
| 9. Producing odors | 42.5 (34.6) | 43.5 (8) | 39.1 (10) | |
| 10. Intimacy | 40.0 (33.9) | 40.3 (10) | 34.3 (11) | |
| 11. Financial Difficulties | 39.0 (34.9) | 31.2 (15) | 41.2 (8) | |
| 12. Feeling out of control | 36.2 (31.5) | 41.7 (9) | 31.6 (13) | |
| 13. Attractiveness | 35.3 (32.0) | 34.5 (14) | 31.6 (14) | |
| 14. Perform sexually | 34.7 (35.0) | 35.6 (13) | 29.0 (17) | |
| 15. Dying early | 34.5 (32.7) | 37.7 (11) | 29.9 (16) | |
| 16. Loss of sex drive | 33.2 (35.1) | 29.2 (17) | 33.5 (12) | |
| 17. Feeling alone | 28.1 (30.0) | 21.5 (19) | 30.4 (15) | |
| 18. Feeling dirty/smelly | 27.8 (31.8) | 30.4 (17) | 23.0 (20) | |
| 19. Pass inflammatory bowel disease to others | 26.6 (35.0) | 21.4 (20) | 28.0 (18) | |
| 20. Treated as having a defect | 25.1 (28.9) | 22.6 (18) | 24.6 (19) | |
| 21. Ability to have a child | 23.5 (32.1) | 14.0 (21) | 27.4 (21) | .03 |

Adapted with permission from Drossman, DA. et al. Health related quality of life in inflammatory bowel disease: Functional status and patient worries and concerns. Digestive Diseases and Sciences 1989;34(9):1379–1386.

'having an ostomy bag', 'uncertain nature of the disease', 'energy level' and 'having surgery'. However, Levenstein et al.[63] have recently documented large variability in some aspects of RFIBDPC scores in a study of 2002 patients from eight countries. First, the overall level of concern varied almost threefold across countries. Second, although 'having surgery', 'having an ostomy bag', 'uncertain nature of the disease' were again identified as the most prevalent concerns, the other items were scored markedly differently in different jurisdictions. Patients from southern European countries had the overall greatest degree of concern. The authors speculated that social, cultural or economic factors might be important explanatory variables. One unique observation was that the study was able to clearly determine a relationship between patients' concern regarding access to care and national economic wellbeing. Another interesting observation was made in a study by Moser and colleagues,[60] who demonstrated a strong negative correlation between RFIPC scores and perceived information level regarding IBD. This finding holds out the possibility that interventions designed to provide education to specific individuals may improve HRQL. Although extensive responsiveness testing of the RFIPC has not been performed, a preliminary evaluation in patients with ulcerative colitis indicates that this instrument will not be useful as an evaluative instrument in randomized controlled trials.[61] Nevertheless, the RFIPC may identify individuals who will benefit from directed psychological or educational interventions.

# DISEASE-SPECIFIC MEASUREMENT OF HRQL IN CHILDREN

Very few data are available regarding the HRQL of children with IBD. Several observational studies have suggested that young people experience a wide range of unique problems at various stages of their development.[64–66] However, analogous to the situation in adults prior to the development of the IBDQ and the RFIPC, the field has been limited by the lack of specific methodological tools. Recently, Griffiths and colleagues[67] have developed a disease-specific measure (IMPACT) for use in children with IBD using the methodology popularized by Guyatt. Initial item generation was performed in 82 patients. These items were then ranked by 117 patients (30 with ulcerative colitis, 87 with Crohn's disease) to develop a prototype questionnaire. In an initial study of 147 patients (97 CD, 50 UC) with an average age of 14 years, the questionnaire showed excellent reliability with an intraclass correlation quotation of 0.90.[45] Surprisingly, less than 1% of questions were left uncompleted by the children. Responsiveness was assessed by comparing the mean total scores among patients with quiescent, mildly active and more severe disease. Questionnaire scores were significantly different among these three groups of patients (180 +/− 32 vs 146 +/− 31 vs. 133 +/− 34, P=0.005 in either of the forms, respectively). Subsequently, Loonen and colleagues[68] described a modified version of this questionnaire

(IMPACT II) that they administered to 83 children with IBD. Validity and reliability testing were performed and demonstrated the modified instrument to be valid and stable in unchanged patients. The ICC for the six domains of the questionnaire ranged from 0.57 to 0.86. Although limited large-scale validation data from controlled clinical trials are currently available, both versions of the IMPACT questionnaire have great promise for future use in pediatric IBD research.

## POTENTIAL APPLICATIONS FOR HRQL ASSESSMENT

HRQL evaluation has many purposes.[69,70] Questionnaires are frequently used as outcomes measures in clinical trials. Epidemiological studies employ these instruments to document the burden of disease, to compare the relative effects on HRQL of different diseases, and to identify specific patient problems that lead to poor quality of life. Interventions can then be designed to determine whether these problems are modifiable. Easily administered instruments such as the SIBDQ may have value as practice management tools in the care of individual patients. Finally, utility estimation is essential for the performance of the cost–utility analyses that are the foundation of pharmacoeconomic comparisons in IBD. The remainder of this chapter reviews the present and future use of HRQL instruments in these areas.

## THE USE OF HRQL ASSESSMENTS IN CLINICAL TRIALS

A strong rationale exists for including HRQL assessments in randomized controlled trials.[71] Potential benefits include the opportunity to identify treatment effects not detectable by conventional measures of disease activity, to quantify negative aspects of drug therapy such as adverse drug reactions, to identify specific subgroups of patients who are more likely to respond to treatment, and to obtain essential information for pharmacoeconomic analyses. However, despite this wealth of potential, the value realized through the use of HRQL measures in clinical trials in IBD has been modest.

In 1990 Martin and colleagues[72] first reported use of an HRQL outcome in a randomized controlled trial that compared prednisone to 5-ASA in patients with active Crohn's disease. Following their initial experience with the IBDQ this instrument became accepted as a standard for use in comparative drug studies. Subsequent trials that evaluated 5-ASA,[73,74] budesonide,[75,76] cyclosporin,[47] methotrexate[52,53] and infliximab[2,30] all included IBDQ assessments. For the most part the results obtained in these studies were consistent. Effective medical therapy rapidly improved IBDQ scores. Typically, patients with active Crohn's disease have scores of approximately 120–130 at the baseline assessment. Following treatment with an effective drug, average scores increase to approximate 170–190 if a clinical response is observed. The magnitude of the change in mean IBDQ scores closely parallels that observed in mean CDAI scores (Fig. 31.5, A & B).[52] Although this observation is not surprising, given that the two measures are highly correlate,[17,55] it does call into question the incremental benefit of including the IBDQ as an efficacy measure in these studies.

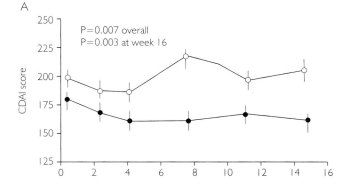

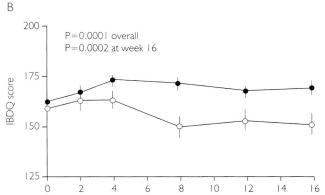

**Fig. 31.5** (A) The change in mean CDAI scores over 16 weeks in corticosteroid-dependent patients treated with either methotrexate or placebo in the NACSG. (Feagan BG, Rochon J, Fedorak RN et al. Methotrexate for the treatment of Crohn's disease. N Engl J Med 1995;332:292–297.) In the study trial prednisone was tapered from 20 mg to 0 mg. Note the increase in CDAI scores that occurs in the placebo group, whereas the average score in methotrexate-treated patients approaches remission = 150. (B) The corresponding IBDQ scores in the same patients. Note the 'mirror image' effect due to the high degree of inverse correlation between the IBDQ and CDAI. (Adapted from Feagan et al. N Engl J Med 1995;332:292–297.)

No example is available where a discordance has been identified between the results obtained using the CDAI and the IBDQ. Furthermore, it is has not yet been possible to characterize the adverse effects of investigational treatments using this instrument. Subgroup analyses based on assessment of IBDQ dimensional scores have also been disappointing. Generally, following administration of effective treatment, all four dimensional scores increase in a similar manner. Moreover, the greatest degree of change is consistently shown by the physical dimensions (bowel function, systemic symptoms) of the questionnaire that show the greatest degree of correlation with the CDAI score. Finally, no subgroup analysis of any clinical trial data has shown that an IBDQ-defined population of patients is more or less likely to respond to a drug of known efficacy.

These observations might lead some to call for a moratorium on the use of the IBDQ as an outcome measure in clinical trials. Although this may be an appropriate conclusion on the basis of the existing data, it is probably premature. Several characteristics of the IBDQ offer important advantages for use in randomized controlled trials. Namely, the IBDQ can be administered repeatedly, with a minimum of respondent burden and without the requirement for a physical examination or laboratory testing.

Thus IBDQ has repeatedly demonstrated a consistently high degree of correlation with the CDAI[17,55,74,76,77] and is of intrinsic relevance to patients. For these reasons the IBDQ remains attractive as an outcome measure for use in clinical trials. Furthermore, the extensive experience acquired over the past decade has familiarized investigators, clinicians and regulatory agencies with this outcome. For these reasons it is unlikely that the IBDQ will disappear from the clinical trial scene in the near future. However, more discriminating use of this measure is probably warranted. The IBDQ appears particularly well suited to the performance of long-term studies that require an instrument that is relatively inexpensive and easy to administer on multiple occasions.

Very limited experience is available with other HRQL instruments, with the exception of the SF-36, which has been utilized in a small number of studies.[30,78] Notably, in the ACCENT I trial the SF-36 detected a clinically meaningful improvement in health status following treatment with infliximab[30,79] (see Fig. 31.2). Although formal analyses of the operating properties of the SF-36 have not been performed, this finding indicates that this generic measure may be useful for inclusion in future studies.

## HRQL ASSESSMENTS IN DESCRIPTIVE EPIDEMIOLOGICAL STUDIES

Cohen[80] has performed a systematic review that evaluated epidemiological studies of HRQL in patients with a confirmed diagnosis of Crohn's disease. The analyses were restricted to studies that evaluated adult patients and were published as manuscripts in English. Studies that exclusively evaluated surgical treatments were not included.

The author concluded that the collective data indicate that HRQL is impaired in patients with Crohn's disease compared with healthy individuals. However, only one of the three comparative studies included in this analysis used a generic measure of HRQL. Two of the studies employed the IBDQ which, not surprisingly, demonstrated inferior scores in patients with Crohn's disease compared to healthy individuals.[50,81]

Many studies ($n = 9$)[11,15,44,60,82–86] were identified that compared the HRQL of patients with Crohn's disease to that of

patients with other disorders. Most of the studies compared patients with Crohn's disease to those with ulcerative colitis. The differences in IBDQ scores demonstrated between the two diseases was relatively small, but many of the studies indicated that patients with Crohn's disease had inferior HRQL than those with ulcerative colitis. A handful of studies used generic measures to compare the HRQL of patients with IBD to other chronic diseases. Patrick and Deyo[21] utilized the Sickness Impact Profile to create a league table of scores for various disorders. Again, patients with ulcerative colitis had better HRQL than those with Crohn's disease. However, patients with Crohn's disease had superior HRQL to those with rheumatoid arthritis, chronic renal failure and chronic obstructive lung disease. Gregor and colleagues[33] measured Standard Gamble scores in a convenience sample of patients with Crohn's disease and compared these scores to published data derived from patients with other diseases. Patients with active Crohn's disease had higher Standard Gamble scores than those with chronic renal failure receiving hemodialysis, but lower scores than patients with severe angina pectoris (Fig. 31.6). Although these results are interesting, such comparative studies should be interpreted with caution. No studies have been performed utilizing a random sample from a carefully defined population of patients. It is particularly difficult to compare severity of disease across different disorders; therefore, some of the comparisons described by these studies may be invalid. Furthermore, in the case of utility studies wide variations in measurement techniques and the choice of instruments may confound such comparisons.

Cohen identified eight studies[17,33,55,77,81,86–88] that compared the HRQL of patients with inactive and active disease. Despite the fact that a wide range of instruments was utilized in these studies, consistent results were obtained. Patients with active disease had inferior HRQL to those with disease in remission. Figure 31.3 shows the results of the previously mentioned study of Gregor and colleagues[33] that measured utility scores in 180 consecutive patients with Crohn's disease attending an outpatient clinic at a tertiary care center. In this study disease activity, defined by the CDAI, was the greatest predictor of HRQL as measured by the Standard Gamble. Surprisingly, even patients in remission had relatively poor utility scores. This inverse relationship between disease activity and HRQL has been consistently confirmed by other studies.

Finally, Cohen also reviewed four studies[81,89–91] that compared patients who received medical treatment to those who underwent surgery. Two of these studies provided unique information. Casellas and colleagues[81] compared 29 patients who underwent a bowel resection to 42 with active Crohn's disease and 48 with a medically induced remission. Patients completed the IBDQ and a psychological assessment, the Psychological General Well-Being Index. These investigators demonstrated impaired HRQL in patients with active disease compared to patients in remission; however, no difference was demonstrated between a medical or a surgically induced remission. They concluded that the type of treatment received by patients is not an independent determinant of HRQL. Tillinger and colleagues[90] prospectively followed 16 patients from the time of surgery to 24 months after the operation. During this interval multiple HRQL assessments (Time Trade-off, RFIPC, Beck Depression Inventory) and CDAI scores were obtained. Patients who entered remission ($n = 12$) showed an improvement in HRQL, whereas those with disease that remained chronically active ($n = 4$) continued to experience poor HRQL despite having

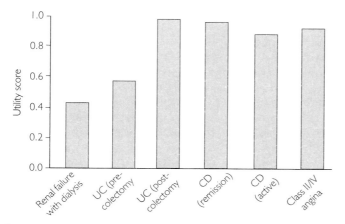

**Fig. 31.6** The Standard Gamble scores obtained from six different health states. A score of 0.0 means death, whereas 1.0 indicates perfect health. (Adapted with permission from Gregor et al. Inflamm Bowel Dis 1997;3:265–276.)

undergone surgery. Again, these data support the notion that disease activity is the dominant known predictor of HRQL in patients with Crohn's disease.

In summary, published epidemiological studies performed with valid HRQL instruments have generated an abundance of useful information. Patients with IBD have worse HRQL than healthy individuals, and those with Crohn's disease seem to fare worse than those with ulcerative colitis. Disease activity is highly correlated with HRQL, and interventions that control symptoms rapidly improve HRQL. Several areas of investigation are likely to be fertile in the future. First, the performance of population-based surveys of HRQL[50] would provide more valid information than that available in the current literature, which is for the most part based on convenience samples originating from tertiary care centers. Second, identification of factors that predict poor HRQOL in patients with relatively low disease activity might be productive. Preliminary data from studies that have utilized the RFIPC for this purpose suggest that many patients have important concerns that are not related to physical symptoms. In some patients interventions to treat these concerns may improve HRQL. Finally, population-based utility surveys will provide invaluable information for use in pharmacoeconomic analyses.

## HRQL ASSESSMENT AS A TOOL FOR PATIENT MANAGEMENT

Very few studies have been performed to explore the potential of HRQL assessment in the usual care of patients. However, the results of several recent investigations suggest that these instruments may have a beneficial role in management. Loudoun and colleagues[92] enrolled 12 sedentary patients with Crohn's disease to a 12-week aerobic exercise program. Participants walked approximately three times a week for an average of just over 30 minutes. Statistically significant improvements from baseline were shown in the body mass index, Harvey–Bradshaw score and an HRQL measure. These findings suggest that HRQL measurement may have a role in measuring the outcomes of targeted interventions. In another study Robinson et al.[93] randomly assigned 203 patients with ulcerative colitis to a patient-centered self-management training program with follow-up on request, or to usual care. The primary outcome measure was the interval between the onset of a relapse and the initiation of therapy. Patients who were assigned to the self-management group initiated therapy approximate 1.5 days faster than those in the control group and required, on average, two fewer visits to the hospital per patient managed. Surprisingly, HRQL scores were unchanged in the two treatment groups, which holds out the possibility that the intervention might have worsened HRQL in some patients. Although the results of this clinical trial do not support the use of HRQL monitoring as a guide to patient management, they illustrate the possibility of using quality of life assessment as one component of an integrated disease management program. Finally, data from a study by Borgaonkar and colleagues[94] highlight the need for controlled studies of interventions designed to improve HRQL. These investigators randomly assigned 59 patients to receive either an IBD-specific educational booklet or usual care. Following exposure to the intervention IBDQ scores were slightly but significantly lower in the group who received education. The authors concluded that the use of educational booklets in a tertiary care center is not beneficial and may worsen short-term HRQL outcomes. However, they also speculated that a different result might have been obtained by using this intervention in a population of newly diagnosed patients.

The studies suggest that sequential monitoring of HRQL using easily administered questionnaires may have a role to play in usual practice. From the perspective of large institutions, such as health maintenance organizations, collection of these data may be useful for quality assurance programs and to identify areas where additional resources are required. However, as two of the previously described studies demonstrate, the use of behavioural interventions and HRQL assessments may have the potential to worsen psychological wellbeing. Thus, controlled studies are required before these measurements are introduced into usual practice.

## THE ECONOMIC BURDEN OF IBD AND PHARMACOECONOMIC ANALYSES

A new era in the therapy of IBD has begun. Over the past decade several new therapies have been developed that have the potential to benefit patients. The introduction of targeted biologic therapy for rheumatoid arthritis and Crohn's disease has greatly advanced patient care. Nevertheless, monoclonal antibodies and recombinant human cytokines are expensive treatments and their addition to already strained pharmacy budgets has potential to create a crisis in many healthcare systems. In the near future many additional biopharmaceuticals will become available. Because resources are finite, sound decisions must be made regarding the funding of new drugs. Is society obtaining good value for money? How can we provide the best care at the lowest cost? To answer these questions comprehensive information regarding the cost of IBD and the relative effects of new treatments on patient outcomes are required.

## ESTIMATING THE ECONOMIC BURDEN OF IBD

Inflammatory bowel disease has a large economic impact for several reasons. First, daily drug therapy is necessary for many patients. Consequently, high lifetime drug acquisition costs are incurred. Second, many patients require surgery. Although an operation is usually effective in the short term, bowel resection may also cause considerable morbidity and, rarely, death. Moreover, in the case of Crohn's disease, disease recurrence frequently develops. Similarily, patients with ulcerative colitis who undergo the pelvic pouch procedure may develop pouchitis. Third, patients with IBD are typically young at the time of diagnosis, and lifelong treatment is usually required. Fourth, although conventional medical treatments, such as glucocorticoids and immunomodulatory drugs, are moderately effective, they also cause adverse reactions and require frequent monitoring by laboratory tests. Finally, and most importantly, patients with IBD have impaired HRQL despite current therapies.

Because the cost of inflammatory bowel disease is high in both humanistic and monetary terms it is vital to understand both the cost and the consequences of new treatments. Hence the rationale for performance of pharmacoeconomic analyses.

# CLASSIFICATION OF PHARMACOECONOMIC ANALYSES

Four unique types of pharmacoeconomic analysis can be performed. A common feature of all is that they relate expenditures, expressed in dollars, to specific outcomes. The key differences between the methods are the choice of outcome to which costs are linked.

The most basic technique is cost-minimization analysis, which is utilized when equivalent clinical outcomes result from two competing treatments.[95] Logically, the least expensive treatment is preferred, given that no clinically relevant difference in efficacy is measurable between the two alternatives. Although the simplicity of this approach is attractive, it is rarely useful in practice as the usual situation is that a new drug is both more expensive and more effective than a standard therapy. Even in the rare situation where two treatments show truly equivalent clinical efficacy other secondary differences usually exist, such as convenience of administration or side-effect profile, which make cost minimization analysis inappropriate. Thus more sophisticated types of pharmacoeconomic comparison are usually necessary.

The most commonly used method to assess the value of drug treatments is cost-effectiveness analysis.[96] This procedure relates the cost of a therapy to the achievement of a discrete, clinically relevant outcome. The incremental cost of a new therapy in comparison to usual care can be expressed in terms of dollars expended per beneficial outcome attained or negative outcome prevented. Cost-effectiveness analysis is particularly appropriate for the assessment of conditions such as cardiovascular disease, where robust, highly meaningful clinical endpoints occur frequently (i.e. death or myocardial infarction).[97–99] As these events have a distinct meaning to both healthcare providers and patients, the concept of expressing the cost of therapy in terms of dollars expended per adverse outcome avoided is easily understood and therefore attractive. However, cost-effectiveness analysis has important limitations. Foremost, it does not consider all of the potential health consequences of an intervention. This is an important issue for chronic diseases such as IBD, where the primary benefit of treatment is to control symptoms rather than to prevent death or major complications.

Another type of procedure, cost–benefit analysis,[100] relies on the 'human capital approach' to measure the relative values of different treatments. Differences in outcomes from two competing treatments are translated into monetary terms (as for the costs).[101,102] As this maneuver converts both expenditures and outcomes into the common unit of dollars, the comparison between treatments is easily interpreted: the strategy that maximizes value to society (i.e. net dollars gained) is preferred. However, the application of these analyses is of questionable relevance to healthcare applications, because the human capital approach requires relative valuations to be placed on human life and productivity. Such judgments are usually considered inappropriate by healthcare providers.

Finally, the analytical technique that is usually considered most appropriate for use in chronic diseases is cost–utility analysis.[103] As described previously, this method, which is a variant of cost-effectiveness analysis, generates estimates expressed in dollars expended per quality-adjusted life year (QALY) gained.[104] To illustrate this concept, consider the example of a new biologic therapy that improves the Standard Gamble scores of a group of patients with chronically active Crohn's disease by 0.2 points per year (0.7 to 0.9) at a net cost increase over standard therapy of $8,000 per annum. Over a 5-year period the patients treated with the new drug would gain 0.2 x 5 = 1.0 QALY in comparison to those who received standard therapy at a cost of $8,000 x 5 = $40,000. Therefore, the cost per QALY gained is $40,000. Empiric data indicate that society is generally willing to pay for interventions that cost US$60,000 or less per QALY gained.[105]

# MEASURING COSTS

## DIRECT VERSUS INDIRECT

Costs are classified into direct – goods and services consumed in the provision of health care to patients – and indirect – the costs that arise from the deleterious consequences of a disease on the social, economic and physical wellbeing of patients.[106] A distinction must also be made between costs and charges. Both costs and cost to charge ratios are influenced by multiple complex environmental factors and thus vary widely among jurisdictions. For this reason the cost component of pharmacoeconomic analyses is not usually generalizable between countries. Accordingly, it is usually necessary to obtain jurisdiction-specific cost inputs in economic models.

### Measurement of direct costs

The direct costs of IBD include the cost of providing inpatient and outpatient care, medications, and diagnostic testing.[107] Direct costs are readily identifiable and can be estimated using several different methods. The appropriate choice of methodology depends upon the sophistication of the model, the feasibility of acquiring relevant data, and the ultimate application of the results. First, data may be prospectively gathered during the course of a clinical trial or cohort study.[108] This choice generates high-quality information, but the cost estimates obtained may not be generalizable to usual care. A second option is to collect relevant cost data retrospectively from an administrative database.[109] This choice is attractive as it may be less costly than collecting data prospectively. Furthermore, the data may be more generalizable than those obtained from a clinical trial. However, information derived from an administrative dataset may not be in an optimal format. Most commonly the problems occur in linking costs to outcomes that may compromise the validity of the cost estimates derived. Finally, it is possible to generate cost estimates based on expert opinion. Although this approach is logistically simple, the validity of the data generated by this method may be poor. Pharmacoeconomic analyses commonly utilize a combination of these methods and the results are then subjected to appropriate sensitivity analyses.

### Measurement of indirect costs

Sources of indirect costs include absence from work, premature retirement, and the social and psychological effects of chronic morbidity.[110] The most easily quantifiable indirect costs are economic loss from absenteeism in the workplace, and disability and pension benefits resulting from premature retirement. Measurement of other indirect costs is more difficult. Many different types of indirect costs can be identified. IBD affects not only patients but also family members, friends and co-

**Table 31.3  Comparison of costs of inflammatory bowel disease in United States (1990)**

| Medical services | Crohn's disease | | Ulcerative colitis | |
|---|---|---|---|---|
| | Annual cost ($)* | Percentage (%) | Annual cost ($)* | Percentage (%) |
| Diagnostic work-up | 98 | 1.5 | 116 | 7.6 |
| Outpatient services | 192 | 2.9 | 105 | 7.1 |
| Medications | 671 | 10.2 | 125 | 8.4 |
| Surgery | 3,032 | 46.2 | 233 | 15.6 |
| Other inpatient services | 2,209 | 33.7 | 469 | 31.5 |
| Treatment of long-term complications | 358 | 5.5 | 439 | 29.5 |
| Total | 6,561 | 100 | 1,488 | 100 |

Sums are not exact because of rounding.
* In US dollars.
Reprinted with permission from Lippincott Williams & Wilkins from Hay JW, Hay AR. Inflammatory Bowel Disease. Cost of Illness. J Clin Gastroenterology. 1992;14(4):309–317.

workers. Thus illness experience by a single patient may generate an 'economic ripple effect' that influences many others. Accordingly, no standardized methodology for measurement of indirect cost has been universally accepted.[110] Nevertheless, for most diseases indirect costs usually exceed direct costs severalfold. Thus it is important for society to attempt to evaluate these expenditures.

# MEASURING THE COST OF INFLAMMATORY BOWEL DISEASE: COST OF ILLNESS STUDIES

Cost of illness studies are descriptive evaluations that assess the economic burden of a disease and define the relative proportions of total costs allocated to specific areas. These include the cost of diagnostic tests, healthcare professionals, institutions, drugs and social benefits. These studies are frequently used to generate hypotheses regarding the economic consequences of competing treatments. Data from cost of illness studies can identify areas where the efficiency of treatment can be improved. Few of these studies have been performed in IBD, and these investigations vary considerably in design, use of cost versus charge data, year of publication and country of origin.

In 1990 Hay and Hay[107] used data from a health maintenance organization to develop a cost of illness model for ulcerative colitis and Crohn's disease (Table 31.3). Charges obtained from a teaching hospital in San Francisco were multiplied by a cost to charge ratio of 0.65 to derive cost estimates. The model estimated the mean annual medical cost of Crohn's disease at $6,561 per person (Table 31.4) Approximately 20% of patients generated 80% of the total cost of the disease. The cost of ulcerative colitis was significantly lower and was estimated to be $1,488 per annum. Surgery and the provision of other types of care for inpatients were the most important cost sources. Collectively these items were responsible for 79.9% of the average costs of medical services utilized by patients with Crohn's disease, compared to only 57.1% of the corresponding costs for patients with ulcera-

**Table 31.4  Crohn's disease medical decision cost algorithm**

| Medical service | n/%* | Cost/patient | Cost/100 patients |
|---|---|---|---|
| Diagnostic workup† | 100 | $1,172 | $9,766 |
| Surgical intervention/year | | | |
| Colon | 4.46 | 18,614 | 83,016 |
| Small bowel | 5.03 | 20,847 | 104,861 |
| Small and large bowel | 7.04 | 16,380 | 115,315 |
| Medical Therapy | | | |
| Sulfasalazine | 64.80 | 304 | 19,724 |
| Prednisone | 41.73 | 443 | 18,488 |
| Metronidazole | 12.00 | 725 | 8,706 |
| Clindamycin | 5.00 | 3,109 | 15,546 |
| Azathioprine and 6-mercaptopurine | 5.54 | 840 | 4,655 |
| Hospitalisation‡ | 26.00 | 7,594 | 197,453 |
| Annual outpatient care§ | 76.00 | 253 | 19,239 |
| Extraintestinal manifestations (average per annum) | | | |
| Joint (ankylosing spondylitis, sacroiliitis, arthritis) | 3.47 | 261 | 908 |
| Ischemic necrosis of bone w/joint replacement | 0.40 | 18,614 | 7,445 |
| Renal stone disease/surgery | 1.20 | 5,212 | 6,254 |
| Cholelithiasis, cholecystectomy | 1.18 | 3,723 | 4,384 |
| Non-Hodgkin's lymphoma | 0.20 | 37,227 | 7,445 |
| Liver disease | 0.36 | 26,059 | 9,381 |
| **Total per 100 patients** | | | **$656,064** |

* As the sample group includes 100 patients, the percentage equals n.
† Diagnostic workup includes clinic visits, stool culture, stool for ova/parasites, Hemoccult®, upper intestinal radiography, barium enema, CAT scan, CBC, Chem-19, erythrocyte sedimentation rate, endoscopy.
‡ Hospitalisation includes lab tests, X-rays, enteral feedings, line placement.
§ Annual outpatient care includes blood tests, X-rays, office visits.
Reprinted with permission from Lippincott Williams & Wilkins from Hay AR, Hay JW. Inflammatory Bowel Disease: Medical Cost Algorithms. J Clin Gastroenterology. 1992;14(4):318–27.

tive colitis. A relatively small component of the total cost was attributable to drug therapy: 10.2% of the cost of Crohn's disease and 8.4% of the total cost of ulcerative colitis.

Subsequently these investigators modeled their data to estimate the overall cost of IBD to US society. Previously published prevalence estimates and data from the 1990 census were used to populate the model. The annual total direct cost of Crohn's disease was estimated to be $1.0–$1.2 bn annually, compared to $0.4–$0.6 bn for ulcerative colitis. The indirect cost of both diseases, based exclusively on estimates of economic loss in the workplace, was extrapolated to be $0.4–$0.8 bn. Based on these data, the total (direct plus indirect) economic burden for ulcerative colitis and Crohn's disease in the United States was estimated at $1.8–$2.6 bn per year.

Another cost of illness study evaluated reimbursement charges from patients enrolled in a health benefit claims program serving 50 of the largest US employers.[111] Eligible patients were enrolled in their health plan for a minimum of 3 years and had at least one Crohn's disease-related claim during 1994–1995. Patients were retrospectively classified into three mutually exclusive health states: mild disease – patients who were in remission or those with disease requiring less than 6 months of active treatment over the period of observation; moderate disease – patients who required chronic treatment (> 6 months) with prednisone or antimetabolites as outpatients; and severe disease – those patients who required admission to hospital for treatment. A total of 607 eligible patients were evaluable. The average charge per patient was $12,417. Charges for the mild, moderate and severe disease groups were $6,277, $10,033 and $37,135, respectively. As in the preceding study, a minority of the patients (25%) generated 80% of the total charges; 57% of the charges occurred as a result of inpatient care.

Finally, Bernstein and colleagues[112] estimated the direct costs of hospitalization for patients with Crohn's disease and ulcerative colitis who were admitted to a tertiary care hospital in the province of Manitoba, Canada, between 1994 and 1995. These investigators analyzed costs from 275 admissions and determined that the mean cost of Crohn's disease was $3,149 compared with $3,726 for ulcerative colitis. Surgery accounted for 49.8% of all admissions and 60.5% of the total inpatient costs.

## WHAT CONCLUSIONS CAN BE DRAWN FROM THESE STUDIES?

First, two of the studies show that the direct cost of care for Crohn's disease, in the setting of a US HMO during the first half of the 1990s, was approximately $6,600–$8,800 per annum (the first estimate is from Hay and Hay; the latter is derived by adjusting the data of Feagan et al. for a cost to charge ratio of 0.65 and an annual rate of inflation of 3%). Second, these studies demonstrate that provision of inpatient care to a minority of patients – 20–25% – is responsible for the majority of the cost of IBD. Third, the data of Hay and Hay indicate that ulcerative colitis probably has less overall economic impact than Crohn's disease.[107] Finally, the relatively low cost estimates obtained from inpatients in Manitoba, compared to US-derived data, highlights the importance of obtaining jurisdiction-specific cost estimates.

Although these three studies provide unique information they also suffer from the same fundamental flaw: because only highly selected, insured individuals who sought medical treatment were assessed, it is likely that the cost of treatment was overestimated. Ideally, cost data should be obtained from a defined cohort of patients who are residents of a region where health care is readily accessible and a comprehensive administrative database exists which has the capacity to reliably measures costs. Two such studies have been reported, one from Minnesota, the other from Sweden. The former concentrated on direct costs in patients with Crohn's disease, whereas the latter provides us with the only published data regarding indirect costs for both disorders.

## POPULATION-BASED COST ESTIMATES: DIRECT COST ESTIMATES FROM OLMSTED COUNTY

Silverstein et al.[113] retrospectively evaluated the direct costs from a cohort of residents of Olmsted County, Minnesota, diagnosed with Crohn's disease between 1970 and 1993. Patients were classified into one of eight unique health states. A Markov model estimated the duration of time spent in these states over the follow-up period. The transition probabilities between each of these states were estimated based on 2-month cycles. The direct costs of the disease were assigned to the specific health states using 1987–1996 charge data from the Olmsted County Utilization and Expenditure Database. Charges were converted to cost estimates in 1995 US dollars using the Medical Price Index. In this study the average lifetime cost of Crohn's disease was estimated to be $125,404 per patient. This estimate translates into an annual cost of $4,308 per patient per year. In accordance with the results of the previously described cost of illness studies, surgery accounted for 44% of the total costs. Surprisingly, 5-ASA for patients with mild disease accounted for 29 % of all costs.

## SWEDEN

A second population-based study, performed in Sweden, provides unique indirect cost data. Blomqvist and Ekbom identified all cases of Crohn's disease in Sweden during 1994.[114] Because access to health care is universal in Sweden this study is a comprehensive, cross-sectional evaluation of both the direct and the indirect burden of the disease. However, the latter analysis was restricted to economic loss caused by disease-related absence from work. The total direct cost of Crohn's disease, expressed in 1994 US dollars, was estimated to be $27.5 million. Admission to hospital was responsible for 58% of the total. The burden of indirect costs was estimated to be even greater, at $58.4 million. These large indirect costs were attributable to a small group of patients who were permanently disabled, and a significant rate of absenteeism due to illness. The average sick leave in the Swedish patients was more than 40 days.

Taken collectively, these population-based cost of illness studies suggest that the average cost estimates derived from HMO data probably overstate the true direct costs of Crohn's disease. This discordance is probably due to overrepresentation of more severely ill patients in the claims-based HMO datasets. The Swedish study also highlights the large burden of indirect costs. These costs are important from a societal perspective and should be considered when decisions are made regarding payment for new drugs. However, it must be emphasized that social programs differ greatly among countries. Thus further indirect costs studies from a broad sample of jurisdictions should be performed. Nevertheless, for many chronic diseases – and no sound argument exists that IBD is unique in this regard – indirect costs are conservatively estimated to be at least two to three times greater than direct costs.

A potential criticism of these analyses is that they may not reflect more recent trends in therapy, which include the use of newer medical treatments (aminosalicylates, antibiotics, 6-mercaptopurine, azathioprine, methotrexate, infliximab), an increased reliance on outpatient care, and an increased surgery rate for patients with Crohn's disease. Nevertheless, a distinct message emerges. Treatments that reduce the need for admission to hospital, surgery or absenteeism may result in important direct and indirect cost savings. A single study from a tertiary care centre provides support for the notion. Rubenstein et al.[115] have shown that patients with Crohn's disease treated with infliximab had significantly reduced use of surgery, fewer hospital visits and fewer diagnostic tests than their historical use of these services.

## COMBINING COSTS AND OUTCOMES: COST–UTILITY MODELS

Cost–utility analyses are well suited to evaluating new treatments for IBD as therapy is focused on improving patient well-being rather than increasing life expectancy. Given that society must make critical decisions regarding reimbursement for effective yet relatively costly new treatments, these analyses will become increasingly important over the next decade.

## EXAMPLES OF COST–UTILITY ANALYSIS

Very few IBD cost–utility analyses have been described in the literature. The pioneering example of this type of economic modeling was performed by Trallori and Messori,[116] who assessed the incremental cost utility of 5-ASA maintenance therapy for Crohn's disease compared to a no-maintenance treatment strategy. The natural history of the disease was estimated using data from a large-scale survey of Italian gastroenterologists. An estimate of the efficacy of 5-ASA maintenance therapy was derived from a meta-analysis performed by one of the authors. Cost estimates were based on published data obtained from a US health maintenance organization. A 5% annual discount rate was incorporated into the estimates, which were modeled on lifetime and 2-year time horizons. Utility estimates were assigned to five health states (remission in non-operated patients, remission in operated patients, relapse not requiring hospitalization, relapse requiring hospitalization without surgical intervention, and relapse requiring hospitalization and surgical intervention) according to the opinion of a group of 10 gastroenterologists. The model considered two hypothetical groups of 100 patients assigned to the competing strategies.

In this study the lifetime cost per QUALY of maintenance therapy was estimated to be $5,015. The authors concluded that chronic therapy with 5-ASA was associated with a small incremental benefit and costs. Sensitivity analyses indicated that the result was insensitive to differences in utility estimates but highly sensitive to variances in the cost of illness. If the cost of Crohn's disease was decreased by 20% the cost per QUALY gained was increased to $26,436. The effect of varying the efficacy estimates for 5-ASA was not examined.

This landmark study was the first attempt to examine economic and quality of life outcomes for Crohn's disease. It should be emphasized that the authors were limited by the quality of the data available at the time of publication. Since this time, additional information suggests that the marginal cost–utility estimate obtained in this study probably overstates the value of 5-ASA maintenance therapy for several reasons. First, the efficacy of maintenance therapy is probably less than the 12% annual absolute risk reduction used in the model. A subsequent meta-analysis by Camma et al.[117] could not identify a statistically significant effect of maintenance therapy following a medically induced remission. A modest benefit (9% absolute risk reduction per year) was observed following surgery. The authors also assumed that 5-ASA therapy prevented surgery and hospitalization. No data are available to support these assumptions. Second, as noted previously, the cost estimates of Hay and Hay probably overestimate the economic burden of the disease, as they were obtained from a referral population.

The second example of a cost–utility analysis comes from Arseneau and colleagues,[118] who compared ' standard therapy' with 6-MP/metronidazole to the following three infliximab-based strategies in patients with fistulizing Crohn's disease: (1) infliximab as an initial therapy followed by 6-MP/metronidazole for treatment failures; (2) infliximab alone with episodic reinfusion; (3) 6-MP/metronidazole as initial therapy followed by infliximab for failures of treatment with 6-MP/metronidazole. The investigators used a Markov model with a 1-month cycle length over a 12-month time horizon. Clinical data from the study of Present and colleagues and utilities derived from 32 patients with Crohn's disease and 20 healthy individuals were used to populate the model. Cost data were obtained from the University of Virginia administrative database. The investigators estimated an incremental cost–utility ratio of greater than $300,000 per QALY gained for all three infliximab strategies, a figure that indicates that this agreement may be of questionable cost-effectiveness. Although this analysis has been the subject of intense criticism,[119–121] these findings raise important questions regarding the economics of infliximab therapy for this indication.

## SUMMARY AND CONCLUSIONS

Over the past decade new data regarding the pharmacoeconomics of Crohn's disease have emerged. The synthesis of this information has culminated in the publication of the first economic models of the disease. Preliminary cost–utility models have been developed which compare the marginal cost of competing therapies with respect to effects on health-related quality of life. Because the validity of these comparisons is critically dependent upon accurate efficacy, natural history, cost and utility inputs, investigators should strive to identify areas where data are lacking and obtain the necessary information. Through this process, more highly refined and valid models will be developed.

Highly effective, yet costly, new treatments for Crohn's disease will soon be in widespread use. Because societal resources are limited healthcare providers will have to make intelligent choices regarding the introduction of new technologies. Cost–utility models incorporating HRQL data can provide useful guidance to decision-makers. Consideration of these analyses should result in improved patient wellbeing at a cost which is affordable to society.

# REFERENCES

1. Best WR, Becktel JM, Singleton J, Kern F Jr. Development of a Crohn's Disease Activity Index. Gastroenterology 1976;70:439–444.

2. Targan SR, Hanauer SB, van Deventer SJ et al. A short-term study of chimeric monoclonal antibody cA2 to tumor necrosis factor for Crohn's disease. N Engl J Med 1997;337:1029–1035.

3. Ghosh S, Goldin E, Gordon FH et al. Natalizumab for active Crohn's disease. N Engl J Med 2003;348:24–32.

4. Spilker B. Quality of life and pharmacoeconomics in clinical trials, 2nd edn. Philadelphia: Lippincott-Raven; 1996.

5. World Health Organization. Constitution of the World Health Organization, Annex I. 1958. Geneva, WHO. Ten Years of the World Health Organization. 1958.

6. Testa MA, Simonson DC. Assessment of quality-of-life outcomes. N Engl J Med 1996;334:835–840.

7. Edwards FC, Truelove SC. The course and prognosis of ulcerative colitis. Gut 1963;4:299–315.

8. Hendricksen C, Binder V. Social prognosis in patients with ulcerative colitis. Br Med J 1980;281:581–583.

9. Michener WM, Farmer RG, Mortimer EA. Long term prognosis of ulcerative colitis with onset in childhood or adolescence. J Clin Gastroenterol 1979;1:301–305.

10. Bergman L, Krause U. Crohn's disease: a long-term study of the clinical course in 186 patients. Scand J Gastroenterol 1977;12:937–944.

11. Sorenson VZ, Olsen BG, Binder V. Life prospects and quality of life in patients with Crohn's disease. Gut 1987;28:382–385.

12. Binder V, Hendriksen C, Kreiner S. Prognosis in Crohn's disease, based on results from a regional patient group from the county of Copenhagen. Gut 1985;26:146–150.

13. Guyatt G, Mitchell A, Irvine EJ et al. A new measure of health status for clinical trials in inflammatory bowel disease. Gastroenterology 1989;96:804–810.

14. Mitchell A, Guyatt G, Singer J et al. Quality of life in patients with IBD. J Clin Gastroenterol 1988;10:306–310.

15. Drossman DA, Leserman J, Li ZM et al. The Rating Form of IBD Patient Concerns: a new measure of health status. Psychosom Med 1991;53:701–712.

16. Guyatt G, Feeny D, Patrick D. Issues in quality-of-life measurement in clinical trials. Control Clin Trials 1991;12:81S–90S.

17. Irvine EJ, Feagan B, Rochon J et al. Quality of life: a valid and reliable measure of therapeutic efficacy in the treatment of inflammatory bowel disease. Gastroenterology 1994;106:287–296.

18. Deyo RA, Diehr P, Patrick D. Reproducibility and responsiveness of health status measures. Control Clin Trials 1991;12:142S–58S.

19. Guyatt G, Walter S, Norman G. Measuring change over time: assessing the usefulness of evaluative instruments. J Chronic Dis 1987;40:171–178.

20. Fitzpatrick, R. Quality of life measures in health care. Br Med J 1992;305: 74–77.

21. Patrick DL, Deyo RA. Generic and disease-specific measures in assessing health status and quality of life. Med Care 1989;27:S217–S232.

22. Gilson BS, Gilson JS, Bergner M et al. The Sickness Impact Profile. Development of an outcome measure of health care. Am J Public Health 1975;65:1304–1310.

23. Chambers LW, MacDonald LA, Tugwell P, Buchanan WW, Kraag G. The McMaster Health Index Questionnaire as a measure of quality of life for patients with rheumatoid disease. J Rheumatol 1982;9:780–784.

24. Hunt SM, McKenna SP, McEwen J, Williams J, Papp E. The Nottingham Health Profile: subjective health status and medical consultations. Soc Sci Med 1981;15:221–229.

25. Ware JE Jr, Sherbourne CD. The MOS 36-Item Short-Form Health Survey (SF-36). I. Conceptual framework and item selection. Med Care 1992;30:473–483.

26. Ware JE. SF-36 Physical and Mental Health Summary Scales: a user's manual, 3rd edn. Boston: The Health Institute; 1994.

27. Ware JE. SF-36 Health survey manual and interpretation guide. Boston: The Health Institute; 1993.

28. Welch G, Richter J, Kawachi I, Bachwich D. The SF-36 Quality of Life Measure in inflammatory bowel disease: an evaluation of its reliability and validity. Gastroenterology 1995;108:A940.

29. Colombel J-F, Yazdanpanah Y, Laurent F, Houcke P, Delas N, Marquis P. Quality of life in chronic inflammatory bowel disease. Validation of a questionnaire. Gastroenterol Clin Biol 1996;20:1071–1077.

30. Hanauer SB, Feagan BG, Lichtenstein GR and the ACCENT I Study Group. Maintenance infliximab for Crohn's disease: the ACCENT I randomised trial. Lancet 2002;359:1541–1549.

31. Brazier J. The Short Form 36 (SF-36) Health Survey and its use in pharmacoeconomic evaluation. PharmacoEconomics 1995;7:403–415.

32. Torrance GW. Health index and utility models: some thorny issues. Health Serv Res 1973;8:12–14.

33. Gregor JC, McDonald JWD, Klar N et al. An evaluation of the utility measurement in Crohn's disease. Inflamm Bowel Dis 1997;3:265–276.

34. Torrance GW. Utility approach to measuring health-related quality of life. J Chronic Dis 1987;40:593–600.

35. Drummond MF, O'Brien B, Stoddart GL, Torrance GW. Methods for the economic evaluation of health care programmes, 2nd edn. Oxford: Oxford University Press; 1987.

36. Sackett DL, Torrance GW. The utility of different health states as perceived by the general public. J Chronic Dis 1978;31:697–704.

37. Churchill DN, Torrance GW, Taylor DW et al. Measurement of quality of life in end-stage renal disease: the time trade-off approach. Clin Invest Med 1987;10:14–20.

38. Froberg DG, Kane RL. Methodology for measuring health-state preferences – II: Scaling methods. J Clin Epidemiol 1989;42:459–471.

39. Torrance GW, Furlong W, Feeny D, Boyle M. Multiattribute preference functions. Health utilities index. PharmacoEconomics 1995;7:503–520.

40. The EuroQol Group. EuroQol – a new facility for the measurement of health-related quality of life. The EuroQol Group. Health Policy 1990;16:199–208.

41. Boyle M, Furlong W, Feeny D, Torrance GW, Hatcher J. Reliability of the Health Utilities Index – Mark III used in the 1991 Cycle 6 Canadian General Social Survey Health Questionnaire. Qual Life Res 1995;4:249–257.

42. Nord E. EuroQol: Health-related quality of life measurement. Valuations of health states by the general public in Norway. Health Policy 1991;18:25–36.

43. Konig HH, Ulshofer A, Gregro M et al. Validation of the EuroQol questionnaire in patients with inflammatory bowel disease. Eur J Gastroenterol Hepatol 2002;14:1205–1215.

44. Drossman DA, Patrick DL, Mitchell CD, Zagami EA, Appelbaum MI. Health-related quality of life in inflammatory bowel disease. Dig Dis Sci 1989;34:1379–1386.

45. Otley A, Smith C, Nicholas D et al. The IMPACT questionnaire: a valid measure of health related quality of life in pediatric inflammatory bowel disease. J Pediatr Gastroenterol Nutr 2002;35:557–563.

46. Kirshner B, Guyatt G. A methodological framework for assessing health indices. J Chronic Dis 1985;38:27–36.

47. Feagan BG, McDonald JWD, Rochon J et al. Low-dose cyclosporine for the treatment of Crohn's disease. N Engl J Med 1994;330:1846–1851.

48. Harvey RF, Bradshaw JM. A simple index of Crohn's disease activity. Lancet 1980;1:514.

49. Irvine EJ, Feagan BG, Wong CJ. Does self-administration of a quality of life index for inflammatory bowel disease change the results? J Clin Epidemiol 1996;49:1177–1185.

50. Love JR, Irvine EJ, Fedorak RN. Quality of life in inflammatory bowel disease. J Clin Gastroenterol 1992;14:15–19.

51. Soetikno RM, Mrad R, Pao V, Lenert LA. Quality of life research on the Internet: feasibility and potential biases in patients with ulcerative colitis. J Am Med Inform Assoc 1997;4:426–435.

52. Feagan BG, Rochon J, Fedorak RN et al. Methotrexate for the treatment of Crohn's Disease. N Engl J Med 1995;332:292–297.

53. Feagan BG, Fedorak RN, Irvine EJ et al. A comparison of methotrexate with placebo for the maintenance of remission in Crohn's disease. North American Crohn's Study Group Investigators. N Engl J Med 2000;342:1627–1632.

54. Jaeschke R, Singer J, Guyatt GH. Measurement of health status. Ascertaining the minimal clinically important difference. Control Clin Trials 1989;10:407–415.

55. Irvine EJ, Zhou Q, Thompson AK, CCRPT Investigators. The Short Inflammatory Bowel Disease Questionnaire: a quality of life instrument for community physicians managing inflammatory bowel disease. Am J Gastroenterol 1996;91:1571–1578.

56. Irvine EJ, Levine DS, Lashner BA, Thompson AK, Zhou Q. A Short health-related quality of life instrument for inflammatory bowel disease in clinical practice. Gastroenterology 1997;112:A1003.

57. Han SW, Gregory W, Nylander D et al. The SIBDQ: further validation in ulcerative colitis patients. Am J Gastroenterol 2000;95:145–151.

58. Jowett SL, Seal CJ, Barton JR, Welfare MR. The short inflammatory bowel disease questionnaire is reliable and responsive to clinically important change in ulcerative colitis. Am J Gastroenterol 2001;96:2921–2928.

59. Moran L-A, Guyatt G, Norman GR. Establishing the minimal number of items for a responsive, valid, health-related, quality of life instrument. J Clin Epidemiol 2001;54:571–579.

60. Moser G, Tillinger W, Sachs G et al. Disease-related worries and concerns: a study on out-patients with inflammatory bowel disease. Eur J Gastroenterol Hepatol 1995;7:853–858.

61. Hjortswang H, Strom M, Almeida RT, Almer S. Evaluation of the RFIPC, a disease-specific health-related quality of life questionnaire, in Swedish patients with ulcerative colitis. Scand J Gastroenterol 1997;32:1235–1240.

62. Blondel-Kucharski F, Chircop C, Marquis P et al. Health-related quality of life in Crohn's disease: a prospective longitudinal study in 231 patients. Am J Gastroenterol 2001;96:2915–2920.

63. Levenstein S, Li Z, Almer S et al. Cross-cultural variation in disease-related concerns among patients with inflammatory bowel disease. Am J Gastroenterol 2001;96:1822–1830.

64. MacPhee M, Hoffenberg EJ, Feranchak A. Quality of life factors in adolescent inflammatory bowel disease. Inflamm Bowel Dis 1998;4:6–11.

65. Rabbett H, Elbadri A, Thwaites R et al. Quality of life in children with Crohn's disease. J Pediatr Gastroenterol Nutr 1996;23:528–533.

66. Engstrom I, Lindquist BL. Inflammatory bowel disease in children and adolescents: a somatic and psychiatric investigation. Acta Paediatr Scand 1991;80:640–647.

67. Griffiths AM, Nicholas D, Smith C et al. Development of a quality of life index for pediatric inflammatory bowel disease: dealing with differences related to age and IBD type. J Pediatr Gastroenterol Nutr 1999;28:S46–S52.

68. Loonen HJ, Grootenhuis MA, Last BF, de Haan RJ, Bouquet J, Derkx BH. Measuring quality of life in children with inflammatory bowel disease: the IMPACT -II (NL). Qual Life Res 2002;11:47–56.

69. Wood-Dauphinee S. Assessing quality of life in clinical research: from where have we come and where are we going? J Clin Epidemiol 1999;52:355–363.

70. Spilker B. Introduction. In: Spilker B, ed. Quality of life and pharmacoeconomics in clinical trials, 2nd edn. Philadelphia: Lippincott-Raven; 1996:1–10.

71. Guyatt G, Sackett D, Adachi J et al. A clinician's guide for conducting randomized trials in individual patients. CMAJ 1988;139:497–505.

72. Martin F, Sutherland L, Beck IT et al. Oral 5-ASA versus prednisone in short term treatment of Crohn's disease: a multicentre controlled trial. Can J Gastroenterol 1990;4:452–457.

73. Singleton JW, Hanauer SB, Gitnick GL et al. Mesalamine capsules for the treatment of active Crohn's disease: results of a 16-week trial. Pentasa Crohn's Disease Study Group. Gastroenterology 1994;107:632–633.

74. Singleton JW, Hanauer S, Robinson M. Quality-of-life results of double-blind, placebo-controlled trial of mesalamine in patients with Crohn's disease. Dig Dis Sci 1995;40:931–935.

75. Greenberg GR, Feagan BG, Martin F et al. Oral budesonide for active Crohn's disease. N Engl J Med 1994;331:836–841.

76. Irvine EJ, Greenberg GR, Feagan BG et al. Quality of life rapidly improves with budesonide therapy for active Crohn's disease. Canadian Inflammatory Bowel Disease Study Group. Inflamm Bowel Dis 2000;6:181–187.

77. Lopez-Vivancos J, Casellas FJ, Badia X et al. Validation of the Spanish version of the Inflammatory Bowel Disease Questionnaire on Ulcerative Colitis and Crohn's Disease. Digestion 1999;60:274–280.

78. Smith GD, Watson R, Roger D et al. Impact of a nurse-led counselling service on quality of life in patients with inflammatory bowel disease. J Adv Nurs 2002;38:152–160.

79. Feagan BG, Yan S, Bala M, Boa W, Olson A, Hanauer S. Infliximab (Remicade) maintenance therapy improves health related quality of life in Crohn's disease over 54 weeks. Gastroenterology 2002;122:A615.

80. Cohen RD. The quality of life in patients with Crohn's disease. Aliment Pharmacol 2002;16:1603–1609.

81. Casellas FJ, Lopez-Vivancos J, Badia X, Vilaseca J, Malagelada JR. Impact of surgery for Crohn's disease on health-related quality of life. Am J Gastroenterol 2000;95:177–182.

82. Farmer RG, Easley KA, Farmer J. Quality of life assessment by patients with inflammatory bowel disease. Cleve Clin J Med 1992;59:35–42.

83. Kim WH, Cho YS, Yoo HM et al. Quality of life in Korean patients with inflammatory bowel diseases: ulcerative colitis, Crohn's disease and intestinal Behçet's disease. Int J Colorectal Dis 1999;14:52–57.

84. Verissimo RM-CR, Taylor G. Relationships between alexithymia, emotional control, and quality of life in patients with inflammatory bowel disease. Psychotherapy Psychosom 1998;67:75–80.

85. Drossman DA, Leserman J, Mitchell CM et al. Health status and health care use in persons with inflammatory bowel disease. Dig Dis Sci 1991;36:1746–1755.

86. Drossman DA, Li Z, Leserman J, Patrick DL. Ulcerative colitis and Crohn's disease health status scales for research and clinical practice. J Clin Gastroenterol 1992;15:104–112.

87. Russel MG, Pastoor CJ, Brandon S et al. Validation of the Dutch translation of the Inflammatory Bowel Disease Questionnaire (IBDQ): a health related quality of life questionnaire in inflammatory bowel disease. Digestion 1997;58:282–288.

88. Martin A, Leone L, Fries W et al. Quality of life in inflammatory bowel disease. Ital J Gastroenterol 1995;27:450–454.

89. Thirlby RC, Land JC, Fenster LF et al. Effect of surgery on health-related quality of life in patients with inflammatory bowel disease: a prospective study. Arch Surg 1998;133:826–832.

90. Tillinger W, Mittermaier C, Lochs H, Moser G. Health-related quality of life in patients with Crohn's disease: influence of surgical operation – a prospective trial. Dig Dis Sci 1999;44:932–938.

91. Yazdanpanah Y, Klein O, Gambiez L et al. Impact of surgery on quality of life in Crohn's disease. Am J Gastroenterol 1997;92:1897–1900.

92. Loudon CP, Corroll V, Butcher J, Rawsthorne P, Bernstein CN. The effects of physical exercise on patients with Crohn's disease. Am J Gastroenterol 1999;94:697–703.

93. Robinson A, Thompson DG, Wilkin D, Roberts C. Guided self-management and patient-directed follow-up of ulcerative colitis: a randomised trial. Lancet 22001;358:976–981.

94. Borgaonkar MR, Townson G, Donnelly M, Irvine EJ. Providing disease-related information worsens health-related quality of life in inflammatory bowel disease. Inflamm Bowel Dis 22002;8:264–269.

95. Marra FO, Frighetto LO, Marra CA et al. Cost-minimization analysis of piperacillin/tazobactam versus imipenem/cilastatin for the treatment of serious infections: a Canadian hospital perspective. Ann Pharmacother 1999;33:156–162.

96. Teutsch SM, Murray JF. Dissecting cost-effectiveness analysis for preventive interventions: a guide for decision makers. Am J Manag Care 1999;5:301–305.

97. Mahoney EM, Jurkovitz CT, Chu H et al. Cost and cost-effectiveness of an early invasive vs conservative strategy for the treatment of unstable angina and non-ST-segment elevation myocardial infarction. JAMA 2002;288:1851–1858.

98. Nathoe HM, van Dijk D, Jansen EW et al. A comparison of on-pump and off-pump coronary bypass surgery in low-risk patients. N Engl J Med 2003;348:394–402.

99. Brosa M, Rubio-Terres C, Farr I, Nadipelli V, Froufe J. Cost-effectiveness analysis of enoxaparin versus unfractional heparin in the secondary prevention of acute coronary syndrome. Pharmcoeconomics 2002;20:979–987.

100. Robinson R. Cost–benefit analysis. Br Med J 1993;307:924–926.

101. Jimenez FJ, Guallar-Castillon P, Rubio TC, Guallar E. Cost-benefit analysis of haemophilus influenzae type b vaccination in children in Spain. PharmacoEconomics 1999;15:75–83.

102. Merkesdale S, Ruof J, Schoffski O, Bernitt K, Zeidler H, Mau W. Indirect medical costs in early rheumatoid arthritis: composition of and changes in indirect costs within the first three years of disease. Arthritis Rheum 2001;44:528–534.

103. Gerard K, Smoker I, Seymour J. Raising the quality of cost–utility analyses: lessons learnt and still to learn. Health Policy 1999;46:217–238.

104. Weinstein MC, Stason WB. Foundations of cost-effectiveness analysis for health and medical practices. N Engl J Med 1977;296:716–721.

105. Laupacis A, Feeny D, Detsky AS, Tugwell PX. How attractive does a new technology have to be to warrant adoption and utilization? Tentative guidelines for using clinical and economic evaluations. CMAJ 1992;146:473–481.

106. Brooten D. Methodological issues linking costs and outcomes. Med Care 1997;35:87–95.

107. Hay JW, Hay AR. Inflammatory bowel disease: cost-of-illness. J Clin Gastroenterol 1992;14:309–317.

108. Schulman KA, Ohishi A, Park J, Glick HA, Eisenberg JM. Clinical economics in clinical trials: the measurement of cost and outcomes in the assessment of clinical services through clinical trials. Keio J Med 1999;48:1–11.

109. Steiner C, Elixhauser A, Schnaier J. The healthcare cost and utilization project: an overview. Eff Clin Pract 2002;5:143–151.

110. Jacobs P, Fassbender K. The measurement of indirect costs in the health economics evaluation literature. A review. Int J Technol Assess Health Care 1998;14:799–808.

111. Feagan BG Larson LR, Vreeland MG et al. Annual cost of care for Crohn's disease patients. A claims-based cost of illness evaluation. Gastroenterology 1999;116:G0239.

112. Bernstein CN, Papineau N, Zajaczkowski J, Rawsthorne P, Okrusko G, Blanchard JF. Direct hospital costs for patients with inflammatory bowel disease in a Canadian tertiary care university hospital. Am J Gastroenterol 2000;95:677–683.

113. Silverstein MD, Loftus EV, Sandborn WJ et al. Clinical course and costs of care for Crohn's disease: Markov model analysis of a population-based cohort. Gastroenterology 1999;117:49–57.

114. Blomqvist P, Ekbom A. Inflammatory bowel disease: health care and costs in Sweden in 1994. Scand J Gastroenterol 1997;32:1134–1139.

115. Rubenstein JH, Chong RY, Cohen RD. Infliximab decreases resource use among patients with Crohn's disease. J Clin Gastroenterol 2002;35:151–156.

116. Trallori G, Messori A. Drug treatments for maintaining remission in Crohn's disease. A lifetime cost–utility analysis. PharmacoEconomics 1997;11:444–453.

117. Camma C, Giunta M, Rosselli M, Cottone M. Mesalamine in the maintenance treatment of Crohn's disease: a meta-analysis adjusted for confounding variables. Gastroenterology 2001;113:1465–1473.

118. Arseneau KO, Cohn SM, Cominelli F, Connors AF Jr. Cost–utility of initial medical management for Crohn's disease perianal fistuale. Gastroenterology 2001;120:1640–1656.

119. Cohen RD. Cost utility of initial medical management for Crohn's disease perianal fistula. Gastroenterology 2002;122:1187–1188.

120. Mitton CR. Funding the new biologics – a health economic critique of the CCOHTA report: Infliximab for the Treatment of Crohn's Disease. Can J Gastroenterol 2002;16:873–876.

121. Hilsden R. Funding the new biologics – what can we learn from infliximab? The CCOHTA Report: a gastroenterologist's viewpoint. Can J Gastroenterol 2002;16:865–868.

## CHAPTER 32

# Clinical pharmacology of inflammatory bowel disease therapy

Uma Mahadevan and William J Sandborn

## INTRODUCTION

As our understanding of the immunologic and genetic basis of inflammatory bowel diseases (IBD) grows, potential therapeutic options are being developed at a rapid pace. However, the majority of patients will still require medical therapy with established agents or will use the new drugs in conjunction with existing therapies. For this reason, understanding the mechanism of action and clinical pharmacology of current medical options for Crohn's disease and ulcerative colitis remains important. In this chapter we will review the clinical pharmacology of standard therapies for IBD, including mesalamine, corticosteroids, immunosuppressants and infliximab.

## AMINOSALICYLATES

Sulfasalazine (SAS), a combination of 5-aminosalicylic acid (5-ASA) azo-bound to the antibiotic sulfapyridine, is effective for the treatment of ulcerative colitis and Crohn's disease. Further investigation suggested that it was the 5-ASA component rather than the sulfapyridine moiety that was the therapeutically active compound in UC.[1-4] Thus, SAS is a prodrug. This finding, as well as the high rate of intolerance to sulfasalazine owing to the systemic absorption of sulfapyridine,[1,5] led to the development of alternative 5-ASA delivery systems for the treatment of IBD.

## MECHANISMS OF ACTION

5-ASA differs from salicylic acid by the addition of an amino group at the 5 (meta) position. 5-Aminosalicylate has pharmacological properties that are different from those of other salicylates such as aspirin. Unlike salicylates, which block prostaglandin synthesis by inhibition of the cyclooxygenase enzymes 1 and 2, 5-aminosalicylates such as 5-ASA and sulfasalazine have variable effects on arachidonic acid metabolites.

Higher concentrations of aminosalicylates inhibit production of prostaglandins and prostacyclin,[6,7] whereas lower concentrations increase prostaglandin production.[8,9] It seems clear that modulation of prostaglandin metabolism in the inflamed gut is not the sole therapeutic action of 5-aminosalicylates, as other more potent inhibitors of cyclooxygenase, such as non-steroidal anti-inflammatory agents (NSAIDs), either have no effect or can potentially exacerbate IBD.[10] Both agents also inhibit 5-lipoxygenase and 5-lipoxygenase activating protein, which then block the production of leukotrienes.[11]

Proinflammatory cytokines such as tumor necrosis factor (TNF), interleukin-1 (IL-1) and interferon (IFN)-γ have important roles in the pathogenesis of IBD.[12,13] Sulfasalazine and 5-ASA have multiple anti-inflammatory effects. Both inhibit the production of IL-1 and TNF.[14-16] Additionally, sulfasalazine inhibits TNF binding with its receptor,[17] thereby reducing signaling for further inflammatory responses. Finally, 5-ASA is an antioxidant and free radical scavenger.[18-20] Some of the anti-inflammatory effects of sulfasalazine and 5-ASA may be mediated through the inhibition of activation of nuclear factor-κB (NFκB). The inducible transcription factor NFκB is an important regulator of the expression of immune response genes in the gut.[21-24] Azo-bound 5-aminosalicylates such as sulfasalazine inhibit the activity of NFκB by blocking the inducible degradation of its cytosolic inhibitor IκBα.[25] 5-ASA also inhibits the activity of NFκB,[26,27] possibly by inhibiting phosphorylation of the NFκB protein RelA (p65).[26] A recent in vivo study in patients with ulcerative colitis demonstrated the ability of 5-ASA to downregulate activation of NFκB in actively inflamed mucosa.[28]

## FORMULATION AND PHARMACOKINETICS

Aminosalicylates are intended to have a local or 'topical' effect on the diseased bowel in IBD. Orally administered free 5-ASA is rapidly and nearly complete absorbed in the proximal small intestine, followed by extensive metabolism to N-acetyl-5-ASA by the N-acetyltransferase 1 (NAT1) enzyme in intestinal

## Table 32.1 5-ASA preparations

| Generic name | Proprietary names | 5-ASA delivery mechanism | Sites of delivery | *Absorption (Reference) (%) | Daily dose, range (g) |
|---|---|---|---|---|---|
| Mesalamine | Rowasa Salofalk | Enema suspension | Left colon and rectum | 13[266] | 1–4 |
| Mesalamine | Rowasa | Suppository | Rectum | 24[51] | 0.5–1.5 |
| Mesalamine | Asacol | Eudragit-S coated tablets (release at pH>7) | Terminal ileum, colon | 23[40] 24[267] 31[41] | 1.6–4.8 |
| Mesalamine | Salofalk, Mesasal, Claversal | Mesalamine in sodium/glycerine buffer coated with Eudragit-L (release at pH >6) | Distal jejunum, proximal ileum | 40[268] 54[41] | 1.5–4 |
| Mesalamine | Pentasa | Ethylcellulose coated microgranules (time- and pH-dependent release) | Entire small bowel, colon | 30[38] 36[41] | 2–4 |
| Sulfasalazine | Azulfidine | 5-ASA azo bound to sulfapyridine | Colon | 11[40] | 1–4 |
| Olsalazine | Dipentum | 5-ASA dimer, linked by azo bond | Colon | 10[40] 17[267] 22[41] | 1–3 |
| Balsalazide | Colazal | 5-ASA azo bound to inert carrier | Colon | 20–25[269] | 2–6.75 |

*Absorption is estimated from cumulative urinary excretion of 5-ASA + acetyl-5-ASA, expressed as a % of total administered dose.

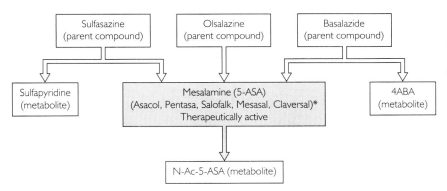

Fig. 32.1 Pharmacologic fate of the different oral formulations of 5-ASA. *Asacol, Pentasa, Salofalk, Mesasal and Claversal deliver 5-ASA via delayed- and controlled-release formulations. Arrows represent metabolic pathways. N-Ac-5-ASA = acetylated 5-aminosalicylic acid. 4-ABA = 4-aminobenzoyl-β-alanine.

epithelial cells and the liver, and is then excreted in the urine as a mixture of free 5-ASA and N-acetyl-5-ASA.[29–31] A variety of formulations have been developed that 'protect' 5-ASA from release, absorption and metabolism in the stomach and proximal small bowel. These formulations either deliver the drug orally as delayed-release tablets, controlled-release microgranules and prodrug tablets, or rectally as enemas or suppositories (Table 32.1). Figure 32.1 illustrates the manner in which each drug is released and metabolized in the gut. pH-dependent resins protect 5-ASA from release in the acidic proximal small bowel, resulting in 'delayed release' of 5-ASA when the intestinal pH rises above a certain threshold, theoretically permitting targeted delivery to a specific intestinal site based on luminal pH. Eudragit S-coated 5-ASA (Asacol) releases at pH 7 in the terminal ileum. Eudragit L-coated 5-ASA (Salofalk, Mesasal, Claversal) releases at pH 5–6 in the mid-small intestine. Ethyl cellulose coated microgranules containing 5-ASA (Pentasa) slowly dissolve throughout the small intestine and colon independent of pH, resulting in 'controlled release' of 5-ASA. Approximately 75% of the Pentasa microgranules pass into the colon. Azo-bound 5-ASA prodrugs (sulfasalazine, olsalazine, balsalazide) are metabolized in the colonic lumen by bacterial azo-reductase enzymes, resulting in the release of free 5-ASA in the colon.[32,33] Approximately 85% of sulfasalazine is metabolized by intestinal bacteria to sulfapyridine and 5-ASA, and 15% is absorbed as the parent compound. Sulfapyridine is then systemically absorbed from the colon and transported to the liver, where it is metabolized via acetylation to form

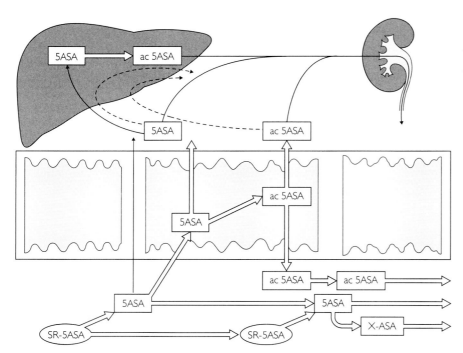

**Fig. 32.2** Elimination pathways of 5-ASA following release of sustained-release drug. SR-5-ASA = sustained release 5-ASA. ac 5-ASA = N-acetyl-5-ASA. 5-ASA = 5-aminosalicylic acid. X – ASA = other metabolites/not defined. (Reproduced with permission from Bondesen S. Pharmacol Toxicol 1997;8:1–28.)

N-acetylsulfapyridine. Acetylator status is genetically determined.[34] Fast acetylators have a mean plasma half-life of sulfapyridine of 10.4 hours, and slow acetylators 14.8 hours. Sulfapyridine can also be metabolized to 5-hydroxysulfapyridine and N-acetyl-5-hydroxysulfapyridine[35] and then excreted in the urine.

A significant portion of the free 5-ASA released topically by the various oral 5-ASA formulations and prodrugs is absorbed into the colonic epithelium, where it undergoes extensive metabolism to N-acetyl-5-ASA by the enzyme NAT1[36] (Fig. 32.2). From the colonic epithelium, N-acetyl-5-ASA is either absorbed systemically and excreted in the urine, or secreted back into the lumen by the membrane-bound drug efflux pump P-glycoprotein and excreted in the feces.[37-39] Although some authors have reported that the azo-bound 5-ASA prodrugs result in lower systemic absorption of 5-ASA than with the delayed- and controlled-release 5-ASA formulations,[40-42] a recent systematic review suggested that the systemic absorption of 5-ASA from sulfasalazine, olsalazine and balsalazide is comparable to that of Asacol and Pentasa.[43]

Factors that may theoretically affect the delivery of orally administered 5-ASA to the site of disease in IBD patients include variations in transit time and luminal pH, use of antibiotics etc. However, in practice it has been difficult to detect clinically significant differences in efficacy between the newer oral 5-ASA formulations compared to each other or to sulfasalazine, though the 5-aminosalicylates lacking sulfapyridine are better tolerated than sulfasalazine.[44] Pharmacological and efficacy comparisons between doses of azo-bound aminosalicylates and free aminosalicylates should be made on the basis of molar content of 5-ASA; thus, 1 g of sulfasalazine contains approximately 0.4 g of 5-ASA, 1 g of olsalazine contains 1 g of 5-ASA, and 1 g of balsalazide contains approximately 0.36 g of 5-ASA.

Rectal administration of 5-ASA as a suppository, liquid or foam enema provides a high concentration of drug at the site of disease in distal ulcerative colitis. Suppositories can only be expected to release medication in the rectum (approximately the last 10 cm of the colon).[45,46] 5-ASA enemas will reach the ascending colon/splenic flexure in approximately 80–90% of patients with ulcerative colitis.[47-50] The effectiveness and absorption of rectally administered 5-ASA depend on the patient's ability to retain the drug, which can be difficult for individuals with active disease. The mean absorption of rectal 5-ASA is approximately 20% of the administered dose.[51]

## ADVERSE EFFECTS

Adverse events in IBD patients treated with sulfasalazine occur in up to 45% of cases[52] and are usually dose related. Table 32.2 lists the adverse events associated with sulfasalazine and non-sulfa 5-ASA formulations. Early reports associated the occurrence of these side effects with genetic acetylator status and the sulfapyridine moiety;[5,52] however, recent reports in the rheumatology literature have not consistently supported this observation.[53-55] Dose-related side effects include nausea, vomiting, dyspepsia, anorexia and headache.[1,5] The inhibition of folate by the sulfapyridine moiety leads to anemia and reversible abnormalities in sperm counts, morphology and motility.[56] Hypersensitivity reactions to sulfasalazine include anaphylaxis, agranulocytosis, fever, hepatotoxicity, pulmonitis, pancreatitis, autoimmune hemolysis, transient reticulosis, aplastic anemia, leukopenia, systemic lupus erythematosus, pustular drug eruptions, sulphonamide-induced toxic epidermal necrolysis and the Stevens–Johnson syndrome.[1,5] Sulfasalazine therapy may rarely cause a paradoxical worsening of diarrhea in patients with ulcerative colitis.[57] In general, patients with significant hypersensitivity reactions, such as anaphylaxis, agranulocytosis, worsening colitis, pancreatitis, hepatitis or pulmonitis, should not be rechallenged with other 5-ASA formulations. Dose-related adverse events, on the other hand, can be accommodated by a reduction in sulfasalazine dose or a switch to a different 5-ASA formulation.

Up to 80–90% of patients intolerant to sulfasalazine will be able to use non-sulfa-containing 5-ASA preparations; however,

## Table 32.2. Adverse events associated with 5-ASA formulations[56]

|  | Sulfasalazine | 5-Aminosalicylates |
|---|---|---|
| Dose Dependent | Nausea<br>Vomiting<br>Malaise<br>Dyspepsia<br>Headache<br>Folate-dependent anemia<br>Abnormal semen quality | Nephrotoxicity<br>Olsalazine-associated<br>secretory diarrhea |
| Hypersensitivity | Anaphylaxis<br>Fever<br>Pustular drug eruptions<br>Toxic epidermal necrolysis<br>Stevens–Johnson syndrome<br>Hematologic (agranulocytosis, autoimmune hemolysis,<br>transient reticulosis, aplastic anemia, leukopenia)<br>Hepatotoxicity<br>Pancreatitis<br>Systemic lupus erythematosus<br>Pulmonitis<br>Exacerbation of colitis | Fever<br>Rash<br>Skin eruptions<br>Pancreatitis<br>Pulmonitis<br>Hepatotoxicity<br>Drug-induced<br>connective tissue disease<br><br>Exacerbation of colitis<br>Pericarditis |

10–20% will have similar reactions to both agents.[56] In general, adverse reactions to 5-ASA are mild, reversible, and allergic in nature. In most of the efficacy trials, the frequency of drug reactions severe or serious enough to warrant discontinuation was similar in the 5-ASA and placebo groups (3–4% each). The most frequently reported side effects of 5-ASA include dizziness, fever, headache, abdominal pain, nausea and rash.[58,59] Rare but serious adverse events associated with 5-ASA include pulmonary toxicity, pericarditis, hepatitis, pancreatitis, aplastic anemia, leukopenia and thrombocytopenia.[60–63] Some investigators have reported that there is greater systemic absorption of 5-ASA from delayed-release or sustained-release oral formulations (although, as discussed above, it is not clear that these observations are correct), and have implied that greater systemic absorption of 5-ASA may theoretically lead to nephrotoxicity.[40–42] Several case series of interstitial nephritis in patients treated with 5-ASA have been reported.[64,65] However, other studies have shown that the frequency of renal insufficiency was low in large safety and pharmacovigilance databases for Asacol and Pentasa,[66,67] that the glomerular filtration rate does not change during maintenance therapy with 5-ASA or olsalazine,[68] and that renal tubular proteinuria correlates with the activity of the inflammatory bowel disease.[69–71] Taken together, these studies suggest that 5-ASA at the doses used in clinical practice does not have clinically important effects on renal function. A minority of patients will experience worsening diarrhea and abdominal pain because of a hypersensitivity reaction to 5-ASA.[72] The 5-ASA dimer, olsalazine, leads to worsened diarrhea resulting from ileal secretion in some patients,[73] particularly in the setting of active ulcerative colitis.[74]

## OPTIMIZATION OF THERAPY

Most clinical trials of 5-ASA for ulcerative colitis have demonstrated a dose response. For active ulcerative colitis, doses in the range of 2.4–4.8 g/day were more efficacious than 1.6 g or

placebo.[58,59] Initially, studies comparing oral and rectal 5-ASA for distal ulcerative colitis suggested that combination therapy was superior to monotherapy with either oral or rectal 5-ASA.[75–77] However, a subsequent study demonstrated that equimolar doses of oral or combination therapy 5-ASA led to similar clinical outcomes.[78]

Studies investigating mucosal drug concentrations have been instructive. Patients with higher mucosal concentrations of 5-ASA had significantly lower endoscopic activity scores.[75,79] Taken together, these data support the concept that the optimum use of aminosalicylates in active IBD demands the highest tolerated dose, whether administered orally, rectally, or in combination. In maintenance of quiescent disease, lower doses may be more tolerable to the patient and are less costly, although again, there is the general theme of dose response.

5-ASA is metabolized primarily by N-acetylation. Of the two N-acetyltransferase isoenzymes, NAT1 has much greater affinity for 5-ASA than NAT2.[80] NAT1 is highly expressed in the epithelium of the small bowel and colon.[81] The NAT1 gene is polymorphic, and inactivating mutations are associated with a phenotype of decreased enzymatic activity.[82] It has been hypothesized that slow acetylators to NAT1 may have increased response to mesalamine, whereas slow acetylators to NAT2 may have increased toxicity to sulfasalazine. However, in clinical practice, a study of 77 patients found that the clinical response rate was not statistically different among patients who were rapid acetylator and slow acetylator genotypes for NAT1.[83] Similarly, the toxicity rates among patients treated with sulfasalazine were no different between the slow and fast acetylator NAT2 genotypes. This study suggests that determination of NAT1 and NAT2 genotypes is not useful in predicting clinical response or toxicity to mesalamine and sulfasalazine.

Finally, apart from a direct benefit to patients with active ulcerative colitis, 5-ASA agents may increase mean 6-thioguanine nucleotide levels in patients treated with azathioprine or

6-mercaptopurine (see below), possibly enhancing the efficacy as well as the toxicity of purine analogs.[84,85]

# GLUCOCORTICOIDS

Glucocorticoids are effective for the treatment of ulcerative colitis and Crohn's disease, but frequently cause side effects. Strategies to reduce side effects have included altering the chemical structure of the steroid and/or topical delivery to the small intestine and colon in order to reduce systemic steroid exposure through first-pass hepatic metabolism or poor absorption.

## MECHANISMS OF ACTION

Corticosteroids are lipophilic hormones that diffuse across cell membranes and bind to the glucocorticoid receptor. In the unbound state, the glucocorticoid receptor (GR) resides in the cytoplasm and is complexed with heat-shock protein 90, cyclophilin and other proteins.[86] There are two highly homologous isoforms of glucocorticoid receptor, GRα and GRβ, resulting from alternative splicing of the mRNA transcript for GR.[87] When GRα binds a glucocorticoid hormone a conformational change occurs, heat-shock protein 90 and other proteins are released, and the hormone/GRα complex translocates to the nucleus. In the nucleus, two hormone/GRα complexes combine to form a dimer.[88] This dimer then interacts with the glucocorticoid-response element (GRE), allowing the hormone/GRα complex to alter the transcription of glucocorticoid-sensitive genes (transactivation).[86] GRα also acts to inhibit various transcription factors, such as activator protein-1 (AP-1) (via protein–protein interaction), NFκB (via induction of an inhibitor of NFκB [I-κB]), and the signal transduction and activation of transcription (STAT) family (transrepression).[86] In contrast to GRα, GRβ does not bind glucocorticoid hormones and is transcriptionally inactive. GRβ acts to competitively bind to the GRE (thereby inhibiting the transcription activation effects of GRα)[89] (Fig. 32.3).

Thus, the molecular mechanisms of action of glucocorticoids result from modulation of gene expression. Effects of glucocorticoids include inhibition of the production of proinflammatory cytokines such as TNF and IL-1, and chemokines such as IL-8; repression of the transcription of the genes for certain enzymes such as inducible nitric oxide synthase, phospholipase $A_2$ and cyclooxygenase II; blockade of adhesion molecule expression; yet induction of protective IkBα.[90–94] These molecular actions of glucocorticoids lead to reduced leukocyte migration and function, and inhibition of numerous mediators of inflammation.

The anti-inflammatory and immune-modulating effects of glucocorticoids in patients with IBD have been studied to a limited extent. Nitric oxide is elevated in the inflamed mucosa of patients with active IBD[95] and, in vitro, the production of nitric oxide by the inducible form of nitric oxide synthase in mucosal biopsy specimens is inhibited by glucocorticoids. In vivo, glucocorticoid treatment of severe ulcerative colitis does not downregulate immunoreactive nitric oxide synthase.[96] In patients with active Crohn's disease, prednisolone, but not budesonide, inhibits neutrophil and peripheral blood lymphocyte expression of activation markers and the proinflammatory cytokines IL-1 and TNF.[97] Similarly, expression of the adhesion molecules intracellular adhesion molecule-3 and $\beta_2$ integrin by peripheral blood lymphocytes was reduced in patients with Crohn's disease and ulcerative colitis treated with prednisone.[98] Oral and rectal prednisolone decreased the luminal concentrations of the arachidonic acid metabolites prostaglandin-$E_2$ and

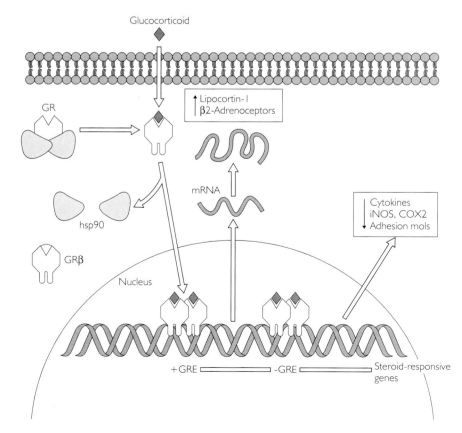

**Fig. 32.3** Mechanism of action of corticosteroids. Corticosteroids enter the cell and bind to cytoplasmic glucocorticoid receptors (GR) complexed to heat-shock protein (hsp90). GR translocates to the nucleus, where the dimmer binds to a glucocorticoid recognition element (GRE) on the 5'-upstream promoter sequence of steroid-responsive genes. GREs increase transcription, but negative GREs (nGREs) may decrease transcription, resulting in alterations in the levels of messenger RNA (mRNA) and protein synthesis. An isoform of GR, GR-β, binds to DNA but is not activated by corticosteroids. (Reproduced with permission from Barnes PJ. Allergy 2001;56:928–936.)

leukotriene-B$_4$.[98] Treatment with prednisolone appears to inhibit the activation of NFκB in the gut mucosa.[21,22] Dexamethasone inhibits the activation of TNF and downregulates that of chemokines such as IL-8, growth-related α, β and γ as well as monocyte chemotactic protein 1, and macrophage inflammatory protein 1β.[99] Overall, these human studies provide evidence that the effects of glucocorticoids on expression of the genes for many proinflammatory cytokines underlie their in vivo anti-inflammatory effects.

## FORMULATION AND PHARMACOKINETICS

Glucocorticoids evaluated for the treatment of IBD are shown in Table 32.3. The naturally occurring glucocorticoid cortisone and the synthetic glucocorticoid prednisone are inactive pro-drugs that are metabolized in the liver to the active glucocorticoid compounds hydrocortisone and prednisolone. Chronic liver disease may impair this process,[100] and therefore prednisolone may be preferable to prednisone in patients with advanced liver disease. Prednisolone and methylprednisolone have similar glucocorticoid and anti-inflammatory activity to hydrocortisone but less mineralocorticoid activity. Systemic steroid therapy is usually achieved with oral administration of cortisone, prednisone or prednisolone, or intravenous administration of prednisolone, methylprednisolone or corticotropin. Both prednisone and prednisolone are well absorbed after oral administration and bioavailability is high, averaging over 70%. However, absorption of prednisolone may be decreased in patients with Crohn's disease of the small bowel,[101,102] and in patients with severe ulcerative colitis in whom oral administration of prednisolone resulted in a lower peak plasma concentration and a slower rate of decrease in the plasma concentration than in healthy volunteers.[103] In contrast to oral administration, intravenous administration of prednisolone in patients with ulcerative colitis resulted in serum concentrations similar to those in healthy volunteers.[104] In this latter study, continuous infusion of prednisolone resulted in greater mean serum concentrations over time compared to bolus intravenous dosing; and both intravenous dosing strategies resulted in greater mean serum concentrations than oral dosing.[104]

Formulations designed to administer topical glucocorticoids directly to the site of disease, either as a rectal enema or a suppository, or orally via an ileal or colonic release formulation, have been developed with the goal of reducing glucocorticoid toxicity.

Hydrocortisone enemas are a systemically active steroid administered directly to the distal colon. Systemic absorption of hydrocortisone from enemas is less than from oral administration, with rectal bioavailability ranging from 15 to 30%;[105,106] nevertheless, the absorption is sufficient to suppress adrenal steroid production. Similarly, significant systemic absorption with adrenal axis suppression occurs following rectal administration of prednisolone, methylprednisolone and betamethasone. Thus, the potential for a reduction in glucocorticoid-related side effects when these steroid compounds are administered rectally compared to intravenous or oral systemic glucocorticoid therapy is modest.

In an effort to further improve the therapeutic window, the glucocorticoids with the additional characteristics of poor absorption or first-pass hepatic metabolism can be administered topically. A poorly absorbed derivative of prednisolone, prednisolone metasulfobenzoate, has also been administered as an enema to patients with distal ulcerative colitis.[107,108] However, studies of adrenal function and bone turnover demonstrated that prednisolone metasulfobenzoate enemas do result in significant systemic glucocorticoid activity when used to treat distal ulcerative colitis.[109,110] Finally, glucocorticoids with extensive first-pass hepatic metabolism and high affinities for glucocorticoid receptors can be administered topically to the ileum or colon via delayed- or sustained-release delivery systems, resulting in a predominantly non-systemic effect. Budesonide is a synthetic analog of prednisolone that has proven efficacy as oral enteric release capsules (Entocort, Budenofalk) in ileal and right-sided Crohn's disease, and as an enema in distal ulcerative colitis. Budesonide has high topical potency, with affinity to the glucocorticoid receptor 15 and 200 times greater than that of prednisolone and hydrocortisone, respectively.[111] A 16α, 17α-acetyl side chain increases the intrinsic activity but allows increased metabolic inactivation in the liver.[112] A controlled ileal release (CIR) formulation of budesonide consists of hard gelatin capsules containing microgranules of budesonide sprayed with an insoluble polymer allowing time-dependent rate controlled release. Each 1 mm microgranule is then coated with Eudragit L, an acrylic resin that dissolves above pH 5.5. First-pass inactivation of budesonide in the liver is 90%, resulting in 10% systemic bioavailability,[112] with the majority of absorption occurring in the distal small bowel. Luminal concentrations of budesonide after intake of CIR capsules are high and intracellular esterification retains the drug at the site of action and may extend duration of action.[112] Systemic exposure of budesonide is still

**Table 32.3 Comparison of the potency, bioavailability and common doses of oral and rectal glucocorticoid preparations used in inflammatory bowel disease**

| Drug | Anti-inflammatory potency | Bioavailability (%) | Usual maximum dose, mg/day |
|---|---|---|---|
| Hydrocortisone | 1 | Oral: >50 Rectal: 16–30 | 100–200 |
| Prednisone | 4 | Oral: >50 | 40–80 |
| Prednisolone | 5 | Oral: >50 Rectal, as metasulfobenzoate: <10 | 70–80 |
| Budesonide CIR | 200 | Oral: 10 Rectal: 16 | 9–15 |

CIR, controlled ileal release.

sufficient to suppress adrenal steroid production, but at lower levels than with equivalent doses of prednisolone.[113,114] For rectal delivery, budesonide is formulated as a suspension enema. Rectal administration of budesonide produces dose-dependent suppression of adrenal function.[115] Thus, with both the oral and rectal formulations of budesonide, adrenal suppression does occur but the magnitude of the effect is less than that observed with conventional glucocorticosteroids.

Other glucocorticoids with extensive first-pass hepatic metabolism and high glucocorticoid receptor affinity include tixicortol pivalate, beclomethasone and fluticasone. Tixocortol pivalate and beclomethasone enemas administered to patients with active distal colitis have revealed efficacy and little adrenal suppression.[116–118] Fluticasone is a high-potency fluorinated corticosteroid with extensive first-pass inactivation, leading to systemic bioavailability of less than 1%. Preliminary studies have demonstrated that oral fluticasone is not effective for the treatment of Crohn's disease and ulcerative colitis.[119,120]

## ADVERSE EFFECTS

Corticosteroid toxicity occurred frequently in patients with active Crohn's disease treated with prednisone at an initial dose of approximately 60 mg/day tapered over 17 weeks.[121] Toxicities observed included a moon face in 47%, acne in 30%, infection in 27%, ecchymoses in 17%, hypertension in 15%, hirsutism in 7%, petechial subcutaneous bleeding in 6%, and striae in 6%.[121] A similar short-term toxicity profile can be expected in patients with ulcerative colitis. Prolonged corticosteroid therapy can result in multiple serious side effects, including hypertension, new-onset diabetes mellitus, infection, osteonecrosis, steroid-associated osteoporosis, myopathy, psychosis, cataracts and glaucoma.[122,123] Table 32.4 lists a number of potential side effects of corticosteroid therapy.

## OPTIMIZATION OF THERAPY

A study of outpatients with active ulcerative colitis demonstrated that prednisolone doses of 40 mg/day and 60 mg/day had similar efficacy, and both were superior to 20 mg/day.[124] Another study demonstrated that administration of the total daily dose as a single dose had similar efficacy to 4 times daily dosing, with fewer side effects.[125] In Crohn's disease, efficacy has been demonstrated for prednisone adjusted on a sliding scale according to disease activity: moderate to severe disease 0.75 mg/kg (52.5 mg for a 70 kg patient); mild to moderate disease 0.5 mg/kg (35 mg for a 70 kg patient); and mild inflammation 0.25 mg/kg (17.5 mg for a 70 kg patient).[126] Another study demonstrated efficacy for 6-methylprednisolone 48 mg/day.[127] One study comparing the duration of tapering regimens found no difference in outcome between a 2-month steroid taper and a 4-month steroid taper in patients with Crohn's disease.[128] In North America, the usual initial prednisone dosing regimen is 40 mg/day administered as a single dose. The optimal tapering strategy has not been determined, but experienced clinicians will typically treat the patient with prednisone 40 mg/day for 2–4 weeks, then taper by 5 mg/week to a daily dose of 20 mg/day, then slow the taper to 2.5 mg/week until the drug is discontinued. European physicians frequently initiate therapy with prednisolone 1 mg/kg.[129]

Several potential genetically determined mechanisms for resistance to corticosteroid therapy in patients with IBD have been described, including an increase in the expression of the inactive membrane receptor GRβ[130] and increased expression of the multidrug resistance-1 gene (*MDR1*). The latter results in an increased expression of the membrane-based drug efflux pump P-glycoprotein 170, which pumps corticosteroids out of cells, thereby lowering the intracellular concentration.[131]

### Table 32.4 Adverse effects associated with systemic corticosteroid therapy

| | |
|---|---|
| Cutaneous | Atrophy, striae, vascular effects, purpura, alopecia, pigmentation, acne, easy bruising |
| Cardiovascular | Hypertension, edema, atherosclerosis |
| Gastrointestinal | Nausea, vomiting, intestinal perforation, pancreatitis, esophagitis |
| Gynecological/obstetrical | Amenorrhea, gestational diabetes, adrenal suppression of infant |
| Neuropsychiatric | Psychosis, peripheral neuropathy, pseudotumor cerebri, depression/mood disorders, impaired cognitive function, seizures, insomnia, irritability |
| Metabolic | Hyperglycemia, hyperlipidemia, obesity, hypocalcemia, hypokalemia, buffalo hump |
| Musculoskeletal | Osteoporosis/osteopenia, aseptic necrosis, growth retardation, muscle atrophy, myopathy |
| Hematological | Leukocytosis, lymphopenia, eosinophenia, infection, immunosuppression, impaired fibroplasia, decreased mitotic rate |
| Ophthalmalogical | Cataracts, glaucoma, infection, exophthalmoses, hemorrhage |
| Endocrine | Hypothalamopituitary–adrenal axis suppression, hirsutism, moon facies |
| Pediatric | Growth retardation |

Adapted from Yang and Lichtenstein.[270]

# AZATHIOPRINE AND 6-MERCAPTOPURINE

6-Mercaptopurine (6-MP) and its prodrug azathioprine are purine antimetabolite drugs demonstrated to be effective for the treatment of ulcerative colitis and Crohn's disease.

## MECHANISM OF ACTION

The exact mechanism of action of azathioprine and 6-MP is not known; however, it is the 6-thioguanine nucleotides that are believed to mediate the biological actions of these drugs. Intracellular accumulation of 6-thioguanine nucleotides causes inhibition of the pathways of purine nucleotide metabolism and DNA synthesis and repair, resulting in inhibition of cell division and proliferation.[132] Proposed mechanisms of action include inhibition of purine nucleotide synthesis and conversion by the intermediate metabolite thioinosinic acid, with resulting inhibition of the DNA synthetic phase of the cell cycle;[133] interference with the antigenic triggering of lymphocytes leading to the inhibition of the mixed lymphocyte reaction;[133,134] reduction in natural killer cell cytotoxicity;[135] and reduction in plasma cells in the rectal lamina propria and a fall in the peripheral lymphocyte count.[135,136] More recently, Tiede and Neurath have reported that azathioprine and 6-MP induce apoptosis of T lymphocytes through specific blockade of Rac1 activation via binding of azathioprine-generated 6-thioguanine triphosphate to Rac1 instead of guanine triphosphate.[137] The activation of Rac1 target genes such as MEK, NFKB, and bcl-xL was suppressed by azathioprine, leading to a mitochondrial pathway of apoptosis.

## PHARMACOKINETICS AND PHARMACOGENETICS

Azathioprine is 50% 6-mercaptopurine by molecular weight. Thus, a conversion factor of 2 will convert a dose of 6-mercaptopurine to azathioprine. Azathioprine is a prodrug that is converted to 6-MP by a non-enzymatic nucleophilic attack from glutathione and other sulfhydryl-containing compounds present in intestinal mucosa, the liver, erythrocytes and other tissues.[138,139] 6-Mercaptopurine may then be metabolized by thiopurine methyltransferase to the inactive metabolite 6-methylmercaptopurine, or by xanthine oxidase to the inactive metabolite 6-thiouric acid (Fig. 32.4).[132,140,141] Alternatively, 6-MP may be activated to the putative active metabolite 6-thioguanine nucleotide (6-TGN) via a multistep enzymatic pathway beginning with the enzyme hypoxanthine phosphoribosyl transferase followed by inosine monophosphate dehydrogenase and guanosine monophosphate synthetase.[132,140,141] The activity of the thiopurine methyltransferase enzyme is genetically determined and will be discussed below in detail.[142]

The parent azathioprine and 6-MP molecules are not therapeutically active. The putative active metabolites, the 6-thioguanine nucleotides, have a half-life of several days or more.[141] Steady-state concentrations of the 6-thioguanine nucleotides occur after 2–4 weeks of oral dosing with azathioprine 2.0 mg/kg/day.[143] The delayed time to reach steady-state 6-thioguanine nucleotide kinetics parallels the slow onset of therapeutic benefit of oral azathioprine or 6-MP therapy in IBD, which has been estimated to average 17 weeks.[144] This observation prompted a placebo-controlled trial of an intravenous loading-dose of azathioprine to reduce the time to clinical response in Crohn's disease.[143] In this study, despite initially higher erythrocyte 6-thioguanine nucleotide concentrations in those receiving active intravenous drug, there was no difference in the onset or proportion of clinical response compared to placebo-treated patients. However, the median time to steady-state erythrocyte 6-thioguanine nucleotide concentration and initial clinical improvement was only 4 weeks, suggesting that oral azathioprine may act more quickly than had previously been realized.

The gene for thiopurine methyltransferase is located on the short arm of chromosome 6.[142] Erythrocyte TPMT activity correlates well with the enzyme's activity in other cells and tissues, and is thus a convenient assay for enzyme activity. There is a trimodal distribution for TPMT activity in the general population: 88.6% are homozygous for the wildtype TPMT allele and have an erythrocyte TPMT activity of 14–25 U/mL erythrocytes. Approximately 11.1% of this population is heterozygous for the wildtype allele and have an intermediate enzyme activity that is 5–13.7 U/mL erythrocytes. Finally, 0.3% of individuals have two inactive TPMT alleles and no detectable TPMT activity[142,145] (Fig. 32.5). To date, 10 mutant alleles for TPMT associated with decreased enzyme activity have been isolated (*2, *3A, *3B, *3C, *3D, *4, *5, *6, *7, *10).[146–148] Patients with low or intermediate thiopurine methyltransferase enzyme activity shunt 6-MP away from the 6-methylmercaptopurine metabolite and towards the 6-thioguanine nucleotides. Excess concentrations of 6-thioguanine nucleotides have been associated with leukopenia.[149,150]

## ADVERSE EFFECTS

Adverse effects from azathioprine and 6-MP can be classified as allergic, occurring within the first 3–4 weeks of therapy, or non-allergic, usually dose dependent, generally occurring later in the course of therapy. Allergic reactions include pancreatitis, fever, rash, malaise, nausea, diarrhea, and some cases of hepatitis.[151–153] Approximately 5% of the IBD population beginning treatment

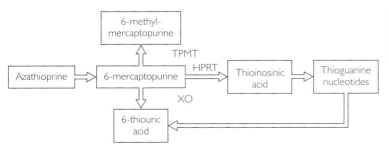

**Fig. 32.4** Metabolism of azathioprine and 6-MP. TPMT, thiopurine methyltransferase; HPRT, hypoxanthine phosphoribosyl transferase; XO, xanthine oxidase. (Reproduced with permission from Chan GL, et al. J Clin Pharmacol 1990;30:358–363.)

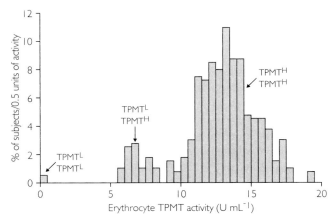

**Fig. 32.5** Frequency distribution of red blood cell (RBC) thiopurine methyltransferase (TPMT) activity in a randomly selected population of 298 adult blood donors. (Reproduced with permission from Weinshilboum R. Am J Hum Genet 1980;32:651–662. © 2003. The University of Chicago Press. All rights reserved.)

with azathioprine or 6-MP will experience an allergic reaction to the drug.[153] Rechallenging patients who experience pancreatitis or significant drug fever with either agent will almost universally lead to recurrent symptoms within one or two doses of either drug, and sometimes within minutes to hours, and is not advised. Cautious rechallenge may be warranted for other side effects. In particular, in patients who experience nausea, which is not an allergic reaction, case reports suggest that those who are intolerant of azathioprine may be successfully switched to 6-MP.[154,155] The intolerance may be partly due to the imidazole ring of azathioprine that is cleaved to release 6-MP.[156]

Non-allergic reactions to azathioprine or 6-MP include bone marrow suppression leading to leukopenia, anemia or thrombocytopenia; opportunistic infection; some cases of hepatitis; and non-Hodgkin's lymphoma. Cytopenias have been reported to develop from 2 weeks to 11 years after beginning therapy, at a cumulative frequency of about 10%.[143,157,158] There are a number of reports of fatal or life-threatening opportunistic infections in leukopenic IBD patients treated with azathioprine or 6-MP. Although the number of patients experiencing opportunistic infections appears to be small compared to the overall number of IBD patients being treated with these drugs, vigilance for such infections is warranted.[153,158] If leukopenia and serious infection develop in a patient receiving azathioprine or 6-MP, reversal of bone marrow suppression is usually possible with temporary discontinuation of the drug and, if necessary, administration of granulocyte colony-stimulating factor (G-CSF).

The risk of malignancy, especially lymphoma, in patients receiving azathioprine/6-MP is controversial. The available evidence suggests that there is no increased baseline risk of lymphoma in patients with IBD who are not using immunosuppressive medications.[159] With respect to patients on 6-MP or azathioprine, one series reported a wide spectrum of malignant neoplasms in IBD patients who had at some point received 6-MP, but the overall rate of 3.1% was low and probably not greater than in the general population.[153] In another series of 755 patients treated with azathioprine for a median of 12.5 years at a dose of 2 mg/kg/day, 31 developed a cancer compared to 24.3 expected cases.[160] The difference was significant only when considering colorectal adenocarcinomas, a recognized complication of IBD. These results were supported by a study of

2204 patients, 626 of who had received azathioprine. No increased risk of cancer following therapy with azathioprine was seen.[161] However, a recent study from the Mayo Clinic found 18 IBD patients in 14 years who developed lymphoma.[162] From 1985 to 1992 there were six patients with lymphoma, none of whom received azathioprine/6-MP and only one of whom had Epstein–Barr virus (EBV) present in the lymphoma cells. From 1993 to 2000 there were 12 patients with lymphoma. Six of the 12 had received azathioprine/6-MP and six were tumor positive for EBV. Five of the six lymphoma patients had received therapy with 6-MP or azathioprine. The association with EBV suggests lymphoproliferation due to reactivation of latent EBV, or newly acquired infection from immunosuppression. Cumulatively, current data suggest that the risk of malignancy, if present, is very small and the overall benefit of azathiprine/6-MP therapy outweighs these risks.

## OPTIMIZING THERAPY

Issues in determining optimal therapy for the use of azathioprine/6-MP involve what dose to use, when to start, how long to continue, and whether TPMT activity and metabolite monitoring should be assessed. Controlled trials have shown that effective doses are azathioprine 2.0–3.0 mg/kg/day and 6-MP 1.0–1.5 mg/kg/day.[144] Although some physicians begin at low doses and titrate upwards, our practice is to begin at the full dose, with careful monitoring of the compete blood count. There is no role for intravenous loading of azathioprine/6-MP.[143] The drug can be initiated to induce remission, to maintain remission and as a steroid-sparing agent.[144] Knowledge of TPMT phenotype or genotype can aid in determining safety and the optimal dosage of azathioprine/6-MP. Low to intermediate levels of TPMT are associated with leukopenia in rheumatoid arthritis[163] and Crohn's disease.[146] Based on these observations, it is recommended that patients with normal TPMT activity receive standard doses of azathioprine or 6-MP. Patients with intermediate activity should receive 50% of the standard dose, and those who have no TPMT activity should not be treated with the drug.[164,165]

The use of metabolite levels (6-TGN and 6-MMP) to gauge optimal dosing of azathioprine/6-MP is controversial. One study prospectively evaluated the association between these metabolites, clinical response and toxicity.[166] Ninety-two patients under 19 years of age who were receiving azathioprine or 6-MP were studied. A Harvey–Bradshaw Index (HBI) score < 4 determined remission in Crohn's disease, and Truelove–Witts criteria were used for ulcerative colitis. A higher mean erythrocyte (RBC) 6-TGN concentration correlated with clinical response, but by quartile analysis was significantly greater only with an RBC 6-TGN >235 pmol/8 × 10⁸. Of the therapeutic failures, 20/70 (27%) had a concentration >235, whereas 69/103 (67%) of responders had a concentration >235 pmol/8 × 10⁸. Thus, approximately 1/4 of failures had adequate concentrations, and 1/3 of responders had concentrations less than 235 pmol/8 × 10⁸ RBC. 6-MMP concentrations did not correlate with disease activity, but concentrations >5700 pmol/8 × 10⁸ RBC were significantly associated with hepatotoxicity (although the robustness of this association is limited by the small sample size of only 16 patients with hepatotoxicity). Although one earlier study supported these results,[167] at least three others have failed to demonstrate a consistent relationship between clinical efficacy and erythrocyte 6-TGN concentrations.[84,143,168] Although metabolite monitoring may be useful in gauging compliance with medical therapy, during concomitant therapy with allopurinol (allopurinol inhibits xanthine oxidase, indirectly increasing 6-TGN), and in patients with intermediate TPMT levels, its utility in standard clinical practice remains to be established.

Predicting who will respond to purine analog therapy is difficult. A recent study found that 37/51 patients who failed to respond to azathioprine/6-MP therapy did not increase their 6-TGN levels with dose escalation, though levels of 6-MMP rose.[169] TPMT activity was not influenced by dose escalation. The results of one retrospective study suggested that the development of mild leukopenia to azathioprine identified Crohn's disease patients with a greater likelihood of a favorable response.[170] Based on this observation, one group of investigators has tried dose escalation in Crohn's disease patients refractory to standard-dose azathioprine. In this uncontrolled study, after increasing the dose of azathioprine from a mean of 2 mg/kg/day to 2.7 mg/kg/day, 14 of 18 patients improved and were able to discontinue steroids.[171] Although no significant leukopenia was observed, two patients developed serious cytomegalovirus infection. Other studies that have examined the relationship between leukocyte count and clinical response during azathioprine and 6-MP therapy for IBD have not supported the concept that leukopenia is associated with efficacy.[84,143]

At present, when initiating therapy with azathioprine/6-MP, we counsel patients about the risk of leukopenia, infection and the theoretical risk of lymphoma. If available, TPMT enzyme activity is determined, and the starting dose is adjusted according to the results. Complete blood counts are checked weekly for approximately 4 weeks, and then every month during therapy. 6-MP metabolite determinations are reserved for special situations.

# METHOTREXATE

Methotrexate (MTX) is a folate analog and inhibitor of dihydrofolate reductase that has demonstrated effectiveness in the treatment of Crohn's disease.

## MECHANISM OF ACTION

The major action of methotrexate is reversible competitive inhibition of dihydrofolate reductase (DHFR), leading to cytotoxicity. Folate receptors bring methotrexate into the cell where, like folate, some of it is metabolized to polyglutamates (MTX-glu) and retained intracellularly.[172] MTX-glu binds DHFR. Dihydrofolate reductase is necessary for regenerating the fully reduced folate cofactors that are required for reactions involving the transfer of one-carbon fragments, such as the production of thymidylate and purines. MTX-glu also has high affinity for enzymes such as thymidylate synthetase (TS) and 5-aminoimidazole-4-carboxamide ribonucleotide (AICAR). Inhibition of TS and AICAR interferes with DNA synthesis and purine metabolism and leads to the release of adenosine into the blood. This increased extracellular adenosine may contribute to the anti-inflammatory effects of MTX[173–176] (Fig. 32.6).

The effects of methotrexate on a number of mediators of inflammation have been evaluated, primarily in patients with rheumatoid arthritis. Methotrexate has been found to decrease the production of proinflammatory monocytic/macrophagic cytokines IL-1,[177] IL-6[178] and TNF;[179] decrease neutrophil pro-

duction of leukotriene $B_4$;[180] increase gene expression of T-helper 2 (Th2) cytokines IL-4 and IL-10;[181] and decrease gene expression of Th1 cytokines IL-2 and IFN-$\gamma$.[181] Methotrexate can also induce lymphocyte apoptosis through an Fas-independent mechanism that requires inhibition of dihydrofolate reductase and thymidylate synthase.[182] The anti-inflammatory effects of methotrexate may also be mediated by the increase in extracellular adenosine. Experiments in tissue culture and animal models of acute inflammation have demonstrated that methotrexate increases extracellular release of adenosine, which inhibits neutrophil adherence to endothelial cells and accumulation at sites of inflammation.[174,183] However, in patients with IBD, adenosine concentrations measured in both plasma and rectal lumen dialysis fluid did not increase after subcutaneous administration of methotrexate at doses of 15–25 mg, suggesting that this is not an important mechanism of action in this disease setting.[184]

## FORMULATION AND PHARMACOKINETICS

Once-weekly dosing of methotrexate in inflammatory diseases such as psoriasis and rheumatoid arthritis has a lower incidence of hepatotoxicity than daily dosing.[185] The doses used ranged from 7.5 to 25 mg/week, usually given orally or by intramuscular injection. When methotrexate was used to treat IBD, this therapeutic regimen was empirically adopted.[186]

The bioavailability of orally administered methotrexate at the low doses (7.5–25 mg/week) used in chronic inflammatory diseases ranges from 50 to 90%.[187–189] In contrast, parenterally administered methotrexate (either intramuscular or subcutaneous) is nearly 100% bioavailable.[190] Patient comfort and ability to self-administer favor the subcutaneous over the intramuscular route. After administration, methotrexate is widely distributed and rapidly cleared, mostly in unchanged form by the kidney. A small fraction of the drug is concentrated in many cell types as polyglutamated methotrexate. In IBD patients receiving weekly injections of methotrexate, the drug accumulates gradually in erythrocytes, reaching steady state at about 8 weeks.[191] Methotrexate is often given with folate supplementation (1 mg/day) to reduce side effects. Co-administration of folate with MTX reduces plasma concentrations of MTX and increases its total clearance.[176,192] In patients with rheumatoid arthritis the addition of folate has been found to reduce side effects, but at the cost of some efficacy, although the authors felt it was of minimal clinical significance.[193]

## ADVERSE EFFECTS

Chronic methotrexate use has the potential for significant toxicity. Up to 18% of patients in IBD series discontinue the drug because of suspected drug-related toxicity.[194,195] Adverse events from methotrexate can be broadly categorized as dose-related antiproliferative effects on bone marrow, gut mucosa and hair follicles; idiosyncratic allergic or hypersensitivity reactions; and hepatic fibrosis/cirrhosis.

The dose-dependent antiproliferative effects of methotrexate, including bone marrow depression, gastrointestinal ulceration, stomatitis and alopecia, occur during high-dose chemotherapy and require 'rescue' with tetrahydrofolate. These antiproliferative adverse events are unusual when methotrexate is used at low doses for the treatment of autoimmune diseases. Idiosyncratic allergic or hypersensitivity reactions to

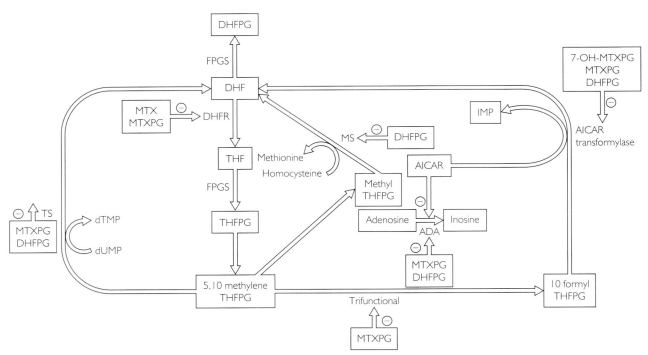

**Fig. 32.6** Methotrexate metabolism. MTX and its polyglutamate metabolites (MTXPG) potently inhibit dihydrofolate reductase (DHFR), impairing production of tetrahydrofolate (THF) and leading to accumulation and polyglutamation of dihydrofolate and oxidized folates (DHFPG). Polyglutamation of MTX confers greatly enhanced inhibitory activity against folate-dependent enzymes distal to DHFR, including thymidylate synthase (TS); the trifunctional enzyme 10-formyltetrahydrofolate synthetase, cyclohydrolase, dehydrogenase; and 5-aminoimidazole-4-carboxamide ribotide (AICAR) transformylase. In addition, DHFPG are potent inhibitors of some folate-dependent enzymes, including TS, AICAR transformylase and methionine synthetase (MS). Polyglutamate derivates of the MTX metabolite, 7-hydroxymethotrexate (7-OH-MTXPG), also inhibit AICAR transformylase. Inhibition of IACAR transformylase leads to accumulation of AICAR, which, like MTXPG and DHFPG, leads to accumulation of adenosine, partly through inhibition of adenosine deaminase (ADA). DHF, dihydrofolate; dtmp, deoxythymidine monophosphate; dump, deoxyuridine monophosphate; FPGS, folylpolyglutamate synthetase; IMP, inosine monophosphate; THFPG, tetrahydrofolate polyglutamate. (Reproduced with permission from Egan et al. Mayo Clin Proc 1996;71:69–80.)

methotrexate primarily consist of rash and pneumonitis. Lung injury occurs in 3–11% of rheumatologic patients treated with low-dose methotrexate.[196] The clinical presentation of methotrexate pneumonitis is characterized by cough, dyspnea, fever, hypoxemia, a restrictive ventilatory defect with impaired gas exchange, and a radiographic picture of a diffuse alveolar/interstitial process. Signs and symptoms usually resolve if methotrexate is discontinued.

Increased serum transaminases are observed in up to 30% of patients treated chronically with methotrexate.[195,197] Elevated transaminases do not correlate well with histologic liver injury. The spectrum of histologic lesions observed in patients treated with chronic methotrexate includes macrovesicular steatosis, hepatocyte necrosis and portal inflammation, which may progress to fibrosis and cirrhosis.[198] Risk factors for liver injury include greater cumulative doses, significant alcohol use, obesity, diabetes[199] and older age.[200]

The frequency of methotrexate-induced liver injury varies according to the treatment indication and use of concomitant hepatotoxins such as alcohol. Patients with psoriasis are at increased risk, and liver biopsies are performed after a cumulative dose of 1.5 g.[201] In contrast, in patients with rheumatoid arthritis the risk of cirrhosis after 5 years of continuous therapy is only 1/1000.[200,202] Thus, liver biopsy in patients with rheumatoid arthritis is only recommended in those with persistent transaminase elevation or a decrease in albumin.[197] Similar to rheumatoid arthritis, patients with IBD appear to have a low risk

of methotrexate liver toxicity.[203,204] One study of 20 IBD patients receiving a mean cumulative MTX dose of 2633 mg found that 95% had mild to no histological abnormalities and only one had hepatic fibrosis. Abnormal liver chemistry tests did not identify the patient with fibrosis.[203] A study of psoriasis patients found that the liver histologic findings demonstrated significant improvement with withdrawal of methotrexate.[199] Based on these data, routine liver biopsies of IBD patients in the absence of other suspicion for liver disease are probably not warranted. Our proposed guidelines for liver monitoring in methotrexate-treated IBD patients are outlined in Table 32.5. We advise patients to refrain from alcohol consumption during methotrexate therapy.

Finally, methotrexate is a known teratogen. Its use is contraindicated in men and women attempting conception, and in women during pregnancy and when breastfeeding. Women should discontinue therapy at least 3 months prior to attempting conception and men 4–6 months prior to attempting conception.[205]

## OPTIMIZATION OF THERAPY

Randomized controlled trials have demonstrated that intramuscular methotrexate 25 mg/week is effective for inducing remission in patients with Crohn's disease,[195] that intramuscular methotrexate 15 mg/week is effective for maintaining remission, and that dose escalation from 15 mg/week to 25 mg/week

**Table 32.5 Guidelines for the prevention and monitoring of hepatotoxicity in IBD**

| Baseline | | Withhold methotrexate |
|---|---|---|
| Liver tests | AST, ALT, ALP, bilirubin | If > 2 x normal |
| | Hepatitis B & C tests | If actively infected |
| Liver biopsy | If abnormal AST, ALT, ALP, bilirubin | If hepatitis, fibrosis or |
| | If clinical suspicion of liver disease | cirrhosis are present |
| *During treatment* | | *Stop or reduce methotrexate* |
| AST | Every 6 weeks | If > 2 x baseline |
| Liver biopsy | If progressive elevation of AST | If hepatitis, fibrosis or |
| | If > 50% of AST tests are high | cirrhosis are present |

AST, aspartate aminotransferase; ALT alanine aminotransferase, ALP alkaline phosphatase.

may be effective in patients who relapse on lower doses.[206] Oral methotrexate 15 mg/week may be effective for maintaining remission as well;[207] however, oral methotrexate 12.5 mg/week is not effective for inducing or maintaining remission in patients with Crohn's disease or ulcerative colitis.[208,209] A randomized pharmacokinetic and dose–response trial comparing subcutaneous methotrexate 15 mg/week and 25 mg/week reported no difference in MTX polyglutamate blood concentrations or clinical response in 32 patients with active IBD, and that patients treated with 15 mg/week who fail to respond may benefit from dose escalation to 25 mg/week.[191] Together, these studies demonstrate that methotrexate 12.5 mg/week is not effective for inducing or maintaining remission in patients with Crohn's disease; that methotrexate 15–25 mg/week given subcutaneously or intramuscularly is effective for Crohn's disease; and that dose escalation from 15 mg/week up to 25 mg/week may be beneficial in patients who fail to respond to 15 mg/week. Therapeutic drug monitoring of methotrexate polyglutamate in erythrocytes is not useful.

Poor outcome with high-dose methotrexate therapy in the hematology/oncology setting is associated with the development of resistance. The competitive absorption of folate and methotrexate may be a contributing factor to MTX resistance in some patients.[176] Increased expression (induction) of the main target enzyme, dihydrofolate reductase, is another proposed mechanism.[210] Finally, lipophilic anion transporter proteins may transport methotrexate out of the cell.[211] It is unknown whether these mechanisms contribute to resistance or loss of response in patients with IBD treated with methotrexate.

# CYCLOSPORIN AND TACROLIMUS (FK506)

Cyclosporin is effective for the treatment of severe ulcerative colitis[212] and tacrolimus is effective for the treatment of fistulizing Crohn's disease.[213]

## MECHANISM OF ACTION

Cyclosporin and tacrolimus are both calcineurin inhibitors with similar mechanisms of immunosuppression and will therefore be discussed together. Sirolimus, a newer calcineurin inhibitor used in organ transplantation, has not been reported in the IBD setting. Cyclosporin is a cyclic lipophilic polypeptide produced by the soil fungus *Tolypocladium inflatum*. Tacrolimus is a macrolide antibiotic. Both tacrolimus and cyclosporin bind to cytoplasmic proteins: cyclosporin to cyclophilin, and tacrolimus to FK-binding protein. These drug–protein complexes inhibit the cytoplasmic phosphatase calcineurin, an enzyme required for activation of the T lymphocyte-specific nuclear factor of activated T cells (NFAT). This transcription factor regulates the rate of transcription of cytokines important in T-lymphocyte activation, including IL-2 and IFN-γ.[214] Thus, cyclosporin and tacrolimus are powerful and specific inhibitors of T-lymphocyte activation. Cyclosporin may also directly inhibit T-cell proliferation by inhibiting other cytoplasmic enzymes within T cells, such as calmodulin and protein kinase C, that appear to be involved in the immune response.[215]

## FORMULATION AND PHARMACOKINETICS

Cyclosporin is formulated in a standard oil (cremaphor)-based formulation (Sandimmune) and as a microemulsion formulation (Neoral). The microemulsion contains polyethylene glycol, castor oil, medium-chain triglycerides and low molecular weight glycols. The original oil-based formulation of cyclosporin is poorly and erratically absorbed, with oral bioavailability of only 20–50% and high interpatient variability.[216] Absorption follows zero-order kinetics (dose independent) and is a function of contact time, which in turn is affected by motility, length and mucosal integrity.[217,218] Cyclosporin absorption is dependent on the presence of bile. In patients with small bowel Crohn's disease absorption may be even lower for these reasons.[219] The increased presence of cytochrome P450IIIA in small bowel mucosa can result in significant first-pass metabolism.[220] Also, grapefruit juice, which inhibits the metabolism of cyclosporin, possibly by inhibition of cytochrome P450, can significantly increase peak concentrations of the drug.[221] Similarly, other drugs that affect the P450 system, such as calcium channel blockers, imidazoles, macrolide antibiotics, rifampin and phenytoin, can alter levels of cyclosporin, and the potential for drug interactions (Table 32.6) should be taken into consideration when prescribing cyclosporin.[222] The newer microemulsion formulation of cyclosporin has an oral bioavailability of 174–239% relative to the standard oral formulation.[223] It is better absorbed from the small bowel and is less dependent on bile for

**Table 32.6 Potential drug interactions of cyclosporin and tacrolimus. Adapted from Kornbluth et al.[222]**

| | |
|---|---|
| Inhibition of cytochrome P450 Increased CSA levels | Calcium channel blockers Bromocriptine Metoclopramide Imidazoles Macrolide antibiotics Methylprednisolone Protease inhibitors Grapefruit juice |
| Induction of cytochrome P450 Decreased cyclosporin levels | Rifampin Phenobarbital Phenytoin Carbamazepine Reverse transcriptase inhibitors St John's Wort |

absorption. One study showed that cyclosporin microemulsion, unlike the standard lipophilic formulation, has similar pharmacokinetic parameters in patients with IBD as in healthy volunteers and those requiring cyclosporin for other disorders.[224]

Tacrolimus is much more potent than cyclosporin. Although oral bioavailability is low, ranging from 21 to 27%, there is less interpatient variability than with oral cyclosporin[225] and it is not dependent on bile or mucosal integrity for absorption.[225,226] However, it has poor aqueous solubility and it increases gastric motility (macrolide antibiotic), both of which can effect absorption. Also, the same P450 system-related drug interactions as cyclosporin affect tacrolimus as well.

## ADVERSE EFFECTS

Both cyclosporin and tacrolimus have significant short- and long-term side-effect profiles. In a report from the Mount Sinai hospital on 111 IBD patients treated with cyclosporin, the most frequent adverse events were paresthesias (51%), hypertension (43%), hypertrichosis (27%), renal insufficiency (23%), infections (20%), gingival hyperplasia (4%), seizures (3%), death (2%) and anaphylaxis (1%).[227] In a similar report from the University of Chicago on 74 patients with IBD treated with cyclosporin, 54% experienced adverse events, including severe events such as *Pneumocystis carinii* pneumonia in two patients, abdominal abscess, *grand mal* seizure, mycotic aneurysm and renal insufficiency.[228] Although non-Hodgkin's lymphoma and post-transplant lymphoproliferative disorder have been reported in the transplantation literature,[229] these conditions have not been reported in patients with IBD treated with cyclosporin or tacrolimus. Nephrotoxicity with cyclosporin is a major concern, as most patients receiving chronic cyclosporin therapy will have a 20% reduction in the glomerular filtration rate without obvious change in the creatinine.[230] Tacrolimus has a comparable side-effect profile to cyclosporin, with similar degrees of nephrotoxicity. However, tacrolimus has a lower incidence of significant hypertension, hypercholesterolemia, hirsutism and gingival hyperplasia, but higher rates of diabetes mellitus, some forms of neurotoxicity (tremor, paresthesias), diarrhea and alopecia.[225]

## OPTIMIZING THERAPY

Prior to initiating therapy with either cyclosporin or tacrolimus, patients should be screened for risk factors for renal disease (including age >50), a history of malignancy, infection, seizure disorder, concomitant medications that may have significant interactions, pregnancy, and non-compliance with medications or drug testing. Blood pressure should be noted and laboratory tests should include creatinine, electrolytes, and cholesterol level.[222] Hypocholesterolemia and hypomagnesemia increase the risk of seizures in patients receiving cyclosporin therapy.[222] Patients treated with cyclosporin are initially started on intravenous cyclosporin 4 mg/kg/day, adjusted to whole blood radioimmune assay (RIA) or high-performance liquid chromatography (HPLC) concentration of 250–350 ng/mL. Tacrolimus is initiated orally at 0.10–0.15 mg/kg twice daily, adjusted to a whole blood tacrolimus trough concentration of 10–20 ng/mL. The patient who responds to therapy should be discharged on oral cyclosporin or continued on oral tacrolimus targeted to the same trough blood concentration levels. Azathioprine or 6-MP should be started as soon as possible and steroids tapered as tolerated. Some authors suggest maintaining prednisone at 20 mg/day for 3–4 months to have an overlap period of triple immunosuppression while the slow-acting agents azathioprine/6-MP are taking effect.[226] Oral cyclosporin and tacrolimus should be discontinued after 3–4 months without tapering. The corticosteroids can then be tapered over the next 4–8 weeks and the patient maintained on azathioprine/6-MP. Blood pressure should be checked twice weekly, and serum creatinine, potassium, glucose and drug concentrations should be monitored every 1 or 2 weeks.

# INFLIXIMAB

Infliximab is effective for induction and maintenance of remission in patients with Crohn's disease,[231,232] and for reduction and maintenance of reduction in the number of draining enterocutaneous fistulae.[233,234]

## FORMULATION AND PHARMACOKINETICS

Infliximab (cA2) is a chimeric mouse–human monoclonal antibody to TNF. It consists of human $IgG_1$ constant regions, human κ light chains, and transplanted monoclonal murine variable regions that recognize TNF with very high affinity.[235] Infliximab binds free and membrane-bound TNF, preventing the cytokine from binding to its cell surface receptor and exerting biological activity. Linkage of the TNF-binding portions to the Fc region of immunoglobulin slows their clearance from plasma and allows for a variety of effector functions related to the immunoglobulin constant regions, such as complement fixation and antibody-mediated cellular cytotoxicity. Infliximab is administered as an intravenous infusion. Pharmacokinetic studies of infliximab demonstrate that the plasma concentrations are linearly proportional to dose, and elimination follows first-order kinetics.[236,237] At therapeutic doses of 5–10 mg/kg, the median terminal half-life of infliximab is in the range of 8–10 days. Crohn's patients receiving maintenance treatment with 5 and 10 mg/kg of infliximab, 20% and 12%, respectively, had undetectable infliximab concentrations 8 weeks following their last infusion.[231,236]

## MECHANISM OF ACTION

TNF is a pivotal cytokine involved in multiple proinflammatory and proliferative pathways of IBD. Monocytes and macrophages are the primary source of secreted TNF, whereas T lymphocytes and monocytes express transmembrane TNF.[238] The biological activity of TNF is mediated by the binding of soluble or membrane-bound TNF to the cell-surface TNF receptors, types I (R1) and II (R2). Both receptors can activate the transcription of NFκB, leading to the transcription of multiple proinflammatory genes.[239-241] TNFR1 has a death domain that initiates programmed cell death, or apoptosis; however, this apoptosis can be prevented by TNF receptor-mediated nuclear translocation of NFκB.[242,243] TNFR2 may be a ligand-passing receptor, binding TNF and transferring it to TNFR1.[241] Patients with IBD have been shown to have elevated levels of TNF in the serum,[244] colonic mucosa[245] and feces.[246]

Immunoglobulin isotype is an important determinant of antibody function. For example, antibodies of the $IgG_1$, but not the $IgG_4$ isotype can stimulate secondary effector mechanisms mediated by the Fc portion of the molecule. Fc receptor binding can result in complement activation and antibody-mediated cellular cytotoxicity.[247] In this regard, infliximab can generate Fc receptor-dependent effector functions resulting in cytotoxicity.[248] This function may in part underlie the effects of infliximab in vivo, and may thus represent an important difference from CDP571, a humanized $IgG_4$ antibody to TNF and etanercept, a fusion protein of the TNFR2, which do not appear to cause complement-mediated or antibody-mediated cytotoxicity and which do not have comparable levels of efficacy to infliximab for the treatment of Crohn's disease.[249,250]

Infliximab binds to soluble and membrane-bound TNF with high affinity, preventing the cytokine from binding to its receptors and thus neutralizing its biological activity.[235,251,252] As a result, serum TNF concentrations may actually increase because binding to the long-residing TNF antagonist molecules slows clearance.[237] In vivo, treatment with infliximab has been demonstrated to downregulate Th1 lymphocyte cytokine production in Crohn's disease mucosa,[253] to decrease the activity of pathways of coagulation and fibrinolysis,[254] and to decrease circulating levels of phospholipase A2. The resulting decrease in inflammation with infliximab helps restore the gut barrier in patients with Crohn's disease.[255]

However, the most important mechanism of action of infliximab in Crohn's disease is probably binding to transmembrane TNF.[241] Binding of infliximab to activated monocytes leads to apoptosis by activation of caspases 8, 9 and 3 via a mitochondrial pathway.[256] T lymphocytes in patients with Crohn's disease are resistant to apoptosis and express low concentrations of the proapoptotic Bax protein.[241,257] Infliximab binding to activated T lymphocytes can increase levels of Bax, resulting in apoptosis.[258] Thus, infliximab probably works by binding both soluble and membrane-bound forms of TNF, leading to a decrease in inflammatory cytokines, apoptosis of activated T lymphocytes and monocytes, and a restoration of more normal gut physiology.

## ADVERSE EFFECTS

Infliximab has been shown to be relatively safe when used as a long-term maintenance therapy. In a study of 573 patients, headache, abdominal pain and upper respiratory tract infection were the most common complications.[259] Integrated safety data from clinical trials of infliximab in Crohn's disease and rheumatoid arthritis noted serious infections in 6.3% of patients versus 6.8% of those given placebo; neurological events such as demyelinating neuropathy (one patient), aggravation of multiple sclerosis (one patient) and peripheral neuropathy (three patients); hematologic events such as anemia (0.4%) and pancytopenia (0.1%); and cardiac failure in seven rheumatoid arthritis patients.[236]

The most worrying adverse events associated with infliximab are infusion reactions, serious infections and the theoretical risk of malignancy. Acute infusion reactions (anaphylactoid, non-IgE mediated) occur in approximately 22% of patients and present with dyspnea, chest tightness, urticaria and headache.[236] Acute infusion reactions occur more commonly in patients positive for antibody to infliximab, and occur less frequently in patients treated concomitantly with immunosuppressive drugs.[259] Severe anaphylactic or anaphylactic-like reactions are rare and are characterized by hypotension, laryngeal edema, bronchospasm etc. Delayed-type hypersensitivity reactions occur 3–12 days after infusion and can be characterized by myalgias, rash, fever, polyarthralgias, pruritus, edema, urticaria, sore throat and dysphagia. The frequency is approximately 2% in patients on maintenance infliximab therapy.[259]

In compiled data from clinical trials, human antichimeric antibodies (HACA) were found in 80/298 (28%) of evaluable patients.[236] The presence of HACA may[260,261] or may not[262] decrease the efficacy of infliximab but, as stated above, does increase the risk of infusion reactions.[259] However, most patients with HACA will not experience an infusion reaction, and these levels do not need to be evaluated prior to therapy. The development of new antinuclear antibodies (44%) and antidouble-stranded DNA (22%) occurred in patients treated with infliximab.[236] This was again reduced by the use of concomitant immunosuppressants. Drug-induced lupus is very rare, occurring in only 1/573 patients in a large maintenance trial.[259]

Infections requiring treatment in clinical studies were reported in 36% of patients receiving infliximab versus 26% of placebo.[236] Respiratory and urinary tract infections are most common. In postmarketing experience severe infections have been reported, including reactivation of latent tuberculosis (>70 cases), pneumonia, sepsis, disseminated coccidiomycoses, histoplasmosis, listeriosis, *Pneumocystis carinii* pneumonia, aspergillosis and disseminated herpes zoster. All patients receiving infliximab should be screened for tuberculosis with a PPD skin test and, if indicated, a chest radiograph. Patients with active tuberculosis should be treated accordingly and should not receive infliximab until the infection is cleared. Patients with evidence of latent tuberculosis should be treated according to the American Thoracic Society guidelines[263] and may start infliximab after the completion of therapy. Patients in areas endemic for other opportunistic infections should be screened appropriately, and all patients should be watched closely for signs of infection.

Finally, all immunosuppressive agents carry the potential risk of malignancy. There have been 18 solid tumors and six lymphomas in 1372 patients treated with infliximab in clinical trials. The solid tumor rate was similar to what was expected in the patient-years of follow-up. Four of the lymphomas occurred prior to 1998, and the infrequent occurrence of lymphoma does not appear to be associated with dose or duration of therapy.[236]

## OPTIMIZATION OF THERAPY

An initial dose of 5 mg/kg is more effective[232,234] or as effective[231,233] as 10 mg/kg, and is the initial dose of choice. A three-dose induction regimen at 0, 2 and 6 weeks for both luminal and fistulizing Crohn's disease may decrease the frequency of infusion reactions and the formation of HACA.[262,264] The duration of benefit of a single dose appears to be 8–12 weeks for most patients[265] and, based on the results of clinical trials, an every-8-weeks maintenance regimen has been adopted.

Concomitant immunosuppressives – azathioprine, 6-MP, methotrexate – confer multiple benefits. They reduce the formation of HACA which, as discussed above, results in fewer infusion reactions and potentially maintains efficacy. In the rheumatoid arthritis literature, concomitant methotrexate yields superior clinical results to infliximab alone.[264] This has not been consistently demonstrated in the IBD literature.[232,234,265] Thus, concomitant therapy with azathioprine, 6-MP or methotrexate should be used to prevent infusion reactions and HACA and autoantibody formation in patients receiving repeated infliximab infusions, or as primary maintenance therapy in patients receiving a single course of infliximab or periodic infusions based on clinical need.

## SUMMARY

A great deal has been learned in the last 30 years about the clinical pharmacology of medications for the treatment of IBD. Although the full mechanism of action is not known for most agents, it has become clear that many patients will require chronic single- or multiple-drug therapy to induce and maintain remission of their disease. Understanding the interactions of these medications with the immune system and with genetically programmed metabolic pathways that determine treatment efficacy and adverse events will be critical for optimizing the management of these patients with Crohn's disease and ulcerative colitis.

## REFERENCES

1. Das KM, Eastwood MA, McManus JP, Sircus W. The metabolism of salicylazosulphapyridine in ulcerative colitis. I. The relationship between metabolites and the response to treatment in inpatients. Gut 1973;14:631–641.
2. Klotz U, Maier K, Fischer C, Heinkel K. Therapeutic efficacy of sulfasalazine and its metabolites in patients with ulcerative colitis and Crohn's disease. N Engl J Med 1980;303:1499–1502.
3. Azad Khan AK, Piris J, Truelove SC. An experiment to determine the active therapeutic moiety of sulphasalazine. Lancet 1977;2:892–895.
4. van Hees PA, Bakker JH, van Tongeren JH. Effect of sulphapyridine, 5-aminosalicylic acid, and placebo in patients with idiopathic proctitis: a study to determine the active therapeutic moiety of sulphasalazine. Gut 1980;21:632–635.
5. Taffet SL, Das KM. Sulfasalazine. Adverse effects and desensitization. Dig Dis Sci 1983;28:833–842.
6. Ligumsky M, Karmeli F, Sharon P, Zor U, Cohen F, Rachmilewitz D. Enhanced thromboxane A2 and prostacyclin production by cultured rectal mucosa in ulcerative colitis and its inhibition by steroids and sulfasalazine. Gastroenterology 1981;81:444–449.
7. Sharon P, Ligumsky M, Rachmilewitz D, Zor U. Role of prostaglandins in ulcerative colitis. Enhanced production during active disease and inhibition by sulfasalazine. Gastroenterology 1978;75:638–640.
8. Hawkey CJ, Boughton-Smith NK, Whittle BJ. Modulation of human colonic arachidonic acid metabolism by sulfasalazine. Dig Dis Sci 1985;30:1161–1165.
9. Punchard NA, Boswell DJ, Greenfield SM, Thompson RP. The effects of sulphasalazine and its metabolites on prostaglandin production by human mononuclear cells. Biochem Pharmacol 1992;43:2369–2376.
10. Felder JB, Korelitz BI, Rajapakse R, Schwarz S, Horatagis AP, Gleim G. Effects of nonsteroidal antiinflammatory drugs on inflammatory bowel disease: a case–control study. Am J Gastroenterol 2000;95:1949–1954.
11. Stenson WF, Lobos E. Sulfasalazine inhibits the synthesis of chemotactic lipids by neutrophils. J Clin Invest 1982;69:494–497.
12. MacDonald TT, Monteleone G, Pender SL. Recent developments in the immunology of inflammatory bowel disease. Scand J Immunol 2000;51:2–9.
13. Papadakis KA, Targan SR. Role of cytokines in the pathogenesis of inflammatory bowel disease. Annu Rev Med 2000;51:289–298.
14. Cominelli F ZC, Dinarello CA. Sulfasalazine inhibits cytokine production in human mononuclear cells: A novel anti-inflammatory mechanism. Gastroenterology 1992;96:A96.
15. Mahida YR, Lamming CE, Gallagher A, Hawthorne AB, Hawkey CJ. 5-Aminosalicylic acid is a potent inhibitor of interleukin 1 beta production in organ culture of colonic biopsy specimens from patients with inflammatory bowel disease. Gut 1991;32:50–54.
16. Rachmilewitz D, Karmeli F, Schwartz LW, Simon PL. Effect of aminophenols (5-ASA and 4-ASA) on colonic interleukin-1 generation. Gut 1992;33:929–932.
17. Shanahan F, Niederlehner A, Carramanzana N, Anton P. Sulfasalazine inhibits the binding of TNF alpha to its receptor. Immunopharmacology 1990;20:217–224.
18. Ahnfelt-Ronne I, Nielsen OH, Christensen A, Langholz E, Binder V, Riis P. Clinical evidence supporting the radical scavenger mechanism of 5-aminosalicylic acid. Gastroenterology 1990;98:1162–1169.
19. Aruoma OI, Wasil M, Halliwell B, Hoey BM, Butler J. The scavenging of oxidants by sulphasalazine and its metabolites. A possible contribution to their anti-inflammatory effects? Biochem Pharmacol 1987;36:3739–3742.
20. MacDermott RP. Progress in understanding the mechanisms of action of 5-aminosalicylic acid. Am J Gastroenterol 2000;95:3343–3345.
21. Thiele K, Bierhaus A, Autschbach F et al. Cell specific effects of glucocorticoid treatment on the NF-kappaBp65/IkappaBalpha system in patients with Crohn's disease. Gut 1999;45:693–704.
22. Schreiber S, Nikolaus S, Hampe J. Activation of nuclear factor kappa B inflammatory bowel disease. Gut 1998;42:477–484.
23. Rogler G, Brand K, Vogl D et al. Nuclear factor kappaB is activated in macrophages and epithelial cells of inflamed intestinal mucosa. Gastroenterology 1998;115:357–369.
24. Neurath MF, Pettersson S, Meyer zum Buschenfelde KH, Strober W. Local administration of antisense phosphorothioate oligonucleotides to the p65 subunit of NF-kappa B abrogates established experimental colitis in mice. Nature Med 1996;2:998–1004.
25. Wahl C, Liptay S, Adler G, Schmid RM. Sulfasalazine: a potent and specific inhibitor of nuclear factor kappa B. J Clin Invest 1998;101:1163–1174.
26. Egan LJ, Mays DC, Huntoon CJ et al. Inhibition of interleukin-1-stimulated NF-kappaB RelA/p65 phosphorylation by mesalamine is accompanied by decreased transcriptional activity. J Biol Chem 1999;274:26448–26453.
27. Kaiser GC, Yan F, Polk DB. Mesalamine blocks tumor necrosis factor growth inhibition and nuclear factor kappaB activation in mouse colonocytes. Gastroenterology 1999;116:602–609.
28. Bantel H, Berg C, Vieth M, Stolte M, Kruis W, Schulze-Osthoff K. Mesalazine inhibits activation of transcription factor NF-kappaB in inflamed mucosa of patients with ulcerative colitis. Am J Gastroenterol 2000;95:3452–3457.
29. Haagen Nielsen O, Bondesen S. Kinetics of 5-aminosalicylic acid after jejunal instillation in man. Br J Clin Pharmacol 1983;16:738–740.
30. Myers B, Evans DN, Rhodes J et al. Metabolism and urinary excretion of 5-amino salicylic acid in healthy volunteers when given intravenously or released for absorption at different sites in the gastrointestinal tract. Gut 1987;28:196–200.
31. Vree TB, Dammers E, Exler PS, Sorgel F, Bondesen S, Maes RA. Liver and gut mucosa acetylation of mesalazine in healthy volunteers. Int J Clin Pharmacol Ther 2000;38:514–522.
32. Peppercorn MA, Goldman P. The role of intestinal bacteria in the metabolism of salicylazosulfapyridine. J Pharmacol Exp Ther 1972;181:555–562.
33. Azad Khan AK, Guthrie G, Johnston HH, Truelove SC, Williamson DH. Tissue and bacterial splitting of sulphasalazine. Clin Sci (Lond) 1983;64:349–354.
34. Das KM, Eastwood MA. Acetylation polymorphism of sulfapyridine in patients with ulcerative colitis and Crohn's disease. Clin Pharmacol Ther 1975;18:514–520.
35. Anon. Sulfasalazine. Physician's Desk Reference 2002.
36. Allgayer H, Ahnfelt NO, Kruis W et al. Colonic N-acetylation of 5-aminosalicylic acid in inflammatory bowel disease. Gastroenterology 1989;97:38–41.
37. Zhou SY, Fleisher D, Pao LH, Li C, Winward B, Zimmermann EM. Intestinal metabolism and transport of 5-aminosalicylate. Drug Metab Dispos 1999;27:479–485.
38. Layer PH, Goebell H, Keller J, Dignass A, Klotz U. Delivery and fate of oral mesalamine microgranules within the human small intestine. Gastroenterology 1995;108:1427–1433.
39. Goebell H, Klotz U, Nehlsen B, Layer P. Oroileal transit of slow release 5-aminosalicylic acid. Gut 1993;34:669–675.
40. Stretch GL, Campbell BJ, Dwarakanath AD et al. 5-amino salicylic acid absorption and metabolism in ulcerative colitis patients receiving maintenance sulphasalazine, olsalazine or mesalazine. Aliment Pharmacol Ther 1996;10:941–947.
41. Staerk Laursen L, Stokholm M, Bukhave K, Rask-Madsen J, Lauritsen K. Disposition of 5-aminosalicylic acid by olsalazine and three mesalazine preparations in patients with ulcerative colitis: comparison of intraluminal colonic concentrations, serum values, and urinary excretion. Gut 1990;31:1271–1276.
42. Christensen LA, Fallingborg J, Jacobsen BA et al. Comparative bioavailability of 5-aminosalicylic acid from a controlled release preparation and an azo-bond preparation. Aliment Pharmacol Ther 1994;8:289–294.
43. Sandborn WJ, Hanauer HS. The pharmocokinetic profiles of oral mesulazine formulations used in the managment of ulcerative colitis. Aliment Pharmacol 2003;17:29–72.
44. Sutherland LR, May GR, Shaffer EA. Sulfasalazine revisited: a meta-analysis of 5-aminosalicylic acid in the treatment of ulcerative colitis. Ann Intern Med 1993;118:540–549.

45. Jay M, Beihn RM, Digenis GA, Deland FH, Caldwell L, Mlodozeniec AR. Disposition of radiolabelled suppositories in humans. J Pharm Pharmacol 1985;37:266–268.

46. Williams CN, Haber G, Aquino JA. Double-blind, placebo-controlled evaluation of 5-ASA suppositories in active distal proctitis and measurement of extent of spread using 99mTc-labeled 5-ASA suppositories. Dig Dis Sci 1987;32(Suppl):71S–75S.

47. Tiel-van Buul MM, Mulder CJ, van Royen EA, Wiltink EH, Tytgat GN. Retrograde spread of mesalazine (5-aminosalicylic acid)-containing enema in patients with ulcerative colitis. Clin Pharmacokinet 1991;20:247–251.

48. Campieri M, Lanfranchi GA, Brignola C et al. Retrograde spread of 5-aminosalicylic acid enemas in patients with active ulcerative colitis. Dis Colon Rectum 1986;29:108–110.

49. Chapman NJ, Brown ML, Phillips SF et al. Distribution of mesalamine enemas in patients with active distal ulcerative colitis. Mayo Clin Proc 1992;67:245–248.

50. van Bodegraven AA, Boer RO, Lourens J, Tuynman HA, Sindram JW. Distribution of mesalazine enemas in active and quiescent ulcerative colitis. Aliment Pharmacol Ther 1996;10:327–332.

51. Klotz U. Clinical pharmacokinetics of sulphasalazine, its metabolites and other prodrugs of 5-aminosalicylic acid. Clin Pharmacokinet 1985;10:285–302.

52. Das KM, Eastwood MA, McManus JP, Sircus W. Adverse reactions during salicylazosulfapyridine therapy and the relation with drug metabolism and acetylator phenotype. N Engl J Med 1973;289:491–495.

53. Pullar T, Hunter JA, Capell HA. Effect of acetylator phenotype on efficacy and toxicity of sulphasalazine in rheumatoid arthritis. Ann Rheum Dis 1985;44:831–837.

54. Bax DE, Greaves MS, Amos RS. Sulphasalazine for rheumatoid arthritis: relationship between dose, acetylator phenotype and response to treatment. Br J Rheumatol 1986;25:282–284.

55. Kitas GD, Farr M, Waterhouse L, Bacon PA. Influence of acetylator status on sulphasalazine efficacy and toxicity in patients with rheumatoid arthritis. Scand J Rheumatol 1992;21:220–225.

56. Ardizzone S, Porro GB. Comparative tolerability of therapies for ulcerative colitis. Drug Saf 2002;25:561–582.

57. Shanahan F, Targan S. Sulfasalazine and salicylate-induced exacerbation of ulcerative colitis. N Engl J Med 1987;317:455.

58. Sninsky CA, Cort DH, Shanahan F et al. Oral mesalamine (Asacol) for mildly to moderately active ulcerative colitis. A multicenter study. Ann Intern Med 1991;115:350–355.

59. Schroeder KW, Tremaine WJ, Ilstrup DM. Coated oral 5-aminosalicylic acid therapy for mildly to moderately active ulcerative colitis. A randomized study. N Engl J Med 1987;317:1625–1629.

60. Bitton A, Peppercorn MA, Hanrahan JP, Upton MP. Mesalamine-induced lung toxicity. Am J Gastroenterol 1996;91:1039–1040.

61. Iaquinto G, Sorrentini I, Petillo FE, Berardesca G. Pleuropericarditis in a patient with ulcerative colitis in longstanding 5-aminosalicylic acid therapy. Ital J Gastroenterol 1994;26:145–147.

62. Deltenre P, Berson A, Marcellin P, Degott C, Biour M, Pessayre D. Mesalazine (5-aminosalicylic acid) induced chronic hepatitis. Gut 1999;44:886–888.

63. Fernandez J, Sala M, Panes J, Feu F, Navarro S, Teres J. Acute pancreatitis after long-term 5-aminosalicylic acid therapy. Am J Gastroenterol 1997;92:2302–2303.

64. Brouillard M, Gheerbrant JD, Gheysens Y et al. [Chronic interstitial nephritis and mesalazine: 3 new cases?]. Gastroenterol Clin Biol 1998;22:724–726.

65. Calvino J, Romero R, Pintos E et al. Mesalazine-associated tubulo-interstitial nephritis in inflammatory bowel disease. Clin Nephrol 1998;49:265–267.

66. Hanauer SB V-BC, Regalli G. Renal safety of long-term mesalamine therapy in inflammatory bowel disease (IBD). Gastroenterology 1997;112:A991.

67. Marteau P, Nelet F, Le Lu M, Devaux C. Adverse events in patients treated with 5-aminosalicyclic acid: 1993–1994 pharmacovigilance report for Pentasa in France. Aliment Pharmacol Ther 1996;10:949–956.

68. Mahmud N, O'Toole D, O'Hare N, Freyne PJ, Weir DG, Kelleher D. Evaluation of renal function following treatment with 5-aminosalicylic acid derivatives in patients with ulcerative colitis. Aliment Pharmacol Ther 2002;16:207–215.

69. Fraser JS, Muller AF, Smith DJ, Newman DJ, Lamb EJ. Renal tubular injury is present in acute inflammatory bowel disease prior to the introduction of drug therapy. Aliment Pharmacol Ther 2001;15:1131–1137.

70. Riley SA, Lloyd DR, Mani V. Tests of renal function in patients with quiescent colitis: effects of drug treatment. Gut 1992;33:1348–1352.

71. Schreiber S, Hamling J, Zehnter E et al. Renal tubular dysfunction in patients with inflammatory bowel disease treated with aminosalicylate. Gut 1997;40(6):761–766.

72. Sturgeon JB, Bhatia P, Hermens D, Miner PB Jr. Exacerbation of chronic ulcerative colitis with mesalamine. Gastroenterology 1995;108:1889–1893.

73. Pamukcu R, Hanauer SB, Chang EB. Effect of disodium azodisalicylate on electrolyte transport in rabbit ileum and colon in vitro. Comparison with sulfasalazine and 5-aminosalicylic acid. Gastroenterology 1988;95:975–981.

74. Feurle GE, Theuer D, Velasco S et al. Olsalazine versus placebo in the treatment of mild to moderate ulcerative colitis: a randomised double blind trial. Gut 1989;30:1354–1361.

75. Naganuma M, Iwao Y, Ogata H et al. Measurement of colonic mucosal concentrations of 5-aminosalicylic acid is useful for estimating its therapeutic efficacy in distal ulcerative colitis: comparison of orally administered mesalamine and sulfasalazine. Inflamm Bowel Dis 2001;7:221–225.

76. Frieri G, Pimpo MT, Palumbo GC et al. Rectal and colonic mesalazine concentration in ulcerative colitis: oral vs. oral plus topical treatment. Aliment Pharmacol Ther 1999;13:1413–1417.

77. d'Albasio G, Pacini F, Camarri E et al. Combined therapy with 5-aminosalicylic acid tablets and enemas for maintaining remission in ulcerative colitis: a randomized double-blind study. Am J Gastroenterol 1997;92:1143–1147.

78. Vecchi M, Meucci G, Gionchetti P et al. Oral versus combination mesalazine therapy in active ulcerative colitis: a double-blind, double-dummy, randomized multicentre study. Aliment Pharmacol Ther 2001;15:251–256.

79. Frieri G, Giacomelli R, Pimpo M et al. Mucosal 5-aminosalicylic acid concentration inversely correlates with severity of colonic inflammation in patients with ulcerative colitis. Gut 2000;47:410–414.

80. Hein DW, Doll MA, Rustan TD, Ferguson RJ. Metabolic activation of N-hydroxyarylamines and N-hydroxyarylamides by 16 recombinant human NAT2 allozymes: effects of 7 specific NAT2 nucleic acid substitutions. Cancer Res 1995;55:3531–3536.

81. Hickman D, Pope J, Patil SD et al. Expression of arylamine N-acetyltransferase in human intestine. Gut 1998;42:402–409.

82. Grant DM, Hughes NC, Janezic SA et al. Human acetyltransferase polymorphisms. Mutat Res 1997;376:61–70.

83. Ricart E, Taylor WR, Loftus EV et al. N-acetyltransferase 1 and 2 genotypes do not predict response or toxicity to treatment with mesalamine and sulfasalazine in patients with ulcerative colitis. Am J Gastroenterol 2002;97:1763–1768.

84. Lowry PW, Franklin CL, Weaver AL et al. Measurement of thiopurine methyltransferase activity and azathioprine metabolites in patients with inflammatory bowel disease. Gut 2001;49:665–670.

85. Dewit O, Vanheuverzwyn R, Desager JP, Horsmans Y. Interaction between azathioprine and aminosalicylates: an in vivo study in patients with Crohn's disease. Aliment Pharmacol Ther 2002;16:79–85.

86. Gronemeyer H. Control of transcription activation by steroid hormone receptors. FASEB J 1992;6:2524–2529.

87. Hollenberg SM, Weinberger C, Ong ES et al. Primary structure and expression of a functional human glucocorticoid receptor cDNA. Nature 1985;318:635–641.

88. Giguere V, Hollenberg SM, Rosenfeld MG, Evans RM. Functional domains of the human glucocorticoid receptor. Cell 1986;46:645–652.

89. Bamberger CM, Bamberger AM, de Castro M, Chrousos GP. Glucocorticoid receptor beta, a potential endogenous inhibitor of glucocorticoid action in humans. J Clin Invest 1995;95:2435–2441.

90. Wissink S vHE, van der Burg, et al. A dual mechanism mediates repression of NF-kappa B and not ATF/c-Jun. J Immunol 1998;158:3836–3844.

91. Barnes PJ, Karin M. Nuclear factor-kappaB: a pivotal transcription factor in chronic inflammatory diseases. N Engl J Med 1997;336:1066–1071.

92. Paliogianni F, Raptis A, Ahuja SS, Najjar SM, Boumpas DT. Negative transcriptional regulation of human interleukin 2 (IL-2) gene by glucocorticoids through interference with nuclear transcription factors AP-1 and NF-AT. J Clin Invest 1993;91:1481–1489.

93. Colotta F, Re F, Muzio M et al. Interleukin-1 type II receptor: a decoy target for IL-1 that is regulated by IL-4. Science 1993;261:472–475.

94. Brostjan C, Anrather J, Csizmadia V, Natarajan G, Winkler H. Glucocorticoids inhibit E-selectin expression by targeting NF-kappaB and not ATF/c-Jun. J Immunol 1997;158:3836–3844.

95. Rachmilewitz D, Stamler JS, Bachwich D, Karmeli F, Ackerman Z, Podolsky DK. Enhanced colonic nitric oxide generation and nitric oxide synthase activity in ulcerative colitis and Crohn's disease. Gut 1995;36:718–723.

96. Leonard N, Bishop AE, Polak JM, Talbot IC. Expression of nitric oxide synthase in inflammatory bowel disease is not affected by corticosteroid treatment. J Clin Pathol 1998;51:750–753.

97. Tillinger W, Gasche C, Reinisch W et al. Influence of topically and systemically active steroids on circulating leukocytes in Crohn's disease. Am J Gastroenterol 1998;93:1848–1853.

98. Bernstein CN, Sargent M, Rawsthorne P, Rector E. Peripheral blood lymphocyte beta 2 integrin and ICAM expression in inflammatory bowel disease. Dig Dis Sci 1997;42:2338–2349.

99. Yang SK, Choi MS, Kim OH et al. The increased expression of an array of C-X-C and C-C chemokines in the colonic mucosa of patients with ulcerative colitis: regulation by corticosteroids. Am J Gastroenterol 2002;97:126–132.

100. Powell LW AE. Corticosteroids in liver disease: studies on the biological conversion of prednisone to prenisolone and plasma protein bindnig. Gut 1972;13:690–696.

101. Tanner AR, Halliday JW, Powell LW. Serum prednisolone levels in Crohn's disease and coeliac disease following oral prednisolone administration. Digestion 1981;21:310–315.

102. Shaffer JA, Williams SE, Turnberg LA, Houston JB, Rowland M. Absorption of prednisolone in patients with Crohn's disease. Gut 1983;24:182–186.

103. Elliott PR, Powell-Tuck J, Gillespie PE et al. Prednisolone absorption in acute colitis. Gut 1980;21:49–51.

104. Berghouse LM, Elliott PR, Lennard-Jones JE, English J, Marks V. Plasma prednisolone levels during intravenous therapy in acute colitis. Gut 1982;23:980–983.

105. Cann PA, Holdsworth CD. Systemic absorption from hydrocortisone foam enema in ulcerative colitis. Lancet 1987;1:922–923.

106.  Petitjean O, Wendling JL, Tod M et al. Pharmacokinetics and absolute rectal bioavailability of hydrocortisone acetate in distal colitis. Aliment Pharmacol Ther 1992;6:351–357.

107.  Lee DA, Taylor M, James VH, Walker G. Rectally administered prednisolone – evidence for a predominantly local action. Gut 1980;21:215–218.

108.  McIntyre PB, Macrae FA, Berghouse L, English J, Lennard-Jones JE. Therapeutic benefits from a poorly absorbed prednisolone enema in distal colitis. Gut 1985;26:822–824.

109.  Luman W, Gray RS, Pendek R, Palmer KR. Prednisolone metasulphobenzoate foam retention enemas suppress the hypothalamo–pituitary–adrenal axis. Aliment Pharmacol Ther 1994;8:255–258.

110.  Robinson RJ, Iqbal SJ, Whitaker RP, Abrams K, Mayberry JF. Rectal steroids suppress bone formation in patients with colitis. Aliment Pharmacol Ther 1997;11:201–204.

111.  Spencer CM, McTavish D. Budesonide. A review of its pharmacological properties and therapeutic efficacy in inflammatory bowel disease. Drugs 1995;50:854–872.

112.  Edsbacker S. Budesonide capsules: scientific basis. Drugs of Today 2000;38(Suppl. G):9–23.

113.  Edsbacker S, Nilsson M, Larsson P. A cortisol suppression dose–response comparison of budesonide in controlled ileal release capsules with prednisolone. Aliment Pharmacol Ther 1999;13:219–224.

114.  Rutgeerts P, Lofberg R, Malchow H et al. A comparison of budesonide with prednisolone for active Crohn's disease. N Engl J Med 1994;331:842–845.

115.  Hanauer SB, Robinson M, Pruitt R et al. Budesonide enema for the treatment of active, distal ulcerative colitis and proctitis: a dose-ranging study. US Budesonide Enema Study Group. Gastroenterology 1998;115:525–532.

116.  Campieri M, Cottone M, Miglio F et al. Beclomethasone dipropionate enemas versus prednisolone sodium phosphate enemas in the treatment of distal ulcerative colitis. Aliment Pharmacol Ther 1998;12:361–366.

117.  D'Arienzo A, Manguso F, Castiglione GN et al. Beclomethasone dipropionate (3 mg) enemas combined with oral 5-ASA (2.4 g) in the treatment of ulcerative colitis not responsive to oral 5-ASA alone. Ital J Gastroenterol Hepatol 1998;30:254–257.

118.  Halpern Z, Sold O, Baratz M, Konikoff F, Halak A, Gilat T. A controlled trial of beclomethasone versus betamethasone enemas in distal ulcerative colitis. J Clin Gastroenterol 1991;13:38–41.

119.  Hawthorne AB, Record CO, Holdsworth CD et al. Double blind trial of oral fluticasone propionate v prednisolone in the treatment of active ulcerative colitis. Gut 1993;34:125–128.

120.  Angus P, Snook JA, Reid M, Jewell DP. Oral fluticasone propionate in active distal ulcerative colitis. Gut 1992;33:711–714.

121.  Singleton JW, Law DH, Kelley ML Jr, Mekhjian HS, Sturdevant RA. National Cooperative Crohn's Disease Study: adverse reactions to study drugs. Gastroenterology 1979;77:870–882.

122.  Talar-Williams C, Sneller MC. Complications of corticosteroid therapy. Eur Arch Otorhinolaryngol 1994;251:131–136.

123.  Kusunoki M, Moeslein G, Shoji Y et al. Steroid complications in patients with ulcerative colitis. Dis Colon Rectum 1992;35:1003–1009.

124.  Baron JH, Connell AM, Kanaghinis TG et al. Out-patient treatment of ulcerative colitis. Comparison between three doses of oral prednisone. Br Med J 1962;2:441–443.

125.  Powell-Tuck J, Bown RL, Lennard-Jones JE. A comparison of oral prednisolone given as single or multiple daily doses for active proctocolitis. Scand J Gastroenterol 1978;13:833–837.

126.  Summers RW, Switz DM, Sessions JT Jr et al. National Cooperative Crohn's Disease Study: results of drug treatment. Gastroenterology 1979;77:847–869.

127.  Malchow H, Ewe K, Brandes JW et al. European Cooperative Crohn's Disease Study (ECCDS): results of drug treatment. Gastroenterology 1984;86:249–266.

128.  Brignola C, De Simone G, Belloli C et al. Steroid treatment in active Crohn's disease: a comparison between two regimens of different duration. Aliment Pharmacol Ther 1994;8:465–468.

129.  Modigliani R, Mary JY, Simon JF et al. Clinical, biological, and endoscopic picture of attacks of Crohn's disease. Evolution on prednisolone. Groupe d'Etude Therapeutique des Affections Inflammatoires Digestives. Gastroenterology 1990;98:811–818.

130.  Honda M, Orii F, Ayabe T et al. Expression of glucocorticoid receptor beta in lymphocytes of patients with glucocorticoid-resistant ulcerative colitis. Gastroenterology 2000;118:859–866.

131.  Farrell RJ, Murphy A, Long A et al. High multidrug resistance (P-glycoprotein 170) expression in inflammatory bowel disease patients who fail medical therapy. Gastroenterology 2000;118:279–288.

132.  Lennard L. The clinical pharmacology of 6-mercaptopurine. Eur J Clin Pharmacol 1992;43:329–339.

133.  Szawlowski PW, Al-Safi SA, Dooley T, Maddocks JL. Azathioprine suppresses the mixed lymphocyte reaction of patients with Lesch–Nyhan syndrome. Br J Clin Pharmacol 1985;20:489–491.

134.  Elion GB. Pharmacologic and physical agents. Immunosuppressive agents. Transplant Proc 1977;9:975–979.

135.  Campbell AC, Skinner JM, Maclennan IC et al. Immunosuppression in the treatment of inflammatory bowel disease. II. The effects of azathioprine on lymphoid cell populations in a double blind trial in ulcerative colitis. Clin Exp Immunol 1976;24:249–258.

136.  Campbell AC, Skinner JM, Hersey P, Roberts-Thomson P, MacLennan IC, Truelove SC. Immunosuppression in the treatment of inflammatory bowel disease. I. Changes in

137.  Tiede I, Wirta S, Strand S et al. CD28-Induced RAc-GTP activity is the molecular target of azathioprine in primary human CD4+ T lymphocytes: A mechanism for azathioprine-mediation in IBD based on the induction of T cell apoptosis. Gastroenterology 2002;122:A14.

138.  De MP, Beacham LM III, Creagh TH, Elion GB. The metabolic fate of the methylnitroimidazole moiety of azathioprine in the rat. J Pharmacol Exp Ther 1973;187:588–601.

139.  Chalmers AH. Studies on the mechanism of formation of 5-mercapto-1-methyl-4-nitroimidazole, a metabolite of the immunosuppressive drug azathioprine. Biochem Pharmacol 1974;23:1891–901.

140.  Lennard L. TPMT in the treatment of Crohn's disease with azathioprine. Gut 2002;51:143–146.

141.  Chan GL, Erdmann GR, Gruber SA, Matas AJ, Canafax DM. Azathioprine metabolism: pharmacokinetics of 6-mercaptopurine, 6-thiouric acid and 6-thioguanine nucleotides in renal transplant patients. J Clin Pharmacol 1990;30:358–363.

142.  Weinshilboum RM, Sladek SL. Mercaptopurine pharmacogenetics: monogenic inheritance of erythrocyte thiopurine methyltransferase activity. Am J Hum Genet 1980;32:651–662.

143.  Sandborn WJ, Tremaine WJ, Wolf DC et al. Lack of effect of intravenous administration on time to respond to azathioprine for steroid-treated Crohn's disease. North American Azathioprine Study Group. Gastroenterology 1999;117:527–535.

144.  Pearson DC, May GR, Fick GH, Sutherland LR. Azathioprine and 6-mercaptopurine in Crohn disease. A meta-analysis. Ann Intern Med 1995;123:132–142.

145.  Weinshilboum R. Methyltransferase pharmacogenetics. Pharmacol Ther 1989;43:77–90.

146.  Colombel JF, Ferrari N, Debuysere H et al. Genotypic analysis of thiopurine S-methyltransferase in patients with Crohn's disease and severe myelosuppression during azathioprine therapy. Gastroenterology 2000;118:1025–1030.

147.  Otterness DM, Szumlanski CL, Wood TC, Weinshilboum RM. Human thiopurine methyltransferase pharmacogenetics. Kindred with a terminal exon splice junction mutation that results in loss of activity. J Clin Invest 1998;101:1036–1044.

148.  Yates CR, Krynetski EY, Loennechen T et al. Molecular diagnosis of thiopurine S-methyltransferase deficiency: genetic basis for azathioprine and mercaptopurine intolerance. Ann Intern Med 1997;126:608–614.

149.  Lennard L, Van Loon JA, Weinshilboum RM. Pharmacogenetics of acute azathioprine toxicity: relationship to thiopurine methyltransferase genetic polymorphism. Clin Pharmacol Ther 1989;46:149–154.

150.  Lennard L, Rees CA, Lilleyman JS, Maddocks JL. Childhood leukaemia: a relationship between intracellular 6-mercaptopurine metabolites and neutropenia. Br J Clin Pharmacol 1983;16:359–363.

151.  Cox J, Daneshmend TK, Hawkey CJ, Logan RF, Walt RP. Devastating diarrhoea caused by azathioprine: management difficulty in inflammatory bowel disease. Gut 1988;29:686–688.

152.  Haber CJ, Meltzer SJ, Present DH, Korelitz BI. Nature and course of pancreatitis caused by 6-mercaptopurine in the treatment of inflammatory bowel disease. Gastroenterology 1986;91:982–986.

153.  Present DH, Meltzer SJ, Krumholz MP, Wolke A, Korelitz BI. 6-Mercaptopurine in the management of inflammatory bowel disease: short- and long-term toxicity. Ann Intern Med 1989;111:641–649.

154.  Boulton-Jones JR, Pritchard K, Mahmoud AA. The use of 6-mercaptopurine in patients with inflammatory bowel disease after failure of azathioprine therapy. Aliment Pharmacol Ther 2000;14:1561–1565.

155.  Bowen DG, Selby WS. Use of 6-mercaptopurine in patients with inflammatory bowel disease previously intolerant of azathioprine. Dig Dis Sci 2000;45:1810–1813.

156.  McGovern DP, Travis SP, Duley J, Shobowale-Bakre el M, Dalton HR. Azathioprine intolerance in patients with IBD may be imidazole-related and is independent of TPMT activity. Gastroenterology 2002;122:838–839.

157.  Bouhnik Y, Lemann M, Mary JY et al. Long-term follow-up of patients with Crohn's disease treated with azathioprine or 6-mercaptopurine. Lancet 1996;347:215–219.

158.  Connell WR, Kamm MA, Ritchie JK, Lennard-Jones JE. Bone marrow toxicity caused by azathioprine in inflammatory bowel disease: 27 years of experience. Gut 1993;34:1081–1085.

159.  Lewis JD, Bilker WB, Brensinger C, Deren JJ, Vaughn DJ, Strom BL. Inflammatory bowel disease is not associated with an increased risk of lymphoma. Gastroenterology 2001;121:1080–1087.

160.  Connell WR, Kamm MA, Dickson M, Balkwill AM, Ritchie JK, Lennard-Jones JE. Long-term neoplasia risk after azathioprine treatment in inflammatory bowel disease. Lancet 1994;343:1249–1252.

161.  Fraser AG, Orchard TR, Robinson EM, Jewell DP. Long-term risk of malignancy after treatment of inflammatory bowel disease with azathioprine. Aliment Pharmacol Ther 2002;16:1225–1232.

162.  Dayharsh GA, Loftus EV Jr, Sandborn WJ et al. Epstein–Barr virus-positive lymphoma in patients with inflammatory bowel disease treated with azathioprine or 6-mercaptopurine. Gastroenterology 2002;122:72–77.

163.  Black AJ, McLeod HL, Capell HA et al. Thiopurine methyltransferase genotype predicts therapy-limiting severe toxicity from azathioprine. Ann Intern Med 1998;129:716–718.

164. Snow JL, Gibson LE. A pharmacogenetic basis for the safe and effective use of azathioprine and other thiopurine drugs in dermatologic patients. J Am Acad Dermatol 1995;32:114–116.

165. Snow JL, Gibson LE. The role of genetic variation in thiopurine methyltransferase activity and the efficacy and/or side effects of azathioprine therapy in dermatologic patients. Arch Dermatol 1995;131:193–197.

166. Dubinsky MC, Lamothe S, Yang HY et al. Pharmacogenomics and metabolite measurement for 6-mercaptopurine therapy in inflammatory bowel disease. Gastroenterology 2000;118:705–713.

167. Cuffari C, Theoret Y, Latour S, Seidman G. 6-Mercaptopurine metabolism in Crohn's disease: correlation with efficacy and toxicity. Gut 1996;39:401–406.

168. Belaiche J, Desager JP, Horsmans Y, Louis E. Therapeutic drug monitoring of azathioprine and 6-mercaptopurine metabolites in Crohn disease. Scand J Gastroenterol 2001;36:71–76.

169. Dubinsky MC, Yang H, Hassard PV et al. 6-MP metabolite profiles provide a biochemical explanation for 6-MP resistance in patients with inflammatory bowel disease. Gastroenterology 2002;122:904–915.

170. Colonna T, Korelitz BI. The role of leukopenia in the 6-mercaptopurine-induced remission of refractory Crohn's disease. Am J Gastroenterol 1994;89:362–366.

171. Barbe LM, Lemann M et al. Dose raising of azathioprine beyond 2.5 mg/kg/day in Crohns' disease patients who fail to improve with a standard dose. Gastroenterology 1998;14:A925.

172. Baugh CM, Krumdieck CL, Nair MG. Polygammaglutamyl metabolites of methotrexate. Biochem Biophys Res Commun 1973;52:27–34.

173. Gruber HE, Hoffer ME, McAllister DR et al. Increased adenosine concentration in blood from ischemic myocardium by AICA riboside. Effects on flow, granulocytes, and injury. Circulation 1989;80:1400–1411.

174. Cronstein BN, Eberle MA, Gruber HE, Levin RI. Methotrexate inhibits neutrophil function by stimulating adenosine release from connective tissue cells. Proc Natl Acad Sci USA 1991;88:2441–2445.

175. Baggott JE, Morgan SL, Ha TS, Alarcon GS, Koopman WJ, Krumdieck CL. Antifolates in rheumatoid arthritis: a hypothetical mechanism of action. Clin Exp Rheumatol 1993;11 (Suppl 8):S101–105.

176. Cutolo M, Sulli A, Pizzorni C, Seriolo B, Straub RH. Anti-inflammatory mechanisms of methotrexate in rheumatoid arthritis. Ann Rheum Dis 2001;60:729–735.

177. Thomas R, Carroll GJ. Reduction of leukocyte and interleukin-1 beta concentrations in the synovial fluid of rheumatoid arthritis patients treated with methotrexate. Arthritis Rheum 1993;36:1244–1252.

178. Crilly A, McInness IB, McDonald AG, Watson J, Capell HA, Madhok R. Interleukin 6 (IL-6) and soluble IL-2 receptor levels in patients with rheumatoid arthritis treated with low dose oral methotrexate. J Rheumatol 1995;22:224–226.

179. Seitz M, Zwicker M, Loetscher P. Effects of methotrexate on differentiation of monocytes and production of cytokine inhibitors by monocytes. Arthritis Rheum 1998;41:2032–2038.

180. Sperling RI, Benincaso AI, Anderson RJ, Coblyn JS, Austen KF, Weinblatt ME. Acute and chronic suppression of leukotriene B4 synthesis ex vivo in neutrophils from patients with rheumatoid arthritis beginning treatment with methotrexate. Arthritis Rheum 1992;35:376–384.

181. Miossec P, Briolay J, Dechanet J, Wijdenes J, Martinez-Valdez H, Banchereau J. Inhibition of the production of proinflammatory cytokines and immunoglobulins by interleukin-4 in an ex vivo model of rheumatoid synovitis. Arthritis Rheum 1992;35:874–883.

182. Genestier L, Paillot R, Fournel S, Ferraro C, Miossec P, Revillard JP. Immunosuppressive properties of methotrexate: apoptosis and clonal deletion of activated peripheral T cells. J Clin Invest 1998;102:322–328.

183. Cronstein BN, Naime D, Ostad E. The antiinflammatory mechanism of methotrexate. Increased adenosine release at inflamed sites diminishes leukocyte accumulation in an in vivo model of inflammation. J Clin Invest 1993;92:2675–2682.

184. Egan LJ, Sandborn WJ, Mays DC, Tremaine WJ, Lipsky JJ. Plasma and rectal adenosine in inflammatory bowel disease: effect of methotrexate. Inflamm Bowel Dis 1999;5:167–173.

185. Dahl MG, Gregory MM, Scheuer PJ. Methotrexate hepatotoxicity in psoriasis – comparison of different dose regimens. Br Med J 1972;1:654–656.

186. Kozarek RA, Patterson DJ, Gelfand MD, Botoman VA, Ball TJ, Wilske KR. Methotrexate induces clinical and histologic remission in patients with refractory inflammatory bowel disease. Ann Intern Med 1989;110:353–356.

187. Teresi ME, Crom WR, Choi KE, Mirro J, Evans WE. Methotrexate bioavailability after oral and intramuscular administration in children. J Pediatr 1987;110:788–792.

188. Oguey D, Kolliker F, Gerber NJ, Reichen J. Effect of food on the bioavailability of low-dose methotrexate in patients with rheumatoid arthritis. Arthritis Rheum 1992;35:611–614.

189. Jundt JW, Browne BA, Fiocco GP, Steele AD, Mock D. A comparison of low dose methotrexate bioavailability: oral solution, oral tablet, subcutaneous and intramuscular dosing. J Rheumatol 1993;20:1845–1849.

190. Egan LJ, Sandborn WJ, Mays DC, Tremaine WJ, Fauq AH, Lipsky JJ. Systemic and intestinal pharmacokinetics of methotrexate in patients with inflammatory bowel disease. Clin Pharmacol Ther 1999;65:29–39.

191. Egan LJ, Sandborn WJ, Tremaine WJ et al. A randomized dose–response and pharmacokinetic study of methotrexate for refractory inflammatory Crohn's disease and ulcerative colitis. Aliment Pharmacol Ther 1999;13:1597–1604.

192. Bressolle F, Kinowski JM, Morel J, Pouly B, Sany J, Combe B. Folic acid alters methotrexate availability in patients with rheumatoid arthritis. J Rheumatol 2000;27:2110–2114.

193. Griffith SM, Fisher J, Clarke S et al. Do patients with rheumatoid arthritis established on methotrexate and folic acid 5 mg daily need to continue folic acid supplements long term? Rheumatology (Oxford) 2000;39:1102–1109.

194. Chong RY, Hanauer SB, Cohen RD. Efficacy of parenteral methotrexate in refractory Crohn's disease. Aliment Pharmacol Ther 2001;15:35–44.

195. Feagan BG, Rochon J, Fedorak RN et al. Methotrexate for the treatment of Crohn's disease. The North American Crohn's Study Group Investigators. N Engl J Med 1995;332:292–297.

196. Goodman TA, Polisson RP. Methotrexate: adverse reactions and major toxicities. Rheum Dis Clin North Am 1994;20:513–528.

197. Kremer JM, Alarcon GS, Lightfoot RW Jr et al. Methotrexate for rheumatoid arthritis. Suggested guidelines for monitoring liver toxicity. American College of Rheumatology. Arthritis Rheum 1994;37:316–328.

198. Podurgiel BJ, McGill DB, Ludwig J, Taylor WF, Muller SA. Liver injury associated with methotrexate therapy for psoriasis. Mayo Clin Proc 1973;48:787–792.

199. Newman M, Auerbach R, Feiner H et al. The role of liver biopsies in psoriatic patients receiving long-term methotrexate treatment. Improvement in liver abnormalities after cessation of treatment. Arch Dermatol 1989;125:1218–1224.

200. Walker AM, Funch D, Dreyer NA et al. Determinants of serious liver disease among patients receiving low-dose methotrexate for rheumatoid arthritis. Arthritis Rheum 1993;36:329–335.

201. Said S, Jeffes EW, Weinstein GD. Methotrexate. Clin Dermatol 1997;15:781–797.

202. Lewis JH, Schiff E. Methotrexate-induced chronic liver injury: guidelines for detection and prevention. The ACG Committee on FDA-related matters. American College of Gastroenterology. Am J Gastroenterol 1988;83:1337–1345.

203. Te HS, Schiano TD, Kuan SF, Hanauer SB, Conjeevaram HS, Baker AL. Hepatic effects of long-term methotrexate use in the treatment of inflammatory bowel disease. Am J Gastroenterol 2000;95:3150–3156.

204. Lemann M, Zenjari T, Bouhnik Y et al. Methotrexate in Crohn's disease: long-term efficacy and toxicity [see comments]. Am J Gastroenterol 2000;95:1730–1734.

205. Janssen NM, Genta MS. The effects of immunosuppressive and anti-inflammatory medications on fertility, pregnancy, and lactation. Arch Intern Med 2000;160:610–619.

206. Feagan BG, Fedorak RN, Irvine EJ et al. A comparison of methotrexate with placebo for the maintenance of remission in Crohn's disease. North American Crohn's Study Group Investigators [see comments]. N Engl J Med 2000;342:1627–1632.

207. Arora S, Katkov W, Cooley J et al. Methotrexate in Crohn's disease: results of a randomized, double-blind, placebo-controlled trial. Hepatogastroenterology 1999;46:1724–1729.

208. Oren R, Moshkowitz M, Odes S et al. Methotrexate in chronic active Crohn's disease: a double-blind, randomized, Israeli multicenter trial. Am J Gastroenterol 1997;92:2203–2209.

209. Oren R, Arber N, Odes S et al. Methotrexate in chronic active ulcerative colitis: a double-blind, randomized, Israeli multicenter trial. Gastroenterology 1996;110:1416–1421.

210. Gorlick R, Goker E, Trippett T, Waltham M, Banerjee D, Bertino JR. Intrinsic and acquired resistance to methotrexate in acute leukemia. N Engl J Med 1996;335:1041–1048.

211. Chen ZS, Lee K, Walther S et al. Analysis of methotrexate and folate transport by multidrug resistance protein 4 (ABCC4): MRP4 is a component of the methotrexate efflux system. Cancer Res 2002;62:3144–3150.

212. Lichtiger S, Present DH, Kornbluth A et al. Cyclosporin in severe ulcerative colitis refractory to steroid therapy. N Engl J Med 1994;330:1841–1845.

213. Sandborn WJ PD, Isaccs KL. Tacrolimus (FK506) for the treatment of perianal and enterocutaneous fistulas in patients with Crohn' disease: a randomized, double-blind, placebo-controlled trial. Gastroenterology 2002;122:A81.

214. Flanagan WM, Corthesy B, Bram RJ, Crabtree GR. Nuclear association of a T-cell transcription factor blocked by FK-506 and cyclosporin A. Nature 1991;352:803–807.

215. Hess AD. Mechanisms of action of cyclosporin: considerations for the treatment of autoimmune diseases. Clin Immunol Immunopathol 1993;68:220–228.

216. Brynskov J, Freund L, Campanini MC, Kampmann JP. Cyclosporin pharmacokinetics after intravenous and oral administration in patients with Crohn's disease. Scand J Gastroenterol 1992;27:961–967.

217. Kahan BD. Cyclosporine. N Engl J Med 1989;321:1725–1738.

218. Drewe J, Beglinger C, Kissel T. The absorption site of cyclosporin in the human gastrointestinal tract. Br J Clin Pharmacol 1992;33:39–43.

219. Fluckiger SS, Schmidt C, Meyer A, Kallay Z, Johnston A, Kutz K. Pharmacokinetics of orally administered cyclosporin in patients with Crohn's disease. J Clin Pharmacol 1995;35:681–687.

220. Sandborn W. A critical review of cyclosporin therapy in inflammatory bowel disease. Inflamm Bowel Dis 1995;1:48–63.

221. Hollander AA, van Rooij J, Lentjes GW et al. The effect of grapefruit juice on cyclosporin and prednisone metabolism in transplant patients. Clin Pharmacol Ther 1995;57:318–324.

222. Kornbluth A, Present DH, Lichtiger S, Hanauer S. Cyclosporin for severe ulcerative colitis: a user's guide. Am J Gastroenterol 1997;92:1424–1428.

223. Mueller EA, Kovarik JM, van Bree JB, Tetzloff W, Grevel J, Kutz K. Improved dose linearity of cyclosporin pharmacokinetics from a microemulsion formulation. Pharm Res 1994;11:301–304.

224. Latteri M, Angeloni TG, Silveri NG, Manna R, Gasbarrini G, Navarra P. Pharmacokinetics of cyclosporin microemulsion in patients with inflammatory bowel disease. Clin Pharmacokinet 2001;40:473–483.

225. Plosker GL, Foster RH. Tacrolimus: a further update of its pharmacology and therapeutic use in the management of organ transplantation. Drugs 2000;59:323–389.

226. Sandborn WJ. Cyclosporin in ulcerative colitis: state of the art. Acta Gastroenterol Belg 2001;64:201–204.

227. Sternthal M GJ, Kornbluth A. Toxicity associated with the use of cyclosporin in patients with inflammatory bowel disease. Gastroenterology 1996;110:A1019.

228. Cohen RD, Stein R, Hanauer SB. Intravenous cyclosporin in ulcerative colitis: a five-year experience. Am J Gastroenterol 1999;94:1587–1592.

229. Penn I. Cancers following cyclosporin therapy. Transplantation 1987;43:32–35.

230. Tegzess AM, Doorenbos BM, Minderhoud JM, Donker AJ. Prospective serial renal function studies in patients with nonrenal disease treated with cyclosporin A. Transplant Proc 1988;20:530–533.

231. Hanauer SB, Feagan BG, Lichtenstein GR et al. Maintenance infliximab for Crohn's disease: the ACCENT I randomised trial. Lancet 2002;359:1541–1549.

232. Targan SR, Hanauer SB, van Deventer SJ et al. A short-term study of chimeric monoclonal antibody cA2 to tumor necrosis factor alpha for Crohn's disease. Crohn's Disease cA2 Study Group. N Engl J Med 1997;337:1029–1035.

233. Sands BE, van Deventer S, Bernstein C et al. Longterm treatment of fistulizing Crohn's disease: response to infliximab in the ACCENT II trial through 54 weeks. Gastroenterology 2002;122:A81.

234. Present DH, Rutgeerts P, Targan S et al. Infliximab for the treatment of fistulas in patients with Crohn's disease. N Engl J Med 1999;340:1398–1405.

235. Knight DM, Trinh H, Le J et al. Construction and initial characterization of a mouse–human chimeric anti-TNF antibody. Mol Immunol 1993;30:1443–1453.

236. Anon. Infliximab (Remicade). Physician's Desk Reference 2002.

237. Wagner C, Mace K, De Woody K et al. Infliximab treatment benefits correlate with pahrmacodynamic parameters in Crohn's disease patients. Digestion 1998;Suppl 3:124–125.

238. Aversa G, Punnonen J, de Vries JE. The 26-kD transmembrane form of tumor necrosis factor alpha on activated CD4+ T cell clones provides a costimulatory signal for human B cell activation. J Exp Med 1993;177:1575–1585.

239. Rothe M, Sarma V, Dixit VM, Goeddel DV. TRAF2-mediated activation of NF-kappa B by TNF receptor 2 and CD40. Science 1995;269:1424–1427.

240. Liu ZG, Hsu H, Goeddel DV, Karin M. Dissection of TNF receptor 1 effector functions: JNK activation is not linked to apoptosis while NF-kappaB activation prevents cell death. Cell 1996;87:565–576.

241. van Deventer SJ. Transmembrane TNF-alpha, induction of apoptosis, and the efficacy of TNF-targeting therapies in Crohn's disease. Gastroenterology 2001;121:1242–1246.

242. Wang CY, Mayo MW, Korneluk RG, Goeddel DV, Baldwin AS Jr. NF-kappaB antiapoptosis: induction of TRAF1 and TRAF2 and c-IAP1 and c-IAP2 to suppress caspase-8 activation. Science 1998;281:1680–1683.

243. Beg AA, Baltimore D. An essential role for NF-kappaB in preventing TNF-alpha-induced cell death. Science 1996;274:782–784.

244. Murch SH, Lamkin VA, Savage MO, Walker-Smith JA, MacDonald TT. Serum concentrations of tumour necrosis factor alpha in childhood chronic inflammatory bowel disease. Gut 1991;32:913–917.

245. Reinecker HC, Steffen M, Witthoeft T et al. Enhanced secretion of tumour necrosis factor-alpha, IL-6, and IL-1 beta by isolated lamina propria mononuclear cells from patients with ulcerative colitis and Crohn's disease. Clin Exp Immunol 1993;94:174–181.

246. Braegger CP, Nicholls S, Murch SH, Stephens S, MacDonald TT. Tumour necrosis factor alpha in stool as a marker of intestinal inflammation. Lancet 1992;339:89–91.

247. Suitters AJ, Foulkes R, Opal SM et al. Differential effect of isotype on efficacy of anti-tumor necrosis factor alpha chimeric antibodies in experimental septic shock. J Exp Med 1994;179:849–856.

248. Scallon BJ, Trinh H, Nedelman M, Brennan FM, Feldmann M, Ghrayeb J. Functional comparisons of different tumour necrosis factor receptor/IgG fusion proteins. Cytokine 1995;7:759–770.

249. Sandborn WJ, Hanauer SB, Katz S et al. Etanercept for active Crohn's disease: a randomized, double-blind, placebo-controlled trial. Gastroenterology 2001;121:1088–1094.

250. Sandborn WJ FB, Hanauer SB. An engineered human antibody to TNF (CDP571) for active Crohn's disease: a randomized double-blind placebo-controlled trial. Gastroenterology 2001;120:1330–1338.

251. Siegel SA, Shealy DJ, Nakada MT et al. The mouse/human chimeric monoclonal antibody cA2 neutralizes TNF in vitro and protects transgenic mice from cachexia and TNF lethality in vivo. Cytokine 1995;7:15–25.

252. Scallon BJ, Moore MA, Trinh H, Knight DM, Ghrayeb J. Chimeric anti-TNF-alpha monoclonal antibody cA2 binds recombinant transmembrane TNF-alpha and activates immune effector functions. Cytokine 1995;7:251–259.

253. Plevy SE, Landers CJ, Prehn J et al. A role for TNF-alpha and mucosal T helper-1 cytokines in the pathogenesis of Crohn's disease. J Immunol 1997;159:6276–6282.

254. Hommes DW, van Dullemen HM, Levi M et al. Beneficial effect of treatment with a monoclonal anti-tumor necrosis factor-alpha antibody on markers of coagulation and fibrinolysis in patients with active Crohn's disease. Haemostasis 1997;27:269–277.

255. Suenaert P, Bulteel V, Lemmens L et al. Anti-tumor necrosis factor treatment restores the gut barrier in Crohn's disease. Am J Gastroenterol 2002;97:2000–2004.

256. Lugering A, Schmidt M, Lugering N, Pauels HG, Domschke W, Kucharzik T. Infliximab induces apoptosis in monocytes from patients with chronic active Crohn's disease by using a caspase-dependent pathway. Gastroenterology 2001;121:1145–1157.

257. Itoh J, de La Motte C, Strong SA, Levine AD, Fiocchi C. Decreased Bax expression by mucosal T cells favours resistance to apoptosis in Crohn's disease. Gut 2001;49:35–41.

258. ten Hove T, van Montfrans C, Peppelenbosch MP, van Deventer SJ. Infliximab treatment induces apoptosis of lamina propria T lymphocytes in Crohn's disease. Gut 2002;50:206–211.

259. Hanauer S, Lichtenstein G, Columbel JF et al. Maintenance infliximab (Remicade) is safe, effective and steroid-sparing in Crohn's disease: preliminary results of the Accent I trial. Gastroenterology 2001;120:A–21.

260. Farrell RJ, Alsahli M, Falchuk KR et al. Human anti-chimeric antibody levels correlate with lack of response and infusion reactions following infliximab therapy. Gastroenterology 2001;120:A69.

261. Norman M BF, Vermeire S. Post infusion infliximab levels determine duration of response in Crohn's disease and are directly related to infusion reactions. Gastroenterology 2002;122:A100.

262. Wagner C, Olson A, Ford J et al. Effects of antibodies to infliximab on safety and efficacy of infliximab treatment in patient's with Crohn's disease. Gastroenterology 2002;122:A613–614.

263. Targeted tuberculin testing and treatment of latent tuberculosis infection. American Thoracic Society. MMWR Recomm Rep 2000;49(RR-6):1–51.

264. Maini RN, Breedveld FC, Kalden JR et al. Therapeutic efficacy of multiple intravenous infusions of anti-tumor necrosis factor alpha monoclonal antibody combined with low-dose weekly methotrexate in rheumatoid arthritis. Arthritis Rheum 1998;41:1552–1563.

265. Rutgeerts P, D'Haens G, Targan S et al. Efficacy and safety of retreatment with anti-tumor necrosis factor antibody (infliximab) to maintain remission in Crohn's disease. Gastroenterology 1999;117:761–709.

266. Almer S, Norlander B, Strom M, Osterwald H. Steady-state pharmacokinetics of a new 4-gram 5-aminosalicylic acid retention enema in patients with ulcerative colitis in remission. Scand J Gastroenterol 1991;26:327–335.

267. Gionchetti P, Campieri M, Venturi A et al. Systemic availability of 5-aminosalicylic acid: comparison of delayed release and an azo-bond preparation. Aliment Pharmacol Ther 1996;10:601–605.

268. Norlander B, Gotthard R, Strom M. Pharmacokinetics of a 5-aminosalicylic acid enteric-coated tablet in patients with Crohn's disease or ulcerative colitis and in healthy volunteers. Aliment Pharmacol Ther 1990;4:497–505.

269. Anon. Balsalazide. Physician's Desk Reference 2002.

270. Yang YX, Lichtenstein GR. Corticosteroids in Crohn's disease. Am J Gastroenterol 2002;97:803–823.

## CHAPTER 33

# Medical therapy for ulcerative colitis

Stephen B Hanauer

## INTRODUCTION

Since the previous edition of this book there have been few novel insights into the pathogenesis of ulcerative colitis[1] and, likewise, the evolution of medical therapy for ulcerative colitis has been incremental rather than revolutionary.[2] Once again, both indications for, and optimization of, therapy are increasingly supported by better evidence. Progress related to the classification of ulcerative colitis into subgroups remains enigmatic and, despite newer serologic criteria for diagnosis, these advances have yet to translate into clinical utility.[3–5] Meanwhile, therapy for ulcerative colitis can continue to be 'staged' initially into inductive and then maintenance therapy, with additional considerations for the treatment of refractory disease and, if necessary, surgery. The continuum of medical therapy for ulcerative colitis now extends beyond surgery to the prevention of, and treatment for, pouchitis, which is discussed in Chapter 46. Whereas the vast majority of patients with ulcerative colitis require long-term medical treatment, continuation of medical therapy must be balanced against the potential for a 'curative colectomy' with cognizance of the short- and long-term impact on the patient's quality of life.

## EVALUATION OF THE PATIENT

### GENERAL PRINCIPLES

The clinical features, differential diagnosis and assessment of disease activity are discussed in Chapters 19, 25 and 30. However, relevant aspects pertaining to patient evaluation prior to initiating medical therapy are reviewed below (Tables 33.1, 33.2). In the absence of pathognomonic features, the diagnosis of ulcerative colitis remains clinical, based upon history, endoscopic and histologic features. Throughout the course an important differential diagnosis will remain the possibility of Crohn's disease, as a significant proportion of patients present with inde-

terminate features. In particular, an increasingly number of children with IBD are presenting at very young ages with primarily colitis, and it is increasingly recognized that patients presenting with fulminate or partially treated colitis may have evidence of focal inflammatory changes during treatment. This has long been recognized in patients with 'relative rectal sparing' who have been receiving topical (rectal) therapy. Most recently, patients undergoing colectomy and ileoanal anastomoses are recognized to have Crohn's disease only months, or years, after surgery. Unfortunately, in these settings serologic studies, including pANCA and ASCA, remain either non-specific (pANCA) or insensitive (ASCA).[4,5] In the future, the distinction between ulcerative colitis and Crohn's disease may be classified according to specific genetic or pathophysiologic markers, which may include patterns of serologic findings similar to the evolving recognition of genetic and serologic patterns in Crohn's disease[6] (Chapter 29). At present continued observation and reassessment of patients over time is the most likely means of defining changes in an individual's clinical pattern of disease. Throughout the disease course it remains essential to monitor for factors that can exacerbate disease activity, as well as for complications related to both chronic inflammation and medical therapies. In addition, the treating physician should be alert to the psychosocial impact of ulcerative colitis in order to optimize compliance[7] and to assist with the patient's and family's adaptation to chronic illness (Chapter 24).

The longitudinal extent and severity of colitis within the affected colon are the two most important factors to define prior to initiating therapy or when assessing the effectiveness of treatment. The disease extent is important from the therapeutic standpoint now that topical (rectal) therapies have become an option for both inductive and maintenance therapies, as long as the formulation reaches the proximal extent of disease.[8] Mucosal extent is also important when considering the long-term risk of dysplasia/cancer and affects recommendations for surveillance (Chapter 43). The severity of colitis is relevant to the intensity of anti-inflammatory therapy (and the risks of treatment)

| Table 33.1 Patient assessment |
| --- |
| Extent |
| Severity |
| Chronicity |
| Response to treatment |
| Complications |
| Intestinal |
| Extraintestinal |
| Disease modifiers |
| Acute infections |
| Smoking |
| NSAIDs |
| IBS |
| Pregnancy |
| Menstrual cycle |
| Stress |

| Table 33.2 Initial evaluation |
| --- |
| History |
| Familial IBD |
| Travel |
| Epidemic gastroenteritis |
| Smoking |
| NSAIDs |
| Extraintestinal manifestations |
| Physical examination |
| Vital signs |
| Nutritional status |
| Abdominal examination |
| Bowel sounds |
| Distension |
| Tenderness/guarding |
| Perianal disease |
| Extraintestinal features |
| Laboratory evaluation |
| Complete blood count and differential |
| Prothrombin time |
| Electrolytes |
| BUN, creatinine |
| Liver enzymes |
| ESR, CRP (fulminant disease) |
| Stool examination for pathogens, ova and parasites, *C. difficile* |
| Endoscopy |
| Flexible sigmoidoscopy |
| Colonoscopy (when stable) |
| Imaging studies |
| Plain abdominal radiograph (severe disease) |
| Leukocyte scan (severe disease) |

required to induce remissions or treat refractory disease. The interpretation of disease extent is somewhat controversial when considering how extent is determined via radiography, endoscopy or histology. From a clinical and a therapeutic standpoint, the diagnostic study is less relevant than from a prognostic standpoint. For instance, the identification of a periappendiceal (cecal) 'patch' of inflammation in patients with distal colitis has not been determined[9] as it pertains to risk of dysplasia/cancer. Likewise, there is no single definition of disease that has served both recommendations for initiating therapy and for regulatory authorities for drug approval (Chapter 30). The original classification by Truelove and Witts[10] is clinically useful and offers simple working definitions that have been used to establish clinical guidelines for initiating treatment for active ulcerative colitis.[11] A modification of the Truelove and Witts criteria, to include severe and fulminant disease, is presented in Table 33.3. Patients with mild disease present with fewer than four to six bloody bowel movements per day (although often there are frequent morning trips to the toilet for the passage of gas or mucus) without signs of systemic toxicity. Moderate disease is characterized by more than four stools per day with minimal systemic signs. Patients with severe disease have more than 6–10 bloody stools per day and evidence of fever, anemia and abdominal tenderness. Fulminant disease pertains to patients with evidence of transmural colitis with elevated white blood cell counts, anemia requiring transfusion, and abdominal tenderness with or without a dilated colon. Toxic megacolon is characterized by fulminant colitis with evidence of colonic dilatation.

Additional features that influence the therapeutic approach are the chronicity of disease, response to prior therapies, and complications of the disease or therapy. Additional, critical, considerations when approaching a patient with ulcerative colitis are factors known to influence the course of ulcerative colitis, such as cigarette smoking, the use of NSAIDs, and stress.

## Mucosal extent

The majority of patients with ulcerative colitis will have disease limited to the distal colon. The extent tends to remain constant throughout the course of the illness, although it may progress or regress with flare-ups or during the course of treatment.[12] It is not uncommon for patients to develop more proximal disease during a severe flare-up and then heal the proximal area sooner than the distal colon. The routine use of colonoscopy and biopsy of normal and abnormal-appearing mucosa has demonstrated that the microscopic extent usually exceeds the endoscopic extent, which exceeds radiographic evidence of disease.[13] Colonoscopic evaluations have also demonstrated the frequent finding of isolated periappendiceal inflammation in the cecum in patients with proctitis or left-sided colitis.[9,14] The significance of these findings remains unknown.[13] The mucosal extent also is an important risk factor for the development of dysplasia and cancer[15] (see Chapter 43).

## Severity

The severity of ulcerative colitis is relevant to acute complications and treatment approaches but not to the risk of eventual neoplasia. Disease severity is based upon composites of clinical and endoscopic criteria discussed in Chapter 30. Although several different activity indices have been employed in clinical trials, the simple categorical scale initially developed by Truelove and Witts remains the most clinically useful estimate of clinical severity used in practice (Table 33.3). It needs to be emphasized that the absence of a relationship between mucosal extent and the severity of inflammation within that extent commonly leads to the recognition that patients with severe distal colitis are often more ill than patients with mild extensive disease. Furthermore, there is no currently agreed upon definition of 'remission',[16] making it important to review individual entry criteria for

## Table 33.3 Classification of colitis*

| Variable | Mild disease | Severe disease | Fulminant disease |
|---|---|---|---|
| Stools (per day) | <4 | >6 | >10 |
| Blood in stool | Intermittent | Frequent | Continuous |
| Temperature (°C) | Normal | >37.5 | >37.5 |
| Pulse | Normal | >90 | >90 |
| Hemoglobin | Normal | <75% of normal | Transfusion required |
| ESR (mm/h) | <30 | >30 | >30 |
| Radiographic features | Normal gas pattern | Edematous colon wall, thumbprinting | Dilated colon |
| Clinical examination | Normal bowel sounds, non-tender abdomen | Tender abdomen, no rebound tenderness | Distended abdomen, decreased bowel sounds, ± rebound tenderness |

*Modified from[10, 12]

'maintenance of remission' ('prevention of relapse') clinical trials. At present, draft guidelines from the FDA continue to define remission based on 'the resolution of clinical symptoms attributed to ulcerative colitis *and* endoscopically documented mucosal healing …(the regeneration of an intact mucosa *without* ulceration, granularity, or friability)'.[17] Histologic activity also can be quantified, but scales have not been reproduced or validated that correlate well with endoscopic or clinical disease activity (Chapter 30).[12]

The laboratory features of ulcerative colitis are non-specific (see Chapter 19) and reflect aspects of inflammation in general (e.g. elevated erythrocyte sedimentation rate, leukocytosis, or increase in acute-phase reactants), complications of diarrhea (e.g. hypokalemia or other electrolyte imbalances), or pathophysiologic consequences of colitis (e.g. iron deficiency anemia, hypoproteinemia). Serologic studies evaluating the presence of perinuclear antineutrophil cytoplasmic antibodies (pANCA) appear to reflect an inflammatory subtype rather than correlating with disease severity.[4]

Therefore, the assessment of severity requires a clinical judgment of the impact of the inflammation and sequelae upon the individual patient. No two patients with the same description of bowel activity, endoscopic appearance and laboratory findings are likely to describe themselves as equally 'sick'. The ultimate measure of disease activity may be the impact on a patient's quality of life (Chapter 31), which also requires knowledge of the patient, family support and social influences (see Chapter 24).

## Chronicity

Assessments of the disease course in ulcerative colitis have demonstrated that, at any time, a significant proportion of patients continue with chronically active symptoms (Chapter 19). At any given time approximately 50% of patients are in clinical remission, but 90% are expected to have a relapsing course, primarily in the first years after diagnosis, when nearly two-thirds will have relapses and nearly one-fifth will have activity every year. One can predict the long-term course based on the first 2 years of disease. Patients with chronic ongoing activity can be considered *refractory to acute therapy* (failure to induce remission), whereas those who relapse frequently are *refractory to maintenance therapy* (failure to maintain remission).[18]

## Complications

The complications of ulcerative colitis are discussed in Chapters 19 and 43–45. Complications directly related to the activity of colitis, such as anemia, electrolyte abnormalities, hypoalbuminemia etc., affect the requisite intensity of medical therapy, as do many of the extraintestinal manifestations, including arthritis or skin lesions. Several of the extraintestinal manifestations also require therapies that are independent of the treatment for colitis per se. Arthritic manifestations, both central and peripheral (Chapter 45), require an individualized therapeutic approach to maximize antiarthritic properties without the use of NSAIDs. In addition, arthritis as well as cutaneous complications (i.e. erythema nodosum, pyoderma gangrenosum), and primary sclerosing cholangitis are risk factors for the development of pouchitis after colectomy and ileoanal anastomosis (Chapter 46). The presence of pANCA, although not recognized as a specific complication, also predicts an increase likelihood of refractory left-sided disease[19] and pouchitis after colectomy and ileoanal anastomosis.[20]

## Exogenous factors

Additional factors that influence the course of colitis or affect the efficacy of treatment are discussed in Chapters 10, 11 and 30. Intercurrent infections have been recognized to initiate flare-ups of IBD,[21] as has travelers' diarrhea.[22] Patients with newly diagnosed ulcerative colitis or presenting with acute exacerbations should be evaluated for the possibility of a complicating enteric infection.[18] Infections with organisms such as *Clostridium difficile* should be treated but may initiate flare-ups that subsequently require specific therapy for ulcerative colitis.

It is important to differentiate non-inflammatory from inflammatory symptoms in ulcerative colitis. Dietary factors influence bowel habits in the general population and will certainly influence bowel habits in the setting of colitis. A review of the patient's 'diet history' is important to identify possible aggravating components. There is no increased risk of lactose intolerance in IBD; however, the impact of lactose on patients with impaired colonic absorptive 'reserve' can induce symptoms in those who were otherwise tolerant. Similarly, the consumption of large quantities of other non-absorbed carbohydrates, such as sorbitol or artificial fats (e.g. Olestra), can produce symptoms of gas, bloating or diarrhea. Conversely, patients with proctitis often present with constipation and will benefit from the addition of additional dietary fiber. In today's environment of health consciousness and interest in non-traditional approaches to health care, a careful review of non-prescription vitamins, health foods, homeopathic agents or herbs may identify factors contributing to changes in bowel habits that are independent from the colitis. Complementary therapies are used by approximately half of adult patients[23] and children or young adults[24] with IBD, emphasizing the frustration related to side effects and/or lack of efficacy with conventional approaches, and requiring careful inquiries regarding potential side effects (e.g. diarrhea or liver toxicity) or drug interactions.

Coexistent irritable bowel syndrome is equally prevalent in patients with IBD as it is in the general population.[18,25] Patients presenting with abdominal cramping, diarrhea or constipation in the absence of rectal bleeding should be evaluated for the presence of fecal leukocytes or undergo an endoscopic assessment to differentiate IBS from active colitis. Similarly, many patients with mild colitis suffer from concurrent IBS symptoms that can respond to antispasmodics, antidiarrheals, fiber supplementation or low doses of tricyclic antidepressants (see below). Although the usual stress of day-to-day living does not affect the activity of IBD (Chapter 24), every practitioner and many patients will identify stressful aspects of life that are associated with, if not a cause for, worsening of disease activity in individual settings.

In women with ulcerative colitis, flare-ups or altered bowel activity are commonly associated with the menstrual cycle.[26] There is a spectrum of impact in individual woman and the use of NSAIDs may contribute to menstrual-related symptoms. Nevertheless, treating physicians should be aware of temporal associations and modify treatment schedules accordingly. Examples include temporarily 'holding' a tapering schedule of steroids during the menstrual period in women who repeatedly 'flare' with menses or, rarely, chronically ablating the menstrual cycle with progesterone or leuprolide. To date it has not been established that oral contraceptives are associated with the onset or worsening of ulcerative colitis, and we usually continue these for patients who so wish. Pregnancy may also have an impact – as often positive as negative – on the course of ulcerative colitis (Chapter 23).

Cigarette smoking has a major impact on ulcerative colitis.[27,28] Whereas concurrent smoking protects against the development of colitis, ex-smokers have a worse course, and are more likely to develop refractory disease and to require immune modulation or colectomy.[29] We have also found that ex-smokers may account for the later 'age of onset' peak in patients with ulcerative colitis (Hanauer SB and Cho J, personal communication). Cigarette smoking also can influence the course and complications of ulcerative colitis by protecting against sclerosing cholangitis[30,31] yet increasing the risk for osteoporosis in women with the disease.[32]

Non-steroidal anti-inflammatory drugs (NSAIDs) are well recognized to exacerbate ulcerative colitis.[1] Similar to conventional NSAIDs, the specific COX-2 agents are negative factors in experimental models and can worsen disease activity, at least in some patients.[33,34] The use and availability of conventional NSAIDs, both over the counter and by prescription, and the increasing use of the newer COX-2-specific agents by primary care physicians or specialists, requires specific questioning in patients with new onset or flare-ups of ulcerative colitis to exclude a contributing factor to the initiation or perpetuation[18] of disease activity.

## INITIAL EVALUATIONS (Table 33.2)

### History

Patients presenting with newly diagnosed ulcerative colitis or with flare-ups need to be evaluated for potential exposure to enteric infections (travel, epidemic gastroenteritis, well water) and antibiotics (C. difficile). A family history of IBD in a patient presenting with diarrhea and or rectal bleeding should raise the suspicion of idiopathic IBD. Additional relevant history includes smoking (including a distant history of smoking cessation) and exposure to NSAIDs, including specific questioning for over-the-counter formulations and COX-2 agents. Although rarely a primary event, the patient's psychosocial background may be relevant regarding stressful life-events and the individual's coping mechanisms and family support.

Focused elements to determine disease activity include constitutional symptoms such as fevers, chills, night sweats and weight loss. Although inquiries into the number of bowel movements, trips to the toilet and degree of rectal bleeding might appear obvious, at times it is important to consider using different terminology to comprehend the nature of the patient's stooling patterns. Diarrhea and bowel movements have different implications in various settings and to different individuals. Patients with extensive colitis may have more diarrhea than bleeding, whereas patients with proctitis are often constipated (passing infrequent, formed stools) yet describe multiple, urgent trips to the toilet to pass blood and mucus. Patients with an inflamed distal colon are often reluctant to pass gas without using the toilet because of the fear of incontinence, which often leads to an increased sense of bloating or increased abdominal cramping. Other patients may describe remaining on the toilet for long periods for a single 'bowel movement'. An assessment of nocturnal bowel movements, the relative 'urgency' to evacuate stool, the degree of tenesmus and episodes of incontinence are important to assess the impact on a patient's quality of life. Patients presenting with chronic symptoms should be questioned regarding the impact on activities of daily living, such as work, social functioning, sexual functioning etc.

Patients should be questioned regarding the degree of weight loss and potential extraintestinal manifestations, including ocular involvement (patients may have a distant history of iritis), articular and skin manifestations. A history of liver enzyme abnormality may precede the diagnosis of ulcerative colitis in patients with primary sclerosing cholangitis.

### Physical examination

Vital signs reflect the severity of disease, including the presence of tachycardia, hypotension, tachypnea or fever. The level of hydration and nutritional status and degree of pallor are critical initial determinations. Specific examinations of the head include the eyes for inflammatory changes (or cataracts in steroid-treated patients), and the mouth for oral ulcerations or thrush (related to steroids) and periodontal disease (also steroid related).

The abdominal examination should assess the presence and nature of bowel sounds, abdominal distension and tenderness. In most situations ulcerative colitis does not induce guarding or rebound tenderness unless the disease is transmural and becoming fulminant. Examination of the perianal region is essential as the vast majority of patients with ulcerative colitis have a normal examination without external hemorrhoids, skin tags or fistulae.

The presence of anything other than a typical, common hemorrhoid or posterior fissure should suggest the presence of Crohn's disease. Rectal examination is relevant to assess the anal canal, sphincter tone and the presence of gross or occult blood.

Examination of the spine and extremities should document the presence or absence of ankylosing spondylitis, arthritis, skin lesions or clubbing (another sign of Crohn's disease).

## Endoscopy (see Chapter 26)

Unless the patient is severely ill either a flexible sigmoidoscopy or a colonoscopy should be performed to define the mucosal extent and severity of disease, and can be used to obtain stool for examination to exclude enteric pathogens and histologic confirmation in new cases.[35] The performance of invasive procedures in patients presenting with severe or fulminant disease is usually avoided to prevent possible perforation or the induction of toxic megacolon. In these settings, a minimal proctoscopic or limited sigmoidoscopic examination can assess the degree of mucosal inflammation, and an immediate postprocedure abdominal X-ray can outline the extent of colitis (see below).

Mucosal biopsies should be performed in newly diagnosed patients to rule out other forms of colitis (e.g. NSAID-induced colitis, infectious (including C. *difficile*) or Crohn's disease). Stains for CMV infection are important for immunocompromised patients or those treated with high doses of steroids (Chapter 27).

## Imaging studies

Plain abdominal radiographs can be extremely useful assessments for patients presenting with severe or fulminant colitis. In addition to excluding free air in the peritoneum and colonic dilatation, a plain radiograph demonstrates the extent of colitis by virtue of the presence or absence of haustrations in the proximal colon and the amount of feces. In active colitis the lumen usually does not contain fecal material that remains proximal to the margin of disease.

Contrast radiography is not commonly employed to diagnose ulcerative colitis, but may at times be useful to differentiate it from Crohn's disease in the setting of focal strictures or fistulae. Leukocyte scanning can be quite helpful in severe colitis to define the extent of inflammation when endoscopy is deemed too risky (Chapter 28). If steroid therapy is anticipated or ongoing an assessment of bone density is important to define long-term management pertaining to osteoporosis.

## Laboratory studies

At presentation, hemoglobin, hematocrit, white blood cell count and differential as well as platelet count should be performed, whereas clotting factors are primarily relevant in patients with severe disease. Electrolytes, kidney function and liver enzymes are additional routine baseline studies. Patients with more severe disease should be assessed for magnesium and cholesterol if cyclosporin therapy is considered (see below). The erythrocyte sedimentation rate and CRP are not uniformly helpful but can be useful as a predictive factor in patients with severe disease.[35–37]

Stool examination for enteric pathogens, ova and parasites and C. *difficile* should be ordered for newly diagnosed patients, patients with unanticipated or atypical flare-ups (e.g. after other illnesses or antibiotic exposure), or at the time of admission of hospitalized patients. Stool examinations should be repeated after several days in hospitalized patients who are not responding to treatment.

# SUPPORTIVE THERAPIES

There are two distinct approaches to the treatment of ulcerative colitis. Whereas the most important is the treatment of inflammatory activity, many of the symptoms of ulcerative colitis can be treated separately from specific anti-inflammatory therapies. These approaches should be individualized according to symptoms and clinical disease state. No single approach suits all patients. A thorough discussion of the nature of ulcerative colitis, the prognosis and proposed therapeutic modalities with the patient and family will gain their involvement and commitment to the therapeutic goals and foster adherence with the recommended therapeutic program.

## ANTISPASMODICS AND ANTIDIARRHEALS

There remains no evidence base to substantiate the use of symptomatic therapies in ulcerative colitis, as clinical trials have been directed at the treatment of inflammatory signs and symptoms. Nevertheless, antispasmodics – primarily anticholinergic agents – are frequently prescribed to treat the cramping abdominal discomfort or symptoms of irritable bowel syndrome that accompany inflammatory manifestations. Once active inflammation has been excluded, or in the setting of mild disease activity, dicyclomine hydrochloride, clidinium bromide, hyoscyamine, propantheline or belladonna alkaloids have been utilized on an empirical basis by experienced clinicians. These, as well as antidiarrheal agents, should be avoided in the setting of severe disease so as to not further paralyze colonic musculature and contribute to the evolution of toxic megacolon.

Antidiarrheal preparations, such as diphenoxylate, loperamide, codeine etc., can be utilized in patients with mild or moderate ulcerative colitis to reduce the frequency of bowel movements and rectal urgency.[38] These agents are more helpful for patients with extensive colitis. Conversely, patients with distal ulcerative colitis are more likely to have impaired proximal colonic motility and right colonic transit, such that antimotility agents may worsen symptoms of bloating, distension and constipation, despite rectal urgency due to diminished rectal compliance. The abnormal motility pattern in patients with distal disease can be improved with the addition of dietary fiber and treatment of distal inflammation.[39] Antimotility agents should be avoided in severe or fulminant disease because of the risk of inducing toxic megacolon.[40]

## ANXIOLYTIC AND ANTIDEPRESSANT THERAPY

There is neither a predisposing psychiatric profile of patients with ulcerative colitis (Chapter 24) nor a routine role for sedative, anxiolytic, antidepressant or antipsychotic therapy. Occasionally, low-dose therapy with tricyclic antidepressants can be used to ameliorate irritable bowel syndrome symptoms in ulcerative colitis patients, but there is no standardized approach. In general, psychopharmacological therapies are reserved for individual settings after consultation with a psychiatrist.

Antidepressants or anxiolytics are sometimes indicated for the treatment of steroid-induced or aggravated underlying cyclothymia or psychosis, and are best prescribed with the assistance of appropriate consultation.

## ANALGESICS

There is rarely a need for analgesia to treat ulcerative colitis, as the inflammation is limited to the superficial mucosa and does not involve pain receptors located in the serosa or peritoneum. Therefore, colonic pain in ulcerative colitis is related either to irritability and muscle spasm or to transmural inflammation. The former is treated with antispasmodics and the latter with specific anti-inflammatory therapy. Narcotics should be avoided outside the perioperative setting because of the potential of inducing toxic megacolon or masking perforation in the setting of transmural disease.[40]

Arthralgias commonly accompany ulcerative colitis and are alleviated by NSAIDs. However, prescription of these agents should be strongly discouraged and patients should be warned against their use on an over-the-counter basis owing to the risk of exacerbating the underlying colitis[1,17,32–33] and the possible development of refractory disease.[39] In the setting of accompanying arthropathy, either intensifying the treatment of underlying colitis or the addition of alternative antiarthritic agents such as sulfasalazine, methotrexate or hydroxychloroquine should be considered (see Chapter 45).

# ANTI-INFLAMMATORY THERAPIES

## AMINOSALICYLATES

The 5-aminosalicylic acid (5-ASA) derivatives of sulfasalazine are the primary therapies for mild or moderate ulcerative colitis.[1,11] These agents have a long history of clinical use and have been extensively studied in clinical trials.[8,41–43] Sulfasalazine, the prototype aminosalicylate formulation, was initially developed with the concept of providing both an antibacterial (sulfapyridine) and an anti-inflammatory (5-ASA, mesalamine, mesalazine) agent into the connective tissues.[44] However, although it is still the benchmark for comparison, recognition that the 5-ASA moiety accounts for the preponderance of therapeutic benefits and sulfapyridine the majority of side effects has allowed the development of a series of sulfa-free aminosalicylates (Chapter 32). 5-ASA drugs are now available in a variety of oral and rectal formulations (Chapter 32) and are summarized in Table 33.4.

### Clinical experience

*Mild or moderate colitis*
Recent meta-analyses of assessments of the pharmacokinetics of the oral aminosalicylates suggest that there is minimal difference in the systemic exposure to mesalamine from the various formulations.[45] Furthermore, the oral aminosalicylates have been

**Table 33.4 Aminosalicylate preparations***

| Preparation | Formulation | Delivery | Dosing |
|---|---|---|---|
| Oral agents | | | |
| *Azo-bond* | | | |
| Sulfasalazine (500 mg) (Azulfidine) | Sulfapyridine carrier | Colon | 3–6 g/day |
| Olsalazine (250 mg) (Dipentum) | 5-ASA dimer | Colon | 1–3 g/day |
| Balsalazide (750 g) (Colazide) | Aminobenzoyl-alanine carrier | Colon | 6 g/day |
| *Delayed release* | | | |
| Asacol (400, 800 mg) | Eudragit S (pH 7) | Distal ileum–colon | 2.4–4.8 g/day (inductive) 0.8–4.8 g/day (maintenance) |
| Claversal/Mesasal/ Salofalk (250, 500 mg) | Eudragit L (pH 6) | Ileum–colon | 1.5–3 g/day (inductive) 0.75–3 g/day (maintenance) |
| *Sustained release* | | | |
| Pentasa (250, 500, 1000 mg) | Ethylcellulose granules | Stomach–colon | 2–4 g/day (inductive) 1.5–4 g/day (maintenance) |
| Rectal agents | | | |
| Mesalamine suppository (400, 500, 1000 mg) | | Rectum | 1–1.5 g/day (inductive) 500 mg–1 g/day (maintenance) |
| Mesalamine enema (1, 4 g) | 60 mL, 100 mL suspension | Rectum–splenic flexure | 1–4 g/day (acute) 1 g q.d.– t.i.w. (maintenance) |

*\* Not all preparations are available in every market.*

equally effective for both proximal and distal colitis,[46] whereas the topical agents are efficacious for distal colitis as long as the formulation reaches the proximal extent of disease.[8] A dose response for the oral aminosalicylates is well defined in the setting of active disease,[41] but is less obvious for the maintenance of remission.[42] In contrast, there does not appear to be an increasing benefit from topical formulations (suppositories, foams or enemas) above 1 g daily.[8] In comparison trials between sulfasalazine and the alternative agents there is no advantage of one compound over another from a therapeutic standpoint, as long as equal amounts of 5-ASA are provided.[41,42] Interestingly, all trials comparing sulfasalazine to alternative, sulfa-free aminosalicylates have demonstrated a numeric, but not a statistical, advantage in favor of sulfasalazine.[40,41] In contrast, there have been relatively few trials comparing different sulfa-free 5-ASA formulations. Several recent trials have suggested the possibility, based on secondary (not primary) outcomes, that azo-bond compounds may offer advantages over mesalamine in distal ulcerative colitis.[47–49] This remains a hypothesis requiring clinical trials adequately powered to demonstrate superiority as a primary endpoint.[46] At present the majority of data argue for equivalence between the available oral aminosalicylates when comparable amounts of 5-ASA are released.[45] There are no data to evaluate delayed- versus continuous-release formulations, although it appears that the dose response in active disease is more relevant than the delivery system.[16]

The clinical response (improvement or remission) to sulfasalazine or an alternative aminosalicylate ranges between 40 and 80%, but varies considerably between clinical trials owing to differing patient populations and endpoint definitions.[41,50] There is a dose response for sulfasalazine between 1 and 4 g/day[40] and doses up to 6 g have been used in clinical trials.[51] A dose response for individual mesalamine formulations between 1.5 g/day and 4.8 g/day has also been observed in clinical trials,[52–54] although the body of evidence is only sufficient to 'suggest' a dose response above 2.4 g/day.[41,50,55] The azo-bond compounds olsalazine[56] and balsalazide[48,49,57–59] have been tested in doses up to 3 g/day and 6.75 g/day (comparable to 3 g and 2.4 g of mesalamine, respectively). With both sulfasalazine and olsalazine, increasing dose-related side effects offset the dose response: intolerance with sulfasalazine and diarrhea with olsalazine.[41,50,60,61] In contrast to the azo-bond formulations sulfasalazine and olsalazine, a potential advantage of the mesalamine formulations is that the dose response within the therapeutic range tested has not been compromised by dose-related side effects. Whether balsalazide can be used at doses higher than 6.75 g/day, or whether there are consistent advantages over mesalamine in subtypes of ulcerative colitis,[46,62] remains to be determined.

Rectal (topical) mesalamine formulations have been highly effective as first-line treatment for patients with mild/moderately active distal ulcerative colitis.[8,43] Mesalamine suppositories reach the upper rectum (approximately 20 cm), and enemas or foams (foams are not currently available in the US) up to the splenic flexure or into the distal transverse colon[8,50,61] (Chapter 32). In contrast to the oral aminosalicylates there does not appear to be a dose response for topical agents between 1 and 4 g/day.[8] Compared to oral therapy with aminosalicylates, topical mesalamine has been more effective for both proctitis[63] and distal colitis,[64] although therapy with oral and topical treatment may be combined[65] and can offer superior results to either therapy alone.[64]

### Severe colitis

Few studies have assessed aminosalicylates for more than mild/moderate colitis. A single trial compared the combination of sulfasalazine with low-dose prednisone and hydrocortisone enemas in outpatients.[66] In this study sulfasalazine actually reduced the response to steroids and so, because of the frequency of gastrointestinal intolerance and the small risk of worsening colitis,[60] and also its inferior anti-inflammatory properties compared to corticosteroids, it is not recommended until patients have stabilized and are receiving a full oral diet.[11,40] These recommendations have been substantiated by a trial demonstrating a greater degree of intolerance to sulfasalazine in moderate/severe disease compared to balsalazide,[57] although neither agent was compared to placebo. Similarly, only a single trial comparing mesalamine to balsalazide enrolled patients with moderate/severe disease,[48] and although balsalazide was better tolerated overall, there were insufficient numbers of patients to conclude that either aminosalicylate has a substantial role in patients with more than mild/moderate disease. Similar to sulfasalazine, alternative aminosalicylates should be withheld in patients with severe colitis until the disease activity has quieted and they are able to tolerate oral diets without manifestations of severe disease. Furthermore, in contrast to corticosteroid enemas, rectal mesalamine formulations have not been evaluated in the setting of severe disease, and clinical experience suggests that, in this setting, mesalamine enemas are less well tolerated than rectal corticosteroids (personal observations).

## Maintenance therapy

Maintenance of clinical remission (prevention of relapse) has been the primary indication for all aminosalicylates in ulcerative colitis,[11,16] as clinical trials have demonstrated a dose response for all of the oral agents.[42] However, there remains no consensus on the 'optimal' maintenance dose.[50,55,67] All of the non-sulfa-containing formulations provide comparable efficacy to sulfasalazine when equimolar doses of 5-ASA are administered in the setting of quiescent disease,[42,50] but there is insufficient clinical trial 'evidence' to support any formulation over another. Historically, the maintenance dose for sulfasalazine was reduced by 50% compared to the amount prescribed for active disease,[68] but this was based on the balance between efficacy and side effects, as a significant proportion of patients were not compliant with prescribed doses of sulfasalazine, presumably owing to dose-related side effects.[16,50] Although the author has personally abandoning this 'dogma' with reference to the non-sulfa- containing aminosalicylates in favor of continuing the same maintenance dose as that employed to induce remission,[16] it must be recognized that, although maintenance studies have evaluated doses of 5-ASA up to 4.4 g/day, adequate dose-ranging trials have not been performed to document a maintenance benefit above 2.4 g of mesalamine daily.[50] Nevertheless, in the absence of dose-related side effects up to 4.8 g of mesalamine daily, it may be prudent to continue the same maintenance dose for patients responding to an aminosalicylate, in particular for those who have recently achieved remission or those who relapse with any dose reduction.

In distal ulcerative colitis (both proctitis and left-sided) rectal formulations of mesalamine are effective at preventing relapse and are more efficacious than oral agents.[8,69] However, compliance and quality of life issues may affect patient preference, tolerance and adherence to continuation of long-term treatment with rectal therapies. Although the continuation of daily rectal therapy is 'optimal' from an efficacy standpoint, a reduction of the dosing intervals on a weekly basis,[70] interval dosing each month[71] or combinations of oral and rectal dosing[72,73] have been shown to be effective. Although a substantial number of patients who require rectal mesalamine to achieve remission will require continued rectal dosing, eventual substitution of an oral aminosalicylate is possible, and preferable, for most patients. Clinical experience suggests that higher doses of an oral aminosalicylate may be required for 'refractory' patients requiring rectal mesalamine;[18] however, these empiric observations have not, as yet, been evaluated in controlled clinical trials.

## CORTICOSTEROIDS

Corticosteroids are the mainstay of acute therapy for moderate to severe and fulminant ulcerative colitis. However, in contrast to the evolution and proliferation of aminosalicylate formulations, and despite the development of more potent glucocorticoids with first-pass hepatic metabolism (e.g. budesonide for Crohn's disease; see Chapter 32), there have been few new applications of corticosteroid therapy for ulcerative colitis over the past several decades. From a mechanistic standpoint, corticosteroids remain quite complex in their mode of action, which is now understood to include the inhibition of NFκB and subsequent downstream translation of cytokines, as well as directly affecting and inhibiting circulating inflammatory cells (see Chapter 32).

### Systemic corticosteroids

Oral administrations of corticosteroids (prednisone, prednisolone, methylprednisolone, prednisolone metasulfobenzoate) are indicated for the treatment of outpatients with moderate or severe ulcerative colitis.[1,11,16] Over the past 40 years there have been few clinical trials to clarify optimal doses or dosing schedules. Since the pioneering trial of Truelove and Witts in 1955 utilizing 100 mg of oral cortisone daily[10] there has been a general consensus among experienced clinicians (rather than an extensive evidence base) favoring prednisone or prednisolone because of their pharmacokinetic profile and ease of administration on a daily to q.i.d. regimen.[61] A dose response for prednisone has been documented between 20 and 60 mg daily, although the modest benefits of higher doses are offset by increasing steroid-related side effects.[77,78] The only trial to date that compared daily dosing with 40 mg of prednisolone versus a schedule of 10 g q.i.d. did not identify a short-term (2-week) difference in responses.[79] Overall, the remission or improvement rates for oral steroid therapy equivalent to 40 mg of prednisone daily ranges from 50 to 70%.[66,77,78,80,81] With these limitations in data, clinical experience does suggest that, although most patients will benefit from once-daily dosing, there may be settings where divided dosing throughout the day is beneficial. Indications for divided dosing may include continued symptoms, particularly nocturnal bowel movements, with once-daily dosing; or during the transition period between intravenous steroids for severe colitis and oral dosing prior to tapering as outpatients.

Oral corticosteroids are neither effective nor indicated in preventing the relapse of quiescent ulcerative colitis.[11,16] In clinical trials, prednisone in doses up to 15 mg daily have failed to maintain remission,[82] although in a single, 24-patient crossover trial of 3 months' duration high-dose (40 mg) prednisolone, on an alternate-day basis, in addition to sulfasalazine was superior to placebo in reducing relapse.[83] However, the overall consensus has long held that their limited efficacy, unlike their well-known adverse effects, contraindicates the use of steroids to prevent relapse.[1,11,16] Yet, whereas the defined role for corticosteroids in ulcerative colitis is for *acute* rather than *maintenance* therapy, the lack of evidence for maintenance is often confused with the clinical observation of 'steroid dependency'.[16] The latter term pertains to individual patients who are unable to taper off steroids without developing recurrent symptoms, in contrast to maintenance therapy, which prevents relapse in a population of patients. Steroid dependency refers to a separate subgroup of patients[81] and provides a specific maintenance indication that often requires an individualized approach (see below, Management of refractory ulcerative colitis).

Parenteral corticosteroids remain the mainstay of therapy for hospitalized patients with severe/fulminant ulcerative colitis. In view of a consistent body of empiric support for the use of parenteral corticosteroids for the treatment of severe ulcerative colitis,[84–86] placebo-controlled trials would be considered unethical. Instead, in addition to observational series, several comparative trials have evaluated the efficacy of parenteral hydrocortisone with ACTH (corticotropin)[87–89] and, most recently, intravenous methylprednisolone with intravenous cyclosporin.[90] The response to intravenous steroids (hydrocortisone 300–400 mg/day or methylprednisolone 40 mg/day) for severe ulcerative colitis is approximately 50% (range ~45–80%), depending upon levels of severity and definitions of response.[86,90] Higher doses of methylprednisolone do not appear to provide improved results,[91] and recently clinical investigators have described the use of pulse dosing of dexamethasone that requires confirmation in controlled settings.[92] The evidence base to recommend an 'optimal' approach with steroids in severe colitis is inadequate.[93] Although the administration of ACTH may have a small advantage for steroid-naive patients, the availability of parenteral formulations has been inconsistent, the majority of hospitalized patients will have had recent exposure to steroids, and most clinicians currently employ either intravenous hydrocortisone, prednisolone or methylprednisolone. The author prefers methylprednisolone as a continuous infusion (40 mg over 24 hours) because of its improved potassium sparing (versus hydrocortisone), the ease and cost savings of a single intravenous set-up, and the theoretical advantage of maintained plasma and tissue concentrations.[77]

## TOPICAL AND NON-SYSTEMIC STEROIDS

Rectal (topical) administration of corticosteroids has been an important component of medical therapy for distal ulcerative colitis for many decades since the early experience in the UK with hydrocortisone and prednisolone.[43] More recently, developments in corticosteroid pharmacology have led to a series of glucocorticoid derivatives with enhanced mucosal potency and less systemic activity that include prednisolone-metasulfobenzoate, beclomethasone diproprionate, tixocortol pivalate and budesonide[61,94–96] (see also Chapter 32). Hydrocortisone or prednisolone enemas have continued to provide a therapeutic option as a primary therapy for patients with distal ulcerative

## Table 33.5 Rectal steroid formulations

| Glucocorticoid | Dose |
| --- | --- |
| Hydrocortisone | 80–100 mg (suppository, foam, enema) |
| Prednisolone-21-phosphate | 20–40 mg (suppository, enema) |
| Prednisolone metasulfobenzoate | 20 mg (enema) |
| Betamethasone | 5–20 mg (enema) |
| Tixocortol pivalate | 250 mg (enema) |
| Beclomethasone diproprionate | 0.5–3 mg (enema) |
| Budesonide | 2 mg (enema) |

colitis,[43] and have been incorporated as an adjunctive therapy for the treatment of severe colitis.[84] Budesonide has been a primary alternative compound to conventional steroids marketed in many parts of the world.[95,97] Clinical trials comparing equal systemic loads of 'non-systemic' topical steroids to conventional oral steroids provide evidence that the topical and systemic effects of glucocorticoids can be divorced and with equal therapeutic benefits,[95,98–101] thus ameliorating the potential systemic impact from absorption of conventional steroids (Chapter 32). However, as first-line therapies even the potent non-systemic glucorticoids are less effective than the aminosalicylates,[43] and raising the dose of budesonide to 2 mg b.i.d. has not proved any more efficacious than 2 mg/day despite increasing adrenal suppression.[102]

There are a variety of topical steroid formulations available worldwide, including suppositories, foams and enemas.[95] Physician and patient preferences are different according to available products and local customs. In general, suppositories are useful for the treatment of proctitis, whereas foams and enemas reach more extensive disease up to or beyond the splenic flexure, according to the volume and activity of colitis.[61,103] In some situations patients prefer suppositories or foams to enema formulations.[43,104] Currently available formulations are listed in Table 33.5.

Non-systemic glucocorticoids are also being developed for oral administration in ulcerative colitis.[105–108] However, obtaining sufficient spread or coating of the inflamed colonic sites and prevention of bacterial metabolism (inactivation) of the steroid molecule remains an obstacle to the development of oral–colonic delivery of non-systemic steroids in ulcerative colitis. To date, the oral delivery systems have not been as effective as conventional, systemically active steroids.

## Clinical experience

The primary use of corticosteroids in ulcerative colitis is to treat active disease. Topical formulations are beneficial to patients with proctitis or left-sided colitis as a primary therapy for mild or moderate disease, and as an adjunct to oral or parenteral steroids for patients with moderate to severe disease. However, neither oral nor topical corticosteroids have maintenance benefits, thus requiring transition to an aminosalicylate to prevent relapse after the induction of clinical remission. In clinical practice topical steroids are often used in conjunction with oral aminosalicylates for patients with distal disease that flares despite maintenance therapy. When topical steroids are prescribed, treatment should be continued until the patient achieves a clinical remission (no bleeding, diarrhea or rectal urgency). Because there is no controlled trial experience to

dictate the rate of withdrawal of topical steroids, clinical judgment is required to gradually taper the frequency of rectal administrations according to the time frame required to achieve the desired clinical response. Patients receiving prolonged rectal administration of steroids require monitoring for steroid-related side effects, including adrenal insufficiency and osteoporosis.[60,94] Despite the lack of maintenance benefits from topical steroids, some patients will become steroid dependent.

Moderate to severe colitis requires therapy with a systemically active corticosteroid. Outpatients are treated with prednisone or prednisolone. Initial doses are between 40 and 60 mg daily as a single morning dose. European centers often begin with a somewhat higher (1 mg/kg) dose.[93] The initial dose is continued until the patient is passing normal bowel movements without blood or urgency. Some clinicians prefer to divide the dose four times daily. The initial dose should be continued until the patient has a complete response or is deemed a failure owing to the absence of clinical improvement over 2–4 weeks. Clinical remission is expected for nearly 90% of patients with mild/moderate disease, but is less for those with more severe disease (~50–70%).[109] Reducing the dose prior to achieving a clinical remission will doom the patient to treatment failure or prolong the overall course of steroid therapy. Likewise, there is no advantage to start at a low dose of prednisone, as patients whose symptoms remit rapidly (e.g. within a few weeks) can taper by 5–10 mg/week. Those who are slower to respond or who have a history of rapid relapses require a more gradual tapering schedule. Below 20 mg daily the dose is generally tapered by 2.5–5 mg/week. There are no clinical trial data to define an optimal schedule for steroid tapering. Aminosalicylate maintenance therapy can be initiated once a clinical remission is achieved.

Patients with severe or fulminant colitis, or those failing outpatient therapy with full doses of steroids, require hospitalization and intravenous steroids.[11,93,110] Either hydrocortisone 300–400 mg/day, in divided doses, or 40–60 mg/day of prednisolone or methylprednisolone, either in divided doses or as a continuous infusion, is initiated. There has been no demonstrable benefit from higher doses of steroids, which can be complicated by increased adverse effects.[91] A few clinicians continue to favor ACTH, 80–120 units/day, as a continuous intravenous infusion for patients who have not recently received steroids.[11] Parenteral administration is continued until the patient has a complete clinical response. Success rates for intravenous steroid therapy are less than for mild/moderate disease and approximate 60% (see above). An important observation is that patients who do not respond within the first 5–7 days are not likely to do so[37] and should be considered candidates for colectomy or an alternative medical approach (either cyclosporin or an investigational agent). Continuation of ineffective steroid therapy is unlikely to produce a remission and risks further morbidity due to progressive disease, complications of colitis or iatrogenic complications such as infection.[36]

## Maintenance therapy

Corticosteroids are not indicated for maintenance therapy of ulcerative colitis.[11,16] Controlled clinical trials have failed to demonstrate a safe and effective formulation or dose that prevents relapses, and the continuation of steroids (parenteral, oral or topical) risks short- and long-term sequelae, including adrenal suppression. As previously mentioned, the concept of steroid dependence differs from that of a maintenance benefit.

Maintenance therapies demonstrate a dose response in a population of patients, whereas steroid dependence pertains to individual patients who are unable to wean below a specific dose without flaring.[16] Patients who are unable to taper steroids despite optimal maintenance strategies (see Refractory colitis, below) need to be constantly reassessed to balance the quality of life and the long-term health risks versus potential surgical cure. The long-term risk of osteoporosis is a particular concern,[60,111,112] such that a DEXA scan should be performed, and adequate calcium and vitamin D supplementation is essential for patients on chronic steroids. There are evolving data regarding the benefits of bisphosphonates or calcitonin[112] (see Chapter 50).

## CONTROVERSIES REGARDING STEROID THERAPY FOR ULCERATIVE COLITIS

The evidence base regarding the use of corticosteroids for ulcerative colitis remains incomplete and there have been no new trials assessing dose, dose intervals or formulations of conventional steroids over the past several years. The relatively small population of ulcerative colitis patients and the lack of proprietary interest has impeded the implementation of trials to assess optimization of treatment with non-patentable formulations. A number of controversies remain regarding therapy with corticosteroids. These include: how to predict which patients will respond; how to optimize therapy between formulations; how to optimize doses and dosing schedules for individual for individual formulations; and whether oral formulations of 'nonsystemic' steroids can be efficacious in extensive or distal colitis.

Assessing and predicting responses (or failure) to corticosteroid therapy is an extremely important issue. At present there are few clinical clues to predict, prior to initiating therapy, which patients are likely to respond, in particular to parenteral steroids for severe disease. Furthermore, definitions of response, including steroid resistance (steroid refractory), have primarily been employed in a retrospective manner.[37,81,113] From a clinical standpoint, patients with a short duration of disease, prior use of steroids, elevated temperature, elevated C-reactive protein and hypoalbuminemia are more likely to be associated with failure of therapy.[113,114] Although clinical response to the introduction of oral steroids has usually been determined after 1 month,[81] it is possible to determine within the first week whether patients are likely to fail parenteral steroid therapy.[37,113] Patients with persisting diarrhea, bleeding requiring transfusions, and persistently elevated C-reactive protein within 5–7 days of initiating intravenous steroids are unlikely to respond. These retrospective observations were confirmed in the trial comparing intravenous cyclosporin in addition to intravenous steroids for patients who had failed at least 1 week of high-dose steroids.[115] None of the patients randomized to receive continuation of intravenous hydrocortisone, alone, improved over the ensuing week. These observations are extremely important in recognizing that the 'critical pathway' for decision-making in severe ulcerative colitis should benchmark a 5–7-day response time before recommending more intensive medical therapy or colectomy, and thus avoid prolonged exposure to an ineffective treatment with an increased likelihood of disease-related or iatrogenic complications.

Recent research is also beginning to evaluate cellular and molecular mechanisms of drug resistance to corticosteroids in ulcerative colitis and other inflammatory diseases.[116] Steroid resistance in ulcerative colitis has been associated with a decreased antiproliferative effect of dexamethasone on the phytohemagglutinin responses of peripheral T lymphocytes,[117] despite the presence of increased glucocorticoid receptors.[118] These observations suggest a change in the nature of glucocorticoid receptors or affinity in patients with active ulcerative colitis that has been demonstrated by investigators, who describe an increased proportion of patients with glucocorticoid receptor β (in contrast to the more predominant α receptor) does not bind to the steroid ligand in 83% of steroid-resistant patients compared to less than 10% of steroid-responsive patients.[119] However, additional mechanisms are likely to account for steroid unresponsiveness, including interference with transcription factors such as NFκB, which may be overexpressed in intestinal epithelial cells from patients with active IBD and inhibits the transcription of glucocorticoid receptor α.[120–122] Thus, there is apparent crosstalk between activated epithelium in IBD and the infiltrating inflammatory cells that may affect responsiveness to systemic or topical steroids.[123]

As far as optimization of parenteral steroid administration is concerned, we favor continuous infusions based on our observations regarding patients who have failed therapy with intermittent infusions, and the rationale of maintaining adequate tissue levels.[77] At present it also remains to be proven whether non-systemic steroids can be formulated to improve the outcome of distal or extensive ulcerative colitis compared to conventional steroids. Although clinical trials to assess optimal tapering schedules for patients responding to steroid therapy would be most helpful, these are not likely to be performed because of the heterogeneity of patients and the lack of priority sponsorship from industry or other funding sources. Thus, at present the optimization of steroid therapy for ulcerative colitis remains in many ways as much art as science.

## IMMUNOMODULATORS

Despite an incomplete understanding of the immunopathogenesis of ulcerative colitis and foundational differences between ulcerative colitis and Crohn's disease (where immune modulators have been well intercalated into the therapeutic scheme; Chapter 33) the utility of immune modulating therapies for ulcerative colitis has continued to gain both mechanistic[124] and clinical evidence. In previous years, the general acceptance of potential 'cure' of ulcerative colitis via proctocolectomy with an ileostomy or ileoanal anastomosis was a deterrent to potential long-term immune suppression. To date there is considerable controversy regarding the role of potent immune suppression with cyclosporin or tacrolimus rather than surgery, owing to recognized iatrogenic complications (infection and rare deaths) from prolongation of medical therapy. However, evolving recognition of complications from surgical therapy (i.e. chronic pouchitis, unrecognized Crohn's disease, or fertility issues in women) and the increased experience in both short- and long-term immunomodulatory therapy clearly provide a role for immunomodulators in both the induction and the maintenance of remission in ulcerative colitis.

## PURINE ANTIMETABOLITES

Azathioprine and 6-mercaptopurine (6-MP) have been utilized for ulcerative colitis for over 30 years.[125,126] During this time the purine analogs have primarily been employed, successfully as maintenance rather than inductive therapies. The longer-term role was predicted by the initial Oxford experience, where azathioprine at 2.5 mg/kg/day, as an adjunct to corticosteroids, offered no benefits in the initial month. However, the relapse rate for responding patients maintained on azathioprine was reduced by nearly 50% compared to placebo.[127] Subsequent studies also suggested a steroid-sparing benefit of azathioprine in ulcerative colitis.[128,129] More recent clinical trials have confirmed the role of azathioprine as an adjunctive maintenance agent to sulfasalazine for patients who require steroids to achieve remission.[130–132] In the trials by Sood et al.,[131,132] relapse rates for patients maintained on azathioprine and sulfasalazine were significantly reduced for both steroid-dependent and newly diagnosed (steroid-induced) patients compared to patients maintained on sulfasalazine alone. One-year remission rates for patients maintained on azathioprine after steroid induction range between 60 and 75%,[130,132] and although these trials did not assess the adjunctive value of aminosalicylates combined with azathioprine compared with azathioprine alone, a recent retrospective analysis of 82 patients with ulcerative colitis treated with azathioprine for at least 6 months did not observe a benefit for adjunctive 5-ASA treatment.[133] The controlled trials mentioned above support large clinical series from New York[134,135] and Oxford,[125] where remission rates (off steroids) for patients treated with azathioprine or 6-MP approximated 60% and, of the responders, nearly 90% remained in remission at 1 year. In contrast, discontinuing azathioprine or 6-MP was associated with relapse in up to two-thirds of patients within 5 years.[125,134,135]

Another increasingly defined role for the purine analogs is to maintain remission after cyclosporin therapy. Our center originally described the benefits of concomitant azathioprine or 6-MP after cyclosporin-induced remissions,[136] and these observations have been supported by other clinical investigators,[137,138] such that it is now recommended that patients responding to cyclosporin therapy (see below) receive maintenance therapy with azathioprine or 6-MP.

Since the initial trials with azathioprine for ulcerative colitis it has been apparent that treatment must usually be continued for 3–6 months before efficacy can be assessed.[125,126] The Mayo Clinic group has begun to explore the potential to hasten the response with intravenous loading of azathioprine (20–40 mg/kg) in hospitalized patients with ulcerative colitis.[139] Five of nine patients responded within 4 weeks, although two developed transient leukopenia and one had hepatotoxicity. This experience needs to be placed into context with the efficacy and safety of induction therapy with cyclosporin, followed by maintenance azathioprine. To date there have been no adequate dose-ranging trials for azathioprine or 6-MP and, similar to the experience in Crohn's disease, there is no standard guideline for using these in ulcerative colitis. Although low-dose therapy may be efficacious and potentially less toxic,[140] prospective trials to assess whether dosing should be according to weight, white blood cell count or 6-MP metabolite levels are needed to establish better guidelines[126] (see Chapter 32).

The expanding experience with the purine analogs in both North America and Europe are reassuring regarding the long-term safety of these agents.[125,126,141,142] The short-term toxicity is quite modest and includes bone marrow suppression (primarily leukopenia) related to dose and thiopurine methyltransferase activity, and idiosyncratic hypersensitivity reactions[126,141] (see Chapter 32). Contrary to previous concerns there does not appear to be an increased risk of neoplasia for patients with ulcerative colitis treated with purine analogs,[143,144] although the risk of Epstein–Barr-related non-Hodgkins lymphomas, although quite small, may be increased.[144,145]

## RECOMMENDATIONS FOR USE

Azathioprine or 6-MP are appropriate maintenance therapies for steroid-dependent ulcerative colitis (i.e. patients who respond to steroid therapy but are unable to taper despite optimization of treatment with oral and/or topical aminosalicylates). Although some experienced clinicians advocate these agents for steroid-refractory ulcerative colitis[134,135] there are few prospective data regarding this group and, because of the slow onset of action (>1 month, up to 3–6 months), alternative approaches to induce remission, such as cyclosporin, are probably more appropriate in this setting. Again, there is no standard approach in ulcerative colitis. Whereas some investigators require preassessment of thiopurine methyltransferase activity (TPMT), we do not routinely advocate such testing as there have been many decades of successful treatment by beginning at low doses with gradual titration upwards. Thus, TPMT activity can be assessed and, if normal, azathioprine can be initiated at 2.5 mg/kg/day or 6-MP at 1.5 mg/kg/day. Patients with low or nil TPMT activity can still be treated, but with markedly reduced dosing and closer monitoring of 6-thioguanine nucleotide levels and the WBC. Our regimen, over the past decades, has been to initiate, at either 50 or 100 mg doses (depending on the patient's weight), and gradually increase by 25 mg every 2 weeks until the WBC begins to drop as steroids are held steady. When the WBC is below 10 000 we hold the dose as steroids are tapered. If patients are unable to taper off steroids the dose is increased to the point of WBC <4–5000 or 6-thioguanine level >250. There are no evidence-based data regarding preference of one agent over another. Azathioprine may be less expensive as a generic agent but is less potent on a gram-per-gram basis. Some patients who develop intolerance side effects from azathioprine (e.g. nausea or abdominal pain) can be transferred to 6-MP,[146,147] and vice versa. However, patients who develop pancreatitis or more severe allergic reactions should not be challenged with the sister compound. Baseline CBC and liver enzymes should be obtained. The CBC, primarily WBC, is monitored biweekly until a stable dose is achieved. If patients are not able to taper off steroids within 6 months despite modest leukopenia (WBC ~3000) the author considers treatment to be ineffective and considers alternative approaches, usually colectomy. Liver enzymes should be reevaluated within the first 3 months, after 6 months, and then yearly. If liver transaminases increase without concomitant decreases in the WBC it usually implies high, functional TPMT levels and preferential conversion to 6-methyl-mercaptopurine metabolites, with a low likelihood of response to azathioprine or 6-MP.[148,149] Thioguanine, which is thought to be the active metabolite, has been tried in pilot trials of Crohn's disease,[148] but it remains to be determined whether this product will be safe and effective in ulcerative colitis.[150]

There is a growing body of data to support the safety of treating patients with the purine analogs through pregnancy[151] (see Chapter 23). Patients on long-term treatment should be entered into a more aggressive colonoscopic surveillance program because of the continued risk of dysplasia or colon cancer.[143] Generally, treatment is continued indefinitely, as relapses can occur after discontinuation,[125,135] although the ultimate duration of long-term treatment has yet to be defined.

# CYCLOSPORIN

The use of cyclosporin for ulcerative colitis has been described since pioneering efforts by Lichtiger and Present[152] and has been a dramatic and highly debated option for the management of severe or refractory colitis over the past decade.[153-155] The initial, uncontrolled experience with cyclosporin for severe, refractory ulcerative colitis[152] has been followed by a small, controlled clinical trial[115] and a large number of substantiating clinical series.[136,138,154,156-162] Intravenous cyclosporin has consistently benefited the short-term management of severe, steroid-refractory ulcerative colitis in 50–80% of patients. Most recently, the Belgian group has described the potential for treating severe, steroid-naive ulcerative colitis with intravenous cyclosporin alone, without corticosteroids.[90] Although there is little debate regarding the short-term efficacy of intravenous cyclosporin for severe colitis, there remain a series of issues regarding the optimal management strategies (dosing, safety, requisite for concomitant steroids) as well as the long-term benefits and safety.[153-155]

Although the initial clinical experience described 'high-dose' intravenous cyclosporin (i.e. 4 mg/kg/day) as a continuous infusion,[115,152] subsequent clinicians have suggested that lower doses can be equally efficacious,[160,163,164] and a dose response between 2 and 4 mg/kg/day has not been established. Our initial experience led to the production of a 'user's guide' to cyclosporin for severe ulcerative colitis,[165] but to date there is a poor correlation between response and blood or tissue levels, or a strong correlation between blood levels and toxicity.[164] As an example, despite adequate tissue levels in the colon, enema applications of cyclosporin have not been effective in controlled trials.[166] In addition, the complex clinical pharmacology of oral cyclosporin[155] has led to the development of microemulsion formulations with improved absorption and more consistent bioavailability[61,149,155,167] that have begun to be evaluated for the outpatient treatment of refractory ulcerative colitis.[168,169] The preliminary results are promising, with similar short-term responses to those reported for intravenous therapy in hospitalized patients.[168-170] Similarly, tacrolimus, which has more reliable oral clinical pharmacokinetics, has been evaluated in a small number of hospitalized adults treated intravenously[171] and steroid-refractory pediatric outpatients[172] treated with oral therapy.

Predictive factors for response (or failure) to cyclosporin therapy have been difficult to identify.[163] High 'band' counts at presentation correlated with both initial response and long-term colectomy rates. Similar to the experience with corticosteroids, patients failing to respond to cyclosporin within the first 5–7 days are not likely to do so, and are at risk for greater toxicity.[37]

A major concern regarding therapy with cyclosporin (or tacrolimus) pertains to its short- and long-term safety,[155] in particular for practitioners outside major medical centers with transplantation expertise[153,154,165] (see Chapter 32). The major toxicities include nephrotoxicity and opportunistic infections. The former can manifest as hypertension or with elevations in creatinine.[165] It has been estimated that up to 20% of IBD patients treated with cyclosporin have a 33% decrease in glomerular filtration rates and a significant likelihood of irreversible histologic nephropathy,[173] although the histologic changes do not necessarily translate into clinically significant, long-term nephrotoxicity.[174,175]

Cyclosporin also has been associated with an increased risk of opportunistic infections, including *Pneumocystis carinii* pneumonia[176] and other uncommon infections.[175] However, it is important to recognize that *Pneumocystis* infections can occur in patients treated with steroids alone,[177] and that we have not seen a case since instituting routine prophylaxis with sulfamethoxazole/trimethoprim for patients on more than one immunosuppressant.[165] Furthermore, the only death in the randomized controlled trial of cyclosporin in severe ulcerative colitis was related to CMV infection in an elderly woman who was randomized to receive steroids alone, without cyclosporin.[115]

A final controversy regards the ultimate, long-term benefit of cyclosporin (or tacrolimus) for severe or refractory ulcerative colitis compared to immediate colectomy and ileostomy or ileoanal anastomosis. Although there may be some benefit from 'delaying' an eventual colectomy (e.g. to allow the patient and or family to adjust and become educated regarding surgical outcomes, or to modulate the disease activity such that an ileoanal anastomosis could be performed in one operation, or to avoid staging) it would be helpful to demonstrate that the risks of short-term cyclosporin therapy for ulcerative colitis lead to a change in the eventual prognosis. It is reassuring to note that several series have not identified worse outcomes for patients undergoing colectomy after cyclosporin therapy.[170,178,179] In addition, we have demonstrated that successful therapy with cyclosporin can lead to an improved quality of life, compared to immediate colectomy for severe ulcerative colitis.[180] In contrast, critics of cyclosporin therapy argue that because only 40–50% of responders achieved long-term benefits (avoided eventual colectomy),[153,159,162] such therapy does not warrant the risk of potential toxicities for a potentially curable disease. However, with the recognition that more patients can be 'salvaged' on a long-term basis when transitioned to maintenance therapy with a purine analog,[136-138,165] the long-term prognosis for maintaining remissions after cyclosporin therapy can be improved to more than 60% 5-year colectomy-free survival with excellent quality of life.[180]

## RECOMMENDATIONS FOR USE

The majority of the experience with cyclosporin or tacrolimus in ulcerative colitis has been in patients who have failed therapy with oral or intravenous steroids. The recent trial by D'Haens et al., comparing cyclosporin with intravenous steroids, suggests that these agents can be effective without steroids.[90] However, at present the primary indications for cyclosporin or tacrolimus are for hospitalized patients receiving concurrent corticosteroids, hospitalized patients for whom corticosteroids are contraindicated or refused, or for steroid-refractory outpatients.

Prior to initiating cyclosporin therapy discussion with the patient and family should focus on the potential benefits and risks, as well as the alternative surgical approach, i.e. colectomy. Patients should be informed about the risks of cyclosporin on the kidneys and blood pressure, as well as the risk of opportunistic infections. Patients with low cholesterol (<100 mg/dL) are at increased risk of grand mal seizures and should be warned and placed on 'seizure precautions'.[165] We usually administer cyclosporin through a large vein, via either a central vein or a PICC line to avoid chemical phlebitis and irritation of smaller, peripheral veins.

The issue of whether to begin at 4 mg/kg/day and titrate down, or 2 mg/kg/day and titrate up, is not very important as cyclosporin blood levels will dictate ongoing dosing.[165] Neither way is likely to produce more side effects over the initial few days. Our process has been to begin infusions at 4 mg/kg continuously over 24 hours in the majority of patients. In those with low cholesterol we will begin with 1 mg/kg and gradually advance the dose according to whole blood levels. We aim for whole blood trough cyclosporin levels between 200 and 400 μg/mL, although there is not a good correlation between blood levels and efficacy or toxicity. In the only controlled trial patients with higher trough levels seemed to respond more favorably.[115] The blood levels are determined after 1–2 days, and subsequently every 3 days, with adjustments in the daily dose. The dose is adjusted according to the blood level and concurrent determination of the BUN and serum creatinine. We lower the dose by approximately 25% for elevations of BUN or creatinine above normal, or for diastolic blood pressure >90. Less than 20% of patients require antihypertensives, in which case a calcium channel blocker is the first choice. The average time to begin responding is 3–5 days, and most patients will respond within the first 7 days. The average time to complete response (forming stools without diarrhea, blood or urgency) is 7–10 days.

Once a patient has a complete response we change to oral steroids and cyclosporin. The daily dose of cyclosporin is doubled and administered b.i.d. In addition, sulfamethoxazole/trimethoprim double-strength tablets are prescribed three times weekly to prevent *Pneumocystis pneumonia* while patients are on more than one immunosuppressant. An oral aminosalicylate is added when the patient is on a full diet, and (although there are no data to determine whether oral aminosalicylates play an adjunctive role in this clinical setting) azathioprine or 6-MP are prescribed as long-term maintenance therapy (unless contraindicated owing to previous toxicity). Trough levels of cyclosporin are determined once weekly, along with weekly BUN and creatinine over the first month, then biweekly. The daily dose is modified according to the clinical response (upward to achieve levels closer to 400 μg/mL if patients are losing response) and complications (i.e. downward in the presence of increased blood pressure, BUN or creatinine), rather than the actual trough levels.

Therapy with cyclosporin in the setting of severe ulcerative colitis and administered with concurrent therapies can be quite complex. Cyclosporin is metabolized by CYP3A4, an enzyme present in both the liver and enterocytes[181] (see Chapter 32). Cyclosporin is highly lipophilic and dependent on bile for absorption, although the newer, microemulsion formulation (Neoral) is less dependent upon bile or influenced by administration with meals.[167] Drug interactions are common and can increase or decrease cyclosporin levels.[182,183] Administration with grapefruit juice can also increase cyclosporin levels owing to the presence of flavonoids that inhibit its metabolism by cytochrome P450.[184] Common drug interactions are listed in Table 33.6.

Once the patient has tapered off of steroids and is maintaining a clinical remission the cyclosporin dose is tapered over several weeks. There is no role for chronic cyclosporin therapy in ulcerative colitis. If patients continue to develop flare-ups despite maintenance therapy with aminosalicylates and/or azathioprine/6-MP, a colectomy is warranted.

## METHOTREXATE

Despite early optimism from uncontrolled clinical experience with methotrexate[185] there remains limited evidence to support

### Table 33.6 Drug interactions with cyclosporin

| Drugs that increase cyclosporin concentrations | Drugs that decrease cyclosporin concentrations |
|---|---|
| *Calcium channel blockers* | *Antibiotics* |
| Diltiazem | Nafcillin |
| Nicardipine | Rifampin |
| Verapamil | Trimethoprim |
| Felodipine | *Anticonvulsants* |
| *Antifungals* | Carbamzepine |
| Fluconazole | Phenobarbitol |
| Itraconazole | Phenytoin |
| Ketoconazole | *Other drugs* |
| *Antibiotics* | Octreotide |
| Clarithromycin | Ticlopidine |
| Erythromycin | |
| *Glucocorticoids* | |
| Methylprednisolone | |
| *Other drugs* | |
| Allopurinol | |
| Metoclopramide | |
| Chloroquine | |

its use in ulcerative colitis.[186,187] Debate continues about whether the controlled trials used optimal doses or endpoints,[188,189] as a recent retrospective trial identified similar results in patients treated with methotrexate for ulcerative colitis as in those with Crohn's disease, at comparable doses, with maintenance of remission at 1, 2 and 3 years of 90%, 73% and 51%, respectively, for patients who had completed at least 3 months of therapy.[190] However, when compared to placebo in a small study population, oral methotrexate at 15 mg/week was not as efficacious at achieving or maintaining remissions in steroid-dependent patients.[191] Thus, although larger controlled trials of parenteral methotrexate in ulcerative colitis at doses employed for Crohn's disease (i.e. 25 mg/week) have not been completed,[192,193] the overall utility of methotrexate does not appear to be comparable in the two diseases. Nevertheless, similar to findings in the early reports of Kozarek et al.,[185,188] in our experience with a few patients who failed or could not tolerate therapy with purine antimetabolites and declined colectomy, methotrexate is sometimes beneficial at doses of 25 mg/week subcutaneously. However, its short- and long-term efficacy is unpredictable, there is no strict evidence base to support its use, and methotrexate is not included in recent practice guidelines for the treatment of ulcerative colitis.[11]

## ANTIBIOTICS

Despite continued interest in a bacterial role in the initiation or perpetuation of inflammatory bowel disease[1] there remains a lack of evidence in favor of antibacterial therapy for the treatment of ulcerative colitis, and current 'practice guidelines' limit recommendations to its 'empiric use' in fulminant or toxic colitis.[11] Controlled trials have failed to demonstrate a role for oral vancomycin,[194] intravenous metronidazole[195] or ciprofloxacin[196] in conjunction with intravenous corticosteroids in the setting of severe colitis. Additional controlled clinical trials have failed to demonstrate evidence in favor of antibiotic therapy for the treatment of active disease or as maintenance therapy.[197,198] A recent large, multicenter controlled trial of oral ciprofloxacin failed to support a preliminary Finnish trial[199] suggesting steroid-sparing benefits (Hanauer, S. personal communication).

In the absence of definitive controlled trials, and based upon their empiric use in experienced centers, antibiotics continue to remain a component of the 'intensive intravenous therapy' for patients presenting with fulminant colitis or toxic megacolon.[84,85] In these settings the addition of short-term broad-spectrum antibiotics can be justified on the basis of preoperative prophylaxis, as prevention against systemic bacteremia due to translocation in more permeable, severely inflamed colons.[40]

## PROBIOTICS

Although the concept of pre- or probiotic therapy for ulcerative colitis remains appealing[4,200] the only controlled trials to date have evaluated the maintenance role of the Nissle strain of a 'non-pathogenic' E. coli.[201,202] In these two studies the probiotic was compared to 'low-dose' mesalamine (e.g. 1.5 g/day) and demonstrated therapeutic 'equivalence' after 3 months in patients entering clinical remission[201] and at 1 year after a combination inductive regimen of steroids and gentamicin.[202] In the latter trial, remission rates at 1 year of 27–33% for the probiotic or mesalamine question the overall utility of therapy (or dosage) in patients requiring steroids to control active disease. Additional trials are required to clarify the potential role of probiotics (or prebiotics) in active or quiescent disease. The role of probiotic therapy for the prevention or treatment of pouchitis is discussed in Chapter 46.

## MISCELLANEOUS THERAPIES

A number of therapeutic classes of agents are currently under investigation or have been evaluated in specific clinical scenarios but, as yet, do not have a defined therapeutic role for ulcerative colitis. Those approaches that have undergone preliminary trials in ulcerative colitis are described below, whereas developing, currently investigational agents are discussed in Chapter 37.

### NICOTINE

The protective role of cigarette smoking against the development of ulcerative colitis[1,28,203,204] has led to the evaluation of nicotine as an adjunctive therapy.[204] We initially performed an 'n of 1' trial using nicotine gum and found symptomatic improvement in ex-smokers, although the gum was poorly tolerated by non-smokers.[205] Subsequently, a series of trials utilizing nicotine patches has supported a role for nicotine in the symptomatic management of ulcerative colitis,[206–210] but patches have not been as effective as aminosalicylates at maintaining remission in quiescent colitis,[211,212] or as efficacious as steroid therapy at inducing remission.[213] Pilot studies are under way to test novel delivery systems of nicotine, including topical (enema) formulations[214–217] and delayed-release preparations.[218,219] Although some centers consider the addition of nicotine patches as a therapeutic option for refractory ulcerative colitis[220] most do not accept nicotine as a proven therapy,[221] and although nicotine patches may be useful as an adjunct for the subgroup of patients who develop ulcerative colitis after smoking cessation, the nicotine has not been proposed in the recently developed American

College of Gastroenterology 'practice guidelines'.[11] There remain numerous questions regarding the role of cigarette smoking and nicotine in ulcerative colitis, including mechanisms of action,[204] potential delivery systems, and the clinical observation that resumption of smoking may be a therapeutic alternative for refractory ulcerative colitis in ex-smokers after a risk–benefit assessment in individual cases.[29]

## FATTY ACIDS AND LEUKOTRIENE INHIBITORS

Because colonocytes utilize short-chain fatty acids as a primary energy source, both the early experience with short-chain fatty acids in diversion colitis[222] and a potential metabolic defect in colonocyte $\beta$-oxidation[223,224] have led to a series of investigations regarding the role of mixed short-chain fatty acids[225–228] or butyrate[229–231] alone in ulcerative colitis. Despite positive benefits in some small trials[232] and evidence for anti-inflammatory properties of butyrate related to inhibition of reactive oxygen species[233] and NF$\kappa$B,[234] these therapies have yet to be developed into proprietary formulations or found a role in routine clinical practice.

Similarly, arachidonic acid metabolites exert both proinflammatory and anti-inflammatory properties as well as cytotoxic effects that may affect the pathogenesis of ulcerative colitis.[235,236] Accordingly, omega-3 fatty acids, which are often derived from fish oil and are recognized to inhibit the synthesis of leukotriene $B_4$, have been evaluated in a series of trials for refractory ulcerative colitis[237–242] or as maintenance therapies.[240,243,244] Despite their ability to alter membrane phospholipid profiles and trends in favor of benefit, the degree of inhibition of proinflammatory mediators has been modest and clinical benefits have failed to overcome patient intolerance to fishy odors.

The inhibitory effects of sulfasalazine and mesalamine on 5-lipoxygenase, leukotriene $B_4$ and thromboxane synthetase[235] have led to therapeutic trials of specific 5-lipoxygenase[245,246] or thromboxane synthetase[247] inhibitors in ulcerative colitis. Neither class of agents has proved effective, suggesting that the benefits of the aminosalicylates are likely to be pluripotent and not specific to these arachidonic acid metabolic pathways.

## HEPARINS

Likewise, from the standpoint of pluripotent inhibition of inflammation, few compounds have the spectrum of potential anti-inflammatory effects of heparin.[248,249] However, it was an original observation of a 'paradoxical' improvement in colitis in patients requiring heparin for venous thromboses by Gaffney[250] that led to a series of small trials of either unfractionated[251–254] or low-molecular weight heparin[255,256] for ulcerative colitis. Pending confirmatory results from a larger, multicenter trial of low-molecular weight heparin the role of heparin remains limited to the treatment of thrombotic complications of ulcerative colitis. It remains to be determined where heparin therapy will ultimately fall within the armamentarium, and whether unfractionated or low-molecular weight heparin will provide similar therapeutic potential.[257]

## BIOLOGIC THERAPIES

We have entered into a new era of therapeutic possibilities in the treatment of IBD in general, and ulcerative colitis in particular.[2,258,259] Elucidation of the immunophysiologic cascades and recognition of cellular messengers, including nuclear factors, interferon, cytokines, chemokines and adhesion molecules, will afford novel targets. Additional targets also include cell-surface markers of specific lymphocyte populations.

The introduction of infliximab for the treatment of Crohn's disease has been a major therapeutic advance (Chapter 34) and has afforded the potential to study the role of TNF in ulcerative colitis. Based upon theoretical differences in Th1 and Th2 cytokine profiles between ulcerative colitis and Crohn's disease,[1,2, 236, 260] one would not anticipate identical therapeutic responses to therapy targeting TNF. Nevertheless, given the multiplicity of cytokine interactions it is conceivable that there may be an anti-TNF responsive 'phase,' or subpopulations of patients with ulcerative colitis who would be more likely to respond to infliximab or another agents targeting TNF. Since the introduction of infliximab into the US market there have been several case series describing its potential efficacy in adult[261-264] and pediatric[265,266] patients with ulcerative colitis. A small, uncontrolled trial of an investigational anti-TNF antibody (CDP571) also demonstrated consistent clinical and laboratory benefits in 15 patients over 2 weeks.[267] These reports must be interpreted with caution, with specific questions regarding case selection, diagnoses, and short- and long-term outcomes,[268,269] as, in contrast to the optimistic uncontrolled reports, a small controlled trial that enrolled 11 hospitalized patients with severe ulcerative colitis demonstrated equivocal short-term benefits, with about 50% of patients responding to infliximab doses between 5 and 20 mg/kg (four of eight responded to infliximab vs. none of three randomized to placebo). Preliminary results from a controlled trial performed in Europe with infliximab 5 mg/kg in 42 hospitalized, steroid-dependent patients were not as optimistic (6-week remission rates of 36% vs. 30% with placebo), although the final reports of the study have yet to be published.[270] One consistency between the controlled and uncontrolled experience with infliximab for ulcerative colitis has been the poor response in steroid-refractory adults. In the reports by both Su[264] and Probert[270] remissions in the steroid-refractory patients ranged between 33 and 36% – much less impressive than the response rates in Crohn's disease.[271] Therefore, we eagerly await the results from two large multicenter trials that are currently in progress.

Monoclonal antibodies also have been developed to target cell adhesion molecules. Two versions have been evaluated in early-phase clinical trials for ulcerative colitis. In a small trial, natalizumab, a humanized monoclonal antibody against $\alpha_4$ integrin, was administered as a single 3 mg/kg infusion to 10 patients with ulcerative colitis. Five patients responded at 2 weeks and another at 4 weeks. However, only one patient remained in remission at 12 weeks.[272] The $\alpha_4\beta_7$ integrins may be more specific to the intestinal endothelium,[258] and in a report from a small, double-blind ascending-dose study of LDP-02 for patients with moderately severe ulcerative colitis, endoscopic improvement was observed in equal numbers of patients receiving active drug and placebo. The most pessimistic aspect of the later trial was the finding that despite saturation of the $\alpha_4\beta_7$ receptors for up to 30 days, no difference was observed between LDP-02 and placebo.[273]

Additional potential targets and biological therapies for ulcerative colitis include IL-2 inhibition (monoclonal antibodies directed at IL-2 receptor), anti-CD3 and anti-CD4 antibodies, growth factors (epidermal growth factor, fibroblast factor 7, keratinocyte growth factor-2) and interferons, reviewed by Sands[259] and Sandborn and Targan.[258] Chapter 37 also describes novel approaches to therapy, including small therapeutic molecules that include eicosanoids, nitric oxide, peroxisome proliferator-activated receptor $\gamma$ stimulation, phosphodiesterase inhibitors, TNF-$\alpha$ converting enzyme inhibitors, and signal transduction inhibitors (e.g NF$\kappa$B, JNK pathways and MAP kinases).[274] Meanwhile, as we continue to search for genetic-environmental underpinnings and eventual targets for the treatment of ulcerative colitis, patients continue to demonstrate frustration with current therapeutic limitations by seeking alternative (complementary) approaches to treatment.[24,275] However, the overall approach to the medical treatment of ulcerative colitis is effective for the vast majority of patients, and the sequential approach to applying and optimizing current treatment is described below.

## CLINICAL APPROACHES

The following discussion describes the overall approach to the management of ulcerative colitis and the sequencing from inductive to maintenance therapy. Initial therapeutic decisions are based on the extent and severity of colitis and the prior response to therapy, and involve thorough discussions with the patient regarding options and alternatives. Before initiating therapy it is essential to perform a comprehensive review of the patient's history, current symptoms, complications of the disease and/or therapy, and an assessment of the individual's and family's adaptation to illness. It should be recognized that the original categorization of disease, including the diagnosis, and the patient's status are neither static nor permanent.[13,276] Therefore, the diagnosis should be confirmed either by a personal review of endoscopic reports and histology slides, or by repetition of studies, as indicated, owing to an important change in status or extended interval between examinations. It is also important to review or update the nutritional, metabolic and hematological status of the patient, along with endoscopic and histological data. Particular attention should be paid to factors that contribute to exacerbations of activity[18] or refractoriness to therapy (e.g. concomitant medications (NSAIDs, antibiotics), intercurrent infections (e.g. C. *difficile*), menstruation, and dietary or lifestyle changes).[39] One should listen to what the patient believes contributes to their disease and illness and involve the patient and family in the decision-making process after extensive discussions focusing on optimistic outcomes, therapeutic expectations and reassurance regarding the potential for maintenance of quality of life.

## ULCERATIVE PROCTITIS

The most common symptoms of ulcerative proctitis are rectal bleeding and tenesmus. Diarrhea is less often a problem than constipation, necessitating inquiry into the nature of bowel movements and trips to the toilet. Often, patients will describe frequent evacuations of blood and/or mucopus with longer intervals between the passage of 'constipated' stool. The inability to distinguish flatus from stool often contributes to descriptions of constipation, bloating or a change in the odor of gas. Although patients with ulcerative colitis are rarely seriously ill, they can develop chronic problems related to iron deficiency anemia or complications of prolonged steroid therapy. In both the inductive and the maintenance phases the advantages of topical therapies are balanced against the patient's preference for oral or topical treatment.

## INDUCTION OF REMISSION

Topical aminosalicylate therapy is the most effective initial approach for the treatment of distal ulcerative colitis.[8] Depending upon the local availability of different mesalamine formulations, therapy can be initiated with mesalamine suppositories, enemas or foam. The initial dose is between 500 and 1500 mg administered nightly or in divided doses for suppositories or foam. Alternatives to topical mesalamine are topical corticosteroids, again administered as suppository, enema or foam. Foam preparations are easier to retain and better tolerated, allowing maintenance of daily activities despite twice-daily administration.[104] In general there is therapeutic equivalence between marketed steroid preparations although the 'non-systemic' formulations (budesonide, beclomethasone, prednisone-metasulfobenzoate) have the advantage of fewer side effects and less potential for adrenal suppression (Chapter 32).

Oral aminosalicylates are less effective than topical therapies for ulcerative proctitis,[63] probably owing to proximal colonic stasis in distal colitis and reduced delivery of 5-ASA to the spastic, irritable rectum that is usually devoid of fecal material when inflamed. Nevertheless, oral aminosalicylates have been used for decades in patients with mild/moderate symptoms of proctitis. There have been no comparative trials of different oral aminosalicylates specifically in the setting of ulcerative proctitis, such that the dose response is extrapolated from therapeutic trials of more proximal disease. Sulfasalazine, 2–6 g/day in divided doses, is the least expensive alternative, but is frequently compromised by dose-related side effects. An alternative non-sulfa containing formulation is preferable for patients with a history of sulfa allergy or for those who develop sulfa-related intolerance or toxicity. In the absence of a response to oral aminosalicylates over several weeks, a topical mesalamine or steroid formulation should be added. Rectal instillation of combinations of mesalamine and steroids is most efficacious[277] but is not yet available in proprietary preparations.

It is rare that an oral steroid will be necessary to treat ulcerative proctitis. All attempts should be made to optimize topical therapy prior to initiating oral steroids. These measures include administration of a rectal mesalamine up to 4 g/daily, or utilizing combinations of topical mesalamine and steroids. Therapy is continued until the patient is asymptomatic, clinically manifest by the ability to pass flatus without the need to use the toilet. Depending upon the chronicity of symptoms a complete response may require 4–12 weeks.

## MAINTENANCE OF REMISSION

The usual requisite for maintenance therapy of ulcerative proctitis is not different from that for more extensive colitis. Relapse rates after discontinuation of therapy are similar;[8] however, owing to the 'milder' nature of the condition there is debate whether every newly diagnosed patient must be treated with maintenance therapy versus treatment 'as needed' for new attacks. It remains to be determined whether maintenance therapy for proctitis prevents the more proximal extension of colitis.[278] A pragmatic approach for newly treated patients once remission is achieved is to gradually taper off therapy according

to the initial response (i.e. taper more quickly if patients respond rapidly, more slowly for prolonged attacks). Few dose–response trials have been performed in ulcerative proctitis, but the small amount of evidence[73] and empiric observations suggest that patients respond best with maintenance therapy utilizing the same doses as in inductive treatment. If rectal mesalamine was used, continuation of the same dose will provide the highest likelihood of preventing relapse. In general, continuation of mesalamine suppositories on a nightly basis, with gradual tapering to every second then every third night, will maintain the majority of patients.[279] Some individuals may require only a weekly suppository or enema to maintain remission. It may also be possible to teach patients 'self-management' to treat themselves according to symptoms and thereby minimize flare-ups and physician visits.[280] Few studies have evaluated transitioning from rectal to oral mesalamine in ulcerative proctitis. It does appear that rectal therapy is more efficacious (at similar doses) than oral mesalamine,[63] and many patients who require rectal therapy to obtain remission will require continued topical therapy. Many patients prefer transitioning to an oral aminosalicylate as a maintenance therapy. There are no comparisons of oral versus topical maintenance therapy in ulcerative proctitis, oral dose-ranging trials, or comparative trials of different aminosalicylate formulations. If patients continue to develop flare-ups they should begin to receive an oral aminosalicylate up to 4.8 g daily, in conjunction with rectal mesalamine. Patients initially treated with topical steroid therapy should be given an oral aminosalicylate and gradually tapered off the topical steroid; if the disease is not responding, a reassessment of the proximal extent of colitis is desirable to exclude IBD above the original level of disease.[278]

Additional advice for patients with ulcerative proctitis includes the avoidance of NSAIDs and awareness of early signs of constipation. Changes in the odor of flatus, bloating or constipation often herald a flare-up and should signal the need to resume regular topical therapy to abort a pending acute exacerbation. Patients with a tendency toward constipation should increase the intake of dietary fiber and fluids.

# LEFT-SIDED COLITIS

## INDUCTION OF REMISSION

Patients with proctosigmoiditis or colitis extending to the splenic flexure have an intermediate presentation and a course between proctitis and extensive colitis. Proximal progression is not uncommon and should be considered if the clinical pattern worsens.[276] Conversely, the disease can become more limited and then be managed as proctitis. Thus, documentation of the proximal level of inflammation is helpful in assessing and following therapy for patients with left-sided disease. As with proctitis, left-sided colitis affords the potential for topical or oral therapy according to the severity of symptoms, the initial therapeutic response, and tolerance of topical therapy.[11,16] Again, despite the advantages of topical treatment over oral therapy[8] many patients prefer an oral regimen.

### Mild to moderate disease

The most effective therapy for left-sided colitis is topical mesalamine[69] and there does not appear to be a dose response between 1 and 4 g daily.[8,281] Depending upon the available formulations, either suppositories, foam or enemas can be used to treat disease extending to the sigmoid[282] or the splenic flexure.[283,284] An alternative to mesalamine is rectal instillation of a steroid enema[43] or foam. The foam preparations are better tolerated than enemas and can be used twice daily, but may not reach the same proximal extent.

Oral aminosalicylates are equally efficacious in left-sided and extensive colitis[52] but are not as effective as topical mesalamine for distal disease.[64,71,285] Nevertheless, many patients prefer initiating therapy with an oral agent, which are effective in 40–80% of patients;[50] improvement generally is noted within 2–4 weeks. There is approximate equivalence among the oral aminosalicylates for distal colitis,[41,50] although a few studies suggested benefit for azo-bond conjugates over delayed-release formulations.[48,57,59] However, the primary determinant of efficacy remains the quantity of oral 5-ASA delivered.[46] Sulfasalazine remains the most cost-effective therapy but is limited by dose-related intolerance and sulfa-related toxicity.[281]

## Severe disease

Patients with left-sided colitis occasionally present with severe symptoms, including toxic megacolon (see later discussion) and extraintestinal manifestations.[281] Moderate to severe symptoms, in the absence of fever, abdominal tenderness, orthostasis, vomiting and profound anemia, may be managed with an ambulatory program, including oral steroids to induce remission, particularly if a preliminary trial with an oral aminosalicylate and rectal therapy with mesalamine or steroid enemas is insufficient to gain control of the flare-up. Despite a history of distal disease, patients with severe symptoms (fever, abdominal tenderness or distension) should not undergo extensive invasive studies. A limited sigmoidoscopy and/or a plain abdominal radiograph will provide an approximation of the extent and severity of colitis. Severe left-sided UC requires treatment with systemic steroids as indicated for extensive colitis (see later discussion).

## MAINTENANCE THERAPY

Treatment for acute disease is continued until the patient achieves a clinical remission (normal bowel movements without bleeding, urgency, tenesmus or inability to evacuate flatus). Subsequently patients are transitioned into a maintenance regimen. Neither oral nor topical steroids are effective at maintaining remissions, whereas both oral and topical aminosalicylates can be used according to the response to inductive therapy and patient preference. Patients who have responded to rectal mesalamine are more likely to remain in remission with continuation of topical therapy than by transferring to oral treatment,[285] and, similar to inductive therapy, combining oral and topical mesalamine has advantages over either therapy alone to prevent relapse,[72] particularly in patients with a high likelihood of relapse.

Oral aminosalicylates remain the mainstay of therapy for ulcerative colitis extending beyond the rectum.[11] Again, dose response correlates with efficacy of maintenance therapy with oral aminosalicylates, whereas the dosing frequency/interval is more relevant with topical mesalamine.[8] Oral aminosalicylates are added as topical therapy is gradually tapered. If patients relapse, the dose of the aminosalicylate should be increased to the maximum tolerated (up to 4.8 g of mesalamine). Again, clinical trials have suggested (but not confirmed) that azo-bond formulations may have some advantage over delayed-release

mesalamine as maintenance therapy.[47,286] If patients continue to relapse despite high-dose oral therapy, it may be necessary to maintain some frequency or interval therapy with topical mesalamine. After inductive therapy with rectal steroids the enemas should be gradually tapered after the introduction of an oral aminosalicylate. The enema frequency should be reduced according to the time course of response. Patients who have required systemic steroids should be maintained on an oral aminosalicylate, with or without topical mesalamine, as necessary, to prevent relapse. There is some concern from controlled trials that conventional 'maintenance' doses of mesalamine (e.g. 1.2–1.5 g/day) may not be effective at maintaining steroid-induced remissions in ulcerative colitis,[201,202] and higher doses, up to 4.8 g, may be necessary. Patients should be educated to discern early symptoms of relapse (e.g. urgency, bleeding, nocturnal bowel movements) and to treat them aggressively with either an increase in oral therapy or, if already maximal, a resumption of topical mesalamine to prevent full-blown exacerbations.[280]

Dietary advice depends upon the baseline symptoms. Iron replacement may be required for patients with anemia, and calcium supplementation should be prescribed for patients treated with steroids. Symptomatic therapy with antispasmodics, antidiarrheals or bulk-forming agents may be useful for patients with accompanying IBS. Loperamide or small quantities of deodorized tincture of opium can be useful for patients unable to retain nightly enemas.

# EXTENSIVE COLITIS

Ulcerative colitis proximal to the splenic flexure accounts for a disproportionate number of patients who develop complications, and who require hospitalization and/or colectomy.[287] Nevertheless, the majority of patients have a good long-term prognosis and quality of life.[288] It is important, however, to gain control over symptoms as prolonged flare-ups forecast continued activity. It is also important to reassess patients at the time of a flare-up, as regression to a more distal colitis is not unusual[276,287] and can be treated, as discussed above, with topical therapies. Because of the increased risk of extraintestinal manifestations and the systemic complications of extensive colitis patients should undergo complete hematologic and metabolic assessments.

## INDUCTION OF REMISSION

### Mild to moderate colitis

Patients with extensive colitis presenting with mild symptoms are managed as outpatients. Oral aminosalicylate therapy is the first line of therapy for patients with extensive colitis, but may be supplemented with topical mesalamine or steroids.[11,16] The dose response for oral aminosalicylates is more relevant than the specific preparation used.[41,46] Antispasmodics or antidiarrheals may be added for symptomatic relief. Response rates up to 80% can be anticipated with 4–6 g of sulfasalazine or 2–4.8 g of a mesalamine formulation, with approximately half of the patients achieving remission.[41,109] Therapy should be continued as long as the patient is improving to the point of clinical remission (normal bowel movements without blood or rectal urgency). If improvement is incomplete, the dose should be increased up to 4.8 g of mesalamine.

If the patient does not demonstrate rapid and consistent improvement, or if there is any evidence of clinical deterioration, steroid therapy (prednisone, 40–60 mg/day) is added. Patients should be treated with effective doses from the outset to assure a rapid and complete response, after which the dose can be tapered according to the time course of improvement. There is rarely value in starting with 'low-dose' prednisone, as failure to respond results in dose escalation and prolongation of steroid exposure. The initial prednisone dose is maintained until the patient is clinically well (as described earlier) – generally 2–4 weeks. There is no controlled trial evidence to determine optimal strategies for steroid tapering. Empirically, prednisone is decreased by approximately 5 mg every week, usually not below 20 mg for 4–8 weeks. Below 20 mg of prednisone, taper by 2.5–5 mg every 1–2 weeks.[11,16] Aminosalicylate therapy is continued as steroids are tapered.

Patients who are unable to lower prednisone despite optimal aminosalicylate therapy are candidates for azathioprine or 6-MP.[11,16] Because it may require up to 3–6 months for these agents to demonstrate therapeutic benefits, steroids are maintained at the lowest doses that prevent recurrence of symptoms. If steroid therapy is prolonged for more than several months, supplementation with calcium and vitamin D is indicated to prevent metabolic bone disease. If there is evidence of reduced bone density, then additional therapy with a bisphosphonate, estrogen replacement in postmenopausal women, calcitonin or parathyroid hormone may be indicated.[111,112]

## Moderate to severe colitis

Patients with moderate to severe colitis span a spectrum of illness between outpatient and inpatient management. Individuals presenting with frequent bowel movements, urgency and mild extraintestinal symptoms (ocular inflammation, arthritis or arthralgias, cutaneous manifestations) who are compliant, have a supportive home environment and are able to maintain close contact with the physician can be treated on an ambulatory basis with oral steroids, as described earlier. Those with significant weight loss, fever, disabling extraintestinal manifestations, frequent nocturnal bowel movements, severe anemia or a rapidly deteriorating course require hospitalization. Similarly, patients who do not improve within several weeks of introducing adequate doses of oral steroids (equivalent to 40–60 mg/day of prednisone) for mild to moderate disease should be hospitalized.

The diet for moderately ill patients is modified to reduce diarrhea and abdominal cramping. In general, a low-residue diet should reduce bowel frequency. These patients should be evaluated for a history of lactose intolerance, and non-digestible carbohydrates, such as sorbitol, should be avoided. However, either the physician or a dietitian should provide counseling regarding the requisite intake of protein and calories to counter the catabolic influence of active inflammation and steroids. Supplementation with calcium 1.2–1.5 g/day and vitamin D 400 iu/day should be encouraged for patients receiving steroids, and many will require iron supplements to treat or avoid anemia. Cautious use of antispasmodics or antidiarrheals is acceptable as long as the patient is carefully monitored for worsening symptoms, particularly fever, abdominal distension or tenderness.

Intravenous steroids are indicated for patients who are febrile, orthostatic or hypotensive, dehydrated, passing more than 10–12 stools daily, incontinent, hemorrhaging, protein depleted, edematous, or with evidence of abdominal tenderness or distension.[11,16] In addition, the initial management of patients with severe colitis includes the prompt institution of general resuscitative measures to correct fluid and electrolyte imbalances, and blood transfusions to maintain a normal hematocrit.[93,110] In these situations, anticholinergics, antidiarrheals and narcotic analgesics should be withheld, as they may induce colonic dilatation or mask peritoneal signs in debilitated patients (especially those on steroids).[40]

Patients with severe colitis are treated with an intensive intravenous steroid regimen of either prednisolone (40–60 mg/day), methylprednisolone (32–48 mg/day) or hydrocortisone (300–400 mg/day), either in divided doses or as a continuous infusion.[40,93,110] We and other experienced clinicians[289] prefer a continuous infusion because of the reliability of blood levels, ease of administration (single intravenous bag, or incorporation into parenteral solution) and lower cost. There is no advantage to higher-dose steroid therapy,[11,91] which may run the risk of additional immunosuppression, opportunistic infection or osteonecrosis. A few clinicians continue to advocate infusions of intravenous ACTH (120 units daily) for patients who have not recently received corticosteroids,[11] but practice is on the decline, as is the availability of ACTH formulations. However, a rectal steroid preparation (e.g. 100 mg hydrocortisone) is often added for patients with rectal urgency or tenesmus.[84,289] Aminosalicylates should be discontinued to avoid the potential intolerant effects and/or the rare instances when 5-ASA can worsen colitis.[60] In addition, there is no role for antibiotic therapy in the management of patients with moderate to severe UC. In the absence of severe pain, nausea and vomiting, patients are allowed to continue on a minimal- or low-residue diet. There are no objective data supporting bowel rest for the treatment of UC[11] (see Chapter 36), although many patients are afraid to eat, fearing abdominal pain or rectal urgency, and many are unable to consume adequate diets. Therefore, supplemental parenteral nutrition may be required to ensure sufficient caloric intake.

The intensive intravenous regimen can be continued for up to 7–10 days as long as the patient is improving. However, patients who are not beginning to respond within the first 5–7 days have a poor prognosis.[37,114] Once clinical improvement has been established by normalization of vital signs, improved nutrition, stabilization of the hematocrit and blood counts, and the ability to tolerate a full diet with formation of bowel movements without blood or urgency, the patient can be advanced to an oral regimen. Full-dose therapy with an aminosalicylate is resumed, and intravenous steroids are replaced with oral steroids, often by dividing the oral dose of prednisone to mimic the intravenous schedule as outpatients gradually move back to once-daily dosing.

If the patient is not improving within the first week of intensive intravenous steroid therapy, the likelihood of future improvement is small.[37,114] By some estimates, the failure rate for patients with severe colitis treated with intravenous steroids is nearly 40%[86] and correlates with the severity of diarrhea, transfusion requirements, hypoalbuminemia[114] and the presence of deep mucosal ulcerations.[290] Therefore, if patients are not considerably improved within the first week of therapy they should be considered candidates for either surgery or the addition of cyclosporin. In our center, the decision to proceed with cyclosporin or colectomy is often determined within the first 5 days of intensive therapy.

Intravenous cyclosporin therapy has been the most important advance in the therapy of severe UC as well as one of the most controversial management issues.[153–156] Consistent benefits

**Table 33.7 Outpatient monitoring of cyclosporin**

History and physical examination
  Weekly for 1 month, then biweekly for 1 month, then monthly until cyclosporin discontinued
Cyclosporin level
  With each visit as above
  Once weekly after any change in dosing
Complete blood count
  With each visit as above
  Two weeks after any change in azathioprine/6-mercaptopurine
Serum creatinine/BUN and electrolytes
  With each visit as above
  With each cyclosporin level
Liver enzymes
  Every 4 weeks for first 3 months

have been reported using intravenous cyclosporin for severe UC, with up to 80% of refractory patients responding within 7–10 days.[115,155,159] There are few factors that predict responsiveness to cyclosporin therapy, although high 'band counts',[163] deep colonic ulcerations[93] and poor overall status of the patient[114] have been associated with treatment failures. Most centers proceed with an initial dose of 4 mg/kg/24 hours as a continuous infusion, although some have reported equal results with 2 mg/kg.[160] It probably makes little difference whether cyclosporin therapy is initiated at higher doses and titrated down, or at lower doses and increased according to blood levels.[155] Prior to initiating therapy with cyclosporin, the patient should be informed of the potential benefits and risks, including immunosuppression, nephrotoxicity and cost, as well as the risk of relapse after the intravenous phase. The cholesterol level should be above 100 mg/dL to limit the risk of seizures, although hypocholesterolemia is a relative contraindication, as we have treated some patients with low cholesterol beginning with 1 mg/kg and following blood levels. Cyclosporin therapy is monitored and adjusted according to the guidelines published by Kornbluth and colleagues[165](Table 33.7).

Desirable whole blood levels of cyclosporin are between 200 and 400 ng/mL by high-performance liquid chromatography (HPLC), although there is poor correlation between efficacy and side effects within this range.[61,155] Minor side effects, such as headache, nausea or paresthesiae, rarely require discontinuation of therapy.[175] The development of hypertension is treated with calcium channel blockers, but care must be taken as these can increase cyclosporin blood levels.[61,165]

Patients should begin to respond within the first 4 or 5 days. Those who do not respond by the first week are not likely to improve and should proceed to colectomy.[37] In experienced centers, surgical morbidity is not altered by prior cyclosporin therapy.[178,179] Once the patient is in clinical remission (formed bowel movements without blood or urgency), the intravenous regimen is replaced with oral cyclosporin and prednisone. The daily dose of cyclosporin is doubled and administered in two divided oral doses (e.g. if the patient was receiving 200 mg daily the oral dosing is 200 mg twice each day).[11,61] In order to prevent the high relapse rate when aminosalicylates are used alone after cyclosporin, we now recommend the addition of azathioprine or 6-MP as maintenance therapy for virtually all

patients responding to cyclosporin.[136,138,155] In addition, double-strength sulfamethoxazole/trimethoprim is added three times weekly as prophylaxis against *Pneumocystis* pneumonia.[136,155] Thus, at discharge the typical patient will be receiving prednisone 40 mg, cyclosporin twice a day, mesalamine 4.8 g in divided doses, azathioprine 100 mg and sulfamethoxazole/trimethoprim every other day.

Ambulatory monitoring of these complicated patients is outlined in Table 33.7. The patient is scheduled to return to the outpatient department in approximately 1 week. Cyclosporin levels and laboratory studies are repeated weekly for the first month and then at increased intervals. Dose reductions of 25% are made in the setting of elevated blood pressure or decreasing renal function. The dose is increased to achieve trough cyclosporin levels greater than 200–400 ng/mL. Prednisone tapering begins after the first or second visit, as just described. After the patient is off steroids (generally 8–12 weeks), cyclosporin is tapered over the next month and the patient is maintained on an aminosalicylate and azathioprine or 6-MP.

## MAINTENANCE OF REMISSION

The maintenance strategy for extensive ulcerative colitis is determined by the intensity of induction therapy necessary to achieve remission. In addition, as has been emphasized in previous sections of this chapter, it is critical to prevent relapse: the patient must be in clinical remission before tapering inductive therapy. One of the most common errors in management is the premature withdrawal of acute therapy, before a patient is in clinical remission, thereby compromising maintenance therapies. The second most common error is to mistake steroid dependency for a maintenance effect.[16] A third type of error is to withdraw maintenance therapy, or to fail to educate patients regarding the likelihood of relapse with dose reduction or cessation of treatment. We see many patients referred for flare-ups who were never told to continue medications after their (acute) symptoms resolved. Occasionally, patients with extensive colitis will develop exacerbations limited to the distal colon.[276] Therefore, any recurrence of symptoms requires a reassessment of the disease extent and severity as well as a search for aggravating factors, such as intercurrent enteric infections, antibiotic exposure, NSAIDs, or cessation of cigarette smoking.[18]

When aminosalicylate therapy alone has been sufficient to induce remission, continuation of the same dosage throughout maintenance therapy is optimal. A dose response for maintenance therapy with aminosalicylates has been demonstrated for both sulfasalazine and mesalamine.[42] In the past, a reduction from the inductive dose to an intermediate dose of sulfasalazine was often recommended as a compromise between efficacy and tolerance. The advantages of the non-sulfa containing aminosalicylates are the absence of dose-related toxicity and the ability to continue maintenance therapy without the need for dose reduction to minimize side effects. Thus, the only reasons to lower dosage recommendations for maintenance therapy would be to reduce cost or improve compliance. Unfortunately, it is not possible to prospectively predict the lowest dose of a maintenance therapy for each individual patient. Some degree of empiricism, over time, as well as communication and education of the patient, is necessary to define an optimal, individualized approach.[280] There are no evidence-based guidelines for the hematological or biochemical monitoring of patients on long-term aminosalicylates.[60] One approach is to perform a complete blood count and basic metabolic profile 3 and 6 months after inducing remission, and thereafter on a yearly basis.

Similarly, patients who needed steroids to achieve remission require an individualized approach to maintenance therapy. Steroids do not prevent relapse but steroid dependency remains a common problem (see discussion under Refractory colitis). In general, the rate of steroid tapering after induction of remission is determined by the rapidity of response. Patients whose symptoms flare as steroids are tapered should be placed on maximized doses of an aminosalicylate (see Table 33.4). Only after the patient has been off steroids for at least a year should tapering of the aminosalicylate dose be considered.

Patients on azathioprine or 6-MP are also continued on maximized aminosalicylate therapy (assuming the indication for the immunomodulator was not 5-ASA intolerance), although there is some debate regarding the necessity for aminosalicylates when patients are maintained on purine antimetabolites.[132,291] Neither the ultimate duration (years) of azathioprine or 6-MP use[125] nor the optimization of dosing has been clarified. Similarly, it has not been established whether leukopenia is necessary to prevent relapse.[291] Individuals maintained on the purine antagonists require quarterly monitoring of the blood count because of the risk of delayed bone marrow suppression.[292,293]

The ultimate duration of maintenance therapy for individuals in long-term remission (more than 2 years without relapse) has not been established. Therapy with aminosalicylates can be continued indefinitely at the lowest dose that prevents relapse, and immunomodulators can be given at least for 1–2 years after discontinuation of steroids[134] and indefinitely if patients relapse and require steroids.

# FULMINANT COLITIS AND TOXIC MEGACOLON

Fulminant colitis, with or without colonic dilatation, is a medical emergency. Fortunately, with advances in medical and surgical therapies the risk of death from acute ulcerative colitis is rare. Morbidity, however, is increased by delay in surgical therapy owing to the prolongation of futile medical treatment, vascular complications (i.e. pulmonary emboli) or opportunistic infections. To minimize disease-related and iatrogenic complications, fulminant colitis or toxic megacolon is best managed by an experienced team of gastroenterologists and surgeons. Patients presenting with fulminant colitis manifest by high fever, abdominal tenderness, abdominal distension and hemorrhage requiring transfusions with or without colonic dilatation require 24-hour monitoring of vital signs, in addition to frequent auscultation of the abdomen for indications of decreasing peristalsis or high-pitched bowel sounds. Daily abdominal radiographs should be reviewed for evidence of impending dilatation or free air beneath the diaphragm, along with daily determinations of complete blood count and serum electrolytes in these unstable patients.

Fulminant colitis represents transmural extension of inflammation to the serosa and is manifest by abdominal tenderness in addition to systemic toxicity.[294] Peritoneal irritation and perforation can occur in the absence of dilatation. Toxic megacolon, caused by the sudden progression of inflammation through the bowel wall to the serosa, is associated with clinical signs of rebound tenderness, indistinguishable from a localized or free perforation. At times the condition is accompanied by a paradoxical diminution of diarrhea, or by the passage of blood clots devoid of stool, associated with progressive abdominal distension and hollow, hypoactive bowel sounds. Toxic megacolon most commonly occurs in the setting of extensive colitis, but has been documented in left-sided colitis or in the presence of coexisting infections (e.g. CMV or C. *difficile*).[40] Additional predisposing factors for toxic megacolon include medications, such as anticholinergics, antidiarrheals and opiates; electrolyte abnormalities, particularly hypokalemia; and invasive diagnostic testing, such as colonoscopy or barium enema.[110]

The diagnosis should be suspected in any seriously ill colitis patient who manifests abdominal wall tenderness associated with distension.[295] High-dose steroids may mask findings, particularly in malnourished or elderly patients. Abdominal radiographs confirm the presence of a distended, haustral gas-filled colon (devoid of fecal material in the segment of colitis) with associated 'thumbprinting,' 'islands' of residual mucosa surrounded by extensive ulceration, or pneumatosis. Serial measurements demonstrating a dilated (usually > 6 cm) colon[296] with features of severe ulceration that do not improve or worsen, in association with clinical symptoms and signs of toxicity, are sufficient to classify the patient as 'toxic'.[297]

The medical management of fulminant colitis or toxic megacolon is the same as that described for severe colitis, with several modifications: intensive monitoring with gastroenterological and surgical consultation is mandatory; support with fluid and electrolytes, whole blood transfusions and fresh frozen plasma (in the presence of clotting abnormalities) and human albumin is essential.[40,110,289] Intravenous steroids are continued and, despite the absence of controlled evidence, broad-spectrum antibiotic coverage is added.[40,110,289] The rationale for antibiotics includes a presumption of transmural extension of disease, the risk of microperforation, systemic bacteremia, and as potential perioperative prophylaxis for patients with a high risk of emergent colectomy.

Patients with fulminant colitis or toxic megacolon do not receive oral fluids or food until clinically improved. The presence of small bowel ileus is a poor prognostic sign[295] necessitating placement of a nasogastric tube. Several additional maneuvers have been proposed to reduce distension by allowing the redistribution and passage of colonic gas per rectum. These patients tend to remain supine and motionless in bed (to avoid movement that stimulates an urgent or painful bowel movement). Therefore, air tends to fill and distend the (superior-when-supine) transverse colon. Encouraging the patient to mobilize, or at least to roll from side-to-side, the insertion of a rectal tube, or the assumption of the 'knee–elbow' position while prone may help to redistribute or dispel colonic gas and reduce distension.[289,298]

The role of cyclosporin in fulminant colitis or toxic megacolon is controversial. There are no clinical trials in this situation, although some experienced tertiary centers use cyclosporin in selected cases after considerable review of the potential risks and benefits with the patient and the family.[289] Both rapid clinical improvement and progressive deterioration have been observed in such circumstances. Too often, patients are transferred to specialty centers, already toxic, when the earlier window of opportunity to intervene has been closed. Patients who fail to improve within the first week of intensive steroid therapy[37,113,114] should be considered candidates for cyclosporin, offered colectomy, or transferred to an experienced tertiary center.

Signs of perforation are an immediate indication for colectomy[299] (Chapters 38 and 39). Likewise, any deterioration is indication for emergency colectomy, with the understanding that the complication of perforation greatly increases the morbidity rate and the potential for death from a curable disease. Failure to improve within 24–72 hours is another indication for abandonment of medical treatment, as rapid surgical intervention minimizes the risk of complications and has reduced the mortality rate to less than 6% in these critically ill patients (Chapter 40). With aggressive medical management a medically induced remission can be achieved in 40–50% of patients, with an acceptable morbidity rate and very low mortality rate. However, the long-term 'viability' of the damaged colon remains in question. Many of these patients are destined for complications or resistant disease, including recurrent toxic megacolon.[86,297]

# REFRACTORY ULCERATIVE COLITIS

The definition of refractory ulcerative colitis continues to evolve as therapeutic options and efficacy improve. In concert with the concepts of induction of remission and maintenance of remission, it is useful to examine refractoriness from the perspectives of *failure to induce* remission and *failure to maintain* remission. 'Steroid resistance' pertains to the former and 'steroid dependence' to the latter. In either setting, both endogenous and exogenous factors contributing to symptoms or inflammation should be examined.[18,39] Endogenous factors include hormonal variations in women during the menstrual cycle[26] and pregnancy (Chapter 23). Coexistent IBS is common in ulcerative colitis and often accounts for residual symptoms after the resolution of inflammatory features. Exogenous factors that affect the therapeutic response include cigarette smoking, NSAIDs and concurrent enteric pathogens, including C. *difficile* and CMV.[300] Finally, the diagnosis of ulcerative colitis, particularly in the setting of severe disease,[301] is based on non-specific clinical,

endoscopic and histologic findings. Without a pathognomonic diagnostic test, the possibility of Crohn's disease should be considered if the clinical course changes or new findings (e.g. perianal fistulae or abscess) develop, particularly in smokers or patients with a family history of Crohn's disease.

# INDUCTION FAILURES

As described in previous sections, the optimization of inductive therapy assumes adequate dosing that may be higher than 'marketed' dosages and duration of therapy for each individual agent. Table 33.8 provides estimated ranges of therapeutic response for each inductive agent.

In addition to adequate dosing, sufficient time must be allotted for a response to occur. The time frame will necessarily depend upon the severity of disease, its impact on quality of life, and tolerance of the therapeutic agent. Patients with mild to moderate colitis may prefer to 'trade off' prolongation of mild symptoms for the longer duration required for efficacy of an aminosalicylate to avoid the side effects of steroids. In some settings (e.g. distal colitis) it may take several months for symptoms to resolve completely.[302] In the setting of more severe disease treated with intensive intravenous therapy a response should be anticipated within 7–10 days.[37]

Topical mesalamine has been the most efficacious therapy for distal UC. Approximately 80% of patients refractory to oral aminosalicylates, oral steroids or topical steroids respond to topical mesalamine as long as the formulation reaches the upper extent of disease. Some patients are unable to retain mesalamine enemas owing to hypertonicity or intolerance to an antioxidant stabilizer in the enema formulations. A trial of mesalamine suppositories (devoid of antioxidants) will determine whether the patient is able to tolerate 5-ASA. Often, healing the rectum will allow a patient subsequently to retain an enema. Rarely, colitis is worsened by mesalamine. When this is suspected, all aminosalicylates are discontinued. If patients do not respond to topical mesalamine alone, then the combination of rectal mesalamine with a rectal steroid may be effective.[277] The intensive intravenous steroid regimen also has been helpful for patients with

## Table 33.8 Response to individual therapies for active ulcerative colitis

| Drug | Response range | Notes |
| --- | --- | --- |
| Sulfasalazine | 64–80% | Mild/moderate disease, clinical improvement or remission (improved efficacy >3 g/day) |
| Non-sulfa aminosalicylates | 40–74% | Mild/moderate disease, clinical improvement or remission (improved efficacy >2 g/day) |
| Topical mesalamine | 60–89% | Mild/moderate distal disease (no dose response >1 g/day) |
| Topical corticosteroids | 41–89% | Mild/moderate distal disease (less effective than topical mesalamine) |
| Systemic corticosteroids | 45–90% | Moderate/severe disease, clinical remission or improvement (dose response up to equivalent of oral prednisone 40–60 mg/day, no dose–response data for IV steroids) |
| Azathioprine/6-MP | 29–78% | Steroid dependence, reduced dose or cessation of steroids (?steroid resistance) |
| Cyclosporin | 60–80% | Severe disease, spared immediate colectomy (with or without steroids?) |
| Placebo | 16–52% | Mild/moderate disease, clinical improvement |

distal disease refractory to oral steroid therapy.[84] Alternative approaches that may be useful in individual patients include the administration of short-chain fatty acid or nicotine enemas, nicotine patches, or the resumption of cigarette smoking.

Patients with extensive colitis failing inductive therapy with maximal doses of oral aminosalicylates and steroids should be treated with steroids *alone* to determine whether 5-ASA paradoxically aggravates colitis. Azathioprine or 6-MP have been reported to be beneficial in steroid-resistant ulcerative colitis but require several months, making the option less acceptable than induction of remission with inpatient management and initiation of maintenance (steroid-sparing) therapy. Nicotine patches can be helpful in reducing symptoms, particularly in ex-smokers. A more reliable treatment is resumption of cigarette smoking,[303] an approach that has yet to be given serious consideration compared to treatment with long-term steroids or immunomodulators. It should be recalled that ex-smokers often have a more refractory course of colitis, are more likely to require steroids or immunomodulators and have a higher incidence of pouchitis after colectomy.[303] Therefore, the risk/benefits of resumption of smoking small amounts may be favorable in selected patients. Finally, if outpatient therapy is not effective, hospitalization with intensive intravenous steroid therapy is indicated, with or without cyclosporin.

## MAINTENANCE FAILURES

There are a number of additional considerations for patients who fail maintenance therapy. Expected therapeutic outcomes are listed in Table 33.9. Patients who develop recurrent disease activity despite maintenance therapy should be evaluated for the same exogenous and endogenous factors described previously. Occasionally, women who flare with each menstrual cycle will respond to hormonal manipulation, such as oral contraceptives or even temporary disruption of menstruation with progesterone or leuprolide. Examination of stool for enteric infections is important for patients with unanticipated disease exacerbation, and a re-examination of the colon is important to rule out IBS when diarrhea, abdominal cramping or irregular bowel habits are disproportionate to mucosal inflammation. Finally, compliance with therapy is an important issue.[7] Physicians must recognize that this is a chronic disease and that human nature dictates that most patients will take the fewest number of pills (suppositories or enemas) that keep them well. Often patients who fail maintenance therapy have reduced their medications below the 'threshold' of effective dosages.

Steroids have never been effective at preventing relapse in ulcerative colitis. Steroid dependency pertains to individual patients who achieve remissions on steroids but are unable to taper without the disease flaring.[16] There are several approaches to steroid dependency in ulcerative colitis. The first is to maximize oral and topical aminosalicylate therapy according to Table 33.4. If this fails, there is general acceptance for the addition of azathioprine or 6-MP.[11] Finally, consider the possibility that 5-ASA intolerance may be obscured by steroid therapy and unmasked as steroids are tapered.

## CHRONIC ULCERATIVE COLITIS
### NEOPLASIA (see Chapter 43)

Colon cancer is a well-recognized risk and long-term complication of ulcerative colitis. Continuation of maintenance therapy with aminosalicylates appears to have some protective effects,[304] as may folic acid supplementation in patients receiving sulfasalazine.[305] Other chemopreventive strategies are currently being evaluated.[15]

## EXTRAINTESTINAL MANIFESTATIONS
(see Chapter 45)

The treatment of extraintestinal manifestations of ulcerative colitis is reviewed in Chapter 45.

## PREGNANCY AND LACTATION (see Chapter 23)

The management of ulcerative colitis in pregnancy is described in Chapter 23.

## INDICATIONS FOR SURGERY (see Chapters 38–40)

Ulcerative colitis can be cured by colectomy. In past decades, surgical cure (proctocolectomy and ileostomy) was compromised by the cosmetic consequences of an external appliance. With the advent of sphincter-saving procedures, the 'cure' is potentially compromised by pouchitis, pouch dysfunction or dysplasia. Nevertheless, the quality of life after surgery for UC is, in general, excellent. In the absence of controlled trials comparing medical and surgical therapy, debate continues as to whether or not the quality of life after an attack of severe colitis is better with medical or surgical therapy.[180] Indications for colectomy in UC are either emergent or elective and are discussed more completely in Chapters 38–40.

## Table 33.9 Response to maintenance therapy for ulcerative colitis

| Drug | Response | Comments |
|------|----------|----------|
| Sulfasalazine | 71–88% | 6-month remission, dose response 1–4 g/day |
| Oral aminosalicylate | 54–80 | 6–12 month remission, dose response 800 mg–4.8g(?) equivalent of 5-ASA |
| Topical mesalamine | 74–80% | 12 month remission, dosing interval more important than daily dose |
| Azathioprine/6-MP | 50–64% | 12-month remission at 100 mg/day (?need for 5-ASA and no dose–response data) |
| Placebo | 25–51% | 6–12-month remission in clinical trials |

# CONCLUSION

The medical therapy of ulcerative colitis is a major challenge requiring the attributes of an astute and humanitarian clinician to guide patients through chronic illness. It is imperative to comprehend and empathize with the perspectives and concerns of patients and family members confronted with a chronic, medically incurable, socially embarrassing and potentially disfiguring condition. Patients require reassurance that, despite the absence of known causation, medical therapy is usually effective, and surgical techniques have improved to the point that both longevity and quality of life are preserved. It may take several visits to complete initial and subsequent communications with the patient and family to allow them to assimilate their comprehension and questions regarding the prognosis and therapeutic options and expectations. Patience, optimism and empathy are required to balance the concerns and misinformation that surround the disease and the guilt associated with the misconceptions that this is a 'neurotic', 'psychologic' or 'self-induced' disorder.

The physician must be a resource for quality medical care, information and support, in addition to coordinating the ancillary care and professional consultation necessary to manage the patient and reassure the family over years. Additional support is available through national organizations, such as the Crohn's and Colitis Foundation of America (CCFA). Not only is the printed material useful but, through videotapes, patient support groups and the internet (www.CCFA.com), and the professional journal *Inflammatory Bowel Diseases*, the organization is a valuable resource for both patients and physicians.

# REFERENCES

1. Podolsky DK. Inflammatory bowel disease. N Engl J Med 2002;347:417–429.
2. Rutgeerts P. A critical assessment of new therapies in inflammatory bowel disease. J Gastroenterol Hepatol 2002;17 :S176–185.
3. Sandborn WJ, Loftus EV Jr, Colombel JF et al. Evaluation of serologic disease markers in a population-based cohort of patients with ulcerative colitis and Crohn's disease. Inflamm Bowel Dis 2001;7:192–201.
4. Shanahan F. Inflammatory bowel disease: immunodiagnostics, immunotherapeutics, and ecotherapeutics. Gastroenterology 2001;120:622–635.
5. Joossens S, Reinisch W, Vermeire S et al. The value of serologic markers in indeterminate colitis: a prospective follow-up study. Gastroenterology 2002;122:1242–1247.
6. Landers CJ, Cohavy O, Misra R et al. Selected loss of tolerance evidenced by Crohn's disease-associated immune responses to auto- and microbial antigens. Gastroenterology 2002;123:689–699.
7. Kane SV, Cohen RD, Aikens JE, Hanauer SB. Prevalence of nonadherence with maintenance mesalamine in quiescent ulcerative colitis. Am J Gastroenterol 2001;96:2929–2933.
8. Cohen RD, Woseth DM, Thisted RA, Hanauer SB. A meta-analysis and overview of the literature on treatment options for left-sided ulcerative colitis and ulcerative proctitis. Am J Gastroenterol 2000;95:1263–1276.
9. D'Haens G, Geboes K, Peeters M, Baert F, Ectors N, Rutgeerts P. Patchy cecal inflammation associated with distal ulcerative colitis: a prospective endoscopic study. Am J Gastroenterol 1997;92:1275–1279.
10. Truelove SC, Witts LJ. Cortisone in ulcerative colitis. Final report on a therapeutic trial. Br Med J 1955;4947:1041–1048.
11. Kornbluth A, Sachar DB. Ulcerative colitis practice guidelines in adults. American College of Gastroenterology, Practice Parameters Committee. Am J Gastroenterol 1997;92:204–211.
12. Geboes K, Dalle I. Influence of treatment on morphological features of mucosal inflammation. Gut 2002;50:III37–42.
13. Bernstein CN. On making the diagnosis of ulcerative colitis [editorial]. Am J Gastroenterol 1997;92:1247–1252.
14. Bernstein CN, Shanahan F, Weinstein WM. Histological patchiness and sparing of the rectum in ulcerative colitis: refuting the dogma [letter; comment]. J Clin Pathol 1997;50:354–355.
15. Itzkowitz SH. Cancer prevention in patients with inflammatory bowel disease. Gastroenterol Clin North Am 2002;31:1133–1144.
16. Hanauer SB. Review articles: drug therapy: inflammatory bowel disease. N Engl J Med 1996;334:841–848.
17. Fredd S. Standards for approval of new drugs for IBD. Inflamm Bowel Dis 1995;1:284–294.
18. Miner PB Jr. Factors influencing the relapse of patients with inflammatory bowel disease. Am J Gastroenterol 1997;92:1S–4S.
19. Sandborn WJ, Landers CJ, Tremaine WJ, Targan SR. Association of antineutrophil cytoplasmic antibodies with resistance to treatment of left-sided ulcerative colitis: results of a pilot study [see comments]. Mayo Clin Proc 1996;71:431–436.
20. Sandborn WJ, Landers CJ, Tremaine WJ, Targan SR. Antineutrophil cytoplasmic antibody correlates with chronic pouchitis after ileal pouch–anal anastomosis. Am J Gastroenterol 1995;90:740–747.
21. Koutroubakis I, Manousos ON, Meuwissen SG, Pena AS. Environmental risk factors in inflammatory bowel disease. Hepatogastroenterology 1996;43:381–393.
22. Schumacher G, Sandstedt B, Kollberg B. A prospective study of first attacks of inflammatory bowel disease and infectious colitis. Clinical findings and early diagnosis. Scand J Gastroenterol 1994;29:265–274.
23. Hilsden RJ, Scott CM, Verhoef MJ. Complementary medicine use by patients with inflammatory bowel disease. Am J Gastroenterol 1998;93:697–701.
24. Heuschkel R, Afzal N, Wuerth A et al. Complementary medicine use in children and young adults with inflammatory bowel disease. Am J Gastroenterol 2002;97:382–388.
25. Bayless TM, Harris ML. Inflammatory bowel disease and irritable bowel syndrome. Med Clin North Am 1990;74:21–28.
26. Kane SV, Sable K, Hanauer SB. The menstrual cycle and its effect on inflammatory bowel disease and irritable bowel syndrome: a prevalence study. Am J Gastroenterol 1998;93:1867–1872.
27. Rubin DT, Hanauer SB. Smoking and inflammatory bowel disease. Eur J Gastroenterol Hepatol 2000;12:855–862.
28. Odes HS, Fich A, Reif S et al. Effects of current cigarette smoking on clinical course of Crohn's disease and ulcerative colitis. Dig Dis Sci 2001;46:1717–1721.
29. Fraga XF, Vergara M, Medina C, Casellas F, Bermejo B, Malagelada JR. Effects of smoking on the presentation and clinical course of inflammatory bowel disease. Eur J Gastroenterol Hepatol 1997;9:683–687.
30. Loftus EV Jr, Sandborn WJ, Tremaine WJ et al. Primary sclerosing cholangitis is associated with nonsmoking: a case–control study [see comments]. Gastroenterology 1996;110:1496–1502.
31. Mitchell SA, Thyssen M, Orchard TR, Jewell DP, Fleming KA, Chapman RW. Cigarette smoking, appendectomy, and tonsillectomy as risk factors for the development of primary sclerosing cholangitis: a case control study. Gut 2002;51:567–573.
32. Silvennoinen JA, Lehtola JK, Niemela SE. Smoking is a risk factor for osteoporosis in women with inflammatory bowel disease. Scand J Gastroenterol 1996;31:367–371.
33. Mahadevan U, Loftus EV Jr, Tremaine WJ, Sandborn WJ. Safety of selective cyclooxygenase-2 inhibitors in inflammatory bowel disease. Am J Gastroenterol 2002;97:910–914.
34. Bonner GF. Using COX-2 inhibitors in IBD: anti-inflammatories inflame a controversy. Am J Gastroenterol 2002;97:783–785.
35. Rizzello F, Gionchetti P, Venturi A, Amadini C, Romagnoli R, Campieri M. Review article: monitoring activity in ulcerative colitis. Aliment Pharmacol Ther 2002;16:3–6.
36. Chakravarty BJ. Predictors and the rate of medical treatment failure in ulcerative colitis. Am J Gastroenterol 1993;88:852–855.
37. Travis SP, Farrant JM, Ricketts C et al. Predicting outcome in severe ulcerative colitis. Gut 1996;38:905–910.
38. Urayama S, Chang EB. Mechanisms and treatment of diarrhea in inflammatory bowel diseases. Inflamm Bowel Dis 1997;3:114–131.
39. Griffin mg, Miner PB. Review article: refractory distal colitis – explanations and options. Aliment Pharmacol Ther 1996;10:39–48.
40. Stein R, Hanauer SB. Life-threatening complications of IBD: How to handle fulminant colitis and toxic megacolon. J Crit Illness 1998;13:518–525.
41. Sutherland L, Roth D, Beck P, May G, Makiyama K. Oral 5-aminosalicylic acid for inducing remission in ulcerative colitis. Cochrane Database Syst Rev 2000;2.
42. Sutherland L, Roth D, Beck P, May G, Makiyama K. Oral 5-aminosalicylic acid for maintaining remission in ulcerative colitis. Cochrane Database Syst Rev 2000;2.
43. Marshall JK, Irvine EJ. Rectal corticosteroids versus alternative treatments in ulcerative colitis: a meta-analysis. Gut 1997;40:775–781.
44. Svartz N. Sulfasalazine: II. Some notes on the discovery and development of salazopyrin. Am J Gastroenterol 1988;83:497–503.
45. Sandborn WJ, Hanauer SB. A metaanalysis of the pharmacokinetics of 5-aminosalicylic acid products. Aliment Pharmacol Ther 2003; (in press).
46. Sandborn WJ. Rational selection of oral 5-aminosalicylate formulations and prodrugs for the treatment of ulcerative colitis. Am J Gastroenterol 2002;97:2939–2941.
47. Courtney MG, Nunes DP, Bergin CF et al. Randomised comparison of olsalazine and mesalazine in prevention of relapses in ulcerative colitis [see comments]. Lancet 1992;339:1279–1281.
48. Green JR, Lobo AJ, Holdsworth CD et al. Balsalazide is more effective and better tolerated than mesalamine in the treatment of acute ulcerative colitis. The Abacus Investigator Group. Gastroenterology 1998;114:15–22.

49. Levine DS, Riff DS, Pruitt R et al. A randomized, double blind, dose–response comparison of balsalazide (6.75 g), balsalazide (2.25 g), and mesalamine (2.4 g) in the treatment of active, mild-to-moderate ulcerative colitis. Am J Gastroenterol 2002;97:1398–1407.

50. Gisbert JP, Gomollon F, Mate J, Pajares JM. Role of 5-aminosalicylic acid (5-ASA) in treatment of inflammatory bowel disease: a systematic review. Dig Dis Sci 2002;47:471–488.

51. Margolin ML, Krumholz MP, Fochios SE, Korelitz BI. Clinical trials in ulcerative colitis: II. Historical review. Am J Gastroenterol 1988;83:227–243.

52. Hanauer S, Schwartz J, Robinson M et al. Mesalamine capsules for treatment of active ulcerative colitis: results of a controlled trial. Pentasa Study Group. Am J Gastroenterol 1993;88:1188–1197.

53. Schroeder KW, Tremaine WJ, Ilstrup DM. Coated oral 5-aminosalicylic acid therapy for mildly to moderately active ulcerative colitis. A randomized study. N Engl J Med 1987;317:1625–1629.

54. Riley SA, Mani V, Goodman MJ, Herd ME, Dutt S, Turnberg LA. Comparison of delayed release 5 aminosalicylic acid (mesalazine) and sulphasalazine in the treatment of mild to moderate ulcerative colitis relapse. Gut 1988;29:669–674.

55. Riley SA. What dose of 5-aminosalicylic acid (mesalazine) in ulcerative colitis? Gut 1998;42:761–763.

56. Meyers S, Sachar DB, Present DH, Janowitz HD. Olsalazine sodium in the treatment of ulcerative colitis among patients intolerant of sulfasalazine. A prospective, randomized, placebo-controlled, double-blind, dose-ranging clinical trial. Gastroenterology 1987;93:1255–1262.

57. Green JR, Mansfield JC, Gibson JA, Kerr GD, Thornton PC. A double-blind comparison of balsalazide, 6.75 g daily, and sulfasalazine, 3 g daily, in patients with newly diagnosed or relapsed active ulcerative colitis. Aliment Pharmacol Ther 2002;16:61–68.

58. Mansfield JC, Giaffer MH, Cann PA, McKenna D, Thornton PC, Holdsworth CD. A double-blind comparison of balsalazide, 6.75 g, and sulfasalazine, 3 g, as sole therapy in the management of ulcerative colitis. Aliment Pharmacol Ther 2002;16:69–77.

59. Pruitt R, Hanson J, Safdi M et al. Balsalazide is superior to mesalamine in the time to improvement of signs and symptoms of acute mild-to-moderate ulcerative colitis. Am J Gastroenterol 2002;97:3078–3086.

60. Cunliffe RN, Scott BB. Monitoring for drug side-effects in inflammatory bowel disease. Aliment Pharmacol Ther 2002;16:647–662.

61. Schwab M, Klotz U. Pharmacokinetic considerations in the treatment of inflammatory bowel disease. Clin Pharmacokinet 2001;40:723–751.

62. Pruitt R, Hanson J, Safdi M et al. Balsalazide is superior to mesalamine in the time to improvement of signs and symptoms of acute mild-to-moderate ulcerative colitis. Am J Gastroenterol 2002;97:3078–3086.

63. Gionchetti P, Rizzello F, Venturi A et al. Comparison of oral with rectal mesalamine in the treatment of ulcerative proctitis. Dis Colon Rectum 1998;41:93–97.

64. Safdi M, DeMicco M, Sninsky C et al. A double-blind comparison of oral versus rectal mesalamine versus combination therapy in the treatment of distal ulcerative colitis. Am J Gastroenterol 1997;92(10):1867–1871.

65. Vecchi M, Meucci G, Gionchetti P, Beltrami M, Di Maurizio P, Beretta L et al. Oral versus combination mesalazine therapy in active ulcerative colitis: a double-blind, double-dummy, randomized multicentre study. Aliment Pharmacol Ther 2001;15:251–256.

66. Lennard-Jones JE. An assessment of prednisone, salazopyrine, and topical hydrocortisone hemisuccinate used as outpatient treatment for ulcerative colitis. Gut 1960;1:217–222.

67. Mulder CJ, van den Hazel SJ. Drug therapy: dose–response relationship of oral mesalazine in inflammatory bowel disease. Mediators Inflamm 1998;7:135–136.

68. Azad Khan AK, Howes DT, Piris J, Truelove SC. Optimum dose of sulphasalazine for maintenance treatment in ulcerative colitis. Gut 1980;21:232–240.

69. Marshall JK, Irvine EJ. Putting rectal 5-aminosalicylic acid in its place: the role in distal ulcerative colitis. Am J Gastroenterol 2000;95:1628–1636.

70. Miner P, Daly R, Nester T et al. The effect of varying dose intervals of mesalamine enemas for the prevention of relapse in distal ulcerative colitis. 10th World Congress of Gastroenterology 1994;1.

71. d'Albasio G, Tralloni G, Ghetti A et al. Intermittent therapy with high-dose 5-aminosalicylic acid enemas for maintaining remission in ulcerative proctosigmoiditis. Dis Colon Rectum 1990;33:394–397.

72. d'Albasio G, Pacini F, Camarri E et al. Combined therapy with 5-aminosalicylic acid tablets and enemas for maintaining remission in ulcerative colitis: a randomized double-blind study. Am J Gastroenterol 1997;92:1143–1147.

73. d'Albasio G, Paoluzi P, Campieri M et al. Maintenance treatment of ulcerative proctitis with mesalazine suppositories: a double-blind placebo-controlled trial. The Italian IBD Study Group. Am J Gastroenterol 1998;93:799–803.

74. Nikolaus S, Folscn U, Schreiber S. Immunopharmacology of 5-aminosalicylic acid and of glucocorticoids in the therapy of inflammatory bowel disease. Hepatogastroenterology 2000;47:71–82.

75. Angeli A, Masera RG, Sartori ML et al. Modulation by cytokines of glucocorticoid action. Ann NY Acad Sci 1999;876:210–220.

76. Refojo D, Liberman A, Holsboer F, Arzt E. Transcription factor-mediated molecular mechanisms involved in the functional cross-talk between cytokines and glucocorticoids. Immunol Cell Biol 2001;79:385–394.

77. Lennard-Jones JE. Toward optimal use of corticosteroids in ulcerative colitis and Crohn's disease. Gut 1983;24:177–181.

78. Baron JH. Outpatient treatment of ulcerative colitis. Br Med J 1962;2:441–444.

79. Powell-Tuck J, Bown RL, Lennard-Jones JE. A comparison of oral prednisolone given as single or multiple daily doses for active proctocolitis. Scand J Gastroenterol 1978;13:833–837.

80. Kjeldsen J. Treatment of ulcerative colitis with high doses of oral prednisolone. The rate of remission, the need for surgery, and the effect of prolonging the treatment. Scand J Gastroenterol 1993;28:821–826.

81. Faubion WA Jr, Loftus EV Jr, Harmsen WS, Zinsmeister AR, Sandborn WJ. The natural history of corticosteroid therapy for inflammatory bowel disease: a population-based study. Gastroenterology 2001;121:255–260.

82. Lennard-Jones JE, Misiewicz JJ, Connell AM, Baron JH, Jones FA. Prednisone as maintenance treatment for ulcerative colitis in remission. 1965;i:188–189.

83. Powell-Tuck J, Bown RL, Chambers TJ, Lennard-Jones JE. A controlled trial of alternate day prednisolone as a maintenance treatment for ulcerative colitis in remission. Digestion 1981;22:263–270.

84. Jarnerot G, Rolny P, Sandberg-Gertzen H. Intensive intravenous treatment of ulcerative colitis. Gastroenterology 1985;89:1005–1013.

85. Truelove SC, Willoughby CP, Lee EG, Kettlewell MG. Further experience in the treatment of severe attacks of ulcerative colitis. Lancet 1978;2:1086–1088.

86. Kornbluth A, Marion JF, Salomon P, Janowitz HD. How effective is current medical therapy for severe ulcerative and Crohn's colitis? An analytic review of selected trials. J Clin Gastroenterol 1995;20:280–284.

87. Kaplan HP, Portnoy B, Binder HJ, Amatruda T, Spiro H. A controlled evaluation of intravenous adrenocorticotropic hormone and hydrocortisone in the treatment of acute colitis. Gastroenterology 1975;69:91–95.

88. Powell-Tuck J, Buckell NA, Lennard-Jones JE. A controlled comparison of corticotropin and hydrocortisone in the treatment of severe proctocolitis. Scand J Gastroenterol 1977;12:971–975.

89. Meyers S, Sachar DB, Goldberg JD, Janowitz HD. Corticotropin versus hydrocortisone in the intravenous treatment of ulcerative colitis. A prospective, randomized, double-blind clinical trial. Gastroenterology 1983;85:351–357.

90. D'Haens G, Lemmens L, Geboes K et al. Intravenous cyclosporin versus intravenous corticosteroids as single therapy for severe attacks of ulcerative colitis. Gastroenterology 2001;120:1323–1329.

91. Rosenberg W, Ireland A, Jewell DP. High-dose methylprednisolone in the treatment of active ulcerative colitis. J Clin Gastroenterol 1990;12:40–41.

92. Sood A, Midha V, Sood N, Awasthi G. A prospective, open-label trial assessing dexamethasone pulse therapy in moderate to severe ulcerative colitis. J Clin Gastroenterol 2002;35:328–331.

93. Daperno M, Sostegni R, Rocca R et al. Review article: medical treatment of severe ulcerative colitis. Aliment Pharmacol Ther 2002;16:7–12.

94. Hamedani R, Feldman RD, Feagan BG. Review article: Drug development in inflammatory bowel disease: budesonide – a model of targeted therapy. Aliment Pharmacol Ther 1997;11:98–107; discussion 107–108.

95. Richter F, Scheppach W. Innovations in topical therapy. Baillières Clin Gastroenterol 1997;11:97–109.

96. Campieri M, Cottone M, Miglio F et al. Beclomethasone dipropionate enemas versus prednisolone sodium phosphate enemas in the treatment of distal ulcerative colitis. Aliment Pharmacol Ther 1998;12:361–366.

97. Nos P, Hinojosa J, Gomollon F, Ponce J. [Budesonide in inflammatory bowel disease: a meta-analysis]. Med Clin (Barc) 2001;116:47–53.

98. Hamilton I, Pinder IF, Dickinson RJ, Ruddell WS, Dixon MF, Axon AT. A comparison of prednisolone enemas with low-dose oral prednisolone in the treatment of acute distal ulcerative colitis. Dis Colon Rectum 1984;27:701–702.

99. Lofberg R, Ostergaard Thomsen O et al. Budesonide versus prednisolone retention enemas in active distal ulcerative colitis [published erratum appears in Aliment Pharmacol Ther 1995;9:213]. Aliment Pharmacol Ther 1994;8:623–629.

100. Lee DA, Taylor M, James VH, Walker G. Rectally administered prednisolone – evidence for a predominantly local action. Gut 1980;21:215–218.

101. McIntyre PB, Macrae FA, Berghouse L, English J, Lennard-Jones JE. Therapeutic benefits from a poorly absorbed prednisolone enema in distal colitis. Gut 1985;26:822–824.

102. Lindgren S, Lofberg R, Bergholm L et al. Effect of budesonide enema on remission and relapse rate in distal ulcerative colitis and proctitis. Scand J Gastroenterol 2002;37:705–710.

103. Mulder CJ, Tytgat GN. Review article: topical corticosteroids in inflammatory bowel disease. Aliment Pharmacol Ther 1993;7:125–130.

104. Ruddell WSJ, Dickinson RJ, Dixon MF, Axon ATR. Treatment of distal ulcerative colitis (proctosigmoiditis) in relapse: comparison of hydrocortisone enemas and rectal hydrocortisone foam. Gut 1980;21:885–889.

105. Thiesen A, Thomson AB. Review article: older systemic and newer topical glucocorticosteroids and the gastrointestinal tract. Aliment Pharmacol Ther 1996;10:487–496.

106. Lofberg R, Danielsson A, Suhr O et al. Oral budesonide versus prednisolone in patients with active extensive and left-sided ulcerative colitis [see comments]. Gastroenterology 1996;110:1713–1718.

107. Keller R, Stoll R, Foerster E, Gutsche N, Domschke W. Oral budesonide therapy for steroid-dependent ulcerative colitis: a pilot trial. Aliment Pharmacol Ther 1997;11:1047–1052.

108. Rizzello F, Gionchetti P, D'Arienzo A et al. Oral beclometasone dipropionate in the treatment of active ulcerative colitis: a double-blind placebo-controlled study. Aliment Pharmacol Ther 2002;16:1109–1116.

109. Kornbluth AA, Salomon P, Sacks HS, Mitty R, Janowitz HD. Meta-analysis of the effectiveness of current drug therapy of ulcerative colitis. J Clin Gastroenterol 1993;16:215–218.

110. Blomberg B, Jarnerot G. Clinical evaluation and management of acute severe colitis. Inflamm Bowel Dis 2000;6:214–227.

111. Valentine JF, Sninsky CA. Prevention and treatment of osteoporosis in patients with inflammatory bowel disease. Am J Gastroenterol 1999;94:878–883.

112. Lichtenstein GR. Management of bone loss in inflammatory bowel disease. Semin Gastrointest Dis 2001;12:275–283.

113. Lindgren SC, Flood LM, Kilander AF, Lofberg R, Persson TB, Sjodahl RI. Early predictors of glucocorticosteroid treatment failure in severe and moderately severe attacks of ulcerative colitis. Eur J Gastroenterol Hepatol 1998;10:831–835.

114. Gelbmann CM. Prediction of treatment refractoriness in ulcerative colitis and Crohn's disease – do we have reliable markers? Inflamm Bowel Dis 2000;6:123–131.

115. Lichtiger S, Present DH, Kornbluth A et al. Cyclosporin in severe ulcerative colitis refractory to steroid therapy [see comments]. N Engl J Med 1994;330:1841–1845.

116. Franchimont D, Belaiche J, Geenen V. [Corticosteroid sensitivity, dependence and resistance in inflammatory and immunologic diseases. Physiopathologic review]. Rev Med Liege 1998;53:33–37.

117. Hearing SD, Norman M, Probert CS, Haslam N, Dayan CM. Predicting therapeutic outcome in severe ulcerative colitis by measuring in vitro steroid sensitivity of proliferating peripheral blood lymphocytes. Gut 1999;45:382–388.

118. Schottelius A, Wedel S, Weltrich R et al. Higher expression of glucocorticoid receptor in peripheral mononuclear cells in inflammatory bowel disease. Am J Gastroenterol 2000;95:1994–1999.

119. Honda M, Orii F, Ayabe T et al. Expression of glucocorticoid receptor β in lymphocytes of patients with glucocorticoid-resistant ulcerative colitis. Gastroenterology 2000;118:859–866.

120. Bantel H, Domschke W, Schulze-Osthoff K. Molecular mechanisms of glucocorticoid resistance. Gastroenterology 2000;119:1178–1179.

121. Bantel H, Schmitz ML, Raible A, Gregor M, Schulze-Osthoff K. Critical role of NFκB and stress-activated protein kinases in steroid unresponsiveness. FASEB J 2002;16:1832–1834.

122. Raddatz D, Toth S, Schworer H, Ramadori G. Glucocorticoid receptor signaling in the intestinal epithelial cell lines IEC-6 and Caco-2: evidence of inhibition by interleukin-1β. Int J Colorectal Dis 2001;16:377–383.

123. Lamberts SW, Bruining HA, de Jong FH. Corticosteroid therapy in severe illness. N Engl J Med 1997;337:1285–1292.

124. Monteleone I, Vavassori P, Biancone L, Monteleone G, Pallone F. Immunoregulation in the gut: success and failures in human disease. Gut 2002;50:11160–11164.

125. Fraser AG, Orchard TR, Jewell DP. The efficacy of azathioprine for the treatment of inflammatory bowel disease: a 30 year review. Gut 2002;50:485–489.

126. Su CG, Stein RB, Lewis JD, Lichtenstein GR. Azathioprine or 6-mercaptopurine for inflammatory bowel disease: do risks outweigh benefits? Dig Liver Dis 2000;32:518–531.

127. Jewell DP, Truelove SC. Azathioprine in ulcerative colitis: final report on controlled therapeutic trial. Br Med J 1974;4:627–630.

128. Rosenberg JL, Wall AJ, Levin B, Binder HJ, Kirsner JB. A controlled trial of azathioprine in the management of chronic ulcerative colitis. Gastroenterology 1975;69:96–99.

129. Kirk AP, Lennard-Jones JE. Controlled trial of azathioprine in chronic ulcerative colitis. Br Med J 1982;284:1291–1292.

130. Hawthorne AB, Logan RF, Hawkey CJ et al. Randomised controlled trial of azathioprine withdrawal in ulcerative colitis. Br Med J 1992;305:20–22.

131. Sood A, Midha V, Sood N, Kaushal V. Role of azathioprine in severe ulcerative colitis: one-year, placebo-controlled, randomized trial. Indian J Gastroenterol 2000;19:14–16.

132. Sood A, Kaushal V, Midha V, Bhatia KL, Sood N, Malhotra V. The beneficial effect of azathioprine on maintenance of remission in severe ulcerative colitis. J Gastroenterol 2002;37:270–274.

133. Campbell S, Ghosh S. Effective maintenance of inflammatory bowel disease remission by azathioprine does not require concurrent 5-aminosalicylate therapy. Eur J Gastroenterol Hepatol 2001;13:1297–1301.

134. George J, Present DH, Pou R, Bodian C, Rubin PH. The long-term outcome of ulcerative colitis treated with 6-mercaptopurine. Am J Gastroenterol 1996;91:1711–1714.

135. Adler DJ, Korelitz BI. The therapeutic efficacy of 6-mercaptopurine in refractory ulcerative colitis. Am J Gastroenterol 1990;85:717–722.

136. Cohen RD, Stein R, Hanauer SB. Intravenous cyclosporin in ulcerative colitis: a five-year experience. Am J Gastroenterol 1999;94:1587–1592.

137. Actis GC, Bresso F, Astegiano M et al. Safety and efficacy of azathioprine in the maintenance of ciclosporin-induced remission of ulcerative colitis. Aliment Pharmacol Ther 2001;15:1307–1311.

138. Fernandez-Banares F, Bertran X, Esteve-Comas M et al. Azathioprine is useful in maintaining long-term remission induced by intravenous cyclosporin in steroid-refractory severe ulcerative colitis. Am J Gastroenterol 1996;91:2498–2499.

139. Mahadevan U, Tremaine WJ, Johnson T et al. Intravenous azathioprine in severe ulcerative colitis: a pilot study. Am J Gastroenterol 2000;95:3463–3468.

140. Shanahan F, Bernstein CN. Safety of low-dose purine analogues in inflammatory bowel disease. Gastroenterology 1994;107:1905–1906.

141. Sandborn WJ. Azathioprine: state of the art in inflammatory bowel disease. Scand J Gastroenterol 1998;225:92–99.

142. Martinez F, Nos P, Pastor M, Garrigues V, Ponce J. Adverse effects of azathioprine in the treatment of inflammatory bowel disease. Rev Esp Enferm Dig 2001;93:769–778.

143. Connell WR, Kamm MA, Dickson M, Balkwill AM, Ritchie JK, Lennard-Jones JE. Long-term neoplasia risk after azathioprine treatment in inflammatory bowel disease. Lancet 1994;343:1249–1252.

144. Farrell RJ, Ang Y, Kileen P et al. Increased incidence of non-Hodgkin's lymphoma in inflammatory bowel disease patients on immunosuppressive therapy but overall risk is low. Gut 2000;47:514–519.

145. Dayharsh GA, Loftus EV Jr, Sandborn WJ et al. Epstein–Barr virus-positive lymphoma in patients with inflammatory bowel disease treated with azathioprine or 6-mercaptopurine. Gastroenterology 2002;122:72–77.

146. Boulton-Jones JR, Pritchard K, Mahmoud AA. The use of 6-mercaptopurine in patients with inflammatory bowel disease after failure of azathioprine therapy. Aliment Pharmacol Ther 2000;14:1561–1565.

147. Bowen DG, Selby WS. Use of 6-mercaptopurine in patients with inflammatory bowel disease previously intolerant of azathioprine. Dig Dis Sci 2000;45:1810–1813.

148. Dubinsky MC, Yang H, Hassard PV et al. 6-MP metabolite profiles provide a biochemical explanation for 6-MP resistance in patients with inflammatory bowel disease. Gastroenterology 2002;122:904–915.

149. Armstrong VW, Oellerich M. New developments in the immunosuppressive drug monitoring of cyclosporin, tacrolimus, and azathioprine. Clin Biochem 2001;34:9–16.

150. Baert F, Rutgeerts P. 6-Thioguanine: a naked bullet? (Or how pharmacogenomics can make old drugs brand new). Inflamm Bowel Dis 2001;7:190–191.

151. Polifka JE, Friedman JM. Teratogen update: azathioprine and 6-mercaptopurine. Teratology 2002;65:240–261.

152. Lichtiger S, Present DH. Preliminary report: cyclosporin in treatment of severe active ulcerative colitis [see comments]. Lancet 1990;336:16–19.

153. Atkinson KA, McDonald JW, Lamba B, Feagan BG. Intravenous cyclosporin for severe attacks of ulcerative colitis: a survey of Canadian gastroenterologists. Can J Gastroenterol 1997;11:583–587.

154. Hyde GM, Thillainayagam AV, Jewell DP. Intravenous cyclosporin as rescue therapy in severe ulcerative colitis: time for a reappraisal? Eur J Gastroenterol Hepatol 1998;10:411–413.

155. Sandborn WJ. Cyclosporin in ulcerative colitis: state of the art. Acta Gastroenterol Belg 2001;64:201–204.

156. Carbonnel F, Boruchowicz A, Duclos B et al. Intravenous cyclosporin in attacks of ulcerative colitis: short-term and long-term responses. Dig Dis Sci 1996;41:2471–2476.

157. Santos J, Baudet S, Casellas F, Guarner L, Vilaseca J, Malagelada JR. Efficacy of intravenous cyclosporin for steroid refractory attacks of ulcerative colitis. J Clin Gastroenterol 1995;20:285–289.

158. Treem WR, Cohen J, Davis PM, Justinich CJ, Hyams JS. Cyclosporin for the treatment of fulminant ulcerative colitis in children. Immediate response, long-term results, and impact on surgery. Dis Colon Rectum 1995;38:474–479.

159. Van Gossum A, Schmit A, Adler M et al. Short- and long-term efficacy of cyclosporin administration in patients with acute severe ulcerative colitis. Belgian IBD Group. Acta Gastroenterol Belg 1997;60:197–200.

160. Actis GC, Ottobrelli A, Pera A et al. Continuously infused cyclosporin at low dose is sufficient to avoid emergency colectomy in acute attacks of ulcerative colitis without the need for high-dose steroids. J Clin Gastroenterol 1993;17:10–13.

161. Stack WA, Long RG, Hawkey CJ. Short- and long-term outcome of patients treated with cyclosporin for severe acute ulcerative colitis. Aliment Pharmacol Ther 1998;12:973–978.

162. Wenzl HH, Petritsch W, Aichbichler BW, Hinterleitner TA, Fleischmann G, Krejs GJ. Short-term efficacy and long-term outcome of cyclosporin treatment in patients with severe ulcerative colitis. Zeitschr Gastroenterol 1998;36:287–293.

163. Rowe FA, Walker JH, Karp LC, Vasiliauskas EA, Plevy SE, Targan SR. Factors predictive of response to cyclosporin treatment for severe, steroid-resistant ulcerative colitis. Am J Gastroenterol 2000;95:2000–2008.

164. Lowry PW, Franklin CL, Weaver AL et al. Leucopenia resulting from a drug interaction between azathioprine or 6-mercaptopurine and mesalamine, sulphasalazine, or balsalazide. Gut 2001;49:656–664.

165. Kornbluth A, Present DH, Lichtiger S, Hanauer S. Cyclosporin for severe ulcerative colitis: a user's guide. Am J Gastroenterol 1997;92:1424–1428.

166. Sandborn WJ, Tremaine WJ, Schroeder KW, Steiner BL, Batts KP, Lawson GM. Cyclosporin enemas for treatment-resistant, mildly to moderately active, left-sided ulcerative colitis [see comments]. Am J Gastroenterol 1993;88:640–645.

167. Freeman D, Grant D, Levy G et al. Pharmacokinetics of a new oral formulation of cyclosporin in liver transplant recipients. Ther Drug Monit 1995;17:213–216.

168. Actis GC, Aimo G, Priolo G, Moscato D, Rizzetto M, Pagni R. Efficacy and efficiency of oral microemulsion cyclosporin versus intravenous and soft gelatin capsule cyclosporin in the treatment of severe steroid-refractory ulcerative colitis: an open-label retrospective trial. Inflamm Bowel Dis 1998;4:276–279.

169. Navazo L, Salata H, Morales S et al. Oral microemulsion cyclosporin in the treatment of steroid-refractory attacks of ulcerative and indeterminate colitis. Scand J Gastroenterol 2001;36:610–614.

170. Pinna-Pintor M, Arese P, Bona R et al. Severe steroid-unresponsive ulcerative colitis: outcomes of restorative proctocolectomy in patients undergoing cyclosporin treatment. Dis Colon Rectum 2000;43:609–613; discussion 613–614.

171. Fellermann K, Ludwig D, Stahl M, David-Walek T, Stange EF. Steroid-unresponsive acute attacks of inflammatory bowel disease: immunomodulation by tacrolimus (FK506). Am J Gastroenterol 1998;93:1860–1866.

172. Bousvaros A, Kirschner BS, Werlin SL et al. Oral tacrolimus treatment of severe colitis in children. J Pediatr 2000;137:794–799.

173. Feutren G, Mihatsch MJ. Risk factors for cyclosporin-induced nephropathy in patients with autoimmune diseases. International Kidney Biopsy Registry of Cyclosporin in Autoimmune Diseases [see comments]. N Engl J Med 1992;326:1654–1660.

174. Mahedevan U KA, Goldstein E, George J, Lichtiger S, Present DH. Is cyclosporin induced nephrotoxicity permanent or progressive in patients with inflammatory bowel disease? Gastroenterology 1997;112:A1030.

175. Stein R CR, Hanauer S. Complications during cyclosporin therapy for inflammatory bowel disease. Gastroenterology 1997;112:A1096.

176. Quan VA, Saunders BP, Hicks BH, Sladen GE. Cyclosporin treatment for ulcerative colitis complicated by fatal *Pneumocystis carinii* pneumonia. Br Med J 1997;314:363–364.

177. Bernstein CN, Kolodny M, Block E, Shanahan F. *Pneumocystis carinii* pneumonia in patients with ulcerative colitis treated with corticosteroids. Am J Gastroenterol 1993;88:574–577.

178. Fleshner PR, Michelassi F, Rubin M, Hanauer SB, Plevy SE, Targan SR. Morbidity of subtotal colectomy in patients with severe ulcerative colitis unresponsive to cyclosporin. Dis Colon Rectum 1995;38:1241–1245.

179. Hyde GM, Jewell DP, Kettlewell MG, Mortensen NJ. Cyclosporin for severe ulcerative colitis does not increase the rate of perioperative complications. Dis Colon Rectum 2001;44:1436–1440.

180. Cohen RD, Brodsky AL, Hanauer SB. A comparison of the quality of life in patients with severe ulcerative colitis after total colectomy versus medical treatment with intravenous cyclosporin. Inflamm Bowel Dis 1999;5:1–10.

181. Wu CY, Benet LZ, Hebert MF et al. Differentiation of absorption and first-pass gut and hepatic metabolism in humans: studies with cyclosporin. Clin Pharmacol Ther 1995;58:492–497.

182. Lake K, Canafax D. Important interactions of drugs with immunosuppressive agents used in transplant recipients. J Antimicrob Chemother 1995;36:11–22.

183. Yee GC, McGuire TR. Pharmacokinetic drug interactions with cyclosporin (Part I). Clin Pharmacokinet 1990;19:319–332.

184. Yee GC, Stanley DL, Pessa LJ et al. Effect of grapefruit juice on blood cyclosporin concentration [see comments]. Lancet 1995;345:955–956.

185. Kozarek RA, Patterson DJ, Gelfand MD, Botoman VA, Ball TJ, Wilske KR. Methotrexate induces clinical and histologic remission in patients with refractory inflammatory bowel disease [see comments]. Ann Intern Med 1989;110:353–356.

186. Baron TH, Truss CD, Elson CO. Low-dose oral methotrexate in refractory inflammatory bowel disease. Dig Dis Sci 1993;38:1851–1856.

187. Oren R, Arber N, Odes S et al. Methotrexate in chronic active ulcerative colitis: a double-blind, randomized, Israeli multicenter trial [see comments]. Gastroenterology 1996;110:1416–1421.

188. Kozarek RA. Methotrexate and ulcerative colitis: wrong drug? Wrong dose? Or wrong disease? [editorial; comment]. Gastroenterology 1996;110:1652–1656.

189. Egan LJ, Sandborn WJ. Methotrexate for inflammatory bowel disease: pharmacology and preliminary results [see comments]. Mayo Clin Proc 1996;71:69–80.

190. Fraser AG, Morton D, McGovern D, Travis S, Jewell DP. The efficacy of methotrexate for maintaining remission in inflammatory bowel disease. Aliment Pharmacol Ther 2002;16:693–697.

191. Mate-Jimenez J, Hermida C, Cantero-Perona J, Moreno-Otero R. 6-mercaptopurine or methotrexate added to prednisone induces and maintains remission in steroid-dependent inflammatory bowel disease. Eur J Gastroenterol Hepatol 2000;12:1227–1233.

192. Egan LJ, Sandborn WJ, Tremaine WJ et al. A randomized dose–response and pharmacokinetic study of methotrexate for refractory inflammatory Crohn's disease and ulcerative colitis. Aliment Pharmacol Ther 1999;13:1597–1604.

193. Vandell AG, DiPiro JT. Low-dosage methotrexate for treatment and maintenance of remission in patients with inflammatory bowel disease. Pharmacotherapy 2002;22:613–620.

194. Dickinson RJ, HJ OC, Pinder I, Hamilton I, Johnston D, Axon AT. Double blind controlled trial of oral vancomycin as adjunctive treatment in acute exacerbations of idiopathic colitis. Gut 1985;26:1380–1384.

195. Chapman RW, Selby WS, Jewell DP. Controlled trial of intravenous metronidazole as an adjunct to corticosteroids in severe ulcerative colitis. Gut 1986;27:1210–1212.

196. Mantzaris GJ, Petraki K, Archavlis E et al. A prospective randomized controlled trial of intravenous ciprofloxacin as an adjunct to corticosteroids in acute, severe ulcerative colitis. Scand J Gastroenterol 2001;36:971–974.

197. Lobo AJ, Burke DA, Sobala GM, Axon AT. Oral tobramycin in ulcerative colitis: effect on maintenance of remission. Aliment Pharmacol Ther 1993;7:155–158.

198. Mantzaris GJ, Archavlis E, Christoforidis P et al. A prospective randomized controlled trial of oral ciprofloxacin in acute ulcerative colitis. Am J Gastroenterol 1997;92:454–456.

199. Turunen UM, Farkkila MA, Hakala K et al. Long-term treatment of ulcerative colitis with ciprofloxacin: a prospective, double-blind, placebo-controlled study [see comments]. Gastroenterology 1998;115:1072–1078.

200. Madsen KL. The use of probiotics in gastrointestinal disease. Can J Gastroenterol 2001;15:817–822.

201. Kruis W, Schutz E, Fric P, Fixa B, Judmaier G, Stolte M. Double-blind comparison of an oral *Escherichia coli* preparation and mesalazine in maintaining remission of ulcerative colitis. Aliment Pharmacol Ther 1997;11:853–858.

202. Rembacken BJ, Snelling AM, Hawkey PM, Chalmers DM, Axon AT. Non-pathogenic *Escherichia coli* versus mesalazine for the treatment of ulcerative colitis: a randomised trial [see comments]. Lancet 1999;354:635–639.

203. Thomas GA, Rhodes J, Green JT. Inflammatory bowel disease and smoking – a review. Am J Gastroenterol 1998;93:144–149.

204. Sandborn WJ. Nicotine therapy for ulcerative colitis: a review of rationale, mechanisms, pharmacology, and clinical results. Am J Gastroenterol 1999;94:1161–1171.

205. Lashner BA, Hanauer SB, Silverstein MD. Testing nicotine gum for ulcerative colitis patients. Experience with single-patient trials. Dig Dis Sci 1990;35:827–832.

206. Pullan RD, Rhodes J, Ganesh S et al. Transdermal nicotine for active ulcerative colitis [see comments]. N Engl J Med 1994;330:811–815.

207. Guslandi M, Tittobello A. Pilot trial of nicotine patches as an alternative to corticosteroids in ulcerative colitis. J Gastroenterol 1996;31:627–629.

208. Sandborn WJ, Tremaine WJ, Offord KP et al. Transdermal nicotine for mildly to moderately active ulcerative colitis. A randomized, double-blind, placebo-controlled trial [see comments]. Ann Intern Med 1997;126:364–371.

209. Guslandi M, Frego R, Viale E, Testoni PA. Distal ulcerative colitis refractory to rectal mesalamine: role of transdermal nicotine versus oral mesalamine. Can J Gastroenterol 2002;16:293–296.

210. Guslandi M. Long-term effects of a single course of nicotine treatment in acute ulcerative colitis: remission maintenance in a 12-month follow-up study. Int J Colorectal Dis 1999;14:261–262.

211. Thomas GA, Rhodes J, Mani V et al. Transdermal nicotine as maintenance therapy for ulcerative colitis. N Engl J Med 1995;332:988–992.

212. Bonapace CR, Mays DA. The effect of mesalamine and nicotine in the treatment of inflammatory bowel disease. Ann Pharmacother 1997;31:907–913.

213. Thomas GA, Rhodes J, Ragunath K et al. Transdermal nicotine compared with oral prednisolone therapy for active ulcerative colitis. Eur J Gastroenterol Hepatol 1996;8:769–774.

214. Green JT, Thomas GA, Rhodes J et al. Nicotine enemas for active ulcerative colitis – a pilot study. Aliment Pharmacol Ther 1997;11:859–863.

215. Green JT, Thomas GA, Rhodes J et al. Pharmacokinetics of nicotine carbomer enemas: a new treatment modality for ulcerative colitis. Clin Pharmacol Ther 1997;61:340–348.

216. Green JT, Rhodes J, Thomas GA et al. Nicotine carbomer enemas--pharmacokinetics of a revised formulation. Ital J Gastroenterol Hepatol 1998;30:260–265.

217. Sandborn WJ, Tremaine WJ, Leighton JA et al. Nicotine tartrate liquid enemas for mildly to moderately active left-sided ulcerative colitis unresponsive to first-line therapy: a pilot study. Aliment Pharmacol Ther 1997;11:663–671.

218. Zins BJ, Sandborn WJ, Mays DC et al. Pharmacokinetics of nicotine tartrate after single-dose liquid enema, oral, and intravenous administration. J Clin Pharmacol 1997;37:426–436.

219. Green JT, Evans BK, Rhodes J et al. An oral formulation of nicotine for release and absorption in the colon: its development and pharmacokinetics. Br J Clin Pharmacol 1999;48:485–493.

220. Tremaine WJ, Sandborn WJ, Loftus EV et al. A prospective cohort study of practice guidelines in inflammatory bowel disease. Am J Gastroenterol 2001;96:2401–2406.

221. Kennedy LD. Nicotine therapy for ulcerative colitis. Ann Pharmacother 1996;30:1022–1023.

222. Edwards CM, George B, Warren B. Diversion colitis – new light through old windows. Histopathology 1999;34:1–5.

223. Kim YI. Short-chain fatty acids in ulcerative colitis. Nutr Rev 1998;56:17–24.

224. Chapman MA. The role of the colonic flora in maintaining a healthy large bowel mucosa. Ann Roy Coll Surg Engl 2001;83:75–80.

225. Vernia P, Marcheggiano A, Caprilli R et al. Short-chain fatty acid topical treatment in distal ulcerative colitis. Aliment Pharmacol Ther 1995;9:309–313.

226. Scheppach W. Treatment of distal ulcerative colitis with short-chain fatty acid enemas. A placebo-controlled trial. German–Austrian SCFA Study Group. Dig Dis Sci 1996;41:2254–2259.

227. Patz J, Jacobsohn WZ, Gottschalk-Sabag S, Zeides S, Braverman DZ. Treatment of refractory distal ulcerative colitis with short chain fatty acid enemas. Am J Gastroenterol 1996;91:731–734.

228. Breuer RI, Soergel KH, Lashner BA et al. Short chain fatty acid rectal irrigation for left-sided ulcerative colitis: a randomised, placebo controlled trial. Gut 1997;40:485–491.

229. Scheppach W, Sommer H, Kirchner T et al. Effect of butyrate enemas on the colonic mucosa in distal ulcerative colitis [see comments]. Gastroenterology 1992;103:51–56.

230. Vernia P, Cittadini M, Caprilli R, Torsoli A. Topical treatment of refractory distal ulcerative colitis with 5-ASA and sodium butyrate. Dig Dis Sci 1995;40:305–307.

231. Vernia P, Monteleone G, Grandinetti G et al. Combined oral sodium butyrate and mesalazine treatment compared to oral mesalazine alone in ulcerative colitis: randomized, double-blind, placebo-controlled pilot study. Dig Dis Sci 2000;45:976–981.

232. Sandborn WJ. Are short-chain fatty acid enemas effective for left-sided ulcerative colitis? Gastroenterology 1998;114:218–219.

233. Liu Q, Shimoyama T, Suzuki K, Umeda T, Nakaji S, Sugawara K. Effect of sodium butyrate on reactive oxygen species generation by human neutrophils. Scand J Gastroenterol 2001;36:744–750.

234. Luhrs H, Gerke T, Muller JG et al. Butyrate inhibits NFκB activation in lamina propria macrophages of patients with ulcerative colitis. Scand J Gastroenterol 2002;37:458–466.

235. Hawkey CJ, Mahida YR, Hawthorne AB. Therapeutic interventions in gastrointestinal disease based on an understanding of inflammatory mediators. Agents Actions 1992;Spec:C22–26.

236. Fiocchi C. Inflammatory bowel disease: etiology and pathogenesis. Gastroenterology 1998;115:182–205.

237. Lorenz R, Weber PC, Szimnau P, Heldwein W, Strasser T, Loeschke K. Supplementation with n-3 fatty acids from fish oil in chronic inflammatory bowel disease – a randomized, placebo-controlled, double- blind cross-over trial. J Intern Med Suppl 1989;225:225–232.

238. Aslan A, Triadafilopoulos G. Fish oil fatty acid supplementation in active ulcerative colitis: a double-blind, placebo-controlled, crossover study. Am J Gastroenterol 1992;87:432–437.

239. Greenfield SM, Green AT, Teare JP et al. A randomized controlled study of evening primrose oil and fish oil in ulcerative colitis. Aliment Pharmacol Ther 1993;7:159–166.

240. Hawthorne AB, Daneshmend TK, Hawkey CJ et al. Treatment of ulcerative colitis with fish oil supplementation: a prospective 12 month randomised controlled trial. Gut 1992;33:922–928.

241. Salomon P, Kornbluth AA, Janowitz HD. Treatment of ulcerative colitis with fish oil n-3-omega-fatty acid: an open trial. J Clin Gastroenterol 1990;12:157–161.

242. Dichi I, Frenhane P, Dichi JB et al. Comparison of omega-3 fatty acids and sulfasalazine in ulcerative colitis. Nutrition 2000;16:87–90.

243. Loeschke K, Ueberschaer B, Pietsch A et al. n-3 fatty acids only delay early relapse of ulcerative colitis in remission. Dig Dis Sci 1996;41:2087–2094.

244. Middleton SJ, Naylor S, Woolner J, Hunter JO. A double-blind, randomized, placebo-controlled trial of essential fatty acid supplementation in the maintenance of remission of ulcerative colitis. Aliment Pharmacol Ther 2002;16:1131–1135.

245. Hawkey CJ, Dube LM, Rountree LV, Linnen PJ, Lancaster JF. A trial of zileuton versus mesalazine or placebo in the maintenance of remission of ulcerative colitis. The European Zileuton Study Group For Ulcerative Colitis. Gastroenterology 1997;112:718–724.

246. Roberts WG, Simon TJ, Berlin RG et al. Leukotrienes in ulcerative colitis: results of a multicenter trial of a leukotriene biosynthesis inhibitor, MK-591. Gastroenterology 1997;112:725–732.

247. Tytgat GN, Van Nueten L, Van De Velde I, Joslyn A, Hanauer SB. Efficacy and safety of oral ridogrel in the treatment of ulcerative colitis: two multicentre, randomized, double-blind studies. Aliment Pharmacol Ther 2002;16:87–99.

248. Korzenik J. IBD: a vascular disorder? The case for heparin therapy. Inflamm Bowel Dis 1997;3:87–94.

249. Michell NP, Lalor P, Langman MJ. Heparin therapy for ulcerative colitis? Effects and mechanisms. Eur J Gastroenterol Hepatol 2001;13:449–456.

250. Gaffney PR, Doyle CT, Gaffney A, Hogan J, Hayes DP, Annis P. Paradoxical response to heparin in 10 patients with ulcerative colitis. Am J Gastroenterol 1995;90:220–223.

251. Folwaczny C, Wiebecke B, Loeschke K. Unfractioned heparin in the therapy of patients with highly active inflammatory bowel disease. Am J Gastroenterol 1999;94:1551–1555.

252. Dwarakanath AD, Yu LG, Brookes C, Pryce D, Rhodes JM. 'Sticky' neutrophils, pathergic arthritis, and response to heparin in pyoderma gangrenosum complicating ulcerative colitis. Gut 1995;37:585–588.

253. Panes J, Esteve M, Cabre E et al. Comparison of heparin and steroids in the treatment of moderate and severe ulcerative colitis. Gastroenterology 2000;119:903–908.

254. Ang YS, Mahmud N, White B et al. Randomized comparison of unfractionated heparin with corticosteroids in severe active inflammatory bowel disease. Aliment Pharmacol Ther 2000;14:1015–1022.

255. Dotan I, Hallak A, Arber N et al. Low-dose low-molecular weight heparin (enoxaparin) is effective as adjuvant treatment in active ulcerative colitis: an open trial. Dig Dis Sci 2001;46:2239–2244.

256. Vrij AA, Jansen JM, Schoon EJ, de Bruine A, Hemker HC, Stockbrugger RW. Low molecular weight heparin treatment in steroid refractory ulcerative colitis: clinical outcome and influence on mucosal capillary thrombi. Scand J Gastroenterol Suppl 2001:41–47.

257. Pineo GF, Hull RD. Unfractionated and low-molecular-weight heparin. Comparisons and current recommendations. Med Clin North Am 1998;82:587–599.

258. Sandborn WJ, Targan SR. Biologic therapy of inflammatory bowel disease. Gastroenterology 2002;122:1592–1608.

259. Sands BE. Biological therapies for ulcerative colitis. Acta Gastroenterol Belg 2001;64:205–209.

260. Blam ME, Stein RB, Lichtenstein GR. Integrating anti-tumor necrosis factor therapy in inflammatory bowel disease: current and future perspectives. Am J Gastroenterol 2001;96:1977–1997.

261. Chey WY. Infliximab for patients with refractory ulcerative colitis. Inflamm Bowel Dis 2001;7:S30–33.

262. Chey WY, Hussain A, Ryan C, Potter GD, Shah A. Infliximab for refractory ulcerative colitis. Am J Gastroenterol 2001;96:2373–2381.

263. Kaser A, Mairinger T, Vogel W, Tilg H. Infliximab in severe steroid-refractory ulcerative colitis: a pilot study. Wien Klin Wochenschr 2001;113:930–933.

264. Su C, Salzberg BA, Lewis JD et al. Efficacy of anti-tumor necrosis factor therapy in patients with ulcerative colitis. Am J Gastroenterol 2002;97:2577–2584.

265. Serrano MS, Schmidt-Sommerfeld E, Kilbaugh TJ, Brown RF, Udall JN Jr, Mannick EE. Use of infliximab in pediatric patients with inflammatory bowel disease. Ann Pharmacother 2001;35:823–828.

266. Mamula P, Markowitz JE, Brown KA, Hurd LB, Piccoli DA, Baldassano RN. Infliximab as a novel therapy for pediatric ulcerative colitis. J Peciatr Gastroenterol Nutr 2002;34:307–311.

267. Evans RC, Clarke L, Heath P, Stephens S, Morris AI, Rhodes JM. Treatment of ulcerative colitis with an engineered human anti-TNF-α antibody CDP571. Aliment Pharmacol Ther 1997;11:1031–1035.

268. Present DH. Infliximab therapy for ulcerative colitis: many unanswered questions. Am J Gastroenterol 2001;96:2294–2296.

269. Rutgeerts P. Infliximab for ulcerative colitis: the need for adequately powered placebo-controlled trials. Am J Gastroenterol 2002;97:2488–2489.

270. Probert CS, Hearing SD, Schreiber S, Kuhbacher T, Ghosh S, Forbes A. Infliximab in steroid-resistant ulcerative colitis: A randomised controlled trial. Gastroenterology 2002;122:A722.

271. Sandborn WJ, Hanauer SB. Infliximab in the treatment of Crohn's disease: a user's guide for clinicians. Am J Gastroenterol 2002;97:2962–2972.

272. Gordon FH, Hamilton MI, Donoghue S et al. A pilot study of treatment of active ulcerative colitis with natalizumab, a humanized monoclonal antibody to α₄ integrin. Aliment Pharmacol Ther 2002;16:699–705.

273. Feagan BG, McDonald J, Greenberg G et al. An ascending dose trial of a humanized α₄β₇ antibody in ulcerative colitis. Gastroenterology 2000;118:A4851.

274. van Deventer SJ. Small therapeutic molecules for the treatment of inflammatory bowel disease. Gut 2002;50:11147–11153.

275. Hilsden RJ, Meddings JB, Verhoef MJ. Complementary and alternative medicine use by patients with inflammatory bowel disease: An Internet survey. Can J Gastroenterol 1999;13:327–332.

276. Langholz E, Munkholm P, Davidsen M, Nielsen OH, Binder V. Changes in extent of ulcerative colitis: a study on the course and prognostic factors. Scand J Gastroenterol 1996;31:260–266.

277. Mulder CJJ, Fockens P, van der Heide H, Tytgat GNJ. A controlled randomized trial of beclomethasone dipropionate (3 mg) versus 5-aminosalicylic acid (1 g) versus the combination of both as retention enemas in active distal ulcerative colitis. Gastroenterology 1994;106:A739.

278. Meucci G, Vecchi M, Astegiano M et al. The natural history of ulcerative proctitis: a multicenter. retrospective study. Gruppo di Studio per le Malattie Infiammatorie Intestinali (GSMII). Am J Gastroenterol 2000;95:469–473.

279. Marteau P, Crand J, Foucault M, Rambaud JC. Use of mesalazine slow release suppositories 1 g three times per week to maintain remission of ulcerative proctitis: a randomised double blind placebo controlled multicentre study. Gut 1998;42:195–199.

280. Robinson A, Thompson DG, Wilkin D, Roberts C. Guided self-management and patient-directed follow-up of ulcerative colitis: a randomised trial. Lancet 2001;358:976–981.

281. Ardizzone S, Porro GB. A practical guide to the management of distal ulcerative colitis. Drugs 1998;55:519–542.

282. Gionchetti P, Rizzello F, Venturi A et al. Comparison of mesalazine suppositories in proctitis and distal proctosigmoiditis. Aliment Pharmacol Ther 1997;11:1053–1057.

283. Campieri M, Corbelli C, Gionchetti P et al. Spread and distribution of 5-ASA colonic foam and 5-ASA enema in patients with ulcerative colitis. Dig Dis Sci 1992;37:1890–1897.

284. Gionchetti P, Venturi A, Rizzello F et al. Retrograde colonic spread of a new mesalazine rectal enema in patients with distal ulcerative colitis. Aliment Pharmacol Ther 1997;11:679–684.

285. Andreoli A, Spinella S, Levenstein S, Prantera C. 5-ASA enema versus oral sulphasalazine in maintaining remission in ulcerative colitis. Ital J Gastroenterol 1994;26:121–125.

286. Green JR, Gibson JA, Kerr GD et al. Maintenance of remission of ulcerative colitis: a comparison between balsalazide 3 g daily and mesalazine 1.2 g daily over 12 months. ABACUS Investigator group. Aliment Pharmacol Ther 1998;12:1207–1216.

287. Farmer RG, Easley KA, Rankin GB. Clinical patterns, natural history, and progression of ulcerative colitis. A long-term follow-up of 1116 patients. Dig Dis Sci 1993;38:1137–1146.

288. Langholz E, Munkholm P, Davidsen M, Binder V. Course of ulcerative colitis: analysis of changes in disease activity over years [see comments]. Gastroenterology 1994;107:3–11.

289. Marion JF, Present DH. The modern medical management of acute, severe ulcerative colitis. Eur J Gastroenterol Hepatol 1997;9:831–835.

290. Carbonnel F, Gargouri D, Lemann M et al. Predictive factors of outcome of intensive intravenous treatment for attacks of ulcerative colitis. Aliment Pharmacol Ther 2000;14:273–279.

291. Campbell S, Ghosh S. Is neutropenia required for effective maintenance of remission during azathioprine therapy in inflammatory bowel disease? Eur J Gastroenterol Hepatol 2001;13:1073–1076.

292. Connell WR, Kamm MA, Ritchie JK, Lennard-Jones JE. Bone marrow toxicity caused by azathioprine in inflammatory bowel disease: 27 years of experience. Gut 1993;34:1081–1085.

293. Colombel JF, Ferrari N, Debuysere H et al. Genotypic analysis of thiopurine S-methyltransferase in patients with Crohn's disease and severe myelosuppression during azathioprine therapy. Gastroenterology 2000;118:1025–1030.

294. Record C. Case records of the Massachusetts General Hospital. Weekly clinicopathological exercises. Case 36-1997. A 58-year-old man with recurrent ulcerative colitis, bloody diarrhea, and abdominal distention [clinical conference]. N Engl J Med 1997;337:1532–1540.

295. Latella G, Vernia P, Viscido A et al. GI distension in severe ulcerative colitis. Am J Gastroenterol 2002;97:1169–1175.

296. Caprilli R, Vernia P, Latella G, Torsoli A. Early recognition of toxic megacolon. J Clin Gastroenterol 1987;9:160–164.

297. Sheth SG, LaMont JT. Toxic megacolon. Lancet 1998;351:509–513.

298. Panos MZ, Wood MJ, Asquith P. Toxic megacolon: the knee–elbow position relieves bowel distension [see comments]. Gut 1993;34:1726–1727.

299. Berg DF, Bahadursingh AM, Kaminski DL, Longo WE. Acute surgical emergencies in inflammatory bowel disease. Am J Surg 2002;184:45–51.

300. Cottone M, Pietrosi G, Martorana G et al. Prevalence of cytomegalovirus infection in severe refractory ulcerative and Crohn's colitis. Am J Gastroenterol 2001;96:773–775.

301. Swan NC, Geoghegan JG, O'Donoghue DP, Hyland JM, Sheahan K. Fulminant colitis in inflammatory bowel disease: detailed pathologic and clinical analysis. Dis Colon Rectum 1998;41:1511–1515.

302. Biddle WL, Miner PB Jr. Long-term use of mesalamine enemas to induce remission in ulcerative colitis. Gastroenterology 1990;99:113–118.

303. Green JT, Rhodes J, Ragunath K et al. Clinical status of ulcerative colitis in patients who smoke. Am J Gastroenterol 1998;93:1463–1467.

304. Eaden J, Abrams K, Ekbom A, Jackson E, Mayberry J. Colorectal cancer prevention in ulcerative colitis: a case–control study. Aliment Pharmacol Ther 2000;14:145–153.

305. Lashner BA, Provencher KS, Seidner DL, Knesebeck A, Brzezinski A. The effect of folic acid supplementation on the risk for cancer or dysplasia in ulcerative colitis. Gastroenterology 1997;112:29–32.

## CHAPTER 34

# Medical therapy for Crohn's disease

William J Sandborn

## INTRODUCTION

The optimal medical treatment of patients with Crohn's disease requires that the treating physician obtain a history and perform any necessary diagnostic procedures, and then prescribe an appropriate medication regimen based on a knowledge of clinical pharmacology and the evidence from controlled clinical trials. This chapter reviews the results from clinical trials that assessed the efficacy of medications used to treat Crohn's disease and then provides an integrated therapeutic approach to the medical treatment of specific clinical settings for patients with Crohn's disease.

## PRETREATMENT EVALUATION OF THE PATIENT

Prior to initiating or altering a medical treatment regimen for Crohn's disease, the physician should evaluate the patient.[1] This evaluation begins with a medical history to determine the age of onset, the duration of disease, the anatomic location of disease, the disease course over time, prior and current medication use (including duration and dose), previous responses to each intervention, prior surgical resections, and the symptoms currently being experienced by the patient. At the time of diagnosis, patients should undergo colonoscopy with mucosal biopsy and small bowel X-ray to provide a baseline characterization of the disease and to exclude ulcerative colitis. Infectious and medication-associated causes of colitis should be excluded. In cases where there is an established diagnosis of Crohn's disease it is useful to repeat these tests when patients relapse and fail to respond to empiric therapy with sulfasalazine, 5-aminosalicylates or corticosteroids, prior to instituting immune modifier or biologic therapy or referring the patient for surgery. Adherence to this methodical approach allows the treating physician to make observations that would lead to a change in therapy, such as a change in the anatomic location of the disease; endoscopic findings of severe enteritis or colitis; endoscopic or radiographic findings of complications, such as stricturing with mechanical obstruction, fistulization and the presence of an abscess; infectious enteritis or colitis; medication-associated enteritis or colitis; and patients with Crohn's disease in endoscopic and radiographic remission who may be experiencing symptoms of concomitant irritable bowel syndrome.

The frequency of involvement in different segments of the gastrointestinal tract in patients with Crohn's disease is shown in Figure 34.1.[2] Patients are typically classified according to their anatomic location of involvement as having one of the following clinical patterns: ileocolic; small intestine; colon; anorectal.[3] Determining the anatomic location of involvement is important because 5-aminosalicylate-based medications and some corticosteroid (budesonide) preparations are delivered topically, and do not distribute uniformly throughout the small intestine and colon at a high concentration. The expected sites of drug delivery for various topically delivered 5-aminosalicylate and corticosteroid (budesonide) formulations are shown in Table 34.1.

In clinical practice, the American College of Gastroenterology working definitions of Crohn's disease activity may be used to classify disease activity and specifically to identify patients with severe disease activity (Table 34.2).[4] This assessment of disease severity is important in determining whether or not to hospitalize the patient and whether intravenous steroid therapy is necessary. The Crohn's disease activity index (CDAI) is a research tool that is more useful for distinguishing patients with remission, mildly active disease and moderately active disease for the purposes of assessing the efficacy of medical therapy (Table 34.3).[5,6] For patients whose symptoms are primarily those of perianal fistulae, the fistulae can be classified anatomically as high (involving the anal sphincter) or low (superficial to the anal sphincter), or functionally as being 'open' or 'closed'.[6,7]

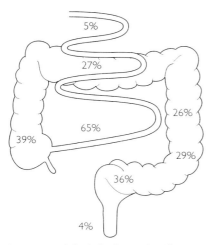

**Fig. 34.1** The frequency of Crohn's disease in different segments of the gastrointestinal tract at diagnosis in 373 patients . (Reprinted from Incidence and prevalence of Crohn's disease in the coutry of Copenhagen, 1962–87 by Munkholm et al from Scand J Gastroenterol, www.tandf.no/gastro, 1992, 27, 609–14, by permission of Taylor & Francis AS).

## GOALS OF TREATMENT

The primary goals of medical therapy are to induce and then maintain significant clinical improvement or remission, resulting in a reduction or resolution of the signs and symptoms of active Crohn's disease draining fistulae. A secondary goal, which often occurs in parallel with clinical changes, is the induction of endoscopic or radiographic improvement and remission. The efficacy of various medical therapies in achieving these endpoints in patients with Crohn's disease is reviewed in the following sections.

## 5-AMINOSALICYLATE-BASED MEDICATIONS

Sulfasalazine, oral mesalamine (Pentasa, Asacol, Salofalk, Mesasal, Claversal) and olsalazine are all drugs that deliver 5-aminosalicylate to the small intestine and colon (Table 34.1). The clinical pharmacology of these medications is reviewed in detail in Chapter 32.

### SULFASALAZINE

In 1942 Svartz[8] reported on both the therapeutic results and the toxic effects of a novel sulfanilamide preparation, sulfasalazine, in patients with ulcerative colitis. Sulfasalazine is comprised of 5-aminosalicylate linked to sulfapyridine by an azo bond. Placebo-controlled trials demonstrated that sulfasalazine administered orally at doses of 3–6 g/day was effective in inducing remission in patients with mildly to moderately active Crohn's disease.[9–12] In the two larger studies, the benefit of sulfasalazine was limited to those patients with active colonic or ileocolonic disease, and there were trends towards sulfasalazine being less effective and slower in onset of action than prednisone or 6-methylprednisolone.[10,11] A comparative study of sulfasalazine 3 g/day versus metronidazole 0.8 g/day demonstrated similar remission rates in patients with active Crohn's disease.[13,14] Studies evalu-

ating sulfasalazine 3–5 g/day as an adjunctive therapy to prednisone 0.25–0.75 mg/kg/day adjusted according to disease activity, or 6-methylprednisolone 40 mg/day in patients with active Crohn's disease, did not demonstrate adjunctive or steroid-sparing benefits for sulfasalazine,[11,15] whereas studies evaluating prednisone 30 mg/day or 6-methylprednisolone 48 mg/day as an adjunctive therapy to sulfasalazine 3–6 g/day in active Crohn's disease did demonstrate an additive benefit for prednisone or 6-methylprednisolone (this additive effect was probably due to the superior efficacy of the corticosteroids, and could probably been achieved with the corticosteroid monotherapy, see above).[11,16] Additional placebo-controlled trials demonstrated that sulfasalazine at doses of 1.5–3 g/day was not effective in maintaining remission in patients with Crohn's disease in either medically[10,11,17] or surgically induced remission.[10,18–20] Approximately 10–20% of orally administered sulfasalazine is absorbed systemically, with the remainder passing unaltered to the colon.[21] Sulfasalazine undergoes metabolism in the colon by bacterial azo reductase enzymes to 5-aminosalicylate and sulfapyridine.[22,23] The active moiety of sulfasalazine in patients with ulcerative colitis was determined to be the poorly absorbed molecule 5-aminosalicylate and not the well absorbed molecule sulfapyridine.[21,24–27]

Adverse events occurring in patients with inflammatory bowel diseases treated with sulfasalazine include headache, epigastric pain, nausea and vomiting, cyanosis, skin rash, fever, hepatitis, autoimmune hemolysis, aplastic anemia, leukopenia, agranulocytosis, folate deficiency, pancreatitis, systemic lupus erythematosus, sulphonamide-induced toxic epidermal necrolysis, Stevens–Johnson syndrome, pulmonary dysfunction and male infertility.[28,29] For the most part, the side effects of sulfasalazine can be attributed to the systemic absorption of sulfapyridine, and they occur more commonly in patients who are genetically predisposed to 'slow' acetylation of sulfapyridine to N-acetylsulfapyridine in the liver.[28] Headache, nausea and vomiting, and epigastric pain often appear to be related to the sulfasalazine dose, and it is frequently possible to desensitize patients by discontinuing the drug for 1–2 weeks and then restarting at 0.125–0.25 g/day and increasing by 0.125 g/week up to a maintenance dose of 2 g/day.[29] Sulfasalazine therapy may also lead to a paradoxical worsening of diarrhea in patients with ulcerative colitis.[30]

## ORAL MESALAMINE (5-AMINOSALICYLATE)

After it was demonstrated that mesalamine (5-aminosalicylate) was the active moiety of sulfasalazine in patients with ulcerative colitis (discussed above), oral drug delivery systems were devised to avoid the absorption of mesalamine in the proximal small intestine, instead targeting the distal small bowel and colon as the site of drug release. One small placebo-controlled study with Asacol 3.2 g/day and another with Pentasa 4 g/day demonstrated the efficacy of mesalamine for active Crohn's disease.[31,32] In contrast, three placebo-controlled trials of Pentasa 1–2 g/day and two larger trials of Pentasa 4 g/day failed to demonstrate efficacy.[33–36] Two small comparative trials suggested similar efficacy of Pentasa 4 g/day versus ciprofloxacin 1000 mg/day, and of Asacol 4 g/day versus 6-methylprednisolone 40 mg/day in patients with active Crohn's disease,[37,38] whereas a large comparative trial demonstrated that Pentasa 4 g/day was inferior to budesonide 9 mg/day.[39] Thus, placebo-controlled trials of oral mesalamine for active Crohn's disease have not consis-

## Table 34.1 5-Aminosalicylate and budesonide topical preparations

| Generic name | Proprietary name | Formulation | Sites of delivery | Unit strength | Daily dose Active Crohn's disease | Maintenance of remission in Crohn's disease |
|---|---|---|---|---|---|---|
| Mesalamine | Asacol | Eudragit-S coated tablets (release at pH ≥ 7.0) | Terminal ileum, colon | 400 mg | 1.6–4.8 g | 0.8–4.8 g |
| Mesalamine | Salofalk Mesasal Claversal | Eudragit-L coated tablets (release at pH ≥ 6.0) | Distal jejunum, proximal ileum | 250 mg 500 mg | 1.5–4 g | 0.75–4 g |
| Mesalamine | Pentasa[1,2] | Ethylcellulose-coated microgranules (time dependent release) available as a tablet, capsule, or sachet | Duodenum jejunum ileum colon | 250 mg and 5000 mg tablets, 250 mg capsules, 1000 mg sachets | 2–4 g | 1.5–4 g |
| Olsalazine | Dipentum | 5-ASA dimer linked by azo-bond, available as a gelatin capsule | Colon | 250 mg | 2–3 g | 1 g |
| Sulfasalazine | Azulfidine | 5-ASA linked to sulfapyridine by azo-bond available as a tablet | Colon | 500 mg (200 mg 5ASA) | 2–4 g (0.8–1.6 g 5ASA) | 2–4 g |
| Sulfasalazine | Azulfidine EN-tabs | 5-ASA linked to sulfapyridine by azo-bond, available as a tablet coated with cellulose acetate phthalate | Colon | 500 mg (200 mg 5ASA) | 2–4 g (0.8–1.6 g 5ASA) | 2–4 g |
| Budesonide | Entocort | Micronized budesonide in an ethylcellulose matrix (time dependent release) coated with Edragit L (release at pH > 5.5). First pass hepatic metabolism 90%. Available as a hard gelatin capsule | Terminal ileum and right colon | 3 mg | 9 mg | 3–6 mg |
| Budesonide | Budenofalk | Budesonide microgranules coated with Eudragit (release at pH > 6.4) First-pass hepatic metabolism 90% Available as a gelatin capsule | Terminal ileum and right colon | 3 mg | 9 mg | 3–6 mg |

United States Pentasa[1]: 250 mg capsule. Non-United States Pentasa[4]: 250 mg and 500 mg tablets, and 1000 mg sachet.

tently demonstrated efficacy (unlike sulfasalazine, which has consistently been shown to be effective). Additional placebo-controlled trials in patients with medically induced remission showed either a small but statistically significant maintence benefit with Asacol 2.4 g/day,[40] Pentasa 2 g/day[41] or Salofalk/Claversal 1 g/day,[42] or no significant maintenance benefit with Asacol 2.4 g/day,[43] Pentasa 2–4 g/day[41,44–46] or Salofalk/Mesasal/Claversal 1.5–3 g/day.[47–49] Likewise, placebo-controlled trials in patients with surgically induced remission showed either a small but statistically significant postoperative maintence benefit with Asacol 2.4 g/day[50] or Salofalk 3 g/day,[51] or no significant maintenance benefit with Pentasa 3–4 g/day[46,52,53] or Claversal 3 g/day.[54] A meta-analysis demonstrated that the pooled difference in risk of symptomatic relapse for mesalamine versus placebo was –4.7% (95% CI –10% to 3%, number needed to treat = 20) for patients with medically induced remission and –10% (95% CI –17% to –3%, number needed to treat = 10) for patients with surgically induced remission.[55,56]

## OLSALAZINE

Olsalazine is a dimer comprised of two 5-aminosalicylate molecules linked by an azo bond. Placebo-controlled trials with olsalazine have not been conducted in patients with active Crohn's disease. A single placebo-controlled trial of olsalazine 2 g/day for the maintenance of medically induced remission in patients with Crohn's disease did not demonstrate efficacy but rather a trend towards a greater dropout rate in patients treated with olsalazine for worsened diarrhea.[57] The worsened diarrhea is a result of ileal secretion.[58]

## Table 34.2 American College of Gastroenterology working definitions for Crohn's disease activity

Remission

Remission refers to patients who are asymptomatic or without inflammatory sequelae and includes those who have responded to acute medical intervention or have undergone surgical resection without gross evidence o f residual disease. Patients requiring steroids to maintain wellbeing are considered to be 'steroid dependent' and are usually not considered to be 'in remission'

Mild to moderate disease

Mild/moderate Crohn's disease applies to ambulatory patients able to tolerate oral alimentation without manifestations of dehydration, toxicity (high fevers, rigors, prostration), abdominal tenderness, painful mass, obstruction, or > 10% weight loss

Moderate/severe disease

Moderate/severe disease applies to patients who have failed to respond to treatment for mild/moderate disease or those with more prominent symptoms of fevers, significant weight loss, abdominal pain or tenderness, intermittent nausea or vomiting (without obstructive findings), or significant anemia

Severe/fulminant disease

Severe/fulminant disease refers to patients with persisting symptoms despite the introduction of steroids as outpatients, or individuals presenting with high fever, persistent vomiting, evidence of intestinal obstruction, rebound tenderness, cachexia or evidence of an abscess

Reprinted with permission from: Hanauer SB, Sandborn W. The Practice Parameters Committee of the American College of Gastroenterology. Management of Crohn's disease in adults. Am J Gastroenterol 2001;96:635–643.

## Table 34.3 Crohn's disease activity index (CDAI)

| Variable no. | Variable description | Multiplier | Total |
|---|---|---|---|
| 1 | No. of liquid or soft stools (each day for 7 days) | 2 | |
| 2 | Abdominal pain, sum of seven daily ratings (0=none, 1 = mild, 2 = moderate, 3 = severe) | 5 | |
| 3 | General wellbeing, sum of seven daily ratings (0 = generally well, 1 = slightly under par, 2 = poor, 3 = very poor, 4 = terrible) | 7 | |
| 4 | Number of listed complications 9arthritis or arthralgia, iritis or uveitis, erythema nodosum or pyoderma gangrenosum or aphthous stomatitis, anal fissure or fistula or abscess, other fistula, fever over 37.8°C (100°F)) | 20 | |
| 5 | Use of diphenoxylate or loperamide for diarrhea (0 = no, 1 = yes) | 30 | |
| 6 | Abdominal mass (0 = no, 2 = questionable, 5 = definite) | 10 | |
| 7 | Hematocrit (males: 47-Hct (%), females: 42-Hct (%)) | 6 | |
| 8 | Body weight (1 – weight/standard weight) x 100 (add or subtract according to sign) | 1 | |
| CDAI score | | | |

* Disease activity can be classified according to the CDAI score using the following definitions: remission = CDAI of < 150, mildly active = CDAI score of 150–219, moderately active = CDAI score of 220–450, severely active = CDAI score of > 450.
(Adapted with permission from: Best WR, Becktel JM, Singleton JW, Kern F Jr. Development of a Crohn's disease activity index. National Cooperative Crohn's Disease Study. Gastroenterology 1976;70:439–444.)

# TOXICITY OF MESALAMINE AND OLSALAZINE

Adverse events attributable to 5-aminosalicylates occur infrequently in patients with inflammatory bowel disease treated with mesalamine and olsalazine. Rare but serious events include pulmonary toxicity, pericarditis, hepatitis and pancreatitis.[59-62] Interstitial nephritis has been reported in patients treated with mesalamine, but whether the mesalamine causes the renal lesion is unclear.[63-66] Several studies have demonstrated that renal tubular proteinuria may be related to the disease activity of the inflammatory bowel disease,[67,68] and one study reported that interstitial nephritis is an extraintestinal manifestation of Crohn's disease.[69] Hanauer reported on the safety of Asacol in 2940 patients with ulcerative colitis at doses up to 7.2 g/day for up to 5.2 years and concluded that there were no clinically significant dose or duration effects on renal function.[70] A similar low frequency of clinically significant renal events has been reported for patients with inflammatory bowel disease treated with Pentasa.[71] A minority of patients will experience worsening diarrhea and abdominal pain owing to a hypersensitivity reaction to 5-aminosalicylate, and treatment with olsalazine will lead to an ileal secretory diarrhea in some patients, as discussed above.[72]

# CORTICOSTEROID-BASED MEDICATIONS

Cortisone is produced by the adrenal cortex. Endogenously secreted or exogenously administered cortisol and exogenously administered prednisone must be activated in the liver to hydrocortisone and prednisolone, respectively. Prednisolone and methylprednisolone have the same glucocorticoid and anti-inflammatory activity as hydrocortisone but less mineralocorticoid activity. Oral administration of cortisone, prednisone and prednisolone, and intravenous administration of prednisolone, methylprednisolone and corticotropin, are methods of delivering corticosteroids for a systemic effect (Table 34.4). In contrast to systemically administered corticosteroids, oral administration of fluticasone and controlled ileal release budesonide are methods of delivering corticosteroids directly to the distal ileum and colon for a non-systemic effect (Table 34.4). Topical administration of fluticasone or budesonide to the ileum or colon results in a predominately non-systemic effect because these newer corticosteroids have high affinities for the glucocorticoid receptors and undergo extensive first pass hepatic metabolism.

# ORAL CORTICOSTEROIDS (SYSTEMIC EFFECT)

Placebo-controlled trials have demonstrated that prednisone administered at doses of 0.25–0.75 mg/kg (17.5–52.5 mg for a 70 kg patient) according to disease activity, and a tapering dose of 6-methylprednisolone beginning at 48 mg/day, are effective in inducing remission in patients with mildly to severely active Crohn's disease.[10,11] Steroids act more rapidly and are more effective than sulfasalazine[10,11] and total enteral nutrition.[73-84] Studies evaluating sulfasalazine 3–5 g/day as an adjunctive therapy to prednisone 0.25–0.75 mg/kg/day adjusted according to disease activity, or 6-methylprednisolone 48 mg/day, in patients with active Crohn's disease did not demonstrate adjunctive benefits for sulfasalazine,[11,15] whereas studies evaluating prednisone 30 mg/day or 6-methylprednisolone 48 mg/day as an adjunctive therapy to sulfasalazine 3–6 g/day in active Crohn's disease did demonstrate an additive benefit for combination therapy with prednisone or 6-methylprednisolone (this additive effect was probably due to the superior efficacy of the corticosteroids, and could probably been achieved with corticosteroid monotherapy, see above).[11,16] Small comparative trials tended towards a greater efficacy of prednisone 30 mg/day versus ciprofloxacin 1 g/day combined with metronidazole 1 g/day, and a similar efficacy of 6-methylprednisolone 40 mg/day versus Asacol 4 g/day in patients with active Crohn's disease.[38,85] Larger comparative trials tended towards a greater efficacy of prednisolone 40 mg/day versus budesonide 9 mg/day,[86-90] with superior efficacy for prednisolone demonstrated by meta-analysis.[91] A dose-ranging study of prednisone or other corticosteroids has not been performed in patients with active

## Table 34.4 Corticosteroid preparations

| Generic name | Potency | Mineralocorticoid | Formulation effect | Sites of delivery | Site and mechanism of action | Daily dose | Indication |
|---|---|---|---|---|---|---|---|
| Hydrocortisone | 1 | ++ | IV | Blood | Systemic | 200 mg | Severe CD |
| Hydrocortisone | 1 | ++ | Oral | Duodenum | Systemic | | Active CD |
| Prednisone | 4 | + | | Duodenum | Systemic | | Active CD |
| Prednisonolone | 4 | + | | Duodenum | Systemic | | Active CD |
| Methyl-prednisolone | 5 | – | IV | Blood | Systemic | | Severe CD |
| 6-Methyl prednisolone | 5 | – | Oral | Duodenum | Systemic | | Active CD |
| Budesonide | 200 | – | Enteric release | Distal ileum, right colon | Non-systemic, first pass metabolism | 6–9 mg/day | Active CD |
| Adreno corticotropic hormone | NA | NA | IV | Blood | Systemic | | Severe CD |

CD, Crohn's disease; NA, not applicable.

Crohn's disease. Many North American physicians administer prednisone at doses of 40–60 mg/day (based on the controlled trials outlined above and extrapolation of dose-response data from ulcerative colitis[92]). In contrast, French and many other European as well as South African physicians often administer prednisolone 1 mg/kg based on the reported high response rates in uncontrolled studies.[45,93–95] The optimal tapering regimen for corticosteroids has not been determined. One controlled trial demonstrated no difference in outcome at 6 months for patients with active Crohn's disease treated with 6-methylprednisolone 40 mg/day tapered over 7 weeks compared to tapering over 15 weeks.[96]

Additional placebo-controlled trials demonstrated that lower doses of oral corticosteroids (prednisone 0.25 mg/kg, 7.5 mg/day or 5–15 mg/day, or 6-methylprednisolone 8 mg/day) were not effective for maintenance in patients with Crohn's disease in either medically[10,11] or surgically induced remission.[18,97] Nevertheless, it is recognized clinically that many patients who initially respond to corticosteroid therapy and who relapse with tapering can be maintained in an asymptomatic state by long-term therapy with prednisone 10–30 mg/day or its equivalent.[98,99] Such patients are termed 'steroid dependent' and have been recognized in population-based natural history studies of steroid therapy in patients with Crohn's disease.[98,99] One placebo-controlled study did demonstrate efficacy for low-dose corticosteroid maintenance therapy with 6-methylprednisolone 0.25 mg/kg/day in asymptomatic patients with elevated laboratory markers of inflammation, with the clinical benefit being attributed to the suppression of active subclinical inflammation, rather than maintenance of remission.[100] Thus, although low-dose corticosteroids are not effective as maintenance therapy in unselected patients, they are effective in suppressing symptoms in a subset of patients with ongoing subclinical inflammation. However, because of the toxicity associated with long-term corticosteroid use, this form of maintenance therapy is not acceptable in clinical practice.

## INTRAVENOUS CORTICOSTEROIDS AND CORTICOTROPIN (ACTH)

Patients with severe Crohn's disease and ulcerative colitis and those refractory to oral corticosteroids are hospitalized and treated with intravenous corticosteroids. The rationale for this practice is altered corticosteroid absorption and metabolism in patients with Crohn's disease and ulcerative colitis. Oral administration of prednisolone 20 mg resulted in lower absorption in patients with Crohn's disease than in volunteers.[101] In contrast, intravenous administration of prednisolone to patients with severe acute Crohn's disease, indeterminate colitis or ulcerative colitis resulted in serum concentrations similar to those in volunteers.[101,102] Continuous infusion of prednisolone resulted in greater mean serum concentrations over time compared to bolus intravenous dosing; and both intravenous dosing strategies resulted in greater mean serum concentrations than oral dosing.[102] Uncontrolled studies have reported that approximately 60–76% of patients hospitalized for severe ulcerative colitis or Crohn's disease will respond to intravenous corticosteroid therapy.[103–106] Dosing strategies have included prednisolone 60 mg/day in four divided doses,[103,106] betamethasone 3 mg twice daily[105] and hydrocortisone 300–400 mg/day.[107–110] Many clinicians prefer methylprednisolone 40–60 mg/day because it has minimal mineralocorticoid effect. There was no apparent advantage in increasing the dose of methylprednisolone to 1000 mg/day in patients with ulcerative colitis.[111] No placebo-controlled trials of intravenous corticosteroid therapy for severe ulcerative colitis or Crohn's disease have been performed. A comparative study of intravenous corticotropin (adrenal corticotropin hormone, ACTH) 120 U/day and hydrocortisone 300 mg/day demonstrated a similar overall benefit in hospitalized patients with active Crohn's disease.[110]

## ORAL CORTICOSTEROIDS (NON-SYSTEMIC EFFECT)

After it was demonstrated that systemically active corticosteroids were effective in patients with active Crohn's disease (discussed above), oral drug delivery systems were devised to provide the efficacy of corticosteroid therapy without the associated corticosteroid toxicity. One such strategy is to administer a corticosteroid with high first-pass hepatic metabolism, budesonide, directly as a topical therapy to the distal small bowel and right colon. A placebo-controlled study demonstrated that controlled ileal release (CIR) budesonide 9 mg/day is effective for the treatment of mild-to-moderately active Crohn's disease and results in an increased quality of life and a second placebo-controlled trial showed a similar trend.[112–114] A large comparative trial demonstrated that CIR budesonide 9 mg/day is more effective than Pentasa 4 g/day in patients with active Crohn's disease and results in an increased quality of life.[39,115] Other large comparative trials tended towards a greater efficacy of prednisolone 40 mg/day versus CIR budesonide or oral pH-modified release budesonide 9 mg/day in patients with active Crohn's disease,[86–90] with superior efficacy for prednisolone demonstrated by meta-analysis.[91] A study evaluating the combination of both metronidazole 1 g/day and ciprofloxacin 1 g/day as an adjunctive therapy to CIR budesonide 9 mg/day in patients with active Crohn's disease did not demonstrate an adjunctive benefit for the addition of metronidazole and ciprofloxacin.[116] The optimal dose of CIR budesonide or oral pH-modified release budesonide for induction of remission is 9 mg once daily, with 3–6 mg/day being less effective,[112,117] 4.5 mg b.i.d. tending towards being less efficacious[88,113] and 15–18 mg/day having similar efficacy and greater adrenal suppression.[112,117]

Additional placebo-controlled trials in patients with medically induced remission showed that CIR budesonide 6 mg/day significantly increases the time to relapse but does not meet the conventional criteria for maintenance of remission at 1 year,[118–121] findings that were confirmed in a combined analysis.[122] CIR budesonide 3 mg/day did not significantly prolong the time to relapse or maintain remission.[118–120] CIR budesonide 6 mg/day is more effective than placebo or mesalamine 3 g/day for maintenance of remission in patients with steroid-dependent Crohn's disease,[123,124] and oral pH-modified release budesonide 6–18 mg/day is effective for the short-term maintenance of remission in patients with prednisolone-induced remission.[125] Maintenance therapy with a variable dose of CIR budesonide dose 0–9 mg/day to maintain symptomatic remission results in similar control of disease activity as CIR budesonide at a fixed dose of 6 mg/day[126] or prednisolone 0–40 mg/day adjusted to disease activity.[127] Maintenance therapy with CIR budesonide 6–9 mg/day resulted in a similar clinical remission rate at 1 year as with azathioprine 2.2 mg/kg/day, but azathioprine resulted in greater endoscopic remission.[128] CIR budesonide and oral pH-modified release budesonide 3–6 mg/day were not effective for postoperative maintenance of remission in patients with surgically induced remission.[129,130] A study comparing another non-systemic steroid, fluticasone, administered orally at a dose of 20 mg/day with prednisolone 40 mg/day tapered to 15 mg/day in patients with active Crohn's disease, showed greater benefit and a more rapid response in the prednisolone group.[131]

## TOXICITY OF CORTICOSTEROIDS

Corticosteroid toxicity occurred frequently in patients with active Crohn's disease treated with prednisone at an initial dose of 60 mg/day tapered over 17 weeks. Toxicities observed included a moon face in 47%, acne in 30%, infection in 27%, ecchymoses in 17%, hypertension in 15%, hirsutism in 7%, petechial bleeding in 6% and striae in 6%.[132]

Prolonged corticosteroid therapy at low to intermediate doses (doses frequently utilized in patients with steroid-dependent Crohn's disease) is associated with the potential for multiple serious side effects.[133] Hypertension occurs in up to 20% of patients.[134] New-onset diabetes mellitus requiring initiation of hypoglycemic therapy occurs at a frequency 2.23 times greater than in the general population.[135] Infection occurs at a frequency of 13–20%.[136] Osteonecrosis occurs at a frequency of approximately 5%.[137] The frequency of steroid-associated osteoporosis may be as high as 50%.[138] Neurologic side effects occur often and can include myopathy at a frequency of 7% and psychosis at a frequency of 3–5%.[139] Ophthalmologic side effects also occur often and can include cataracts at a frequency of 22% (dose dependent) and glaucoma (frequency unclear, response genetically determined).[140,141]

Corticosteroid side effects in patients undergoing induction treatment with budesonide 9 mg/day occur at a frequency similar to that of placebo or Pentasa 4 g/day[39,112,113] and at a lower frequency than with prednisolone 40 mg/day.[86–89] Similarly, corticosteroid side effects in patients undergoing maintenance treatment with budesonide 6 mg/day occur at a frequency similar to that of placebo.[118–121] Budesonide maintenance therapy for 2 years at doses of 0–9 mg/day adjusted to control disease activity did not result in a decrease in bone density.[127]

## ANTIBIOTICS

Given the attractive but unsubstantiated hypothesis that Crohn's disease may be a specific infectious enteritis or colitis, studies evaluating treatment with antibiotics were logical.

## METRONIDAZOLE

Two small placebo-controlled studies with metronidazole 1 g/day and metronidazole 0.8 g/day in combination with cotrimoxazole did not demonstrate efficacy of metronidazole for active Crohn's disease.[142,143] Subsequently, a larger dose-ranging study of metronidazole 10 and 20 mg/day in patients with active Crohn's disease demonstrated a significant decrease in the median CDAI scores for metronidazole 20 mg/day compared with placebo, but failed to demonstrate efficacy as assessed by the more conventional criterion of induction of remission.[144] In this study there was a trend towards greater efficacy of metronidazole in patients with colonic disease. Two small comparative trials demonstrated a trend towards greater efficacy of prednisone 30 mg/day versus ciprofloxacin 1 g/day combined with metronidazole 1 g/day,[85] and similar efficacy of metronidazole 0.8 g/day and sulfasalazine

3 g/day in patients with active Crohn's disease.[14] A study evaluating metronidazole 1 g/day combined with ciprofloxacin 1 g/day as an adjunctive therapy to budesonide 9 mg/day in patients with active Crohn's disease did not demonstrate an adjunctive benefit for metronidazole combined with ciprofloxacin.[116] There was a trend towards efficacy of metronidazole combined with ciprofloxacin in patients with colonic disease. A controlled trial of metronidazole 20 mg/kg for postoperative maintenance of remission in patients with surgically induced remission demonstrated efficacy for reduction in the frequency of severe endoscopic recurrence at 12 weeks, but failed to demonstrate efficacy for maintenance of clinical remission at 1 year by intent-to-treat analysis.[145] Uncontrolled studies have suggested that metronidazole 20 mg/day is beneficial in patients with perianal Crohn's disease,[146] and that relapse rates are high when metronidazole is discontinued.[147] No controlled trials of metronidazole for perianal Crohn's disease have been performed. Thus, although metronidazole is widely used in clinical practice for the treatment of Crohn's disease, controlled trials have not consistently demonstrated efficacy.

## CIPROFLOXACIN

One small placebo-controlled study with ciprofloxacin 1 g/day demonstrated efficacy in active Crohn's disease.[148] Two small comparative trials demonstrated a trend towards greater efficacy of prednisone 30 mg/day versus ciprofloxacin 1 g/day combined with metronidazole 1 g/day,[85] and similar efficacy of ciprofloxacin 1 g/day and Pentasa 4 g/day[37] in patients with active Crohn's disease. A study evaluating metronidazole 1 g/day combined with ciprofloxacin 1 g/day as an adjunctive therapy to budesonide 9 mg/day in patients with active Crohn's disease did not demonstrate adjunctive benefits for metronidazole combined with ciprofloxacin.[116] There was a trend towards efficacy of metronidazole combined with ciprofloxacin in patients with colonic disease. Another study of ciprofloxacin 1–1.5 g/day as an adjunctive therapy to corticosteroids combined with metronidazole did not demonstrate an adjunctive benefit for ciprofloxacin.[149] Uncontrolled studies have suggested that ciprofloxacin 1 g/day, either alone[150] or in combination with metronidazole 1 g/day,[151] is beneficial in patients with perianal Crohn's disease. No controlled trials of ciprofloxacin for perianal Crohn's disease have been performed. Thus, although ciprofloxacin is widely used in clinical practice for the treatment of Crohn's disease, efficacy data from controlled trials supporting this treatment approach are extremely limited.

## ANTIMYCOBACTERIAL THERAPY

Two small placebo-controlled trials of antimycobacterial therapy in combination with a tapering course of corticosteroids demonstrated efficacy in the maintenance phase (following corticosteroid withdrawal) for clofazimine monotherapy and for a combination of ethambutol, clofazimine, dapsone and rifampicin in patients with active Crohn's disease.[152,153] In contrast, five placebo-controlled trials in which antimycobacterial therapy was administered without corticosteroids failed to demonstrate efficacy for varying combinations of ethambutol, rifampin, isoniazid, sulphadoxine, pyrimethamine and rifabutin in patients with active Crohn's disease.[154–159] These results are summarized in a meta-analysis.[160] Based on the nearly uniform negative outcome of these studies, antimycobacterial antibiotic therapy has no role in the treatment of Crohn's disease.

## PROBIOTIC THERAPY

One placebo-controlled study failed to demonstrated efficacy of *Lactobacillus* GG for postoperative maintenance of remission in patients with surgically induced remission.[161] Similarly, a small placebo-controlled trial of *Saccharomyces boulardii* was not effective for maintence of medically induced remission in patients with Crohn's disease, but did decrease stool frequency.[162]

# IMMUNOSUPPRESSIVE MEDICATIONS

The antimetabolite mediators 6-mercaptopurine, its prodrug azathioprine, and methotrexate, the calcineurin inhibitors cyclosporin and tacrolimus (FK506), and the T-cell inhibitor mycophenolate mofetil are all medications with immunosuppressive activity. The clinical pharmacology of these medications is reviewed in detail elsewhere in this book.

## AZATHIOPRINE AND 6-MERCAPTOPURINE

Azathioprine is 50% 6-mercaptopurine (6-MP) by molecular weight. Thus, a dose of 6-MP must be doubled to calculate an equivalent dose of azathioprine. Six placebo-controlled trials have evaluated azathioprine at doses of 2–3 mg/kg/day or 6-MP 50 mg/day up to 1.5 mg/kg/day for the treatment of active Crohn's disease.[10,95,163–168] Five of these studies reported on the subset of patients with fistulae.[163,164,166,167,169] Most of the studies demonstrated an induction benefit for induction of remission of luminal disease and for fistula closure, results confirmed by a meta-analysis.[170] An uncontrolled study also reported that 6-MP is of clinical benefit for closing fistulae.[171] A placebo-controlled trial showed no benefit of pretreatment with intravenous azathioprine 40 mg/kg loading over standard therapy with oral azathioprine 2.0 mg/kg in patients with active Crohn's disease.[172] Eight placebo-controlled trials evaluated azathioprine at doses of 1.0–2.5 mg/kg or 6-MP 1.5 mg/kg/day for maintenance of medically induced remission and steroid sparing in patients with Crohn's disease.[10,95,167–169,173–175] Most of these studies demonstrated a maintenance benefit for azathioprine and 6-MP, a result confirmed by a meta-analysis.[170] A small comparative controlled trial demonstrated that azathioprine 2.2 mg/kg/day was more effective than budesonide 6–9 mg/day for inducing endoscopic remission in patients with Crohn's disease, and there was a trend towards a greater rate of clinical remission in azathioprine-treated patients at 1 year.[128] Another small comparative trial demonstrated that 6-MP was more effective than mesalamine 3 g/day in maintaining steroid-induced remission.[176] Once patients begin maintenance treatment with azathioprine or 6-MP it should be continued for at least 4 years and perhaps indefinitely.[175,177] One small trial that compared a low dose of 6-MP (50 mg/day), Pentasa 3 g and placebo for postoperative maintenance of remission in patients with surgically induced remission showed a modest benefit for 6-MP.[178] Additional trials for this indication using higher doses of azathioprine or 6-MP are needed. Overall, these controlled studies demonstrate that 6-MP and azathioprine are effective for induction of remission, fistula closure, maintenance of medically induced remission, steroid sparing, and possibly postoperative maintenance of remission in patients with chronically active and treatment-refractory or fistulizing Crohn's disease.

Adverse events occurring in patients with inflammatory bowel diseases treated with 6-MP and azathioprine include pancreatitis (3%), fever, rash, arthralgias, malaise, nausea, diarrhea, leukopenia (2–5%), thrombocytopenia, infection, and hepatitis.[179–181] It appears that there is not an increased risk of solid malignancies when AZA/6-MP is used as monotherapy in inflammatory bowel disease.[179,182] The risk of non-Hodgkin's lymphoma is uncertain: in three large series only one lymphoma occurred among 1308 patients,[177,179,182] whereas another study reported six Epstein–Barr virus-associated non-Hodgkin's lymphomas among approximately 1200 patients treated with azathioprine or 6-MP for inflammatory bowel disease.[183]

## METHOTREXATE

Three placebo-controlled trials have evaluated methotrexate at doses of 25 mg/week intramuscularly and 12.5–15 mg/week orally for the treatment of active and steroid-dependent Crohn's disease.[168,184,185] Intramuscular methotrexate 25 mg/week was effective for inducing remission and steroid sparing, and there was a trend towards the 15 mg/week oral dose also being effective for active Crohn's disease.[184,185] In contrast, 12.5 mg/week orally was not more effective than placebo or low-dose 6-MP (50 mg/day) in active Crohn's disease. An uncontrolled study has reported that methotrexate may be of some benefit in closing fistulae.[186] One placebo-controlled trial demonstrated that methotrexate 15 mg/week intramuscularly was effective for maintaining remission in patients who were previously steroid dependent,[187] and a small comparative trial demonstrated that oral methotrexate 15 mg/week was more effective than mesalamine 3 g/day in maintaining steroid-induced remission.[176] Subcutaneous administration of methotrexate at doses of 15–25 mg/week appears to result in therapeutic blood and mucosal concentrations as well as clinical benefit,[188] and patients failing to respond to or maintain remission with 15 mg methotrexate may benefit from dose escalation to 25 mg.[187,188] Overall, these controlled studies demonstrate that parenterally administered methotrexate is effective for induction of remission, maintenance of medically induced remission, and steroid sparing in patients with chronically active and treatment refractory Crohn's disease.

Adverse events occurring in patients with Crohn's disease treated with methotrexate include elevation of serum transaminases (5%), nausea (4%), skin rash (1%) and *Mycoplasma* pneumonia (1%).[184] Dose-limiting nausea may be more frequent with oral methotrexate therapy.[185] Other forms of toxicity reported to occur during methotrexate treatment of autoimmune diseases such as psoriasis and rheumatoid arthritis include diarrhea, mucositis, headache, central nervous system effects, hypersensitivity pneumonitis, bone marrow suppression, hepatic fibrosis/cirrhosis and lymphoma.[189,190] In patients with psoriasis, treatment with methotrexate led to hepatic fibrosis/cirrhosis in 0–21%,[191] and a meta-analysis showed a 7% overall risk of developing severe hepatic fibrosis/cirrhosis.[192] In contrast, in patients with rheumatoid arthritis the risk of severe fibrosis/cirrhosis after treatment with methotrexate is much lower, at approximately 1%.[193] Other factors which appear to increase the risk for fibrosis/cirrhosis in methotrexate-treated patients include a history of excessive alcohol use, abnormal baseline serum transaminases, concomitant diabetes and obesity, a cumulative dose of methotrexate > 1500 mg, and daily administration of methotrexate.[189,191–193] Two small preliminary studies have suggested that the risk of methotrexate hepatotoxicity in patients with inflammatory bowel diseases is low.[194,195] Elevation of serum transaminases up to three times normal during treatment with MTX occurs in 20–31% of patients.[189,193] These elevations are poor predictors of the severity of liver histopathology and are of concern only if they persist.

## CYCLOSPORIN AND TACROLIMUS

Cyclosporin and tacrolimus (FK506) are both calcineurin inhibitors. One placebo-controlled trial demonstrated that standard-dose oral cyclosporin (mean dose 7.6 mg/kg/day) was effective for the treatment of active Crohn's disease.[196] In contrast, three placebo-controlled trials of low-dose oral cyclosporin (5 mg/kg/day) failed to demonstrate efficacy for induction or remission and/or maintenance of remission in patients with Crohn's disease.[197–199] One controlled trial demonstrated efficacy of oral tacrolimus 0.2 mg/kg/day for treatment of Crohn's disease perianal fistulae.[200] Uncontrolled studies of high-dose intravenous cyclosporin (4 mg/kg/day, equivalent to 12–16 mg/kg/day assuming 25–33% oral bioavailability)[201–210] and oral tacrolimus 0.2–0.3 mg/kg/day[211–214] have suggested a clinical benefit in patients with Crohn's disease fistulae. Overall, these studies demonstrate that low-dose oral cyclosporin is not effective for the induction or maintenance of remission in patients with Crohn's disease, whereas oral tacrolimus, and possibly high-dose intravenous cyclosporin, is effective for the treatment of actively draining fistulae.

Adverse events occurring in patients with inflammatory bowel diseases treated with cyclosporin include hypertension, headaches, paresthesias, seizures, gingival hyperplasia, hypertrichosis, anaphylaxis, opportunistic infection and renal insufficiency.[215–218] There is an increased risk of opportunistic infection in hospitalized patients with severe steroid-refractory ulcerative colitis or Crohn's disease treated with intravenous cyclosporin combined with corticosteroids and azathioprine or 6-MP; *Pneumocystis carinii* pneumonia, invasive apergillosis, lung abscess, mycotic aneurysm, cytomegalovirus and overwhelming sepsis have all been reported, with death rates ranging from 1 to 2% in larger series.[215,217–221] There does not appear to be an increase in perioperative morbidity or mortality in patients with ulcerative colitis who receive intravenous cyclosporin and then require colectomy within a short period.[222] Another study reported that 20% of 99 patients with inflammatory bowel diseases treated with intravenous cyclosporin had a decrease in estimated renal function greater than 30%.[223] Results from a previous study in patients with autosomal disease suggest that treatment with high-doseoral cyclosporin results in a significant likelihood of having histological evidence of irreversible nephrotoxicity on renal biopsy (to date, similar data have not been generated in patients with inflammatory bowel diseases).[224]

Adverse events observed in patients with Crohn's disease treated with tacrolimus include headache, increased serum creatinine, insomnia, leg cramps, paresthesias and tremor.[200,212–214] Opportunistic infection has not been reported in this treatment setting. Similar to patients treated with cyclosporin, an increased frequency of striped interstitial nephritis and arteriolar alterations on renal biopsy has been observed in patients with tacrolimus-associated nephrotoxicity,[225] and it is reasonable to speculate that high-dose tacrolimus therapy or a significant rise in serum creatinine from baseline in tacrolimus-treated patients may lead to important renal pathology.

## MYCOPHENOLATE MOFETIL

A single small controlled trial reported that mycophenolate mofetil 15 mg/kg/day had similar efficacy to azathioprine 2.5 mg/kg/day in patients with chronically active Crohn's disease.[226] Uncontrolled studies reported variable benefit and high rates of drug intolerance in patients with active Crohn's disease.[227–232] There is insufficient evidence at present to recommend that patients with Crohn's disease be treated with mycophenolate mofetil.

# ANTITUMOR NECROSIS FACTOR AGENTS

Infliximab, etanercept, CDP571, onercept, CDP870, adalimumab, CNI-1493 and thalidomide are all medications that have anti-TNF activity. The clinical pharmacology of these medications is reviewed in detail in Chapter 32.

## INFLIXIMAB

Infliximab is a mouse/human chimeric $IgG_1$ monoclonal antibody to TNF. Two placebo-controlled trials have demonstrated that infliximab at doses of 5, 10 and 20 mg/kg is effective for the treatment of active Crohn's disease unresponsive to conventional therapy.[233,234] The recommended induction regimen is three doses of 5 mg/kg administered at 0, 2 and 6 weeks.[234–236] One of these studies demonstrated efficacy in patients with actively draining fistulae.[234] In addition, three placebo-controlled trials demonstrated that infliximab 5 and 10 mg/kg every 8 weeks is effective for prolongation of time to loss of clinical response and prolongation of time to loss of fistula improvement, for maintenance of clinical remission and maintenance of fistula closure, and for steroid sparing in patients who previously responded to infliximab.[235,237,238] Thus, the indications for infliximab in patients with chronically active and treatment refractory or fistulizing Crohn's disease include induction of remission, fistula closure, maintenance of infliximab-induced remission, maintence of fistula closure, and steroid sparing. Infliximab is also effective for the treatment of ankylosing spondylitis associated with Crohn's disease.[239]

Human antichimeric antibodies (HACA), also known as antibodies to infliximab (ATI), occurred in 28% of patients who received a single induction dose of infliximab compared to 6–9% of patients who received three induction doses followed by maintenance dosing every 8 weeks.[235] Concomitant therapy with an immunosuppressive agent was also protective.[235] These findings have been confirmed by other studies using a different assay for HACA that demonstrated independent protective effects from immunosuppressive therapy, multiple induction doses, and pretreatment with 200 mg of intravenous hydrocortisone.[240,241] Patients who developed HACA had an increased rate of infusion reactions and a shortening of the duration of benefit by 50%.[240,241] In order to minimize the chance of HACA formation, it is recommended that patients have three induction doses of infliximab and receive concomitant therapy with azathioprine, 6-MP or methotrexate.[240,242]

Side effects from infliximab reported in patients with Crohn's disease in an integrated safety data set of 771 patients and in a large maintenance trial include infusion reactions; delayed-type hypersensitivity reactions; formation of autoantibodies; drug-induced lupus; reactivation of latent tuberculosis; serious infections; and possibly non-Hodgkin's lymphoma.[235,243] Infusion reactions are defined as adverse events that occur during or within 2 hours following an infusion of infliximab. Most infusion reactions include symptoms of urticaria, dyspnea and/or hypotension. Overall, infusion reactions occur in 17% of infliximab-treated patients compared to 7% of placebo-treated patients.[243] In addition, a syndrome of delayed hypersensitivity (myalgia and/or arthralgia with fever and/or rash, and in some patients pruritus, facial, hand or lip edema, dysphagia, urticaria, sore throat and headache) was reported in up to 25% of patients retreated with infliximab after a drug holiday of 2–4 years.[244] However, in another long-term treatment trial, and in clinical practice, delayed hypersensitivity appears to occur at a much lower rate of ≤ 3%.[235,245] Patients with Crohn's disease treated with infliximab in clinical trials develop new antinuclear antibodies in 34% of cases and new antidouble-stranded DNA antibodies in 9%.[243] Another study reported that the cumulative frequency of developing a new positive ANA was 50%.[246] In rare circumstances, some of these patients may develop features of drug-induced lupus.[243,245] Non-Hodgkin's lymphoma appears to be relatively rare but has been reported in some patients with Crohn's disease and rheumatoid arthritis treated with infliximab.[235,243,245,247–249] A causal link between treatment with infliximab and the occurrence of non-Hodgkin's lymphoma has not been established. Serious infections may occur after treatment with infliximab, including sepsis, reactivation of latent tuberculosis or histoplasmosis, listeriosis and aspergillosis.[243,250–252] Tuberculin skin testing and chest radiography before treatment with infliximab are recommended.[243,250,253]

## CDP571

CDP571 is a humanized IgG$_4$ monoclonal antibody to TNF. Two phase II trials suggested a benefit of intravenous CDP571 for active Crohn's disease,[254,255] but a large phase III trial failed to confirm efficacy.[256] Similarly, a phase II trial suggested a benefit of intravenous CDP571 for steroid sparing,[257] but a large phase III trial failed to confirm efficacy (Celltech press release 2002).

## CDP870

CDP870 is a PEGylated humanized FAB fragment to TNF. A phase II trial of subcutaneous CDP870 for active Crohn's disease demonstrated efficacy at the highest dose level, particularly in patients with elevated C-reactive protein.[258] Another phase II trial of intravenous CDP870 for active Crohn's disease failed to demonstrate a benefit.[259] A phase III trial of subcutaneous CDP870 in patients with active Crohn's disease is planned.

## ADALIMUMAB (D2E7)

Adalimumab (D2E7) is a fully human IgG$_1$ monoclonal antibody to TNF. Subcutaneous adalimumab is effective for the treatment of rheumatoid arthritis.[260,261] Phase II trials of subcutaneous adalimumab in patients with active Crohn's disease and medically induced remission are under way.

## ONERCEPT

Onercept is a recombinant human soluble p55 tumor necrosis factor receptor that binds TNF. A small phase II study of subcutaneous onercept suggested a benefit in active Crohn's disease.[262] The results of a larger phase II study of subcutaneous onercept in patients with active Crohn's disease are expected in the near future.

## ETARNECEPT

Etanercept is a p75 soluble TNF receptor:FC fusion protein that binds TNF. A pilot study of subcutaneous etanercept in patients with active Crohn's disease suggested benefit,[263] but a phase II controlled trial failed to demonstrate efficacy.[264]

## MAP KINASE INHIBITORS (CNI-1493 AND BIRB796)

CNI-1493 is a guanylhydrazone small molecule that inhibitors the mitogen-activated protein kinases (MAP kinases) JNK and p38, thereby indirectly inhibiting the production of TNF. A small phase II study of intravenous CNI-1493 suggested a benefit for active Crohn's disease.[265] A larger phase II trial of intravenous CNI-1493 for active Crohn's disease is under way. BIRB796 is a small molecule inhibitor of the MAP kinase p38 that can be administered orally.[266,267] A large phase II trial of BIRB796 in patients with active Crohn's disease is under way.

## THALIDOMIDE

Thalidomide is a small molecule with anti-inflammatory properties that include inhibiting the production of TNF. Three small pilot studies suggested a benefit of thalidomide for both active Crohn's disease and maintenance of medically induced remission.[268–270] However, the significant toxicity associated with thalidomide, including teratogenicity, excessive sedation and peripheral neuropathy, will probably limit its widespread use for the treatment of Crohn's disease.

# OTHER BIOTECHNOLOGY AGENTS

## NATALIZUMAB

Natalizumab is a humanized IgG$_4$ monoclonal antibody to $\alpha$4 integrin that selectively inhibits leukocyte adhesion. A small phase II trial of intravenous natalizumab suggested a benefit in patients with active Crohn's disease,[271] and efficacy was confirmed in a large phase II trial.[272] Large phase III trials of intravenous natalizumab in patients with active Crohn's disease and medically induced remission are under way.

## LDP-02

LDP-02 is a humanized IgG$_1$ monoclonal antibody to $\alpha_4\beta_7$ integrin that selectively inhibits leukocyte adhesion in mucosa. A phase II trial of intravenous LDP-02 failed to achieve the primary endpoint of clinical improvement, but did show efficacy for remission at the highest dose studied.[273]

## ALICAFORSEN (ISIS 2302, ANTISENSE TO ICAM-1)

Alicaforsen (Isis 2302) is a 20-base phosphorothioate oligodeoxynucleotide designed to hybridize to a sequence in the 39 untranslated region of the human ICAM-1 message. The oligonucleotide–RNA heterodimer so formed serves as a substrate for the ubiquitous nuclease RNase-H, with subsequent cleavage and reduction in cell-specific message content and consequent reduction in ICAM-1 expression. A small phase II trial suggested a benefit of intravenous alicaforsen for active Crohn's disease,[274] but a large phase III trial failed to confirm efficacy.[275]

Similarly, a phase II trial failed to demonstrate efficacy of subcutaneous alicaforsen for active Crohn's disease.[276] Subgroup analysis suggested that patients with high blood levels of alicaforsen had a better response,[275] and a dose-ranging pilot study identified a higher dose of intravenous alicaforsen that could achieve high blood levels.[277] Two phase III trials of high-dose intravenous alicaforsen in patients with Crohn's disease are under way (Isis Pharmaceuticals press releases 2002).

## INTERLEUKIN-10

Interleukin-10 (IL-10), a T-helper (Th) type 2 cytokine, suppresses the production of IL-2 and interferon-γ by Th1 cells[278] and decreases IL-12 production and the expression of major histocompatibility molecules by innate immune cells. A small phase II study of intravenous IL-10 in patients with active Crohn's disease suggested benefit.[279] Subsequently, phase II trials of subcutaneous IL-10 in patients with mild to moderately active Crohn's disease[280] and postoperative remission,[281] and phase III trials in patients with chronically active Crohn's disease,[282,283] failed to demonstrate efficacy.

## ANTI-CD4 ANTIBODIES

cM-T412, MAX.16H5 and BF-5 are all monoclonal antibodies to CD4. Pilot studies in patients with active Crohn's disease have suggested some benefit from their use.[284–290] However, no controlled trials have been performed in patients with Crohn's disease.

## INTERFERON-α

The interferon-αs are produced naturally by virally infected cells to induce resistance of the cells to viral infection. Recombinant interferon-$\alpha_{2a}$, interferon-$\alpha_{2b}$ and interferon-$\alpha_n$ are used clinically to treat HIV-related Kaposi's sarcoma, melanoma, chronic hepatitis B infection and chronic hepatitis C infection.[291] Pilot studies with interferon-$\alpha_{2a}$ and interferon-$\alpha_{2b}$ reported benefit in patients with active Crohn's disease.[292–296] Treatment of hepatitis C with interferon-α in patients with Crohn's disease does not lead to relapse or worsening of the disease.[297]

## INTERFERON-$\beta_{1A}$

Interferon-β is produced naturally by virally infected cells to induce resistance of the cells to viral infection. Recombinant interferon-β is used clinically to treat multiple sclerosis.[291] A pilot study of interferon-β in patients with active Crohn's disease reported a beneficial effect.[298] A phase II trial in patients with active Crohn's disease is under way.

## ANTI-INTERFERON-γ ANTIBODY

Increased production of interferon-γ by Th1 cells is part of the process of polarization towards a Th1 immunologic response that is typical of Crohn's disease. Recombinant interferon-γ is used to enhance the killing of phagocytosed bacteria in chronic granulomatous disease.[291] Theoretically, the administration of interferon-γ to patients with Crohn's disease could result in disease exacerbation. However, small pilot studies with intravenous or subcutaneous low-dose recombinant interferon-γ did not result in disease exacerbation.[299,300] On the other hand, a phase II study of huzaf, a monoclonal antibody to interferon-γ, did not show a clear benefit in patients with active Crohn's disease.[301] A larger phase II study of huzaf in patients with active Crohn's disease is under way.

## GRANULOCYTE COLONY-STIMULATING FACTOR (FILGRASTIM) AND GRANULOCYTE–MACROPHAGE COLONY-STIMULATING FACTOR (SARGRAMOSTIM)

Genetic syndromes associated with intestinal inflammation that is phenotypically similar to Crohn's disease include chronic granulomatous disease, glycogen storage disease and Chediak–Higashi syndrome.[302,303] Pilot studies have suggested that filgrastim (human granulocyte colony-stimulating factor, also know as recombinant methionyl human granulocyte colony-stimulating factor, or r-metHuG-CSF) and sargramostim (human granulocyte–macrophage colony-stimulating factor, also known as recombinant human granulocyte–macrophage colony-stimulating factor or RhuGM-CSF) may have a beneficial effect in patients with active and fistulizing Crohn's disease, perhaps through an immunostimulant effect on neutrophils.[304,305] A phase II trial with sargramostim in patients with active Crohn's disease is under way.

## BACILLE CALMETTE–GUÉRIN VACCINE

Bacille Calmette–Guérin (BCG) is an immunostimulant that is used to vaccinate against tuberculosis and to treat transitional cell carcinoma of the bladder. Two placebo-controlled trials of BCG vaccine as a treatment for active Crohn's disease failed to demonstrate efficacy.[306,307]

## HUMAN GROWTH HORMONE

Growth hormone (GH) is a regulatory peptide that increases amino acid and electrolyte uptake by the intestines, decreases intestinal permeability and induces the expression of insulin-like growth factor I, which in turn stimulates collagen synthesis. The rationale for the use of growth hormone in Crohn's disease is to reverse the catabolic process associated with inflammation. A small placebo-controlled trial of recombinant human growth hormone (somatropin) plus a high-protein diet in patients with active Crohn's disease demonstrated a greater decrease in the mean CDAI score for somatropin-treated patients than for placebo-treated patients.[308] The rates of remission were not reported. Additional controlled trials are needed.

## INTERLEUKIN-11

Interleukin-11 (IL-11) is a cytokine produced by cells of mesenchymal origin with multiple biologic effects, including thrombocytopoiesis and enhancement of the barrier function of intestinal mucosa. Two placebo-controlled trials of subcutaneous IL-11 in patients with active Crohn's disease failed to clearly demonstrate efficacy.[309,310] IL-11 is stable in the gastrointestinal lumen and an oral formulation has been developed.[311] A phase II study of oral IL-11 in patients with active Crohn's disease is under way.

## MISCELLANEOUS AGENTS

### LEVAMISOLE

Levamisole is an antihelminthic agent. It also has immunostimulatory properties and is used as an adjuvant therapy with 5-fluorouracil for the treatment of colorectal cancer. Five placebo-controlled trials of levamisole in patients with active Crohn's disease failed to demonstrate efficacy.[312–31]

## DISODIUM CROMOGLYCATE

Disodium cromoglycate is a mast cell stabilizer that is used to treat allergic diseases. Three placebo-controlled trials failed to demonstrate efficacy of disodium cromoglycate for the treatment of active Crohn's disease.[317–319]

## ZINC

A controlled trial of zinc failed to demonstrate efficacy for the treatment of active Crohn's disease.[320]

## APHERESIS

A controlled trial of lymphapheresis in patients with active Crohn's disease was negative.[321] Apheresis columns and techniques have subsequently advanced, with reported success in ulcerative colitis. Pilot studies with these newer apheresis columns have reported benefit in patients with active Crohn's disease.[322–325] Sham-controlled trials are needed.

## FISH OIL

Fish oil (eicosapentanoic acid and docosahexenoic acid) inhibits 5-lipoxygenase and other enzymes involved in arachidonate metabolism. Small controlled trials of oral ω-3 fatty acids and omega-3 fatty acids failed to demonstrate a benefit for fish oil in patients with active Crohn's disease or medically induced remission.[326,327] In contrast, two placebo-controlled trials of enteric-coated fish oil (enteric coating improves tolerability) demonstrated efficacy in patients with Crohn's disease and both medically induced remission and postoperative remission.[328,329] Two large phase III trials in patients with Crohn's disease in medically induced remission are under way.

# TREATMENT INDICATIONS AND ALGORITHM AND SPECIFIC TREATMENT APPROACHES

The indications for therapy in patients with Crohn's disease are summarized in Table 34.5 and suggested treatment algorithms for induction of remission in patients with mild to moderately active disease, refractory disease, perianal fistula and postoperative remission are proposed in Figures 34.2–34.6. The specific approaches to induction and maintenance of remission in patients with mild to moderately active Crohn's disease, refractory disease including steroid-dependent disease, severely active disease, perianal fistulizing disease and postoperative remission are each reviewed separately below.

## TRADITIONAL NON-EVIDENCE BASED APPROACH TO INDUCTION AND MAINTENANCE OF REMISSION IN MILD TO MODERATE CROHN'S DISEASE

As discussed above, oral mesalamine and antibiotics have not consistently demonstrated efficacy in controlled trials. Nevertheless, current practice guideline recommend a stepwise approach that includes these agents for induction and maintenance of remission in patients with mild to moderately active Crohn's disease, beginning with oral mesalamine or sulfasalazine, adding antibiotics such as metronidazole or ciprofloxacin, then progressing to budesonide, and finally using oral corticosteroids in patients who fail to respond to the initial first line-therapies.[4]

### Table 34.5 Crohn's disease: evidence-based indications for treatment

| Drug | Mildly to moderately active | | Refractory and severely active | | Perianal fistulae | | Postoperative maintenance |
|---|---|---|---|---|---|---|---|
| | Induction | Maintenance | Induction | Maintenance | Induction | Maintenance | |
| Sulfasalazine | Yes | No | No | No | No data | No data | No |
| Oral mesalamine | No[1] | No[1] | No data | No | No data | No data | No[1] |
| Olsalazine | No data | No | No data | No data | No data | No data | No data |
| Oral corticosteroids | Yes | No | Yes | No | No data | No data | No |
| Intravenous corticosteroids | No data | No data | Yes | No data | No data | No data | No data |
| Budesonide | Yes | No[2] | No data | Yes[2] | No data | No data | No |
| Antibiotics | No[1] | No data | No data | No data | Yes[3] | No data | No[4] |
| Azathioprine/ 6-mercaptopurine | No[5] | No[6] | No[5] | Yes | No[5] | Yes | Yes |
| Methotrexate | No data | No data | No[5] | Yes | No data | No data | No data |
| Cyclosporin | No data | No data | No | No | Yes[7] | No data | No data |
| Tacrolimus | No data | No data | No data | No data | Yes | No data | No data |
| Infliximab | No data | No data | Yes | Yes | Yes | Yes | No data |

1 Recommended in current practice guidelines and widely used in clinical practice. Evidence for controlled clinical trials does not consistently support efficacy.
2 Budesonide 6 mg/day significantly increases the time to relapse but does not meet the conventional criteria for maintenance of remission at 1 year in patients with medically induced remission. Budesonide 6 mg is effective as a steroid-sparing agent in patients who are dependent of prednisone or prednisolone.
3 Recommended in current practice guidelines and widely used in clinical practice. Evidence is based on uncontrolled studies only, no controlled trials ever performed.
4 Studies have showed short-term reduction in recurrence of severe endoscopic lesions, no difference in clinical remission rates at 1 year.
5 Slow onset of action precludes use as induction agent.
6 Toxicity profile of agent precludes use for this indication.
7 Evidence is based on uncontrolled studies only, no controlled trials ever performed.

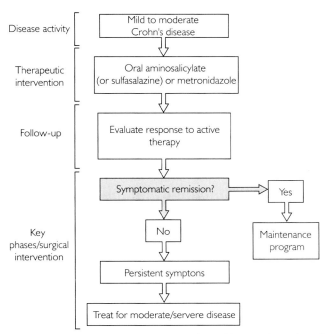

Fig. 34.2 Suggested treatment algorithm for mild to moderately active Crohn's disease using the traditional approach to induction.

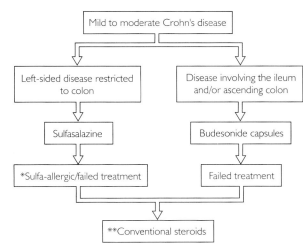

Fig. 34.3 Suggested treatment algorithm for mild to moderately active Crohn's disease using the new evidence-based approach to induction. * Indicates metronidazole and/or ciprofloxacin as a possible alternative if the patient is intolerant of or fails sulfasalazine, although evidence is based on only a few small studies. ** Indicates that if the patient is not improving, need to reclassify as moderate to severe disease and evaluate for treatment with infliximab, immunomodulators or surgery.

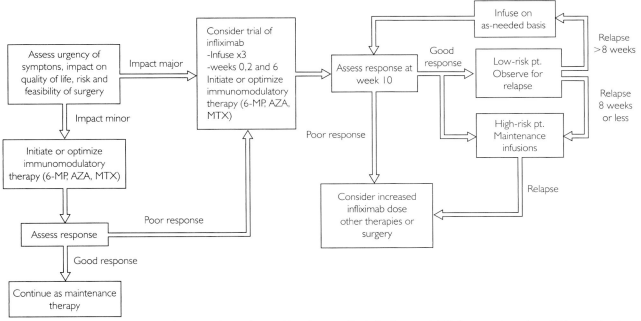

Fig. 34.4 Suggested treatment algorithm for managing patients with refractory Crohn's disease. 6-MP, 6-mercaptopurine; AZA, azathioprine; MTX, methotrexate. Reproduced with permission from Sands BE. Therapy of inflammatory bowel disease. Gastroenterology 2000;118:S68–S82.

The following paragraph outlines this traditional approach to treatment (Fig. 34.2).

Oral mesalamine 3.2–4.0 g/day or sulfasalazine 3–6 g/day are used as first-line treatments for active disease. Sulfasalazine therapy is associated with more side effects and requires activation in the colon, but is less expensive than oral mesalamine. Pentasa should be given to those patients with extensive small bowel Crohn's disease, as it delivers 5-aminosalicylate throughout the small bowel and colon, whereas Asacol, Salofalk, Mesasal and Claversal only deliver 5-aminosalicylate to the distal ileum and colon. No trials have ever demonstrated efficacy for oral mesalamine at doses less than 3.2 g/day in patients with active Crohn's disease. Therefore, if oral mesalamine is selected patients should always be treated at a dose greater than or equal to 3.2 g/day. When treatment with one of these agents has failed, then metronidazole 750–1500 mg/day (10–20 mg/kg) or ciprofloxacin 1000 mg/day is added to the oral mesalamine or sulfasalazine (this approach may be considered more strongly in those patients with colonic involvement). For patients with Crohn's disease involving the terminal ileum and/or right colon

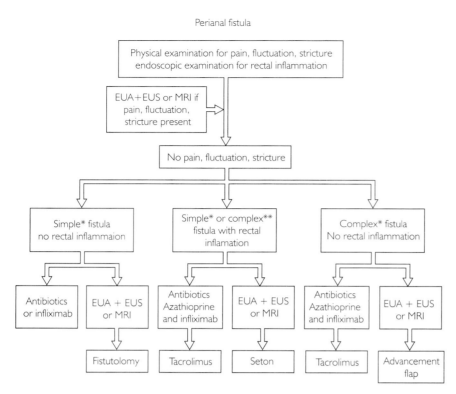

Perianal fistula

Fig. 34.5 Suggested treatment algorithm for managing patients with Crohn's perianal fistulae. EUA, examination under anesthesia; EUS, anorectal endoscopic ultrasound; MRI, pelvic magnetic resonance imaging. A simple fistula* is low, has a single external opening, and does not have associated perianal abscess, rectovaginal fistula, anorectal stricture or macroscopically evident rectal inflammation. A complex fistula** is high and/or has multiple external openings, perianal abscess, rectovaginal fistula, anorectal stricture or macroscopic evidence of rectal inflammation.

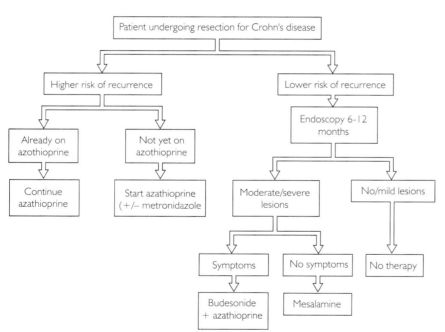

Fig. 34.6 Suggested treatment algorithm for the approach to patients operated on for Crohn's disease using the new evidence-based approach.

who continue to have active symptoms, budesonide can be added at a dose of 9 mg/day for 8–16 weeks and then discontinued over 2–4 weeks by tapering in 3 mg increments. When treatment with all of these agents has failed, then oral prednisone is added to the oral mesalamine or sulfasalazine and the antibiotic. Budesonide should be discontinued without tapering if prednisone therapy is initiated. The preferred initial prednisone dosing regimen is 40–60 mg/day (North American approach) or prednisolone 1 mg/kg/day (European approach) administered as a single dose. The optimal tapering strategy has not been determined, but experienced clinicians will typically treat the patient with prednisone 40 mg/day for 2–4 weeks, then taper by 5 mg/week to a daily dose of 20 mg/day, then slow the taper to 2.5 mg/week until prednisone is discontinued. There is no evidence that a more prolonged taper over 4–6 months improves the long-term outcome, and such an approach leads to greater steroid exposure.[96]

Once the patient has achieved clinical remission, a long-term maintenance strategy is undertaken to avoid relapse. Oral therapy with a drug that delivers 5-aminosalicylate to the colon is the first-line treatment. The results of placebo-controlled trials of oral mesalamine for maintenance of medically induced remission have been mixed, with some studies showing efficacy for Asacol 2.4 g/day, Pentasa 2 g/day and Salofalk/Claversal 1 g/day, and other studies showing no benefit for Asacol 2.4 g/day, Pentasa 2–4 g/day, and Salofalk/Mesasal/Claversal 1.5–3 g/day. Similarly, the results of placebo-controlled trials of sulfasalazine at doses of 1.5–3.0 g/day for maintenance of medically induced remission have uniformly shown no benefit. These disparate results make dose selection for maintenance of remission difficult. Clinicians typically use oral mesalamine at doses of 2.4–4.8 g/day and sulfasalazine 2–4 g/day as first-line maintenance treatments. Sulfasalazine therapy is associated with more side effects but is less expensive than oral mesalamine. There is no agreement among expert clinicians as to whether patients with Crohn's disease should taper oral mesalamine or sulfasalazine to the lowest effective dose, or instead continue maintenance therapy with the same dose required to induce remission. The former strategy is less expensive and may improve patient compliance by reducing the amount and frequency of medication administered, whereas the latter may result in effective maintenance of remission in a larger proportion of patients. There are no controlled trials of antibiotics as maintenance therapy for patients with Crohn's disease in medically induced remission. Nevertheless, long-term treatment with metronidazole 500–750 mg/day or ciprofloxacin 500–1000 mg/day is often undertaken in those patients in whom induction of remission therapy with an antibiotic was deemed successful. Patients treated with metronidazole maintenance therapy should be warned about the risk of peripheral neuropathy and instructed to report any compatible symptoms immediately. Clinical trials have demonstrated that oral corticosteroids at low to moderate doses are not effective for maintaining remission. Nevertheless, some patients who respond to higher doses of prednisone will relapse with steroid tapering and can be maintained nearly asymptomatic by increasing the prednisone dose back to 10–30 mg/day. These patients are classified as steroid dependent. Because of the toxicity associated with long-term corticosteroid use this is not an acceptable form of maintenance therapy, and such patients should be treated for refractory disease as described below. Similarly, clinical trials have demonstrated that budesonide 6 mg prolongs the time to relapse but is not effective for maintaining remission at 1 year. Nevertheless, some patients who respond to budesonide 9 mg relapse with budesonide tapering and can be maintained by increasing the budesonide dose back to 6–9 mg/day. According to the traditional, non-evidence based view of treatment for mild to moderately active Crohn's disease, these patients are also classified as steroid dependent and treated similarly to prednisone-dependent patients.

## NEW EVIDENCE-BASED APPROACH TO INDUCTION AND MAINTENANCE OF REMISSION IN MILD TO MODERATE CROHN'S DISEASE

As discussed above, controlled trials with sulfasalazine 3–6 g/day in patients with mild to moderately active Crohn's disease have consistently demonstrated modest efficacy, with subgroup analysis demonstrating that this benefit is limited to patients with colonic involvement. In contrast, oral mesalamine at doses up to 4 g/day and antibiotics in patients with mild to moderately active Crohn's disease have not consistently demonstrated efficacy in controlled trials, whereas controlled trials of budesonide 9 mg/day in patients with ileal and/or right colonic

involvement have consistently demonstrated efficacy compared with both placebo and oral mesalamine 9 mg/day. Based on these results, a new evidence-based treatment algorithm can be developed which may be preferable to the current non-evidence based treatment guidelines (Fig. 34.3). The following paragraph outlines this new approach to induction treatment.

Budesonide 9 mg/day and sulfasalazine 3–6 g/day are used as first-line treatments for active disease. Sulfasalazine therapy is associated with more side effects and requires activation in the colon (subgroup analysis suggests that efficacy is largely limited to patients with colonic involvement) but is less expensive than budesonide. Sulfasalazine is used as induction therapy for up to 16 weeks. Budesonide is only effective in patients with terminal ileal and/or right colon involvement. Budesonide is used at a dose of 9 mg/day for 8–16 weeks and then discontinued over 2–4 weeks by tapering in 3 mg increments. Oral mesalamine and antibiotics are never used because they are not effective. When treatment with one of these agents has failed, then oral prednisone should be initiated. Sulfasalazine should be discontinued if prednisone is initiated because controlled trials have shown no adjunctive value of sulfasalazine in prednisone-treated patients.[11,15] Similarly, budesonide should be discontinued without tapering because it is a steroid, and there is no evidence of a dose response above the starting dose of prednisone or prednisolone. The preferred initial prednisone dosing regimen is 40–60 mg/day (North American approach) or 1 mg/kg/day (European approach) administered as a single dose. The optimal tapering strategy has not been determined, but experienced clinicians will typically treat the patient with prednisone 40 mg/day for 2–4 weeks, then taper by 5 mg/week to a daily dose of 20 mg/day, then slow the taper to 2.5 mg/week until the drug is discontinued. There is no evidence that a more prolonged taper over 4–6 months improves the long-term outcome, and such an approach leads to greater steroid exposure.[96]

As discussed above, controlled trials with sulfasalazine 1.5–3 g/day uniformly showed no benefit in patients with Crohn's disease in medically induced remission, and controlled trials of oral mesalamine 1.0–3.0 g/day have not consistently demonstrated efficacy, with most studies showing no benefit. No maintenance trials with antibiotics have been performed. Clinical trials have demonstrated that budesonide 6 mg prolongs the time to relapse but is not effective for maintaining remission at 1 year, and that oral corticosteroids at low to moderate doses are not effective for maintaining remission. Maintenance therapy with azathioprine, 6-MP, methotrexate and infliximab may not be appropriate in this patient population because of their respective toxicity profiles. Based on these results, a new evidence-based treatment algorithm can be developed which may be preferable to the current non-evidence based treatment guidelines. The following paragraph outlines this new approach to maintenance treatment.

Following successful induction treatment with sulfasalazine, budesonide or prednisone, all therapy is discontinued after a total of 8–16 weeks. Patients are instructed to report any recurrence of clinical symptoms, and are observed off therapy. If patients relapse early, within 6–12 months after discontinuation of sulfasalazine or prednisone, they should receive another cycle of induction therapy and begin maintenance treatment with one of the slow onset of action immunosuppressive agents azathioprine, 6-MP or methotrexate, as described below in the section on refractory disease. Patients who relapse during taper of prednisone but can be maintained nearly asymptomatic by increasing the dose back to 10–30 mg/ day are classified as steroid dependent. Because of the toxicity associated with long-term corticosteroid use this is not an acceptable form of maintenance therapy, and such patients should also be started on immunosuppressive maintenance therapy with azathioprine, 6-MP or methotrexate. As an alternative to long-term immunosuppressive therapy, these patients can also be switched to maintenance therapy with budesonide 6 mg/day (see below). Patients who relapse early, within 6–12 months after discontinuation of budesonide, and patients who relapse during taper of budesonide but can be maintained by increasing the dose to 6–9 mg/day, may be handled differently from those treated with sulfasalazine or prednisone. Controlled trials have demonstrated that budesonide 6 mg/day prolongs the time to relapse and is effective for maintaining remission in steroid-dependent patients (which includes budesonide-dependent patients), that budesonide adjusted from 0 to 9 mg/day according to disease activity can maintain remission in a majority of patients, and that long-term treatment with budesonide 6–9 mg/day is safe and does not result in osteoporosis. Thus, long-term treatment with budesonide 6–9 mg/day may be an alternative to long-term immunosuppressive therapy in budesonide-treated patients who experience an early relapse or who become budesonide dependent. If patients have a late relapse (more than 6–12 months after discontinuation of sulfasalazine, budesonide or prednisone) then they should receive another cycle of induction therapy without necessarily beginning maintenance therapy.

## REFRACTORY CROHN'S DISEASE

Patients with mild to moderately active Crohn's disease who fail to respond to oral prednisone at dose of 40–60 mg/day can be considered to have moderately active refractory Crohn's disease. It is important to exclude high-grade partial obstruction, internal fistulae complicated by abdominal abscess, or non-inflammatory conditions such as irritable bowel syndrome and bile acid-induced diarrhea following ileal resection as the cause of symptoms. An algorithm of the treatment approach to refractory disease is shown in Figure 34.4. One potential approach to treatment is hospitalization for intravenous administration of corticosteroids. The rationale for this approach is a clinical trial that demonstrated greater mean serum prednisolone concentrations with intravenous than with oral dosing.[102]

The mainstay of treatment in patients who have failed therapy with oral corticosteroids is azathioprine, 6-MP or methotrexate. The prodrug azathioprine is approximately 50% 6-MP by molecular weight, requiring a conversion factor of 2 to convert a dose of azathioprine to a therapeutically equivalent dose of 6-MP. The doses of azathioprine and 6-MP shown to be effective for Crohn's disease in controlled trials are 2.0–3.0 mg/kg/day and 1.5 mg/kg/day, respectively. For patients with normal azathioprine and 6-MP metabolism (based on normal thiopurine methyltransferase (TPMT) activity or genotype), a starting azathioprine dose of 2.0–2.5 mg/kg/day or 6-MP 1.0–1.5 mg/kg/day is recommended (see Chapter 32 for further details). Patients with decreased TPMT activity or intermediate TPMT activity genotype should have their starting azathioprine or 6-MP dose reduced by 50% to 1.0–1.25 mg/kg/day and 0.5–0.75 mg/kg/day, respectively. Patients with absent TPMT activity should not be treated with azathioprine or 6-MP. The

dose of methotrexate shown to be effective for inducing remission and steroid discontinuation in patients with active steroid-treated Crohn's disease in controlled trials is 25 mg/week administered intramuscularly or subcutaneously. After 16 weeks of methotrexate therapy at 25 mg/week, tapering to 15 mg/week (again administered intramuscularly or subcutaneously) for long-term maintenance therapy can be attempted. For patients who relapse on methotrexate 15 mg/week, another induction cycle of prednisone combined with an increase in the methotrexate dose to 25 mg/week, and continuation of methotrexate at 25 mg/week for the long term, can be attempted. Azathioprine, 6-MP and methotrexate are slow-acting antimetabolite drugs, requiring at least 1–2 months, and perhaps 3–4 months for azathioprine and 6-MP and 6-8 weeks for methotrexate, to reach the full clinical effect. Thus, concomitant therapy with corticosteroids should not be tapered below a dose of 15–20 mg/day for 2–3 months in patients who are beginning azathioprine or 6-MP and 1.5–2 months in patients who are beginning methotrexate. Concomitant therapy with mesalamine or sulfasalazine, and/or antibiotics should be discontinued in most cases because there is no evidence that these agents have any adjunctive benefit in patients treated with immunosuppressives. Measurement of a total leukocyte count every 1–2 months as long as patients are receiving azathioprine, 6-MP or methotrexate is mandatory to monitor for leukopenia. Measurement of liver transaminase enzymes every 1–1.5 months as long as patients are receiving methotrexate is mandatory to monitor for hepatotoxicity. Patients without risk factors for methotrexate hepatotoxicity (obesity, excessive alcohol use, diabetes) who have normal liver transaminase values do not need liver biopsy. Patients who do have risk factors for methotrexate hepatotoxicity should undergo liver biopsy prior to treatment with methotrexate and after every 1.5 g of cumulative methotrexate. Patients without risk factors who have elevated liver transaminase values at baseline or who develop persistently elevated liver transaminase values during treatment should also undergo liver biopsy. Indications for treatment with azathioprine or 6-MP in patients with Crohn's disease include maintenance of remission in those who have failed maintenance therapy with first-line agents (sulfasalazine, oral mesalamine or antibiotics) or observation; induction of remission in steroid-refractory disease and steroid sparing in steroid-dependent disease; fistula closure and maintenance of fistula closure; and maintenance of postoperative remission in high-risk patients (previously failed postoperative maintenance therapy with sulfasalazine, oral mesalamine or antibiotics; multiple surgeries; smokers; extensive resection) or patients who develop severe endoscopic recurrence under observation. Indications for methotrexate include maintenance of remission in patients who have failed maintenance therapy with first-line agents (sulfasalazine, oral mesalamine or antibiotics) or observation, induction of remission in steroid-refractory disease, and steroid sparing in steroid-dependent disease.

Infliximab should primarily be used in patients with active Crohn's disease refractory to corticosteroids and immunosuppressive agents. The recommended induction regimen for infliximab is three doses of 5 mg/kg administered at 0, 2 and 6 weeks. Once infliximab is initiated, the relapse rate following discontinuation is approximately 80% at 1 year and, as noted below, discontinuation of infliximab leads to an increased rate of HACA formation that may limit the benefit and tolerability of future therapy. Thus, patients should be carefully selected for initiation of infliximab therapy, and in most instances, once infliximab is initiated it should be continued indefinitely in responding patients as an every-8-week 5 mg/kg maintenance therapy. Patients who initially respond to infliximab 5 mg/kg and later lose their response may benefit from dose escalation by either increasing the dose to 10 mg/kg or shortening the interval for a 5 mg/kg dose to every 4–6 weeks. Concomitant therapy with mesalamine or sulfasalazine, antibiotics, budesonide and prednisone should be discontinued in most patients treated with infliximab because there is no evidence that these agents have any adjunctive benefit. Infliximab is immunogenic, and a strategy to minimize HACA formation, thereby minimizing the risk of loss of response and infusion reactions, should be employed in every patient treated. Treatment for a clinically relevant period of time with azathioprine or 6-MP (2–3 months) or methotrexate (1.5–2 months) prior to initiating infliximab, and subsequent long-term continuation of the same immunosuppressive agent as concomitant therapy, is protective against HACA formation and is recommended in all patients who can tolerate one of the available immunosuppressive agents. Three-dose induction therapy followed by maintenance therapy, and pretreatment with 200 mg intravenous hydrocortisone, is also protective against HACA formation. No specific toxicity monitoring is required for infliximab, but clinicians should be vigilant for serious infections, including unusual opportunistic infections such as fungal infections and tuberculosis. Indications for treatment with infliximab in patients with chronically active and treatment-refractory or fistulizing Crohn's disease include induction of remission, closure of abdominal and perianal enterocutaneous fistulae, maintenance of infliximab-induced remission, maintence of enterocutaneous fistula closure, and steroid sparing.

## SEVERE CROHN'S DISEASE

Severe Crohn's disease can include severely active or toxic enteritis or colitis, and complications of megacolon, small bowel obstruction and abdominal abscess. Severely active enteritis or colitis presents variably as severe abdominal pain and/or severe diarrhea complicated by tachycardia, dehydration, severe anemia and fever. Toxic enteritis or colitis results from transmural inflammation, presenting as severe disease with the additional finding of focal visceral tenderness to deep palpation, with guarding and rebound. Megacolon is defined as dilatation of the colon (5–6 cm or more) demonstrated by X-ray and presenting clinically as abdominal distension, decreased or absent bowel sounds, and in some cases decreased stool frequency. Small bowel obstruction can result from fibrosis or adhesions, presenting as nausea, vomiting, abdominal distension and abdominal pain. Abdominal abscess resulting from a contained perforation or internal fistula from bowel affected by Crohn's disease presents variably as a tender palpable abdominal mass, abdominal pain, fever and sepsis. Hospitalization is mandatory in patients with suspected severe or toxic enteritis or colitis, megacolon, small bowel obstruction or abdominal abscess. For patients with severe or toxic enteritis or colitis, the treatment regimen outlined by Shepherd and Jewell,[106] consisting of intravenous fluids, electrolyte supplements, bowel rest, transfusion if indicated, intravenous antibiotics and intravenous corticosteroids, remains in use today. Infliximab is often used in patients with severe disease who fail intravenous corticosteroids, although published data are lacking. Patients with bowel obstruction should undergo exploratory laparotomy and patients with abdominal abscess should undergo CT or ultrasound-guided drainage, with subsequent bowel resection in most instances.

Some patients hospitalized with severe Crohn's disease can continue to receive a normal diet. However, patients with toxic colitis or enteritis, megacolon and small bowel obstruction should be made nil by mouth because of the potential for imminent surgical intervention. Peripheral or central intravenous nutrition should be instituted if there is evidence of malnutrition. The goal of intravenous nutrition is primarily to replace nutritional deficits, although bowel rest may occasionally be therapeutic. Factors that have been implicated in the development of toxic megacolon should be avoided in patients with severe Crohn's colitis, including barium enema, narcotic antidiarrheals (codeine, tincture of opium, loperamide and diphenoxylate), anticholinergic agents, antidepressants and electrolyte imbalance. Patients should be monitored frequently. Abdominal X-ray may be indicated daily in patients with severe Crohn's colitis and twice daily in patients with megacolon. Frequent physical examination by both an experienced gastroenterologist and a surgeon is also of great importance, as is frequent monitoring of the complete blood count, electrolytes and nutritional parameters.

Mesalamine and sulfasalazine should usually be temporarily discontinued in patients hospitalized with severe or toxic Crohn's enteritis or colitis because of the possibility of a drug-induced exacerbation of Crohn's disease, which can be indistinguishable from a flare of Crohn's disease. No controlled clinical trials of antibiotics in the treatment of severe Crohn's enteritis or colitis have been performed. Many authorities advocate broad-spectrum antibiotic therapy with either a combination of metronidazole, an aminoglycoside and a broad-spectrum penicillin, or with a third-generation cephalosporin. Intravenous corticosteroid therapy should be initiated with hydrocortisone 300–400 mg/day or methylprednisolone 40–60 mg/day. There are no controlled data to determine the frequency of administration, but a pharmacokinetic study showed that corticosteroid blood levels are better maintained within the presumptive therapeutic range when administered as a continuous infusion rather than as intermittent bolus therapy. There is no advantage of intravenous ACTH over conventional corticosteroids in patients with Crohn's disease. Patients with severe Crohn's enteritis or colitis who fail to respond to 7–10 days of intravenous corticosteroid therapy, and who fail the addition of infliximab after approximately 5 days, should undergo surgical resection.

## PERIANAL FISTULIZING CROHN'S DISEASE

In addition to perianal fistulae, a variety of other fistulae may occur in patients with Crohn's disease, including enteroenteric, enterocutaneous, enterovesical and rectovaginal fistulae; the medical management of these other types is discussed elsewhere (see Chapter 49). Perianal fistulae can be classified as simple or complex. Simple perianal fistulae are low, have a single external opening, and do not have associated perianal abscess, rectovaginal fistula, anorectal stricture or macroscopically evident rectal inflammation, whereas complex fistulae are high and/or have multiple external openings, perianal abscess, rectovaginal fistula, anorectal stricture, or macroscopic evidence of rectal inflammation.

The treatment goal for patients with simple fistulae should be cure, without the requirement for long-term maintenance therapy administered primarily to suppress fistula recurrence. Potential treatments for simple fistulae include antibiotics, infliximab and surgical fistulotomy (Fig. 34.5). Antibiotics are widely used to treat simple fistulae, and are recommended in practice guidelines and previous treatment algorithms[4,7] but have not been evaluated in placebo-controlled trials. Infliximab has been proved effective in placebo-controlled trials both to reduce the number of draining fistulae and to maintain that reduction; however, concomitant immunosuppressive therapy is required to prevent the formation of HACA, and serious infections may occur. Surgeons frequently treat simple fistulae by fistulotomy: this procedure results in a high rate of durable healing. However, surgical series have been small, there are no controlled trials comparing fistulotomy to sham operation or medical therapy, and some patients fail to heal and may require proctectomy. There is insufficient evidence to make an unequivocal recommendation as to whether antibiotics, infliximab or fistulotomy is the best strategy for simple fistulae. Azathioprine and 6-MP are not appropriate for simple fistulae because they act slowly and are primarily maintenance rather than induction drugs. Likewise, tacrolimus and cyclosporin are not appropriate for simple fistulae because of toxicity.

The treatment goal for patients with complex fistulae is typically fistula closure and then suppression of recurrence. Potential treatments for complex fistulae include antibiotics, azathioprine and 6-MP, infliximab, tacrolimus and cyclosporin, and surgery (dilation of anal strictures, placement of non-cutting setons, endorectal advancement flap, repair of rectovaginal fistulae, fecal diversion and proctectomy (see Fig. 34.4). Antibiotics are widely used to treat complex fistulae, and are recommended in practice guidelines and treatment algorithms[4,7] but have not been evaluated in placebo-controlled trials. Relapse rates for complex fistulae are high after antibiotic therapy is discontinued, and their use is adjunctive in combination with other medical agents in this setting. Similarly, the immunosuppressive medications azathioprine and 6-MP have been used to treat complex fistulae, and are recommended in practice guidelines[4] but have not been evaluated in placebo-controlled trials where treatment of fistulae was the primary endpoint. These agents are slow acting, and thus are of more use for maintaining fistula closure than for the initial reduction in the number of draining fistulae. In contrast to antibiotics and immunosuppressive medications, infliximab has been proved effective in placebo-controlled trials for reducing the number of draining fistulae and maintenance of that reduction; although concomitant immunosuppressive therapy to prevent the formation of HACA is required and serious infections may occur, these factors are of less consequence in patients with complex perianal fistulae, who have an otherwise poor prognosis. Tacrolimus and cyclosporin can be used on a limited basis in patients with complex fistulae who have failed other medical therapies, including infliximab.[4] However, these agents should be used with caution because of the risk of nephrotoxicity. Surgical therapy for complex perianal disease is palliative. Perianal abscesses should be drained and anal strictures dilated. Non-cutting setons can be placed in fistula tracts and endorectal advancement flap procedures for high perianal fistulae and rectovaginal fistulae can be performed. The recurrence rates following removal of non-cutting setons and endorectal advancement flap procedures are relatively high. Setons can be left in place indefinitely, but many patients dislike

this option. Because infliximab therapy can completely close all fistula tracks in many patients with complex fistulae, this is now the initial treatment of choice. Routine surgical examination under anesthesia and seton placement prior to initiating infliximab therapy is not required, although such an approach may improve treatment outcomes. Patients with complex fistulae who fail treatment with infliximab should undergo pelvic imaging with anorectal endoscopic ultrasound or pelvic MRI, as well as examination under anesthesia with placement of setons as indicated, while continuing treatment with infliximab, azathioprine or 6-MP and antibiotics. Tacrolimus or cyclosporin can be considered in patients who fail this multimodality approach. As a last resort, fecal diversion or proctectomy may be undertaken.

## POSTOPERATIVE MAINTENANCE OF REMISSION

As discussed above, oral mesalamine, antibiotics and 6-MP have not consistently demonstrated clinically relevant efficacy (maintenance of clinical remission) in controlled trials of maintenance therapy following ileocolonic resection. Nevertheless, current practice guidelines recommend these agents for postoperative maintenance of remission.[4] The following paragraph outlines this traditional approach to treatment.

Oral therapy with a drug that delivers 5-aminosalicylate to the terminal ileum and colon is the first-line treatment. The results of placebo-controlled trials of oral mesalamine for postoperative maintenance remission have been mixed, with some studies showing efficacy for Asacol 2.4 g/day or Salofalk 3 g/day, and other studies showing no benefit for Pentasa 3–4 g/day and Claversal 3 g/day. Similarly, the results of placebo-controlled trials of sulfasalazine at doses of 1.5–3.0 g/day for postoperative maintenance of remission have uniformly shown no benefit. These disparate results make dose selection difficult. Clinicians typically use oral mesalamine at doses of 3.0–4.8 g/day and sulfasalazine 2–4 g/day as first-line maintenance treatments. Sulfasalazine therapy is associated with more side effects but is less expensive than oral mesalamine. The only controlled trial of antibiotics for postoperative maintenance of remission evaluated metronidazole 1500 mg/day for 3 months compared to placebo and demonstrated a significantly reduced rate of severe endoscopic recurrence at 3 months but no difference in clinical relapse rates after 1 year. Nevertheless, long-term treatment with metronidazole 500–750 mg/day or ciprofloxacin 500–1000 mg/day is often undertaken as postoperative maintenance therapy. Patients treated with metronidazole maintenance therapy should be warned about the risk of peripheral neuropathy and instructed to report any compatible symptoms immediately. Clinical trials have demonstrated that oral corticosteroids at low to moderate doses and budesonide 6 mg are not effective for maintaining postoperative remission. A single small controlled trial demonstrated that 6-MP 50 mg/day was more effective than placebo or oral mesalamine 4 g/day for postoperative maintenance. However, when adjusted for multiple statistical comparisons, these results were not significant. Nevertheless, long-term treatment with azathioprine 2.0–3.0 mg/kg/day or 6-MP 1.0–1.5 mg/kg/day is often undertaken as postoperative maintenance therapy, particularly in patients deemed to be at high risk for recurrence or for significant sequelae from subsequent surgical resection (previously failed postoperative maintenance therapy with sulfasalazine, oral mesalamine or antibiotics; multiple surgeries; internal fistulae, smokers; extensive resection). Given the lack of controlled evidence that any of these therapies is effective for postoperative maintenance, a new alterative management strategy that is more evidence based is to discontinue all medical therapy after surgical resection and perform a follow-up colonoscopy at 6–12 months to evaluate for findings of severe endoscopic recurrence (Fig. 34.6). Patients previously treated with azathioprine, patients who become symptomatic, and asymptomatic patients with findings of severe endoscopic recurrence at the follow-up colonoscopy[330] can be treated with azathioprine or 6-MP.

## CONCLUSIONS

Initial treatment of mild to moderately active Crohn's disease may be sulfasalazine, budesonide or oral corticosteroids. Patients with persistent mild-to-moderate symptoms of Crohn's disease despite these therapies (treatment refractory) may require azathioprine, 6-MP or methotrexate, and in some cases infliximab or intravenous corticosteroids. Patients with severely active Crohn's disease should be treated with intravenous corticosteroids, and infliximab in those who do not respond. Patients who relapse following discontinuation of induction therapy should be maintained with azathioprine, 6-MP or methotrexate, and in some cases with budesonide or infliximab. Perianal fistulae should be treated with antibiotics, azathioprine, 6-MP, infliximab or perianal surgery, and in some cases cyclosporin or tacrolimus. Patients undergoing ileocolonic resection should discontinue medications postoperatively; those already taking azathioprine, those with severe endoscopic recurrence at 6–12 months, and those judged to be at high risk should be treated with azathioprine or 6-MP.

## REFERENCES

1. Tremaine WJ, Sandborn WJ. Practice guidelines for inflammatory bowel disease: an instrument for assessment. Mayo Clin Proc 1999;74:495–501.
2. Munkholm P, Langholz E, Nielsen OH, Kreiner S, Binder V. Incidence and prevalence of Crohn's disease in the county of Copenhagen, 1962–87: a sixfold increase in incidence. Scand J Gastroenterol 1992;27:609–614.
3. Farmer RG, Hawk WA, Turnbull RB Jr. Clinical patterns in Crohn's disease: a statistical study of 615 cases. Gastroenterology 1975;68:627–635.
4. Hanauer SB, Sandborn W. The Practice Parameters Committee of the American College of Gastroenterology. Management of Crohn's disease in adults. Am J Gastroenterol 2001;96:635–643.
5. Best WR, Becktel JM, Singleton JW, Kern F Jr. Development of a Crohn's disease activity index. National Cooperative Crohn's Disease Study. Gastroenterology 1976;70:439–444.
6. Sandborn WJ, Feagan BG, Hanauer SB et al. A review of activity indices and efficacy endpoints for clinical trials of medical therapy in adults with Crohn's disease. Gastroenterology 2002;122:512–530.
7. Schwartz DA, Pemberton JH, Sandborn WJ. Diagnosis and treatment of perianal fistulae in Crohn disease. Ann Intern Med 2001;135:906–918.
8. Svartz N. Salazopyrin, a new sulfanilamide preparation: A. Therapeutic results in rheumatic polyarthritis. B. Therapeutic results in ulcerative colitis. C. Toxic manifestations in treatment with sulfanilamide preparation. Acta Med Scand 1942;110:557–590.
9. Anthonisen P, Barany F, Folkenborg O et al. The clinical effect of salazosulphapyridine (Salazopyrin r) in Crohn's disease. A controlled double-blind study. Scand J Gastroenterol 1974;9:549–554.
10. Summers RW, Switz DM, Sessions JT Jr et al. National Cooperative Crohn's Disease Study: results of drug treatment. Gastroenterology 1979;77:847–869.
11. Malchow H, Ewe K, Brandes JW et al. European Cooperative Crohn's Disease Study (ECCDS): results of drug treatment. Gastroenterology 1984;86:249–266.
12. Van Hees PA, Van Lier HJ, Van Elteren PH et al. Effect of sulphasalazine in patients with active Crohn's disease: a controlled double-blind study. Gut 1981;22:404–409.
13. Rosen A, Ursing B, Alm T et al. A comparative study of metronidazole and sulfasalazine for active Crohn's disease: the cooperative Crohn's disease study in Sweden. I. Design and methodologic considerations. Gastroenterology 1982;83:541–549.
14. Ursing B, Alm T, Barany F et al. A comparative study of metronidazole and sulfasalazine for active Crohn's disease: the cooperative Crohn's disease study in Sweden. II. Result. Gastroenterology 1982;83:550–562.
15. Singleton JW, Summers RW, Kern F Jr et al. A trial of sulfasalazine as adjunctive therapy in Crohn's disease. Gastroenterology 1979;77:887–897.
16. Rijk MC, van Hogezand RA, van Lier HJ, van Tongeren JH. Sulphasalazine and prednisone compared with sulphasalazine for treating active Crohn disease. A double-blind, randomized, multicenter trial. Ann Intern Med 1991;114:445–450.
17. Lennard-Jones JE. Sulphasalazine in asymptomatic Crohn's disease. A multicentre trial. Gut 1977;18:69–72.
18. Bergman L, Krause U. Postoperative treatment with corticosteroids and salazosulphapyridine (Salazopyrin) after radical resection for Crohn's disease. Scand J Gastroenterol 1976;11:651–656.
19. Wenckert A, Kristensen M, Eklund AE et al. The long-term prophylactic effect of salazosulphapyridine (Salazopyrin) in primarily resected patients with Crohn's disease. A controlled double-blind trial. Scand J Gastroenterol 1978;13:161–167.
20. Ewe K, Herfarth C, Malchow H, Jesdinsky HJ. Postoperative recurrence of Crohn's disease in relation to radicality of operation and sulfasalazine prophylaxis: a multicenter trial. Digestion 1989;42:224–232.
21. Das K, Eastwood M, McManus J, Sircus W. The metabolism of salicylazosulphapyridine in ulcerative colitis. II. The relationship between metabolites and the progress of the disease studied in out-patients. Gut 1973;14:637–641.
22. Peppercorn MA, Goldman P. The role of intestinal bacteria in the metabolism of salicylazosulfapyridine. J Pharmacol Exp Ther 1972;181:555–562.
23. Azad Khan AK, Guthrie G, Johnston HH, Truelove SC, Williamson DH. Tissue and bacterial splitting of sulphasalazine. Clin Sci (Lond) 1983;64:349–354.
24. Das K, Eastwood MA, McManus JP, Sircus W. The metabolism of salicylazosulphapyridine in ulcerative colitis. I. The relationship between metabolites and the response to treatment in inpatients. Gut 1973;14:631–641.
25. Azad Khan AK, Piris J, Truelove SC. An experiment to determine the active therapeutic moiety of sulphasalazine. Lancet 1977;2:892–895.
26. van Hees PA, Bakker JH, van Tongeren JH. Effect of sulphapyridine, 5-aminosalicylic acid, and placebo in patients with idiopathic proctitis: a study to determine the active therapeutic moiety of sulphasalazine. Gut 1980;21:632–635.
27. Klotz U, Maier K, Fischer C, Heinkel K. Therapeutic efficacy of sulfasalazine and its metabolites in patients with ulcerative colitis and Crohn's disease. N Engl J Med 1980;303:1499–1502.
28. Das KM, Eastwood MA, McManus JP, Sircus W. Adverse reactions during salicylazosulfapyridine therapy and the relation with drug metabolism and acetylator phenotype. N Engl J Med 1973;289:491–495.
29. Taffet SL, Das KM. Sulfasalazine. Adverse effects and desensitization. Dig Dis Sci 1983;28:833–842.
30. Shanahan F, Targan S. Sulfasalazine and salicylate-induced exacerbation of ulcerative colitis. N Engl J Med 1987;317:455.
31. Tremaine WJ, Schroeder KW, Harrison JM, Zinsmeister AR. A randomized, double-blind, placebo-controlled trial of the oral mesalamine (5-ASA) preparation, Asacol, in the treatment of symptomatic Crohn's colitis and ileocolitis. J Clin Gastroenterol 1994;19:278–282.
32. Singleton JW, Hanauer SB, Gitnick GL et al. Mesalamine capsules for the treatment of active Crohn's disease: results of a 16-week trial. Pentasa Crohn's Disease Study Group. Gastroenterology 1993;104:1293–1301.
33. Mahida YR, Jewell DP. Slow-release 5-amino-salicylic acid (Pentasa) for the treatment of active Crohn's disease. Digestion 1990;45:88–92.
34. Rasmussen SN, Lauritsen K, Tage-Jensen U et al. 5-Aminosalicylic acid in the treatment of Crohn's disease. A 16-week double-blind, placebo-controlled, multicentre study with Pentasa. Scand J Gastroenterol 1987;22:877–883.
35. Singleton J. Second trial of mesalamine therapy in the treatment of active Crohn's disease. Gastroenterology 1994;107:632–633.
36. Hanauer SB, Stromberg U. Efficacy of oral Pentasa 4 g/day in treatment of active Crohn's disease: a meta-analysis of double-blind, placebo-controlled trials. Gastroenterology 2001;120:A-453.
37. Colombel JF, Lemann M, Cassagnou M et al. A controlled trial comparing ciprofloxacin with mesalazine for the treatment of active Crohn's disease. Groupe d'Etudes Therapeutiques des Affections Inflammatoires Digestives (GETAID). Am J Gastroenterol 1999;94:674–678.
38. Prantera C, Cottone M, Pallone F et al. Mesalamine in the treatment of mild to moderate active Crohn's ileitis: results of a randomized, multicenter trial. Gastroenterology 1999;116:521–526.
39. Thomsen OO, Cortot A, Jewell D et al. A comparison of budesonide and mesalamine for active Crohn's disease. International Budesonide–Mesalamine Study group. N Engl J Med 1998;339:370–374.
40. Prantera C, Pallone F, Brunetti G, Cottone M, Miglioli M. Oral 5-aminosalicylic acid (Asacol) in the maintenance treatment of Crohn's disease. The Italian IBD Study Group. Gastroenterology 1992;103:363–368.
41. Gendre JP, Mary JY, Florent C et al. Oral mesalamine (Pentasa) as maintenance treatment in Crohn's disease: a multicenter placebo-controlled study. Groupe d'Etudes Therapeutiques des Affections Inflammatoires Digestives (GETAID). Gastroenterology 1993;104:435–439.

42. Arber N, Odes HS, Fireman Z et al. A controlled double blind multicenter study of the effectiveness of 5-aminosalicylic acid in patients with Crohn's disease in remission. J Clin Gastroenterol 1995;20:203–206.

43. Bresci G, Parisi G, Banti S. Long-term therapy with 5-aminosalicylic acid in Crohn's disease: is it useful? Our four years experience. Int J Clin Pharmacol Res 1994;14:133–138.

44. Brignola C, Iannone P, Pasquali S et al. Placebo-controlled trial of oral 5-ASA in relapse prevention of Crohn's disease. Dig Dis Sci 1992;37:29–32.

45. Modigliani R, Colombel JF, Dupas JL et al. Mesalamine in Crohn's disease with steroid-induced remission: effect on steroid withdrawal and remission maintenance. Groupe d'Etudes Therapeutiques des Affections Inflammatoires Digestives. Gastroenterology 1996;110:688–693.

46. Sutherland LR, Martin F, Bailey RJ et al. A randomized, placebo-controlled, double-blind trial of mesalamine in the maintenance of remission of Crohn's disease. Canadian Mesalamine for Remission of Crohn's Disease Study Group. Gastroenterology 1997;112:1069–1077.

47. International Mesalazine Study Group. Coated oral 5-aminosalicylic acid versus placebo in maintaining remission of inactive Crohn's disease. Aliment Pharmacol Ther 1990;4:55–64.

48. Thomson AB, Wright JP, Vatn M et al. Mesalazine (Mesasal/Claversal) 1.5 g b.d. vs. placebo in the maintenance of remission of patients with Crohn's disease. Aliment Pharmacol Ther 1995;9:673–683.

49. de Franchis R, Omodei P, Ranzi T et al. Controlled trial of oral 5-aminosalicylic acid for the prevention of early relapse in Crohn's disease. Aliment Pharmacol Ther 1997;11:845–852.

50. Caprilli R, Andreoli A, Capurso L et al. Oral mesalazine (5-aminosalicylic acid; Asacol) for the prevention of post-operative recurrence of Crohn's disease. Gruppo Italiano per lo Studio del Colon e del Retto (GISC). Aliment Pharmacol Ther 1994;8:35–43.

51. McLeod RS, Wolff BG, Steinhart AH et al. Prophylactic mesalamine treatment decreases postoperative recurrence of Crohn's disease. Gastroenterology 1995;109:404–413.

52. Brignola C, Cottone M, Pera A et al. Mesalamine in the prevention of endoscopic recurrence after intestinal resection for Crohn's disease. Italian Cooperative Study Group. Gastroenterology 1995;108:345–349.

53. Lochs H, Mayer M, Fleig WE et al. Prophylaxis of postoperative relapse in Crohn's disease with mesalamine: European Cooperative Crohn's Disease Study VI. Gastroenterology 2000;118:264–273.

54. Florent C, Cortot A, Quandale P et al. Placebo-controlled clinical trial of mesalazine in the prevention of early endoscopic recurrences after resection for Crohn's disease. Groupe d'Etudes Therapeutiques des Affections Inflammatoires Digestives (GETAID). Eur J Gastroenterol Hepatol 1996;8:229–233.

55. Camma C, Giunta M, Rosselli M, Cottone M. Mesalamine in the maintenance treatment of Crohn's disease: a meta-analysis adjusted for confounding variables. Gastroenterology 1997;113:1465–1473.

56. Sutherland LR. Mesalamine for the prevention of postoperative recurrence: is nearly there the same as being there? Gastroenterology 2000;118:436–438.

57. Mahmud N, Kamm MA, Dupas JL et al. Olsalazine is not superior to placebo in maintaining remission of inactive Crohn's colitis and ileocolitis: a double blind, parallel, randomised, multicentre study. Gut 2001;49:552–556.

58. Pamukcu R, Hanauer SB, Chang EB. Effect of disodium azodisalicylate on electrolyte transport in rabbit ileum and colon in vitro. Comparison with sulfasalazine and 5-aminosalicylate. Gastroenterology 1988;95:975–981.

59. Bitton A, Peppercorn MA, Hanrahan JP, Upton MP. Mesalamine-induced lung toxicity. Am J Gastroenterol 1996;91:1039–1040.

60. Iaquinto G, Sorrentini I, Petillo FE, Berardesca G. Pleuropericarditis in a patient with ulcerative colitis in longstanding 5-aminosalicylic acid therapy. Ital J Gastroenterol 1994;26:145–147.

61. Deltenre P, Berson A, Marcellin P, Degott C, Biour M, Pessayre D. Mesalazine (5-aminosalicylic acid) induced chronic hepatitis. Gut 1999;44:886–888.

62. Fernandez J, Sala M, Panes J, Feu F, Navarro S, Teres J. Acute pancreatitis after long-term 5-aminosalicylic acid therapy. Am J Gastroenterol 1997;92:2302–2303.

63. Brouillard M, Gheerbrant JD, Gheysens Y et al. [Chronic interstitial nephritis and mesalazine: 3 new cases?]. Gastroenterol Clin Biol 1998;22:724–726.

64. Calvino J, Romero R, Pintos E et al. Mesalazine-associated tubulo-interstitial nephritis in inflammatory bowel disease. Clin Nephrol 1998;49:265–267.

65. Colombel JF, Brabant G, Gubler MC et al. Renal insufficiency in infant: side-effect of prenatal exposure to mesalazine? Lancet 1994;344:620–621.

66. Corrigan G, Stevens PE. Review article: interstitial nephritis associated with the use of mesalazine in inflammatory bowel disease. Aliment Pharmacol Ther 2000;14:1–6.

67. Riley SA, Lloyd DR, Mani V. Tests of renal function in patients with quiescent colitis: effects of drug treatment. Gut 1992;33:1348–1352.

68. Schreiber S, Hamling J, Zehnter E et al. Renal tubular dysfunction in patients with inflammatory bowel disease treated with aminosalicylate. Gut 1997;40:761–766.

69. Izzedine H, Simon J, Piette AM et al. Primary chronic interstitial nephritis in Crohn's disease. Gastroenterology 2002;123:1436–1440.

70. Hanauer SB, Verst-Brasch C, Regalli G. Renal safety of long-term mesalamine therapy in inflammatory bowel disease (IBD). Gastroenterology 1997;112:A991.

71. Marteau P, Nelet F, Le Lu M, Devaux C. Adverse events in patients treated with 5-aminosalicylic acid: 1993–1994 pharmacovigilance report for Pentasa in France. Aliment Pharmacol Ther 1996;10:949–956.

72. Sturgeon JB, Bhatia P, Hermens D, Miner PB Jr. Exacerbation of chronic ulcerative colitis with mesalamine. Gastroenterology 1995;108:1889–1893.

73. O'Morain C, Segal AW, Levi AJ. Elemental diet as primary treatment of acute Crohn's disease: a controlled trial. Br Med J (Clin Res Ed) 1984;288:1859–1862.

74. Saverymuttu S, Hodgson HJ, Chadwick VS. Controlled trial comparing prednisolone with an elemental diet plus non-absorbable antibiotics in active Crohn's disease. Gut 1985;26:994–998.

75. Sanderson IR, Udeen S, Davies PS, Savage MO, Walker-Smith JA. Remission induced by an elemental diet in small bowel Crohn's disease. Arch Dis Child 1987;62:123–127.

76. Malchow H, Steinhardt HJ, Lorenz-Meyer H et al. Feasibility and effectiveness of a defined-formula diet regimen in treating active Crohn's disease. European Cooperative Crohn's Disease Study III. Scand J Gastroenterol 1990;25:235–244.

77. Lochs H, Steinhardt HJ, Klaus-Wentz B et al. Comparison of enteral nutrition and drug treatment in active Crohn's disease. Results of the European Cooperative Crohn's Disease Study. IV. Gastroenterology 1991;101:881–888.

78. Lindor KD, Fleming CR, Burnes JU, Nelson JK, Ilstrup DM. A randomized prospective trial comparing a defined formula diet, corticosteroids, and a defined formula diet plus corticosteroids in active Crohn's disease. Mayo Clin Proc 1992;67:328–333.

79. Gonzalez-Huix F, de Leon R, Fernandez-Banares F et al. Polymeric enteral diets as primary treatment of active Crohn's disease: a prospective steroid controlled trial. Gut 1993;34:778–782.

80. Belli DC, Seidman E, Bouthillier L et al. Chronic intermittent elemental diet improves growth failure in children with Crohn's disease. Gastroenterology 1988;94:603–610.

81. Gorard DA, Hunt JB, Payne-James JJ et al. Initial response and subsequent course of Crohn's disease treated with elemental diet or prednisolone. Gut 1993;34:1198–1202.

82. Zoli G, Care M, Parazza M et al. A randomized controlled study comparing elemental diet and steroid treatment in Crohn's disease. Aliment Pharmacol Ther 1997;11:735–740.

83. Ruuska T, Savilahti E, Maki M, Ormala T, Visakorpi JK. Exclusive whole protein enteral diet versus prednisolone in the treatment of acute Crohn's disease in children. J Pediatr Gastroenterol Nutr 1994;19:175–180.

84. Griffiths AM, Ohlsson A, Sherman PM, Sutherland LR. Meta-analysis of enteral nutrition as a primary treatment of active Crohn's disease. Gastroenterology 1995;108:1056–1067.

85. Prantera C, Zannoni F, Scribano M et al. An antibiotic regimen for the treatment of active Crohn's disease: a randomized, controlled clinical trial of metronidazole plus ciprofloxacin. Am J Gastroenterol 1996;91:328–332.

86. Rutgeerts P, Lofberg R, Malchow H et al. A comparison of budesonide with prednisolone for active Crohn's disease. N Engl J Med 1994;331:842–845.

87. Gross V, Andus T, Caesar I. Oral pH-modified release budesonide versus 6-methylprednisolone in active Crohn's disease. German/Austrian Budesonide Study Group. Eur J Gastroenterol Hepatol 1996;8:905–909.

88. Campieri M, Ferguson A, Doe W, Persson T, Nilsson LG. Oral budesonide is as effective as oral prednisolone in active Crohn's disease. The Global Budesonide Study Group. Gut 1997;41:209–214.

89. Bar-Meir S, Chowers Y, Lavy A et al. Budesonide versus prednisone in the treatment of active Crohn's disease. The Israeli Budesonide Study Group. Gastroenterology 1998;115:835–840.

90. D'Haens G, Verstraete A, Cheyns K, Aerden I, Bouillon R, Rutgeerts P. Bone turnover during short-term therapy with methylprednisolone or budesonide in Crohn's disease. Aliment Pharmacol Ther 1998;12:419–424.

91. Kane SV, Schoenfeld P, Sandborn WJ, Tremaine W, Hofer T, Feagan BG. The effectiveness of budesonide therapy for Crohn's disease. Aliment Pharmacol Ther 2002;16:1509–1517.

92. Baron JH, Connell AM, Kanaghinis TG, Lennard-Jones JE, Avery Jones F. Out-patient treatment of ulcerative colitis. Comparison between three doses of oral prednisone. Br Med J 1962;2:441–443.

93. Modigliani R, Mary JY, Simon JF et al. Clinical, biological, and endoscopic picture of attacks of Crohn's disease. Evolution on prednisolone. groupe d'Etude Therapeutique des Affections Inflammatoires Digestives. Gastroenterology 1990;98:811–818.

94. Landi B, Anh TN, Cortot A et al. Endoscopic monitoring of Crohn's disease treatment: a prospective, randomized clinical trial. Groupe d'Etudes Therapeutiques des Affections Inflammatoires Digestives. Gastroenterology 1992;102:1647–1653.

95. Candy S, Wright J, Gerber M, Adams G, Gerig M, Goodman R. A controlled double blind study of azathioprine in the management of Crohn's disease. Gut 1995;37:674–678.

96. Brignola C, De Simone G, Belloli C et al. Steroid treatment in active Crohn's disease: a comparison between two regimens of different duration. Aliment Pharmacol Ther 1994;8:465–468.

97. Smith RC, Rhodes J, Heatley RV et al. Low dose steroids and clinical relapse in Crohn's disease: a controlled trial. Gut 1978;19:606–610.

98. Munkholm P, Langholz E, Davidsen M, Binder V. Frequency of glucocorticoid resistance and dependency in Crohn's disease. Gut 1994;35:360–362.

99. Faubion WJ, Loftus EJ, Harmsen WS, Zinsmeister AR, Sandborn WJ. The natural history of corticosteroid therapy for inflammatory bowel disease: a population-based study. Gastroenterology 2001;121:255–260.

100. Brignola C, Campieri M, Farruggia P et al. The possible utility of steroids in the prevention of relapses of Crohn's disease in remission. A preliminary study. J Clin Gastroenterol 1988;10:631–634.

101. Shaffer JA, Williams SE, Turnberg LA, Houston JB, Rowland M. Absorption of prednisolone in patients with Crohn's disease. Gut 1983;24:182–186.

102. Berghouse LM, Elliott PR, Lennard-Jones JE, English J, Marks V. Plasma prednisolone levels during intravenous therapy in acute colitis. Gut 1982;23:980–983.

103. Truelove SC, Jewell DP. Intensive intravenous regimen for severe attacks of ulcerative colitis. Lancet 1974;1:1067–1070.

104. Truelove SC, Willoughby CP, Lee EG, Kettlewell MG. Further experience in the treatment of severe attacks of ulcerative colitis. Lancet 1978;2:1086–1088.

105. Jarnerot G, Rolny P, Sandberg-Gertzen H. Intensive intravenous treatment of ulcerative colitis. Gastroenterology 1985;89:1005–1013.

106. Shepherd HA, Barr GD, Jewell DP. Use of an intravenous steroid regimen in the treatment of acute Crohn's disease. J Clin Gastroenterol 1986;8:154–159.

107. Powell-Tuck J, Buckell NA, Lennard-Jones JE. A controlled comparison of corticotropin and hydrocortisone in the treatment of severe proctocolitis. Scand J Gastroenterol 1977;12:971–975.

108. Kaplan HP, Portnoy B, Binder HJ, Amatruda T, Spiro H. A controlled evaluation of intravenous adrenocorticotropic hormone and hydrocortisone in the treatment of acute colitis. Gastroenterology 1975;69:91–95.

109. Meyers S, Sachar DB, Goldberg JD, Janowitz HD. Corticotropin versus hydrocortisone in the intravenous treatment of ulcerative colitis. A prospective, randomized, double-blind clinical trial. Gastroenterology 1983;85:351–357.

110. Chun A, Chadi RM, Korelitz BI et al. Intravenous corticotrophin vs. hydrocortisone in the treatment of hospitalized patients with Crohn's disease: a randomized double-blind study and follow-up. Inflamm Bowel Dis 1998;4:177–181.

111. Ireland A, Rosenberg W, Jewell DP. High dose methylprednisolone in the treatment of active ulcerative colitis. Gastroenterology 1988;29:A1466.

112. Greenberg GR, Feagan BG, Martin F et al. Oral budesonide for active Crohn's disease. Canadian Inflammatory Bowel Disease Study Group. N Engl J Med 1994;331:836–841.

113. Tremaine WJ, Hanauer SB, Katz S et al. Budesonide CIR capsules (once or twice daily divided-dose) in active Crohn's disease: a randomized placebo-controlled study in the United States. Am J Gastroenterol 2002;97:1748–1754.

114. Irvine EJ, Greenberg GR, Feagan BG et al. Quality of life rapidly improves with budesonide therapy for active Crohn's disease. Canadian Inflammatory Bowel Disease Study Group. Inflamm Bowel Dis 2000;6:181–187.

115. Thomsen OO, Cortot A, Jewell D et al. Budesonide and mesalazine in active Crohn's disease: a comparison of the effects on quality of life. Am J Gastroenterol 2002;97:649–653.

116. Steinhart AH, Feagan BG, Wong CJ et al. Combined budesonide and antibiotic therapy for active Crohn's disease: A randomized controlled trial. gastroenterology 2002;123:33–40.

117. Gross V, Caesar I, Andus T et al. and German/Austrian Budesonide Study Group. Dose-finding study or oral budesonide in patients with active Crohn's ileocolitis. Gastroenterology 1997;112:A986.

118. Greenberg GR, Feagan BG, Martin F et al. Oral budesonide as maintenance treatment for Crohn's disease: a placebo-controlled, dose-ranging study. Canadian Inflammatory Bowel Disease Study Group. Gastroenterology 1996;110:45–51.

119. Lofberg R, Rutgeerts P, Malchow H et al. Budesonide prolongs time to relapse in ileal and ileocaecal Crohn's disease. A placebo controlled one year study. Gut 1996;39:82–86.

120. Ferguson A, Campieri M, Doe W, Persson T, Nygard G. Oral budesonide as maintenance therapy in Crohn's disease – results of a 12-month study. Global Budesonide Study Group. Aliment Pharmacol Ther 1998;12:175–183.

121. Hanauer SB, Sandborn WJ, Levine JG, Persson A, Persson T. Budesonide modified release capsules as maintenance treatment in mild to moderate Crohn's disease. Am J Gastroenerol 2001;96:S151.

122. Sandborn WJ, Feagan B, Rutgeerts P et al. Maintenance budesonide capsules for prolongation of time to relapse in Crohn's disease patients with medically induced remission: a pooled analysis of 4 randomized, double-blind, placebo-controlled trials in 380 patients with medically induced remission. Gastroenterology 2003;124:A381.

123. Cortot A, Colombel JF, Rutgeerts P et al. Switch from systemic steroids to budesonide in steroid dependent patients with inactive Crohn's disease. Gut 2001;48:186–190.

124. Mantzaris GJ, Petraki K, Sfakianakis M et al. A comparison of the effect of budesonide and mesalamine on the quality of life in patients with steroid-dependent Crohn's disease. Clin Gastroenterol and Hepatol 2003;1:122–128.

125. Gross V, Caesar I, Andus T et al. Replacement of systemic steroids by oral budesonide in patients with post-active or chronic Crohn's ileocolitis – a dose finding study. Gastroenterology 1997;112:A987.

126. Green JR, Lobo AJ, Giaffer M, Travis S, Watkins HC. Maintenance of Crohn's disease over 12 months: fixed versus flexible dosing regimen using budesonide controlled ileal release capsules. Aliment Pharmacol Ther 2001;15:1331–1341.

127. Schoon E, Bollani S, Mills P et al. Budesonide versus prednisolone: effect on bone mineral density in patients with ileo-cecal Crohn's disease. Am J Gastroenterol 2001;97:272.

128. Mantzaris GJ, Petraki K, Chadio-Iordanides H et al. Maintenance therapy with azathioprine is superior to budesonide in healing endoscopic lesions and improving histology in clinically quiescent Crohn's disease. Gastroenterology 2002;122:A-81.

129. Hellers G, Cortot A, Jewell D et al. Oral budesonide for prevention of postsurgical recurrence in Crohn's disease. The IOIBD Budesonide Study Group. Gastroenterology 1999;116:294–300.

130. Ewe K, Bottger T, Buhr HJ. Ecker KW, Otto HF. Low-dose budesonide treatment for prevention of postoperative recurrence of Crohn's disease: a multicentre randomized placebo-controlled trial. German Budesonide Study Group. Eur J Gastroenterol Hepatol 1999;11:277–282.

131. Wright JP, Jarnum S, Schaffalitzky de Muckadell O, Keech ML, Lennard-Jones JE. Oral fluticasone proprianate compared with prednisolone in treatment of active Crohn's disease: a randomized double-blind multicentre study. Eur J Gastroenterol Hepatol 1993;5:499–503.

132. Singleton JW, Law DH, Kelley ML Jr, Mekhjian HS, Sturdevant RA. National Cooperative Crohn's Disease Study: adverse reactions to study drugs. Gastroenterology 1979;77:870–882.

133. Talar-Williams C, Sneller MC. Complications of corticosteroid therapy. Eur Arch Otorhinolaryngol 1994;251:131–136.

134. Whitworth JA. Mechanisms of glucocorticoid-induced hypertension. Kidney Int 1987;31:1213–1224.

135. Gurwitz JH, Bohn RL, Glynn RJ, Monane M, Mogun H, Avorn J. Glucocorticoids and the risk for initiation of hypoglycemic therapy. Arch Intern Med 1994;154:97–101.

136. Stuck AE, Minder CE, Frey FJ. Risk of infectious complications in patients taking glucocorticosteroids. Rev Infect Dis 1989;11:954–963.

137. Mankin HJ. Nontraumatic necrosis of bone (osteonecrosis). N Engl J Med 1992;326:1473–1479.

138. Lukert BP, Raisz LG. Glucocorticoid-induced osteoporosis. Rheum Dis Clin North Am 1994;20:629–650.

139. Lacomis D, Samuels MA. Adverse neurologic effects of glucocorticosteroids. J Gen Intern Med 1991;6:367–377.

140. Urban RC Jr, Dreyer EB. Corticosteroid-induced glaucoma. Int Ophthalmol Clin 1993;33:135–139.

141. Urban RC Jr, Cotlier E. Corticosteroid-induced cataracts. Surv Ophthalmol 1986;31:102–110.

142. Blichfeldt P, Blomhoff JP, Myhre E, Gjone E. Metronidazole in Crohn's disease. A double blind cross-over clinical trial. Scand J Gastroenterol 1978;13:123–127.

143. Ambrose NS, Allan RN, Keighley MR et al. Antibiotic therapy for treatment in relapse of intestinal Crohn's disease. A prospective randomized study. Dis Colon Rectum 1985;28:81–85.

144. Sutherland L, Singleton J, Sessions J et al. Double blind, placebo controlled trial of metronidazole in Crohn's disease. Gut 1991;32:1071–1075.

145. Rutgeerts P, Hiele M, Geboes K et al. Controlled trial of metronidazole treatment for prevention of Crohn's recurrence after ileal resection. Gastroenterology 1995;108:1617–1621.

146. Bernstein LH, Frank MS, Brandt LJ, Boley SJ. Healing of perineal Crohn's disease with metronidazole. Gastroenterology 1980;79:357–365.

147. Brandt LJ, Bernstein LH, Boley SJ, Frank MS. Metronidazole therapy for perineal Crohn's disease: a follow-up study. Gastroenterology 1982;83:383–387.

148. Arnold GL, Beaves MR, Pryjdun VO, Mook WJ. Preliminary study of ciprofloxacin in active Crohn's disease. Inflamm Bowel Dis 2002;8:10–15.

149. Turunen U, Farkkila M, Hakala K et al. Ciprofloxacin treatment combined with conventional therapy in Crohn's disease. A prospective, double blind, placebo controlled study. Gut 1995;37:A193.

150. Turunen U. Farkkila M, Valtonen V. Long-term outcome of ciprofloxacin treatment in severe perianal or fistulous Crohn's disease. Gastroenterology 1993;104:A793.

151. Solomon MJ, McLeod RS, O'Connor BI, Steinhart AH, Greenberg GR, Cohen Z. Combination ciprofloxacin and metronidazole in severe perianal Crohn's disease. Can J Gastroenterol 1993;7:571–573.

152. Afdhal NH, Long A, Lennon J, Crowe J, O'Donoghue DP. Controlled trial of antimycobacterial therapy in Crohn's disease. Clofazimine versus placebo. Dig Dis Sci 1991;36:449–453.

153. Prantera C, Kohn A, Mangiarotti R, Andreoli A, Luzi C. Antimycobacterial therapy in Crohn's disease: results of a controlled, double-blind trial with a multiple antibiotic regimen. Am J Gastroenterol 1994;89:513–518.

154. Shaffer JL, Hughes S, Linaker BD, Baker RD, Turnberg LA. Controlled trial of rifampicin and ethambutol in Crohn's disease. Gut 1984;25:203–205.

155. Swift GL, Srivastava ED, Stone R et al. Controlled trial of anti-tuberculous chemotherapy for two years in Crohn's disease. Gut 1994;35:363–368.

156. Thomas GA, Swift GL, Green JT et al. Controlled trial of antituberculous chemotherapy in Crohn's disease: a five year follow up study. Gut 1998;42:497–500.

157. Elliott PR, Burnham WR, Berghouse LM, Lennard-Jones JE, Langman MJ. Sulphadoxine-pyrimethamine therapy in Crohn's disease. Digestion 1982;23:132–134.

158. Basilisco G, Ranzi T, Campanini MC, Piodi L, Bianchi PA. Controlled trial of rifabutin in Crohn's disease. Curr Ther Res Clin Exp 1989;46:245–250.

159. Rutgeerts P, Geboes K, Vantrappen G et al. Rifabutin and ethambutol do not help recurrent Crohn's disease in the neoterminal ileum. J Clin Gastroenterol 1992;15:24–28.

160. Borgaonkar MR, MacIntosh DG, Fardy JM. A meta-analysis of antimycobacterial therapy for Crohn's disease. Am J Gastroenterol 2000;95:725–729.

161. Prantera C, Scribano ML, Falasco G, Andreoli A, Luzi C. Ineffectiveness of probiotics in preventing recurrence after curative resection for Crohn's disease: a randomised controlled trial with *Lactobacillus GG*. Gut 2002;51:405–409.

162. Plein K, Hotz J. Therapeutic effects of *Saccharomyces boulardii* on mild residual symptoms in a stable phase of Crohn's disease with special respect to chronic diarrhea – a pilot study. Z Gastroenterol 1993;31:129–134.

163. Rhodes J, Bainton D, Beck P, Campbell H. Controlled trial of azathioprine in Crohn's disease. Lancet 1971;2:1273–1276.

164. Klein M, Binder HJ, Mitchell M, Aaronson R, Spiro H. Treatment of Crohn's disease with azathioprine: a controlled evaluation. Gastroenterology 1974;66:916–922.

165. Ewe K, Press AG, Singe CC et al. Azathioprine combined with prednisolone or monotherapy with prednisolone in active Crohn's disease. Gastroenterology 1993;105:367–372.

166. Present DH, Korelitz BI, Wisch N, Glass JL, Sachar DB, Pasternack BS. Treatment of Crohn's disease with 6-mercaptopurine. A long-term, randomized, double-blind study. N Engl J Med 1980;302:981–987.

167. Willoughby JM, Beckett J, Kumar PJ, Dawson AM. Controlled trial of azathioprine in Crohn's disease. Lancet 1971;2:944–947.

168. Oren R, Moshkowitz M, Odes S et al. Methotrexate in chronic active Crohn's disease: a double-blind, randomized, Israeli multicenter trial. Am J Gastroenterol 1997;92:2203–2209.

169. Rosenberg JL, Levin B, Wall AJ, Kirsner JB. A controlled trial of azathioprine in Crohn's disease. Am J Dig Dis 1975;20:721–726.

170. Pearson DC, May GR, Fick GH, Sutherland LR. Azathioprine and 6-mercaptopurine in Crohn disease. A meta-analysis. Ann Intern Med 1995;123:132–142.

171. Korelitz BI, Present DH. Favorable effect of 6-mercaptopurine on fistulae of Crohn's disease. Dig Dis Sci 1985;30:58–64.

172. Sandborn WJ, Tremaine WJ, Wolf DC et al. Lack of effect of intravenous administration on time to respond to azathioprine for steroid-treated Crohn's disease. North American Azathioprine Study Group. Gastroenterology 1999;117:527–535.

173. O'Donoghue DP, Dawson AM, Powell-Tuck J, Bown RL, Lennard-Jones JE. Double-blind withdrawal trial of azathioprine as maintenance treatment for Crohn's disease. Lancet 1978;2:955–957.

174. Markowitz J, Grancher K, Kohn N, Lesser M, Daum F. A multicenter trial of 6-mercaptopurine and prednisone in children with newly diagnosed Crohn's disease. Gastroenterology 2000;119:895–902.

175. Lemann M, Bouhnik Y, Colombel JF et al. Randomized, double-blind, placebo-controlled, multicenter, azathioprine (AZA) withdrawal trial in Crohn's disease (CD). Gastroenterology 2002;122:A23.

176. Mate-Jimenez J, Hermida C, Cantero-Perona J, Moreno-Otero R. 6-mercaptopurine or methotrexate added to prednisone induces and maintains remission in steroid-dependent inflammatory bowel disease. Eur J Gastroenterol Hepatol 2000;12:1227–1233.

177. Bouhnik Y, Lemann M, Mary JY et al. Long-term follow-up of patients with Crohn's disease treated with azathioprine or 6-mercaptopurine. Lancet 1996;347:215–219.

178. Korelitz B, Hanauer SB, Rutgeerts P, Present DH, Peppercorn M, Workgroup CS. Postoperative prophylaxis with 6-MP, 5-ASA or placebo in Crohn's disease: a 2 year multicenter trial. Gastroenterology 1998;114:A1011.

179. Present DH, Meltzer SJ, Krumholz MP, Wolke A, Korelitz BI. 6-Mercaptopurine in the management of inflammatory bowel disease: short-and long-term toxicity. Ann Intern Med 1989;111:641–649.

180. Connell WR, Kamm MA, Ritchie JK, Lennard-Jones JE. Bone marrow toxicity caused by azathioprine in inflammatory bowel disease: 27 years of experience. Gut 1993;34:1081–1085.

181. Kirschner BS. Safety of azathioprine and 6-mercaptopurine in pediatric patients with inflammatory bowel disease. Gastroenterology 1998;115:813–821.

182. Connell WR, Kamm MA, Dickson M, Balkwill AM, Ritchie JK, Lennard-Jones JE. Long-term neoplasia risk after azathioprine treatment in inflammatory bowel disease. Lancet 1994;343:1249–1252.

183. Dayharsh GA, Loftus EV Jr, Sandborn WJ et al. Epstein–Barr virus-positive lymphoma in patients with inflammatory bowel disease treated with azathioprine or 6-mercaptopurine. Gastroenterology 2002;122:72–77.

184. Feagan BG, Rochon J, Fedorak RN et al. Methotrexate for the treatment of Crohn's disease. The North American Crohn's Study Group Investigators. N Engl J Med 1995;332:292–297.

185. Arora S, Katkov W, Cooley J et al. Methotrexate in Crohn's disease: results of a randomized, double-blind, placebo-controlled trial. Hepatogastroenterology 1999;46:1724–1729.

186. Mahadevan U, Marion J, Present D. The place of methotrexate in the treatment of refractory Crohn's disease. Gastroenterology 1997;112:A1031.

187. Feagan BG, Fedorak RN, Irvine EJ et al. A comparison of methotrexate with placebo for the maintenance of remission in Crohn's disease. North American Crohn's Study Group Investigators. N Engl J Med 2000;342:1627–1632.

188. Egan LJ, Sandborn WJ, Tremaine WJ et al. A randomized dose–response and pharmacokinetic study of methotrexate for refractory inflammatory Crohn's disease and ulcerative colitis. Aliment Pharmacol Ther 1999;13:1597–1604.

189. Goodman TA, Polisson RP. Methotrexate: adverse reactions and major toxicities. Rheum Dis Clin North Am 1994;20:513–528.

190. Egan LJ, Sandborn WJ. Methotrexate for inflammatory bowel disease: pharmacology and preliminary results. Mayo Clin Proc 1996;71:69–80.

191. Roenigk HH Jr, Auerbach R, Maibach HI, Weinstein GD. Methotrexate in psoriasis: revised guidelines. J Am Acad Dermatol 1988;19:145–156.

192. Kremer JM, Alarcon GS, Lightfoot RW Jr et al. Methotrexate for rheumatoid arthritis. Suggested guidelines for monitoring liver toxicity. American College of Rheumatology. Arthritis Rheum 1994;37:316–328.

193. Whiting-O'Keefe QE, Fye KH, Sack KD. Methotrexate and histologic hepatic abnormalities: a meta-analysis. Am J Med 1991;90:711–716.

194. Kozarek RA, Bredfeldt JE, Rosoff LE, Patterson DJ, Fenster LF. Does methotrexate (MTX) cause liver toxicity when used for refractory inflammatory bowel disease (IBD)? Gastroenterology;100:A221.

195. Te HS, Schiano TD, Kuan SF, Hanauer SB, Conjeevaram HS, Baker AL. Hepatic effects of long-term methotrexate use in the treatment of inflammatory bowel disease. Am J Gastroenterol 2000;95:3150–3156.

196. Brynskov J, Freund L, Rasmussen SN et al. A placebo-controlled, double-blind, randomized trial of cyclosporin therapy in active chronic Crohn's disease. N Engl J Med 1989;321:845–850.

197. Feagan BG, McDonald JW, Rochon J et al. Low-dose cyclosporin for the treatment of Crohn's disease. The Canadian Crohn's Relapse Prevention Trial Investigators. N Engl J Med 1994;330:1846–1851.

198. Jewell D, Lennard-Jones J and the Cyclosporin Study Group of Great Britain and Ireland. Oral cyclosporin for chronic active Crohn's disease: a multicentre controlled trial. Eur J Gastroenterol Hepatol 1995;5:499–505.

199. Stange EF, Modigliani R, Pena AS, Wood AJ, Feutren G, Smith PR. European trial of cyclosporin in chronic active Crohn's disease: a 12-month study. The European Study Group. Gastroenterology 1995;109:774–782.

200. Sandborn WJ, Present DH, Isaacs KL et al. Tacrolimus (FK506) for the treatment of perianal and enterocutaneous fistulae in patients with Crohn's disease: a randomized, double-blind, placebo-controlled trial. Gastroenterology 2002;122:A81.

201. Fukushima T, Sugita A, Masuzawa S, Yamazaki Y, Tsuchiya S. Effects of cyclosporin A on active Crohn's disease. Gastroenterol Jpn 1989;24:12–15.

202. Lichtiger S. Cyclosporin therapy in inflammatory bowel disease: open-label experience. Mt Sinai J Med 1990;57:315–319.

203. Hanauer SB, Smith MB. Rapid closure of Crohn's disease fistulae with continuous intravenous cyclosporin A. Am J Gastroenterol 1993;88:646–649.

204. Present DH, Lichtiger S. Efficacy of cyclosporin in treatment of fistula of Crohn's disease. Dig Dis Sci 1994;39:374–380.

205. Markowitz J, Rosa J, Grancher K, Aiges H, Daum F. Long-term 6-mercaptopurine treatment in adolescents with Crohn's disease. Gastroenterology 1990;99:1347–1351.

206. Abreu-Martin J, Vasiliauskas E, Gaiennie J, Voigt B, Targan SR. Continuous infusion cyclosporin is effective for acute severe Crohn's disease... but for how long? Gastroenterology 1996;110:A851.

207. O'Neill J, Pathmakanthan S, Goh J et al. Cyclosporin A induces remission in fistulous Crohn's disease but relapse occurs upon cessation of treatment. Gastroenterology 1997;112:A1056.

208. Hinterleitner TA, Petritsch W, Aichbichler B, Fickert P, Ranner G, Krejs GJ. Combination of cyclosporin, azathioprine and prednisolone for perianal fistulae in Crohn's disease. Z Gastroenterol 1997;35:603–608.

209. Egan LJ, Sandborn WJ, Tremaine WJ. Clinical outcome following treatment of refractory inflammatory and fistulizing Crohn's disease with intravenous cyclosporin. Am J Gastroenterol 1998;93:442–448.

210. Gurudu SR, Griffel LH, Gialanella RJ, Das KM. Cyclosporin therapy in inflammatory bowel disease: short-term and long-term results. J Clin Gastroenterol 1999;29:151–154.

211. Sandborn WJ. Preliminary report on the use of oral tacrolimus (FK506) in the treatment of complicated proximal small bowel and fistulizing Crohn's disease. Am J Gastroenterol 1997;92:876–879.

212. Fellermann K, Ludwig D, Stahl M, David-Walek T, Stange EF. Steroid-unresponsive acute attacks of inflammatory bowel disease: immunomodulation by tacrolimus (FK506). Am J Gastroenterol 1998;93:1860–1866.

213. Lowry PW, Weaver AL, Tremaine WJ, Sandborn WJ. Combination therapy with oral tacrolimus (FK506) and azathioprine or 6-mercaptopurine for treatment-refractory Crohn's disease perianal fistulae. Inflamm Bowel Dis 1999;5:239–245.

214. Ierardi E, Principi M, Rendina M et al. Oral tacrolimus (FK 506) in Crohn's disease complicated by fistulae of the perineum. J Clin Gastroenterol 2000;30:200–202.

215. Cohen RD, Stein R, Hanauer SB. Intravenous cyclosporin in ulcerative colitis: a five-year experience. Am J Gastroenterol 1999;94:1587–1592.

216. Sandborn WJ. A critical review of cyclosporin therapy in inflammatory bowel disease. Inflamm Bowel Dis 1995;1:48–63.

217. Stein R, Cohen R, Hanauer S. Complications during cyclosporin therapy for inflammatory bowel disease. Gastroenterology 1997;112:A1096.

218. Sternthal M, George J, Kornbluth A, Present DH. Toxicity associated with the use of cyclosporin in patients with inflammatory bowel disease (IBD). Gastroenterology 1996;110:A1019.

219. Scott AM, Myers GA, Harms BA. *Pneumocystis carinii* pneumonia postrestorative proctocolectomy for ulcerative colitis: a role for perioperative prophylaxis in the

cyclosporin era? Report of a case and review of the literature. Dis Colon Rectum 1997;40:973–976.

220. Quan VA, Saunders BP, Hicks BH, Sladen GE. Cyclosporin treatment for ulcerative colitis complicated by fatal *Pneumocystis carinii* pneumonia. Br Med J 1997;314:363–364.

221. Papadakis KA, Tung JK, Binder SW et al. Outcome of cytomegalovirus infections in patients with inflammatory bowel disease. Am J Gastroenterol 2001;96:2137–2142.

222. Fleshner PR, Michelassi F, Rubin M, Hanauer SB, Plevy SE, Targan SR. Morbidity of subtotal colectomy in patients with severe ulcerative colitis unresponsive to cyclosporin. Dis Colon Rectum 1995;38:1241–1245.

223. Mahadaven U, Kornbluth AA, Goldstein E, George J, Lichtiger S, Present DH. Is cyclosporin (CS) induced nephrotoxicity permanent or progressive in patients with inflammatory bowel disease (IBD)? Gastroenterology 1997;112:A1030.

224. Feutren G, Mihatsch MJ. Risk factors for cyclosporin-induced nephropathy in patients with autoimmune diseases. International Kidney Biopsy Registry of Cyclosporin in Autoimmune Diseases. N Engl J Med 1992;326:1654–1660.

225. Randhawa PS, Shapiro R, Jordan ML, Starzl TE, Demetris AJ. The histopathological changes associated with allograft rejection and drug toxicity in renal transplant recipients maintained on FK506. Clinical significance and comparison with cyclosporin. Am J Surg Pathol 1993;17:60–68.

226. Neurath MF, Wanitschke R, Peters M, Krummenauer F, Meyer zum Buschenfelde KH, Schlaak JF. Randomised trial of mycophenolate mofetil versus azathioprine for treatment of chronic active Crohn's disease. Gut 1999;44:625–628.

227. Hafraoui S, Dewit O, Marteau P et al. [Mycophenolate mofetil in refractory Crohn's disease after failure of treatments by azathioprine or methotrexate]. Gastroenterol Clin Biol 2002;26:17–22.

228. Skelly MM, Logan RF, Jenkins D, Mahida YR, Hawkey CJ. Toxicity of mycophenolate mofetil in patients with inflammatory bowel disease. Inflamm Bowel Dis 2002;8:93–97.

229. Miehsler W, Reinisch W, Moser G, Gangl A, Vogelsang H. Is mycophenolate mofetil an effective alternative in azathioprine-intolerant patients with chronic active Crohn's disease? Am J Gastroenterol 2001;96:782–787.

230. Hassard PV, Vasiliauskas EA, Kam LY, Targan SR, Abreu MT. Efficacy of mycophenolate mofetil in patients failing 6-mercaptopurine or azathioprine therapy for Crohn's disease. Inflamm Bowel Dis 2000;6:16–20.

231. Fellermann K, Steffen M, Stein J et al. Mycophenolate mofetil: lack of efficacy in chronic active inflammatory bowel disease. Aliment Pharmacol Ther 2000;14:171–176.

232. Fickert P, Hinterleitner TA, Wenzl HH, Aichbichler BW, Petritsch W. Mycophenolate mofetil in patients with Crohn's disease. Am J Gastroenterol 1998;93:2529–2532.

233. Targan SR, Hanauer SB, van Deventer SJ et al. A short-term study of chimeric monoclonal antibody cA2 to tumor necrosis factor α for Crohn's disease. Crohn's Disease cA2 Study Group. N Engl J Med 1997;337:1029–1035.

234. Present DH, Rutgeerts P, Targan S et al. Infliximab for the treatment of fistulae in patients with Crohn's disease. N Engl J Med 1999;340:1398–1405.

235. Hanauer SB, Feagan BG, Lichtenstein GR et al. Maintenance infliximab for Crohn's disease: the ACCENT I randomised trial. Lancet 2002;359:1541–1549.

236. Remicade (infliximab) for IV injection. Package Insert 2003.

237. Rutgeerts P, D'Haens G, Targan S et al. Efficacy and safety of retreatment with anti-tumor necrosis factor antibody (infliximab) to maintain remission in Crohn's disease. Gastroenterology 1999;117:761–769.

238. Sands B, Van Deventer S, Bernstein C et al. Long-term treatment of fistulizing Crohn's disease: response to infliximab in the ACCENT II trial through 54 weeks. Gastroenterology 2002;122:A81.

239. Braun J, Brandt J, Listing J et al. Treatment of active ankylosing spondylitis with infliximab: a randomised controlled multicentre trial. Lancet 2002;359:1187–1193.

240. Baert F, Norman M, Vermeire S et al. Influence of immunogenicity on the long-term efficacy of infliximab in Crohn's disease. N Engl J Med 2003;348:601–608.

241. Farrell RJ, Alsahli M, Jeen YTJ, Falchuk KR, Peppercorn MA, Michetti P. Intravenous hydrocortisone premedication to prevent antibodies to infliximab in Crohn's disease: a randomized controlled trial. Gastroenterology 2003;124:917–924.

242. Sandborn WJ, Hanauer SB. Infliximab for the treatment of Crohn's disease: a user's guide. Am J Gastroenterol 2002;97:2962–2972.

243. Schaible TF. Long term safety of infliximab. Can J gastroenterol 2000;14:29C–32C.

244. Hanauer S, Rutgeerts P, Targan S et al. Delayed hypersensitivity to infliximab (Remicade) re-infusion after a 2–4 year interval without treatment. Gastroenterology 1999;116:A731.

245. Colombel JF, Loftus EV Jr, Tremaine WJ et al. The safety profile of infliximab for Crohn's disease in clinical practice: the Mayo Clinic experience in 500 patients. Gastroenterology 2003;124:A7.

246. Vermeire S, Norman M, Van Assche G et al. Autoimmunity associated with antitumor necrosis factor alpha treatment in Crohn's disease: a prospective cohort study. Gastroenterology 2003;125:32–38.

247. Bickston SJ, Lichtenstein GR, Arseneau KO, Cohen RB, Cominelli F. The relationship between infliximab treatment and lymphoma in Crohn's disease. Gastroenterology 1999;117:1433–1437.

248. Sachmechian A, Vasiliauskas E, Abreu M et al. Malignancy following Remicade therapy: incidence and characteristics. Gastroenterology 2001;120:A619.

249. Brown SL, Greene MH, Gershon SK, Edwards ET, Braun MM. Tumor necrosis factor antagonist therapy and lymphoma development: twenty-six cases reported to the Food and Drug Administration. Arthritis Rheum 2002;46:3151–3158.

250. Keane J, Gershon S, Wise RP et al. Tuberculosis associated with infliximab, a tumor necrosis factor alpha-neutralizing agent. N Engl J Med 2001;345:1098–1104.

251. Warris A, Bjorneklett A, Gaustad P. Invasive pulmonary aspergillosis associated with infliximab therapy. N Engl J Med 2001;344:1099–1100.

252. Lee JH, Slifman NR, Gershon SK et al. Life-threatening histoplasmosis complicating immunotherapy with tumor necrosis factor alpha antagonists infliximab and etanercept. Arthritis Rheum 2002;46:2565–2570.

253. Diagnostic Standards and Classification of Tuberculosis in Adults and Children. This official statement of the American Thoracic Society and the Centers for Disease Control and Prevention was adopted by the ATS Board of Directors, July 1999. This statement was endorsed by the Council of the Infectious Disease Society of America, September 1999. Am J Respir Crit Care Med 2000;161:1376–1395.

254. Stack WA, Mann SD, Roy AJ et al. Randomised controlled trial of CDP571 antibody to tumour necrosis factor-alpha in Crohn's disease. Lancet 1997;349:521–524.

255. Sandborn WJ, Feagan BG, Hanauer SB et al. An engineered human antibody to TNF (CDP571) for active Crohn's disease: a randomized double-blind placebo-controlled trial. Gastroenterology 2001;120:1330–1338.

256. Sandborn W, Feagan B, Radford-Smith G, Kovacs A, Enns R, Patel J. A randomized, placebo-controlled trial of CDP571, a humanized monoclonal antibody to TNF-α, in patients with moderate to severe Crohn's disease. Gastroenterology 2003;124:A61.

257. Feagan BG, Sandborn WJ, Baker J et al. A randomized, double-blind, placebo-controlled, multi-center trial of the engineered human antibody to TNF (CDP571) for steroid sparing and maintenance of remission in patients with steroid-dependent Crohn's disease. Gastroenterology 2000;118:A655.

258. Schreiber S, Rutgeerts P, Fedorak R, Khaliq-Kareemi M, Kamm MA, Patel J and the CDP870 Crohn's Disease Study Group. CDP870, a humanized anti-TNF antibody fragment, induces clinical response with remission in patients with active Crohn's disease (CD). Gastroenterology 2003;124:A61.

259. Winter T, Wright J, Ghosh S, Jahnsen J, Patel J. Intravenous CDP870, a humanized anti-TNF antibody fragment, in patients with active Crohn's disease – an exploratory study. Gastroenterology 2003;124:A377.

260. den Broeder A, van de Putte L, Rau R et al. A single dose, placebo controlled study of the fully human anti-tumor necrosis factor-alpha antibody adalimumab (D2E7) in patients with rheumatoid arthritis. J Rheumatol 2002;29:2288–2298.

261. Weinblatt ME, Keystone EC, Furst DE et al. Adalimumab, a fully human anti-tumor necrosis factor alpha monoclonal antibody, for the treatment of rheumatoid arthritis in patients taking concomitant methotrexate: The ARMADA trial. Arthritis Rheum 2003;48:35–45.

262. Rutgeerts P, Lemmens L, Van Assche G, Noman M, Borghini-Fuhrer I, Goedkoop R. Treatment of active Crohn's disease with onercept (recombinant human soluble p55 tumour necrosis factor receptor): results of a randomized, open-label, pilot study. Aliment Pharmacol Ther 2003;17:185–192.

263. D'Haens G, Swijsen C, Noman M et al. Etanercept in the treatment of active refractory Crohn's disease: a single-center pilot trial. Am J Gastroenterol 2001;96:2564–2568.

264. Sandborn WJ, Hanauer SB, Katz S et al. Etanercept for active Crohn's disease: a randomized, double-blind, placebo-controlled trial. Gastroenterology 2001;121:1088–1094.

265. Hommes D, Van Den Blink B, Plasse T et al. Inhibition of stress-activated MAP kinases induces clinical improvement in moderate to severe Crohn's disease. Gastroenterology 2002;122:7–14.

266. Pargellis C, Tong L, Churchill L et al. Inhibition of p38 MAP kinase by utilizing a novel allosteric binding site. Nature Struct Biol 2002;9:268–272.

267. Regan J, Breitfelder S, Cirillo P et al. Pyrazole urea-based inhibitors of p38 MAP kinase: from lead compound to clinical candidate. J Med Chem 2002;45:2994–3008.

268. Vasiliauskas EA, Kam LY, Abreu-Martin MT et al. An open-label pilot study of low-dose thalidomide in chronically active, steroid-dependent Crohn's disease. Gastroenterology 1999;117:1278–1287.

269. Ehrenpreis ED, Kane SV, Cohen LB, Cohen RD, Hanauer SB. Thalidomide therapy for patients with refractory Crohn's disease: an open-label trial. Gastroenterology 1999;117:1271–1277.

270. Sabate JM, Villarejo J, Lemann M, Bonnet J, Allez M, Modigliani R. An open-label study of thalidomide for maintenance therapy in responders to infliximab in chronically active and fistulizing refractory Crohn's disease. Aliment Pharmacol Ther 2002;16:1117–1124.

271. Gordon FH. Lai CW, Hamilton MI et al. A randomized placebo-controlled trial of a humanized monoclonal antibody to α4 integrin in active Crohn's disease. Gastroenterology 2001;121:268–274.

272. Ghosh S, Goldin E, Gordon FH et al. Natalizumab for active Crohn's disease. N Engl J Med 2003;348:24–32.

273. Feagan BG, Greenberg G, Wild G et al. Efficacy and safety of a humanized α4β7 antibody in active Crohn's disease (CD). Gastroenterology 2003;124:A25–26.

274. Yacyshyn BR, Bowen-Yacyshyn MB. Jewell L et al. A placebo-controlled trial of ICAM-1 antisense oligonucleotide in the treatment of Crohn's disease. Gastroenterology 1998;114:1133–1142.

275. Yacyshyn BR, Chey WY, Goff J et al. Double blind, placebo controlled trial of the remission inducing and steroid sparing properties of an ICAM-1 antisense oligodeoxynucleotide, alicaforsen (ISIS 2302), in active steroid dependent Crohn's disease. Gut 2002;51:30–36.

276. Schreiber S, Nikolaus S, Malchow H et al. Absence of efficacy of subcutaneous antisense ICAM-1 treatment of chronic active Crohn's disease. Gastroenterology 2001;120:1339–1346.

277. Yacyshyn BR, Barish C, Goff J et al. Dose ranging pharmacokinetic trial of high-dose alicaforsen (intercellular adhesion molecule-1 antisense oligodeoxynucleotide) (ISIS 2302) in active Crohn's disease. Aliment Pharmacol Ther 2002;16:1761–1770.

278. Fiorentino DF, Bond MW, Mosmann TR. Two types of mouse T helper cell. IV. Th2 clones secrete a factor that inhibits cytokine production by Th1 clones. J Exp Med 1989;170:2081–2095.

279. van Deventer SJ, Elson CO, Fedorak RN. Multiple doses of intravenous interleukin 10 in steroid-refractory Crohn's disease. Crohn's Disease Study Group. Gastroenterology 1997;113:383–389.

280. Fedorak RN, Gangl A, Elson CO et al. Recombinant human interleukin 10 in the treatment of patients with mild to moderately active Crohn's disease. The Interleukin 10 Inflammatory Bowel Disease Cooperative Study Group. Gastroenterology 2000;119:1473–1482.

281. Colombel JF, Rutgeerts P, Malchow H et al. Interleukin 10 (Tenovil) in the prevention of postoperative recurrence of Crohn's disease. Gut 2001;49:42–46.

282. Schreiber S, Fedorak RN, Nielsen OH et al. Safety and efficacy of recombinant human interleukin 10 in chronic active Crohn's disease. Crohn's Disease IL-10 Cooperative Study Group. Gastroenterology 2000;119:1461–1472.

283. Fedorak R, Nielsen O, Williams N et al. Human recombinant interleukin-10 is safe and well tolerated but does not induce remission in steroid dependent Crohn's disease. Gastroenterology 2001;120:A127.

284. Deusch K, Reiter C, Mauthe B, Riethmuller G, Classen M. Chimeric monoclonal anti-CD4 antibody therapy proves effective for treating inflammatory bowel disease. Gastroenterology 1992;102:A615.

285. Deusch K, Mauthe B, Reiter C, Riethmuller G, Classen M. CD4-antibody treatment of inflammatory bowel disease: one-year follow up. Gastroenterology 1993;104:A691.

286. Stronkhorst A, Radema S, Yong SL et al. CD4 antibody treatment in patients with active Crohn's disease: a phase 1 dose finding study. Gut 1997;40:320–327.

287. Emmrich J, Seyfarth M, Fleig WE, Emmrich F. Treatment of inflammatory bowel disease with anti-CD4 monoclonal antibody. Lancet 1991;338:570–571.

288. Emmrich J, Seyfarth M, Fleig WE, Emmrich F. Treatment of inflammatory bowel diesease with anti-CD4 monoclonalantibody. Gastroenterology 1992;102:A620.

289. Emmrich J, Seyfarth M, Liebe S, Emmrich F. Anti-CD4-antibody treatment in inflammatory bowel disease without a long CD4+-cell depletion. Gastroenterology 1995;108:A815.

290. Canva-Delcambre V, Jacquot S, Robinet E et al. Treatment of severe Crohn's disease with anti-CD4 monoclonal antibody. Aliment Pharmacol Ther 1996;10:721–727.

291. Baron S, Tyring SK, Fleischmann WR Jr et al. The interferons. Mechanisms of action and clinical applications. JAMA 1991;266:1375–1383.

292. Hanauer S, Baert F, Robinson M. Interferon treatment in mild to moderate active Crohn's disease: preliminary results of an open label pilot study. Gastroenterology 1994;106:A696.

293. Hadziselimovic F, Schaub U, Emmons LR. Interferon alpha-2A (roferon) as a treatment of inflammatory bowel disease in children and adolescents. Adv Exp Med Biol 1995;6:1323–1326.

294. Wirth HP, Zala G, Meyenberger C, Jost R, Ammann R, Munch R. [Alpha-interferon therapy in Crohn's disease: initial clinical results]. Schweiz Med Wochenschr 1993;123:1384–1388.

295. Davidsen B, Munkholm P, Schlichting P, Nielsen OH, Krarup H, Bonnevie-Nielsen V. Tolerability of interferon alpha-2b, a possible new treatment of active Crohn's disease. Aliment Pharmacol Ther 1995;9:75–79.

296. Gasche C, Reinisch W, Vogelsang H et al. Prospective evaluation of interferon-alpha in treatment of chronic active Crohn's disease. Dig Dis Sci 1995;40:800–804.

297. Cottone M, Magliocco A, Trallori G et al. Clinical course of inflammatory bowel disease during treatment with interferon for associated chronic active hepatitis. Ital J Gastroenterol 1995;27:3–4.

298. Vantrappen G, Coremans G, Billiau A, De Somer P. Treatment of Crohn's disease with interferon. A preliminary clinical trial. Acta Clin Belg 1980;35:238–242.

299. Yoshida T, Higa A, Sakamoto H et al. Immunological and clinical effects of interferon-gamma on Crohn's disease. J Clin Lab Immunol 1988;25:105–108.

300. Debinski H, Forbes A, Kamm MA. Low dose interferon gamma for refractory Crohn's disease. Ital J Gastroenterol Hepatol 1997;29:403–406.

301. Rutgeerts P, Reinisch W, Colombel JF et al. Preliminary results of a phase I/II study of Huzaf, an anti-INF-gamma monoclonal antibody, in patients with moderate to severe active Crohn's disease. Gastroenterology 2002;122:A61.

302. Korzenik JR, Dieckgraefe BK. Is Crohn's disease an immunodeficiency? A hypothesis suggesting possible early events in the pathogenesis of Crohn's disease. Dig Dis Sci 2000;45:1121–1129.

303. Dieckgraefe BK, Korzenik JR, Husain A, Dieruf L. Association of glycogen storage disease 1b and Crohn's disease: results of a North American survey. Eur J Pediatr 2002;161:S88–92.

304. Dieckgraefe BK, Korzenik JR. Treatment of active Crohn's disease with recombinant human granulocyte–macrophage colony-stimulating factor. Lancet 2002;360:1478–1480.

305. Korzenik J, Dieckgraefe B. Immunostimulation in Crohn's disease: results of a pilot study of G-CSF (R-Methug-CSF) in mucosal and fistulizing Crohn's disease. Gastroenterology 2000;118:A874.

306. Burnham WR, Lennard-Jones JE, Hecketsweiler P, Colin R, Geffroy Y. Oral BCG vaccine in Crohn's disease. Gut 1979;20:229–233.

307. Rahban S, Sherman JH, Opelz G et al. BCG treatment of Crohn's disease. Am J Gastroenterol 1979;71:196–201.

308. Slonim AE, Bulone L, Damore MB, Goldberg T, Wingertzahn MA, McKinley MJ. A preliminary study of growth hormone therapy for Crohn's disease. N Engl J Med 2000;342:1633–1637.

309. Sands BE, Bank S, Sninsky CA et al. Preliminary evaluation of safety and activity of recombinant human interleukin 11 in patients with active Crohn's disease. Gastroenterology 1999;117:58–64.

310. Sands BE, Winston BD, Salzberg B et al. Randomized, controlled trial of recombinant human interleukin-11 in patients with active Crohn's disease. Aliment Pharmacol Ther 2002;16:399–406.

311. Cotreau MM, Stonis L, Schwertschlag US. A phase 1, randomized, double-blind, placebo-controlled, dose-escalating, safety, tolerability, pharmacokinetic, and pharmacodynamic study of oral recombinant human interleukin eleven (O-rhIL-11) in normal healthy subjects. Gastroenterology 2003;124:A377.

312. Segal AW, Levi AJ, Loewi G. Levamisole in the treatment of Crohn's disease. Lancet 1977;2:382–385.

313. Wesdorp E, Schellekens PT, Weening RS, Meuwissen SG, Tytgat GN. Levamisole in Crohn's disease – a double-blind controlled trial. Digestion 1978;18:186–191.

314. Sachar DB, Rubin KP, Gumaste V. Levamisole in Crohn's disease: a randomized, double-blind, placebo-controlled clinical trial. Am J Gastroenterol 1987;82:536–539.

315. Vicary FR, Chambers JD, Dhillon P. Double-blind trial of the use of transfer factor in the treatment of Crohn's disease. Gut 1979;20:408–413.

316. Modigliani R, Pieddeloup C, Hecketsweiler P et al. [Effect of levamisole on the prevention of developmental flare-ups in quiescent Crohn's disease: a prospective multicenter controlled trial in 155 patients]. Gastroenterol Clin Biol 1983;7:683–692.

317. Williams SE, Grundman MJ, Baker RD, Turnberg LA. A controlled trial of disodium cromoglycate in the treatment of Crohn's disease. Digestion 1980;20:395–398.

318. Binder V, Elsborg L, Greibe J et al. Disodium cromoglycate in the treatment of ulcerative colitis and Crohn's disease. Gut 1981;22:55–60.

319. Franchi F, Meneghelli S, Seminara P, Spadini M, Bonomo R. [Failure of disodium cromoglycate in the treatment of 17 patients with chronic inflammatory diseases of the intestine. An occasion to review the pathogenetic problems of ulcerative rectocolitis and Crohn's disease]. Minerva Dietol Gastroenterol 1982;28:285–291.

320. Van de Wal Y, Van der Sluys Veer A, Verspaget HW et al. Effect of zinc therapy on natural killer cell activity in inflammatory bowel disease. Aliment Pharmacol Ther 1993;7:281–286.

321. Lerebours E, Bussel A, Modigliani R et al. Treatment of Crohn's disease by lymphocyte apheresis: a randomized controlled trial. Groupe d'Etudes Therapeutiques des Affections Inflammatoires Digestives. Gastroenterology 1994;107:357–361.

322. Kawamura A, Saitoh M, Yonekawa M et al. New technique of leukocytapheresis by the use of nonwoven polyester fiber filter for inflammatory bowel disease. Ther Apher 1999;3:334–337.

323. Kosaka T, Sawada K, Ohnishi K et al. Effect of leukocytapheresis therapy using a leukocyte removal filter in Crohn's disease. Intern Med 1999;38:102–111.

324. Sawada K, Ohnishi K, Kosaka T et al. Leukocytapheresis therapy with leukocyte removal filter for inflammatory bowel disease. J Gastroenterol 1995;30:124–127.

325. Sawada K, Ohnishi K, Fukui S et al. Leukocytapheresis therapy, performed with leukocyte removal filter, for inflammatory bowel disease. J Gastroenterol 1995;30:322–329.

326. Lorenz R, Weber PC, Szimnau P, Heldwein W, Strasser T, Loeschke K. Supplementation with n-3 fatty acids from fish oil in chronic inflammatory bowel disease – a randomized, placebo-controlled, double-blind cross-over trial. J Intern Med 1989;225:225–232.

327. Lorenz-Meyer H, Bauer P, Nicolay C et al. Omega-3 fatty acids and low carbohydrate diet for maintenance of remission in Crohn's disease. A randomized controlled multicenter trial. Study Group Members (German Crohn's Disease Study Group). Scand J Gastroenterol 1996;31:778–785.

328. Belluzzi A, Brignola C, Campieri M, Pera A, Boschi S, Miglioli M. Effect of an enteric-coated fish-oil preparation on relapses in Crohn's disease. N Engl J Med 1996;334:1557–1560.

329. Belluzzi A, Campieri M, Belloli C et al. A new enteric coated preparation of omega-3 fatty acids for preventing post-surgical recurrence in Crohn's disease. Gastroenterology 1997;112:A930.

330. Rutgeerts P, geboes K, Vantrappen G, Beyls J, Kerremans R, Hiele M. Predictability of the postoperative course of Crohn's disease. Gastroenterology 1990;99:956–963.

## CHAPTER 35

# Medical and nutritional therapy for pediatric inflammatory bowel disease

Kent C Williams and George D Ferry

## INTRODUCTION

The medical management of inflammatory bowel disease (IBD) in pediatric patients presents many challenges. Although the clinical manifestations and severity of IBD vary from patient to patient, having a chronic disease interferes almost universally with family function. Moreover, the complexity of IBD is often magnified in the growing and developing pediatric patient.

Clinically, Crohn's disease (CD) and ulcerative colitis (UC) may present with problems that are specific to children, such as growth failure, with or without malnutrition.[1-4] In addition, Crohn's disease, and to a lesser extent, ulcerative colitis, can cause pubertal delay, bone demineralization and impaired psychological development in adolescence. Medical treatment itself may have adverse affects in each of these areas. Corticosteroids are strongly disliked by children and parents because of their negative effect on growth, and cosmetic side effects such as moon face, acne and general body appearance.[5] In a cross-cultural study, 53 British and 117 Canadian children were asked to rank their top 50 disease-related concerns. Being concerned or upset about how they looked due to their bowel condition and its treatment was number 5 for the British children and number 14 for the Canadian children (see Table 35.1).[6]

A chronic disease such as IBD greatly affects the social, psychological and emotional development of children.[7,8] Children may refuse to sleep over at a peer's house, or may be unable to engage in sports owing to a lack of energy, abdominal pain or diarrhea.[9] Studies have documented increased school absences, social problems and disruptions in the lives of other family members of pediatric IBD patients.[9-11]

This chapter will deal with medical and nutritional therapy in pediatric IBD, but all of the above issues must be borne in mind when treating children with IBD. The primary goals in pediatric patients are the same as for adults: to induce and maintain clinical remission, alleviate gastrointestinal and systemic symptoms, and avoid complications. Pediatric gastroenterologists also focus on maintaining or restoring linear growth and development, avoiding bone mineral loss, encouraging psychological, emotional and social development, and providing strong family support.

## EVALUATION OF THE PEDIATRIC PATIENT

Although the basic evaluation of a patient with suspected IBD is similar at any age in terms of ruling out infection, localizing the extent of disease, and characterizing extraintestinal manifestations, there are additional items that are essential in children. Evaluation of linear growth at the time of diagnosis, along with growth percentiles and body mass index (BMI), is important in establishing therapeutic goals. Obtaining prior growth data and parental height is valuable in predicting a child's true growth potential, an important issue in therapeutic strategy. Because adult bone mineral density is directly related to deposition of bone calcium during adolescence, evaluation for osteopenia or osteoporosis should be considered, even when exposure to corticosteroids is minimal. These and other issues are outlined in Table 35.2.

## PHARMACOLOGICAL AGENTS USED IN PEDIATRIC PATIENTS

Most of the clinical trials evaluating medical therapy of IBD have been performed in adults and the results extrapolated to pediatric patients. This section will review the different pharmacological agents used to treat children with both Crohn's disease (CD) and ulcerative colitis (UC). Although there are relatively few clinical trials in pediatric IBD, those studies that are available will be discussed. Our approach to the actual use of these

**Table 35.1 Top 15 of 50 disease-related concerns of 117 children from Canada with IBD***

| 1 | Feeling bothered by having to take medicines |
|---|---|
| 2 | Feeling worried about the possibility of having a flare-up |
| 3 | Feeling upset that your bowel condition is a lifelong condition |
| 4 | Being concerned about your weight |
| 5 | Feeling worried about health problems you might have in the future |
| 6 | Feeling bothered about your height |
| 7 | Feeling bothered about the stomach pains or cramps |
| 8 | Feeling you have to give up doing things because of your bowel condition |
| 9 | Feeling that you don't have the energy to do the things you want |
| 10 | Feeling that it is unfair that you have IBD |
| 11 | Stomach pains or cramps |
| 12 | Feeling tired |
| 13 | Feeling frustrated because of your bowel condition |
| 14 | Being concerned or upset about the way you look because of your bowel condition or its treatment |
| 15 | Feeling worried about needing surgery |

*From Richardson G et al. J Pediatr J Gastroenterol Nutr 2001;32:573–578.

**Table 35.2 Evaluation of the pediatric patient with IBD**

Establish disease location – important for long-term management. Should include a UGI/small bowel series and colonoscopy. An upper endoscopy should be performed in patients with upper intestinal symptoms

Evaluate growth with current and prior heights and weights – use growth charts, and when necessary, growth velocity charts

Evaluate nutrition and use BMI (body mass index) charts

Include use of complementary and alternative therapy in initial evaluation and follow-up

Evaluate puberty and growth potential with Tanner staging and, when needed, bone age films

Evaluate bone density, especially with a history of corticosteroid use

Evaluate social history, family dynamics and school performance

---

agents, individually and in combination, is discussed in later sections for both Crohn's disease and ulcerative colitis.

## AMINOSALICYLATES

Sulfasalazine was the first aminosalicylate to be used in the treatment of IBD.[12] Because sulfasalazine reaches the colon intact, where the colonic bacteria reduce and break down the azo bond between the sulfa and 5-aminosalicylic acid moieties, the anti-inflammatory properties of the 5-ASA component are best utilized in inflammation in the large intestine. Sulfasalazine is also effective against CD, as long as the majority of the affected intestine is located in the colon. Two large multicenter trials of primarily adult patients showed that sulfasalazine induced remission better than a placebo in Crohn's patients whose disease was located in the ileocolon and colon, but was ineffective if the disease was isolated in the small bowel.[13,14]

No trials have ever looked directly at the use of sulfasalazine in children with IBD. However, sulfasalazine has been compared to other aminosalicylates – mesalamine and olsalazine – in pediatric trials. Sulfasalazine 500–1000 mg and mesalamine (Asacol) 400–800 mg daily, were equally effective in maintaining remission in a majority of 67 children with both CD and UC, but nausea and vomiting were significantly more common with sulfasalazine.[15] In a multicenter, randomized double-blind study, 56 children with mild to moderate UC were divided into two groups of 28; one group received sulfasalazine and the other received olsalazine.[16] After 3 months, 79% of those taking sulfasalazine showed clinical improvement, whereas only 39% of the group on olsalazine improved clinically (Table 35.3). Most children achieved this response by the end of the first month.

Although sulfasalazine may achieve a good clinical response in adult and pediatric trials, studies in both populations have shown that sulfasalazine causes a high incidence of side effects. Adult studies have reported that 45% of patients experience adverse effects, with the most common being nausea, vomiting, headaches and anorexia.[17] Rare, but more serious, side effects include allergic reactions, skin rash, bone marrow suppression, suppressed sperm count, neurotoxicity and hepatotoxicity. Unfortunately, no studies have been carried out in young children to evaluate the minimum effective dose of sulfasalazine needed to achieve the maximum therapeutic response with minimal side effects.

Pediatric studies, as in adult studies, have shown that the sulfa-free aminosalicylates are better tolerated than sulfasalazine. Fewer side effects have also been associated with olsalazine, but it has not been shown to be as efficacious as sulfasalazine in the pediatric population.[16,16] Barden et al.[15] reported that 73% of 45 pediatric patients who previously took sulfasalazine preferred a delayed-release formulation of mesalamine, Asacol, because of the ease of administration and the reduction in gastrointestinal side effects. Although a few patients (6 of 45) who were unable to tolerate mesalamine because of headache or nausea were successfully treated with sulfasalazine, the overall incidence of side effects was less with mesalamine. Although uncommon, and less frequent than with sulfasalazine, there are case reports of mesalamine inducing symptoms of colitis, including bloody diarrhea and abdominal pain, in both adult and pediatric patients.[18,21]

Although sulfasalazine is still considered an excellent drug, mesalamine in various formulations is often used to avoid potential side effects. For young children who cannot swallow tablets, sulfasalazine has an advantage in that it can be mixed as a suspension at 50 mg/mL in seven parts methylcellulose to three parts cherry syrup and stored at room temperature for 60 days.[22] Although there are no dose-ranging studies for 5-ASA drugs in children, generally accepted therapeutic doses are shown in Table 35.4.

## CORTICOSTEROIDS

Corticosteroids remain the primary therapy in moderate to severe Crohn's disease and ulcerative colitis because of their rapid onset of action and generally favorable clinical response. Although the use and dosing of corticosteroids in pediatric patients is based primarily on adult studies,[14,23] their efficacy in fulminant colitis in children is well documented.[24] Because corticosteroids do not maintain remission or prevent clinical relapses, and side effects increase significantly when they are used over several months, every effort is made to limit the amount and duration of their use.[13,14,23,25] In children the chronic use of corticosteroids has the added risk of impaired growth and permanent alteration in bone mineral density.[13,14,26–28]

**Table 35.3 Clinical response to olsalazine and sulfasalazine**

| | Olsalazine (n = 28) 30 mg/kg/day (maximum 2 g/day) | | | Sulfasalazine (n = 28) 60 mg/kg/day (maximum 4 g/day) | | |
|---|---|---|---|---|---|---|
| | I mo. | 2 mos. | 3 mos. | I mo. | 2 mos. | 3 mos. |
| Clinical improvement | | | | | | |
| Asymptomatic | 4 | 5 | 4 | 6 | 8 | 9 |
| Improved | 9 | 9 | 7 | 15 | 14 | 13 |
| Total | 13 (46%)[a] | 14 (50%)[b] | 11 (39%)[c] | 21 (75%)[a] | 22 (79%)[b] | 22 (79%)[c] |

[a] P = 0.034 (Fisher's exact test).
[b] P = 0.03 (Fisher's exact test).
[c] P = 0.03 (Fisher's exact test).
(From Ferry G et al. J Pediatr Gastroenterol Nutr 1993;17:32–38, with permission from Lippincott Williams & Wilkins.)

Adolescence is the time in life when accretion of bone calcium is at a maximum, and interfering with this process by using long-term or repeated courses of corticosteroids runs the risk of permanent loss of bone mineral density.[29]

In spite of the above concerns and limitations, and the reluctance to use corticosteroids in children, on a short-term basis corticosteroids can rapidly reduce inflammation and symptoms and improve appetite, leading to rapid weight gain and improved growth. These early effects aid in improving the nutritional status and growth of a child or adolescent who presents with malnourishment and decreased physical development secondary to IBD.

Once a decision is made to use corticosteroids, it is best to start with a full therapeutic dose (1–2 mg/kg/day, up to 60 mg/day), tapering off as soon as is clinically feasible. Starting with too low a dose can prolong the time to response and lead to greater corticosteroid exposure.

The most commonly used corticosteroids are prednisone and methylprednisolone, and both possess similar profiles of efficacy and adverse events. As already mentioned, impaired growth and bone metabolism derangements are two of the most detrimental side effects in the pediatric population. Height and weight should be closely monitored with each clinic visit or prolonged hospitalization for early signs of growth failure. Bone density measurements may be helpful in monitoring for signs for osteopenia or osteoporosis. Other serious side effects seen in children include aseptic necrosis of joints, adrenal suppression, psychosis, pseudotumor cerebri, glaucoma, poor wound healing, and increased risk of infection. Of course, some of the undesirable physical manifestations of corticosteroids (i.e. cushingoid facies, obesity, acne, hirsutism) can profoundly affect a child's or adolescent's psychosocial development. A clinician should also consider the effect steroids have on an adolescent's behavior when a parent or patient reports an increase in emotional outbursts, and not just dismiss these episodes as typical teenage behavior.

Newer corticosteroids have been developed in an effort to decrease the adverse side effects of steroid therapy. Budesonide is a second-generation corticosteroid that has less systemic bioavailability than prednisone owing to an increased first-pass hepatic metabolism.[30] European and Canadian multicenter adult trials have shown budesonide to be more effective in inducing remission than placebo or mesalamine while producing less systemic side effects than prednisone.[30–32] A randomized, double blind multicenter trial in Europe of children aged 6–16 with CD compared budesonide to prednisone. Twenty-two children received budesonide and 26 received prednisone. Remission was achieved in 55% of the budesonide group and in 71% of the prednisone group, which was not statistically significant. However, glucocorticoid side effects were significantly lower in the budesonide group than in the prednisone group, as determined by measuring morning cortisol levels at 8 weeks (200 nmol/L vs. 98nmol/L), incidence of moon facies (23% vs. 60%) and incidence of acne (23% vs. 36%).[33]

A small maintenance trial looking at budesonide 6 mg/day in 32 children 11–17 years of age suggested that this dose may inhibit linear growth. Although five of the six children receiving this dose were free of symptoms, growth was only 2.3 ± 1.0 cm/year, well below the normal of 5 cm/year.[31]

## ANTIBIOTICS

Because of growth and other problems related to corticosteroids, there is a strong desire on the part of pediatric gastroenterologists to avoid steroids. Antibiotics are often used in children with mild to moderate Crohn's disease, but there are no clinical trials to show which antibiotic or combination of antibiotics is best and under what circumstances. It is also unclear how long to use antibiotics and what, if any, role they have in maintenance therapy.

Metronidazole has shown some benefit in treating perianal complications of Crohn's disease in adults.[34] A study of 21 patients treated with metronidazole reported complete healing of perianal disease in 48% of cases.[35] However, a follow-up study 2 years later reported that only 28% of the patients studied were able to stop metronidazole completely.[36] Common side effects of metronidazole are nausea, headaches and a metallic aftertaste, which all resolve with stopping the medication. However, a more significant complication from long-term administration of metronidazole is peripheral neuropathy. In a study of 13 pediatric patients who received metronidazole for 4–11 months, 11 (85%) showed signs of peripheral sensory neuropathy.[37] Complete resolution or improvement occurred in eight of the nine patients examined 5–13 months after discontinuing the medication.

Studies in Europe and Canada have reported that the combination of metronidazole and ciprofloxacin may be comparable

## Table 35.4 Pharmacologic agents for inflammatory bowel disease

| Agent and route | Dose | |
|---|---|---|
| **Aminosalicylates/5-ASA** | | |
| Sulfasalazine | 25–50 mg/kg/day (divided in 2–4 doses) (maximum dose: 4 g/day) | PO |
| Mesalamine (Asacol) | 30–60 mg/kg/day (divided in 2–4 doses) (maximum dose: 4.8 g/day) | PO |
| Mesalamine (Pentasa) | 50–60 mg/kg/day (divided in 2–4 doses) (maximum dose: 3.0 g/day) | PO |
| Mesalamine enema | 2.0–4.0 g q 12–24 h | PR |
| Mesalamine suppository | 500 mg q 12–24 h | PR |
| Balsalazide | 750 mg – 2.25 g tid | PO |
| **Corticosteroids** | | |
| Prednisone | 1–2 mg/kg/day (divided in 1–2 doses) (maximum: 60–80 mg/day) | PO |
| Methylprednisolone | 1–2 mg/kg/day (divided in 1–4 doses) (maximum: 60–80 mg/day) | IV |
| Budesonide | 9 mg/day divided into 3 doses | PO |
| Hydrocortisone enemas | 50–100 mg qhs PR | |
| Hydrocortisone foam | 80 mg qhs PR | |
| **Immunomodulators** | | |
| 6-meracaptopurine (6-MP) | 1.0–1.5 mg/kg/day | PO |
| Azathioprine | 1.5–2.0 mg/kg/day | PO |
| Cyclosporin | 2.0–4.0 mg/kg/day | IV |
| | 3.0–6.0 mg/kg/day (note: doses must be adjusted according to blood levels) | PO |
| Methotrexate | Starting dose: 5 mg/week; can increase to 20 mg/week (10–20 mg/m$^2$/week) | SC |
| **Antibiotics** | | |
| Metronidazole | 10–20 mg/kg/day (divided in 2–3 doses) | PO |
| Ciprofloxacin | 20–30 mg/kg/day (divided in 2 doses) (maximum dose: 750 mg bid) | PO |
| **Biological agents** | | |
| Infliximab (anti-TNF) | 5 mg/kg every at 0, 2 and 6 weeks then as needed at 4–8 weeks | IV |

Kim S, Ferry G et al. Current problems in pediatrics and adolescents. Inflammatory Bowel Disease in Children, Vol 32, No. 4 April 2002:
With permission from the American Gastroenterology Association)

in efficacy to corticosteroid therapy for colonic Crohn's disease.[37–39] However, it should be noted that a large randomized controlled trial comparing monotherapy with budesonide 9 mg/day to combination therapy with budesonide 9 mg/day, metronidazole and ciprofloxacin showed no benefit for combination therapy (Sheinhart H, et al. Gastroenterology 2002). Many pediatric clinicians have previously been reluctant to use ciprofloxacin because of abnormal cartilage growth in experimental animals. However, no joint toxicity or arthritis was found in a retrospective surveillance study of 1733 children who received at least one prescription of ciprofloxacin.[40] Ciprofloxacin may cause diarrhea and a rash, but these symptoms resolve with discontinuation of the drug.

Current practice is to use either metronidazole 10–15 mg/kg/day up to 250 tid to 500 mg bid, or ciprofloxacin 500 mg bid, or both, for induction of remission. Both antibiotics are often used for several months.

# IMMUNOMODULATORS

## Thioguanine derivatives

Pediatric trials have reported azathioprine (AZA) and 6-mercaptopurine (6-MP) to be effective adjunctive therapy in resolving IBD symptoms and reducing steroid use.[41–44] 6-MP not only aided in achieving remission in CD, but has also shown potential in maintaining remission.[45,46] Markowitz et al. studied the remission rates and steroid-sparing potential of 6-MP in 36 adolescents with intractable CD.[41] All of the patients had previously received corticosteroids, aminosalicylates and antibiotics for 3–8 years. Eighty per cent of them were able to discontinue steroid use after 1 year of treatment with 6-MP.

Another study looked at 6-MP plus prednisone versus prednisone alone in 55 pediatric patients with newly diagnosed moderate to severe Crohn's disease (Table 35.5).[42] The patients in the 6-MP group required a shorter duration of steroid therapy,

**Table 35.5 6-mercaptopurine in pediatric Crohn's disease***

| Remission | Corticosteroids plus 6-mercaptopurine n = 27 | Controls (corticosteroids alone) n = 28 |
|---|---|---|
| 30 days | 25 (93%) | 22 (79 %) |
| 90 days | 24 (89%) | 25 (89 %) |
| Relapse of those in remission | | |
| Within 180 days | 1 (4%) | 7 (28%) |
| Within 548 days | 2 (9%) | 13 (47%) |

*From Markowitz J et al. Gastroenterology 2000;119:895–902.
With permission from the American Gastroenterology Association)

had less overall corticosteroid exposure, and the rate of relapse was significantly lower in those who achieved remission with 6-MP (9%) than in the controls who received only steroids (47%). Many pediatric clinicians now recommend starting 6-MP in newly diagnosed pediatric patients with moderate to severe Crohn's to minimize the use of corticosteroids and potential adverse effects.

In growing children, having a target range for therapeutic blood levels of 6-MP is considered a real advantage, especially with the variability in metabolism of 6-MP and AZA. Dubinsky et al.[47] sought to determine optimal therapeutic dosing of 6-MP in 92 pediatric patients by measuring the metabolites of 6-MP, the 6-thioguanine nucleotides (6-TGN) and 6-methylmercaptopurine (6-MMP), and the genotype for the enzyme, thiopurine methyltransferase (TPMT), which controls the metabolism of 6-MP to 6-MMP. The results showed that the frequency of response increased with 6-TG levels above 235 pmol/$8 \times 10^8$ erythrocytes, hepatotoxicity correlated with levels of 6-MP above 5700 pmol/$8 \times 10^8$, leukopenia was associated with increased levels of 6-TGN, and patients heterozygous for TPMT had higher 6-TGN levels and had a better response to therapy. The authors concluded that measuring 6-MP metabolites and determining TPMT genotype could help optimize therapeutic response to 6-MP and identify individuals at risk for drug toxicity.[47] However, a study of 101 children failed to show correlation with 6-TGN levels greater than 235 and remission, but did suggest benefit in using 6-TGN levels to adjust dose in patients with ongoing active disease.[48] An added benefit of measuring metabolite levels in children is determining whether failure of medical therapy could be due to non-compliance.

It is now common practice to start children on 1.0–1.5 mg/kg/day of 6-MP and 2.0 mg/kg/day for azathioprine. The dose can be followed clinically for efficacy and adverse events, and drug levels can be checked at 4–6 weeks if suggested by CBC, aminotransferases or poor response. Close monitoring of the white cell count and aminotransferases is important.

## Methotrexate

Adult clinical studies have clearly shown the benefit of parenteral methotrexate in patients with steroid-dependent or -resistant Crohn's disease.[49-51] The efficacy of methotrexate has also been shown in both adult and adolescent patients who did not respond to 6-MP/AZA and steroids.[49,50,52,53] Improvement was seen with weekly parenteral methotrexate in 9 of 14 (64%) adolescents who had failed (11 patients) or had been intolerant

of (3 patients) 6-MP treatment.[53] Six of the 11 patients who had failed previous treatments showed a response to methotrexate, and all three who had developed pancreatitis from 6-MP improved. Steroid use was reduced in those patients who continued on methotrexate for 12 months.

Although studies in pediatric IBD are limited, there is an extensive body of knowledge in pediatric rheumatology where methotrexate is a main-line therapy in children with JRA resistant to NSAIDs.[54-56] Pediatric trials have shown that low-dose methotrexate (5–20 mg/m²/week) has generally been a safe treatment with very little liver toxicity.[55,57] Hashkes et al. reported in a retrospective study that of 25 pediatric patients with juvenile rheumatoid arthritis who underwent liver biopsy because of abnormal liver enzymes or prolonged use of methotrexate (>28 months), only five showed mild to moderate histological changes, and none showed significant fibrosis.[57]

Nausea, oral stomatitis and diarrhea are the most common side effects of methotrexate and these can limit patient acceptance and tolerance. More serious side effects include bone marrow suppression and alopecia. Folic acid (1–2 mg/day) can prevent some of these side effects. Methotrexate in adolescent females post menarche must be used with extreme caution because of its known teratogenic effects.

Some pediatric patients are unwilling to accept weekly injections, but most are comfortable once they find out these injections are not particularly painful, especially if given subcutaneously. Methotrexate is usually started at a dose of 15 mg/m²/week and increased, if necessary, up to a maximum weekly dose of 20 mg/m². This can be divided into two doses on two different days if nausea is a major problem.

## Cyclosporin

Cyclosporin use in pediatric IBD has primarily been in children with steroid-refractory fulminant colitis.[58-60] The decision to use cyclosporin is most often entertained when the next option is a total colectomy. Intravenous cyclosporin may be started at 2–4 mg/kg/day and adjusted to achieve serum trough levels of 150–200 ng/mL (in adult patients, trough levels are often adjusted to 250–300 ng/mL).[61] Clinical response usually occurs within 1–2 weeks of starting therapy. Oral cyclosporin can begin once the patient is taking adequate enteral nutrition. Even though the initial response to cyclosporin may be favorable, in one series eight of 11 patients who responded initially still went on to colectomy within 12 months.[60]

Cyclosporin possesses a narrow therapeutic window and close monitoring of serum drug levels is required. Most side effects are dose dependent and reversible upon reduction or discontinuation of the medication. Potential adverse affects include nephrotoxicity, which may present either as acute renal failure or chronic renal insufficiency; neurological sequelae such as headaches, seizures, paresthesias or tremors; opportunistic infections due to immunosuppression; hypertension secondary to renal insufficiency; hepatotoxicity; and anaphylaxis.

## Tacrolimus

Because cyclosporin possesses the potential for many serious side effects, tacrolimus may provide an alternative immunomodulator for refractory Crohn's and ulcerative colitis. Tacrolimus has been shown to be more potent and better absorbed in an inflamed intestine than cyclosporin.[62-65] Previous adult studies have shown some promise in the use of intravenous and oral tacrolimus in refractory IBD, including fulminant colitis and fistulizing Crohn's disease.[66-68]

In a multicenter open label trial looking at tacrolimus in children with severe ulcerative colitis, 13 children who had not responded to conventional therapy with intravenous corticosteroids were started on 0.1 mg/kg of tacrolimus twice a day and doses were adjusted to maintain blood levels of 10–15 ng/mL.[63] Nine of the 13 responded within 14 days and were discharged home after between 7 and 38 days. Two of these nine relapsed within a month after being discharged. The other seven were started on 6-MP or ASA at 4–6 weeks after the tacrolimus had been started. Tacrolimus was discontinued after 2–3 months in all of the responders, except for one who continued to receive it for 11 months. At 1 year, five of the original 13 (38%) patients remained in remission on maintenance therapy.

## BIOLOGICAL AGENTS

### Infliximab

Many adult studies have demonstrated the success of infliximab in treating refractory and steroid-dependent Crohn's disease.[69-74] Cohen et al. reported that more than 90% of 129 patients were able to taper their steroids, with 54% being able to discontinue them soon after a second infusion.[69] Improvement of clinical status was higher in those patients who were also receiving 6-MP. A report from The Netherlands showed that 73% of 57 patients with luminal disease and 100% of 16 patients with fistulous disease were able to taper off steroids.[70]

Pediatric studies also have supported the steroid-sparing benefits of infliximab.[75-77] Hyams et al. studied 19 patients ranging in age from age 9 to 19 years over 12 weeks. Seven had shown no response to 5-ASA and/or immunosuppressive therapy, and 12 were steroid dependent. Over the 12 weeks, the daily prednisone dose decreased from $28 \pm 14$ mg to $8 \pm 12$ mg.[75] Kugathasan et al. studied 15 pediatric patients with refractory Crohn's disease:[76] 14 reported a significant improvement, with 10 patients achieving complete remission by 10 weeks. Daily corticosteroid use decreased from more than 40 mg/day to less than 10 mg/day by 10 weeks. Kugathasan et al. compared patients who had a shorter history of Crohn's disease ($10.8 \pm 6.5$ months) with those who had a prolonged history ($42.5 \pm 10.9$ months) and found that three of six patients with early disease maintained clinical improvement for 12 months, whereas all seven patients with long-standing disease relapsed within 12 months.

Common side effects from infliximab include headache, fatigue, fever, rash, nausea and upper respiratory infections. Infliximab has also been associated with activating latent tuberculosis, histoplasmosis and coccidioidomycosis infections.[78,79] Because infliximab is a chimeric monoclonal antibody that is 25% murine and 75% human, drug sensitivity reactions can occur. Anaphylactic reactions are rare, but have been reported.[80,81] Assessment of the long-term safety of repeated infliximab use in young patients is ongoing.

## CDP571

A more humanized antibody to TNF-α, CDP571, has been developed with the goal of decreasing adverse effects. CDP571 has been studied in three adult clinical trials for the treatment of Crohn's disease and one for ulcerative colitis.[82-84] The results of these trials indicate that CDP571 may cause fewer adverse events than, but may not be as efficacious as, infliximab. However, no trials directly comparing CDP571 with infliximab have been reported. Multicenter pediatric trials studying CDP571 are ongoing.

# NUTRITIONAL THERAPY

Optimal nutrition is important in any chronic disease but is especially important for children and adolescents with IBD. At the time of the initial diagnosis most pediatric patients are consuming only 40–80% of their daily caloric requirements, partly because eating increases the symptoms of abdominal pain or diarrhea.[85-88] The potential for decreased oral intake, malabsorption and increased nutrient losses, combined with the increased needs of growth and development, predisposes a child with IBD to multiple nutritional deficiencies. Around 30% of pediatric Crohn's patients and 5–10% of pediatric ulcerative colitis patients present with impaired growth.[1-4] Delayed sexual maturation is also often found in conjunction with growth failure.[2,88] As growth is a constant concern in children, maintenance of adequate nutritional status is a vital part of the medical management of IBD.

Pediatric patients should be encouraged to choose a nutritious diet as tolerated to support linear growth and development, and restrictive diets are not recommended. However, symptoms may be made worse by dairy products (in lactose-intolerant individuals), hot spices or high-fiber foods. In addition, some patients may find the restriction of caffeine beneficial during severe diarrhea. In lactose-intolerant patients special consideration should be made to encourage the use of lactose-free dairy products or fortified soy products, so that adequate protein and calcium consumption is achieved. A daily multivitamin and mineral supplement is recommended. In addition, therapeutic doses of iron, calcium, zinc, vitamin $B_{12}$ and folic acid may be necessary. The primary goal of nutritional therapy in children is to provide adequate energy for growth and development and to prevent nutritional deficiencies.

## ENTERAL NUTRITION AS PRIMARY THERAPY IN CROHN'S DISEASE

In addition to treating malnutrition and growth failure, enteral nutrition may also be offered as an alternative primary therapy for active Crohn's disease. The interest in enteral therapy comes from the desire to avoid the complications of medications such as corticosteroids, plus the recognition that nutrition is critical to achieve normal growth in children and adolescents. Various adult and pediatric studies have claimed that elemental or polymeric diets were as effective as corticosteroids in achieving remission in active Crohn's disease.[89–91,94]

Meta-analyses of clinical trials of enteral feeding found that enteral nutrition was not as effective as corticosteroids in treating active Crohn's disease, but did provide therapeutic benefit (53–82%) when compared to the placebo response rates (18–42%) in most controlled clinical trials.[95,97] There appears to be no difference in efficacy between elemental and nonelemental formulas.[96] Studies on additives such as transforming-growth factor-$\beta$ and $\omega$3-polyunsaturated fatty acids in specially formulated liquid formulas have shown potential in increasing mucosal healing and reducing inflammation.[98,99] However, further studies are needed to validate these findings.

A variety of techniques for inducing and maintaining remission with enteral nutrition have been attempted. When we choose this form of therapy, we provide 100% of daily intake as a single polymeric or monomeric formula for 2–4 weeks, and then gradually increase the amount of food allowed over the next month. We may continue long-term daily supplementation with the same formula to provide up to 25% of the daily energy requirements. If needed, we also may repeat a month of mostly enteral formula feeds to maintain remission. There are some children who can follow this regimen by taking everything by mouth, but many need nighttime supplementation via a nasogastric tube to achieve adequate caloric and nutritional intake while on a mostly liquid diet. Although some may not tolerate nasogastric feeds, other children prefer this treatment to corticosteroids and will pass their own tube each night with no difficulty. In children who have experienced major side effects from corticosteroids (psychological, neurological, or severe loss of bone mineral density) enteral feeds are particularly useful and better tolerated.

# COMPLEMENTARY AND ALTERNATIVE THERAPIES

Children with a chronic medical condition are twice as likely to have used complementary and alternative therapies as those without.[100] In a recent evaluation of the use of complementary medicine (CAM) in children and young adults with IBD, the frequency of use was 41%.[101] The most common CAM were megavitamin therapy (19%), dietary supplements (17%) and herbal medicine (14%). Parental CAM use and the number of adverse effects from conventional medicines were found to be independent predictors of CAM use. Because some complementary and alternative therapies have the potential for adverse effects as well as drug interactions, their use should be thoroughly evaluated in an ongoing basis in all children and adolescents with IBD.

# TREATMENT REGIMENS FOR CROHN'S DISEASE IN CHILDREN

(Table 35.6)

The approach to treating Crohn's disease in children is based on disease site, severity of disease, and the presence or absence of growth failure. Younger children may not be able to take tablets or capsules as needed, and children at any age may have significant side effects and/or aversion to corticosteroids. Many parents have great concerns about giving corticosteroids to their children, and it often takes considerable discussion to help them understand the need. With the newer therapies now available, corticosteroids are not always the only choice for newly diagnosed children or children with an acute flare.

## MILD TO MODERATE DISTAL DISEASE

For distal disease (ileocolonic) of mild or moderate severity, 5-ASA drugs are most commonly used and are well tolerated in children. Pediatric doses are shown in Table 35.4. Although the doses of mesalamine in Table 35.4 show a maximum of 60 mg/kg/day, we are beginning to use higher doses, up to 90 mg/kg/day (maximum 4.8–5.0 g/day), without adverse events. For those who cannot swallow tablets or capsules, there are several alternatives. One is to make a suspension of 250 mg/teaspoon of sulfasalazine, or to open a 5-ASA capsule and sprinkle the contents on to a soft food, such as apple sauce. This requires that the child swallow without chewing. 5-ASA enemas may be useful in distal disease with diarrhea and urgency. Although it can be a challenge to get young children and some adolescents to accept enemas, for the most part they are well tolerated. In more moderately ill children we also add antibiotics, such as metronidazole and/or ciprofloxacin to induce remission. These may be continued for several months, depending on the response. If there is no response or remission is not achieved, a course of prednisone may be needed. If the disease is limited to the ileum and proximal colon, budesonide may be used in place of prednisone to induce remission. 6-Mercaptopurine or azathioprine can be added or used in place of antibiotics if patients do not respond to the above regimen or are corticosteroid dependent. For moderately ill patients infliximab might also be considered when response is poor or there is intolerance to other therapies. In cases where there is intolerance to other therapy, partial response, dependence or a strong aversion to corticosteroids, we would consider an elemental or monomeric liquid diet either as a supplement to drugs or as a replacement for other therapy. As this often requires nighttime nasogastric tube feeding to provide adequate nutrition, we do not routinely use these diets as a sole source of nutrition.

## MODERATE TO SEVERE DISTAL DISEASE

In spite of their side effects corticosteroids remain the standard therapy for most children with more severe disease, both new onset and disease flares. Depending on disease severity, prednisone or prednisolone may be needed intravenously along with bowel rest and total parenteral nutrition. For disease limited to the ileum and ascending colon, budesonide may be a reasonable substitute for outpatients. 5-ASA drugs and/or antibiotics are often combined with the corticosteroids. Although it is not yet routine in pediatrics to start 6-mercaptopurine or azathioprine along with corticosteroids, it is becoming more common in patients who are quite sick, especially if they have extensive disease. If there is no response, an incomplete response, drug intolerance or corticosteroid dependence, infliximab and/or methotrexate should be considered. Although an elemental or monomeric liquid diet may be additive, we rarely use this approach in the very ill child.

Maintenance therapy for patients with moderate to severe distal disease will depend on what was used to induce remission

**Table 35.6 Treatment of pediatric Crohn's disease.** Drugs generally are listed in the order used in children, but choices may be combined or modified, depending on length of disease, symptoms, complications and tolerance

| Disease location | Mild to moderate disease | Moderate to severe disease |
|---|---|---|
| Distal disease: terminal ileum, ileocolonic, colonic | Active disease:<br>5-ASA[a] (oral and/or enemas) or antibiotics – metronidazole, Ciprofloxacin, or both<br>Corticosteroids orally<br>Budesonide for terminal ileal/cecal disease<br>6-MP/AZA[b]<br>Infliximab if no response or intolerance to above treatment<br>Methotrexate<br>Elemental or monomeric liquid feeds<br>Maintenance therapy:<br>5-ASA[a], 6-MP/AZA[b]<br>Infliximab if used for active disease and relapse occurs on other therapy<br>Methotrexate<br>Antibiotics can be used for several months, but side effects often limit long term use<br>Partial or intermittent elemental or monomeric liquid feeds | Active disease:<br>Corticosteroids orally or IV<br>Budesonide for terminal ileal/cecal disease<br>5-ASA[a] (oral and/or enemas) or antibiotics – metronidazole, Ciprofloxacin, or both<br>6-MP/AZA[b]<br>Infliximab if no response or intolerance to above treatment<br>Methotrexate if no response or intolerant to 6-mercaptopurine or azathioprine<br>Elemental or monomeric liquid feeds<br>Maintenance therapy: Same as for mild to moderate disease |
| Proximal disease | Active disease:<br>Corticosteroids orally<br>6-MP/AZA[b]<br>Infliximab if no response or intolerance to above treatment<br>Methotrexate<br>Proton pump inhibitor for gastric/esophageal disease<br>Maintenance therapy:<br>6-MP/AZA[b]<br>Infliximab if no response or intolerance to above treatment<br>Methotrexate<br>Proton pump inhibitor | Active disease:<br>Corticosteroids orally or IV<br>6-MP/AZA[b]<br>Infliximab if no response or intolerance to above treatment<br>Methotrexate<br>Maintenance therapy: Same as for mild to moderate disease |
| Perianal disease | Active and maintenance therapy:<br>Antibiotics – metronidazole, ciprofloxacin or both<br>Infliximab<br>6-MP/AZA[b]<br>Combinations of above | Active and maintenance therapy:<br>Antibiotics– metronidazole, ciprofloxacin or both<br>Infliximab<br>6-MP/AZA[b]<br>Cyclosporin or tacrolimus if no response to above<br>Combinations of above |

[a]Aminosalicylic acid.
[b]6-Mercaptopurine/azathioprine.

and the response. 5-ASA drugs, 6-mercaptopurine or azathioprine can be used. We have used methotrexate in some cases for both induction and maintenance of remission, although experience is limited. If infliximab is needed to induce remission, it also may be needed to maintain remission. We generally use an immunosuppressive agent along with infliximab to reduce allergic reactions. To date it is not clear how long patients might require infliximab and with what frequency. The requirement for maintenance doses varies in our experience from 6- to 12-week intervals.

## PROXIMAL DISEASE (MILD, MODERATE OR SEVERE)

For disease involving the duodenum, jejunum and ileum, corticosteroids and 6-mercaptopurine or azathioprine remain the primary treatment. If there is no response, or corticosteroids or 6-mercaptopurine/azathioprine cannot be used or are not tolerated, infliximab and/or methotrexate are our next choices. For more severe disease IV corticosteroids or infliximab may be required, along with bowel rest and total parenteral nutrition. Maintenance therapy will require one of the immunosuppressive drugs in most cases. In gastric or esophageal disease, a proton pump inhibitor is often helpful in reducing symptoms.

## PERIANAL DISEASE

Disease involving the anal sphincter with fissuring and/or fistulae may respond to antibiotics, either singly or in combination, or to 6-mercaptopurine or azathioprine. In more severe disease infliximab is used either initially or if other therapy fails. We use corticosteroids where there is active bowel disease along with perianal disease. Combinations of the above are often necessary, and response is variable. Cyclosporin and tacrolimus also have been used to close fistulae, but are not considered long-term maintenance therapy because of their potential toxicity. We have maintained children on long-term antibiotics, but side effects, especially peripheral neuropathy with metronidazole, dictate dose minimization if possible, or stopping after 6 months.

# TREATMENT REGIMENS FOR ULCERATIVE COLITIS IN CHILDREN

(Table 35.7)

The treatment of ulcerative colitis in children, as in adults, is based on the knowledge that a colectomy is always an option in fulminant or long-standing disease. Although the majority of children present with pancolitis, the extent of disease does not necessarily predict the severity of symptoms and many children with pancolitis have mild disease.[16]

The 5-ASA drugs remain our choice for initial therapy for mild to moderate disease (see Table 35.4 for doses). Either 5-ASA enemas or corticosteroid enemas can be added if there are symptoms of urgency and tenesmus or response to oral 5-ASA is slow. In cases that do not respond, or in patients who present with more acute symptoms, oral corticosteroids can be added, starting with 1–2 mg/kg/day up to 60 mg/day and tapering, as tolerated, over 6–12 weeks. If there is incomplete response or corticosteroids cannot be weaned, 6-mercaptopurine or azathioprine can be started to further the induction of remission. Both 5-ASA drugs and 6-mercaptopurine or azathioprine can be used for maintenance of remission. In patients who are intolerant of 6-mercaptopurine or azathioprine, or who relapse and continue to have mild to moderate disease, weekly subcutaneous injections of methotrexate are potentially an option (although it should be noted that the only placebo-controlled trial of oral methotrexate 12.5 mg/week for induction and maintenance of remission in adults with ulcerative colitis failed to demonstrate efficacy) (Oren Gastroenterology 1994). Although we have seen a good response to methotrexate, our experience in ulcerative colitis is limited. In cases where methotrexate is required to maintain remission, we discuss the potential side effects versus elective colectomy with the patients and their families so they can help make this choice.

For more severe disease, including fulminant colitis, hospitalization with IV corticosteroids may be indicated. In these cases we routinely start total parenteral nutrition to provide protein and other essential nutrients. In the presence of fever or other complications (impending toxic megacolon) broad-spectrum antibiotics may also be needed. If there is improvement on corticosteroids (decreased bleeding, diarrhea, transfusion requirements) we may continue high-dose corticosteroids for 1–2 weeks before considering alternative therapy. Although colectomy is an option, and at times the only one in fulminant colitis, generally we will try either cyclosporin or tacrolimus after 5–7 days of no response to IV corticosteroids. In these cases we ask pediatric surgeons to help monitor progress and the potential need for colectomy. If there is no improvement by 2 weeks, or worsening of the colitis, a colectomy is strongly considered. Infliximab is being used with increasing frequency in severe and fulminant ulcerative colitis in place of cyclosporin, but at the time of writing there are insufficient data to make a formal recommendation.

Isolated proctitis is relatively uncommon in children, but localized treatment with 5-ASA enemas or suppositories, or corticosteroid enemas or foam, may bring about remission. Unfortunately, most children require ongoing therapy and often want to try oral 5-ASA drugs rather than enemas nightly or every second or third night. In our experience, oral 5-ASA work

**Table 35.7 Treatment of pediatric ulcerative colitis.** Drugs generally are listed in the order used in children, but choices may be combined or modified, depending on length of disease, symptoms, complications and tolerance

| Disease location | Mild to moderate disease | Moderate to severe disease |
|---|---|---|
| Left-sided and pancolitis | Active disease:<br>5-ASA[a] orally and/or 5-ASA[a] or corticosteroid enema<br>Oral corticosteroids<br>6-MP/AZA[b]<br>Infliximab if no response or intolerance to above treatment<br>Methotrexate if no response or intolerant to 6-MP/AZA (efficacy not established with controlled data in adults or children)[b]<br>Maintenance therapy:<br>5-ASA[a] orally or 5-ASA[a] enemas<br>6-MP/AZA[b]<br>Methotrexate if no response or intolerant to 6-MP/AZA (efficacy not established with controlled data in adults or children)[b] | Active disease:<br>Corticosteroids orally or IV<br>5-ASA[a] orally and/or 5-ASA[a] enemas<br>6-MP/AZA[b]<br>Infliximab if no response or intolerance to above treatment<br>Cyclosporin or Tacrolimus<br><br>Methotrexate if no response or intolerant to 6-MP/AZA (efficacy not established with controlled data in adults or children)[b]<br>Maintenance therapy:<br>above |
| Proctitis | Active disease:<br>5-ASA[a] or corticosteroid enema or suppository<br>5-ASA[a] orally<br>Maintenance therapy:<br>5-ASA[a] enema or suppository<br>5-ASA[a] orally | Active disease:<br>Same as for mild to moderate disease<br>Corticosteroid orally<br>Maintenance therapy:<br>Same as for mild to moderate disease |

[a]Aminosalicylic acid.
[b]6-Mercaptopurine/azathioprine.

for some patients, but the amount of drug reaching the rectum may be inadequate and ineffective.

## PSYCHOSOCIAL ISSUES

Crohn's disease and ulcerative colitis are chronic diseases. In spite of many therapeutic options, the course of both is repeated relapse and remission, and with any chronic disease there often is a negative impact on quality of life for patients and their families. The coping mechanisms of an entire family are strained when each member may have to make sacrifices: a parent may have to give up a career to provide homebound schooling for a child; family finances may be limited because only one parent is working and because of recurring medical expenses; and healthy siblings receive less parental attention. Adding to these stresses are delays in the physical, social and psychological development of children, leading to truancy, social isolation, and antisocial and dependent behaviors.

Different standardized questionnaires and indices have been developed to assess how a child is adapting to a life with IBD. Although the different models include different formats and response scales, they assess common basic categories: network for social support (i.e. family and friends); coping skills; the performance of daily activities of living (school); and issues of self-perception. Current multicenter studies are trying to develop and validate a comprehensive pediatric IBD quality of life questionnaire that will help clinicians assess the goals of promoting a child's psychosocial development and providing adequate family support. Having this information may enhance the physician's ability to return children and adolescents to productive, healthy lives even with intermittently or chronically active IBD.

Achieving all of the goals to return children and adolescents to a normal life often requires the efforts of a multidisciplinary team that includes physicians, nurses, social workers, psychologists and teachers. Many pediatric IBD centers sponsor educational meetings and support groups and provide written materials, videos, and even web sites to help educate and support their patients and families. Many of these pediatric IBD centers also coordinate summer camps, often supported by local sponsors, so that any child with IBD can attend regardless of their ability to pay. This combined medical, social and psychological support offers growing and developing children the best chance of coping with the many problems brought about by IBD.

## REFERENCES

1. Rosenthal SR, Snyder JD, Hendricks KM et al. Growth failure and inflammatory bowel disease: approach to treatment of a complicated adolescent problem. Pediatrics 1983;72:481–490.
2. Motil KJ, Grand RJ, Davis-Kraft L et al. Growth failure in children with inflammatory bowel disease: a prospective study. Gastroenterology 1993;105:681–691.
3. Sentongo TA, Semeao EJ, Piccoli DA et al. Growth, body composition, and nutritional status in children and adolescents with Crohn's disease. J Pediatr Gastroenterol Nutr 2000;31:33–40.
4. Ruemmele FM, Roy CC, Levy E et al. Nutrition as primary therapy in pediatric Crohn's disease: fact or fantasy? J Pediatr 2000;136:285–291.
5. Allen DB. Growth suppression by glucocorticoid therapy. Endocrinol Metab Clin North Am 1996;25:699–717.
6. Richardson G, Griffiths AM, Miller V et al. Quality of life in inflammatory bowel disease: a cross-cultural comparison of English and Canadian children. J Pediatr Gastroenterol Nutr 2001;32:573–578.
7. Gortmaker SL, Walker DK, Weitzman M et al. Chronic conditions, socioeconomic risks, and behavioral problems in children and adolescents. Pediatrics 1990;85:267–276.
8. Seigel WM, Golden NH, Gough JW et al. Depression, self-esteem, and life events in adolescents with chronic diseases. J Adolesc Health Care 1990;11:501–504.
9. Rabbett H, Elbadri A, Thwaites R et al. Quality of life in children with Crohn's disease. J Pediatr Gastroenterol Nutr 1996;23:528–533.
10. Engstrom I, Lindquist BL. Inflammatory bowel disease in children and adolescents: a somatic and psychiatric investigation. Acta Paediatr Scand 1991;80:640–647.
11. Wood B, Watkins JB, Boyle JT et al. Psychological functioning in children with Crohn's disease and ulcerative colitis: implications for models of psychobiological interaction. J Am Acad Child Adolesc Psychiatry 1987;26:774–781.
12. Svartz N. Sulfasalazine: II. Some notes on the discovery and development of salazopyrin. Am J Gastroenterol 1988;83:497–503.
13. Malchow H, Ewe K, Brandes JW et al. European Cooperative Crohn's Disease Study (ECCDS): results of drug treatment. Gastroenterology 1984;86:249–266.
14. Summers RW, Switz DM, Sessions JT Jr. et al. National Cooperative Crohn's Disease Study: results of drug treatment. Gastroenterology 1979;77:847–869.
15. Barden L, Lipson A, Pert P et al. Mesalazine in childhood inflammatory bowel disease. Aliment Pharmacol Ther 1989;3:597–603.
16. Ferry GD, Kirschner BS, Grand RJ et al. Olsalazine versus sulfasalazine in mild to moderate childhood ulcerative colitis: results of the Pediatric Gastroenterology Collaborative Research Group Clinical Trial. J Pediatr Gastroenterol Nutr 1993;17:32–38.
17. Schroder H, Evans DA. Acetylator phenotype and adverse effects of sulphasalazine in healthy subjects. Gut 1972;13:278–284.
18. Fardy JM, Lloyd DA, Reynolds RP. Adverse effects with oral 5-aminosalicyclic acid. J Clin Gastroenterol 1988;10:635–637.
19. Iofel E, Chawla A, Daum F et al. Mesalamine intolerance mimics symptoms of active inflammatory bowel disease. J Pediatr Gastroenterol Nutr 2002;34:73–76.
20. Kapur KC, Williams GT, Allison MC. Mesalazine induced exacerbation of ulcerative colitis. Gut 1995;37:838–839.
21. Sturgeon JB, Bhatia P, Hermens D et al. Exacerbation of chronic ulcerative colitis with mesalamine. Gastroenterology 1995;108:1889–1893.
22. McCrea J, Rappaport P, Stansfield S, Baker D, Dupuis LL, James G. Extemporaneous oral liquid dosage preparations. Toronto: Canadian Society of Hospital Pharmacists, 1988.
23. Brignola C, De Simone G, Belloli C et al. Steroid treatment in active Crohn's disease: a comparison between two regimens of different duration. Aliment Pharmacol Ther 1994;8:465–468.
24. Werlin SL, Grand RJ. Severe colitis in children and adolescents: diagnosis. Course, and treatment. Gastroenterology 1977;73:828–832.
25. Munkholm P, Langholz E, Davidsen M et al. Frequency of glucocorticoid resistance and dependency in Crohn's disease. Gut 1994;35:360–362.
26. Nesbitt LT Jr. Minimizing complications from systemic glucocorticosteroid use. Dermatol Clin 1995;13:925–939.
27. Hyams JS, Moore RE, Leichtner AM et al. Relationship of type I procollagen to corticosteroid therapy in children with inflammatory bowel disease. J Pediatr 1988;112:893–898.
28. Valentine JF, Sninsky CA. Prevention and treatment of osteoporosis in patients with inflammatory bowel disease. Am J Gastroenterol 1999;94:878–883.
29. Bonjour JP, Theintz G, Buchs B et al. Critical years and stages of puberty for spinal and femoral bone mass accumulation during adolescence. J Clin Endocrinol Metab 1991;73:555–563.
30. Greenberg GR, Feagan BG, Martin F et al. Oral budesonide for active Crohn's disease. Canadian Inflammatory Bowel Disease Study Group. N Engl J Med 1994;331:836–841.
31. Kundhal P, Zachos M, Holmes JL et al. Controlled ileal release budesonide in pediatric Crohn disease: efficacy and effect on growth. J Pediatr Gastroenterol Nutr 2001;33:75–80.
32. Rutgeerts P. The use of budesonide in the treatment of active Crohn's disease is good clinical practice. Inflamm Bowel Dis 2001;7:60–61.
33. Escher JC, Lindquist B, Hildebrand H et al. Budesonide capsules versus prednisolone in children with active Crohn's disease: Results of a European multicenter trial. Gastroenterology 2002;122 (Suppl 1):A12.
34. Janowitz HD, Croen EC, Sachar DB. The role of the fecal stream in Crohn's disease: an historical and analytic review. Inflamm Bowel Dis 1998;4:29–39.
35. Bernstein LH, Frank MS, Brandt LJ et al. Healing of perineal Crohn's disease with metronidazole. Gastroenterology 1980;79:357–365.
36. Brandt LJ, Bernstein LH, Boley SJ et al. Metronidazole therapy for perineal Crohn's disease: a follow-up study. Gastroenterology 1982;83:383–387.
37. Duffy LF, Daum F, Fisher SE et al. Peripheral neuropathy in Crohn's disease patients treated with metronidazole. Gastroenterology 1985;88:681–684.
38. Greenbloom SL, Steinhart AH, Greenberg GR. Combination ciprofloxacin and metronidazole for active Crohn's disease. Can J Gastroenterol 1998;12:53–56.
39. Prantera C, Zannoni F, Scribano ML et al. An antibiotic regimen for the treatment of active Crohn's disease: a randomized, controlled clinical trial of metronidazole plus ciprofloxacin. Am J Gastroenterol 1996;91:328–332.
40. Jick S. Ciprofloxacin safety in a pediatric population. Pediatr Infect Dis J 1997;16:130–133.
41. Markowitz J, Rosa J, Grancher K et al. Long-term 6-mercaptopurine treatment in adolescents with Crohn's disease. Gastroenterology 1990;99:1347–1351.

42. Markowitz J, Grancher K, Kohn N et al. A multicenter trial of 6-mercaptopurine and prednisone in children with newly diagnosed Crohn's disease. Gastroenterology 2000;119:895–902.

43. Verhave M, Winter HS, Grand RJ. Azathioprine in the treatment of children with inflammatory bowel disease. J Pediatr 1990;117:809–814.

44. Kader HA, Mascarenhas MR, Piccoli DA et al. Experiences with 6-mercaptopurine and azathioprine therapy in pediatric patients with severe ulcerative colitis. J Pediatr Gastroenterol Nutr 1999;28:54–58.

45. Pearson DC, May GR, Fick GH et al. Azathioprine and 6-mercaptopurine in Crohn disease. A meta-analysis. Ann Intern Med 1995;123:132–142.

46. Sandborn W, Sutherland L, Pearson D et al. Azathioprine or 6-mercaptopurine for inducing remission of Crohn's disease. Cochrane Database Syst Rev 2000;(2):CD000545.

47. Dubinsky MC, Lamothe S, Yang HY et al. Pharmacogenomics and metabolite measurement for 6-mercaptopurine therapy in inflammatory bowel disease. Gastroenterology 2000;118:705–713.

48. Gupta P, Gokhale R, Kirschner BS. 6-mercaptopurine metabolite levels in children with inflammatory bowel disease. J Pediatr Gastroenterol Nutr 2001;33:450–454.

49. Chong RY, Hanauer SB, Cohen RD. Efficacy of parenteral methotrexate in refractory Crohn's disease. Aliment Pharmacol Ther 2001;15:35–44.

50. Feagan BG, Fedorak RN, Irvine EJ et al. A comparison of methotrexate with placebo for the maintenance of remission in Crohn's disease. North American Crohn's Study Group Investigators. N Engl J Med 2000;342:1627–1632.

51. Yang YX, Lichtenstein GR. Methotrexate for the maintenance of remission in Crohn's disease. Gastroenterology 2001;120:1553–1555.

52. Feagan BG, Rochon J, Fedorak RN et al. Methotrexate for the treatment of Crohn's disease. The North American Crohn's Study Group Investigators. N Engl J Med 1995;332:292–297.

53. Mack DR, Young R, Kaufman SS et al. Methotrexate in patients with Crohn's disease after 6-mercaptopurine. J Pediatr 1998;132:830–835.

54. Athreya BH, Cassidy JT. Current status of the medical treatment of children with juvenile rheumatoid arthritis. Rheum Dis Clin North Am 1991;17:871–889.

55. Giannini EH, Brewer EJ, Kuzmina N et al. Methotrexate in resistant juvenile rheumatoid arthritis. Results of the USA–USSR double-blind, placebo-controlled trial. The Pediatric Rheumatology Collaborative Study Group and The Cooperative Children's Study Group. N Engl J Med 1992;326:1043–1049.

56. Ilowite NT. Current treatment of juvenile rheumatoid arthritis. Pediatrics 2002;109:109–115.

57. Hashkes PJ, Balistreri WF, Bove KE et al. The relationship of hepatotoxic risk factors and liver histology in methotrexate therapy for juvenile rheumatoid arthritis. J Pediatr 1999;134:47–52.

58. Hyams JS, Treem WR. Cyclosporin treatment of fulminant colitis. J Pediatr Gastroenterol Nutr 1989;9:383–387.

59. Ramakrishna J, Langhans N, Calenda K et al. Combined use of cyclosporin and azathioprine or 6-mercaptopurine in pediatric inflammatory bowel disease. J Pediatr Gastroenterol Nutr 1996;22:296–302.

60. Treem WR, Hyams JS. Cyclosporin therapy for gastrointestinal disease. J Pediatr Gastroenterol Nutr 1994;18:270–278.

61. Lichtiger S, Present DH, Kornbluth A et al. Cyclosporin in severe ulcerative colitis refractory to steroid therapy. N Engl J Med 1994;330:1841–1845.

62. Randomised trial comparing tacrolimus (FK506) and cyclosporin in prevention of liver allograft rejection. European FK506 Multicentre Liver Study Group. Lancet 1994;344:423–428.

63. Bousvaros A, Kirschner BS, Werlin SL et al. Oral tacrolimus treatment of severe colitis in children. J Pediatr 2000;137:794–799.

64. Fellermann K, Herrlinger KR, Witthoeft T et al. Tacrolimus: a new immunosuppressant for steroid refractory inflammatory bowel disease. Transplant Proc 2001;33:2247–2248.

65. McDiarmid SV, Wallace P, Vargas J et al. The treatment of intractable rejection with tacrolimus (FK506) in pediatric liver transplant recipients. J Pediatr Gastroenterol Nutr 1995;20:291–299.

66. Fellermann K, Ludwig D, Stahl M et al. Steroid-unresponsive acute attacks of inflammatory bowel disease: immunomodulation by tacrolimus (FK506). Am J Gastroenterol 1998;93:1860–1866.

67. Lowry PW, Weaver AL, Tremaine WJ et al. Combination therapy with oral tacrolimus (FK506) and azathioprine or 6-mercaptopurine for treatment-refractory Crohn's disease perianal fistulae. Inflamm Bowel Dis 1999;5:239–245.

68. Sandborn WJ. Preliminary report on the use of oral tacrolimus (FK506) in the treatment of complicated proximal small bowel and fistulizing Crohn's disease. Am J Gastroenterol 1997;92:876–879.

69. Cohen RD, Tsang JF, Hanauer SB. Infliximab in Crohn's disease: first anniversary clinical experience. Am J Gastroenterol 2000;95:3469–3477.

70. Hommes DW, van de Heisteeg BH, van der SM et al. Infliximab treatment for Crohn's disease: one-year experience in a Dutch academic hospital. Inflamm Bowel Dis 2002;8:81–86.

71. Lichtenstein GR. Treatment of fistulizing Crohn's disease. Gastroenterology 2000;119:1132–1147.

72. Present DH, Rutgeerts P, Targan S et al. Infliximab for the treatment of fistulas in patients with Crohn's disease. N Engl J Med 1999;340:1398–1405.

73. Rutgeerts P, D'Haens G, Targan S et al. Efficacy and safety of retreatment with anti-tumor necrosis factor antibody (infliximab) to maintain remission in Crohn's disease. Gastroenterology 1999;117:761–769.

74. Targan SR, Hanauer SB, van Deventer SJ et al. A short-term study of chimeric monoclonal antibody cA2 to tumor necrosis factor alpha for Crohn's disease. Crohn's Disease cA2 Study Group. N Engl J Med 1997;337:1029–1035.

75. Hyams JS, Markowitz J, Wyllie R. Use of infliximab in the treatment of Crohn's disease in children and adolescents. J Pediatr 2000;137:192–196.

76. Kugathasan S, Werlin SL, Martinez A et al. Prolonged duration of response to infliximab in early but not late pediatric Crohn's disease. Am J Gastroenterol 2000;95:3189–3194.

77. Serrano MS, Schmidt-Sommerfeld E, Kilbaugh TJ et al. Use of infliximab in pediatric patients with inflammatory bowel disease. Ann Pharmacother 2001;35:823–828.

78. Keane J, Gershon S, Wise RP et al. Tuberculosis associated with infliximab, a tumor necrosis factor alpha-neutralizing agent. N Engl J Med 2001;345:1098–1104.

79. Nakelchik M, Mangino JE. Reactivation of histoplasmosis after treatment with infliximab. Am J Med 2002;112:78.

80. Lankarani KB. Mortality associated with infliximab. J Clin Gastroenterol 2001;33:255–256.

81. Diamanti A, Castro M, Papadatou B et al. Severe anaphylactic reaction to infliximab in pediatric patients with Crohn's disease. J Pediatr 2002;140:636–637.

82. Evans RC, Clarke L, Heath P et al. Treatment of ulcerative colitis with an engineered human anti-TNFalpha antibody CDP571. Aliment Pharmacol Ther 1997;11:1031–1035.

83. Sandborn WJ, Feagan BG, Hanauer SB et al. An engineered human antibody to TNF (CDP571) for active Crohn's disease: a randomized double-blind placebo-controlled trial. Gastroenterology 2001;120:1330–1338.

84. Stack WA, Mann SD, Roy AJ et al. Randomised controlled trial of CDP571 antibody to tumour necrosis factor-alpha in Crohn's disease. Lancet 1997;349:521–524.

85. Kelts DG, Grand RJ, Shen G et al. Nutritional basis of growth failure in children and adolescents with Crohn's disease. Gastroenterology 1979;76:720–727.

86. Kirschner BS, Klich JR, Kalman SS et al. Reversal of growth retardation in Crohn's disease with therapy emphasizing oral nutritional restitution. Gastroenterology 1981;80:10–15.

87. Motil KJ, Altchuler SI, Grand RJ. Mineral balance during nutritional supplementation in adolescents with Crohn disease and growth failure. J Pediatr 1985;107:473–479.

88. Oliva MM, Lake AM. Nutritional considerations and management of the child with inflammatory bowel disease. Nutrition 1996;12:151–158.

89. Gonzalez-Huix F, de Leon R, Fernandez-Banares F et al. Polymeric enteral diets as primary treatment of active Crohn's disease: a prospective steroid controlled trial. Gut 1993;34:778–782.

90. Gorard DA, Hunt JB, Payne-James JJ et al. Initial response and subsequent course of Crohn's disease treated with elemental diet or prednisolone. Gut 1993;34:1198–1202.

91. Teahon K, Bjarnason I, Pearson M et al. Ten years' experience with an elemental diet in the management of Crohn's disease. Gut 1990;31:1133–1137.

92. Papadopoulou A, Rawashdeh MO, Brown GA et al. Remission following an elemental diet or prednisolone in Crohn's disease. Acta Paediatr 1995;84:79–83.

93. Ruuska T, Savilahti E, Maki M et al. Exclusive whole protein enteral diet versus prednisolone in the treatment of acute Crohn's disease in children. J Pediatr Gastroenterol Nutr 1994;19:175–180.

94. Thomas AG, Taylor F, Miller V. Dietary intake and nutritional treatment in childhood Crohn's disease. J Pediatr Gastroenterol Nutr 1993;17:75–81.

95. Fernandez-Banares F, Cabre E, Esteve-Comas M et al. How effective is enteral nutrition in inducing clinical remission in active Crohn's disease? A meta-analysis of the randomized clinical trials. JPEN J Parenter Enteral Nutr 1995;19:356–364.

96. Griffiths AM, Ohlsson A, Sherman PM et al. Meta-analysis of enteral nutrition as a primary treatment of active Crohn's disease. Gastroenterology 1995;108:1056–1067.

97. Griffiths AM. Inflammatory bowel disease. Nutrition 1998;14:788–791.

98. Belluzzi A, Boschi S, Brignola C et al. Polyunsaturated fatty acids and inflammatory bowel disease. Am J Clin Nutr 2000;71(1 Suppl):339S–342S.

99. Fell JM, Paintin M, Arnaud-Battandier F et al. Mucosal healing and a fall in mucosal pro-inflammatory cytokine mRNA induced by a specific oral polymeric diet in paediatric Crohn's disease. Aliment Pharmacol Ther 2000;14:281–289.

100. Clawson D. Prevalence and nature of CAM use in children under 18 years in the United States. Paper presented at the International Scientific Conference on Complementary, Alternative and Integrative Medical Research, Boston, MA 2002.

101. Heuschkel R, Afzal N, Wuerth A et al. Complementary medicine use in children and young adults with inflammatory bowel disease. Am J Gastroenterol 2002;97:382–388.

## CHAPTER 36

# Nutrition in inflammatory bowel disease

Herbert Lochs

## INTRODUCTION

Patients with inflammatory bowel disease (IBD) frequently suffer from malnutrition and food-associated symptoms. Therefore, it is obvious to doctors and patients that nutrition is an important factor in the course of inflammatory bowel disease. In this chapter different aspects of nutrition in IBD will be analyzed. First, the question has to be discussed, is there evidence for a causative role of specific dietary habits for the development of inflammatory bowel disease? If so, the possibility of a disease-preventing diet would be of interest. Second, as specific nutritional deficiencies and even gross malnutrition occur frequently in the course of inflammatory bowel disease, the role of nutritional intervention in the prevention and therapy of nutritional deficits will be evaluated. Third, nutrition is itself an effective treatment for the active phase of IBD. This chapter will discuss the scientific basis for the role of nutrition in the different indications and then give practical recommendations for the clinical use of nutritional therapy.

## NUTRITION AS CAUSE OF INFLAMMATORY BOWEL DISEASE

Epidemiological studies show that IBD is more frequent in Western countries than in developing countries or in Asia. This finding suggests that the Western lifestyle might play a role in the development of IBD. One obvious factor to investigate was dietary habits. Several studies have therefore compared nutritional habits of IBD patients before the onset of their disease and during its course with the nutritional habits of the general population. Obviously such studies are difficult to perform, as the dietary habits of patients have to be evaluated retrospectively with a delay of up to several years. Despite these problems some of these studies found significant differences between patients and controls matched for age, gender and social group,

indicating a higher carbohydrate and sugar intake in IBD patients before the onset of their disease. However, in subsequent studies these differences could not be confirmed.[1-3] Similarly, other nutrients, such as *trans* fatty acids, which can be found in margarine, were suspected of inducing IBD, but none of these hypotheses could eventually be proved. At present there is no evidence that specific dietary components play a causative role in inflammatory bowel disease.

An alternative pathogenetic model is based on the observation of increased intestinal permeability in IBD patients and families. Therefore, more nutritional antigens could pass the intestinal barrier and induce a chronic immune reaction. Although this hypothesis explains some findings in IBD patients it still lacks proof.

*Mycobacterium paratuberculosis*, which can be found especially in milk, has also been discussed as a further possible etiologic factor (see Chapters 10 and 34 for additional details). In fact, several studies showed M. paratuberculosis more frequently in the stool and mucosa of IBD patients than in healthy controls, but it is not clear whether mycobacteria play a pathogenetic role.

In summary, the role of nutrition as a causative factor for IBD appears to be limited. Neither a specific preventive diet can be recommended, nor do the scientific data support special processing of food to eliminate possible contamination with M. paratuberculosis. Although such considerations about a disease-preventing diet might not be important for the general population, they could be useful for risk groups such as the relatives of IBD patients. Indeed, family members of IBD patients frequently ask for advice about preventive measures. However, with current knowledge no specific diet can be recommended to such persons.

## NUTRITIONAL STATUS IN IBD

### Effect of inflammatory bowel disease on nutritional status

Table 36.1 shows the frequencies of different nutritional deficiencies in IBD patients. Although there seems to be a

**Table 36.1 Frequency of different nutritional deficiencies in inflammatory bowel disease**

| Type of deficiency | Frequency of deficiency (%) | References |
|---|---|---|
| Growth retardation | 20–40 | |
| Final height below 5th percentile | 7–30 | 4–11 |
| Weight loss (active phase) | 75 | 12–13, 22 |
| Loss of muscle mass, fat mass | 60 | |
| Osteopenia | 45 | 19 |
| <Iron, Anemia | 70 | 24 |
| Vitamin D | ~ 50 | 19 |
| K, Ca, PO$_4$, Mg | described | 14, 15, 16, 17, 18 |
| Fat-soluble Vit, Vit B$_{12}$ | described | 19, 20, 21, 22, 23 |
| Folic acid | described | |

difference between Crohn's disease and ulcerative colitis, many deficits develop in both diseases. In general, loss of muscle mass and gross malnutrition are more frequent in Crohn's disease, whereas anemia and iron deficiency are more prevalent in ulcerative colitis. Interestingly, the location of the disease does not appear to play a major role in the development of malnutrition. A difference between small bowel and colonic CD regarding frequency and type of malnutrition could not be shown, with the exception of vitamin B$_{12}$ deficiency, which is more frequent in patients with disease of the terminal ileum.

In adults severe malnutrition is dependent on disease activity, and in the active phase of IBD it is quite common. Up to 75% of hospitalized patients with Crohn's disease suffer from weight loss. If body composition is analyzed with bioimpedance or other specific methods reduction of muscle mass as well as body fat can be detected in 60% of patients with active CD. Besides the general protein–energy malnutrition a number of deficits, such as anemia, low serum albumin or vitamin deficits, are seen in active CD. However, because patients frequently are dehydrated as a result of diarrhea, hypoalbuminemia may not be detected until patients are infused parenterally to replace their fluid losses.

In remission protein–energy malnutrition is only seen in patients with severe stenoses or extensive bowel resections. In contrast, specific deficits such as trace element, vitamin and electrolyte deficits are frequent even in patients with quiescent Crohn's disease. These deficits have long been ignored for the treatment of these patients; however, adequate supplementation may improve quality of life and reduce the risk of complications such as osteoporosis and fractures.

Specific risk groups for different nutritional deficiencies have been described. Patients with chronic active CD or frequent relapses, as well as patients on long-term steroid treatment, are at higher risk to develop calcium and vitamin D deficiencies and may need supplementation.[25] An increased risk of bone fractures has been described in these patients.[26,27]

In patients with involvement or resection of the terminal ileum vitamin B$_{12}$ deficiency is frequent. Sulfasalazine interferes with the absorption of folic acid. This can lead to folic acid deficiency.[21]

Bile acid-binding resins such as cholestyramine, which are prescribed to control diarrhea in some patients, can lead to steatorrhea and might lead to malabsorption of fat-soluble vitamins.

Iron deficiency and anemia are seen in both Crohn's disease and ulcerative colitis. Recent studies have shown that in the majority of IBD patients anemia is a consequence of chronic blood loss and reduced iron absorption rather than anemia of chronic disease. Up to 80% of IBD patients react with an increase in hemoglobin and improvement of their quality of life if they are supplemented with oral or intravenous iron.[28,29]

In children, IBD can lead to specific malnutrition problems, such as growth retardation and delayed sexual development. Malnutrition frequently precedes the development of intestinal symptoms. Up to 90% of children with Crohn's disease fall below the 5th percentile of the normal growth rate before the diagnosis is established. Seven to 30% of these patients will fail to reach their height potential despite treatment of disease activity with steroids.[30] Decreased growth hormone levels occur in these children as a secondary phenomenon, and growth hormone therapy is not indicated unless and until adequate nutrition has been provided.

## PATHOGENESIS OF MALNUTRITION

The development of nutritional deficiencies in IBD is multifactorial, with reduced intake, increased intestinal losses, some degree of malabsorption and increased energy expenditure. However, it appears that reduced dietary intake due to anorexia is the most important factor.

In active Crohn's disease most patients are anorectic because of food-associated symptoms and as a consequence of the inflammatory state. In several studies a reduced oral intake has been found in these patients. Treatment with steroids increases intake; however, owing to the catabolic effect of steroids, patients still remain in negative nitrogen balance until the steroid dose can be reduced because of diminished disease activity.

Dietary habits in adults with quiescent Crohn's disease have been less well investigated. One study[31] reported a daily intake of approximately 2800 kcal, which still was not enough for the patients to maintain their optimal body weight. This shows that besides inadequate dietary intake, increased intestinal losses and/or an increased metabolic rate might contribute to malnutrition. Increased intestinal protein losses have been found in the majority of IBD patients by measuring the excretion of $\alpha_1$-antitrypsin.[32] As mentioned above, despite these protein losses only few patients have low serum albumin levels. However, this finding is an artifact resulting from concomitant dehydration, and can lead to the erroneous conclusion that patients have no protein deficit. Studies measuring total body protein and total body potassium, a reliable parameter for the body cell mass, showed a reduction of the body cell mass and protein in the majority of IBD patients.

In children malnutrition does not appear to be limited to the active phases of the disease. Once patients suffer from growth retardation during the active phase, they usually do not grow enough while in remission to make up for the deficit, unless they are treated with an aggressive nutritional supplementation program such as nocturnal tube feeds.

Clinically apparent steatorrhea is infrequently seen in IBD patients. However, fat malabsorption may occur in patients with small bowel disease. This can lead to calcium malabsorption, which then leads to the formation of calcium soaps and increased reabsorption of oxalate. Clinical consequences are osteopenia and the development of kidney stones. In patients with resections of the terminal ileum bile acid-induced diarrhea may also occur.

## METABOLIC CHANGES

IBD-specific metabolic changes have not been described. However, energy expenditure is slightly increased during the active phase of disease.[33-35] There is also increased fat oxidation and reduced carbohydrate oxidation.

These changes are not specific for IBD but rather reflect the inflammatory process and reduced fat mass. Metabolism quickly normalizes when disease activity is reduced and nutritional status improved. Moreover, the slightly increased energy expenditure does not explain the weight loss in IBD patients.

Energy requirements may therefore be calculated using standard formulas. Usually 25–30 kcal/kg/day are adequate. A normal relation of the different substrates, protein, fat and carbohydrate, should be used for dietary calculation in IBD patients.

## CLINICAL RELEVANCE OF MALNUTRITION

Metabolic derangements and malnutrition are important prognostic factors. In one study fluid deficits, electrolyte disturbances and protein–energy malnutrition were key factors associated with mortality in IBD patients.[35a] Furthermore, postoperative complications are higher in patients with preoperative weight loss and low serum albumin.[44] These patients also have longer hospital stays.[35b]

## NUTRITIONAL THERAPY

### DIETARY PREVENTION OF IBD

Based on the early findings that specific dietary habits predispose to the development of IBD the question has been raised if a specific preventive diet should be recommended to a population at risk. This would mainly be relatives of IBD patients. Low carbohydrate intake, reduction of refined sugar intake, as well as reduction of the sulfur content of the diet, have been discussed. However, there is no scientific evidence that such dietary changes may have any preventive effect on the development of IBD[36] and they can therefore not be recommended.

## THERAPY OF MALNUTRITION

Prevention and therapy of malnutrition is most urgent in children with IBD, as after the end of the growing period growth retardation can no longer be treated. It is important to diagnose growth retardation as early as possible. As soon as the growth velocity decreases the cause should be investigated. This allows children to be treated before they have developed a large growth deficit. In IBD growth retardation is a problem of inadequate substrate availability rather than of catabolism due to the chronic inflammatory process. Therefore, an increase in dietary intake does result in increased body weight and growth velocity. However, this cannot be achieved by dietary counseling, and in most instances not even by improving intake with anti-inflammatory therapy. In early studies children were treated either with parenteral nutrition, in addition to their normal diet, or even with total parenteral nutrition.[37] This did result in weight gain and increased growth, but because of the high rate of complications parenteral nutrition is no longer used for this indication. Instead, the best overall results (considering both efficacy and safety) have been achieved with supplementary tube feeding besides the standard oral diet.[38,39] Because constant nasogastric tube feeding is socially difficult to accept, many children are treated with intermittent enteral nutrition, mainly administered overnight. Different methods have been used. Special tubes have been constructed with an olive at the end which fits into the nose. The tube can be swallowed so far in the morning that the olive is hidden in the nostril and the tube is not visible during the day. In the evening, with slight pressure to the nose the end of the tube can be pulled out and connected to the infusion line. Percutaneous endoscopic gastrostomy has also been used for long-term enteral nutrition in children with Crohn's disease with no increased risk of fistula development.[40]

An even easier approach has been investigated in two studies. Children can quickly adjust to swallowing a nasogastric tube every evening and receiving up to 1000 kcal tube feeding overnight. In the morning the tube is removed and the child can lead a normal life and eat their normal diet.[38,39] With this treatment children can make up for their growth deficit and reach a normal height. Such additional tube feeding may be necessary for months or even years.

In addition to improvement of the nutritional status intermittent enteral nutrition seems to prolong remission.[41] However, these effects have not been adequately investigated in a prospective manner.

Similarly, adults with Crohn's disease and malnutrition do not appear to be able to increase their food intake except if they are provided with liquid diets via tube or sip oral feeding. The addition of 500 mL of a standard liquid diet for 2 months caused a weight gain of 3 kg in a group of malnourished Crohn's patients.[31] Preliminary results indicate that this might also have a steroid-sparing effect in patients with chronic active Crohn's disease.[42]

Standard enteral diets appear to be sufficient for this supplementary enteral nutrition. No advantage of elemental diets or diets containing specific substrates such as omega-3 fatty acids or glutamine has been shown.

Clinically apparent vitamin and mineral deficiencies are uncommon in IBD patients; however, a larger number will have subclinical deficiencies, which can only be diagnosed by laboratory tests. As mentioned above depletion of fat-soluble vitamins, vitamin $B_{12}$, iron and calcium is most frequently seen. Patients at risk should be periodically tested for these deficiencies and be supplemented. Regular intramuscular injection of vitamins A, D, E and K may be necessary in patients with fat malabsorption and resection of the terminal ileum.

Special emphasis should be given to iron deficiency. The majority of patients with Crohn's disease and ulcerative colitis suffer from iron depletion and frequently even from anemia. This is partly due to inadequate intake and to increased losses via the intestine. Oral iron supplementation is not well tolerated by many patients and in most cases therefore does not improve iron status. However, parenteral iron supplements with three to five infusions of 100–200 mg iron/day led to an increase in hemoglobin of more than 2 g/dL in up to 80% of patients. Patients not reacting to intravenous iron may be given erythropoietin. Iron supplementation also improved the quality of life of IBD patients.[28,29,43]

Patients with fat malabsorption and those with chronic active disease and long-term steroid treatment do need calcium and vitamin D supplementation. Vitamin D should be injected parenterally specifically during the winter, whereas calcium can be supplemented orally. The increased bone fracture risk of these patients can be reduced by adequate supplementation. Owing to the high frequency of lactose intolerance in IBD patients milk, which is the major calcium source in standard diets, may not be advisable as calcium supplementation.

## PREOPERATIVE NUTRITIONAL SUPPORT

A history of recent weight loss of more than 10% of the standard weight and/or the finding of a serum albumin concentration below 3.5 g/dL are both risk factors for an increased incidence of postoperative complications.[35b,44] Patients fulfilling these criteria should be treated with preoperative nutritional support, even if the operation is delayed. There are no clear data as to what would be the optimal duration of preoperative nutrition; however, generally enteral nutrition or total parenteral nutrition is performed for 5–7 days before operation in malnourished patients to stabilize the metabolic parameters.

## NUTRITION AS PRIMARY TREATMENT OF INFLAMMATORY BOWEL DISEASE

Early observations demonstrated that patients who failed standard medical therapy and were then treated by parenteral nutrition achieved remission in some instances. These initial uncontrolled observations led to the conduct of controlled studies on the effect of nutrition as primary therapy of the inflammatory process.

## CROHN'S DISEASE

Enteral nutrition was compared to steroid therapy for active Crohn's disease. Initially elemental diets (Vivonex) were compared to steroids and found to be similarly effective at inducing remission.[45] However, these studies were limited by small patient numbers. Therefore, larger studies were subsequently performed comparing steroids with tube feeding or even

**Table 36.2 Randomized studies comparing enteral nutrition with steroids in active CD**

| Study | n | Diet | Mode of delivery | % Remission EN | Steroids |
|---|---|---|---|---|---|
| O'Morain[45] | 21 | Elemental | Oral/tube | 82 | 80 |
| Lindor[46] | 19 | Semi-elemental | Oral/tube | 22 | 50 |
| Gonzalez[47] | 32 | Polymeric | Tube | 80 | 88 |
| Malchow[48] | 95 | Semi-elemental | Oral | 41 | 73 |
| Lochs[49] | 107 | Semi-elemental | Tube | 55 | 85 |
| Seidmann[50] | 78 | Semi-elemental | Tube | 75 | 90 |
| Gorard[51] | 42 | Elemental | Oral/tube | 45 | 85 |
| Seidmann[52] | 19 | Elemental | Tube | 80 | 67 |

sip feeding. In summary, these studies showed that enteral nutrition is an effective therapy for the active phase of CD. Approximately 60% of patients with active Crohn's disease do achieve remission by enteral nutrition as sole therapy within 4–6 weeks. Although the effect of enteral nutrition has never been directly compared to placebo, it is known from studies on drug therapy that about 20–30% of patients achieve remission with placebo. This suggests that enteral nutrition may be more effective than placebo; however, enteral nutrition is less effective than steroids. A higher percentage of patients reach remission in a shorter time with steroids than with enteral nutrition (Table 36.2).

These findings limit the role of enteral nutrition as primary therapy to those patients who want to avoid the side effects of long-term or repeated steroid therapy, those who are not willing to take steroids, or those who do not tolerate steroids. For this group, however, enteral nutrition represents a valid alternative, as was concluded in a recent meta-analysis.[53] The duration of remission achieved by enteral nutrition does not appear to be different from that achieved with steroids.

Whereas it was initially assumed that only elemental diets may be used in active Crohn's disease, further studies compared different elemental diets, semi-elemental diets, standard polymeric diets and diets with special compositions. It was shown that standard polymeric diets are as effective as elemental diets.[54–56] Furthermore, specific compositions, such as omega-3 fatty acid- or glutamine-containing diets, do not appear to have an advantage.[57–59] Different compositions of the fat component were also investigated but no clear advantage of specific diets could be shown.

Recently, a milk-based diet containing higher amounts of TGF-β has been investigated in children with Crohn's disease and the authors showed a quick reduction of mucosal inflammation as well as of clinical activity. However, adequate studies comparing this diet with standard polymeric diets or steroids are lacking.[60]

Some studies indicated that disease location might play a role, with enteral nutrition being more effective in patients with small bowel disease rather than colonic CD, but this could not be confirmed by other studies.

In the treatment of active CD enteral nutrition should be delivered via a nasogastric or nasoduodenal tube, with continuous infusion of 25–30 kcal/kg body weight/day. When using elemental diets nasoduodenal tubes are preferred, as the patients sense less of the unpleasant taste of these diets than when they are infused into the stomach. Specific starter regimens do not appear to be necessary. Infusion rates should be increased as individually tolerated. Infusion rates up to 120 mL/h are usually tolerated. Bolus application caused more side effects such as diarrhea, bloating and fullness, which disappeared when continuous infusion was used. Usually, enteral nutrition is given for 4–6 weeks.

Studies investigating the possibility of sip feeding instead of tube feeding failed because of the lack of patient compliance.[48] Tube feeding is therefore the adequate route of nutrition in the treatment of active Crohn's disease.

The mechanism by which enteral nutrition reduces inflammation in the active phase of Crohn's disease is not known. Initially it was assumed that total bowel rest and reduction of luminal antigens might play a role; however, some studies, where patients were allowed to eat a standard diet besides enteral nutrition, showed similar effects to enteral nutrition alone.[61,62] Moreover, total parenteral nutrition, which provides total bowel rest, is not superior to enteral nutrition. The lack of an advantage of elemental diets over polymeric diets also speaks against total bowel rest as an important mechanism.

Improvement of the nutritional status has also been discussed as a possible mechanism of action. This is supported by results from a study showing that those patients who achieved a positive nitrogen balance by enteral nutrition had the best long-term results. It might therefore be possible that induction of anabolism is a key mechanism by which enteral nutrition reduces inflammation in the intestine.[56]

In summary, enteral nutrition can be recommended as an alternative treatment for the active phase of Crohn's disease for all patients who are reluctant to take steroids, and specifically for malnourished patients. Whether a combination of both enteral nutrition and steroids would lead to an additive or a synergistic effect has not been investigated; however, such combinations are frequently used in clinical practice.

## PARENTERAL NUTRITION

Parenteral nutrition has also been used in active Crohn's disease, specifically for patients resistant to steroid treatment. Response rates up to 90% have been reported.[63] Although these were not randomized studies comparing parenteral nutrition to any other treatment, they still demonstrate that even in steroid-resistant patients parenteral nutrition might be an effective therapy.

Compared to enteral nutrition, parenteral nutrition bears a higher risk of complications and is more expensive. It would therefore be justified only if it were more efficacious than enteral nutrition. Several studies have compared parenteral and enteral nutrition in the treatment of active Crohn's disease and found no significant difference regarding the effect on disease activity.[61,62,64] Therefore, enteral nutrition should be preferred over parenteral nutrition in the treatment of active Crohn's disease. Indications for parenteral nutrition are limited to patients who do not tolerate enteral nutrition, such as those with ileus, severe sepsis etc.

In earlier studies a course of home parenteral nutrition for 12 weeks was used in patients with very severe Crohn's disease who were too sick to be operated on; 80% of these patients eventually reached remission, and surgery could even be avoided. However, owing to the introduction of new treatments for Crohn's disease, this indication has become rare.[65–67]

## NUTRITION AS PRIMARY TREATMENT FOR ACTIVE ULCERATIVE COLITIS

Unlike Crohn's disease, active ulcerative colitis does not appear to respond to nutritional support. In several studies providing parenteral nutrition in addition to steroid therapy to patients with severe ulcerative colitis, surgery could not be avoided.[68–70] However, it has to be mentioned that parenteral nutrition was not used as sole treatment in these patients.

Studies comparing parenteral and enteral nutrition in addition to steroids in active ulcerative colitis also showed no difference between the two groups regarding remission rates and need for colectomy. However, complications were higher in the parenteral nutrition group. Because of the lower risk of complications and the lower costs, enteral nutrition should be preferred in these patients. However, it appears that patients do suffer from more diarrhea even on enteral nutrition than with parenteral nutrition, which might make parenteral nutrition preferable.

In general the role of both parenteral and enteral nutrition in ulcerative colitis is limited to adjunctive therapy in fulminant colitis or toxic megacolon to avoid further nutritional deterioration.

## NUTRITION AS MAINTENANCE THERAPY IN IBD

The value of specific diets to maintain remission in Crohn's disease and ulcerative colitis has been extensively studied. Some dietary recommendations, such as the reduction of total carbohydrate intake or reduction of refined sugar intake, were not based on strong scientific evidence. In a 2-year multicenter study[36] a low-carbohydrate diet was compared to standard diets and a diet with increased intake of omega-3 fatty acids. Patients were asked to limit their carbohydrate intake to a maximum of 8 units/day, which is equivalent to 100 g. It turned out that only a minority of patients were able to comply with this dietary recommendation. On the intention to treat basis no advantage of carbohydrate reduction could be shown. This diet is therefore not recommended.

An elimination diet was successfully investigated in several studies. The development of such individualized diets, however, may be troublesome. Patients who achieve remission on enteral nutrition add one new food item to their diet every few days. They will then experience symptoms after a few food items and note this in a diary. Together with the physician they will eliminate those food items from their future diet. Studies showed that most patients are intolerant of one or two food items only. In prospective randomized studies it could be shown that such an elimination diet reduces the likelihood of relapse of Crohn's disease even compared to long-term low-dose steroid treatment.[71,72]

Omega-3 fatty acids have been investigated in Crohn's disease as well as in ulcerative colitis, with controversial results. In the multicenter study mentioned above[36] with carbohydrate reduction the third arm were patients with increased intake of omega-3 fatty acids. They had a similar rate of recurrence as the group with standard diet. In an Italian study, however, a special preparation of omega-3 fatty acids caused a significant reduction of recurrences in Crohn's disease;[73] however, these data have not been reproduced in other studies. Omega-3 fatty acids are therefore not currently recommended as maintenance treatment in Crohn's disease.

Similarly, several studies have investigated the effect of omega-3 fatty acids in ulcerative colitis. A reduction of endoscopic and histologic inflammation, as well as of disease activity, was shown by several investigators,[74–76] but the effects were not clinically meaningful enough to support a recommendation for long-term treatment.

### Probiotics

Probiotics might be taken as food, for example in the form of yoghurt or as tablets. As a result of new data indicating a crucial role of the intestinal flora in the pathogenesis of IBD, specific emphasis has been put on the possibility of altering the intestinal flora. The use of probiotic bacteria was based on data showing that probiotics reduce the adherence of other bacteria to the mucosa. Furthermore, a reduction of intestinal inflammation has been demonstrated by some probiotic preparations. Studies have investigated the effect of probiotics in the therapy of both ulcerative colitis and Crohn's disease.

Several studies showed that the application of *E. coli* Nissle was as effective as mesalazine in maintaining remission in ulcerative colitis.[77,78] A mixture of eight probiotic bacteria called VSL-3 successfully prevented relapse of pouchitis in patients with pouches after proctocolectomy for severe ulcerative colitis.[79] This finding has been supported by animal studies, demonstrating a clear reduction of intestinal inflammation in IL-10 knockout mice when they were fed with VSL-3.[80]

In Crohn's disease only preliminary data exist about a relapse preventing effect of *E. coli* Nissle1917.

Several studies are ongoing to further investigate the clinical effect of probiotics. At present data support an effect of *E. coli* Nissle in the maintenance of ulcerative colitis and an effect of VSL-3 in the maintenance of chronic pouchitis. For other indications and other probiotics data are not sufficient to support clear indications. There are no adequate data to support the use of probiotic foods as therapeutic agents in IBD.

Not all probiotic bacteria appear to be equivalent. An Italian study showed an increased rate of postoperative recurrences after the application of *Lactobacillus GG* compared to placebo.[81]

## NUTRITION AS ADJUVANT THERAPY FOR COMPLICATIONS OF INFLAMMATORY BOWEL DISEASE

### Nutritional therapy of fistulae

Fistulae in patients with Crohn's disease may have different causes. Postoperatively fistulae may develop as a result of leaks from the anastomosis or leaks caused by drainage tubes. Such fistulae may not be specific for Crohn's disease and may therefore be treated like any postoperative fistula, with a high probability of closure when the patients are put on bowel rest.

However, Crohn's-specific fistulae have a completely different prognosis. They may develop between different parts of the intestine, enterocutaneously, or perianally. Several groups have studied the effect of total parenteral nutrition and bowel rest on fistula healing: 30–70% of fistulae were reported to heal primarily, but with a high rate of recurrence when normal nutrition was reinstituted. Long-term closure has been reported in 20–30% of patients only.[82–85]

In patients with high-output fistulae or with fistulae bypassing major parts of the small intestine, preoperative parenteral nutrition might be important to correct nutritional deficiencies and metabolic imbalances.

Enteral nutrition has also been used in patients with Crohn's fistulae, but the results were not encouraging.

In patients with fistulae from the stomach or the duodenum a feeding tube can be passed beyond the fistula and the patient can thereby still be nourished via the gastrointestinal tract.

In summary, nutritional therapy is not effective as primary treatment of fistulae but rather as additive therapy to improve nutritional status before surgery is performed.

## SHORT BOWEL SYNDROME

Crohn's disease patients may develop short bowel syndrome owing to repeated small bowel resections. These patients do then need home parenteral nutrition (PN). Long-term observation of relatively large groups of CD patients on home PN has been performed in several countries.[86] These studies showed that Crohn's patients have a good prognosis on home PN compared to patients on home PN for other indications. However, there is still a considerable morbidity, with a risk of catheter-related sepsis and catheter occlusions as well as central venous thrombosis. Despite extensive monitoring, phases of dehydration and electrolyte disorders have been described. Complications of long-term parenteral nutrition are metabolic bone disease and cholestatic liver disease. In many patients some cholestasis will be noted initially which improves despite continuation of parenteral nutrition; however, in patients with a very short small intestine and a resection of the whole colon, cholestatic liver cirrhosis develops in a high percentage and can eventually be fatal.

From national registries it can be concluded that home parenteral nutrition is definitely a life-saving therapy for Crohn's patients with short bowel syndrome that allows considerable medical and social rehabilitation.

## REFERENCES

1. Thornton JR, Emmett PM, Heaton KW. Diet and Crohn's disease: characteristics of the pre-illness diet. Br Med J 1979;2:762–764.
2. Reif S, Klein I, Lubin F, Farbstein M, Hallak A, Gilat T. Pre-illness dietary factors in inflammatory bowel disease. Gut 1997;40:754–760.
3. Riordan AM, Ruxton CH, Hunter JO. A review of associations between Crohn's disease and consumption of sugars. Eur J Clin Nutr 1998;52:229–238.
4. Motil KJ, Grand RJ, Maletskos CJ, Young VR. The effect of disease, drug, and diet on whole body protein metabolism in adolescents with Crohn disease and growth failure. J Pediatr 1982;101:345–351.
5. Kanof ME, Lake AM, Bayless TM. Decreased height velocity in children and adolescents before the diagnosis of Crohn's disease. Gastroenterology 1988;95:1523–1527.
6. Seidman EG. Nutritional management of inflammatory bowel disease. Gastroenterol Clin North Am 1989;18:129–155.
7. Seidman E, LeLeiko N, Ament M et al. Nutritional issues in pediatric inflammatory bowel disease. J Pediatr Gastroenterol Nutr 1991;12:424–438.
8. Hildebrand H, Karlberg J, Kristiansson B. Longitudinal growth in children and adolescents with inflammatory bowel disease. J Pediatr Gastroenterol Nutr 1994;18:165–173.
9. Rosenberg IH, Bengoa JM, Sitrin MD. Nutritional aspects of inflammatory bowel disease. Annu Rev Nutr 1985;5:463–484.
10. Markowitz J, Grancher K, Rosa J, Aiges H, Daum F. Growth failure in pediatric inflammatory bowel disease. J Pediatr Gastroenterol Nutr 1993;16:373–380.
11. Kirschner BS. Growth and development in chronic inflammatory bowel disease. Acta Paediatr Scand 1990;366:98–104.
12. Heatley RV. Assessing nutritional state in inflammatory bowel disease. Gut 1986;27:61–66.
13. Beeken WL, Busch HJ, Sylwester DL. Intestinal protein loss in Crohn's disease. Gastroenterology 1972;62:207–215.
14. Lashner BA. Red blood cell folate is associated with the development of dysplasia and cancer in ulcerative colitis. J Cancer Res Clin Oncol 1993;119:549–554.

15. Sjogren A, Floren CH, Nilsson A. Evaluation of magnesium status in Crohn's disease as assessed by intracellular analysis and intravenous magnesium infusion. Scand J Gastroenterol 1988;23:555–561.

16. Chan AT, Fleming CR, O'Fallon WM, Huizenga KA. Estimated versus measured basal energy requirements in patients with Crohn's disease. Gastroenterology 1986;91:75–78.

17. Rath HC, Caesar I, Roth M, Scholmerich J. [Nutritional deficiencies and complications in chronic inflammatory bowel diseases]. Med Klin 1998;93:6–10.

18. Maier-Dobersberger T, Lochs H. Enteral supplementation of phosphate does not prevent hypophosphatemia during refeeding of cachectic patients. J Parenter Enteral Nutr 1994;18:182–184.

19. Vogelsang H, Schofl R, Tillinger W, Ferenci P, Gangl A. 25-hydroxyvitamin D absorption in patients with Crohn's disease and with pancreatic insufficiency. Wien Klin Wschr 1997;109:678–682.

20. Schoon EJ, Muller MC, Vermeer C, Schurgers LJ, Brummer RJ, Stockbrugger RW. Low serum and bone vitamin K status in patients with longstanding Crohn's disease: another pathogenetic factor of osteoporosis in Crohn's disease? Gut 2001;48:473–477.

21. Franklin JL, Rosenberg IH. Impaired folic acid absorption in inflammatory bowel disease: effects of salicylazosulfapyridine (azulfidine). Gastroenterology 1973;64:517.

22. Greenling BJ, Badart-Smook A, Stockbrugger RW, Brummer RJ. Comprehensive nutritional status in recently diagnosed patients with inflammatory bowel disease compared with population controls. Eur J Clin Nutr 2000;54:514–521.

23. Behrend C, Jeppesen PB, Mortensen PB. Vitamin B12 absorption after ileorectal anastomosis for Crohn's disease: effect of ileal resection and time span after surgery. Eur J Gastroenterol Hepatol 1995;7:397.

24. Thomson ABR, Brust R, Ali MAM et al. Iron deficiency in inflammatory bowel disease. Diagnosis: efficacy of serum ferritin. Am J Dig Dis 1978;23:705.

25. Schoon EJ, van Nunen AB, Wouters RS, Stockbrugger RW, Russel MG. Osteopenia and osteoporosis in Crohn's disease: prevalence in a Dutch population-based cohort. Scand J Gastroenterol 2000;232:43–47.

26. Loftus EV Jr, Crowson CS, Sandborn WJ, Tremaine WJ, O'Fallon WM, Melton LJ 3rd. Long-term fracture risk in patients with Crohn's disease: a population-based study in Olmsted County, Minnesota. Gastroenterology 2002;123:468–475.

27. Klaus J, Armbrecht G, Steinkamp M et al. High prevalence of osteoporotic vertebral fractures in patients with Crohn's disease. Gut 2002;51:654–658.

28. Gasche C, Dejaco C, Waldhoer T et al. Intravenous iron and erythropoietin for anemia associated with Crohn disease. A randomized, controlled trial. Ann Intern Med 1997;126:782–787.

29. Schreiber S, Howaldt S, Schnoor M et al. Recombinant erythropoietin for the treatment of anemia in inflammatory bowel disease. N Engl J Med 1996;334:619–623

30. Motil KJ, Grand RJ, Davis-Kraft L, Ferlic LL, Smith EO. Growth failure in children with inflammatory bowel disease: a prospective study. Gastroenterology 1993;105:681–691.

31. Harries AD, Jones LA, Danis V et al. Controlled trial of supplemented oral nutrition in Crohn's disease. Lancet 1983;1:887–890.

32. Florent C, L'Hirondel C, Desmazures C et al. Evaluation of ulcerative colitis and Crohn's disease activity by measurement of $\alpha_1$-antitrypsin intestinal clearance. Gastroenterol Clin Biol 1981;5:193.

33. Schneeweiss B, Lochs H, Zauner C et al. Energy and substrate metabolism in patients with active Crohn's disease. J Nutr 1999;129:844–848.

34. Azcue M, Rashid M, Griffiths A, Pencharz PB. Energy expenditure and body composition in children with Crohn's disease: effect of enteral nutrition and treatment with prednisolone. Gut 1997;41:203–208.

35. Barot LR, Rombeau JL, Feurer ID, Mullen JL. Caloric requirements in patients with inflammatory bowel disease. Ann Surg 1982;195:214–218.

35a. Cucino C, Sonnenberg A. Cause of death in patients with inflammatory bowel disease. Inflamm Bowel Dis 2001;7:250–255.

35b. Higgens CS, Keighley MR, Allan RN. Impact of preoperative weight loss and body composition changes on postoperative outcome in surgery for inflammatory bowel disease. Gut 1984;25:732–736.

36. Lorenz-Meyer H, Bauer P, Nicolay C et al. Omega-3 fatty acids and low carbohydrate diet for maintenance of remission in Crohn's disease. A randomised controlled multicenter trial. Study Group Member's (German Crohn's Disease Study Group). Scand J Gastroenterol 1996;31:778–785.

37. Kirschner BS, Klich JR, Kalman SS, de Favaro MV, Rosenberg IH. Reversal of growth retardation in Crohn's disease with therapy emphasing oral nutritional restitution. Gastroenterology 1981;80:10–15.

38. Belli DC, Seidman E, Bouthillier L et al. Chronic intermittent elemental diet improves growth failure in children with Crohn's disease. Gastroenterology 1988;94:603–610.

39. Aiges H, Markowitz J, Rosa J, Daum F. Home nocturnal supplemental nasogastric feedings in growth-retarded adolescents with Crohn's disease. Gastroenterology 1989;97:905–910.

40. Israel DM, Hassall E. Prolonged use of gastrostomy for enteral hyperalimentation in children with Crohn's disease. Am J Gastroenterology 1995;90:1084.

41. Wilschanski M, Sherman P, Pencharz P et al. Supplementary enteral nutrition maintains remission in pediatric Crohn's disease. Gut 1996;38:543.

42. Verma S, Holdsworth CD, Giaffer MH. Does adjuvant nutritional support diminish steroid dependence in Crohn's disease? Scand J Gastroenterol 2001;36:383–388.

43. Gasche C, Waldhoer T, Feichtenschlager T et al. and Austrian Inflammatory Bowel Diseases Study Group. Prediction of response to iron sucrose in inflammatory bowel disease-associated anemia. Am J Gastroenterol 2001;96:2382–2387.

44. Lindor KD, Fleming CR, Ilstrup DM. Preoperative nutritional status and other factors that influence surgical outcome in patients with Crohn's disease. Mayo Clin Proc 1985;60:393–396.

45. O'Morain C, Segal AW, Levi AJ. Elemental diet as primary treatment of acute Crohn's disease: a controlled trial. Br Med J (Clin Res Ed) 1984;288:1859–1862.

46. Lindor KD, Fleming CR, Burnes JU, Nelson JK, Ilstrup DM. A randomized prospective trial comparing a defined formula diet, corticosteroids, and a defined formula diet plus corticosteroids in active Crohn's disease. Mayo Clin Proc 1992;67:328–333.

47. Gonzalez-Huix F, de Leon R, Fernandez-Banares F et al. Polymeric enteral diets as primary treatment of active Crohn's disease: a prospective steroid controlled trial. Gut 1993;34:778–782.

48. Malchow H, Steinhardt HJ, Lorenz-Meyer H et al. Feasibility and effectiveness of a defined-formula diet regimen in treating active Crohn's disease. European Cooperative Crohn's Disease Study III. Scand J Gastroenterol 1990;25:235–244.

49. Lochs H, Steinhardt HJ, Klaus-Wentz B et al. Comparison of enteral nutrition and drug treatment in active Crohn's disease. Results of the European Cooperative Crohn's Disease Study. IV. Gastroenterology 1991;101:881–888.

50. Seidman E, Griffiths A, Jones A, Issenman R. Semielemental diet versus prednisone in the treatment of active Crohns´s disease in children and adolescents. Gastroenterology 1993;104:A778 (Abstract).

51. Gorard DA, Hunt JB, Payne-James JJ et al. Initial response and subsequent course of Crohn's disease treated with elemental diet or prednisolone. Gut 1993;34:1198–1202.

52. Seidmann EG, Lohoues MJ, Turgeon J, Bouthillier L, Morin CL. Elemental diet versus prednisone as initial therapy in Crohn's disease: early and long-term results (Abstract). Gastroenterology 1991;100:250A.

53. Zachos M, Tondeur M, Griffiths AM. Enteral nutritional therapy for inducing remission of Crohn´s disease. Cochrane Database System Review 2001;(3):CD 000542.

54. Raouf AH, Hildrey V, Daniel J et al. Enteral feeding as sole treatment for Crohn's disease: controlled trial of whole protein v amino acid based feed and a case study of dietary challenge. Gut 1991;32:702–707.

55. Rigaud D, Cosnes J, Le Quintrec Y, Rene E, Gendre JP, Mignon M. Controlled trial comparing two types of enteral nutrition in treatment of active Crohn's disease: elemental versus polymeric diet. Gut 1991;32:1492–1497.

56. Royall D, Jeejeebhoy KN, Baker JP et al. Comparison of amino acid v peptide based enteral diets in active Crohn's disease: clinical and nutritional outcome. Gut 1994;35:783–787.

57. Den Hond E, Hiele M, Peeters M, Ghoos Y, Rutgeerts P. Effect of long-term oral glutamine supplements on small intestinal permeability in patients with Crohn's disease. J Parenter Enteral Nutr 1999;23:7–11.

58. Akobeng AK, Miller V, Stanton J, Elbadri AM, Thomas AG. Double-blind randomized controlled trial of glutamine-enriched polymeric diet in the treatment of active Crohn's disease. J Pediatr Gastroenterol Nutr 2000;30:78–84.

59. Gassull MA, Fernandez-Banares F, Cabre E et al. Fat composition may be a clue to explain the primary therapeutic effect of enteral nutrition in Crohn's disease: results of a double blind randomised multicentre European trial. Gut 2002;51:164–168.

60. Fell JM, Paintin M, Arnaud-Battandier F et al. Mucosal healing and a fall in mucosal pro-inflammatory cytokine mRNA induced by a specific oral polymeric diet in paediatric Crohn's disease. Aliment Pharmacol Ther 2000;14:281–289.

61. Lochs H, Meryn S, Marosi L, Ferenci P, Hörtnagl H. Has total bowel rest a beneficial effect in the treatment of Crohn's Disease? Clin Nutr 1983;2:61–64.

62. Greenberg GR, Fleming CR, Jeejeebhoy KN, Rosenberg IH, Sales D, Tremaine WJ. Controlled trial of bowel rest and nutritional support in the management of Crohn's disease. Gut 1988;29:1309–1315.

63. Sales DJ, Rosenberg IH. Total parenteral nutrition in inflammatory bowel disease. Prog Gastroenterol 1983;4:299.

64. Muller JM, Keller HW, Erasmi H et al. Total parenteral nutrition as the sole therapy in Crohn's disease – a prospective study. Br J Surg 1983;70:40.

65. Kushner RF, Shapir J, Sitrin MD. Endoscopic, radiographic, and clinical response to prolonged bowel rest and home parenteral nutrition in Crohn's disease. J Parenter Enteral Nutr 1986;10:568.

66. Lerebours E, Messing B, Chevalier B et al. An evaluation of total parenteral nutrition in the management of steroid-resistant patients with Crohn's disease. J Parenter Enteral Nutr 1986;10:274.

67. Dickinson RJ, Ashton MG, Axon ATR et al. Controlled trial of intravenous hyperalimentation and total bowel rest as an adjunct to the routine therapy of acute colitis. Gastroenterology 1980;79:1199.

68. McIntyre PB, Powell-Tuck J, Wood SR et al. Controlled trial of bowel rest in the treatment of severe acute colitis. Gut 1986;27:481.

69. Gonzalez-Huix F, Fernandez-Banares F, Esteve-Comas M et al. Enteral versus parenteral nutrition as adjunct therapy in acute ulcerative colitis. Am J Gastroenterol 1993;88:227–232.

70. Riordan AM, Hunter JO, Cowan RE et al. Treatment of active Crohn's disease by exclusion diet: East Anglian multicentre controlled trial. Lancet 1993;342.1131.

71. Jones VA, Dickinson RJ, Workman E et al. Crohn's disease: maintenance of remission by diet. Lancet 1985;2:177.

72. Belluzzi A, Brignola C, Campieri M et al. Effect of an enteric-coated fish-oil preparation on relapses in Crohn's disease. N Engl J Med 1996;334:1557.

73. Hawthorne AB, Daneshmend TK, Hawkey CJ et al. Treatment of ulcerative colitis with fish oil supplementation: a prospective 12 month randomised controlled trial. Gut 1992;33:922–928.

74. Stenson WF, Cort D, Rodgers J et al. Dietary supplementation with fish oil in ulcerative colitis. Ann Intern Med 1992;116:609–614.

75. Loeschke K, Ueberschaer B, Pietsch A et al. n-3 fatty acids only delay early relapse of ulcerative colitis in remission. Dig Dis Sci 1996;41:2087–2094.

76. Kruis W, Schutz E, Fric P, Fixa B, Judmaier G, Stolte M. Double-blind comparison of an oral *Escherichia coli* preparation and mesalazine in maintaining remission of ulcerative colitis. Aliment Pharmacol Ther 1997;11:853–858.

77. Rembacken BJ, Snelling AM, Hawkey PM, Chalmers DM, Axon AT. Non-pathogenic *Escherichia coli* versus mesalazine for the treatment of ulcerative colitis: a randomised trial. Lancet 1999;21:635–639.

78. Gionchetti P, Rizzello F, Venturi A et al. Oral bacteriotherapy as maintenance treatment in patients with chronic pouchitis: a double-blind, placebo-controlled trial. Gastroenterology 2000;119:305–309.

79. Madsen K, Cornish A, Soper P et al. Probiotic bacteria enhance murine and human intestinal epithelial barrier function. Gastroenterology 2001;121:580–591.

80. Prantera C, Scribano ML, Falasco G, Andreoli A, Luzi C. Ineffectiveness of probiotics in preventing recurrence after curative resection for Crohn's disease: a randomised controlled trial with *Lactobacillus GG*. Gut 2002;51:405–409.

81. Lashner BA, Evans AA, Hanauer SB. Preoperative total parenteral nutrition for bowel resection in Crohn's disease. Dig Dis Sci 1989;34:741.

82. Fukuci S, Seeburger J, Parquet P et al. Nutrition support of patients with enterocutaneous fistulae. Nutr Clin Pract 1998;13:59.

83. Voitk AJ, Echave V, Brown RA et al. Elemental diet in the treatment of fistulae of the alimentary tract. Surg Gynecol Obstet 1973;137:68.

84. Calam J, Crooks PE, Walker RJ. Elemental diets in the management of Crohn's perianal fistulae. J Parenter Enteral Nutr 1980;4:4–8.

85. Howard L, Ament M, Fleming CR et al. Current use and clinical outcome of home parenteral and enteral nutrition therapies in the United States. Gastroenterology 1995;109:355.

86. Messing B, Crenn P, Beau P, Boutron-Ruault MC, Rambaud JC, Matuchansky C. Long-term survival and parenteral nutrition dependence in adult patients with the short bowel syndrome. Gastroenterology 1999;117:1043–1050.

## CHAPTER 37

# New therapeutic drugs for inflammatory bowel disease

Sander JH van Deventer

## INTRODUCTION

Current medical therapy for inflammatory bowel disease is based on the use of broad-acting anti-inflammatory or immuno-suppressive drugs. With these drugs, in many patients disease activity can be adequately suppressed, and in general the safety of sulfasalazine, mesalazine, azathioprine and methotrexate and short courses (8–12 weeks) of corticosteroids is acceptable.[1] Surgery remains an attractive option for selected patients with refractory disease, such as ulcerative pancolitis or complicated ileitis. Anti-TNF-α therapies such as infliximab have augmented the therapeutic possibilities in patients with therapy-refractory Crohn's disease, are steroid sparing, and significantly improve the quality of life.[2,3] Nevertheless, despite these improvements, for several reasons new drugs for inflammatory bowel disease are needed. About half of all patients admitted with severe ulcerative colitis will eventually undergo colectomy, and a significant minority of Crohn's disease patients do not respond to standard medical therapies, including TNF-α neutralizing antibodies, or suffer from significant side effects. Finally, recurrence of disease activity following remission is frequent in both ulcerative colitis and Crohn's disease, and there is an unmet need for effective maintenance strategies.

During the past two decades many attempts have been made to identify new therapeutic targets for therapy of inflammatory bowel disease. Initial efforts yielded small molecules inhibiting peripheral inflammatory events such as platelet-activating factor, leukotrienes, NO production and thromboxane, but unfortunately this did not translate into effective therapies.[4] Recent insight into the pathogenesis of inflammatory bowel disease, acquired mainly from animal models, has enabled the characterization of the molecular interactions that are critical for the induction of mucosal inflammatory responses, and this has directed drug development in recent years. This chapter will review new medical tools and targets that are relevant for the therapy of inflammatory bowel disease. We then briefly review compounds that are currently in preclinical or clinical development for Crohn's disease or ulcerative colitis.

## NEW THERAPEUTIC TARGETS

### DENDRITIC CELLS AND T CELLS

The currently prevailing hypothesis of the pathogenesis of Crohn's disease is that mucosal inflammation results from an inadequately controlled T cell-driven immune response that is driven by antigens present in the intestinal lumen.[5,6] According to this view, the interaction between the antigen-presenting mucosal (dendritic) cell and a gut-homing naive T lymphocyte within a mesenterial lymph node is a pivotal event that would provide many possibilities for therapeutic intervention. The normal intestinal mucosa already contains a large number of dendritic cells (DC), and the inflamed mucosa is literally packed with activated DC. It has been reported that DC are able to protrude extensions between epithelial cells into the gut lumen that are thought to be involved in the continuous antigen uptake.[7] Originally considered an inert innate immune cell, it is now clear that the DC orchestrates adaptive immune responses, making decisions with respect to activation and differentiation of T-cell subpopulations, or the induction of tolerance. DC are activated and mature after contact with cytokines and certain 'danger' signals. This is partly dependent on the expression and activation of Toll-like membrane receptors, and probably intracellular NOD receptors, that recognize specific patterns associated with microbial pathogens (PAMP) such as Gram-negative bacterial lipopolysaccharides, peptidoglycans and bacterial CpG DNA motifs.[8,9] Research in this field is progressing rapidly and it is likely that the mechanisms that lead to abnormal activation of DC in inflammatory bowel disease will become clear within the coming years. Although at present no therapeutic approaches in inflammatory bowel disease are directly targeted at these early events, it is likely that this will become an interesting field of research. For example, there is increasing evidence that some probiotic therapies act at the dendritic cell level (Braat H, van Deventer SJH, unpublished results 2002).

Once matured and activated, dendritic cells in their turn activate T lymphocytes by presenting antigenic peptide/HLA molecule complexes to the T-cell receptor. Activation of T cells requires additional expression of co-stimulatory molecules by dendritic cells that bind to specific ligands on T cells (i.e. B7-CD28 and ICOS-ICOS), as well as the production of cytokines such as IL-12 and IL-18.[10–14] Recent observations have indicated that at least two different mucosal subpopulations exist that are characterized by mutual expression of either the adhesion molecule ligand DC-SIGN and production of IL-18, or by expression of the differentiation marker CD83 and production of IL-12 (te Velde A et al., manuscript submitted). Activation of T lymphocytes within the periphery, and certainly within the mucosal compartment, needs to be tightly controlled in order to prevent chronic inflammation and tissue damage. Apart from anergy, which occurs when the T-cell receptor is engaged in the absence of co-stimulatory signals, peripheral tolerance is dependent upon the induction of apoptosis of activated T lymphocytes and on the activity of 'regulatory' T lymphocytes.[15] In Crohn's disease, but not in ulcerative colitis, lamina propria T cells are abnormally resistant to the induction of apoptosis, and this potentially increases their lifespan as well as their ability to replicate.[16–18] Hence, targeted induction of apoptosis of activated lamina propria T cells is an attractive therapeutic goal, and there is increasing evidence that infliximab therapy causes the induction of apoptosis in activated monocytes as well as T lymphocytes.[19,20]

'Regulatory' T lymphocytes are functional subsets of T cells that downregulate adaptive immune responses by interfering with the activation of dendritic cells and proliferation of T cells. These subsets include 'Th3' cells that mainly produce TGF-β, 'Tr1' cells, which are dependent upon IL-10 production, and thymus-derived CD4+CD25+ regulatory cells that produce both TGF-β and IL-10.[21–23] From experimental work it is now clear that these regulatory T-cell subsets play a critical role in maintaining immune homeostasis, and several therapeutic approaches are targeted at the induction of regulatory T cells in order to control mucosal inflammation.

## THE EPITHELIUM

At present, the role of adaptive immune responses in ulcerative colitis is less well defined. In ulcerative colitis lamina propria T cells are activated, but cytokine production by these cells differs from the Th1-type pattern (IFN-γ, TNF-α) observed in Crohn's disease. Activation of the humoral arm of the immune response is more prominent in ulcerative colitis than in Crohn's disease, and several autoantibodies (recognizing epithelial antigens and neutrophil-associated antigens) are associated with ulcerative colitis.[24–26] Recently, a series of observations has implicated colonic epithelial cells as a primary target for new therapies. Epithelial cells from ulcerative colitis patients in complete clinical and endoscopic remission produce increased amounts of chemokines such as IL-8 that are able to recruit neutrophils from the circulation into the mucosa.[27–29] This abnormal epithelial chemokine production is controlled by both NFκB and MAP kinases, which are normally controlled by the nuclear receptor PPARγ.[30] Recent studies suggest that in patients with ulcerative colitis epithelial PPARγ expression may be lost, which may

explain their sensitivity to activation of either NFκB or MAP kinases. The stimuli responsible for the activation of these signal transduction pathways have not been completely characterized, but it has been speculated that this may proceed through Toll-like receptors (TLR). Indeed, the inflamed intestinal epithelium is able to express several TLR.[31–33] These are early data but, if confirmed, would indicate that control of activation of the intestinal epithelium would be a major primary goal in ulcerative colitis.

Increased epithelial permeability is a feature of both Crohn's disease and ulcerative colitis, and this has been suggested to cause immune stimulation by antigenic overload. Some, but not all, mice that were genetically engineered to have increased intestinal permeability indeed show mucosal inflammation. However, none of the therapeutic interventions that were primarily aimed at restoring intestinal permeability have shown significant therapeutic effect in animal models or clinical trials. Conversely, potent anti-inflammatory interventions rapidly restore mucosal integrity, and it is therefore likely that increased permeability is a consequence rather than a cause of inflammatory bowel disease.

## SIGNAL TRANSDUCTION PATHWAYS

The expression of many genes involved in inflammation, including cytokines, cell adhesion proteins, and proteins involved in cell proliferation and apoptosis, is controlled by either NFκB or MAP kinases.[34,35] Moreover, the secondary responses resulting from engagement of several cytokine receptors depend on the same signal transduction pathways, which have consequently become important targets for anti-inflammatory therapies. One of the major advantages of these candidate drugs is that these are small molecules that generally can be administered orally. MAP kinases are a large family of serine/threonine kinases (20 isoforms have been described) that constitute evolutionary well-conserved pathways that convey growth and stress signals from membrane receptors to the cell nucleus. Activation of these pathways is dependent on a series of subsequent phosphorylations, eventually leading to the formation of an active transcription factor (i.e. the jun-fos heterodimer AP-1) that recognizes specific DNA-binding sites present in many genes involved in inflammation. The three major mammalian MAP kinase pathways are ERK1/2, p38 and JNK. ERK1 and ERK2 (also known as the p42/p44 MAP kinases) have classically been associated with cell growth and proliferation, but it has recently been shown that this pathway is rapidly activated in low-dose human endotoxemia.[36] Moreover, ERK1-deficient mice have reduced T-cell receptor expression and decreased thymocyte maturation.[37] Although these observations suggest that ERK1 is necessary for adaptive immune responses, inhibition of this pathway would be expected to have many side effects because of the ubiquitous role of ERK1/2 in cell proliferation. The three JNK MAP kinases, also known as stress-activated protein kinases (SAPK), are involved in immune activation and apoptosis, and JNK2-deficient T lymphocytes produce greatly reduced amounts of IFN-γ. JNK1 is overexpressed in the mucosa of both ulcerative colitis and Crohn's disease patients, and therefore is an attractive therapeutic candidate.[38,39] p38 MAP kinases (four MAP p38 kinase isoforms, α–δ, are known) are activated by a wide range of proinflammatory cytokines as well as bacterial toxins (through several Toll-like receptors) and have attracted major attention as therapeutic targets.[40] p38 MAP kinases regulate the transcription of many genes involved in inflammation, and in addition activate MAPKAP kinase 2, which is necessary for derepression of mRNA encoding TNF-α.[41] Hence, in the case of TNF-α, p38 regulates protein production at the transcriptional as well as the post-transcriptional level. It should be recognized that there is extensive crosstalk between the various MAP kinase pathways, as well as with other signal transduction cascades such as the IKK-NFκB route. Several pharmaceutical companies have generated small molecules that more or less specifically interfere with MAP kinase signaling, and some of these have potent anti-inflammatory properties.

NFκB signal transduction factors are homo- or dimeric proteins of the Rel family. These proteins are bound within the cytoplasm by IκB, that is phosphorylated and degraded in the proteasome upon activation of receptors for pro-inflammatory cytokines, thereby allowing the NFκB protein to enter the nucleus.[42] Within the nucleus, NFκB binds to a specific motif present in the promoter of many genes involved in inflammation and immune activation. Activation of NFκB occurs within immune cells present in the inflamed lamina propria, but also within epithelial cells. In the latter situation, NFκB is known to drive production of chemokines that are upregulated in ulcerative colitis, and activation of NFκB in lamina propria immune cells precedes TNF-α production and clinical relapse in Crohn's disease.

Two other signal transduction pathways may become future therapeutic targets in inflammatory bowel disease. STAT-1 is part of the interferon signaling chain, and STAT-1 expression is upregulated in ulcerative colitis.[43] STAT-1 signaling is antago-nized by the a class of intracellular proteins known as suppressors of cytokine signaling (SOCS), but no clinically useful specific inhibitors are available. Smad proteins regulate signaling through the TGF-β receptor family, and Smad7, a potent inhibitor of TGF-β signal transduction, is upregulated in Crohn's disease. Indeed, blockade of Smad7 restored the ability of TGF-β to inhibit the secretion of proinflammatory cytokines, suggesting that this strategy might be used to store immune homeostasis in Crohn's disease.[44]

Recently, a novel signal transduction pathway in T lymphocytes was found to be important for the pathogenesis of Crohn's disease. The transcription factor T-bet has been shown to be of great importance for the functional differentiation of T lymphocytes, controlling the mucosal IFN-γ/IL-4 ration as well as the production of the regulatory cytokine TGF-β.[45,46]

# NEW THERAPEUTIC TOOLS (Table 37.1)

## MONOCLONAL ANTIBODIES, RECEPTOR FUSION MOLECULES AND SOLUBLE RECEPTOR ANTAGONISTS

For several reasons, monoclonal antibodies have become important research and therapeutic tools in inflammatory bowel disease. First, monoclonal antibodies against a wide variety of inflammatory proteins can be easily generated, allowing rapid characterization of the importance of these proteins in experimental models of mucosal inflammation. Following the

**Table 37.1 New biological therapies**

| System | Mechanism of action | (Expected) side effects | Stage of development | Investigations in inflammatory bowel disease? |
|---|---|---|---|---|
| Monoclonal antibodies | Bind to soluble proteins (cytokines) or to membrane associated molecules | Immunogenicity, induction of anti-dsDNA antibodies (anti-TNFα mAbs), infusion reactions | Several antibodies approved for clinical use | Many studies ongoing |
| Antisense oligonucleotides | Bind to mRNA, which is degraded by RNAse H | High doses inhibit coagulation activation and may induce complement activation. Subcutaneous injection causes lymph node swelling | One antisense oligonucleotide is approved for clinical use | ICAM-1 and NFκB p65 targeting oligonucleotides in clinical studies |
| Gene therapy | Viral or non-viral vectors are used to deliver a gene to a target cell. Gene can be integrated in the host genome or expressed outside the nucleus. Time of expression varies from days to years | Specific toxicities associated with vector technology. Immunogenicity of adenovirus vectors. Hepatotoxicity of high-dose adenovirus. Potential carcinogenicity by random insertion of genes in host genome | Many clinical studies in cancer and hemophilia No approved drugs | Ex vivo transduction of human T lymphocytes with human IL-10 gene Clinical intrarectal administration of cytokine-encoding plasmids. Clinical administration of IL-10 producing lactococcus |
| mRNA loading of dendritic cells | mRNA is amplified ex vivo and electroporated into monocyte-derived DCs, which are used as a vaccine | Potential autoimmunity | Several studies in cancer No approved drugs | |
| RNA interference | dsRNA silences gene transcription by several mechanisms (see text) | ? | Works in cell systems and in lower animals (C. elegans) | |

identification of a potential therapeutic target in mouse models, high-affinity monoclonal antibodies against the human homolog can be rapidly generated. Mouse monoclonal antibodies rapidly induce immunogenic responses (in particular human antimouse antibodies; HAMA) that preclude repetitive administration. This problem can be tackled by the generation of mouse/human chimeric antibodies (i.e. infliximab; 30% mouse protein, binds TNF-α), by further humanizing the antibody (i.e. CDP571; 5% mouse protein, binds TNF-α) or by generating completely human antibodies (i.e. D2E7, completely human, binds TNF-α). The clinical efficacy of a therapeutic monoclonal antibody is dependent on binding properties, which are defined by the affinity as well as the irreversibility of binding (also referred to as the 'off' rate). Other important factors are the ability to bind the target protein in various conformations and the effector functions mediated by the antibody heavy chain. For example, TNF-α circulates as a homotrimer, but membrane-expressed TNF-α consists of monomers, dimers and trimers, and not all antibodies recognize these different conformations equally well. Apart from antibodies, several designer molecules have been made with the specific purpose of interfering with the biological function of a specific cytokine, etanercept (composed of the TNF p75 receptor fused to an $IgG_1$ tail) being an example. An important difference between an antibody and a receptor fusion protein is that the former is usually able to bind to two target molecules, thereby potentially cross-linking membrane-associated proteins, whereas the latter generally binds a single molecule. The choice of the IgG tail is also relevant in view of the fact that the mode of action of some antibodies has been linked to activation of complement ($IgG_1$, but not $IgG_4$, activates complement), whereas other antibodies mediated killing of target cells by antibody-dependent killer T-cell activity. Target cells may also be killed by linking the antibody to a toxin such as ricin. Other modifications of therapeutic antibodies are F(ab)2 or F(ab)1 fragment, which may be PEG linked in order to increase half-life. Clearly, F(ab)1 fragments only bind a single target molecule and have an IgG tail to induce effector functions.

Cytokine receptor antagonists are natural proteins that bind to a cytokine receptor without causing signal transduction, such as IL-1 receptor antagonist, which blocks IL-1β signaling.[47] Decoy receptors are either membrane-associated or soluble cytokine-binding proteins that do not induce signaling, such as IL-18-binding protein.[48] The advantage of these naturally occurring proteins is that even large doses generally do not induce immune responses; their disadvantage is that, in general, large doses are needed, because effective competition with high-affinity receptor binding requires high concentrations.

## PROTEINS AND PEPTIDES

Large foreign proteins usually are too immunogenic to be used therapeutically, but some exceptions exist. For example, neutrophil inhibitory factor (NIF) is a 41 kDa protein derived from the hookworm that can be clinically used to block CD11b-dependent adhesion of neutrophils.[49,50] NIF is currently in clinical trials in stroke patients, but interference with neutrophil influx would obviously be a valid therapeutic goal in patients with fulminant colitis. Many therapeutic peptides have a short half-life and are vulnerable to cleavage by peptidases. These problems can be overcome by designing peptides that associate with carrier proteins (i.e. albumin) or with lipoproteins, and several newly designed (circular) peptides cannot be cleaved by peptidases and

have demonstrated efficacy in animal models.[51] Interestingly, some of these new therapeutic peptides also have a very good oral bioavailability. In combination, the rapid evolution in the design of therapeutic peptides has made the development of orally available compounds feasible.

## ANTISENSE DNA OLIGONUCLEOTIDES, mRNA LOADING AND RNAi

DNA oligonucleotides that are complementary to certain mRNA sequences are able to enter cells and subsequently cause a shutdown of the production of the mRNA-encoded protein. Initially it was thought that the antisense DNA oligonucleotides would physically interfere with the translation process, but it has now been established that the mRNA/DNA heterodimer is destroyed by RNAse H.[52,53] Many antisense DNA oligonucleotides that specifically target cytokines, adhesion molecules and signal transduction proteins have been designed. A general problem with antisense oligonucleotides is that sufficient intracellular concentrations often require local delivery. Subcutaneous administration frequently causes side effects, and systemic administration of high doses has been reported to cause inhibition of the intrinsic pathway of blood coagulation.[54] Clinical trials using antisense ODN targeting ICAM-1 and NFκB p65 have been started in inflammatory bowel disease.

RNA is rapidly becoming an important therapeutic tool. Certain RNA (ribozymes) have a catalytic activity that can be directed at specific RNA transcripts. Clinical studies with HIV transcript-cleaving ribozymes have been initiated in HIV-infected patients, but the technology could be adapted to target a large range of (exogenous or endogenous) transcripts involved in inflammation or carcinogenesis. mRNA can also be used as a source for antigenic peptides that are presented by dendritic cells. It has been demonstrated that peripheral blood monocyte-derived dendritic cells can be effectively loaded with mRNA, and immunization with these mRNA-loaded cells results in cytotoxic T-cell responses.[55] At present the technology is mainly suited for cancer vaccination programs, but it is expected that the indications can be extended to antiviral therapies and even the induction of tolerance.

A new and exciting discovery is the finding that double-stranded RNA can cause post-transcriptional gene silencing (RNA interference, or RNAi; for a review see[56]). This development was initiated by the finding that double-stranded RNA is able to silence gene expression in plants and in the worm *Caenorhabditis elegans*.[57] Initially thought to be a result of post-transcriptional interference, the precise mechanism of action is still under investigation, and may involve DNA methylation and chromatin remodeling. The importance of these findings in plants and worms for the development of new therapeutics in humans became clear when it was found that RNAi is also functional in mammalian cells, and has become feasible by the development of a dsRNA expression system that enables expression of dsRNA in mammalian cells.

## GENE THERAPY

The goal of gene therapy is the expression of a therapeutic gene by specific cells. Injection of naked DNA plasmids into muscle can result in the uptake and expression of the plasmid-encoded genes by muscle cells, and expression of plasmids in other tissues can be achieved by packaging in liposomes. However, efficient uptake and long-term expression of therapeutic genes generally requires delivery by 'vectors', which are modified viral particles containing the genes of interest.[58] The most commonly used vectors are derived from adenovirus, retrovirus and adeno-associated virus (AAV).[59] Adenoviral vectors are relatively easy to produce and accommodate large genes, but virtually all currently available vectors are rather immunogenic, restricting their use to a limited series of administrations. Genes encoded by adenoviral vectors do not integrate into the host genome, and their expression is transient. Another disadvantage of these vectors is the limited target cell specificity, which is mainly dictated by the restricted expression of the Coxsackie adenoviral receptor (CAR).[60] Adenoviral as well as other vectors can be modified to target specific cells by modification of the outer proteins (the adenoviral knob proteins, and the retroviral envelope proteins). Most studies with adenoviral vectors have been conducted in patients with cancer. Retroviral vectors are based on mouse leukemia viruses that are non-pathogenic in humans and integrate into the host genome, resulting in long-term expression. These vectors are best suited to target lymphocytes, but may be modified to transduce other cells.[61] A major disadvantage is that the nuclear membrane of the target cells only becomes permeable for retroviral vectors when the cells divide, and resting cells are not transduced. Integration of retroviral constructs within the host DNA occurs randomly, and this may cause disruption of genes involved in regulation of cell differentiation and replication. Indeed, rearrangements in the chromosome 11q23 region have been reported in a child that developed leukemia following gene therapy with a retroviral vector.[62] In contrast to retroviral vectors, lentiviral vectors transduce resting cells. Finally, AAV-based vectors are considered to be non-immunogenic and integrate into the host genome, resulting in long-term expression of the vector-encoded genes.[63,64] A disadvantage of AAV is their inability to accommodate large genes, and these vectors are difficult to produce.

No clinical studies have been initiated using gene therapy in inflammatory bowel disease, but preclinical studies have indicated the feasibility of several approaches. For example, mucosal expression of regulatory cytokines can be achieved by genetically modified lymphocytes or by oral administration of genetically modified bacteria. Long-term expression of the β-galactose gene within the small bowel of rats has been reported using an AAV-based system, and even short-term adenoviral-based approaches have shown efficacy in experimental colitis.[65–67]

# NEW THERAPEUTIC APPROACHES IN INFLAMMATORY BOWEL DISEASE

## TAMING THE DENDRITIC CELL

Both IL-12 and IL-18 are upregulated in the mucosa of patients with active Crohn's disease, but not in ulcerative colitis, and these cytokines are involved in differentiating T lymphocytes into a Th1 direction (characterized by increased production of IL-2, IFN-γ and TNF-α).[68–72] It should be noted that IL-12 is a heterodimeric protein containing a p35 α chain and a p40 β chain. The p40 β chain is shared with two other biologically active cytokines, i.e. p40/p40 homodimers, and the p19/p40 heterodimer known as IL-23. In experimental colitis in mice,

p40/p40 homodimers are protective and IL-23 primarily stimulates the subfraction of T lymphocytes that contains memory cells (CD4+CD45RB$^{low}$).[73–75] Most anti-IL-12 antibodies are directed against the p40 chain, and are therefore expected to neutralize all three p40-containing cytokines. Anti-IL-12 p40 antibodies have important therapeutic effects in the TNBS mouse model of Th1-biased colitis, and a clinical trial has been initiated.[76] However, it should be borne in mind that these antibodies block three cytokines (p40 homodimers, IL-23 and IL-12) simultaneously. The production of IL-12 is greatly increased by activation of the CD40 receptor expressed by DC through interaction with CD40 ligand on T lymphocytes, and interference with this pathway is known to interfere with Th1-biased immune responses. There is a wealth of data that both anti-CD40 and anti-CD40L (CD154) therapies are effective in diseases characterized by T-lymphocyte activation, and clinical studies in transplantation and autoimmune disease have been initiated.[77,78]

IL-18 is a monomeric member of the IL-1 family of cytokines that binds to a specific dimeric receptor mainly expressed by T lymphocytes. Similar to IL-12, IL-18 can direct T-lymphocyte differentiation into a Th1 direction. In mice and humans, IL-18 is antagonized by a naturally occurring binding protein (IL-18BP), a situation reminiscent of the IL-1β/soluble IL-1 receptor and TNF-α/soluble TNF receptor systems, the main difference being that there is no membrane-associated IL-18 BP.[48] IL-18 and IL-18BP are dramatically upregulated in the mucosa of patients with Crohn's disease,[79] and therapeutic administration of IL-18BP reduced TNF-α expression and the severity of experimental colitis.[80] Similar results have been reported using IL-18-binding antibodies.[81]

The binding of CD28 to either B7.1 (CD80) or B7.2 (CD86) expressed by antigen-presenting cells is an important co-stimulatory and survival signal for T lymphocytes, and is downregulated by expression of an alternative inhibitory B7 ligand, CTLA-4.[82] A fusion protein consisting of the CTLA-4-binding domain and IgG$_1$ has been shown to downregulate T lymphocyte-dependent inflammation in various animal models of chronic inflammation, including colitis, and is currently undergoing clinical testing in psoriasis and bone marrow transplantation.[83] Obviously, CTLA-4 Ig would be an interesting therapeutic candidate in Crohn's disease. However, it should be noted that engagement of CD28 is necessary for the maintenance of regulatory T lymphocytes in the periphery, and long-term blockade of CD28 may cause a loss of regulatory cells that are necessary for the maintenance of mucosal immune homeostasis.[84]

ICOS is a protein with significant homology to CD28, and the ICOS gene is located in the CD28/CTLA-4/ICOS gene cluster in chromosome 2q23.[11,85] ICOS is expressed on (CD28/T cell receptor) activated T lymphocytes, but not on resting cells. In humans and in mice, T lymphocytes in the Peyer's patches express ICOS. In humans, the ligand for the ICOS receptor, ICOS-L, is expressed by B lymphocytes, monocytes and monocyte-derived DC, all known to be antigen-presenting cells. Engagement of ICOS increases the production of both Th1 and Th2 cytokines but, in contrast to CD28, the ICOS pathway is important for IL-10 production by T lymphocytes. Interference with ICOS signal transduction by the administration of soluble ICOS in mouse models has indicated that this pathway is more important for Th2 (reducing production of IL-4 and IL-13) than for Th1 responses.[86] This would make ICOS blockade a candidate for ulcerative colitis rather than for Crohn's disease.

## KILLING OR SUPPRESSING ACTIVATED T LYMPHOCTES

Immune tolerance is based on the ability of the immune system to differentiate between self and non-self (for reviews see[87,88]). Central thymus-dependent tolerance is a consequence of apoptosis of T lymphocytes that bind to antigens expressed by the thymus epithelium with a high affinity.[89] In addition, some T lymphocytes that show high-affinity recognition of self-antigens are educated to become CD4+CD25+ regulatory cells that are of critical importance for peripheral tolerance.[90,91] Peripheral tolerance, in particular in the gut mucosa, is importantly dependent on peripheral mechanisms, in part because the mucosal immune system should not mount immune responses towards commensal intestinal bacteria. Obviously, peripheral tolerance only occurs after birth and bacterial colonization of the gut. Mucosal peripheral mechanisms is dependent on at least two mechanisms, apoptosis and the functions of regulatory T lymphocytes, which in many systems are dependent on IL-10 and TGF-β. The importance of T-lymphocyte apoptosis as a regulatory mechanism is emphasized by the observation that defects in this mechanism (for example caused by mutations in signaling through the Fas death receptor) lead to widespread inflammation and have a high chance of developing lymphoma.[92,93] Apoptosis of T lymphocytes can be induced by activation of the Fas receptor (CD95) by Fas ligand in an autocrine (suicide) or paracrine (fratricide) fashion. Activation of the Fas receptor causes recruitment of a number of proteins to the membrane, resulting in the formation of the death-inducing signaling complex (DISC), which is able to activate procaspase 8, which in its turn activates procaspase 3, resulting in apoptosis.[94] Apart from this direct pathway, caspase 8 also can activate proteins of the Bcl-2 family, which regulate mitochondrial permeability, resulting in an altered ratio of Bax/Bak (increased permeability) on the one hand and Bcl-2/Bcl$_{XL}$ (decreased permeability) on the other.[94] Cytochrome C, leaking from permeable mitochondria, can form a multiprotein complex with APAF-1 and caspase 9, known as the apoptosome, that is able to induce activation of downstream apoptotic events.[95] It is now known that lamina propria T lymphocytes from patients with Crohn's disease, but not from ulcerative colitis patients, are abnormally resistant to apoptosis induction, which is related to a low intracellular expression of Bax and a low Bax/Bcl-2 ratio.[16,17,96,97] In addition, it was found that binding of the anti-TNF-α antibody infliximab to membrane-expressed TNF-α on activated monocytes and lymphocytes resulted in an increase of the Bax/Bcl-2 ratio, and increased apoptosis of activated T lymphocytes ex vivo.[98] Moreover, administration of infliximab to Crohn's disease patients resulted in a rapid (within 24 hours) increase of the number of apoptotic lamina propria lymphocytes.[20] These observations suggest that the efficacy of infliximab is at least partly dependent on the activation of apoptosis of activated lamina propria T lymphocytes. Interestingly, the resistance of mucosal T lymphocytes in an animal model of colitis was demonstrated to be dependent on activation of the IL-6 receptor, and could be overcome by the administration of soluble IL-6R.[99] Taken together, these observations indicate that strategies that specifically induce apoptosis of activated T lymphocytes would have great potential therapeutic effects in Crohn's disease.

In several mouse models, but most strikingly in the CD4+CD45$^{RBhigh}$ transfer model, the mucosal inflammatory response can be controlled by regulatory T lymphocytes producing IL-10.[22,100] This finding has not directly translated into a clinically useful therapy, because systemic IL-10 administration did not sufficiently reduce disease activity in Crohn's disease, presumably because of low mucosal bioavailability and the activation of systemic immune responses by high-dose IL-10.[101–103] However, two new approaches, both aiming at mucosal delivery of IL-10, may revive the interest in this regulatory cytokine. The first approach used genetically modified bacteria (*Lactococcus lactis*) that secrete IL-10, and oral administration of these bacteria reduced inflammation in mouse models of colitis.[104] A clinical study using this approach has begun. The second approach aims to generate regulatory T lymphocytes ex vivo by using an MMLV-based vector to introduce the human IL-10 gene into T lymphocytes. Indeed, this approach has been reported to generate cells with regulatory properties that can specifically 'home' to the gut mucosa and protect against colitis in the CD45RB$^{high}$ transfer model.[105,106]

## PREVENTING ACTIVATION OF THE EPITHELIUM

The intestinal epithelium is an important victim of inflammation, but it may also have a primary role in activating immune responses. This has been well established in the case of infections with pathogenic bacteria, where the initial immune response is initiated by increased production of chemokines by epithelial cells.[107] Ulcerative colitis is associated with increased chemokine production by epithelial cells, which can even be detected in patients in complete endoscopic remission.[108] Several of these chemokines, including IL-8 and gro-α, are known to be able to recruit neutrophils from the circulation into the intestinal mucosal.[27,109,110] The activation pathways causing increased chemokine production have been incompletely characterized, but both MAP kinase and NFκB-dependent signal transduction pathways have been implicated.[111–114] These observations suggest that inhibition of these signal transduction pathways may have therapeutic effects, and interventions in animal models have supported this hypothesis. For example, the administration of an NFκB-p65-specific antisense oligonucleotide reduced inflammation in experimental colitis, and a clinical trial using this approach has been started.[115] New and interesting data concerning the regulation of these proinflammatory signal transduction pathways have recently emerged. The nuclear receptor PPARγ downregulates both pathways, and mice deficient in both PPARγ and RXR (an another 'orphan' nuclear receptor) have increased inflammatory responses.[30,116] Because PPARγ also seems to be downregulated in the epithelial cells of ulcerative colitis patients, the efficacy of stimulation of this receptor using rosiglitazone is currently under clinical investigation.[117]

## REDIRECTING CELL TRAFFICKING

Activation of innate and adaptive immune responses can only result in significant inflammation when the immune response is augmented by recruitment of white blood cells such as neutrophils, lymphocytes and monocytes. It has long been known that such recruitment is a multistep process that is dependent on sequential receptor–ligand interactions between the inflamed endothelium and the white blood cell. Neutrophils are initially slowed down by L-selectin-mediated 'rolling' over the endothelial surface, and become activated by chemokines and platelet-activating factor (PAF) bound to endothelial heparan sulfate, which leads to a greatly increased affinity of the neutrophil CD11b/CD18 integrin for its endothelial ligand ICAM-1.[118–121] This interaction causes the firm adhesion that is necessary for subsequent transmigration. In many animal models of inflammation it has been well established that interference with this sequence of events can have anti-inflammatory effects, targeting of ICAM-1 being the most popular approach. It should be noted that this approach interferes not only with neutrophil recruitment, but also with adhesion of lymphocytes to the endothelium (see later). In mouse models of inflammatory bowel disease an ICAM-1-specific antisense oligonucleotide reduced inflammation, and an initial clinical trial in Crohn's disease reported a beneficial effect.[122,123] Unfortunately, this has not been corroborated in subsequent larger controlled clinical trials, possibly because the intravenous and subcutaneous administration routes used did not result in sufficient mucosal concentrations.[124] A small controlled trial in ulcerative colitis patients, in which the compound was delivered as an enema, resulted in high mucosal concentrations, and this caused a dose-dependent reduction of clinical and endoscopic endpoints (van Deventer SJ et al., 2002; submitted for publication).

As discussed, lymphocytes have a pivotal role in inflammatory bowel disease. As with neutrophils, the entrance of lymphocytes at local sites of inflammation is a multistep process, but the ligand–receptor interactions differ.[125–127] Specific homing of lymphocytes to the gut mucosa is a result of specific binding of the $\alpha_4\beta_7$ integrin to the mucosal addressin MAdCAM-1, and interference with this interaction by administration of $\alpha_4$-binding antibodies is beneficial in animal models (including colitis in primates).[128–131] Two monoclonal $\alpha_4$-binding antibodies are in clinical trials in Crohn's disease and ulcerative colitis, with promising results.[132] Such antibodies may have additional functional effects, because $\alpha_4\beta_1$, which is also expressed by lymphocytes, is needed for binding of transmigrated lymphocytes to stromal fibronectin, and this provides a survival signal.[133] Finally, it is important to note that recruitment of both T and B cells is targeted by interfering with $\alpha_4$-mediated lymphocyte–endothelial interactions.

## INHIBITION OF SIGNAL TRANSDUCTION

As has already been discussed, signal transduction through NFκB proteins is pivotal for activation of the innate and adaptive immune systems, and for chemokine production by epithelial cells. Although this pathway has long been known, and studies using p65 antisense oligonucleotides are under way, there is a surprising lack of small molecules that specifically interfere with NFκB signaling and that are clinically useful (NFκB antisense oligonucleotides were discussed earlier). It is possible that specific foodstuffs, such as curcumin, have NFκB-inhibiting effects.[113]

MAP kinases have been identified more recently, and pharmaceutical companies have generated a rapidly expanding array of more or less specific small molecular inhibitors. Some of these compounds have a good oral bioavailability, and significantly reduce LPS-induced proinflammatory responses in humans.[134] Clinical development of these compounds is ongoing in Crohn's disease and rheumatoid arthritis, mainly with MAP p38 kinase-specific inhibitors, or dual inhibitors of JNK and MAP p38 kinases.[39] This does make sense in view of the finding that both MAP p38α and JNK-1 are activated in the intestinal mucosa of patients with active Crohn's disease. Indeed, a small study in patients with severe Crohn's disease reported beneficial effects of treatment with a dual MAP p38 and JNK1 inhibitor.[39] In this study important mucosal healing was observed, as well as a reduction of mucosal TNF-α production that correlated with a reduction of JNK, but not p38, phosphorylation. At present, the role of MAP kinase activation in inflammatory bowel disease is incompletely understood, and interference with p38 activation significantly worsened the severity of TNBS-induced colitis in mice.[135]

## CONCLUSION

The pathogenesis of mucosal inflammation in Crohn's disease and ulcerative colitis has become much better known in the last decade, and this has led to the identification of a wealth of new targets for therapeutic interventions. Understandably, the clinical development of therapies lags behind results obtained in cell culture and in animal models, and the first clinical successes have been obtained using technology that was state-of-the-art more than a decade ago, i.e. chimeric or humanized monoclonal antibodies. Some monoclonal antibodies have been very effective in inflammatory bowel disease, and TNF-α-neutralizing antibodies are an important new addition to the therapeutic options in Crohn's disease. However, there are some problems associated with the long-term administration of monoclonal antibodies, immunogenicity being a major point of concern. Small molecules that inhibit MAP kinase signal transduction and which can be orally administered have been shown to have potent anti-inflammatory properties and are undergoing clinical testing. The initial results are encouraging, but larger controlled studies are needed, and in view of the involvement of this signal transduction pathway in many cellular processes, long-term toxicity may occur. However, if safe and effective, many patients would prefer such a therapy to repeated infusions.

Finally, new technologies have resulted in alternative therapeutic approaches, some of which have made it to the clinic (antisense oligonucleotides), whereas others (gene therapy, RNA interference) are expected to follow.

## REFERENCES

1. Harrison J, Hanauer SB. Medical treatment of Crohn's disease. Gastroenterol Clin North Am 2002;31:167–184.
2. Van Balkom BP, Schoon EJ, Stockbrugger RW et al. Effects of anti-tumour necrosis factor-alpha therapy on the quality of life in Crohn's disease. Aliment Pharmacol Ther 2002;16:1101–1107.
3. Hanauer SB, Feagan BG, Lichtenstein GR et al. Maintenance infliximab for Crohn's disease: the ACCENT I randomised trial. Lancet 2002;359:1541–1549.
4. van Deventer SJ. Small therapeutic molecules for the treatment of inflammatory bowel disease. Gut 2002;50:III47–III53.
5. Elson CO. Genes, microbes, and T cells – new therapeutic targets in Crohn's disease. N Engl J Med 2002;346:614–616.
6. Strober W, Fuss IJ, Blumberg RS. The immunology of mucosal models of inflammation. Annu Rev Immunol 2002;20:495–549.
7. Rescigno M, Urbano M, Valzasina B et al. Dendritic cells express tight junction proteins and penetrate gut epithelial monolayers to sample bacteria. Nature Immunol 2001;2:361–367.
8. Medzhitov R, Janeway C Jr. Innate immunity. N Engl J Med 2000; 343:338–344.
9. Janeway CA Jr, Medzhitov R. Innate immune recognition. Annu Rev Immunol 2002; 20:197–216.

10. Sharpe AH, Freeman GJ. The B7-CD28 superfamily. Nature Rev Immunol 2002;2:116–126.

11. Carreno BM, Collins M. The B7 family of ligands and its receptors: new pathways for costimulation and inhibition of immune responses. Annu Rev Immunol 2002;20:29–53.

12. Camoglio L, Juffermans NP, Peppelenbosch M et al. Contrasting roles of IL-12p40 and IL-12p35 in the development of hapten-induced colitis. Eur J Immunol 2002;32:261–269.

13. MacDonald TT, Monteleone G. IL-12 and Th1 immune responses in human Peyer's patches. Trends Immunol 2001;22:244–247.

14. Kanai T, Watanabe M, Okazawa A, Sato T, Hibi T. Interleukin-18 and Crohn's disease. Digestion 2001;63:37–42.

15. Van Parijs L, Abbas AK. Homeostasis and self-tolerance in the immune system: turning lymphocytes off. Science 1998;280:243–248.

16. Itoh J, de La Motte C, Strong SA, Levine AD, Fiocchi C. Decreased Bax expression by mucosal T cells favours resistance to apoptosis in Crohn's disease. Gut 2001;49:35–41.

17. Ina K, Itoh J, Fukushima K et al. Resistance of Crohn's disease T cells to multiple apoptotic signals is associated with a Bcl-2/Bax mucosal imbalance. J Immunol 1999;163:1081–1090.

18. Sturm A, Fiocchi C. Life and death in the gut: more killing, less Crohn's. Gut 2002;50:148–149.

19. Lugering A, Schmidt M, Lugering N, Pauels HG, Domschke W, Kucharzik T. Infliximab induces apoptosis in monocytes from patients with chronic active Crohn's disease by using a caspase-dependent pathway. Gastroenterology 2001;121:1145–1157.

20. ten Hove T, van Montfrans C, Peppelenbosch MP, van Deventer SJ. Infliximab treatment induces apoptosis of lamina propria T lymphocytes in Crohn's disease. Gut 2002;50:206–211.

21. Maloy KJ, Powrie F. Regulatory T cells in the control of immune pathology. Nature Immunol 2001;2:816–822.

22. Singh B, Read S, Asseman C et al. Control of intestinal inflammation by regulatory T cells. Immunol Rev 2001;182:190–200.

23. Weiner HL. Oral tolerance: immune mechanisms and the generation of Th3-type TGF-beta-secreting regulatory cells. Microbes Infect 2001;3:947–954.

24. Shashaty GG. Hemolytic anemia and ulcerative colitis. Dig Dis Sci 1980;25:154–155.

25. Rump JA, Scholmerich J, Gross V et al. A new type of perinuclear anti-neutrophil cytoplasmic antibody (p-ANCA) in active ulcerative colitis but not in Crohn's disease. Immunobiology 1990;181:406–413.

26. Das KM, Vecchi M, Sakamaki S. A shared and unique epitope(s) on human colon, skin, and biliary epithelium detected by a monoclonal antibody. Gastroenterology 1990;98:464–469.

27. Masuda H, Iwai S, Tanaka T, Hayakawa S. Expression of IL-8, TNF-alpha and IFN-gamma m-RNA in ulcerative colitis, particularly in patients with inactive phase. J Clin Lab Immunol 1995;46:111–123.

28. Raab Y, Gerdin B, Ahlstedt S, Hallgren R. Neutrophil mucosal involvement is accompanied by enhanced local production of interleukin-8 in ulcerative colitis. Gut 1993;34:1203–1206.

29. Ina K, Kusugami K, Yamaguchi T et al. Mucosal interleukin-8 is involved in neutrophil migration and binding to extracellular matrix in inflammatory bowel disease. Am J Gastroenterol 1997;92:1342–1346.

30. Desreumaux P, Dubuquoy L, Nutten S et al. Attenuation of colon inflammation through activators of the retinoid X receptor (RXR)/peroxisome proliferator-activated receptor gamma (PPARgamma) heterodimer. A basis for new therapeutic strategies. J Exp Med 2001;193:827–838.

31. Hornef MW, Frisan T, Vandewalle A, Normark S, Richter-Dahlfors A. Toll-like receptor 4 resides in the Golgi apparatus and colocalizes with internalized lipopolysaccharide in intestinal epithelial cells. J Exp Med 2002;195:559–570.

32. Abreu MT, Vora P, Faure E, Thomas LS, Arnold ET, Arditi M. Decreased expression of Toll-like receptor-4 and MD-2 correlates with intestinal epithelial cell protection against dysregulated proinflammatory gene expression in response to bacterial lipopolysaccharide. J Immunol 2001;167:1609–1616.

33. Cario E, Podolsky DK. Differential alteration in intestinal epithelial cell expression of Toll-like receptor 3 (TLR3) and TLR4 in inflammatory bowel disease. Infect Immun 2000;68:7010–7017.

34. Schreiber S, Nikolaus S, Hampe J. Activation of nuclear factor kappa B inflammatory bowel disease. Gut 1998;42:477–484.

35. Dong C, Davis RJ, Flavell RA. MAP kinases in the immune response. Annu Rev Immunol 2002;20:55–72.

36. van den Blink B, Branger J, Weijer S, Deventer SH, van der Poll T, Peppelenbosch MP. Human endotoxemia activates p38 MAP kinase and p42/44 MAP kinase, but not c-Jun N-terminal kinase. Mol Med 2001;7:755–760.

37. Bettini M, Xi H, Milbrandt J, Kersh GJ. Thymocyte development in early growth response gene 1-deficient mice. J Immunol 2002;169:1713–1720.

38. Waetzig GH, Seegert D, Rosenstiel P, Nikolaus S, Schreiber S. p38 mitogen-activated protein kinase is activated and linked to TNF-alpha signaling in inflammatory bowel disease. J Immunol 2002;168:5342–5351.

39. Hommes D, Van Den Blink B, Plasse T et al. Inhibition of stress-activated MAP kinases induces clinical improvement in moderate to severe Crohn's disease. Gastroenterology 2002;122:7–14.

40. Ulevitch RJ. New therapeutic targets revealed through investigations of innate immunity. Crit Care Med 2001;29:S8–12.

41. Kotlyarov A, Neininger A, Schubert C et al. MAPKAP kinase 2 is essential for LPS-induced TNF-alpha biosynthesis [see comments]. Nature Cell Biol 1999;1:94–97.

42. Ghosh S, Karin M. Missing pieces in the NF-kappaB puzzle. Cell 2002;109:S81–96.

43. Schreiber S, Rosenstiel P, Hampe J et al. Activation of signal transducer and activator of transcription (STAT) 1 in human chronic inflammatory bowel disease. Gut 2002;51:379–385.

44. Monteleone G, Kumberova A, Croft NM, McKenzie C, Steer HW, MacDonald TT. Blocking Smad7 restores TGF-beta1 signaling in chronic inflammatory bowel disease. J Clin Invest 2001;108:601–609.

45. Neurath MF, Weigmann B, Finotto S et al. The transcription factor T-bet regulates mucosal T cell activation in experimental colitis and Crohn's disease. J Exp Med 2002;195:1129–1143.

46. Weigmann B, Neurath MF. T-bet and mucosal Th1 responses in the gastrointestinal tract. Gut 2002;51:301–303.

47. Arend WP, Malyak M, Guthridge CJ, Gabay C. Interleukin-1 receptor antagonist: role in biology. Annu Rev Immunol 1998;16:27–55.

48. Novick D, Kim SH, Fantuzzi G, Reznikov LL, Dinarello CA, Rubinstein M. Interleukin-18 binding protein: a novel modulator of the Th1 cytokine response. Immunity 1999;10:127–136.

49. Meenan J, Hommes DW, Mevissen M et al. Attenuation of the inflammatory response in an animal colitis model by neutrophil inhibitory factor, a novel beta2-integrin antagonist. Scand J Gastroenterol 1996;31:786–791.

50. Moyle M, Foster DL, McGrath DE et al. A hookworm glycoprotein that inhibits neutrophil function is a ligand of the integrin CD11b/CD18. J Biol Chem 1994;269:10008–10015.

51. Woodruff TM, Strachan AJ, Dryburgh N et al. Antiarthritic activity of an orally active C5a receptor antagonist against antigen-induced monarticular arthritis in the rat. Arthritis Rheum 2002;46:2476–2485.

52. Giles RV, Tidd DM. The direction of ribonucleases H by antisense oligodeoxynucleotides. Meth Mol Biol 2001;160:157–182.

53. Faria M, Spiller DG, Dubertret C et al. Phosphoramidate oligonucleotides as potent antisense molecules in cells and in vivo. Nature Biotechnol 2001;19:40–44.

54. Sheehan JP, Phan TM. Phosphorothioate oligonucleotides inhibit the intrinsic tenase complex by an allosteric mechanism. Biochemistry 2001;40:4980–4989.

55. Sullenger BA, Gilboa E. Emerging clinical applications of RNA. Nature 2002;418:252–258.

56. Hannon GJ. RNA interference. Nature 2002;418:244–251.

57. Tijsterman M, Ketting RF, Plasterk RH. The genetics of RNA silencing. Annu Rev Genet 2002;36:489–519.

58. Pfeifer A, Verma IM. Gene therapy: promises and problems. Annu Rev Genomics Hum Genet 2001;2:177–211.

59. Wagner JA. Gene therapy. N Engl J Med 1996;334:332–333.

60. Bergelson JM, Cunningham JA, Droguett G et al. Isolation of a common receptor for Coxsackie B viruses and adenoviruses 2 and 5. Science 1997;275:1320–1323.

61. Abe A, Chen ST, Miyanohara A, Friedmann T. In vitro cell-free conversion of noninfectious Moloney retrovirus particles to an infectious form by the addition of the vesicular stomatitis virus surrogate envelope G protein. J Virol 1998;72:6356–6361.

62. Buckley RH. Gene therapy for SCID – a complication after remarkable progress. Lancet 2002;360:1185–1186.

63. Wang L, Nichols TC, Read MS, Bellinger DA, Verma IM. Sustained expression of therapeutic level of factor IX in hemophilia B dogs by AAV-mediated gene therapy in liver [see comments]. Mol Ther 2000;1:154–158.

64. Flotte TR, Carter BJ. Adeno-associated virus vectors for gene therapy. Gene Ther 1995;2:357–362.

65. During MJ, Xu R, Young D, Kaplitt MG, Sherwin RS, Leone P. Peroral gene therapy of lactose intolerance using an adeno-associated virus vector. Nature Med 1998;4:1131–1135.

66. Lindsay J, Van Montfrans C, Brennan F et al. IL-10 gene therapy prevents TNBS-induced colitis. Gene Ther 2002;9:1715–1721.

67. Lindsay JO, Ciesielski CJ, Scheinin T, Hodgson HJ, Brennan FM. The prevention and treatment of murine colitis using gene therapy with adenoviral vectors encoding IL-10. J Immunol 2001;166:7625–7633.

68. Monteleone G, Biancone L, Marasco R et al. Interleukin 12 is expressed and actively released by Crohn's disease intestinal lamina propria mononuclear cells. Gastroenterology 1997;112:1169–1178.

69. Kanai T, Watanabe M, Okazawa A et al. Interleukin 18 is a potent proliferative factor for intestinal mucosal lymphocytes in Crohn's disease. Gastroenterology 2000;119:1514–1523.

70. Monteleone G, Trapasso F, Parrello T et al. Bioactive IL-18 expression is up-regulated in Crohn's disease. J Immunol 1999;163:143–147.

71. Pizarro TT, Michie MH, Bentz M et al. IL-18, a novel immunoregulatory cytokine, is up-regulated in Crohn's disease: Expression and localization in intestinal mucosal cells. J Immunol 1999;162:6829–6835.

72. Barbulescu K, Becker C, Schlaak JF, Schmitt E, Meyer zum Buschenfelde KH, Neurath MF. IL-12 and IL-18 differentially regulate the transcriptional activity of the human

IFN-gamma promoter in primary CD4+ T lymphocytes. J Immunol 1998;160:3642–3647.

73. Camoglio L, Juffermans NP, Peppelenbosch M et al. Contrasting roles of IL-12p40 and IL-12p35 in the development of hapten-induced colitis. Eur J Immunol 2002;32:261–269.

74. Frucht DM. IL-23: a cytokine that acts on memory T cells. Sci STKE 2002;2002:E1.

75. Oppmann B, Lesley R, Blom B et al. Novel p19 protein engages IL-12p40 to form a cytokine, IL-23, with biological activities similar as well as distinct from IL-12. Immunity 2000;13:715–725.

76. Neurath MF, Fuss I, Kelsall BL, Stuber E, Strober W. Antibodies to interleukin 12 abrogate established experimental colitis in mice. J Exp Med 1995;182:1281–90.

77. Yamada, Sayegh MH. The CD154-CD40 costimulatory pathway in transplantation. Transplantation 2002;73:S36–39.

78. Burkly LC. CD40 pathway blockade as an approach to immunotherapy. Adv Exp Med Biol 2001;489:135–152.

79. Corbaz A, ten Hove T, Herren S et al. IL-18-binding protein expression by endothelial cells and macrophages is up-regulated during active Crohn's disease. J Immunol 2002;168:3608–3616.

80. Ten Hove T, Corbaz A, Amitai H et al. Blockade of endogenous IL-18 ameliorates TNBS-induced colitis by decreasing local TNF-alpha production in mice. Gastroenterology 2001;121:1372–1379.

81. Siegmund B, Fantuzzi G, Rieder F et al. Neutralization of interleukin-18 reduces severity in murine colitis and intestinal IFN-gamma and TNF-alpha production. Am J Physiol Regul Integr Comp Physiol 2001;281:R1264–1273.

82. Salomon B, Bluestone JA. Complexities of CD28/B7: CTLA-4 costimulatory pathways in autoimmunity and transplantation. Annu Rev Immunol 2001;19:225–252.

83. Liu Z, Geboes K, Hellings P et al. B7 interactions with CD28 and CTLA-4 control tolerance or induction of mucosal inflammation in chronic experimental colitis. J Immunol 2001;167:1830–1838.

84. Salomon B, Lenschow DJ, Rhee L et al. B7/CD28 costimulation is essential for the homeostasis of the CD4+CD25+ immunoregulatory T cells that control autoimmune diabetes. Immunity 2000;12:431–440.

85. Dong C, Juedes AE, Temann UA et al. ICOS co-stimulatory receptor is essential for T-cell activation and function. Nature 2001;409:97–101.

86. Gonzalo JA, Tian J, Delaney T et al. ICOS is critical for T helper cell-mediated lung mucosal inflammatory responses. Nature Immunol 2001;2:597–604.

87. Medzhitov R, Janeway CA Jr. Decoding the patterns of self and nonself by the innate immune system. Science 2002;296:298–300.

88. Matzinger P. The danger model: a renewed sense of self. Science 2002;296:301–305.

89. Durkin HG, Waksman BH. Thymus and tolerance. Is regulation the major function of the thymus? Immunol Rev 2001;182:33–57.

90. Shevach EM. CD4+ CD25+ suppressor T cells: more questions than answers. Nature Rev Immunol 2002;2:389–400.

91. Shevach EM. Regulatory T cells in autoimmunity. Annu Rev Immunol 2000;18:423–449.

92. Ramenghi U, Bonissoni S, Migliaretti G et al. Deficiency of the Fas apoptosis pathway without Fas gene mutations is a familial trait predisposing to development of autoimmune diseases and cancer. Blood 2000;95:3176–3182.

93. Avila NA, Dwyer AJ, Dale JK et al. Autoimmune lymphoproliferative syndrome: a syndrome associated with inherited genetic defects that impair lymphocytic apoptosis – CT and US features. Radiology 1999;212:257–263.

94. Krammer PH. CD95's deadly mission in the immune system. Nature 2000;407:789–795.

95. Salvesen GS, Renatus M. Apoptosome: the seven-spoked death machine. Dev Cell 2002;2:256–257.

96. Neurath MF, Finotto S, Fuss I, Boirivant M, Galle PR, Strober W. Regulation of T-cell apoptosis in inflammatory bowel disease: to die or not to die, that is the mucosal question. Trends Immunol 2001;22:21–26.

97. Boirivant M, Marini M, Di Felice G et al. Lamina propria T cells in Crohn's disease and other gastrointestinal inflammation show defective CD2 pathway-induced apoptosis. Gastroenterology 1999;116:557–565.

98. ten Hove T, van Deventer SJH. Anti-TNF antibody Ca2 induces apoptosis in CD3/CD28 stimulated Jurkat cells: A potent immunomodulatory mechanism. Gastroenterology 1999;116:A739.

99. Atreya R, Mudter J, Finotto S et al. Blockade of interleukin 6 trans signaling suppresses T-cell resistance against apoptosis in chronic intestinal inflammation: evidence in Crohn's disease and experimental colitis in vivo. Nature Med 2000;6:583–588.

100. Asseman C, Mauze S, Leach MW, Coffman RL, Powrie F. An essential role for interleukin 10 in the function of regulatory T cells that inhibit intestinal inflammation. J Exp Med 1999;190:995–1004.

101. Fedorak RN, Gangl A, Elson CO et al. Recombinant human interleukin 10 in the treatment of patients with mild to moderately active Crohn's disease. The Interleukin 10 Inflammatory Bowel Disease Cooperative Study Group. Gastroenterology 2000;119:1473–1482.

102. Schreiber S, Fedorak RN, Nielsen OH et al. Safety and efficacy of recombinant human interleukin 10 in chronic active Crohn's disease. Gastroenterology 2000;119:1461–1472.

103. Tilg H, van Montfrans C, van Den Ende A et al. Treatment of Crohn's disease with recombinant human interleukin 10 induces the proinflammatory cytokine interferon gamma. Gut 2002;50:191–195.

104. Steidler L, Hans W, Schotte L et al. Treatment of murine colitis by Lactococcus lactis secreting interleukin-10. Science 2000;289:1352–1355.

105. Van Montfrans C, Hooijberg E, Rodriguez Pena MS et al. Generation of regulatory gut-homing human T lymphocytes using ex vivo interleukin 10 gene transfer. Gastroenterology 2002;123:1877–1888.

106. Van Montfrans C, Rodriguez Pena MS, Pronk I, ten Kate FJ, Te Velde AA, Van Deventer SJ. Prevention of colitis by interleukin 10-transduced T lymphocytes in the SCID mice transfer model. Gastroenterology 2002;123:1865–1876.

107. Eckmann L, Smith JR, Housley MP, Dwinell MB, Kagnoff MF. Analysis by high density cDNA arrays of altered gene expression in human intestinal epithelial cells in response to infection with the invasive enteric bacteria Salmonella. J Biol Chem 2000;275:14084–14094.

108. van Deventer SJ. Review article: Chemokine production by intestinal epithelial cells: a therapeutic target in inflammatory bowel disease? Aliment Pharmacol Ther 1997;11:116–120; discussion 120–121.

109. Mitsuyama K, Toyonaga A, Sasaki E et al. IL-8 as an important chemoattractant for neutrophils in ulcerative colitis and Crohn's disease. Clin Exp Immunol 1994;96:432–436.

110. MacDermott RP, Sanderson IR, Reinecker HC. The central role of chemokines (chemotactic cytokines) in the immunopathogenesis of ulcerative colitis and Crohn's disease. Inflamm Bowel Dis 1998;4:54–67.

111. Lahde M, Korhonen R, Moilanen E. Regulation of nitric oxide production in cultured human T84 intestinal epithelial cells by nuclear factor-kappa B-dependent induction of inducible nitric oxide synthase after exposure to bacterial endotoxin. Aliment Pharmacol Ther 2000;14:945–954.

112. Brand S, Sakaguchi T, Gu X, Colgan SP, Reinecker HC. Fractalkine-mediated signals regulate cell-survival and immune-modulatory responses in intestinal epithelial cells. Gastroenterology 2002;122:166–177.

113. Jobin C, Bradham CA, Russo MP et al. Curcumin blocks cytokine-mediated NF-kappa B activation and proinflammatory gene expression by inhibiting inhibitory factor I-kappa B kinase activity. J Immunol 1999;163:3474–3483.

114. Jobin C, Hellerbrand C, Licato LL, Brenner DA, Sartor RB. Mediation by NF-kappa B of cytokine induced expression of intercellular adhesion molecule 1 (ICAM-1) in an intestinal epithelial cell line, a process blocked by proteasome inhibitors. Gut 1998;42:779–787.

115. Neurath MF, Pettersson S, Meyer zum Buschenfelde KH, Strober W. Local administration of antisense phosphorothioate oligonucleotides to the p65 subunit of NF-kappa B abrogates established experimental colitis in mice. Nature Med 1996;2:998–1004.

116. Su CG, Wen X, Bailey ST et al. A novel therapy for colitis utilizing PPAR-gamma ligands to inhibit the epithelial inflammatory response. J Clin Invest 1999;104:383–389.

117. Lewis JD, Lichtenstein GR, Stein RB et al. An open-label trial of the PPAR-gamma ligand rosiglitazone for active ulcerative colitis. Am J Gastroenterol 2001;96:3323–3328.

118. Kadono T, Venturi GM, Steeber DA, Tedder TF. Leukocyte rolling velocities and migration are optimized by cooperative L-selectin and intercellular adhesion molecule-1 functions. J Immunol 2002;169:4542–4550.

119. Hafezi-Moghadam A, Thomas KL, Prorock AJ, Huo Y, Ley K. L-selectin shedding regulates leukocyte recruitment. J Exp Med 2001;193:863–872.

120. Simon SI, Hu Y, Vestweber D, Smith CW. Neutrophil tethering on E-selectin activates beta 2 integrin binding to ICAM-1 through a mitogen-activated protein kinase signal transduction pathway. J Immunol 2000;164:4348–4358.

121. Steeber DA, Tang ML, Green NE, Zhang XQ, Sloane JE, Tedder TF. Leukocyte entry into sites of inflammation requires overlapping interactions between the L-selectin and ICAM-1 pathways. J Immunol 1999;163:2176–2186.

122. Bennett CF, Kornbrust D, Henry S et al. An ICAM-1 antisense oligonucleotide prevents and reverses dextran sulfate sodium-induced colitis in mice. J Pharmacol Exp Ther 1997;280:988–1000.

123. Yacyshyn BR, Bowen-Yacyshyn MB, Jewell L et al. A placebo-controlled trial of ICAM-1 antisense oligonucleotide in the treatment of Crohn's disease. Gastroenterology 1998;114:1133–1142.

124. Schreiber S, Nikolaus S, Malchow H et al. Absence of efficacy of subcutaneous antisense ICAM-1 treatment of chronic active Crohn's disease. Gastroenterology 2001;120:1339–1346.

125. Stein JV, Soriano SF, M'Rini C et al. CCR7-mediated physiological lymphocyte homing involves activation of a tyrosine kinase pathway. Blood 2002;28:28.

126. Tang ML, Steeber DA, Zhang XQ, Tedder TF. Intrinsic differences in L-selectin expression levels affect T and B lymphocyte subset-specific recirculation pathways. J Immunol 1998;160:5113–5121.

127. Chao CC, Jensen R, Dailey MO. Mechanisms of L-selectin regulation by activated T cells. J Immunol 1997;159:1686–1694.

128. Berlin C, Berg EL, Briskin MJ et al. Alpha 4 beta 7 integrin mediates lymphocyte binding to the mucosal vascular addressin MAdCAM-1. Cell 1993;74:185–195.

129. Hamann A, Andrew DP, Jablonski-Westrich D, Holzmann B, Butcher EC. Role of alpha 4-integrins in lymphocyte homing to mucosal tissues in vivo. J Immunol 1994;152:3282–3293.

130. Kato S, Hokari R, Matsuzaki K et al. Amelioration of murine experimental colitis by inhibition of mucosal addressin cell adhesion molecule-1. J Pharmacol Exp Ther 2000;295:183–189.

131. Podolsky DK, Lobb R, King N et al. Attenuation of colitis in the cotton-top tamarin by anti-alpha 4 integrin monoclonal antibody. J Clin Invest 1993;92:372–380.

132. Gordon FH, Hamilton MI, Donoghue S et al. A pilot study of treatment of active ulcerative colitis with natalizumab, a humanized monoclonal antibody to alpha-4 integrin. Aliment Pharmacol Ther 2002;16:699–705.

133. Tchilian EZ, Owen JJ, Jenkinson EJ. Anti-alpha 4 integrin antibody induces apoptosis in murine thymocytes and staphylococcal enterotoxin B-activated lymph node T cells. Immunology 1997;92:321–327.

134. Branger J, van den Blink B, Weijer S et al. Anti-inflammatory effects of a p38 mitogen-activated protein kinase inhibitor during human endotoxemia. J Immunol 2002;168:4070–4077.

135. ten Hove T, van Den Blink B, Pronk I, Drillenburg P, Peppelenbosch MP, van Deventer SJ. Dichotomal role of inhibition of p38 MAPK with SB 203580 in experimental colitis. Gut 2002;50:507–512.

# SURGICAL THERAPY

## CHAPTER 38

# Indications for surgery in inflammatory bowel disease from the gastroenterologist's point of view

James F Marion and Daniel H Present

## INTRODUCTION

The interaction between a surgeon and a gastroenterologist in the management of the patient with inflammatory bowel disease often determines the quality of the outcome for that patient. This collaboration requires that the gastroenterologist understands the surgical procedures and possible consequences of surgery, and the surgeon understands the increasingly complex medical regimens that can precede surgery. The importance of the interaction between surgeon and gastroenterologist should be established during residency and fellowship training. Surgical residents rounding with GI fellows and GI fellows accompanying their patients to the operating room would set the stage for improved communication from the earliest stage of training. The advantages and limitations of both the medical and the surgical approach would be better appreciated by trainees setting the foundation for a trusting, close working relationship.

Most patients with Crohn's disease and many with ulcerative colitis will require surgery in their lifetime. Improved surgical techniques and careful screening of surgical candidates have made surgery less of a perceived 'defeat' than it was in years past. In addition, careful combining of early aggressive medical therapy prior to surgical therapy can ensure better outcomes for these patients. The purpose of this chapter is to provide an outline of disease behavior and an algorithm of medical therapy that, we think, should precede surgery in a patient with inflammatory bowel disease. We will review the more standard recommendations, and later in the chapter elaborate on some more unique, and even controversial, areas regarding indications for surgery in IBD.

## CROHN'S DISEASE

Most patients (70–75%) with Crohn's disease will confront the issue of surgery at some point in the course of their illness.

Crohn's disease is a chronic, lifelong recurrent illness that cannot be cured by surgery. The decision to operate for Crohn's disease can be difficult in certain cases. The current medical armamentarium is evolving rapidly, and the increased and earlier use of immunomodulator agents and biological therapies has further complicated the algorithm leading up to surgery. Decisions regarding the timing of surgery depend heavily upon disease behavior and the anatomic location of the patient's disease, i.e. whether it be inflammatory, cicatrizing, fistulizing, and predominantly small bowel, colonic or perineal.[1] Finally, the response of the disease to conventional medical therapy adds to the decision-making process.

## ABSOLUTE INDICATIONS FOR SURGERY

All gastroenterologists and surgeons would agree that surgical intervention is absolutely indicated in Crohn's disease in the presence of a free perforation, uncontrollable hemorrhage, and persistent complete bowel obstruction not responding to medical therapy. Fortunately, the two former indications are rare but the last occurs frequently. Furthermore, the presence of high-grade dysplasia, or cancer, in Crohn's colitis is another indication for surgery that is unlikely to produce controversy.[2]

### Inflammatory disease

Relative indications for surgery, more likely to stir disagreement among clinicians, include refractoriness to medical therapy, steroid dependence or resistance, chronic low-grade partial small bowel obstruction, or a desire to avoid immunosuppressive therapy.[3] Patient preference will often drive these decisions. The gastroenterologist's goal should always be an improved quality of life for the patient, and therefore it is the physician's role to educate the patient as to how to best reach an informed decision to reach the highest level of quality of life possible. Extent, anatomic location and severity of disease further determine the value of surgical intervention. For example, in the patient with inflammatory disease of a limited extent in the terminal ileum there are certain social situations, such as a young patient about to go to college or a new job or about to be married, where aggressive immunomodulatory or biological therapy might not be desired by the patient or their family. Surgery in this instance should not be considered a defeat or a 'last resort', but can usually be performed laparoscopically by a surgeon skilled in laparoscopic techniques in inflammatory bowel disease patients. In this situation, surgery can be a means of returning the patient to school or work rapidly. For other patients with more extensive disease that requires more extensive resection, an aggressive approach medically up to, and including, immunomodulatory therapy or biological therapies should be considered prior to recommending surgery. The presence of accompanying active perineal disease should always push the clinician toward immunomodulatory therapy and away from proximal surgical resection, as patients can experience an exacerbation of perineal disease postoperatively.

For most patients, especially younger ones, the possibility of needing an ostomy appliance, whether temporarily or permanently, can greatly influence a decision about surgery. Consideration of the risks and benefits of what is regarded as a disfiguring intervention must be made carefully and mindfully to ensure that the patient is not left with a clinically successful but psychologically devastating result.

In the pediatric population, growth failure can be an important indicator of the effectiveness of medical therapy. Children with inflammatory bowel disease – more often Crohn's disease than ulcerative colitis – may have significant growth failure if undiagnosed or inadequately treated. The chronic use of prednisone in this population may also contribute to their developmental delay. Aggressive, effective medical therapy and steroid avoidance will usually resolve the growth issue.[4] Should these fail, then surgical intervention must be considered.

## Fibrostenotic disease

Stricturing disease poses several problems in management. Most important to recognize is the degree of overlap between inflammatory and fibrostenotic disease. Patients may not strictly adhere to their category and will present clinically with symptoms produced by inflammatory activity producing obstruction. Aggressive use of medical therapy such as steroids, antibiotics, and even infliximab may effectively treat their obstruction. Patients with fibrostenotic disease will often present with the acute onset of obstructive symptoms (including pain, bloating, nausea and vomiting), which for the most part resolve spontaneously. Immediate surgical intervention is usually not required. Obstruction may often be managed conservatively, with resolution of the obstructive episode following nasogastric decompression, bowel rest, IV fluids or antibiotics. Steroids are 'rarely' (or, in the opinion of the editors, 'not always') required for acute obstruction and should not be used indiscriminately. Furthermore, steroids may alter the clinical findings (e.g. fever, white blood cell count), leading to confusion regarding the clinical status.

Plain film radiographic series can be helpful in monitoring the patient's progress but usually lag behind the clinical status. Patients with chronic partial small bowel obstruction may have few symptoms, but significant dilatation can be apparent on radiologic evaluation. The patient's symptomatology should guide the clinician in these situations. Patients with recurrent obstructions who do not respond to dietary modification may require surgery. The presence of adhesions from previous operations can also confound the evaluation of an obstructed patient with Crohn's disease. Careful contrast radiographic evaluation of the small bowel can usually distinguish recurrent disease from residual adhesive disease. Barium, not Gastrografin, is the contrast medium of choice. Barium obstruction will not occur in small bowel strictures, only with colonic narrowing.

In contrast to patients with ongoing active inflammation, some with endoscopic and radiographic stenotic disease may have long symptom-free intervals. Patients who present with recurrent obstructive symptoms may require surgical treatment of the obstruction. Symptomatic strictures are treated with surgical resection of the affected area and restoration of bowel continuity. Patients with multiple short small bowel strictures can usually be treated with stricturoplasty, thereby obviating the need for extensive bowel resection.[5] Operative intervention, especially in cases of long-standing fibrostenotic disease, is eventually required. This subgroup of disease often proves refractory to medical therapy and can recur quite rapidly following surgery.[6,7]

The goal of the surgeon and gastroenterologist must be bowel preservation. Multiple resections can lead to short bowel syndrome and TPN dependence. The improved methods and results of intestinal transplantation offer an investigational option for such extreme and admittedly rare cases (this option must be approached very cautiously because of the significant risk of peri- and post-transplant mortality).[8] More often, the process of evaluation for intestinal transplantation leads to an optimization of the patient's medical regimen, thereby obviating the need for transplantation.[9]

Long-standing small bowel Crohn's disease is a strong relative risk factor for small bowel adenocarcinoma (although the absolute risk remains small). Such cancers remain a rare complication of Crohn's but should be borne in mind, especially when an older patient or one with 'long-standing' disease presents with clinical and radiographic obstruction.[10]

A specific gene that contributes to a patient's susceptibility to developing Crohn's disease has recently been found.[11] The genotype, which can be found in approximately 32% of patients with Crohn's disease, may be linked to an innate immune response to intestinal bacterial flora. The genotype has also been associated with the phenotype of fibrostenotic disease but does not appear to predict response to infliximab.[12,13] Genetic testing may in the future influence the timing and type of medical versus surgical therapy offered to Crohn's disease patients.

### Endoscopic therapy for fibrostenotic Crohn's disease

Fibrostenotic disease does not respond to medical therapy, and there are few alternatives to surgical resection. Patients with recurrent stricture formation at an ileocolonic anastomosis may be candidates for endoscopic therapy (see Chapter 26 for more details). Increasingly, therapeutic endoscopic dilatation of strictures in Crohn's disease has been performed using hydrostatic through-the-scope (TTS) balloons.[14] Strictures with a luminal diameter of less than 1 cm often require therapeutic intervention. These flexible balloon catheters can be passed through a standard endoscopic channel and positioned without the aid of fluoroscopy or a guidewire. Endoscopic treatment is feasible in up to 90% of cases. A long-term prospective uncontrolled trial involving 55 patients with ileocolonic strictures suggests that complete symptomatic relief can be achieved in 62% of patients, if up to three dilatation procedures are allowed for.[15] Eventually, surgery had to be performed in 38% of the patients. Interestingly, no significant correlation between disease activity and successful treatment was found. The procedure is associated with a relatively high rate of perforation (up to 11%), mainly in patients with ileosigmoid or ileorectal anastomotic strictures. Dilatation should be considered and can be attempted prior to surgery, but with full awareness and careful discussion about the risk of perforation. An experienced surgeon should be available in case perforation occurs. Patients with documented strictures but without a previous surgical history are rarely candidates for endoscopic therapy. Despite the interest in endoscopic therapy most patients with symptomatic Crohn's strictures are treated with surgical resection of the affected area.

## Fistulizing disease

Internal fistulizing Crohn's disease that eventually progresses to an intra-abdominal abscess almost always requires surgery. Percutaneous drainage preoperatively can, however, facilitate the surgical procedure. The simple presence of an internal fistula does not require surgical therapy unless the symptoms dictate. Aggressive therapy using antibiotics, immunomodulatory therapy (6-mercaptopurine (6-MP), azathioprine, methotrexate), biological therapy (infliximab), or even cyclosporin (CSA) or tacrolimus can be attempted prior to consideration of surgical intervention for symptomatic fistulae.

Perineal fistulae should be considered separately (see Chapter 49 for more details). Abscesses must be detected and drained prior to attempting medical therapy. A careful examination under anesthesia by an experienced rectal surgeon or an MRI scan of the perineum can rule out most clinically significant abscesses. Once perianal abscesses are drained, the efficacy of infliximab and immunosuppressant agents such as CSA/tacrolimus and 6-MP in the treatment of perineal and fistulizing disease requires that they be tried before further surgical intervention is considered. Local incision and drainage procedures, and possibly repeated placement of non-cutting setons in the absence of immunotherapy, may over time compromise the rectal musculature, producing a loss of continence, and is less likely to offer lasting relief. A combination of aggressive medical and surgical therapies up to and including rectal advancement flaps can sometimes benefit patients with intractable perineal disease.[16]

Rectovaginal fistulae represent an especially difficult clinical challenge (see Chapter 49 for more details). Management should consist of combination medical therapy (immunosuppressive and/or antibiotics and/or biological therapy). Surgical repair, often with a temporary diversion ostomy, can be attempted if medical therapy fails. Unfortunately, because of frequent recurrence, long-term outcomes remain poor.[17]

## POSTOPERATIVE PREVENTION

In the past, the promise of a postoperative, medicine-free existence often accompanied an explanation of the surgical procedure by the surgeon.[18] Although the data remain somewhat controversial, many physicians discussing surgery with a patient with predominantly inflammatory disease recommend postoperative prevention, with mesalamine, 6-MP or metronidazole (see Chapter 47 for additional details). Postoperative prevention for stenotic disease that might develop over many years is probably ineffective. The controversy about postoperative prevention persists because of our inability to predict the future clinical behavior more precisely from the time of surgery.

Reports suggest that recurrence occurs more quickly in fistulizing disease and that systemic immunomodulatory therapy, such as 6-MP or metronidazole prophylaxis, is likely to be more effective. On the other hand, prevention using 5-ASA may be more likely to benefit patients with more superficial or mucosal inflammatory disease.

## CONTROVERSIES IN THE SURGICAL MANAGEMENT OF CROHN'S DISEASE

Since Crohn's disease was described in 1932 there have been several phases of surgical management, both minimalistic and preservative, as well as aggressive with more extensive bowel resections. With the availability of newer medical therapies controversies still persist and now take on other forms. For example, with active localized ileal disease should surgery be an earlier choice rather than treating with medications and waiting for complications? Proponents for early surgery would argue that it will eventually be required in over three-quarters of patients, and that when questioned retrospectively the majority of patients would have preferred earlier surgical intervention.[19] Quality of life is restored rapidly after surgery and recurrence rates can possibly be lowered with postoperative medical prevention. Arguing against earlier intervention in localized ileal disease, experts would note that thus far there are no prospective randomized clinical trials indicating that earlier surgery can alter the natural history of localized ileocolic disease.[20] Adding to the controversy is the fact that laparoscopic ileocolic resection may hold significant advantages over open surgical resection. It has been stated that some patients with Crohn's are not candidates for laparoscopic resection, because of either prior surgical procedures or complicating fistula and abscess. Recent literature would suggest that as expertise is acquired the vast majority of complications can be overcome, and laparoscopic techniques can be utilized in a high percentage of patients.[21]

It is the authors' opinion that laparoscopic treatment for Crohn's disease is feasible in the vast majority of patients without requiring conversion to open resection or without increasing the complication rate.[22] We currently lean towards recommending earlier intervention laparoscopically, especially when there is evidence of fixed stenosis and early obstructive symptoms (audible bowel sounds, distension at the end of the day, and/or weight loss).

In a similar manner, although troublesome duodenal Crohn's is uncommon it may produce early symptoms of obstruction, and rather than use a variety of potent medications, such as steroids or immunomodulating agents, a laparoscopic gastroenterostomy is associated with a short hospital stay, rapid relief of the obstruction and long-lasting improvement in quality of life.[23]

It is quite clear that not all Crohn's disease is the same, and the decision between early or late surgical intervention will vary from patient to patient. In one study with a 96% postoperative follow-up it was demonstrated that the cumulative probability of requiring reoperation was determined by whether or not the patient had fistulizing rather than non-fistulizing disease. The fistulizing (or perforating group) had a median time between the two operations of less than 2 years, whereas the interval in the non-perforating group was 9.9 years ($P = 0.0002$).[24] When reviewing Crohn's patients with diffuse jejunoileitis and the role of stricturoplasty it was shown that patients with a short duration of disease and a short interval since the last surgery are at a higher risk of accelerated recurrence. Patients with diffuse disease are not at any higher risk for recurrence than patients with more limited disease.[25] These studies raise the important issue as to whether we should be more aggressive in the use of immunomodulatory agents in patients who are moderate to severely ill, and who have either had surgery in the recent past or have had a short duration of disease complicated by fistulization. Prospective trials are indicated using agents such as 6-MP/azathioprine, methotrexate and/or infliximab in combinations in order to avoid surgery as well as early recurrences. It should be pointed out that despite the fact that immunomodulators are effective in healing fistulae, patients with asymptomatic internal fistulae (ileosigmoid, ileoileal, ileocolic, ileovesical) do not routinely require immunomodulators.

Despite its efficacy in treating active Crohn's disease with fistulization, the role of infliximab remains uncertain. A recent study suggested that despite its efficacy in perianal disease, enterocutaneous fistulae did not do well after the use of infliximab and still required surgery. An enterovesical fistula closed completely during this study.[26] There have been conflicting reports as to the role of infliximab in the treatment of Crohn's disease with strictures or partial obstruction. One series suggested that after improving the inflammatory response, further stricturing leading to obstruction might occur in fewer than 10% of patients. More recent studies looking at larger series could not confirm that infliximab produced stricturing requiring an increased need for surgical intervention.[27]

The management of internal abscesses and the timing of surgery remain to be clarified, as does the concomitant use of immunomodulatory agents. Standard surgical procedure in a patient with Crohn's disease who presents with an abscess would be to drain the cavity and then electively perform a resection of the diseased bowel. A current alternative would be to drain the abscess and then to treat with infliximab followed by 6-MP/azathioprine. In selected cases this might result in healing without the ultimate need for surgery. Anecdotally, after infliximab is used for the treatment of internal fistulae surgery may be technically somewhat easier, which may be because of the significant improvement in the inflammatory reaction.

Severe hemorrhage is unusual in Crohn's disease and thus far there are no prospective studies looking at the use of rapidly acting inductive agents such as infliximab or steroids to stop gastrointestinal hemorrhage and avoid surgery.

The standard management of clinically obstructing Crohn's is surgical resection. The role of balloon dilatation in long-term management has not been enthusiastically pursued, especially because of the relatively high complication rate.[14,15] A common error made by gastroenterologists is to perform a colonoscopy and find that the terminal ileum cannot be intubated. This is often thought to represent obstruction; however, what occurs in the retrograde manner is not necessarily related to what occurs antegrade when food or barium travels down the gastrointestinal tract. Despite the findings on endoscopy, clinical obstruction requires nausea, vomiting, abdominal pain, distension, audible bowel sounds, and often weight loss and confirmatory radiographic findings. 'Intestinal obstruction remains a clinical and radiographic diagnosis, not an endoscopic diagnosis.'

Recent studies have suggested that surveillance colonoscopy is required in extensive Crohn's colitis, as the incidence of dysplasia and cancer is similar to that seen in ulcerative colitis.[28,29] What is less certain is the type of surgery to be performed if dysplasia is observed. The choice would rest between a segmental resection or a subtotal colectomy.[30] Likewise, the same issue would arise when a stricture prevents adequate surveillance of the more proximal colon. We currently suggest that each case be individualized, and if there is extensive and active disease throughout the rest of the colon then a subtotal colectomy and ileoproctostomy or ileosigmoidostomy should be the procedures of choice, whereas with minimal activity, localized disease and stricturing a segmental resection would best preserve bowel function and quality of life. On the other hand, total proctocolectomy should be avoided if possible because of the high incidence of complications, especially delayed perineal wound healing (13–35%), as well as stomal complications in approximately 15%. A recent study suggested that young male patients are at high risk for recurrence after total proctocolectomy.[31]

An area of current controversy is that of whether or not an ileal pouch–anal anastomosis should be performed for colorectal Crohn's disease. As clinical recurrence is seen in over half of the patients 10 years after having an ileorectal anastomosis it was felt that the ileoanal pouch anastomosis is inappropriate for patients with Crohn's disease. Early experience noted that 34% of patients initially diagnosed as having ulcerative colitis and undergoing colectomy with ileoanal pouch, in whom Crohn's disease was subsequently diagnosed, required excision of their pouch or were permanently defunctionalized.[32] A more recent study[33] looked at 41 patients with Crohn's colitis who had no evidence of perianal disease or small bowel involvement. Follow-up 10 years later indicated that Crohn's disease-related complications occurred in 35%, and pouch excision was required in only 10%. Functional results were similar to those seen in ulcerative colitis patients having undergone ileal pouch–anal anastomosis. Several patients received azathioprine, although it is unclear as to the timing of the introduction of this agent or the exact dose. None of the patients received infliximab. At present it would appear that ileal pouch–anal anastomosis should be further investigated for selected Crohn's patients, but cannot yet be advocated as routine practice. The postoperative use of prophylactic 6-MP or azathioprine must be considered in these patients, and if a complication does occur, early institution of infliximab may be indicated.

Even more uncertain is the long-term outcome in patients with indeterminate colitis after ileal pouch–anal anastomosis. In an initial report, with a mean follow-up of 5 years after surgery, patients with indeterminate colitis appeared to fail somewhat more frequently than those with ulcerative colitis; however, at 5 years the long-term functional results were similar to those in patients with ulcerative colitis.[53] A follow-up report from the same institution at 10 years reported a higher incidence of pelvic abscess, pouch fistulae and pouch failure seen in indeterminate colitis patients. If the patients did not go on to develop Crohn's disease then the long-term outcome in indeterminate colitis was similar to that seen in ulcerative colitis.[34,35] Once again it is our opinion that patients with indeterminate colitis should be offered ileal pouch–anal anastomosis provided they are made fully aware of the potentially higher complication rate.

The final area of controversy is the appropriate management of perianal Crohn's disease. This requires close coordination between gastroenterologist and surgeon. The incidence of fistula ranges from as low as 17% to as high as 50%, depending on the definition of fistula. In about 9–17% proctectomy has been required. In 170 patients developing an abscess for the first time it was shown that only 37% developed a fistula and 10% developed a recurrent abscess.[36] Therefore, incision and drainage alone was recommended. The cumulative incidence of fistula occurring in Olmsted County was 38%.[37] Diagnosis of fistula can be made either by examination under anesthesia, by MRI or by endoanal ultrasound. The latter cannot be performed when there is significant anal stricturing. If a fistula persists, medical therapy using antibiotics and/or 6-MP is the treatment of choice.[38] For complicating fistulae or recurrent abscesses, placement of setons is required to allow medical therapy to be effective. The most potent and effective medications for fistula closure are infliximab[39] or cyclosporin.[40] Closure is initially seen in 55% of the former patients and about 60% of the latter. Fistula closure can be maintained with administration of infliximab every 8 weeks.[41] Although it is effective acutely cyclosporin is not a good maintenance agent and 6-MP/azathioprine should be initiated soon after cyclosporin has been given. The surgical procedures, as noted above, consist of placing non-cutting setons and drainage of all abscesses. Although diversion of the fecal stream was thought to be effective most surgeons have abandoned this technique, as efficacy did not last long and continuity has almost never been restored. If ostomy is required then a proctectomy is indicated. Advancement flaps have been tried and are an effective method of repair for both anorectal and rectovaginal fistulae. However, in a recent study the primary rate of healing was only 64%, whereas reports in the literature have been quite variable.[42] A randomized control trial of fibrin glue versus conventional treatment for anal fistula showed no advantage of the glue over fistulotomy for simple fistulae. However, the glue healed more complex fistulae than did conventional treatment, with good patient satisfaction.[43] Finally, as regards perianal disease, it must be pointed out that carcinomas may complicate anorectal fistulae and can be very difficult to diagnose. A flexible sigmoidoscopy is usually not adequate in these patients with strictured rectums, and annual examination under anesthesia is indicated in patients with long-standing perianal fistula. Parenthetically it should be noted that anal strictures should not always be dilated, especially in those who have had an ileorectal or ileosigmoid anastomosis, as in these patients with watery stools the stricture may be helpful in maintaining continence. Dilatation should only be performed if the patient has symptomatic obstruction or surveillance cannot be completed.

A recent study has been completed looking at the efficacy of tacrolimus in the treatment of Crohn's perianal fistula. The placebo-controlled trial showed efficacy, but nephrotoxicity was quite high and precludes the routine use of this agent.[44] Lower doses should be evaluated for efficacy and toxicity.

# ULCERATIVE COLITIS

It has been stated many times that ulcerative colitis is nominally a surgically 'curable' condition. However, advances in the modern medical therapy of ulcerative colitis have made it important that patients be treated medically with aggressive immunosuppressive therapy prior to being considered for surgery. Strong biases against medical therapy exist in the surgical community, mostly due to lack of experience with and unfounded fears of immunomodulatory therapies. Most ulcerative colitis patients are treated as outpatients and never require the services of a colorectal surgeon, whereas surgeons usually meet patients with ulcerative colitis in the acute setting or the immediate preoperative period.

# INDICATIONS FOR SURGERY

Absolute indications for surgery in ulcerative colitis include free perforation, colonic obstruction secondary to stricture, the presence of high-grade dysplasia or carcinoma and/or uncontrolled hemorrhage.[45,46] Less certain indications for surgery include steroid refractoriness, steroid complications, intractable extraintestinal manifestations (e.g. pyoderma gangrenosum) and side effects from immunomodulatory therapy. Failure of medical therapy, particularly immunomodulatory therapy, is, however, a clearer indication for surgery.

Hospitalization is mandatory for patients with acute severe ulcerative colitis to ensure adequate intravenous fluid replacement with careful monitoring of fluid output and serum electrolytes. Patients should be instructed in self-charting their stool frequency, urgency, consistency, and the presence or absence of gross blood. Frequent abdominal examinations to exclude signs of peritoneal irritation and evidence of toxic dilation are essential. Initial blood tests should include a complete blood count, serum electrolytes, liver function tests, BUN and creatinine. A serum magnesium and cholesterol should be obtained if cyclosporin is likely to be used. Stool studies, including culture and sensitivity, *Clostridium difficile* toxin assay (A and B) and stool examination for ova and parasites, should be performed. Abdominal X-rays – supine and upright films with visualization of both diaphragms – should be urgently performed to detect the presence of excess small bowel gas or colonic dilation.

Advances in medical therapy have made it less likely that these patients with toxic megacolon or fulminant colitis will require surgery. Nevertheless, surgical consultation should be obtained at the time of admission of a patient with fulminant colitis. In a large representative series, colectomy was required in 37% of patients presenting with their first attack of fulminant disease.[47] A coordinated effort by a team of experienced gastroenterologists and surgeons can reduce mortality in these patients.[46] Patients admitted to hospital with severe ulcerative colitis should be stabilized and toxic dilatation ruled out prior to giving them food or liquids by mouth. These patients can be fed a low-residue lactose-free diet. There is no evidence to suggest that bowel rest and total parenteral nutrition are effective, and three controlled trials examining this therapeutic modality have failed to demonstrate any benefit.[48–50] In fact, in the McIntyre study[49] the patients with ulcerative colitis who were fed appeared to respond to medical therapy and avoided surgery more often than those kept nil by mouth. Total parenteral nutrition should be reserved for severe ulcerative colitis patients who have evidence of profound, long-standing nutritional depletion.

Rolling the patient with megacolon, in addition to aggressive immunomodulatory therapy, can also spare patients colectomy.[51] Intravenous cyclosporin is 80% effective in inducing remission, and in combination with either azathioprine or 6-MP can spare 70% of patients colectomy.[52,53] However, as discussed in Chapter 34, there is a short- to intermediate-term mortality of up to 1% with this therapeutic strategy (primarily due to opportunistic infection), and thus both the benefits and the potential risks of cyclosporin therapy must be discussed with the patient and family. Flexible sigmoidoscopy with biopsy should be performed in non-responders to rule out the presence of CMV. Long-term use of 6-MP or azathioprine appears to be safe for most patients.[52–56]

The 'surgical cure' remains an imperfect one. Total procto-colectomy with ileostomy is disfiguring and is rejected by most patients. Few surgeons perform the continent ileostomy (Kock pouch) today. The ileal pouch–anal anastomosis has several potential drawbacks, including multiple surgical stages, frequent postoperative complications, decreased fecundity, the possibility of sexual dysfunction, frequent bowel movements, nocturnal stools or leakage, incontinence and recurrent pouchitis.[57]

## DYSPLASIA AND ULCERATIVE COLITIS

It has long been appreciated that long-standing UC is associated with an increased risk of colorectal carcinoma. Most clinicians would agree that patients with extensive UC of at least 8–10 years' duration should undergo annual to biannual colonoscopic surveillance with multiple biopsies. One of the most contentious areas of debate in the field concerns the meaning of dysplasia and adenomatous polyps in the setting of colitic mucosa. Few disagree that there is an increased risk of colon carcinoma in patients with both extensive ulcerative colitis of greater than 8–10 years' duration and low-grade dysplasia or adenomatous changes found on surveillance colonoscopy. The disagreement stems from a lack of understanding of the biology of these 'precancerous' lesions and a clear sense of the true risk of progression to cancer. The age of the patient, the extent and severity of disease, age at diagnosis, family history of colon cancer, the presence of polyps in areas of colitis or the finding of dysplasia in truly flat mucosa all factor into the decision to pursue colectomy.[58]

Avoiding surgery in patients with long-standing ulcerative colitis, and findings of either low-grade dysplasia or adenomatous polyps, requires careful, vigilant surveillance. The decision to pursue colonoscopic surveillance should be made with the patient's fully informed participation.[59,60] Prior to performing surveillance colonoscopy, the patient should be well prepared and have little or no disease activity. Colonoscopic surveillance should involve at least 32–40 biopsy samples at 10 cm intervals throughout the colon. These biopsies should be placed in separate specimen bottles to enable localization of any abnormal area. Dysplastic areas may be difficult to visualize endoscopically. Areas of normal-appearing shiny mucosa are rarely dysplastic. Featureless or atrophic areas should be targeted and biopsied.

Particular attention should be paid to areas with raised irregular mucosa, frond-like mucosa and irregular strictures. Dysplasia may also arise in a raised lesion or mass. In ulcerative colitis patients these endoscopic findings, in combination with the histologic finding of dysplasia, have been associated with a high risk of colorectal carcinoma.[61] Pseudopolyps are commonly seen in patients with ulcerative colitis. These are characteristically small and glistening and consist of regenerating mucosa or inflammatory nodules. Sometimes these pseudopolyps can grow quite large and cause luminal obstruction or intussusception. Biopsies from any suspicious lesion should reveal the correct diagnosis. Once dysplasia has been identified, an independent review of the biopsy slides by an expert pathologist is mandatory prior to referral for surgery.

The finding of adenomatous polyps in the right colon of a patient with left-sided colitis or the finding of a single low-grade dysplasia presents a difficult management issue. We treat these patients with endoscopic polypectomy and surveillance biopsies throughout the colon. Surveillance intervals should be shortened to every 3–6 months, depending on the age of the patient or the number of adenomas found. India ink marking of suspicious areas may improve the yield of follow-up surveillance. For polyps not amenable to endoscopic management, segmental laparoscopic resection can be facilitated with tattooing as well.

Similar colon cancer rates have been observed in patients with UC and Crohn's colitis of similar duration and extent.[28,62] Physicians should treat patients with Crohn's colitis of more than 10 years' duration and involvement of more than one-third of the colonic mucosa with the same vigilant surveillance as their UC patients.[29]

## CONTROVERSIES IN THE SURGICAL MANAGEMENT OF ULCERATIVE COLITIS

It would seem on the surface that surgery in ulcerative colitis patients would be less controversial and more straightforward than in those with Crohn's disease. Patients are often advised by surgeons that undergoing a colectomy will allow them to be 'cured' of their disease. In seeking to avoid a standard Brooke ileostomy, colorectal surgeons have enthusiastically supported the ileal pouch–anal anastomosis, which is now considered the gold standard. However, this does have its drawbacks. It usually requires two, not one, surgical procedures, as one-stage ileoanals are performed in only 10% or less of patients. Also after closure of the ostomy 9–10% or more of patients develop obstruction and approximately half require surgical intervention to relieve the obstruction. Approximately 5% of all patients will develop surgical complications and may require even a third operation to reconstruct or excise the pouch. Overall, the worldwide failure rate of ileal pouch–anal anastomosis is about 10%.[63]

In contrast to the older literature, several recent studies have suggested that one-stage ileoanals may have fewer total complications than the two-stage procedure. However, this issue remains controversial, and most colorectal surgeons view a one-stage ileoanal pouch as investigational. Even in the best hands the complication rate is significant, with a leak rate of approximately 10% and pelvic infections seen in 5% of all patients.[64,65]

Actual functional results must be given to patients. A recent paper indicates a bowel frequency of about seven times daily, with at least one nocturnal bowel movement.[66] Major nocturnal incontinence was worse in 22% of patients followed over 10 years, and major daytime incontinence was worse in 18% of patients. The authors concluded that a small number of patients continue to improve over 10 years, but a large number suffer deterioration that is measurable, and this can occur 12 or more years after the initial surgery. These functional results are acceptable to the majority of ulcerative colitis patients who come to surgery for chronic activity. However, for patients who require surgery for dysplasia and have been totally asymptomatic there will be a significant diminution in quality of life.

Knowledge of the natural history and outcome in ulcerative colitis patients after medical therapy should play an important role in trying to avoid surgical intervention. Recent studies from the Mayo Clinic have indicated that in ulcerative colitis patients who require steroids for activity, only half are in remission off steroids at 1 year.[67] This would strongly suggest that if steroids are required to induce an remission, then 6-MP or azathioprine should be added at the same time steroids are initiated. Such a strategy would probably avoid a colectomy in many patients. There has been some fear that immunosuppressive drugs may increase the rate of postoperative complications, but a recent study[68] has shown that there are no increased surgical complications with azathioprine/6-MP, but rather that postoperative complications occur at a higher rate when patients are taking steroids.[68]

Many young patients have opted for colectomy and ileal pouch–anal anastomosis in order to return to good health and bear children. A recent study has revealed that surgery significantly reduced female fecundity compared with a reference population sample, decreasing to 0.20 ($P<0.0001$).[69] This information provides another reason for earlier intervention with immunomodulatory drugs. Likewise, it raises the controversial issue as to whether the initial surgical procedure of choice should be a subtotal colectomy and ileostomy, and after the patient has recovered to try and have their families before ileoanal pouch anastomosis is undertaken.

In specific instances alternatives to ileal pouch–anal anastomosis are available. Ileal rectal anastomosis is an uncomplicated one-stage procedure which maintains good sexual function and no loss of fertility. Bowel movements occur on an average of four to five times daily (less than the average with ileal pouch–anal anastomosis). However, the procedure cannot be performed unless the rectum is distensible, which can be shown with a barium enema. Also, the rectum will probably require continued topical therapy, and there is a cancer risk that is approximately 6% at 20 years and 20% at 30 years. However, in looking at a large series[70] 79% of 145 patients were well with a mean postoperative follow-up of over 8 years. Only one of the patients had gone on to develop cancer.

The continent ileostomy (Kock pouch) preceded the ileal pouch–anal anastomosis and was an excellent operation apart from the problem of nipple slippage, which occurred in 20–25% of patients.[71] New valve designs are currently being developed in order to avoid this complication. Failed ileal pouch-anal anastomoses can also be turned into Kock pouches.

Later complications are also observed with ileal pouch–anal anastomosis, namely pouchitis. A single episode has been observed in 30–60% of patients, and this incidence increases with increased duration from the time of surgery. Chronic pouchitis complicates 8–10% of patients and requires continuous therapy, usually with antibiotics. Both ciprofloxacin and metronidazole are effective therapies, but some patients may require immunomodulatory drugs, and most recently probiotic therapy with VSL-3 has been used to maintain remission once it has been induced with antibiotics (see Chapter 46 for more details).[72]

An interesting new entity has been described, namely of that of the irritable pouch syndrome.[73] This appears to represent irritable bowel syndrome occurring in patients having undergone an ileal pouch–anal anastomosis. As 10–15% of the population has irritable bowel syndrome it clearly should have been expected that the same frequency would be observed in patients having undergone a colectomy. The irritable pouch syndrome should be differentiated from pouchitis and cuffitis, as well as a fistula. Treatment will probably be required with antidiarrheals, anticholinergics or antidepressants. Newly available agents such as alosetron require study in these patients.

It is worth emphasizing what was noted earlier, namely that fulminant colitis and toxic megacolon can be treated medically in the vast majority of cases. High doses of intravenous steroids are effective, but 30% of patients will still require colectomy while in hospital. Cyclosporin can be offered if a patient does not show a significant response in 4–7 days.[52] Cyclosporin will induce remission in approximately 80% of patients, but carries a small risk of serious opportunistic infection. Cyclosporin can be administered to severe ulcerative colitis patients if they have not been receiving steroids, and the response rate appears to be similar to that of steroids alone.[74] Adequate and rapid use of immunomodulators will allow patients to avoid colectomy long term in well over 50% of cases. Toxic megacolon per se is not an absolute indication for surgery, and decompression can be rapidly obtained with the passage of a long tube and the rolling technique, in which patients are placed on their abdomen for 10 minutes every 2 hours.[51] This allows the movement of gas through the colon, which can be passed out as flatus and result in decompression. A frequent cause of failure to respond to adequate medical therapy is superimposed C. *difficile* and, less commonly, cytomegalovirus infection. These should be ruled out prior to surgical intervention.

Laparoscopic technique can be used for ulcerative colitis, as well as for Crohn's disease. A recent case–control study[75] showed a significantly earlier return of bowel function and a shorter hospital stay; however, this technique increased hospital costs. Ileal pouch–anal anastomosis can also be performed laparoscopically with a better cosmetic outcome and less postoperative pain, but will certainly increase the duration of the surgical procedure.

The final controversy regarding ulcerative colitis is related to surveillance and the development of dysplasia and/or cancer. This was outlined earlier in the chapter. However, it should be re-emphasized that surveillance should be performed by experienced gastroenterologists who are capable of distinguishing between true polyps and dysplasia-associated lesions or masses and pseudopolyps. Surveillance is very time intensive and performing just a few random biopsies is not acceptable as an adequate surveillance procedure. Benign polyps in the right side of the colon in patients with left-sided colitis should be treated as polyps similar to those in patients without colitis. They should be completely removed, with adequate follow-up surveillance in the future. More difficult is distinguishing benign polyps in colitic mucosa from dysplastic masses associated with colitis. This requires total removal and four quadrant biopsies around the base of the polyp. If any of these biopsies shows dysplasia then a colectomy would be indicated. Negative biopsies allow continued surveillance.

Although it is quite clear that high-grade dysplasia warrants colectomy, some studies have suggested that low-grade dysplasia may not be an 'early' precursor of the development of cancer. In a recent paper[76] 60 patients with low-grade dysplasia were followed for a mean of 10 years. Only three went on to develop high-grade dysplasia or cancer. We have had a similar experience, and this suggests that an alternative to removal of the colon for a single finding of low-grade dysplasia would be to intensify the frequency of surveillance follow-up. After finding unifocal low-grade dysplasia we recommend that a surveillance be performed every 3–4 months for the next year. If no further dysplasia is found, then patients can return to an interval of 1 year. We have also had an anecdotal experience of performing segmental resections in several ulcerative colitis patients who had recurrent low-grade dysplasia which could not be removed through the colonoscope. No surgical complications were observed. The issue of surveillance intervals and low-grade dysplasia continues to be a problem that requires further extensive study.

## CONCLUSION

The decision to go to surgery can be quite complicated for patients with inflammatory bowel disease. All patients should have clear expectations of the likely outcome of any surgery prior to undergoing the procedure. The gastroenterologist should assume the mantle of an empathetic, educated, experienced escort through the surgical process. Careful collaboration on the part of the gastroenterologist and the surgeon is crucial in ensuring that the patient's wishes are truly honored and their best interests served.

## References

1. Sachar DB, Andrews HA, Farmer RG et al. Proposed classification of patient subgroups in Crohn's disease. Gastroenterol Int 1992;5:141.
2. Friedman S, Rubin PH, Bodian C, Goldstein E, Harpaz N, Present DH. Screening and surveillance colonoscopy in chronic Crohn's colitis. Gastroenterology. 2001;120:820–826.
3. Kornbluth A, Marion J, Salomon P et al. How effective is current medical therapy for severe ulcerative colitis and Crohn's colitis? J Clin Gastroenterol 1995;20:280.
4. Saha MT, Ruuska T, Laippala P et al. Growth of prepubertal children with inflammatory bowel disease. J Pediatr Gastroenterol Nutr 1998;26:310–314.
5. Fazio VW, Galandiuk S, Jagelman DG et al. Stricturoplasty in Crohn's disease. Ann Surg 1989;210:621.
6. Stebbing JF, Jewell DP, Kettlewell MGW et al. Long-term results of recurrence and reoperation after strictureplasty for obstructive Crohn's disease. Br J Surg 1995;82:1471.
7. Ozuner G, Fazio VW, Lavery IC et al. How safe is strictureplasty in the management of Crohn's disease? Am J. Surg 1996;171:57.
8. Krupnick AS, Morris JB. The long-term results of resection and multiple resections in Crohn's disease. Semin Gastrointest Dis 2000;11:41–51.
9. Fishbein T, Schiano T, LeLeiko N et al. An integrated approach to intestinal failure: results of a new program with total parenteral nutrition, bowel rehabilitation and transplantation. J Gastrointest Surg 2002;6:544–562.
10. Kaerlev L, Teglbjaerg PS, Sabroe S et al. Medical risk factors for small-bowel adenocarcinoma with focus on Crohn's disease: a European population-based case–control study. Scand J Gastroenterol 2001;36:641–646.
11. Ogura Y, Bonen DK, Inohara N et al. A frameshift mutation in NOD2 associated with susceptibility to Crohn's disease. Nature 2001;411:537–539.
12. Abreu MT, Taylor KD, Lin YC. Mutations in NOD2 are associated with fibrostenosing disease in patients with Crohn's disease. Gastroenterology 2002;123:679–688.
13. Vermeire S, Louis F, Rutgeerts P et al. NOD2/CARD15 does not influence response to infliximab in Crohn's disease. Gastroenterology 2002;123:106–111.
14. Dear KLE, Hunter JO. Hydrostatic balloon dilatation of Crohn's strictures: a five year review [abstract]. Gut 1998;42: A49.
15. Couckuyt H, Gevers AM, Coremans G et al. Efficacy and safety of hydrostatic balloon dilatation of ileocolonic Crohn's strictures: a prospective long term analysis. Gut 1995;36:577–580.
16. Makowics F, Jehle EC, Becker HD, Starlinger M. Clinical course after transanal advancement flap repair of perianal fistula in patients with Crohn's disease. Br J Surg 1995;82:603–606.
17. Edwards CM, George BD, Jewell DP et al. Role of defunctioning stoma in the management of large bowel Crohn's disease. Br J Surg 2000;87:1063–1066.
18. Sachar DB. The problem with postoperative recurrence of Crohn's disease. Med Clin North Am 1990;74:183.
19. Scott NA, Hughes LE. Timing of ileocolonic resection for symptomatic Crohn's disease: the patient's view. Gut 1994;35:652.
20. Windsor ACJ, Farthing MJG. Ileal disease is best treated by surgery. Gut 2002;51:11.
21. Evans J, Poritz L, Macrae H. Influence of experience on laparoscopic ileocolic resection for Crohn's disease. Dis Colon Rectum 2002;45:1595.
22. Gurland BH, Wexner SD. Laparoscopic surgery for inflammatory bowel disease: results of the past decade. Inflamm Bowel Dis 2002;8:46.
23. Salky B. Severe gastroduodenal Crohn's disease – surgical treatment. Inflamm Bowel Dis 2003; (in press).
24. Aeberhard P, Berchtold W, Riedtmann HJ et al. Surgical recurrence of perforating and non-perforating Crohn's disease. Dis Colon Rectum 1996;39:80.
25. Dietz DW, Fazio VW, Leureti S et al. Strictureplasty in diffuse Crohn's jejunoileitis. Dis Colon Rectum 2002;45:764.
26. Poritz LS, Rowe WA, Kolten WA. Remicade does not abolish the need for surgery in fistulizing Crohn's disease. Dis Colon Rectum 2002;45:771.
27. Toy LS, Scherl EJ, Present DH. Complete bowel obstruction following initial response to infliximab therapy for Crohn's disease. Gastroenterology 2000;85:69.
28. Sachar DB. Cancer in Crohn's disease: dispelling the myths. Gut 1994:1507–1508.
29. Friedman S, Rubin PH, Bodian C, Goldstein E, Harpaz N, Present DH. Screening and surveillance colonoscopy in chronic Crohn's colitis. Gastroenterology 2001;120:820–826.
30. Andersson P, Olaison G, Hallbook O. Segmental resection on subtotal colectomy in Crohn's colitis. Dis Colon Rectum 2002;45:47.
31. Yamamoto T, Allan RN, Keighley RB. Audit of single stage proctocolectomy for Crohn's disease. Dis Colon Rectum 2000;43:249.
32. Phillips RS. Ileal pouch–anal anastomosis of Crohn's disease. Gut 1998;43:303.
33. Regimbeau JM, Panis Y, Pocard M et al. Long term results of ileal pouch–anal anastomosis for colorectal Crohn's disease. Dis Colon Rectum 2001;44:769.
34. McIntyre PB, Pemberton JH, Wolff BG et al. Indeterminate colitis, long term outcome after ileal pouch–anal anastomosis. Dis Colon Rectum 1995;38:51.
35. Yu CS, Pemberton JH, Larson D. Ileal pouch–anal anastomosis in patients with indeterminate colitis. Dis Colon Rectum 2000;43:1487.
36. Kari Pekko J, Hamalainen P, Saino P. Incidence of fistulae after drainage for acute anorectal abscess. Dis Colon Rectum 1998;41:13597.
37. Schwartz DA, Loftus EV, Tremaine WJ et al. The natural history of fistulizing Crohn's disease in Olmsted County, Minnesota. Gastroenterology 2002;122:875.
38. Korelitz BI, Present DH. Favorable effect of 6 mercaptopurine on fistulae of Crohn's disease. Dig Dis Sci 1985;30:58.
39. Present DH, Rutgeerts P, Targan S et al. Infliximab for the treatment of fistula in patients with Crohn's disease. N Engl J Med 1999;340:1398.
40. Present DH, Lichtiger S. Efficacy of cyclosporin in the treatment of fistula of Crohn's disease. Dig Dis Sci. 1994;39:374.
41. Sands B, Vandeventer S, Bernstein C. Long term treatment of fistulizing Crohn's disease response to infliximab in the Accent II trial through 54 weeks. Gastroenterology 2002;122:A81.
42. Sonoda T, Hull T, Piedmont MA et al. Outcomes of primary repair of anorectal and rectovaginal fistula using the endorectal advancement flap. Dis Colon Rectum 2002;45:1622.
43. Lindsey I, Smilgin-Humphies MM, Cunningham C et al. A randomized control trial of fibrin glue versus conventional treatment for anal fistula. Dis Colon Rectum 2002;45:1608.
44. Sandborn WJ, Present DH, Isaacs KL et al. Tacrolimus (FK506) for the treatment of perianal and endocutaneous fistulae in patients with Crohn's disease: a randomized double blind placebo control trial. Gastroenterology 2002;122:A81.
45. Robert, JH, Sachar DB, Aufses AH Jr et al. Management of severe hemorrhage in ulcerative colitis. Am J Surg 1990;159:550.
46. Jewell DP, Caprilli R, Mortensen N et al. Indications and timing of surgery for severe ulcerative colitis (Working Team Report). Gastroenterol Int 1991;4:161.
47. Janerot G, Rolny P, Sandberg-Gertzen H. Intensive intravenous treatment of ulcerative colitis. Gastroenterology 1985;89:1005–1013.
48. Dickinson RJ, Ashton MG, Axon ATR, Smith RC, Yeung CK, Hill GL. Controlled trial of intravenous hyperalimentation and total bowel rest as an adjunct to the routine therapy of acute colitis. Gastroenterology 1980;79:1199–1204.
49. McIntyre PB, Powell-Tuck J, Wood SR et al. Controlled trial of bowel rest in the treatment of acute severe colitis. Gut 1986;27:481–485.
50. Gonzales-Huix F, Fernandez-Banares F, Esteve-Comas M et al. Enteral versus parenteral nutrition as adjunct therapy in acute ulcerative colitis. Am J Gastroenterol 1993;88:227–232.
51. Present DH, Wolfson D, Gelernt IM et al. Medical decompression of toxic megacolon by 'rolling'. A new technique of decompression with favorable long term follow-up. J Clin Gastroenterol 1988;10:485–490.
52. Lichtiger S, Present DH, Kornbluth A et al. Cyclosporin in severe ulcerative colitis refractory to steroid therapy. N Engl J Med 1994;330:1841.
53. Marion JF, Present DH. The modern medical management of acute, severe ulcerative colitis. Eur J Gastroenterol Hepatol 1997;9:831.
54. George J, Present DH, Pou R et al. The long-term outcome of ulcerative colitis treated with 6 mercaptopurine. Am J Gastroenterol 1996;91:1711.
55. Sternthal M, George J, Kornbluth A et al. Toxicity associated with the use of cyclosporin in patients with inflammatory bowel disease [abstract]. Gastroenterology 1996;110:A1019.
56. Sandborn WJ. A critical review of cyclosporin therapy in inflammatory bowel disease. Inflamm Bowel Dis 1995;1:48.
57. Marion JF, Present DH Complications of ileal pouch anal anastomosis: pouchitis. Acta Endosc 1999;29:1–7.
58. Connell WR, Lennard-Jones JE, Williams CB et al. Factors affecting the outcome of colonoscopic surveillance for cancer in ulcerative colitis. Gastroenterology 1994;107:934.

59. Engelsgjerd M, Farraye FA, Odze RD et al. Polypectomy may be adequate treatment for adenoma-like dysplastic lesion in chronic ulcerative colitis. Gastroenterology 1999;117:1288–1294.

60. Rubin PH, Friedman S, Harpaz N et al. Colonoscopic polypectomy in chronic colitis: conservative management after endoscopic resection of dysplastic polyps. Gastroenterology 1999;117:1295–1300.

61. Blackstone M, Riddell R, Rogers B, Levin B. Dysplasia associated lesion or mass (DALM) detected by colonoscopy in longstanding ulcerative colitis: an indication for colectomy. Gastroenterology 1981;80:366.

62. Gillen CD, Walmsley RS, Prior P et al. Ulcerative colitis and Crohn's disease: a comparison of the colorectal cancer risk in extensive colitis. Gut 1994;35:1590–1592.

63. Heuscheun UA , Hinz U, Allemeyer EN et al. One or two-stage procedure for restorative proctocolectomy. Ann Surg 2001;237:788.

64. Pemberton JH. The long term results with ileal anal pouch in advanced therapy of inflammatory bowel diseases. In: Bayless T, Hanauers DC, eds. Advanced therapy in inflammatory bowel disease. London: Marcel Decker; 2001:203.

65. Meagher AP, Farouk R, Dozois RR et al. Ileal pouch–anal anastomosis for chronic ulcerative colitis. Complications and outcomes in 1310 patients. Br J Surg 1990;85:100.

66. Bullard KM, Maroff RD, Gemlo BT. Is ileoanal pouch function stable with time? Dis Colon Rectum 2002;45:299.

67. Faubion WA, Loftus EV, Harmson WS et al. The natural history of corticosteroid therapy for inflammatory bowel disease: a population based study. Gastroenterology 2001;121:355.

68. Mahadevan U, Loftus EV, Tremaine WS et al. Azathioprine or 6 mercaptopurine before colectomy for ulcerative colitis is not associated with increased postoperative complications. Inflamm Bowel Dis 2002;8:311.

69. Olsen KO, Svend J, Berndtsson I et al. Ulcerative colitis: female fecundity before diagnosis, during disease, and after surgery compared with a population sample. Gastroenterology 2002;122:15.

70. Lavery IC. Ileorectal anastomosis in advanced therapy of inflammatory bowel disease. In: Bayless T, Hanauer BC, eds. Advanced therapy in inflammatory bowel disease. London; Marcel Decker; 2001:237.

71. Parc YR, Radice E, Dozois RR et al. Surgery for ulcerative colitis – historical perspective. Dis Colon Rectum 2002;45:299.

72. Gionchetti P, Rizzelo F, Venturi A et al. Prophylaxis of pouchitis onset with probiotic therapy. A double blind placebo control trial. Gastroenterology 2000;118:A190.

73. Shen B, Achkar JP, Lashner BA et al. Irritable pouch syndrome: a new category of diagnosis of symptomatic patients with ileal pouch–anal anastomosis. Am J Gastroenterol 2002;97:972.

74. D'Haensgeert G, Lemmons L, Geboes K et al. Intravenous cyclosporin versus intravenous corticosteroids as single therapy for severe attacks of ulcerative colitis. Gastroenterology 2001;120:1323.

75. Marcello PW, Milsom JW, Wong SK et al. Laparoscopic total colectomy for acute colitis – a case–control study. Dis Colon Rectum 2001;44:1441.

76. Befrits R, Ljung T, Jaramillo E et al. Low grade dysplasia in extensive longstanding inflammatory bowel disease. A follow up study. Dis Colon Rectum 2002;45:615.

## CHAPTER 39

# Indications for surgery: a surgeon's opinion

Alessandro Fichera and Fabrizio Michelassi

## INTRODUCTION

Crohn's disease, ulcerative colitis and the rare forms of true indeterminate colitis represent a disease spectrum with protean manifestations and complications. Although as many as half of patients with inflammatory bowel disease require at least one surgical procedure during their lifetime, the decision to operate is rarely an easy one and should be the result of a thorough collaboration between the gastroenterologist and the surgeon, assisted by the radiologist and the pathologist. Factors to take into consideration include the duration of the disease and the treatment offered to that point; the extent of the disease and the length of grossly normal intestine; the specific complication in regard to the available treatment options; and the patient's specific goals and expectations.

The purpose of this chapter is to explain the surgeon's algorithm in the treatment of patients with inflammatory bowel disease. The indications for surgery are different in Crohn's disease and ulcerative colitis; therefore, these diseases will be discussed in separate sections. The section on Crohn's disease will present the most common indications for surgical treatment, followed by special considerations that relate to the specific sites of gastrointestinal tract involvement. The latter part of the chapter will be devoted to indications for surgical treatment of ulcerative colitis.

## CROHN'S DISEASE

### INDICATIONS FOR SURGERY IN CROHN'S DISEASE

The chronic, unrelenting and recurrent nature of Crohn's disease brings patients to the attention of the gastroenterologist during the early phases of the disease.[1] Most patients present with uncomplicated disease and are initially treated with medical therapy, but although medical therapy has become more sophis-ticated with the adoption of new biologic agents, it still fails to significantly change the natural history of the disease.[2,3] Patients tend to require surgery as time progresses: after 20 and 30 years of symptoms, 78% and 90% of patients, respectively, require surgery.[4]

The indications for surgical intervention in Crohn's disease (Table 39.1) have evolved over past decades based on a better understanding of the disease entity. Crohn's disease is pan-intestinal and surgery is not curative; therefore, surgery should be employed only to treat complications, and bowel conservation should be practiced.

As many as half of the patients require surgery because of failure of medical treatment. Medical treatment fails (a) when maximal medical treatment proves inadequate; (b) for those patients who may be asymptomatic while on maximal induction medical therapy, but who develop recurrence of symptoms with tapering of those induction medications that do not have an acceptable safety profile for use as maintenance therapy; (c) when disease progresses with worsening symptoms or a complication arises while the patient is receiving maximal medical therapy; and (d) in the presence of significant treatment-related complications, including steroid-induced cushingoid features, cataracts, glaucoma, hypertension, aseptic necrosis of the head of the femur, myopathy, vertebral body fractures, myelo-suppression, anaphylactic reaction or growth retardation in children.[5] In our series failure of medical therapy was the primary indication for surgery in 33.6% of patients.[6]

A significant number of patients with Crohn's disease present with septic complications as the first presentation or recurrence.[7] Not all septic complications are an absolute indication for surgery, but are rather a marker of a severe and aggressive form of the disease. Fistulae are identified in one-third of Crohn's disease patients[6] but they are rarely the primary indication for surgery. Specific fistulae requiring surgical treatment include enterocutaneous and enterovaginal fistulae, where the enteric drainage becomes a matter of personal embarrassment for the patient;[8] enterovesical or colovesical fistulae, where the con-

**Table 39.1 Indications for surgery in Crohn's disease. (Adapted from Michelassi F, Milsom J, eds. Operative strategy in inflammatory bowel disease . London: Springer Verlag; 150–153.)**

Failure of medical treatment
    Persistence of symptoms despite corticosteroid therapy for longer than 6 months
    Recurrence of symptoms when high-dose corticosteroids tapered
    Worsening symptoms or new onset of complications with maximal medical therapy
    Occurrence of steroid-induced complications (cushingoid features, cataracts, glaucoma, systemic
    hypertension, aseptic necrosis of the head of the femur, myopathy, or vertebral body fractures)
Obstruction
    Intestinal obstruction (partial or complete)
Septic complications
    Fistula if
        Drainage causes personal embarrassment (e.g. enterocutaneous, enterovaginal fistula, fistula
        in ano)
        Fistula communicates with the genitourinary system (e.g. entero- or colovesical fistula)
        Fistula produces functional or anatomic bypass of a major segment of intestine with consequent
        malabsorption and/or profuse diarrhea (e.g. duodenocolic or enterorectosigmoid fistula)
Inflammatory mass or abscess (intra-abdominal, pelvic, perineal)
Free perforation
    Hemorrhage
    Carcinoma
    Fulminant colitis with or without toxic megacolon
    Growth retardation

nection of the intestine to the genitourinary system causes repeated urinary tract infections and eventually impairment of renal function;[9] and those enteroenteric fistulae that produce functional and anatomic bypass of a major segment of intestine, with consequent malabsorption and/or profuse diarrhea. Inflammatory masses and abscesses occur in as many as 20% of patients.[6,10] These patients should be treated with antibiotics, the abscesses drained percutaneously, if feasible, and surgery should be postponed until a definitive procedure can be safely performed. Primary free perforation is a very unusual complication of Crohn's disease: usually the severity of the transmural inflammation leads to the formation of adhesions, which wall off the perforation, resulting in an abscess. Primary free perforation or the secondary rupture of an abscess into the abdominal cavity requires prompt surgical intervention.

As many as 22% of patients present to the surgeon with worsening obstipation.[6] Symptoms are caused by a single or multiple strictures or a lengthy diseased segment, and differ depending on the location of the disease in the gastrointestinal tract: delayed gastric emptying in gastroduodenal disease; postprandial cramps in jejunoileitis; distension, pain and diarrhea in colonic disease; laborious defecation in perianal Crohn's disease. Intestinal obstruction, even when complete, is rarely an indication for urgent surgery. In general, it is advisable to let the obstruction, even if complete, resolve with nasogastric decompression, intravenous hydration and medical therapy, and to postpone surgery until after resolution of the obstruction to allow for a definitive procedure, i.e. strictureplasty or resection.

Other less frequent complications requiring surgical treatment include gastrointestinal hemorrhage, cancer and toxic megacolon. Massive hemorrhage is an extremely rare complication, occurring in less than 1% of patients.[1,11] Preoperative localization studies are mandatory to minimize the length of intestine to be resected in the presence of multiple disease locations.

Cancer has been described in the small bowel,[12] in the colon,[13] in bypassed loops[14–17] and at strictureplasty sites.[18,19] The risk of cancer correlates with duration of the disease and may be higher in bypassed loops. Surgery for cancer in Crohn's disease patients follows the same oncologic principles as for sporadic cancers. Fulminant colitis with or without toxic megacolon is a known entity in inflammatory bowel disease.[20,21] The surgical treatment of this complication will be discussed in more detail in the ulcerative colitis section.

Growth retardation occurs in 26% of children affected by Crohn's disease.[22] If this persists despite adequate medical and nutritional therapy, prompt surgical treatment should be carried out before puberty or meaningful longitudinal growth will not occur, owing to epiphyseal closure.[23] Specific indications for surgery in the pediatric population also include intractability (20%), fistulae (30%) and perianal disease, fulminant colitis with or without toxic megacolon (20%), obstruction, abdominal abscess or mass (12–30%), free perforation and massive bleeding (2%).[22]

## INDICATIONS FOR SURGERY ACCORDING TO INTESTINAL LOCATION

The clinical manifestations and complications of Crohn's disease vary with the location of the disease. This section analyzes indications for surgical treatment of Crohn's disease according to its location in the gastrointestinal tract. In all locations, failure of medical treatment, as described above, may be an indication for surgical treatment.

## Crohn's diseases of the stomach and duodenum

About 2–4% of Crohn's disease patients present with involvement of the stomach or duodenum, but only one-third require surgical treatment.[24] Obstruction is by far the most common indication for surgical treatment.[25] Indeed, in a recent review of 108 patients, 83% underwent surgery for this complication.[26] Patients complain of upper abdominal postprandial distension with a prolonged gastric emptying time, nausea and, eventually, vomiting.

The duodenum at times can be the site of ileoduodenal or coloduodenal fistulae, with the fistula originating from the diseased ileocolonic segment and draining into the duodenum. Treatment follows the principle of resection of the primary disease and closure of the defect in the target organ. Acute massive gastroduodenal hemorrhage from major gastroduodenal vessels is a rare indication for surgery. Acute pancreatitis may develop in the presence of duodenal disease,[27] probably as a result of duodenal contents refluxing into the pancreatic duct. When other more common causes of pancreatitis have been excluded, a gastrojejunostomy is indicated to prevent recurrent attacks of pancreatitis.

## Crohn's disease of the small bowel

The jejunum and ileum, not including the terminal ileum, are affected by Crohn's disease in 3–10% of patients.[6,28] Obstruction is the most common indication for surgical treatment; sepsis, massive hemorrhage and carcinoma are much less common. Chronic, high-grade small bowel obstruction may be caused by single or multiple, short or long strictures. These patients present with postprandial abdominal pain, nausea and vomiting, and often progress to a high-grade obstruction. When multiple tight strictures are present the small bowel is transformed into a sequence of dilated saccular segments separated by tight, ring-like strictures. The dilated segments, which contain partially digested food particles, become the ideal environment for bacterial overgrowth. Bacterial overgrowth and stagnation cause occasional diarrhea, malabsorption and vitamin $B_{12}$ deficiency.

Septic complications such as an inflammatory mass, an abscess and, occasionally, a fistula are also indications for surgical treatment of small bowel Crohn's disease. Septic complications will be discussed in further details in the section on Crohn's disease of the terminal ileum.

The first case of a carcinoma of the small bowel in Crohn's disease was described by Ginzburg in 1956.[29] Since then there have been more than 100 cases described in the literature,[19,29–31] including several reported in bypassed loops[14–17] and two originating at a previous strictureplasty site.[18,19] Most cancers are adenocarcinomas,[31] but they differ from de novo cancers in many respects: they present at a younger age, are more common in the distal small bowel, and may be multifocal or diffuse.[14]

## Crohn's disease of the terminal ileum

The terminal ileum is the most common gastrointestinal location requiring surgery in Crohn's disease (approximately 40%).[1] Classically, patients present with obstructive symptoms or with septic features suggesting either a contained perforation or an abscess with or without a fistula. Cancer and hemorrhage are infrequent indications for surgical resection.

Obstruction, characterized by postprandial abdominal crampy pain and distension, is a very common indication for surgery for Crohn's disease of the terminal ileum. Unremitting, chronic obstructive symptoms or an episode of high-grade obstruction indicate that the degree of cicatricial stenosis is such

that medical treatment is unlikely to be successful and surgical treatment is necessary.

Abscesses are relatively common complications of Crohn's disease of the terminal ileum. Their occurrence may influence the timing of surgery and significantly increase its complexity. When feasible, these patients should be managed with image-guided drainage and antibiotics, with elective resection at a later time. This approach is feasible in approximately 50% of patients.[32] If percutaneous drainage is not successful or in the presence of a secondary free rupture of the abscess in the peritoneal cavity, open surgical exploration is necessary.

Psoas abscess occurs as a result of a retroperitoneal perforation of the ileocecal region. Clinical manifestations vary from mild sepsis to severe psoas spasm with hip pain, flexion and external rotation of the thigh associated with an abdominal mass. The retroperitoneal process can compress the ureter and cause right hydronephrosis. Resection of the inflammatory mass and drainage of the abscess usually relieves the compression on the ureter and cures the hydronephrosis.

Fistulae are common in Crohn's disease of the terminal ileum, but they rarely represent the only indication for surgical treatment. In our series of 639 patients undergoing operation for Crohn's disease 331 had disease in the terminal ileum. Of these, 217 (65.6%) were found to harbor 285 intra-abdominal fistulae; yet these fistulae represented the primary indication for surgical treatment in only 6.3% of cases.[33]

Enterocutaneous fistulae usually drain through a previous abdominal scar or through the umbilicus.[34] At times they result from surgical incision and drainage of a subcutaneous abscess complicating severe intra-abdominal disease, or from percutaneous drainage of an abdominal abscess.[32] The presence of an enterocutaneous fistula does not necessarily dictate the need for immediate surgical intervention.[8,34] Patients may be reluctant to undergo surgical treatment when the enterocutaneous fistula has a minimal output and the underlying disease is under satisfactory control. However, in most cases the difficulty in maintaining personal hygiene, the fear of social embarrassment, the troublesome symptoms associated with the severely diseased segment that led to the formation of the fistula, and the skin excoriation that invariably forms around the cutaneous opening of the fistula, become factors in indicating the need for surgical treatment.

Enterovesical fistulae occur in 2–5% of patients with Crohn's disease.[35,36] There is some controversy about the timing of surgical intervention in their presence, but most surgeons and gastroenterologists agree that the consequences of chronic urinary tract infections on renal function, in addition to the symptoms of the intestinal tract itself, are an indication for operation. Enterovaginal fistulae are rare complications of Crohn's disease and most often occur in women who have undergone a previous hysterectomy. The vaginal discharge is cause for discomfort, social and sexual embarrassment, and difficulty in maintaining personal hygiene. Most patients readily accept surgical intervention.

Enteroduodenal, enteroenteric and enterocolic fistulae usually are asymptomatic and often discovered only during a careful radiological study or at abdominal exploration, or upon inspection of the resected specimen.[37] We consider these fistulae to be an indication for surgical treatment only if they cause massive diarrhea because of the bypass of a sizable length of intestine.

Massive intestinal hemorrhage is a rare complication of terminal ileitis.[38] Because the hemorrhage originates from active disease, patients with Crohn's disease are likely to have repeated episodes that will ultimately require surgical intervention. If the extent of the disease is limited, as assessed by contrast radiography, an elective resection should be considered after two episodes of self-limited hemorrhage. In the presence of an ongoing, unrelenting hemorrhage an angiogram should be obtained to localize the source of bleeding, especially in the presence of multiple sites of disease involvement.[11] The possibility of a life-threatening hemorrhage in Crohn's disease patients should not be underestimated, as four cases of exsanguinating gastrointestinal hemorrhage have been reported in the literature.[39]

Malignant transformation of the terminal ileum is, fortunately, rare. Its treatment is based on oncologic principles and it has been described in the previous section.

## Crohn's disease of the colorectum

The colon is affected by Crohn's disease in up to 30% of patients.[1,6,40] The involvement can be limited to a segment or extend to the entire colon and rectum; furthermore, patients may present with associated anorectal or small bowel disease.

The most common indication for surgery in patients with disease localized primarily to the colon is failure of medical therapy.[6,41] These patients present with persistent and often bloody diarrhea and abdominal pain not responding to medical therapy. With worsening conditions, toxic colitis with or without megacolon may develop. This complication is less frequently associated with Crohn's disease than ulcerative colitis, but it carries similar mortality rates (14–16%) in both conditions. Factors that affect mortality include age (30% for patients over 40 years old, versus 5% for those younger than 40), gender (21% in women versus 13% in men) and the occurrence of colonic perforation (44% for cases with perforation versus only 2% in those without).[21] In the absence of overt perforation, initial therapy consists of high-dose steroids, bowel rest and antibiotics. Lack of improvement over a short period of time or any signs of worsening condition are indications for an urgent operation to avoid colonic perforation.

Septic complications occur in the form of inflammatory masses or, more infrequently, fistulae or abscesses. Inflammatory masses can be found with equal frequency in any segment of the colon and rectum. Occasionally transverse colon disease fistulizes into the stomach. A common location for abscesses to occur is the descending colon at the junction with the sigmoid colon. These abscesses, which form in the left parietocolic gutter and lie over the psoas muscle, may be confused with diverticular abscesses. Usually, the age of the patient and other manifestations of Crohn's disease help in reaching the correct diagnosis. Percutaneous drainage and intravenous antibiotic treatment have obviated the need for urgent laparotomy in many of these patients. However, even if sepsis is controlled, surgery usually is indicated because of concomitant significant symptoms or the insurgence of a colocutaneous fistula in the vast majority of patients.[42]

The risk of colorectal cancer is increased in Crohn's colitis between four- and 20-fold,[43,44] with an incidence between 1.4 and 1.8%.[8,19,29,30,45,46] Carcinoma can arise in long-standing benign strictures, probably due to chronic inflammation.[47] Routine surveillance colonoscopies should be considered after 7–10 years of disease duration, with the recommendation to proceed with resection in the presence of dysplasia. Prophylactic segmental resection or colectomy should be performed for tight strictures not allowing passage of the endoscope, thereby interfering with a complete colonoscopy; a stricture that is difficult to survey; multiple pseudopolyps rendering surveillance difficult; and, as mentioned earlier, the presence of an excluded intestinal segment (retained rectal stump). Surgery for adenocarcinoma in Crohn's colitis should be based on oncologic principles and on the extent of the luminal disease.

## Perianal Crohn's disease

Anorectal Crohn's disease may manifest with edematous skin tags, fissures, ulcers, abscesses, fistulae, strictures and, as a complication of chronic, long-standing inflammation, anal cancer. The reported incidence of perianal Crohn's disease requiring surgery varies between 25 and 34%.[48,49] Crohn's colitis is much more frequently associated with anal lesions than Crohn's disease of the small bowel (52 % vs. 14 %).

Skin tag, fissures and ulcers rarely require surgical treatment. The most common indications for surgery in perianal Crohn's disease are septic in nature (abscess, fistula in ano, anovaginal fistula). Anovaginal fistulae occur as a complication of anorectal Crohn's disease in about 10% of patients[50,51] and require special mention. In approximately half of cases the discharge through the vagina is so minimal that patients tolerate it and do not require operative treatment. In the remainder the discharge is sufficient to cause difficulty in maintaining personal hygiene and sexual inhibition. These patients may require a transanal advancement flap or a proctectomy, depending on the absence or presence of Crohn's rectal disease or concomitant additional perianal manifestations of Crohn's.

Anorectal complications also include stenosis and cancer. Anal strictures occur in fewer than 5% of patients with Crohn's disease. Cancer may develop from the diseased anorectal mucosa, a chronic fistula in ano or a retained rectal stump.

# ULCERATIVE COLITIS

The majority of ulcerative colitis patients presents with bloody diarrhea, urgency and fatigue; during an acute flare they may present with fever and, possibly, abdominal distension. In the absence of absolute indications for immediate surgery, such as perforation or carcinoma, the patient is treated initially with medical therapy.[52-54] However, a definitive treatment plan should be formulated after complete diagnostic evaluation, taking into account the extent and duration of the disease, the presence of dysplasia or cancer, medical therapy used, presence of side effects due to the medical treatment, and the patient's general conditions and expectations. As in Crohn's disease an optimal treatment plan requires input from the patient as well as the surgeon and the gastroenterologist, assisted by the radiologist and pathologist.

## INDICATIONS FOR SURGERY FOR ULCERATIVE COLITIS

The most common indication for the surgical treatment of ulcerative colitis in our experience (Table 39.2) is failure of medical therapy,[55] considered as such when maximal medical therapy

**Table 39.2 Indications for surgery in ulcerative colitis. (Adapted from Michelassi F, Milsom J, eds. Operative strategy in inflammatory bowel disease . London: Springer Verlag; 150–153.)**

Failure of medical treatment
  Persistence of symptoms despite corticosteroid therapy
  Recurrence of symptoms when high-dose corticosteroids are tapered
  Worsening symptoms or new onset of complications while on maximal medical therapy
  Occurrence of steroid-induced complications (cushingoid features, weight gain, systemic
    hypertension, diabetes, steroid myopathy, osteopenia, compression fractures, aseptic necrosis of
    femoral head, increased irritability, cataracts)
Malignant transformation
  Suspicious mass on colonoscopy
  Dysplasia
  DALM
  Carcinoma
Fulminant colitis with acute abdomen
  Without toxic megacolon
  With toxic megacolon
  With walled-off perforation
  With free perforation
Hemorrhage

proves inadequate; or for those patients who may be asymptomatic while on maximal induction medical therapy but who develop recurrence of symptoms with tapering of those induction medications that do not have an acceptable safety profile for use as maintenance therapy; when the disease progresses with worsening symptoms while the patient is receiving maximal medical therapy; and when the patient develops significant treatment-related complications.

Other indications for surgical treatment include the presence of a suspicious mass at colonoscopy, dysplasia on colonic biopsy, the association of dysplasia with a mass (DALM), and the occurrence of a carcinoma. Colonoscopic detection of mucosal dysplasia is considered the best available surveillance tool for the detection of cancer. Synchronous cancer has been reported in 10–20% of patients with low-grade dysplasia. When high-grade dysplasia is present this risk increases to 30–40%. If the dysplasia is associated with a mass (DALM), the risk of carcinoma is as high as 40–60%.[56] Yet, because the correlation between dysplasia and cancer is not constant, when dysplasia is found on surveillance colonoscopy some suggest immediate colectomy, whereas others opt for continued surveillance. Gorfine et al.[57] recently reviewed the pathology reports of 590 patients who underwent total proctocolectomy or restorative proctocolectomy for ulcerative colitis and found that cancers were significantly more common among specimens with dysplastic changes. Specimens with dysplasia of any grade were 36 times more likely to harbor invasive carcinoma. More importantly, tumor stage did not correlate with dysplasia grade. They concluded that even though dysplasia is an unreliable marker for the detection of synchronous carcinoma, when dysplasia of any grade is discovered at colonoscopy the probability of a coexistent carcinoma is high. We believe that a histopathologic diagnosis of dysplasia, confirmed by an experienced pathologist, is an indication for colectomy.

Carcinoma was the indication for surgery in 2% of our series.[55] Patients with ulcerative colitis are known to have an increased risk of colorectal cancer[58,59] which increases with the extent and duration of the colitis. Gyde et al.[60] reported an overall eightfold increase in the risk of cancer in these patients, with a fourfold increase in the left-sided colitis and proctitis group and a 19-fold increase in the pancolitis group. In addition, the pancolitis group had a cumulative risk of 7.2% at 20 years and 16.5% at 30 years from diagnosis.

Acute fulminant colitis with or without an acute abdomen develops in about 13% of patients.[55] About 60% of these fail to respond to medical therapy[52,61] or develop persistent abdominal pain, distension, diffuse abdominal tenderness, rebound, tachycardia, fever and leukocytosis, suggesting an acute abdomen. The latter may be due to the development of a toxic megacolon, often triggered by the administration of narcotic, antidiarrheal, anticholinergic or antidepressant medications. Diffuse abdominal pain and tenderness, tachycardia, increasing colonic dilatation with thumbprinting (suggestive of edema of the colonic wall) or pneumatosis indicate impending perforation. These patients should undergo emergency surgical intervention after appropriate volume resuscitation.

Free perforation is rare and usually represents the end result of an untreated toxic megacolon. At times a perforation is walled off by neighboring structures or by the lateral abdominal wall: it usually manifests itself with persistent localized tenderness, fever and elevated white blood cell count. Both free and walled-off perforations require surgical treatment.

Massive hemorrhage occurs in up to 4% of patients[55] and is another indication for urgent surgery. Persistent hemorrhage despite maximal medical treatment is a manifestation of severe disease. The hemorrhage originates from extensive mucosal ulcerations, rather than a definite arterial source. Because of this, an abdominal colectomy is necessary to remove the majority of the bleeding surface. A primary anastomosis should be avoided in favor of an ileostomy and closure of the rectal stump. With fecal diversion, postoperative rectal bleeding from the retained rectum is rare. When it happens it usually responds to increased doses of systemic steroids, or the administration of topical steroids or intrarectal tamponade with gauzes soaked in a dilute epinephrine solution. Preservation of the rectum maintains the option for a subsequent restorative procedure.

# REFERENCES

1. Farmer RG, Hawk WA, Turnbull RB Jr. Clinical patterns in Crohn's disease: a statistical study of 615 cases. Gastroenterology 1975;68:627–635.

2. Rhodes J, Bainton D, Beck P, Campbell H. Controlled trial of azathioprine in Crohn's disease. Lancet 1971;2:1273–1276.

3. Cohen RD, Tsang JF, Hanauer SB. Infliximab in Crohn's disease: first anniversary clinical experience. Am J Gastroenterol 2000;95:3469–3477.

4. Mekhjian HS, Switz DM, Melnyk CS, Rankin GB, Brooks RK. Clinical features and natural history of Crohn's disease. Gastroenterology 1979;77:898–906.

5. Motil KJ, Grand RJ, Davis-Kraft L, Ferlic LL, Smith EO. Growth failure in children with inflammatory bowel disease: a prospective study. Gastroenterology 1993;105:681–691.

6. Michelassi F, Balestracci T, Chappell R, Block GE. Primary and recurrent Crohn's disease. Experience with 1379 patients. Ann Surg 1991;214:230–238.

7. Greenstein RJ, Greenstein AJ. Is there clinical, epidemiological and molecular evidence for two forms of Crohn's disease? Mol Med Today 1995;1:343–348.

8. Keighley M, Heyen F, Winslet MC. Entero-cutaneous fistulae and Crohn's disease. Acta Gastroenterol Belg 1987;50:580–600.

9. Yamamoto T, Keighley MR. Enterovesical fistulae complicating Crohn's disease: clinicopathological features and management. Int J Colorectal Dis 2000;15:211–215.

10. Keighley MR, Eastwood D, Ambrose NS, Allan RN, Burdon DW. Incidence and microbiology of abdominal and pelvic abscess in Crohn's disease. Gastroenterology 1982;83:1271–1275.

11. Homan WP, Tang CK, Thorbjarnarson B. Acute massive hemorrhage from intestinal Crohn disease. Report of seven cases and review of the literature. Arch Surg 1976;111:901–905.

12. Hordijk ML, Shivananda S. Risk of cancer in inflammatory bowel disease: why are the results in the reviewed literature so varied? Scand J Gastroenterol 1989;170(Suppl):70–74.

13. Keighley MR, Thompson H, Alexander-Williams J. Multifocal colonic carcinoma and Crohn's disease. Surgery 1975;78:534–537.

14. Frank JD, Shorey BA. Adenocarcinoma of the small bowel as a complication of Crohn's disease. Gut 1973;14:120–124.

15. Greenstein AJ, Sachar D, Pucillo A et al. Cancer in Crohn's disease after diversionary surgery. A report of seven carcinomas occurring in excluded bowel. Am J Surg 1978;135:86–90.

16. Ribeiro MB, Greenstein AJ, Heimann TM, Yamazaki Y, Aufses AH Jr. Adenocarcinoma of the small intestine in Crohn's disease. Surg Gynecol Obstet 1991;173:343–349.

17. Senay E, Sachar DB, Keohane M, Greenstein AJ. Small bowel carcinoma in Crohn's disease. Distinguishing features and risk factors. Cancer 1989;63:360–363.

18. Jaskowiak NT, Michelassi F. Adenocarcinoma at a strictureplasty site in Crohn's disease: report of a case. Dis Colon Rectum 2001;44:284–287.

19. Marchetti F, Fazio VW, Ozuner G. Adenocarcinoma arising from a strictureplasty site in Crohn's disease. Report of a case. Dis Colon Rectum 1996;39:1315–1321.

20. Mortensen NJ, Ritchie JK, Hawley PR, Todd IP, Lennard-Jones JE. Surgery for acute Crohn's colitis: results and long term follow-up. Br J Surg 1984;71:783–784.

21. Greenstein AJ, Sachar DB, Gibas A et al. Outcome of toxic dilatation in ulcerative and Crohn's colitis. J Clin Gastroenterol 1985;7:137–143.

22. Telander RL, Schmeling DJ. Current surgical management of Crohn's disease in childhood. Semin Pediatr Surg 1994;3:19.

23. Homer DR, Grand RJ, Colodny AH. Growth course and prognosis after surgery for Crohn's disease in children and adolescents. Pediatrics 1997;59:717

24. Murray JJ, Schoetz DJ Jr, Nugent FW, Coller JA, Veidenheimer MC. Surgical management of Crohn's disease involving the duodenum. Am J Surg 1984;147:58–65.

25. Yamamoto T, Allan RN, Keighley MR. An audit of gastroduodenal Crohn disease: clinicopathologic features and management. Scand J Gastroenterol 1999;34:1019–1024.

26. Reynolds HL Jr, Stellato TA. Crohn's disease of the foregut. Surg Clin North Am 2001;81:117–35, viii.

27. Legge DA, Hoffman HN II, Carlson HC. Pancreatitis as a complication of regional enteritis of the duodenum. Gastroenterology 1971;61:834–838

28. Tan WC, Allan RN. Diffuse jejunoileitis of Crohn's disease. Gut 1993;34:1374–1378.

29. Greenstein AJ. Cancer in inflammatory bowel disease. Mt Sinai J Med 2000;67:227–240.

30. Gyde SN, Prior P, Macartney JC, Thompson H, Waterhouse JA, Allan RN. Malignancy in Crohn's disease. Gut 1980;21:1024–1029.

31. Michelassi F, Testa G, Pomidor WJ, Lashner BA, Block GE. Adenocarcinoma complicating Crohn's disease. Dis Colon Rectum 1993;36:654–661.

32. Sahai A, Belair M, Gianfelice D, Cote S, Gratton J, Lahaie R. Percutaneous drainage of intra-abdominal abscesses in Crohn's disease: short and long-term outcome. Am J Gastroenterol 1997;92:275–278.

33. Michelassi F, Stella M, Balestracci T, Giuliante F, Marogna P, Block GE. Incidence, diagnosis, and treatment of enteric and colorectal fistulae in patients with Crohn's disease. Ann Surg 1993;218:660–666.

34. Blackett RL, Hill GL. Postoperative external small bowel fistulae: a study of a consecutive series of patients treated with intravenous hyperalimentation. Br J Surg 1978;65:775–778.

35. Liu CH, Chuang CK, Chu SH et al. Enterovesical fistula: experiences with 41 cases in 12 years. Changgeng Yi Xue Za Zhi 1999;22:598–603.

36. Heyen F, Ambrose NS, Allan RN, Dykes PW, Alexander-Williams J, Keighley MR. Enterovesical fistulae in Crohn's disease. Ann Roy Coll Surg Engl 1989;71:101–104.

37. Wilk PJ, Fazio V, Turnbull RB Jr. The dilemma of Crohn's disease: ileoduodenal fistula complicating Crohn's disease. Dis Colon Rectum 1977;20:387–392.

38. Farmer RG. Lower gastrointestinal bleeding in inflammatory bowel disease. Gastroenterol Jpn 1991;26 (Suppl 3):93–100.

39. Cirocco WC, Reilly JC, Rusin LC. Life-threatening hemorrhage and exsanguination from Crohn's disease. Report of four cases. Dis Colon Rectum 1995;38:85–95.

40. Hurst RD, Molinari M, Chung TP, Rubin M, Michelassi F. Prospective study of the features, indications, and surgical treatment in 513 consecutive patients affected by Crohn's disease. Surgery 1997;122:661–667.

41. Fazio VW, Wu JS. Surgical therapy for Crohn's disease of the colon and rectum. Surg Clin North Am 1997;77:197–210.

42. Greenstein AJ, Kark AE, Dreiling DA. Crohn's disease of the colon. I. Fistula in Crohn's disease of the colon, classification, presenting features and management in 63 patients. Am J Gastroenterol 1974;63:419–425.

43. Hamilton SR. Colorectal carcinoma in patients with Crohn's disease. Gastroenterology 1985;89:398–407.

44. Weedon DD, Shorter RG, Ilstrup DM, Huizenga KA, Taylor WF. Crohn's disease and cancer. N Engl J Med 1973;289:1099–1103.

45. Green S, Stock RG, Greenstein AJ. Rectal cancer and inflammatory bowel disease: natural history and implications for radiation therapy. Int J Radiat Oncol Biol Phys 1999;44:835–840.

46. Ribeiro MB, Greenstein AJ, Sachar DB et al. Colorectal adenocarcinoma in Crohn's disease. Ann Surg 1996;223:186–193.

47. Yamazaki Y, Ribeiro MB, Sachar DB, Aufses AH Jr, Greenstein AJ. Malignant colorectal strictures in Crohn's disease. Am J Gastroenterol 1991;86:882–885.

48. Hurst RD, Crucitti P, Melis M, Rubin M, Gottlieb L, Michelassi F. Primary myocutaneous flap closure of the perineal wound following proctectomy for perineal complications of Crohn's disease: a prospective feasibility study. Surgery (in press).

49. Williams DR, Coller JA, Corman ML, Nugent FW, Veidenheimer MC. Anal complications in Crohn's disease. Dis Colon Rectum 1981;24:22–24.

50. Radcliffe AG, Ritchie JK, Hawley PR, Lennard-Jones JE, Northover JM. Anovaginal and rectovaginal fistulae in Crohn's disease. Dis Colon Rectum 1988;31:94–99.

51. Williamson PR, Hellinger MD, Larach SW, Ferrara A. Twenty-year review of the surgical management of perianal Crohn's disease. Dis Colon Rectum 1995;38:389–392.

52. Lichtiger S, Present DH, Kornbluth A et al. Cyclosporine in severe ulcerative colitis refractory to steroid therapy. N Engl J Med 1994;330:1841–1845.

53. Veidenheimer MC, Nugent FW. Treatment of chronic ulcerative colitis. Surg Clin North Am 1968;48:559–565.

54. Van Rosendaal GM. Inflammatory bowel disease. CMAJ 1989;141:113–123.

55. Hurst RD, Finco C, Rubin M, Michelassi F. Prospective analysis of perioperative morbidity in one hundred consecutive colectomies for ulcerative colitis. Surgery 1995;118:748–754.

56. Blackstone MO, Radial RH, Rogers BHG et al. Dysplasia-associated lesion or mass (DALM) detected by colonoscopy in long-standing ulcerative colitis: an indication for colectomy. Gastroenterology 1981;80:366–370

57. Gorfine SR, Bauer JJ, Harris MT, Kreel I. Dysplasia complicating chronic ulcerative colitis: is immediate colectomy warranted? Dis Colon Rectum 2000;43:1575–1581.

58. Langholz E, Munkholm P, Davidsen M, Binder V. Colorectal cancer risk and mortality in patients with ulcerative colitis. Gastroenterology 1992;103:1444–1451.

59. Lindberg B, Persson B, Veress B, Ingelman-Sundberg H, Granqvist S. Twenty years' colonoscopic surveillance of patients with ulcerative colitis. Detection of dysplastic and malignant transformation. Scand J Gastroenterol 1996;31:1195–1204.

60. Gyde SN, Prior P, Allan RN et al. Colorectal cancer in ulcerative colitis: a cohort study of primary referrals from three centres. Gut 1988;29:206–217.

61. Kirsner JB. Current medical and surgical opinions on important therapeutic issues in inflammatory bowel disease. A special 1979 survey. Am J Surg 1980;140:391–395.

## CHAPTER 40

# Surgical management of ulcerative colitis

Robert R Cima and John H Pemberton

## INTRODUCTION

Chronic ulcerative colitis (CUC) is an inflammatory bowel disease limited to the mucosa of the rectum and colon. This process is characterized by contiguous inflammation beginning in the rectum and progressing for variable distances proximally. The etiology of the disease is unknown. The natural history is one of a chronic inflammatory state, characterized by intermittent flares of disease activity. In a small number of patients the initial presentation of chronic ulcerative colitis is of a fulminant nature, which can be fatal. Medical therapy is directed at control of symptoms or at the underlying inflammatory process. Medications are not curative for the either the intestinal or the extraintestinal manifestations of CUC. However, surgical removal of the colon and rectum cures the intestinal manifestations of the disease and eliminates or markedly reduces the associated risk of malignancy in long-standing CUC.

The indications for surgical intervention in CUC are divided into two categories (Table 40.1). First, emergency surgery is usually necessary for patients with fulminant disease, toxic megacolon or massive hemorrhage. In this situation, the operative strategy needs to be tailored to the situation to allow the patient to recover from the inciting event without precluding a future restorative procedure or definitive therapy to remove all diseased tissue. Second, the chronic nature of ulcerative colitis leads to a number of complications requiring surgical intervention in an urgent or elective fashion. These include failure of medical management to control symptoms; complications associated with side effects of medications; stricture formation or obstruction; mucosal dysplasia, dysplasia-associated lesion or mass (DALM), or malignancy; extraintestinal manifestations of CUC; and growth retardation in children.

There are four surgical options for the treatment of CUC: proctocolectomy with an end (Brooke) ileostomy; total abdominal colectomy and ileorectal anastomosis; proctocolectomy with construction of a continent ileostomy or Kock pouch; and proc-

tocolectomy with ileal pouch–anal anastomosis. The choice needs to be individualized to the patient, based on their underlying physical and medical condition as well as their social and psychological situation. In selected patients a proctocolectomy with end ileostomy or a colectomy with an ileorectal anastomosis may be a better alternative, given certain circumstances. The Kock pouch, although it is a continent ileostomy, does not allow for normal defecation through the anus, requiring instead intermittent intubation of an abdominal wall stoma to empty the small bowel reservoir. Although there was initial enthusiasm for the Kock pouch, it has fallen out of favor because it is a technically difficult operation to perform and is associated with an almost unacceptably high incidence of pouch dysfunction requiring frequent operative repair. It is of mainly historical interest and will not be discussed further in this chapter. Today, the preferred operation is proctocolectomy with ileal pouch–anal anastomosis (IPAA) because it removes the diseased colon while preserving fecal continence and nearly normal defecation through the anus. In almost all series of patients who have had an IPAA, the majority report good functional results and a high degree of satisfaction with quality of life, which is stable over time. The adaptation of newer technologies such as laparoscopic surgery to this procedure might further increase patient satisfaction and decrease morbidity.

## INDICATIONS FOR SURGERY IN ULCERATIVE COLITIS

### EMERGENCY SURGERY

#### Fulminant colitis

Although CUC is commonly a chronic disease that permits deliberate and coordinated care, occasionally it presents fulminantly. This is the initial presentation in approximately 10% of patients.[1] Fulminant disease is characterized by the sudden onset of severe frequent bloody bowel movements (more than 10 per

| Table 40.1 Indications for surgery in ulcerative colitis |
| --- |

**Emergency surgery**
Fulminant colitis
Acute toxic megacolon
Acute toxic megacolon with perforation
Massive hemorrhage
Acute intractable colitis
**Non-emergency surgery**
Intractable symptoms on maximal medical therapy
Side effects of medications
Stricture formation/obstruction
Dysplasia or mass lesion
Colon/rectal cancer
Growth retardation in children
Extraintestinal manifestations

day), abdominal pain, dehydration and anemia. The Truelove and Witts criteria for fulminant colitis include the above and at least two of the following conditions: tachycardia, body temperature higher than 38.6°C, leukocytosis (more than 10.5 K) and hypoalbuminemia.[2] These patients are extremely ill and require rapid aggressive medical therapy. Medical therapy consists of fluid resuscitation and correction of electrolyte abnormalities. Blood transfusions may be necessary. The patient should be given nothing by mouth. Nasogastric tube decompression may be required if colonic distension is a component of the presentation. If the patient is known to have CUC, then high-dosage intravenous steroids should be initiated. Stool cultures should be obtained. If no prior diagnosis of CUC has been made, the patient should undergo expeditious endoscopic evaluation of the gastrointestinal tract, and of the colon in particular. An experienced endoscopist using minimal air insufflation should perform the colonic endoscopy. Many physicians are concerned about performing endoscopy during an episode of acute colitis because of the risk of perforation; however, although there are scattered reports of perforation occurring after endoscopy in this setting, this is actually quite rare. Urgent endoscopy is not meant to evaluate the entire colon but only to visualize the rectal and distal colonic mucosa. If the examination is obviously consistent with CUC, then the endoscope can be withdrawn without evaluating the remainder of the entire colon. If the patient is clinically stable, there is no indication for antibiotic therapy. However, if the patient is very ill or has a high fever or leukocytosis, appropriate broad-spectrum antibiotics should be initiated after cultures are obtained. The patient should be observed closely for 24–48 hours while on maximal medical therapy. If there is no improvement, or if their condition deteriorates, then surgery is advised. If there is evidence of peritonitis, profound hemodynamic instability or perforation the patient should be operated upon immediately.

## Toxic megacolon

Another surgical emergency in patients with ulcerative colitis, toxic megacolon is thankfully rarely seen today. This process may be the initial presentation of ulcerative colitis or may represent a flare in a patient with long-standing disease. The entire colon or an isolated segment of it (usually transverse or the left colon) is involved. Toxic megacolon is a *clinical* diagnosis. However, the strict radiographic definition of toxic megacolon is dilatation of the transverse colon greater than 5.5 cm on a supine abdominal film. The medical treatment of toxic megacolon is similar to that used for patients with fulminant colitis, namely, nothing given by mouth, nasogastric tube decompression, correction of fluid deficits and electrolyte abnormalities, high-dose steroids, and antibiotics if there is fever or elevated leukocyte count. Some physicians advocate rolling the patient from supine to a prone position every hour to prevent the accumulation of air in the transverse colon. Emergency surgery is indicated if the patient's clinical or radiographic status worsens, if there is evidence of perforation, or if there is no improvement 24–36 hours after beginning aggressive medical therapy. Delaying surgery increases the risk of perforation, which raises the mortality from less than 5% to nearly 30%.[1]

## Other surgical emergencies

Other surgical emergencies in CUC patients are perforation and severe hemorrhage. Perforation outside the setting of toxic megacolon occurs infrequently. A patient presenting with a perforation without megacolon should raise concern that the actual diagnosis could be Crohn's disease, or that there is another cause for the perforation, such as a gastric or duodenal ulcer related to steroid use. Whatever the cause, there is no role for conservative therapy and the patient should immediately undergo exploration.

Profuse hemorrhage is another indication for surgical intervention. Hemorrhage resulting in hemodynamic instability is an unusual complication. Decisions regarding intervention are made after consultation with the treating gastroenterologist. Initial treatment should be aggressive fluid and blood-product resuscitation. Any electrolyte or clotting deficiencies should be corrected. Identification of another possible source of bleeding should be aggressively sought by endoscopy. Evaluation should include both upper and lower endoscopy. Upper endoscopy should be performed to exclude a possible gastric or duodenal ulcer as the bleeding source. The timing of operation is determined by the clinical situation. If the patient is hemodynamically unstable even after effective resuscitation, then operation is indicated because medical therapy takes too long to decrease the mucosal inflammation responsible for the bleeding. If there is slow but continuing hemorrhage that does not cause hemodynamic instability or symptoms, then a trial of high-dose steroids may be instituted. If there is no improvement after 48–72 hours of medical therapy, then the patient should proceed to surgery.

## ELECTIVE SURGERY

Elective surgical intervention in CUC is prompted by intractability of symptoms and treatment of dysplasia or for suspected or known malignancies. Intractability is a clinical definition occurring in both the acute and chronic states of CUC. During an acute flare, intractability refers to the inability to control a patient's symptoms on maximal medical therapy; intractability in a patient with long-standing CUC refers to either the inability to taper steroids to a reasonable maintenance dose or the development of severe drug-related side effects. Some centers recommend the initiation of intravenous or oral cyclosporin for patients suffering from an acute flare of CUC not responding to intravenous steroid therapy. Several small series investigating cyclosporin for patients with intractable CUC reported hopeful initial results; however, more recent reports with larger numbers of patients and longer follow-up showed that nearly 50% of all patients subsequently required colectomy within 1 year.[3] Therefore, our policy is usually to treat acute flares with intravenous steroid therapy for 7–10 days. If there is no clinical improvement, then elective surgery is recommended. The type of surgical procedure performed in that specific setting depends on a number of patient-related factors, including age and overall medical condition.

The development of malignancy in the setting of CUC has been well described. The estimated risk of colon cancer in a patient with CUC has been estimated to be anywhere from 2% at 20 years after onset of CUC to 43% at 35 years.[4] Most clinicians agree that the risk for developing colon cancer is between 10 and 20% after 20 years of disease. A patient's individual risk for colon cancer is probably increased if there is evidence of high-grade dysplasia on random colon biopsies, or if there is a dysplasia-associated lesion or mass (DALM). Also, any colonic stricture, whether it appears benign on endoscopy or is significant enough to cause obstructive symptoms, should be considered to harbor a malignancy and the patient should proceed to surgery.

If there is a suspected or known malignancy, oncologic principles drive the surgical decision-making process. A colectomy is indicated if there is either high-grade dysplasia or a DALM. In most patients, except for those with low rectal cancers or metastatic disease, total colectomy with IPAA is an acceptable surgical treatment modality. The presence of low-grade dysplasia on random biopsy is a more difficult clinical situation: most clinicians recommend colectomy,[5] although some recommend increasing the frequency of surveillance colonoscopies and not surgery. There is controversy regarding the need for a mucosectomy in these patients, the aim of which is to remove all tissue at risk for dysplasia in the future. However, there have been reports of dysplasia and of adenocarcinomas arising at the pouch–anal anastomosis after either mucosectomy or stapled anastomosis.[6–9] Our recommendation is that any patient who undergoes an IPAA for CUC, regardless of how the anastomosis was performed, should have lifelong surveillance of both the pouch and the anastomosis.

# SURGICAL PROCEDURES FOR ULCERATIVE COLITIS

The choice of operation is dependent upon a number of factors that must be individualized to the patient's clinical condition. Currently, there are three operative approaches used in the treatment of ulcerative colitis. These are proctocolectomy with an end ileostomy; total colectomy with ileal pouch–anal anastomosis (IPAA); and total abdominal colectomy with ileorectal anastomosis. Ileorectal anastomosis is rarely performed, particularly because a large amount of diseased mucosa is left in situ. However, it should be considered an option in patients who refuse an ileostomy or for those who have medical conditions in which a stoma is relatively contraindicated, such as portal hypertension or ascites. In general, the operative approach used is dictated by the presentation of the disease requiring either emergency or elective operation. Table 40.2 illustrates the process of choosing an operation depending upon the clinical situation. For those patients who require emergency surgery or are in poor medical condition because of their underlying disease, a three-stage procedure is performed. Stage I is total abdominal colectomy with a Hartman pouch and an end ileostomy. This allows the majority of diseased colon to be removed, thus improving the patient's clinical condition while they are being tapered off of any immunosuppressive medications. Once the patient is recovered and clinically ready for another operation, again depending upon their condition, stage II entails either a completion proctectomy with end ileostomy or an IPAA with diverting loop ileostomy. In the latter situation the patient will have to undergo a third stage to reverse the ileostomy. The reason for not performing a proctectomy in an emergency is that by leaving the rectum in place, a restorative operation can be performed in the future without having disturbed the dissection planes in the pelvis. In addition, an emergency proctectomy is associated with a higher risk of bleeding and injury to the nerves of the pelvic floor, bladder and genitalia. Usually the small amount of diseased tissue left behind does not present a clinical problem. In the non-emergency setting the procedure of choice in appropriate patients is the ileal pouch–anal anastomosis with a diverting loop ileostomy.

## Table 40.2 Choice of operations for patients with ulcerative colitis

| Patient presentation | Preferred procedures |
| --- | --- |
| Fulminant ulcerative colitis, toxic megacolon, acute intractable colitis, perforation, massive hemorrhage | Total abdominal colectomy with Hartman pouch or venting mucous fistula. Subsequent surgery depending upon clinical condition and circumstance. |
| CUC in non-emergency circumstances | a) Total proctocolectomy with ileal pouch– anal anastomosis and diverting loop ileostomy for patients under 65 years of age in good health and continent<br>b) Total proctocolectomy with end ileostomy in older patients or patients with poor continence |
| CUC with malignancy | Same as above, but oncologic considerations dictate the operation selected. For rectal cancers, mucosectomy is recommended |

Reprinted with permission from: Cima RR, Pemberton JH. Surgical management of inflammatory bowel disease. Curr Treatment Options Gastroenterol 2001;4:215–225.

# ILEAL POUCH–ANAL ANASTOMOSIS

Ileal pouch–anal anastomosis (IPAA) is considered the standard elective surgical therapy for the treatment of chronic ulcerative colitis. Parks and Nichols first described the procedure in 1978.[10,11] The decision to proceed with operations other than IPAA is based upon individual patient circumstances or pre-existing medical or physiologic conditions that are a contraindication for this type of restorative procedure. IPAA is the ideal operation for the treatment of CUC because it removes the entire diseased organ while simultaneously preserving the normal anatomic route for defecation. Construction of the ileal pouch is the key to the success of this operation, as it provides an adequate fecal reservoir to allow voluntary defecation, albeit at a higher (but manageable) daily frequency than in patients with a normal rectum.

Since the introduction of IPAA in the early 1980s, the surgical technique used at the Mayo Clinic has been refined. The procedure continues to evolve with the application of new technologies such as laparoscopic surgery. Whereas every surgeon and institution that performs IPAA has a different technique or preference, the operation basically involves four phases: removal of the intra-abdominal colon; dissection and removal of the rectum, sparing the pelvic nerves and the anal sphincter mechanism; construction of an ileal reservoir; and anastomosis of the ileal reservoir to the anal canal. The general techniques used at the Mayo Clinic are described here. The anesthetized patient, who will have undergone a complete bowel preparation, including oral antibiotics, the night before, is positioned in a modified lithotomy position. During different phases of the operation the patient will need to be placed in Trendelenburg to facilitate the rectal dissection. This positioning allows easy access to the abdomen and perineum for a single surgical team, or for a second team to operate simultaneously.

The abdomen is entered through a midline vertical incision and is thoroughly explored to determine whether there are any technical or pathologic contraindications to proceeding with the total colectomy and IPAA. Starting with the cecum, the entire colon is mobilized from its retroperitoneal attachments. The transverse colon is freed from the greater omentum, which is preserved if it is of good quality and quantity. Once the intra-abdominal colon has been mobilized, the terminal ileum is divided from the right colon adjacent to the ileocecal junction using a linear stapling device. The mesentery is divided as close to the right colon as possible to avoid injuring the ileocolic vessels supplying the terminal ileum. Once the right colon has been mobilized, the remainder of the colon is divided from its mesentery in a routine fashion. When the intra-abdominal colon has been fully mobilized and the mesentery divided, the patient is placed in steep Trendelenburg to facilitate the pelvic dissection of the rectum, which is freed down to the pelvic floor. The mesorectum is mobilized from the presacral fascia in the avascular plane. Great care is taken to avoid the pelvic nerves that lie in the interface between the mesorectum and the presacral fascia. Although the posterior dissection is similar to that of a dissection for a rectal cancer, the lateral dissection of the rectum should be performed closer to the rectum to preserve the small terminal nerve branches that innervate the pelvic floor and urinary bladder. The rectum is divided at the pelvic floor with a stapling device. The entire colon and rectum is then sent for pathologic evaluation.

After the colon has been removed, the ileal pouch is constructed. The small bowel mesentery is completely mobilized from the retroperitoneum up to the inferior border of the pancreas. It is important to perform this mobilization completely to ensure adequate length for the ileal pouch to reach the pelvic floor. Also to increase the length, the visceral peritoneum should be scored along the right side of the superior mesenteric vessel. Once the mesentery has been mobilized, the pouch is fashioned. It has become our practice to use a J-shaped reservoir constructed from the last 30–35 cm of the terminal ileum (Fig. 40.1). This is simpler to construct, uses less intestinal length, and is associated with fewer complications related to pouch emptying problems than the W- and S-shaped pouches. Also, there is no difference in clinical reservoir capacity or function as measured by bowel movement frequency among the pouch designs. To ultimately achieve a reservoir capacity of approximately 400 mL, the pouch is constructed by folding the terminal ileum into a J shape. The hook of the J should be approximately 15 cm in length (Fig.40.1). This efferent limb of the J is then loosely secured to the afferent limb of the small bowel. Prior to forming the reservoir, adequate length of small bowel has to be determined. To ensure that the pouch will reach the pelvic floor and the region of the anastomosis without tension, the apex of the pouch should be able to be pulled 3–5 cm below the upper aspect of the pubic symphysis. If after full mesenteric mobilization and scoring of the visceral peritoneum the pouch does not easily reach the pelvic floor, it may be necessary to divide either the ileocolic vessel or one of the

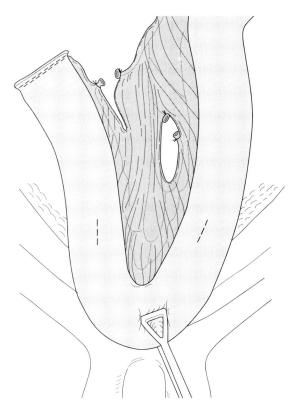

Fig. 40.1 Two 15-cm limbs of terminal ileum are used to construct the J pouch. The apex is approximately 15 cm from the cut end of the terminal ileum. Note that the ileocolic vessels have been taken and a mesenteric window created.

proximal branches of the superior mesenteric artery. When there is a concern that the J-shaped reservoir will not reach the pelvic floor satisfactorily, one may alternatively construct an S- or W-shaped pouch. If the J pouch will reach the pelvic floor, the reservoir is constructed by two firings of the 75-mm linear cutting stapling device from the apex of the pouch dividing the common wall between the two limbs of the J pouch. Prior to bringing the pouch down to the anus it is important to verify that the small intestine from the ligament of Treitz to the ileal pouch is not twisted. At this point in the operation, one of two options is available to perform the anastomosis. The pouch may be secured to the anal canal by performing a double-stapled technique in which the head of the EEA stapling device is secured in the apex of the pouch with a pursestring suture (Fig. 40.2). The stapling device is then placed into the anus and the attachment pin is placed through the staple line where the rectum was divided at the level of the pelvic floor. The pouch is then brought down into the pelvis, maintaining the proper orientation, and the stapled anastomosis is performed.

The other option is to perform a mucosectomy of the anal canal and lower rectal remnant. To perform the mucosectomy, the dentate line area is exposed using two Gelpi retractors placed at right-angles to one another. A dilute solution of epinephrine is then injected into the submucosa to facilitate circumferential excision of the anal canal mucosa, leaving the muscularis propria intact. The excision is carried proximal to the level of the stapled rectum. Once the staple line is reached, the full thickness of the rectal wall is divided, allowing removal of the intact lower rectal remnant and the anal canal mucosa. A

long Babcock clamp is placed into the pelvis through the anal opening and the pouch apex is brought down to the level of the dentate line. A side-to-end handsewn anastomosis between the apex of the pouch and the dentate line is performed with absorbable sutures (Fig. 40.3) The choice of anastomotic technique depends on the clinical situation and surgeon preference and will be discussed later. However, if the procedure is being performed with a known cancer or high-grade dysplasia in the rectum our preference is to do a mucosectomy to remove as much of the diseased mucosa as possible.

Once the anastomosis is complete, one or two closed suction drains are placed behind the pouch and brought out of separate left abdominal stab-wounds. In the majority of patients we construct a loop ileostomy in the right lower abdomen. The need for an ileostomy will be discussed later. The wound is then closed in the standard fashion. The patient is resumed on a diet when there is evidence of bowel function through the ileostomy. The drains are removed when the patient is ready to leave. Approximately 2–3 months after the original operation, the patient has a proctoscopic evaluation of the pouch and a barium study through the anus to detect a pouch leak. If the reservoir and the anastomosis have healed completely then the loop ileostomy can be reversed during a second operation. Often, the ileostomy can be closed by mobilizing it through a small transverse biconvex incision around the stoma. The loop of ileum is then fully mobilized and an end-to-end or a side-to-side functional end-to-end anastomosis can be performed without re-entering the abdomen through the previous midline incision.

## OPERATIVE CONTROVERSIES

As discussed above, how the ileal pouch–anal anastomosis is constructed is usually left to the operating surgeon's preference.

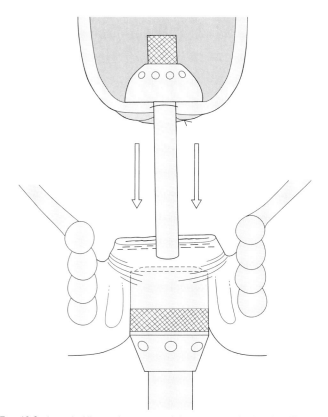

**Fig. 40.2** A stapled ileoanal anastomosis is constructed using the EEA stapler. The TA-30 stapler has been used to staple across the anal canal *below* the anorectal ring. At the termination of the ileoanal stapling procedure, the distance between the dentate line and the staple line should be less than 1 cm.

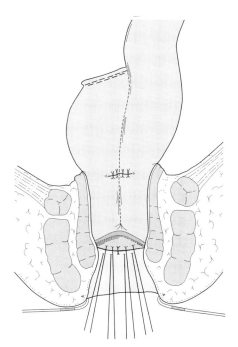

**Fig. 40.3** The apex of the J pouch has been pulled through an almost non-existent rectal cuff. The mucosa of the anal canal (the anal transition zone) has been removed. The anastomosis is made by suturing the full thickness of the pouch to the internal anal sphincter.

The relative value of performing a mucosectomy or a double-stapled anastomosis continues to be debated. The purpose of the mucosectomy is to remove all of the diseased or at-risk mucosa. However, even after a complete mucosectomy the risk that residual tissue might undergo malignant transformation is not entirely eliminated, as there have been reported cases of adenocarcinomas occurring at the anastomosis or in the transition zone.[7,8] The fate of the anal canal mucosa after mucosectomy has been evaluated. In the Mayo Clinic experience, anal canal specimens obtained from patients who had to have their pouches removed within 4 years of their IPAA underwent histologic evaluation.[12,13] Even with complete mucosectomy, small islands of rectal mucosa could be found buried in the fibrous tissue between the rectal muscularis and the serosa of the ileal pouch. However, none of the specimens revealed any evidence of rectal mucosa regeneration or dysplasia. Whether this relatively short follow-up is long enough to determine that these small islands of rectal mucosa represent benign findings is unclear. Those surgeons who advocate a double-stapled pouch–anal anastomosis at the level of the pelvic floor believe that the remaining 1.5–2.0 cm of anal mucosa proximal to the dentate line improves the functional result by improving anal canal sensation. In a randomized prospective trial performed at the Mayo Clinic in 41 patients with CUC, there was no significant difference in functional outcomes as measured by stool frequency or episodes of fecal incontinence at 6 months after ileostomy closure.[14] However, there was a higher resting sphincter pressure as measured by manometry and a trend toward less nocturnal incontinence in those patients who had a double-stapled anastomosis. Follow-up needs to be performed to see if there is a difference in function after a longer period. In a small subset of patients recently reported by the University of Minnesota after 12 years of follow-up, the investigators were unable to state conclusively that there was a significant change in function between the two groups.[15]

Although IPAA has become the surgical treatment of choice for chronic ulcerative colitis, occasionally it is not feasible because of technical or intraoperative findings. At the Mayo Clinic from 1981 to 1995 IPAA was attempted in 1789 patients with CUC and FAP.[16] Intraoperative abandonment occurred in 74 out of 1789 patients for an overall rate of 4.1%. The most common reason for abandonment was technical factors: either inability to make the pouch reach the anus without tension, or pouch ischemia after lengthening maneuvers. The technical abandonment group was older and more likely to be male. Mesenteric obesity was specifically noted in 44% of patients in the abandonment group. The second most common reason for abandoning an IPAA was the intraoperative diagnosis of Crohn's disease. In this series, 27 patients out of 1581 thought to have CUC were found to have Crohn's disease on intraoperative pathologic evaluation. The majority of patients who had their IPAA abandoned underwent proctocolectomy and ileostomy. The remainder had sphincter-preserving procedures. During the preoperative discussion it is important to inform patients that there is a small but definable risk of operative abandonment and permanent ileostomy, especially in older men or obese patients.

## COMPLICATIONS AFTER IPAA

Total proctocolectomy with ileal pouch–anal anastomosis is a technically demanding procedure. The patient commonly has to endure two and sometimes three operations. There are a number of short- and long-term complications associated with the IPAA procedure that can influence the function of the pouch and which could eventually result in loss of the pouch. A number of centers have reported upon these complications.[17–21] The most commonly encountered short-term complications are small bowel obstruction, anastomotic stricture, pouch leak and pelvic abscess. Long-term complications include small bowel obstruction, pouch fistulae and pouchitis. Chronic pouch dysfunction, fistulae and chronic pouchitis contribute to pouch failure that may require revision or excision.

The most common short-term complication after IPAA is small bowel obstruction. The incidence of perioperative small bowel obstruction in the Mayo Clinic series of 1310 patients was 15%.[17] In the 195 patients who developed a small bowel obstruction during the perioperative period 47 (24%) required laparotomy to relieve the obstruction. Other groups have reported a similar incidence of postoperative small bowel obstruction, although the reoperative rates tended to be lower.[20,23] Anastomotic stricture is another common complication after IPAA. In our experience, of the 114 patients that required reoperative treatment for pouch-related complications 42 (37%) had symptomatic anastomotic strictures.[24] Initially, these strictures were treated by dilatation under anesthesia. However, more than 50% of patients had recurrent strictures that had to be treated one or more times.

The pouch leak and associated pelvic sepsis rates in large series have been reported as ranging from 5 to 14%.[17,25–27] In our experience, sepsis occurred in 74 patients out of 1310 (6%), of whom 73 had pelvic sepsis as the result of the pouch procedure.[17] The majority of these patients (63%) required operative intervention, whereas the remainder were treated with either antibiotics or a combination of antibiotics and CT-guided drainage. It should be noted that in this large series spanning a 13-year period the rate of pelvic sepsis and leak declined as experience with the procedure increased. During the first 4 years of the study the pelvic sepsis rate was 7%, but by the last 4 years it had fallen to 3%.

## LATE COMPLICATIONS AND POUCH FAILURE

The late complications associated with IPAA include small bowel obstruction (SBO), fistula and pouchitis. MacLean and colleagues' review of the literature on the incidence of late small bowel resection after IPAA revealed a reported incidence of 12–35% with varying lengths of follow-up from many studies.[20] In their institution's evaluation of late small bowel obstructions in 1178 patients after IPAA, there was a 1-year SBO rate of 18%. The cumulative risk increased to 27% at 5 years and 31% at 10 years. The majority of patients responded to conservative management, but the rate of operative treatment increased from 2.7% at 1 year to 7.5% at 10 years. Operative findings in those patients who required exploration for relief of the SBO were most commonly pelvic adhesions (32%), followed by adhesions to the ileostomy closure site (20%). In the multivariate analysis for late small bowel obstructions, performance of a diverting ileostomy and pouch reconstruction both led to a higher risk of a bowel obstruction.

## FISTULA

Fistulae after IPAA are difficult postoperative complications to treat. Pouch–vaginal fistulae and, rarely, pouch–perineal fistulae can occur either in the perioperative period or years later. Early pouch fistulae are most likely the result of a technical error or the complication of a pouch leak or pelvic abscess. The occurrence of late fistulae is worrying in Crohn's disease. Most fistulae are low and originate at the level of the anastomosis. They have been reported with equal frequency in both handsewn and double-stapled anastomosis. The reported incidence of pouch–vaginal fistulae ranges from 4 to 12%.[23,28–32] If the fistula occurs prior to closure of a protecting ileostomy, then closure should be delayed. In addition, prior to any surgery, an examination under anesthesia and biopsies should be performed to rule out the presence of Crohn's disease. Principles of management include local control of any septic process and repair of the fistula by the interposition of healthy tissue between the pouch and the vagina or perineal opening. Many authors have reported transanal, transvaginal, transperineal and transabdominal approaches to pouch–vaginal fistulae, with rates of successful closure ranging from 10 to 78%.[28,29,31–33] However, simple interventions, such as the use of seton fistulotomy, can be used to successfully manage pouch–perineal or pouch–vaginal fistulae.[28] The most important considerations in managing a post-pouch fistula are to rule out Crohn's disease and to initiate treatment by a surgeon experienced in treating these complications. In cases where the fistula cannot be closed and the patient is symptomatic, pouch excision and end ileostomy may be the only recourse.

## POUCHITIS

Pouchitis is a late complication of the IPAA for which there is no clear etiology. It is an acute inflammatory process of the pouch which in a minority of patients can become chronic. Chronic pouchitis may eventually lead to pouch failure requiring pouch excision, which is fortunately quite rare. It occurs very rarely, if at all, in those patients who had an IPAA procedure for FAP, and may thus represent an element of immune dysfunction in ulcerative colitis patients. Supporting this is the finding that pouchitis occurs more frequently in ulcerative colitis patients who have extraintestinal manifestations than in those without them.[34] Measuring the exact incidence of pouchitis is difficult because of varying presentations and different diagnostic criteria. Most series report an incidence between 12 and 50%.[15,17,22, 35–38] In the Mayo Clinic series the cumulative risk of suffering at least one episode was 18% at 1 year and 48% at 10 years. We fully recognize the probability that the incidence of pouchitis in our series was overestimated, because diagnoses are most often on clinical grounds alone.[17,22] In those patients who had an episode of pouchitis, the probability of suffering a second episode was 64%. Age, sex, anastomotic technique, the use of a diverting ileostomy or postoperative sepsis did not influence the risk of developing pouchitis. Pouchitis should be suspected in any patient who experiences abdominal cramps, increased stool frequency, watery or bloody diarrhea and flu-like symptoms. Although many patients are treated on clinical grounds alone, accurate diagnosis requires endoscopic visualization of the pouch and histologic evaluation. The combination of clinical symptoms, degree of endoscopic inflammation and acute histologic inflammation has been used to develop a severity index that can be used to measure effectiveness of different treatment protocols.[39]

Although the exact cause of pouchitis is unclear, the successful use of antibiotics, particularly metronidazole, in the treatment of acute and chronic pouchitis lends support to a theory that an interaction between pouch bacteria levels and the mucosal immune system is important. The pouch stasis–bacterial overgrowth theory as a cause of pouchitis is unlikely to be correct because FAP patients with pouches very rarely have episodes of pouchitis. After the diagnosis of pouchitis is made, most patients respond to a short course of antibiotics, the main one used being metronidazole over a 7–10-day course. If the patient is intolerant to metronidazole, then other broad-spectrum antibiotics such as ciprofloxacin, augmentin, erythromycin or tetracycline may be used. Other agents that may be used include those medications used to treat the colitis originally, including steroids, both oral and enema formulations, and oral immunosuppressive agents. Less than 8% of patients who have an IPAA will go on to develop chronic pouchitis, and about half will require pouch excision.[22,34]

## POUCH FAILURE

In nearly all series of patients who have undergone an IPAA the majority report either good or excellent functional results.[17,18,21,22,35–37] However, early technical complications or later severe pouch dysfunction due to either Crohn's disease, dysfunction or chronic pouchitis may lead to failure rates reportedly ranging from 1% to approximately 20%.[17–19,21] Pouch failure may be treated with either a proximal diverting ileostomy, pouch excision and end ileostomy, or pouch revision. In the Mayo Clinic's experience with 1310 pelvic pouches, 134 patients (10%) were considered to have pouch failure.[17] Eighty-four pouches had to be excised and 50 had formation of defunctioning ileostomies. Pouch ischemia was the most common cause of perioperative pouch excision. The most common cause of pouch failure within the first 2 years ($n=40$) after IPAA was chronic sepsis, manifest as recurrent pelvic abscess with or without fistulae. The next most common cause was poor functional outcome ($n=20$), as noted by increased stool frequency with incontinence and perineal irritation. Korsgen and Keighley[19] reported similar findings in their review of pouch failures in 180 IPAA patients. The overall pouch failure rate was 17.2%, with twice as many failures in those patients who had pouches for inflammatory bowel disease compared to those performed for FAP. There was a significant association between pouch failure and a history of pelvic sepsis. Multiple regression analysis showed pelvic sepsis and recurrent pouchitis to be independent factors of pouch failure.

A few centers with a large experience in pouch surgery have reported good results in 'salvage' surgery for pouch dysfunction due to mechanical causes or from prior episodes of pelvic sepsis.[24,38,40,41] A number of different techniques may be used to address pouch complications. Pouch-related complications can be divided into four groups: anastomotic strictures; perianal abscess or fistula; intra-abdominal fistula or abscess; or functional pouch problems. In the Mayo Clinic experience the most common complication that required reoperation was anastomotic stricture, which is often treated with dilatation under anesthesia.[24] However, 52% of these patients had recurrent strictures that required intervention, with 14% eventually requiring pouch excision. In those patients who had poor pouch function and required reconstruction, postreconstruction functional results were reported as satisfactory in 60%. Overall, in all patients who required some type of reoperation for pouch-related complications, 70% reported good to excellent clinical outcomes. However, pouch excision with permanent ileostomy was required in 20% of cases.

## ILEAL POUCH–ANAL ANASTOMOSIS WITHOUT ILEAL DIVERSION

To address the concerns about complications associated with staged procedures, some institutions have investigated performing proctocolectomy and IPAA without a temporary ileostomy. The majority of large series have included a 'protecting' ileostomy to divert the fecal stream from the pouch while the pouch staple line and anastomosis heal.[22,23,38,43] The idea is that the rate of pelvic sepsis decreases, which will avoid the long-term detrimental functional consequences of a leak from an unprotected pouch. On the other hand, supporters of a one-stage procedure believe that an IPAA can be performed without an increased risk of pelvic sepsis.[36,37,44–47] Also, a one-stage procedure avoids an ileostomy and a second hospitalization and operation, lowers the total cost, and results in a shorter hospital stay and perhaps a decreased incidence of small bowel obstruction. In the large single-institution study reported by Sugerman et al. 201 patients underwent a stapled IPAA in which 196 were done without a diverting ileostomy.[36] In the one-stage group, 178 were patients with CUC and 81% of these were on prednisone at the time of surgery. In this series, 23 (12%) patients developed anastomotic leaks but only nine required a return to the operating room for diverting ileostomies. There was no increase in anastomotic leak in those patients on steroids. The long-term functional results and late complications were also evaluated, and no differences were found between those that did and those that did not have leaks. Cohen and colleagues reported their experience in performing IPAA procedures without a diverting ileostomy with similar findings, except for a leak rate for patients on steroids, but the majority were treated conservatively and had no long-term functional problems.[25] In the only randomized controlled trial addressing this issue, 45 patients were randomized at the end of the IPAA to having either a one- or a two-stage procedure.[48] The decision to enroll the patient into the study was based upon the operating surgeon's intraoperative opinion that the conduct of the procedure was uneventful and that all anastomoses were intact. A total of 59 patients were eligible for the study, but only 45 were randomized to loop ileostomy ($n=23$) or no ileostomy ($n=22$). The majority of the patients were being operated on for chronic ulcerative colitis. Postoperatively, there were two anastomotic leaks, one in each group. Short-term analysis of pouch function did not show any difference between the two groups once the loop ileostomies were closed. Although some authors believe that a one-stage operation may be performed with comparable complication rates, one study suggested that the severity of complications was greater in those patients without a protecting ileostomy.[49] In 100 consecutive IPAA procedures, patients either had a one-stage or a two stage procedure. The decision as to which to perform was left up to the operating surgeon at the completion of the IPAA. Factors that influenced the decision were urgent operation, a technically imperfect anastomosis, a malnourished patient, or a patient on high-dose prednisone. Whereas the incidence of morbidity was similar in both groups of patients, life-threatening complications were much more common in the patients who underwent a one-stage procedure. Pelvic sepsis developed in seven of the patients with an ileostomy and in 11 patients without. However, the seven patients with an ileostomy were all successfully treated with intravenous antibiotics. In contrast, seven of the 11 patients without an ileostomy required operative drainage and the creation of a diverting ileostomy. It is clear that as experience with this technically demanding operation has increased the rate of complications has declined. In properly selected patients who have uncomplicated procedures performed by experienced surgeons a one-stage IPAA might be appropriate. However, the surgeon and patient care team must be vigilant for the early signs of pelvic sepsis, aggressively investigating the possibility of a pouch or an anastomotic leak and intervening as needed.

## ELDERLY PATIENTS AND IPAA

The majority of patients suffering from chronic ulcerative colitis are younger, and unless there are unusual circumstances they should be offered proctocolectomy and IPAA. However, CUC is known to have a bimodal age distribution and older patients are being referred for surgical evaluation. Whereas many institutions have reported their long-term results with IPAA, few have regularly performed IPAA in elderly patients. In the Mayo Clinic survey of 1386 patient who underwent IPAA the median age at time of operation was 32, with a range from 5 to 65 years.[22] Only 16% were over 45 years of age, and none was older than 65. The functional outcomes as noted by nocturnal stool frequency, daytime and nocturnal incontinence, and need for constipating medications were all significantly higher in patients who were over 45 at the time of the IPAA. These relatively poorer functional results have led us to not routinely recommend IPAA in older patients (age >65). However, Tan and colleagues have evaluated their experience with IPAA patients from the age of 50 to more than 70 years.[50] Twenty-eight of 227 patients were older than 50 when the IPAA was performed; of those 28, 10 were between 60 and 70 years old and five were between the ages of 70 and 80. In the over-50 age group, 86% of the patients were taken to surgery because of medically refractory illness or complications related to CUC. The incidence of perioperative complications and the long-term functional results were analyzed. When the elderly patients operated on for chronic ulcerative colitis were compared to younger patients with CUC, there were no significant differences between the groups for the major complications of pelvic sepsis, pouch related fistula or anastomotic leak. Pouch–anal stenosis was, however, significantly more common in the older patient group. In regard to functional outcome, including frequency of daytime and nighttime bowel movements, use of pads, and incontinence episodes, there were no significant differences. However, patients over 70 tended to have slightly higher bowel movement frequencies. Interestingly, the incidence of pouchitis and chronic pouchitis was less in the elderly group with CUC than in the younger patients, although this difference was not significantly different. Overall, advanced age is not an absolute contraindication to IPAA. The data would seem to suggest that healthy older patients with good sphincter tone might have functional results similar to those of younger patients.

# SEXUALITY, FERTILITY AND PREGNANCY AFTER SURGERY FOR ULCERATIVE COLITIS

Many men and women are first diagnosed or surgically treated for their CUC during their peak years of sexual activity and reproduction. The issue of sexual activity has been reported in a few studies of such patients.[22,51,52] In our series, 16% of patients reported complete abstinence and 20% had reduced sexual activity prior to surgery.[22] After IPAA, 25% reported an improvement in the quality of their sexual life, 56% had no change, and 16% reported that their sexual activity was mildly restricted. At 10-year follow-up, retrograde or no ejaculation was reported in 3% of men and 8% of women reported dyspareunia. Earlier studies have suggested that fertility is not affected in women with ulcerative colitis.[53,54] In female patients with inactive or medically controlled CUC there is no increased risk of pregnancy-related complications. However, there is an increase risk of fetal death in patients with CUC-related complications that require surgical intervention during pregnancy.[55]

The impact of surgery for ulcerative colitis on fertility and the course of a subsequent pregnancy has been evaluated by a number of investigators.[22,51,55–58] Patients who have had a proctocolectomy and end ileostomy or Kock pouch can expect to have a normal pregnancy and delivery. The decision as to type of delivery, either vaginal or cesarean section, should be based on obstetric issues. Although these women may have uneventful pregnancies and deliveries, they often may have stoma or Kock pouch dysfunction. Gopal et al. surveyed 66 female ostomates who had 82 pregnancies:[56] 29% reported stoma dysfunction during their pregnancies, including difficulty with appliance leakage, stomal obstruction, bowel obstruction and stomal prolapse.

Fertility and pregnancy in women who have had IPAA has been evaluated in a few studies.[22,51,58] In the Mayo Clinic series of 546 women evaluated after their IPAA, 85 had a pregnancy and vaginal delivery.[22] The women tended to be significantly younger than those who did not have any pregnancies. Whereas older studies looked at the course of pregnancies and complications that arose after IPAA, the specific issue of fertility after IPAA has not been thoroughly investigated. In a recent analysis of the rate of pregnancy after IPAA, there was shown to be a significant reduction in postoperative fertility.[57] Two hundred and fifty-eight Swedish women with ulcerative colitis were followed. The birth rate in this cohort was compared to the expected pregnancy and birth rate for age-matched women in Sweden. There was a no difference in the expected birth rate in women during the period from the onset of ulcerative colitis to the time of colectomy:120 births versus an expected 131. However, there was a significant reduction in births after IPAA: 34 versus 69 expected ($P<0.001$). More importantly, of the post-IPAA patients who became pregnant, 29% occurred after in vitro fertilization compared to the expected 1% of all births in Sweden during the study period. The basis of this decreased fertility is unknown, but the authors believe that anatomical changes in the pelvis may be a contributor to the problem. Until further studies are done to confirm and clarify these findings, women considering undergoing IPAA should be informed of the possibility of decreased fertility.

Once a woman who has had an IPAA is pregnant, there appears to be no increased risk to the pregnancy or with complications after delivery.[58,59] In the Mayo Clinic series of 43 woman who became pregnant after IPAA, there was a slight increase in stool frequency, incontinence and pad usage during the pregnancy.[58,60] However, all the patients returned to their baseline pouch function after delivery. There was a higher rate of cesarean sections in post-IPAA patients compared to other studies that reported on modes of fetal delivery in patients with Kock pouches and end ostomies. However, it is unclear whether this increase was due to uncertainty about how these patients would fare after vaginal deliveries, because less than 50% of these cesarean sections were performed for obstetric indications. Overall, there appeared to be no contraindication to vaginal delivery, although the authors suggest that women who have a scarred, stiff perineum might avoid vaginal delivery.

# IPAA AND CANCER

IPAA has become the surgical treatment of choice for both CUC and FAP. Both of these diseases have an associated risk of cancer developing while the colon remains in situ. Between 1 and 9% of patients who present for IPAA will have a colorectal cancer at the time of surgery.[61–64] If an IPAA can be performed without compromising oncologic results, then there are few reasons to deny the patient the benefits of this operation. There are concerns, however, about performing an IPAA in this situation. One is that the presence of the pouch may compromise adjuvant chemoradiation therapy, because the function of the pouch may deteriorate or be permanently compromised by the adjuvant treatments. The Mayo Clinic has reported on the use of IPAA in both FAP and CUC patients who had a concomitant malignancy.[64] In the 1616 patient who had undergone an IPAA for either CUC or FAP, 77 (4.8%) had an adenocarcinoma of the colon, rectum or both at the time of surgery. The majority of patients had either stage I or stage II disease, but 29% had stage III disease. In those patients who required adjuvant therapy, 15% required dose reduction or interruption of therapy because of complications related to the chemotherapy. Evaluation of the functional results was made separately for CUC and FAP patients. In those patients with cancer, compared to their respective cohort of patients without cancer, there were no significant differences in postoperative complications or functional outcomes. However, there was an overall higher pouch failure rate requiring reoperation than in the patients without cancer – 16% and 7%, respectively. Oncologically, results for IPAA patients are similar to those reported for non-IPAA patients. The overall long-term survival was 84%. For patients with stages II and III disease, the overall recurrence rate for IPAA patients, 32%, was similar to that for non-IPAA patients. In general, if oncologic principles are not compromised then an IPAA can be performed without deleterious impact on oncologic outcome or long-term IPAA function.

# FUNCTIONAL RESULTS OF IPAA

Even though a large number of different surgeons and institutions have reported their experience with IPAA, the functional results are surprisingly and gratifyingly quite similar.[15,17,18,21–23,25,36–38,43]

The majority of patients report good to excellent function with their ileal pouch. The markers of function that are most often recorded are the number of bowel movements during the day and the night, episodes of soiling, episodes of incontinence, and use of medications to control bowel activity. In the Mayo Clinic series the average number of daytime bowel movements at the time of discharge after closure of the ileostomy was six, and the average number of nocturnal bowel movements was 1.[17,22] During the day, 79% of patients reported complete continence, 19% had occasional incontinence and 2% had frequent incontinence episodes. During the night, 59% had no incontinence episodes and 49% report occasional nocturnal incontinence. Nearly 50% of patients were discharged home on some type of medication to slow their bowels or to provide dietary bulk. After a mean follow-up of 6.5 years, the number of daily bowel movements had declined to five per day and the number of nocturnal bowel movements remained at one. In those patients who had had their ileal pouch for more than 10 years, stool frequency and continence were remarkably stable over time. On average, the number of daytime and nighttime bowel movements was unchanged. Episodes of incontinence had increased slightly in all patients. Among 300 patients followed for more than 10 years the percentage reporting complete continence decreased from 80% at 1 year to 73% at 10 years. The only significant change that occurred over time was in those patients who initially reported frequent nocturnal incontinence. In that group the incidence went from 2% at 1 year to 8% at 10 years. In a similar study of the long-term functional results after IPAA, the University of Minnesota reported on 154 patients followed for a median of 12 years (range 8–19 years).[15] They reported no change in the frequency of bowel movements either during the day or during the night. However, they did find a significant increase in the incidence of major and minor daytime and nocturnal incontinence. This change was greatest in the patients who had had their pouch for more than 12 years. The authors reported that even with the significant decline in functional results seen in nearly a quarter of their patients, the majority reported a high degree of satisfaction with their ileal pouch. This level of satisfaction with the IPAA procedure and the functional results over time is similar to that reported by other authors.[65,66]

IPAA has become the procedure of choice for the majority of patients with ulcerative colitis because it removes the diseased colon, markedly reduces the risk of cancer, and maintains anal defecation. As previously discussed, most patients report a high degree of satisfaction with the functional result. Fazio and colleagues have shown that the quality of life after IPAA is comparable to the norms for the general healthy United States population.[67] However, it is unclear whether this complex procedure results in an improved quality of life because the diseased bowel was removed, or because they could control their stools. The literature on this subject is mixed. Some authors report that quality of life measures after an IPAA are better than after an end or continent ileostomy.[68–70] However, other authors have shown that quality of life improves no matter what procedure is performed, and is probably due to eradication of the disease.[71–73] Although it is generally accepted that avoiding an abdominal stoma will improve quality of life by maintaining body image, it is unclear if the relative change in bowel emptying with a pouch causes enhanced quality of life relative to a stoma. A recent study by O'Bichere and colleagues using specific and generic quality of life questionnaires, and a survey instrument which estimated the monetary value for continuing disability, found that patients with an IPAA had much better body image than those with a Brooke or Kock ileostomy.[74] However, patients were awarded equal amounts of compensation for the relative disability resulting from the different operations. Surprisingly, on ranking the impact of altered bowel emptying on quality of life and disability, the patients with pelvic pouches were found to rank altered bowel emptying as a significantly worse area than those patients with stomas. This finding was even demonstrated in patients who evaluated their quality of life before and after their diverting stomas were reversed as part of their IPAA procedure. The authors suggested that existing quality of life measurement tools may not completely address all of the important parameters influenced by these procedures. Ideally, further technical or medical approaches that might improve bowel habits after IPAA may further increase the already high patient satisfaction with the procedure.

## LAPAROSCOPIC SURGERY FOR ULCERATIVE COLITIS

Although patient satisfaction with the IPAA procedure is high, the application of newer technologies, such as laparoscopic surgery, might reduce the morbidity of the procedure. This might then lead to earlier acceptance of surgery, faster resumption of normal activity, and possibly decreased costs. Of course, laparoscopic approaches would have to demonstrate similar functional results. Other potential advantages of laparoscopic surgery are decreased surgical stress in immunocompromised patients and decreased adhesion formation, making future operations easier. Laparoscopy also improves the cosmetic outcome and patients' perceptions of their illness and quality of life. As surgeons have become more comfortable with laparoscopic colon surgery, and as the instrumentation has improved, there are an increasing number of institutions reporting their results with laparoscopic IPAA.[75–77] Laparoscopic total colectomy and IPAA have evolved over time. Initially the procedure was performed using multiple ports and a Pfannenstiel incision. Currently, the technique developed at Mayo uses four incisions: two 5-mm port sites, a stoma site, and a 4-cm periumbilical incision.[78] In the case-matched series reported by Dunker and colleagues, a laparoscopic-assisted IPAA resulted in similar functional results and quality of life outcome measurements.[75] The only significant difference between the laparoscopic-assisted and conventional IPAA was improved cosmetic outcome. Continued refinement in the techniques and prospective evaluation are needed to better define the possible benefits of laparoscopic IPAA.

## CONCLUSIONS

Ulcerative colitis is an inflammatory disease of unknown etiology that is limited to the colonic mucosa. Surgical removal of the colon and rectum results in cure of the intestinal manifestations of the disease. The timing of surgical intervention needs to be closely coordinated between the surgeon and the gastroenterologist to ensure that the diagnosis is correct and that appropriate medical therapy has been used. Two commonly used definitive surgical procedures for chronic ulcerative colitis are total proctocolectomy with end ileostomy, and proctocolectomy with ileal pouch–anal anastomosis (IPAA). Patient characteristics and overall medical condition determine which procedure is selected. IPAA has become the procedure of choice in the majority of patients requiring colectomy because it cures the disease, avoids a permanent abdominal wall stoma and maintains the normal route of defecation. IPAA is a technically demanding operation that has a relatively high rate of morbidity even in experienced hands. However, the majority of patients report a high degree of satisfaction with the functional results, which appear to be stable over time, as is the level of patient satisfaction. The application of newer techniques such as laparoscopic surgery might further improve patient satisfaction and decrease morbidity.

# REFERENCES

1. Becker JM. Surgical therapy for ulcerative colitis and Crohn's disease. Gastroenterol Clin North Am 1999;28:371–390.
2. Truelove SC, Witts LF. Cortisone in ulcerative colitis: final report on a therapeutic trial. Br Med J 1955;2:1041–1048.
3. Gurudu SR, Griffel LH, Gialanell RJ et al. Cyclosporin therapy in inflammatory bowel disease: short-term and long-term results. J Clin Gastroenterol 1999;29:151–154.
4. Lewis JD, Deren JJ, Lichenstein GR. Cancer risk in patients with inflammatory bowel disease. Gastroenterology Clinics of North America 1999;28(2):459–477.
5. Gorfine SR, Bauer JJ, Harris MT et al. Dysplasia complicating chronic ulcerative colitis: is immediate colectomy warranted? Dis Colon Rectum 2000;43:1575–1581.
6. O'Riordain MG, Fazio VW, Lavery IC et al. Incidence and natural history of dysplasia of the anal transitional zone after ileal pouch–anal anastomosis: results of a five-year to ten-year follow-up. Dis Colon Rectum 2000;43:1600–1665.
7. Laureti S, Ugolini F, D'Errico A et al. Adenocarcinoma below ileoanal anastomosis for ulcerative colitis: report of a case and review of the literature. Dis Colon Rectum 2002;45:418–421.
8. Rodriguez-Sanjuan JC, Polavieja MG, Naranjo A et al. Adenocarcinoma in an ileal pouch for ulcerative colitis. Dis Colon Rectum 1995;38:779–780.
9. Sequens R. Cancer in the anal canal (transitional zone) after restorative proctocolectomy with stapled ileal pouch–anal anastomosis. Int J Colorectal Dis 1997;12:254–255.
10. Parks AG, Nichols RJ. Proctocolectomy without ileostomy for ulcerative colitis. Br Med J 1978;2:85–88.
11. Parks AG, Nichols RJ, Belliveau P. Proctocolectomy with ileal reservoir and anal anastomosis. Br J Surg 1980;67:533–538.
12. Heppell J, Weiland LH, Perrault J et al. Fate of the rectal mucous after rectal mucosectomy and ileoanal anastomosis. Dis Colon Rectum 1983;26:768–771.
13. O'Connell PR, Pemberton JH, Weiland LH et al. Does rectal mucus regenerate after ileoanal anastomosis? Dis Colon Rectum 1987;30:1–5.
14. Reilly WT, Pemberton JH, Wolff BG et al. Randomized prospective trial comparing ileal pouch–anal anastomosis performed by excising the anal mucosa to ileal pouch–anal anastomosis performed by preserving the anal mucosa. Ann Surg 1997;225:666–677.
15. Bullard KM, Madoff RD, Gemlo BT. Is ileoanal pouch function stable with time? Results of a prospective audit. Dis Colon Rectum 2002;45:299–304.
16. Browning SM, Nivatvongs S. Intraoperative abandonment of ileal pouch to anal anastomosis – the Mayo Clinic experience. J Am Coll Surg 1998;186:441–446.
17. Meagher AP, Farouk R, Dozois RR et al. J ileal pouch–anal anastomosis for chronic ulcerative colitis: complications and long-term outcome in 1310 patients. Br J Surg 1998;85:800–803.
18. Dayton MT, Larsen KP. Outcomes of pouch-related complications after ileal pouch–anal anastomosis. Am J Surg 1997;174:728–732.
19. Korsgen S, Keighley MRB. Causes of failure and life expectancy of the ileoanal pouch. Int J Colorect Dis 1997;12:4–8.
20. Maclean AR, Cohen Z, MacRae HM et al. Risk of small bowel obstruction after the ileal pouch–anal anastomosis. Ann Surg 2002;235:200–206.
21. Romanos J, Samarasekera DN, Stebbing JF et al. Outcomes of 200 restorative proctocolectomy operations: the John Radcliffe Hospital experience. Br J Surg 1997;84:814–818.
22. Farouk R, Pemberton JH, Wolff BG et al. Functional outcomes after ileal pouch–anal anastomosis for chronic ulcerative colitis. Ann Surg 2000;231:919–926.
23. Fazio VW, Ziv Y, Church JM et al. Ileal pouch–anal anstomoses complications and function in 1005 patients. Ann Surg 1995;222:120–127.
24. Galandiuk S, Scott NA, Dozois RR et al. Ileal pouch–anal anastomosis: reoperation for pouch-related complications. Ann Surg 1990;212:446–454.
25. Cohen Z, McLeod RS, Stephen W et al. Continuing evolution of the pelvic pouch procedure. Ann Surg 1992;216:506–511.
26. Marcello PW, Robert PL, Schoetz DJ Jr et al. Long-term results of ileoanal pouch procedure. Arch Surg 1993;128:500–503.
27. Keighley MRB, Grobler S, Bain I. An audit of restorative proctocolectomy. Gut 1993;34:690–684.
28. Keighly MRB, Gobler SP. Fistula complicating restorative proctocolectomy. Br J Surg 1993;80:1065–1067.
29. Wexner SD, Rothenberger DA, Jensen L et al. Ileal pouch vaginal fistulas: incidence, etiology, and management. Dis Colon Rectum 1989;32:460–465.
30. Paye F, Penna C, Chiche L et al. Pouch-related fistulas following restorative proctocolectomy. Br J Surg 1996;83:1574–1577.
31. Groom JS, Nicholls RJ, Hawley PR et al. Pouch–vaginal fistulas. Br J Surg 1993;80:936–940.
32. Lee PY, Fazio VW, Church JM et al. Vaginal fistula following restorative proctocolectomy. Dis Colon Rectum 1997;40:752–759.
33. Burke D, van Laarhoven JHM, Herbst F et al. Transvaginal repair of pouch–vaginal fistula. Br J Surg 2001;88:241–245.
34. Lohmuller JL, Pemberton JH, Dozois RR et al. Pouchitis and extraintestinal manifestations of inflammatory bowel disease after ileal pouch–anal anastomosis. Ann Surg 1990;211:622–629.
35. McCourtney JS, Finlay IG. Totally stapled restorative proctocolectomy. Br J Surg 1997;84:808–812.
36. Sugarman HJ, Sugerman EL, Meador JG et al. Ileal pouch anal anastomosis without ileal diversion. Ann Surg 2000;232:530–541.
37. Heuschen UA, Hinz U, Allemeyer EH et al. One- or two-stage procedure for restorative proctocolectomy: rationale for a surgical strategy in ulcerative colitis. Ann Surg 2001;234:788–794.
38. Pemberton JH, Kelly KA, Beart RW et al. Ileal pouch–anal anastomosis for chronic ulcerative colitis: long-term results. Ann Surg 1987;206:504–513.
39. Sandborn WJ, Tremaine WJ, Batts KP et al. Pouchitis after ileal pouch–anal anastomosis: a pouchitis disease activity index. Mayo Clinic Proc 1994;69:409–415.
40. Fonkalsrud EW, Bustorff-Silva J. Reconstruction for chronic dysfunction of ileoanal pouches. Ann Surg 1999;229:197–204.
41. Fazio VW, Wu JS, Lavery IC. Repeat ileal pouch–anal anastomosis to salvage septic complications of pelvic pouches: clinical outcomes and quality of life assessment. Ann Surg 1998;228:588–597.
42. Sagar PM, Dozois RR, Wolff BG et al. Disconnection, pouch revision, and reconnection of the ileal pouch–anal anastomosis. Br J Surg 1996;83:1401–1405.
43. Becker JM, McGrath KM, Meager MP et al. Late functional adaptation after colectomy, mucosal proctectomy, ileal pouch–anal anastomosis. Surgery 1991;110:718–725.
44. Hosie KB, Grobler SP, Keighley MR. Temporary loop ileostomy following restorative proctocolectomy. Br J Surg 1992;79:33–34.
45. Tjandra JJ, Fazio VW, Milsom JW et al. Omission of temporary diversion in restorative proctocolectomy – is it safe? Dis Colon Rectum 1993;36:1007–1014.
46. Matikainen M, Santavirta J, Hiltunen K. Ileoanal anastomosis without a covering ileostomy. Dis Colon Rectum 1990;33:384–388.
47. Sugerman HJ, Newsome HH, Decosta G et al. Stapled ileoanal anastomosis for ulcerative colitis and familial polyposis without a temporary diverting ileostomy. Ann Surg. 1991;213:606–619.
48. Grobler SP, Hosie KB, Keighly MRB. Randomized trial of loop ileostomy in restorative proctocolectomy. Br J Surg 1992;79:903–906.
49. Williamson MER, Lewis WG, Sagar PM et al. One-stage restorative proctocolectomy without temporary ileostomy for ulcerative colitis: a note of caution. Dis Colon Rectum 1997;40:1019–1022.
50. Tan HT, Connolly AB, Morton D et al. Results of restorative proctocolectomy in the elderly. Int J Colorectal Dis 1997;12:319–322.
51. Metcalf AM, Dozios RR, Kelly KA. Sexual function after proctocolectomy. Ann Surg 1986;204:624–627.
52. Ambrick M, Fazio VW, Hull TL et al. Sexual function after restorative proctocolectomy in women. Dis Colon Rectum 1996;39:610–614.
53. Korelitz BI. Inflammatory bowel disease in pregnancy. Gastroenterol Clin North Am 1992;21:827–834.
54. Sorokin JJ, Levin SM, Pregnancy and inflammatory bowel disease: a review of the literature. Obstet Gynecol 1983;62:247–252.
55. Anderson JB, Turner GM, Williamson RC. Fulminant ulcerative colitis in late pregnancy and the puerperium. J Roy Soc Med 1987;80:492–494.
56. Gopal KA, Amshel AI, Shonberg IL et al. Ostomy and pregnancy. Dis Colon Rectum 1985;28:912–916.
57. Olsen Ko, Joelsson M, Laurberg S et al. Fertility after ileal pouch–anal anastomosis in women with ulcerative colitis. Br J Surg 1999;86:493–495.
58. Juhasz ES, Fozard B, Dozois RR et al. Ileal pouch–anal anastomosis function following childbirth: an extended evaluation. Dis Colon Rectum 1995;38:159–165.
59. Scott HJ, McLeod RS, Blair J et al. Ileal pouch–anal anastomosis: pregnancy, delivery and pouch function. Int J Colorectal Dis 1996;11:84–87.
60. Nelson H, Dozois RR, Kelly KA et al. The effect of pregnancy and delivery on ileal pouch–anal anastomosis functions. Dis Colon Rectum 1989;32:384–388.
61. Ziv Y, Fazio VW, Strong SA et al. Ulcerative colitis and coexisting colorectal cancer: recurrence rate after restorative proctocolecomy. Ann Surg Oncol 1994;1:512–515.
62. Ohman U. Colorectal carcinoma in patients with ulcerative colitis. Am J Surg 1982;144:344–349.

63. Wiltz O, Hashmi HF, Schoetz DJ Jr et al. Carcinoma and ileal pouch–anal anastomosis. Dis Colon Rectum 1991;34:805–809.

64. Radice E, Nelson H, Devine RM et al. Ileal pouch–anal anastomosis in patients with colorectal cancer: long-term functional and oncologic outcomes. Dis Colon Rectum 1998;41:11–17.

65. Brunel M, Penna C, Tiret E et al. Restorative proctocolectomy for distal ulcerative colitis. Gut 1999;45:542–545.

66. Martin A, Dinca M, Leone L et al Quality of life after proctocolectomy and ileo-anal anastomosis for severe ulcerative colitis. Am J Gastroenterol 1998;93:166–169.

67. Fazio VW, O'Riordan MG, Lavery IC et al. Long-term functional outcome and quality of life after stapled restorative proctocolectomy. Ann Surg 1999;230:575–584.

68. Kohler LW, Pemberton JH, Zinsmeister AR et al. Quality of life after proctocolectomy. A comparison of Brooke ileostomy, Kock pouch, ileal pouch–anal anastomosis. Gastroenterology 1991;101:679–684.

69. Pemberton JH, Phillips SF, Ready RR et al. Quality of life after Brooke ileostomy and ileal pouch–anal anastomosis: comparision of performance status. Ann Surg 1989;209:620–626.

70. Pezim ME, Nicholls RJ. Quality of life after restorative proctocolectomy with pelvic ileal reservoir. Br J Surg 1985;72:31–33.

71. Jimmo B, Hyman NH. Is ileal pouch–anal anastomosis really the procedure of choice for patients with ulcerative colitis? Dis Colon Rectum 1998;41:41–45.

72. McLeod RS, Churchill DN, Lock AM et al. Quality of life of patients with ulcerative colitis preoperatively and postoperatively. Gastroenterology 1991;101:1307–1313.

73. Weinryb RM, Gustavsson JP, Liljeqvist L et al. A prospective study of the quality of life after pelvic pouch operation. J Am Coll Surg 1995;180:589–595.

74. O'Bichere A, Wilkinson K, Rumbles S et al. Functional outcomes after restorative panproctocolectomy for ulcerative colitis decreases an otherwise enhanced quality of life. Br J Surg 2000;87:802–807.

75. Dunker MS, Bemelman WA, Slors JFM et al. Functional outcome, quality of life, body image, and cosmesis in patients after laparoscopic-assisted and conventional restorative proctocolectomy: a comparative study. Dis Colon Rectum 2001;44:1800–1807.

76. Reissman P, Salky BA, Pfeifer J et al. Laparoscopic surgery in the management of inflammatory bowel disease. Am J Surg 1996;171:47–50.

77. Santoro E, Carlini M, Carboni F et al. Laparoscopic total proctocolectomy with ileal J pouch–anal anastomosis. Hepatogastroenterology 1999;46:894–899.

78. Young-Fadok TM, Dozois EJ, Sandborn WJ et al. A case-matched study of laparoscopic proctocolectomy and ileal pouch anal anastomosis (PC-IPAA) versus open PC-IPAA for ulcerative colitis. Gastroenterology (Suppl 1) 2001;120:A452.

## CHAPTER 41

# Surgery for Crohn's disease

Robin S McLeod

## INTRODUCTION

Crohn's disease is a panintestinal disease that may affect any part of the gastrointestinal tract. Although modern medical therapy is effective, surgical therapy will be required in approximately 80% of patients at some time during their disease process.[1] However, the need for surgery should not be perceived as a failure of medical therapy. Rather, one should view the treatment of Crohn's disease as being multimodal – i.e. including both surgical and medical therapies – and each is required at different times.

Although surgery is usually effective in treating complications and improving quality of life in the short term, it is not curative as the disease may recur elsewhere in the gut. This fact should be considered when deciding whether to operate on the patient, the timing of surgery and the procedure to be performed. Similarly, both the short- and the long-term consequences of surgery must always be considered. Inappropriate surgical therapy may lead to improved outcome in the short term but impaired long-term outcome and quality of life. Also, whereas surgery is usually very effective in improving outcome, its limitations must also be accepted and it may not be the best therapeutic option, especially for patients with recurrent or extensive disease.

The technical aspects of Crohn's disease may be challenging. The disease may occur at variable sites and the clinical manifestations may vary. The course may be slow and indolent, or acute and rapidly progressive. Finally, associated findings such as the presence of an abscess, generalized peritonitis from a free perforation, or a cancer may affect the operative decision-making. Thus, the surgical approach may be quite variable and must often be individualized.

## GENERAL CONSIDERATIONS

### PREOPERATIVE EVALUATION AND MANAGEMENT

Before surgery the patient's medical status should be optimized and the gastrointestinal tract fully evaluated. This may not be possible because of the urgent need for surgery or the status of the underlying disease. However, even in an emergency there are certain measures, such as correction of fluid and electrolyte abnormalities, administration of antibiotics and thromboembolic prophylaxis and stoma marking, that should be undertaken. The latter is particularly important in the emergency situation, where there may be unanticipated findings necessitating the construction of a temporary stoma. Although most patients with Crohn's disease are young and therefore do not have associated comorbidities, other medical conditions should be corrected preoperatively.

### PREOPERATIVE ASSESSMENT OF THE GASTROINTESTINAL TRACT

Preoperatively, the entire gastrointestinal tract should be examined radiologically with a small bowel enema (enteroclysis) and colonoscopy. These examinations are preferred to a gastrointestinal follow-through examination and barium enema because they are more sensitive in detecting earlier mucosal disease.[2] Although the bowel may be assessed intraoperatively, preoperative information about the extent and site of the disease and the presence of complications (such as a fistula) may be helpful in planning the surgery, as well as discussing the planned procedure with the patient. Also, it may not always be possible intraoperatively to assess the distal colon and rectum, and decisions regarding the extent of the resection and whether to create an anastomosis may be difficult to make. Furthermore, many gastroenterologists are now basing their recommendations about the need for maintenance therapy on the postoperative endoscopic appearance of the bowel.[3] If this is the case, then a preoperative baseline assessment is required.

In patients with known Crohn's disease, ultrasound may be useful to detect the extent and location of disease in the small bowel. The advantage of this method is that it is non-invasive. Parente and colleagues[4] reported that ultrasound had a sensitivity and specificity of over 90% in detecting skip lesions in a series of 296 patients who underwent ultrasound examination of the bowel. However, in patients who are being considered for surgery, information on whether the bowel is strictured or whether there is a fistula present is usually more helpful, and this can be ascertained better with a small bowel enema. It may be less important to know preoperatively whether there are skip lesions because these can be detected intraoperatively. Obviously, this technique is also dependent on the experience of the radiologist.

## MANAGEMENT OF INTRA-ABDOMINAL ABSCESSES

Abdominal abscesses may complicate Crohn's disease in 10–28% of patients. Patients presenting with a fever or abdominal mass should have a CT scan performed preoperatively to assess whether there is an intra-abdominal abscess or phlegmon. If so, it should be percutaneously drained if possible. Improvements in imaging and the ability to drain abscesses percutaneously have had a major impact on the surgical management of patients with Crohn's disease.[5,6] Although most patients will ultimately require surgery, percutaneous drainage of the abscess reduces the morbidity of the operation and obviates the need for a multiple-stage operation and a temporary stoma.[5] Patients in whom an abscess is drained should also receive broad-spectrum antibiotics. Following percutaneous drainage, surgery should usually be delayed a week or more until the inflammatory mass has resolved both clinically and radiologically. During this time the patient may require enteral or parenteral nutrition, depending on their nutritional status, whether there is an obvious fistula, and whether they can tolerate an oral diet.

Gervais and colleagues[6] reported their experience in 32 patients with Crohn's disease in whom 53 abscesses were drained. This included 19 patients who had spontaneous abscesses and 13 in whom an abscess occurred postoperatively. The abscesses were drained successfully 96% of the time. In the 19 patients who had abscesses related to their disease process, 69% avoided surgery within the first month following abscess drainage. The presence of a fistula was a predictor of success: 80% of patients with a documented fistula required early surgery, compared with 36% of patients in whom a fistula was not visualized. However, in the long term only 15% of patients with a spontaneous abscess did not require surgical intervention for their Crohn's disease.

Whereas most intra-abdominal abscesses may be successfully drained percutaneously, the chance of successfully draining a psoas abscess percutaneously is smaller. Most often these patients require operative intervention, at which time the diseased bowel can be resected, the abscess drained and the cavity curetted.

## OPTIMIZATION OF THE NUTRITIONAL STATUS AND RESTORATION OF PHYSIOLOGICAL DEFICITS

There is little evidence to support a course of preoperative total parenteral nutrition (TPN). However, most reports are small and retrospective. Afonso and Rombeau[7] reviewed the literature and found that most reports showed positive changes in nutritional parameters but no difference in postoperative complications. Despite this, in some situations it may be worth delaying surgery and instituting a course of TPN. These include patients with septic complications in whom an abscess has been drained or a phlegmon has been treated with antibiotics. Postponement of the surgery for up to several weeks may allow resolution of the inflammation and make surgery easier to perform. Similarly, patients who are severely malnourished may benefit. Alternately, enteral feeds may be instituted if they are tolerated.

## BOWEL PREPARATION

Traditionally, a mechanical bowel preparation and prophylactic antibiotics have been employed in all patients undergoing small bowel and colonic surgery. However, recent evidence suggests that septic complications may actually be increased in patients having a mechanical bowel preparation. Guenga[8] performed a meta-analysis under the auspices of the Cochrane Collaboration. Six randomized controlled trials with almost 1000 patients were included. The wound infection rate was not significantly different between the groups: 8.4% in the mechanical bowel preparation group (MBP) compared with 7.2% in the group not having MBP. However, the anastomotic leak rate was significantly higher (5.2%) in the MBP group than in the non-MBP group (0.3%). Thus, data from a relatively small number of patients suggest that MBP is not only unnecessary but potentially harmful. However, further studies may be warranted to determine the role of MBP in certain situations, such as left-sided resections and surgery for inflammatory bowel disease. In the emergency situation other factors besides fecal loading may affect the risk of an anastomotic leak. Thus, decision-making may have to be individualized with regard to whether it is safe to reanastomose the bowel or whether a stoma should be created. This may be particularly true if the bowel is obstructed and edematous or there are associated septic complications.

There is level I evidence to support the use of perioperative antibiotics in colon surgery.[9] Song and Glenny[9] performed a meta-analysis which included 147 trials comparing over 70 different antibiotic regimens. Because of the diversity of the regimens, it was difficult to make comparisons. However, single doses or short-term use of an antimicrobial agent appears to be as efficacious as long-term postoperative use (OR –1.17, 95% CI 0.89–1.54 for the risk of a surgical wound infection following pooling of 17 trials). Generally, monotherapy is less effective. There appears to be no additional benefit with the addition of oral antibiotics to parenteral antibiotics. None of these studies, however, was limited to patients with inflammatory bowel disease. These patients appear to be at higher risk for septic complications, possibly because of the presence of septic complications at surgery, the inflammatory nature of the diseases, and the fact that many patients have stomas. However, other than stating that some type of antibiotic prophylaxis is necessary, it is not possible to make a specific recommendation on the most efficacious regimen.

## STOMA SITE MARKING

An ileostomy, either permanent or temporary, is frequently required in patients with Crohn's disease. Preoperative marking of the stoma is essential, as how well the stoma functions may have a profound effect on outcome and the patient's acceptance of it.[10] Stomas should be placed away from scars and creases and in a location where the patient can visualize it adequately when sitting or lying. If not, the patient may have difficulty changing the appliance. Both stoma placement and siting of incisions are extremely important in patients with Crohn's disease. These patients will often have multiple operations, possibly require stoma revisions in the future, and may have significant weight gain or loss in the future. Thus, not only must the stoma be placed well initially but other sites, say in the left lower quadrant, should be preserved. For this reason, midline incisions are preferred.

Temporary ileostomies may be constructed in a number of situations. If surgery is performed in an emergency because of a free perforation, abscess or obstruction, it may be unwise to perform an anastomosis because of the risk of it not healing. In this situation, the proximal end can be brought out as an ileostomy or colostomy, or the anastomosis can be performed with a proximal defunctioning ileostomy. Loop ileostomies are often indicated in patients who have severe perianal disease unresponsive to more conservative surgical procedures or medical therapy. Although it is unusual for it to be possible to close the stoma in the future, it will allow the perianal sepsis to settle before performing a proctectomy. Psychologically patients may not be willing to have a permanent stoma initially, but may be more accepting knowing that there is a possibility, albeit remote, of its being temporary. In the past, Harper and colleagues[11] advocated performing a split ileostomy so that medication could be delivered to the defunctioned colon through the distal limb of the ileostomy. However, that approach has failed to gain acceptance at other centers and there is little evidence to support its use.

## COUNSELING AND PATIENT EDUCATION

Patient education is an important aspect of surgical management. Patients require psychological as well as physical preparation for surgery. Many patients are well educated about their disease and its treatment because they have had the disease for many years and may have family members with it. However, many will have misinformation, gathered from sources such as the Internet. Others may fear surgery and have concerns about their postoperative status, including loss of bowel control and frequent bowel movements and weight loss, as well as concerns about body image. A team approach is often required, with assistance from an enterostomal therapist and a psychiatrist. Also, many helpful publications are available from the Crohn's and Colitis Foundations and the United Ostomy Association, as well as others.

## EFFECT OF MEDICAL THERAPIES ON SURGERY

Preoperatively many patients may be taking various drugs, including immunosuppressants and anti-inflammatory agents. Antibiotics and the 5-aminosalicylics can be continued or discontinued and have no impact on the type of surgical procedure performed or the timing of surgery. On the other hand, the operative procedure may have to be modified if patients are on high doses of steroids because of concerns related to wound healing. Not only should the dose of steroids be considered, but also the general and nutritional status of the patient. Patients on high doses of steroids may require a temporary stoma rather than an anastomosis. Brown and Buie[12] reviewed the literature regarding the need for perioperative steroid coverage in patients on or with a history of taking steroids. They concluded that there is no evidence that supraphysiologic doses of corticosteroids are necessary to prevent hemodynamic instability secondary to adrenal insufficiency in the perioperative period. They recommended that patients on steroids preoperatively should continue on the same dose of steroids throughout the perioperative period. Only critically ill patients requiring vasopressors should

be started on high doses of steroids and at the same time be tested for adrenal insufficiency.

There has been concern about whether immunosuppressive agents affect surgical outcome. There are few data to suggest that imuran has a deleterious effect and it generally does not need to be stopped preoperatively. Brezezinski and colleagues[13] reviewed the Cleveland Clinic surgical experience with 35 patients who received infliximab in the perioperative period: 22 patients received infliximab preoperatively and 13 postoperatively. Surgery was classified as major or minor, and complications as major or minor. Although this was a small series, there did not appear to be an increased risk of surgical complications in these patients compared to a group of historical controls.

## LAPAROSCOPIC SURGERY FOR CROHN'S DISEASE

Crohn's disease is an ideal indication for the laparoscopic approach because it is a benign disease and the concerns related to cancer recurrence do not apply.[14-21] In addition, it may have an improved cosmetic result, which is an important consideration in this often young and single patient population. There tends to be less pain and higher patient satisfaction with laparoscopic procedures. On the other hand, there is no consistent evidence that hospital stays are shortened significantly and that the return to work occurs earlier following laparoscopy.

As laparoscopic techniques have become more widely adopted, the indications have widened. Laparoscopic resections may be more difficult in patients who have had previous surgery and have multiple adhesions or have a large inflammatory mass, abscess or fistula. Nevertheless, Poulin and colleagues[14] reported a conversion rate of only 7% in 31 patients having disease complicated by a fistula, and no increase in postoperative stay or complication rate. Evans and colleagues[15] reported on 84 patients who had ileocolic resections: 49 were considered to be complex cases because of the presence of fistulae, abscesses, masses or previous resections. The conversion rate was 18%. Overall, the complication rate was 13%.[15] Schmidt and colleagues[16] reported a series of 110 patients with Crohn's disease who had surgery laparoscopically. The conversion rate was quite high at 40%, which may be an indicator of the complexity of the disease. The reasons for conversion were adhesions in 21, extent of the inflammation or disease in nine, an inflammatory mass in seven, inability to dissect a fistula in five, and inability to assess the anatomy in three.

Most procedures in patients with Crohn's disease can now be attempted laparoscopically. The laparoscopic approach for creating a defunctioning stoma offers real advantages over an open approach. It can be performed easily, with the stoma being brought out through one of the port sites. Currently, terminal ileal and right colon resections, segmental resections of the small and large bowel, proctectomy, and reconstruction of the gastrointestinal tract following a Hartmann procedure are being performed. Some surgeons are performing subtotal colectomies and pouch procedures laparoscopically, but the benefit of this approach is less obvious because of the increased time taken to perform them. Most proponents advocate performing laparoscopic-assisted resections so that the bowel is exteriorized through a small incision at one of the port sites and the mesentery, which is often thickened, is divided extracorporeally.

Several studies have compared outcome in patients having laparoscopic rather than open ileocolic resections. There are four studies comparing the results of surgery to either historical or concurrent controls who had open surgery.[17–20] Obviously, in interpreting the results of these studies one must be cautious because almost certainly those cases with more favorable anatomy and disease were selected for laparoscopic surgery. In these studies, the complication rates were generally comparable at approximately 10%. However, length of stay was significantly decreased, with savings of 2–5 days in the laparoscopic group. As a result, two studies reported a savings in direct hospital costs.[17,20] There is one randomized controlled trial comparing open to laparoscopic ileocolic resection. Milson and colleagues[21] randomized 31 patients to laparoscopic and 29 to the conventional surgery group. The time to flatus and first bowel movement were a median of 3 and 4 days, respectively, after laparoscopic surgery, and 3.3 and 4 days, respectively, after conventional surgery. The median length of stay was 5 days after laparoscopic and 6 days after conventional surgery. There was no significant difference in the rate of major complications, but there were significantly more minor complications in the conventional surgery group. Two patients in the laparoscopic group were converted to an open procedure. Despite the differences being statistically insignificant, the authors concluded that the laparoscopic approach results in fewer complications and a shorter length of stay.

Dunker and colleagues[22] administered a questionnaire to 11 patients who had open resections and 11 who had a laparoscopic-assisted resection. Questions pertained to body image, hospital experience and quality of life. The cosmesis score was significantly higher in the laparoscopic group. Body image correlated strongly with cosmesis and quality of life. Interestingly, the hospital experiences of the laparoscopic and open groups were similar. Thus, although enthusiasts may hail the benefits of the laparoscopic approach in terms of a savings of time in hospital, there is little convincing evidence to support this. The real advantage appears to be in patient satisfaction and improved body image, which are not insignificant variables in this patient population.

# SURGERY FOR GASTRODUODENAL DISEASE

Gastroduodenal disease is rarely seen in isolation. Yamamoto et al.[23] reported that gastroduodenal disease occurred in association with disease elsewhere in 96% of patients. The most common and significant complication of gastroduodenal Crohn's disease is stricture formation. Most patients with a stricture will not respond to medical therapy and will require surgery. Whereas in the past the preferred option for gastroduodenal disease was a bypass procedure (usually gastrojejunostomy), strictureplasty is the preferred option now where it is technically possible. The advantage of strictureplasty is that the pylorus is preserved and hopefully there is slower transit time and less diarrhea. This is an important consideration in this patient population, who frequently have had resection of other parts of their small bowel or colon. Because surgery for gastroduodenal Crohn's is performed infrequently, the reported series are small. Yamamoto and colleagues reported the results of 10 patients who had a strictureplasty for duodenal obstruction.[23] In four patients the strictureplasty included a pyloroplasty. Eight patients had a good result, one required a Roux-en-Y duodenojejunostomy because of anastomotic breakdown, and one required a gastrojejunostomy for persistent symptoms of obstruction.

When strictureplasty is not possible, gastrojejunostomy is the procedure of choice.[24,25] Because of the risk of marginal ulceration with long-term follow-up, vagotomy has been advocated. With the availability of proton pump inhibitors and $H_2$ blockers vagotomy may not be necessary, but there are no data to make recommendations for or against its addition.

Fistulae to the duodenum most commonly occur secondary to Crohn's disease elsewhere.[26] Fistulae arising from the colon or from a previous ileocolonic anastomosis are the most common owing to the proximity of these structures to the duodenum. Because the duodenum is usually not involved with disease, the duodenum and colon and ileum may be separated and the fistula closed primarily. There is often associated induration, so it is important to mobilize the duodenum widely and excise the surrounding tissue before attempting closure. Results are excellent in most patients. Wilk and colleagues[27] have advocated bringing up a loop of proximal jejunum to the duodenum and performing a side-to-side duodenojejunostomy. This has not been required in our experience but may be an option where there is considerable reaction around the duodenal defect.

# SURGERY FOR SMALL BOWEL CROHN'S DISEASE

Although Crohn's disease may affect any part of the small bowel, the terminal ileum is most frequently involved. At the other end of the spectrum there may be multiple skip lesions throughout the small bowel. The pattern of disease may also vary, with some patients having primarily fibrostenotic, inflammatory or fistulizing disease. In a review of 500 patients operated on at the Cleveland Clinic between 1966 and 1973, Farmer and colleagues observed that obstruction was the indication for surgery in 55% and intestinal fistula and abscess in 32% of patients with small bowel disease.[28] The indications in patients with ileocolic disease were similar. With the increased use of immunosuppressive agents it may be difficult to know whether surgery or immune modifier therapy with azathioprine or 6-mercaptopurine should be recommended for patients with steroid-resistant or -dependent disease. Kennedy and colleagues[29] performed a decision analysis to explore this question: both strategies appeared to be reasonable in this setting. The preferred treatment strategy was highly dependent on the quality of life that could be expected after each treatment option. Thus, in this setting, therapeutic decisions must be individualized taking into consideration the disease pattern and activity and the patient's preferences for or against the treatment options.

Depending on the site of the disease and the indication for surgery, the surgical approach may vary. However, resection is preferred in most patients with small bowel or ileocolic disease. Although strictureplasty is used in only selected patients it has been a valuable addition to the surgical armamentarium in Crohn's disease. Bypass procedures (the so-called Eisenhower procedure) were popular in the 1960s but they are rarely performed now because of the high rate of recrudescence of the disease in the short term and the increased risk of small bowel cancer in the long term. At present, the only indication for a bypass procedure would be a gastrojejunostomy for duodenal Crohn's disease. In the unusual situation where the surgeon felt it was unsafe to resect small intestinal disease, a defunctioning ileostomy would be preferable to a bypass procedure. However, this situation is rarely encountered today because of improved imaging techniques and the ability to drain abscesses percutaneously before surgery.

Patients with multiple skip lesions throughout the small bowel are often challenging. It is estimated that only 5% of all patients with small bowel disease present in this way.[30] However, their prognosis seems to be worse, although these data come from older reports. Surgery is usually required for obstructive symptoms, rarely for fistulae and abscesses. Andrews and Allan[31] reported on 27 patients with diffuse jejunoileitis: nine patients (33%) died, three from small bowel carcinoma, four from sepsis, one from thromboembolism and one from metabolic causes.

If the skip lesions are relatively few in number and close together, then resection is usually the preferred option, assuming the patient has not previously had a significant resection. If so, a side-to-side isoperistaltic bypass procedure, as discussed later, might be an alternative.[32] However, if the lesions are multiple and scattered throughout the bowel, then strictureplasties should be performed. Dietz and colleagues[33] reported a series of 123 patients with diffuse jejunoileitis treated with strictureplasty. In total, 701 strictureplasties were performed with a median of five per patient (range 2–19). Seventy per cent had a synchronous bowel resection. The morbidity and need for reoperation did not differ compared to the larger series of patients having strictureplasties performed at the Cleveland Clinic. Five per cent developed septic complications and 29% required reoperation. Yamamoto[34] reported on the experience from Birmingham of 46 patients who had strictureplasties for diffuse jejunoileal disease. After 15 years' follow-up, 39 of the 43 required reoperation but only two experienced short bowel syndrome. Three patients had died: one from postoperative sepsis, one from small bowel cancer and one from bronchogenic cancer.

## BOWEL RESECTION

Resection of the involved bowel is the most common surgical procedure performed for small bowel Crohn's disease, especially if there is ileal or ileocolic disease. For disease involving the terminal ileum the resection usually encompasses the terminal ileum and cecum, as the disease usually extends to or into the cecum. The decision as to whether a primary anastomosis should be performed will depend on whether the procedure is performed electively or as an emergency; the status of the patient, including his/her nutritional status, whether he or she is on high doses of steroids or immunosuppressive agents; and the local conditions of the bowel, including whether it is obstructed or whether there is an abscess present. In suboptimal conditions it may be prudent to bring out the proximal end of the bowel as an ileostomy or to perform an anastomosis and a proximal defunctioning ileostomy, with the plan being to reanastomose the bowel at a later date.

Recognizing that recurrence following surgery is a significant problem, surgeons have looked at various maneuvers that might decrease the risk. There are conflicting data regarding the effect of microscopic disease at the resection margin.[35] However, given that Crohn's disease is a panintestinal disease, that it is focal in distribution, and that histological abnormalities have been demonstrated in segments of bowel which appear to be grossly normal, the significance of microscopic disease at the resection margin is questionable.

The length of the resection margin has also generated conflicting and controversial results. In the 1970s Krause and Bergman[36] advocated a radical approach of excising 10–30 cm of normal bowel proximal and distal to the affected area. This was based on a retrospective study with follow-up ranging from 7 to 19 years, where recurrence rates of 29% and 84%, respectively, were reported in patients having radical or limited surgery. However, the two approaches were performed at different hospitals, so the possibility of selection bias is real. Fazio and colleagues published the results of a randomized controlled trial where 152 patients were randomized to one of two groups: proximal resection margins of 2 or 12 cm in length.[37] After a mean follow-up of 56 months, the recurrence rate (as defined by the need for a further resection) was 25% in the limited resection group compared to 18% in the extended resection group, a difference which was not statistically significant. Thus, the approach accepted by most surgeons is to resect the bowel which is grossly involved plus a margin of several centimeters of normal bowel. Frozen sections are usually unnecessary.

Although there is theoretical concern that obstruction to the fecal stream may be important in the recurrence of Crohn's disease preanastomotically, at present there is little evidence to suggest that the type of anastomosis alters the risk. Two trials have addressed this issue. Cameron and colleagues randomized 86 patients who had an ileocolic resection to an end-to-end or an end-to-side anastomosis.[38] After a mean follow-up of 47 months the recurrence rates in the two groups were similar, at 23% and 31%, respectively.

Ikeuchi and colleagues[39] randomized 33 patients to a hand-sewn end-to-end anastomosis and 30 to a stapled functional end-to-end (using the 60 mm linear stapler) or circular stapled anastomosis. There was a variety of anastomotic sites, including ilealileal, ileocolic, colocolic and ileorectal. Recurrence was based on the need for another operation for disease recurrence. The recurrence rate was significantly lower in the stapled group (18.9%) than in the hand-sewn group (37.8%) after a median follow-up of 87 months.

It is hypothesized that a side-to-side anastomosis may be wider and therefore lead to less fecal stasis than an end-to-end anastomosis. There are no trials comparing side-to-side and end-to-end anastomoses. Munoz-Juarez and colleagues[40] reviewed the experience of 138 patients who had ileocolic resections at the Mayo Clinic and Birmingham General Hospital. There were 69 patients who had stapled side-to-side anastomoses and they were age and gender matched to 69 who had end-to-end sutured anastomoses. The groups were similar with the exception of mean follow-up (20 vs. 35 months), which may account for the difference in symptomatic recurrence rates of 18% in the stapled and 48% in the sutured group. Two other studies have reported similar findings.[41,42] On the other hand, two other studies have found no difference in recurrence rates when the data were analyzed actuarially.[43,44] The discrepancies in the reports may be due to the studies being retrospective, with variable anastomotic techniques and criteria for diagnosing recurrence, and finally, follow-up may differ between the groups.

## STRICTUREPLASTY

Strictureplasty was first advocated in the 1980s for the treatment of fibrotic strictures in Crohn's disease.[45] Although resection of the diseased segment is still the preferred surgical option for most patients, strictureplasty has been used with increasing frequency, especially in patients who have multiple skip lesions or have had multiple resections in the past. As a consequence, the largest experience has been with strictureplasties performed in the small bowel. However, they may also be performed for strictures involving a previous ileocolic anastomosis, as well as those in the duodenum and colon. Strictureplasty is less applicable to strictures in the colon, as there is usually involvement of the rest of the colon which requires resection. Also, one must always be cautious that a stricture in the colon is not cancerous.

Two types of strictureplasty have been described, the so-called Heinicke–Mickulitz (41.1–41.2), which is performed for short strictures, and the Finney for longer strictures (Figs. 41.3–41.4). In performing a strictureplasty, a longitudinal incision the length of the stricture is made. The base of the strictureplasty should be biopsied to ensure it is not malignant. Our preference is to suture the bowel using a single-layer continuous absorbable suture. Because the bowel is usually thickened and fibrotic, there is a risk of fracture if a stapler is used.

Recently Michalessi et al.[32] described a side-to-side isoperistaltic strictureplasty (SSIS) for the management of a long segment of disease or multiple strictures in the mid small bowel. The bowel is divided and a side-to-side anastomosis performed, thereby avoiding a resection, a blind loop or a bypassed segment. Their recent report documents the results in 21 patients. One patient had a postoperative bleed. After follow-up of up to 7.5 years there was evidence of regression of disease in all patients. Another recent report from Poggioli et al.[46] described a strictureplasty where a side-to-side anastomosis is performed between the diseased terminal ileum and the right colon. This technique has been used in only five patients, and therefore its utility is also yet to be determined.

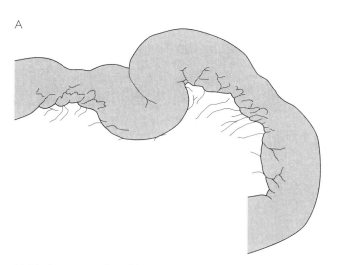

Fig. 41.1A  A segment of small bowel showing a short Crohn's stricture.

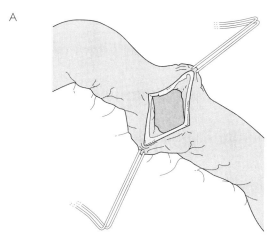

Fig. 41.2A  Once the enterotomy or incision is made, the bowel may be inspected and the base biopsied to ensure that the stricture is benign and not caused by an unrecognized cancer. The incision is then closed transversely.

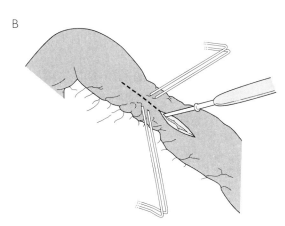

Fig. 41.1B  To perform a Heinicke–Mickulitz strictureplasty, a longitudinal incision is made on the antimesenteric border of the involved segment of bowel. Two holding sutures may facilitate closure of the strictureplasty.

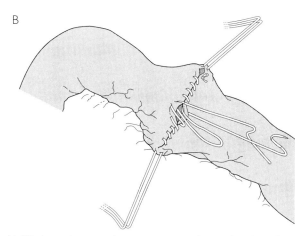

Fig. 41.2B  A one layer continuous suture may be used to close the enterotomy although some surgeons prefer to perform the anastomosis with interrupted sutures. Generally, strictureplasties should not be performed using a stapler because the tissue is scarred and may fracture with the stapler.

A

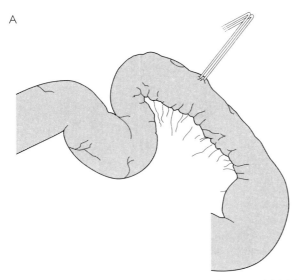

Fig. 41.3A Long strictures are not amenable to performing a Heinicke–Mickulitz strictureplasty.

B

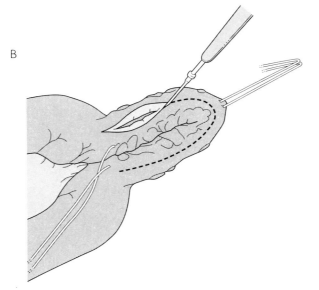

Fig. 41.3B A Finney strictureplasty may be performed for long strictures. As shown here, the bowel is folded on itself. Like a Heinicke–Mickulitz strictureplasty, an enterotomy is made on the anti-mesenteric surface of the involved bowel. Again, a biopsy of the base of the stricture should be taken.

Despite the concerns regarding anastomosing diseased bowel, the short-term complication rate following strictureplasty is low, ranging from 1 to 14% as shown in Table 41.1.[47–59] In our own series of 43 patients in whom 154 strictureplasties were performed between 1985 and 1994, there was only one confirmed leak and one other suspected leak.[53] The largest series reported to date is from the Cleveland Clinic.[47] They reported on 314 patients in whom 1224 strictureplasties were performed. A median of two strictureplasties were performed in each patient, with a range of 1–19. Sixty-six per cent of patients had a synchronous bowel resection. Eighteen per cent had complications, with 5% having septic complications. Preoperative weight loss and older age were predictors of complications. With a median follow-up of 7.5 years, 34% of their patients have required further surgery for symptomatic

A

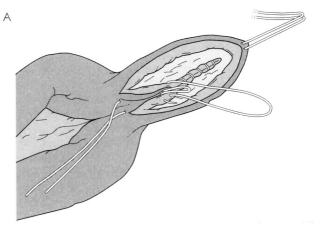

Fig. 41.4A The strictureplasty is closed with a running continuous suture beginning with the posterior wall of the bowel.

B

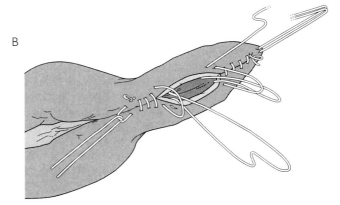

Fig. 41.4B The strictureplasty is completed by suturing the anterior wall of the bowel.

Crohn's disease. Hurst and Michelassi reported recurrence rates, defined as need for reoperation, of 15 +/– 6% at 1 year and 22 +/– 10% at 5 years.[51] In our series, 14 of 43 patients (33%) required reoperation after a mean follow-up of 55 months.[53] However, in most of these patients there was progression of disease elsewhere and the original strictureplasties were still patent. Stebbing et al., reporting on the experience at Oxford, also noted that only 3.7% of strictureplasty sites restenosed and required reoperation.[54] In Hurst's series, 5% of strictureplasty sites had evidence of recurrence. In our own series, the type of strictureplasty, the number of previous operations, the site of the stricture and whether a resection was performed in conjunction with the strictureplasty had an effect on the long-term outcome. Yamamoto[50] found that young age at surgery (<37 years) was a poor prognostic variable, as did Dietz and colleagues.[47] Tichansky et al.[59] reviewed 15 series containing 506 patients in whom 1825 strictureplasties were performed. They found a lower reoperative rate in those patients who had Finney rather than Heineke–Mikulicz strictureplasties (80% were Heineke–Mikulicz strictureplasties), in whom the disease was not active and there was no preoperative weight loss.

There are three reports of adenocarcinoma arising at or adjacent to a strictureplasty site, occurring on average 7 years following the surgery.[60–62] One patient presented with anemia and the other presented with obstructive symptoms. Two patients had long-standing Crohn's disease and were somewhat

**Table 41.1 Results of strictureplasty**

| | Years | No. of patients | % resected | No. of strictureplasties | Complications | Mean follow-up | Recurrence | Reoperation |
|---|---|---|---|---|---|---|---|---|
| Dietz 2001 | 1984–1999 | 314 | 66 | 1124 | 18% | 7.5 years | | 34% |
| Broering 2001 | 1987–1996 | 29 | 21 | 35 | 16.1% | 70 months | | 36% |
| Cristaldi 2000 | 1993–1999 | 50 | 30 | 97 | 3/50 | 36 months | | N/A |
| Yamamato 1999 | 1980–1997 | 87 | 49 | 245 | 7/87 | 104 months | 56% | 44% |
| Hurst 1998 | 1989–1997 | 57 | 67 | 109 | 12% | 38 months | | 12% |
| Sasaki 1996 | | 3 | 0 | 4 | 0 | N/A | | |
| Serra 1995 | 1985–1994 | 43 | 74 | 154 | 2/43 | 54.4 months | | 33% |
| Stebbing 1995 | 1978–1994 | 52 | 65 | 241 | 19% | 49.5 months | | 36% |
| Spencer 1994 | 1985–1991 | 35 | 67 | 71 | 14% | 36 months | 20% | 17% |
| Quandalle 1994 | 1985–1991 | 22 | 68 | 107 | | 36 months | 41% | 23% |
| Pritchard 1990 | 1982–1989 | 12 | 31 | 52 | | 24 months | 60% | 31% |
| Kendall 1986 | N/A | 9 | 66 | 45 | | 20 months | 77 | 44% |
| Lee 1986 | 1979–1982 | 9 | 89 | 9 | | 25 months | 33% | 11% |

older (47 and 78 years of age). Both were treated with resection. The details of the other patient were not reported.[62]

Given that the procedure can be performed safely and that a conservative approach to Crohn's disease is advocated, strictureplasty has an important role in the surgical management of the disease. However, at present its use is generally limited to those patients who have multiple skip lesions or who have previously had multiple resections. Tichansky[59] reported that obstruction was the indication for surgery in 92% of patients. It is contraindicated in patients with long strictures, abscesses or fistulizing disease. In the future, however, further evaluation of this procedure compared with resection is warranted, especially with respect to long-term outcome. Broering and colleagues[63] performed an interesting study comparing patients who had a strictureplasty to those who had had a resection. There was no significant difference in the mean scores of the IBDQ in the two cohorts of patients.

Another question that remains unanswered is whether these patients should receive maintenance therapy. There are no data from randomized controlled trials and opinion seems to be divided on this question. However, as most of these patients do have extensive disease, it has been our practice recently to advise prophylaxis with an immunosuppressant such as azathioprine or 6-mercaptopurine.[64]

# SURGERY FOR LARGE BOWEL DISEASE

The pattern of involvement in Crohn's colitis is quite variable, with some patients having predominantly right-sided involvement, possibly with small bowel involvement, others having colonic involvement with sparing of the rectum, and others having pancolitis. Furthermore, the disease may be complicated by the presence of perianal disease. As a result, the indications for surgery may vary as well as the surgical procedure. Most patients requiring surgery for colonic disease will require a resection. If there is sparing of the rectum and no or minimal perianal disease, then a colectomy and ileorectal or ileosigmoid anastomosis can be performed. Proctocolectomy and ileostomy

will be required for patients with pancolitis or those with severe perianal disease. The obvious advantage of performing an anastomosis is that a stoma is avoided. However, the reported recurrence rates are significantly higher in those in whom a colectomy and anastomosis is performed. Andrews et al.[65] reported recurrence rates of 46% and 60% at 5 and 10 years, respectively, in patients who had ileorectal anastomoses, compared with 10 and 21% in those who had a proctocolectomy and ileostomy. Patients with limited disease of the colon may have a segmental resection. Strictureplasty is rarely an option for patients with Crohn's colitis.

Farmer et al.[28] reported that the indication for surgery in patients with colonic Crohn's disease was poor response to medical therapy in 26%, the presence of internal fistulae and abscesses in 23%, toxic megacolon in 20% and perianal disease in 19%. Recently, Andersson and colleagues[66] reported on the changes in surgical management of Crohn's colitis in Sweden between 1970 and 1997. There were 211 patients followed during this period, of whom 84 underwent surgery. The indications for and outcome of surgery were compared during the time periods 1977–1990 and 1991–1997. In the early time period active disease was the indication for surgery in 64% of patients, compared to 25% in the more recent period. With this, there was a concomitant increase in stricture as the indication for surgery (9% compared to 50%). Also, the median time from diagnosis to operation increased significantly, from 3.5 to 11.5 years between the two periods. Proctocolectomy or colectomy as the primary procedure fell from 69% to 10%, whereas segmental resection increased from 31% to 90%. Only 7% of patients were on postoperative maintenance therapy in the early time period, compared to 70% more recently.

## STRICTUREPLASTY

Broering and colleagues[48] reported on a relatively large series of patients with Crohn's colitis treated by resection or strictureplasty. The indications for surgery in the strictureplasty group were symptomatic strictures and obstruction in 81%, fistulae in 16% and abscess in 3%. The strictureplasty sites were generally in the sigmoid colon or at a previous anastomosis. Ten sites where strictureplasties were performed were stenotic areas with fistulae. It is unclear whether these sites were primarily involved with Crohn's disease. Quality of life was assessed using the IBDQ and was found to be similar to that of patients who had had a resection. At a median follow-up of 70 months, recurrence was observed in 36% of patients treated with a strictureplasty and 24% in those who had had a resection.

## SEGMENTAL RESECTION

The role of segmental resection in Crohn's colitis is controversial. Segmental colonic disease occurs uncommonly, and so most reported series are small and it is difficult to draw conclusions and treatment may have to be individualized. However, recently Andersson and colleagues reported on a small series of 31 patients who had a segmental resection and compared them to a group of 26 patients who had a subtotal colectomy followed over a 27-year period.[67] Twelve of the patients in the segmental resection group had ileocolic anastomoses. In the cohort of patients who had a subtotal colectomy there were 12 who had limited disease where it would have been possible to perform a segmental resection. Bowel continuity was established in all patients in the colectomy group. There was no significant difference in the re-resection rates. At 10 years, the cumulative risk of re-resection was 55.3% in the segmental resection group compared to 41.4% in the subtotal colectomy group. Patients who had a segmental resection reported significantly fewer symptoms, fewer loose stools and better anorectal function.

Martel and colleagues[68] reported on 84 patients who had a segmental resection. Of these, 55% had a right segmental colectomy, 40% had a left segmental colectomy and 5% had a right- and left-sided resection. A stoma was constructed in 27%. Thirty-six of the 84 patients (43%) required reoperation at a mean time of 4.5 years. Twenty-six had a colonic recurrence and required a colectomy or another segmental resection. Overall, function was good in these patients.

Although these results are promising, the series are small. Most surgeons would agree that segmental resection of right-sided disease is the preferred option. It is less clear in patients with segmental disease involving the left side, or where there is a segment of active disease but quiescent or minimal disease elsewhere in the bowel. The decision-making in these situations is difficult and patients must be carefully selected. However, as shown by the study of Andersson and colleagues, there has been a trend toward more conservative resections in patients with Crohn's colitis.[66]

## COLECTOMY AND ILEORECTAL ANASTOMOSIS

Despite the higher recurrence rates, colectomy and ileorectal anastomosis (IRA) has an important role in the management of patients with Crohn's disease, as many patients are young and would prefer to avoid having an ileostomy. However, patients must be carefully selected. Patients who have significant perianal disease or severe rectal disease are not candidates. Longo et al.[69] reviewed 131 patients who underwent colectomy and ileorectal anastomosis at the Cleveland Clinic and found that the presence of small bowel disease preoperatively was the only predictive factor of the need for further surgery. The age at surgery, duration of disease, steroid use, presence of proctitis and perianal disease did not affect outcome. However, it is quite

likely that this was a highly selected group of patients, and those with significant rectal or perianal disease would not have been included. From the results of reported series it can be anticipated that approximately 50–65% of patients will have recurrence of their disease. In some patients the recurrence may be confined to the small bowel, so a further resection and anastomosis is possible. Thus, the Cleveland Clinic reported that 86% of their patients had a functioning IRA at 5 years and 48% at 10 years.[69] Similarly, Buchmann and colleagues[70] reported that 70% of their 105 patients had a functioning IRA at 7 years, and Ambrose et al.[71] reported that 66% of their patients had a functioning IRA at 9.5 years. Recently, Cattan and colleagues reported the risk of clinical recurrence after IRA to be 58% at 5 years and 83% at 10 years.[72] However, at 5 years 70% of patients had a preserved rectum and at 10 years 63% had a preserved rectum. Interestingly, maintenance therapy with 5-ASA was associated with a lower rate of failure. Patients with extraintestinal manifestations were more likely to require proctectomy. Patients with ileal involvement preoperatively were more likely to have recurrence of ileal disease.

## PROCTOCOLECTOMY AND ILEOSTOMY

Proctocolectomy is the procedure of choice for patients with pancolitis or extensive perianal disease. In those with perianal disease with associated sepsis it may be prudent to perform a subtotal colectomy and ileostomy, and to perform the proctectomy later, when the sepsis has settled. This may minimize the risk of an unhealed perineal wound. The major complication of this operation is the risk of an unhealed perineal wound, which has been reported to occur in up to 20% of patients. Pelvic nerve injury is a rare but important complication. As stated previously, the recurrence rates following proctocolectomy and ileostomy are lower than with colectomy and ileorectal anastomosis.

At the time of surgery measures to decrease the potential for sepsis should be employed, including prophylactic antibiotics. Tapering of steroids and improving the general status of the patient with parenteral nutrition may be helpful. An intersphincteric dissection of the anorectum along anatomical planes and meticulous hemostasis are also important in preventing the perineal wound problems that are frequent complications after proctectomy in patients with Crohn's disease.

## ILEAL POUCH PROCEDURE

The ileal pouch–anal anastomosis has become the surgical procedure of choice for most patients with ulcerative colitis. When it was first introduced there was a high complication rate, but today it can be performed safely with relatively few complications, a low failure rate and good functional results. However, it has generally been performed only in patients with ulcerative colitis and familial adenomatous polyposis. Crohn's disease has been considered a contraindication because of the risk of small bowel and perianal involvement. Also, failure rates of 30–50% have been reported in small series of patients with Crohn's disease.[73–76] In our own review, the failure rate among 36 patients who were diagnosed with Crohn's disease (only one diagnosed preoperatively) was 56%. Only one recent report has suggested that the procedure can be performed safely in patients with Crohn's disease with a complication rate similar to that in patients with ulcerative colitis.[77] Regimbeau and colleagues performed ileal pouches in 41 patients with Crohn's disease who had no evidence of associated anoperineal or small bowel disease. After a mean follow up of 10 years 27% had experienced CD-related complications; however, only three (7%) required a definitive ileostomy.

Although this report suggests that selected Crohn's disease patients may have a satisfactory outcome with a pouch procedure, one must be somewhat cautious in the interpretation of these results. Because perianal disease frequently complicates Crohn's colitis these patients are a highly selected group, or alternatively may have indeterminate colitis. Others have reported satisfactory results in patients with indeterminate colitis.[76,78] Thus, generally Crohn's disease remains a contraindication to performing a pouch procedure. However, in patients where there is uncertainty about the diagnosis, this procedure may be considered. Patients must be carefully selected and fully informed that their risk of complications and failure may be higher. Also, maintenance medical therapy may be considered if the diagnosis of Crohn's disease is suspected. However, although there is theoretical appeal to this strategy, at present there is little evidence to support the use of maintenance therapy. Another option would be to perform a subtotal colectomy and ileostomy and delay construction of the pouch for several years, possibly allowing delineation of the disease pattern before embarking on a pouch procedure. However, even with this approach one must recognize that recurrence of Crohn's disease may not occur for many years.

In patients who subsequently develop features of Crohn's disease a range of medical therapies, including antibiotics, have been used. Recently, the Mayo Clinic reported a complete response in six patients and a partial response in one with active Crohn's disease complicating an IPAA.[79] However, follow-up was short and the long-term outcome is unknown.

## SPECIFIC PROBLEMS AND COMPLICATIONS

### MANAGEMENT OF FISTULAE AND ABSCESSES

Approximately 25% of patients may have evidence of a fistula at the time of surgery.[80] There may be special concerns related to the surgical management of fistulae and abscesses. Hopefully, as discussed above, abscesses will have been recognized and drained percutaneously preoperatively. If not, anastomosis of the bowel is not advised unless there is a small contained abscess within the mesentery of the resected bowel. The most common fistulae are enterocolonic or enteroenteric, often occurring in segments of bowel which are otherwise normal. Other sites of fistulization are the bladder, skin, vagina and, less commonly, the stomach and duodenum.[81–84] In our experience, about one-third of patients have multiple fistulae.[81]

Most fistulae do not close with medical therapy, although recent reports suggest that infliximab may be successful in closing 50–70% of internal fistulae.[85] On the other hand, many isolated enteroenteric fistulae are asymptomatic unless there are associated obstructive or septic complications. Many are not recognized preoperatively. The presence of a fistula in itself is not an indication for surgery. When surgery is performed, resection of the involved segment of Crohn's disease is always required

and in many instances the fistula can be removed in continuity with the Crohn's disease. However, if it is into a segment of bowel remote from the Crohn's disease, the bowel may be repaired or a short segment may have to be resected, depending on the amount of surrounding reaction. The resected bowel may then be primarily anastomosed, unless there is associated sepsis. In our series only 22% of patients required an ileostomy, with those having multiple fistulae being more likely to require a defunctioning ileostomy.[81]

Fistulae into the bladder usually do require surgery. Most often patients present with gastrointestinal symptoms.[86–88] Pneumaturia and fecaluria are infrequent, but some patients may have recurrent bladder infections and it is for this reason that surgery is usually advised. They are often associated with other fistulae. Preoperatively, cystoscopy and CT scanning may be performed, but often no evidence of the fistula is seen. At surgery, the affected loop of bowel can be pinched off the bladder and resected, as discussed previously. Often the fistula opening into the bladder is small and the defect can be repaired with one or a few sutures. For a large defect, omentum may be laid over the bladder repair. Resection of the bladder defect is discouraged. Prolonged catheter drainage is recommended, as is a cystogram prior to removal of the catheter. However, recurrence is rare.

Enterovaginal fistulae can be especially troublesome to females, and most want the fistula eradicated. Enterovaginal fistulae may arise from the ileum, colon or rectum. Often they occur in females who have had a previous hysterectomy. Treatment differs depending on whether the fistula arises from the intraperitoneal bowel or extraperitoneal rectum. Fistulae arising from the intraperitoneal bowel may be treated similar to other fistulae by resection of the diseased bowel and closure of the fistula.

## FREE PERFORATION OF THE SMALL BOWEL

Free perforation of the small bowel occurs in less than 1% of patients with Crohn's disease.[89] Depending on the amount of peritoneal contamination, the segment can be resected and reanastomosed, or resected with construction of an ileostomy. In most instances the latter will be required. Even if the perforation occurs proximally in the bowel, an anastomosis should not be performed in suboptimal conditions where there is a high risk of anastomotic breakdown. If a high ileostomy or jejunostomy is constructed, patients may require intravenous supplements or TPN in addition to antidiarrheal agents and acid inhibitors. However, most patients can be discharged home and readmitted in a few months to have their gastrointestinal tract reanastomosed when the sepsis has settled. We have reported a high satisfaction rate and low complication rate in patients requiring prolonged home TPN.[90] Greenstein[89] reported a 41% mortality rate with simple suture closure of perforations and a 4% mortality with resection.

## HEMORRHAGE

Hemorrage is an extremely unusual complication of both small and large bowel Crohn's disease. Generally, management should follow the principles of management of bleeding from any source in the gastrointestinal tract. This includes adequate resuscitation of the patient and localization of the site of bleeding. One should not forget that patients with Crohn's disease may bleed from other causes, especially peptic ulcer disease, particularly if they are on steroids for treatment of their disease or NSAIDs for treatment of arthritis. Localization with nuclear scanning and mesenteric angiography may be useful if there is profuse bleeding. If surgery is required, resection of the involved bowel is indicated. Bleeding is unusual in Crohn's colitis unless the patient has fulminant disease. Subtotal colectomy and ileostomy are usually sufficient in this situation, and proctectomy in the emergency situation should usually be avoided.

## TOXIC MEGACOLON

Although toxic megacolon is a potentially fatal condition, in recent times it has become an extremely rare complication of both ulcerative colitis and especially Crohn's colitis. Supportive measures, including adequate fluid resuscitation, antibiotics and medical therapy for the disease, should be instituted. Should there be signs of sepsis, systemic instability or failure of response to treatment, then surgery will be required. Patients with fulminant colitis or toxic megacolon should always be treated by both medical and surgical teams and therapeutic decisions made jointly.

Should surgery be required, subtotal colectomy and ileostomy is the preferred option. If the bowel is quite friable, the sigmoid colon should be divided and exteriorized. Otherwise, the rectum can be divided and left intra-abdominally. In either situation it is unnecessary to divide the rectum below the sacrum. The disease will settle and patients will be able to discontinue their medications if the colon is divided at or above the sacral promontory. In addition, subsequent surgery will be easier, with less risk to the pelvic structures.

## MALIGNANCY

There is an increased risk of cancer complicating both small and large bowel Crohn's disease, as discussed later in this book. Adenocarcinoma affecting the small bowel in Crohn's disease should be managed as it would if the patient did not have Crohn's disease. The tumor should be widely resected with adequate margins and removal of the lymphovascular pedicle. As many adenocarcinomas are present in bypassed segments, the whole bypassed segment should be removed.

Decision-making may be difficult in patients with Crohn's colitis. Generally, all of the diseased colon should be resected, given that synchronous cancers and areas of dysplasia remote from the cancer can occur. Thus, if there is pancolitis the patient would probably require a total proctocolectomy; if there is lesser extent of involvement, then a smaller resection could be performed. However, individual factors such as the age of the patient, the activity of the disease and patient preferences must be considered.

## OUTCOME

### POSTOPERATIVE COMPLICATIONS

Postoperative death occurs very rarely following surgery for Crohn's disease. On the other hand, complications occur frequently. Major abdominal procedures are usually performed in patients with Crohn's disease and therefore the complications encountered are similar to those observed after any gastrointestinal surgery. Recent reports comparing laparoscopic to open procedures fairly consistently report overall complication rates of 10–15%.[14–21] These include general complications such as cardiac and respiratory complications as well as specific abdominal complications. Septic complications occur in approximately 5% of patients, with a smaller proportion having anastomotic leaks. Although anastomotic leaks can be life threatening, especially if they manifest as generalized peritonitis, more often they present with localized signs of peritonitis and with imaging the diagnosis can be made. If there is a localized leak and abscess, it can often be treated successfully with antibiotics, percutaneous drainage of the abscess and a course of TPN. Postoperative enterocutaneous fistulae can also be treated in a similar fashion.

Several complications somewhat unique to surgery for Crohn's disease warrant further discussion. Following proctectomy or proctocolectomy, problems related to healing of the perineal wound may occur in 15–20% of patients.[91] Predisposing factors include perianal sepsis, poor nutritional status and steroid use. In patients with severe perianal sepsis it is worth staging the procedure by first performing a subtotal colectomy and ileostomy and subsequently performing a proctectomy. In addition to improving the local conditions, this usually allows the patient to improve his or her nutritional status, and steroids and other medications can be discontinued. Local procedures such as unroofing of fistulae and draining abscesses can be performed when the colectomy is performed. When the proctectomy is performed, an intersphincteric dissection is preferred for patients with inflammatory bowel disease, as it will result in a smaller wound and a dead space where hematomas can collect. In most instances the wound can be closed primarily. If the perianal disease is extensive this may not be possible, and the wound can be packed and allowed to heal by secondary intention or a myocutaneous flap can be used. The latter has been advocated by Hurst and colleagues with good results. However, one must select patients carefully to minimize septic complications and the risk of sloughing of the flap.[92]

Despite the above measures, many patients will develop first a perineal wound infection and subsequently a chronic unhealed perineal wound. By definition, the latter is a wound that has not healed by 6 months. In most patients it will be minimally symptomatic, manifesting as persistent drainage and skin irritation. Often nothing needs to be done about it. However, a few patients will have a large amount of drainage and persistent severe pelvic pain. In such cases it is prudent to perform a small bowel study to ensure that there is no communication with the gastrointestinal tract. If there is not, one can curette the cavity, and this is often successful in decreasing the amount of drainage, although it is rarely effective in completely closing the wound. The problem is that the sinus tract is usually long, often extending to the sacral promontory, and the cavity is surrounded by a thick fibrous capsule. Eradication usually requires complete excision of the tract and capsule. The defect can be covered with a split-thickness skin graft or a myocutaneous flap.[93,94] It is a rather large procedure, and unless the symptoms are severe most patients do not opt for further treatment.

Patients requiring stomas frequently encounter skin problems such as irritation, allergic reactions and yeast infections.[95,96] An enterostomal therapist is an essential part of the team looking after Crohn's disease patients, and these problems are best handled by them. More severe problems may be encountered in approximately 20% of patients, and some 5–10% may require a revision of their stoma. Some of the complications include retraction of the stoma, parastomal herniation, pyoderma gangrenosum and peri-ileostomy ulcers, and peristomal fistulae. In some cases the complication may be associated with recurrence of Crohn's disease, whereas in others it is due to local problems. Treatment will vary depending on the symptoms, especially whether the patient is able to maintain an appliance, and whether there is recurrence of disease.

## RECURRENCE OF CROHN'S DISEASE

Although surgery is often successful in treating the complications of the disease and improving patients' quality of life, recurrence of the disease is frequent and therefore a major concern. Recurrence rates vary depending on the criteria used to define recurrence.[97] Thus, endoscopic recurrence rates varying from 29 to 93% at 1 year have been reported.[98–100] The reported clinical or symptomatic recurrence rates, which are probably most relevant, range from 6 to 16% per year.[97] In our own study of 76 patients who were followed prospectively, the symptomatic recurrence rate was approximately 12% at 1 year and 47% at 3 years.[100] Bernell and colleagues studied a population-based cohort of 907 subjects who had ileocecal resections. The clinical relapse rates were 28% and 36% at 5 and 10 years, respectively, following the first resection.[101]

Various patient factors may affect the recurrence rate. The site of disease is a predictor of recurrence. Lock and colleagues[102] reported a recurrence rate (defined as the need for a second surgical resection) of 31.2% at 8 years. For ileocolonic disease it was 44% at 10 years, for small bowel disease 33% and for colonic disease 23%. Other reports have failed to show a difference in recurrence rates between ileocolic and small bowel disease.[104] However, there are consistent reports of lower recurrence rates in patients with disease limited to the colon.

Greenstein et al.[104] reviewed 770 patients and classified them as those having fistulizing disease or an obstructive pattern of disease. The recurrence rate was significantly higher in those with fistulizing disease than in those with non-fistulizing or obstructive disease. Furthermore, these authors also found that patients who developed a recurrence tended to manifest with a similar pattern of disease.[105] Others have not been able to confirm this pattern.[106–108] Furthermore, Steinhart and colleagues[109] performed an interesting study which showed there was a lack of agreement in classifying the disease even among experts. Twelve cases with clinical information, radiology and surgical pathology reports were presented to 20 experts. The inter-rater agreement was poor, with a κ of 0.353.

With regard to factors that can be modified, there are few data to suggest that length or proximal margin length or anastomotic type make a difference.[37,35] On the other hand, there are some data to support the use of 5-ASA, antibiotics or immunosuppressive therapy with azathioprine or 6-mercaptopurine as postoperative maintenance therapy.[110–114] Perhaps the most important factor affecting recurrence which can be modified is smoking.[115,116] There are fairly striking data documenting an increased risk of Crohn's disease in smokers compared to non-smokers, with the relative risk being between 1.33 and 4.99.[115] This same effect has been shown with respect to recurrence following surgery. Cottone and colleagues[116] found a difference in clinical recurrence between smokers and non-smokers of 73 versus 40%, 70 versus 35% in endoscopic recurrence and 24 versus 8% in surgical recurrence. A dose–response rate was also observed.

Other factors, such as age of onset of disease, gender, number of previous resections, previous blood transfusions, the presence of granulomas and length of the resection have been implicated as risk factors for predicting recurrence, but in fact the data are conflicting.[103,106]

## QUALITY OF LIFE FOLLOWING SURGERY

There are several studies documenting outcome in patients both preoperatively and postoperatively using validated instruments that measure quality of life. All have consistently reported significantly improved outcome postoperatively compared with the preoperative status.

Thirlby and colleagues[117] studied 63 patients who had surgery for inflammatory bowel disease; of these, 36 had Crohn's disease and all had intractable disease as the indication for surgery. Outcome was measured preoperatively and at 3 months postoperatively using the Medical Outcomes Health Status Questionnaire (SF-36). In this cohort, health-related quality of life (HRQL) was low preoperatively, with scores in all eight scales being below those of the general population, whereas scores were significantly improved postoperatively and equal to those of the general population in most cases.

Yazdanpanah and colleagues[118] examined HRQL in 26 patients who had an elective ileocolonic resection for Crohn's disease using a questionnaire comprised of the SF-36 to which was added the Rating Form of Inflammatory Bowel Disease Patients Concerns (RFIPC), a sleep module and three questions of pertinence to the French population. This was administered immediately preoperatively and 3 months postoperatively. Again these investigators found that HRQL was significantly better postoperatively, although patients' concerns about having an ostomy bag, surgery, energy level, uncertainty about the disease, and pain or suffering were unchanged.

Tillinger and colleagues[119] studied 16 patients preoperatively and at 3, 6 and 24 months postoperatively using the time trade-off technique and direct questioning of objectives (DQO) to ascertain utilities for their HRQL, as well as administering the Crohn's Disease Activity Index (CDAI), RFIPC and Beck Depression Index. Again, using these instruments there was a significant improvement in all patients at 3 and 6 months preoperatively. However, at 24 months four patients had developed recurrent disease and their scores were similar to those obtained preoperatively, whereas the other 12 patients continued to have significantly improved scores.

Casellas and colleagues[120] performed a cross-sectional study which included four cohorts of patients: 29 in remission following surgical resection; 48 with a medically induced remission; 42 with clinically active disease; and a control group of 63 healthy individuals. HRQL was measured using the Inflammatory Bowel Disease Questionnaire (IBDQ), the Psychological General Well Being Index (PGWBI) and the EuroQol. Patients with active Crohn's disease had significantly poorer scores on the IBDQ, PGWBI and EuroQol. Both cohorts of patients with inactive disease (whether it was surgically or medically induced) had better scores on the three instruments than those with active disease, but there was no significant difference between the two cohorts.

Thus, these studies indicate that quality of life is consistently improved following surgery for Crohn's disease. However, quality of life appears to correlate with disease activity. Thus, patients appear to have equally good HRQL whether they are in remission due to surgery or to medical treatment. Furthermore, patients who have had a surgical resection continue to have excellent HRQL until the disease recurs, when their quality of life again deteriorates.

# PERIANAL DISEASE

There is great variation in the reported frequency of perianal lesions. These discrepancies are probably due to differences in the intensity of the search made for anal lesions and in the definition of what constitutes perianal Crohn's disease. In addition, most reviews have been performed retrospectively. Rates ranging from 32 to 80% have been reported.[121–124] Although the rates vary from series to series, there is consistency in reporting a higher frequency of perianal lesions with colonic or rectal disease.

There is also a wide range of perianal manifestations. Buchmann and Alexander-Williams[125] classified perianal disease into the following categories: skin lesions, anal canal lesions, and abscesses and fistulae. Skin lesions include maceration, erosion, ulceration, superficial abscess formation and skin tags. Anal canal lesions include fissures, ulcers and stenosis of the anal canal.

Outcome is also variable. In a series of 224 patients with anorectal manifestations Michelassi et al.[126] reported that only 38% required proctectomy. Patients with associated rectal disease were more likely to require proctectomy than those with rectal sparing (77.6% vs. 13.6%), as were those with multiple complications: 23% compared to 10% with single complications. The indication for proctectomy was rectal disease (66/85), extensive fistular disease (15/85), fecal incontinence (2/85) and anal stenosis (1/85).

## MANAGEMENT OF SKIN LESIONS

These lesions are usually due to diarrhea and local irritation, resulting in maceration and subsequent ulceration and subcutaneous abscess formation. Non-operative management only is required.

## MANAGEMENT OF ANAL ULCERS AND FISSURES

Fissures tend to be broad based and deep, with undermining of the edges. There may be associated large skin tags and a cyanotic hue to the surrounding skin. They may be multiple and placed eccentrically around the anal canal. Fissures or ulcers such as these are often associated with rectal disease. Medical therapy aimed at both the perianal and the gastrointestinal disease is indicated. Anal surgery should be avoided. Occasionally, patients with Crohn's disease develop what appears to be an idiopathic fissure without evidence of the classic features of a Crohn's fissure or any associated rectal disease. These fissures may be difficult to treat, but even in this situation surgery should be avoided. If the patient is having frequent bowel movements these should be controlled with management of the proximal disease or, in the absence of disease, by antidiarrheal agents. Local therapies including nitroglycerin or diltiazem ointment may be used. However, sphincterotomy and anal dilatation should be avoided because of the concerns about non-healing of the wound and subsequent problems with continence.

# MANAGEMENT OF FISTULAE AND ABSCESSES

Fistulae can be further subdivided into simple and complex fistulae involving the anus only, or rectovaginal fistulae. Abscesses and fistulae often require a combined medical and surgical approach. Fistulae tend to be the most difficult perianal lesions to treat, and often both medical and surgical modalities must be employed. Initial treatment will depend on the symptoms, the complexity of the fistula, and whether there is associated rectal disease.

Abscesses always require drainage. They should be suspected in patients who have perianal disease and who complain of pain in previously asymptomatic fissures and fistulae. In these cases one should not hesitate to perform an examination while the patient is under anesthesia. This may be helpful in assessing the extent of disease and determining whether there is an abscess. Treatment of abscesses should consist of incision, unroofing and drainage. Primary fistulotomy should usually be avoided. There is no role for treating abscesses with antibiotics alone, although combination metronidazole and ciprofloxacin therapy may be a useful adjunct to surgical drainage, especially if there is cellulitis.[127] Although both the diagnosis can be made and the patient treated by performing an examination under anesthesia, a transanal ultrasound or MRI may be helpful in some patients where the abscess is not obvious or complex disease is suspected.[128–132]

## SIMPLE FISTULAE

Simple fistulae are generally those that are low lying with only one external opening. They are usually seen in patients without rectal involvement. Even in Crohn's disease they make up the majority of fistulae. Although many gastroenterologists treat simple fistulae with repeated courses of antibiotics when the patient becomes symptomatic, these fistulae are usually amenable to fistulotomy and the fistula can be eradicated without risk of incontinence or delayed wound healing. Several series have reported excellent results, with healing rates of 70–100% and low rates of recurrence.[133–137] It is important that the extent of fistulous disease and the presence of associated sepsis be properly evaluated by means of an examination with the patient under anesthesia, and the rectum be evaluated by means of an endoscopic examination before undertaking fistulotomy.

## COMPLEX FISTULAE

Although simple fistulae can usually be treated definitively by means of surgical intervention, complex fistulae or those occurring in the presence of active rectal disease must be approached differently. These include fistulae with multiple external openings or tracts, as well as those that are high. It is unusual that they can be eradicated surgically without leading to significant morbidity, especially problems with continence. However, before undertaking any form of therapy an examination with the patient under anesthesia should be undertaken to carefully evaluate the extent of disease and the presence of associated sepsis. Undetected abscesses may be drained. Some patients with multiple fistulae may have less complex disease, with all the tracts emanating from one internal opening. In these cases the fistula may be treated definitively, with excellent results. If the fistula is complex, the tracts should be identified and unroofed and curetted of all infected granulation tissue. This tissue should be sent for histological assessment to rule out the rare association of cancer with Crohn's disease fistulae. Although these measures may not necessarily allow for complete healing of the fistula, they may lead to partial healing of the tracts and significantly decreased drainage. Drains and setons can be inserted on a long-term basis to allow drainage and prevent the reaccumulation of pus (see Chapter 49). Even if healing does not occur, prolonged palliation may be obtained and if necessary local surgical measures may be repeated.

Patients with high fistulae without associated rectal disease and complex tracts may have significant continence problems if a fistulotomy is performed. In these patients a long-term seton may be inserted or, alternatively, there have been reports of transposing the internal opening of the fistula tract distally to simplify definitive surgical therapy, or performing a flap advancement procedure (see Chapter 49, Figures 3, 4, and 5). Although the results of these techniques are encouraging, the number of patients in each series is small.[138–140]

Where definitive surgical therapy is not possible or advisable, medical therapy may be an alternative. Most medical therapies, such as antibiotics and immunosuppressants, are of little benefit in healing perianal disease. The major role of antibiotics is to control sepsis and thus minimize symptoms. With the introduction of infliximab there may be effective medical therapy. Present and colleagues[85] performed a randomized controlled trial on 94 adult patients with abdominal or perianal fistulae who were randomized to infliximab 5 mg/kg or 10 mg/kg, or placebo. Almost 90% of the patients included in the trial had perianal fistulae. There was complete healing of 38–55% of fistulae in the infliximab groups compared to 13% of patients in the placebo group. Subsequently, van Bodegraven and colleagues reported a series of eight patients with perianal and vaginal or perineal fistulae treated with infliximab. Despite clinical evidence of improvement all of the patients had ultrasonographic evidence of the fistulous tracts.[141] Poritz and colleagues also reported that although there was complete or partial improvement in 68% of 26 patients with fistulae, more than half of them went on to require surgery with a mean follow-up of 6 months.[142] However, infliximab appeared to be most effective in perianal fistulae: only four of nine (44%) required surgery. Obviously, longer-term follow-up will be required to determine the role of infliximab. Infliximab may decrease the drainage from fistulae, as do antibiotics, but may fail to cause complete healing. If so, long-term outcome may not be changed.

Should medical measures fail, be refused by a patient or be contraindicated, other measures may be required. Construction of a loop or split ileostomy to divert the fecal stream may be of benefit in some patients.[143,144] Although initial improvement in the local perianal disease usually occurs, the ileostomy does not produce a change in the natural history of the disease. Relapse is common and it is often not possible to restore intestinal continuity. In our series of 12 patients treated with a diverting ileostomy for proctitis or anorectal sepsis, all had temporary remission of their disease.[143] Five required proctocolectomy because of exacerbation of their disease. None has had successful closure of the ileostomy. Similar experiences have been reported by others. In another series reported by Zelas and Jagelman, 22 patients underwent ileostomy for anorectal disease and six remained well for 3–5 years.[144] Harper and colleagues reported that 21 (72%) of 29 patients with anorectal Crohn's disease treated with split ileostomy had early improvement.[11] However, only six patients had intestinal continuity restored, eight underwent a proctocolectomy and 15 remained diverted. Despite this, there may be some merit in constructing a diverting ileostomy. First, the general status, including the nutritional status, of the patient often improves and the perianal sepsis resolves to some extent. Therefore, at least in theory, a subsequent proctectomy or other definitive procedure can be performed with less morbidity. Second, some patients may be loathe to have definitive surgery as an initial procedure, and a loop or split ileostomy allows them to adjust psychologically to a stoma without committing themselves to a permanent one.

Proctectomy may be necessary in patients who are refractory to other medical and surgical measures. It is unusual for proctectomy to be required to treat perianal disease alone. Patients almost always have associated severe rectal involvement. Farmer et al.[28] reported that perianal disease was a significant indication for surgery in only 12–19% of patients with ileocolonic or colonic Crohn's disease. Before performing a proctectomy, it is important that the patient be in optimal condition because this operation is associated with a relatively high morbidity, particularly perianal wound problems. Thus, preoperative measures to decrease local sepsis and improve healing should be undertaken. To decrease local sepsis, a staged procedure may be planned. This may mean a subtotal colectomy or defunctioning ileostomy initially.

## RECTOVAGINAL FISTULAE

The presence of a rectovaginal fistula is often an ominous sign indicating severe rectal disease. Thus, in most instances proctectomy or proximal diversion is necessary. However, in very selected patients local repair of the fistula may be undertaken. Medical treatment alone is usually unsuccessful in the treatment of these fistulae because it is a short tract which epithelializes. Similarly, spontaneous closure virtually never occurs. Medical treatment may have a role in inducing a remission of the rectal disease so that a local repair can be undertaken, or improving the consistency of stool so there is less discharge through the fistula opening.

The choice of treatment depends on two factors: patient symptoms and the disease status of the rectum. If the fistula is small and low lying the patient may experience relatively minor symptoms and no treatment other than medical management of any rectal disease is indicated, although spontaneous closure of the fistula for long periods would be unusual. However, if the patient has persistent fecal or purulent discharge from the vagina or has gross incontinence, treatment is indicated.

A local repair of the fistula should be undertaken only when the disease is in remission and the rectal tissue is healthy. In the Cleveland Clinic experience 40% of patients were amenable to local repair of the rectovaginal fistula.[145] In these patients, repair was successful after one attempt in 54% and in 68% overall. The type of repair performed depends largely on the preference of the individual surgeon. Our preference, where possible, is to perform a mucosal flap advancement via the rectum (see Chapter 49, Figure 6). Meticulous surgical technique is mandatory. We also recommend temporary fecal diversion with a loop ileostomy in most patients, although in the Cleveland Clinic series protection with a stoma did not affect outcome. If patients are carefully selected, excellent results may be achieved.

# CONCLUSIONS

Surgery plays an important role in the management of Crohn's disease and will probably continue to do so until the etiology of the disease is elucidated and more specific medical therapies are available. In most instances surgery leads to an improvement in quality of life and allows patients to regain normal physical well-being without experiencing the side effects and dysutility of taking medication. Thus, the need for surgery should not be considered a failure of management. Instead, there is a role for both medical and surgical therapy. Because of the variable patterns of disease seen in Crohn's disease, as well as the individual concerns of patients, treatment may have to be individualized. Optimally, care should be given with a team approach including gastroenterologists, surgeons, and paramedical personnel such as nurses, enterostomal therapists and psychiatrists. Also, care should be provided as a continuum. However, in order to achieve excellent results, patients require careful preoperative evaluation and management and surgeons must be familiar with the various patterns of disease and the complications that they may encounter.

# REFERENCES

1. Binder V, Both H, Hansen PK, Hendriksen C, Kreiner S, Torp-Pedersen K. Incidence and prevalence of ulcerative colitis and Crohn's disease in the county of Copenhagen 1962 to 1978. Gastroenterology 1982;83:563–568.

2. Freeney PC. Crohn's disease and ulcerative colitis. Evaluation with double contrast barium enema examination and endoscopy. Postgrad Med 1986;80:139–156.

3. Rutgeerts P, Gebbes K, Vantrappen G, Beys J, Kerremaus R, Ahiele M. Predictability of the postoperative course of Crohn's disease. Gastroenterology 1990;99:956–963.

4. Parente F, Maconi G, Bollani S et al. Bowel ultrasound in assessment of Crohn's disease and detection of related small bowel strictures: a prospective comparative study versus X-ray and intraoperative findings. Gut 2002;50:490–495.

5. Doemeny JM, Burke DR, Meranze SG. Percutaneous drainage of abscesses in patients with Crohn's disease. Gastrointest Radiol 1988;13:237–241.

6. Gervais DA, Hahn PF, O'Neill MJ, Mueller PR. Percutaneous abscess drainage in Crohn's disease: technical success and short and long-term outcomes during 14 years. Radiology 2002;222:645–651.

7. Afonso JJ, Rombeau JL. Parenteral nutrition for patients with inflammatory bowel disease. In: Rombeau JL, Caldwell M, eds. Parenteral nutrition, 2nd edn. Philadelphia: WB Saunders; 1993.

8. Guenaga KF. Preoperative bowel cleansing. Semin Colon Rect Surg 2002;13:53–61.

9. Song F, Glenny AM. Antimicrobial prophylaxis in colorectal surgery: a systematic review of randomized controlled trials. Health Technology Assessment 2(7). National Coordinating Centre for Health Technology Assessment (NCCHTA) 13665278. 1998;110.

10. McLeod RS, Lavery IC, Leatherman JR et al. Factors affecting quality of life with a conventional ileostomy. World J Surg 1986;10:474–480.

11. Harper PH, Truelove SC, Lee ECG, Kettlewell MGW, Jewell DP. Split ileostomy and ileocolostomy for Crohn's disease of the colon and ulcerative colitis: a 20 year survey. Gut 1983;24:106–113.

12. Brown CJ, Buie WD. Perioprative stress dose steroids: do they make a difference? J Am Coll Surg 2001;193:678–685.

13. Brezezinski A, Armstrong A, Del Real GA, Parsi M, Lashner B, Achkar JP. Infliximab does not increase the risk of complications in the perioperative period in patients with Crohn's disease. Gastroenterology 2002;122:A617.

14. Poulin EC, Schlachta CM, Mamazza J, Seshadri. Should enteric fistulae from Crohn's disease or diverticulitis be treated laparoscopically or by open surgery? A matched cohort study. Dis Colon Rectum 2000;43:621–626.

15. Evans J, Poritz L, MacRae HM. Influence of experience on laparoscopic ileocolic resection for Crohn's disease. Dis Colon Rectum (accepted for publication).

16. Schmidt SM, Talamini MA, Kaufman HS, Lillemoe KD, Learn P, Bayless T. Laparoscopic surgery for Crohn's disease: Reasons for conversion. Ann Surg 2001;233:733–739.

17. Duepree HJ, Senagore AJ, Delaney CP, Brady KM, Fazio VW. Advantages of laparoscopic resection for ileocecal Crohn's disease. Dis Colon Rectum 2002;45:605–610.

18. Bemelman WA, Slors JFM, Dunker MS et al. Laparoscopic-assisted vs open ileocolic resection for Crohn's disease. Surg Endosc 2000;14:721–725.

19. Tabet J, Hong D, Kim CW, Wong J, Goodacre R, Anvari M. Laparoscopic versus open bowel resection for Crohn's disease. Can J Gastroenterol 2001;15:237–242.

20. Young-Fadok TM, Hall Long K, McConnell EJ, Gomez Rey G, Cabanela RL. Advantages of laparoscopic resection for ileocolic Crohn's disease. Improved outcomes and reduced costs. Surg Endosc 2001;15:450–454.

21. Milsom JW, Hammerhofer KA, Bohm B, Marcello P, Elson P, Fazio VW. Prospective, randomized trial comparing laparoscopic vs. conventional surgery for refractory ileocolic Crohn's disease. Dis Colon Rectum 2001;44:1–9.

22. Dunker MS, Stiggelbout AM, van Hogezand RA, Ringers J, Griffioen G, Bemelman WA. Cosmesis and body image after laparoscopic-assisted and open ileocolic resection for Crohn's disease. Surg Endosc 1998;12:1334–1340.

23. Yamamoto T, Allan RN, Keighley MRB. An audit of gastroduodenal Crohn disease: clinicopathologic features and management. Scand J Gastroenterol 1999;34:1019–1024.

24. Ross TM, Fazio VW, Farmer RG. Long-term results of surgical treatment for Crohn's disease of the duodenum. Ann Surg 1983;197:399–406.

25. Murray JM, Schoetz DJ, Nugent FW, Coller JA, Veidenheimer MC. Surgical management of Crohn's disease involving the duodenum. Am J Surg 1984;147:58–65.

26. Jacobson IM, Schapiro RH, Warshaw AL. Gastric and duodenal fistulae in Crohn's disease. Gastroenterology 1985;89:1347–1352.

27. Wilk PJ, Fazio VW, Turnbull RB Jr. Ileoduodenal fistula complicating Crohn's disease. Dis Colon Rectum 1977;20:387.

28. Farmer RG, Hawk WA, Turnbull RB. Indications for surgery in Crohn's disease. Gastroenterology 1976;71:245–250.

29. Kennedy ED, Urbach DR, Krahn MD, Steinhart AH, Cohen Z, McLeod RS. Azathioprine or ileocolic resection for steroid dependent terminal ileal Crohn's disease? A decision analysis. Submitted for publication.

30. Cooke WT, Swan CH. Diffuse jejunoileitis of Crohn's disease. QJ Med 1974; 72:583.

31. Andrews HA, Allan RN. Crohn's disease of the small intestine. In: Allan RN, Keighley MRB, Alexander-Williams J et al., eds. Inflammatory bowel disease, 2nd edn. Edinburgh: Churchill Livingstone; 1990.

32. Michelassi F, Hurst RD, Melis M et al. Side-to-side isoperistaltic strictureplasty in extensive Crohn's strictures: a prospective longitudinal study. Ann Surg 2000;232:401–408.

33. Dietz DW, Fazio VW, Laureti S et al. Strictureplasty in diffuse Crohn's jejunoileitis. Safe and durable. Dis Colon Rectum 2002; 45:764–770.

34. Yamamoto T, Allan RN, Keighley MRB. Long-term outcome of surgical management for diffuse jejunoileal Crohn's disease. Surgery 2001;129:96–102.

35. Wolff BG. Factors determining recurrence following surgery for Crohn's disease. World J Surg 1998;22:364–369.

36. Krause U, Bergman L, Norlen BJ. Crohn's disease: a clinical study based on 186 patients. Scand J Gastroenterol 1984;6:97.

37. Fazio VW, Marchetti F, Church JM et al. Effect of resection margins on the recurrence of Crohn's disease in the small bowel. Ann Surg 1996;224:563–573.

38. Cameron JL, Hamilton SR, Coleman J, Sitzman JV, Bayless TM. Patterns of ileal recurrence in Crohn's disease. Ann Surg 1992;215:546–552.

39. Ikeuchi H, Kusunoki M, Yamamura T. Long-term results of stapled and hand-sewn anastomoses in patients with Crohn's disease. Dig Surg 2000;17:493–496.

40. Munoz-Juarez M, Yamamoto T, Wolff BG, Keighley MRB. Wide lumen stapled anastomosis versus conventional end-to-end anastomosis in the treatment of Crohn's disease. (in press).

41. Hashemi M, Novell JR, Lewis AA. Side-to-side anastomosis may delay recurrence in Crohn's disease. Dis Colon Rectum 1998;41:1293–1296.

42. Kusunoki M, Ikeuchi H, Yanagi H, Shoji Y, Yamamura T. A comparison of stapled and hand-sewn anastomosis in Crohn's disease. Dig Surg 1998;15:679–682.

43. Scott NA, Sue-Ling HM, Hughes LM. Anastomotic configuration does not affect recurrence of Crohn's disease after ileocolonic resection. Int J Colorectal Dis 1995;10:67–69.

44. Moskovicz D, McLeod RS, Greenberg GR, Cohen. Operative and environmental risk factors for recurrence of Crohn's disease. Int J Colorectal Dis 1999;14:224–226.

45. Lee ECG, Papaioannou N. Minimal surgery for chronic obstruction in patients with extensive or universal Crohn's disease. Ann Roy Coll Surg 1982;64:519–521.

46. Poggioli G, Stocchi L, Laureti S et al. Conservative surgical management of terminal ileitis. Dis Colon Rectum 1997;40:234–239.

47. Dietz DW, Laueti S, Strong SA et al. Safety and longterm efficacy of strictureplasty in 314 patients with obstructing small bowel Crohn's disease. J Am Coll Surg 2001;192:330–337.

48. Broering DC, Eisenberger CF, Koch A et al. Strictureplasty for large bowel stenosis in Crohn's disease: quality of life after surgical therapy. Int J Colorectal Dis 2001;16:81–87.

49. Cristaldi M, Sampietro GM, Danelli PG, Bollani S, Bianchi Porro G, Taschieri AM. Long-term results and multivariate analysis of prognostic factors in 138 consecutive patients operated on for Crohn's disease using "bowel-sparing" techniques. Am J Surg 2000;179:266–270.

50. Yamamoto T, Keighley MRB. Factors affecting the incidence of postoperative septic complications and recurrence after strictureplasty for jejunoileal Crohn's disease. Am J Surg 1999;178:240–245.

51. Hurst RD, Michelassi F. Strictureplasty for Crohn's disease: techniques and long-term results. World J Surg 1998;20:359–363.

52. Sasaki I, Funayama Y, Naito H, Fukushima K, Shibata C, Matsuno S. Extended strictureplasty for multiple short skipped strictures of Crohn's disease. Dis Colon Rectum 1996; 39:342–344.

53. Serra J, Cohen Z, McLeod RS. Natural history of strictureplasty in Crohn's disease: 9-year experience. Can J Surg 1995;38:481–485.

54. Stebbing JF, Jewell DP, Kettlewell GW, Mortensen NJ. Long-term results of recurrence and reoperation after strictureplasty for obstructive Crohn's disease. Br J Surg 1995;82:1471–1474.

55. Spencer MP, Nelson H, Wolff BG, Dozois RR. Strictureplasty for obstructive Crohn's disease: the Mayo experience. Mayo Clin Proc 1994;69:33–36.

56. Quandolle P, Gambiez L, Cocombel JF, Paris JC, Cortot A. Long-term follow up of strictureplasties in Crohn's disease. Acta Gastroenterol Belg 1994;57:314–322.

57. Pritchard TJ, Schoetz DJ, Cushaj FP et al. Stictureplasty of the small bowel in patients with Crohn's disease: an effective surgical option. Arch Surg 1990;125:715–717.

58. Kendall GP, Hawley PR, Nicholls RJ, Lennard-Jones JE. Strictureplasty: a good operation for small bowel Crohn's disease? Dis Colon Rectum 1986;29:312–316.

59. Tichansky D, Cagir B, Yoo E, Marcus SM, Fry RD. Strictureplasty for Crohn's disease. Meta-analysis. Dis Colon Rectum 2000;43:911–919.

60. Marchetti F, Fazio VW, Ozuner G. Adenocarcinoma arising from a strictureplasty site in Crohn's disease. Report of a case. Dis Colon Rectum 1996;39:1315–1321.

61. Jaskowiak NT, Michelassi F. Adenocarcinoma at a strictureplasty site in Crohn's disease. Report of a case. Dis Colon Rectum 2001;44:284–286.

62. Alexander-Williams J, Haynes IG. Up-to-date management of small-bowel Crohn's disease. Adv Surg 1987;20:245–264.

63. Broering DC, Eisenberger CF, Koch A, Bloechle C, Knoefel WT, Izbicki JR. Quality of life after surgical therapy of small bowel stenosis in Crohn's disease. Dig Surg 2001;18:124–130.

64. Cuillerier E, LeMann M, Bouhnik Y, Allez M, Rambaud JC, Modigliani R. Azathiprine for prevention of post recurrence on Crohn's disease. A retrospective study. Eur J Gastroenterol Hepatol 2001;13:1277–1279.

65. Andrews HA, Lewis P, Allan RN. Prognosis after surgery for colonic Crohn's disease. Br J Surg 1989;76:1184–1190.

66. Andersson P, Olaison G, Bodemar G, Nystrom PO, Sjodahl R. Surgery for Crohn colitis over a twenty-eight year period: fewer stomas and the replacement of total colectomy by segmental resection. Scand J Gastroenterol 2002;37:68–73.

67. Andersson P, Olaison G, Hallbook O, Sjodahl R. Segmental resection or subtotal colectomy in Crohn's colitis? Dis Colon Rectum 2002;45:47–53.

68. Martel P, Betton PO, Gallot D, Malafosse M. Crohn's colitis: experience with segmental resections. Results in a series of 84 patients. J Am Coll Surg 2002;194:448–453.

69. Longo WE, Oakley JR, Lavery IC, Church JM, Fazio VW. Outcome of ileorectal anastomosis for Crohn's colitis. Dis Colon Rectum 1992;35:1066–1071.

70. Buchmann P, Weterman IT, Keighley MR et al. The prognosis of ileorectal anastomosis in Crohn's disease. Br J Surg 1981;68:7–10.

71. Ambrose NS, Keighley MR, Alexander-Williams J, Allan RN. Clinical impact of colectomy and ileorectal anastomosis in the management of Crohn's disease. Gut 1984;25:223–227.

72. Cattan P, Bonhomme N, Panis Y et al. Fate of the rectum in patients undergoing total colectomy for Crohn's disease. Br J Surg 2002;89:454–459.

73. Hyman NH, Fazio VW, Tukson WB, Lavery IC. Consequences of ileal pouch–anal anastomosis for Crohn's colitis. Dis Colon Rectum 1991;34:653–657.

74. Grobler SP, Hosie KB, Affie E, Thompson H, Keighley MRB. Outcome of restorative proctocolectomy when the diagnosis is suggestive of Crohn's disease. Gut 1993;34:1384–1388.

75. Peyregne V, Francois Y, Gilly F-N, Descos J-L, Flourie B, Vignal J. Outcome of ileal pouch after secondary diagnosis of Crohn's disease. Int J Colorectal Dis 2000;15:49–53.

76. Brown CJ, MacLean AR, Asano T et al. Crohn's disease and indeterminate colitis and the IPAA: Outcomes and patterns of failure. (Submitted for publication)

77. Regimbeau JM, Panis Y, Pocard M et al. Long-term results of ileal pouch–anal anastomosis for colorectal Crohn's disease. Dis Colon Rectum 2001;44:769–778.

78. Pezim ME, Pemberton JH, Beart RW et al. Outcome of 'indeterminate' colitis following ileal pouch anal anastomosis. Dis Colon Rectum 1989;32:653–658.

79. Ricart E, Panaccione R, Loftus EV, Tremaine WJ, Sandborn WJ. Successful management of Crohn's disease of the ileoanal pouch with infliximab. Gastroenterology 1999;117:429–432.

80. Michelassi F, Stella M, Balestracci T, Giuliant F, Marogna P, Block GE. Incidence, diagnosis and treatment of enteric and colorectal fistulae in patients with Crohn's disease. Ann Surg 1993;218:660–666.

81. Waly A, McLeod RS, O'Connor BI, Cohen Z. Intestinal fistulae complicating Crohn's disease. (unpublished)

82. Saint-Marc O, Tiret E, Vaillant JC, Frileux P, Parc R. Surgical management of internal fistulae in Crohn's disease. J Am Coll Surg 1996;183:97–100.

83. Fazio VW, Wilk PJ, Turnbull RB Jr et al. Ileosigmoidal fistula complicating Crohn's disease. Dis Colon Rectum 1977; 20:381.

84. Young-Fadok TM, Wolff BG, Meagher A et al. Surgical management of ileosigmoid fistulae in Crohn's disease. Dis Colon Rectum 1997;40:558.

85. Present DH, Rutgeerts P, Targan S et al. Infliximab for the treatment of fistulae in patients with Crohn's disease. N Engl J Med 1999; 340:13980–1405.

86. McNamara MJ, Fazio VW, Lavery IC et al. Surgical treatment of enterovesical fistulae in Crohn's disease. Dis Colon Rectum 1990;33:271.

87. Schraut WM, Chapman C, Abraham VS. Operative treatment of Crohn's ileocolitic complicated by ileosigmoid and ileovesical fistulae. Ann Surg 1988;207:48.

88. Ikeuchi H, Yamamura T. Management of fistulae in Crohn's disease. Dig Surg 2002;19:36–39.

89. Greenstein AJ, Sachar DB, Mann D et al. Spontaneous free perforation and perforated abscess in 30 patients with Crohn's disease. Ann Surg 1987; 205:72.

90. Evans J, Steinhart AH, Cohen Z, McLeod RS. Temporary home TPN. JOGS Accepted for publication.

91. McLeod RS, Cohen Z, Langer B, Taylor B. Primary perineal wound closure following excision of the rectum. Can J Surg 1983;26:122–124.

92. Hurst RD, Gottlieb JL, Crucitti P, Melis M, Rubin M, Michelassi F. Primary closure of complicated perineal wounds with myocutaneous and fasciocutaneous flaps after proctectomy from Crohn's disease. Surgery 2001;130:767–773.

93. McLeod RS, Palmer JA, Cohen Z. Management of chronic perineal sinus by wide excision and split thickness skin grafting. Can J Surg 1985;28:315–318.

94. Back SM, Greenstein A, McElhinney AJ, Aufses AH. The gracilis myocutaneous flap for persistent perineal sinus following proctocolectomy. Surg Gynecol Obstet 1981;153:713–716.

95. McLeod RS, Lavery IC, Leatherman JR et al. Patient evaluation of the conventional ileostomy. Dis Colon Rectum 1985;28:152–154.

96. Leong APK, Londonmo-Schimmer EE, Phillips RKS. Life-table analysis of stomal complications following ileostomy. Br J Surg 1994;81:727–729.

97. McLeod RS. Resection margins and recurrent Crohn's disease. Hepatogastroenterology 1990;37:63–66.

98. Rutgeerts P, Geobes K, Vantrappen G, Kerremans R, Coengrachts JL, Coremans G. Natural history of recurrent Crohn's disease at the ileocolonic anastomosis after curative surgery. Gut 1984;25:665–672.

99. Olaison G, Smedh K, Sjodahl R. Natural course of Crohn's disease after ileocolic resection: Endoscopically visualized ileal ulcers preceding symptoms. Gut 1992;33:331–335.

100. McLeod RS, Wolff BG, Steinhart AH et al. Risk and significance of endoscopic radiological evidence of recurrent Crohn's disease. Gastroenterology 1997;113:1823–1827.

101. Bernell O, Lapidus A, Hellers G. Risk factors for surgery and recurrence in 907 patients with primary ileocaecal Crohn's disease. Br J Surg 2000;87:1697–1701.

102. Lock MR, Fazio VW, Farmer RG et al. Recurrence and reoperation for Crohn's disease. N Engl J Med 1981;304:1586–1588.

103. Borley NR, Mortensen NJ, Jewell DP. Preventing postoperative recurrence of Crohn's disease. Br J Surg 1997;84:1493–1502.

104. Greenstein AJ, Lachman P, Sachar DB et al. Perforating and non-perforating indications for repeated operations in Crohn's disease: evidence for two clinical forms. Gut 1988;29:588–592.

105. Sachar DB, Subramani K, Mauer K et al. Patterns of postoperative recurrence in fistulizing and stenotic Crohn's disease. J Clin Gastroenterol 1996;22:114–116.

106. Williams JG, Wong WD, Rothenberger DA, Goldberg SM. Recurrence of Crohn's disease after resection. Br J Surg 1991;78:10–19.

107. McDonald PJ, Fazio VW, Farmer RG et al. Perforating and non-perforating Crohn's disease. Dis Colon Rectum 1989;32:117–120.

108. Aeberhard P, Berchtold W, Riedtmann HJ et al. Surgical recurrence of perforating and non-perforating Crohn's disease. Dis Colon Rectum 1996;39:80–87.

109. Steinhart AH, Girgrah N, McLeod RS. Reliability of a Crohn's disease clinical classification scheme based on disease behavior. Inflamm Bowel Dis 1998;4:228–234.

110. McLeod RS, Wolff BG, Steinhart AH et al. Prophylactic mesalamine treatment decreases postoperative recurrence of Crohn's disease. Gastroenterology 1995;109:404–413.

111. Korelitz B, Hanauer S, Rutgeerts P et al. Postoperative prophylaxis with 6-MP, 5-ASA or placebo in Crohn's disease: a 2-year multicenter trial. Gastroenterology 1998;114:A1011 (abstract).

112. Rutgeerts P, Hiele M, Geboes K et al. Controlled trial of metronidazole treatment in the prevention of Crohn's recurrence after ileal resection. Gastroenterology 1996;108:1617–1621.

113. Lochs H, Mayer M, Fleig WE et al. Prophylaxis of postoperative relapse in Crohn's disease with mesalamine: European Cooperative Crohn's Disease Study VI. Gastroenterology 2000;118:264–273.

114. Camma C, Guinta M, Rosselli M, Rosselli M, Cottone M. Mesalamine in the maintenance treatment of Crohn's disease: A meta-analysis adjusted for confounding variables. Gastroenterology 1997;113:1465–1473.

115. Benoni C, Nilsson A. Smoking and inflammatory bowel disease: Comparison with systemic lupus erythematosus. A case control study. Scand J Gastroenterol 1990;25:751–755.

116. Thomas GAO, Rhodes J, Green JT. Inflammatory bowel disease and smoking – a review. Am J Gastroenterol 1998;93:144–149.

117. Thirlby RC, Land JC, Fenster LF et al. Effect of surgery on health-related quality of life in patients with inflammatory bowel disease; a prospective study. Arch Surg 1998;133:826–832.

118. Yazdanpanah Y, Klein O, Gambiez et al. Impact of surgery on quality of life in Crohn's disease. Am J Gastroenterol 1997;92:1897–2000.

119. Tillinger W, Mittermaier C, Lochs H et al. Health-related quality of life in patients with Crohn's disease. Dig Dis Sci 1999;44:932–938.

120. Casellas F, Lopez-Ivancos J, Badia X et al. Impact of surgery for Crohn's disease on health-related quality of life. Am J Gastroenterol 2000;95:177–182.

121. Hobbiss JH, Schofield PF. Management of perianal Crohn's disease. J Roy Soc Med 1982;75:414–417

122. Fielding JF. Perineal lesions in Crohn's disease. J Roy Coll Surg Edin 1972;17:27–32.

123. Rankin GB, Watts HD, Melnyk CS et al. National Cooperative Crohn's Disease Study: extraintestinal manifestations and perianal complications. Gastroenterology 1979;77:914–920.

124. Marks CG, Ritchie JK, Lockhart-Mummery HE. Anal fistulae in Crohn's disease. Br J Surg 1981;68:525–527.

125. Buchmann P, Alexander-Williams J. Classification of perianal Crohn's disease. Clin Gastroenterol 1980;9:323–330.

126. Michelassi F, Melis M, Rubin M, Hurst RD. Surgical treatment of anorectal complications in Crohn's disease. Surgery 2000;128:597–603.

127. Solomon MJ, McLeod RS, O'Connor BI, Steinhart AH, Greenberg GR, Cohen Z. Combination ciprofloxacin and metronidazole in severe perianal Crohn's disease. Can J Gastroenterol 1993;7:571–573.

128. Van Outryve MJ, Pelckmans PA, Michielsen PP, Van Maercke YM. Value of transrectal ultrasonography in Crohn's disease. Gastroenterology 1991;101:1171–1177.

129. Solomon MJ, McLeod RS, Cohen EK, Cohen Z. Anal wall thickness under normal and inflammatory conditions of the anorectum as determined by endoluminal ultrasonography. Am J Gastroenterol 1995;90:574–578.

130. Haggett PJ, Moore NR, Shearman JD, Travis SP, Jewell DP, Mortensen NJ. Pelvic and perineal complications of Crohn's disease: assessment using magnetic resonance imaging. Gut 1995;36:407–410.

131. Jenss H, Starlinger M, Skaleij M. Magnetic resonance imaging in perianal Crohn's disease. Lancet 1992;340:1286.

132. Lunniss PJ, Barker PG, Sultan AH et al. Magnetic resonance imaging of fistula-in-ano. Dis Colon Rectum 1994;37:708–718.

133. Bergstrand O, Ewerth S, Hellers G, Holmstrom B, Ullman J, Wallberg P. Outcome following treatment of anal fistulae in Crohn's disease. Acta Chir Scand 1980;500:43–44.

134. Bernard D, Morgan S, Tasse D. Selective surgical management of Crohn's disease of the anus. Can J Surg 1986;29:318–321.

135. Sohn N, Korelitz BI. Local operative treatment of anorectal Crohn's disease. J Clin Gastroenterol 1982;4:395–399.

136. Sohn N, Korelitz BI, Weinstein MA. Anorectal Crohn's disease: definitive surgery for fistulae and recurrent abscesses. Am J Surg 1980;139:394–397.

137. Nordgren S, Fasth S, Hulten L. Anal fistulae in Crohn's disease: incidence and outcome of surgical treatment. Int J Colorectal Dis 1992;7:214–218.

138. Williams JG, MacLeod CA, Rothenberger DA, Goldberg SM. Seton treatment of high anal fistulae. Br J Surg 1991;78:1159–1161.

139. Matos D, Lunniss PJ, Phillips RK. Total sphincter conservation in high fistula in ano: results of a new approach. Br J Surg 1993;80:802–804.

140. Winter AM, Banks PA, Petros JG. Healing of transsphincteric perianal fistulae in Crohn's disease using a new technique. Am J Gastroenterol 1993;88:2022–2025.

141. Van Bodegraven AA, Sloots CEJ, Felt-Bersma RJF, Meuwissen SGM. Endosconographic evidence of persistence of Crohn's disease associated fistulae after infliximab treatment, irrespective of clinical response. Dis Colon Rectum 2002; 45:39–46.

142. Poritz LS, Rowe WA, Koltun WA. Remicade does not abolish the need for surgery in fistulizing Crohn's disease. Dis Colon Rectum 2002;45:771–775.

143. Grant DR, Cohen Z, McLeod RS. Loop ileostomy for anorectal Crohn's disease. Can J Surg 1986;29:32–35.

144. Zelas P, Jagelman DG. Loop ileostomy in the management of Crohn's colitis in the debilitated patient.

145. Hull TL, Fazio VW. Surgical approaches to low anovaginal fistula in Crohn's disease. Am J Surg 1997;173:95–98.

## CHAPTER 42

# Care of the patient with a fecal diversion

Janice C Colwell

## INTRODUCTION

Enterostomal therapy is an advanced practice nursing specialty, one that has its roots in the 1950s at Cleveland Clinic under the tutelage of Dr Rupert Turnbull. It was recognized then, as it is today, that adjustment to a stoma is a complex process with three important aspects: stoma placement, stoma location, and in-depth consultation and support. Living with a stoma means the patient must be psychologically prepared before the surgery (if possible); the stoma site must be chosen prior to the surgical procedure; the stoma should protrude 2 cm above the skin surface; and the patient must be supported postoperatively by being given the skills to take control over the stoma and helped to gain confidence to procede with activities of normal living. A certified nursing specialty, the Wound, Ostomy and Continence Nurses' Society provides a comprehensive educational program in ostomy management (as well as wound and continence care), leading to certification. Previously referred to as the Enterostomal Therapy Nurse or ET nurse, a new title has been adopted to reflect the entire scope of the advanced practice nurse in wound, ostomy and continence: the WOC nurse. The WOC nurse brings to the healthcare team knowledge of appliance systems, wound and skin care techniques, and skills to assist the patient in living with a stoma.[1] The WOC nurse, working collaboratively with the surgical team, is an important resource to any patient who is learning to live with a stoma.

## PREOPERATIVE CONSIDERATIONS

Surgical intervention in inflammatory bowel disease patients frequently results in the creation of an abdominal stoma. Once surgery has been identified as a possible treatment option, information regarding stoma care should be provided. Patients are often ignorant about stoma issues, or have fears that are un-justified. Once the creation of an ostomy is considered as one option for treatment, written information, consultation with the WOC nurse and/or a meeting with a person with a stoma should be arranged.[2] Information about living with a stoma will help the patient make an appropriate decision.

Preoperative patient assessment should include the reading ability of the patient, their physical abilities, the presence or absence of physical and emotional support, the source of reimbursement for supplies, and the patient's home location to determine whether outpatient follow-up with the WOC nurse will be an option. Most educational materials are written in pamphlet or booklet form, at approximately eighth-grade level. If reading is not an option, several companies distribute videos that review the same material as the literature. Much of the printed information is also available in several languages, such as Spanish and Japanese.

Assessing the ability of the patient to provide self-ostomy care is important.[3] While a family member might assist the patient in changing the ostomy pouch once or twice a week, it is important that the patient is able to empty the pouch themselves. Bringing a pouch and clamp to the preoperative teaching session can provide the patient with the visual explanation of how the stoma will be managed, and the instructor will see how the patient is able to manipulate the pouch adhesive and the clamp. Pouch emptying is done four or five times a day; if the patient is not able to empty the pouch independently, this may put a strain on family resources.

Family or significant other support should also be identified preoperatively. Inclusion of the identified persons in the early lessons can contribute to smooth adjustment and adaptation. Ostomy pouches and skin products can be a costly expense to patients and their families. The source of reimbursement (or lack of it) is important, as product choices may be altered depending on the financial situation. All patients should have the ongoing support of a WOC nurse: referrals can be initiated soon after surgery if the current WOC nurse will not be able to follow the patient after discharge.

Topics in the preoperative stoma teaching session include: how the GI tract functions and how the stoma will alter that function; where the stoma will be located; the physical appearance of the stoma; the care and management of the appliance system; dietary issues; and psychosocial adjustment. The big fears of most people anticipating living with a stoma are odor and visibility of the appliance to others. These fears should be addressed as soon as possible.

Two factors are critical to living with a stoma: stoma location and stoma construction. A poorly located stoma will interfere with the appliance seal, the appliance system will not adhere securely to the peristomal skin, and the patient will have skin and leakage problems. A stoma that does not protrude adequately into the ostomy appliance will discharge the output under the adhesive seal, causing it to leak.

The location for the stoma is selected preoperatively.[4] The stoma should be located away from any dominant skin folds and creases, and the proposed site should be surrounded by 5–5.5 cm of relatively flat skin.[5] Bringing the stoma through the rectus muscle will help to prevent herniation. If possible, the stoma location should not be at the patient's belt line, which should be identified while the patient is wearing street clothes. Many individuals are short waisted and wear the belts of their clothes significantly below the waistline. If possible, the stoma should be located below the belt line, as the appliance can then be concealed under the undergarments. An appliance worn above the belt line may be constricted by the belt, preventing the flow of effluent into the appliance, and will be obvious under most clothes. Finally, the stoma site should be within the patient's line of vision, to facilitate changing and emptying the appliance.

Choosing the stoma site requires that the patient sit in an upright position, feet flat on the ground. It is recommended that the person have street clothes on, preferably with a belt, when the site is chosen. The belt line is identified and marked with a felt tip marker. A 2–2.5 inch round firm disc is used to determine possible stoma sites. If no disc is available, using the skin barrier from a two-piece appliance system is an option. The rectus muscle and the quadrant of the abdomen where the stoma will be located are identified. An ileostomy is most comfortably located in the right lower abdominal quadrant; however, if circumstances dictate (clearly no good sites on the right side), the left side might be considered after consultation with the surgeon. Colostomy placement will be dictated by the procedure to be performed. Using the disc or skin barrier, an initial site is chosen and the patient leans forward to permit assessment of any additional skin folds or creases. This procedure is continued until the criteria for stoma placement are met. The one criterion that can be flexible is belt line; however, placing a stoma at or above the belt line will mean changing clothing preferences or the use of suspenders. Once the proposed stoma site is chosen, it must be marked with dye that will remain on the skin until surgery. A permanent skin marker pen is used and the area covered with a moisture/vapor-permeable dressing (i.e. Tegaderm, Biocclusive). These dressings are water resistant and prevent clothes from rubbing the mark from the skin. If the dressing loosens prior to surgery, the patient is advised to remove the dressing, reinforce the mark with the pen and reapply a new dressing. An alternative method for stoma site marking is an India ink tattoo. The site is chosen, cleansed with alcohol, and a drop of India ink placed at the site. Using a sterile 25 gauge needle, the skin is punctured three times through the drop of ink. The India ink will be absorbed into the punctures, leaving a permanent tattoo.[6] This may not be a good option for a patient who goes to surgery without 100% assurance that they will receive a stoma, as the mark is permanent.

Stoma construction will contribute to the success of wearing an appliance.[7] The idea height of any abdominal stoma is 2–2.5 cm. above the skin level. This protrusion will allow the effluent to pass out of the stoma, over the skin barrier located on the peristomal skin and into the pouch. A flush stoma will discharge the stool under the stoma appliance seal, and a barely protruding stoma will evacuate the output directly on to the appliance seal, weakening it within a short period of time. Excessive protrusion maybe a source of stomal trauma: the stoma can rub on the flange of the appliance, causing bleeding and ulceration. A long stoma may also be difficult to camouflage under clothing. It was once thought that colostomy stomas should be created flush to the skin level, as the output would be semiformed and would not contribute to pouch failure.[8] However, given the nature of inflammatory bowel disease, patients may have shortened bowel length and resultant loose output even from a left-sided stoma. Therefore, all fecal stomas in a patient identified as having inflammatory bowel disease should protrude adequately above the skin level.

Loop stomas require support under the intestine at the time of creation. To secure a pouch seal around the stoma, the rod or support bridge should not protrude from under the stoma. Rods that protrude from below the stoma on to the peristomal skin create difficulties in fitting the pouch skin barrier around the stoma and the rod, leading to denuded peristomal skin and potential pouch failure. It is recommended that a 20 Fr red rubber catheter be placed under the stoma and brought up over it, and the ends sutured together. Sutures can be placed at the stoma–skin junction to prevent dislodgment of the rod. A rod placed in this manner allows the skin barrier of the pouch to be placed directly up to the stoma, protecting the peristomal skin from the effluent.[9] It is advisable to leave the support bridge in place under a stoma in a patient who has been receiving high-dose corticosteroids and who is nutritionally deplete for as long as 3 weeks postoperatively. Using the above-noted rod placement does not cause the patient hardship at home managing the stoma with the red rubber rod.

Double-barrelled stomas may be created for bowel perforation, bowel rest, or when complete diversion is required. The proximal and distal stomas must be separated by at least 8 cm to allow for placing an appliance only over the proximal stoma. The distal stoma, or mucous fistula, will usually reduce in size as the postoperative edema subsides. A small pad with a water-soluble ointment is placed over the mucous fistula. The pad will protect the patient's clothes from the mucous output and the ointment will prevent the mucus from sticking to the skin and stoma. For a non-elective surgical event, where bowel cleansing is not achieved preoperatively, there may be several days during the postoperative period when retained fecal material will pass from the distal stoma. It is advisable to place an appliance over the mucous fistula for a few days until the bowel is emptied. After 2 days of no output the appliance is removed and the dressing instituted.

## Table 42.1 Ostomy product listing*

| Products | Purpose | Manufacturer |
|---|---|---|
| Solid skin barrier | Protects skin from effluent, provides adhesive seal. | ConvaTec Stomahesive & Durahesive<br>Hollister Hollihesive & Premium Barrier<br>Eakin Cohesive Seal |
| Liquid skin barrier | Provides a film barrier for skin protection. | Bard Protective Barrier<br>ConvaTec AllKare Wipe<br>Hollister Skin Gel Wipes<br>Smith & Nephew No Sting Skin Prep |
| Skin barrier paste | Caulks solid skin barrier, fills in uneven areas. | ConvaTec Stomahesive Paste<br>Hollister Hollihesive & Premium Pastes<br>Coloplast Paste |
| Skin barrier powder | Absorbs moisture on peristomal skin. | ConvaTec Stomahesive Powder<br>Hollister Premium Powder |
| One-piece drainable pouch | Collects fecal drainage, allows for emptying via pouch tail, skin barrier attached. | ConvaTec**<br>Hollister**<br>Coloplast**<br>NuHope** |
| Two-piece drainable pouch | Collects fecal drainage, allows for emptying via pouch tail, attaches to skin barrier. | ConvaTec**<br>Hollister**<br>Coloplast**<br>NuHope** |
| Waterproof tape | To secure skin barrier for prolonged water activities. | Hy-Tape Surgical Tape<br>Perma-Type Pink Tape |
| Deodorizer | Decreases fecal odor. | Hollister M 9 liquid Deodorant |
| Ostomy pouch belt | Supports use of convex skin barrier. | ConvaTec<br>Hollister |
| Fistula pouches | Cut to fit pouches of various sizes to accommodate drainage from fistula. | ConvaTec Wound Manager<br>Hollister Wound Drainage Collector<br>NuHope Custom Fistula Pouches |

*Examples of various manufacturers, not meant to be inclusive.
**Various brand names.

# POSTOPERATIVE STOMA CARE

A stoma appliance should be fitted in the operating room at the conclusion of the operation. A clear, drainable one-piece appliance with a solid, cut-to-fit skin barrier is used (Table 42.1). A transparent appliance will allow for assessment of the stoma mucosa. Stoma assessment should be performed every 8 hours for the first 48 hours postoperatively. All postoperative appliances must be drainable, as the output will be closely monitored every 4–8 hours, and the appliance will be drained of stool and flatus through the bottom. Because the output of most fecal stomas following surgery will be liquid and between 800 and 1200 mL/24 hours, a solid, cut-to-fit skin barrier on the back of the appliance is recommended. The skin barrier is cut to fit the stoma, protecting the peristomal skin from the liquid output.

Patient teaching regarding ostomy self-management is begun as soon as the person is able to participate in care, generally 1–2 days postoperatively. The patient is first instructed on how to empty the appliance and master using the clamp. They are taught to empty the appliance when it is one-third full, to wipe the outer and inner edges of the appliance with tissue, and to replace the clamp. Once the emptying procedure is mastered, appliance changing is the next step. The one-piece appliance is used in the postoperative period for up to 3 weeks, especially if a support rod is in place. The alternative is to use a two-piece appliance system, but until recently most two-piece systems had flange seals to secure the appliance to the skin adhesive. This type of seal necessitates pressure against the abdomen, a procedure not advised on a new surgical wound, especially one that has a support rod sutured under the stoma. The two-piece system is discussed further below.

Patient teaching topics prior to discharge include:

- Appliance changing schedule: generally every 3–4 days until the postoperative edema subsides;
- Treatment of peristomal skin irritation: the use of skin barrier powder, maintenance of an adequate peristomal seal;
- Nutritional advice, diet advancement, education regarding foods that thicken output;
- Appliance purchasing information, insurance issues;
- Support group information.

# POSTOPERATIVE COMPLICATIONS

Mucocutaneous separation – separation of the stoma and skin junction – can occur in patients receiving high-dose corticosteroids. When noted, the separation should be probed for integrity of the wound base. If no tunneling or abscess tracts are identified, the area of separation is filled to skin level with a skin barrier powder and covered with a solid skin barrier. The appliance system is changed every 2–3 days until the area begins to decrease in size and show evidence of healing.

An edematous stoma may make the passage of the effluent difficult. If necessary, an 18 Fr red rubber catheter is passed approximately 3 inches into the stoma and left to drain into the stoma appliance. This can relieve cramping at the stoma site and facilitate drainage. As the edema subsides, the peristaltic action will push the tube out of the stoma.

Stoma necrosis is most common in the first 3 days following surgery. If necrosis is suspected, the stoma can be gently intubated with a lubricated test tube and illuminated with a penlight to ascertain the level of diminished blood flow. An appliance with an access window can allow direct visualization of the stoma at frequent intervals.

# APPLIANCE SYSTEMS

Appliance systems are the products used to manage an abdominal stoma and consist of two parts: the skin barrier/adhesive seal and the appliance/collection device. The critical part is the skin barrier/adhesive seal: the skin barrier must protect the peristomal skin from the effluent as well as maintain the seal of the system to the skin for a predictable amount of time. Security in wearing an appliance system is based upon intact peristomal skin and the knowledge that the seal will be maintained despite activity for a set wear time.

Skin barriers protect the skin by acting as a barrier between the skin and stoma output, and are available in several configurations: solids, liquids, pastes and powders.[10] All patients with a fecal stoma must use an appliance system with a solid skin barrier. Solid skin barriers are hydrocolloids containing pectin, carboxymethylcellulose and tacifers (adhesives). Hydrocolloids absorb skin moisture while maintaining a skin seal. The appliance side of the skin barrier (upon which the effluent drains) has a thin film that slows erosion. Thus the solid skin barrier protects the peristomal skin and creates the seal of the appliance system. Solid skin barriers are available in standard or extended wear types. Standard wear skin barriers maintain a seal for at least 3 days; the integrity of the skin barrier is dependent upon the amount and consistency of the output, as well as the location of the stoma lumen. A stoma lumen that allows the effluent to drain directly upon the solid skin barrier (a stoma with minimal protrusion) 'melts' the skin barrier more quickly than one with adequate protrusion (i.e. that discharges the output directly into the appliance). Extended wear skin barriers contain special additives that achieve a stronger adhesive seal and resist breakdown. The seal of the extended wear skin barrier has the potential to last up to 7 days. Extended wear adhesives can assist the patient with a high liquid output or a flush stoma to maintain a longer seal compared to a standard wear skin barrier.

Solid skin barriers are available in several configurations: flat or convex, cut-to-fit or pre-cut. A flat skin barrier is appropriate for the person with a protruding stoma and few or no skin creases or folds in the direct peristomal area. A convex skin barrier is used to enhance the seal for a person with a retracted stoma, a stoma that discharges the effluent at the skin surface, or to flatten out the area around the stoma that has significant creases or folds. Convexity, the outward curving of the skin barrier, begins at the stoma–skin junction and is available in several depths. A deep convex skin barrier may be indicated for a stoma that 'disappears' into a deep fold. The barrier will flatten out the fold and cause the stoma output to discharge into the appliance.

Cut-to-fit skin barriers are generally preferred, especially after surgery. As the postoperative edema subsides, the skin barrier opening can be altered to fit the stoma, allowing no skin to be exposed to fecal output. If a stoma is round, a measuring guide is fitted over it and the corresponding size cut in the skin barrier. If the stoma is not round, a clear plastic sheet is held over the stoma, a felt tip marker used to trace its exact size, and a custom template is made. Skin barriers are heat and pressure sensitive; a solid skin barrier is applied by using firm pressure around the stoma.

Liquid skin barriers are copolymers with alcohol as the carrier. The alcohol will cause stinging if it comes in contact with denuded peristomal skin and must be avoided if a break in the skin integrity is encountered. Two companies now manufacture a 'no-sting' skin barrier that can be used on denuded skin. Liquid skin barriers are used to 'prepare' the peristomal skin, providing a smooth, clean dry surface to adhere the appliance system. Liquid skin barriers can be used if a mild peristomal skin sensitivity is encountered; preparing the skin will provide a barrier between the sensitive skin and the product.

There are several products that can be used to enhance the seal of the solid skin barrier. Skin barrier pastes are used to 'caulk' the cut edge of the solid skin barrier, or can be used to fill in dips or depressions in the peristomal skin area. The paste will prevent the migration of the stool under the seal – important if the stoma does not protrude well into the appliance. Skin barrier pastes contain alcohol and will cause stinging if placed on denuded skin. Pastes do not dry and become solid; they will become adherent to the solid skin barrier, but are not effective alone as a skin barrier. Solid skin barrier is also available in strips and washers used on the appliance system to further enhance the seal. A belt can be used to apply pressure to the skin barrier when achieving a seal is an issue. Figure 42.1 illustrates skin barrier options.

Skin barrier powders are used on denuded skin to absorb small amounts of moisture and assist in maintaining the seal of the ostomy appliance. The peristomal skin is cleansed and dried, a small amount of skin barrier powder is sprinkled on the denuded area, rubbed gently into the skin, and the excess brushed off. The solid skin barrier is then placed over the powdered area. If necessary a no-sting liquid skin barrier can be placed over the powder to enhance the appliance seal.

When ostomy appliances were first developed they were constructed of rubber and held in place with a double-faced adhesive disc, or cement and a belt. The seal was dependent on the amount of pressure the belt could apply, the appliances were bulky, not odor resistant, and were cleaned and reused. Technology has advanced the management of stomas to the point

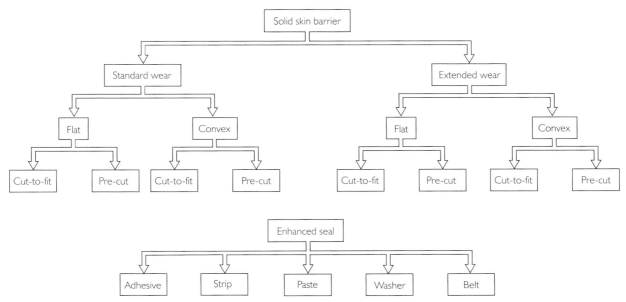

Fig. 42.1 Skin barrier options.

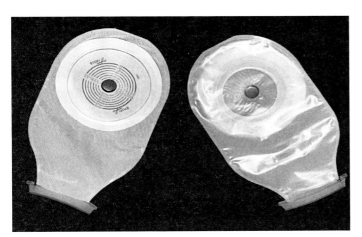

Fig. 42.2 One-piece pouches.

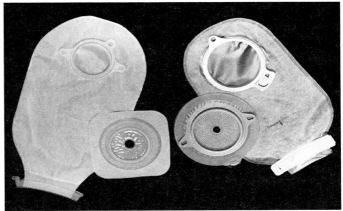

Fig. 42.3 Two-piece pouches.

where all appliances are odor resistant, disposable, and available in many sizes, shapes and configurations. Systems can be classified into one- and two-piece varieties. A one-piece appliance is all-inclusive: the solid skin barrier and the appliance are integrated (Fig. 42.2). A two-piece system includes the solid skin barrier and the appliance as separate components.

Appliances are available in various lengths, with an appliance film that is either transparent or opaque. Fabric backing on one or two sides is an option (recommended for patients who encounter moisture build-up between the appliance system and the skin).

Two-piece appliances utilize a solid skin barrier surrounded with a water-resistant adhesive and a flange that accepts an appliance (Fig. 42.3). The appliance attaches to the flange on the skin barrier wafer. This attachment varies depending on the manufacturer's product, the most common being a snapping of the appliance to the flange, by applying pressure to the attachment device against the patient's abdomen. A variation of this attachment is a flange/appliance attachment system that has a 'floating' flange, allowing the appliance to be attached by pinching the flange between fingers and not applying pressure to the abdomen. Considerations for using a two-piece system include: appliance changing as often as necessary without disturbing the adhesive seal (popping off a 12-inch appliance, popping on a 9-inch appliance which might accommodate a certain activity); the ability to utilize an opaque appliance and see the stoma when attaching the skin barrier seal (place the skin barrier seal on first and then attach the appliance); or changing the angle of the appliance to facilitate emptying. Figure 42.4 illustrates appliance system options.

Criteria for choice of appliance are ease of use for the wearer, affordability, and adaptability of the system to the wearer's lifestyle.[11] The choice of the skin barrier will be made with the WOC nurse and the criterion should be a seal that maintains the peristomal skin integrity and provides a predictable wear time. The patient should try several types of appliance system under the supervision of the WOC nurse. The pros and cons of the various systems can be evaluated and a product decided on. The cost involved with the use of an ostomy system can vary, depending on the length of time the system is worn,

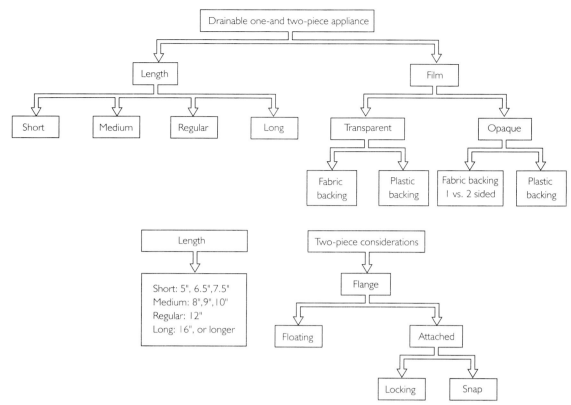

**Fig. 42.4** Drainable appliance options.

the type of skin barrier chosen (extended wear barriers costing more than standard barriers) and the accessories needed (pastes, belts etc.). Reimbursement issues are covered below.

## ISSUES OF DAILY LIVING

Concealing an appliance is a major issue for most patients with ostomies. The appliance system is worn under form-fitting undergarments; this will flatten the appliance against the abdomen, causing the effluent to be equally distributed through the length of the appliance, maintaining a flat profile. The undergarments will support the weight of the appliance, offering additional security for the seal. Outer clothes can be worn loose or snug: snug clothing will not prevent the output from draining from the stoma. If the stoma is located at the belt line of pants, and the belt is key to keeping the pants in place, suspenders may need to be considered. If a snug belt is worn over the appliance the effluent may not drain, causing overflow and appliance leakage.

All appliances are odor resistant. The adhesive seal is snug against the peristomal skin and the clamp secures the appliance end, preventing air (odor) escape. If the patient encounters odor this means that the seal is not secure, and evaluation of the system is necessary. When a patient empties the appliance (sitting back on the commode, emptying between the legs into the bowl) the effluent is drained into the toilet and the toilet flushed to decrease odor. Odor when emptying the appliance is unavoidable; liquid deodorant can be used (putting 10 drops into the appliance after each emptying), interacting with the fecal output and reducing odor before the appliance is opened. Oral agents that can reduce odors include chlorophyllin copper complex, 100–200 mg daily, and bismuth subgallate, 1–2 tablets four times daily. These agents can darken (green) and thicken the output and should not be started until normal bowel function has returned.

The appliance system adhesive seal is water resistant, allowing the person to shower, bathe or swim while wearing it. For patients who enjoy water sports and may spend prolonged periods of time immersed, several types of waterproof tape are manufactured that can be placed around the appliance adhesive in a picture-frame fashion. Bathing or showering can be done with the appliance on or without it: water and soap will not harm the stomal mucosa and may facilitate adhesive removal.

Diet is a concern of most patients with inflammatory bowel disease. Postoperative advice for ostomy patients includes the avoidance of high-fiber foods for 6–8 weeks. Stomal and intestinal edema can cause cramping and difficulty in passing fibrous materials. Once the edema has subsided, previously restricted foods are introduced slowly to monitor response. Gas can be a concern, as it becomes trapped in the appliance causing it to bulge. Gas is emptied from the bottom of the appliance, or can be 'burped' if a two-piece appliance is worn. A hole should not be made in the appliance to allow gas to escape, as this will allow odor to escape as well. Gas filters are integrated into some appliance, but their effectiveness to filter odor is questionable because, once moistened, they no longer vent gas. Patients who note excessive gas in the ostomy appliance upon awakening in the morning are encountering air that was swallowed while they were asleep. They are advised to take simethicone preparations before sleeping. Simethicone preparations can also be taken following meals if daytime gas is a problem.

Sexual activity can be resumed when the patient's physical healing is complete. Patients may require emotional support to feel comfortable participating in intimate activities. First, the patient should recognize that the appliance seal is secure and will not loosen during sexual activity. Next, both the patient and their partner need to understand that pressure will not hurt the stoma or cause pain. Some patients feel more comfortable if the appliance is covered or concealed with a cover that resembles lingerie. Many companies manufacture such covers. A mini appliance (2.5 inches in length when closed) can be snapped on to the two-piece skin barrier and will lie flat against the skin barrier and not be obtrusive. Resumption of sexual activity should be discussed with patients prior to discharge and in the outpatient clinic.[12]

Ostomy equipment can be a financial burden for many patients. Appliance systems vary from $4.50 to $10.50 per change, and the average ostomy system is changed every 4–6 days. In the postoperative period the patient and family should make inquiries about reimbursement by their healthcare coverage program. Some programs insist on the purchase of supplies at identified suppliers; other programs, such as Medicare, have identified the amount and type of supplies that will be reimbursed on a monthly basis. Reimbursement issues can be a deciding factor as to the type of appliance system used. These should be identified early in the postoperative period.

## COMPLICATIONS/PROBLEM SOLVING

One of the most frequently encountered problems for a person with a fecal diversion is peristomal skin breakdown. The appliance system fails to seal adequately to the peristomal skin, allowing the effluent to contact the skin and causing epidermal loss. There are a variety of causes for this, and a thorough stoma evaluation must be carried out to determine the cause and solution.

The stoma changes size significantly in the postoperative period, and the opening in the skin barrier must be adjusted to its current size. If the stoma is not round, a custom pattern or template is made to assist the patient in achieving a tight seal. The stoma and peristomal skin should be evaluated in a sitting position. The stoma is assessed for height above the skin, and the lumen evaluated for position. A stoma should protrude 2–2.5 cm above the skin, and the ideal location for the lumen is in the center of the stoma; if both characteristics are present the effluent will evacuate directly into the appliance. A stoma lumen at the skin level will discharge the effluent under the solid skin barrier seal, causing loss of the peristomal skin and appliance failure. The peristomal skin should be assessed for skin folds, creases and firmness. A sitting position frequently demonstrates a concave peristomal area, or the presence of creases or folds not present in the preoperative period because of the effects of long-term corticosteroid administration and resultant abdominal weight distribution. One solution for a slightly uneven peristomal area is the use of skin barrier paste. This can be used around the cut edge of the solid skin barrier and will fill in uneven areas to assist in maintaining the appliance seal. For deep creases and folds in the peristomal area, and to assist in getting the stoma to protrude above the skin edges, the use of a convex appliance system is recommended.[13] Convexity will assist in flattening the peristomal skin and apply even pressure around the stoma, causing it to protrude above the skin. Convexity is avail-able in both one- and two-piece appliance systems, and various degrees of convexity are also an option. All convex products should be used with a belt that will provide pressure to the convexity to enhance the appliance seal.

Once the etiology of the skin breakdown is determined and the appliance system chosen to correct the problem, the peristomal skin integrity is addressed. Denuded skin with minimal skin loss can be dusted lightly with a skin barrier powder, sealed with a no-sting liquid skin barrier and covered with the solid skin barrier of the appliance system. Severely involved peristomal skin can be treated with a steroid spray, which will not interfere with the appliance seal. When treating denuded peristomal skin, the appliance system generally needs to be changed every 2–3 days because the moisture generated by the peristomal skin breakdown will erode the adhesive seal.

Peristomal candidiasis is common at ostomy sites. The dark, moist area, together with the use of systemic corticosteroids and antibiotic therapy, can predispose the patient with an ostomy to an overgrowth of *Candida* on the peristomal skin. Achieving an adequate appliance seal is the first intervention, followed by the use of an antifungal powder to the affected area. Use of creams or ointments is contraindicated in the peristomal area as they will interfere with the appliance seal. The antifungal powder is sprinkled liberally on to the area, rubbed into the skin and the excess brushed off. The appliance system is applied and changed every 3 days until the peristomal skin has healed.

An uncommon but difficult peristomal problem is the development of pyoderma gangrenosum. The patient presents with very painful, irregularly shaped small ulcers, usually with purple margins. Tunneling from one ulcer to another may be present. Treatment may include pulsed systemic steroids, cyclosporin, infliximab, and topical preparations such as steroid pastes or tacrolimus ointment to decrease the inflammatory response.[14] The ulcers can be covered with a hydrofiber dressing and/or a small piece of thin hydrocolloid to assist in maintaining an appliance seal. The ulcers are full thickness and, once the involved area heals, scarring may produce an uneven scar in the peristomal area.

## ENTEROCUTANEOUS FISTULA

Enterocutaneous fistula presents a challenging clinical management situation. The fistula orifice is generally located below the skin surface, expelling output under or at the skin surface, causing skin breakdown and discomfort. If the amount of output from the fistula exceeds 100 mL/24 hours and contains a strong odor, it is recommended that the fistula be managed with an appliance system. The appliance system will collect drainage and protect the perifistular skin, allow for measurement of the drainage and control odor. Many of the appliances described above can be used to manage a fistula. Several companies manufacture appliances with solid extended wear skin barriers that allow customization to accommodate several irregularly shaped fistula openings. For high-output small bowel fistulae suction can be added to the appliance system to wick away the effluent and maintain the seal.

## SUMMARY

Achieving a successful outcome in patients with a fecal diversion requires a team approach; team members should include the patient and family, the surgeon, gastroenterologist, nutritional support staff, and the certified ostomy care nurse. By addressing the variables of stoma placement and construction and offering the patient the tools to manage and control the ostomy, the pieces should be in place to incorporate the ostomy into the patient's daily routine.

# RESOURCES

Wound, Ostomy and Continence Nurses Society
4700 W. Lake Avenue
Glenview, Illinois 60025, USA
1-888-224-WOCN
www.wocn.org
Resources available: certified WOC nursing educational programs, clinical fact sheets, clinical guidelines, WOC nurse referral database.

United Ostomy Association
36 Executive Park, Suite 120
Irvine, California 92714-6744, USA
1-800-826-0826
www.uoa.org
Resources: A volunteer-based health organization dedicated to assisting people who have had or will have intestinal or urinary diversions. Provides local support and educational chapters and satellites throughout the United States. Publishes the *Ostomy Quarterly* magazine. Offers preoperative and postoperative patient visiting and support and ostomy publications. Participates in advocacy activities and national, state and regional conferences.

Appliance manufacturers
Coloplast
1955 West Oak Circle
Marietta, GA 30062-2249, USA
1-800-533-0464
www.coloplast.com

ConvaTec
PO Box 5254
Princeton, NJ 08543-5254, USA
1-800-631-5244
www.convatec.com

Hollister Incorporated
2000 Hollister Drive
Libertyville, IL 60048, USA
1-800-323-4060
www.hollister.com

HyTape Surgical Products Corporation
772 McLean Avenue
Younkers, NY 10704, USA
1-800-248-0101

NuHope Laboratories Inc.
PO Box 331150
Pacoima, CA 91333, USA
1-800-899-5017
www.nu-hope.com

# References

1. Doughty D. Role of the enterostomal therapy nurse in ostomy patient rehabilitation. Cancer 1992;70:1390–1392.
2. Bryant RA. Ostomy patient management: care that engenders adaptation. Cancer Invest 1993;11:565–577.
3. O'Shea HS. Teaching the adult ostomy patient. J Wound Ostomy Continence Nursing 2001;28:47–54.
4. Bass EM, Del Pino A, Tan A et al. Does preoperative stoma marking and education by the enterostomal therapist affect outcome? Dis Colon Rectum1997;49:440–442.
5. Abcarian H, Pearl RK. Stomas. Surg Clin North Am 1988.68:1295–1305.
6. Erwin-Toth P, Barrett P. Stoma site marking: a primer. Ostomy/Wound Mgt 1997;43:18–23.
7. Pearl RK, Prasad ML, Orsay CP et al. A survey of technical considerations in the construction of intestinal stomas. Am Surg 1985;51:462–465.
8. Stephenson BM, Myers, C, Phillips RK. Minimally raised end colostomy. Int J Colorectal Dis 1995;10:232–233.
9. Colwell JC, Hurst RD. Ileostomy support bridge. Abstract presentation at Wound Ostomy and Continence Nurses Meeting, Nashville, TN, 1997.
10. Colwell, JC, Goldberg M, Carmel J. The state of the standard diversion. J Wound, Ostomy Continence Nursing 2001;28:6–17.
11. Wound, Ostomy and Continence Nurses Society. Guidelines for management: caring for a patient with an ostomy. Glenview (IL): The Society; 1998.
12. Golis AM. Sexual issues for the person with an ostomy. J Wound Ostomy Continence Nursing 1996;23:33–37.
13. Rolstad BS, Boarini J. Principles and techniques in the use of convexity. Ostomy/Wound Mgt 1996; 42:24–32.
14. Sheldon DB, Sawchuck LL, Kozarek RA, Thirlby RC. Twenty cases of peristomal pyoderma gangrenosum. Diagnostic implications and clinical management. Arch Surg 2000:135:568–569.

# SURGICAL THERAPY

## CHAPTER 43

# Cancer in inflammatory bowel disease – clinical considerations

Anders Ekbom and Robert Löfberg

## INTRODUCTION

Cancer morbidity and mortality are consistently increased in patients with inflammatory bowel disease in almost all published studies.[1-8] This is due almost entirely to an excess risk of intestinal cancers.[1,2,4,6-7] There is also an excess risk of smoking-related cancers in patients with Crohn's disease.[2] This is not surprising, bearing in mind that smoking is a risk factor[9] as well as a negative prognostic factor for Crohn's disease.[10] Thus, in addition to the beneficial effects of smoking cessation to the natural course of Crohn's disease, help from the treating physician towards a smoke-free life will have an impact on the overall cancer risk. This chapter will, however, focus on the clinical considerations with regard to gastrointestinal cancers in patients with ulcerative colitis and Crohn's disease.

## CHOLANGIOCARCINOMA

Around 4% of patients with extensive ulcerative colitis will eventually develop a clinically overt primary sclerosing cholangitis (PSC).[11] There is also reason to believe that patients with colonic Crohn's disease are at risk, although precise risk estimates are lacking.[12] In some instances a diagnosis of PSC will precede the diagnosis of ulcerative colitis. The duration of either ulcerative colitis or Crohn's disease does not seem to affect the risk of PSC. Patients with PSC are at risk for a malignant transformation of the bile ducts. There are reports that the cumulative incidence for such a malignant transformation is as high as 10% 10 years after a diagnosis of PSC.[13] The presence of a substantial cumulative risk is further underlined by the fact that there were malignant or premalignant changes in the bile duct in 30% of patients who underwent liver transplant for PSC.[14] The risk for cholangiocarcinoma is present both in patients in whom the disease is confined to the small bile ducts and in those where the disease has spread to the entire bile duct system.[14] A history of colectomy does not seem to affect the risk of cholangiocarcinoma.[13,14] However, there are indications that patients with prior malignancy or dysplasia in the colorectal tract are at an even higher risk for cholangiocarcinoma.[13] This could imply that there is a genotype in these patients, making them especially vulnerable for malignant transformation in areas with chronic inflammation, such as the colon or bile ducts.

In a clinical setting the treating physician should be aware of the risk of cholangiocarcinoma in patients with PSC. There are no known preventive measures, although there are some indications that long-term treatment with ursodeoxycholic acid (UDCA) may have a protective effect. Follow-up studies are in progress.[15] It is of the utmost importance that a liver transplant is considered early in patients with PSC in the case of any suspicion of malignant changes in the bile ducts. Special emphasis should probably be placed on patients with a history of prior colorectal malignancy. One can also discuss to what extent a prophylactic proctocolectomy is indicated in patients subjected to a liver transplant.

## CANCER OF THE SMALL INTESTINE

Cancer of the small intestine is a known complication in patients with Crohn's disease.[2,16-18] The relative risk estimate is as high as for cholangiocarcinoma in patients with ulcerative colitis[18] but, similar to cholangiocarcinoma, the cumulative incidence overall is small. The attributable fraction, on the other hand, for Crohn's disease in patients with cancer of the small intestine is high and has been assessed at around 20%;[19] it is the underlying reason for these high relative risk estimates. There are strong indications that a malignant transformation in the small intestine will occur in affected inflammatory areas, and it has been repeatedly proposed that a bypass procedure should make such patients especially vulnerable.[16] However, this is the result of a series of case reports and no observational data exist that have assessed to what extent a bypass procedure is an independent risk factor. Moreover, there are indications of a higher relative risk in the United States than in Sweden[3] or Israel.[20] It is therefore of interest that bypass procedures are less common in Sweden and Israel than in the US. Another area that deserves to be studied is to what extent the risk of small bowel cancer in patients with Crohn's disease is further aggravated following cholecystectomy. Cholecystectomy has recently been shown to be associated with an increased risk of small bowel cancer, and there is a gradient with a decreasing risk with increasing distance from the duodenum, indicating that exposure to bile or bile products is important for a malignant transformation.[21] Another area of concern is to what extent the introduction of minor surgery, including strictureplasty, as opposed to resection of the small intestine will lead to an even higher risk of cancer of the small intestine in patients with Crohn's disease. There is therefore a need for follow-up studies encompassing a long duration – perhaps more than 20 years – in order to evaluate this fairly new surgical approach.

In a clinical setting, the treating physician should be aware of the risk of malignant transformation in Crohn's disease patients with involvement of the small intestine. If indications of an aggravated disease, either clinically or on barium double-contrast follow-through, the cancer alternative should be considered. The potential role in screening/surveillance using the new small bowel endoscopic capsule device in the setting of Crohn's disease located to this area of the gut remains to be evaluated.

# ULCERATIVE COLITIS AND COLORECTAL CANCER

Colorectal cancer is the most important cause of the excess long-term mortality in patients with ulcerative colitis.[1,22] This was demonstrated in 1971 by Devroede et al. from the Mayo Clinic[22] and has since been confirmed in other studies. The study from the Mayo Clinic demonstrated that patients who underwent proctocolectomy had a substantially better long-term prognosis than patients left with an intact colon. Prophylactic proctocolectomy was therefore frequently advocated, and also sometimes performed in patients with ulcerative colitis during the 1970s and 1980s, but nowadays there is only limited support for this from patients and physicians. Great efforts have been made to identify those patients at the highest risk in order to identify subgroups where the option of a prophylactic proctocolectomy would be advocated. The following exposures have been addressed in different studies.

## TIME PERIOD

The literature shows a clear tendency for the risk estimates of malignant transformation to have changed over time. The highest risk estimates were in earlier studies.[22–24] The most recent studies, dealing with patients diagnosed during the 1970s, have consistently lower risk estimates,[25,26] the extreme being the patient groups followed up in Copenhagen.[25] This could be the result of methodological problems, as the earlier studies were probably more prone to selection bias. Another reason could be that surveillance programs where patients with precancerous changes are identified will have an impact on the risk of cancer. Data from Sweden, however, indicate that this is not the case, as only a minority of patients with ulcerative colitis are enrolled in surveillance programs.[27] Data from the Department of Pathology, Karolinska Hospital, have also demonstrated that the occurrence of combined ulcerative colitis/colorectal cancer has decreased over time after a peak during the 1950s and 1960s.[28] The notion that there are changes in the risk over time further emphasizes the need to identify correct comparison groups when assessing the risk of cancer in specific subgroups and to evaluate different types of intervention.

## EXTENT OF DISEASE

Extent of disease at the time of diagnosis is probably the most important risk factor for colorectal cancer patients with ulcerative colitis.[29–31] There are reasons to believe that the maximum extent of disease would probably be an even better predictor, but because of methodological problems this exposure has not been assessed as an independent factor. Another interesting notion is that the risk estimates for extent of disease are derived almost exclusively from patient groups where the extent was assessed by barium enema, which has a much lower sensitivity than endoscopy either alone or combined with histopathological examinations of the mucosa. Future follow-up studies of patient groups where the assessment of extent has been made by endoscopy, or even by histology, will therefore be of great interest and possibly lead to a better means of identifying patients at the highest risk.

Patients with proctitis do not seem to differ significantly in the risk of colorectal cancer compared to the general population, even after analyzing rectal cancer as an entity per se.[29] This indicates that it is not the inflammation as such, but that some additional exposure or factor is needed for a malignant transformation. This could be interpreted as meaning that proctitis is a disease with its own natural history that differs from a more extensive inflammation. In the case of left-sided colitis it is also obvious that the risk of a malignant transformation is lower than that for patients with pancolitis[29,31] and, as in the case of proctitis, also in the rectum. The increased risk of cancer in left-sided colitis could also be because left-sided colitis comprises different subgroups, of which one constitutes those patients in whom the disease will progress to pancolitis.

## DURATION

In all studies, with the exception of the experience from Copenhagen,[25] an increase in excess risk has been found by duration since diagnosis. The first 10 years after onset are not associated with any clinically relevant increase, but thereafter the risk of colorectal cancer emerges as a clinically relevant problem. There are very few studies with long follow-up (more than 30–40 years) and these have a low precision in their risk estimates because of low statistical power.[22,29] There are, however, indications that the longer the follow-up, the higher the risk estimates in both relative and absolute terms, because cumulative incidence of colorectal cancer of 30–40% has been demonstrated in at least two studies with a follow-up of 30–40 years.[22,29] It is also uncertain to what extent we can extrapolate the results of patients diagnosed during the 1940s and 1950s to those diagnosed during the 1970s and 1980s. The latter have a much better long-term survival,[32] and patients surviving during the last 20–30 years may have different characteristics with regard to the risk of malignant transformation than those diagnosed in the 1940s and 1950s.

There is therefore a great need to obtain a better assessment of the magnitude of the long-term risk, and this is an arena where future clinical research should be focused.

## AGE AT ONSET

In the study by Devroede et al.[22] the study base was confined to patients under 15 years of age at the time of diagnosis. In this subgroup there was a cumulative incidence of colorectal cancer of 43% 35 years after diagnosis, very similar to the results from a study from Sweden, where a cumulative incidence of 40% was found 35 years after diagnosis in the same age group.[29] No other age group has been found to have such a cumulative risk, and this indicates that young age at diagnosis could possibly be an independent risk factor. One alternative explanation for this high risk estimate could be that patients diagnosed with pancolitis at such a young age are not diluted by other subgroups of patients with a phenotype similar to that of ulcerative colitis. Furthermore, young age at onset will also lead to a longer duration of ulcerative colitis. If the risk of malignant transformation is mainly due to duration of disease, this patient group will, when they reach the cancer-prone age (over the age of 60), belong to a group that should be targeted for vigilant surveillance. Although it has been proposed that patients with ulcerative colitis reach a maximum risk for developing colorectal cancer at the age of approximately 50,[33] there are very few data to support such a hypothesis. On the contrary, results both from Sweden and the United States indicate that even after the age of 70, patients with long-standing ulcerative colitis have an increased risk compared to the general population in both absolute and relative terms.[29,31]

## PRIMARY SCLEROSING CHOLANGITIS

As mentioned above, primary sclerosing cholangitis constitutes a special clinical problem, including implications as to the risk of colorectal cancer. Already at the beginning of the 1990s there were reports that there was a high risk for both dysplasia and colorectal cancer in patients with ulcerative colitis and primary sclerosing cholangitis compared to patients with ulcerative colitis only.[34,35] Such an association has been confirmed in later studies[36,37] with one exception.[38] The absence of a positive association in that study could be the result of historical comparison groups which, as mentioned above, can skew the results. Although an underestimation of the duration of the disease could, to some extent, explain the high risk estimates in patients with primary sclerosing cholangitis, this patient group warrants special monitoring, for the potential of cancer not only in the bile ducts but also in the colorectal tract.

## FAMILY HISTORY OF COLORECTAL CANCER

Both animal studies[39] and observational studies[40,41] have demonstrated that a family history of colorectal cancer is an independent risk factor for malignant transformation in both ulcerative colitis and Crohn's disease. This seems to be of a magnitude of a twofold increase, but is even higher if a patient has a first-degree relative with colorectal cancer diagnosed under the age of 50.[41] On the other hand, a family history of inflammatory bowel disease does not seem to affect the risk.[42] Thus, an assessment of a family history of colorectal cancer should be included in normal clinical practice in patients with IBD, and those with such a history should be of special concern.

## PHARMACOTHERAPY

In the 1980s researchers in Israel speculated that the low incidence of colorectal cancer in their patients could be due to maintenance therapy with sulfasalazine.[43] A similar explanation has also been proposed from Copenhagen, where patients have been subjected to an extremely thorough follow-up clinically, also characterized by a consistent maintenance therapy mainly with sulfasalazine.[25] In a study where the effects of colonoscopic surveillance programs in the UK were evaluated[44] the authors found that 'A review of the notes of our cancer patients suggests that virtually none of them were taking disease suppressive drugs, such as sulfasalazine, regularly or at all.'

The hypothesis that anti-inflammatory therapies such as sulfasalazine may act as a protective factor against malignant transformation has been put to the test in three independent observational studies.[45–47] The results have been consistent, with a substantially lower risk following maintenance therapy with compounds such as sulfasalazine or mesalazine. Similar results have also been demonstrated in the United States, where sulfa allergy has been found to be an independent risk factor for malignant transformation in patients with ulcerative colitis.[48]

## CLINICAL IMPLICATIONS

The treating physician facing the problem of colorectal cancer in patients with ulcerative colitis has, in essence, three different options: prophylactic proctocolectomy; watchful waiting, monitoring the clinical course of the patient and being aware that new symptoms could be the result of the underlying malignancy; or colonoscopic surveillance. In discussing the last option, one must start by stating the obvious: there is no point in performing surveillance colonoscopy if the patient will refuse to have a proctocolectomy if the test is positive. Using the surveillance approach, patients selected for a prophylactic proctocolectomy will only be those who would subsequently develop colorectal cancer. The goal of a surveillance program is to decrease colorectal cancer morbidity and eliminate the excess mortality due to this malignancy.[49]

Premalignant polypoid changes associated with colorectal cancer in ulcerative colitis were recognized as early as the late 1950s[50] and were subsequently also described in flat mucosa.[51] Cellular atypia and certain structural changes, particularly villous changes in the surface epithelium, were considered the most important findings. A detailed definition and grading classification of these epithelial changes, designated dysplasia, were performed in 1983.[52] Dysplasia, defined as 'unequivocal neoplastic changes' of the epithelium, is subclassified as indefinite or definite (i.e. low- or high-grade dysplasia, LGD or HGD) based on the extent and severity of the epithelial lesions.[52] The concept of dysplasia incorporates the assumption that there is a stepwise neoplastic transformation of the epithelium, from early changes via LGD and HGD into invasive carcinoma. The presence of macroscopic lesions, i.e. sessile-type or raised plaque-like or nodular lesions, in dysplastic mucosa (so called DALM – dysplasia-associated lesion or mass) in ulcerative colitis has been found to be associated with the presence or subsequent findings of invasive carcinoma.[53] Mucosal dysplasia has been found in up to 80% of patients with ulcerative colitis who later develop colorectal cancer,[54] and the likelihood of finding dysplasia in flat mucosa or solitary or widespread lesions preceding the development of invasive carcinoma in ulcerative colitis forms the mainstay of colonoscopic surveillance.

There are no randomized clinical trials comparing surveillance programs with other options, and the evaluation of the impact of such programs has to rely on observational data and case series. There are some methodological problems with such an approach:

1. **'The healthy worker effect'.** Patients enrolled into surveillance programs have been subjected to clinical evaluation including barium enema and/or colonoscopy before entering such a program. This is probably to a lesser extent true for patients choosing not to participate or who are being left outside a surveillance program. This means that patients within the surveillance program will consist of those who are healthy survivors until the time of recruitment, creating difficulties in comparing those within with those outside surveillance programs.
2. **Surveillance bias.** In such a setting as described above it is impossible to assess the prevalence of neoplastic lesions or early-stage colon cancer which has not manifested itself with any symptoms in the non-surveillance group. Thus, any comparison in the frequency of neoplastic lesions in the surveillance group compared to the non-surveillance group will be biased and misleading.
3. **Selection bias.** As mentioned above, maintenance therapy with anti-inflammatory drugs such as sulfasalazine or mesalazine seems to lower the risk of malignant transformation. There is reason to believe that compliance with maintenance therapy is higher in patients who stay within a surveillance program than in those outside such a program.

The first program for surveillance of high-risk patients was pioneered in the early 1970s at St Mark's Hospital[55] and was followed by several other programs in Europe and the US. There have, however, been great differences in the number of patients included, the completeness of colonoscopy, biopsy sampling, criteria for colectomy, length and completeness of follow-up, and also in patient compliance. All these factors have rendered evaluation and direct comparisons among the programs difficult. Table 43.1 presents the sensitivities and specificities from 11 large programs.[56–66] Sensitivity is defined as the proportion of patients with cancer who survived following colectomy, and specificity is

defined as the proportion of patients without cancer who did not develop dysplasia. From this table one can conclude that the specificity from surveillance programs is approximately 85%. Sensitivity is much harder to assess owing to the low number of cancers in these programs, but in most instances it exceeds 50%.

The search for alternative markers to replace (or enhance) dysplasia has hitherto failed to find a tool that is better, more sensitive, more reliable, and early in the course of neoplastic transformation of the colorectal mucosa in UC. The findings of gross chromosomal changes – aneuploidy – in cell nuclei using flow cytometry has been proved more reliable and associated with less observer variability than dysplasia assessed by pathologists. However, this method is technically more demanding and single findings are difficult to interpret. Other methods, including immunohistochemistry (e.g. P53 staining, proliferation markers), gene analyses or various enzyme assessments (e.g. sphingomyelinase) are still experimental.

Another attempt to evaluate the impact of colonoscopy surveillance in ulcerative colitis was made in Sweden, where exposure to a colonoscopic surveillance program was associated with a substantially reduced risk of death in colorectal cancer.[27] The results of decision analysis studies also indicate that if the threshold for surgery is low-grade dysplasia the surveillance will convey the same life expectancy as an early prophylactic colectomy.[67] Although those types of study have obvious limitations, they still indicate that surveillance is the most appropriate approach to decrease the increased risk of colorectal cancer, but then expedient action has to be taken if definite dysplasia is detected.

In conclusion, if colonoscopic surveillance is selected as the preferred method the optimal time to initiate such a program is around 10 years after onset. Patients should be fully informed about the possible consequences of a finding of dysplasia. It is also important to adhere to a strict protocol with predefined criteria for surgery, such as the finding of high-grade dysplasia, DALM or repeated low-grade dysplasia in multiple biopsy locations.

## COLORECTAL CANCER IN CROHN'S DISEASE

The risk of colorectal cancer in patients with Crohn's disease has previously been regarded as less of a problem than in patients

**Table 43.1 The sensitivity and specificity of 11 large colorectal cancer surveillance programs in ulcerative colitis patients**

|  | Year | Number | Sensitivity | Specificity |
|---|---|---|---|---|
| University of Leeds[56] | 1980 | 43 | 2/2 (100%) | 34/41 (83%) |
| Cleveland Clinic[57] | 1985 | 248 | 6/7 (86%) | 194/241 (80%) |
| University of Chicago[58] | 1989 | 99 | 4/8 (50%) | 73/91 (80%) |
| Karolinska Institutet[59] | 1990 | 72 | 2/2 (100%) | 54/70 (77%) |
| Lahey Clinic[60] | 1991 | 213 | 4/10 (40%) | 171/203 (84%) |
| Helsinki University[61] | 1991 | 66 | 0/0 — | 57/66 (86%) |
| Lennox Hill Hospital[62] | 1992 | 121 | 4/7 (57%) | 91/114 (80%) |
| St. Mark's Hospital[63] | 1994 | 284 | 13/17 (76%) | 205/267 (77%) |
| Ornskoldsvik Hospital[64] | 1994 | 131 | 2/4 (50%) | 103/127 (81 %) |
| Tel Aviv Medical Center[65] | 1995 | 154 | 3/4 (75%) | 41/150 (94%) |
| University of Bologna[66] | 1995 | 65 | 4/4 (100%) | 58/61 (95%) |

with ulcerative colitis. However, one should bear in mind that Crohn's disease, especially the colonic variety, is a relatively new disease and there are strong indications that the risk profile for patients with colonic Crohn's disease is very similar to that for patients with ulcerative colitis. Duration of disease, age at onset and extent seem to be independent risk factors.[8,68–70] Thus there are reasons to believe that colorectal cancer in patients with Crohn's disease is an emerging clinical problem that will increase during the decades to come, and further research is urgently needed in order to identify these patients and also to assess the impact of different screening procedures and to what extent anti-inflammatory pharmacotherapy will have an impact on the risk.

## CLINICAL IMPLICATIONS

In 1994, Sachar[71] stated in an editorial in *Gut* that 'Whatever you choose to do for your patients with ulcerative colitis, do no differently for those with Crohn's colitis with similar duration and extent.' There is, however, one problem with such an approach: the sequence dysplasia–cancer. This has been reported to be less frequent in Crohn's disease than in ulcerative colitis, and the presence of strictures can complicate the examination to an extent which is not common in patients with ulcerative colitis.[72]

In conclusion, gastrointestinal cancer as a complication in patients with inflammatory bowel disease is a problem facing any physician responsible for this patient group. Future research is needed to better identify the characteristics of such patients, but there is reason to believe that continuous maintenance and anti-inflammatory therapy should be recommended, and so far, apart from proctocolectomy, colonoscopic surveillance is the only strategy that will have any impact on the risk of colorectal cancer.

## References

1. Ekbom A, Helmick CG, Zack M, Holmberg L, Adami HO. Survival and causes of death in patients with inflammatory bowel disease: a population-based study. Gastroenterology 1992;103:954–960.
2. Persson PG, Karlen P, Bernell O et al. Crohn's disease and cancer: a population-based cohort study. Gastroenterology 1994;107:1675–1679.
3. Ekbom A, Helmick C, Zack M, Adami HO. Extracolonic malignancies in inflammatory bowel disease. Cancer 1991;67:2015–2019.
4. Fielding JF, Prior P, Waterhouse JA, Cooke WT. Malignancy in Crohn's disease. Scand J Gastroenterol 1972;7:3–7.
5. Greenstein J, Gennuso R, Sachar DB et al. Extraintestinal cancers in inflammatory bowel disease. Cancer 1985;56:2914–2921.
6. Mir-Madjlessi SH, Farmer RG, Easly KA, Beck GJ. Colorectal cancer and extra-colonic malignancies in ulcerative colitis. Cancer 1986;58:1569–1574.
7. Prior P, Gyde S, Macartney JC, Thompson H, Waterhouse JAH, Allan RN. Cancer morbidity in ulcerative colitis. Gut 1982;23:490–497.
8. Gyde SN, Prior P, Macartney JC, Thompson H, Waterhouse JAH, Allan RN. Malignancy in Crohn's disease. Gut 1980;21:1024–1029.
9. Benoni C, Nilsson Å. Smoking habits in patients with inflammatory bowel disease. Scand J Gastroenterol 1987;125:445–452.
10. Cottone M, Rosselli M, Orlando A et al. Smoking habits and recurrence in Crohn's disease. Gastroenterology 1994;106:643–648.
11. Olsson R, Danielsson Å, Järnerot G et al. Prevalence of primary sclerosing cholangitis in patients with ulcerative colitis. Gastroenterology 1991;100:1319–1323.
12. Choi PM, Nugent FW, Zelig MP, Munson JL, Schoetz DJ. Cholangiocarcinoma and Crohn's disease. Dig Dis Sci 1994;39:667–670.
13. Kornfeld D, Ekbom A, Ihre T. Survival and risk of cholangiocarcinoma in patients with primary sclerosing cholangitis – a population-based study. Scand J Gastroenterol 1997;32:1042–1045.
14. Broomé U, Olsson R, Lööf L et al. Natural history and prognostic factors in 305 Swedish patients with primary sclerosing cholangitis. Gut 1996;38:610–615.
15. Olsson R. Ursodeoxycholic acid for the treatment of cholestatic liver disease. Resulting delay in disease progression inspires hope. Läkartidningen 2002;99:1325–1330.
16. Senay E, Sachar DB, Keohane M, Greenstein AJ. Small bowel carcinoma in Crohn's disease. Distinguishing features and risk factors. Cancer 1989;63:360–363.
17. Greenstein AJ, Sachar DB, Smith H, Janowitz HD, Aufses AH. A comparison of cancer risk in Crohn's disease and ulcerative colitis. Cancer 1981;48:2742–2745.
18. Munkholm P, Langholz E, Davidsen M, Binder V. Intestinal cancer risk and mortality in patients with Crohn's disease. Gastroenterology 1993;105:1716–1723.
19. Chen CC, Neugut AI, Rotterdam H. Risk factors for adenocarcinomas and malignant carcinoids of the small intestine: preliminary findings. Cancer Epidemiol Biomarkers Prev 1994;3:205–207.
20. Fireman Z, Grosman A, Lilos P et al. Intestinal cancer in patients with Crohn's disease. A population study in central Israel. Scand J Gastroenterol 1989;24:346–350.
21. Lagergren J, Ye W, Ekbom A. Intestinal cancer after cholecystectomy: is bile involved in carcinogenesis? Gastroenterology 2001;121:542–547.
22. Devroede GJ, Taylor WF, Saucer WG, Jackman RJ, Stickler GB. Cancer risk and life expectancy of children with ulcerative colitis. N Engl J Med 1971;285:17–21.
23. Edwards FC, Truelove SC. The course and prognosis of ulcerative colitis. IV. Carcinoma of the colon. Gut 1964;5:15–22.
24. Kewenter J, Ahlman H, Hulten L. Cancer risk in extensive ulcerative colitis. Ann Surg 1978;188:824–828.
25. Langholtz E, Munkholm P, Davidsen M, Binder V. Colorectal cancer risk and mortality in patients with ulcerative colitis. Gastroenterology 1992;103:1444–1451.
26. Mellemkjaer L, Olsen JH, Frisch M, Johansen C, Gridley G, McLaughlin JK. Cancer in patients with ulcerative colitis. Int J Cancer 1995;60:330–333.
27. Karlén P, Kornfeld D, Broström O, Löfberg R, Persson PG, Ekbom A. Is colonoscopic surveillance reducing colorectal cancer mortality in ulcerative colitis? A population-based case–control study. Gut 1998;42:711–714.
28. Rubio CA, Befrits R, Ljung T, Jaramillo E, Slezak P. Colorectal carcinoma in ulcerative colitis is decreasing in Scandinavian countries. Anticancer Res 2001;21:2921–2924.
29. Ekbom A, Helmick C, Zack M, Adami HO. Ulcerative colitis and colorectal cancer. A population-based study. N Engl J Med 1990;323:1228–1233.
30. Stewenius J, Adnerhill I, Anderson H et al. Incidence of colorectal cancer and all cause mortality in non-selected patients with ulcerative colitis and indeterminate colitis in Malmö, Sweden. Int J Colorectal Dis 1995;10:117–122.
31. Sugita A, Sachar DB, Bodian C, Aufses AH Jr, Greenstein AJ. Colorectal cancer in ulcerative colitis. Influence on anatomical extent and age at onset on colitis–cancer interval. Gut 1991;32:167–169.
32. Edwards FC, Truelove SC. The course and prognosis of ulcerative colitis. Part I. Short-term prognosis. Gut 1963;4:299–308.
33. Gyde SN, Prior P, Allan RN et al. Colorectal cancer in ulcerative colitis: a cohort study of primary referrals from three centres. Gut 1988;29:206–217.
34. Broomé U, Lindberg G, Löfberg R. Primary sclerosing cholangitis in ulcerative colitis: a risk factor for the development of dysplasia and DNA-aneuploidy? Gastroenterology 1992;102:1877–1880.
35. D'Haens GR, Lashner BA, Hanauer SB. Pericholangitis and sclerosing cholangitis are risk factors for dysplasia and cancer in ulcerative colitis. Am J Gastroenterol 1993;88:1174–1178.
36. Brentnall TA, Haggitt RC, Rabinovitch PS et al. Risk and natural history of colonic neoplasia in patients with primary sclerosing cholangitis and ulcerative colitis. Gastroenterology 1996;110:331–338.
37. Kornfeld D, Ekbom A, Ihre T. Is there an excess risk for colorectal cancer in patients with ulcerative colitis and concomitant primary sclerosing cholangitis? A population based study. Gut 1997;41:522–525.
38. Loftus EV Jr, Sandborn WJ, Tremaine WJ et al. Risk of colorectal neoplasia in patients with primary sclerosing cholangitis. Gastroenterology 1996;110:432–440.
39. Bertone ER, Giovannucci EL, King NW Jr, Petto AJ, Johnson LD. Family history as a risk factor for ulcerative colitis-associated colon cancer in cotton-top tamarin. Gastroenterology 1998;114:669–674.
40. Nuako KW, Ahlquist DA, Mahoney DW, Schaid DJ, Siems DM, Lindor NM. Familial predisposition for colorectal cancer in chronic ulcerative colitis: a case–control study. Gastroenterology 1998;115:1079–1083.
41. Askling J, Dickman PW, Karlén P et al. Family history as a risk factor for cancer in inflammatory bowel disease. Gastroenterology 2001;120:1356–1362.
42. Askling J, Dickman PW, Karlén P et al. Colorectal cancer rates among first-degree relatives of patients with inflammatory bowel disease: a population-based cohort study. Lancet 2001;357:262–266.
43. Odes HS, Fraser D. Ulcerative colitis in Israel: epidemiology, morbidity and genetics. Public Health Rev 1989–1990;17:297–319.
44. Lynch DAF, Lobo AJ, Sobala GM, Dixon MF, Axon ATR. Failure of colonoscopic surveillance in ulcerative colitis. Gut 1993;34:1075–1080.
45. Pinczowski D, Ekbom A, Baron J, Yuen J, Adami HO. Risk factors for colorectal cancer among patients with ulcerative colitis – a case–control study. Gastroenterology 1994;107:117–120.
46. Moody GA, Jayanthi V, Probert CS, Mac Kay H, Mayberry JF. Long-term therapy with sulphasalazine protects against colorectal cancer in ulcerative colitis: a retrospective study

of colorectal cancer risk and compliance with treatment in Leicestershire. Eur J Gastroenterol Hepatol 1996;8:1179–1183.

47. Eaden J, Abrams K, Ekbom A, Jackson E, Mayberry J. Colorectal cancer prevention in ulcerative colitis: a case–control study. Aliment Pharmacol Ther 2000;14:145–153.

48. Lashner BA, Heidenreich PA, Su GL, Kane SV, Hanauer SB. Effect of folate supplementation on the incidence of dysplasia and cancer in chronic ulcerative colitis. A case–control study. Gastroenterology 1989;97:255–259.

49. Zack MM, Ekbom A, Persson PG, Adami HO. Evaluation of surveillance programs for colorectal cancer in ulcerative colitis patients by case–control studies: Methodological considerations. J Med Screening 1997;4:137–141.

50. Dawson IMP, Pryse-Davies J. The development of carcinoma in the large intestine in ulcerative colitis. Br J Surg 1959;47:113–128.

51. Morson BC, Pang LSC. Rectal biopsy as an aid to cancer control in ulcerative colitis. Gut 1967; 8:423–434.

52. Riddell RH, Goldman H, Ransohoff DF et al. Dysplasia in inflammatory bowel disease. Standardized classification with provisional clinical applications. Hum Pathol 1983;14:931–966.

53. Blackstone MO, Riddell RH, Rogers BHG, Levin B. Dysplasia associated lesion or mass (DALM) detected by colonoscopy in longstanding ulcerative colitis. An indication for colectomy. Gastroenterology 1981;80: 366–374.

54. Connell WR, Talbot IC, Harpaz N et al. Clinicopathological characteristics of colorectal carcinoma complicating ulcerative colitis. Gut 1994;35:1419–1423.

55. Lennard-Jones JE, Misiewicz JJ, Parrish JA, Ritchie JK, Swarbrick ET, Williams CB. Prospective study of outpatients with extensive colitis. Lancet 1974;i:1065–1067.

56. Dickenson RJ, Dixon MF, Axon ATR. Colonoscopy and the detection of dysplasia in patients with longstanding ulcerative colitis. Lancet 1980;2:620–622.

57. Rosenstock E, Farmer RG, Petras R, Sivak MV, Rankin GB, Sullivan BH. Surveillance for colonic carcinoma in ulcerative colitis. Gastroenterology 1985;89:1342–1346.

58. Lashner BA, Silverstein MD, Hanauer SB. Hazard rates for dysplasia and cancer in ulcerative colitis: results from a surveillance program. Dig Dis Sci 1989;34:1536–1541.

59. Lofberg R, Brostrom O, Karlen P, Tribukait B, Ost A. Colonoscopic surveillance in long-standing ulcerative colitis – a 15-year follow-up study. Gastroenterology 1990;99:1021–1031.

60. Nugent FW, Haggitt RC, Gilpin PA. Cancer surveillance in ulcerative colitis. Gastroenterology 1991;100:1241–1248.

61. Leidenius M, Kellokumpu I, Husa A, Riihela M, Sipponen P. Dysplasia and carcinoma in longstanding ulcerative colitis: an endoscopic and histologic surveillance program. Gut 1991;32:1521–1525.

62. Woolrich AJ, DaSilva MD, Korelitz BI. Surveillance in the routine management of ulcerative colitis: the predictive value of low-grade dysplasia. Gastroenterology 1992;103:431–438.

63. Connell WR, Lennard-Jones JE, Williams CD, Talbot IC, Price AB, Wilkinson KH. Factors affecting the outcomes of endoscopic surveillance for cancer in ulcerative colitis. Gastroenterology 1994;107:934–944.

64. Jonsson B, Ahsgren L, Andersson LO, Sterling R, Rutegard J. Colorectal cancer survival in patients with ulcerative colitis. Br J Surg 1994;81:689–691.

65. Rozen P, Baratz M, Fefer F, Gilat T. Low incidence of significant dysplasia in a successful endoscopic surveillance program of patients with ulcerative colitis. Gastroenterology 1995;108:1361–1370.

66. Biasco G, Brandi G, Paganelli GM et al. Colorectal cancer in patients with ulcerative colitis: A prospective cohort study in Italy. Cancer 1995;75:2045–2050.

67. Provenzale D, Kowdley KV, Arora S, Wong JB. Prophylactic colectomy or surveillance for chronic ulcerative colitis? A decision analysis. Gastroenterology 1995;109:1188–1196.

68. Ekbom A, Helmick C, Zack M, Adami HO. Increased risk of large bowel cancer in Crohn's disease with colonic involvement. Lancet 1990;336:357–359.

69. Gillen CD, Andrews HA, Prior P, Allan RN. Crohn's disease and colorectal cancer. Gut 1994; 35:651–655.

70. Choi PM, Zelig MP. Similarity of colorectal cancer in Crohn's disease and ulcerative colitis: implications for carcinogenesis and prevention. Gut 1994;35:950–954.

71. Sachar D. Cancer in Crohn's disease: dispelling the myths. Gut 1994;35:1507–1508.

72. Yamazaki Y, Ribeiro MB, Sachar DB, Aufses AH Jr, Greenstein AJ. Malignant colorectal strictures in Crohn's disease. Am J Gastroenterol 1991;86:882–885.

## CHAPTER 44

# Primary sclerosing cholangitis

Paul Angulo and Keith D Lindor

## INTRODUCTION

Primary sclerosing cholangitis (PSC) is a chronic cholestatic liver disease of unknown etiology that is frequently associated with inflammatory bowel disease (IBD). PSC is characterized by diffuse inflammation and fibrosis of the biliary tree and usually leads to biliary cirrhosis, which may be complicated by portal hypertension and liver failure. PSC was first described in 1924, and prior to the widespread availability of endoscopic retrograde cholangiography (ERC) in the late 1970s it was considered to be a rare disease.[1,2] PSC is one of the most common chronic cholestatic liver diseases in adults and is increasingly being diagnosed in children and adolescents.[3] The recognized common association of PSC with IBD, along with the screening of IBD patients with liver tests, has probably increased the frequency with which the diagnosis of PSC is made today. This greater recognition of the disease and increased experience has led to a better understanding of the natural history of PSC, although its pathogenesis remains hypothetical and the identification of specific beneficial therapies have eluded investigators so far.

## PREVALENCE

The true prevalence of PSC is unknown and the worldwide geographic distribution is still undefined. Based on a number of past cross-sectional studies PSC is found in 2.4–7.8% of patients with ulcerative colitis and in 1–3.4% of patients with Crohn's disease[4–9] (Table 44.1). More than 70% of patients with PSC reported from the United States and western European countries suffer also from IBD[9–19] (Table 44.2). However, about 50% of patients with PSC reported from other countries, such as Italy, Spain and India, suffer also from IBD, whereas the prevalence of IBD is as low as 20% among Japanese patients with PSC (Table 44.2). Hence, the prevalence of PSC can be estimated based on its association with IBD. The prevalence of ulcerative colitis ranges from 400 to 2200 cases per million.[20] We can then use these ranges to estimate the prevalence of PSC to be 10–165 cases per million in the United States population. An epidemiologic study from Norway[16] reported an annual incidence of 13 cases of PSC per million population and a point prevalence of 85 cases of PSC per million population. A study from Sweden[12] reported 75 cases per million population. These figures, however, clearly underestimate the real prevalence of PSC, as some cases can occur with normal alkaline phosphatase levels and hence may be subclinical.[21,22] Furthermore, many patients with PSC will not have IBD and hence would not be captured with these estimates.

Crohn's disease involving only the small bowel has not been reported in patients with PSC. There is no clear-cut temporal association between the diagnosis of PSC and the diagnosis of IBD, although in general the diagnosis of IBD is usually established before the liver disease is evident. Certainly there are well-documented cases of IBD occurring years after a diagnosis of PSC has been established. Similarly, patients have developed PSC many years after a proctocolectomy for colitis. The bowel disease pattern in patients with colitis and PSC is one of relatively quiescent disease; however, it is important to point out that the risk of developing colon cancer in patients with ulcerative colitis and PSC seems to be substantially greater than if patients did not have PSC. There has been no association between the severity of the bowel disease and the severity of the liver disease, and treatment of the bowel disease does not affect the liver disease. The most aggressive treatment for the bowel disease, proctocolectomy, has had no effect on PSC.

## CLINICAL FEATURES

### CLINICAL MANIFESTATIONS

PSC can affect any age range and has been described in most ethnic groups. It usually occurs in men twice as commonly as in

**Table 44.1 Prevalence of primary sclerosing cholangitis among patients with inflammatory bowel disease**

| Region | Author (ref.) | Year | Inflammatory bowel disease (n) | Prevalence of PSC in ulcerative colitis(%) | Crohn's disease(%) |
|---|---|---|---|---|---|
| Norway | Schrumpf[4] | 1980 | 336 | 4.0 | – |
| United Kingdom | Shepherd[5] | 1983 | 681 | 2.4 | – |
| South Africa | Tobias[6] | 1983 | 414 | 3.0 | 1.2 |
| Sweden | Olsson[7] | 1991 | 1500 | 3.7 | – |
| Denmark | Rasmussen[8] | 1997 | 262 | – | 3.4 |
| United States | Angulo[9] | 2002 | 3285 | 7.8 | 1.0 |

PSC, primary sclerosing cholangitis.

**Table 44.2 Prevalence of inflammatory bowel disease among patients with primary sclerosing cholangitis**

| Region | Author (ref.) | Year | Primary sclerosing cholangitis(n) | Inflammatory bowel disease(%) |
|---|---|---|---|---|
| United Kingdom | Chapman[10] | 1980 | 29 | 72 |
| Spain | Escorsell[11] | 1994 | 43 | 47 |
| Sweden | Broome[12] | 1996 | 305 | 81 |
| Italy | Okolicsanyi[13] | 1996 | 117 | 54 |
| India | Kockbar[14] | 1996 | 18 | 50 |
| Japan | Takikawa[15] | 1997 | 192 | 21 |
| Norway | Boberg[16] | 1998 | 17 | 71 |
| Germany | Stiehl[17] | 2002 | 106 | 66 |
| Western Europe | Boberg[18] | 2002 | 330 | 83 |
| Sweden | Bergquist[19] | 2002 | 604 | 79 |
| United States | Angulo[9] | 2002 | 434 | 70 |

women.[10,23,24] The average age of diagnosis is in the 30s to early 40s, with a wide range from 1 to 90 years. PSC is often identified in asymptomatic patients who come to attention solely because of abnormal liver tests. In symptomatic patients the most common symptoms are fatigue and abdominal pain, although some patients complaint of itching, fever and weight loss. Jaundice or manifestations of portal hypertension found in advanced stages of liver disease are uncommon presenting manifestations. Physical examination may be unrevealing. Hepatomegaly, splenomegaly, hyperpigmentation and excoriations can be found, but patients now are coming to medical attention earlier, with a diagnosis established before some of the physical findings of more advanced liver disease have developed. Health-related quality of life is significantly impaired in patients with PSC compared to a normal population, although it is similarly affected as in other chronic liver diseases such as PBC and chronic hepatitis B or C virus infection.[25,26] PSC in patients with IBD is not significantly different from that found in those who do not suffer from IBD. A variety of diseases, mostly with an autoimmune basis apart from inflammatory bowel disease, have been associated with patients with PSC, as listed in Table 44.3.

## LABORATORY ABNORMALITIES

Chronic cholestasis of at least 6 months' duration is the biochemical hallmark. However, the biochemical findings are non-

**Table 44.3 Disease associated with primary sclerosing cholangitis**

| | |
|---|---|
| Inflammatory bowel disease | Acute pancreatitis |
| Chronic pancreatitis | Celiac disease |
| Rheumatoid arthritis | Retroperitoneal fibrosis |
| Peyronie's disease | Riedel's thyroiditis |
| Bronchiectasis | Sjögren's sclerosis |
| Autoimmune chronic active hepatitis | Glomerulonephritis |
| Systemic lupus erythematosus | Pseudotumor of the orbit |
| Vasculitis | Autoimmune hemolytic anemia |
| Immune thrombocytopenic purpura | Angioimmunoblastic lymphadenopathy |
| Histiocytosis X | Cystic fibrosis |
| Gallbladder disease | Eosinophilia |
| Intra-abdominal lymphadenopathy | Sarcoidosis |
| Systemic mastocytosis | Polymyositis |
| Alopecia universalis | Pyostomatitis vegetans |
| Thymoma | Ankylosing spondylitis |

specific. Alkaline phosphatase and γ-glutamyl transferase (GGT) are the most commonly elevated liver tests and are often more prominently elevated than aminotransferase levels. However, the occasional patient with well-documented PSC but with normal alkaline phosphatase levels has been described.[21,22] Mildly to moderately elevated aminotransferase levels are frequently found. Serum bilirubin levels and prothrombin time are usually normal, but they may be slightly elevated in some patients, or reach very high levels in patients with advanced disease and in those with dominant stricturing of the main bile ducts. Low serum albumin levels suggest that a more advanced liver disease with cirrhosis is present.

PSC in children may occur with features of autoimmune hepatitis,[27,28] and sometimes with markedly elevated levels of serum aminotransferases. Furthermore, the serum alkaline phosphatase activity may be in the normal range in a quarter[29] to a half[28] of children with PSC; an invasive cholangiography is therefore mandatory for diagnostic purposes. Interestingly, GGT is elevated in almost all children with PSC who present with normal alkaline phosphatase activity,[29] suggesting that GGT may be a more reliable biochemical abnormality than alkaline phosphatase in children with PSC. The overlap of PSC and autoimmune hepatitis is an uncommon finding in adults with PSC, occurring in less than 10% of patients.[30–32]

## IMMUNOLOGIC TESTING

Hypergammaglobulinemia occurs in about 25% of patients, with IgM levels being the most commonly elevated component.[23] PSC is associated with a high proportion of non-organ specific autoantibodies whose relevance in the pathogenesis of PSC remains uncertain.[33] The most common autoantibodies found in patients with PSC are antineutrophil nuclear antibody with a peripheral nuclear labeling (pANNA), formerly named atypical perinuclear antineutrophil cytoplasmic antibody (atypical pANCA). These antibodies are found in 33%[34] to 88%[35] of patients with PSC. The target antigen for this antibody has recently being recognized as being a neutrophil nuclear envelope protein with a molecular mass of approximately 50 kDa, and thus it has been recommended that these antibodies be referred to as pANNA instead of pANCA.[36] pANNA are not specific for PSC: they are found in 60–87% of patients with ulcerative colitis alone, in 5–25% of patients with Crohn's disease, in 50–96% of patients with autoimmune hepatitis, and in 5% of patients with primary biliary cirrhosis. Antinuclear antibodies are found in a half of patients with PSC, whereas antismooth muscle antibodies are found in about 15% of patients.[33,37,38] Interestingly, about two-thirds of patients with PSC have anticardiolipin antibodies in serum.[33] Antimitochondrial antibodies which are seen in patients with primary biliary cirrhosis are almost never found in patients with PSC.[3,33]

## RADIOLOGIC FINDINGS

Visualization of the biliary tree is essential for establishing the diagnosis of PSC. Invasive cholangiography, i.e. ERC and/or percutaneous transhepatic cholangiography (PTC), is the diagnostic test of choice (Fig. 44.1). Percutaneous approaches can be used, but because of the frequently sclerotic intrahepatic bile ducts, gaining access to the intrahepatic biliary system via the percutaneous route can be challenging. Recently, magnetic resonance cholangiography (MRC) has shown to be reasonably sensitive and specific for the detection of PSC and may be a more cost-effective alternative for establishing the diagnosis in patients with suspected PSC (Fig. 44.2).[39–41] Typical cholangiographic findings of PSC include multifocal stricturing and beading, usually involving

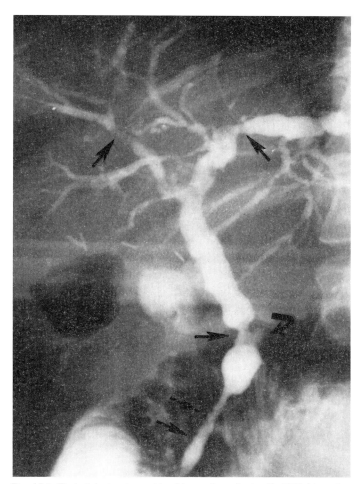

**Fig. 44.1** Typical cholangiographic picture of a patient with PSC. Note the extensive extra- and intrahepatic involvement.

both the intrahepatic and extrahepatic biliary systems (Fig. 44.1). Involvement of the intrahepatic tree alone may be found in up to 20% of patients, whereas about 5% of patients have only extrahepatic involvement. Often the strictures are diffusely distributed and are short and annular in appearance. Cystic duct and gallbladder involvement can be seen in up to 15% of patients.[42] In patients with PSC about a half of gallbladder polyps are malignant, suggesting that cholecystectomy should be performed in all patients with PSC who have polyps in the gallbladder.[43] Polypoid masses in the bile ducts should raise the suspicion of cholangiocarcinoma, although the diagnosis of cholangiocarcinoma can be difficult to establish.[44] Cholangiocarcinoma appears to affect 1/100–200 patients with PSC per year.[44–47] Biliary cytology and biopsies are insensitive and may be positive in only 30–60% of cases of complicating cholangiocarcinoma.[48–50]

## LIVER HISTOLOGY

Liver biopsy findings are usually not diagnostic for patients with PSC. Histological features in PSC include periductal inflammation and fibrosis, portal edema and fibrosis, fibro-obliterative cholangitis, 'onion-skin' fibrosis, ductular proliferation, ductopenia, increased copper deposition, periportal inflammation and fibrosis, septal fibrosis and cirrhosis.[51] The classic onion-skin fibrosis may be seen in fewer than 15% of biopsy specimens from patients with PSC, but when seen is highly suggestive of PSC (Fig. 44.3).[51] The most commonly used histologic grading system,

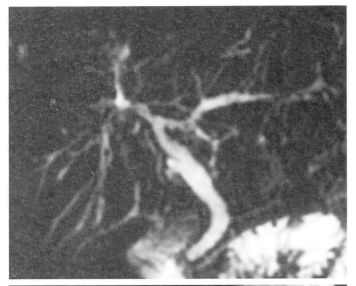

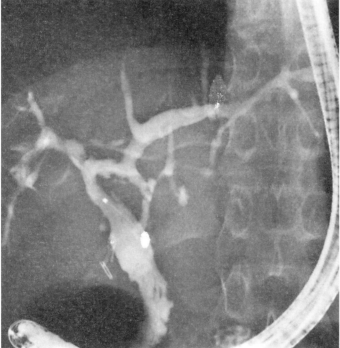

Fig. 44.2 Comparison of ERC and MRC from the same patient with PSC. MRC provides a more complete visualization of bile ducts distal to the multiple stricturing.

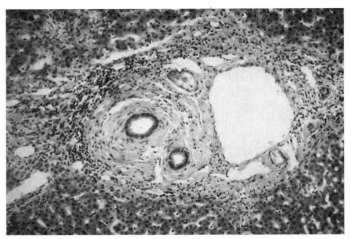

Fig. 44.3 Characteristic fibro-obliterative or 'onion-skin' fibrosis surrounding the bile duct on liver biopsy in a patient with PSC. This lesion is highly suggestive of PSC but is not commonly found.

proposed by Ludwig et al., includes four stages: stage 1 represents cholangitis or portal hepatitis; stage 2 represents periportal hepatitis with or without periportal fibrosis; stage 3 represents septal fibrosis; and stage 4 represents cirrhosis. Unfortunately, the histologic changes in patients with PSC seem to be quite varied from segment to segment of the same liver at any given point in time. In fact, histologic staging has not been seen as a necessary component of the most recently developed survival models.

## PATHOGENESIS

The pathogenesis of PSC has remained poorly understood since the earliest description of the disease. Most current think-

ing remains hypothetical, as the mechanism or mechanisms are still being worked out. A number of immunologic and non-immunologic avenues have been explored.

## ASSOCIATION OF PSC WITH THE INFLAMED COLON

Any proposed hypotheses for the pathogenesis of PSC will need to take into consideration its strong association with IBD. In this regard, much interest has been paid to the potential role of an inflamed colonic mucosa in causing the liver disease.[7,8,10,52] It is thought that the inflamed colon may increase permeability to various intraluminal products, leading to liver injury. Bacteria or bacterial toxins have been considered, but have not been convincingly demonstrated as playing a pathogenic role in patients with PSC.[53,54] Abnormal bile acids generated by bacterial action in the diseased colon and then directly absorbed through the inflamed colon into the portal system have been suggested as possibly being involved in the etiology of PSC, but no direct evidence in support of this theory has been forthcoming.[55,56]

In an animal model for PSC, inflammatory bacterial peptides led to portal inflammation and histologic changes suggestive of PSC in humans.[57,58] A variety of agents in the model were useful in blocking this response, including antibiotics, antibodies to a bacterial cell wall product, or an inhibitor of tumor necrosis factor-alpha (TNF-α). However, medications with anti-TNF-α activity, such as pentoxifylline[59] and etanercept,[60] were of no benefit in patients with PSC, casting some doubt on the value of this model in understanding the human disease. Furthermore, the finding that PSC can develop in many patients with normal colons, the lack of association between the severity of the colonic disease and the likelihood of developing PSC on the severity of the liver disease, and the temporal dissociation between the liver and colonic disease, all argue against an essential role of the inflamed colon and portal bacteremia in the development of this liver condition.[61,62]

## VIRAL INFECTIONS

The usual hepatotrophic viruses, hepatitis A, B and C, have been excluded. Cytomegalovirus (CMV) can cause changes suggestive of PSC in patients with acquired immunodeficiency states, but in immunocompetent patients no evidence of CMV infection has been found.[63,64] Reovirus type 3 was considered a possible causative agent, but further work excluded this as a cause for PSC.[65,66] At present there is no convincing evidence of a viral or other microbial cause of PSC, although newer, more sensitive techniques should certainly be applied.

## GENETIC SUSCEPTIBILITY

Several lines of evidence, such as family occurrence[67,68] and a strong association with some HLA haplotypes, suggest that PSC occurs in the context of a genetic predisposition. There has been an association between PSC and various HLA haplotypes, including B8, DR3, DR2, and A1, B8, DR3.[69–71] Disease associated with DR4 appears to have a more aggressive course, although this association has not been universally found.[72,73] More recently, PSC has been associated with polymorphisms in the TNF-α receptor, which may also indicate a possible genetic link.[74] A significant association between possession of the TNF2 allele (a G to A substitution at position –308 in the TNF-α gene) and susceptibility to PSC has been reported.[74] The increase in frequency of the TNF2 allele in PSC, however, occurs only in the presence of DR3 and B8A. Stromelysin polymorphisms (MMP-3) may influence susceptibility and disease progression in PSC as well.[75] Similarly, the MICA 002 allele seems to significantly reduce the risk of PSC, whereas the MICA 008 allele seems to increase the risk of developing PSC independently of other HLA haplotypes associated with PSC.[76] More recent data indicate that PSC is associated with the extended B8-MICA5.1-MICB24-DR3 haplotype.[77]

## IMMUNE MECHANISMS

Immune-mediated damage of bile ducts in PSC seems like the most plausible, but yet unproven, mechanism leading to development of PSC. Abnormalities of the immune system include the presence of hypergammaglobulinemia, particularly IgM levels; high prevalence of non-organ specific autoantibodies, including antinuclear, antismooth muscle, anticolonic, pANNA, anticardiolipin; circulating immune complexes; complement activation; and the reported sharing of a specific epitope on human colonic and biliary epithelial cells.[33,37,38,78–82]

Abnormalities of the cellular immune system have been described and include a decrease in circulating total T cells owing to a decrease in CD8 (suppressor/cytotoxic cells), an increase in circulating B cells, increased γδ cells, and T cells with preferential use of the Vβ3 gene of the T-cell receptor in lymphocytes infiltrating the liver.[83–86]

Aberrant expression of HLA class II antigens on the biliary epithelial cells may help to target an immune response to the biliary cells, but may also be an epiphenomenon related to bile duct inflammation as a causative factor.[87,88] The presence of intracellular adhesion molecule 1 (ICAM-1), which serves as a ligand for the leukocyte function-associated antigen (LFA-1), may help form connections between T lymphocytes and antigen-presenting cells. Increased levels of ICAM-1 have been described both in bile duct epithelial cells and the serum.[89,90] LFA-1 also appears to be overexpressed by intrahepatic lymphocytes, but this expression may simply be induced by proinflammatory cytokines.[91] The role of various cytokines in the pathogenesis of PSC has not been well worked out, and further work is certainly needed to elucidate the potential immunologic mechanisms that might underlie this disease.

| Table 44.4 Diagnostic criteria for primary sclerosing cholangitis |
|---|
| Typical cholangiographic abnormalities involving any part of the biliary tree |
| Compatible clinical (i.e. history of IBD, cholestatic symptoms) and biochemical findings (i.e. two- to threefold increases in serum alkaline phosphatase for longer than 6 months) |
| Exclusion of identifiable causes of secondary sclerosing cholangitis |
|    AIDS cholangiopathy |
|    Bile duct neoplasm (unless diagnosis of PSC previously established) |
|    Biliary tract surgery, trauma |
|    Choledocholithiasis |
|    Congenital abnormalities of biliary tract |
|    Caustic sclerosing cholangitis |
|    Ischemic stricturing of bile ducts |
|    Toxicity/stricturing of bile ducts related to intra-arterial infusion of fluoxuridine |

## DIAGNOSIS

The diagnostic criteria for primary sclerosing cholangitis include the absence of previous surgical trauma to the biliary tree, absence of stones in the gallbladder and common bile duct, stenosis involving the majority of the hepatobiliary system, and the exclusion of malignant disease (Table 44.4). In most series, the typical patient with PSC has both intrahepatic and extrahepatic involvement of bile ducts on cholangiography; although some have only extrahepatic involvement of bile ducts, some others show only intrahepatic involvement.[24] However, given the progressive nature of PSC, many patients with only localized bile duct abnormalities at the time of diagnosis will show more extensive involvement of bile ducts during follow-up. MRC as a screening test for patients with suspected PSC makes non-invasive diagnosis now possible.[40] MRC has a sensitivity of 83%, a specificity of 98% and an accuracy of 93% in the correct diagnosis of PSC compared to invasive cholangiography (ERC and/or PTC). In patients with high-grade stricturing of bile ducts, MRC provides a more complete visualization of the distal biliary tree than that obtained by ERC or PTC;[40] furthermore, MRC provides additional diagnostic information, such as identification of masses, organomegaly, and findings of portal hypertension such as ascites and the development of a portosystemic collateral circulation.[40]

The diagnostic criteria for PSC include typical cholangiographic abnormalities involving any part of the biliary tree, compatible clinical and biochemical findings (typically prolonged cholestasis), and exclusion of other causes of secondary sclerosing cholangitis, such as previous biliary tract surgery, bile duct neoplasm, AIDS cholangiopathy, choledocholithiasis, congenital abnormalities, history of caustic sclerosis of the bile ducts, ischemic strictures secondary to hepatic artery injury, or caustic/chemical injury to the bile ducts via infusion. Bile duct obstruction cased by choledocholithiasis or tumors should be ruled out as a cause of secondary sclerosing cholangitis.

PSC must be distinguished from other hepatobiliary disorders that may present with chronic cholestasis, such as primary biliary cirrhosis, drug-induced cholestasis, alcoholic hepatitis, and cases of autoimmune hepatitis or viral hepatitis that present with a predominantly cholestatic profile. Liver biopsy has been used in the past to help confirm the diagnosis, although the diagnostic specificity and sensitivity of the biopsy has come under question and histologic findings are not always found to be of value in the most recently developed prognostic scoring systems for patients with PSC.[12,18,92–94] Liver biopsy, however, is useful in a patient with suspected PSC but a normal cholangiogram, as well as in those PSC patients who present with clinical and laboratory abnormalities of autoimmune hepatitis overlapping with PSC. A liver biopsy in the setting of IBD may show typical changes of sclerosing cholangitis. In patients with chronic cholestasis in the clinical setting of IBD the finding of a normal cholangiogram but a compatible biopsy has been termed small-duct PSC,[95] and comprises 6% of all cases of histologically confirmed PSC.[9]

## OVERLAP OF PSC WITH OTHER AUTOIMMUNE LIVER DISEASES

Patients with PSC may present with clinical and biochemical features of autoimmune hepatitis overlapping with PSC.[27,28,30–32,96,97] Two large clinical experiences have recently been reported.[31,32] The group from the Mayo Clinic[31] assessed the revised international scoring system for diagnosis of autoimmune hepatitis in 211 patients with cholangiography-confirmed PSC; of these, three (1.4%) patients met the 'definite' diagnosis and 13 (6%) met the 'probable' diagnosis of autoimmune hepatitis. As would be anticipated, those with features of both PSC and AIH tended to have higher ratios of aspartate aminotransferase to alkaline phosphatase, higher titers of autoantibodies and immunoglobulins, and more interface hepatitis. A similar study from Rotterdam[32] looked at 108 cases of PSC and found that nine (8%) met the diagnosis of 'definite' autoimmune hepatitis. Differences in patient populations and referral patterns may be among the explanations for these different proportions.

Reports in children suggest that the association of PSC and autoimmune hepatitis is more common than in adults. In an early series of 13 children with PSC[27] all but one had antismooth muscle and/or antinuclear antibodies; five patients had a marked degree of portal and periportal inflammation suggestive of autoimmune hepatitis. In a subsequent study of 32 children with radiological and histological features of PSC[28] over half of the patients showed a raised IgG and positive antismooth muscle or antinuclear antibodies. In a more recent report from the Mayo Clinic[96] 6% of 52 children with cholangiography-proven PSC met the diagnosis of 'definite' autoimmune hepatitis, whereas 31% met the diagnosis of 'probable' autoimmune hepatitis overlapping with PSC using the international scoring system for diagnosis of autoimmune hepatitis. In a report from London,[97] 17 of 34 children with positive autoimmune serology had cholangiographic changes of PSC at presentation. These studies together suggest that the expression of PSC in children is skewed towards a hepatic presentation, perhaps owing to changes in immune homeostasis with maturity.

## NATURAL HISTORY

PSC is usually a progressive disease. In a study of 174 patients, the median survival from the time of diagnosis was about 12 years.[98] A large study from Sweden estimated the median survival to be 12 years.[12] However, an Italian study suggested that the screening and early diagnosis of PSC is associated with a longer apparent survival owing to a presumed lead time bias.[13] Patients with PSC who present with symptoms of chronic cholestasis have a long-term survival significantly shorter than that in PSC patients who do not have symptoms.[12,99] However, survival in asymptomatic patients is still significantly shorter than that expected in age- and gender-matched populations.[99] Patients with small-duct PSC have a significantly better long-term survival than patients with classic PSC.[9] Patients with small-duct PSC have a normal life expectancy compared to age- and gender-matched populations. Nevertheless, some patients with small-duct PSC progress to classic PSC and end-stage liver disease over time, whereas in some others the disease remains stable for many years.[9] The aggregate of all of this information does suggest that PSC is a progressive disease, and that if suitable therapy were available its use early in the course of the disease would seem warranted.

## PROGNOSTIC SURVIVAL MODELS

Given the uncertainty of natural history studies, prognostic models based on actual data obtained from patients at a given point in time have been developed to help more accurately predict an individual patient's prognosis[12,18,92–94,98,100] (Table 44.5). Cox multivariable regression analysis has been most widely used to define the variables for these models. Based on these models several mathematical formulae have been developed, as shown in Table 44.6. Age and bilirubin appear in nearly all of these models. Obviously, models that do not require a liver biopsy have the advantage of patient convenience and safety, and obviate concerns about sampling variability from the liver of patients with PSC as noted above. Recently, a time-dependent Cox regression model was reported and shown to be superior to a time-fixed model in estimating short-term prognosis in patients with PSC.[18] Some of the shortcomings of these prognostic models is that all use retrospective data; although some have been validated, none has been evaluated prospectively; they do not take into account quality of life and cannot predict the development of complications such as cancer or complications of portal hypertension, which clearly affect the long-term prognosis of patients with PSC.

## COMPLICATIONS OF PSC AND ITS MANAGEMENT

### COMPLICATIONS OF CHRONIC CHOLESTASIS

#### Pruritus

Although not common, pruritus can be disabling and associated with a diminished quality of life. The pathogenesis of pruritus in cholestasis is unknown, although endogenous opioids or retention of factors usually excreted in the bile have been considered.[101–103] The severity of the pruritus does not seem to parallel the severity of the liver disease, and pruritus may diminish as the liver disease progresses. Cholestyramine or antihistamines and rifampin, as well as opiate receptor antagonists, have all been used with varying results in patients with cholestatic pruritus.[103–105] The usual doses of these medications is as

**Table 44.5 Independent clinical predictors of survival used in selected natural history models for PSC**

| Mayo Clinic[98] (n=174) | King's Cambridge[92] (n=126) | Multicenter[100] (n=426) | Swedish[12] (n=305) | New Mayo model[94] (n=405) | Time-dependent model[18] (n = 330) |
|---|---|---|---|---|---|
| Age | Age | Age | Age | Age | Age |
| Bilirubin | Hepatomegaly | Bilirubin | Bilirubin | Bilirubin | Bilirubin |
| Histologic stage | Histologic stage | Histologic stage | Histologic stage | AST | Albumin |
| Hemoglobin | Splenomegaly | Splenomegaly | | Variceal bleed | |
| Inflammatory bowel disease | Alkaline phosphatase | | | Albumin | |

**Table 44.6 Prognostic index formulae for selected natural history models in PSC**

| Model | Formulae |
|---|---|
| Mayo[98] | R = 0.06 × (age in years) + 0.85 × log (minimum [bilirubin in mg/dL or 10]) − 4.39 × log (minimum [hemoglobin in g/dL or 12]) + 0.51 × (biopsy stage) + 1.59 × (indicator for inflammatory bowel disease) |
| King's Cambridge[92] | R = 1.81 × (presence of hepatomegaly) + 0.88 × (presence of splenomegaly) + 2.66 × log (alkaline phosphatase) + 0.58 × (histologic stage) + 0.04 × (age in years) |
| Multicenter[100] | R = 0.535 × log (bilirubin in mg/dL) + 0.486 × (histologic stage) + 0.041 × (age in years) + 0.705 × (presence of splenomegaly) |
| New Mayo Model[94] | R = 0.03 (age in years) + 0.54 × log (bilirubin in mg/dL) + 0.54 × log (aspartate aminotransferase in U/L) + 1.24 (history of variceal bleeding) − 0.84 × (albumin in g/dL) |

follows: cholestyramine 4 g three to four times daily; naltrexone 50 mg by mouth daily; rifampin 150–300 mg by mouth twice daily; in some patients ursodeoxycholic acid may improve pruritus of cholestasis.

It is important to remember that rifampin, which may relieve pruritus in 3–5 days, can be associated with a reversible hepatotoxicity in about 15% of cases. Therefore, it is important to monitor liver tests closely if this drug is used.

## Fat-soluble vitamin deficiency

Fat-soluble vitamin deficiency is relatively common in patients with PSC, particularly as they progress towards liver transplantation.[106] Up to 40% of patients in some series are vitamin A deficient, whereas vitamin D and vitamin E deficiencies were seen in 14% and 2% of patients, respectively. Vitamin K deficiency is uncommon. If suspected, a short trial of water-soluble vitamin K can be considered and if the prothrombin time responds after a few doses, long-term therapy should be recommended. Vitamin E deficiency is rare and, unfortunately, once established can be very difficult to correct with replacement therapy. The usual doses of replacement therapy with these vitamins is as follows: vitamin A 25–50 000 units two to three times per week; vitamin D 25–50 000 units two to three times per week; vitamin E 100 units twice daily; and vitamin K 5 mg daily.

## Bone disease

Osteopenic bone disease, usually due to osteoporosis rather than osteomalacia, is relatively common and an important complication in patients with PSC.[107,108] A large clinical experience showed that osteopenia, as defined by a t-score (number of standard deviations from the mean peak bone mass) below −1 is found in about half of patients with PSC at the time of referral or diagnosis of the liver disease, whereas osteoporosis as defined by a t-score below −2.5 is found in about 15% of patients.[108] Osteoporosis occurs 23.8 times (95% CI 4.6–122.8) more commonly in patients with PSC than would be expected in the general population.[108] Several risk factors have been recognized to increase the risk for osteoporosis in patients with PSC, such as the underlying cholestatic liver disease and IBD per se, the use of corticosteroids for the treatment of IBD, celiac disease when present, and hypogonadism in more advanced liver disease. Unfortunately, there is no proven specific therapy that will help these patients. Hormone replacement therapy can be considered in postmenopausal women. Calcitonin does not appear to be useful in patients with osteoporosis in PBC, although it has not been tested in patients with PSC. Bisphosphonates have been used with varying results in patients with PBC, but have not been tested in patients with PSC.[109,110] Patients with PSC and IBD on long-term corticosteroid therapy for the bowel disease may benefit from oral administration of vitamin D and calcium and potentially a bisphosphonate, particularly those with bone density in the range of osteopenia or osteoporosis.

## Lipid metabolism abnormalities

Abnormalities in lipid metabolism are common in patients with chronic cholestasis. These have not been as well described in patients with PSC as they have been in PBC, but elevated cholesterol levels with deposition of cholesterol in the skin as xanthelasma have been found.

## Steatorrhea

Steatorrhea may occur in patients with PSC. This can be due to diminished delivery of bile acids to the bowel or to chronic pancreatitis or celiac disease, all of which should be considered in patients with steatorrhea in the setting of PSC.[111] The latter two should be particularly thought of in those patients with steatorrhea but without evidence of advanced liver disease.

## COMPLICATIONS SPECIFIC TO PSC

Specific complications of PSC include cholelithiasis, dominant strictures with recurrent cholangitis, malignancy (cholangiocarcinoma, colon cancer) and peristomal varices in patients with an ileostomy after colectomy for colitis.

## Gallstones

Gallstones involving the gallbladder or bile ducts (choledocholithiasis) can occur in up to approximately a third of patients with PSC. This is because chronic cholestasis predisposes to the formation of cholesterol gallstones, and bile stasis with bacterial cholangitis will lead to the formation of pigment stones. These patients with PSC may form choledocholithiasis, leading to acute deterioration of liver function if the bile duct becomes obstructed. This possibility should be considered in patients with PSC who develop evidence of rapidly developing jaundice or bacterial cholangitis. Frequently, choledocholithiasis can be treated endoscopically at the same time the diagnosis is made.

## Biliary strictures

Dominant biliary strictures requiring endoscopic or percutaneous dilation can occur in patients with PSC. In the largest series reported to date, this occurred in only 7% of patients when followed for up to 10 years.[112] These dominant strictures are usually in the extrahepatic biliary system and may be associated with jaundice, pruritus or recurrent bacterial cholangitis. If any of these symptoms occur in patients with PSC, cholangiography should be considered. If a dominant stricture is found brush cytology should be obtained, although this is an insensitive technique for the detection of malignancy. Often these strictures can be dilated endoscopically by a balloon catheter. Short-term biliary stenting has been suggested by some to be of value in improving the prognosis of the liver disease,[113] whereas other series using biliary stents show that these stented patients run an increased risk of complications.[112] Direct surgical intervention for strictures is seldom applied and may predispose patients to recurrent ascending cholangitis because of the widely patent surgical anastomosis and make future liver transplantation more technically demanding.

Prophylaxis for bacterial cholangitis should be considered in patients with PSC undergoing biliary manipulation such as diagnostic or therapeutic ERC. Ciprofloxacin or other broad-spectrum antibiotics are frequently administered both immediately before and for 1–2 days after the procedure.

## Cholangiocarcinoma

Cholangiocarcinoma represents the most feared complication of patients with PSC. Tumors arise most commonly around the common hepatic duct and its bifurcation. The prevalence of the tumor in PSC varies from 4% to 20%; however, about a third of patients with PSC will develop cholangiocarcinoma if follow-up is extended long enough. The prevalence in autopsy series varies between 30 and 42%, whereas the prevalence of hepatobiliary malignancy, in particular cholangiocarcinoma in explanted livers of patients undergoing liver transplantation, varies from 0 to 44% (overall mean 6.8%; 49 of 711 patients reported) despite an exhaustive pretransplantation diagnostic approach.[3] The annual incidence of cholangiocarcinoma is 0.5–1.5%. The development of cholangiocarcinoma does not correlate with the severity of liver disease. No clear risk factors are associated with developing cholangiocarcinoma in PSC. Smoking and the presence of inflammatory bowel disease have been suggested by several groups as predisposing conditions, although these associations are controversial. The diagnosis of cholangiocarcinoma in the setting of PSC represents a difficult challenge. Serum markers for early detection for cholangiocarcinoma have so far been unhelpful. CA19-9 levels are usually elevated in patients with cholangiocarcinoma and PSC, but often patients with the elevated levels have advanced malignant disease.[114-116] A threshold value of 100 U/mL is 89% sensitive and 86% specific in detecting cholangiocarcinoma in PSC.[114] Serological screening with an index =400 for the two tumor markers, CA19-9 and carcinoembryonic antigen (CEA) (CA19-9 + (CEA X 40)), is 86% accurate in detecting cholangiocarcinoma and has a 100% specificity, but with a sensitivity of only 67%.[117] The prognosis of patients with cholangiocarcinoma is very poor, with a reported survival less than 12 months from the time of diagnosis in almost all cases.[118] About half of patients with cholangiocarcinoma have advanced disease at the time of diagnosis, which does not allow successful surgical resection. Liver transplantation is not an effective therapy for most patients because of the high probability of tumor recurrence shortly after transplantation. Nevertheless, patients with incidental microscopic cholangiocarcinoma found in the explanted liver in whom the spread to regional lymph nodes has been carefully excluded during the transplant procedure may experience a similar long-term survival to transplanted patients without cholangiocarcinoma.[119] Patients with PSC may also develop hepatocellular cancer. In one series, 25% of the hepatobiliary malignancies occurring in patients with PSC were due to hepatocellular cancer.[120]

## Colorectal dysplasia/cancer

PSC has been found in several series to be an independent risk factor for the development of colorectal dysplasia and cancer. The cumulative risk for development of colorectal cancer has been reported to increase five times in patients with PSC plus ulcerative colitis than in patients with ulcerative colitis alone.[121] Another historical cohort study[122] found that the relative risk of colorectal cancer in patients with PSC plus ulcerative colitis is elevated 10-fold compared to the general population, but not in patients with PSC without ulcerative colitis. Although this evidence suggests that PSC increases significantly the risk of development of colorectal cancer in patients with ulcerative colitis, this has not been a universal experience.[123,124] Conversely, ulcerative colitis per se does not seem to be a risk factor for the development of cholangiocarcinoma in the absence of PSC.

## Portal hypertension

The development of portal hypertension with its consequent complications in PSC patients does not differ from other end-stage liver diseases. However, a special complication of portal hypertension is the development of peristomal varices, which may occur in patients with ileostomy after proctocolectomies for underlying IBD.[125] The bleeding can be severe and refractory to local measures, including ileostomy revision and injection of sclerosants. TIPS or portocaval shunt can be considered, although many of these patients with bleeding peristomal varices have severe liver disease with portal hypertension and should be considered for liver transplantation.

# TREATMENT

## MEDICAL THERAPY

A variety of drugs have been tested, as listed in Table 44.7, but to date none has been found to be useful. Penicillamine was the first drug tested in patients with PSC in a randomized trial, but was ineffective.[126] Colchicine, methotrexate and ursodeoxycholic acid in a dose of 13–15 mg/kg/day all have also been ineffective in randomized controlled trials.[127–130] Other drugs that have been tested in small-scale studies, sometimes in open-label trials, have included nicotine, pirfenidone, cyclosporin, silymarin, pentoxifylline and budesonide.[59,131–134] Azathioprine combined with prednisone and ursodeoxycholic acid appeared promising.[135] The combination of colchicine and corticosteroids led to some transient biochemical improvement,[136] but the combination of ursodiol and methotrexate was not successful in an open-label trial in patients with PSC.[137] Tacrolimus appeared promising in a small open-label pilot study, but these results need confirmation.[138] Ursodeoxycholic acid in higher doses of 20–30 mg/kg/day has appeared most promising, and large-scale randomized trials are being undertaken with higher doses of this drug.[139,140]

## ENDOSCOPIC AND SURGICAL THERAPY

Most patients with PSC present with diffuse involvement of the bile ducts; however, some may present with clinical and biochemical deterioration of cholestasis owing to a dominant stricture that involves the larger extrahepatic bile ducts. Such lesions may be amenable to balloon dilation with or without sphincterotomy and short-term stenting via the endoscopic or percutaneous approach. The impact of endoscopic therapy in survival in PSC is uncertain. Two recent studies[141,142] reported an improved survival in patients with PSC treated endoscopically with[141] or without[142] ursodeoxycholic acid compared to the expected survival as predicted by the Mayo risk score. Prospective randomized trials are necessary to better define the impact of endoscopic therapy in the natural course of PSC.

The role of biliary surgery in PSC has diminished considerably with the growing success of liver transplantation. Biliary reconstruction has been suggested as helpful,[143] but this aggressive approach has not been validated in prospective controlled studies. Patients with extensive extrahepatic dominant strictures in which concerns about cholangiocarcinoma cannot otherwise be addressed may be among the few in whom non-transplant surgery should be contemplated.

## LIVER TRANSPLANTATION

The greatest pressing need for patients with PSC at present is for effective medical therapy for the underlying disease. Until this occurs, liver transplantation is the only option for patients with advanced disease. The results of liver transplantation for patients with PSC has steadily improved, such that the 1- and 5-year survival rates are now reported to be 90–97% and 85–88%, respectively.[119,144,145] Complications after liver transplantation for PSC include an increased risk of infection as well as acute and chronic rejection, the development of biliary strictures, hepatic artery thrombosis, and lymphoproliferative diseases due to the immunosuppressive agents. PSC recurs after liver transplantation and, as follow-up is extended, a greater risk of recurrence seems to occur, although, fortunately, to date the recurrent disease has been mild.[146,147] Patients with PSC and CUC who have undergone transplantation seem to be at a particularly higher risk for developing colon cancers if they have a remaining colon, and require close screening with annual visits and 6-monthly colonoscopy with surveillance biopsies.[148]

# References

1. Delbet P. Retrecissement du choledoque cholecystoduodenostomie. Bull Mem Soc Chir Paris 1924;50:1144–1146.
2. Brantigan CO, Brantigan OC. Primary sclerosing cholangitis: case report and review of literature. Am Surg 1973;39:191–198.
3. Angulo P, Lindor KD. Primary sclerosing cholangitis. Hepatology 1999;30:325–332.
4. Schrumpf E, Elgjio O, Fausa E et al. Sclerosing cholangitis in ulcerative colitis. Scand J Gastroenterol 1980;15:689–697.
5. Shepherd HA, Selby WS, Chapman RWG et al. Ulcerative colitis and persistent liver dysfunction. Q J Med 1983;208:503–513.
6. Tobias R, Wright JP, Kottler RE et al. Primary sclerosing cholangitis associated with inflammatory bowel disease in Cape Town, 1975–1981. S Afr Med J 1983;63:229–235.
7. Olsson R, Danielsson A, Jarnerot G et al. Prevalence of primary sclerosing cholangitis in patients with ulcerative colitis. Gastroenterology 1991;100:1319–1323.
8. Rasmussen HH, Fallingborg JF, Mortensen PB et al. Hepatobiliary dysfunction and primary sclerosing cholangitis in patients with Crohn's disease. Scand J Gastroenterol 1997;32:604–610.
9. Angulo P, Maor-Kendler Y, Lindor KD. Small-duct primary sclerosing cholangitis: a long-term follow-up study. Hepatology 2002;35:1494–1500.
10. Chapman RWG, Arborgh BA, Rhodes JM et al. Primary sclerosing cholangitis: a review of its clinical features, cholangiography, and hepatic histology. Gut 1980;21:870–877.
11. Escorsell A, Pares A, Rodes J et al. Epidemiology of primary sclerosing cholangitis in Spain. Spanish association for study of the liver. J Hepatol 1994;21:787–791.
12. Broome U, Olsson R, Loof L et al. Natural history and prognostic factors in 305 Swedish patients with primary sclerosing cholangitis. Gut 1996;38:610–615.
13. Okolicsanyi L, Fabris L, Viaggi S et al. Primary sclerosing cholangitis: clinical presentation, natural history and prognostic variables: an Italian multicentre study. Eur J Gastroenterol Hepatol 1996;8:685–691.
14. Kockbar R, Goenka MK, Das K et al. Primary sclerosing cholangitis: an experience from India. J Gastroenterol Hepatol 1996;11:429–433.
15. Takikawa H, Manabe T. Primary sclerosing cholangitis in Japan – analysis of 192 cases. J Gastroenterol Hepatol 1997;32:134–137.

## Table 44.7 Medical therapies tested to date

| | | |
|---|---|---|
| Penicillamine | Colchicine | Azathioprine |
| Cyclosporin | Methotrexate | Ursodeoxycholic acid |
| Pentoxifylline | Budesonide | |
| Nicotine | Pirfenidone | |

16. Boberg KM, Aadland E, Jahnsen J et al. Incidence and prevalence of primary biliary cirrhosis, primary sclerosing cholangitis and autoimmune hepatitis in a Norwegian population. Scand J Gastroenterol 1998;33:99–103.

17. Stiehl A, Rudolph G, Kloters-Plachky P et al. Development of dominant bile duct stenoses in patients with primary sclerosing cholangitis treated with ursodeoxycholic acid: outcome after endoscopic treatment. J Hepatol 2002;36:151–156.

18. Boberg KM, Rocca G, Egeland T et al. Time-dependent cox regression model is superior in prediction of prognosis in primary sclerosing cholangitis. Hepatology 2002;35:652–657.

19. Bergquist A, Ekbom A, Olsson R et al. Hepatic and extrahepatic malignancies in primary sclerosing cholangitis. J Hepatol 2002;36:321–327.

20. Stonnington CM, Phillips SF, Melton LJI et al. Chronic ulcerative colitis: incidence and prevalence in a community. Gut 1987;28:402–409.

21. Balasubramanian K, Wiesner RH, LaRusso NF. Primary sclerosing cholangitis with normal serum alkaline phosphatase activity. Gastroenterology 1988;95:1395–1398.

22. Clements D, Rhodes JM, Elias E. Severe bile duct lesions without biochemical evidence of cholestasis in a case of sclerosing cholangitis. J Hepatol 1986;3:72–74.

23. Wiesner RH, LaRusso NF. Clinicopathologic features of the syndrome of primary sclerosing cholangitis. Gastroenterology 1980;79:200–206.

24. MacCarty RL, LaRusso NF, Wiesner RH, Ludwig J. Primary sclerosing cholangitis: findings on cholangiography and pancreatography. Radiology 1983;149:39–44.

25. Kim WR, Lindor KD, Malinchoc M et al. Reliability and validity of the NIDDK-QA instrument in the assessment of QOL in ambulatory patients with cholestatic liver disease. Hepatology 2000;32:924–929.

26. Younossi ZM, Boparai N, Price LL et al. Health related quality of life in chronic liver disease. Am J Gastroenterol 2001;96:2199–2205.

27. El-Shabrawi M, Wilkinson ML, Portmann B et al. Primary sclerosing cholangitis in childhood. Gastroenterology 1987;92:1226–1235.

28. Wieschansei M, Chait P, Wade JA. Primary sclerosing cholangitis in 32 children: clinical, laboratory, and radiographic features, with survival analysis. Hepatology 1995;22:1415–1422.

29. Feldstein A, Angulo P, El-Youssef M et al. Overlap with autoimmune hepatitis in pediatric patients with primary sclerosing cholangitis. Gastroenterology 2002;122:202.

30. McNair ANB, Moloney M, Portmann BC et al. Autoimmune hepatitis overlapping with primary sclerosing cholangitis in five cases. Am J Gastroenterol 1998;93:777–784.

31. Kaya M, Angulo P, Lindor KD. Overlap of autoimmune hepatitis and primary sclerosing cholangitis: an evaluation of a modified scoring system. J Hepatol 2000;33:537–542.

32. van Burren HR, van Hoogstraten HJF, Terkivatan T. High prevalence of autoimmune hepatitis among patients with primary sclerosing cholangitis. J Hepatol 2000;33:543–548.

33. Angulo P, Peter JB, Gershwin ME et al. Serum autoantibodies in patients with primary sclerosing cholangitis. J Hepatol 1999;32:182–187.

34. Peen E, Sundquist T, Skogh T. Leucocyte activation by anti-lactoferrin antibodies bound to vascular endothelium. Clin Exp Immunol 1996;103:403–407.

35. Seibold F, Weber P, Klein P et al. Clinical significance of antibodies against neutrophils in patients with inflammatory bowel disease and primary sclerosing cholangitis. Gut 1992;33:657–662.

36. Terjung B, Spengler U, Sauerbruch T et al. 'Atypical p-ANCA' in IBD and hepatobiliary disorders react with a 50 kD nuclear envelop protein of neutrophils and myeloid cell lines. Gastroenterology 2000;119:310–322.

37. Zauli D, Schrumpf E, Crespi C et al. An autoantibody profile in primary sclerosing cholangitis. J Hepatol 1987;5:14–18.

38. Duerr RH, Targan SR, Landers CJ et al. Neutrophil cytoplasmic antibodies: a link between primary sclerosing cholangitis and ulcerative colitis. Gastroenterology 1991;100:1385–1391.

39. Soto JA, Barish MA, Yucel EK et al. Magnetic resonance cholangiography: comparison with endoscopic retrograde cholangiopancreatography. Gastroenterology 1996;110:589–597.

40. Angulo P, Pearce DH, Johnson CD et al. Magnetic resonance cholangiography in patients with biliary disease: its role in primary sclerosing cholangitis. J Hepatol 2000;33:520–527.

41. Talwalkar JA, Angulo P, Johnson CD et al. Cost-minimization analysis of MRC vs ERCP in patients with biliary disease: its role in primary sclerosing cholangitis (PSC). Hepatology 2000;32:175A.

42. Brandt DJ, MacCarty RL, Charboneau JW et al. Gallbladder disease in patients with primary sclerosing cholangitis. Am J Roentgenol 1988;150:571–574.

43. Buckles DC, Lindor KD, LaRusso NF et al. In primary sclerosing cholangitis, gallbladder polyps are frequently malignant. Am J Gastroenterol 2002;97:1138–1142.

44. de Groen PC, Gores GJ, LaRusso NF et al. Biliary tract cancers. N Engl J Med 1999;341:1368–1378.

45. Berquist A, Glaumann H, Persson B et al. Risk factors and clinical presentation of hepatobiliary carcinoma in patients with primary sclerosing cholangitis: a case–control study. Hepatology 1998;27:311–316.

46. Kornfeld D, Ekbom A, Ihre T. Survival and risk of cholangiocarcinoma in patients with primary sclerosing cholangitis. Scand J Gastroenterol 1997;32:1042–1045.

47. Chalasai N, Baluyut A, Ismail A et al. Cholangiocarcinoma in patients with primary sclerosing cholangitis: a multicenter case–control study. Hepatology 2000;31:7–11.

48. Foutch PG, Kerr DM, Harlan JR et al. Endoscopic retrograde wire-guided brush cytology for diagnosis of patients with malignant obstruction of the bile duct. Am J Gastroenterol 1990;85:791–795.

49. Kurzawinski TR, Deery A, Sooley JS et al. A prospective study of biliary cytology in 100 patients with bile duct strictures. Hepatology 1993;18:1399–1403.

50. Fleming KA, Boberg KM, Glaumann H et al. Biliary dysplasia as a marker of cholangiocarcinoma in primary sclerosing cholangitis. J Hepatol 2001;34:360–365.

51. Ludwig J, Barham SS, LaRusso NF et al. Morphologic features of chronic hepatitis associated with primary sclerosing cholangitis or chronic ulcerative colitis. Hepatology 1981;1:632–640.

52. Schrumpf E, Fausa O, Elgio K et al. Hepatobiliary complications of inflammatory bowel disease. Semin Liver Dis 1988;8:201–209.

53. Eade MN, Brooke BN. Portal bacteremia in cases of ulcerative colitis submitted to colectomy. Lancet 1969;1:1008–1009.

54. Palmer KR, Duerden BJ, Holdworth CD. Bacteriological and endotoxin studies in cases of ulcerative colitis submitted to surgery. Gut 1980;21:851–854.

55. Dew MJ, van Berge Henegouwen GP, Huybregts AWM et al. Hepatotoxic effect of bile acids in inflammatory bowel disease. Gastroenterology 1980;78:1393–1401.

56. Holzbach RT, Marsh ME, Freedman MR et al. Portal vein bile acids in patients with severe inflammatory bowel disease. Gut 1980;21:428–435.

57. Hobson CH, Butt TJ, Ferry DM et al. Enterohepatic circulation of bacterial chemotactic peptide in rats with experimental colitis. Gastroenterology 1988;94:1006–1013.

58. Lichtman SN, Sartor RB, Keku J et al. Hepatic inflammation in rats with experimental small intestinal bacterial overgrowth. Gastroenterology 1990;98:414–423.

59. Bharucha AE, Jorgensen RA, Lichtman SN et al. A pilot study of pentoxifylline for the treatment of PSC. Am J Gastroenterol 2000;95:2338–2342.

60. Epstein MP, Kaplan MM. A trial of etanercept in the treatment of primary sclerosing cholangitis. Gastroenterology 2002;122:202A.

61. Cangemi JR, Wiesner RH, Beaver SJ et al. Effect of proctocolectomy for chronic ulcerative colitis on the natural history of primary sclerosing cholangitis. Gastroenterology 1989;96:790–794.

62. Steckman M, Drossman DA, Lesesne HR. Hepatobiliary disease that precedes ulcerative colitis. J Clin Gastroenterol 1984;6:425–428.

63. Finegold MJ, Carpenter RJ. Obliterative cholangitis due to cytomegalovirus: a possible precursor of paucity of intrahepatic bile ducts. Hum Pathol 1982;13:662–665.

64. Mehal WZ, Hattersley AT, Chapman RW et al. A survey of cytomegalovirus (CMV) DNA in primary sclerosing cholangitis (PSC) liver tissues using a sensitive polymerase chain reaction (PCR) based assay. J Hepatol 1992;15:396–399.

65. Morecki R, Glaser JH, Cho S et al. Biliary atresia and reovirus type 3 infection. N Engl J Med 1982;307:481–484.

66. Minuk GY, Rascanin N, Paul RW et al. Reovirus type 3 infection in patients with primary biliary cirrhosis and primary sclerosing cholangitis. J Hepatol 1987;5:8–13.

67. Quigley EMM, LaRusso NF, Ludwig J et al. Familial occurrence of primary sclerosing cholangitis and ulcerative colitis. Gastroenterology 1983;85:1160–1165.

68. Jorge AD, Esley C, Ahumada J. Family incidence of primary sclerosing cholangitis associated with immunological diseases. Endoscopy 1987;19:114–117.

69. Chapman RW, Varghese Z, Gaul R et al. Association of primary sclerosing cholangitis with HLA-B8. Gut 1983;24:38–41.

70. Schrumpf E, Fausa O, Forre O et al. HLA antigens and immunoregulatory T cells in ulcerative colitis associated with hepatobiliary disease. Scand J Gastroenterol 1982;17:187–191.

71. Donaldson PT, Farrant JM, Wilkinson ML et al. Dual association of HLA DR2 and DR3 with primary sclerosing cholangitis. Hepatology 1991;13:129–133.

72. Mehal WZ, Lo D-M, Wordsworth PD et al. HLA DR4 is a marker for disease progression in primary sclerosing cholangitis. Gastroenterology 1994;106:160–167.

73. Olerup O, Olsson R, Hultcrantz R et al. HLA-DR and HLA-DQ are not markers for rapid disease progression in primary sclerosing cholangitis. Gastroenterology 1995;108:870–878.

74. Mitchell SA, Grove J, Spurkland A et al. Association of the tumour necrosis factor A-308 but no the interleukin 10-627 promoter polymorphism with genetic susceptibility to primary sclerosing cholangitis. Gut 2001;49:288–294.

75. Santsangi J, Chapman RW, Haldar N et al. A functional polymorphism of the stromelysin gene (MMP-3) influences susceptibility to PSC. Gastroenterology 2001;121:124–130.

76. Norris S, Kondeatis E, Collins R et al. Mapping MHC-encoded susceptibility and resistance in primary sclerosing cholangitis: the role of MICA polymorphism. Gastroenterology 2001;120:1475–1482.

77. Wiecke K, Spurkland A, Schrumpf E et al. Primary sclerosing cholangitis is associated with an extended B8-DR3 haplotype including particular MICA and MICB alleles. Hepatology 2001;34:625–630.

78. Bodenheimer HC Jr, LaRusso NF, Thayer WR Jr et al. Elevated circulating immune complexes in primary sclerosing cholangitis. Hepatology 1983;3:150–154.

79. Senaldi G, Donaldson PT, Magrin S et al. Activation of the complement system in primary sclerosing cholangitis. Gastroenterology 1989;97:1430–1434.

80. Minuk GY, Angus M, Brickman CM et al. Abnormal clearance of immune complexes from the circulation of patients with primary sclerosing cholangitis. Gastroenterology 1985;88:166–170.

81. Das KM, Vecchi M, Sakamakis S. A shared and unique epitope(s) on human colon, skin and biliary epithelium detected by monoclonal antibody. Gastroenterology 1990;98:464–469.

82. Mandal A, Dasgupta A, Jeffers L et al. Autoantibodies in sclerosing cholangitis against a shared peptide in biliary and colon epithelium. Gastroenterology 1994;106:185–192.

83. Whiteside TL, Lasky S, Si L et al. Immunologic analysis of mononuclear cells in liver tissues and blood of patients with primary sclerosing cholangitis. Hepatology 1985;5:468–474.

84. Lindor KD, Wiesner RH, Katzmann JA et al. Lymphocyte subsets in primary sclerosing cholangitis. Dig Dis Sci 1987;32:720–725.

85. Martins EBG, Graham AK, Chapman RW et al. Elevation of γδ T lymphocytes in peripheral blood and livers of patients with primary sclerosing cholangitis and other autoimmune liver diseases. Hepatology 1996;23:988–993.

86. Broome U, Grunewald J, Scheynius A et al. Preferential Vβ3 usage by hepatic T lymphocytes in patients with primary sclerosing cholangitis. J Hepatol 1997;26:527–534.

87. Broome U, Glaumann H, Hultcrantz R et al. Distribution of HLA-DR, HLA-DP, and HLA-DQ antigens in liver tissue from patients with primary sclerosing cholangitis. Scand J Gastroenterol 1990;25:54–58.

88. van Milligen de Wit AW, van Deventer SJ, Tytgat GN. Immunogenetic aspects of primary sclerosing cholangitis: implications for therapeutic strategies. Am J Gastroenterol 1995;90:893–900.

89. Adams DH, Hubscher SG, Shaw J et al. Increased expression of intercellular adhesion molecule 1 on bile ducts in primary biliary cirrhosis and primary sclerosing cholangitis. Hepatology 1991;14:426–431.

90. Bloom S, Fleming K, Chapman R. Adhesion molecule expression in primary sclerosing cholangitis and primary biliary cirrhosis. Gut 1995;36:604–609.

91. Broome U, Hultcrantz R, Scheynius A. Lack of concomitant expression of ICAM-1 and HLA-DR on bile duct cells from patients with primary sclerosing cholangitis and primary biliary cirrhosis. Scand J Gastroenterol 1993;28:126–130.

92. Farrant JM, Hayllar KM, Wilkinson ML et al. Natural history and prognostic variables in primary sclerosing cholangitis. Gastroenterology 1991;100:1710–1717.

93. Shetty K, Rybicki L, Carey WD. The Child–Pugh classification as a prognostic indicator for survival in primary sclerosing cholangitis. Hepatology 1997;25:1049–1053.

94. Kim WR, Therneau TM, Poterucha JJ et al. A revised natural history model for primary sclerosing cholangitis obviates the need for liver histology. Mayo Clin Proc 2000;75:688–694.

95. Wee A, Ludwig J. Pericholangitis in chronic ulcerative colitis: primary sclerosing cholangitis of the small bile ducts? Ann Intern Med 1985;102:581–587.

96. Feldstein A, Angulo P, El-Youssef M et al. Primary sclerosing cholangitis in children: a long-term follow-up study. Gastroenterology 2002;122:A645–646.

97. Gregorio GV, Portmann V, Karani J et al. Autoimmune hepatitis/sclerosing cholangitis overlap syndrome in childhood: a 16-year prospective study. Hepatology 2001;33:544–553.

98. Wiesner RH, Grambsch PM, Dickson ER et al. Primary sclerosing cholangitis: natural history, prognostic factors, and survival analysis. Hepatology 1989;10:430–436.

99. Porayko MK, Wiesner RH, LaRusso NF et al. Patients with asymptomatic primary sclerosing cholangitis frequently have progressive disease. Gastroenterology 1990;98:1594–1602.

100. Dickson ER, Murtaugh PA, Wiesner RH et al. Primary sclerosing cholangitis: refinement and validation of survival models. Gastroenterology 1992;103:1893–1901.

101. Bergasa NV, Jones EA. The pruritus of cholestasis: potential pathogenic and therapeutic implications of opioids. Gastroenterology 1995;108:1582–1588.

102. Spivey JR, Jorgensen RA, Gores GJ et al. Methionin–enkephalin concentrations correlate with stage of disease but not pruritus in patients with primary biliary cirrhosis. Am J Gastroenterol 1994;89:2028–2032.

103. Jones EA, Bergasa NV. The pruritus of cholestasis. Hepatology 1999;29:1003–1006.

104. Bachs L, Pares A, Elena M et al. Effects of long-term rifampicin administration in primary biliary cirrhosis. Gastroenterology 1992;102:2077–2080.

105. Wolfhagen FHJ, Sternieri E, Hop WCJ et al. Oral naltrexone treatment of cholestatic pruritus: a double-blind, placebo-controlled study. Gastroenterology 1997;113:1264–1269.

106. Jorgensen RA, Lindor KD, Sartin JS et al. Serum lipid and fat-soluble vitamin levels in primary sclerosing cholangitis. J Clin Gastroenterol 1995;20:215–219.

107. Angulo P, Therneau TM, Jorgensen RA et al. Bone disease in patients with primary sclerosing cholangitis: prevalence, severity and prediction of progression. J Hepatol 1998;29:729–735.

108. Angulo P, Fong D, Keach JC et al. Predictors and rate of progression of bone disease in patients with primary sclerosing cholangitis. Hepatology 2000;32:308A.

109. Lindor KD, Jorgensen RA, Tiegs RD et al. Etidronate for osteoporosis in PBC: a randomized trial. J Hepatol 2000;33:878–882.

110. Pares A, Guanabens N, Alvarez L et al. Alendronate is more effective than etidronate for increasing bone mass in osteopenic patients with primary biliary cirrhosis. Hepatology 1999;30:472A.

111. Lanspa SJ, Chan ATH, Bell JS et al. Pathogenesis of steatorrhea in primary biliary cirrhosis. Hepatology 1985;5:837–842.

112. Kaya M, Petersen BT, Angulo P et al. Balloon dilatation compared to stenting of dominant strictures in primary sclerosing cholangitis. Am J Gastroenterol 2001;96:1059–1066.

113. Ponsioen CY, Lam K, van Milligen de Wit AWM et al. Four years experience with short-term stenting in primary sclerosing cholangitis. Am J Gastroenterol 1999;94:2403–2407.

114. Nichols JC, Gores GJ, LaRusso NF et al. Diagnostic role of serum CA 19-9 for cholangiocarcinoma in patients with primary sclerosing cholangitis. Mayo Clin Proc 1993;68:874–879.

115. Maestranzi S, Przemioslo R, Mitchell H et al. The effect of benign and malignant liver disease on the tumour markers CA 19-9 and CEA. Ann Clin Biochem 1998;35:99–103.

116. Fisher A, Theise ND, Min A et al. CA 19-9 does not predict cholangiocarcinoma in patients with primary sclerosing cholangitis undergoing liver transplantation. Liver Transplant Surg 1995;1:94–98.

117. Ramage JK, Donagly A, Farrant JM et al. Serum tumor markers for the diagnosis of cholangiocarcinoma in primary sclerosing cholangitis. Gastroenterology 1995;108:865–869.

118. Rosen CB, Nagorney DM, Wiesner RH et al. Cholangiocarcinoma complicating primary sclerosing cholangitis. Ann Surg 1991;213:21–25.

119. Gross JA, Shackelton CR, Farmer DG et al. Orthotopic liver transplantation for primary sclerosing cholangitis. A 12-year single center experience. Ann Surg 1997;225:472–483.

120. Harnois DM, Gores GJ, Ludwig J et al. Are patients with cirrhotic stage primary sclerosing cholangitis at risk for the development of hepatocellular cancer? J Hepatol 1997;27:512–516.

121. Broome U, Lofberg R, Veress R et al. Primary sclerosing cholangitis and ulcerative colitis: indicator of increase neoplastic potential. Hepatology 1995;22:1404–1408.

122. Loftus EV, Sandborn WJ, Tremaine WJ et al. Risk of colorectal neoplasia in patients with primary sclerosing cholangitis. Gastroenterology 1996;110:432–440.

123. Choi PM, Nugent FW, Rossi RL. Relationship between colorectal neoplasia and primary sclerosing cholangitis in ulcerative colitis. Gastroenterology 1992;103:1707–1708.

124. Nuako KW, Ahlquist DA, Sandborn WJ et al. Primary sclerosing cholangitis and colorectal carcinoma in patients with chronic ulcerative colitis. Cancer 1998;82:822–826.

125. Wiesner RH, LaRusso NF, Dozois RR et al. Peristomal varices after proctocolectomy in patients with primary sclerosing cholangitis. Gastroenterology 1986;90:316–322.

126. LaRusso NF, Wiesner RH, Ludwig J et al. Prospective trial of penicillamine in primary sclerosing cholangitis. Gastroenterology 1988;95:1036–1042.

127. Olsson R, Broome U, Danielsson A et al. Colchicine treatment of primary sclerosing cholangitis. Gastroenterology 1995;108:1199–1203.

128. Stiehl A, Raedsch R, Theilmann L et al. The effect of ursodeoxycholic acid (UDCA) in primary sclerosing cholangitis (PSC). Gastroenterology 1989;96:A664.

129. Lindor KD. Ursodiol for primary sclerosing cholangitis. N Engl J Med 1997;336:691–695.

130. Beuers U, Spengler U, Kruis W et al. Ursodeoxycholic acid for treatment of primary sclerosing cholangitis: a placebo-controlled trial. Hepatology 1992;16:707–714.

131. Angulo P, Bharucha AE, Jorgensen RA et al. Oral nicotine in the treatment of primary sclerosing cholangitis. Dig Dis Sci 1999;44:602–607.

132. Angulo P, Lindor KD, Wiesner RH et al. Pirfenidone in the treatment of primary sclerosing cholangitis. Dig Dis Sci 2002;47:157–161.

133. van Hoogstraten HJF, Vleggaar FP, Boland GJ et al. Budesonide or prednisone in combination with ursodeoxycholic acid in primary sclerosing cholangitis: a randomized double-blind pilot study. Am J Gastroenterol 2000;95:2015–2022.

134. Angulo P, Batts KP, Jorgensen RA et al. Oral budesonide in the treatment of primary sclerosing cholangitis. Am J Gastroenterol 2000;95:2333–2337.

135. Schramm C, Schirmacher P, Helmreich-Becker I et al. Combined therapy with azathioprine, prednisolone, and ursodiol in patients with primary sclerosing cholangitis. Ann Intern Med 1999;131:943–946.

136. Lindor KD, Wiesner RH, Colwell LJ et al. The combination of prednisone and colchicine in patients with primary sclerosing cholangitis. Am J Gastroenterol 1991;85:57–61.

137. Lindor KD, Jorgensen RA, Anderson ML et al. Ursodeoxycholic acid and methotrexate for primary sclerosing cholangitis: a pilot study. Am J Gastroenterol 1996;91:511–515.

138. van Thiel DH, Carroll P, Abu-Elmagd K et al. Tacrolimus (FK506), a treatment for primary sclerosing cholangitis: results of an open-label preliminary trial. Am J Gastroenterol 1995;90:455–459.

139. Harnois DM, Angulo PA, Jorgensen RA et al. High-dose ursodeoxycholic acid as therapy for patients with primary sclerosing cholangitis. Am J Gastroenterol 2001;96:1558–1562.

140. Mitchell SA, Bansi DS, Hunt N et al. A preliminary trial of high-dose ursodeoxycholic acid in primary sclerosing cholangitis. Gastroenterology 2001;121:900–907.

141. Stiehl A, Rudolph G, Sauer P et al. Efficacy of ursodeoxycholic acid treatment and endoscopic dilation of major duct stenoses in primary sclerosing cholangitis. J Hepatol 1997;26:560–566.

142. Baluyut AR, Sherman S, Lehman GA et al. Impact of endoscopic therapy on the survival of patients with primary sclerosing cholangitis. Gastrointest Endosc 2001;53:308–312.

143. Pitt HA, Thompson HH, Tompkins RK et al. Primary sclerosing cholangitis: results of an aggressive surgical approach. Ann Surg 1982;196:259–266.

144. Narumi S, Roberts JP, Emond JC et al. Liver transplantation for sclerosing cholangitis. Hepatology 1995;22:451–457.

145. Graziadei IW, Wiesner RH, Marotta PJ et al. Long-term results of patients undergoing liver transplantation for primary sclerosing cholangitis. Hepatology 1999;30:1121–1127.

146. Sheng R, Campbell WL, Zajko AB, Baron RL. Cholangiographic features of biliary strictures after liver transplantation for primary sclerosing cholangitis: evidence of recurrent disease. AJR 1996;166:1109–1113.

147. Graziadei IW, Wiesner RH, Marotta PJ et al. Strong evidence for recurrence of primary sclerosing cholangitis after liver transplantation. Hepatology 1997;26:176A.

148. Knechtle SJ, D'Allesandro AM, Harms BA, Pirsch JD, Belzer FO, Kalayoglu M. Relationships between sclerosing cholangitis, inflammatory bowel disease, and cancer in patients undergoing liver transplantation. Surgery 1995;118:615–620.

## CHAPTER 45

# Extraintestinal manifestations: skin, joints and mucocutaneous manifestations

Timothy R Orchard and Derek P Jewell

## INTRODUCTION

Inflammatory bowel disease is associated with a number of complications outside the gastrointestinal tract, including organs such as the skin, eyes, joints, blood, kidney and biliary tract. Some of these manifestations appear to be related to the activity of the underlying gut inflammation, whereas others may be secondary to abnormalities of intestinal function, which may be due to disease activity or surgery.

Although many conditions have been reported in association with IBD, the commonest problems relate to the eyes and joints, along with some skin manifestations such as erythema nodosum (EN) and pyoderma gangrenosum (PG). Other conditions appear much less common and have been reported in small case series only, such as Sweet's syndrome and pyostomatitis vegetans, and some conditions have only been reported in case reports. This chapter deals with the common complications and those reported in case series, and which are probably present at an increased incidence in patients with IBD compared to the general population. Because of the relatively small numbers involved, even in the common conditions management options are not based on data from controlled trials, but largely on the experience of large centers specializing in IBD.

The mechanisms involved in the pathogenesis of extraintestinal manifestations of IBD are not clear, but the relationship of many of them to active gut disease suggests that the increased gut permeability during active disease may allow luminal antigens to be presented to the systemic immune system. As there is already activation of immune and inflammatory responses this may lead to significant inflammatory responses elsewhere in the body. The reasons for certain systems being targeted, such as the joints, is not clear, but the finding of T cells bearing $\beta_7$ integrins (a molecule essential for homing of T cells to the lamina propria) in the synovial fluid[1] suggests a direct link between intestinal and extraintestinal inflammation.

An exhaustive list of extraintestinal manifestations (EIM) reported in IBD is shown in Table 45.1.

## COMMON EXTRAINTESTINAL MANIFESTATIONS

### MUCOCUTANEOUS

Many different mucocutaneous manifestations have been reported in IBD, of which erythema nodosum, oral ulceration and pyoderma gangrenosum are by far the most common. Other manifestations are rare, but probably occur more often in IBD than in the general population.

#### Erythema nodosum (EN)

EN is the most common skin manifestation of IBD. Its prevalence varies widely between studies, depending upon the nature of the study population and the type of study. It is reported in 1–9% of UC patients[2–4] and 6–15% of Crohn's disease patients,[5–8] although the most comprehensive study suggests a prevalence at the lower end of this range. However, all studies show a marked female preponderance, with a female to male ratio of about 5:1.[3,7]

EN consists of painful tender raised erythematous nodules. These are classically non-ulcerating but may be up to 3 cm in diameter. They are found predominantly on the extensor surfaces, nearly always in the pretibial region, as shown in Figure 45.1. A number of studies have demonstrated an association with other EIM of IBD, particularly arthritis and uveitis (see below). It is associated with active bowel disease in over 90% of cases, but the site and extent of the inflammatory bowel disease do not seem to influence EN. The majority of patients suffer a single episode, which occurs at or before the diagnosis of IBD in 53% of patients, but up to 30% of patients will suffer from recurrent episodes. In a large study from Oxford the

## Table 45.1 Extraintestinal manifestations previously reported in inflammatory bowel disease

| | |
|---|---|
| **Musculoskeletal** | **Cardiac** |
| Peripheral arthritis | Pleuropericarditis |
| Granulomatous arthritis and synovitis | Cardiomyopathy |
| Rheumatoid arthritis | Endocarditis |
| Sacroiliitis | Myocarditis |
| Ankylosing spondylitis | **Hematologic** |
| Clubbing | Anemia – iron deficiency |
| Osteoporosis and osteomalacia | Vitamin $B_{12}$ deficiency |
| Rhabdomyolysis | Anemia of chronic diseases |
| Relapsing polychondritis | Autoimmune hemolytic anemia |
| **Skin and mucous membranes** | Hyposplenism |
| Oral ulceration | Anticardiolipin antibody |
| Cheilitis | Takayasu's arteritis |
| Pyostomatitis vegetans | Wegener's arteritis |
| Erythema nodosum | **Renal and genitourinary** |
| Pyoderma gangrenosum | Nephrolithiasis |
| Sweet's syndrome | Retroperitoneal fibrosis |
| Metastatic Crohn's disease | Fistula formation |
| Psoriasis | Glomerulonephritis |
| Epidermolysis bullosa acquisita | Renal amyloidosis |
| Perianal skin tags | Drug-related nephrotoxicity |
| Polyarteritis nodosa | **Hepatopancreaticobiliary** |
| Cutaneous vasculitis | Primary sclerosing cholangitis |
| **Ocular** | (PSC) |
| Conjunctivitis | Small-duct PSC |
| Uveitis, iritis | Cholangiocarcinoma |
| Episcleritis | Cholelithiasis |
| Scleritis | Autoimmune hepatitis |
| Retrobulbar neuritis | Primary biliary cirrhosis |
| Crohn's keratopathy | Pancreatitis |
| **Bronchopulmonary** | Ampullary Crohn's disease |
| Chronic bronchitis with bronchiectasis | Granulomatous pancreatitis |
| Fibrosing alveolitis | **Endocrine and metabolic** |
| Pulmonary vasculitis | Growth failure |
| Interstitial lung disease | Thyroiditis |
| Sarcoidosis | Osteoporosis, osteomalacia |
| Tracheal obstruction | **Neurologic** |
| | Peripheral neuropathy |
| | Meningitis |
| | Vestibular dysfunction |
| | Pseudotumor cerebri |

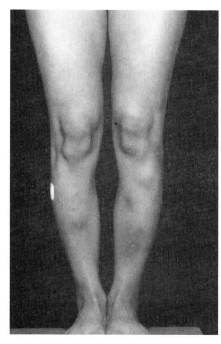

Fig. 45.1 Erythema nodosum. These are the typical raised erythematous painful lesions of EN. They are normally found on the extensor surfaces of the leg, as in this case, and occur with active gut disease. They normally resolve spontaneously with treatment of the gut disease.

median length of each episode was 4 weeks, with a range of 1–12 weeks. Rarely the lesions may recur frequently and very occasionally they may ulcerate; however, they normally heal without significant scarring.[7]

Histological examination of EN demonstrates a septal panniculitis. There is initially an acute inflammatory infiltrate in the lower dermis and subcutaneous tissue, with edema and extravasation of red blood cells and a range of leukocytes, including lymphocytes and histiocytes. There is subsequently swelling and fragmentation of collagen fibers, with fibrinoid necrosis. However, the clinical picture of EN is usually so typical that histologic confirmation is not required, and biopsies are now rarely performed.

The pathogenetic mechanisms involved in EN remain unknown. Because of its association with active disease, it has been suggested that it is triggered by bacteria or other foreign antigens, but no clear pathogenic influences have been determined. Some investigators have suggested that EN is part of an autoimmune reaction to an isoform of tropomyosin found in the gut, skin, joints and eyes,[9] but the evidence for this is currently weak. More recently genetic associations have been described in EN with the HLA region on chromosome 6, suggesting that at least part of the susceptibility to EN is inherited. These include weak associations with HLA-B.[10] However, recently an association with a polymorphism in the neighboring TNF-α gene has been described in EN associated with sarcoid,[11] and a stronger association has been described in IBD-associated EN with a slightly different polymorphism, with 70% of EN patients possessing the −1031c polymorphism compared to 37% of IBD controls.[12] Although this may not be the primary genetic influence, it is clear that genes in this region may play an important role in determining the presence of EN.

The diagnosis of EN is essentially a clinical one, with the appearance of characteristic nodules associated with active bowel disease. Occasionally, particularly in Crohn's disease, there may be little in the way of overt bowel disease, but inflammatory markers are usually raised. EN in the absence of active bowel disease or which is very persistent should raise the possibility of another cause of EN. The commonest cause in the Western world is sarcoidosis, but other causes, such as poststreptococcal infection and drugs such as the oral contraceptive pill, should be considered. Other forms of panniculitis, such as those seen in lymphoproliferative disorders, infections and vasculitis, may also need to be excluded in these cases by histologic examination of lesions by an experienced pathologist. Because of the tendency of EN to occur at the onset of IBD, the diagnosis of IBD should be considered in any patient presenting with apparently isolated EN.

The most effective treatment for EN is that of the underlying bowel disease, although up to 25% of patients will heal spontaneously. Symptomatic relief is therefore the goal, and analgesia is the mainstay of treatment. Ideally non-steroidal anti-inflammatory drugs should be avoided because of the risk of worsening the bowel disease,[13,14] and combination analgesics involving paracetamol and opiates may be used. However, in some cases NSAIDs may be unavoidable and will usually provide effective relief of pain in EN. In cases which are resistant oral prednisolone may be required, and very occasionally immunosuppressants such as methotrexate or azathioprine. However, in cases that require this treatment the diagnosis should be confirmed histologically and a dermatological review may be appropriate to exclude other diagnoses.

The prognosis for EN is good, the disease being largely self-limiting. Thirty per cent will have more than one episode, but these subsequent episodes also remain self-limiting. A small number of patients may have prolonged and frequent attacks and this group may require immunosuppression. There is an overlap with the arthritis and uveitis associated with IBD, which may also cause problems.[6,15,16]

## Pyoderma gangrenosum

Pyoderma gangrenosum (PG) is a less common but more troublesome skin manifestation associated with IBD. It is present in between 0.5 and 2% of both UC and Crohn's disease patients,[2,4,5] although some authors suggest it may be more common in UC. It is often unrelated to the activity of the bowel disease, although in some cases severe pyoderma gangrenosum is associated with severe relapse of the IBD. The site and extent of the IBD do not influence the PG. PG may also be found in other systemic diseases, including lymphoproliferative disorders and rheumatological disorders. In the former it is not associated with active disease, but in rheumatological conditions it is usually associated with severe, active and advanced disease. The reasons for this apparent difference are not clear.

The lesions of PG are ulcerating and are characteristically found on the lower limbs. However, they may occur at multiple sites and away from the limbs, and these cases are particularly associated with underlying systemic disease such as IBD. The lesions start as painful areas on the skin and then develop into pustules, before becoming sterile abscesses. They then break down to leave a necrotic central portion with a violaceous coloration around the edges, which undermines the adjacent healthy tissue (Fig. 45.2). The lesions also exhibit pathergy – they can be induced or extended by trauma. This phenomenon is also seen in other neutrophilic dermatoses such as Sweet's syndrome (see below). The ulcers are normally less than 4 cm across, but very occasionally may be quite extensive.[2] The lesions may last for many months, and up to 35% of patients will have recurrent episodes.[4]

Histologically there are no pathognomonic features of PG, but biopsies demonstrate an intense neutrophilic infiltrate in the dermis and subcutaneous tissues, with the presence of epithelioid granulomata in some patients. There may be fibrinoid necrosis and hemorrhage, but no other evidence of vasculitis or infection. The etiology of the lesions remains unknown.

The diagnosis of PG is a clinical one, but a biopsy is recommended if there is any question regarding the diagnosis to exclude vasculitis and infection (keeping in mind that the pathergy associated with the biopsy may extend the lesion). Biopsies must include deep tissue from the borders of the ulcers

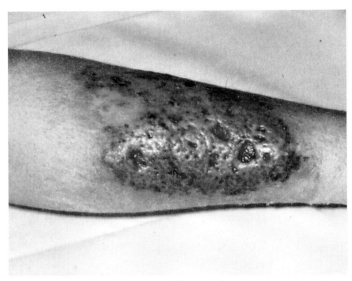

**Fig. 45.2** Pyoderma gangrenosum. This normally occurs on the lower limbs in IBD and the lesions start as painful areas on the skin and then develop into pustules, before becoming sterile abscesses. They then break down to leave a necrotic central portion with a violaceous coloration around the edges, which undermines the adjacent healthy tissue.

and should be stained for bacteria, mycobacteria and fungi, in addition to normal histopathological processing.

### Management

PG may be very troublesome. In some cases lesions may resolve spontaneously, but this may take many months and the risk of secondary infection, and the severe pain necessitates early treatment.

### Medical

Medical treatments are generally immunosuppressive in nature. First-line treatment is with corticosteroids, either as oral prednisolone (0.5–1 mg/kg) or pulsed intravenous methylprednisolone (10–15 mg/kg) for 3 days followed by oral prednisolone. Pulsed intravenous steroids may produce quite marked pain relief and healing. Intralesional steroid injections have been used in some instances.

Steroid-sparing agents should be used early in those who are not responding, or who require high doses of steroids. In mild cases dapsone or thalidomide may work in combination with prednisolone. In more severe cases other agents should be introduced, the most effective of which are probably calcineurin inhibitors such as cyclosporin and tacrolimus.[17] These can be used together with prednisolone, and in refractory cases azathioprine or mycophenolate may also be introduced.[18] However, this is a very potent immunosuppressive regimen and, if used, prophylaxis against *Pneumocystis carinii* pneumonia should also be used, such as co-trimoxazole 960 mg three times weekly.

In patients who cannot tolerate the calcineurin inhibitors, or who have persistent disease, azathioprine or mycophenolate may be used in combination with prednisolone. More recently small studies have suggested that treatment with monoclonal antibody to TNF-α infliximab may be effective in resistant cases, and this may obviate the necessity for potent combinations of corticosteroids and immune suppressants.[19]

Surgery for PG is difficult because PG exhibits pathergy. However, in patients who have responded to medical treatment, surgery to debride the lesions or plastic reconstruction may be undertaken, although these procedures are not without risk.[20] Surgery for the underlying bowel disease has also been used as a treatment for PG: in a series from the Cleveland Clinic the PG healed well after surgery, but recurred at the ileostomy site in 3/14 (21%) patients.[4]

The prognosis of PG is variable. It is certainly the most severe skin manifestation associated with IBD and can be very prolonged, but will usually come under control with medical therapy. However, in the most severe cases this may need to involve a combination of corticosteroids and immunosuppressants. Very occasionally surgical debridement or skin grafting may be required.

## Oral ulceration

Oral ulceration is very common, particularly in Crohn's disease, where up to 20 or 30% of patients may suffer.[6] The appearances are of superficial aphthous ulcers in the buccal mucosa. They tend to occur in crops around the oral cavity. Active oral ulceration is almost always associated with active bowel disease. Patients who develop recurrent oral ulceration are at increased risk of developing other extraintestinal manifestations, such as EN, ocular inflammation and arthritis, and recent small studies have suggested there may be a genetic predisposition, localized to the HLA region. Interestingly, this group of patients may share clinical features with Behçet's disease, raising the intriguing possibility of clinically overlapping syndromes.[21] Occasionally aggressive oral ulceration may occur as a result of treatment with methotrexate. This is easily distinguishable from aphthous ulceration as the ulcers are large and deep.

### Treatment

Ulcers usually heal with treatment of the underlying bowel disease. In severe or persistent cases topical steroid preparations may be helpful. One approach is to spray a dose of corticosteroids from a canister designed for asthma inhalation on to the affected mucosa (rather than inhaling it). Patients may also gain symptomatic relief from proprietary gel treatments for oral ulcers containing a local anesthetic such as lidocaine. Treatment with dapsone may also be of benefit in refractory cases. Methotrexate-induced ulceration responds promptly to stopping treatment and to folinic acid.

## JOINTS

Joint complications are the most common extraintestinal manifestations of inflammatory bowel disease and were recognized as long ago as the 1920s. Both axial and peripheral joint complications are recognized.

## Axial arthropathies

### Ankylosing spondylitis

Ankylosing spondylitis (AS) is a seronegative inflammatory arthropathy that affects the vertebral column, characterized by sacroiliitis and progressive ankylosis (fusion) of the vertebral facet joints, and is the classic condition of the seronegative spondyloarthropathy group. AS is normally defined by the modified New York criteria.[22] This definition relies upon the presence of radiographic sacroiliitis associated with inflammatory back pain, but there is some overlap with the more general term of spondyloarthropathy as defined by the European study group on spondyloarthropathy.[23] This relies on a combination of inflam-

matory low back pain and a number of other factors, including associated conditions such as urethritis, IBD or enteric infection, and the term includes postdysenteric reactive arthritis, psoriatic arthritis and posturethritis arthritis. The prevalence of AS in the general population is 0.25–1%,[24,25] but in IBD this is increased to 1–6%, depending on the study population and the methodology used.[26–28] Idiopathic AS is more common in males, with a M:F ratio of 3:1, whereas in IBD the M:F ratio is 1:1.

The central lesion of AS is sacroiliitis, and this is associated with inflammatory low back pain. This is characterized by an insidious onset over months, morning stiffness, and exacerbation of pain by rest, along with pain radiating into the buttocks (rather than central back pain). It tends to occur in patients under 40 years of age. As the disease progresses there is increasing immobility in the spine and there may be ankylosis of the spine, leading to the so-called 'bamboo spine' appearance on plain radiographs. This may be associated with other complications such as respiratory embarrassment secondary to poor lung expansion and upper lobe lung fibrosis, and the aortic root is often dilated.

The progress of AS associated with IBD is independent of the bowel disease, and most authors suggest it is identical to idiopathic AS. However, there has been some suggestion that IBD-associated AS runs a more benign clinical course, although this has yet to be established.[29]

AS is associated with other features, including peripheral arthritis in about 30% of patients and uveitis in up to 25% of patients.

There has been much research into the etiology of ankylosing spondylitis, based on the original observation that the condition is strongly associated with possession of HLA-B*27.[30] Research has concentrated on both the underlying genetic predisposition and environmental factors that might trigger AS. In addition, there have been a number of studies of the role of intestinal inflammation in AS and other spondyloarthropathies.

Genetics and environmental factors

Idiopathic AS is strongly associated with possession of HLA-B*27, with 94% of northern European patients being HLA-B*27 positive compared to 10% of healthy controls.[30,31] This genetic predisposition is also evident in patients with IBD-associated AS, but is considerably weaker, with between 50 and 80% of patients being HLA-B*27 positive.[32–34] Conversely, however, 50% of IBD patients who are HLA-B*27 positive have AS, compared to between 1 and 11% of B*27-positive people in the general population. Other genes in the HLA region have also been implicated in numerous small studies, including HLA-DR1,[35,36] TAP[37–39] and LMP,[40–42] but none of these has been definitive. Many studies have been performed to try to elucidate a mechanism through which HLA-B*27 itself might cause AS, but none of these has been conclusive. Putative mechanisms include B*27 presenting peptide from luminal bacteria, or self-protein causing an inflammatory response, or B*27 acting as a source of peptide to be presented to the immune system by other antigen presentation systems such as HLA-DR.[43] Central to these theories is the concept of a triggering bacterial antigen, although it is not clear what this antigen is. It has been suggested that idiopathic ankylosing spondylitis is associated with antibodies to *Klebsiella* species,[44] and that an abnormal immune response involving HLA-B27 is of pathogenetic importance. The less prominent HLA-B27 association in AS associated with IBD might suggest that in the presence of an inflamed gut, with increased permeability, more pathogenic antigen may be presented, allowing other HLA-B alleles to act pathogenically (see below). However, in IBD no associations between AS and bacteria have been demonstrated, and in idiopathic AS the evidence in favor of *Klebsiella* as opposed to other gut flora is unconvincing.

Further information about the role of bacteria in initiating arthritis in the presence of gut inflammation has been gained from the study of the HLA-B27 transgenic animal models. Although the rat and mouse models differ in some respects they provide useful working models. These animals spontaneously develop a colitis and axial and peripheral arthritis when reared under normal conditions.[45,46] However, if they are reared in a germ-free environment the gut and joint inflammation is abrogated.[46] Furthermore, Rath and colleagues have demonstrated that different bacteria induce gut and joint inflammation with differing efficiencies, with *Bacteroides vulgatus* and a cocktail of bacteria isolated from Crohn's disease patients being the most efficient, whereas *Escherichia coli* is ineffective.[45,47]

Thus it appears likely that bacteria are important in the pathogenesis of IBD-associated AS, but the mechanisms by which they interact with the immune system are unclear.

What is clear is that there is a strong genetic component in AS, which is conferred either by HLA-B*27 or by a gene in linkage with it.

### Role of intestinal inflammation in AS

There is a clear and obvious link between joint and gut inflammation in postenteric reactive arthritis, but recent work has demonstrated an important possible association in other spondyloarthropathies, including AS. Mielants and colleagues[48,49] performed ileocolonoscopy on 217 patients with spondyloarthropathies and took ileal biopsies. They found inflammatory lesions in 68% of patients (23% were acute and 45% chronic). The proportion with ileal inflammation was similar in AS and reactive arthritis (ReA), and the subsequent evolution of the articular disease to remission was similar in groups with or without initial gut inflammation. Eight patients went on to develop overt IBD (seven Crohn's disease and one UC) and all of these had gut inflammation initially (seven chronic and one acute).[50]

A potential confounding factor in studies of this sort is that most patients with spondyloarthropathy are treated with NSAIDs, which may themselves cause gastrointestinal inflammation. NSAID enteropathy may be difficult to distinguish from other inflammatory lesions of the gut; however, its distribution is characteristically more proximal than that associated with spondyloarthropathy, and it is rarely present in the terminal ileum.[51,52] Stricturing lesions due to NSAIDs have a typical diaphragmatic appearance and there may also be an increase in the number of apoptotic cells in the intestinal mucosa.[53,54] By these methods it is normally possible to diagnose NSAID enteropathy, although it may coexist with IBD or spondyloarthropathy-associated enteropathy in the same patient. Under these circumstances it may be very difficult to assess the contribution of each to the ongoing symptoms. In Mielants' study a subgroup of 49 patients, all of whom were treated with NSAIDs, underwent further colonoscopies between 2 and 9 years later.[50] At review 16 (32%) were found to be in clinical remission from their locomotor symptoms. None of these patients had inflammatory gut lesions at review. Thirty-three patients (68%) had persistent locomotor inflammation, 14 of whom had persistent inflammatory gut lesions and six had developed overt IBD. Of patients with non-AS spondyloarthropathy initially, seven of 19 developed AS, and all had persistent inflammatory gut lesions. Thus it appears that intestinal inflammation may be important in idiopathic as well as IBD-associated AS, possibly by allowing an increased antigenic load across the inflamed mucosa.

### Idiopathic versus IBD-associated AS

Clinically the AS seen in IBD appears similar to idiopathic AS. There has been a suggestion that it may follow a more benign course than idiopathic AS, but there is no current consensus on this.[29] The reasons for the difference in the prevalence of B*27 in the two types of AS may reflect the degree of intestinal inflammation seen in the two conditions. In overt IBD the intestinal mucosa is markedly damaged, whereas in idiopathic AS any intestinal mucosal changes tend to be more subtle. Thus a much higher antigenic load may be delivered to the immune system through the gut in IBD, and a higher proportion of B*27-positive subjects develop AS. In addition, the increased antigenic load may provoke disease in B*27-negative individuals, overriding the inherent genetic predisposition provided by HLA-B*27 or a closely linked gene.[55] The most widely accepted clinical criteria for the diagnosis of AS are the modified New York criteria,[56] which include low back pain for more than 3 months, relieved by exercise and not improved by rest; limited spinal movement in two planes; and decreased chest expansion. If any of these clinical features is present in association with bilateral grade 2–4 or unilateral grade 3–4 sacroiliitis then a definite diagnosis of AS can be made. In clinical practice the combination of inflammatory low back pain and morning stiffness, decreased spinal mobility and radiographic sacroiliitis is the characteristic feature. Inflammatory low back pain tends to occur in the morning, after rest, and to improve with exercise. It is often central and may radiate into the buttocks, and may occur in young people. In contrast, mechanical low back pain tends to worsen with exercise, improves with rest, and occurs in older people. A simple method of assessing spinal mobility in two planes is shown in Table 45.2. Patients with abnormal spinal mobility and pain should undergo radiological examination of the sacroiliac joints and HLA testing.

The traditional method of radiological assessment is by plain radiology of the sacroiliac joints, where sclerosis and erosion of the sacroiliac joints may be seen either unilaterally or bilaterally. Magnetic resonance (MR) scanning has been demonstrated to have a higher sensitivity in detecting sacroiliac abnormalities, although in the absence of symptoms their significance is sometimes unclear, but the lack of radiation means that this is now the gold standard investigation in patients with suspected sacroiliitis.

The management of AS consists of analgesia, physiotherapy to maintain spinal mobility, and disease-modifying drugs to try and slow down progression of the disease. All patients should be managed jointly by a gastroenterologist and rheumatologist.

### Analgesia

Simple analgesics should be used if possible. NSAIDs are the drugs of choice in idiopathic AS, and if there is active spinal disease in the absence of active IBD then it is reasonable to use them. However, NSAIDs may cause enterocolitis in their own right, and may trigger or exacerbate relapse of the pre-existing IBD, and they should be stopped if the IBD flares up.[13,14,54] The recent advent of cyclooxygenase-2 (COX-2)-specific NSAIDs

**Table 45.2 Methods for asessing spinal mobility**

| Test | Normal values |
|---|---|
| Lumbar flexion (modified Schober test): Mark the skin 5 cm below and 10 cm above the dimples of Venus. Ask the patient to flex forward fully and measure the distance between the two marks | The distance between the two marks should increase to ≥21 cm |
| Lateral flexion: From a vertical position the patient should slide each arm in turn down their leg. The distance moved by the fingertips should be measured and the mean calculated | The fingertips should move ≥14 cm, or to touch the joint line of the knee each side |
| Chest expansion: Measured in the fourth intercostal space | ≥5 cm |

Any decrease in the above not accounted for by pre-existing conditions should be regarded as reflecting decreased spinal mobility, and merits further investigation.

has raised the prospect of fewer unwanted gastrointestinal problems, particularly in the stomach. A recent open study suggested that COX-2-specific NSAIDs may improve the tolerability of these drugs in IBD patients, and they can be tried as an alternative to traditional NSAIDs.[57]

Physical therapies
Physical therapies are of particular importance and all patients should take regular exercise to maintain the mobility of the spine. This may include swimming and spinal exercises, with regular physiotherapy if necessary. These forms of exercise should also be recommended to patients with sacroiliitis associated with any form of low back pain or decreased spinal mobility. For patients with severely reduced spinal mobility or severe low back pain a period of intensive inpatient physiotherapy, often combined with injection of steroid into the sacroiliac joints, may help.

Drug therapies
Sulfasalazine can be used for both the IBD and the joint symptoms, but it is most effective in patients with associated peripheral joint problems. Other 5-ASA drugs are not as effective, as it is thought to be the sulfapyridine component that confers the articular effects, rather than the 5-ASA.

Corticosteroids and immunomodulators
Injection of the sacroiliac joints with steroids may provide relief, although this may be short-lived, particularly if not combined with aggressive physiotherapy. Oral corticosteroids may have a beneficial effect on the spine if used for active bowel disease, but should be used long term for control of spinal disease alone.

Methotrexate may be used to treat spinal disease alone,[58] although recent studies have suggested that it is more effective in peripheral than axial joint disease,[59] or for both spinal and bowel disease, and should be considered as a first-line immunosuppressant in patients with active IBD and AS, particularly in Crohn's disease.

There are now small studies demonstrating that infliximab is effective in patients with active ankylosing spondylitis,[60,61] and it may also be effective in patients with IBD-related spondyloarthropathies.[62] This treatment should certainly be considered

early in Crohn's disease patients with active bowel disease and difficult spinal disease.

## Isolated sacroiliitis

In addition to ankylosing spondylitis, isolated sacroiliitis is also associated with IBD. In these cases there is inflammation in the sacroiliac joints without evidence of progressive spinal disease. Although some may develop low back pain, many patients with sacroiliitis may be asymptomatic. Because of this its prevalence is largely dependent upon the means of diagnosis.

Radiographic surveys suggest a prevalence of up to 18%,[26] but more recent studies have suggested a higher prevalence. Diagnosis on radiographic grounds alone is hampered by a large degree of inter- and intraobserver error.[63] CT imaging studies have detected sacroiliitis in 32% of patients with IBD,[64] and studies using radioisotope scintigraphy have found uptake abnormalities in up to 52% of patients with Crohn's disease and 42% of those with UC.[65] However, the significance of these findings is not clear, and long-term follow-up studies to establish what proportion progress to AS have not been undertaken. It may be that in the majority of patients this is a non-progressive condition.

### Aetiology
The genetic predisposition to sacroiliitis is much less clear than in AS, partly because it is not clear what proportion of patients with sacroiliitis have early progressive disease (and will ultimately develop AS), and what proportion have true isolated sacroiliitis. Large follow-up studies are required to address this question.

The only study of sacroiliitis performed so far is a small study in 136 patients with Crohn's disease, which looked at patients with symptomatic back pain.[66] This demonstrated that 29% of these patients had evidence of sacroiliitis, including 7% who had AS. Those patients with sacroiliitis in the absence of AS were less likely to be HLA-B*27 positive. However, a full clinical assessment was not undertaken to differentiate inflammatory from mechanical back pain, and the study did not examine patients with asymptomatic sacroiliitis. A smaller study of 45 patients with Crohn's disease for 5–10 years' duration showed the presence of AS in 8% and isolated sacroiliitis in 22%; 30% of patients with isolated sacroiliitis were asymptomatic, and in this study HLA-B*27 appeared to be associated with sacroiliitis rather than progressive disease.[67] Only larger long-term follow-up studies will decide this issue.

In clinical practice diagnosis is usually by plain abdominal radiograph or radiography of the sacroiliac joints. In the majority of patients it is detected incidentally, and the patients do not complain of low back pain. However, in a proportion of patients it is found on X-ray or MRI for investigation of back pain. All patients with radiological evidence of sacroiliitis should have spinal mobility assessed and HLA status measured.

Patients who are symptomatic should have spinal mobility exercises, and analgesia as for patients with AS (see above). Mobility exercises should also be given to patients with restriction of spinal mobility or who are HLA-B*27 positive, as these are at high risk of developing progressive spinal disease. It would seem sensible in these groups of patients to assess spinal mobility periodically. Patients who are asymptomatic, have no restriction of spinal mobility and who are HLA-B*27 negative require no specific treatment.

## Peripheral arthritis

Peripheral arthritis has been reported in association with IBD for many years, but it was only in 1958 that the arthritis was proved to be inflammatory and quite distinct from classic rheumatoid, being seronegative for rheumatoid factor.[15]

### Prevalence

The prevalence of peripheral arthritis in IBD has been reported as between 10 and 20%.[27,68,69] However, the definitions of arthritis vary between studies, and often arthralgia in the absence of objective evidence of inflammation has been included. This is certainly common, and may relate to steroid reduction, or the commencement of immunosuppressants such as azathioprine. Many studies have noted a wide range of articular involvement, including a large joint oligoarthritis and a polyarthritis,[6,70,71] but recently this has been formalized by studying only patients with objective evidence of joint swelling.[16] This study demonstrated two distinct types of arthropathy with different natural histories and articular distributions.

**Type 1 (pauciarticular)** affects fewer than five joints, including a weightbearing joint. The swelling is acute and self-limiting, and associated with relapse of the IBD in the majority of cases.

**Type 2 (polyarticular)** affects five or more and a wide range of joints, but particularly the metacarpophalangeal (MCP) joints. It may cause persistent problems, with a median duration of 3 years.

The onset of arthritis may occur at any time during the course of the IBD, or before it becomes clinically manifest. It is not related to disease extent in UC, but in Crohn's disease it is reportedly more common in colonic disease. In both types of arthropathy there is little or no joint destruction and patients are seronegative.

In this series of 1459 patients the prevalence of type 1 was 3.6% in UC and 6.0% in Crohn's disease, and for type 2 was 2.5% in UC and 4.0% in Crohn's disease. A further 5.3% of UC patients and 14.3% of Crohn's disease patients complained of arthralgia.[16] These figures may underestimate the true prevalence, but it seems clear that the prevalence of all forms of peripheral arthritis in UC is between 5 and 10%, and significantly more in Crohn's disease – perhaps 10–20%.

As in AS the etiology of peripheral arthritis in IBD is likely to be a combination of genetic susceptibility and luminal factors.

### Genetics

Until recently there has been little evidence for the involvement of genetic factors such as HLA in the peripheral arthritis of IBD. Small serological studies performed in the 1970s failed to detect any HLA associations, and a small study of IBD patients undergoing restorative proctocolectomy[72] showed that 27% of patients who suffered arthritis possessed the rare allele HLA-DR103, compared to 3% of healthy controls.

The apparent lack of associations is surprising, given the strong HLA-B*27 association seen in reactive arthritis associated with acute bacterial gastroenteritis. This is a pauciarticular arthritis clinically very similar to type 1 IBD peripheral arthritis. However, recent studies using PCR-based techniques in larger groups of patients have demonstrated quite clear HLA associations in IBD arthritis. The association with HLA-DR103 is solely with type 1, which is also associated with HLA-B*27, whereas type 2 is associated with HLA-B44 (Table 45.3).[73]

Further evidence for a role for the MHC region on chromosome 6 comes from the finding that type 2 arthritis is associated

**Table 45.3 HLA associations reported with extraintestinal manifestations of inflammatory bowel disease**

| Manifestation | HLA antigen | Affected patients (% with HLA) | IBD controls (% with HLA) |
|---|---|---|---|
| Type 1 arthritis | HLA-B27 | 26 | 7 |
| | HLA-B35 | 33 | 15 |
| | HLA-DR103 | 35 | 3 |
| Type 2 arthritis | HLA-B44 | 62 | 31 |
| Ankylosing spondylitis | HLA-B27 | 60 | 7 |
| Uveitis | HLA-B27 | 33 | 7 |
| | HLA-B58 | 13 | 3 |
| | HLA-DR103 | 20 | 3 |
| Erythema nodosum | HLA-B62 | 28 | 11 |

in some studies with MICA (MHC class I chain-like gene A), a non-classic HLA gene which is found close to HLA-B.[74]

### Environmental factors

The role of luminal factors in the etiology of peripheral arthritis is an area of debate. Postenteric reactive arthritis is associated with Gram-negative enterobacteria such as *Salmonella*, *Escherichia coli*, *Yersinia*, *Klebsiella* and *Campylobacter*, and bacterial antigens may be isolated from the affected joints. These postenteric arthritides are clinically very similar to the type 1 peripheral arthritis seen in IBD, and so it seems likely that presentation of bacterial antigen may be important in the initiation of type 1 IBD arthritis. This is plausible, given the association between type 1 arthritis and active disease. In these circumstances the gut is inflamed and therefore more permeable, a similar situation to that which pertains in acute bacterial enterocolitis. Proliferative T-cell responses to the relevant bacteria have been demonstrated from the synovial fluid of patients with reactive arthritis, but interestingly most of these appear to be HLA-DR restricted rather than HLA-B restricted.[75–77] This suggests that the HLA class II alleles may be more important than HLA-B*27 in this group of conditions.

As in AS, animal models may hold the key to understanding the interaction between bacteria and the immune system to cause peripheral arthritis in the presence of intestinal inflammation. The HLA-B*27 transgenic animal models develop peripheral arthritis and colitis when reared under normal conditions.[45,46] However, if reared in a germ-free environment the gut and joint inflammation is abrogated.[46] Furthermore, Rath and colleagues have demonstrated that different bacteria induce gut and joint inflammation with differing efficiencies, with *Bacteroides vulgatus* and a cocktail of bacteria isolated from Crohn's disease patients being the most efficient in HLA-B*27 transgenic rats, whereas *E. coli* is ineffective.[45,47] However, in other animal models, such as the IL-10 knockout mouse, it is other bacteria, such as *E. coli*, that cause inflammation.

Thus it appears likely that bacteria are important in the pathogenesis of the type 1 peripheral arthritis of IBD, but the mechanisms by which they interact with the immune system are unclear, and host genetic background may well be important.

The exact site within the gut where this interaction occurs is also a matter for debate, and in this area animal models may provide some useful information.

Rath et al. have demonstrated in the HLA-B*27 transgenic rat that diversion of the fecal stream away from the cecum abrogates distant inflammation while leaving the colitis unaffected.[78] They have postulated a role for bacterial overgrowth in the cecum in the pathogenesis of extracolonic inflammation. In humans the cecum is relatively much smaller than in the rat, and so these data cannot be extrapolated directly. However, in a study of 434 patients with Crohn's disease there was a significant decrease in the incidence of new joint complications after resection of the ileocecal region – from one complication for every 89 years of follow-up to one complication every 701 years of follow-up.[79] This is a highly significant difference, even when correcting for the time spent in remission from Crohn's disease after surgery. Although this study provides circumstantial evidence that the ileocecal region may be important in the development of arthritis in IBD it does not help determine whether it is stasis proximal to the ileocecal valve or cecal bacteria that are of importance, and clearly this is an area where further research is required.

### Clinical features

Type 1 arthritis tends to affect large weightbearing joints, particularly the knees, wrists and ankles. It never involves more than four joints at any one time, and tends to run an acute self-limiting course associated with relapse of the IBD. The median duration is 5 weeks, with a maximum of 10 weeks. However, as with reactive arthritis, 10–20% will develop persistent problems; 25–40% of patients will have more than one episode of arthritis, and there is also an increased risk of erythema nodosum and uveitis with this form of arthritis. On examination, the joint will be hot, painful, and there may be an effusion.

Type 2 arthritis is a symmetrical polyarthritis and may occur at any time, irrespective of the activity of the bowel disease. It runs a more chronic course than type 1, with a median duration of 3 years. The small joints of the hands are the most commonly affected, but it may affect a wide range of joints. It is associated with uveitis, but not erythema nodosum.

The diagnosis of peripheral arthritis in IBD is clinical. Radiology is usually normal, as the arthritis does not characteristically cause joint erosion or deformity. Laboratory tests may show high inflammatory markers reflecting the inflammatory nature of the arthritis, or underlying activity of the IBD. Anyone with persistent or severe disease should have rheumatoid factor checked to exclude seropositive rheumatoid arthritis, and anyone with erosions on radiology should be referred to a rheumatologist for an expert opinion, as these are signs that the arthritis is not simply secondary to the IBD. In the presence of a single acutely inflamed joint, joint aspiration should be undertaken to exclude either gout or septic arthritis. Some patients may also have other radiological signs of seronegative arthritis spondyloarthropathies, such as calcaneal spurs and sacroiliitis. Patients with incidental sacroiliitis should be managed as recommended above.

### Management

Type 1 arthritis is usually self-limiting, and so treatment is largely symptomatic.

Resting the joint is important, and the use of a walking stick or splint to take pressure off the joint may lead to a significant improvement. Range of movement exercises should be performed to minimize any periarticular muscle atrophy and to prevent contractures. In severe cases formal physiotherapy may be required to improve function.

Analgesia should be with simple analgesia and, as type 1 arthritis is usually associated with active bowel disease, NSAIDs should not be used. A good, but relatively seldom used, therapy is intra-articular injection of steroid. This may provide very effective symptom relief and may remove the requirement for other treatments. This may be done in the outpatient clinic, where a combination of local anesthetic such as lidocaine and a steroid such as methylprednisolone may be injected into large joints such as the knee. If oral steroids are used to treat the active bowel disease then these will normally treat the arthritis effectively. If not, an empirical change of 5-ASA drug to sulfasalazine may give good symptom relief. In this clinical circumstance, sulfasalazine is the first-line 5-ASA because of the beneficial effects of the sulfapyridine on the arthritis. If sulfasalazine fails then a lower dose of oral steroid specifically for the joint disease may be effective (10–15 mg of prednisolone, rather than 30–40 mg), but this should not be prolonged for more than a few weeks.

Long-term treatment is not usually required, although maintenance with sulfasalazine as the 5-ASA of choice may be appropriate, particularly in patients at risk of recurrent disease, such as those who are HLA-DR103 positive. In the minority of patients with persistent problems the treatment options are those of type 2 arthritis (see below).

Type 2 arthritis patients generally have persistent problems and may require long-term treatment. Again, as the disease is usually non-erosive and non-deforming symptomatic relief is the major aim.

Again, splinting of affected joints and rest are important components of management, but the persistent and polyarthritic nature of this condition makes this harder to achieve than in type 1 arthritis.

Simple analgesia should be tried initially. NSAIDs should only be considered in patients with quiescent disease unresponsive to simple or combination analgesia, and if there is any evidence of an increase in the activity of the bowel disease they should be stopped immediately.

For patients with persisting problems sulfasalazine or low-dose prednisolone (10–15 mg daily) may be used; however, prolonged courses of oral steroids should be avoided. In patients with active bowel disease, concurrent arthritis is a good indication for the use of methotrexate as the first-line immunosuppressant rather than azathioprine, in order to treat both gut and joints.

Patients who have evidence of erosive joint disease, a positive rheumatoid factor, or who do not respond to the measures outlined above should be managed jointly with a rheumatologist.

## OCULAR INFLAMMATION

Ocular inflammation in IBD was first documented by Crohn in 1925.[80] If left untreated it is a potential cause of blindness, but prompt treatment with topical steroids can minimize this risk.

### Prevalence

The prevalence of ocular inflammation varies widely between studies – from 2 to 13%, depending on the population and methodology used.[6,8,81] The manifestations range from con-junctivitis to more significant inflammation. This usually affects the anterior chamber, but may include iritis, episcleritis, scleritis and anterior uveitis. In a large retrospective study of 1459 patients (976 UC and 483 Crohn's disease patients) 3% of UC and 5% of Crohn's disease patients had these more serious eye complications.[7] The commonest were iritis (60%), episcleritis (30%) and uveitis (10%). The conditions affect females more than males, with a ratio of approximately 3:1, and in about 30% of cases the patients suffered from recurrent episodes. Posterior segment eye disease has been described, including serous choroidoretinopathy and retinal detachment, but these are very rare, and it is not clear whether there is an increased incidence in IBD above that seen in the general population.[82,83]

## Pathophysiology

### Genetics

Acute anterior uveitis may occur alone or in association with other conditions such as AS and IBD. The condition appears clinically identical in these conditions, but different from the uveitis of Behçet's disease, which characteristically affects the posterior chamber of the eye.[84] Idiopathic acute anterior uveitis has been demonstrated to be associated with HLA-B*27 in a number of small studies,[84] and recently a large retrospective study in IBD demonstrated associations between ocular inflammation and several HLA alleles, including HLA–B*27 (40% vs. 9% in IBD controls; $P<0.0001$), HLA-B*58 (12% vs. 1%; $P=0.002$) and HLA-DR*103 (20% vs. 8%; $P=0.001$).[10] Thus it appears that HLA genes may have an important role in the ocular complications of IBD.

Other hypotheses for the etiology of uveitis in IBD have included an autoimmune reaction to an antigenic form of tropomyosin expressed in both gut and eye.[9] However, the proposed antigen is expressed in the ciliary body (which is rarely affected) and not in the iris (which is often affected).

### Clinical features

Patients present with a gritty feeling in the eye, associated with perikeratic (corneal) injection. This may be the extent of the symptoms in conjunctivitis, but patients with uveitis will usually complain of an acute painful red eye and there may be blurring of vision and decreased visual acuity. It is usually unilateral, but may occasionally affect both eyes. It is associated with activity of the IBD in over 70% of cases. If left untreated the condition may lead to permanent damage to the eye, and even blindness. An example of uveitis is shown in Figure 45.3.

### Diagnosis

Cases of mild conjunctivitis may be diagnosed clinically, but for accurate diagnosis patients should undergo a full ophthalmologic assessment, including slit-lamp examination with dilated pupils. This may detect keratic precipitates on the cornea, cells in the anterior and posterior chambers, and posterior synechiae and pigment on the lens. Thus early referral to an ophthalmologist is important.

### Management

Treatment normally consists of topical steroid treatment, initially frequently (hourly) but subsequently reducing, although a 6–8-week course is usual. A cycloplegic agent such as atropine is often added to prevent the formation of posterior synechiae. Occasionally periocular injection or oral steroids may be required for acute anterior uveitis, and often in scleritis. Oral or topical

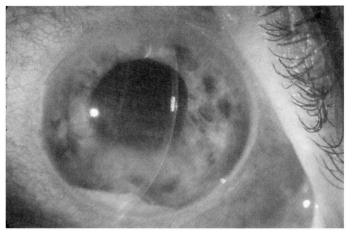

**Fig. 45.3** Uveitis. The uvea is one of the inner layers of the eye and comprises the iris, ciliary body and choroid. Inflammation of any one or all of these structures is generically termed 'uveitis'; more specific terms would include iritis, intermediate uveitis or choroiditis, respectively. This example is from a patient with inflammatory bowel disease and demonstrates a red eye, an irregularly shaped pupil, and most notably a hypopyon inferiorly. The pupil has been pharmacologically dilated, but adhesions between the iris and the lens capsule related to the iritis prevent dilation. The hypopyon represents a layering of the inflammatory white cells and is present only in the most severe cases of uveitis. Photo courtsey of James Garrity, MD, Mayo Clinic, Rochester, MN.

NSAIDs may be useful in anterior scleritis, but have no role in anterior uveitis. Their use carries a risk of triggering the IBD, as described above.

Posterior chamber inflammation is uncommon in IBD, but necessitates more aggressive therapy as topical agents do not penetrate effectively into the posterior chamber. Intraocular injection of corticosteroid may be effective, but usually oral corticosteroids are required. These may need to be continued for up to 4 weeks before a gradual reduction when the eye disease is under control. In patients who have a poor response immunosuppressants such as azathioprine, methotrexate or cyclosporin may be required in addition to the corticosteroids.

### Drug-induced ocular inflammation

Patients who are treated with systemic corticosteroids with or without immunosuppressants are at increased risk of opportunistic infection. Candidal infection of the eye should always be considered in patients who present with acute ocular inflammation, and slit-lamp examination should be performed by an ophthalmologist before initiation of treatment. Topical antifungal therapy is usually adequate for treatment of candidal infections, but oral therapy may sometimes be required.

Thus all patients with acute ocular inflammation with IBD should have a rapid assessment by an ophthalmologist, who should guide their treatment, which normally consists of topical or oral corticosteroid therapy. Failure to treat the inflammation effectively may lead to long-term complications or even blindness, although these situations are rare.

# MULTIPLE EXTRAINTESTINAL MANIFESTATIONS

Many of the studies on EIM have described the occurrence of more than one in the same patient. This overlap is particularly obvious between peripheral arthritis, EN and uveitis. Within this group both EN and uveitis are associated with type 1 (large joint) arthritis, whereas only uveitis is associated with type 2 arthritis, and there is no independent association between EN and uveitis. A number of hypotheses have been suggested to account for this overlap. The first suggests that the EIM are due to an autoimmune reaction to an antigen expressed in eye, skin, joint and colon. This antigen could be an isoform of tropomyosin.[9] However, although this antigen was found in the target organs it was not found in the components that became inflamed. Thus it was expressed in chondrocytes but not synovium, and in ciliary muscles but not the iris. In addition, this hypothesis fails to explain why in some patients ocular inflammation, EN or arthritis occur as single manifestations, and in others as part of a complex of extraintestinal manifestations.

A second hypothesis which may explain the clinical characteristics more easily is a genetic one. As described above, all of these EIM have distinct associations with genes in the HLA region. If each is determined by a gene or genes in this region the overlap between them could be explained by the phenomenon of linkage disequilibrium. In this hypothesis the different EIM are determined by different genes located close together in the HLA region. Because of this they are more likely to be inherited together than would be predicted by chance, and thus some patients may inherit the genes for more than one EIM. Much further work is required to establish whether this is the case by clarification of the nature of the genetic associations in this region; however, it does appear that genes in the HLA region may play an important part in the etiology of several of the EIM associated with IBD.

## LESS COMMON EXTRAINTESTINAL MANIFESTATIONS

Extraintestinal manifestations have been reported in a wide variety of organ systems that appear to have less clinical impact than those described above. These include rare skin manifestations, blood disorders including hemolytic anemia and thrombotic disorders, vasculitis, cardiac and pulmonary manifestations, and renal manifestations.

## RARE MUCOCUTANEOUS MANIFESTATIONS

### REACTIVE MANIFESTATIONS

**Sweet's syndrome** is a neutrophilic dermatosis which is rarely associated with IBD. It may also be associated with inflammatory connective tissue disorders and hematologic malignancy. It presents as painful urticarial lesions, predominantly on the head, neck and arms. Lesions normally resolve with corticosteroids, thalidomide or dapsone treatment.[85]

### VESICULOPUSTULAR ERUPTIONS

**Pyostomatitis vegetans** is a condition that affects the oral cavity and is characterized by friable erythematous plaques, which may be associated with aseptic abscesses.[86] It is thought to represent a mucosal form of pyoderma gangrenosum, and may be mistaken for a variant of pemphigus (pemphigus vegetans). This should

be excluded by histologic and immunofluorescence studies. The condition may be caused in some patients by zinc deficiency, and zinc replacement may improve it. Otherwise corticosteroids may be effective.[87]

**Bowel-associated dermatosis–arthritis syndrome** was first described in patients who had undergone intestinal bypass surgery, but it has been reported in association with IBD. The skin lesions of this condition are characterized by a characteristic pustular and purpuric rash. It is associated with a fever and oligoarthritis, which is usually mild.[88] It is thought to be due to circulating immune complexes caused by bacterial overgrowth in the gut.[89] Histologic examination demonstrates a heavy neutrophilic infiltrate which may extend subcutaneously. There may be an associated vaculitis. Treatment with dapsone is usually effective in combination with antibiotics to treat the underlying bacterial overgrowth.[90]

**Vasculitis** is a superficial vasculitis that may sometimes complicate IBD. The vessels affected are normally superficial cutaneous vessels only. The condition presents with purpura, which may be palpable or non-palpable on the lower extremities. The vasculitis may rarely be the presenting feature of the IBD, but it is usually associated with activity of the underlying bowel disease. Involvement of the viscera in the vasculitic process is exceptional. The diagnosis should be confirmed by histologic and immunofluorescent examination of skin biopsies in order to exclude other causes, such as Henoch–Schönlein purpura or IgA vasculitis. Some authors have suggested that vasculitis of larger vessels may be associated with IBD, but this remains controversial. Treatment is by controlling the underlying bowel disease, and oral corticosteroids. Adjuvant therapy with immunosuppressants may be required.[91]

## GRANULOMATOUS CONDITIONS

### CUTANEOUS CROHN'S DISEASE

The commonest manifestation of cutaneous Crohn's disease is perianal disease, which is discussed elsewhere. This may present with discharging sinuses, ulceration and skin tags, and tends to reflect the activity of the underlying bowel disease. Metastatic Crohn's disease is characterized by granulomatous skin lesions away from the perineum. It is rare, and most commonly affects the lower extremities, where it presents as nodules or plaques which may ulcerate.[92,93] The clinical course of the lesions tends to be independent of that of the underlying bowel disease. Diagnosis is usually made on biopsy of the lesions. Treatment may be difficult and may require a combination of medicines, including immunosuppressants and anti-inflammatory drugs. Good responses have been reported with oral corticosteroids in combination with either azathioprine, mycophenolate mofetil, cyclosporin or thalidomide. In very persistent cases infliximab may cause improvement, although repeated infusions may be required.

### OROFACIAL GRANULOMATOSIS

This is a granulomatous condition that presents with inflammation and cobblestone ulceration of the mouth, and thus could be considered as oral Crohn's disease. It often presents in young people before there is evidence of disease in other parts of the gut, and is more common in males than females.[94] It may occur as an isolated condition or as a complication of sarcoidosis, and this condition should be actively excluded. Histologic examination reveals inflammation, edema and non-caseating granulomata.

Treatment is often unrewarding, and there are no large-scale trials to guide therapy. The simplest treatments include dietary manipulations, concentrating especially on food additives, but these work in only a minority of patients. In a study of 79 patients 58% went into remission with topical corticosteroid therapy, and in 50% of the remainder systemic corticosteroids with or without azathioprine were successful.[94] The condition relapsed after treatment in 57% of cases. Thus first-line treatment should probably consist of topical steroid therapy with anti-inflammatories and local anesthetic gels. If these are unsuccessful, oral steroids alone or in combination with azathioprine may be effective. Other immunosuppressants may be more effective, but currently there is no evidence on which to base treatment.

# NUTRITIONAL DEFICIENCY STATES

Patients who have had extensive surgery for Crohn's disease or who have had severe active disease for a long period may develop a number of nutritional deficiencies which may manifest as cutaneous conditions, including pyostomatitis vegetans (see above). The commonest is a form of necrolytic migratory erythema. This scaling erythematous condition usually affects the perineal region and around the mouth, and is more usually associated with glucagonoma. The pathogenesis is thought to be due to zinc deficiency and hypoaminoacidemia as a result of malabsorption and chronic diarrhea. A similar condition has been reported in IBD, and responds to control of active disease along with zinc and amino acid replacement.[95]

# OTHERS

## EPIDERMOLYSIS BULLOSA ACQUISITA

This is a blistering condition of the skin and mucous membranes. It has been reported rarely in IBD,[96] including rather localized epidermolysis bullosa and cases restricted to the esophagus.[97] The lesions often heal with scarring, and the condition is associated with possession of autoantibodies to type VII collagen, which is a component of the basement membrane in stratified squamous epithelium. Treatment is with oral corticosteroids and immunosuppressants. In severe cases, or those with laryngeal or esophageal blistering, this should include cyclophosphamide.[98]

# HEMATOLOGIC MANIFESTATIONS

The commonest hematologic abnormalities reported in IBD are thromboembolic events and autoimmune hemolytic anemia. Other forms of anemia may be seen, including iron deficiency secondary to blood loss and vitamin $B_{12}$ deficiency in patients with terminal ileal Crohn's disease.

Clinical studies suggest that venous thromboembolism occurs in between 1 and 6% of IBD patients,[99–101] although postmortem studies have found higher prevalences. Arterial thrombosis has also been reported, particularly in Crohn's disease, but is much less common, although there is clearly an increase risk of cerebrovascular accident from arterial thromboembolism.[102,103] Venous thrombosis is most common in the deep veins of the legs, followed by pulmonary embolism, but sagittal sinus and cavernous sinus thromboses have been reported, as has thrombosis of mesenteric, portal and hepatic veins.

Patients over the age of 60 have the greatest absolute risk of thrombosis, but the relative risk is highest in patients under the age of 40, whose risk of thromboembolism is five times that of the age-matched healthy population.[99] Thrombosis may occur in patients with quiescent or limited bowel disease, but in most cases it is associated with extensive and active disease: 50–70% of patients overall have active disease,[100,104] and in Crohn's disease it may be as many as 90%.[105]

The pathogenesis of thrombotic complications probably relates to the generalized activation of a systemic inflammatory response. Increased circulating levels of Factor V, Factor VIII and fibrinogen have been described,[101,103] as well as increased Factor VII coagulant activity and the reactive thrombocytosis typically seen in active IBD.[106] In addition, circulating levels of free protein S have been noted to be decreased in Crohn's disease, again indicating a procoagulant state.[107]

Recently a number of studies have examined the question of whether inherited abnormalities in the clotting pathway could be of pathogenic significance. Some studies have found a small increase in Factor V Leiden mutations in patients with IBD,[108–110] particularly in Crohn's disease, but generally studies have been contradictory, and no association has been found with activated protein C resistance, methylenetetrahydrofolate reductase polymorphisms (associated with homocysteinemia), prothrombin gene mutations, or the presence of anticardiolipin antibodies.[104,111–115]

Clearly, patients suffering venous thromboembolism should be anticoagulated for an appropriate period and, given the relatively high risk of recurrent thrombosis, patients with active bowel disease thereafter should be prophylactically anticoagulated while the disease is active.

A less common but widely reported complication of IBD is autoimmune hemolytic anemia. This is almost exclusively associated with ulcerative colitis, where the prevalence is around 1%,[116–118] although there is a single case report of hemolytic anemia complicating Crohn's disease.[119] It may be subclinical, with the incidental finding of a positive direct Coombs' test, or may lead to significant hemolysis. This is usually associated with active disease,[116] and the majority of patients have a total or subtotal colitis.[118] It is important to remember that sulfasalazine is a cause of hemolytic anemia, and this may be responsible in patients taking this drug.[118,120,121]

The mainstay of treatment is corticosteroids with or without the use of immunosuppression. Any drugs that could be causing or exacerbating the condition should be withdrawn, particularly sulfasalazine. In most cases this is sufficient, but in a minority splenectomy may be required, often at the same time as a proctocolectomy for active disease.[116,118]

# VASCULITIS

Inflammation of blood vessels of all sizes has been reported in IBD, although largely as case reports rather than series. As mentioned above a cutaneous vasculitis may occur, and polyarthritis nodosa and retinal vasculitis have also been reported in Crohn's disease[122-124] and UC.[125] There have also been several case reports of medium and large vessel vasculitis, including large cerebral vessels[126] and the aorta. This includes cases with predominantly vaso-occlusive disease and cases of Takayasu's arteritis with arterial aneurysm formation.[127-129] These cases require full treatment as for systemic vasculitis, and are often linked to activity of the underlying bowel disease. The nature of the association between IBD and vasculitis is unknown. It has been suggested that there may be a common immunologic trigger in some patients, and in Japanese populations the association between UC and large vessel arteritis appears to occur most often in patients with HLA-B*52, DR52 haploptypes,[130] suggesting a common genetic predisposition.

## PULMONARY MANIFESTATIONS

Clinically significant pulmonary manifestations are rare in IBD, but prospective studies have suggested that a significant proportion of IBD patients have abnormalities of pulmonary function.

The largest prospective registry of clinically significant pulmonary problems demonstrated a number of clinical patterns.[131] These included airway inflammation, including chronic bronchitis, bronchiectasis and chronic bronchiolitis; and interstitial lung disease, particularly bronchiolitis obliterans with organizing pneumonia (BOOP) and pulmonary infiltrates with eosinophilia, and necrotic parenchymal nodules. Other authors have also reported parenchymal nodules, which need to be carefully distinguished from Wegener's granulomatosis.[132]

Most of the respiratory complications developed after the onset of the IBD and did not appear to be related to either smoking or drug therapy.[131,133] Both 5-ASA and sulfasalazine are known to cause pulmonary fibrosis. The respiratory complications are generally highly steroid responsive, although occasionally more aggressive immunosuppression may be required.[131]

Pathogenetically one of the most interesting reported pulmonary associations in IBD is with sarcoidosis. Much has been written about the relationship between IBD and pulmonary sarcoid, and certainly sarcoid has been reported in both UC and Crohn's disease.[134-137] It is well recognized that a response to the Kveim test can be elicited in IBD patients,[138] and it has been reported that the CD4:CD8 ratio in bronchoalveolar lavage fluid is similar in Crohn's to that seen in pulmonary sarcoid.[139] Other extraintestinal manifestations seen in IBD are also seen in sarcoidosis, such as arthropathy and EN, again suggesting similarities in etiology. Interestingly, EN in both sarcoidosis and Crohn's disease is associated with polymorphisms of the TNF-α gene promoter, which lead to increased production of TNF-α. However, the polymorphism associated is different in the two diseases, with the –308 locus being associated with sarcoidosis[11,140] and the –1031 locus being associated with Crohn's disease.[141] This suggests that, although they are similar, there are genetic differences between sarcoidosis and Crohn's disease.

Measurements of pulmonary function tests have been performed in a number of small (10–100 patients) cohorts of asymptomatic IBD patients and have demonstrated significant decreases in a variety of parameters,[133,142-144] although some series have found no significant abnormalities.[145] The most consistent finding is a decrease in the transfer factor (TLCO), which does not appear to relate to smoking status, and suggests interstitial lung disease.[133,142] If these observations are confirmed in

larger cohorts they will serve to emphasize the systemic nature of the inflammation in IBD, but they are unlikely to represent a significant clinical problem.

## CARDIAC DISEASE

Cardiac disease was been reported in inflammatory bowel disease as far back as 1929,[146] when seven cases of endocarditis were found in 693 patients. However, clinically significant cardiac disease as an association of IBD appears to be quite rare. The commonest form of disease reported is pericarditis or pleuropericarditis. It may occur when the bowel disease is quiescent, but rarely may be very severe, with tamponade.[147-149] Generally the pericarditis responds well to salicylates or NSAIDs (although these may exacerbate the bowel disease). In severe cases corticosteroid therapy may be required, and is usually effective. The pericarditis may on occasion be caused by the drugs used to treat IBD, and several case reports of mesalamine-induced pericarditis exist.[150-152] Patients with IBD also appear to at a higher risk of myocarditis than healthy controls, but the risk is still low at 4.6 cases per 100 000 years of risk.[153]

The relative risk of developing bacterial endocarditis is quite significantly higher in IBD patients – 44 times that of the healthy population. The reasons for this may be multiple, including increased bowel permeability during active disease, the relative frequency of invasive bowel investigations, and the use of immunosuppressive drugs.[154]

## CONDITIONS ASSOCIATED WITH IBD

In addition to complications considered as extraintestinal manifestations of IBD there are a number of conditions that may occur more frequently in IBD than in the general population. These may be secondary to surgery or due to poor intestinal function resulting from the bowel disease. The commonest are nutritional deficiencies, renal disease including renal stones and amyloidosis, and gallstones.

### NUTRITIONAL DEFICIENCIES

Patients who have had extensive small bowel surgery may suffer from a large number of nutritional deficiencies associated with the short bowel syndrome, and these are discussed elsewhere. The most significant are the excessive loss of water, and loss of essential elements such as calcium and magnesium. The most common nutritional deficiency is that of vitamin $B_{12}$, which occurs as a result of a failure to absorb $B_{12}$ in the terminal ileum, secondary to either active disease or surgery. It may manifest itself as anemia, or may rarely cause peripheral neuropathy, dementia and subacute combined degeneration of the spinal cord.

Deficiencies of specific nutrients may also cause problems, one of which is zinc deficiency, which is associated with pyostomatitis vegetans and migratory necrolytic erythema (both of which are discussed above).

### RENAL DISEASE

The most common renal manifestation is that of nephrolithiasis – renal stones. This may occur in up to 19% of IBD patients[6,155,156] and is particularly associated with Crohn's disease after small bowel resection or ileostomy formation.[156] The most common type of stone is oxalate, which form because of the increased oxalate absorption seen in IBD patients. This is thought to be because less oxalate is bound to luminal calcium in IBD as the calcium preferentially binds to unabsorbed fatty acids in the gut lumen. This in turn leads to a decrease in the insoluble calcium oxalate and an increase in colonic absorption of oxalate. The oxalate then precipitates out in the renal tract, leading to stone formation.[155-157] Uric acid stones may also form, but these tend to occur largely in patients with ileostomies and a high ileostomy output. This is because the loss of a large volume of alkaline fluid from the stoma gives rise to a low-volume acidic urine which favors the precipitation of uric acid, and hence stone formation.[155-157] Strategies to avoid nephrolithiasis include increased fluid intake, a low-oxalate diet, and substituting medium-chain fatty acids for fats in the diet.

Renal amyloidosis occurs in about 1% of Crohn's disease patients and less than 0.1% of UC patients, although postmortem studies suggest a higher prevalence. It does not become apparent until an average of 15 years after the IBD is diagnosed, and is more common in males than females. Resection of affected gut may be of therapeutic benefit, but experience is limited and patients may progress to renal failure.[158]

Other complications in the renal tract may occur, but are probably a direct result of inflammation in the surrounding bowel, including fistulization and periureteric fibrosis, which may occasionally lead to an obstructive uropathy.

## CHOLELITHIASIS

There is an increased prevalence of cholelithiasis in IBD, particularly terminal ileal Crohn's disease, and gallstones may be present in 10–34% of patients after ileal resection or bypass.[159] It is generally thought that this is largely due to interruption of the enterohepatic circulation of bile salts. This leads to increased bile salt loss from the bowel and depletion of the bile salt pool, allowing cholesterol to crystallize in the gallbladder and biliary tree.[160] This may account for most cases, but radiolucent stones are also common in Crohn's disease, suggesting that other mechanisms may also be important.[161]

## SUMMARY

Both ulcerative colitis and Crohn's disease may be associated with a number of manifestations outside the gut. By far the most common are those involving the joints, eyes and skin, and these are probably caused by the presentation of luminal antigens to the systemic immune system in genetically susceptible hosts via the leaky inflamed gut. Others, including venous thromboembolism and pulmonary manifestations, may be manifestations of the systemic nature of the inflammation seen in IBD, and yet other complications such as nephrolithiasis and cholelithiasis are secondary to intestinal absorptive failure, which may be disease or surgery related.

## REFERENCES

1. Elewaut D, De Keyser F, Van Den Bosch F et al. Enrichment of T cells carrying beta7 integrins in inflamed synovial tissue from patients with early spondyloarthropathy, compared to rheumatoid arthritis. J Rheumatol 1998;25:1932–1937.
2. Schorr-Lesnick B, Brandt LJ. Selected rheumatologic and dermatologic manifestations of inflammatory bowel disease. Am J Gastroenterol 1988;83:216–223.
3. Johnson ML, Wilson HTH. Skin lesions in ulcerative colitis. Gut 1969;10:255–263.
4. Hossein Mir-Madjlessi S, Taylor JS, Farmer RG. Clinical course and evolution of erythema nodsum and pyoderma gangrenosum in chronic ulcerative colitis: A study of 42 patients. Am J Gastroenterol 1985;80:615–620.
5. Bernstein CN, Blanchard JF, Rawsthorne P, Yu N. The prevalence of extraintestinal diseases in inflammatory bowel disease: A population based study. Am J Gastroenterol 2001;96:1116–1122.
6. Greenstein A, Janowitz H, Sachar D. Extra-intestinal complications of Crohn's disease and ulcerative colitis. Medicine 1976;55:401–412.
7. Orchard TR, Chua C, Cheng H, Jewell DP. Clinical features of erythema nodosum (EN) and uveitis associated with inflammatory bowel disease. Gastroenterology 2000;118:755.
8. Veloso FT, Carvalho J, Magro F. Immune-related systemic manifestations of inflammatory bowel disease. A prospective study of 792 patients. J Clin Gastroenterol 1996;23:29–34.
9. Bhagat S, Das KM. A shared and unique peptide in the human colon, eye, and joint detected by a monoclonal antibody. Gastroenterology 1994;107:103–108.
10. Orchard TR, Dhar A, Simmons JD, Welsh KI, Jewell DP. Phenotype determining genes in the HLA region may determine the presence of uveitis and erythema nodosum (EN) in inflammatory bowel disease. Gastroenterology 2000;118:A4832.
11. Labunski S, Posern G, Ludwig S, Kundt G, Brocker EB, Kunz M. Tumour necrosis factor-alpha promoter polymorphism in erythema nodosum. Acta Dermatol Venereol 2001;81:18–21.
12. Orchard TR, Ahmad T, Welsh KI, Jewell DP. Extra-intestinal manifestations of inflammatory bowel disease and polymorphisms in the TNF-alpha gene: Further evidence for phenotype determining genes in the MHC region on chromosome 6. Gastroenterology 2001;120:2320.
13. Felder JB, Korelitz BI, Rajapakse R, Schwarz S, Horatagis AP, Gleim G. Effects of nonsteroidal antiinflammatory drugs on inflammatory bowel disease: a case-control study. Am J Gastroenterol 2000;95:1949–1954.
14. Evans JM, McMahon AD, Murray FE, McDevitt DG, MacDonald TM. Non-steroidal anti-inflammatory drugs are associated with emergency admission to hospital for colitis due to inflammatory bowel disease. Gut 1997;40:619–622.
15. Bywaters E, Ansell B. Arthritis associated with ulcerative colitis: a clinical and pathological study. Ann Rheum Dis 1958;17:169–183.
16. Orchard T, Wordsworth B, Jewell D. The peripheral arthropathies of inflammatory bowel disease: their articular distribution and natural history. Gut 1998;42:387–391.
17. D'Inca R, Fagiuoli S, Sturniolo GC. Tacrolimus to treat pyoderma gangrenosum resistant to cyclosporine. Ann Intern Med 1998;128:783–784.
18. Nousari HC, Lynch W, Anhalt GJ, Petri M. The effectiveness of mycophenolate mofetil in refractory pyoderma gangrenosum. Arch Dermatol 1998;134:1509–1511.
19. Tan MH, Gordon M, Lebwohl O, George J, Lebwohl MG. Improvement of pyoderma gangrenosum and psoriasis associated with Crohn's disease with anti-tumour necrosis factor alpha monoclonal antibody. Arch Dermatol 2001;137:930–933.
20. Rozen SM, Nahabedian MY, Manson PN. Management strategies for pyoderma gangrenosum: case studies and a review of the literature. Ann Plast Surg 2001;47:310–315.
21. Ahmad T, Mulcahy-Hawes K, Bunce M et al. Recurrent oral ulceration (ROU) in inflammatory bowel disease (IBD): The clinical hallmark of a molecularly defined IBD/Behcet's (BD) overlap group. Gut 2002;50:170.
22. van der Linden S, Valkenburg HA, Cats A. Evaluation of diagnostic criteria for ankylosing spondylitis. A proposal for modification of the New York criteria. Arthritis Rheum 1984;27:361–368.
23. Dougados M, Linden S, Juhlin R et al. The European Spondyloarthropathy Study Group preliminary criteria for the classification of spondyloarthropathy. Arthritis Rheum 1991;34:1218–1227.
24. Calin A. Ankylosing spondylitis. In: Maddison P, Isenberg D, Woo P, Glass D, eds. Oxford textbook of rheumatology. Oxford: Oxford University Press; 1998:1058–1070.
25. van der Linden S, van der Heijde DM. Clinical and epidemiologic aspects of ankylosing spondylitis and spondyloarthropathies. Curr Opin Rheumatol 1996;8:269–274.
26. Wright V, Watkinson G. Sacroiliitis and ulcerative colitis. Br Med J 1965;2:675–680.
27. Dekker-Saeys B, Meuwissen S, VandenBerg-Loonen E, De Haas W, Agenant D, Tytgat G. Prevalence of peripheral arthritis, sacroiliitis and ankylosing spondylitis in patients suffering from inflammatory bowel disease. Ann Rheum Dis 1978;37:33–35.
28. de Vlam K, Mielants H, Cuvelier C, De Keyser F, Veys EM, De Vos M. Spondyloarthropathy is underestimated in inflammatory bowel disease: prevalence and HLA association. J Rheumatol 2000;27:2860–2865.
29. Helliwell PS, Hickling P, Wright V. Do the radiological changes of classic ankylosing spondylitis differ from the changes found in the spondylitis associated with inflammatory bowel disease, psoriasis, and reactive arthritis? Ann Rheum Dis 1998;57:135–140.
30. Brewerton D, Caffery M, Hart F, James D, Nichols A, Sturrock R. Ankylosing spondylitis and HLA-27. Lancet 1973;i:904–907.
31. Brown MA, Pile KD, Kennedy LG et al. HLA class I associations of ankylosing spondylitis in the white population in the United Kingdom. Ann Rheum Dis 1996;55:268–270.
32. Brewerton D, Caffery M, Nicholls A, Walters D, James D. HLA-27 and arthropathies associated with ulcerative colitis and psoriasis. Lancet 1974;i:956–958.
33. Dekker-Saeys B, Meuwissen S, Berg-Loonen EVD et al. Clinical characteristics and results of histocompatibitility typing (HLA B27) in 50 patients with both ankylosing spondylitis and inflammatory bowel disease. Ann Rheum Dis 1978;37:36–41.

34. Mallas EG, Mackintosh P, Asquith P, Cooke WT. Histocompatibility antigens in inflammatory bowel disease. Their clinical significance and their association with arthropathy with special reference to HLA-B27 (W27). Gut 1976;17:906–910.

35. Sanmarti R, Ercilla MG, Brancos MA, Cid MC, Collado A, Rotes-Querol J. HLA class II antigens (DR, DQ loci) and peripheral arthritis in ankylosing spondylitis. Ann Rheum Dis 1987;46:497–500.

36. Brown MA, Kennedy LG, Darke C et al. The effect of HLA-DR genes on susceptibility to and severity of ankylosing spondylitis. Arthritis Rheum 1998;41:460–465.

37. Fraile A, Collado MD, Mataran L, Martin J, Nieto A. TAP1 and TAP2 polymorphism in Spanish patients with ankylosing spondylitis. Exp Clin Immunogenet 2000;17:199–204.

38. Konno Y, Numaga J, Mochizuki M, Mitsui H, Hirata R, Maeda H. TAP polymorphism is not associated with ankylosing spondylitis and complications with acute anterior uveitis in HLA-B27-positive Japanese. Tissue Antigens 1998;52:478–483.

39. Maksymowych WP, Tao S, Li Y, Wing M, Russell AS. Allelic variation at the TAP 1 locus influences disease phenotype in HLA-B27 positive individuals with ankylosing spondylitis. Tissue Antigens 1995;45:328–332.

40. Maksymowych WP, Tao S, Vaile J, Suarez-Almazor M, Ramos-Remus C, Russell AS. LMP2 polymorphism is associated with extraspinal disease in HLA-B27 negative Caucasian and Mexican Mestizo patients with ankylosing spondylitis. J Rheumatol 2000;27:183–189.

41. Fraile A, Nieto A, Vinasco J, Beraun Y, Martin J, Mataran L. Association of large molecular weight proteasome 7 gene polymorphism with ankylosing spondylitis. Arthritis Rheum 1998;41:560–562.

42. Maksymowych WP, Adlam N, Lind D, Russell AS. Polymorphism of the LMP2 gene and disease phenotype in ankylosing spondylitis: no association with disease severity. Clin Rheumatol 1997;16:461–465.

43. Sieper J, Braun J. Pathogenesis of spondyloarthropathies: persistent bacterial antigen, autoimmunity or both? Arthritis Rheum 1995;38:1547–1554.

44. Ebringer A. Ankylosing spondylitis is caused by Klebsiella. Evidence from immunogenetic, microbiologic, and serologic studies. Rheum Dis Clin North Am 1992;18:105–121.

45. Rath H, Herfath H, Ikeda J et al. Normal luminal bacteria, especially bacteroides species, mediate chronic colitis, gastritis and arthritis in HLA-B27/Human b2 microglobulin transgenic rats. J Clin Invest 1996;98:945–953.

46. Taurog JD, Richardson JA, Croft JT et al. The germ-free state prevents development of gut and joint inflammation in HLA B27 transgenic rats. J Exp Med 1994;180:2359–2364.

47. Rath H, Schulta M, Grenther W et al. Colitis, gastritis and antibacterial Imphocyte responses in HLA-B27 transgenic rats monoinnoculated wityh Bacteroides vulgatus or Escherichia coli . Gastroenterology 1997;112:A1068.

48. Mielants H, Veys E, Vos MD et al. The evolution of spondyloarthropathies in relation to gut histology. I. Clinical Aspects. J Rheumatol 1995;22:2266–2272.

49. Mielants H, Veys E, Cuvelier C et al. The evolution of spondyloarthropathies in relation to gut histology. II. Histological aspects. J Rheumatol 1995;22:2273–2278.

50. Mielants H, Veys E, Cuvelier C et al. The evolution of spondyloarthropathies in relation to gut histology. III. Relation between gut and joint. J Rheumatol 1995;22:2279–2284.

51. Bjarnason I, Zanelli G, Smith T et al. Nonsteroidal antiinflammatory drug induced intestinal inflammation in humans. Gastroenterology 1987;93:480–489.

52. Bjarnason I, Peters T. Influence of anti-rheumatic drugs on gut permeability and on the gut associated lymphoid tissue. Baillière's Clin Rheumatol 1996;10:165–176.

53. Bjarnason I, Price A, Zanelli G et al. Clinicopathological features of nonsteroidal antiinflammatory drug-induced small intestinal strictures. Gastroenterology 1988;94:1070–1074.

54. Lang J, Price A, Levi A, Burke M, Gumpel J, Bjarnason I. Diaphragm disease: pathology of disease of the small intestine induced by non-steroidal anti-inflammatory drugs. J Clin Pathol 1988;41:516–526.

55. Smale S, Natt RS, Orchard TR, Russell AS, Bjarnason I. Inflammatory bowel disease and spondylarthropathy. Arthritis Rheum 2001;44:2728–2736.

56. van der Linden S, Valkenburg HA, Cats A. Evaluation of diagnostic criteria for ankylosing spondylitis. A proposal for modification of the New York criteria. Arthritis Rheum 1984;27:361–368.

57. Mahadevan U, Loftus EV Jr, Tremaine WJ, Sandborn WJ. Safety of selective cyclooxygenase-2 inhibitors in inflammatory bowel disease.  Am J Gastroenterol 2002;97:783–785.

58. Sampaio-Barros PD, Costallat LT, Bertolo MB, Neto JF, Samara AM. Methotrexate in the treatment of ankylosing spondylitis. Scand J Rheumatol 2000;29:160–162.

59. Altan L, Bingol U, Karakoc Y, Aydiner S, Yurtkuran M. Clinical investigation of methotrexate in the treatment of ankylosing spondylitis. Scand J Rheumatol 2001;30:255–259.

60. Braun J, Brandt J, Listing J et al. Treatment of active ankylosing spondylitis with infliximab: a randomised controlled multicentre trial. Lancet 2002;359:1187–1193.

61. Maksymowych WP, Jhangri GS, Lambert RG et al. Infliximab in ankylosing spondylitis: a prospective observational inception cohort analysis of efficacy and safety. J Rheumatol 2002;29:959–965.

62. Van den Bosch F, Kruithof E, De Vos M, De Keyser F, Mielants H. Crohn's disease associated with spondyloarthropathy: effect of TNF-alpha blockade with infliximab on articular symptoms. Lancet 2000;356:1821–1822.

63. Hollingsworth P, Cheah P, Dawkins R, Owen E, Calin A, Wood P. Observer variation in grading sacroiliac radiographs in HLA-B27 positive individuals. J Rheumatol 1983;10:247–254.

64. McEniff N, Eustace S, McCarthy C, O'Malley M, Morain C, Hamilton S. Asymptomatic sacroiliitis in inflammatory bowel disease. Assessment by computed tomography. Clin Imag 1995;19:258–262.

65. Agnew JE, Pocock DG, Jewell DP. Sacroiliac joint uptake ratios in inflammatory bowel disease: relationship to back pain and to activity of bowel disease. Br J Radiol 1982;55:821.

66. Steer S, Jones H, Hibbert J, Gibson T, Sanderson J. CT defined sacroiliitis and HLA-B27 in Crohn's disease. Gut 1999;44:A41.

67. Orchard TR, Holt H, Bradley L et al. Prevalence of sacroiliitis in Crohn's disease, and its correlation with clinical, radiologic and genotypic parameters. Gastroenterology 2002;122:W1298.

68. Gravalese E, Kantrowitz F. Arthritic manifestations of inflammatory bowel disease. Am J Gastro 1988;83:703–709.

69. Moll J. Inflammatory bowel disease. In: Panayi G, ed. Clinics in rheumatic diseases. Philadelphia: WB Saunders; 1985:87–105.

70. Wright V, Watkinson G. The arthritis of ulcerative colitis. Br Med J 1965;2:670–675.

71. Edwards F, Truelove S. The course and prognosis of ulcerative colitis. III. Complications. Gut 1964;5:1–15.

72. Roussomoustakaki M, Satsangi J, Welsh KI et al. Genetic markers may predict disease behaviour in patients with ulcerative colitis. Gastroenterology 1997;112:1645–1653.

73. Orchard TR, Thiyagaraja S, Welsh KI, Wordsworth BP, Hill Gaston JS, Jewell DP. Clinical phenotype is related to HLA genotype in the peripheral arthropathies of inflammatory bowel disease. Gastroenterology 2000;118:274–278.

74. Orchard TR, Dhar A, Simmons JD, Vaughan R, Welsh KI, Jewell DP. MHC class I chain-like gene A (MICA) and its associations with inflammatory bowel disease and peripheral arthropathy. Clin Exp Immunol 2001;126:437–440.

75. Gaston J, Life P, Granfors K et al. Synovial T lymphocyte recognition of organisms that trigger reactive arthritis. Clin Exp Immunol 1989;76:348–353.

76. Hermann E, Fleischer B, Mayet WJ, Poralla T, Meyer zum Buschenfelde KH. Response of synovial fluid T cell clones to Yersinia enterocolitica antigens in patients with reactive Yersinia arthritis. Clin Exp Immunol 1989;75:365–370.

77. Hermann E, Yu D, zum Buschenfelde K, Fleischer B. HLA-B27-restricted CD8 T cells derived from synovial fluids of patients with reactive arthritis and ankylosing spondylitis. Lancet 1993;342:646–650.

78. Rath H, Ikeda J, Wilson K, Sartor R. Varying cecal bacterial loads influences colitis and gastritis in HLA-B27 transgenic rats. Gastroenterology 1997;112:A1068.

79. Orchard TR, Jewell DP. The importance of ileocaecal integrity in the arthritic complications of Crohn's disease. Inflamm Bowel Dis 1999;5:92–97.

80. Crohn BB. Ocular lesions complicating ulcerative colitis. Am J Med Sci 1925;169:260.

81. Salmon JF, Wright JP, Murray AD. Ocular inflammation in Crohn's disease. Ophthalmology 1991;98:480–484.

82. Schreiber JB, Lakhanpal V, Nasrallah SM. Crohn's disease complicated by idiopathic central serous chorioretinopathy with bullous retinal detachment. Dig Dis Sci 1989;34:118–122.

83. Ernst BB, Lowder CY, Meisler DM, Gutman FA. Posterior segment manifestations of inflammatory bowel disease. Ophthalmology 1991;98:1272–1280.

84. Lyons JL, Rosenbaum JT. Uveitis associated with inflammatory bowel disease compared with uveitis associated with spondyloarthropathy. Arch Ophthalmol 1997;115:61–64.

85. Becuwe C, Delaporte E, Colombel JF, Piette F, Cortot A, Bergoend H. Sweet's syndrome associated with Crohn's disease. Acta Dermatol Venereol 1989;69:444–445.

86. VanHale HM, Rogers RS III, Zone JJ, Greipp PR. Pyostomatitis vegetans. A reactive mucosal marker for inflammatory disease of the gut. Arch Dermatol 1985;121:94–98.

87. Ficarra G, Cicchi P, Amorosi A, Piluso S. Oral Crohn's disease and pyostomatitis vegetans. An unusual association. Oral Surg Oral Med Oral Pathol 1993;75:220–224.

88. Gregory B, Ho VC. Cutaneous manifestations of gastrointestinal disorders. Part II. J Am Acad Dermatol 1992;26:371–383.

89. Jorizzo JL, Schmalstieg FC, Dinehart SM et al. Bowel-associated dermatosis-arthritis syndrome. Immune complex-mediated vessel damage and increased neutrophil migration. Arch Intern Med 1984;144:738–740.

90. Delaney TA, Clay CD, Randell PL. The bowel-associated dermatosis-arthritis syndrome. Australas J Dermatol 1989;30:23–27.

91. Zlatanic J, Fleisher M, Sasson M, Kim P, Korelitz BI. Crohn's disease and acute leukocytoclastic vasculitis of skin. Am J Gastroenterol 1996;91:2410–2413.

92. Kafity AA, Pellegrini AE, Fromkes JJ. Metastatic Crohn's disease. A rare cutaneous manifestation. J Clin Gastroenterol 1993;17:300–303.

93. Marotta PJ, Reynolds RP. Metastatic Crohn's disease. Am J Gastroenterol 1996;91:373–375.

94. Plauth M, Jenss H, Meyle J. Oral manifestations of Crohn's disease. An analysis of 79 cases. J Clin Gastroenterol 1991;13:29–37.

95. Sercki P, Janssen F, Vignon-Pennamen MD. [Cutaneous manifestations of zinc deficiency in Crohn disease]. Ann Dermatol Venereol 1990;117:833–834.

96. Raab B, Fretzin DF, Bronson DM, Scott MJ, Roenigk HH Jr, Medenica M. Epidermolysis bullosa acquisita and inflammatory bowel disease. JAMA 1983;250:1746–1748.

97. Schattenkirchner S, Lemann M, Prost C et al. Localized epidermolysis bullosa acquisita of the esophagus in a patient with Crohn's disease. Am J Gastroenterol 1996;91:1657–1659.

98. Woodley DT, Briggaman RA, Gammon WT. Review and update of epidermolysis bullosa acquisita. Semin Dermatol 1988;7:111–122.

99. Bernstein CN, Blanchard JF, Houston DS, Wajda A. The incidence of deep venous thrombosis and pulmonary embolism among patients with inflammatory bowel disease: a population-based cohort study. Thromb Haemost 2001;85:430–434.

100. Conlan MG, Haire WD, Burnett DA. Prothrombotic abnormalities in inflammatory bowel disease. Dig Dis Sci 1989;34:1089–1093.

101. Talbot RW, Heppell J, Dozois RR, Beart RW Jr. Vascular complications of inflammatory bowel disease. Mayo Clin Proc 1986;61:140–145.

102. Johns DR. Cerebrovascular complications of inflammatory bowel disease. Am J Gastroenterol 1991;86:367–370.

103. Schneiderman JH, Sharpe JA, Sutton DM. Cerebral and retinal vascular complications of inflammatory bowel disease. Ann Neurol 1979;5:331–337.

104. Novacek G, Miehsler W, Kapiotis S, Katzenschlager R, Speiser W, Vogelsang H. Thromboembolism and resistance to activated protein C in patients with inflammatory bowel disease. Am J Gastroenterol 1999;94:685–690.

105. Jackson LM, O'Gorman PJ, O'Connell J, Cronin CC, Cotter KP, Shanahan F. Thrombosis in inflammatory bowel disease: clinical setting, procoagulant profile and factor V Leiden. Q J Med 1997;90:183–188.

106. Hudson M, Chitolie A, Hutton RA, Smith MS, Pounder RE, Wakefield AJ. Thrombotic vascular risk factors in inflammatory bowel disease. Gut 1996;38:733–737.

107. Aadland E, Odegaard OR, Roseth A, Try K. Free protein S deficiency in patients with Crohn's disease. Scand J Gastroenterol 1994;29:333–335.

108. Nagy Z, Nagy A, Karadi O et al. Prevalence of the factor V Leiden mutation in human inflammatory bowel disease with different activity. J Physiol Paris 2001;95:483–487.

109. Over HH, Ulgen S, Tuglular T et al. Thrombophilia and inflammatory bowel disease: does factor V mutation have a role? Eur J Gastroenterol Hepatol 1998;10:827–829.

110. Haslam N, Standen GR, Probert CS. An investigation of the association of the factor V Leiden mutation and inflammatory bowel disease. Eur J Gastroenterol Hepatol 1999;11:1289–1291.

111. Heneghan MA, Cleary B, Murray M, O'Gorman TA, McCarthy CF. Activated protein C resistance, thrombophilia, and inflammatory bowel disease. Dig Dis Sci 1998;43:1356–1361.

112. Helio T, Wartiovaara U, Halme L et al. Arg506Gln factor V mutation and Val34Leu factor XIII polymorphism in Finnish patients with inflammatory bowel disease. Scand J Gastroenterol 1999;34:170–174.

113. Papa A, De Stefano V, Gasbarrini A et al. Prevalence of factor V Leiden and the G20210A prothrombin-gene mutation in inflammatory bowel disease. Blood Coag Fibrinol 2000;11:499–503.

114. Vecchi M, Sacchi E, Saibeni S et al. Inflammatory bowel diseases are not associated with major hereditary conditions predisposing to thrombosis. Dig Dis Sci 2000;45:1465–1469.

115. Aichbichler BW, Petritsch W, Reicht GA et al. Anti-cardiolipin antibodies in patients with inflammatory bowel disease. Dig Dis Sci 1999;44:852–856.

116. Gumaste V, Greenstein AJ, Meyers R, Sachar DB. Coombs-positive autoimmune hemolytic anemia in ulcerative colitis. Dig Dis Sci 1989;34:1457–1461.

117. Poulsen LO, Freund L, Lylloff K, Grunnet N. Positive Coombs' test associated with ulcerative colitis. A prevalence study. Acta Med Scand 1988;223:75–78.

118. Giannadaki E, Potamianos S, Roussomoustakaki M, Kyriakou D, Fragkiadakis N, Manousos ON. Autoimmune hemolytic anemia and positive Coombs test associated with ulcerative colitis. Am J Gastroenterol 1997;92:1872–1874.

119. Hochman JA. Autoimmune hemolytic anemia associated with Crohn's disease. Inflamm Bowel Dis 2002;8:98–100.

120. van Hees PA, van Elferen LW, van Rossum JM, van Tongeren JH. Hemolysis during salicylazosulfapyridine therapy. Am J Gastroenterol 1978;70:501–505.

121. Teplitsky V, Virag I, Halabe A. Immune complex haemolytic anaemia associated with sulfasalazine. Br Med J 2000;320:1113.

122. Gudbjornsson B, Hallgren R. Cutaneous polyarteritis nodosa associated with Crohn's disease. Report and review of the literature. J Rheumatol 1990;17:386–390.

123. Ruby AJ, Jampol LM. Crohn's disease and retinal vascular disease. Am J Ophthalmol 1990;110:349–353.

124. Duker JS, Brown GC, Brooks L. Retinal vasculitis in Crohn's disease. Am J Ophthalmol 1987;103:664–668.

125. Silverman MH. Polyarteritis nodosa associated with ulcerative colitis. J Rheumatol 1984;11:377–379.

126. Nelson J, Barron MM, Riggs JE, Gutmann L, Schochet SS Jr. Cerebral vasculitis and ulcerative colitis. Neurology 1986;36:719–721.

127. Miwa Y, Nagasako K, Sasaki H et al. Aortitis syndrome associated with ulcerative colitis: report of a case. Gastroenterol Jpn 1979;14:492–495.

128. Lenhoff SJ, Mee AS. Crohn's disease of the colon with Takayasu's arteritis. Postgrad Med J 1982;58:386–389.

129. Sakhuja V, Gupta KL, Bhasin DK, Malik N, Chugh KS. Takayasu's arteritis associated with idiopathic ulcerative colitis. Gut 1990;31:831–833.

130. Morita Y, Yamamura M, Suwaki K et al. Takayasu's arteritis associated with ulcerative colitis; genetic factors in this association. Intern Med 1996;35:574–578.

131. Camus P, Piard F, Ashcroft T, Gal AA, Colby TV. The lung in inflammatory bowel disease. Medicine (Baltimore) 1993;72:151–183.

132. Stebbing J, Askin F, Fishman E, Stone J. Pulmonary manifestations of ulcerative colitis mimicking Wegener's granulomatosis. J Rheumatol 1999;26:1617–1621.

133. Kuzela L, Vavrecka A, Prikazska M et al. Pulmonary complications in patients with inflammatory bowel disease. Hepatogastroenterology 1999;46:1714–1719.

134. Fries W, Grassi SA, Leone L et al. Association between inflammatory bowel disease and sarcoidosis. Report of two cases and review of the literature. Scand J Gastroenterol 1995;30:1221–1223.

135. Fellermann K, Stahl M, Dahlhoff K, Amthor M, Ludwig D, Stange EF. Crohn's disease and sarcoidosis: systemic granulomatosis? Eur J Gastroenterol Hepatol 1997;9:1121–1124.

136. Dumot JA, Adal K, Petras RE, Lashner BA. Sarcoidosis presenting as granulomatous colitis. Am J Gastroenterol 1998;93:1949–1951.

137. Barr G, Shale D, Jewell D. Ulcerative colitis and sarcoidosis. Postgrad Med J 1986;62:341–345.

138. Hurley TH, Sullivan JR, Hurley JV. Reaction to Kveim test material in sarcoidosis and other diseases. Lancet 1975;1:494–496.

139. Bewig B, Manske I, Bottcher H, Bastian A, Nitsche R, Folsch UR. Crohn's disease mimicking sarcoidosis in bronchoalveolar lavage. Respiration 1999;66:467–469.

140. Grutters JC, Sato H, Pantelidis P et al. Increased frequency of the uncommon tumor necrosis factor-857T allele in British and Dutch patients with sarcoidosis. Am J Respir Crit Care Med 2002;165:1119–1124.

141. Orchard TR, Ahmad T, Welsh KI, Jewell DP. Extraintestinal manifestations of inflammatory bowel disease (IBD) and polymorphisms in the TNF alpha gene: Further evidence for phenotype determining genes in the MHC region on chromosome 6. Gastroenterology 2001;120:2320.

142. Herrlinger KR, Noftz MK, Dalhoff K, Ludwig D, Stange EF, Fellermann K. Alterations in pulmonary function in inflammatory bowel disease are frequent and persist during remission. Am J Gastroenterol 2002;97:377–381.

143. Fireman Z, Osipov A, Kivity S et al. The use of induced sputum in the assessment of pulmonary involvement in Crohn's disease. Am J Gastroenterol 2000;95:730–734.

144. Mansi A, Cucchiara S, Greco L et al. Bronchial hyperresponsiveness in children and adolescents with Crohn's disease. Am J Respir Crit Care Med 2000;161:1051–1054.

145. Tzanakis N, Bouros D, Samiou M et al. Lung function in patients with inflammatory bowel disease. Respir Med 1998;92:516–522.

146. Bargen JA. Complications and sequelae of chronic ulcerative colitis. Ann Intern Med 1929:335–352.

147. Abid MA, Gitlin N. Pericarditis - an extraintestinal complication of inflammatory bowel disease. West J Med 1990;153:314–315.

148. Goodman MJ, Moir DJ, Holt JM, Truelove SC. Pericarditis associated with ulcerative colitis and Crohn's disease. Am J Dig Dis 1976;21:98–102.

149. Patwardhan RV, Heilpern RJ, Brewster AC, Darrah JJ. Pleuropericarditis: an extraintestinal complication of inflammatory bowel disease. Report of three cases and review of literature. Arch Intern Med 1983;143:94–96.

150. Ishikawa N, Imamura T, Nakajima K et al. Acute pericarditis associated with 5-aminosalicylic acid (5-ASA) treatment for severe active ulcerative colitis. Intern Med 2001;40:901–904.

151. Iaquinto G, Sorrentini I, Petillo FE, Berardesca G. Pleuropericarditis in a patient with ulcerative colitis in longstanding 5-aminosalicylic acid therapy. Ital J Gastroenterol 1994;26:145–147.

152. Gujral N, Friedenberg F, Friedenberg J, Gabriel G, Kotler M, Levine G. Pleuropericarditis related to the use of mesalamine. Dig Dis Sci 1996;41:624–626.

153. Sorensen HT, Fonager KM. Myocarditis and inflammatory bowel disease. A 16-year Danish nationwide cohort study. Dan Med Bull 1997;44:442–444.

154. Kreuzpaintner G, Horstkotte D, Heyll A, Losse B, Strohmeyer G. Increased risk of bacterial endocarditis in inflammatory bowel disease. Am J Med 1992;92:391–395.

155. Banner MP. Genitourinary complications of inflammatory bowel disease. Radiol Clin North Am 1987;25:199–209.

156. McLeod RS, Churchill DN. Urolithiasis complicating inflammatory bowel disease. J Urol 1992;148:974–978.

157. Fukushima T, Ishiguro N, Matsuda Y, Takemura H, Tsuchiya S. Clinical and urinary characteristics of urolithiasis in ulcerative colitis. Am J Gastroenterol 1982;77:238–242.

158. Greenstein AJ, Sachar DB, Panday AK et al. Amyloidosis and inflammatory bowel disease. A 50-year experience with 25 patients. Medicine (Baltimore) 1992;71:261–270.

159. Williams SM, Harned RK. Hepatobiliary complications of inflammatory bowel disease. Radiol Clin North Am 1987;25:175–188.

160. Heaton KW, Read AE. Gall stones in patients with disorders of the terminal ileum and disturbed bile salt metabolism. Br Med J 1969;3:494–496.

161. Hutchinson R, Tyrrell PN, Kumar D, Dunn JA, Li JK, Allan RN. Pathogenesis of gall stones in Crohn's disease: an alternative explanation. Gut 1994;35:94–97.

## CHAPTER 46

# Pouchitis

William J Tremaine

## DEFINITION AND CLINICAL FEATURES

The most frequent complication of the ileal pouch–anal anastomosis for treatment of ulcerative colitis (UC) is acute non-specific inflammation of the pouch, known as pouchitis.[1] The term was first used by Kock in 1977 in reference to the continent ileal reservoir following proctocolectomy for UC,[2] and the definition has since been broadened to include the similar disorder that occurs in some patients following the ileal pouch–anal procedure. Pouchitis is a unique phenotype of inflammatory bowel disease (IBD). Identification of the cause of this postoperative complication will provide clues to the causes of the other forms of IBD.

## DEFINITION AND CLINICAL FEATURES

Pouchitis is a syndrome of symptoms, endoscopic abnormalities and histologic abnormalities.[3-5] Symptoms include one or more of the following: an increased stool frequency (or increased ileostomy output for the continent ileal reservoir), rectal urgency, fecal incontinence, rectal bleeding, abdominal cramping, fever and malaise. The diarrhea can be mild, with one or two more stools per day than usual, or severe with hourly watery stools and dehydration. In the normal pouch, the staple line created by the side-to-side anastomosis of the two ileal segments is visible as a linear ridge (Fig. 46.1). Endoscopic mucosal findings in pouchitis include one or more of the following: erythema, edema, mucus exudate, contact bleeding, spontaneous bleeding, aphthous ulcers, and focal deep ulcers that may be round or serpiginous. The endoscopic abnormalities can be patchy or diffuse and confluent (Fig. 46.2). There is usually a sharp demarcation from the involved pouch mucosa to normal-appearing mucosa in the afferent ilea limb, known as the prepouch ileum. Also, the blind end of an ileal J pouch is often normal in appearance, even in the presence of abnormal adjacent mucosa, perhaps because of lack of direct contact with the stool on the mucosa in the blind end. Histology findings are acute inflammatory changes that include one or more of the following: polymorphonuclear cell infiltration, crypt abscesses and ulcers (Fig. 46.3). The Pouchitis Disease Activity Index (PDAI) is a 19-point scoring system that incorporates several criteria for diagnosis, including symptoms, endoscopic findings and histology findings, with pouchitis defined as a score of ≥ 7 (Table 46.1).[5] The PDAI is most useful as a research tool for documenting the presence or absence of active pouchitis and quantitatively measuring change in pouchitis activity with medical therapy. Histologic changes of chronic inflammation are usually found in the pouch mucosa even in the absence of symptoms or endoscopic abnormalities,[3] so the histologic presence of chronic inflammation is not a reliable indicator of pouchitis activity. The components of the PDAI – the symptom, endoscopy and histology scores – appear to be independent measures of pouchitis activity and each is important to the diagnosis.[6] Pouchitis cannot be diagnosed reliably based on symptoms alone, as one-quarter of patients with high symptom scores may not fulfill the criteria for pouchitis as diagnosed by the PDAI, which necessitates endoscopic and histologic confirmation of pouchitis as a form of inflammatory bowel disease.[6] Pouchitis is subdivided into two types: acute, with one or more discrete episodes that resolve with therapy, and chronic, with persistent disease activity despite therapy, or disease that responds to therapy but which recurs promptly when therapy is discontinued. Chronic pouchitis has also been defined by the duration of symptoms, with persistent symptoms for more than 4 weeks[7] or for longer than 3 months.[8,9]

## OTHER DIAGNOSTIC STUDIES

A retrograde pouch X-ray contrast study, known as a pouchogram, using water-soluble contrast, is useful for delineating the size and shape of the pouch and identifying fistulae or strictures[10-12] (Fig. 46.4). Scintigraphic scanning can be used to quantify pouch volume and the fraction of the pouch contents spontaneously emptied,[13] but it has not been a useful test for assessment of pouchitis as there is no correlation between the

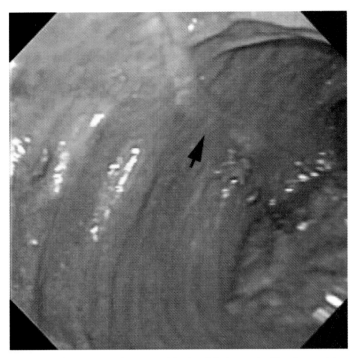

Fig. 46.1 Endoscopy of a normal ileal pelvic J pouch. The linear ridge (arrow) is created by the staple line joining the two ileal limbs to create the ileal reservoir.

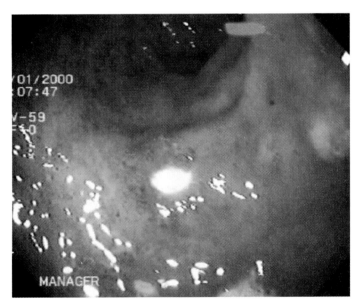

Fig. 46.2 Endoscopy of an ileal J pouch with pouchitis. The mucosa is erythematous and edematous, with focal shallow ulcers.

pouch emptying fraction and the risk of pouchitis. [111]In-labeled granulocyte scanning and 4-day fecal collections for [111]In-labeled granulocyte excretion can be used to quantify the severity of inflammation in pouchitis.[14] Fecal $\alpha_1$-antitrypsin activity has also been used as a quantitative index of disease activity.[15]

# FREQUENCY AND NATURAL HISTORY

The frequency of pouchitis in recent series ranges from 23 to 51% for pelvic pouches,[1,16–18] and was 34% in a series of patients

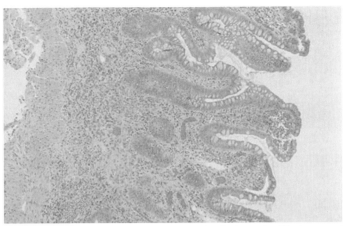

Fig. 46.3 Endoscopic mucosal biopsy from the ileal pouch with changes of acute inflammation.

## Table 46.1 Pouchitis Disease Activity Index

| Criteria | Score |
|---|---|
| **Clinical** | |
| *Stool frequency* | |
| Usual postoperative stool frequency | 0 |
| 1–2 stools/day > postoperative usual | 1 |
| Three or more stools/day > postoperative usual | 2 |
| *Rectal bleeding* | |
| None or rare | 0 |
| Present daily | 1 |
| *Fecal urgency or abdominal cramps* | |
| None | 0 |
| Occasional | 1 |
| Usual | 2 |
| *Fever (temperature >37.8°C)* | |
| Absent | 0 |
| Present | 1 |
| **Endoscopic inflammation** | |
| Edema | 1 |
| Granularity | 1 |
| Friability | 1 |
| Loss of vascular pattern | 1 |
| Mucous exudate | 1 |
| Ulceration | 1 |
| **Acute histologic inflammation** | |
| *Polymorphonuclear leukocyte infiltration* | |
| Mild | 1 |
| Moderate + crypt abscess | 2 |
| Severe + crypt abscess | 3 |
| *Ulceration per low-power field (mean)* | |
| <25% | 1 |
| 25 to 50% | 2 |
| >50% | 3 |

*Pouchitis is defined as a total score of ≥ 7 points

with a continent ileostomy[4] (Table 46.2). In a Swedish study, the risk of developing pouchitis was highest during the first 6 months after closure of the temporary ileostomy (23.1%), and the frequency decreased during the next 6 months to 11.4%, dropping to 3.1% during the subsequent 6 months.[16] The cumulative risk

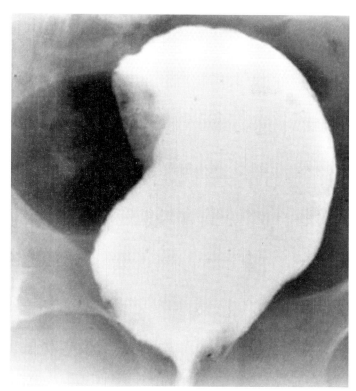

Fig. 46.4 Pouchogram using water-soluble contrast of an ileal J pouch to anal anastomosis.

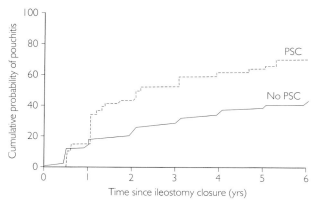

Fig. 46.5 Cumulative risk of developing pouchitis after closure of the temporary diverting ileostomy in patients with pelvic pouch following surgery for ulcerative colitis. (From Penna C, Dozois R, Tremaine W et al. Pouchitis after ileal pouch–anal anastomosis for ulcerative colitis occurs with increased frequency in patients with associated primary sclerosing cholangitis. Gut 1996;38:234–239, with permission.)

continues to rise with prolonged follow-up[19] (Fig. 46.5). In a series of 1310 patients from the Mayo Clinic, the cumulative probability of suffering at least one episode of pouchitis was 18% at 1 year and 48% at 10 years after surgery.[1] In a recent German study there was a similar cumulative risk of pouchitis of 50% at 8 years among 210 patients with ulcerative colitis.[9] Patients who have a single episode of pouchitis during the first 2 years after pelvic pouch surgery have a cumulative probability of suffering one or more additional episodes of 64%.[1] A single episode of pouchitis is an indicator of a poorer long-term outcome. In a study of 120 patients at the University of Chicago there were 50 patients with at least one episode of pouchitis and 70 with no history of pouchitis.[20] Those with a history of pouchitis were more likely to have a higher stool frequency, less formed stools, and have more incontinence and the need to wear a protective pad during the day than the patients who had never had pouchitis.[20] The rates of chronic pouchitis, using definitions of persistent symptoms for more than 3 months, or the need for chronic antibiotic therapy, range from 4.5 to 21.5%.[9,16,21]

As illustrated in the data from three referral centers, only a minority of patients undergo pouch excision because of pouchitis. In the Mayo Clinic series of 1310 patients, pouchitis was the cause of pouch failure requiring excision of the pouch or diverting ileostomy in three patients.[1] Among 104 consecutive patients who underwent pelvic pouch surgery for ulcerative colitis at the University of Chicago, two required pouch removal owing to chronic pouchitis.[22] In a Swedish series of 149 patients, two underwent pouch removal and permanent ileostomy for chronic pouchitis.[16]

## DIFFERENTIAL DIAGNOSIS

The differential diagnosis includes causes of secondary pouchitis that mimic the symptoms or endoscopic findings of idiopathic pouchitis, or worsen the severity of established idiopathic pouchitis[9] (Table 46.3). Strictures at the ileal pouch–anal anastomosis can occur as a consequence of postoperative anastomotic leakage and abscess formation. An anastomotic stricture can also develop as a result of ischemia caused by tension at the anastomosis, from pulling down into the pelvis a relatively short mesentery to make the connection of the pouch to the anus.[23] Because of the stricture there is increased stasis of stool in the pouch, with bacterial overgrowth and inflammation. Dilating the stricture under anesthesia and then instructing the patient in self-dilatation of the anastomosis with a 12–16 mm diameter

| Table 46.2 Frequency of pouchitis in recent series | | | | | | |
|---|---|---|---|---|---|
| Author | Location | Year | No. of UC operated | Procedure | Follow-up (months) | % with pouchitis |
| Svaninger 1993 | Goteberg, Sweden | 1993 | 180 | Kock pouch | 102 | 34 |
| Keränen 1997 | Helsinki, Finland | 1997 | 291 | IPAA | 56 | 22 |
| Romanos 1997 | Oxford, UK | 1997 | 177 | IPAA | 27 | 24 |
| Meagher 1998 | Rochester, MN, USA | 1998 | 1310 | IPAA | 78 | 43 |
| Heuschen 2001 | Heidelberg, Germany | 2001 | 210 | IPAA | 48 | 23 |
| Madiba 2001 | Edinburgh, UK | 2001 | 139 | IPAA | | 34 |

**Table 46.3 Differential diagnosis of pouch symptoms**

Idiopathic pouchitis
Secondary pouchitis
   Anastomotic stricture with bacterial stasis
Anastomotic abscess
Fecal incontinence due to anal sphincter dysfunction
Specific infection
   Cytomegalovirus
Intestinal malabsorption
Pancreatic maldigestion
Irritable pouch syndrome
Cuffitis
Crohn's disease

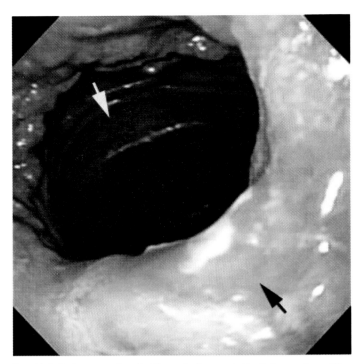

**Fig. 46.6** Endoscopy of an ileal J pouch demonstrating inflammation of the anal transition zone mucosa, known as 'cuffitis', in the lower right (black arrow), with normal ileal J-pouch mucosa in the upper left (white arrow).

Hegar dilator two to three times weekly can keep the stricture open and resolve the pouchitis.[24]

Pouchitis due to cytomegalovirus (CMV) infection has been reported in three patients with severe diarrhea and systemic symptoms, including fever, myalgias and malaise.[25,26] CMV pouchitis can occur in immunocompetent patients who have not received recent treatment with immunomodulators or corticosteroids.[26] The endoscopic findings in CMV pouchitis are indistinguishable from those of severe idiopathic pouchitis. The diagnosis is made by the identification of CMV inclusion bodies identified with routine hematoxylin and eosin staining, or immunofluorescence staining for CMV antigen using monoclonal antibodies.[27] Treatment with intravenous ganciclovir 10 mg/kg/day or, more recently, oral valganciclovir for 10–21 days, has been effective.[26] Common bacterial pathogens that cause infectious colitis, such as *Campylobacter* and *Clostridium difficile*, have not been reported to cause pouchitis.[28] Intestinal malabsorption and pancreatic maldigestion should be considered in the differential diagnosis of diarrhea in patients with a dysfunctional ileoanal pouch. Serum total and low-density lipoprotein cholesterol absorption is significantly impaired in patients with an ileal pelvic pouch,[29] raising the possibility of malabsorption of other fats in some patients. In addition, unrelated causes of diarrhea and weight loss should be considered in patients with ileal pouches, particularly if the pouch examination is normal or minimally abnormal, for example gluten-sensitive enteropathy or pancreatic insufficiency. The term irritable pouch syndrome has been applied to patients with normal or near-normal ileal pouch mucosa by endoscopy and biopsy, but with increased stool frequency, urgency and abdominal pain.[30] The underlying disorder could be a condition resembling irritable bowel syndrome. In a series of 61 consecutive symptomatic patients with pouchitis, 26 (42.6%) had irritable pouch syndrome and 12 of the 26 responded to therapy with anticholinergics, antidiarrheal and antidepressant therapies.[30] Cuffitis is the term applied to inflammation of the anal and sometimes the rectal mucosa that is retained after a stapled ileal pouch–anal anastomosis (Fig. 46.6). In two reports from the Cleveland Clinic the frequency of symptomatic cuffitis was 14.7% in a series of 217 patients,[31] and in another series reported 5 years later cuffitis occurred in four of 61 (6.5%).[30] In a series of 113 patients from the UK, symptomatic cuffitis occurred in 9%.[32] Patients with cuffitis may respond to topical hydrocortisone or mesalamine,[30] and refractory patients require mucosec-

tomy of the retained rectal and anal mucosa with advancement of the pouch and hand sewing of the new ileoanal anastomosis. Crohn's disease is often suspected in patients with pelvic pouch inflammation, but uncommonly found.[33] In a retrospective study of 32 patients with refractory pouchitis, including 16 Kock pouches and eight pelvic pouches, the pathology slides from colectomy were reviewed blindly and clinical features prior to colectomy were compared with matched controls. The patients with refractory pouchitis were no more likely to have Crohn's disease than controls.[33] Crohn's disease cannot be distinguished from pouchitis by the endoscopic appearance of the pouch mucosa. In patients with or without ileal pouches, the presence of granulomas is useful in making the diagnosis of Crohn's disease. For example, the chance of finding granulomas on colonoscopic biopsies of known Crohn's colitis is 25 %.[34] However, granulomas are rarely found in the ileal pouch. The diagnosis of Crohn's disease in a patient with a continent ileostomy or pelvic pouch is dependent on characteristic findings of Crohn's disease elsewhere than in the pouch, such as in the afferent ileal limb (prepouch ileum). Pouch–cutaneous or pouch–vaginal fistulae may be due to Crohn's disease, but must be distinguished from perioperative anastomotic leakage with abscess and fistula formation (Fig. 46.7).[35]

## POSSIBLE ETIOLOGIES

The cause of pouchitis is unknown, and theories are based on laboratory and clinical observations. Intraluminal bacteria, particularly anaerobes, appear to be an important element in the development of pouchitis. The role of anaerobes is highlighted by the efficacy of antibiotics that have anaerobic coverage, such as metronidazole. However, pouchitis is not simply a conse-

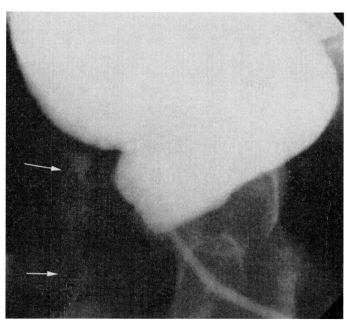

**Fig. 46.7** Pouchogram using water-soluble contrast demonstrating a pouch–vaginal fistula (arrows).

quence of fecal stasis and bacterial overgrowth: all patients with an ileal pouch have increased bacterial concentrations compared to patients with end ileostomies, but not all develop pouchitis.[28,36,37] Pouchitis rarely occurs in patients with a history of familial adenomatous polyposis, even though bacterial concentrations in the pouch are similar to those of patients with a history of ulcerative colitis.[28]

Injury from degraded bile acids has been postulated as a cause of pouchitis. Patients with continent ileostomies and pelvic pouches have deconjugated and dehydroxylated bile acids present,[28,38,39] unlike patients with end ileostomies, who have mainly conjugated primary bile acids.[39] The deconjugated and dehydroxylated bile acids are potentially cytotoxic and could injure the pouch mucosa.[40] There is no difference in the total bile acid concentration in the ileal pouch in patients with and those without pouchitis.[28] Bile acids may cause the chronic inflammatory changes seen on pouch mucosal biopsies, but not the acute changes of symptomatic pouchitis.

A deficiency of intraluminal short-chain fatty acids (SCFA) is another hypothesis for the cause of pouchitis. SCFA, produced by intracolonic bacteria, are the primary nutrient source for colonic epithelial cells. As the ileal mucosal cells in the pouch undergo morphologic changes towards an appearance of colonic epithelium, it has been hypothesized that these ileal cells now require SCFA, which are relatively lacking in the pouch. However, ileal pouch SCFA levels do not consistently correlate with the presence of pouchitis.[28,41]

Mucosal ischemia of the pouch, possibly due to decreased mesenteric vascular perfusion,[42] has been hypothesized as a potential cause of pouchitis. However, the profound differences in the occurrence of pouchitis in patients with FAP compared to ulcerative colitis, despite an identical surgical procedure, make this explanation unlikely.

Clinical and laboratory findings indicate that pouchitis is due to the underlying process that initially caused ulcerative colitis. Pouchitis is seen almost exclusively in patients who have had

ulcerative colitis, and rarely in patients with FAP.[43] Patients with extraintestinal manifestations of colitis are more likely to develop pouchitis.[44,45] Pouchitis is more common with a history of extensive ulcerative colitis,[46] but it does not correlate with the presence of backwash ileitis.[46] Cigarette smoking is correlated with a lower risk of pouchitis, just as it correlates with a lower risk of symptomatic ulcerative colitis.[47] In addition, there are a number of immunological changes in pouchitis that are also found in ulcerative colitis, as well as other immune changes, as noted below.

# IMMUNOLOGIC FEATURES OF POUCHITIS

A number or characteristics of immune function have been reported in patients with pouchitis. The presence of the perinuclear cytoplasmic antibody pANCA, found in about 60% of individuals with ulcerative colitis, is associated with the development of chronic pouchitis.[48] The expression of pANCA reflects an immune response to the antigen products of enteric bacteria.[49,50] In a study of 95 patients with ulcerative colitis who had pANCA measurements at the time of ileal pouch–anal anastomosis, 60 were pANCA positive. Pouchitis developed in 42% of these 60 and in 20% of the pANCA-negative patients.[51] Among those with a high titer of pANCA, with more than 100 ELISA units, the cumulative risk of pouchitis was 56%, and the risk in patients who had lower titers was no greater than in pANCA-negative patients.[51]

Mucosal inflammation in pouchitis is associated with an increase in proinflammatory cytokines, including interleukins-1 (IL-1), -6 (IL-6), -8 (IL-8), interferon-γ (IFN-γ), and tumor necrosis factor-α (TNF-α). IL-1 and IL-8 concentrations in whole gut lavage fluid are higher in pouchitis patients than in those without pouchitis.[52] In a study of proinflammatory cytokine IL-8 and the anti-inflammatory cytokine IL-10, the mucosal mRNA levels of IL-8 and IL-10 were similar in patients with and without pouchitis, but the IL-10/IL-8 ratio was significantly lower in patients with pouchitis than in those without.[53] The IL-1 receptor antagonist gene allele 2 is more common in patients with ulcerative colitis, particularly extensive disease, and it is also found more commonly in patients with pouchitis.[54] In both ulcerative colitis and pouchitis there is an increased state of activation of T cells, with expression of CD25 on CD4+ cells that is more pronounced than on CD8+ cells.[55] In pouchitis there is an increased CD4:CD8 ratio in the mucosal lymphocytes, and there is an increased number of IFN-γ-producing mononuclear cells.[55]

Degradation of the extracellular matrix (ECM), a key step in tissue destruction, is accomplished by a number of proteases, including the matrix metalloproteinases (MMP). MMP-1 and MMP-2 are increased in both pouchitis and ulcerative colitis.[56] MMP levels fall with treatment of pouchitis.[57]

Abnormal regulation of apoptosis may also play a role in the development of pouchitis. Increased epithelial cell apoptosis correlates with the degree of villous atrophy in patients with pouchitis, which may in turn predispose the host to infection by otherwise commensal (non-pathogenic) organisms in the ileal pouch.[58]

Cyclooxygenase-2 (COX-2) and nitric oxide synthase-2 (NOS-2) mRNA are increased in both healthy ileal pouches and in pouchitis, suggesting that a latent inflammatory process is always present in the ileal reservoir in patients with a history of ulcerative colitis.[59] The severity of inflammation in the pouch correlated with the mRNA levels.[59] NOS-2 is the inducible form of the enzyme, and NOS-3 is the endothelial form. High levels of NOS-2 correlate with acute inflammation in the pouch mucosa, whereas NOS-3 levels are increased in pouchitis, with or without acute inflammation.[60] Nitric oxide levels decrease with effective treatment of pouchitis.[57]

## RISK OF MALIGNANCY

Patients with a history of ulcerative colitis have several risk factors to develop malignancy in association with the pelvic pouch. After either rectal mucosectomy and handsewn anastomosis or double-stapled pouch anal anastomosis rectal mucosa is left intact. This retained mucosa carries a risk of adenocarcinoma in long-standing disease and has been reported in a few patients.[61,62] Periodic surveillance endoscopy with biopsies of the remaining rectal cuff mucosa is recommended in patients with the double-stapled pouch–anal anastomosis. In a patient who undergoes surgery because of dysplasia in the rectum, mucosectomy and a handsewn anastomosis or an end ileostomy should be performed, to minimize the amount of rectal mucosa retained.[62]

Rarely, adenocarcinoma may also arise from atrophic ileal mucosa. There are two case reports of carcinoma in the distal ileum following an end ileostomy,[63,64] and single case reports of carcinoma in a Kock pouch[65] and in an ileal pelvic pouch.[66] Patients with severe pouchitis, which has been termed type C[67] with chronic severe mucosal atrophy, are at risk for the development of dysplasia.[67,68] Dysplasia was found in five of seven patients with long-standing type C pouchitis, compared to none in 14 patients with no atrophy or only slight atrophy (type A).[68] DNA aneuploidy is also a feature of long-standing type C pouchitis.[69] Despite these concerns, the overall risk of malignancy in patients with chronic pouchitis appears to be low. Among 106 patients with ileal pouches selected because of risk factors for malignancy, including chronic pouchitis, a pelvic pouch for ≥ 12 years' duration, a Kock pouch for ≥ 14 years' duration, and neoplasia in the colectomy specimen, only one had dysplasia.[70] DNA aneuploidy was found in this patient and two others.[70] To date, no guidelines for screening for dysplasia in ileal pouches have been established.

One patient was reported with chronic pouchitis who developed large cell lymphoma in the ileal pelvic pouch in the absence of immunosuppressive therapy.[71]

## TREATMENT

### MEDICAL

Broad-spectrum antibiotics have been the mainstay of treatment for pouchitis (Fig. 46.8). Metronidazole was effective in two small controlled trials.[72,73] In a placebo-controlled crossover study, 11 of 13 patients completed the study and received

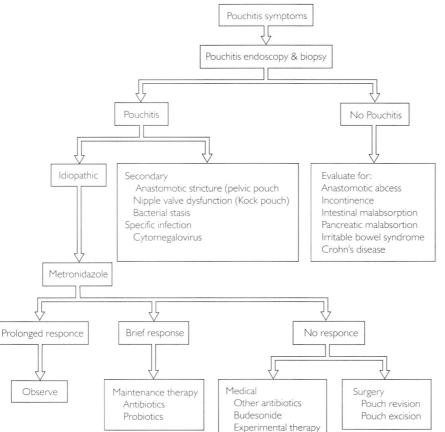

**Fig. 46.8** Algorithm for management of pouch symptoms.

metronidazole three times daily for 7 days, with improvement in eight of the 11 (73%).[72] In an 'n of 1' trial, a patient with a continent ileostomy took metronidazole 250 mg once daily for 14 days for five courses, alternating randomly with five courses of placebo, and improved while on the drug.[73] Two recent studies evaluated metronidazole and ciprofloxacin (Cipro) for the treatment of pouchitis.[74,75] In a study from the Cleveland Clinic, 16 patients with acute pouchitis with symptoms for 4 weeks or less were randomized to a 2-week course of Cipro 1 g/day or metronidazole 20 mg/kg/day. All seven patients in the Cipro group achieved remission with no adverse effects, and six of nine (67%) of the metronidazole-treated patients achieved remission with side effects in one-third, including nausea, vomiting, dysgeusia and paresthesias.[74] In an open-label multicenter European study, 36 of 44 (82%) patients with recurrent or chronic pouchitis were treated with a combination of metronidazole 400 or 500 mg twice daily and Cipro 500 mg twice daily for 28 days.[75] The patients who did not achieve remission were older, with a longer history of pouchitis, and were more likely to have chronic pouchitis.[75] Metronidazole given as an enema also appeared effective in an open-label trial.[76] In an Italian study, Cipro 500 mg twice daily was given in combination with the non-absorbable antibiotic rifaximin 1 g daily for 15 days for chronic, treatment-resistant pouchitis, with remission in six of 18 patients and improvement in 10.[77] Other antibiotics have been beneficial for pouchitis in open-label use, including amoxicillin-clavulanate, erythromycin and tetracycline.[78] There are no long-term maintenance studies of antibiotics for chronic pouchitis. Some patients appear to develop resistance to metronidazole or Cipro over months of use. Anecdotally, these patients can sometimes be managed by alternating between two broad-spectrum antibiotics at 2-week intervals.

Bismuth has both antimicrobial and antidiarrheal activity and appears useful in the treatment of ulcerative colitis;[79] it has also been used in a trial of pouchitis. An uncontrolled study of bismuth enema in patients with treatment-resistant pouchitis showed benefit,[80] but a placebo-controlled study was negative.[81] An uncontrolled trial suggested benefit from chewable bismuth subsalicylate tablets for chronic pouchitis.[82]

Probiotics have been proposed as a logical treatment for pouchitis, in view of the importance of the fecal flora in the development of pouchitis and the beneficial effects of antibiotics.[83] A placebo-controlled trial of an oral probiotic preparation, VSL #3, containing four strains of lactobacilli, three strains of Bifidobacterium and one strain of Streptococcus was effective in maintaining remission of chronic pouchitis in a study of 40 patients, after induction of remission with an oral antibiotic.[84]

During the 9 months of treatment, three of 20 patients who received the probiotic mixture relapsed, compared to all 20 patients who received placebo (Fig. 46.9).[84] Fecal concentrations of the probiotic bacterial strains increased, and there was no change in the concentrations of fecal anaerobes, including Bacteroides. Once-daily dosing with VSL#3 also appears effective in maintaining remission in chronic pouchitis.[85]

Based on the hypothesis that pouchitis is due to specific nutrient deficiencies, short-chain fatty acid (SCFA) enemas, butyrate suppositories and glutamine suppositories have been used in small trials.[86–88] The benefit of these therapies is unclear.

A double-blind double-dummy controlled trial of budesonide enemas versus metronidazole in 26 patients with acute pouchitis showed a similar benefit with the two treatments over 4 weeks.[89] Adverse effects occurred in 25% of patients who received budesonide enemas and in 57% of patients on metronidazole.[89]

Other anti-inflammatory and immunomodulator therapies used for ulcerative colitis and Crohn's disease have been tested in pouchitis, with mixed results. Small trials and case reports using mesalamine enemas,[90] mesalamine and budesonide suppositories,[91] oral 5-aminosalicylic acid,[92] prednisone,[93] cyclosporin enemas,[94] azathioprine and tacrolimus[95] have all shown some activity, but efficacy has not been confirmed in controlled trials.

Allopurinol has been used for the treatment of active pouchitis with some success in a small, uncontrolled trial,[42] but it was not effective as prophylaxis.[96]

Infliximab appears effective for the treatment of Crohn's disease of the ileal pouch, for both inflammatory and fistulizing disease,[35] but it has not been reported for the treatment of pouchitis.

## SURGICAL TREATMENT OF POUCHITIS

Secondary causes of pouchitis, including pouch–anal anastomotic strictures with outlet obstruction and pouch–anal fistula, can be treated surgically (Fig. 46.7).[9,97] For inflammation of the retained rectal mucosa following double-stapled anastomosis, known as cuffitis,[31,32] mucosectomy with advancement of the pouch towards the dentate line is an option.

Rarely, patients require pouch excision or a diverting ileostomy because of a poor quality of life due to chronic pouchitis.[1]

## SUMMARY

Pouchitis is the most common complication of the continent ileostomy (Kock pouch) and the ileal pelvic pouch, with a cumulative frequency of about 30–50% with 5–10 years' follow-up. Pouchitis is a syndrome of unknown cause that includes symptoms and also endoscopic and histologic abnormalities of the pouch. Idiopathic pouchitis must be distinguished from pouch inflammation due to an anastomotic stricture, infection due to cytomegalovirus or other specific pathogen, inflammation in retained rectal mucosa known as cuffitis, and irritable pouch syndrome. Possible etiologies for pouchitis include fecal stasis, injury from bile acid metabolites, short-chain fatty acid or other nutritional deficiencies, ischemia, or reactivation or continuation of

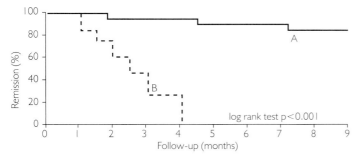

**Fig. 46.9** Kaplan-Meier estimates of relapse of chronic pouchitis comparing a probiotic (A), with placebo (B) over 9 months [Gionchetti, 2000 #6].

the underlying disorder that caused ulcerative colitis. Patients with long-standing chronic pouchitis appear to have an increased risk of malignancy and require regular follow-up with pouch mucosal biopsies. Broad-spectrum antibiotics, particularly metronidazole, are the most common treatments, and probiotics and budesonide are other options.

# REFERENCES

1. Meagher AP, Farouk R, Dozois RR et al. J ileal pouch–anal anastomosis for chronic ulcerative colitis: complications and long-term outcome in 1310 patients. Br J Surg 1998;85:800–803.
2. Kock NG, Darle N, Hulten L et al. Ileostomy. Curr Probl Surg 1977;14:1–52.
3. Moskowitz RL, Shepherd NA, Nicholls RJ. An assessment of inflammation in the reservoir after restorative proctocolectomy with ileoanal ileal reservoir. Int J Colorectal Dis 1986;1:167–174.
4. Svaninger G, Nordgren S, Oresland T et al. Incidence and characteristics of pouchitis in the Kock continent ileostomy and the pelvic pouch. Scand J Gastroenterol 1993;28:695–700.
5. Sandborn WJ, Tremaine WJ, Batts KP et al. Pouchitis after ileal pouch–anal anastomosis: a Pouchitis Disease Activity Index. Mayo Clin Proc 1994;69:409–415.
6. Shen B, Achkar JP, Lashner BA et al. Endoscopic and histologic evaluation together with symptom assessment are required to diagnose pouchitis. Gastroenterology 2001;121:261–267.
7. Sandborn WJ. Pouchitis following ileal pouch–anal anastomosis: definition, pathogenesis, and treatment. Gastroenterology 1994;107:1856–1860.
8. Stallmach A, Moser C, Hero-Gross R et al. Pattern of mucosal adaptation in acute and chronic pouchitis. Dis Colon Rectum 1999;42:1311–1317.
9. Heuschen UA, Autschbach F, Allemeyer EH et al. Long-term follow-up after ileoanal pouch procedure: algorithm for diagnosis, classification, and management of pouchitis. Dis Colon Rectum 2001;44:487–499.
10. Tsao JI, Galandiuk S, Pemberton JH. Pouchogram: predictor of clinical outcome following ileal pouch–anal anastomosis. Dis Colon Rectum 1992;35:547–551.
11. Malcolm PN, Bhagat KK, Chapman MA et al. Complications of the ileal pouch: is the pouchogram a useful predictor? Clin Radiol 1995;50:613–617.
12. Hillard AE, Mann FA, Becker JM et al. The ileoanal J pouch: radiographic evaluation. Radiology 1985;155:591–594.
13. Woolfson K, McLeod RS, Walfisch S et al. Pelvic pouch emptying scan: an evaluation of scintigraphic assessment of the neorectum. Int J Colorectal Dis 1991;6:29–32.
14. Kmiot WA, Hesslewood SR, Smith N et al. Evaluation of the inflammatory infiltrate in pouchitis with 111In-labeled granulocytes. Gastroenterology 1993;104:981–988
15. Boerr LA, Sambuelli AM, Sugai E et al. Faecal alpha 1-antitrypsin concentration in the diagnosis and management of patients with pouchitis. Eur J Gastroenterol Hepatol 1995;7:129–133.
16. Stahlberg D, Gullberg K, Liljeqvist L et al. Pouchitis following pelvic pouch operation for ulcerative colitis. Incidence, cumulative risk, and risk factors. Dis Colon Rectum 1996;39:1012–1018.
17. Heuschen UA, Heuschen G, Autschbach F et al. Adenocarcinoma in the ileal pouch: late risk of cancer after restorative proctocolectomy. Int J Colorectal Dis 2001;16:126–130.
18. Madiba TE, Bartolo DC. Pouchitis following restorative proctocolectomy for ulcerative colitis: incidence and therapeutic outcome. J Roy Coll Surg Edin 2001;46:334–337.
19. Penna C, Dozois R, Tremaine W et al. Pouchitis after ileal pouch–anal anastomosis for ulcerative colitis occurs with increased frequency in patients with associated primary sclerosing cholangitis. Gut 1996;38:234–239.
20. Hurst RD, Chung TP, Rubin M et al. The implications of acute pouchitis on the long-term functional results after restorative proctocolectomy. Inflamm Bowel Dis 1998;4:280–284.
21. Keranen U, Luukkonen P, Jarvinen H. Functional results after restorative proctocolectomy complicated by pouchitis. Dis Colon Rectum 1997;40:764–769.
22. Hurst RD, Molinari M, Chung TP et al. Prospective study of the incidence, timing and treatment of pouchitis in 104 consecutive patients after restorative proctocolectomy. Arch Surg 1996;131:497–500; discussion 501–502.
23. Smith L, Friend WG, Medwell SJ. The superior mesenteric artery. The critical factor in the pouch pull-through procedure. Dis Colon Rectum 1984;27:741–744.
24. Tremaine WJ. Diagnosis and management of pouchitis. Semin Colon Rectal Surg 2001;12:49–54.
25. Moonka D, Furth EE, MacDermott RP et al. Pouchitis associated with primary cytomegalovirus infection. Am J Gastroenterol 1998;93:264–266.
26. Munoz-Juarez M, Pemberton JH, Sandborn WJ et al. Misdiagnosis of specific cytomegalovirus infection of the ileoanal pouch as refractory idiopathic chronic pouchitis: report of two cases. Dis Colon Rectum 1999;42:117–120
27. Theodossiou C, Temeck B, Vargas H et al. Cytomegalovirus enteritis after treatment with 5-fluorouracil, leukovorin, cisplatin, and alpha-interferon. Am J Gastroenterol 1995;90:1174–1176.

28. Sandborn WJ, Tremaine WJ, Batts KP et al. Fecal bile acids, short-chain fatty acids, and bacteria after ileal pouch–anal anastomosis do not differ in patients with pouchitis. Dig Dis Sci 1995;40:1474–1483.
29. Hakala K, Vuoristo M, Luukkonen P et al. Impaired absorption of cholesterol and bile acids in patients with an ileoanal anastomosis. Gut 1997;41:771–777.
30. Shen B, Achkar JP, Lashner BA et al. Irritable pouch syndrome: a new category of diagnosis for symptomatic patients with ileal pouch–anal anastomosis. Am J Gastroenterol 2002;97:972–977.
31. Lavery IC, Sirimarco MT, Ziv Y et al. Anal canal inflammation after ileal pouch–anal anastomosis. The need for treatment. Dis Colon Rectum 1995;38:803–806.
32. Thompson-Fawcett MW, Mortensen NJ, Warren BF: "Cuffitis" and inflammatory changes in the columnar cuff, anal transitional zone, and ileal reservoir after stapled pouch–anal anastomosis. Dis Colon Rectum 1999;42:348–355.
33. Subramani K, Harpaz N, Bilotta J et al. Refractory pouchitis: does it reflect underlying Crohn's disease? Gut 1993;34:1539–1542.
34. Potzi R, Walgram M, Lochs H et al. Diagnostic significance of endoscopic biopsy in Crohn's disease. Endoscopy 1989;21:60–62.
35. Ricart E, Panaccione R, Loftus EV et al. Successful management of Crohn's disease of the ileoanal pouch with infliximab. Gastroenterology 1999;117:429–432.
36. O'Connell PR, Rankin DR, Weiland LH et al. Enteric bacteriology, absorption, morphology and emptying after ileal pouch–anal anastomosis. Br J Surg 1986;73:909–914.
37. Kmiot WA, Youngs D, Tudor R et al. Mucosal morphology, cell proliferation and faecal bacteriology in acute pouchitis. Br J Surg 1993;80:1445–1449.
38. Kay RM, Cohen Z, Siu KP et al. Ileal excretion and bacterial modification of bile acids and cholesterol in patients with continent ileostomy. Gut 1980;21:128–132.
39. Natori H, Utsunomiya J, Yamamura T et al. Fecal and stomal bile acid composition after ileostomy or ileoanal anastomosis in patients with chronic ulcerative colitis and adenomatosis coli. Gastroenterology 1992;102:1278–1288.
40. Merrett MN, Owen RW, Jewell DP et al. Ileal pouch dialysate is cytotoxic to epithelial cell lines, but not to CaCo-2 monolayers. Ileal pouches: adaptation and inflammation. Eur J Gastroenterol Hepatol 1997;9:1219–1226.
41. Clausen MR, Tvede M, Mortensen PB. Short-chain fatty acids in pouch contents from patients with and without pouchitis after ileal pouch–anal anastomosis. Gastroenterology 1992;103:1144–1153.
42. Levin KE, Pemberton JH, Phillips SF et al. Role of oxygen free radicals in the etiology of pouchitis. Dis Colon Rectum 1992;35:452–456.
43. Dozois RR, Kelly KA, Welling DR et al. Ileal pouch–anal anastomosis: comparison of results in familial adenomatous polyposis and chronic ulcerative colitis. Ann Surg 1989;210:268–271; discussion 272–273.
44. Oresland T, Fasth S, Nordgren S et al. The clinical and functional outcome after restorative proctocolectomy. A prospective study in 100 patients. Int J Colorectal Dis 1989;4:50–56.
45. Lohmuller JL, Pemberton JH, Dozois RR et al. Pouchitis and extraintestinal manifestations of inflammatory bowel disease after ileal pouch–anal anastomosis. Ann Surg 1990;211:622–627; discussion 627–629.
46. de Silva HJ, de Angelis CP, Soper N et al. Clinical and functional outcome after restorative proctocolectomy. Br J Surg 1991;78:1039–1044.
47. Merrett MN, Mortensen N, Kettlewell M et al. Smoking may prevent pouchitis in patients with restorative proctocolectomy for ulcerative colitis. Gut 1996;38:362–364.
48. Sandborn WJ, Landers CJ, Tremaine WJ et al. Antineutrophil cytoplasmic antibody correlates with chronic pouchitis after ileal pouch–anal anastomosis. Am J Gastroenterol 1995;90:740–747.
49. Seibold F, Brandwein S, Simpson S et al. pANCA represents a cross-reactivity to enteric bacterial antigens. J Clin Immunol 1998;18:153–160.
50. Cohavy O, Bruckner D, Gordon LK et al. Colonic bacteria express an ulcerative colitis pANCA-related protein epitope. Infect Immun 2000;68:1542–1548.
51. Fleshner PR, Vasiliauskas EA, Kam LY et al. High level perinuclear antineutrophil cytoplasmic antibody (pANCA) in ulcerative colitis patients before colectomy predicts the development of chronic pouchitis after ileal pouch–anal anastomosis. Gut 2001;49:671–677.
52. Evgenikos N, Bartolo DC, Hamer-Hodges DW et al. Assessment of ileoanal pouch inflammation by interleukin 1beta and interleukin 8 concentrations in the gut lumen. Dis Colon Rectum 2002;45:249–255.
53. Bulois P, Tremaine WJ, Maunoury V et al. Pouchitis is associated with mucosal imbalance between interleukin-8 and interleukin-10. Inflamm Bowel Dis 2000;6:157–164.
54. Carter MJ, Di Giovine FS, Cox A et al. The interleukin 1 receptor antagonist gene allele 2 as a predictor of pouchitis following colectomy and IPAA in ulcerative colitis. Gastroenterology 2001;121:805–811.
55. Stallmach A, Schafer F, Hoffmann S et al. Increased state of activation of CD4 positive T cells and elevated interferon gamma production in pouchitis. Gut 1998;43:499–505.
56. Stallmach A, Chan CC, Ecker KW et al. Comparable expression of matrix metalloproteinases 1 and 2 in pouchitis and ulcerative colitis. Gut 2000;47:415–422.
57. Ulisse S, Gionchetti P, D'Alo S et al. Expression of cytokines, inducible nitric oxide synthase, and matrix metalloproteinases in pouchitis: effects of probiotic treatment. Am J Gastroenterol 2001;96:2691–2699.
58. Coffey JC, Bennett MW, Wang JH et al. Upregulation of Fas-Fas-L (CD95/CD95L)-mediated epithelial apoptosis – a putative role in pouchitis? J Surg Res 2001;98:27–32.

59. Leplingard A, Brung-Lefebvre M, Guedon C et al. Increase in cyclooxygenase-2 and nitric oxide-synthase-2 mRNAs in pouchitis without modification of inducible isoenzyme heme-oxygenase-1. Am J Gastroenterol 2001;96:2129–2136.

60. Vento P, Kiviluoto T, Jarvinen HJ et al. Expression of inducible and endothelial nitric oxide synthases in pouchitis. Inflamm Bowel Dis 2001;7:120–127.

61. Stern H, Walfisch S, Mullen B et al. Cancer in an ileoanal reservoir: a new late complication? Gut 1990;31:473–475.

62. Rotholtz NA, Pikarsky AJ, Singh JJ et al. Adenocarcinoma arising from along the rectal stump after double-stapled ileorectal J-pouch in a patient with ulcerative colitis: the need to perform a distal anastomosis. Report of a case. Dis Colon Rectum 2001;44:1214–1217.

63. Bedetti CD, DeRisio VJ. Primary adenocarcinoma arising at an ileostomy site. An unusual complication after colectomy for ulcerative colitis. Dis Colon Rectum 1986;29:572–575.

64. Smart PJ, Sastry S, Wells S. Primary mucinous adenocarcinoma developing in an ileostomy stoma. Gut 1988;29:1607–1612.

65. Cox CL, Butts DR, Roberts MP et al. Development of invasive adenocarcinoma in a long-standing Kock continent ileostomy: report of a case. Dis Colon Rectum 1997;40:500–503.

66. Vieth M, Grunewald M, Niemeyer C et al. Adenocarcinoma in an ileal pouch after prior proctocolectomy for carcinoma in a patient with ulcerative pancolitis. Virchows Arch 1998;433:281–284.

67. Veress B, Reinholt FP, Lindquist K et al. Long-term histomorphological surveillance of the pelvic ileal pouch: dysplasia develops in a subgroup of patients. Gastroenterology 1995;109:1090–1097.

68. Gullberg K, Stahlberg D, Liljeqvist L et al. Neoplastic transformation of the pelvic pouch mucosa in patients with ulcerative colitis. Gastroenterology 1997;112:1487–1492.

69. Gullberg K, Lindforss U, Zetterquist H et al. Cancer risk assessment in long-standing pouchitis. DNA aberrations are rare in transformed neoplastic pelvic pouch mucosa. Int J Colorectal Dis 2002;17:92–97.

70. Thompson-Fawcett MW, Marcus V, Redston M et al. Risk of dysplasia in long-term ileal pouches and pouches with chronic pouchitis. Gastroenterology 2001;121:275–281.

71. Nyam DC, Pemberton JH, Sandborn WJ et al. Lymphoma of the pouch after ileal pouch–anal anastomosis: report of a case. Dis Colon Rectum 1997;40:971–972.

72. Madden MV, McIntyre AS, Nicholls RJ. Double-blind crossover trial of metronidazole versus placebo in chronic unremitting pouchitis. Dig Dis Sci 1994;39:1193–1196.

73. McLeod RS, Taylor DW, Cohen Z et al. Single-patient randomised clinical trial. Use in determining optimum treatment for patient with inflammation of Kock continent ileostomy reservoir. Lancet 1986;1:726–728.

74. Shen B, Achkar JP, Lashner BA et al. A randomized clinical trial of ciprofloxacin and metronidazole to treat acute pouchitis. Inflamm Bowel Dis 2001;7:301–305.

75. Mimura T, Rizzello F, Helwig U et al. Four-week open-label trial of metronidazole and ciprofloxacin for the treatment of recurrent or refractory pouchitis. Aliment Pharmacol Ther 2002;16:909–917.

76. Nygaard K, Bergan T, Bjorneklett A et al. Topical metronidazole treatment in pouchitis. Scand J Gastroenterol 1994;29:462–467.

77. Gionchetti P, Rizzello F, Venturi A et al. Antibiotic combination therapy in patients with chronic, treatment-resistant pouchitis. Aliment Pharmacol Ther 1999;13:713–718.

78. Scott AD, Phillips RK. Ileitis and pouchitis after colectomy for ulcerative colitis. Br J Surg 1989;76:668–689.

79. Pullan RD, Ganesh S, Mani V et al. Comparison of bismuth citrate and 5-aminosalicylic acid enemas in distal ulcerative colitis: a controlled trial. Gut 1993;34:676–679.

80. Gionchetti P, Rizzello F, Venturi A et al. Long-term efficacy of bismuth carbomer enemas in patients with treatment-resistant chronic pouchitis. Aliment Pharmacol Ther 1997;11:673–678.

81. Tremaine WJ, Sandborn WJ, Wolff BG et al. Bismuth carbomer foam enemas for active chronic pouchitis: a randomized, double-blind, placebo-controlled trial. Aliment Pharmacol Ther 1997;11:1041–1046.

82. Tremaine W, Sandborn W, Kenan ML. Bismuth subsalicylate tablets for chronic antibiotic-resistant pouchitis. Gastroenterology 1998;114:A1101.

83. Campieri M, Gionchetti P. Probiotics in inflammatory bowel disease: new insight to pathogenesis or a possible therapeutic alternative? Gastroenterology 1999;116:1246–1249.

84. Gionchetti P, Rizzello F, Venturi A et al. Oral bacteriotherapy as maintenance treatment in patients with chronic pouchitis: a double-blind, placebo-controlled trial. Gastroenterology 2000;119:305–309.

85. Mimura T, Rizzello F, Schreiber S et al. Once daily high dose probiotic therapy maintains remission and improved quality of life in patients with recurrent or refractory pouchitis: a randomised, placebo-conrolled, double-blind trial. Gastroenterology 2002;122:A81.

86. den Hoed PT, van Goch JJ, Veen HF et al. Severe pouchitis successfully treated with short-chain fatty acids. Can J Surg 1996;39:168–169.

87. de Silva HJ, Ireland A, Kettlewell M et al. Short-chain fatty acid irrigation in severe pouchitis. N Engl J Med 1989;321:1416–1417.

88. Wischmeyer P, Pemberton JH, Phillips SF. Chronic pouchitis after ileal pouch–anal anastomosis: responses to butyrate and glutamine suppositories in a pilot study. Mayo Clin Proc 1993;68:978–981.

89. Sambuelli A, Boerr L, Negreira S et al. Budesonide enema in pouchitis—a double-blind, double-dummy, controlled trial. Aliment Pharmacol Ther 2002;16:27–34.

90. Miglioli M, Barbara L, Di Febo G et al. Topical administration of 5-aminosalicylic acid: a therapeutic proposal for the treatment of pouchitis. N Engl J Med 1989;320:257.

91. Belluzzi A, Campieri M, Gionchetti P. Acute pouchitis: 5-aminosalicylic acid and budesonide suppositories effectiveness on inflammatory mediator production. Gastroenterology 1993;104:A665.

92. Meuwissen SG, Hoitsma H, Boot H et al. Pouchitis (pouch ileitis). Neth J Med 1989;35:S54–66.

93. Knobler H, Ligumsky M, Okon E et al. Pouch ileitis – recurrence of the inflammatory bowel disease in the ileal reservoir. Am J Gastroenterol 1986;81:199–201.

94. Winter TA, Dalton HR, Merrett MN et al. Cyclosporin A retention enemas in refractory distal ulcerative colitis and 'pouchitis'. Scand J Gastroenterol 1993;28:701–704.

95. Zins BJ, Sandborn WJ, Penna CR et al. Pouchitis disease course after orthotopic liver transplantation in patients with primary sclerosing cholangitis and an ileal pouch–anal anastomosis. Am J Gastroenterol 1995;90:2177–2181.

96. Joelsson M, Andersson M, Bark T et al. Allopurinol as prophylaxis against pouchitis following ileal pouch–anal anastomosis for ulcerative colitis. A randomized placebo-controlled double-blind study. Scand J Gastroenterol 2001;36:1179–1184.

97. Nicholls RJ, Banerjee AK. Pouchitis: risk factors, etiology, and treatment. World J Surg 1998;22:347–351.

## CHAPTER 47

# Postoperative recurrence of Crohn's disease

Geert D'Haens and Paul Rutgeerts

## INTRODUCTION

The management of Crohn's disease is predominantly medical, although surgical resection remains necessary to treat complications such as stenosis or abscess formation. Following surgical resection, Crohn's disease usually recurs after months to years. New lesions almost invariably develop in the previously unaffected mucosa of the neoterminal ileum, proximal to the ileocolonic anastomosis. This situation offers an excellent opportunity to study the earliest pathophysiological events of this disease, the etiology of which is still unknown. Based on this model, it has been established that the 'culprit' inciting chronic Crohn's inflammation is most likely a component of the fecal stream, probably of bacterial origin.

The clinical pattern of recurrent Crohn's disease often resembles that of the preoperative disease. A number of follow-up studies that have identified risk factors for early and severe recurrence will be discussed.

Several medical therapies to prevent postoperative recurrence have been looked at. The benefit from mesalamine therapy has been rather limited, but immunosuppressive agents and nitroimidazole antibiotics appear more efficacious. The answer to whether all patients operated on for Crohn's disease need prophylactic treatment depends on a number of variables and strategies, which will be discussed in the last part of the chapter.

## INCIDENCE OF CROHN'S RECURRENCE IN THE NEOTERMINAL ILEUM

The cumulative probability of surgery for Crohn's disease is high.[1] Based on follow-up studies, Farmer and colleagues[2] demonstrated that surgical resection was most often necessary in ileocolonic Crohn's disease (92%), followed by small intes-

tinal disease (66%) and the least frequently in colonic disease (58%). Following intestinal resection, clinical recurrence of Crohn's disease is observed in 10–20% of all patients per year postoperatively.[3,4] The definition of clinical recurrence is the appearance of symptoms caused by new intestinal lesions following 'curative resection' (all inflamed tissue removed). Olaison and colleagues even reported clinical recurrence in one-third of their patients as early as 3 months after surgery.[5] These numbers, however, are based on older studies from an era when immunosuppressive medication was less frequently used.

The diagnosis of recurrent Crohn's disease on purely clinical grounds is often not evident, especially early after surgery. The symptoms of recurrent disease are not always easily distinguishable from symptoms due to the postoperative state and to cholerrheic diarrhea. The clinical index CDAI (Crohn's Disease Activity Index) is an instrument which is not really reliable and is possibly even invalid in the postoperative setting. In addition, the variability in individual perception and interpretation of symptoms is often significant.

The need for repeated surgery gives an idea about so-called 'surgical recurrence'. Reoperation rates at 10 years have varied from 16 to 65%.[2,6] Again, these numbers may have changed owing to the advent of more potent medical therapy. A few studies have used radiologic criteria to document recurrence ('radiologic recurrence') and reported cumulative recurrence rates of 41–60% at 10 years.[7,8] In recent years, however, ileocolonoscopy has been the most sensitive method to detect the earliest mucosal changes, with signs of 'endoscopic recurrence' in 50–75% of patients at 3 months and in 50–90% at 12 months after surgery.[5,9–11] Clearly, the appearance of recurrent tissue lesions precedes the appearance of recurrent symptoms. The severity and extent of endoscopic lesions determines the further clinical disease course.[11] Patients without lesions in the neoterminal ileum, or presenting with only a few aphthous ulcers, are not at risk for early symptomatic relapse, but more than half of patients with diffuse ileitis or ulcerative ileitis will have symptomatic recurrence within 1–3 years after operation. Patients with ulcers confined to the immediate anastomotic region are probably prone to develop fibrostenosis of the anastomosis.[9] The relationship between endoscopic abnormalities and clinical relapse was also studied in the above-mentioned work by Olaison. Whereas 1 year postoperatively 93% of his patients had endoscopic recurrence, only 37% had symptomatic disease. The proportion of patients with endoscopic disease increased to 94% at 2 years and even 100% at 3 years after surgery, with symptomatic relapse rates in these patients of 82% and 86% at 2 and 3 years, respectively, again showing that symptomatic disease lags behind the development of endoscopic lesions.[5]

# PATHOPHYSIOLOGY OF CROHN'S RECURRENCE IN THE NEOTERMINAL ILEUM

At a microscopic level, the inflammatory events in recurrent Crohn's disease begin within the first few days following resection with ileocolonic anastomosis. As long as the fecal stream is diverted, however, the mucosa in the neoterminal ileum remains unaffected. As a consequence, the presence of ileal fluid seems to be mandatory in order for recurrence to develop. The combined presence of bacteria and bile acids, a break in the mucosa of the suture, reflux of colonic content and a disturbance in the organization of mucosal immune cells may be contributing factors. We studied the potential deleterious effects of the intestinal luminal content in patients who underwent a two-step ileal resection.[12] Because of extensive fistulization to the rectum a temporary stoma was considered necessary. After 'curative' resection and ileocolonic anastomosis, a terminal ileostomy was constructed 25–35 cm proximally to the ileocolonic anastomosis, excluding the neoterminal ileum, the anastomosis and the colon from the fecal stream. Six months later endoscopy with biopsies of the excluded ileum and the ileocolonic anastomosis was normal. The ileostomy fluid was then infused through a tube introduced in the efferent limb of the loop ileostomy for 7 days. On the eighth day the patients underwent a new endoscopy of the excluded neoterminal ileum and colon. Biopsies were obtained in the excluded ileum and in the remaining small intestine. Subsequently the normal continuity was surgically restored and the loop ileostomy closed. All biopsies were examined with routine histology, immunohistochemistry using antibodies directed against monocyte/macrophage cells, antigen-presenting cells and adhesion molecules, and with electron microscopy.

The hematoxylin–eosin (H&E)-stained preinfusion biopsies were completely normal. After 7 days of infusion epithelial and inflammatory changes were observed in each patient in the excluded segment, but in none of the biopsies in the afferent (proximal) small intestine. The lesions showed a focal distribution and included villous architectural changes, limited patchy surface epithelial cell damage, and necrosis and accumulation of eosinophils and mononuclear cells in the lamina propria in the top of the villi. Further characterization of mononuclear cells using monoclonal antibodies showed increased macrophage activation (KP1-CD 68), antigen presentation (B7-1, HLA DR), epithelioid transformation (RFD9), and active transendothelial lymphocyte recruitment (ICAM-1, LFA-1) into the mucosal compartment. Electron microscopic examination revealed damage to the epithelial cells with dilation of the rough endo-

plasmic reticulum and Golgi apparatus, and the presence of basally located transport vesicles.[12]

In an earlier, larger study we also demonstrated that recurrent Crohn's lesions in the neoterminal ileum did not appear as long as the fecal stream was diverted. The majority of patients (53/75, i.e. 71%) developed mucosal lesions 6 months after intestinal continuity had been restored.[13] An identical phenomenon was observed in an Oxford study in which ileal fluid was infused into defunctioned colon previously affected by Crohn's disease.[14] Signs of recurrent inflammation did not develop when this ileal effluent was first ultrafiltered, suggesting that intact bacteria or certain large dietary particles ($>0.22$ μm) had to be present for inflammation to develop.[15] Among potential antigenic candidates *Bacteroides* species seemed particularly important, given their markedly increased concentrations in Crohn's disease ileal resection specimens.[16] In addition, reduction of the load of anaerobes with nitroimidazole antibiotics led to less severe endoscopic recurrences in human Crohn's disease.[17,18] All this indirect evidence suggests a potential role of bacteria or bacterial molecules, most likely from anaerobic bacteria, in the induction of Crohn's disease recurrence.

Other experiments focused on dietary components as a factor in luminal-content induced recurrence. Ubiquitous titanium dioxide and aluminosalicylate particles used as food and pharmaceutical additives, for instance, induce persistent intestinal injury.[19] It has also been suggested that increased intestinal permeability, leading to enhanced penetration of antigens, may be a basic feature of Crohn's disease.[20] In a French study, however, a significant correlation between enhanced permeability and endoscopic recurrence 6 weeks postoperatively could not be established.[21]

Early intestinal inflammation is characterized by a disturbance of the delicate balance of mucosal cytokines. The inflamed mucosa of chronic Crohn's disease is characterized by a typical Th1 pattern of cytokines, with an abundance of tumor necrosis factor (TNF), interleukin-1 (IL-1) and interferon-γ (IFN-γ). This pattern is different from the one observed in early ileal Crohn's lesions, where low levels of IFN-γ and high levels of IL-4, a typical immunoregulatory Th2 cytokine, were demonstrated.[22] IL-4 attenuates the barrier function of the intestinal epithelium and may permit enhanced penetration of noxious agents. In addition, incubation of monocytes/macrophages with IL-4 stimulates IL-12 and TNF production by these cells, and may explain a switch from a Th2 towards a more typical Th1 response.[23] Following this work, the same group of investigators also demonstrated that ileal Crohn's disease recurrence was associated with an enhanced IL-5 and immunoglobulin E (IgE) production accompanied by eosinophilic infiltration, a finding which suggested the involvement of an allergic mechanism.[24] Most recently, low mucosal levels of IL-10, a typical anti-inflammatory cytokine, have been found to correlate with severe postoperative recurrence.[25]

It remains unclear why postoperative recurrence of Crohn's disease develops preferentially in the ileum immediately proximal to the ileocolonic anastomosis. Scanning electron-microscopic studies have shown that a triad of mucosal architectural alterations, epithelial bridge formation and goblet cell hyperplasia can be found in the majority of biopsies taken from resection specimens, both in the affected area and in the unaffected proximal ileum. Macroscopic recurrence of Crohn's disease would merely represent a transition from (electron-)

microscopic towards endoscopically visible disease.[26] In an interesting study looking at the predictive value of endoscopically visible lesions in the remnant small intestine observed during surgery, Esaki and colleagues,[27] however, demonstrated that the presence of such lesions did not correlate with clinical postoperative recurrence. Furthermore, reflux of colonic content, stasis and bacterial overgrowth after removal of the ileocecal valve could also play a part in the development of recurrence. In the absence of a classic ileocolonic anastomosis, e.g. with primary ileostomies, the risk of severe recurrence is indeed much lower.[28] The reflux hypothesis is not supported, however, by the observation that clinical and surgical recurrence occurs less frequently in patients having undergone a wide-lumen stapled anastomosis (allowing more reflux) rather than a conventional sutured end-to-end anastomosis.[29]

An alternative explanation has been sought in the inflammatory changes often encountered in the enteric nervous system. Even in the absence of microscopic inflammation in the ileal resection margins, subtle inflammation surrounding neural structures is commonly observed and may 'guide' the inflammation to the more proximal ileal segments.[30] We recently showed that the presence and severity of 'neuritis' in the ileal section margin were predictive of recurrent Crohn's disease.[31]

# CHARACTERISTICS OF CROHN'S DISEASE RECURRENCE

There is convincing evidence that the evolution of Crohn's disease in patients with postoperative recurrence mimics the natural evolution of the disease at its onset. The clinical presentation of recurrent Crohn's ileitis is, in other words, often strikingly similar to the preoperative presentation. In 1971 de Dombal et al.[32] suggested that there might be several subtypes of Crohn's disease: an 'indolent' one, which tends to recur slowly, and an 'aggressive' one, recurring soon after the surgical intervention. This impression was confirmed by a retrospective analysis at the Mount Sinai Hospitals in New York, in which patients were classified into a subgroup with 'perforating' Crohn's disease (presenting with fistulae and abscesses) and a 'non-perforating' or fibrostenotic subgroup. A second surgical intervention for perforating problems was performed more often among cases whose surgical indication had been perforation initially. In addition, reoperation for perforating disease ('aggressive type') was required about twice as soon as for non-perforating Crohn's disease ('indolent type') (4.7 versus 8.8 years, $P<0.001$). The interval between the second and the third operation was only 2.3 years in patients with a perforating disease behavior, versus 5.2 years in patients with non-perforating disease ($P<0.005$).[33]

Aberhardt and colleagues in Switzerland investigated the same hypothesis in a cohort of 101 patients followed for a median of more than 13 years after their first operation. Their analysis showed that the only variable affecting the time to reoperation was disease behavior. The median interval between first and second operation was only 1.7 years for patients with perforating disease, versus 13 years in patients with fibrostenotic or non-perforating disease.[34] Again, these numbers were recorded between 1970 and 1985, when the use of immunomodulating medication was still very limited. We have not been able to reproduce these findings in a group of North American patients in whom recurrence was defined radiologically and not based on

reoperation. In this study, we studied the length of ileal inflammation on small bowel radiologic studies in 23 patients before resection and at the time of symptom recurrence, and found a striking correlation between both ($r= 0.70$, $P<0.001$). Moreover, in seven patients who had sequential small bowel studies without intervening surgery, the length of measured inflammation correlated with $r= 0.995$ ($P<0.001$), which demonstrated that the extent of disease rarely changes once it is established.[35]

# RISK FACTORS FOR POSTOPERATIVE RECURRENCE OF CROHN'S DISEASE

(Table 47.1)

## PATIENT-RELATED FACTORS: AGE, SMOKING AND PARITY

The age at the time of diagnosis of Crohn's disease would not affect the rate of postoperative recurrence. Recurrence rates are probably higher, however, in patients operated on at a younger age than in those undergoing a resection at an older age.[36] Patients with a preoperative disease history of more than 10 years at the time of surgical intervention do better than those with a shorter disease history.[37] The Aeberhard study could not confirm either of these observations.[34] Additional multivariate analyses have looked at many other factors, such as gender, first or subsequent resection, and use of oral contraceptives, blood transfusions or a positive family history, and failed to demonstrate an enhanced risk recurrence depending on these factors.[38,39]

Generally speaking, cigarette smoking has a deleterious effect on Crohn's disease. The effect of cigarette smoking on the development of postoperative Crohn's recurrence has been examined thoroughly. Many well-designed studies have demonstrated that smoking is associated with higher recurrence rates, particularly in female patients. In a survey by Sutherland and co-workers the need for repeat surgery at 5 and 10 years after the first intervention was significantly lower in non-smokers (20% and 41%) than in smokers (36% and 70%). The risk was particularly high in female smokers with small bowel disease (odds ratio (OR) 9.2).[40] In an Italian series by Cottone et al. in 1994 the 6-year clinical recurrence-free rate was 60% for non-smokers, 41% for ex-smokers and 27% for smokers (OR 2.2, 95% CI 1.2–38).[41] Hence, all operated patients (as well as non-operated ones) should be dissuaded from smoking. The risk of excisional surgery associated with smoking may only be increased in smokers who do not use immunosuppressive drugs, as shown by the French GETAID (Groupe d'Etudes Thérapeutiques des Affections Inflammatoires Digestives).[42]

Recent data have demonstrated that the need for second and third resections after the initial surgical intervention may also be influenced by the number of pregnancies. The authors hypothesized that pregnancy could influence the natural history of Crohn's disease, either by decreasing immune responsiveness or by retarding fibrous stricture formation.[43]

## DISEASE-RELATED FACTORS: DURATION, LOCATION, INFLAMMATORY ACTIVITY

Patients with a preoperative disease history of more than 10 years at the time of surgical intervention appear to do better than those with a shorter disease history.[37] This is in agreement with the observation that patients with 'early' recurrence had a shorter

**Table 47.1 Risk factors for postoperative recurrence of CD**

| Predictive factors | Strong risk factors | Weak/questionable risk factors |
| --- | --- | --- |
| Patient-related | Smoking | Younger age<br>Fewer pregnancies |
| Disease-related | Behavior<br>Perforating > fibrostenotic<br>Indication for surgery<br>intractability<br>Location<br>Ileocolitis > ileitis > colitis | Shorter disease history |
| Surgery-related | Type of intervention<br>Ileorectal/ileocolonic anastomosis<br>> ileal resection >> ileostomy | |

history of symptoms at operation than those with 'late' recurrence.[44] The impact of the location of the disease is also striking. Patients with combined ileocolonic disease suffer higher recurrence rates than those with isolated colonic disease.[45] Additional risk factors are related to the subtype and the inflammatory activity of Crohn's disease. As mentioned before, the virulence of the inflammatory activity is indeed often comparable before and after surgery. Hence, resections should, if at all possible, be avoided if the disease appears clinically active.

## SURGERY-RELATED FACTORS

The postoperative recurrence rates of Crohn's disease are much lower after surgical resection with ileostomy than after resection with ileocolonic anastomosis.[46–48] Moreover, a recent review of 182 patients with an end ileostomy for Crohn's disease revealed that the site of initial disease played a part in recurrence in the neoterminal ileum proximal to the ileostomy: estimated overall cumulative probabilities of recurrence 20 years after the construction of the ileostomy was 64% in the patients with ileocolitis as initial presentation, versus 15% in the patients with colitis alone ($P<0.001$).[49] At the ileal side of the ileocolonic anastomosis no signs of Crohn's recurrence appear as long as the ileum remains 'protected' from the fecal stream by a proximal (diverting) ileostomy.[13] Surprisingly, Crohn's disease also recurs in the ileum after right colonic resection with ileocolonic anastomosis even when the ileum was not diseased prior to surgery. Conversely, some patients develop Crohn's proctitis after ileocolonic resection, even when the rectum had previously been unaffected.[50]

The location of the inflammation and the type of surgical resection may affect recurrence rates as well. Puntis et al., in a follow-up study in Birmingham, demonstrated that the need for reoperation is lower in patients who underwent resection of the distal ileum alone (30–40% at 10 years) than in those who had also part of their right colon and ileocecal valve resected (45–55% at 10 years).[51]

The number of interventions seems to be of little importance with regard to recurrence. In a Swedish study the cumulative recurrence rates at 10 years were 65% after the second intervention versus 60% after the third one. Again, this supports the hypothesis that the disease behavior remains unchanged throughout the patient's history. The same study reported that an ileorectal anastomosis may carry an increased risk for postoperative recurrence – up to 70% at 10 years.[15] Two surgical techniques for the construction of an ileocolonic anastomosis have been com-

pared and it was demonstrated that recurrence rates did not differ between an end-to-end anastomosis and an end-to-side.[52]

Contrary to what was originally believed, the pathological features of the section margins and of the resected bowel loops do not affect the incidence of recurrence. Neither the presence of granulomas in the resection specimen nor the presence or absence of 'disease-free' resection margins (i.e. with or without inflammatory activity) has been shown to influence recurrence rates or severity.[53,54]

## DIAGNOSIS OF RECURRENT CROHN'S DISEASE

As outlined above, endoscopic examinations have been the most sensitive tool to document early recurrence, and a reliable correlation between endoscopic abnormalities in the neoterminal ileum and the development of symptomatic relapse has been established.[11] The majority of recurrence prevention trials with various pharmaceutical agents have therefore used endoscopic parameters as an endpoint. Endoscopic recurrence can be classified as 'mild' or 'severe', but a pragmatic score developed by Rutgeerts et al. allows a more detailed classification (Table 47.2, Figs 47.1–47.4).[11]

Recently, several efforts have been made to develop more sensitive methods to detect recurrence and likelihood of recurrence at an even earlier stage. An adjunct to routine endoscopic examination may be offered by endoscopic fluorescence imaging. With this technique (injection of sodium fluorescein and mucosal illumination with blue light), bright fluorescent spots looking normal macroscopically were found to correlate with superficial erosive inflammatory lesions on histological

**Table 47.2 Endoscopic score for recurrent Crohn's disease in the neoterminal ileum[11] ('i' = 'ileal')**

| | |
| --- | --- |
| i0 | absence of any endoscopic lesion |
| i1 | fewer than 5 aphthous ulcers (<5 mm) |
| i2 | more than 5 aphthous ulcers with normal mucosa between the lesions or lesions confined to the ileocolonic anastomosis (< 1 cm), |
| i3 | diffuse aphthous ileitis with diffusely inflamed mucosa |
| i4 | diffuse ileitis with larger ulcers, nodularity and/or narrowing |

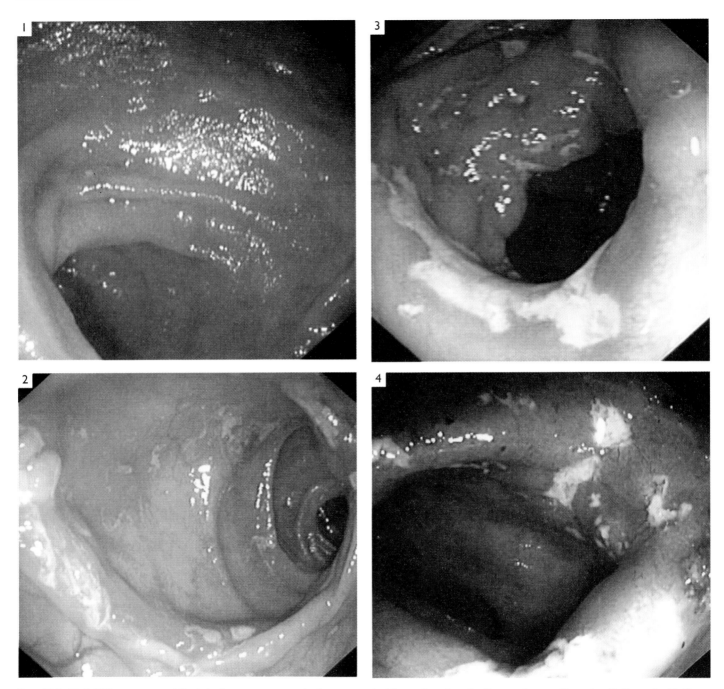

**Figs 47.1–47.4** Different stages of Crohn's disease recurrence in the neoterminal ileum. Based on the Rugeerts' score, Figure 1 = i1, Figure 2 = i2, Figure 3 = i3, Figure 4 = i4.

examination.[55] Alternatively, radiolabeled granulocyte scintigraphy was found to be reliable in the detection of early postoperative recurrence in a small group of patients.[56]

# PREVENTION OF POSTOPERATIVE RECURRENCE OF CROHN'S DISEASE

## RATIONALE AND DIFFICULTIES

Although various operative techniques have been evaluated to reduce the risk of recurrence, none has been shown to be effective apart from the formation of an ostomy. In one trial a wide-stapled ileocolonic anastomosis instead of a classic hand-sutured end-to-end anastomosis led to lower recurrence rates, but other comparable studies failed to demonstrate any benefit based on the type of anastomosis.[57,58]

Because a lot of evidence points towards the persistence of minimal disease in the macroscopically 'healthy' residual gut, medical strategies should try to suppress this minimal inflammation in order to prevent macroscopic lesions leading to symptoms. The evolution from minimal (aphthous) ulcers to larger and deeper lesions causing symptoms has now been well described. Given the correlation between the lesions and the onset of symptoms, it appears logical to prevent the appearance of severe endoscopic lesions if at all possible. The ultimate goal

**Table 47.3 Prevention of postoperative recurrence: most relevant drug trials**

| Authors (ref.) | Drug | Start | Duration (months) | Endpoint | Results at final endpoint | Weakness |
|---|---|---|---|---|---|---|
| Caprilli[64] | Asacol 2.4 g/day | < 15 days | 24 | Endo 6,12,24 mo Clin 6,12,24 mo | 52% vs 85% (P=0.02) 18% vs 41% (P=0.006) | No placebo |
| McLeod[69] | Salofalk 3 g/day | < 8 weeks | 36 | Clin + endo/RX confirmation | Clin 27% vs. 47% | Late start |
| Lochs[66] | Pentasa 4 g/day | < 10 days | 18 | Clin (CDAI) | 24% vs. 31% (NS) | Only clinical parameters |
| Florent[10] | Claversal 3 g/day | < 15 days | 3 | Endo 3 mo | 50% vs. 63% (NS) | No clinical data; short follow-up period |
| Brignola[65] | Pentasa 3 g/day | < 30 days | 12 | Endo 12 mo | Severe 21% vs. 56% (P<0.008) | Few clinical data |
| Rutgeerts[17] | Metronidazole 20 mg/kg/day | < 1 week | 3 treatment 36 follow-up | Endo 3 mo and 36 mo Clin 12, 24, 36 mo | Endo 3 mo: 75% vs. 52% (NS); severe 43% vs.13% (P 0.02) Clin 12 mo: 4% vs. 25% | Poor tolerability |
| Rutgeerts[18] | Ornidazole 500 mg bid | < 1 week | 12 | Endo 3 and 12 mo Clin 12 mo | Endo 12 mo: 64% vs. 94% (P 0.06) Clin 12 mo: 37% vs. 8% (P 0.002) | Toxicity |
| Korelitz[79] | Purinethol 50 mg/day or Pentasa 3 g/day | < 1 week | 24 | Endo, clin 3,6,12,24 mo RX 12 and 24 mo | Endo 24 month: recurrence 68% vs. 80% vs. 90% | Many drop-outs Low-dose 6-MP |

Endo, endoscopic evaluation (ileocolonoscopy); clin/clinical, clinical evaluation; RX, radiographic evaluation. mo = months

---

of recurrence prevention, however, consists of reducing the risk of clinical recurrence and reoperation and improving quality of life compared to untreated patients.

Clinical trials in this field have faced a number of important methodological problems. First, the delay between surgery and clinical recurrence can be very long. Second, clinical symptom scores such as the CDAI are rather unreliable in the postoperative setting. Third, the preventive medication should be initiated early after surgery, and this has not been the case in many trials. Finally, the diagnosis of recurrence should be based on the most sensitive method, this being endoscopy and not radiologic or endosonographic methods.

So far, the medications studied for postsurgical prophylaxis has been roughly the same as those used to maintain remission in active chronic Crohn's disease: aminosalicylates, corticosteroids, antibiotics, the biological agent IL-10, and immunosuppressive drugs such as 6-mercaptopurine (Table 47.3).

One of the most potent 'acute' anti-inflammatory therapies for Crohn's disease, namely corticosteroids, has been ineffective to prevent postoperative recurrence. In a randomized placebo-controlled double-blind study with budesonide, a topical corticosteroid, versus placebo, recurrence rates were no lower in the budesonide group, except when patients operated on for 'active disease' were analyzed separately.[59] Similarly, in a placebo-controlled trial with IL-10, an anti-inflammatory cytokine given subcutaneously for the first 3 months after surgery, no difference between IL-10 treatment and placebo was observed. The latter study, however, had a limited follow-up of only 3 months and comprised a large subgroup of patients operated on for inactive obstructive disease, which is a situation in which recurrence appears later anyway.[60] A significant reduction in recurrence

rates has been observed with aminosalicylates, antibiotics and the thiopurine immunosuppressive drugs.

## SULFASALAZINE AND 5-AMINOSALICYLATES

By far the largest number of recurrence prevention trials have been performed with 5-ASA or mesalamine products. This medication is considered safe and well tolerated but rather expensive when used chronically in appropriate doses. The benefit of aminosalicylates as maintenance therapy for active or inactive chronic Crohn's disease is questionable. Camma and colleagues performed a meta-analysis of all the controlled clinical trials with 5-ASA for maintenance of remission in Crohn's disease and demonstrated that the benefit was rather marginal.[61] The analysis showed that mesalamine therapy significantly reduced the risk of symptomatic relapse by an average of 6%, with the best results in the postsurgical setting, in patients with ileal disease and with prolonged disease duration. These results were somewhat encouraging for the prevention of recurrence post resection, but prevention studies with 5-ASA have, somewhat surprisingly, produced varying results. Possible explanations could be sought in the different pharmacologic preparations that were used in these trials, differences in dosing schedules, and the time when postoperative treatment was initiated (from immediate start up to 12 weeks following surgery).

Ewe and colleagues demonstrated that sulfasalazine was significantly more effective than placebo in the first 2 years following surgery to maintain clinical remission of the disease. Surprisingly, the recurrence rates were higher in the group of patients treated with radical resection than in those with more limited resections. Both strategies were additive: non-radical operation and sulfasalazine had the best prognosis.[62]

In an early Belgian trial Claversal (SmithKline Beecham), an Eudragit-coated mesalamine formulation, was given in a dose of 3 g/day starting 3 months after resection.[63] The results have only been published in abstract form. Clinical and radiological criteria were used to establish the presence of recurrence. A significant difference in the clinical relapse rates or the severity of radiologic lesions at 1 year in the 37 patients (19 on placebo and 18 on 5-ASA) who completed the trial could not be established. A major drawback of this study was that the therapy was only started 3 months postoperatively, whereas many studies have shown that recurrence develops already within these first months.

Caprilli and colleagues studied the effects of another 5-ASA formulation, Asacol, characterized by a Eudragit-S coating and drug release at pH 7.[64] As a consequence, the drug is released more in the right side of the colon than in the terminal ileum The 47 patients randomized to mesalamine therapy received 2.4 g Asacol per day for 2 years following their first intestinal resection, and were compared to 48 comparable control patients who received no therapy at all, not even placebo. All patients underwent an ileocolonoscopy at 6, 12 and 24 months following surgery, with scoring of the lesions as 'normal, mild or severe recurrence,' and were followed clinically to detect signs of 'clinical recurrence'. The compliance with mesalamine use was considered acceptable, with all patients on active drug taking more than 80% of the tablets. Two patients had to discontinue therapy because of severe adverse events (skin rash, epigastric pain, vomiting). In the untreated group, endoscopic recurrence was observed in 29% of patients at 6 months, 56% at 1 year and 85% at 2 years, which was similar to what had been observed in earlier observational studies. The cumulative proportion of endoscopic recurrence at 24 months in mesalamine-treated patients was only 52% and of symptomatic recurrence 18%, versus 41% in untreated patients ($P=0.006$). In summary, Asacol prevented 39% of all recurrences and 55% of the severe recurrences after 2 years. Recurrence rates did not differ among patients operated on for fibrostenotic or perforating disease. The major problem with this trial was, of course, the absence of a proper placebo treatment, which could have led to observer bias.

The next trial was also performed by an Italian group of investigators and published by Brignola.[65] They used the most recent mesalamine formulation, Pentasa, ethylcellulose-encapsulated 5-ASA gradually released throughout the intestinal tract (Ferring, Denmark). Treatment consisted of 3 g/day of this drug, initiated within 1 month following resection with ileocolonic anastomosis. The endpoint was endoscopic and radiological recurrence at 12 months. Severe recurrence was observed in 56% of the placebo patients and in 21% of the Pentasa-treated patients ($P<0.001$).

The Pentasa formulation was also used in a large multicenter trial in Austria, Germany, Denmark, Norway and Switzerland named the European Cooperative Crohn's Disease Study VI.[66] The investigators tried to optimize outcome with three measures:

1. Therapy was initiated within 2 weeks after surgery.
2. They chose the 5-ASA formulation with the highest drug release in the small bowel.
3. They used the highest dose of 5-ASA ever studied in active Crohn's disease, namely 4 g/day.

For various reasons, only 70% of the eligible patients were randomized, 154 to mesalamine and 170 to placebo. Treatment was continued for 18 months, with clinical relapse as the primary outcome measure. Relapse was defined as a CDAI score above 250 or an increase in this score of at least 60 points above the lowest postoperative value *and* a value >200. Endoscopic evaluation was 'recommended' at week 6 and month 18 after the start of therapy or at the time of clinical relapse. The intent-to-treat analysis demonstrated that the cumulative relapse rates after 18 months amounted to $24.5 \pm 3.6\%$ in the mesalamine group and $31.4 \pm 3.7\%$ in the placebo group (NS). In a subgroup analysis relapse rates were recalculated in patients with ileal resection alone (i.e. no colonic involvement). In this group of 124 patients, clinical relapse rates were significantly lower in Pentasa- than in placebo-treated patients ($21.8 \pm 5.6\%$ vs. $39.7 \pm 6.1\%$; $P=0.002$). Variables leading to earlier recurrence included duration of the disease and age of the patient. Unfortunately, only 97 patients were included in the colonoscopy substudy at week 6 and 133 at month 18. A correlation between the severity of the endoscopic lesions and the presence of symptoms could not be established. The incidence of endoscopic recurrence was not significantly lower in mesalamine-treated patients (66% vs. 50% with placebo). The authors concluded that the study failed to demonstrate a protective effect of Pentasa on the development of clinical recurrence, but that patients operated on for small bowel disease alone may benefit from this treatment none the less. An important number of patients did not enter the study in the first weeks after surgery owing to complications. One could argue that precisely these patients, with more complicated and possibly more aggressive disease, would have the greatest benefit from anti-inflammatory therapy. In an accompanying editorial, Sutherland added this trial to the meta-analysis by Camma, which demonstrated that the number-needed-to-treat (NNT) with mesalamine to prevent one recurrence was 13. Adding the ECCDS IV led to an NNT of 25. When the trial by Caprilli, which had not used a placebo drug, was withdrawn from the analysis, the NNT became 100![67]

In addition to these European trials, two Canadian trials were also included in the Camma meta-analysis. A large Canadian multicenter trial (163 patients) with an appropriate placebo group again confirmed the rather limited benefit of mesalamine.[68] Treatment consisted of 1.5 g mesalamine twice daily (Salofalk) or placebo started within 8 weeks after curative resection. The maximum follow-up period was 72 months. The endpoint chosen by the investigators was 'symptomatic recurrence', defined as symptoms plus endoscopic and/or radiographic confirmation. The overall 3-year symptomatic recurrence amounted to 31% in the active treatment group and 41% in the control group ($P=0.031$). The relative risk of developing recurrence was 0.628 for those in the mesalamine group. Only one severe adverse event occurred (pancreatitis) in a patient taking mesalamine. The most important limitation of this study was the time point at which therapy was initiated: 8 weeks after surgery some patients undoubtedly already had microscopic (and endoscopic) signs of recurrence. Based on the placebo results in this study one could argue that 53% of the patients received unnecessary treatment for 3 years.

A second Canadian prevention study treated patients with both medically and surgically induced remission (the latter comprising 26% of the study population) with mesalamine (Pentasa formulation) 750 mg four times per day or placebo for

48 weeks.[69] Patients were examined at regular intervals, with CDAI calculations on every occasion. Patients whose remission was induced by a bowel resection had a lower relapse rate than those who had a medically induced remission ($P=0.003$). For unclear reasons, the effect of mesalamine was more pronounced in women than in men, and in patients with ileocolitis. No benefit could be demonstrated in patients with ileal disease alone. Although conventional statistical significance could not be achieved, the proportion of patients with relapse within 2 years was lower with mesalamine (25%) than with placebo (36%, $P=0.056$). When only the patients with surgical remission were analyzed, the results became more insignificant, probably owing to the small sample size that was left.

Finally, there is a French trial which was carefully designed and performed by GETAID (Groupe d'Etudes Thérapeutiques des Affections Inflammatoires Digestives).[10] The investigators administered the Claversal 5-ASA preparation 1 g three times daily or placebo for 12 weeks, starting as soon as oral feeding was resumed. At week 12 a colonoscopy was performed. Sixty-one patients were included in the 5-ASA group and 61 in the placebo group. Forty-two per cent of the patients treated with Claversal had no signs of recurrence, versus 34% with placebo, a difference which was not statistically significant. In conclusion, this 5-ASA drug affected neither the presence of endoscopic recurrence nor its severity. Patients who had never smoked had a lower recurrence rate.

## NITROIMIDAZOLE ANTIBIOTICS

Based on the evidence discussed above that bacterial agents or components are likely to play an important part in the development of postoperative Crohn's recurrence, it seemed logical to try and prevent recurrence with antibiotics. Because anaerobic bacteria are present in high concentrations in the ileum following ileal resection with ileocolonic anastomosis,[70] and because of the established effects of metronidazole in active Crohn's disease,[71-73] this drug was chosen to perform a first recurrence prevention trial with antibiotics. In addition, metronidazole is not only active against anaerobic bacteria, but it may have immunomodulating properties, as well.[74-76]

Rutgeerts and colleagues performed a controlled trial with metronidazole 20 mg/kg/day or placebo started within a week after the ileal resection for 12 weeks.[17] Thirty patients received active treatment and 30 received placebo. At week 12 all patients underwent an ileocolonoscopy with biopsies. Patients were further followed clinically at 6-month intervals up to 3 years by gastroenterologists unaware of the treatment that the patients had received. At the end of the 3-year follow-up period, all patients underwent a new ileocolonoscopy. Besides the primary endpoints of endoscopic recurrence at week 12 and year 3, the secondary endpoints were the development of clinical relapse at 1, 2 and 3 years after surgery. At week 12, recurrent lesions in the neoterminal ileum were observed in 75% of the placebo-treated patients and in 52% of the metronidazole-treated patients ($P=0.09$). When only *severe* forms of recurrence were looked at, metronidazole treatment reduced their incidence from 43% (placebo) to 13% ($P=0.02$). In addition, and somewhat surprisingly, the effects of this intervention seemed to be prolonged, with a reduction in clinical recurrence rates at 1, 2 and 3 years of 4% versus 25%, 26% versus 43%, and 30% versus 50%, respectively, for metronidazole and placebo.

The difference was only statistically significant at 1 year. Unfortunately, side effects with metronidazole were common and included metallic taste (7/30), paresthesias and polyneuropathy (5/30), gastrointestinal intolerance (5/30), leukopenia (2/30), abnormal liver function tests (1/30) and psychosis (1/30). The authors concluded that metronidazole therapy reduced the incidence of severe endoscopic recurrence and delayed the development of symptomatic recurrence, but also that lower doses and potentially less toxic nitroimidazole components should be tested in this indication.

The next step the same group of investigators then undertook was a similar trial with ornidazole (Tiberal, Roche, Basel), an analog of metronidazole which was considered to be better tolerated with prolonged use.[18] The trial design was almost identical to that of the metronidazole trial, but treatment was continued for a full year in a dose of 500 mg twice daily. At 3 months 59% of placebo-treated patients had severe endoscopic recurrence, versus 34% of the ornidazole-treated patients ($P=0.02$). Clinical recurrence was observed in 8% of the ornidazole-treated patients 1 year after surgery, in 27% at 2 years and in 65% at 3 years. Clinical recurrence rates in placebo-treated patients were 37% ($P=0.002$) at 1 year, 45% at 2 years ($P=0.1$) and 48% ($P=0.27$) at 3 years following surgery. The toxicity of this long-term treatment was also considerable and, in fact, not much different from the toxicity profile observed with metronidazole. At any rate, metronidazole or ornidazole treatment should probably be limited to the first months after surgery, and preferably be combined with other therapies which are safer in the long run.

## IMMUNOSUPPRESSIVES

Azathioprine and 6-mercaptopurine are the most potent agents in the maintenance treatment of Crohn's disease. None the less, the benefit of these agents in preventing postoperative recurrence has so far only been examined in a small number of trials. The reason for this is probably the presumed unfavorable toxicity profile of these antimetabolites when compared to aminosalicylates. If the efficacy were found to be much better, however, this therapy would still offer an important clinical benefit. Cuillerier and colleagues performed a retrospective analysis of 38 patients treated with azathioprine between 1987 and 1996 following subtotal colectomy with ileorectal anastomosis ($n=12$), ileocolonic resection ($n=18$), coloproctectomy with ileoanal anastomosis ($n=4$) or segmental ileal or colonic resection.[77] Twelve patients were already taking azathioprine prior to surgery and continued the medication, and 26 started to take it within 2 months after surgery. With a mean duration a follow-up of 29 months, recurrence rates amounted to 9, 16 and 28% at 1, 2 and 3 years, respectively. The authors concluded that these numbers were lower than what would be expected in untreated patients and recommended further investigation of azathioprine in this indication. In a Spanish study, 39 patients were treated with mesalamine 3 g/day ($n=21$) or azathioprine 50 mg/day ($n=17$).[78] After 2 years no significant differences were observed between groups in terms of clinical or endoscopic recurrence. This study had a number of serious shortcomings, however: the sample size was too small to allow reliable conclusions; the dose of azathioprine was suboptimal, as generally doses of 2–2.5 mg/kg/day are recommended; and, finally, the study was not appropriately randomized and controlled.

These shortcomings were avoided to an important extent in a North American–European prospective double-blind controlled trial with 118 patients randomized postoperatively to treatment with 50 mg 6-mercaptopurine (6-MP) per day, 3 g mesalamine per day or placebo at five academic centers.[79] Patients receiving a certain treatment also received placebo tablets for the alternative treatment (so-called double-dummy design). Treatment and follow-up lasted 2 years, with clinical checks and ileocolonoscopies 6, 12 and 24 months after surgery and small bowel X-rays at months 12 and 24. The dosage of 6-MP was reduced by an independent physician in case of leukopenia. Patients were withdrawn from the study in case of significant clinical recurrence, drug toxicity, serious adverse events, opportunistic infections or their own choice. During the course of this trial, a considerable number of patients dropped out of the study because of adverse events or lack of compliance (16 in the mesalamine group, 16 in the 6-MP group and 11 in the placebo group), but the adverse event rate was not considerably higher with mesalamine than with 6-MP. Intent-to-treat analysis showed an absence of endoscopic relapse in 32% of the patients on 6-MP ($P=0.04$), in 20% of those on mesalamine (NS) and in 10% of the placebo patients at 2 years. *Severe* endoscopic relapse at 2 years was more frequently observed with placebo and mesalamine than with 6-MP ($P=0.01$ vs. placebo and 0.07 vs. mesalamine). The clinical relapse rate was reduced by both mesalamine and 6-MP, but statistical significance was only achieved with 6-MP ($P=0.04$). This study demonstrated that 6-MP is currently the strongest recurrence prevention therapy, but the authors concluded that higher doses may be needed to achieve even lower recurrence rates (1–1.5 mg/kg body weight/day of 6-MP or 2-2.5 mg/kg body weight/day of azathioprine). Further trials to confirm these suggestions are currently being performed.

Besides their efficacy to prevent severe recurrence, immunosuppressives have also been useful in the treatment of established recurrent ileitis, not only to control symptoms but also to induce mucosal healing.[80] Patients who undergo balloon dilatation of an anastomotic stenosis have longer remissions if they are treated with a short course of budesonide CIR and further azathioprine maintenance than if they remain untreated.[81]

## FUTURE MEDICAL THERAPIES

Several potential new candidate drugs are being explored, not only for active Crohn's disease but also for the prevention of postoperative recurrence. Monoclonal antibodies to TNF are highly effective in active Crohn's disease, but trials in the postoperative setting are being awaited. It remains unclear whether this type of therapy can alter the natural history of the disease. Novel delivery forms of IL-10, for instance using viral vectors via genetic manipulation, could prove to be much more effective than subcutaneous administration of this cytokine.

Finally, combination therapies are appealing. We are currently studying a combination of metronidazole for a short time after surgery and azathioprine for maintenance thereafter. Also, the administration of probiotics affecting the fecal flora is a safe, promising and theoretically appealing strategy.

## SURGICAL PROPHYLAXIS OF CROHN'S DISEASE RECURRENCE

Surgeons have looked at various strategies to decrease the risk of postsurgical recurrence. A recent clinical trial performed at the Cleveland Clinic where patients were randomized to 2 or 10 cm margins detected no difference in recurrence rates.[82] The type of anastomosis (end-to-end versus end-to-side ileocolonic anastomosis) also had no effect on the rate of recurrence.[83] In some centers an end-to-end ileocolonic anastomosis is preferred, because anastomotic strictures can more easily be treated endoscopically with this construction. Finally, the presence of microscopic signs of inflammation at the resection margin does not affect recurrence either.[84] Given these findings, resections should be as limited as possible and surgically safe.

# A STRATEGY FOR THE PREVENTION OF ILEAL RECURRENCE OF CROHN'S DISEASE

As outlined above, several clinically relevant risk factors for the development of early and/or severe postoperative recurrence have been identified and allow the selection of patients who will benefit most from immediate prophylactic treatment (Table 47.2). It seems unnecessary to treat *all* patients operated on for Crohn's disease, given the limited gains, the cost of the medication and the potential side effects. Patients undergoing a resection at a young age, for instance, have higher recurrence rates than those operated upon at an older age, and those with perforating disease may suffer from a more aggressive disease course. Multiple studies also demonstrated that smoking is associated with higher recurrence rates, particularly in female patients.

The available treatments for the prevention of postoperative recurrence are limited. Based on all the studies outlined above, we can state that aminosalicylates have rather weak preventive effects, that nitroimidazole antibiotics are definitely effective but are characterized by a high rate of adverse events, and that thiopurines are also effective when given for a sufficient period of time and if tolerated well by the patient.

Given all this information, and knowing that the endoscopic appearance of the neoterminal ileum provides a clue to the clinical evolution, it seems possible to develop an algorithm that can be used in daily practice (Fig. 47.5). Patients with a low risk profile for recurrence (non-smokers, older patients, long disease history, fibrostenotic disease) usually do not need prophylactic treatment, but are advised to undergo an ileocolonoscopy 6–12 months after surgery. If no or only mild endoscopic lesions are found at this time, patients are reassured about the unlikelihood of serious future problems and remain untreated. If more severe endoscopic lesions are present and the patient is still free of symptoms, we institute mesalamine 3–4 g/day. In patients with severe endoscopic lesions and symptoms, we immediately start with a 3-month course of topical corticosteroids (budesonide CIR) in combination with azathioprine 2–2.5 mg/kg/day, the latter of which is continued for at least a number of years.

Patients with a high risk of early recurrence are approached differently. If they undergo a second, third or fourth resection, or if they undergo surgery for medically intractable disease, they will immediately be started on azathioprine, often accompanied by metronidazole 250 mg three times per day or ornidazole 500 mg twice daily in the first 3 months. Patients already taking azathioprine will be continued on it.

Using this strategy, it seems likely that the severity and rapidity of recurrent postoperative Crohn's disease can be decreased

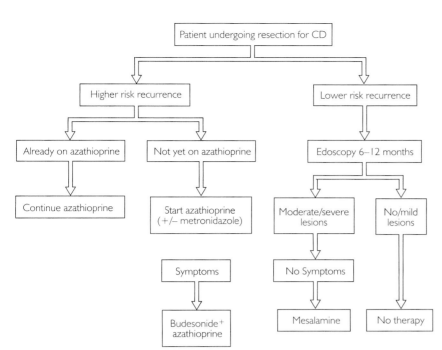

**Fig. 47.5** Algorithm for the prophylaxis of postoperative recurrence of Crohn's disease.

significantly. Prospective studies supporting this hypothesis are strongly recommended.

## CONCLUSION

A large number of studies looking at risk factors for postoperative recurrence of Crohn's disease allow us to estimate the individual risk and to stratify patients with regard to the need for prophylactic treatment. The findings at an early ileocolonoscopy provide relevant information about the further clinical course. In patients with a low risk, recurrence prevention is not always necessary, although maintenance therapy with mesalamine may be of benefit. High-risk patients or early relapsers are preferably treated with immunomodulators such as azathioprine or 6-MP, initially in combination with metronidazole (immediately after surgery) or with budesonide (in the presence of symptoms).

## REFERENCES

1. Mekhijan HS, Switz DM, Watts HD et al. National cooperative Crohn's disease study: factors determining recurrence of Crohn's disease after surgery. Gastroenterology 1979;77:907–913.
2. Whelan G, Farmer RG, Fazio VW, Goormastic M. Recurrence after surgery in Crohn's disease. Gastroenterology 1985;88:1826–1833.
3. Kyle J. Prognosis after ileal resection for Crohn's disease. Br J Surg 1971;58:735–737.
4. Lennard-Jones JE, Stalder GA. Prognosis after resection of chronic regional enteritis. Gut 1967;8:332–336.
5. Olaison G, Smedh K, Sjödahl R. Natural course of Crohn's disease after ileocolic resection: endoscopically visualized ileal ulcers preceding symptoms. Gut 1992;33: 331–335.
6. Greenstein AJ, Sachar DB, Pasternack BS et al. Reoperation and recurrence in Crohn's colitis and ileocolitis. N Engl J Med 1975;293:685–690.
7. Ekberg O, Fork FT. Predictive value of small bowel radiography for recurrent Crohn's disease. AJR 1980;135:1051–1055.
8. Hildell J, Lindstrom C, Wenckert A. Radiographic appearances in Crohn's disease. IV. The new distal ileum after surgery. Acta Radiol Diagn 1980;21:221–229.
9. McLeod RS, Wolff B, Steinhart H et al. Risk and significance of endoscopic/radiological evidence of recurrent Crohn's disease. Gastroenterology 1997;113:1823–1827.
10. Florent C, Cortot A, Quandale P et al. Placebo-controlled clinical trial of mesalazine in the prevention of early endoscopic recurrences after resection for Crohn's disease. Eur J Gastroenterol Hepatol 1996;8:229–233.
11. Rutgeerts P, Geboes K, Vantrappen G et al. Predictability of the postoperative course of Crohn's disease. Gastroenterology 1990;99:956–963.
12. D'Haens G, Geboes K, Peeters M et al. Early lesions of recurrent Crohn's disease caused by infusion of intestinal contents in excluded ileum. Gastroenterology 1998;114:262–267.
13. Rutgeerts P, Geboes K, Peeters M et al. Effect of fecal stream diversion on recurrence of Crohn's disease in the neoterminal ileum. Lancet 1991;338:771–774.
14. Fasoli R, Kettlewell MGW, Mortensen N et al. Response to fecal challenge in defunctioned colonic Crohn's disease: prediction of long-term response. Br J Surg 1990;77:616–617.
15. Harper PH, Lee ECG, Kettlewell MGW et al. Role of fecal stream in the maintenance of Crohn's colitis. Gut 1985;26:279–284.
16. Keighly MR, Arabi Y, Dimock F et al. Influence of inflammatory bowel disease on intestinal microflora. Gut 1978;19:1099–1104.
17. Rutgeerts P, Peeters M, Hiele M et al. Controlled trial of metronidazole treatment for prevention of Crohn's recurrence after ileal resection. Gastroenterology 1995;108:1617–1621.
18. Rutgeerts P, Van Assche G, D'Haens G et al. Ornidazol for prophylaxis of postoperative Crohn's disease: final results of a double blind placebo controlled trial. Gastroenterology 2002;122:A666.
19. Powell JJ, Ainley CC, Mason IM et al. Characterization of inorganic microparticles in pigment cells of human gut associated lymphoid tissue. Gut 1996;38:390–395.
20. Wyatt J, Vogelsang H, Hubl W et al. Intestinal permeability and the prediction of relapse in Crohn's disease. Lancet 1993;341:1437–1439.
21. Klein O, Houdret N, Desreumaux P et al. Intestinal permeability is not predictive of endoscopic recurrence in patients operated on for Crohn's disease. Gastroenterology 1996;112:A1096.
22. Desreumaux P, Brandt E, Gambiez L et al. Distinct cytokine patterns in early and chronic ileal lesions of Crohn's disease. Gastroenterology 1997;113:118–126.
23. D'Andrea A, Ma X, Aste-Amezaga M et al. Stimulatory and inhibitory effects of interleukin-4 and IL-13 on the production of cytokines by human peripheral blood mononuclear cells: priming for IL-12 and TNF production. J Exp Med 1995;181:537–546.
24. Dubucquoi S, Janin A, Klein O et al. Activated eosinophils and interleukin 5 expression in early recurrence of Crohn's disease. Gastroenterology 1995;37:242–246.
25. Meresse B, Rutgeerts P, Malchow H et al. Low ileal interleukin 10 concentrations are predictive of endoscopic recurrence in patients with Crohn's disease. Gut 2002;50:25–28.
26. Nagel E, Bartels M, Pichlmayer R. Scanning electron-microscopic lesions in Crohn's disease: relevance for the interpretation of postoperative recurrence. Gastroenterology 1995;108:376–382.
27. Esaki M, Matsumoto T, Hizawa K et al. Intraoperative enteroscopy detects more lesions but is not predictive of postoperative recurrence in Crohn's disease. Surg Endosc 2001;15:455–459.
28. Cameron JL, Hamilton SR, Coleman J et al. Patterns of ileal recurrence in Crohn's disease. Ann Surg 1992;215:546–551.
29. Munoz-Juarez M, Yamamoto T, Wolff BG et al. Wide-lumen stapled anastomosis vs. conventional end-to-end anastomosis in the treatment of Crohn's disease. Dis Colon Rectum 2001;44:20–25.

30. Geboes K, Rutgeerts P, Ectors N et al. Are section margins useful for the prediction of recurrence of Crohn's disease after all? Gastroenterology 1990;98:A171.

31. D'Haens G, Penninckx F, Rutgeerts P et al. The presence and severity of neural inflammation predict severe postoperative recurrence of Crohn's disease. Gastroenterology 1998;114:A963.

32. de Dombal FT, Burton I, Goligher C. The early and late results of surgical treatment for Crohn's disease. Br J Surg 1971;11:805–816.

33. Greenstein AJ, Lachman P, Sachar DB et al. Perforating and non-perforating indications for repeated operations in Crohn's disease: evidence for two clinical forms. Gut. 1988;29:588–592.

34. Aeberhard P, Berchtold W, Riedtmann HJ et al. Surgical recurrence of perforating and nonperforating Crohn's disease. Dis Colon Rectum 1996;39:80–87.

35. D'Haens G, Baert F, Gasparaitis AE et al. Length and type of recurrent ileitis after ileal resection correlate with presurgical features in Crohn's disease. Inflamm Bowel Dis 1997;3:249–253.

36. Hellers G. Crohn's disease in Stockholm County 1955–1974. A study of epidemiology, results of surgical treatment and long-term prognosis. Acta Chir Scand 1979;490(suppl.):5–81.

37. Baker WNW. The results of ileorectal anastomosis at St. Mark's Hospital from 1953 to 1968. Gut 1970;11:235–239.

38. Wolff BG. Factors determining recurrence following surgery for Crohn's disease. World J Surg 1998;22:364–369.

39. Lautenbach E, Berlin JA, Lichtenstein GR. Risk factors for early postoperative recurrence of Crohn's disease. Gastroenterology 1998;115:259–267.

40. Sutherland LR, Ramcharan S, Bryant H et al. Effect of cigarette smoking on recurrence of Crohn's disease. Gastroenterology 1990;98:1123–1128.

41. Cottone M, Rosselli M, Orlando A et al. Smoking habits and recurrence in Crohn's disease. Gastroenterology 1994;106:643–648.

42. Cosnes J, Carbonnel F, Carrot F et al. Effects of current and former cigarette smoking on the clinical course of Crohn's disease. Aliment Pharmacol Ther 1999;13:1403–1411.

43. Nwokolo CU, Tan WC, Andrews HA et al. Surgical resections in parous patients with distal ileal and colonic Crohn's disease. Gut 1994;35:220–223.

44. Griffiths AM, Wesson DE, Shandling B et al. Factors influencing postoperative recurrence of Crohn's disease in childhood. Gut 1991;32:491–495.

45. de Dombal FT, Burton I, Goligher JC. Recurrence of Crohn's disease after primary excisional surgery. Gut 1971;12:519–527.

46. Sachar DB, Wolfson DM, Greenstein AJ et al. Risk factors for postoperative recurrence of Crohn's disease. Gastroenterology. 1983;85:917–921.

47. Goligher JC. The long-term results of excisional surgery for primary and recurrent Crohn's disease of the large intestine. Dis Colon Rectum 1985;28:51–55.

48. Heimann TM, Greenstein AJ. Lewis B et al. Prediction of early symptomatic recurrence after intestinal resection in Crohn's disease. Ann Surg. 1993;218:294–299.

49. Ho I, Greenstein AJ, Bodian CA et al. Recurrence of Crohn's disease in end ileostomies. IBD 1995;1: 173–178.

50. D'Haens G, Sels F, Peeters M et al. Curative ileal resection of Crohn's disease followed by recurrence in the rectum. Digestion 1998;59 (suppl 3):132.

51. Puntis J, McNeish AS, Allan RN. Long term prognosis of Crohn's disease with onset in childhood and adolescence. Gut 1984;25:329–336.

52. Cameron JL, Hamilton SR, Coleman J et al. Patterns of ileal recurrence in Crohn's disease. Ann Surg. 1992;215:546–551.

53. Wolfson DM, Sachar DB, Cohen A et al. Granulomas do not affect postoperative recurrence rates in Crohn's disease. Gastroenterology. 1982;83:405–409.

54. Kotanagi HH, Kramer K, Fazio VW et al. Do microscopic abnormalities at resection margins correlate with increased anastomotic recurrence in Crohn's disease? Retrospective analysis of 100 cases. Dis Colon Rectum 1991;34:909–916.

55. Maunoury V, Mordon S, Geboes K et al. Endoscopic fluorescence imaging for the study of anastomotic recurrences in Crohn's disease: correlation with histological findings. Gastroenterology 1999;116:A689.

56. Biacone L, Scopinaro F, Ierardi M et al. 99m Tc-HMPOA granulocyte scintigraphy in the early detection of postoperative asymptomatic recurrence of Crohn's disease. Dig Dis Sci 1997;42:1549–1556.

57. Munoz-Juarez M, Yamamoto T, Wolff BG et al. Wide-lumen stapled anastomosis vs. conventional end-to-end anastomosis in the treatment of Crohn's disease. Dis Colon Rectum 2001;44:20–25.

58. de Dombal FT, Burton I, Goligher C. The early and late results of surgical treatment for Crohn's disease. Br J Surg 1971;11:805–816.

59. Hellers G, Cortot A, Jewell D et al. Oral budesonide for prevention of postsurgical recurrence in Crohn's disease. Gastroenterology 1999;116:294–300.

60. Colombel JF, Rutgeerts P, Malchow H et al. Interleukin 10 (Tenovil) in the prevention of postoperative recurrence of Crohn's disease. Gut 2001;49: 42–46.

61. Camma C, Giunta M, Roselli M et al. Mesalamine in the maintenance treatment of Crohn's disease: a meta-analysis adjusted for confounding variables. Gastroenterology 1997;113:1465–1473.

62. Ewe K, Herfarth C, Malchow H et al. Postoperative recurrence of Crohn's disease in relation to radicality of operation and sulfasalazine prophylaxis: a multicentre trial. Digestion 1989;42:224–232.

63. Fiasse R, Fontaine F, Vanheuverzwyn R. Prevention of Crohn's disease recurrences after intestinal resection with Eudragit-L-coated 5-ASA. Gastroenterology 1991;100:A208.

64. Caprilli R, Andreoli A, Capurso L et al. Oral mesalazine (Asacol) for the prevention of postoperative recurrence of Crohn's disease. Eur J Gastroenterol Hepatol 1994;8:35–43.

65. Brignola C, Cottone M, Pera A et al. Mesalamine in the prevention of endoscopic recurrence after intestinal resection for Crohn's disease. Gastroenterology 1995;108:345–349.

66. Lochs H, Mayer M, Fleig WE et al. Prophylaxis of postoperative relapse in Crohn's disease with mesalazine (Pentasa): European Cooperative Crohn's Disease Study VI. Gastroenterology 2000;118:264–273.

67. Sutherland LR. Mesalamine for the prevention of postoperative recurrence: is nearly being there the same as being there? Gastroenterology 2000;118:436–438.

68. Sutherland LR, Martin F, Bailey RJ et al. and the Canadian Mesalamine for Remission Study Group. A randomized, placebo-controlled, double-blind trial of mesalamine in the maintenance of remission of Crohn's disease. Gastroenterology 1997;112:1069–1077.

69. McLeod RS, Wolff BG, Steinhart AH et al. Prophylactic mesalamine treatment decreases postoperative recurrence of Crohn's disease. Gastroenterology 1995;109:404–413.

70. Gorbach SL, Tabaqchali S. Bacteria, bile and the small bowel. Gut 1969;10:963–971.

71. Ursing B, Kamme G. Metronidazole for Crohn's disease. Lancet 1975;i:775–777.

72. Blichfeldt P, Blomhoff JP, Myhre E et al. Metronidazole in Crohn's disease. Scand J Gastroenterol 1978;13:123–127.

73. Sutherland L, Singleton J, Sessions J et al. Double blind, placebo-controlled trial of metronidazole in Crohn's disease. Gut 1991;32:1071–1075.

74. Grove DI, Mahmoud AAF, Warren KS. Suppression of cell-mediated immunity by metronidazole. Int Arch Allergy Appl Immunol 1977;54:422–427.

75. Blair V, Ullman U. The influence of metronidazole and its two main metabolites on murine in vitro lymphocyte transformation. Eur J Clin Microbiol 1983;2:568–570.

76. Arndt H, Palitzsch K, Grisham M, Granger N. Metronidazole inhibits leucocyte–endothelial cell adhesion in rat mesenteric venules. Gastroenterology 1994;106:1271–1276.

77. Cuillerier E, Lemann M, Bouhnik Y. Azathioprine for prevention of postoperative recurrence in Crohn's disease. Eur J Gastroenterol Hepatol 2001;13:1291–1296.

78. Nos P, Hinojosa J, Aguilera V et al. Azathioprine and 5-ASA in the prevention of postoperative recurrence of Crohn's disease. Gastroenterol Hepatol 2000;23:374–378.

79. Korelitz B, Hanauer S, Rutgeerts P et al. Postoperative prophylaxis with 6-MP, 5-ASA or placebo in Crohn's disease: a two year multicenter trial. Gastroenterology 1998;114:A1011.

80. D'Haens G, Geboes K, Ponette E et al. Healing of severe recurrent ileitis with azathioprine therapy in patients with Crohn's disease. Gastroenterology 1997;112:1475–1481.

81. Raedler A, Peters I, Screiber S. Treatment with azathioprine and budesonide prevents reoccurrence of ileocolonic stenosis after endoscopic dilatation in Crohn's disease. Gastroenterology 1997;112:A1067.

82. McLeod RS. Is it possible to prevent recurrent Crohn's disease with medical or surgical interventions? Neth J Med 1996;48:68–70.

83. Cameron JL, Hamilton SR, Coleman J et al. Patterns of ileal recurrence in Crohn's disease. Ann Surg 1992;215:546–551.

84. Kotanagi HH, Kramer K, Fazio VW, Petras RE. Do microscopic abnormalities at resection margins correlate with increased anastomotic recurrence in Crohn's disease? Retrospective analysis of 100 cases. Dis Colon Rectum 1991;34:909–916.

## CHAPTER 48

# Microscopic colitis

Johan Bohr, Curt Tysk and Gunnar Järnerot

## INTRODUCTION

The term microscopic colitis was originally introduced by Read et al. in 1980 to describe a disease with chronic diarrhea of unknown origin with no endoscopic or radiologic lesions, but with a mild, unspecific inflammation in the colonic mucosa.[1] It has since evolved as a collective term for all colitides where the colonic mucosa appears normal macroscopically, but where microscopic examination of mucosal biopsies reveals specific histopathologic features. Collagenous colitis and lymphocytic colitis constitute the two main forms of microscopic colitis. Collagenous colitis was first described by Lindström in 1976.[2] The term lymphocytic colitis was suggested by Lazenby et al. in 1989, as the major distinguishing feature of lymphocytic colitis was an increased number of intraepithelial lymphocytes.[3] The predominant clinical symptom in both diseases is chronic watery diarrhea. Another subtype of microscopic colitis, 'microscopic colitis with giant cells', was recently described and this needs further study.[4]

## EPIDEMIOLOGY

Initially, collagenous colitis was regarded as rare until the first epidemiologic studies showed incidence rates of $1.8/10^5$ and $2.3/10^5$ inhabitants, respectively, and a prevalence of $15.7/10^5$ inhabitants.[5,6] Recent epidemiologic studies, however, show that the incidence of collagenous colitis is even higher, with figures of $5.2/10^5$ and $6.1/10^5$ inhabitants, respectively[7,8] (Table 48.1). Thus, if these figures are representative the incidence of collagenous colitis is close to that of Crohn's disease.[9] Patients with collagenous colitis are typically middle-aged women, the age at diagnosis being around 65 years, and the female:male ratio is around 7:1[5–8] (Fig. 48.1). Only four children below the age of 12 have been reported.[10] However, 25% of 163 patients

were diagnosed before the age of 45 years, and so it must be considered even in younger subjects with chronic watery diarrhea.[11]

Epidemiologic data on lymphocytic colitis are at present available from three different regions in Europe during the 1990s[6–8] (Table 48.1). The data are fairly consistent, and an annual incidence of 3.7–5.7 per $10^5$ inhabitants has been reported. The incidence of lymphocytic colitis is close to that of Crohn's disease, and combined rates for collagenous colitis and lymphocytic colitis even approach the incidence of ulcerative colitis.[9] This illustrates that these conditions are more common than was previously considered, and microscopic colitis may account for about 10% of patients investigated for chronic diarrhea. The onset of symptoms in lymphocytic colitis is around 60–65 years, but the female predominance is less pronounced than with collagenous colitis.

## DISTRIBUTION AND HISTOPATHOLOGY

The histopathologic findings are mainly located in the colon and the rectum. Deposits of subepithelial collagen in the stomach and duodenum, as well as in the terminal ileum in occasional patients with collagenous colitis – so-called collagenous gastritis and collagenous enterocolitis – have been reported.[14–23] Collagenous gastritis is also seen without collagen deposits in the colon, and might be a syndrome on its own.[24] Within the colon and rectum the collagenous layer is most prominent in the proximal part, and may be absent in the rectal mucosa in between 18 and 73% of biopsy specimens.[6,7,25,26]

The following histopathologic features are the hallmarks of collagenous colitis. A diffuse non-continuous thickening of a subepithelial collagen layer is seen beneath the basement membrane (Fig. 48.2). The thickness of the subepithelial layer must

| Region and study period | Collagenous colitis | Lymphocytic colitis |
|---|---|---|
| Örebro, Sweden, 1984–88[5] | 0.8 | |
| Örebro, Sweden, 1989–93[5] | 2.7 | |
| Örebro, Sweden, 1993–95[8] | 3.7 | 3.1 |
| Örebro, Sweden, 1996–98[8] | 6.1 | 5.7 |
| Franche-Comté, France, 1987–92[12] | 0.6 | |
| Uppsala, Sweden, 1992–94[13] | 1.9 | |
| Terrassa, Spain, 1993–97[6] | 2.3 | 3.7 |
| Iceland, 1995–99[7] | 5.2 | 4.0 |

Table 48.1 Annual incidence per $10^5$ inhabitants in epidemiological studies of collagenous and lymphocytic colitis

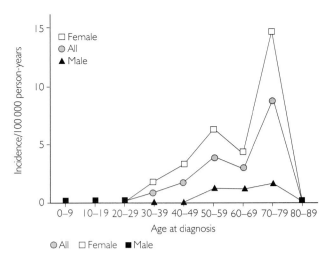

Fig. 48.1 Age- and sex-specific incidence of collagenous colitis. (Reproduced with permission from Gut 1995;37:394–397.)

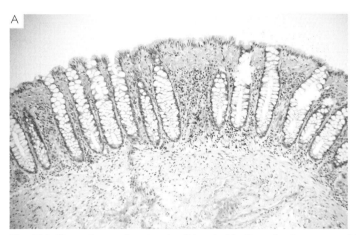

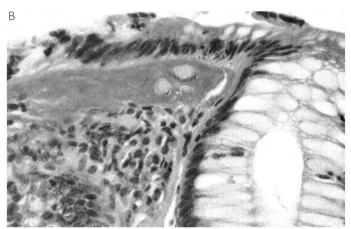

Fig. 48.2 Biopsy from colon showing (A) typical findings of collagenous colitis – increased subepithelial collagen layer, inflammation of lamina propria and (B) epithelial lesions with intraepithelial lymphocytes (van Gieson stain).

be 10 $\mu$m or more on a well-orientated section of the mucosa, compared to 0–3 $\mu$m in normal individuals. An inflammation in the lamina propria is seen, which is dominated by lymphocytes and plasma cells. Eosinophils and mast cells can be found, but neutrophils are rarely seen. Flattening and vacuolization of the epithelial cells and detachment of the surface epithelium are seen. Intraepithelial lymphocyte infiltration may be present, though not as prominently as in lymphocytic colitis.[1–3,27] Cryptitis does not exclude the diagnosis of collagenous colitis.[28] In the matrix containing the thickened collagenous layer collagen types I, III and VI and fibronectin have been identified.[29–31]

The characteristic histopathologic features of lymphocytic colitis are epithelial lesions, an increase in intraepithelial lymphocytes (>20 per 100 epithelial cells), and infiltration of the lamina propria with lymphocytes and plasma cells, whereas no increase of the collagen layer is found[3,32] (Fig. 48.3).

## ETIOLOGY AND PATHOPHYSIOLOGY

The etiology of microscopic colitis is largely unknown. The available data are based on small patient numbers and need further confirmation. Both collagenous and lymphocytic colitis are, at present, supposed to be caused by an abnormal immunologic reaction to different mucosal insults in predisposed individuals.

## GENETICS

Data on genetics are sparse. A small number of familial cases with collagenous and lymphocytic colitis and of mixed collagenous and lymphocytic colitis have been reported.[33–36] Whether these associations are due to genetics, environmental factors or chance cannot be assessed.

## A LUMINAL AGENT AS ETIOLOGIC FACTOR

The finding of an increased number of T lymphocytes in the epithelium has supported the theory that collagenous colitis may be caused by an abnormal immunologic reaction to a luminal agent in predisposed individuals.[37–39] This theory is further supported by the observation that diversion of the fecal stream by an ileostomy normalizes or reduces the characteristic histopathologic changes in collagenous colitis.[40] Recurrence of symptoms and histopathologic changes were seen after ileostomy closure. Furthermore, abnormalities of colonic histology resembling lymphocytic colitis have been reported in untreated celiac disease.[41]

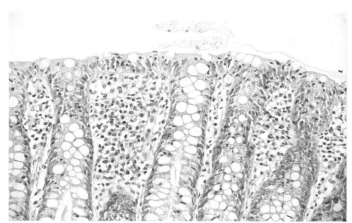

**Fig. 48.3** Biopsy from colon showing typical findings of lymphocytic colitis – epithelial lesions with intraepithelial lymphocytes and inflammation in the lamina propria (Hematoxylin–eosin stain).

| Table 48.2 Drugs reported to be associated with microscopic colitis | |
|---|---|
| **Drug** | **Diagnosis** |
| Ticlopidine[55–60] | Lymphocytic colitis |
| Cyclo 3 Fort[61–64] | Lymphocytic colitis |
| Ranitidine[65] | Lymphocytic colitis |
| Vinburnine[66] | Lymphocytic colitis |
| Tardyferon[67] | Lymphocytic colitis |
| Flutamide[60] | Lymphocytic colitis |
| Acarbose[68] | Lymphocytic colitis |
| Piroxicam[69] | Lymphocytic colitis |
| Levodopa–benserazide[70] | Lymphocytic colitis |
| Carbamazepine[71, 72] | Lymphocytic colitis |
| Lanzoprazole[73] | Lymphocytic colitis |
| Lanzoprazole[74, 75] | Collagenous colitis |
| NSAIDs[53] | Collagenous colitis |
| Cimetidine[76] | Collagenous colitis |

## INFECTIOUS AGENT

As in other forms of inflammatory bowel disease a microbiological origin has been suggested. The sudden onset of the disease in a proportion of patients, and the effect of various antibiotics, support the possibility of an infectious etiology.[11] This is supported by a study where *Yersinia enterocolitica* was detected in three of six patients prior to the diagnosis of collagenous colitis, and by another serologic study which showed that antibodies to *Yersinia* species were more common in collagenous colitis patients than in healthy controls.[42,43] Other microbiologic agents reported in association with microscopic colitis are *Campylobacter jejuni*[44] and *Clostridium difficile*.[45,46] Of special interest in this context is the condition known as 'Brainerd diarrhea', which has been applied to outbreaks of chronic watery diarrhea characterized by acute onset and prolonged duration.[47] Colonic biopsies in these patients show epithelial lymphocytosis similar to microscopic colitis but lack the surface epithelial lesions.

## BILE ACIDS

Data on bile acid malabsorption in microscopic colitis are conflicting. In one study no association was found.[48] Recently, bile acid malabsorption was reported in 27–44% of patients with collagenous colitis and in 9–60% of patients with lymphocytic colitis.[49–51] The coexistence of bile acid malabsorption seems to worsen the diarrhea in patients with collagenous colitis.[49] These observations are the rationale for recommendations of bile acid-binding treatment, which was reported to be effective in a majority of patients with microscopic colitis and concomitant bile acid malabsorption.[49,51] Even patients without bile acid malabsorption may respond to this treatment. This emphasizes the importance of the fecal stream, and the therapeutic effect may possibly be related to binding of luminal toxins.[52]

## DRUGS

There are several reports on drug-induced microscopic colitis, especially on lymphocytic colitis (Table 48.2). Most reports concern ticlopidine and Cyclo 3 Fort. In a case–control study the use of NSAIDs was significantly more common among collagenous colitis patients than in controls, and discontinuation was followed by improvement of the diarrhea in some cases.[53] Others found that use of NSAIDs at presentation was associated with a greater need for 5-ASA and steroid therapy, possibly reflecting a more resistant form of disease, and in that study the withdrawal of NSAIDs did not improve clinical symptoms.[54] The increased use of NSAIDs in collagenous colitis is most likely due to the occurrence of concomitant arthritis. The number of reported cases of drug-induced microscopic colitis is small and a chance association cannot be ruled out. However, it is important to assess concomitant drug use in patients and to consider the withdrawal of drugs that might possibly worsen the condition.

## AUTOIMMUNITY

It has been proposed that an autoimmune pathogenesis in collagenous colitis could be the result of an inflammation initiated by a foreign luminal agent that causes an immunologic cross-reaction with an endogenous antigen.[39,77] The theory is supported by the strong association of collagenous colitis with other autoimmune diseases. A study of autoantibodies and immunoglobulins in collagenous colitis showed that the mean level of IgM in collagenous colitis patients was significantly increased,[78] which might represent a parallel to the increased IgM level in primary biliary cirrhosis. A specific autoantibody in collagenous colitis has not been reported.

## NITRIC OXIDE

Colonic nitric oxide (NO) production is greatly increased in active microscopic colitis, because of an upregulation of inducible nitric oxide synthase (iNOS) in the colonic epithelium.[79–82] The levels of NO correlated with clinical activity and histopathologic status of the colonic mucosa, i.e. patients in histopathologic remission had normal levels of colonic NO, in contrast to increased levels in patients with histologically active disease.[81] The role of NO in microscopic colitis is uncertain. NO is an inflammatory mediator, but whether its role is pro-inflammatory or protective remains unclear. Furthermore, NO may be involved in the pathophysiology of diarrhea, as infusion in the colon of $N^G$-monomethyl-L-arginine, an inhibitor of NOS, reduced colonic net secretion by 70% and the addition of L-arginine increased colonic net secretion by 50%.[83]

## SECRETORY OR OSMOTIC DIARRHEA

The diarrhea in collagenous colitis has been regarded as secretory owing to the epithelial lesions, the inflammatory infiltrate in the lamina propria and the collagenous band, that might be a barrier for reabsorption of electrolytes and water.[84,85] Studies on the influence of fasting on diarrhea in collagenous colitis, however, indicated that osmotic diarrhea was predominant.[86,87] This is in accordance with the experience reported by many patients that fasting reduces their diarrhea.

## CLINICAL FEATURES AND DIAGNOSIS

The main symptom in collagenous colitis is watery diarrhea, and 40% of patients report that the onset of the disease was sudden.[11] It may be accompanied by nocturnal diarrhea, crampy abdominal pain and distension. Initial weight loss of up to 5 kg is common, and occasionally is even more pronounced. Serious dehydration is rare, although 25% of the patients had 10 daily stools or more and stool volumes up to 5 L have been reported. Mucus or blood in the stools is unusual. As a large proportion of patients are over 70 years of age, fecal incontinence is frequent.[11,60]

The course in the majority of cases is chronic, relapsing and benign. The relative risk of developing colorectal cancer in collagenous colitis does not appear to be increased.[88,89] In a follow-up study, 63% of the patients had lasting remission after 3.5 years.[90] Another cohort study showed that all patients were improved 47 months after the diagnosis, and only 29% of these required medication.[91] In a number of collagenous colitis patients, however, remission is difficult to achieve, and such patients have usually tried a large variety of medications in vain.[11,40]

Patients with collagenous colitis often have concomitant diseases. Up to 40% have one or more associated autoimmune diseases. The most common are rheumatoid arthritis, thyroid disorders, celiac disease, asthma/allergy and diabetes mellitus. Crohn's disease or ulcerative colitis concomitant with collagenous colitis have occasionally been reported.[11,92]

The clinical picture of lymphocytic colitis is similar to that of collagenous colitis and the predominant symptom is chronic watery diarrhea. In a recent report, however, it was found that symptoms in lymphocytic colitis were milder and more likely to disappear than in collagenous colitis.[60] Like collagenous colitis, lymphocytic colitis has also been reported in association with autoimmune diseases.[60] The prognosis for lymphocytic colitis seems good. There is no increased mortality and no increased risk of subsequent bowel malignancy reported. Mullhaupt et al.[93] reported a benign course in 27 cases, with resolution of diarrhea and normalization of histology in over 80% of the patients within 38 months.

No blood tests make screening for collagenous colitis possible at present. The erythrocyte sedimentation rate may be mildly elevated. Analyses of pANCA[94] or serum procollagen III propeptide are not of diagnostic value.[95] Stool examinations reveal no pathologic organisms, though increased excretion of fecal leukocytes has been reported in more than half of collagenous colitis patients.[21]

Barium enema and endoscopy are usually normal,[96] though subtle endoscopic changes such as mucosal edema, granularity or erythema may be seen in up to 30% of cases.[11] Pancolonoscopy must be preferred to sigmoidoscopy, as a thickened collagenous layer may be absent in between 18 and 73% of rectal biopsy specimens.

## THERAPY IN MICROSCOPIC COLITIS

Few controlled studies have been conducted in microscopic colitis and recommendations on therapy are mainly based on retrospective reports and uncontrolled data (Table 48.3). As there are no variables that can predict the response to medical therapy, the strategy generally is a 'step-up' treatment according to clinical response and outcome (Fig. 48.4). In a recent retrospective study, however, the degree of lamina propria inflammation was found to predict the response to therapy, and patients with a greater inflammation more often needed corticosteroid therapy.[54]

A careful assessment of concomitant drug use and dietary factors that might worsen the condition is important. Loperamide, bulking agents and cholestyramine have been reported to be of benefit in a majority of collagenous colitis and lymphocytic colitis patients and are recommended as the primary treatment.[11] It was reported that bismuth subsalicylate gave lasting clinical and histopathologic resolution in microscopic colitis.[97,98] A later report on its efficacy in lymphocytic colitis was somewhat less optimistic.[99] Still, bismuth subsalicylate can be recommended together with earlier mentioned drugs as the

**Table 48.3 Treatment responses (%) in retrospective, uncontrolled series of microscopic colitis**

|  | Collagenous colitis[11] (n=163) | Lymphocytic colitis[99] (n=188) |
|---|---|---|
| Antidiarrheals | 71 | 72 |
| Bismuth | – | 69 |
| Sulfasalazine | 34 | 36 |
| Mesalazine | 50 | 41 |
| Cholestyramine | 59 | 59 |
| Corticosteroids | 82 | 70 |
| AZA/6-MP | – | 28 |

In the study by Bohr,[11] figures show percentages of patients with effect of therapy.
In the study by Pardi,[99] figures show percentages of patients with complete or partial response to therapy.
AZA, azathioprine; 6-MP, 6-mercaptopurine.

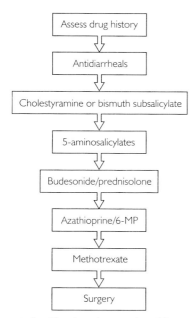

Fig. 48.4 Treatment algorithm for microscopic colitis.

first-line therapy in microscopic colitis. However, bismuth subsalicylate is not available in a number of countries for toxicity reasons.

Sulfasalazine and mesalazine are the next choice if the initial treatment fails. A retrospective assessment of sulfasalazine and mesalazine showed effect in 34–50% of patients,[11,99] and an even greater effect has been reported in an abstract.[100]

Metronidazole and erythromycin were earlier frequently prescribed antibiotic drugs in collagenous colitis and around 60% responded temporarily to one of these treatments. However, antibiotics are seldom used today in our unit in the therapy of these conditions.

Prednisolone is an effective drug with a reported response rate of 70–80%. The effect, however, is generally not sustained after withdrawal, and the dose required to maintain remission is often unacceptably high: more than 20 mg/day.[11] Uncontrolled

data on budesonide show a similar response rate as for prednisolone even in prednisone-refractory patients.[101] Recently, three randomized, placebo-controlled trials of budesonide have been reported in collagenous colitis[102–104] (Table 48.4). The short-term outcome in these studies is significantly better than for placebo. Further controlled studies, however, are required to address the long-term clinical efficacy, as uncontrolled data show that the effect is not sustained after withdrawal, but the dose can often be tapered to 3–6 mg/day.[105] The corticosteroid adverse effects are less frequent than with prednisolone but must be considered during long-term treatment.

For steroid-resistant or steroid-dependent patients there are some other options. An open trial with azathioprine gave partial or complete remission in eight of nine patients with microscopic colitis.[106] Low-dose methotrexate was effective in 10 of 11 patients with prednisolone-refractory collagenous colitis.[107] The required median dose of methotrexate was 7.5 mg/week. An effect of octreotide has been casuistically reported.[108]

If medical therapy fails and alternative diagnoses are ruled out, surgery may be considered in patients with severe microscopic colitis. Split ileostomy was conducted successfully in nine women with collagenous colitis,[40] whereas others have reported a successful outcome in both collagenous colitis and lymphocytic colitis after subtotal colectomy or colectomy with ileoanal pouch.[109–113]

## Collagenous versus lymphocytic colitis

As collagenous colitis and lymphocytic colitis have a similar clinical expression and similar histopathologic features, except for the subepithelial collagenous layer in collagenous colitis, it has been speculated whether they are actually the same disease in different stages of development, or two different but associated conditions. Conversion of lymphocytic colitis to collagenous colitis, or the opposite, has been reported,[114,115] but the fact that conversion happens relatively seldom, and the differences in sex ratio and HLA pattern,[116] makes it more reasonable to consider collagenous colitis and lymphocytic colitis as two separate but related entities.

**Table 48.4 Data from randomized, placebo-controlled studies of budesonide in collagenous colitis**

| Author | Number of cases | Dosage of budesonide and duration of trial | Clinical response in budesonide vs placebo treated cases | Histopathologic response in budesonide vs placebo treated cases | Side effects |
|---|---|---|---|---|---|
| Baert et al[102] | 28 | 9 mg/day for 8 weeks | 8/14 vs 3/14 (p=0.05) | Reduction of lamina propria inflammation in 9/13 vs 4/12 (p<0.001). No difference in collagen layer | Mild No difference between treatment group |
| Miehlke et al[104] | 45* | 9 mg/day for 6 weeks | Remission: 20/23 vs 3/22 (p<0.001) | Improvement in 14/23 vs 1/22 (p<0.001) No difference in collagen layer. | Mild 38% vs 12% P=0.052 |
| Bonderup et al[103] | 20 | 9 mg/day for 8 weeks | 10/10 vs 2/10 (p<0.001) | Reduction of overall inflammation (P<0.01) and of collagen layer in sigmoid colon (P<0.02) | None |

* per protocol analysis, 51 patients were randomized but 6 were withdrawn early due to lack of efficacy or adverse events.

# REFERENCES

1. Read NW, Krejs GJ, Read MG et al. Chronic diarrhea of unknown origin. Gastroenterology 1980;78:264–271.
2. Lindström CG. 'Collagenous colitis' with watery diarrhoea – a new entity? Pathol Eur 1976;11:87–89.
3. Lazenby AJ, Yardley JH, Giardiello FM et al. Lymphocytic ('microscopic') colitis: a comparative histopathologic study with particular reference to collagenous colitis. Hum Pathol 1989;20:18–28.
4. Libbrecht L, Croes R, Ectors N et al. Microscopic colitis with giant cells. Histopathology 2002;40:335–338.
5. Bohr J, Tysk C, Eriksson S et al. Collagenous colitis in Örebro, Sweden, an epidemiological study 1984–1993. Gut 1995;37:394–397.
6. Fernandez-Banares F, Salas A, Forne M et al. Incidence of collagenous and lymphocytic colitis: a 5-year population-based study. Am J Gastroenterol 1999;94:418–423.
7. Agnarsdottir M, Gunnlaugsson O, Orvar KB et al. Collagenous and lymphocytic colitis in Iceland. Dig Dis Sci 2002;47:1122–1128.
8. Olesen M, Bohr J, Eriksson S et al. Epidemiology of microscopic colitis in Örebro, Sweden 1993–1998. Scand J Gastroenterol 2002;37(suppl 235):21.
9. Sandler RS, Eisen GM. Epidemiology of inflammatory bowel disease. In: Kirsner JB, ed. Inflammatory bowel disease, 5th edn. Philadelphia: WB Saunders; 2000:89–112.
10. Gremse DA, Boudreaux CW, Manci EA. Collagenous colitis in children. Gastroenterology 1993;104:906–909.
11. Bohr J, Tysk C, Eriksson S et al. Collagenous colitis: a retrospective study of clinical presentation and treatment in 163 patients. Gut 1996;39:846–851.
12. Raclot G, Queneau PE, Ottignon Y et al. Incidence of collagenous colitis. A retrospective study in the east of France. Gastroenterology 1994;106:A23.
13. Taha Y, Kraaz W, Lööf L. Förekomst av kollagen kolit i biopsier vid kolonoskopi med makroskopiskt normal slemhinna (Swedish). Sv Läkarsällskapets handl Hygiea 1995;104:167.
14. Eckstein RP, Dowsett JF, Riley JW. Collagenous enterocolitis: a case of collagenous colitis with involvement of the small intestine. Am J Gastroenterol 1988;83:767–771.
15. Stolte M, Ritter M, Borchard F et al. Collagenous gastroduodenitis on collagenous colitis. Endoscopy 1990;22:186–187.
16. Lewis FW, Warren GH, Goff JS. Collagenous colitis with involvement of terminal ileum. Dig Dis Sci 1991;36:1161–1163.
17. Meier PN, Otto P, Ritter M et al. [Collagenous duodenitis and ileitis in a patient with collagenous colitis]. Leber Magen Darm 1991;21:231–232.
18. McCashland TM, Donovan JP, Strobach RS et al. Collagenous enterocolitis: a manifestation of gluten-sensitive enteropathy. J Clin Gastroenterol 1992;15:45–51.
19. Chatti S, Haouet S, Ourghi H et al. [Collagenous enterocolitis. Apropos of a case and review of the literature]. Arch Anat Cytol Pathol 1994;42:149–153.
20. Veress B, Löfberg R, Bergman L. Microscopic colitis syndrome. Gut 1995;36:880–886.
21. Zins BJ, Tremaine WJ, Carpenter HA. Collagenous colitis: mucosal biopsies and association with fecal leukocytes. Mayo Clin Proc 1995;70:430–433.
22. Pulimood AB, Ramakrishna BS, Mathan MM. Collagenous gastritis and collagenous colitis: a report with sequential histological and ultrastructural findings. Gut 1999;44:881–885.
23. Freeman HJ. Topographic mapping of collagenous gastritis. Can J Gastroenterol 2001;15:475–478.
24. Lagorce-Pages C, Fabiani B, Bouvier R et al. Collagenous gastritis: a report of six cases. Am J Surg Pathol 2001;25:1174–1179.
25. Tanaka M, Mazzoleni G, Riddell RH. Distribution of collagenous colitis: utility of flexible sigmoidoscopy. Gut 1992;33:65–70.
26. Offner FA, Jao RV, Lewin KJ et al. Collagenous colitis: a study of the distribution of morphological abnormalities and their histological detection. Hum Pathol 1999;30:451–457.
27. Levy AM, Yamazaki K, Van Keulen VP et al. Increased eosinophil infiltration and degranulation in colonic tissue from patients with collagenous colitis. Am J Gastroenterol 2001;96:1522–1528.
28. Jessurun J, Yardley JH, Giardiello FM et al. Chronic colitis with thickening of the subepithelial collagen layer (collagenous colitis): histopathologic findings in 15 patients. Hum Pathol 1987;18:839–848.
29. Birembaut P, Adnet JJ, Feydy P et al. [Collagenous colitis: immunomorphologic approach to the lesion]. Gastroenterol Clin Biol 1982;6:833.
30. Flejou JF, Grimaud JA, Molas G et al. Collagenous colitis. Ultrastructural study and collagen immunotyping of four cases. Arch Pathol Lab Med 1984;108:977–982.
31. Aigner T, Neureiter D, Muller S et al. Extracellular matrix composition and gene expression in collagenous colitis. Gastroenterology 1997;113:136–143.
32. Bogomoletz WV. Collagenous, microscopic and lymphocytic colitis. An evolving concept. Virchows Arch 1994;424:573–579.
33. van Tilburg AJ, Lam HG, Seldenrijk CA et al. Familial occurrence of collagenous colitis. A report of two families. J Clin Gastroenterol 1990;12:279–285.
34. Järnerot G, Hertervig E, Grännö C et al. Familial occurrence of microscopic colitis: a report on five families. Scand J Gastroenterol 2001;36:959–962.

35. Abdo AA, Zetler PJ, Halparin LS. Familial microscopic colitis. Can J Gastroenterol 2001;15:341–343.
36. Freeman HJ. Familial occurrence of lymphocytic colitis. Can J Gastroenterol 2001;15:757–760.
37. Giardiello FM, Lazenby AJ. The atypical colitides. Gastroenterol Clin North Am 1999;28:479–490.
38. Stampfl DA, Friedman LS. Collagenous colitis: pathophysiologic considerations. Dig Dis Sci 1991;36:705–711.
39. Armes J, Gee DC, Macrae FA et al. Collagenous colitis: jejunal and colorectal pathology. J Clin Pathol 1992;45:784–787.
40. Järnerot G, Tysk C, Bohr J et al. Collagenous colitis and fecal stream diversion. Gastroenterology 1995;109:449–455.
41. Fine KD, Lee EL, Meyer RL. Colonic histopathology in untreated celiac sprue or refractory sprue: is it lymphocytic colitis or colonic lymphocytosis? Hum Pathol 1998;29:1433–1440.
42. Mäkinen M, Niemela S, Lehtola J et al. Collagenous colitis and Yersinia enterocolitica infection. Dig Dis Sci 1998;43:1341–1346.
43. Bohr J, Nordfelth R, Järnerot G et al. Yersinia species in collagenous colitis: A serologic study. Scand J Gastroenterol 2002;37:711–714.
44. Perk G, Ackerman Z, Cohen P et al. Lymphocytic colitis: a clue to an infectious trigger. Scand J Gastroenterol 1999;34:110–112.
45. Vesoulis Z, Lozanski G, Loiudice T. Synchronous occurrence of collagenous colitis and pseudomembranous colitis. Can J Gastroenterol 2000;14:353–358.
46. Khan MA, Brunt EM, Longo WE et al. Persistent Clostridium difficile colitis: a possible etiology for the development of collagenous colitis. Dig Dis Sci 2000;45:998–1001.
47. Bryant DA, Mintz ED, Puhr ND et al. Colonic epithelial lymphocytosis associated with an epidemic of chronic diarrhea. Am J Surg Pathol 1996;20:1102–1109.
48. Eusufzai S, Löfberg R, Veress B et al. Studies on bile acid metabolism in collagenous colitis: no evidence of bile acid malabsorption as determined by the SeHCAT test. Eur J Gastroentol Hepatol 1992;4:317–321.
49. Ung KA, Gillberg R, Kilander A et al. Role of bile acids and bile acid binding agents in patients with collagenous colitis. Gut 2000;46:170–175.
50. Ung KA, Kilander A, Willén R et al. Role of bile acids in lymphocytic colitis. Hepatogastroenterology 2002;49:432–437.
51. Fernandez-Banares F, Esteve M, Salas A et al. Bile acid malabsorption in microscopic colitis and in previously unexplained functional chronic diarrhea. Dig Dis Sci 2001;46:2231–2238.
52. Andersen T, Andersen JR, Tvede M et al. Collagenous colitis: are bacterial cytotoxins responsible? Am J Gastroenterol 1993;88:375–377.
53. Riddell RH, Tanaka M, Mazzoleni G. Non-steroidal anti-inflammatory drugs as a possible cause of collagenous colitis: a case–control study. Gut 1992;33:683–686.
54. Abdo A, Raboud J, Freeman HJ et al. Clinical and histological predictors of response to medical therapy in collagenous colitis. Am J Gastroenterol 2002;97:1164–1168.
55. Martinez Aviles P, Gisbert Moya C, Berbegal Serra J et al. [Ticlopidine-induced lymphocytic colitis]. Med Clin (Barc) 1996;106:317.
56. Brigot C, Courillon-Mallet A, Roucayrol AM et al. [Lymphocytic colitis and ticlopidine]. Gastroenterol Clin Biol 1998;22:361–362.
57. Swine C, Cornette P, Van Pee D et al. [Ticlopidine, diarrhea and lymphocytic colitis]. Gastroenterol Clin Biol 1998;22:475–476.
58. Schmeck-Lindenau HJ, Kurtz W, Heine M. [Lymphocytic colitis during ticlopidine therapy]. Dtsch Med Wochenschr 1998;123:479.
59. Berrebi D, Sautet A, Flejou JF et al. Ticlopidine induced colitis: a histopathological study including apoptosis. J Clin Pathol 1998;51:280–283.
60. Baert F, Wouters K, D'Haens G et al. Lymphocytic colitis: a distinct clinical entity? A clinicopathological confrontation of lymphocytic and collagenous colitis. Gut 1999;45:375–381.
61. Ouyahya F, Codjovi P, Machet MC et al. [Diarrhea induced by Cyclo 3 fort and lymphocytic colitis]. Gastroenterol Clin Biol 1993;17:65–66.
62. Pierrugues R, Saingra B. [Lymphocytic colitis and Cyclo 3 fort: 4 new cases]. Gastroenterol Clin Biol 1996;20:916–917.
63. Beaugerie L, Luboinski J, Brousse N et al. Drug induced lymphocytic colitis. Gut 1994;35:426–428.
64. Bouaniche M, Chassagne P, Landrin I et al. [Lymphocytic colitis caused by Cyclo 3 Fort]. Rev Med Interne 1996;17:776–778.
65. Beaugerie L, Patey N, Brousse N. Ranitidine, diarrhoea, and lymphocytic colitis. Gut 1995;37:708–711.
66. Chauveau E, Prignet JM, Carloz E et al. [Lymphocytic colitis likely attributable to use of vinburnine (Cervoxan)]. Gastroenterol Clin Biol 1998;22:362.
67. Bouchet-Laneuw F, Deplaix P, Dumollard JM et al. [Chronic diarrhea following ingestion of Tardyferon associated with lymphocytic colitis]. Gastroenterol Clin Biol 1997;21:83–84.
68. Piche T, Raimondi V, Schneider S et al. Acarbose and lymphocytic colitis. Lancet 2000;356:1246.
69. Mennecier D, Gros P, Bronstein JA et al. [Chronic diarrhea due to lymphocytic colitis treated with piroxicam beta cyclodextrin]. Presse Med 1999;28:735–737.
70. Rassiat E, Michiels C, Sgro C et al. [Lymphocytic colitis due to Modopar]. Gastroenterol Clin Biol 2000;24:852–853.

71. Mahajan L, Wyllie R, Goldblum J. Lymphocytic colitis in a pediatric patient: a possible adverse reaction to carbamazepine. Am J Gastroenterol 1997;92:2126–2127.

72. Linares Torres P, Fidalgo Lopez I, Castanon Lopez A et al. [Lymphocytic colitis as a cause of chronic diarrhea: possible association with carbamazepine]. Aten Primaria 2000; 25:366–367.

73. Ghilain JM, Schapira M, Maisin JM et al. Lymphocytic colitis associated with lansoprazole treatment]. Gastroenterol Clin Biol 2000:24:960–962.

74. Macaigne G, Boivin JF, Simon P et al. [Lansoprazole-associated collagenous colitis]. Gastroenterol Clin Biol 2001;25:1030.

75. Wilcox GM, Mattia A. Collagenous colitis associated with lansoprazole. J Clin Gastroenterol 2002;34:164–166.

76. Duncan HD, Talbot IC, Silk DB. Collagenous colitis and cimetidine. Eur J Gastroenterol Hepatol 1997;9:819–820.

77. Bayless TM, Giardiello FM, Lazenby A et al. Collagenous colitis. Mayo Clin Proc 1987;62:740–741.

78. Bohr J, Tysk C, Yang P et al. Autoantibodies and immunoglobulins in collagenous colitis. Gut 1996;39:73–76.

79. Lundberg JO, Herulf M, Olesen M et al. Increased nitric oxide production in collagenous and lymphocytic colitis. Eur J Clin Invest 1997;27:869–871.

80. Hillingsø J, Nordgaard-Andersen I, Munkholm P et al. Greatly increased mucosal nitric oxide (NO) production in patients with collagenous colitis (CC). Gastroenterology 1997;112:A15.

81. Olesen M, Middelveld R, Bohr J et al. Luminal nitric oxide and epithelial expression of inducible and endothelial nitric oxide synthase in collagenous and lymphocytic colitis. Scand J Gastroenterol 2003;38:66–72.

82. Perner A, Nordgaard I, Matzen P et al. Colonic production of nitric oxide gas in ulcerative colitis, collagenous colitis and uninflamed bowel. Scand J Gastroenterol 2002;37:183–188.

83. Perner A, Andresen L, Normark M et al. Expression of nitric oxide synthases and effects of L-arginine and L-NMMA on nitric oxide production and fluid transport in collagenous colitis. Gut 2001;49:387–394.

84. Rask-Madsen J, Grove O, Hansen MG et al. Colonic transport of water and electrolytes in a patient with secretory diarrhea due to collagenous colitis. Dig Dis Sci 1983;28:1141–1146.

85. Phillips S, Donaldson L, Geisler K et al. Stool composition in factitial diarrhea: a 6-year experience with stool analysis. Ann Intern Med 1995;123:97–100.

86. Giardiello FM, Bayless TM, Jessurun J et al. Collagenous colitis: physiologic and histopathologic studies in seven patients. Ann Intern Med 1987;106:46–49.

87. Bohr J, Järnerot G, Tysk C et al. The effect of fasting on the diarrhoea in collagenous colitis. Digestion 2002;65:30–34.

88. Bonderup OK, Folkersen BH, Gjersoe P et al. Collagenous colitis: a long-term follow-up study. Eur J Gastroenterol Hepatol 1999;11:493–495.

89. Chan JL, Tersmette AC, Offerhaus GJ et al. Cancer risk in collagenous colitis. Inflamm Bowel Dis 1999;5:40–43.

90. Goff JS, Barnett JL, Pelke T et al. Collagenous colitis: histopathology and clinical course. Am J Gastroenterol 1997;92:57–60.

91. Bonner GF, Petras RE, Cheong DM et al. Short- and long-term follow-up of treatment for lymphocytic and collagenous colitis. Inflamm Bowel Dis 2000;6:85–91.

92. Pokorny CS, Kneale KL, Henderson CJ. Progression of collagenous colitis to ulcerative colitis. J Clin Gastroenterol 2001;32:435–438.

93. Mullhaupt B, Guller U, Anabitarte M et al. Lymphocytic colitis: clinical presentation and long term course. Gut 1998;43:629–633.

94. Yang P, Bohr J, Tysk C et al. Antineutrophil cytoplasmic antibodies in inflammatory bowel disease and collagenous colitis: no association with lactoferrin, b-glucuronidase, myeloperoxidase, or proteinase 3. Inflamm Bowel Dis 1996;2:173–177.

95. Bohr J, Jones I, Tysk C et al. Serum procollagen III propeptide is not of diagnostic predictive value in collagenous colitis. Inflamm Bowel Dis 1995;1:276–279.

96. Feczko PJ, Mezwa DG. Nonspecific radiographic abnormalities in collagenous colitis. Gastrointest Radiol 1991;16:128–132.

97. Fine KD, Lee EL. Efficacy of open-label bismuth subsalicylate for the treatment of microscopic colitis. Gastroenterology 1998;114:29–36.

98. Fine K, Ogunji F, Lee E et al. Randomized, double-blind, placebo-controlled trial of bismuth subsalicylate for microscopic colitis. Gastroenterology 1999;116:A880 (abstract).

99. Pardi DS, Smyrk TC, Tremaine WJ et al. Microscopic colitis: a review. Am J Gastroenterol 2002;97:794–802.

100. Kimble J, Taboada C, Randall CW. Mesalazine is effective therapy for the microscopic colitis. Gastroenterology 2001;120:A215.

101. Lanyi B, Dries V, Dienes HP et al. Therapy of prednisone-refractory collagenous colitis with budesonide. Int J Colorectal Dis 1999;14:58–61.

102. Baert F, Schmit A, D'Haens G et al. Budesonide in collagenous colitis: a double-blind placebo-controlled trial with histologic follow-up. Gastroenterology 2002;122:20–25.

103. Bonderup OK, Hansen JB, Birket-Smith L et al. Budesonide treatment of collagenous colitis: a randomised, double blind, placebo controlled trial with morphometric analysis. Gut 2003;52:248–51.

104. Miehlke S, Heymer P, Bethke B et al. Budesonide treatment for collagenous colitis: a randomized, double-blind, placebo-controlled, multicenter trial. Gastroenterology 2002;123:978–84.

105. Bohr J, Olesen M, Tysk C et al. Budesonide and bismuth in microscopic colitis. Gut 1999;45:A202.

106. Pardi DS, Loftus EV Jr, Tremaine WJ et al. Treatment of refractory microscopic colitis with azathioprine and 6-mercaptopurine. Gastroenterology 2001;120:1483–1484.

107. Hillman LC, Ashton C, Chirigakis L et al. Collagenous colitis remission with methotrexate. Gastroenterology 2001;120:A278.

108. Fisher NC, Tutt A, Sim E et al. Collagenous colitis responsive to octreotide therapy. J Clin Gastroenterol 1996;23:300–301.

109. Alikhan M, Cummings OW, Rex D. Subtotal colectomy in a patient with collagenous colitis associated with colonic carcinoma and systemic lupus erythematosus. Am J Gastroenterol 1997;92:1213–1215.

110. Yusuf TE, Soemijarsih M, Arpaia A et al. Chronic microscopic enterocolitis with severe hypokalemia responding to subtotal colectomy. J Clin Gastroenterol 1999;29:284–288.

111. Williams RA, Gelfand DV. Total proctocolectomy and ileal pouch anal anastomosis to successfully treat a patient with collagenous colitis. Am J Gastroenterol 2000;95:2147.

112. Varghese L, Galandiuk S, Tremaine WJ et al. Lymphocytic colitis treated with proctocolectomy and ileal J-pouch–anal anastomosis: report of a case. Dis Colon Rectum 2002;45:123–126.

113. Riaz AA, Pitt J, Stirling RW et al. Restorative proctocolectomy for collagenous colitis. J R Soc Med 2000;93:261.

114. Bowling TE, Price AB, al-Adnani M et al. Interchange between collagenous and lymphocytic colitis in severe disease with autoimmune associations requiring colectomy: a case report. Gut 1996;38:788–791.

115. Tremaine WJ. Collagenous colitis and lymphocytic colitis. J Clin Gastroenterol 2000;30:245–249.

116. Giardiello FM, Lazenby AJ, Yardley JH et al. Increased HLA A1 and diminished HLA A3 in lymphocytic colitis compared to controls and patients with collagenous colitis. Dig Dis Sci 1992;37:496–499.

## CHAPTER 49

# Fistulizing Crohn's disease

Thomas A Judge and Gary R Lichtenstein

## INTRODUCTION

Crohn's disease is a chronic inflammatory disorder that may affect the length of the bowel from mouth to anus. A number of specific disease patterns have been identified, including the development of fistulae, which is a complication common to many patients with Crohn's disease. Fistulae have been a recognized feature of Crohn's disease since the original report in 1932. In their initial description, Crohn and associates noted that six of 14 patients had fistulizing disease affecting various colon segments.[1] Rectovaginal and enterocutaneous fistulae were also observed by these authors. Moreover, one potential mechanism underlying the pathogenesis of these fistulae was suggested in this report: 'As the necrotizing process of mucosa of the ileum progresses through its several coats, the serosa become involved. Any hollow viscus, usually the colon, now becomes adherent to the point of threatened perforation. A slowly progressive perforation is thus walled off, but results in a fistulous tract being formed between the 2 viscera.' Although no perianal fistulae were observed in this initial case series, the association of anal disease and Crohn's enteritis was soon reported by Bissell.[2] Thus, the diagnosis and treatment of fistula complicating Crohn's disease has also been a component of care for these patients since the recognition of this disorder.

As suggested by Crohn, Ginzburg and Oppenheimer in their initial report, the transmural nature of the inflammatory process that underlies Crohn's disease predisposes to fistula formation. The development of a fistula indicates that the inflammatory process has extended into adjacent organs, skin and tissues. The consequences of the fistulous tract are dependent on the nature of the adjacent tissues, the origin and terminus of the fistula, and the potential infectious processes resulting from the transit of enteric microorganisms through the fistula. Classification schemes are based on the origin and terminus of fistula tracts. In general, fistulae may be described as internal when the fistula terminates in a contiguous organ or adjacent mesentery, or external when it terminates on the body surface. Examples of internal fistulae would include enteroenteric, enterovesical and enterovaginal. External fistulae would include enterocutaneous, perianal and peristomal. Whereas external fistulae are commonly associated with local pain, discharge and abscess formation, internal fistulae may be clinically silent and unrecognized. Additional classification of internal fistulae based on the clinical consequences of these connections allows the discrimination of 'major' fistulae (such as a gastrocolic fistula with potential for significant luminal bypass and resulting short-gut syndrome) from 'minor' fistulae (such as an asymptomatic ileocecal fistula). In the case of perianal fistula, identification and classification of specific routes created by fistula tracts is important for determining prognosis and for making therapeutic decisions.

The lifetime risk of fistula development in patients with Crohn's disease has typically been reported to range from 20 to 40%.[3-5] The reported incidence of fistulizing Crohn's disease from referral-based case series has ranged from 17% to as much as 85%.[6] Two population-based studies reporting the natural history of Crohn's-associated fistula have been published to date. Hellers et al. reported a 23% cumulative incidence for perianal fistula in Crohn's disease patients identified in Stockholm County, Sweden, during the years 1955–1974.[7] More recently, Schwartz et al. reported the natural history of fistulizing Crohn's disease in patients from Olmsted County, Minnesota, diagnosed between 1970 and 1993.[8] As in the Swedish experience, the cumulative incidence of perianal fistula in the Olmsted County cohort was 20%. Fistulae of all forms were identified in 35% of the cohort studied. Including all forms of fistula, the cumulative risk for fistula development was 33% at 10 years and 50% after 20 years. The development of fistula may precede or coincide with the diagnosis of Crohn's disease, a feature noted by Gray et al. and confirmed in the population-based studies by Hellers, Schwartz and colleagues.[7-9] Approximately 45% of patients developed fistula at or before the diagnosis of Crohn's disease in these cohorts. The clinical course of fistulae varies with their location and complexity. Complex fistulae rarely heal spontaneously. None the less, complete fistula closure rates of 6% (for unspecified time duration) and 13% (for at least

1 month's duration) have been reported in placebo-treated patients in randomized trials of 6-mercaptopurine and infliximab, respectively, emphasizing the need for controlled trials evaluating therapeutic maneuvers in the management of fistulizing Crohn's disease.[10,11] In addition, small surgical series reported by Buchmann et al. and Halme and Saino have documented spontaneous healing of simple fistula in ano in 50% of patients with Crohn's disease.[12,13] Recurrence of perianal fistula has been frequently reported after medical and surgical therapy. Makowiec and colleagues reported that 47% of patients treated for fistula complicating Crohn's disease developed recurrent fistula, with a risk of 59% at 2 years.[14] Similarly, rates of recurrent fistula in Crohn's patients following discontinuation of medical therapy derived from uncontrolled series have ranged from 71 to 82%.[15–18] However, in contrast, Schwartz and colleagues identified recurrent fistula in only 34% of the Olmsted County cohort.[8]

The treatment of fistulae depends on location, severity of symptoms, number and complexity of the fistula tracts, and the presence or absence of rectal inflammation. Previous local surgeries and anal sphincter function also influence therapeutic decisions regarding conservative medical management or a more aggressive surgical approach. Patients with painful perianal fistula and associated abscess formation require surgical drainage, possible seton placement, and in severe cases proctectomy. In contrast, patients with asymptomatic internal fistulae require no intervention. A variety of measures to induce fistula healing have been advanced in the literature. No well-validated clinical measure of fistula disease activity has been broadly utilized in studies of specific medical or surgical interventions. Most recently, the absence of drainage upon gentle compression of the external fistula orifice has been defined as complete healing.[19] An established time to healing has yet to be standardized, limiting comparison of treatments between studies. Further, most clinical trials to date have been uncontrolled. As a result, treatment decisions have been informed by clinical experience and the few controlled clinical trials published to date.

# MEDICAL THERAPY OF FISTULOUS CROHN'S DISEASE

## AMINOSALICYCLATES

Sulfasalazine and mesalamine derivatives have not been demonstrated to be effective in the healing of fistulae.

## CORTICOSTEROIDS

Corticosteroids have not proved efficacious in the treatment of fistulizing Crohn's disease. In two large uncontrolled clinical trials the use of corticosteroids resulted in an increase incidence of surgical resection.[20,21] In a large 452-patient controlled trial, clinically significant adverse events including death occurred in corticosteroid-treated patients with abdominal masses associated with fistulae.[22]

## ANTIBIOTICS

### Metronidazole

Metronidazole, the antibiotic most frequently utilized in the management of fistulizing perianal Crohn's disease, has been evaluated in several small and uncontrolled clinical trials. In 1975, Ursing and Kamme first reported that metronidazole healed perianal fistulae in three patients.[23] Subsequently, Bernstein and colleagues treated 21 patients with long-standing perianal fistula using metronidazole 20 mg/kg/day in divided doses.[24] A clinical response was noted in 20 of the 21 patients, with complete healing noted in 56% of patients at 8 weeks. Clinical improvement was appreciated by 90% of patients within 2 weeks of therapy. However, a follow-up report presented by Brandt et al. noted symptomatic recurrence in 78% of patients within 4 months following cessation of therapy.[25] Subsequent uncontrolled studies of metronidazole therapy conducted by Jakobovits and Schuster, and a European study conducted by Schneider et al., confirmed healing of perianal Crohn's fistula with closure rates of 50% and 40%, respectively.[26,27] Maintenance therapy with metronidazole appears to be necessary, as a high rate of recurrence has been observed upon cessation of treatment. Metronidazole in combination with an immunomodulatory medication such as azathioprine may be the most cost-effective initial therapy for fistulizing Crohn's disease, based on a recently published cost–utility analysis performed by Arseneau and colleagues.[28] Adverse reactions to high-dose metronidazole include paresthesias, dyspepsia, a metallic taste, and a disulfiram-like response to alcohol ingestion. Peripheral neurologic dysfunction has been demonstrated by physical examination and nerve conduction studies in 85% of treated patients, many of whom were asymptomatic.[29]

### Ciprofloxacin

The potential for adverse effects from long-term use of metronidazole prompted clinical trials of alternate antibiotic regimens in fistulizing Crohn's disease. Ciprofloxacin, a fluoroquinolone with broad-spectrum activity against Gram-negative organisms, has been the subject of two small, uncontrolled trials in severe perineal Crohn's disease. Turunen and colleagues first reported the use of ciprofloxacin in eight patients with perineal Crohn's disease refractory to metronidazole therapy.[30] Patients were treated with 1–1.5 g/day ciprofloxacin in divided doses for 3–12 months. All were reported to show improvement; however, four of eight patients had persistent perineal drainage and 'several' patients required surgical intervention. In a separate trial, Wolf reported resolution of perineal pain in four of five patients with active perineal Crohn's disease within 5 weeks of therapy.[31] No controlled trials of ciprofloxacin for fistulizing Crohn's disease have been reported. As with metronidazole, there is a high rate of recurrence upon cessation of ciprofloxacin therapy.[32] Adverse reactions to ciprofloxacin include headache, nausea, diarrhea and rash.[33] There have also been reports of spontaneous tendon ruptures (including the Achilles tendon) in patients using long-term ciprofloxacin.[34]

### Ciprofloxacin and metronidazole

A single trial has been reported utilizing combination therapy with ciprofloxacin and metronidazole. The rationale for this approach has been the overlapping antimicrobial activity of these agents (metronidazole has activity against anaerobic bacteria; ciprofloxacin is active against Gram-negative organisms). Solomon and colleagues reported an uncontrolled study in 14 patients treated with metronidazole (500–1500 mg/day) and ciprofloxacin (1000–1500 mg/day).[35] The study included nine patients with complex fistulae and one with a rectovaginal fistula. Clinical improvement was noted in nine patients at 12 weeks, with closure of the fistula in three. One patient worsened, necessitating proximal diversion. Recurrent disease was observed following cessation of therapy.

## IMMUNOMODULATORS

### 6-Mercaptopurine and azathioprine

The purine metabolites 6-mercaptopurine (6-MP) and azathio-prine (AZA) are immunomodulatory medications that have demonstrated efficacy in fistulizing Crohn's disease as a second-ary endpoint in controlled clinical trials. AZA and 6-MP are typ-ically discussed interchangeably because AZA is converted to 6-MP in vivo. The first controlled trial evaluating the effect of medical therapy on fistulizing Crohn's disease was reported by Present and colleagues.[36] Patients randomized to receive 6-MP or placebo were assessed for clinical response, fistula healing and corticosteroid dose reduction. Thirty-six patients with a total of 40 fistulae were enrolled in this study. The overall response rate was 55% for patients treated with 6-MP compared to 24% for individuals receiving placebo. Complete fistula healing was observed in nine of 29 patients (31%) in the 6-MP cohort com-pared to one of 17 (6%) in the placebo arm. The study was insufficiently powered to demonstrate a statistically significant difference among treatment groups for the secondary endpoint of fistula closure.

An uncontrolled follow-up article by Present et al. reported the results of 6-MP therapy (1.5 mg/kg/day) in a total of 34 patients.[37] This study included 24 patients with single fistulae and 10 patients with multiple fistulae. A wide variety of fistulae were examined, including perirectal (18), abdominal wall (8), enteroenteric (7), rectovaginal (6) and vulvar (2). The overall response rate was 65%, with complete healing observed in 39% of patients. The median time to clinical response was 3.1 months, but some patients responded to therapy as late as 8 months after therapy was initiated. This study also documented the need for maintenance therapy. Of the 13 patients with complete fistula closure, six remained on therapy with continued fistula closure, whereas five of seven patients who discontinued therapy had a recurrence. Reinstitution of 6-MP therapy healed the fistulae again.

The response of Crohn's fistulae to AZA has also been evalu-ated. An uncontrolled study by O'Brien and colleagues at Johns Hopkins Hospital reported on 26 patients with fistulae treated with AZA.[38] Complete fistula closure was observed in eight patients (31%) and partial healing in an additional 14 (54%). Most recently, Pearson et al. presented a meta-analysis of five controlled trials of AZA and 6-MP for Crohn's disease in which fistula closure was described in detail.[39] A total of 70 patients were included in this assessment. Patients treated with azathio-prine or 6-MP were more likely to respond to treatment (22 of 41) than patients treated with placebo (six of 29); the pooled odds ratio favoring fistula healing with AZA or 6-MP was 4.44.

AZA and 6-MP also appear to be effective in the treatment of some gastrocolic and enterovesicular fistulae. In their review of gastrocolic fistula, Pichney and colleagues noted three patients treated with AZA or 6-MP, all of whom responded to medical therapy.[40] Similarly, Wheeler et al. observed a clinical response of enterovesicular fistula in 18 of 31 patients (58%) treated with 6-MP or AZA, with healing maintained in 12 of 31 patients (39%).[41] These results, although encouraging, are derived from uncontrolled studies. To date, no placebo-controlled trials assessing the utility of AZA/6-MP therapy for gastrocolic or enterovesicular fistulae have been published.

Dosing and administration of azathioprine and 6-mercapto-purine has not been standardized. Controlled trials indicate that azathioprine at doses of 2.0–3.0 mg/kg/day and 6-MP at a dose of 1.5 mg/kg/day is effective for the treatment of Crohn's disease. Clinical practice varies considerably. Frequently, clini-cians initiate therapy with either drug at a dose of 50 mg/day and gradually titrate to effect (mild leukopenia) or to a specified blood 6-thioguanine nucleotide metabolite concentration (6-TGs $> 235$ pM/$10^8$ erythrocytes).[42] The efficacy of this approach in minimizing drug-induced toxicity has not been proven in a prospective, randomized controlled trial. Adverse events are reported to occur in 9–15% of patients receiving aza-thioprine or 6-MP for inflammatory bowel disease. The most commonly encountered serious adverse events are infections (affecting 7% of treated patients), pancreatitis (3%), profound leukopenia (2%), allergic reactions (2%) and drug-induced hepatitis (0.3%).[43]

### Methotrexate

Although methotrexate (MTX) has been demonstrated to be efficacious for induction of remission in patient's with Crohn's disease, initial controlled studies did not assess the effect of MTX therapy on fistula healing. Recently, uncontrolled trials have reported on fistula healing with MTX. Mahadevan et al. examined the efficacy of intramuscular MTX (25 mg/week) on 16 patients with fistulizing Crohn's disease.[44] With treatment, four of 16 had fistula closure and an additional five had partial responses, yielding an overall response rate of 56%. As with other medications, fistula recurrence was noted upon reduction in MTX dose or with conversion to an oral formulation. A second, retrospective study reported by Vandeputte et al. exam-ined the effect of parenteral MTX on 20 patients with refrac-tory Crohn's disease, including eight with fistulae.[45] Although the authors noted induction of remission in 70% of patients treated with MTX, the specific response of patients with fistuliz-ing disease was not reported separately. Adverse events associ-ated with parenteral MTX have been reported in nearly 50% of patients treated for more than 6 months, and include elevation of serum transaminases (affecting 5–20% of patients), nausea (4–12%) and bone marrow suppression (10–20%).[46–48] Hepatic fibrosis was observed in 0–5% of IBD patients who had under-gone liver biopsy after a cumulative MTX dose of $>1500$ mg.[49] Serious adverse events requiring discontinuation of MTX occur in approximately 10% of patients.[46] Less common but poten-tially life-threatening interstitial pneumonitis has been observed in 3–12% of patients treated with long-term low-dose MTX.[48]

### Cyclosporin A

There are no published, randomized placebo-controlled trials specifically designed to evaluate the efficacy of cyclosporin A (CyA) on fistula closure in Crohn's disease. CyA has been demonstrated to be efficacious for induction of remission in patients with luminal Crohn's disease in only one of four placebo-controlled trials. The rapidity with which clinical response is observed (often within 1–2 weeks) makes CyA a potential candidate for fistulizing disease.[50] In an uncontrolled series 16 patients with fistulizing Crohn's, including 10 with fistulae refractory to AZA/6-MP therapy, were treated with intravenous CyA at a daily dose of 4 mg/kg as a continuous infusion.[51] Fourteen patients (88%) responded acutely, with com-plete closure observed in half of the responding patients. Nine of 10 patients with fistulae refractory to AZA/6-MP responded to CyA. The mean time to respond in this series was 7.4 days, confirming the rapidity of clinical response. These results have subsequently been supplemented by a review of the literature including 39 patients with fistulizing Crohn's disease treated with CyA.[52] In this group, 90% of patients responded to intravenous CyA. Relapse in the absence of oral CyA therapy was quite high (82%). Other investigators have demonstrated modest reductions in the rate of fistula recurrence through combined use of CyA, azathioprine, and a tapering schedule of prednisolone for a period of 3 months before cessation of CyA therapy.[53] These results suggest that fistula healing with CyA may necessitate short-term concurrent use of oral CyA with other immunosuppressants (AZA/6-MP, or MTX) to allow adequate time for the latter to take effect. Adverse events observed in patients treated with high-dose cyclosporin include paresthesias (25%), hypertrichosis (13%), hypertension (11%), tremor (7%), renal insufficiency (6%), headache (5%), opportunistic infections (3%), gingival hyperplasia (2%) and seizure (1%).[48]

## Tacrolimus

Tacrolimus is a potent immunosuppressant agent that inhibits transcription of IL-2 in T-helper cells in a manner similar to CyA. It is most frequently used in the prevention of allograft rejection, and case reports and uncontrolled retrospective series have suggested efficacy for the treatment of fistulizing Crohn's disease, including healing of rectovaginal fistula.[54–56] Sandborn and colleagues recently performed the only placebo-controlled trial assessing the efficacy of tacrolimus.[57] Forty-six patients with actively draining Crohn's fistulae (43 had perianal fistulae) were randomized to treatment with placebo or oral tacrolimus at an initial dose of 0.20 mg/kg/day. A clinical response (defined as closure of at least 50% of fistulae present at baseline, maintained for at least 4 weeks) occurred in 43% of tacrolimus-treated patients, compared to 8% of patients treated with placebo ($P=0.004$). However, no significant difference was observed with respect to the complete closure of baseline fistulae that was observed in 10% of tacrolimus-treated patients compared to 8% of placebo-treated patients ($P=0.86$). Adverse events observed in patients treated with tacrolimus include renal insufficiency, tremor, headache, paresthesias, leg cramps, paresthesias and tremor.

## Mycophenolate mofetil

Mycophenolate mofetil, a potent immunosuppressant which inhibits lymphocyte proliferation through blockade of guanosine nucleotide synthesis, has been reported to induce clinical remission of steroid-resistant Crohn's disease in at least one uncontrolled clinical trial.[58] Uncontrolled case series have suggested efficacy in fistulizing Crohn's disease, yet other reports have cast doubt on the efficacy on mycophenolate in the long-term maintenance of remission.[59–61] To date, no well-designed, placebo-controlled trials have been published.

## ANTI-TNF-α THERAPIES

### Infliximab

Infliximab is a chimeric monoclonal antibody that binds and neutralizes human tumor necrosis factor-α (TNF-α). This antibody consists of a murine variable chain directed against human TNF-α combined with human IgG$_1$ constant region. The IgG$_1$ Fc fragment allows activation of complement, and antibody-

dependent cytotoxicity has been demonstrated in vitro against human tumor cell lines expressing transmembrane TNF-α. Cytokines including TNF-α are critical to the inflammatory processes that characterizes Crohn's disease. Mucosal biopsy specimens and mononuclear cells isolated from the lamina propria of patients with Crohn's disease express high levels of TNF-α. Therapy directed against TNF-α through the infusion of infliximab would therefore be anticipated to result in a significant reduction in Crohn's-associated inflammation, as has been confirmed in a number of randomized, placebo-controlled clinical trials.

The efficacy of infliximab in the treatment of fistulizing Crohn's disease was demonstrated in a placebo-controlled multicenter study performed by Present and colleagues.[62] In this study, 94 patients with active abdominal (10%) or perianal (90%) fistulae were randomized to receive either infliximab 5 mg/kg, infliximab 10 mg/kg or placebo. Treatments were administered at weeks 0, 2 and 6, and the patients were monitored for clinical response, which was defined as a 50% reduction in the number of draining fistulae present at baseline examination which was maintained for at least 4 weeks. Sixty-eight per cent of patients who received infliximab 5 mg/kg and 56% of those who received infliximab 10 mg/kg achieved a clinical response, compared to 26% of the patients infused with placebo. Additionally, 55% of patients receiving 5 mg/kg infliximab and 38% of patients receiving 10 mg/kg infliximab had complete closure of all fistulae (defined as an absence of discharge despite gentle compressions for at least 4 weeks), compared to 13% of patients treated with placebo. Thus, infliximab appears to be an effective medical therapy for induction treatment of fistulizing Crohn's disease. However, the median duration of fistula closure following the initial series of infliximab infusions was approximately 3 months, suggesting the need for maintenance therapy in patients responding to infliximab. Eleven per cent of the patients treated with infliximab developed a perianal abscess, possibly due to closure of the cutaneous end of the fistula tract before the rest of it closed. The rate of infections in those on infliximab did not differ from that in patients on placebo.

Sands and colleagues recently presented the results of a second controlled trial confirming the efficacy of infliximab in both induction and maintenance treatment of fistulizing Crohn's disease.[63] This long-term study included 306 patients with actively draining fistulae who received three open doses of infliximab 5 mg/kg at 0, 2 and 6 weeks. Patients who responded to therapy (closure of at least 50% of fistulae present at baseline maintained for at least 4 weeks) were then randomized into two groups 8 weeks after the initial infusion series was completed: group 1 received maintenance doses of placebo every 8 weeks, beginning at week 14; group 2 received maintenance doses of infliximab 5 mg/kg every 8 weeks, beginning at week 14. Patients were monitored for 54 weeks, and the time to loss of clinical response was the primary endpoint of this study. Of 306 patients,195 (69%) had a fistula response at week 14. The median time to loss of response to week 54 was 14 weeks for placebo-treated patients and > 40 weeks for infliximab 5 mg/kg-treated patients ($P < 0.001$).

The long-term efficacy of infliximab in management of fistulizing Crohn's disease has recently been challenged.

Other agents which inhibit TNF-α activity, such as pentoxifylline and etanercept, have failed to demonstrate efficacy in Crohn's disease, whereas two recent open-label studies of thalidomide, a potent inhibitor of TNF-α, have shown efficacy in fistulizing Crohn's disease.[67,68]

Adverse events observed in patients treated with infliximab include infusion reactions; delayed hypersensitivity reactions; the formation of human antichimeric antibodies; formation of anti-double-stranded DNA antibodies; and, in rare cases, drug-induced lupus.[69,70] Infusion reactions were observed in 6% of infliximab infusions in the recently reported ACCENT I maintenance trial.[71] Approximately 3% of patients in the ACCENT I trial developed delayed hypersensitivity reactions, manifest by serum sickness-like symptoms. There is also an increased overall rate of infections and, rarely, serious infections occur, including pneumonia, sepsis, tuberculosis, and infections due to opportunistic organisms such as *Listeria monocytogenes* and *Pneumocystis carinii*.[69,70,72–74] Skin testing with tuberculin purified protein derivative (PPD) is now recommended for all patients prior to treatment with infliximab.[75] In addition to its well-known teratogenic effects, therapy with thalidomide has been complicated by marked somnolence and peripheral neuropathy.[76]

## NOVEL THERAPIES

A number of novel therapies have been advanced for the treatment of fistulizing Crohn's disease. Temporary fecal diversion has been successful in the induction of clinical response in combination with medical therapy. However, fistula recurrence frequently accompanies reversal of the diverting ileostomy.[77–79] More advanced perianal disease has been successfully controlled with proctectomy.[80] In addition, the use of fibrin glue and plasma factor XIII concentrates has been advanced as adjunctive therapy in the management of perianal fistulae.[81–83] Hyperbaric oxygen has also been suggested as an adjunctive measure in healing fistulizing Crohn's disease.[84–86] Although case reports have documented successful healing during therapy, no well-controlled, randomized studies have been performed to confirm these findings. Further study is therefore necessary to assess the role of these therapies in the management of fistulizing Crohn's disease.

## EXTERNAL FISTULAE

## SPONTANEOUS

Spontaneous external abdominal wall fistulae in the absence of previous surgery rarely occur. Reviewing a series of 1500 patients, Greenstein identified only four with spontaneous abdominal wall fistulae, three being coloumbilical and one connecting the ileum to the linea alba.[87]

## POSTOPERATIVE

The majority of external enterocutaneous fistulae occur in the postoperative setting. These classically arise from the ileum or colon and commonly drain through the site of a previous scar. Early enterocutaneous fistulae develop as a result of anastomotic breakdown and frequently present within 1 week of surgery. Fistulae developing at a later stage (> 7–10 days postoperatively) typically result from recurrent Crohn's disease, although some may arise from the site of a contained anastomotic leak.

The standard surgical approach to postoperative fistula has been early fecal diversion in addition to resection of the fistula and anastomosis. More recently, somatostatin analog has been used in selected patients to initiate fistula closure associated with anastomotic breakdown, but this has not been subjected to controlled clinical trials.[88] Late fistulae resulting from recurrent Crohn's disease usually require surgical intervention in addition to aggressive medical therapy. In selected patients with high operative risk and low fistula output, aggressive medical therapy may be the initial treatment of choice.

## PERISTOMAL

Individuals with proctocolectomy and ileostomy may be at risk for two different forms of cutaneous fistula: peri-ileostomy and enteroperitoneal. Peri-ileostomy fistulae may develop either early or late in the postoperative period. Early postoperative fistulae frequently result from excess tension at the site of sutures placed between the abdominal fascia and the bowel serosa that initiates seromuscular damage or injury to the ileostomy within the abdominal wall. These fistulae typically present during hospitalization and require exteriorization of the ileostomy and a second stomal maturation. In contrast, late ileostomy fistulae develop as a result of recurrent Crohn's disease. Therapeutic options for management of these fistulae include primary resection of the neoterminal ileum and the recreation of a neo-end ileostomy or aggressive medical therapy. When abscess or infection complicates the peristomal fistula, relocation of the stoma may be required.

## PERIANAL FISTULA

### Classification

Perianal Crohn's disease has been the subject of a variety of classification systems. A commonly used classification scheme for fistulizing disease was introduced by Parks and colleague (Fig. 49.1).[89] This uses the external anal sphincter as the reference point for description of the fistula tract (Table 49.1 and Fig. 49.2). Although this is useful for surgical management, many complex fistulae associated with Crohn's disease are not easily classified anatomically. As a result, many clinicians define such fistulae as either simple or complex, based on their location in relationship to the anal sphincter, the nature of the fistula track, associated inflammatory lesions such as abscesses, and, most importantly, the presence or absence of active rectal inflammation.

### Simple fistula and fistula in ano

Simple fistula and fistula in ano are classically low-lying lesions with a single external opening. Other fistulae with similar classification include subcutaneous, low-intersphincteric and low-transsphincteric. The feature common to all of these is that the fistula tract lies below the majority of the anal sphincter. These fistulae, which comprise the majority observed in patients with Crohn's disease, typically develop in patients without rectal involvement. Surgical series demonstrate excellent response to fistulotomy in patients without macroscopic rectal inflammation and a low rate of associated fecal incontinence or delayed wound healing.[90–99] Healing rates of 70–100% have been reported, with low rates of recurrence (<20%) and minor incontinence reported in <10% of individuals (Table 49.2). In contrast, simple low

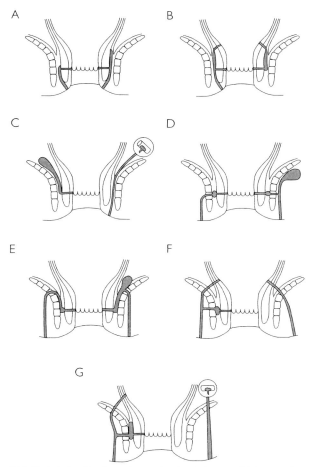

Fig. 49.1 Parks' classification scheme for fistula in ano. (A) Intersphincteric fistula (simple low tract) uncomplicated or with high blind tract; (B) intersphincteric fistula (high tract with rectal opening) with or without perineal opening; (C) intersphincteric fistula with extrarectal extension or secondary to pelvic disease; (D) transsphincteric fistula, uncomplicated or with high blind tract; (E) suprasphincteric fistula, uncomplicated or with high blind tract; (F) extrasphincteric fistula, secondary to transsphincteric fistula or trauma; (G) extrasphincteric fistula, secondary to anorectal disease or pelvic inflammation.

| Table 49.1 Classification of fistula in ano |
| --- |
| Intersphincteric |
|     Simple low tract |
|     High blind tract |
|     High tract with rectal outlet |
|     High fistula without perineal outlet |
|     High fistula with extrarectal or pelvic extension |
| Transsphincteric |
|     Uncomplicated |
|     High blind tract |
| Suprasphincteric |
|     Uncomplicated |
|     High blind tract |
| Extrasphincteric |
|     Secondary to transsphincteric fistula |
|     Secondary to anorectal disease |
| Combined |
| Horseshoe |
|     Intersphincteric |
|     Transsphincteric |

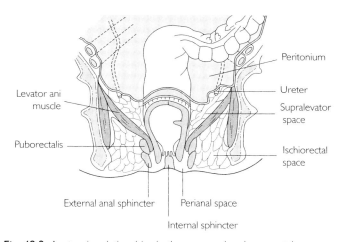

Fig. 49.2 Anatomic relationships in the para-anal and pararectal spaces.

fistulae in patients with active Crohn's proctocolitis should be treated by placement of non-cutting setons rather than fistulotomy, because of poor wound healing in the setting of active rectal inflammation (Fig. 49.3). Nordgren and colleagues noted that healing occurred after fistulotomy in only four of 15 patients (27%) with active Crohn's proctocolitis, compared to 10 of 12 patients (83%) with classic intestinal Crohn's disease.[96] Caution should also be exercised in performing a fistulotomy in patients with diarrhea and in women who have an anterior fistula and a short anal canal. In these settings, the risk of postoperative fecal incontinence following division of the anal sphincter may be substantial. The performance of a partial internal sphincterotomy at the site of the internal fistula orifice has been advanced as an alternative to the classic fistulotomy in selected cases of intersphincteric fistula with associated abscess.[97,100] An intersphincteric abscess is unroofed, but the fistula tract is not opened. This technique removes the source of infection while minimizing the risk of persistent perineal wounds.

The use of an endorectal advancement flap has also been suggested as an alternative to fistulotomy in patients with simple fistula who do not have active rectal inflammation (Fig. 49.4). Sustained fistula closure was reported in 74% of 26 patients with fistulizing Crohn's disease treated with an endorectal advancement flap procedure.[101] As described below, an advancement flap involves incising a flap of tissue around the internal opening of a fistula. The internal opening of the fistula tract is excised, and the flap is pulled down to cover the opening (Fig. 49.4).

## Complex fistulae

Despite the excellent response of simple fistulae to surgical intervention, complex fistulae and those occurring in the presence of active rectal Crohn's disease present a significant challenge. Complex fistulae include fistulae with multiple openings, those with fistula tracts passing high above the bulk of the anal sphincter, those with internal orifices above the dentate line, those with horseshoe tracts, and those with high blind

**Table 49.2 Results of fistulotomy for treatment of simple perianal fistulae in patients with Crohn's disease**

Patients without active proctitis

| Investigator | Year | Wound healed | Incontinence | Recurrence | Proctectomy/ diversion |
|---|---|---|---|---|---|
| Nordgren | 1992 | 6/6 (100%) | 0/6 (0%) | 2/6 (33%) | 0/6 (0%) |
| Hobliss | 1982 | 18/20 (90%) | NA | 4/18 (22%) | 3/20 (15%) |
| Sohn | 1980 | 4/4 (100%) | 0/4 (0%) | 0/4 (0%) | 0/4 (0%) |

Patients with active proctitis

| Investigator | Year | Wound healed | Incontinence | Recurrence | Proctectomy/ diversion |
|---|---|---|---|---|---|
| Michelassi | 2000 | 27/33 (82%) | NA* | NA | NA |
| Platell | 1996 | 40/44 (91%) | 0/44 (0%) | 2/40 (5%) | 0/44 (0%) |
| Sangwan | 1996 | 35/35 (100%) | 0/35 (0%) | 31/35 (89%) | 0/35 (0%) |
| McKee | 1996 | 21/34 (62%) | NA | 4/21 (19%) | 10/34 (29%); 3 diversion |
| Scott | 1996 | 22/27 (81%) | 5/27 (19%) | NA | 5/27 (19%); 2 diversion |
| Williamson | 1995 | 7/26 (27%) | NA | NA | NA |
| Halme | 1995 | 10/10 (100%) | 5/10 (50%) | 4/10 (40%) | 1/10 (10%) |
| Winter | 1993 | 22/26 (85%) | 0/26 (0%) | 3/22 (14%) | 0/26 (0%) |
| Nordgren | 1992 | 2/5 (40%) | 0/5 (0%) | NA | 3/5 (60%) |
| Williams | 1991 | 38/41(93%)** | 7/33 (21%) | NA | 3/33 (9%) |
| Kangas | 1991 | 3/5 (60%) | NA | NA | 2/5 (40%) |
| Levien | 1989 | 29/46 (63%) | NA | 19/29 (41%) | 4/46 (9%) |
| Fuhrman | 1989 | 18/19 (95%) | NA | NA | 2/19 (11%) |
| Morrison | 1989 | 16/17 (94%) | NA | 2/26 (13%) | 1/17 (6%) |
| Fry | 1989 | 13/13 (100%) | NA | NA | 0/13 (0%) |
| Bernard | 1986 | 9/15 (60%) | NA | NA | 1/15 (7%) |
| Keighley | 1986 | 1/12 (8%) | 6/12 (50%) | NA | NA |
| Marks | 1981 | 25/32 (78%) | NA | NA | NA |

*Not addressed in publication.
** Study included 33 patients with total of 41 lesions.

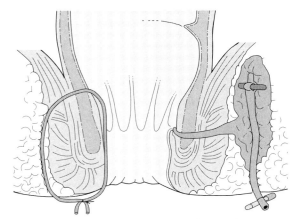

**Fig. 49.3** Management of complex perianal fistulae. Sagittal view of perianal region demonstrates seton drain in place on the left, with catheter drainage of the ischiorectal fossa on the right.

extensions. Additionally, fistulae that recur after fistulotomy, suprasphincteric and extrasphincteric fistulae are classified as complex. In general, these fistulae will not heal with surgical intervention alone without significant postoperative morbidity. A combined medical and surgical approach is critical to the management of these patients. Examination under anesthesia (EUA) is preferred to define the extent of disease and identify abscesses or infectious complications. A recent study by Schwartz and colleagues demonstrated that the addition of either pelvic magnetic resonance imaging (MRI) or endoscopic ultrasound examination increased the accuracy of the diagnostic evaluation of perianal fistulae compared to examination under anesthesia alone.[102] Abscesses detected during examination may be appropriately drained. Moreover, simple fistulae mistakenly diagnosed as complex on initial evaluation may be appropriately diagnosed and treated definitively. Tissue removed from curettage of fistula tracts should be sent for pathologic examination, as carcinoma has been identified on rare occasions in patients with refractory perineal and enterocutaneous fistulae.[103–105] Placement of drains and setons may facilitate drainage of inflammatory debris and prevent the reaccumulation of infectious material (Fig. 49.3). The addition of aggressive medical therapy is frequently helpful in this population once the infected material has been removed.

Patients with high fistulae or complex tracts may experience significant morbidity after surgical sphincterotomy even in the absence of rectal inflammation. Long-term placement of a seton is often preferable in these settings (Fig. 49.3). Recent reports have described transposition of the internal fistula opening distally to enable definitive surgical therapy to be more easily

A

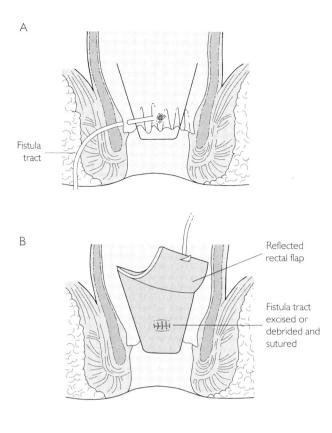

Fistula
tract

B

Reflected
rectal flap

Fistula tract
excised or
debrided and
sutured

C

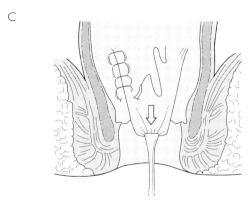

**Fig. 49.4** Rectal advancement flap procedure. This procedure requires a rhomboid-shaped incision of the rectal mucosa extending beyond the internal opening of the fistula and the dentate line (A). After elevating the mucosal flap, the fistula tract is excised and the internal muscular defect is sutured as illustrated (B). The distal portion of the mucosal flap containing the internal opening is excised; the remaining flap is drawn forward over the closed muscular defect and secured in a tension-free manner. (Reproduced with permission from Fazio VW, Strong SA. The surgical management of Crohn's disease. In: Kirsner JB, Shorter RG, eds. Inflammatory bowel disease, 4th edn. Philadelphia: Lippincott; Williams & Wilkins: 1995;830–887.)

performed.[106–108] However, these remain preliminary reports which have included few patients.

## SURGICAL TECHNIQUES

### Non-cutting setons

Long-term placement of non-cutting setons is the procedure of choice for patients with complex fistulae and those with fistulae

associated with local sepsis or rectal Crohn's disease. The fistula tract is defined while the patient is under general anesthesia and a suture or, more commonly, a thin silastic loop, is passed into the cutaneous outlet of the fistula, through the tract and across the internal orifice into the rectum and anal canal (Fig.49.3). The loop, tied loosely around the sphincter, allows continued drainage, resolution of sepsis and decreased pain. Several reports have documented clinical improvement in the vast majority of patients[109–119] (Table 49.3). Pearl and associates evaluated 10 patients with 18 fistulae treated with non-cutting seton placement.[116] Clinical improvement was shown in 90% and none required proctectomy or fecal diversion during follow-up. Similar results were observed by Scott and Northover, who evaluated seton therapy in Crohn's disease patients with perianal fistulae.[110] Clinical improvement, including fistula closure, was noted in 23 of 27 patients in this study, though incontinence ensued in four (12%) necessitating proctectomy. The rate of fistula recurrence is high following removal of the seton in several studies.[109,114,117] The optimal approach to long-term management of these patients is controversial. Some investigators have advocated indefinite retention of setons.[120] Others have suggested combination therapy with medications or more definitive surgical interventions, including fistulotomy or an endorectal advancement flap procedure once local infectious complications have been treated.[109,121] It is important to recall that patients treated with staged fistulotomy or cutting seton remain at significant risk for fecal incontinence.

### Mucosal advancement flap

The use of the mucosal advancement flap technique avoids division of the anal sphincter and is efficacious in those individuals without concurrent rectal inflammation, cavitary ulceration, anal stenosis or a local abscess (Fig. 49.4). It has been used most commonly in patients with complicated anal disease, rectovaginal fistula or perineal fistula. A semicircular incision centered on the internal fistula orifice is performed at the level of the dentate line. A 3–4 cm flap of mucosa, submucosa and smooth muscle is elevated, the internal fistula orifice excised, and the fistula tract curetted and closed. The flap is then advanced to the anoderm below the origin of the fistula and sutured into place. Care is taken to avoid tension on the flap as it is advanced. The external opening is curetted and drained with placement of a small catheter (typically a mushroom-tip catheter). Several surgical series have reported success with this technique, with documented healing rates between 60 and 80%.[101,112,113,122–127] Recurrent fistulae may also be treated with a second procedure. In their series of 26 patients treated with endorectal advancement flap, Joo and associates noted success in four of five patients who underwent a second procedure.[101]

Selected patients with anal canal ulcerations or stricturing may benefit from a rectal sleeve advancement combined with a temporary diverting ileostomy (Fig. 49.5).[128] In contrast to the mucosal advancement flap, this procedure involves circumferential mobilization of the full thickness of the rectum following surgical resection of the strictured or ulcerated region. A proctoanal anastomosis is then performed in conjunction with the proximal diverting ileostomy. Alternative techniques, including flap repair with perianal skin, laser ablation, and fistulectomy with sphincter repair, have been developed and may be beneficial in selected clinical settings.[121,129,130]

**Table 49.3 Response to surgical therapy of complex perianal fistulae in patients with Crohn's disease**

| Investigator | Year | Therapy | Improved | Incontinence | Recurrence | Proctectomy |
|---|---|---|---|---|---|---|
| Faucheron | 1996 | Seton | 36/41 (88%)[1] | 5/41 (12%) | 8/36 (22%) | 5/41 (12%) |
| Scott | 1996 | Seton | 23/27 (85%) | 4/27 (15%) | 4/27 (15%) | 4/27 (15%) |
| Sangwan | 1996 | Seton | 22/24 (92%) | NA | 17/24 (63%) | 7/24 (33%) |
| McKee | 1996 | Seton | 4/7 (57%) | NA | 3/7 (43%) | 2/7 (29%) |
| Williamson | 1995 | Seton | 7/9 (78%) | NA | 2/9 (22%) | NA |
| Sugita | 1995 | Seton | 17/21 (81%)[2] | 1/21 (5%) | 9/17 (53%) | NA |
| Koganei | 1995 | Seton | 10/13 (77%)[3] | 0/13 (0%) | 3/10 (30%) | 1/13 (8%) |
| Pearl | 1993 | Seton | 21/21 (100%) | 0/21 (0%) | 0/21 (0%) | 0/21 (0%) |
| Williams | 1991 | Seton | 20/23 (87%)[4] | 6/23 (26%) | 9/20 (45%) | 5/23 (22%) |
| White | 1990 | Seton | 10/10 (100%) | NA | 2/10 (20%) | 0/10 (0%) |
| Van Donegen | 1986 | Seton | 2/2 (100%) | NA | 0/2 (0%) | 0/2 (0%) |
| McKee | 1996 | Fistulotomy | 2/5 (40%) | 2/5 (40%) | 3/5 (60%) | 2/5 (40%) |
| Nordgren | 1992 | Fistulotomy | 4/10 (40%) | NA | 1/4 (25%) | 6/10 (60%) |
| Morrison | 1989 | Fistulotomy | 3/4 (75%)[5] | NA | NA | 1/4 (25%) |
| Matos | 1993 | Excision/closure | 10/10 (100%) | 5/10 (50%) | 6/10 (60%) | 0/10 (0%) |
| Joo | 1998 | Advancement flap | 19/26 (73%) | NA | 7/26 (27%) | 2/26 (9%) |
| Robertson | 1998 | Advancement flap | 3/6 (50%) | NA | 3/6 (50%) | 0/6 (0%) |
| Marchesa | 1998 | Advancement flap[6] | 8/13 (62%) | NA | 5/13 (38%) | 3/13 (23%) |
| McKee | 1996 | Advancement flap | 1/2 (50%) | NA | 1/2 (50%) | 1/2 (50%) |
| Makowiec | 1995 | Advancement flap | 16/20 (80%) | 0/20 (0%) | 4/20 (20%) | 0/20 (0%) |
| Williamson | 1995 | Advancement flap | 1/4 (25%) | NA | 3/4 (75%) | NA |
| Lewis | 1990 | Advancement flap | 5/6 (83%) | NA | 1/6 (17%) | 0/6 (0%) |
| Fry | 1989 | Advancement flap | 3/3 (100%) | NA | 0/3 (0%) | 0/3 (0%) |
| Jones | 1987 | Advancement flap | 2/6 (33%) | NA | 4/6 (67%) | 1/6 (17%) |

NA, not addressed.
Advancement flap, transanal advancement flap.
[1] Closure of fistula observed in 11 patients (27%).
[2] Closure of fistula observed in 8 patients (38%).
[3] Closure of fistula observed in 8 patients (62%).
[4] Closure of fistula observed in 3 patients (13%).
[5] In addition to fistulotomy, setons were placed in 2 patients.
[6] Sleeve advancement flap.

# INTERNAL FISTULAE

## ENTEROENTERIC FISTULAE

Ileocolic fistulae are the most common type of enteroenteric fistulae. The majority of these are ileocecal or ileosigmoid in location. Rarely, fistulae arising from the ileum may connect to the transverse colon, stomach or duodenum. Enteroenteric fistulae usually present with few symptoms in the absence of obstruction or associated septic complications. They are best demonstrated by radiographic techniques, including enteroclysis, barium enema, computed tomography (CT) scan, MRI and colonoscopy. Enteroenteric fistulae identified in the absence of symptoms or evidence of significant bowel diversion do not require surgical intervention. When symptomatic, internal fistulae are usually indications for surgery. The natural history of enteroenteric fistula was reported by Broe and associates in 1982.[131] Patients with internal fistulae were followed to evaluate the effect of medical therapy. Surgical intervention was necessary within 1 year in 10 of 24 patients; an additional eight ultimately required surgery within a period of 9 years, largely because of intractable disease. The remaining six patients, none of whom had radiographically demonstrable fistulae, did not require surgical intervention, and four of these remained healthy for more than 5 years following diagnosis. Thus, identification of an enteroenteric fistula alone does not warrant surgical intervention.

## RECTOVAGINAL FISTULA

The clinical hallmark of an enterovaginal fistula is the discharge of gas or fecal material from the vagina. In the vast majority of cases this represents an abnormal connection between the anus or rectum and the vagina. Although the true incidence of this disorder is unknown, Radcliffe and colleagues concluded from their series that rectovaginal or anovaginal fistula developed in 9% of women with anal Crohn's disease.[132] Anovaginal fistulae arise from deep ulcerations in the anterior anal canal or, less commonly, from a cryptoglandular abscess. Rectovaginal fistulae have an internal orifice above the anorectal ring and most frequently develop secondary to a deep rectal ulceration in the anterior wall that erodes into the vagina, typically in the mid-portion of the rectovaginal septum. Rarely, in patients who have undergone hysterectomy, ileal or sigmoid Crohn's disease may fistulize to the vagina. Anovaginal fistulae have also been reported as a late complication of restorative proctocolectomy in patients with Crohn's disease.[133,134] In these patients, the fistula has been found both at and below the anastomosis.

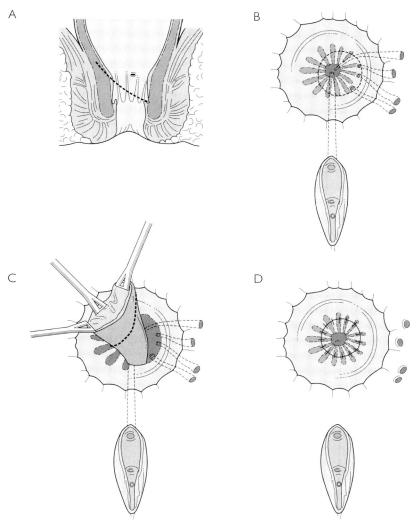

**Fig. 49.5** Rectal sleeve advancement for repair of a highly complex fistula. (A) An asymmetric incision is performed with an increased incisional depth on the involved versus uninvolved side. (B) Outline of incision for proposed sleeve advancement anorectoplasty. (C) Sleeve advancement dissection prior to amputation. The vaginal and external fistula tracks have been detached. The line of amputation is proximal to the diseased tissues (arrows). (D) Restoration of anorectal continuity by full-thickness anastomosis at site of initial incision. The anal transition zone has been retained on the uninvolved side. The vaginal and external tracks are curetted and left open for drainage.

Clinically, symptoms may vary quite broadly. Some women experience dyspareunia, perineal pain and recurrent yeast infections, whereas others may experience drainage of purulent material and the passage of stool or flatus.[134] Diagnosis of these fistulae may be difficult. Initial examination should include an examination under anesthesia, including proctoscopy and vaginoscopy. If the tract cannot be identified, Gastrografin or methylene blue may be infused into the rectum with a tampon in the vagina. Alternatively, rectal insufflation while the vagina is filled with saline may reveal the fistula. More recently, endoluminal MRI or endosonographic imaging with hydrogen peroxide enhancement has been successfully utilized to identify and characterize vaginal fistulae.[135,136]

General principles for the treatment of perianal fistulae apply also to rectovaginal fistulae. Patients with minimal or no symptoms need no intervention. In contrast, patients who have associated abscesses need drainage. The insertion of a mushroom drain or seton allows drainage of purulent material and provides pain relief. Patients with low anovaginal fistula with a superficial tract may be treated with fistulotomy.[132] Those with trans- and extrasphincteric rectovaginal fistulae have been treated with mucosal advancement flaps, with clinical improvement noted in 70–75%, though recurrence rates exceed those documented for anorectal fistulae (Figs 49.4 and 49.6)[101,126,127,136,138–151] (Table 49.4). Long-term success is variable. Makowiec and

colleagues reported a 70% recurrence rate at 24-month follow-up.[151] In contrast, Fry and Kodner reported an 80% healing rate, and Hull and colleagues documented improvement in 60%, although several patients required repeat procedures.[126,149,150] Patients with significant proctitis who cannot be treated with a mucosal flap may be treated with an anocutaneous flap (Fig. 49.7). This approach has been complicated by a 33% recurrence rate at 18 months.[138] An alternative transvaginal approach has been reported to be successful in 93% of patients with no recurrence in one published series with a mean follow-up of 55 months.[139] The use of healthy vaginal tissue may underlie the improved results with this technique. In addition, all patients underwent proximal diverting ileostomy as part of their surgical intervention.

When the fistula results from disease in the ileum or colon, resection of the contiguous bowel should be considered. It is important to define the extent of disease and the origin of the fistula to select the appropriate surgical intervention. Ileal resection should be considered if disease is limited to the small bowel. Similarly, segmental resection of the colon (typically the sigmoid colon) may be considered if the rectum and remainder of the colon are unaffected by Crohn's disease. More extensive resection of the colon with an ileorectal anastomosis is dependent upon the integrity of the anal sphincter. An omental pedicle is commonly interposed between the anastomosis and the vagina

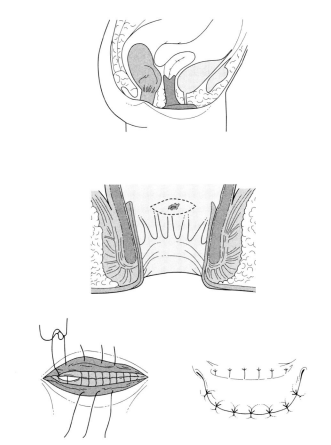

**Fig. 49.6** Transanal repair of midrectovaginal fistula. The rectal mucosa surrounding the fistula opening is excised and the muscular defect in the rectovaginal septum is repaired. A mucosal advancement flap is then advanced and sutured. If the high-pressure zone in the rectum is successfully repaired, a vaginal closure is unnecessary.

if the bowel anastomosis is in the region of the vaginal stump. When closure of a rectovaginal fistula results from proximal fecal diversion, additional medical and surgical therapy is imperative as the fistulae recur frequently following ileostomy reversal in the absence of adjunctive or definitive therapy.[77] Finally, should other options fail or be inappropriate, proctocolectomy may allow healing. A two-stage procedure should be considered in the presence of sepsis or severe rectal inflammation to minimize the risk of a persistent perineal wound.[152] Various surgical techniques, including muscle flap perineal reconstruction procedures, have been applied as therapeutic options for Crohn's patients with persistent perineal sinus tracts refractory to medical therapy.[153–160] The use of adjunctive therapies such as fibrin glue has not been shown to be efficacious when applied to rectovaginal and anovaginal fistulae, presumably owing to the short length of the fistula tract.

Medical therapy may also be useful for the treatment of selected patients with vaginal fistulae. The choice of specific medication should be dictated by the degree to which patients are symptomatic, as well as the likely time of onset of action. Medications that have been applied as therapy for these fistulae include AZA and 6-MP, intravenous CyA and, more recently, infliximab. The efficacy of 6-MP in the treatment of rectovaginal fistula was assessed by Korelitz and Present in Crohn's patients with rectovaginal or vulvar fistulae.[37] Clinical improvement was observed in three of six patients with rectovaginal

fistulae, including two with fistula closure. One of two patients with vulvar fistulae was noted to be improved, though fistula closure was not achieved. A 1993 study reported by Hanauer and Smith evaluating the efficacy of intravenous CyA in refractory Crohn's disease included five patients with a total of 12 fistulae (five enterovaginal, three perianal, three enterocutaneous, and one enterovesical).[161] Complete resolution of drainage was observed in 10 of 12 fistulae after a mean of 7.9 days. Subsequently, recurrent drainage was documented in two perianal and two enterovaginal fistulae. Present and Lichtiger reported an uncontrolled study of 16 patients with fistulizing Crohn's disease treated with a 2-week course of intravenous CyA followed by maintenance therapy with oral CyA.[162] Fistula closure was observed in one of two patients with rectovaginal fistulae after 2 weeks of therapy. However, both patients had recurrence despite continued therapy, and one required surgery. There have been no reported controlled trials of infliximab focusing on the treatment of rectovaginal and anovaginal fistulae. A recent uncontrolled study reported by van Bodegraven and associates failed to demonstrate healing of rectovaginal fistulae in four patients treated with three infliximab infusions (5 mg/kg) at baseline, week 2 and week 6.[163]

## ENTEROVESICAL FISTULAE

Enterovesical fistula, the most common Crohn's-related urinary fistula, affects 2–8% of patients (Fig. 49.8).[164–167] Ileovesical fistulae comprised the majority of enterovesical fistulae (58%) in a large series of patients with IBD reported by Greenstein and colleagues.[165] Enteroureteral, rectourethral, urethrocutaneous and enterourachal fistulae also occur, though less frequently. These fistulae are the result of an extension of inflammation from the small bowel and colon penetrating into adjacent bladder, ureter, urethra, perineum or urachal remnant. Although fistulae most commonly result from penetrating Crohn's disease, they may complicate surgical resection in the setting of anastomotic breakdown. Complex fistulae developing from pelvic abscesses may involve the ileum, colon, vagina and bladder.[166]

Clinically, enterovesical fistulae present with dysuria, recurrent cystitis and the passage of gas and fecal material with urine. *Escherichia coli* and other Enterobacteriaceae species are the most common pathogens, but multibacterial infections may also develop. Dysuria almost always precedes the development of pneumaturia or frank fecaluria. Non-specific complaints, including diarrhea, abdominal pain and nausea, are present in the majority of patients. Physical examination findings are commonly non-specific, but abdominal tenderness may be appreciated in 29% of patients.[168] Whereas an accurate history and positive urinary culture provide a presumptive diagnosis of enterovesical fistula in 95% of cases, diagnosis is frequently delayed, with symptoms being present for weeks to months in most patients.[167,169]

Intravenous pyelograms and retrograde cystograms commonly fail to detect the fistula tract, although a filling defect may be observed in the bladder. Cystoscopy confirms the diagnosis of fistula in 30–67% of patients with urinary symptoms.[167,168,170] An area of bullous edema or mucosal inflammation with purulent (or rarely feculent) exudate characterizes the cystoscopic appearance of a fistula. Multiple small fistulous tracts extending from a perivesical abscess may not be appreciated by cystoscopy but may be diagnosed if intravesical contrast injection results in opacification of an adjacent bowel lumen.[171] Other radiographic

## Table 49.4 Results of surgical therapy for rectovaginal fistulae in patients with Crohn's disease

| Investigator | Year | Therapy | Improved | Proctectomy/diversion |
|---|---|---|---|---|
| Francois | 1993 | Fistulotomy | 9/9 (100%) | 0/9 (0%) |
| Radcliffe | 1988 | Fistulotomy | 6/12 (50%) | 4/12 (33%) |
| Fauloconer | 1975 | Fistulotomy | 0/3 (0%) | 2/3 (67%) |
| Hudson | 1970 | Fistulotomy | 3/5 (60%) | 0/5 (0%) |
| O'Leary | 1998 | Primary closure | 1/2 (50%) | 0/2 (0%) |
| Wiskind | 1992 | Primary closure | 3/3 (100%) | 0/3 (0%) |
| Cohen | 1989 | Primary closure | 3/6 (50%) | 2/6 (33%)[1] |
| Radcliffe | 1988 | Primary closure | 2/4 (50%) | (20%)[2] |
| Bandy | 1983 | Primary closure | 8/9 (89%) | 0/9 (0%) |
| Givel | 1982 | Primary closure | 1/2 (50%) | 0/2 (0%) |
| Tuxen | 1979 | Primary closure | 1/2 (50%) | 02 (0%) |
| Hudson | 1970 | Primary closure | 3/4 (75%) | 0/4 (0%) |
| Michelassi | 2000 | Advancement flap | 4/16 (25%) | 11/16 (69%) |
| O'Leary | 1998 | Advancement flap | 3/6 (50%) | 0/6 (0%) |
| Simmang | 1998 | Advancement flap[3] | 2/2 (100%) | 0/2 (0%) |
| Hull | 1997 | Advancement flap[4] | 21/35 (60%) | 5/35 (14%) |
| Makowiec | 1995 | Advancement flap | 10/12 (83%) | 0/12 (0%) |
| Hesterberg | 1993 | Advancement flap[5] | 7/10 (70%) | 0/10 (0%) |
| Fry | 1989 | Advancement flap | 2/3 (67%) | 0/3 (0%) |
| Jones | 1987 | Advancement flap | 6/10 (60%) | 1/10 (10%) |
| Radcliffe | 1988 | Advancement flap[6] | 7/11 (64%) | (20%)[2] |
| O'Leary | 1998 | Transvaginal flap | 0/1 (0%) | 0/1 (0%) |
| Sher | 1991 | Transvaginal flap | 13/14 (93%) | 1/14 (7%) |

Advancement flap, transanal advancement flap.
[1] One patient treated with diverting ileostomy.
[2] A total of 15 patients were treated with surgical therapy (primary closure or advancement flap); 3/15 required proctectomy.
[3] Sleeve advancement flap procedure.
[4] Includes patients treated with curvilinear (24), linear (6) and sleeve (2) advancement flap procedures.
[5] Transanal anocutaneous flap procedure.
[6] Includes patients treated with anterior (3) and transanal (4) advancement flap procedures.

studies, including barium enema, CT and MRI, may be useful to detect these fistulae. As the ileum is the most commonly involved bowel segment, colonoscopy and barium enema are most useful to identify or exclude associated colonic abnormalities (diverticulitis or colorectal malignancy) which may also fistulize to the bladder. The detection of radio-opaque barium in a centrifuged urine sample collected immediately after barium enema (Bourne test) confirms the presence of a colovesical fistula even when the fistula tract cannot be defined radiographically.[172] Oral charcoal may be similarly administered, and microscopic examination of the urine sediment for charcoal will suggest the presence of an intestinal–urinary fistula.[170] CT and MRI are the most sensitive techniques to detect enterovesical fistulae (Fig. 49.8). They may demonstrate small amounts of air in the bladder which, in the absence of instrumentation or infection, are diagnostic of a fistula. In addition, abnormalities in adjacent organs responsible for fistula formation may be detected. Although MRI has not been systemically compared with CT for efficacy in diagnosing enterovesical fistulae, MRI has the greatest potential for detecting fistulae, as small amounts of fluid in a fistula may be identified as a high signal-intensity tract on $T_2$-weighted images.[173,174] Adjacent perivesical abnormalities

may also be delineated with the use of specialized endoluminal surface coils and pelvic multiarray body coils.

Management of enterovesical fistulae parallels that of other internal fistulae. The primary goals of therapy are reduction of bowel inflammation and treatment of any urinary infections. Medical therapy may be initially utilized in those patients without significant risk for pyelonephritis or sepsis, as some fistulae will close spontaneously. The utility of medical therapy in treatment of enterovesical fistulae has not been evaluated in a controlled fashion. In those patients in whom fistulae persist, surgical intervention is nearly always necessary.[164–167,176–181] (Table 49.5). The most common procedure is resection of the diseased bowel segment, together with curettage and primary closure of the bladder defect. Partial bladder resection is usually not indicated, and if the bladder defect is small it may require no particular repair. Bladder drainage is used postoperatively and the Foley catheter is removed after a cystogram demonstrates no bladder leak. A single-stage approach may be used even in patients with multiple fistulae, but when the fistula is associated with an intra-abdominal abscess (present in 34–47% of cases), a two-stage operative intervention is often necessary.[169] Recurrence of fistulae is uncommon when treated in this fashion.

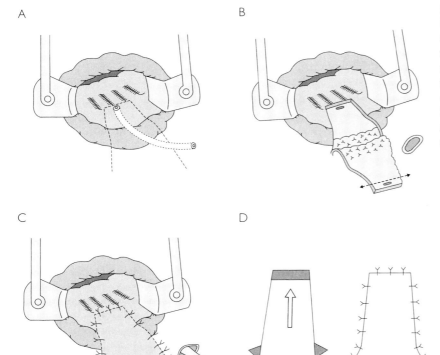

A

B

C

D

**Fig. 49.7** Anocutaneous advancement flap. (A) An inverted U-shaped flap is incised including the internal fistula opening at the level of the dentate line. (B) The flap is elevated and the fistula tract is excised or curetted. The internal mucosal defect is excised. (C) The defect in the internal anal sphincter is sutured closed. The flap is then advanced into the anal canal and approximated to the anal mucosa and underlying internal sphincter muscle proximal to the fistula site. (D) Additional advancement is gained by excising skin from the adjacent base (Burow's triangles).

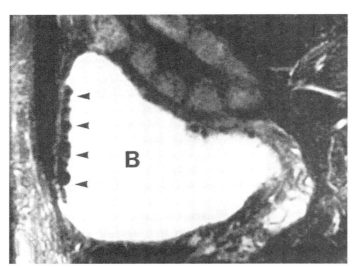

**Fig. 49.8** Enterovesical fistula secondary to Crohn's disease. $T_2$-weighted MR image through the pelvis of a 65-year-old man with pneumaturia. Urine in the bladder displays high signal intensity. On sagittal view, air in the bladder (arrowheads) has risen to the most non-dependent portion of the bladder (patient imaged in the recumbent position).

Postsurgical complications occur in 10–30% of patients and include abscess formation, sepsis, recurrent enterovesical or new enterocutaneous fistula, urine and anastomotic leaks, and bowel obstruction. Whereas urine leaks may seal with prolonged bladder drainage, recurrent or new enteric fistulae necessitate additional surgery. Urinary retention and impotence may develop if extensive pelvic surgery results in damage to preganglionic parasympathetic fibers of the pelvic plexus.

Rectourethral and urethrocutaneous fistulae have also been associated with Crohn's disease. They present with symptoms similar to those of enterovesical fistulae and frequently develop in the setting of multiple perianal and scrotal abscesses that erode into the bulbous urethra.[175] Retrograde urethrography and barium enema may demonstrate the fistula. CT and MRI may also reveal associated perirectal or periurethral fistulae, if present. In selected patients without active proctitis, a transanal rectal advancement flap procedure may be used to close the fistula.[176]

## CONCLUSIONS

The primary goals of the clinician in the management of fistulizing Crohn's disease include defining the anatomy of the fistula, draining any associated infectious material, attempting to eradicate the fistulous tract through medical or surgical therapies, and preventing the recurrence of fistulae. Evaluation and therapeutic decisions require close collaboration between the gastroenterologist and the surgeon. This is particularly true when dealing with perianal disease. Appropriate evaluation should include identification of septic complications, delineation of the fistulous tract, including the origin and terminus of the fistula, and determination of the extent of bowel involvement with active Crohn's disease, in particular the presence or absence of proctitis. Drainage of abscesses and control of septic complications through the placement of drains or setons is essential. Conservative therapy with avoidance of sphincter-cutting procedures is the standard approach typically followed. Preservation of continence and sphincter integrity should be an essential goal of management. When simple fistulae are present surgery is appropriate, as it avoids the potential risk of long-term immunosuppression without a significant risk of fecal incontinence. When complex fistulae are present, surgical intervention should be minimized and medical therapy may be more appropriate.

## Table 49.5 Response of enterovesical fistulae to surgical therapy in patients with Crohn's disease

| Investigator | Year | No. patients | No. treated[1] | Coexistent fistulae | Resolved | Recurrence |
|---|---|---|---|---|---|---|
| Kyle | 1969 | 10 | 10 | NA | 10/10 (100%) | 0/10 (0%) |
| Talamani | 1982 | 14 | 16 | NA | 14/16 (88%) | 1/16 (6%)[2] |
| Van Dongen | 1984 | 14 | 14 | 9 | 7/14 (50%) | 7/14 (50%) |
| Schraut | 1984 | 29 | 29 | 19 | 29/29 (100%)[3] | 0/29 (0%) |
| Greenstein | 1984 | 38 | 36 | 12 | 36/36 (100%) | 0/29 (0%) |
| Glass | 1985 | 16 | 12 | NA | 12/12 (100%)[3] | 0/12 (0%) |
| Margolin | 1986 | 16 | 9 | NA | 9/9 (100%) | 0/9 (0%) |
| Fazio | 1987 | 3 | 3 | 0 | 3/3 (100%)[4] | 0/3 (0%) |
| Heyen | 1988 | 19 | 15 | 4 | 13/15 (87%)[3] | 2/15 (13%) |
| McNamara | 1989 | 63 | 61 | 31 | 60/61 (98%)[5] | 1/61 (2%) |

NA, not addressed in publication.
[1] Patients treated with variety of surgical procedures.
[2] One patient underwent proctectomy for intractable perianal disease during follow-up.
[3] Urine leak complicated postoperative course in one patient.
[4] Three patients with rectourethral fistulae treated with rectal advancement flap.
[5] Urine leak complicated postoperative course in two patients.

When internal fistulae are present, it is important to ascertain the severity of the illness. In acutely ill patients in whom local abscess or sepsis is a concern a surgical approach is often the best option, with subsequent medical maintenance therapy of residual Crohn's disease. In patients with internal fistula who have minimal symptoms, medical therapy initiated with an antibiotic may be appropriate. The appropriate approach to asymptomatic patients is uncertain, as there are few data to indicate whether treatment alters the natural course of disease.

# REFERENCES

1. Crohn BB, Ginzburg L, Oppenheimer GD. Regional ileitis: a pathologic and clinical entity. JAMA 1932;99:1323–1329.
2. Bissell AD. Localized chronic ulcerative colitis. Ann Surg 1934;99:957–966.
3. Steinberg DM, Cooke WT, Alexander-Williams J. Abscess and fistulae in Crohn's disease. Gut 1973;14:865–869.
4. Rankin GB, Watts HD, Melnyk CS, Kelly MI Jr. National cooperative Crohn's disease study: extraintestinal manifestations and perianal complications. Gastroenterology 1979;77:914–920.
5. Farmer RG, Hawk WA, Turnbull RB Jr. Clinical patterns in Crohn's disease: a statistical study of 615 cases. Gastroenterology 1975;68:627–635.
6. Present DH. Management of fistula disease. Inflamm Bowel Dis 1998;4:302–307.
7. Hellers G, Bergstrand O, Ewerth S, Holmstrom B. Occurrence and outcome after primary treatment of anal fistulae in Crohn's disease. Gut 1980;21:525–527.
8. Schwartz DA, Loftus EV Jr, Tremaine WJ et al. The natural history of fistulizing Crohn's disease in Olmsted County, Minnesota. Gastroenterology. 2002;122:875–880.
9. Gray BK, Lockhart-Mummery HE, Morson BC. Crohn's disease of the anal region. Gut 1965;6:515–524.
10. Present DH, Korelitz BI, Wisch N, Glass JL, Sachar DB, Pasternack BS. Treatment of Crohn's disease with 6-mercaptopurine: a long-term randomized double blind study. N Engl J Med 1980;302:981–987.
11. Present DH, Rutgeerts P, Targan S et al. Infliximab for the treatment of fistulae in patients with Crohn's disease. N Engl J Med 1999;340:1398–1405.
12. Buchmann P, Keighley MR, Allan RN, Thompson H, Alexander-Williams J. Natural history of perianal Crohn's disease. Ten year follow-up: a plea for conservatism. Am J Surg 1980;140:642–644.
13. Halme L, Sainio AP. Factors related to frequency, type, and outcome of anal fistulae in Crohn's disease. Dis Colon Rectum 1995;38:55–59.
14. Makowiec F, Jehle EC, Becker HD, Starlinger M. Clinical course after transanal advancement flap repair of perianal fistula in patients with Crohn's disease. Br J Surg 1995;82:603–606.
15. Jakobovits J, Schuster MM. Metronidazole therapy for Crohn's disease and associated fistulae. Am J Gastroenterol 1984;79:533–540.
16. Turunen U, Farkkila M, Seppala K. Long-term treatment of peri-anal or fistulous Crohn's disease with Ciprofloxacin (suppl148). Scand J Gastroenterol 1989;24:144.
17. O'Brien JJ, Bayless TM, Bayless JA. Use of azathioprine or 6-mercaptopurine in the treatment of Crohn's disease. Gastroenterology 1991;101:39–46.
18. Egan LJ, Sandborn WJ, Tremaine WJ. Clinical outcome following treatment of refractory inflammatory and fistulizing Crohn's disease with intravenous cyclosporine. Am J Gastroenterol 1998;93:442–448.
19. Present DH, Rutgeerts P, Targan S et al. Infliximab for the treatment of fistulae in patients with Crohn's disease. N Engl J Med 1999;340:1398–1405.
20. Sparberg M, Kirsner JB. Long-term corticosteroid therapy for regional enteritis: an analysis of 58 courses in 54 patients. Am J Dig Dis 1966;11:865–880.
21. Jones JH, Lennard-Jones JF. Corticosteroids and corticotropin in the treatment of Crohn's disease. Gut 1966;7:181–187.
22. Malchow H, Ewe EK, Brandes JW et al. European cooperative Crohn's disease study (ECCDS): results of drug treatment. Gastroenterology 1984;86:249–266.
23. Ursing B, Kamme C. Metronidazole for Crohn's disease. Lancet 1975;1:775–777.
24. Bernstein LH, Frank MS, Brandt LJ, Boley SJ. Healing of perineal Crohn's disease with metronidazole. Gastroenterology 1980;79:357–365.
25. Brandt LJ, Bernstein LH, Boley SJ. Frank MS. Metronidazole therapy for perineal Crohn's disease: a follow-up study. Gastroenterology 1982;83:383–387.
26. Jakobovits J, Schuster MM. Metronidazole therapy for Crohn's disease and associated fistulae. Am J Gastroenterol 1984;79:533–540.
27. Schneider MU, Laudage G, Guggenmoos-Holzman I, Riemann JF. Metronidazol in der behandlung des morbus Crohn. Dtsch Med Wochenschr 1985;110:1724–1730.
28. Arseneau KO, Cohn SM, Cominelli F, Connors AF Jr. Cost–utility of initial medical management for Crohn's disease perianal fistulae. Gastroenterology 2001;120:1640–1656.
29. Duffy LF, Daum F, Fisher SE et al. Peripheral neuropathy in Crohn's disease patients treated with metronidazole. Gastroenterology 1985;88:681–684.
30. Turunen U, Farkkila M, Seppala K. Long-term treatment of peri-anal or fistulous Crohn's disease with Ciprofloxacin. Scand J Gastroenterol 1989;24 (Suppl 48):144.
31. Wolf J. Ciprofloxacin may be useful in Crohn's disease. Gastroenterology 1990;98:A212 [abstract].
32. Turunen U, Farkkila M, Valtonen V. Long-term outcome of ciprofloxacin treatment in severe perianal or fistulous Crohn's disease. Gastroenterology 1993;104:A793.
33. Davis R, Markham A, Balfour JA. Ciprofloxacin. An updated review of its pharmacology, therapeutic efficacy and tolerability. Drugs 1996;51:1019–1074.
34. Casparian JM, Luchi M, Moffat RE, Hinthorn D. Quinolones and tendon ruptures. South Med J 2000;93:488–491.
35. Solomon M, McLeod R, O'Connor B, Steinhart A, Greenberg G, Cohen Z. Combination ciprofloxacin and metronidazole in severe perianal Crohn's disease. Can J Gastroenterol 1993;7:571–573.
36. Present DH, Korelitz BI, Wisch N, Glass JL, Sachar DB, Pasternack BS. Treatment of Crohn's disease with 6-mercaptopurine: a long-term randomized double blind study. N Engl J Med 1980;302:981–987.
37. Korelitz BI, Present DH. Favorable effect of 6-mercaptopurine on fistulae of Crohn's disease. Dig Dis Sci 1985;30:58–64.
38. O'Brien JJ, Bayless TM, Bayless JA. Use of azathioprine or 6-mercaptopurine in the treatment of Crohn's disease. Gastroenterology 1991;101:39–46.

39. Pearson DC, May GR, Fick GH, Sutherland LR. Azathioprine and 6-mercaptopurine in Crohn disease. A meta-analysis. Ann Intern Med 1995;123:132–142.

40. Pichney LS, Fantry GT, Graham SM. Gastrocolic and duodeno-colic fistulae in Crohn's disease. J Clin Gastroenterol 1992;15:205–211.

41. Wheeler SC, Marion JF, Present DH. Medical therapy, not surgery is the appropriate first line of treatment for Crohn's entero-vesical fistula. Gastroenterology 1998;114:A1113.

42. Cuffari C, Hunt S, Bayless T. Utilisation of erythrocyte 6-thioguanine metabolite levels to optimise azathioprine therapy in patients with inflammatory bowel disease. Gut 2001;48:642–646.

43. Present DH, Meltzer SJ, Krumholtz MP, Wolke A, Korelitz BI. 6-Mercaptopurine in the management of inflammatory bowel disease: short- and long-term toxicity. Ann Intern Med 1989;111:641–649.

44. Muhadevan U, Marion J, Present DH. The place of methotrexate in the treatment of refractory Crohn's disease (abstr). Gastroenterology 1997;112:A1031.

45. Vandeputte L, D'Haens G, Baert F, Rutgeerts P. Methotrexate in refractory Crohn's disease. Inflamm Bowel Dis 1999;5:11–15.

46. Lemann M, Zenjari T, Bouhnik Y et al. Methotrexate in Crohn's disease: long-term efficacy and toxicity. Am J Gastroenterol 2000;95:1730–1734.

47. Feagan BG, Fedorak RN, Irvine EJ et al. A comparison of methotrexate with placebo for the maintenance of remission in Crohn's disease. N Engl J Med 2000;342:1627–1632.

48. Sandborn WJ. A review of immune modifier therapy for inflammatory bowel disease: azathioprine, 6-mercaptopurine, cyclosporine, and methotrexate. Am J Gastroenterol 1996;91:423–433.

49. Te HS, Schiano TD, Kuan SF, Hanauer SB, Conjeevaram HS, Baker AL. Hepatic effects of long-term methotrexate use in the treatment of inflammatory bowel disease. Am J Gastroenterol 2000;95:3150–3156.

50. Stein RB, Hanaper SB. Medical therapy for inflammatory bowel disease. Gastroenterol Clin North Am 1999;28:297–321.

51. Present DH, Lichtiger S. Efficacy of cyclosporine in treatment of fistula of Crohn's disease. Dig Dis Sci 1994;39:374–380.

52. Egan LJ, Sandborn WJ, Tremaine WJ. Clinical outcome following treatment of refractory inflammatory and fistulizing Crohn's disease with intravenous cyclosporine. Am J Gastroenterol 1998; 93:442–448.

53. Hinterleitner TA, Petritsch W, Aichbichler B, Fickert P, Ranner G, Krejs GJ. Combination of cyclosporine, azathioprine and prednisolone for perianal fistulae in Crohn's disease. Zeitschr Gastroenterol 1997;35:603–608.

54. Lowry PW, Weaver AL, Tremaine WJ, Sandborn WJ. Combination therapy with oral tacrolimus (FK506) and azathioprine or 6-mercaptopurine for treatment-refractory Crohn's disease perianal fistulae. Inflamm Bowel Dis 1999;5:239–245.

55. Sandborn WJ. Preliminary report on the use of oral tacrolimus (FK506) in the treatment of complicated proximal small bowel and fistulizing Crohn's disease. Am J Gastroenterol 1997;92:876–879.

56. Fellerman K, Ludwig D, Stahl M, David-Walek T, Stange EF. Steroid-unresponsive acute attacks of inflammatory bowel disease: immunomodulation by tacrolimus (FK506). Am J Gastroenterol 1998;93:1860–1866.

57. Sandborn WJ, Present DH, Isaacs KL et al. Tacrolimus (FK506) for the treatment of perianal and enterocutaneous fistulae in patients with Crohn's disease: a randomized, double-blind, placebo-controlled trial. Gastroenterology 2002;122:A81.

58. Neurath MF, Wanitschke R, Peters M, Krummenauer F, Meyer zum Buschenfelde KH, Schlaak JF. Randomised trial of mycophenolate mofetil versus azathioprine for treatment of chronic active Crohn's disease. Gut 1999;44:625–628.

59. Fickert P, Hinterleitner TA, Wenzl HH, Aichbichler BW, Petritsch W. Mycophenolate mofetil in patients with Crohn's disease. Am J Gastroenterol 1998;93:2529–2532.

60. Miehsler W, Reinisch W, Moser G, Gangl A, Vogelsang H. Is mycophenolate mofetil an effective alternative in azathioprine-intolerant patients with chronic active Crohn's disease? Am J Gastroenterol 2001;96:782–787.

61. Fellermann K, Steffen M, Stein J et al. Mycophenolate mofetil: lack of efficacy in chronic active inflammatory bowel disease. Aliment Pharmacol Ther 2000;14:171–176.

62. Present DH, Rutgeerts P, Targan S et al. Infliximab for the treatment of fistulae in patients with Crohn's disease. N Engl J Med 1999;340:1398–1405.

63. Sands B, Van Deventer S, Bernstein C et al. Long-term treament of fistulizing Crohn's disease: response to infliximab in the ACCENT II trial through 54 weeks. Gastroenterology 2002;122:A81.

64. Poritz LS, Rowe WA, Koltun WA. Remicade does not abolish the need for surgery in fistulizing Crohn's disease. Dis Colon Rectum 2002;45:771–775.

65. Feagan BG, Sandborn WJ, Baker JP et al. A randomized, double-blind, placebo-controlled, multi-center trial of the engineered human antibody to TNF (CDP571) for steroid sparing and maintenance of remission in patients with steroid-dependent Crohn's disease (abstract). Gastroenterology 2000;118:A655.

66. Sandborn WJ, Feagan BG, Hanauer SB et al. CDP571 Crohn's Disease Study Group. An engineered human antibody to TNF (CDP571) for active Crohn's disease: a randomized double-blind placebo-controlled trial. Gastroenterology 2001;120:1330–1338.

67. Ehrenpreis ED, Kane SV, Cohen LB, Cohen RD, Hanaper SB. Thalidomide therapy for patients with refractory Crohn's disease: an open-label trial. Gastroenterology 1999;117:1271–1277.

68. Vasiliauskas EA, Kam LY, Abreu-Martin MT et al. An open-label pilot study of low-dose thalidomide in chronically active, steroid-dependent Crohn's disease. Gastroenterology 1999;117:1278–1287.

69. Schaible TF. Long term safety of infliximab. Can J Gastroenterol 2000;14 Suppl C:29C–32C.

70. Sandborn WJ, Hanauer SB. Antitumor necrosis factor therapy for inflammatory bowel disease: a review of agents, pharmacology, clinical results, and safety. Inflamm Bowel Dis 1999;5:119–133.

71. Hanauer SB, Feagan BG, Lichtenstein GR et al. ACCENT I Study Group. Maintenance infliximab for Crohn's disease: the ACCENT I randomised trial. Lancet 2002;359:1541–1549.

72. Keane J, Gershon S, Wise RP et al. Tuberculosis associated with infliximab, a tumor necrosis factor alpha- neutralizing agent. N Engl J Med 2001;345:1098–1104.

73. Warris A, Bjorneklett A, Gaustad P. Invasive pulmonary aspergillosis associated with infliximab therapy. N Engl J Med 2001;344:1099–1100.

74. Morelli J, Wilson FA. Does administration of infliximab increase susceptibility to listeriosis? Am J Gastroenterol 2000;95:841–842.

75. Remicade (infliximab) for IV injection. Package Insert 2002.

76. Bousvaros A, Mueller B. Thalidomide in gastrointestinal disorders. Drugs 2001;61:777–787.

77. Grant DR, Cohen Z, Mcleod R. Loop ileostomy for anorectal Crohn's disease. Can J Surg 1986;29:32–35.

78. Zelas P, Jagelman DG. Loop ileostomy in the management of Crohn's colitis in the debilitated patient. Ann Surg 1980;191:164–168.

79. Harper PH, Kettlewell MG, Lee EC. The effect of split ileostomy on perianal Crohn's disease. Br J Surg 1982;69:608–610.

80. Farmer RG, Hawk WA, Turnbull RB Jr. Indications for surgery in Crohn's disease: analysis of 500 patients. Gastroenterology 1976;71:245–250.

81. Kirkegaard P, Madsen PV. Perineal sinus after removal of the rectum. Occlusion with fibrin adhesive. J Surg 1983;145:791–794.

82. Abel M, Chiu Y, Russell T, Volpe P. Autologous fibrin glue in the treatment of rectovaginal and complex fistula. Dis Colon Rectum 1993;36:447–449.

83. Oshitani N, Nakamura S, Matsumoto T, Kobayashi K, Kitano A. Treatment of Crohn's disease fistulae with coagulation factor XIII. Lancet 1996;347:119–120.

84. Nelson EW Jr, Bright DE, Villar LF. Closure of refractory perineal Crohn's lesion. Integration of hyperbaric oxygen into case management. Dig Dis Sci 1990;35:1561–1565.

85. Brady CE III. Hyperbaric oxygen and perineal Crohn's disease: a follow-up. Gastroenterology 1993;105:1264.

86. Colombel JF, Mathieu D, Bouault JM et al. Hyperbaric oxygenation in severe perineal Crohn's disease. Dis Colon Rectum 1995;38:609–614.

87. Greenstein AJ. Surgical management and ultimate outcome. In: Haubrich WS, Schaffner F, Berk E, eds. Bockus gastroenterology, 5th edn. Philadelphia: WB Saunders; 1995:1526.

88. Skvarilova M, Nicakova R, Axmann K. New alternatives for the treatment of fistulae in Crohn's disease. Acta Universitatis Palackianae Olomucensis Facultatis Medicae 1994;138:29–31 [abstract].

89. Parks AG, Gordon PH, Hardcastle JD. A classification of fistula-in-ano. Br J Surg 1976;63:1–12.

90. Hobbiss JH, Schofield PF. Management of perianal Crohn's disease. J Roy Soc Med 1982;75:414–417.

91. Marks CG, Ritchie JK, Lockhart-Mummery HE. Anal fistulae in Crohn's disease. Br J Surg 1981;68:525–527.

92. Bergstrand O, Ewerth S, Hellers G, Holmstrom B, Ullman J, Wallberg P. Outcome following treatment of anal fissure in Crohn's disease. Acta Chir Scand 1980;500 (Suppl):43–44.

93. Bernard D, Morgan S, Tasse D. Selective surgical management of Crohn's disease of the anus. Can J Surg 1986;29:318–321.

94. Sohn N, Korelitz BI. Local operative treatment of anorectal Crohn's disease. J Clin Gastroenterol 1982;4:395–399.

95. Sohn N, Korelitz BI, Weinstein MA. Anorectal Crohn's disease: definitive surgery for fistulae and recurrent abscesses. Am J Surg 1980;139:394–397.

96. Nordgren S, Fasth S, Hulten L. Anal fistulae in Crohn's disease: incidence and outcome of surgical treatment. Int J Colorectal Dis 1992;7:214–218.

97. Williams J, Rothenberger D, Nemer F, Goldberg S. Fistula-in-ano in Crohn's disease. Dis Colon Rectum 1991;34:378–384.

98. Fuhrman G, Larach S. Experience with perianal fistulae in patients with Crohn's disease. Dis Colon Rectum 1989;32:847–848.

99. Levien D, Surrell J, Mazier W. Surgical treatment of anorectal fistulae in patients with Crohn's disease. Surg Gynecol Obstet 1989;169:133–136.

100. Williamson P, Hellinger M, Larach S, Ferrara A. Twenty year review of the surgical management of perianal Crohn's disease. Dis Colon Rectum 1995;38:389–392.

101. Joo JS, Weiss EG, Nogueras JJ, Wexner SD. Endorectal advancement flap in perianal Crohn's disease. Am Surg 1998;64:147–150.

102. Schwartz DA, Wiersema MJ, Dudiak KM et al. A comparison of endoscopic ultrasound, magnetic resonance imaging, and exam under anesthesia for evaluation of Crohn's perianal fistulae. Gastroenterology 2001;121:1064–1072.

103. Ying LT, Hurlbut DJ, Depew WT, Boag AH, Taguchi K. Primary adenocarcinoma in an enterocutaneous fistula associated with Crohn's disease. Can J Gastroenterol 1998;12:265–269.

104. Ky A, Sohn N, Weinstein MA, Korelitz BI. Carcinoma arising in anorectal fistulae of Crohn's disease. Dis Colon Rectum 1998;41:992–996.

105. Korelitz BI. Carcinoma arising in Crohn's disease fistulae: another concern warranting another type of surveillance. Am J Gastroenterol 1999;94:2337–2339.

106. Williams JG, Macleod CA, Rothenberger DA, Goldberg SM. Seton treatment of high anal fistulae. Br J Surg 1991;78:1159–1161.

107. Matos D, Lunniss PJ, Phillips RK. Total sphincter conservation in high fistula in ano: results of a new approach. Br J Surg 1993;80:802–804.

108. Winter AM, Banks PA, Petros JG. Healing of transsphincteric perianal fistulae in Crohn's disease using a new technique. Am J Gastroenterol 1993;88:2022–2025.

109. Faucheron JL, Saint-Marc O, Guibert L, Parc R. Long-term seton drainage for high anal fistulae in Crohn's disease – a sphincter-saving operation? Dis Colon Rectum 1996;39:208–211.

110. Scott HJ, Northover JM. Evaluation of surgery for perianal Crohn's fistulae. Dis Colon Rectum 1996;39:1039–1043.

111. Sangwan YP, Schoetz DJ Jr, Murray JJ, Roberts PL, Coller JA. Perianal Crohn's disease. Results of local surgical treatment. Dis Colon Rectum 1996;39:529–535.

112. McKee RF, Keenan RA. Perianal Crohn's disease – is it all bad news? Dis Colon Rectum 1996;39:136–142.

113. Williamson PR, Hellinger MD, Larach SW, Ferrara A. Twenty-year review of the surgical management of perianal Crohn's disease. Dis Colon Rectum 1995;38:389–392.

114. Sugita A, Koganei K, Harada H, Yamazaki Y, Fukushima T, Shimada H. Surgery for Crohn's anal fistulae. J Gastroenterol 1995;30 (Suppl 8):143–146.

115. Koganei K, Sugita A, Harada H, Fukushima T, Shimada H. Seton treatment for perianal Crohn's fistulae. Surg Today 1995;25:32–36.

116. Pearl RK, Andrews JR, Orsay CP et al. Role of the seton in the management of anorectal fistulae. Dis Colon Rectum 1993;36:573–577; discussion 577–579.

117. Williams JG, Rothenberger DA, Nemer FD, Goldberg SM. Fistula-in-ano in Crohn's disease. Results of aggressive surgical treatment. Dis Colon Rectum 1991;34:378–384.

118. White RA, Eisenstat TE, Rubin RJ, Salvati EP. Seton management of complex anorectal fistulae in patients with Crohn's disease. Dis Colon Rectum 1990;33:587–589.

119. van Dongen LM, Lubbers EJ. Perianal fistulae in patients with Crohn's disease. Arch Surg 1986;121:1187–1190.

120. Lunniss PJ, Thomson J. The loose seton. In: Phillips R, Lunnis P, eds. Anal fistula: surgical evaluation and management. London: Chapman & Hall; 1996.

121. Delemarre S. What is new in the treatment of perianal fistulae in Crohn's disease? Neth J Med 1996;48:74–76.

122. Robertson WG, Mangione JS. Cutaneous advancement flap closure: alternative method for treatment of complicated anal fistulae. Dis Colon Rectum 1998;41:884–886; discussion 886–887.

123. Marchesa P, Hull TL, Fazio VW. Advancement sleeve flaps for treatment of severe perianal Crohn's disease. Br J Surg 1998;85:1695–1698.

124. Makowiec F, Jehle EC, Becker HD, Starlinger M. Clinical course after transanal advancement flap repair of perianal fistula in patients with Crohn's disease. Br J Surg 1995;82:603–606.

125. Lewis P, Bartolo DC. Treatment of trans-sphincteric fistulae by full thickness anorectal advancement flaps. Br J Surg 1990;77:1187–1189

126. Fry RD, Shemesh EI, Kodner IJ, Timmcke A. Techniques and results in the management of anal and perianal Crohn's disease. Surg Gynecol Obstet 1989;168:42–48.

127. Jones IT, Fazio VW, Jagelman DG. The use of transanal rectal advancement flaps in the management of fistulae involving the anorectum. Dis Colon Rectum 1987;30:919–923.

128. Simmang CL, Lacey SW, Huber PJ Jr. Rectal sleeve advancement: repair of rectovaginal fistula associated with anorectal stricture in Crohn's disease. Dis Colon Rectum 1998;41:787–789.

129. Matos D, Lunniss PJ, Phillips RK. Total sphincter conservation in high fistula in ano: results of a new approach. Br J Surg 1993;80:802–804.

130. Bodzin JH. Laser ablation of complex perianal fistulae preserves continence and is a rectum-sparing alternative in patients with Crohn's disease. Am Surg 1998;64:627–631.

131. Broe PO, Bayless TM, Cameron JL. Crohn's disease: are enteroenteral fistulae an indication for surgery? Surgery 1982;91:249–253.

132. Radcliffe A, Ritchie J, Hawley P, Lennard-Jones J, Northover J. Anovaginal and rectovaginal fistulae in Crohn's disease. Dis Colon Rectum 1988;31:94–99.

132. Hyman NH, Fazio VW, Tuckson WB, Lavery IC. Consequences of ileal pouch–anal anastomosis for Crohn's colitis. Dis Colon Rectum 1991;34:653–657.

133. Lee PY, Fazio VW, Church JM, Hull TL, Eu KW, Lavery IC. Vaginal fistula following restorative proctocolectomy. Dis Colon Rectum 1997;40:752–759.

134. Givel JC, Hawker P, Allan RN, Alexander-Williams J. Enterovaginal fistulae associated with Crohn's disease. Surg Gynecol Obstet 1982;155:494–496.

135. Sudol-Szopinska I, Jakubowski W, Szczepkowski M. Contrast-enhanced endosonography for the diagnosis of anal and anovaginal fistulae. J Clin Ultrasound 2002;30:145–150.

136. Stoker J, Rociu E, Schouten WR, Lameris JS. Anovaginal and rectovaginal fistulae: endoluminal sonography versus endoluminal MR imaging. Am J Roentgenol 2002;178:737–741.

137. Scott N, Nair A, Hughes L. Anorectal and rectovaginal fistula with Crohn's disease. R J Surg 1992;79:1379–1380.

138. Hesterberg R, Schmidt W, Myller F, Reher HD. Treatment of anovaginal fistulae with an anocutaneous flap in patients with Crohn's disease. Int J Colorectal Dis 1993;8:51–54.

139. Sher M, Bauer J, Gelernt I. Surgical repair of rectovaginal fistulas in patients with Crohn's disease: transvaginal approach. Dis Colon Rectum 1991;34:641–648.

140. Francois Y, Vignal J, Descos L. Outcome of perianal fistulae in Crohn's disease – value of Hughes' pathogenic classification. Int J Colorectal Dis 1993;8:39–41.

141. Faulconer HT, Muldoon JP. Rectovaginal fistula in patients with colitis: review and report of a case. Dis Colon Rectum 1975;18:413–415.

142. Hudson CN. Acquired fistulae between the intestine and the vagina. Ann Roy Coll Surg Engl 1970;46:20–40.

143. O'Leary DP, Milroy CE, Durdey P. Definitive repair of anovaginal fistula in Crohn's disease. Ann Roy Coll Surg Engl 1998;80:250–252.

144. Wiskind AK, Thompson JD. Transverse transperineal repair of rectovaginal fistulae in the lower vagina. Am J Obstet Gynecol 1992;167:694–699.

145. Cohen JL, Stricker JW, Schoetz DJ Jr, Coller JA, Veidenheimer MC. Rectovaginal fistula in Crohn's disease. Dis Colon Rectum 1989;32:825–828.

146. Bandy LC, Addison A, Parker RT. Surgical management of rectovaginal fistulae in Crohn's disease. Am J Obstet Gynecol 1983;147:359–363.

147. O'Leary DP, Milroy CE, Durdey P. Definitive repair of anovaginal fistula in Crohn's disease. Ann Roy Coll Surg Engl 1998;80:250–252.

148. Michelassi F, Melis M, Rubin M, Hurst RD. Surgical treatment of anorectal complications in Crohn's disease. Surgery 2000;128:597–603.

149. Hull TL, Fazio VW. Surgical approaches to low anovaginal fistula in Crohn's disease. Am J Surg 1997;173:95–98.

150. Ozuner G, Hull TL, Cartmill J, Fazio VW. Long-term analysis of the use of transanal rectal advancement flaps for complicated anorectal/vaginal fistulae. Dis Colon Rectum 1996;39:10–14.

151. Makowiec F, Jehle EC, Becker HD, Starlinger M. Clinical course after transanal advancement flap repair of perianal fistula in patients with Crohn's disease. Br J Surg 1995;82:603–606.

152. Ward MWN, Morgan BG, Clark CG. Treatment of persistent perianal sinus with vaginal fistula following proctocolectomy for Crohn's disease: a long-term perspective. Dis Colon Rectum 1982;28:709–711.

153. Anthony JP, Mathes SJ. The recalcitrant perineal wound after rectal extirpation. Application of muscle flap closure. Arch Surg 1990;125:1371–1377.

154. Shaw A, Futrell JW. Cure of chronic perineal sinus with gluteus maximus flap. Surg Gynecol Obstet 1978;147:417–420.

155. Achauer BM, Turpin IM, Furnas DW. Gluteal thigh flap in reconstruction of complex pelvic wounds. Arch Surg 1983;118:18–22.

156. Mann CV, Springall R. Use of muscle graft for unhealed perineal sinus. Br J Surg 1986;73:1000–1001.

157. Bartholdson L, Hulten L. Repair of persistent perineal sinuses by means of a pedicle of musculus gracilis. Scand J Reconstruct Surg 1975;9:74–76.

158. Pezim ME, Wolf BG, Woods JE, Beart RW, Listrup DM. Closure of postproctectomy perineal sinus with gracilis muscle flaps. Can J Surg 1987;30:212–214.

159. Young MRA, Small JO, Leonard AG, McKelvey STD. Rectus abdominis muscle flap for persistent perineal sinus. Br J Surg 1988;75:1228.

160. Cox MR, Parks TG, Hanna WA, Leonard AG. Closure of persistent post-proctectomy perineal sinus using a rectus muscle flap. Aust NZ J Surg 1991;61:67–71.

161. Hanauer SB, Smith MB. Rapid closure of Crohn's disease fistulae with continuous intravenous cyclosporine A. Am J Gastroenterol 1993;88:646–649.

162. Present DH, Lichtiger S. Efficacy of cyclosporine in treatment of fistula of Crohn's disease. Dig Dis Sci 1994;39:374–380.

163. van Bodegraven AA, Sloots CEJ, Felt-Bersma RJF, Meuwissen GM. Endosonographic evidence of persistence of Crohn's disease-associated fistulae after infliximab treatment, irrespective of clinical response. Dis Colon Rectum 2002; 45:39–46.

164. Talamini MA, Broe PJ, Cameron JL. Urinary fistulae in Crohn's disease. Surg Gynecol Obstet 1982;154:553–556.

165. Greenstein AJ, Sachar DB, Tzakis A, Wher L, Heimann T, Aufses AH Jr. Enterovesical fistulae occurring during the course of Crohn's disease. Am J Surg 1984;147:788–792.

166. Heyen F, Ambrose NS, Allan RN, Dykes PW, Alexander-Williams J, Keighley MR. Enterovesical fistulae in Crohn's disease. Ann Roy Coll Surg Engl 1989;71:101–104.

167. McNamara MJ, Fazio VW, Lavery IC, Weakley FL, Farmer RG. Surgical treatment of enterovesical fistulae in Crohn's disease. Dis Colon Rectum 1990;33:271–276.

168. Moss RL, Ryan JA. Management of enterovesical fistulae. Am J Surg 1990;159:514–517.

169. Manganiotis AN, Banner MP, Malkowicz SB. Urologic complications of Crohn's disease. Surg Clin North Am 2001;81:197–215.

170. Pontari MA, McMillen MA, Garvey RH, Ballantyne GH. Diagnosis and treatment of enterovesical fistulae. Am Surg 1992;58:258–263.

171. Shield DE, Lytton B, Weiss RM, Schiff M Jr. Urologic complications of inflammatory bowel disease. J Urol 1976;115:701–706.

172. Amendola MA, Agha FP, Dent TL, Amendola BE, Shirazi KK. Detection of occult colovesical fistula by the Bourne test. Am J Roentgenol 1984;142:715–718.

173. Outwater E, Schiebler ML. Pelvic fistulae: findings on MR images. Am J Roentgenol 1993;160:327–330.

174. Semelka RC, Hricak H, Kim B et al. Pelvic fistulae: appearances on MR images. Abdom Imag 1997;22:91–95.

175. Stamler JS, Bauer JJ, Janowitz HD. Rectourethroperineal fistula in Crohn's disease. Am J Gastroenterol 1985;80:111–112.

176. Fazio VW, Jones IT, Jagelman DG, Weakley FL. Rectourethral fistulae in Crohn's disease. Surg Gynecol Obstet 1987;164:148–150.

177. Kyle J, Murray CM. Ileovesical fistula in Crohn's disease. Surgery 1969;66:497–501.

178. van Dongen LM, Lubbers EJ. Fistulae of the bladder in Crohn's disease. Surg Gynecol Obstet 1984;158:308–310.

179. Schraut WH, Block GE. Enterovesical fistula complicating Crohn's ileocolitis. Am J Gastroenterol 1984;79:186–190.

180. Glass RE, Ritchie JK, Lennard-Jones JE, Hawley PR, Todd IP. Internal fistulae in Crohn's disease. Dis Colon Rectum 1985;28:557–561.

181. Margolin ML, Korelitz BI. The management of entero-vesical fistulae in Crohn's disease. Gastroenterology 1986;90:A1534.

## CHAPTER 50

# Osteoporosis

A Hillary Steinhart

## INTRODUCTION

In many patients with inflammatory bowel disease the extraintestinal features may be prominent on presentation. Although in the past much attention has been paid to the classic extraintestinal manifestations involving the joints, skin, eyes and hepatobiliary tract, there has been increasing recognition over the past decade of the potential importance of altered bone metabolism in patients with ulcerative colitis and Crohn's disease. The most common clinical presentations resulting from this altered metabolism are osteopenia, osteoporosis, and the bone fractures that are the end result of reduced bone mineral content. When bone density is reduced fractures may occur as a result of minimal trauma, or even without obvious trauma, and can result in severe pain, disability and deformity. Fractures often lead to diminished quality of life and can result in morbidity and mortality as a result of the associated pain and immobility. Alterations in bone metabolism and bone mineral content are relatively common and may be a result of genetic factors, disease-related factors, or the adverse consequences of therapy. This chapter will review the pathophysiologic mechanisms contributing to altered bone metabolism in IBD, the commonly available techniques of clinical assessment, the prevalence and natural history of reduced bone mineral content in IBD, and its prevention and treatment.

## DEFINITIONS OF OSTEOPENIA AND OSTEOPOROSIS

Osteopenia is generally defined according to the World Health Organization criteria, which bases the categorization of abnormality in an individual according to the number of standard deviations (SD) below the mean value of bone mineral density (BMD) for a young adult reference population (t-score). A t-score of less than –2.5 (i.e. more than 2.5 SD below the mean) is generally considered to be representative of osteoporosis, whereas a t-score between –1 and –2.5 is representative of osteopenia. A z-score is the number of standard deviations above or below the mean bone mineral density value of an age- and gender-matched reference population. Bone mineral density is usually measured at the hip (representative of cortical bone) and the lumbar spine (representative of cancellous or trabecular bone) using a variety of techniques. In the non-IBD general population bone mineral density has been shown to predict the risk of pathologic fractures.[1,2] The relative risk of a fracture increases by a factor of 2.6 for each standard deviation reduction in bone mineral density.[2] Similar increases in fracture risk have not been specifically demonstrated in the IBD population, but the effect of diminished BMD is generally thought to be similar to that in the postmenopausal population. A population-based study of fractures in the Canadian province of Manitoba has demonstrated an increased fracture risk in the IBD population compared to an age-matched general population.[3]

At present the dual-energy X-ray absorptiometry (DEXA) method is the most commonly used technique for measuring bone mineral density, both in the clinical arena and for the purposes of clinical investigation (Fig. 50.1). Some techniques have been more frequently used in the past (e.g. dual-photon X-ray absorptiometry, DPX) but are no longer commonly used because of issues of radiation exposure, as well as their relatively poor accuracy and predictive value relative to the newer techniques. Other techniques, such as quantitative CT scanning and ultrasound of the calcaneus and other sites,[4,5] have been reported to have advantages in certain situations and may provide information that is complementary to that obtained from DEXA.[6] However, these newer techniques are not used for routine clinical testing and have not been fully evaluated with respect to their value in predicting fracture risk, or in following response to therapy.

An important aspect of fracture risk that is not assessed by DEXA is the quality of the bone formation and the impact this may have on the resistance or susceptibility to fractures.

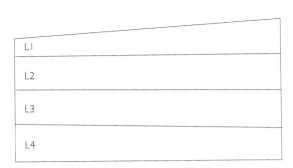

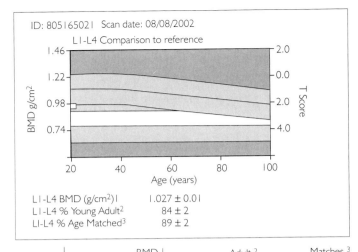

ID: 805165021  Scan date: 08/08/2002

L1-L4 Comparison to reference

| L1-L4 BMD (g/cm²)1 | 1.027 ± 0.01 |
| L1-L4 % Young Adult2 | 84 ± 2 |
| L1-L4 % Age Matched3 | 89 ± 2 |

| | | | | | Large Standard | 274.71 | Scan Mode | Medium |
| Age | 21 | | | | | | | |
| Sex | male | | | | | | | |
| Weight (Kg) | 61 | | | | | | | |
| Height Icm) | 180 | | | | | | | |
| Ethnic | White | | | | | | | |
| System | 2112 | | | | | | | |

| Age | 21 | Large Standard | 274.71 | Scan Mode | Medium |
|---|---|---|---|---|---|
| Sex | male | Medium Standard | 203.92 | Scan type | DPXIQ |
| Weight (Kg) | 61 | Small Standard | 145.62 | Collimation (mm) | 1.68 |
| Height Icm) | 180 | Low keV Air (cps) | 738867 | Sample size (mm) | 1.2 × 1.2 |
| Ethnic | White | High keV Air (cps) | 432233 | Current (μA) | 750 |
| System | 2112 | Rvalue (%Fat) | 1.390 (4.1) | | |

| Region | BMD 1 g/cm² | Young % | Adult 2 T-score | Age % | Matches 3 Z-score |
|---|---|---|---|---|---|
| L1 | 1.p031 | 89 | -1.1 | 94 | -0.5 |
| L2 | 1.066 | 86 | -1.4 | 91 | -09 |
| L3 | 1.030 | 83 | -1.7 | 88 | -1.2 |
| L4 | 0.989 | 80 | -2.1 | 84 | -1.5 |
| L1-L2 | 1.050 | 87 | -1.3 | 93 | -0.8 |
| L1-L3 | 1.042 | 86 | -1.4 | 91 | -1.0 |
| L1-L4 | 1.027 | 84 | -1.6 | 89 | -1.0 |
| L2-L3 | 1.047 | 84 | -1.6 | 89 | -1.2 |
| L2-L4 | 1.025 | 83 | -1.8 | 87 | -1.41 |
| L3-L4 | 1.009 | 81 | -1.9 | 86 | |

1-see appendix on precision and accuracy.
   Statistically 68% of repeat scans will fall within 1 SD. (±0.01 g/cm²)
2-USA  AP Spine Reference Population, Young Adult ages 20-40. See Appendices.
3-Matched for Age, Weight (25-100g), Ethnic.

**Fig. 50.1**  Dual-energy X-ray absorptiometry report of a 21-year-old male with newly diagnosed untreated ileocolic Crohn's disease and 4 weeks of symptoms prior to evaluation. Bone density is reported as absolute amount (g/cm²), t-score (number of standard deviations above or below a young adult standard) and z-score (number of standard deviations above or below an age matched control mean). This report shows evidence of osteopenia of the lumbar spine but normal bone mineral content in the hip (femur).

Although bone mineral density is generally predictive of bone strength and risk of fractures, it is generally accepted that there are other features of bone quality, not measured by DEXA, that may influence resistance to fractures. These features, such as bone microarchitecture, may be captured by other methods of evaluation, such as ultrasound or computerized spectral analysis of bone radiographs,[6,7] but these have yet to be shown to be capable of either replacing DEXA or providing complementary information that can significantly alter clinical practice.

Much of the variation among studies in reporting the prevalence of osteopenia and osteoporosis in inflammatory bowel disease almost certainly relates to the different techniques used to measure bone mineral density, the different sites reported, and how the results were reported (i.e. Crohn's disease alone, ulcerative colitis alone, or all inflammatory bowel disease).

# NORMAL BONE METABOLISM AND PATHOGENESIS OF OSTEOPOROSIS IN IBD

Bone is a metabolically active tissue that undergoes constant remodeling, involving the simultaneous resorption of existing bone and the formation of new bone. Under normal circumstances the balance between resorption and formation is tightly regulated to maintain the normal strength and physical properties of bone. The basic unit of interacting bone cells involved in maintaining the equilibrium is the bone remodeling unit (Fig. 50.2). The remodeling unit consists of osteocytes, osteoblasts and osteoclasts. Remodeling consists of a continuous cycle of resorption, reversal, formation and mineralization. The remodeling process is influenced by a number of factors, such as activity, weight bearing, local and systemic hormonal levels and cytokine levels.

## OSTEOBLASTS

The osteoblasts are the bone-forming cells that synthesize the organic matrix upon which mineralization occurs. The predominant component of the matrix is type I collagen, with a small amount of other proteins, including osteonectin and osteocalcin. As osteoblasts create bone matrix they become trapped within it and transform into osteocytes.

## OSTEOCLASTS

The osteoclasts are large, multinucleated cells derived from monocyte–macrophage stem cell lines. The primary function of osteoclasts is bone resorption through the secretion of acid proteinases, and maintenance of a low pH in the local environment

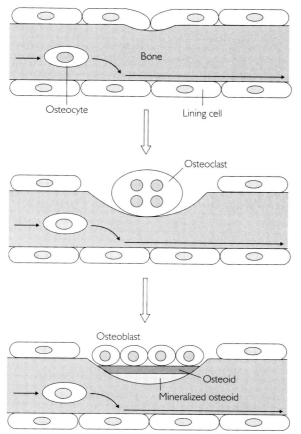

Fig. 50.2 Bone remodeling unit with mature osteoclasts causing bone resorption adjacent to osteoblasts laying down new osteoid (solid area), which becomes mineralized to form mineralized bone (hatched area) containing mature osteocytes.

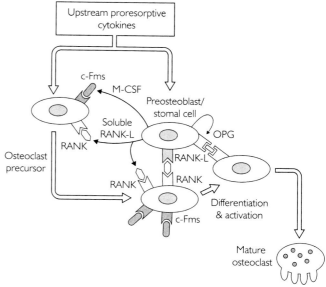

Fig. 50.3 Differentiation of preosteoclasts to mature osteoclasts requires the binding of RANK on the surface of osteoclastic precursor cells to RANK ligand (RANK-L) on the surface of preosteoblastic/stromal cells (membrane bound) or secreted by the same cells (soluble RANK-L). This process also requires the production of M-CSF produced by the preosteoblastic cells. M-CSF binds to its receptor, c-Fms, on the osteoclast precursor cells. Osteoprotegerin (OPG) can block osteoclast development by binding RANK-L and blocking its effect on RANK. Several proresorptive cytokines, such as IL-1 and TNF-α, directly increase RANK-L expression on preosteoblast cells, whereas other cytokines and hormones exert their effect through modulation of OPG production or a combination of altered RANK-L and OPG production. (Reproduced with permission from [11].)

via a proton pump at its cell surface. Proinflammatory cytokines such as IL-1 and IL-6 have been shown to result in increased osteoclast differentiation and function, as discussed below.

## EFFECTS OF HORMONES, CYTOKINES AND CELLULAR MESSENGERS ON BONE FORMATION

Parathyroid hormone (PTH) is thought to be a key mediator of bone metabolism and mineral balance in the body. PTH results in bone resorption through effects mediated via osteoblasts. When preosteoblast stromal cells and osteoblasts are continuously exposed to PTH the production of matrix is inhibited and they are stimulated to produce proteins and cytokines, such as tumor necrosis factor-α (TNF-α), IL-1, IL-6, IL-11, receptor activator of NFκB ligand (RANK-L) and osteoprotegerin (OPG). These cytokines and molecules can influence the differentiation of osteoclast precursors, which ultimately results in increased bone resorption. It is through modulation and alteration of the activity of these molecules and cytokines that chronic systemic inflammatory disorders, such as IBD, are thought to have an effect on bone metabolism.[8] IL-1, IL-6, IL-11 and TNF-α all result in the generation of new osteoclasts, whereas OPG binds to RANK ligand (RANK-L), thereby preventing it from binding to the RANK receptor on preosteoclast macrophages and preventing the development of osteoclasts which, in turn, reduces bone resorption (Fig. 50.3). IL-1 and TNF-α have been shown

to increase the gene expression of RANK-L and can increase bone resorption through its effect on the RANK receptor and osteoclastogenesis.[9] Some of the effects of 1,25-dihydroxyvitamin $D_3$, estrogen and glucocorticoids on bone formation and resorption are mediated, in part, via the OPG/RANK/RANK-L system.[10–13]

Calcitonin is a peptide hormone that binds directly to receptors on osteoclasts, resulting in inhibition of osteoclast activity and a reduction in bone resorption. Gonadal steroid hormones generally result in increased bone formation, and drugs or conditions that interfere with their secretion or action may result in loss of bone mineral density. This is one of the postulated mechanisms whereby glucocorticoids exert a negative effect on bone density.

## EFFECTS OF INFLAMMATORY BOWEL DISEASE ON BONE MINERAL CONTENT

The reduction in bone mineral density that may be seen in patients with IBD is generally felt to be multifactorial and is probably due to a complex interaction between genetic susceptibility, chronic systemic inflammation, dietary changes, changes in sex hormone secretion, altered intestinal absorptive physiology and the deleterious effects of treatments such as glucocorticoids (Fig. 50.4). The relative contribution of the various

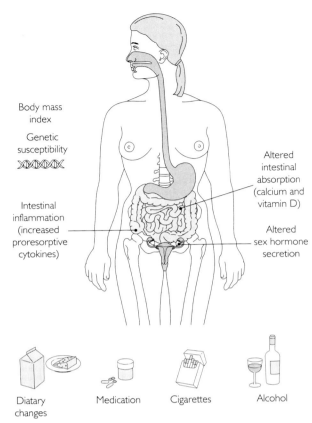

Body mass index

Genetic susceptibility

Intestinal inflammation (increased proresorptive cytokines)

Altered intestinal absorption (calcium and vitamin D)

Altered sex hormone secretion

Diatary changes    Medication    Cigarettes    Alcohol

**Fig. 50.4** Factors that potentially contribute to the loss of bone mineral content in patients with inflammatory bowel disease. The influence of these factors may not be independent of one another (e.g. intestinal inflammation can have direct effects on bone metabolism via proresorptive cytokines, but may also cause abdominal pain, which can alter dietary intake with respect to both quantity and type of foods).

postulated factors has not been precisely determined, but they have each individually been examined and found to be significant predictors of bone mineral density, either in IBD or in other clinical scenarios.

## GENETICS AND BONE MINERAL DENSITY

It has been demonstrated in non-IBD mother–daughter pairs that bone density, as measured by DEXA or calcaneal ultrasound, is partially determined by genetic factors.[14] The estimated heritability of bone density – in other words the proportion of the variability in bone density that is attributable to inherited factors – is between 34% and 63%.[14] However, to some extent markers of bone and mineral metabolism can be altered by interventions such as increased calcium intake, so that individuals who are genetically predisposed to develop osteoporosis may be able to significantly reduce their future risk.[15] The collagen 1A1 (COL1A1) gene has been shown, in non-IBD populations, to predict bone density and strength.[16] Individuals who are 'Ss' heterozygotes at the polymorphic Sp1 binding site have reduced bone strength compared to 'SS' homozygotes.[16] It is likely that changes in the synthesis or degradation of type I collagen is also associated with loss of bone density in the IBD patient population.[17] Other genes that have been postulated as having a role in determining bone mineral density in the non-IBD population include the vitamin D receptor and, in the IBD

population, genes regulating or modulating immune response, such as IL-1, IL-1 receptor antagonist, IL-6 and TNF-α, have been considered as likely candidates for determinants of bone mineral density. This is because increased levels or activities of the proinflammatory cytokines, or decreased levels of the anti-inflammatory cytokines, such as IL-1 receptor antagonist, may result in decreased bone formation and/or increased bone resorption. Where polymorphisms in these genes result in altered levels or biological activity of the protein product it is possible that such polymorphisms may, in turn, affect bone mineral metabolism.

## SYSTEMIC INFLAMMATION AND ALTERED BONE MINERAL DENSITY

As discussed above there are a number of cytokines and inflammatory mediators that may affect bone metabolism. Patients with active Crohn's disease demonstrate higher levels of biochemical markers of bone turnover independent of drug therapy.[18] Indirect evidence that the inflammatory mileu in IBD, with its increased proinflammatory cytokines, can affect bone metabolism is derived from an experimental model in which serum from children with IBD was placed into an in vitro bone model.[19] Serum from patients with Crohn's disease, but not from those with ulcerative colitis, resulted in reduced bone formation in a rat parietal cell culture system. Serum from IBD patients had no effect on bone resorption. Levels of IL-6 did not correlate with measures of bone resorption or formation, suggesting that other unmeasured soluble factors in the serum of IBD patients influence bone metabolism. These factors may also affect bone strength in other ways. In the latter study, histologic examination of the cultured bone showed disorganization between osteoid and mineral and morphologically abnormal osteoblasts when the bone was cultured in the presence of serum from Crohn's disease patients.[19] Proinflammatory cytokines may exert some of their effects on bone metabolism via alterations induced in the osteoprotegerin, RANK and RANK ligand system, which is critical in maintaining appropriately function bone remodeling.[8,9,11]

## NUTRITIONAL EFFECTS

Patients with small intestinal Crohn's disease who have an extensive length of inflamed small bowel, or who have had previous small bowel resections, may have alterations of vitamin or mineral absorption which may, over time, result in diminished bone density. Reduced absorption of calcium, magnesium and vitamin D can all contribute to a reduction in bone mineral content through the resulting increased bone resorption that occurs in order to maintain mineral homeostasis and normal serum and tissue levels of these minerals. Although serum calcium levels are generally normal in patients with inflammatory bowel disease, some studies have found decreased vitamin D levels in a significant proportion of patients.[18,20]

## MEDICAL THERAPY

Of all of the drugs used to treat inflammatory bowel disease, glucocorticoids are the one class of therapy that has been clearly associated with accelerated loss of bone mineral density.[21] There is some evidence from renal transplant patients that cyclosporin may increase bone loss.[22] Other IBD therapies, such as sulfasalazine, 5-aminosalicylic acid, antibiotics, azathioprine,

6-mercaptopurine, methotrexate and infliximab, have not been shown to result in an increased rate of bone loss, either in patients with inflammatory bowel disease or in patients with other disorders. The relationship between glucocorticoid use, disease activity and bone loss is complex, and the interaction among these factors has not been completely defined (see below). Although glucocorticoid therapy can clearly cause loss of bone mineral density it has also been demonstrated that a significant proportion of Crohn's disease patients who have never been treated with glucocorticoids have osteopenia or osteoporosis.[23] In rheumatoid arthritis, where disease activity itself has been shown to produce osteopenia and osteoporosis, the use of glucocorticoids has been shown to be an independent risk factor for loss of bone mass.[24] This loss appears to be most rapid in the first few months of therapy, and doses of prednisone at or below 10 mg/day appear to produce minimal or no loss of bone mass.[24]

There are several purported mechanisms of glucocorticoid action on bone density.[25] These include a direct effect on osteoblasts, osteoclasts and osteocytes, with a net result of decreased bone turnover and repair; reduced intestinal calcium absorption; increased renal calcium excretion; resistance to the effects of PTH; and suppression of gonadal sex hormone secretion. The rate of onset of some of these changes suggest that many are not related to steroid-induced genomic events but are possibly due to direct effects of glucocorticoids on cellular membranes and cell function.[25]

## PREVALENCE OF REDUCED BONE MINERAL DENSITY IN IBD

The prevalence of reduced bone mineral density in patients with IBD is generally higher than that found in an age- and gender-matched population. A great deal of variation exists in the reported prevalence among different cross-sectional studies, but rates as high as 77% have been reported in some populations of patients with inflammatory bowel diseases[18,23,26–49] (Table 50.1). This is probably due to differences in the method of patient recruitment and ascertainment, the differences in the methods of assessing and defining low bone density, and the differences in the populations from which the patients were drawn.

It appears that the prevalence of osteopenia and osteoporosis is higher in Crohn's disease than in ulcerative colitis.[38] Cross-sectional studies have reported the prevalence of reduced bone density to be between 3% and 92% in patients with Crohn's disease,[27–30] and between 0% and 85% in patients with ulcerative colitis.[27,28,36] The majority of patients with low bone mineral content are classified as having osteopenia (t-score between −1 and −2.5). The prevalence of osteoporosis (t-score less than −2.5) has not been reported to be higher than 43% in ulcerative colitis and 59% in Crohn's disease, with all but one study[35] reporting the prevalence of osteoporosis in UC and CD at no more than 18% and 37%, respectively.[27,28,35,37] Despite the occasional outlying studies[35,39] the risk of osteopenia and osteoporosis in ulcerative colitis does not appear to be higher than that of an age- and gender-matched population unless the patient has been treated with glucocorticosteroids.[27] Although indicators of increased bone turnover may be found in ulcerative colitis in the absence of glucocorticoid therapy, osteopenia is usually associated with the use of glucocorticoids.[27] In addition, it appears that patients with ulcerative colitis do not demonstrate reduced

bone mineral content at the time of diagnosis, whereas patients with Crohn's disease have a mean bone mineral content that is lower than that of patients with ulcerative colitis and lower than in the general population.[36] These observations suggest that some feature of Crohn's disease – perhaps the nature or degree of the systemic inflammatory response, or the effect of the disease on mineral or vitamin absorption – results in changes in bone metabolism and bone mineral loss, whereas in ulcerative colitis the different systemic inflammatory response and lack of effect on mineral or vitamin absorption does not lead to such changes.

The reduction in bone mineral content observed in IBD appears to be different between bone sites when examined both within individuals and within patient groups (as mean z-scores or t-scores). Such variation may not be specific to the osteopenia and osteoporosis associated with disease states but may, in fact, be seen in non-IBD populations who are screened for bone mineral loss.[50] This variation between sites within an individual appears to occur more often in females and in the elderly. Some studies have suggested that inflammatory bowel disease results in a preferential reduction in bone mineral content at the hip,[29,51] whereas others have found equivalent prevalence of bone loss at both the hip and the lumbar spine in patients with Crohn's disease.[30,33] Irrespective of the precise frequency of discordance between sites, the frequency of this discrepancy is high enough to warrant evaluation of bone mineral content at both hip and spine in patients with IBD undergoing evaluation for osteopenia or osteoporosis.

## FRACTURE RISK IN IBD

Although it is well documented that IBD patients have a prevalence of bone loss higher than that observed in the general age-matched population, the precise consequence of this, in terms of fracture risk, is not completely known. Data from postmenopausal women with osteoporosis clearly document an increased fracture risk that is proportionate to the decrease in bone mineral content. This risk approximately doubles for every standard deviation reduction in the bone mineral content. However, other factors, such as bone architecture and fragility, patient instability, and type and level of patient activity, contribute to fracture risk. These other factors may not necessarily be the same in the postmenopausal women and in patients with IBD and, as a result, extrapolating the fracture risk data from the postmenopausal to the IBD population may not be applicable, particularly when therapeutic interventions are applied.

In a retrospective survey of 245 patients with IBD the prevalence of fractures was found to be higher than expected.[18] However, in a Canadian population-based study which used an administrative database to identify all patients with IBD and all those with fractures, the patients with IBD had a 40% increase in the risk of fractures compared to a population of individuals matched for gender, age and geographic location.[3] To some these results would represent only a minimal increase in the absolute risk of fracture. However, the absolute increase in risk becomes more significant as patients become older. An important caveat associated with this type of population-based study was the fact that the prevalence of reduced bone mineral content in the IBD population was not reported and, as such, the study could not address the question of whether IBD patients with low bone mineral content have increased fracture risk, or what that risk

## Table 50.1 Studies of prevalence of reduced bone mineral content in IBD

| Study Author (ref) | Number of patients CD/UC/IBD | Method of evaluation | Bone mineral content (t-score#/z-score*) | | Osteopenia (%) | Osteoporosis (%) (*z < −2;#t < −2.5) |
|---|---|---|---|---|---|---|
| | | | Femoral neck | Lumbar spine | | |
| Compston[32] | 46/17/12 | SPA/CT | – | – | – | 30.7 * |
| Clements[31] | 33/17/– | SPA | – | – | – | 12* (CD) 6* (UC) |
| Pigot[61] | 27/34/– | DEXA | CD −0.83* UC −0.70 | CD −1.11* UC −0.93 | – | 23* |
| Ghosh[36] | 15/15/– | DEXA | – | CD −1.06* UC −0.03 | | – |
| Scharla[42] | 15/4/– | DPA | – | −0.6* | – | 0* |
| Abitbol[23] | 34/50/– | DEXA | −0.69* | −0.73 | 43 (t < −1) | – |
| Bernstein[28] | 26/23/– | DEXA | CD −1.5* UC −1.1 | CD −1.1* UC −1.0 | 43–64 (z < −1) | 4–36* |
| Roux[41] | 14/21/– | DEXA | CD −1.01* UC −0.28 | CD −1.12* UC −0.37 | 43 (z < −1) | 20* |
| Silvennoinen[47] | 78/67/7 | DEXA | CD −0.42* UC −0.38 IC 0.47 | CD −0.18* UC 0.36 IC 1.06 | – | 5.3* |
| Bischoff[18] | 61/22/7 | QCT radius | CD −0.76 UC −0.50 (radius) | – | 45 (z < −1) | – |
| Bjarnason[29] | 44/35/– | DEXA | −1.92# | −0.93# | 54–78 (t < −1) | 18–29# |
| Cowan[33] | 21/11/– | DEXA | – | – | 41–47 (z < −1) | – |
| Jahnsen[38] | 60/60/– | DEXA | CD −0.74* UC 0.12 | CD −0.39* UC 0.17 | CD 40 UC 22 (z < −1) | CD 15* UC 8 |
| Staun[48] | 108/–/– | DPA | – | No colectomy −0.51* Colectomy −0.80 | – | 10–23* |
| Robinson[57] | 117/–/– | DEXA | −0.20* | −0.09* | 40 (z < −1) | 11* |
| Schulte[45] | 104/45/– | DEXA | – | – | CD 36 UC 32 (t < −1) | CD 15# UC 7 |
| Andreassen[26] | 113/–/– | DEXA | – | – | – | 3# |
| Dinca[34] | 54/49/– | DEXA | – | CD −0.9* UC −0.63 | CD 48 UC 38 (t < −1) | CD 6# UC 6 |
| Semeao[46] | 119/–/– | DEXA | – | M −1.48* F −1.08 | – | M 39* F 21 |
| Ardizzone[27] | 51/40/– | DEXA | CD −1.80# UC −1.60 | CD −1.49# UC −1.67 | CD 55 UC 67 (t < −1) | CD 37# UC 18 |
| Chinea[30] | 66/–/– | DEXA | – | – | 68–69 (z < −1) | – |
| Dresner-Pollak[35] | 22/14/– | DEXA | CD −2.49# UC −2.09 | CD −2.26# UC −1.6# | – | CD 59# UC 43 |
| Lee[39] | 14/25/– | DEXA | CD 0.03* UC 0.14 | CD −0.61* UC −0.58 | – | CD 0# UC 8 |
| Schoon[44] | 24/44/– | DEXA | – | – | CD 0 UC 0 (at diagnosis) | – |
| Schoon[43] | 119/–/– | DEXA | −0.96# | −0.42# | 45 (t < −1) | 13# |
| Ulivieri[49] | –/43/– | DEXA | – | M −0.59* F −0.05 | – | – |
| Habtezion[37] | 168/–/– | DEXA | −0.78# | −0.87# | 40–45 (t < −1) | 10–11# |

is relative to non-IBD individuals. It is possible that, being a population-based sample of patients, the mean disease severity and use of corticosteroids were relatively low, and as a result these patients may have had better bone mineral content than that found in other study populations. If a significant proportion of the IBD population did, in fact, have normal bone mineral content it would have been difficult to demonstrate an increase in the overall rate of fractures.

Another case–control study of over 15 000 Danish IBD patients found a slightly increased fracture risk in CD but not UC patients both prior to and after diagnosis.[52] Once again, similar arguments about the nature of the population studied and their background bone mineral content become important in interpreting the results of the study and how to apply the results in the clinical setting.

Based on the studies of fracture risk, it seems reasonable to conclude that IBD patients with reduced bone mineral content are at increased risk and, therefore, merit further consideration and intervention, particularly when bone loss is progressive or accelerated.

This may also be particularly important in the pediatric age group, where clinically important fractures have been reported in patients with reduced bone mineral content.[53] It is also important to be aware that the overall increase in fractures in the IBD population is not huge, and efforts toward fracture prevention should be focused upon the patients at highest risk.

## PROGRESSION OF BONE LOSS IN IBD

Although cross-sectional studies of bone mineral content in IBD have suggested that osteopenia and osteoporosis are frequent occurrences, longitudinal studies have not consistently demonstrated progressive loss of bone mineral content over time in IBD patients. There are a number of possible explanations for this apparent dichotomy. First, once bone mineral loss reaches a given point in an individual there may be no further loss, and measures of bone mineral content may be stable thereafter. Second, the longitudinal studies may have been too short in duration of follow-up and/or too small in the number of patients studied to detect a true reduction in bone mineral content. Third, once tested for bone mineral content, both patients and the treating physicians may have become more aware of the problem and may have taken steps to intervene, particularly in the patients with the lowest bone mineral content.

Although aggregate data have suggested that accelerated loss of bone mineral content does not occur in IBD patients, or only at a rate that is only slightly above that of an age- and gender-matched population, clinical experience suggests that there is a subset of patients that progressively loses bone mass at a rapid rate. In some cases it is the effect of glucocorticoid therapy that seems to accelerate bone loss, or at least permits it to occur,[54] but in others there is no obvious underlying predisposing factor other than the bowel disease itself or its metabolic consequences that may play a role in the pathogenesis of osteopenia and osteoporosis.[31,48,55]

Because progressive age-related reduction in mean bone mass is seen universally in healthy populations it would be surprising if it were not observed in the IBD population. Reductions in bone mineral content have been observed in IBD patients when followed over periods averaging 7 years.[31] These reductions were greater in women and, in particular, postmenopausal women. In addition, it was found that normal bone density at initial evaluation does not necessarily guarantee against accelerated bone loss over time.[31] Not all longitudinal studies have confirmed accelerated bone loss in the IBD patient population,[56] and some have demonstrated significant bone mineral loss at specific bone sites (e.g. the femoral neck).[48]

## PREVENTION OF OSTEOPENIA AND OSTEOPOROSIS IN IBD

Although loss of bone mass is, as discussed above, a frequent occurrence in patients with inflammatory bowel disease, a significant proportion of patients do not have abnormally low bone mineral content at the time of diagnosis, and the large majority are not at significantly increased fracture risk at the time of diagnosis. The prolonged preclinical stage of osteopenia and osteoporosis opens the door for potential 'preventative' therapy. Although many patients may demonstrate radiologic evidence of bone mineral loss the clinically relevant endpoint of fracture has yet to occur in most, and can potentially be prevented in these patients.

### RISK STRATIFICATION

The first step in instituting preventative therapy is identifying those patients who are at particularly high risk of future fractures (i.e. those who are higher risk of rapid progression of osteoporosis and those who have existing severe loss of bone mass). There are some specific clinical risk factors that assist in estimating a patient's future risk of osteoporosis and fracture (Table 50.2). Some of these are related to the IBD itself, whereas others are independent of IBD and its activity level. Patients with Crohn's disease appear to be more likely to develop osteoporosis, or to have it at diagnosis, whereas those with ulcerative colitis, in particular those with distal or left-sided disease, are less likely to develop accelerated bone loss.[36,38] Disease extent and location in Crohn's disease may also influence the risk of osteoporosis, with extensive small bowel disease or severe inflammatory disease being important factors.[37] Low body mass index correlates strongly with low bone mineral content.[37] Gender does not appear to be particularly discriminating, and it is well recognized that males with IBD are also at significant risk of developing osteopenia or osteoporosis.[57] Unrecognized, or poorly studied, risk factors possibly related to bone mineral loss in IBD are age of onset of disease, smoking, family history, physical activity level and diet. However, there is evidence from non-IBD populations that physical inactivity, weight loss and low body weight are all predictive of an increased risk of fracture.[58]

Those patients who are deemed to be at high risk of developing osteoporosis, or those who already have abnormal bone mineral content, should undergo formal evaluation of their complete bone metabolism risk profile, as outlined in Table 50.3. These patients require a baseline bone density measurement and modification of any risk factors that can be modified.

### ROLE OF GLUCOCORTICOID THERAPY IN BONE MINERAL LOSS

The precise role of glucocorticoids in the pathogenesis of bone mineral loss in patients with IBD remains to be clearly defined. Although some studies suggest that a history of glucocorticoid use

## Table 50.2 Risk factors for the development of osteoporosis

**Genetic factors**
Family history of osteoporosis
**Disease factors**
Crohn's disease
Ulcerative colitis
Severity of disease activity
Extent of disease
Presence of small intestinal disease
Associated liver disease
**Medication**
Glucocorticoids
**Endocrine**
Postmenopausal status
Amenorrhea or irregular menstrual cycle
Hypogonadism
Hyperthyroidism
Hyperparathyroidism (primary or secondary)
**Diet/nutrition**
Inadequate calcium intake
Inadequate vitamin D intake (with lack of sun exposure)
Low body mass index (malnutrition)
**Lifestyle**
Physical activity
Smoking
Alcohol
**Renal**
Hypercalciuria

## Table 50.3 Initial bone evaluation of IBD patients

**History**
Family history of osteoporosis or fractures
Menstrual history (women)/infertility (men)
Disease history (disease activity, surgical resections)
Medication history (especially glucocorticoids, cyclosporine, hormone replacement therapy/oral contraceptive, antiresorptive therapy)
Lifestyle (activity, alcohol, smoking)
**Physical examination**
Anthropometric measures (height, weight, body mass index, percentage body fat)
Evidence of bony deformity (kyphosis)
**Bone density evaluation**
Dual-energy X-ray absorptiometry (DEXA) of hip and lumbar spine
**Laboratory evaluation**
Complete blood count
Serum electrolytes
Serum creatinine
Serum calcium
Serum phosphorus
Serum alkaline phosphatase
Serum albumin
Serum AST/ALT
**Laboratory evaluation (for patients with demonstrated loss of bone mineral content)**
Serum 25-OH vitamin D
Serum PTH
Serum testosterone (males)
Serum luteinizing hormone (females)
Urinary calcium (24 hour collection)

does not correlate with bone loss in patients with IBD,[36,37,48,51] many others have demonstrated a direct relationship between the use of glucocorticoids – and, where studied, the total dose – and bone loss.[28,32,38,40,41,47,59-61] However, none of these studies has adequately separated the effects of inflammatory disease activity and glucocorticoid therapy on bone mineral content. Because it is quite likely that glucocorticoid therapy is a marker for more severe and more sustained intestinal inflammatory activity, only a prospective study that carefully measures disease activity and glucocorticoid use over time can adequately answer the question of whether glucocorticoid use is an independent risk factor for osteopenia and osteoporosis. Notwithstanding these considerations, it is apparent that in non-IBD populations glucocorticoids are associated with an increase in the rate of bone mineral loss and the development of osteopenia and osteoporosis.[24] There is no reason to believe that the situation would be different in the IBD population, although it is apparent that there is considerable interindividual variability with respect to the effect of glucocorticoid therapy on bone metabolism and bone mineral loss in the IBD patient population. A significant proportion of this variability is probably due to genetic factors.[14,16,62,63]

Irrespective of the precise estimate of the independent risk attributed to the use of glucocorticoids in IBD patients, it is reasonable to suggest that patients receiving glucocorticoids, particularly for extended periods, be considered for preventative or prophylactic therapy and closely monitored for rapid bone mineral loss. Because the most rapid loss of bone mineral content tends to occur in the first 6 months of glucocorticoid therapy, decisions regarding preventative therapy should probably be made as close to the time of start of therapy as possible.

Use of the minimum effective dose has been advocated as an effective means of preventing glucocorticoid-induced osteoporosis.[64] However, the evidence that this is effective preventative therapy in patients with IBD is not strong, and the recommendations have generally been based on indirect lines of evidence such as the association, in some studies, between the use of glucocorticoids or their lifetime dose, and the presence of osteopenia and osteoporosis. This recommendation is also based upon data from the rheumatic disorders, where it has been found that prednisone in doses of 10 mg/day or less are associated with very little or no reduction in bone mineral content.[24] It has also been suggested that the use of newer glucocorticoids, such as budesonide, which are highly topically active in the intestinal mucosa but which undergo high first-pass metabolism in the liver to inactive metabolites, might minimize the bone loss that can be seen in patients receiving conventional systemic glucocorticoids. Randomized trials of non-absorbed inhaled topical glucocorticoids in patients with asthma have generally not shown an effect on bone mineral density.[65] It is not clear whether the use of glucocorticoids that are topically active at the level of the intestinal mucosa in patients with IBD will be as safe as topical respiratory glucocorticoids in asthma. When bone mineral density was examined over the course of 2 years in a group of 48 patients with quiescent CD who were receiving chronic budesonide therapy, the rate of decline of bone mineral density was found to be greater than that observed in patients receiving non-steroid therapy.[66] In addition, the loss of bone mineral density appeared to be greater, although not statistically significantly so, than that observed in a group of 45 patients with quiescent CD receiving chronic prednisone at a mean dose of 10.5 mg daily. This difference occurred despite the fact that significantly more patients on prednisone were taking calcium supplementation than were those on budesonide. Other disease features were not different among the patient groups. However, at the time patients were entered into the study the patients receiving budesonide had been on therapy for a mean of between 4 and 5 months, whereas those in the prednisone group had been on the glucocorticoid therapy for a mean of 3.5 years. As patients in the budesonide group were relatively early on in the course of their therapy they may have still been in the more rapid phase of bone loss, whereas those in the prednisone group were in a more stable phase where bone loss might be expected to be less rapid. These considerations notwithstanding, the study demonstrates that the use of non-systemic glucocorticoids may not be an effective means of preventing glucocorticoid-induced bone loss.

## CALCIUM AND VITAMIN D THERAPY FOR PREVENTION OF OSTEOPOROSIS

Vitamin D levels have been reported to be low in some patients with IBD.[20,67–69] This finding has been more common in the CD population, where up to 65% have been found to have low 25-OH vitamin D levels in serum.[18,20,69,70] Unfortunately, many of the studies did not adequately account for the season in which the samples were drawn and, as a result, the effect of seasonal sunlight on endogenous vitamin D production may have been overlooked. Despite the low serum of levels of vitamin D found in some patients, clinical osteomalacia is a rare occurrence and the vitamin D levels do not necessarily correlate with PTH levels or bone mineral content.[68] When used therapeutically to prevent bone loss, vitamin D at a dose of 1000 IU/day may have a modest effect but, interestingly, in one study the largest benefit was observed in the subgroup of patients with normal serum vitamin D levels.[71] In non-IBD patients the use of vitamin D 50 000 IU/week (plus calcium 1000 mg/day) resulted in a small, but not statistically significant, reduction in the rate of bone loss in the lumbar spine over the first year in patients starting prednisone for the treatment of rheumatoid disease.[72] This effect appeared to be lost between 1 and 3 years of therapy.

For the most part, serum calcium levels are normal in patients with IBD.[18,42] However, many patients have suboptimal dietary intake of calcium and, as a result, have a progressive loss of total body calcium.[73,74] The normal homeostatic mechanisms probably serve to keep the serum calcium levels normal, but this may be at the cost of increased bone resorption.[70] Nevertheless, dietary calcium intake in IBD patients has not been shown to correlate with bone mineral content.[74] In a subset of patients with IBD taking glucocorticoids, dietary calcium has also not been shown to correlate with loss of bone mineral content.[75] In that study the administration of a daily supplement of 1000 mg of calcium and 250 IU of vitamin D produced no improvement in bone mineral content over a period of 1 year.[75] The use of calcium supplementation has not been studied as preventative therapy in patients with IBD who are starting glucocorticoid therapy, but maintenance of adequate calcium intake (1500 mg/day), if necessary through the use of supplementation, is generally advocated. Although there is not sufficient evidence to make a firm recommendation, vitamin D supplementation is also advocated for patients starting glucocorticoid therapy.

## BISPHOSPHONATE THERAPY FOR PREVENTION OF OSTEOPOROSIS

Bisphosphonates, such as alendronate, etidronate and risedronate, are recognized as effective treatments of postmenopausal osteoporosis and have been shown to increase bone mineral content and reduce the risk of fractures in these patients.[76,77] Several studies have also demonstrated that these agents prevent glucocorticoid-induced bone loss in a variety of inflammatory disorders in which the long-term use of glucocorticoids is required.[78–81] These studies have generally included either no patients with IBD or only a small minority with IBD, and as a result no conclusions can be drawn about their safety or efficacy in the IBD population. That notwithstanding, in non-IBD patients the bisphosphonates are considered to be the treatment of choice for the prevention and treatment of glucocorticoid-induced osteoporosis.[82] However, there are concerns about the use of this class of medication in patients with inflammatory bowel disease, given the documented detrimental effects of some bisphosphonates on the upper gastrointestinal mucosa.[83] Despite these concerns the bisphosphonates have not been shown to result in an increase in the frequency or severity of disease flares, nor is there an increased incidence of gastrointestinal side effects in the IBD patient population compared with the non-IBD population. In a randomized placebo controlled trial of alendronate 10 mg daily in 32 patients with Crohn's disease and a *t*-score less than −1 the use of the bisphosphonate medication was not associated with an increase in adverse events or disease exacerbations, and a significant improvement in bone density at the lumbar spine was observed relative to placebo.[84] No information is available on the effect of bisphosphonates on fracture occurrence in IBD patients. The use of bisphosphonates in IBD patients treated with glucocorticoids but who have normal baseline bone mineral content has also not been studied. However, when the baseline bone density is abnormal (i.e. *t*-score below −1) prior to initiation of glucocorticoids the use of a bisphosphonate should be considered as standard preventative therapy.

The safety of bisphosphonates in children and in women of childbearing potential is not known. It is known that bisphosphonates are contraindicated during pregnancy because of their potential deleterious effect on fetal bone formation. The concern that relates to the use of bisphosphonates in young women is that they bind to hydroxyapatite in bone, and that following discontinuation of therapy the bisphosphonate can be released over many months or years as bone turns over, as only 10% of bone is remodeled each year. The bisphosphonate that is released from bone may then be available to the fetus, where it can theoretically produce skeletal abnormalities.

## THERAPY OF ESTABLISHED OSTEOPOROSIS IN IBD

Once osteoporosis is established there may be an opportunity to halt or reverse the process of bone loss. The assessment of the bone metabolism risk profile is similar to that described above (Table 50.3), but extra attention also needs to be paid to the possibility of fractures in the past or at the time of initial evaluation. Where risk factors or causative factors are found they should, if possible, be corrected.

The use of calcium, vitamin D and exercise may reduce the rate of further bone loss, but these measures do not usually reverse already existing bone loss. Maintenance or recovery of a normal body mass index and optimization of nutritional status may also be helpful in minimizing loss of bone mass but, once again, it is not known whether this will result in an increase in bone mineral content.

Control of disease activity, through either medical or surgical means, may halt and reverse loss of bone mineral content through a reduction in the production and release or an increase in degradation of inflammatory cytokines or mediators. In patients with ulcerative colitis who undergo colectomy and ileal pouch–anal anastomosis an increase in bone mineral content of 2.1–2.3% per year can be observed.[85] Similar beneficial responses secondary to small intestinal resection in Crohn's disease have not been observed, but resection is not, by itself, associated with accelerated bone loss.[48] It might be expected that limited small intestinal resection for Crohn's disease may be helpful in reducing the rate of bone loss by controlling disease activity, improving nutritional status and reducing the need for glucocorticoid therapy. However, patients with diffuse small bowel disease and multiple small intestinal resections may be at risk of osteoporosis.[40] This is probably a reflection of the long-term or chronic disease activity and inflammation, and the nutritional or absorptive effects of diffuse small intestinal disease or multiple resections on bone and mineral metabolism. It would seem, therefore, that the effect of small intestinal resection on bone mineral content is a fine balance between the positive effect on the control of inflammatory activity and the negative effect on absorptive capacity and vitamin and mineral metabolism.

The effect of long-term control of disease activity on bone mineral content, through the use of immunomodulatory agents such as azathioprine, 6-mercaptopurine and methotrexate, has not been specifically examined. It might be expected that improved control of disease activity, as is often achieved by immunomodulator therapy, will minimize or prevent the bone loss that occurs as a result of the effects of the systemic inflammation in IBD. However, when the use of these agents has been studied a weak association between their use and the occurrence of bone loss has been found by some investigators,[86] whereas other investigators have found no effect on bone density, either positive or negative.[87] In these studies the use of immunomodulators may have been a surrogate marker for more severe disease activity and inflammation. These factors, and not the medication, may predispose to osteopenia and osteoporosis and, as a result, it can be concluded that there is no convincing evidence to suggest that the use of azathioprine, by itself, increases the risk of osteoporosis.

The use of other therapies that have been used to prevent or treat postmenopausal osteoporosis, such as hormone replacement therapy, calcitonin, fluoride and thiazide diuretics, has not been studied specifically in IBD patients. As discussed above, the use of bisphosphonates is of benefit in reducing the rate of decline, or in producing an increase, in bone mineral content in patients with inflammatory bowel disease who are receiving chronic glucocorticoid therapy. No studies have specifically examined the use of bisphosphonates in reversing bone loss in IBD patients who are not receiving glucocorticoids. However, bisphosphonates are effective agents for producing an increase in bone mass and preventing fractures in a setting in which glucocorticoid use is not a contributing factor – postmenopausal

osteoporosis. As such, it is reasonable to expect that bisphosphonates may also be effective in IBD patients with osteoporosis who are not receiving glucocorticoid therapy, and their use can be considered when other factors that may contribute to bone loss – disease activity, mineral absorption, nutritional status – have been considered and corrected or improved upon.

In postmenopausal IBD patients the use of hormone replacement therapy can be considered to prevent or treat osteoporosis. However, the potential benefit of therapy needs to be weighed against the potential effects on disease activity and thrombogenesis, as well as the increased risk of certain malignancies and, possibly, heart disease.[88] In premenopausal women with IBD menstrual irregularity is not uncommon, particularly when the disease is active. This menstrual irregularity or amenorrhea may be associated with hypoestrogenemia and accelerated bone loss. Attention should be paid to this symptom in IBD patients and the use of the oral contraceptive pill considered if menstrual irregularities persist. A potentially underappreciated cause for bone loss in males with IBD is secondary hypogonadism. In many cases this is probably due to the suppressive effects of systemic glucocorticoids on androgen secretion but, in males with established osteopenia, evaluation of serum testosterone levels and correction of deficiency should be undertaken.

# REFERENCES

1. Kanis JA, Johnell O, Oden A, Dawson A, De Laet C, Jonsson B. Ten year probabilities of osteoporotic fractures according to BMD and diagnostic thresholds. Osteoporos Int 2001;12:989–995.

2. Marshall D, Johnell O, Wedel H. Meta-analysis of how well measures of bone mineral density predict occurrence of osteoporotic fractures. Br Med J 1996;312:1254–1259.

3. Bernstein CN, Blanchard JF, Leslie W, Wajda A, Yu BN. The incidence of fracture among patients with inflammatory bowel disease. A population-based cohort study. Ann Intern Med 2000;133:795–799.

4. Fries W, Dinca M, Luisetto G, Peccolo F, Bottega F, Martin A. Calcaneal ultrasound bone densitometry in inflammatory bowel disease—a comparison with double X-ray densitometry of the lumbar spine. Am J Gastroenterol 1998;93:2339–2344.

5. Robinson RJ, Carr I, Iqbal SJ, al Azzawi F, Abrams K, Mayberry JF. Screening for osteoporosis in Crohn's disease. A detailed evaluation of calcaneal ultrasound. Eur J Gastroenterol Hepatol 1998;10:137–140.

6. Karlsson MK, Duan Y, Ahlborg H, Obrant KJ, Johnell O, Seeman E. Age, gender, and fragility fractures are associated with differences in quantitative ultrasound independent of bone mineral density. Bone 2001;28:118–122.

7. Wigderowitz CA, Paterson CR, Dashti H, McGurty D, Rowley DI. Prediction of bone strength from cancellous structure of the distal radius: can we improve on DXA? Osteoporos Int 2000;11:840–846.

8. Hofbauer LC, Khosla S, Dunstan CR, Lacey DL, Boyle WJ, Riggs BL. The roles of osteoprotegerin and osteoprotegerin ligand in the paracrine regulation of bone resorption. J Bone Miner Res 2000;15:2–12.

9. Hofbauer LC, Lacey DL, Dunstan CR, Spelsberg TC, Riggs BL, Khosla S. Interleukin-1beta and tumor necrosis factor-alpha, but not interleukin-6, stimulate osteoprotegerin ligand gene expression in human osteoblastic cells. Bone 1999;25:255–259.

10. Hofbauer LC, Hicok KC, Chen D, Khosla S. Regulation of osteoprotegerin production by androgens and anti-androgens in human osteoblastic lineage cells. Eur J Endocrinol 2002;147:269–273.

11. Khosla S. Minireview: the OPG/RANKL/RANK system. Endocrinology 2001;142:5050–5055.

12. Hofbauer LC, Gori F, Riggs BL et al. Stimulation of osteoprotegerin ligand and inhibition of osteoprotegerin production by glucocorticoids in human osteoblastic lineage cells: potential paracrine mechanisms of glucocorticoid-induced osteoporosis. Endocrinology 1999;140:4382–4389.

13. Hofbauer LC, Dunstan CR, Spelsberg TC, Riggs BL, Khosla S. Osteoprotegerin production by human osteoblast lineage cells is stimulated by vitamin D, bone morphogenetic protein-2, and cytokines. Biochem Biophys Res Commun 1998;250:776–781.

14. Danielson ME, Cauley JA, Baker CE et al. Familial resemblance of bone mineral density (BMD) and calcaneal ultrasound attenuation: the BMD in mothers and daughters study. J Bone Miner Res 1999;14:102–110.

15. Ulrich CM, Georgiou CC, Snow-Harter CM, Gillis DE. Bone mineral density in mother–daughter pairs: relations to lifetime exercise, lifetime milk consumption, and calcium supplements. Am J Clin Nutr 1996;63:72–79.

16. Mann V, Hobson EE, Li B et al. A COL1A1 Sp1 binding site polymorphism predisposes to osteoporotic fracture by affecting bone density and quality. J Clin Invest 2001;107:899–907.

17. Silvennoinen J, Risteli L, Karttunen T, Risteli J. Increased degradation of type I collagen in patients with inflammatory bowel disease. Gut 1996;38:223–228.

18. Bischoff SC, Herrmann A, Goke M, Manns MP, von zur MA, Brabant G. Altered bone metabolism in inflammatory bowel disease. Am J Gastroenterol 1997;92:1157–1163.

19. Hyams JS, Wyzga N, Kreutzer DL, Justinich CJ, Gronowicz GA. Alterations in bone metabolism in children with inflammatory bowel disease: an in vitro study. J Pediatr Gastroenterol Nutr 1997;24:289–295.

20. Driscoll RH Jr, Meredith SC, Sitrin M, Rosenberg IH. Vitamin D deficiency and bone disease in patients with Crohn's disease. Gastroenterology 1982;83:1252–1258.

21. Lukert BP, Raisz LG. Glucocorticoid-induced osteoporosis: pathogenesis and management. Ann Intern Med 1990;112:352–364.

22. Monegal A, Navasa M, Guanabens N et al. Bone mass and mineral metabolism in liver transplant patients treated with FK506 or cyclosporine A. Calcif Tissue Int 2001;68:83–86.

23. Abitbol V, Roux C, Chaussade S et al. Metabolic bone assessment in patients with inflammatory bowel disease. Gastroenterology 1995;108:417–422.

24. Olbricht T, Benker G. Glucocorticoid-induced osteoporosis: pathogenesis, prevention and treatment, with special regard to the rheumatic diseases. J Intern Med 1993;234:237–244.

25. Patschan D, Loddenkemper K, Buttgereit F. Molecular mechanisms of glucocorticoid-induced osteoporosis. Bone 2001;29:498–505.

26. Andreassen H, Hylander E, Rix M. Gender, age, and body weight are the major predictive factors for bone mineral density in Crohn's disease: a case–control cross-sectional study of 113 patients. Am J Gastroenterol 1999;94:824–828.

27. Ardizzone S, Bollani S, Bettica P, Bevilacqua M, Molteni P, Bianchi PG. Altered bone metabolism in inflammatory bowel disease: there is a difference between Crohn's disease and ulcerative colitis. J Intern Med 2000;247:63–70.

28. Bernstein CN, Seeger LL, Sayre JW, Anton PA, Artinian L, Shanahan F. Decreased bone density in inflammatory bowel disease is related to corticosteroid use and not disease diagnosis. J Bone Miner Res 1995;10:250–256.

29. Bjarnason I, Macpherson A, Mackintosh C, Buxton-Thomas M, Forgacs I, Moniz C. Reduced bone density in patients with inflammatory bowel disease. Gut 1997;40:228–233.

30. Chinea B, Rosa A, Oharriz JJ et al. Osteopenia in Puerto Ricans with Crohn's disease. P R Health Sci J 2000;19:329–333.

31. Clements D, Motley RJ, Evans WD et al. Longitudinal study of cortical bone loss in patients with inflammatory bowel disease. Scand J Gastroenterol 1992; 27:1055–1060.

32. Compston JE, Judd D, Crawley EO et al. Osteoporosis in patients with inflammatory bowel disease. Gut 1987;28:410–415.

33. Cowan FJ, Warner JT, Dunstan FD, Evans WD, Gregory JW, Jenkins HR. Inflammatory bowel disease and predisposition to osteopenia. Arch Dis Child 1997;76:325–329.

34. Dinca M, Fries W, Luisetto G et al. Evolution of osteopenia in inflammatory bowel disease. Am J Gastroenterol 1999;94:1292–1297.

35. Dresner-Pollak R, Karmeli F, Eliakim R, Ackerman Z, Rachmilewitz D. Increased urinary N-telopeptide cross-linked type I collagen predicts bone loss in patients with inflammatory bowel disease. Am J Gastroenterol 2000;95:699–704.

36. Ghosh S, Cowen S, Hannan WJ, Ferguson A. Low bone mineral density in Crohn's disease, but not in ulcerative colitis, at diagnosis. Gastroenterology 1994;107:1031–1039.

37. Habtezion A, Silverberg MS, Parkes R, Mikolainis S, Steinhart AH. Risk factors for low bone density in Crohn's disease. Inflamm Bowel Dis 2002;8:87–92.

38. Jahnsen J, Falch JA, Aadland E, Mowinckel P. Bone mineral density is reduced in patients with Crohn's disease but not in patients with ulcerative colitis: a population based study. Gut 1997;40:313–319.

39. Lee SH, Kim HJ, Yang SK et al. Decreased trabecular bone mineral density in newly diagnosed inflammatory bowel disease patients in Korea. J Gastroenterol Hepatol 2000;15:512–518.

40. Robinson RJ, al Azzawi F, Iqbal SJ et al. Osteoporosis and determinants of bone density in patients with Crohn's disease. Dig Dis Sci 1998;43:2500–2506.

41. Roux C, Abitbol V, Chaussade S et al. Bone loss in patients with inflammatory bowel disease: a prospective study. Osteoporos Int 1995;5:156–160.

42. Scharla SH, Minne HW, Lempert UG et al. Bone mineral density and calcium regulating hormones in patients with inflammatory bowel disease (Crohn's disease and ulcerative colitis). Exp Clin Endocrinol 1994;102:44–49.

43. Schoon EJ, van Nunen AB, Wouters RS, Stockbrugger RW, Russel MG. Osteopenia and osteoporosis in Crohn's disease: prevalence in a Dutch population-based cohort. Scand J Gastroenterol 2000;232 (Suppl):43–47.

44. Schoon EJ, Blok BM, Geerling BJ, Russel MG, Stockbrugger RW, Brummer RJ. Bone mineral density in patients with recently diagnosed inflammatory bowel disease. Gastroenterology 2000;119:1203–1208.

45. Schulte C, Dignass AU, Mann K, Goebell H. Reduced bone mineral density and unbalanced bone metabolism in patients with inflammatory bowel disease. Inflamm Bowel Dis 1998;4:268–275.

46. Semeao EJ, Jawad AF, Zemel BS, Neiswender KM, Piccoli DA, Stallings VA. Bone mineral density in children and young adults with Crohn's disease. Inflamm Bowel Dis 1999;5:161–166.

47. Silvennoinen JA, Karttunen TJ, Niemela SE. Manelius JJ, Lehtola JK. A controlled study of bone mineral density in patients with inflammatory bowel disease. Gut 1995;37:71–76.

48. Staun M, Tjellesen L, Thale M, Schaadt O, Jarnum S. Bone mineral content in patients with Crohn's disease. A longitudinal study in patients with bowel resections. Scand J Gastroenterol 1997;32:226–232.

49. Ulivieri FM, Lisciandrano D, Ranzi T et al. Bone mineral density and body composition in patients with ulcerative colitis. Am J Gastroenterol 2000;95:1491–1494.

50. Phillipov G, Phillips PJ. Skeletal site bone mineral density heterogeneity in women and men. Osteoporos Int 2001;12:362–365.

51. Pollak RD, Karmeli F, Eliakim R, Ackerman Z, Tabb K, Rachmilewitz D. Femoral neck osteopenia in patients with inflammatory bowel disease. Am J Gastroenterol 1998;93:1483–1490.

52. Vestergaard P, Mosekilde L. Fracture risk in patients with celiac disease, Crohn's disease, and ulcerative colitis: a nationwide follow-up study of 16,416 patients in Denmark. Am J Epidemiol 2002;156:1–10.

53. Semeao EJ, Stallings VA, Peck SN, Piccoli DA. Vertebral compression fractures in pediatric patients with Crohn's disease. Gastroenterology 1997;112:1710–1713.

54. Boot AM, Bouquet J, Krenning EP, Muinck Keizer-Schrama SM. Bone mineral density and nutritional status in children with chronic inflammatory bowel disease. Gut 1998;42:188–194.

55. Issenman RM, Atkinson SA, Radoja C, Fraher L. Longitudinal assessment of growth, mineral metabolism, and bone mass in pediatric Crohn's disease. J Pediatr Gastroenterol Nutr 1993;17:401–406.

56. Schulte C, Dignass AU, Mann K, Goebell H. Bone loss in patients with inflammatory bowel disease is less than expected: a follow-up study. Scand J Gastroenterol 1999;34:696–702.

57. Robinson RJ, Iqbal SJ, al Azzawi F, Abrams K, Mayberry JF. Sex hormone status and bone metabolism in men with Crohn's disease. Aliment Pharmacol Ther 1998;12:21–25.

58. Espallargues M, Sampietro-Colom L, Estrada MD et al. Identifying bone-mass-related risk factors for fracture to guide bone densitometry measurements: a systematic review of the literature. Osteoporos Int 2001;12:811–822.

59. Dear KL, Compston JE, Hunter JO. Treatments for Crohn's disease that minimise steroid doses are associated with a reduced risk of osteoporosis. Clin Nutr 2001;20:541–546.

60. Haugeberg G, Vetvik K, Stallemo A, Bitter H, Mikkelsen B, Stokkeland M. Bone density reduction in patients with Crohn disease and associations with demographic and disease variables: cross-sectional data from a population-based study. Scand J Gastroenterol 2001;36:759–765.

61. Pigot F, Roux C, Chaussade S et al. Low bone mineral density in patients with inflammatory bowel disease. Dig Dis Sci 1992;37:1396–1403.

62. Rizzoli R, Bonjour JP, Ferrari SL. Osteoporosis, genetics and hormones. J Mol Endocrinol 2001;26:79–94.

63. Schulte CM, Dignass AU, Goebell H, Roher HD, Schulte KM. Genetic factors determine extent of bone loss in inflammatory bowel disease. Gastroenterology 2000;119:909–920.

64. Valentine JF, Sninsky CA. Prevention and treatment of osteoporosis in patients with inflammatory bowel disease. Am J Gastroenterol 1999;94:878–883.

65. Tattersfield AE, Town GI, Johnell O et al. Bone mineral density in subjects with mild asthma randomised to treatment with inhaled corticosteroids or non-corticosteroid treatment for two years. Thorax 2001;56:272–278.

66. Cino M, Greenberg GR. Bone mineral density in Crohn's disease: a longitudinal study of budesonide, prednisone, and nonsteroid therapy. Am J Gastroenterol 2002;97:915–921.

67. Compston JE, Ayers AB, Horton LW, Tighe JR, Creamer B. Osteomalacia after small-intestinal resection. Lancet 1978;1:9–12.

68. Silvennoinen J. Relationships between vitamin D, parathyroid hormone and bone mineral density in inflammatory bowel disease. J Intern Med 1996;239:131–137.

69. Vogelsang H, Ferenci P, Woloszczuk W et al. Bone disease in vitamin D-deficient patients with Crohn's disease. Dig Dis Sci 1989;34:1094–1099.

70. Andreassen H, Rix M, Brot C, Eskildsen P. Regulators of calcium homeostasis and bone mineral density in patients with Crohn's disease. Scand J Gastroenterol 1998;33:1087–1093.

71. Vogelsang H, Ferenci P, Resch H, Kiss A, Gangl A. Prevention of bone mineral loss in patients with Crohn's disease by long-term oral vitamin D supplementation. Eur J Gastroenterol Hepatol 1995;7:609–614.

72. Adachi JD, Bensen WG, Bianchi F et al. Vitamin D and calcium in the prevention of corticosteroid induced osteoporosis: a 3 year followup. J Rheumatol 1996;23:995–1000.

73. Ryde SJ, Clements D, Evans WD et al. Total body calcium in patients with inflammatory bowel disease: a longitudinal study. Clin Sci (Lond) 1991;80:319–324.

74. Silvennoinen J, Lamberg-Allardt C, Karkkainen M, Niemela S, Lehtola J. Dietary calcium intake and its relation to bone mineral density in patients with inflammatory bowel disease. J Intern Med 1996;240:285–292.

75. Bernstein CN, Seeger LL, Anton PA et al. A randomized, placebo-controlled trial of calcium supplementation for decreased bone density in corticosteroid-using patients with inflammatory bowel disease: a pilot study. Aliment Pharmacol Ther 1996;10:777–786.

76. Liberman UA, Weiss SR, Broll J et al. Effect of oral alendronate on bone mineral density and the incidence of fractures in postmenopausal osteoporosis. The Alendronate Phase III Osteoporosis Treatment Study Group. N Engl J Med 1995;333:1437–1443.

77. Montessori ML, Scheele WH, Netelenbos JC, Kerkhoff JF, Bakker K. The use of etidronate and calcium versus calcium alone in the treatment of postmenopausal osteopenia: results of three years of treatment. Osteoporos Int 1997;7:52–58.

78. Adachi JD, Bensen WG, Brown J et al. Intermittent etidronate therapy to prevent corticosteroid-induced osteoporosis. N Engl J Med 1997;337:382–387.

79. Adachi JD, Saag KG, Delmas PD et al. Two-year effects of alendronate on bone mineral density and vertebral fracture in patients receiving glucocorticoids: a randomized, double-blind, placebo-controlled extension trial. Arthritis Rheum 2001;44:202–211.

80. Eastell R, Devogelaer JP, Peel NF et al. Prevention of bone loss with risedronate in glucocorticoid-treated rheumatoid arthritis patients. Osteoporos Int 2000;11:331–337.

81. Saag KG, Emkey R, Schnitzer TJ et al. Alendronate for the prevention and treatment of glucocorticoid-induced osteoporosis. Glucocorticoid-Induced Osteoporosis Intervention Study Group. N Engl J Med 1998;339:292–299.

82. Boulos P, Ioannidis G, Adachi JD. Glucocorticoid-induced osteoporosis. Curr Rheumatol Rep 2000;2:53–61.

83. Lanza FL, Hunt RH, Thomson AB, Provenza JM, Blank MA. Endoscopic comparison of esophageal and gastroduodenal effects of risedronate and alendronate in postmenopausal women. Gastroenterology 2000;119:631–638.

84. Haderslev KV, Tjellesen L, Sorensen HA, Staun M. Alendronate increases lumbar spine bone mineral density in patients with Crohn's disease. Gastroenterology 2000;119:639–646.

85. Abitbol V, Roux C, Guillemant S et al. Bone assessment in patients with ileal pouch–anal anastomosis for inflammatory bowel disease. Br J Surg 1997;84:1551–1554.

86. Semeao EJ, Jawad AF, Stouffer NO, Zemel BS, Piccoli DA, Stallings VA. Risk factors for low bone mineral density in children and young adults with Crohn's disease. J Pediatr 1999;135:593–600.

87. Floren CH, Ahren B, Bengtsson M, Bartosik J, Obrant K. Bone mineral density in patients with Crohn's disease during long-term treatment with azathioprine. J Intern Med 1998;243:123–126.

88. Risks and benefits of estrogen plus progestin in healthy postmenopausal women: principal results From the Women's Health Initiative randomized controlled trial. JAMA 2002;288:321–333.

# Index

**Abbreviations**
CD – Crohn's disease
CNS – central nervous system
DALM – dysplasia-associated lesion or mass
GI – gastrointestinal
HPA axis – hypothalamopituitary-adrenal axis
IBD – inflammatory bowel disease
IBS – irritable bowel syndrome
IL – interleukin
IPAA – ileal pouch–anal anastomosis

LPS – lipopolysaccharide
MAb – monoclonal antibody
MMP – matrix metalloproteinase
NSAIDs – non-steroidal anti-inflammatory drugs
PG-PS – peptidoglycan-polysaccharide
TGF-β transforming growth factor-β
TNBS – trinitrobenzenesulfonic acid
UC – ulcerative colitis